Life-threatening side effects are emphasized

Subheads indicate specific administration for dosing and routes of administration

High Alert header highlights drugs that pose the greatest risk if administered improperly

Controlled Substance Schedules appear in an easy-to-spot header

Black Box Warnings identify serious and life-threatening adverse effects

968 oxazepam

- To report signs of **anemia**: fatigue, headache, faintness, SOB, irritability
- To report **bleeding**; to avoid use of razors, commercial mouthwash
- To avoid aspirin, ibuprofen, NSAIDs, alcohol; may cause GI bleeding
- To report any changes in breathing, coughing
- To report numbness, tingling in face or extremities, poor hearing, or joint pain or swelling
- Not to receive live virus vaccines during treatment
- **Dysesthesias:** to avoid contact with cold (air, ice, liquid)
- To use contraception during treatment and for 4 mo after; that product may cause infertility

⚠ HIGH ALERT

oxazepam (Rx)
(ox-ay'ze-pam)
Novoxapam ✦, Oxpam ✦, Serax, Zapex ✦
Func. class.: Sedative/hypnotic; antianxiety
Chem. class.: Benzodiazepine, short acting

Controlled Substance Schedule IV

ACTION: Potentiates the actions of GABA, especially in the limbic system and reticular formation

USES: Anxiety, alcohol withdrawal

Unlabeled uses: Insomnia

CONTRAINDICATIONS: Pregnancy, breastfeeding, children <6 yr, hypersensitivity to benzodiazepines, closed-angle glaucoma, psychosis

Precautions: Geriatric patients, debilitated patients, renal/hepatic disease, depression, suicidal ideation, dementia, sleep apnea, seizure disorder

Black Box Warning: Depressants, respiratory depression

DOSAGE AND ROUTES
Anxiety
- **Adult:** PO 10-15 mg tid-qid, max 120 mg/day
- **Geriatric:** PO 10 mg daily-bid, max 60 mg/day tid

Alcohol withdrawal
- **Adult:** PO 15-30 mg tid-qid

Severe anxiety syndrome, agitation, anxiety with depression
- **Adult/child >12 yr:** PO 15-30 mg tid

Available forms: Caps 10, 15, 30 mg
Administer:
- Without regard to food
- Taper product (0.5 mg q3days) before discontinuing

SIDE EFFECTS
CNS: *Dizziness, drowsiness,* confusion, headache, anxiety, tremors, fatigue, depression, insomnia, hallucinations, paradoxical excitement, transient amnesia
CV: *Orthostatic hypotension,* ECG changes, tachycardia, hypotension
EENT: *Blurred vision,* tinnitus, mydriasis
GI: Nausea, vomiting, anorexia, drug-induced hepatitis
HEMA: Leukopenia
INTEG: Rash, dermatitis, itching
SYST: Dependence

PHARMACOKINETICS
Peak 2-4 hr; metabolized by liver; excreted by kidneys; half-life 5-15 hr; crosses placenta, breast milk; protein binding 97%

INTERACTIONS

Black Box Warning: Increase: oxazepam effects, respiratory depression—CNS depressants, alcohol, disulfiram

Decrease: oxazepam effects—oral contraceptives, phenytoin, theophylline, valproic acid
Decrease: effects of levodopa
Drug/Herb
Increase: CNS depression—kava, melatonin, valerian
Drug/Lab Test
Increase: AST, ALT, serum bilirubin
Decrease: WBC

✦ Canada only

☣Rx Genetic warn

Please see the following page for more features.

NURSING CONSIDERATIONS

Assess:
• CBC and LFTs periodically
• B/P (lying, standing), pulse; if systolic B/P drops 20 mm Hg, hold product, notify prescriber

Black Box Warning: Respiratory depression: not to be used in preexisting respiratory depression; use cautiously in severe pulmonary disease; monitor respirations

• Mental status: mood, sensorium, affect, sleeping pattern, drowsiness, dizziness, sedation, suicidal thoughts/behaviors
• **Physical dependency, withdrawal symptoms:** headache, nausea, vomiting, muscle pain, weakness, tremors, seizures (long-term use)
• **Beers:** avoid in older adults; delirium, cognitive impairment may occur
• **Pregnancy/breastfeeding:** assess for pregnancy before use; do not use in pregnancy; do not breastfeed

Evaluate:
• Therapeutic response: decreased anxiety, restlessness, insomnia

Teach patient/family:
• That product may be taken without regard to food
• That medication is not to be used for everyday stress or used >4 mo unless directed by prescriber; not to take more than prescribed dose because product may be habit forming
• To avoid OTC preparations (cough, cold, hay fever) unless approved by prescriber
• To avoid driving, activities that require alertness because drowsiness may occur
• To avoid alcohol, other psychotropic products unless directed by prescriber
• Not to discontinue product abruptly after long-term use
• To rise slowly because fainting may occur, especially among geriatric patients
• That drowsiness may worsen at beginning of treatment
• To notify prescriber if pregnancy is planned or suspected

OXcarbazepine (Rx)
(ox'kar-baz'uh-peen)
Trileptal, Oxtellar XR
Func. class.: Anticonvulsant
Chem. class.: CarBAMazepine ana

Do not confuse:
OXcarbazepine/carBAMazepine

ACTION: May inhibit nerve impulses by limiting influx of sodium ions across cell membrane in motor cortex

USES: Partial seizures
Unlabeled uses: Trigeminal neuralgia, atypical panic disorder, bipolar disord

CONTRAINDICATIONS: Hyp sensitivity
Precautions: Pregnancy, breastfeedi children <4 yr, hypersensitivity to carB Mazepine, renal disease, fluid restriction hyponatremia, abrupt discontinuation suicidal ideation, **⚠** positive for HLA-1502 allele

DOSAGE AND ROUTES
Seizures, adjunctive therapy
• **Adult:** PO 300 mg bid, may be increased by 600 mg/day in divided doses bid at weekly intervals; maintenance 1200 mg/day; ext rel: 600 mg daily × wk, increase weekly in 600 mg/day increments to 1200-2400 mg daily
• **Child 4-16 yr:** PO 8-10 mg/kg/day vided bid; dose determined by weig increase by 5 mg/kg/day q3days, m doses weight dependent
• **Child 2 to <4 yr:** PO 8-10 mg/kg c vided in 2 doses, max 600 mg/day
Conversion to monotherapy for partial seizures
• **Adult:** PO 300 mg bid with reduction in other anticonvulsants; increase OXcarbazepine by 600 mg/day each week over 2-4 wk; withdraw other anticonvulsants over 3-6 wk; max 2400 mg/day
Initiation of monotherapy for partial seizures
• **Adult:** PO 300 mg bid, increase by 300 mg/day q3days to 1200 mg in divided doses bid, max 2400 mg/day

Side effects: *italics* = common; red = life-threatening

Nursing considerations provide guidance throughout the nursing process

Easily confused drug names are located beneath the header

Common unlabeled uses and doses are clearly indicated

Genetic warning icon highlights drugs with genetic contraindications

Mosby's

2021
NURSING
DRUG
REFERENCE

3251 Riverport Lane
St. Louis, Missouri 63043

MOSBY'S 2021 NURSING DRUG REFERENCE,
THIRTY-FOURTH EDITION

ISBN: 978-0-323-75733-1
ISSN: 1044-8470

Notices

Previous editions copyrighted 2020, 2019, 2018, 2017, 2016.
International Standard Book Number: 978-0-323-75733-1

Executive Content Strategist: Sonya Seigafuse
Content Development Manager: Luke Held
Senior Content Development Specialist: Sarah Vora
Publishing Services Manager: Julie Eddy
Senior Project Manager: Jodi M. Willard
Design Direction: Ryan Cook

Printed in the United States of America and China

Last digit is the print number: 9   8   7   6   5   4   3   2   1

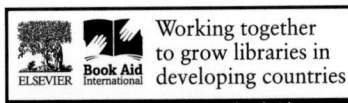

Working together
to grow libraries in
developing countries

www.elsevier.com • www.bookaid.org

Mosby's
2021
NURSING DRUG REFERENCE

34TH EDITION

LINDA SKIDMORE-ROTH, RN, MSN, NP
Consultant
Littleton, Colorado

Formerly, Nursing Faculty
New Mexico State University
Las Cruces, New Mexico
El Paso Community College
El Paso, Texas

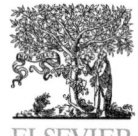
ELSEVIER

Consultants

James Graves, PharmD
Clinical Pharmacist
Inpatient Pharmacy
University of Missouri Health Center
Columbia, Missouri

Kathleen S. Jordan, DNP, MS, FNP-BC, ENP-BC, ENP-C, SANE-P
Nurse Practitioner
Mid-Atlantic Emergency Medicine Associates;
Clinical Assistant Professor
School of Nursing
The University of North Carolina–Charlotte
Charlotte, North Carolina

Janis McMillan, MSN, RN, CNE
Associate Clinical Professor
School of Nursing
Northern Arizona University
Flagstaff, Arizona

Meera K. Shah, PharmD
Clinical Pharmacist
Saint Louis, Missouri

Travis E. Sonnett, PharmD
Inpatient Pharmacy Supervisor
Mann-Grandstaff VA Medical Center
Spokane, Washington;
Residency Program Director
Pharmacy
Washington State University
College of Pharmacy
Spokane, Washington

William Kendall Wyatt, MD, RN, EMT-P
Chief Resident Physician
West Virginia University
Charleston Area Medical Center
Charleston, West Virginia

Preface

Increasingly, patients are relying on nurses to know every detail of health care. More important, nurses are expected to have these answers, especially when it comes to medication. Let *Mosby's 2021 Nursing Drug Reference* be your answer. Our indispensable, yet compact, resource contains hundreds of monographs with several easy-to-use features.

NEW FEATURES

This edition features:
- Over 30 recent FDA-approved drugs located in **Appendix A** (see Contents for a complete list). Included are monographs for:
  esketamine—for depression
  lefamulin—for pneumonia
  selinexor—for complicated cases of multiple myeloma
- **An ebook** with easy-to-use navigation for quick access to monographs of your choice

NEW FACTS

This edition features more than 2000 new drug facts, including:
- New drugs and dosage information
- Newly researched side effects and adverse reactions
- New and revised Black Box Warnings
- The latest precautions, interactions, and contraindications
- IV therapy updates
- Revised nursing considerations
- Updated patient/family teaching guidelines
- Updated BEERS information

ORGANIZATION

This reference is organized into two main sections:
- Individual drug monographs (in alphabetical order by generic name)
- Appendixes (identified by the wide thumb tabs on the edge)
  The guiding principle behind this book is to provide fast, easy access to drug information and nursing considerations. Every detail—the paper, typeface, cover, binding, use of color, and appendixes—has been carefully chosen with the user in mind.

INDIVIDUAL DRUG MONOGRAPHS

This book contains monographs for more than 1300 generic and 4500 trade medications. Common trade names are given for all drugs regularly used in the United States and Canada, with drugs available only in Canada identified by a maple leaf ✤.
  The following information is provided, whenever possible, for safe, effective administration of each drug:
  High-alert status: Identifies high-alert drugs with a label and icon. Visit the Institute for Safe Medication Practices (ISMP) at http://www.ismp.org/tools/highalert-medications.pdf for a list of medications and drug classes with the greatest potential for patient harm if they are used in error.
  Tall man lettering: Uses the capitalization of distinguishing letters to avoid medication errors and is required by the FDA for drug manufacturers.

Pronunciation: Helps the nurse master complex generic names.

Rx/OTC: Identifies prescription or over-the-counter drugs.

Functional and chemical classifications: Allow the nurse to see similarities and dissimilarities among drugs in the same functional but different chemical classes.

Do not confuse: Presents drug names that might easily be confused within each appropriate monograph.

Action: Describes pharmacologic properties concisely.

Uses: List the conditions the drug is used to treat.

Unlabeled uses: Describe drug uses that may be encountered in practice but are not yet FDA approved.

Dosages and routes: List all available and approved dosages and routes for adult, pediatric, and geriatric patients.

Available forms: Include tablets, capsules, extended-release, injectables (IV, IM, SUBCUT), solutions, creams, ointments, lotions, gels, shampoos, elixirs, suspensions, suppositories, sprays, aerosols, and lozenges.

Side effects: Groups these reactions by body system, with common side effects *italicized* and life-threatening reactions (those that are potentially fatal and/or permanently disabling) in red type for emphasis. *It is important to note that in some electronic versions of* Mosby's 2021 Nursing Drug Reference, *the red type may appear as* **black, bold** *print.*

Contraindications: List conditions under which the drug absolutely should not be given.

Precautions: List conditions that require special consideration when the drug is prescribed.

Black Box Warnings: Identify FDA warnings that highlight serious and life-threatening adverse effects.

Pharmacokinetics: Outline metabolism, distribution, and elimination.

Interactions: Include confirmed drug interactions, followed by the drug or nutrient causing that interaction, when applicable.

Drug/herb: Highlights potential interactions between herbal products and prescription or OTC drugs.

Drug/food: Identifies many common drug interactions with foods.

Drug/lab test: Identifies how the drug may affect lab test results.

Nursing considerations: Identify key nursing considerations for each step of the nursing process: Assess, Administer, Evaluate, and Teach Patient/Family. Instructions for giving drugs by various routes (e.g., PO, IM, IV) are included, with route subheadings in bold.

Compatibilities: List syringe, Y-site, and additive compatibilities and incompatibilities. If no compatibilities are listed for a drug, the necessary compatibility testing has not been done and that compatibility information is unknown. To ensure safety, assume that the drug may not be mixed with other drugs unless specifically stated.

Genetic icon ⟩⟨: Highlights drugs with genetic contraindications.

Treatment of overdose: Provides drugs and treatment for overdoses where appropriate.

APPENDIXES

Selected New Drugs: Includes comprehensive information on over 30 key drugs approved by the FDA during the past 12 months.

Ophthalmic, Otic, Nasal, and Topical Products: Provides essential information for more than 80 ophthalmic, otic, nasal, and topical products commonly used today, grouped by chemical drug class.

Vaccines and Toxoids: Features an easy-to-use table with generic and trade names, uses, dosages and routes, and contraindications for over 40 key vaccines and toxoids.
Recently Approved Drugs: Highlights the most recently approved drugs for the market.

I am indebted to the nursing and pharmacology consultants who reviewed the manuscript and thank them for their criticism and encouragement. I would also like to thank Luke Held and Sarah Vora, my editors, whose active encouragement and enthusiasm have made this book better than it might otherwise have been. I am likewise grateful to Jodi Willard for the coordination of the production process and assistance with the development of the new edition. A special "thank-you" to my son, Craig Roth, for completing the electronic files.

Linda Skidmore-Roth

Contents

INDIVIDUAL DRUG MONOGRAPHS, 1

APPENDIXES,

EVOLVE WEBSITE

- Additional Monographs

A HIGH ALERT

abacavir (Rx)

(ah-bak′ah-veer)

Ziagen

Func. class.: Antiretroviral

Chem. class.: Nucleoside reverse
transcriptase inhibitor (NRTI)

ACTION: Inhibitory action against
HIV-1; inhibits replication of the virus
by incorporating into cellular DNA by
viral reverse transcriptase, thereby terminating the cellular DNA chain

USES: In combination with other antiretroviral agents for HIV-1 infection

Unlabeled uses: HIV prophylaxis following occupational exposure

CONTRAINDICATIONS

Black Box Warning: Hypersensitivity,
moderate/severe hepatic disease, lactic
acidosis

Precautions: Pregnancy, breastfeeding,
children <3 mo, granulocyte count
<1000/mm³ or Hgb <9.5 g/dL, severe renal
disease, impaired hepatic function, ☞
HLA B5701+ (black, Caucasian, Asian
patients), abrupt discontinuation; Guillain-
Barré syndrome, immune reconstitution
syndrome, MI, obesity, polymyositis

DOSAGE AND ROUTES

• **Adult and adolescent ≥16 yr: PO** 300
mg bid or 600 mg/day with other antiretrovirals

• **Adolescent <16 yr and child ≥3 mo:**
PO (oral solution) 8 mg/kg bid or 16
mg/kg daily, max 300 mg bid with other
antiretrovirals; tablets 14-19 kg 150 mg
bid or 300 mg daily; 20-24 kg 150 mg
AM and 300 mg PM or 450 mg daily;
≥25 kg 300 mg bid or 600 mg daily

Hepatic dose

• **Adult: PO** (Child-Pugh A [5-6 points])
(oral sol) 200 mg bid; moderate to severe
hepatic disease, do not use

HIV prophylaxis (unlabeled)

• **Adult: PO** 600 mg daily as an alternative

Available forms: Tabs 300 mg; oral sol
20 mg/mL

Administer:

• Give in combination with other antiretrovirals

• May give without regard to food q12hr
around the clock

• Reduce dose in hepatic disease, use
oral sol

• Storage in cool environment; protect
from light; oral sol stored at room temperature; do not freeze

SIDE EFFECTS

CNS: *Fever, headache, malaise, insomnia*

GI: *Nausea, vomiting, diarrhea,
anorexia,* ALT, hepatotoxicity, hepatomegaly with steatosis

INTEG: *Rash,* urticaria, hypersensitivity
reactions

META: Lactic acidosis

OTHER: Fatal hypersensitivity reactions, MI,
fat redistribution, immune reconstitution

PHARMACOKINETICS

Rapid/extensive absorption, distributed
to extravascular space, then erythrocytes; 50% protein binding; extensively
metabolized to inactive metabolites by
the liver; half-life 1½ hr; excreted in
urine, feces (unchanged); onset, peak,
duration unknown

INTERACTIONS

• Do not coadminister with abacavir-
containing products, ribavirin, interferon

• **Increase:** possible lactic acidosis—
ribavirin

Increase: abacavir levels—alcohol

Decrease: abacavir levels—tipranavir

Decrease: levels of—methadone, may
require higher dose of methadone

Drug/Lab Test

Increase: serum glucose, triglycerides,
ALT, AST, amylase, CK

NURSING CONSIDERATIONS
Assess:

• Symptoms of HIV and possible infections; increased temperature baseline and throughout treatment

Black Box Warning: **Lactic acidosis** (elevated lactate levels, increased LFTs), severe hepatomegaly with steatosis, discontinue treatment and do not restart; may have large liver, elevated AST, ALT, lactate levels; women and the obese may be at greater risk; monitor serum lactate levels, LFTs, palpate liver for enlargement

Black Box Warning: **Fatal hypersensitivity reactions:** fever, rash, nausea, vomiting, fatigue, cough, dyspnea, diarrhea, abdominal discomfort; treatment should be discontinued and not restarted; those with ⟐⟐ HLA-B5701 are at great risk for hypersensitivity; obtain genetic testing for HLA-B 5701 before starting treatment, register at the Abacavir Hypersensitivity Registry (1-800-270-0425)

• Renal studies: BUN, serum uric acid, CCr before, during therapy; these may be elevated

Black Box Warning: **Hepatotoxicity:** monitor hepatic studies before and monthly during therapy: bilirubin, AST, ALT, amylase, alk phos, creatine phosphokinase, creatinine

• **Blood counts:** monitor viral load and CD4 counts during treatment; watch for decreasing granulocytes, Hgb; if low, therapy may have to be discontinued and restarted after hematologic recovery; blood transfusions may be required; perform hepatitis B virus (HBr) screening to confirm correct treatment
• **Resistance:** do not use triple antiretrovirals (abacavir, lamivudine, tenofovir) in treatment-naive persons
• **Immune reconstitution syndrome:** may occur anytime during treatment and is a response to CMV, *Mycobacterium avium* infection

• **Fat redistribution:** may occur anytime during treatment; buffalo hump, breast growth, moon face, facial wasting, trunk obesity

Evaluate:

• Therapeutic response: increased CD4 count, decreased viral load, decreased disease progression

Teach patient/family:

• That product is not a cure but will control symptoms; that patient is still infective, may pass HIV virus on to others, not to have sexual contact without condom, needles should not be shared, blood from infected individual should not come in contact with another's mucous membranes
• To carry emergency ID with condition, products taken; not to take other products that contain abacavir
• That body fat redistribution may occur; not to share product
• **Hypersensitivity:** to notify prescriber of sore throat, swollen lymph nodes, malaise, fever; other infections may occur; to stop product and to notify prescriber immediately if skin rash, fever, cough, shortness of breath, GI symptoms occur; to advise all health care providers that allergic reaction has occurred with abacavir
• That follow-up visits must be continued because serious toxicity may occur; blood counts must be done
• **Pregnancy/breastfeeding:** to consider the use of contraception during treatment; identify if pregnancy is planned or suspected; use only if benefits outweigh risk; pregnant patients should enroll in Antiretroviral Pregnancy Registry at 800-258-4263; avoid breastfeeding
• To review and discuss points outlined on Medication Guide and Warning Card
• That other products may be necessary to prevent other infections and that drug is taken with other antiretrovirals
• Not to drink alcohol while taking this product
• To use exactly as prescribed, not to stop product or change dose, not to use with other products unless approved by prescriber

abaloparatide (Rx)

(a-bal-oh-PAR-a-tide)

Tymlos

Func. class.: Parathyroid hormone analog and modifier

ACTION: A synthetic peptide analog of a parathyroid hormone–related protein, which acts as an agonist at the PTH receptors

USES: For the treatment of postmenopausal women with osteoporosis at high risk for fracture

CONTRAINDICATIONS:

Hypersensitivity

Precautions: Breastfeeding, children, pregnancy, radiation, hypercalcemia, hypercalciuria, hyperuricemia, hyperparathyroidism, renal disease, orthostatic hypotension

Black Box Warning: Osteogenic sarcoma, new primary malignancy

DOSAGE AND ROUTES

Postmenopausal women with osteoporosis at high risk for fracture

• **Adult postmenopausal female:** SUBCUT 80 mcg q day

Available forms: Solution for injection 80 mcg/dose

Administer:

SUBCUT route

• Visually inspect for particulate matter and discoloration before use

• Do not use IV/IM

• Needles are not included with the pen; a separate prescription for needles is needed. Use 8-mm, 31-gauge Clickfine needles such as ReliOn, Smart Sense, or TopCare brands

• **Storage:** Before first use, store pen in refrigerator (do not freeze). After first use, store for up to 30 days at room temperature (68-77° F or 20-25° C); do not freeze or expose to heat. Keep cap on when not in use. Do not store with a needle attached. Use pen only for 30 days. Dispose of properly

• Place capped needle straight onto the pen. A click will be heard when attached

• Pull off the outer pen needle cap from the pen needle; pull off the inner pen needle cap

• Prime before first use to remove air bubbles

• Turn dose knob on the pen away from you (clockwise) until it stops. You will see "80" lined up in the dose display window

• Hold the pen with the pen needle pointing up. Tap lightly on the cartridge holder to move air bubbles to the top of the cartridge

• Press the green injection button until it stops. You will see "0" in the dose display window. A drop of liquid should come out of the needle tip. If not, repeat the priming steps

• Set the patient's dose on the pen by turning the knob on the pen away from you (clockwise) until the knob stops and "80" is lined up in the display window

• Choose and clean an injection site in the periumbilical region of the abdomen. Avoid the 2-inch area around the navel. Do not inject into areas where skin is tender, bruised, red, scaly, or hard. Avoid areas with scars or stretch marks

• Insert pen needle straight into patient's skin

• Press the green button until "0" is in the dose display window. Do not move the pen after inserting the needle

• Continue to press the green button while counting to 10. Counting to 10 will allow the full dose to be given

• After counting to 10, release the green button and remove the pen from the site by pulling straight out

• Place the outer needle cap back on the needle. Press on the outer needle cap until it snaps into place

---

Side effects: *italics* = common; red = life-threatening

• Unscrew the used needle. To unscrew the capped needle you may need to turn it 8 or more turns and then pull until the needle comes off. Properly dispose of used needle

• Firmly replace pen cap onto the pen. Keep pen cap on the pen for storage between injections

• Rotate site daily and give at the same time daily

• The first several doses should be given with the patient lying down in case of orthostatic hypotension

SIDE EFFECTS
CNS: Dizziness
META: Hypercalcemia, hyperuricemia
INTEG: Injection site reactions
CV: Orthostatic hypotension

PHARMACOKINETICS
Protein binding approximately 70%; half-life 0.7 hr

INTERACTIONS
None known

NURSING CONSIDERATIONS
Assess:
• **Osteoporosis:** before and during treatment
• **Blood studies:** serum calcium, uric acid baseline and periodically
• **Urolithiasis:** product may increase the risk of urolithiasis in those with recent or current urolithiasis

> Black Box Warning: **Osteosarcoma:** increased risk; use product for <2 yr

• **Pregnancy/breastfeeding:** not indicated for women of reproductive potential
Evaluate:
• Therapeutic response: increased bone mineral density
Teach patient/family:
• Not to try to inject until patient or caregiver receives training
• To receive the first several injections near a place to sit or lie down, until the

effect of the injection is known; blood pressure may drop
• To inject 1 time each day into lower stomach area (abdomen) just under the skin (SUBCUT); to avoid giving the injection within the 2-inch area around the navel; to rotate injection sites daily
• That periodic lab test will be done
• To take at same time each day; that if the dose is forgotten or cannot be taken at the usual time, to take drug as soon as remembered on that day
• Not to share pen or pen needles with others even if the needle has been changed
• **Urolithiasis:** to report painful urination

---

abatacept (Rx)
(ab-a-ta′sept)
Orencia, Orencia ClickJet
Func. class.: Antirheumatic agent (disease modifying)
Chem. class.: Immunomodulator

Do not confuse:
Orencia/Oracea

ACTION: A selective costimulation modulator; inhibits T-lymphocytes, inhibits production of tumor necrosis factor (TNF-α), interferon-γ, interleukin-2, which are involved in immune and inflammatory reactions

USES: Polyarticular juvenile rheumatoid arthritis; moderate to severe rheumatoid arthritis; acute, chronic rheumatoid arthritis that has not responded to other disease-modifying agents; may use in combination with DMARDs; do not use with TNF antagonists (adalimumab, etanercept, inFLIXimab), anakinra

CONTRAINDICATIONS: Hypersensitivity
Precautions: Pregnancy, breastfeeding, children, geriatric patients, recurrent infections, COPD, TB, viral hepatitis,

---

immunosuppression, neoplastic disease, respiratory infection

DOSAGE AND ROUTES

Rheumatoid arthritis/psoriatic arthritis

• **Adult: SUBCUT** 125 mg within 1 day after single IV loading dose, then 125 mg weekly; weekly subcut dose may be initiated without an IV loading dose for those unable to receive an infusion

• **Adult >100 kg (220 lb): IV INFUSION** 1 g over 30 min, give at 2, 4 wk after first infusion, then q4wk

• **Adult 60-100 kg (132-220 lb): IV INFUSION** 750 mg over 30 min, give at 2, 4 wk after first infusion, then q4wk

• **Adult <60 kg (132 lb): IV INFUSION** 500 mg over 30 min, give at 2, 4 wk after first infusion, then q4wk

Juvenile rheumatoid arthritis (JRA)/juvenile idiopathic arthritis (JIA)

• **Adolescent and child ≥6 yr and >100 kg: IV INFUSION** 1 g given over 30 min q2wk × 3 doses, then 1 g given over 30 min q4wk starting at wk 8

• **Adolescent and child ≥6 yr and 75-100 kg: IV INFUSION** 750 mg over 30 min q2wk × 2 doses, then 750 mg given over 30 min q4wk starting at wk 8

• **Adolescent and child ≥6 yr and <75 kg: IV INFUSION** 10 mg/kg given over 30 min q2wk × 3 doses, then 10 mg/kg q4wk starting at wk 8

Moderate/severe polyarticular juvenile idiopathic arthritis as monotherapy with or without methotrexate

• **Child/adolescent ≥2 yr and ≥50 kg: SUBCUT** 125 mg q1wk

• **Child/adolescent ≥2 yr and 25-50 kg: SUBCUT** 87.5 mg q1wk

• **Child/adolescent ≥2 yr and 10-25 kg: SUBCUT** 50 mg q1wk

Available forms: Lyophilized powder, single-use vials 250 mg; sol for subcut inj 125 mg/mL

Administer:

• Storage in refrigerator; do not use expired vials, protect from light, do not freeze

Intermittent IV INFUSION route

• **To reconstitute,** use 10 mL sterile water for injection; insert syringe needle into vial and direct stream of sterile water for inj on the wall of vial; rotate vial until mixed; vent with needle to rid foam after reconstitution (25 mg/mL); **further dilute** in 100 mL NS from a 100-mL infusion bag/bottle; withdraw the needed volume (2 vials remove 20 mL, 3 vials remove 30 mL, 4 vials remove 40 mL); slowly add the reconstituted sol from each vial into the infusion bag/bottle using the same disposable syringe supplied; mix gently; discard unused portions of vials; do not use if particulate is present or discolored; **give** over 30 min; use non–protein-binding filter (0.2-1.2 microns); protect from light

• Do not admix with other sol or medications

SUBCUT route

• Use prefilled syringe for subcut only (do not use for IV); allow to warm to room temperature (30-60 min); do not speed up warming process; the amount of liquid should be between the 2 lines on the barrel; do not use the syringe if there is more or less liquid; inject into fronts of thighs, outer area of upper arm, or abdomen except for 2-inch area around the navel; do not inject into tender, bruised area

• Gently pinch skin and hold firmly; insert needle at 45-degree angle; inject full amount in 125-mg syringe

• Rotate injection sites

• Use ClickJet for subcut only; let warm for 30 min after removal from refrigerator, do not use if damaged or past expiration date, pull cap straight off, push down on skin to unlock, push button and hold for 15 sec, a click will be heard, keep holding until blue indicator stops moving in the window, remove, tip will lock over needle

SIDE EFFECTS

CNS: Headache, asthenia, dizziness
CV: *Hypo/hypertension*
GI: Abdominal pain, dyspepsia, nausea, diarrhea, diverticulitis
GU: UTI, pyelonephritis
MS: Back pain
INTEG: Rash, *inj site reaction,* flushing, urticaria, pruritus
RESP: *Pharyngitis, cough, URI,* non-URI, *rhinitis,* wheezing
SYST: Anaphylaxis, malignancies, serious infections, antibody development

PHARMACOKINETICS

Half-life IV 13 days, subcut 14.3 days, steady state 60 days; clearance increases with increased body weight

INTERACTIONS

• Do not give concurrently with live virus vaccines; immunizations should be brought up to date before treatment
• Do not use with TNF antagonists: adalimumab, etanercept, inFLIXimab; anakinra; infection may occur
• Avoid use with corticosteroids, immunosuppressives, atropine, scopolamine, halothane, nitrous oxide

NURSING CONSIDERATIONS
Assess:
• **RA:** pain, stiffness, ROM, swelling of joints during treatment baseline and periodically
• **TB:** for latent/active TB, viral hepatitis before beginning treatment
• For inj site pain, swelling
• Patient's overall health at each visit; product should not be given with active infections; parenteral product contains maltose, glucose monitoring must be done with glucose-specific testing
• **Infection:** sinusitis, urinary tract infection, influenza, bronchitis; serious infections have occurred; notify prescriber, therapy may need to be changed

• **Pregnancy/breastfeeding:** assess whether pregnancy is planned or suspected; if pregnant, register by calling 877-311-8972; use only if benefits outweigh fetal risk; do not breastfeed
Evaluate:
• Therapeutic response: decreased inflammation, pain in joints
Teach patient/family:
• That product must be continued for prescribed time to be effective, not to use with alcohol
• To use caution when driving; dizziness may occur
• Not to have live virus vaccinations while taking this product or use alcohol, TNF antagonists, other immunosuppressants; bring vaccinations up to date before use of this product
• About patient information included in packaging, including "do not shake"
• How to inject and rotate inj sites
• To immediately report signs of infection: temperature, flu-like symptoms, urinary burning/stinging, sinusitis
• To avoid those with known infections

---

abemaciclib
(uh-beh'-muh-sy'-klib)
Verzenio
Func. class.: Antineoplastic
Chem. class.: Protein kinase inhibitors

ACTION: It is an inhibitor of the cyclin-dependent kinases 4 and 6, a protein kinase inhibitor

USES: For the treatment of HR-positive, HER2-negative advanced or metastatic breast cancer with disease progression following endocrine therapy and prior chemotherapy, as monotherapy, or in combination with fulvestrant

CONTRAINDICATIONS: Hypersensitivity
Precautions: Breastfeeding, contraception requirements, hepatic disease,

---

hepatotoxicity, infertility, neutropenia, pregnancy, pregnancy testing, reproductive risk, thromboembolic disease

DOSAGE AND ROUTES

HR-positive, HER2-negative advanced or metastatic breast cancer disease progression following endocrine therapy and prior chemotherapy, as monotherapy
• **Adult:** PO 200 mg bid until disease progression or unacceptable toxicity

HR-positive, HER2-negative advanced or metastatic breast cancer with disease progression following endocrine therapy, in combination with fulvestrant
• **Adult:** PO 150 mg bid with fulvestrant (500 mg **IM** as two 250-mg [5 mL] injections, 1 injection in each buttock, on days 1, 15, 29, and q month thereafter) until disease progression or unacceptable toxicity. Pre- and perimenopausal women should also be treated with a gonadotropin-releasing hormone agonist

Therapeutic drug monitoring: dosage adjustments for treatment-related toxicities
Interrupt therapy per specific instructions. Restart as appropriate at the following reduced doses:
• **Starting dose:** Monotherapy, 200 mg bid; combination with fulvestrant, 150 mg bid
• **First occurrence:** Monotherapy, 150 mg bid; combination with fulvestrant, 100 mg bid
• **Second occurrence:** Monotherapy, 100 mg bid; combination with fulvestrant, 50 mg bid
• **Third occurrence:** Monotherapy, 50 mg bid; combination with fulvestrant, not applicable

Diarrhea
• **Grade 1:** Begin antidiarrheals, increase oral fluid intake. No change needed
• **Grade 2, first occurrence:** Begin antidiarrheals, increase oral fluid intake. If diarrhea does not resolve to grade ≤1 within 24 hr, hold therapy until resolution. No change needed unless grade 2 diarrhea persists; upon resolution to grade ≤1, resume at next lower dose level
• **Grade 2, recurrent despite maximal supportive measures:** Begin antidiarrheals, increase oral fluid intake. When diarrhea resolves to grade ≤1, resume at next lower dose level
• **Grade 3 or 4, or requires hospitalization:** Begin antidiarrheals, increase oral fluid intake. When diarrhea resolves to grade ≤1, resume at next lower dose level

Hematologic toxicities
• **Grade 3, first occurrence:** Hold; when toxicity resolves to grade ≤2, resume; dose reduction is not needed unless growth factor was needed. If treatment with growth factors is needed, additionally wait for at least 48 hr after the last dose of growth factor before resuming at the next lower dose level
• **Grade 3, recurrent, or grade 4:** Hold; when toxicity resolves to grade ≤2, resume at the next lower dose level. If treatment with growth factors is needed, additionally wait for at least 48 hr after the last dose of growth factor before resuming

Hepatic dose
• **Adult:** PO
Child-Pugh A or B: no change; Child-Pugh C: reduce dosing to once per day; grade 1 (AST/ALT 1.1–3× the upper limit of normal [ULN]), without an increase in total bilirubin above 2× ULN: no change; grade 2, first occurrence (AST/ALT 3.1–5× ULN), without an increase in total bilirubin above 2× ULN: no change; if grade 2 persists, hold; after resolution to baseline or grade 1, resume at the next lower dose level; grade 2, recurrent (AST/ALT 3.1–5× ULN), without an increase in total bilirubin above 2× ULN: hold; after resolution to baseline or grade 1, resume at the next

lower dose level; **grade 2 or 3 (AST/ALT 3.1–20× ULN) with total bilirubin greater than 2× ULN, in the absence of cholestasis:** discontinue; **grade 4 (AST/ALT >20× ULN):** discontinue

Available forms
Tabs 50, 100, 150, 200 mg

Administer
• With food at the same time every day
• Swallow tablets whole; do not chew, crush, or split. Do not take if broken, cracked
• If a dose is missed, do not replace missed dose; resume with the next scheduled daily dose

SIDE EFFECTS

GI: Diarrhea, abdominal pain, anorexia, nausea, vomiting, constipation, stomatitis, weight loss
CNS: Dizziness, drowsiness, fatigue, fever
MS: Arthralgia
INTEG: Rash, alopecia
GU: Renal failure (rare)
HEMA: Anemia, leukemia, neutropenia, thrombocytopenia
MISC: Infection

PHARMACOKINETICS
Protein binding 96.3%; half-life 18.3 hr; fecal excretion 97.1%; metabolized in liver by CYP3A4

INTERACTIONS
• **Increase:** abemaciclib effect—strong or moderate CYP3A4 inhibitors; avoid concomitant use
• **Decrease:** abemaciclib effect—strong or moderate CYP3A4 inducers; avoid concomitant use

NURSING CONSIDERATIONS
Assess:
• **Diarrhea:** at the first sign of loose stools, start antidiarrheal therapy, increase oral fluids
• **Neutropenia:** CBC baseline then q2wk for the first 2 mo, then monthly for the next 2 mo, and as needed
• **Venous thromboembolism:** monitor for signs, symptoms of thrombosis, pulmonary embolism; treat as needed

• **PE:** chest pain worse when breathing deeply or coughing, coughing up blood, dizziness, fainting, tachypnea, rapid heartbeat, irregular heartbeat, shortness of breath
• **Infection:** assess for urinary tract infection, lung infection, pharyngitis, conjunctivitis, sinusitis, vaginal infection, sepsis
• **Hepatotoxicity:** monitor LFTs baseline, then q2wk × 2 mo, monthly × next 2 mo, and then as needed; interruption in therapy or delay in treatment may be needed
• **Pregnancy/breastfeeding:** Avoid in females of reproductive potential during treatment and for at least 3 wk after last dose; can cause fetal harm or death; discontinue breastfeeding during treatment and for 3 wk after final dose. Presence in breast milk unknown. Obtain pregnancy test before treatment

Evaluate:
• Therapeutic outcome: decrease in size of cancerous tumor

Teach patient/family:
• **Infection:** to report the following to health care provider: increased temperature, fever, shaking, chills, cough, sore throat
• **Diarrhea:** to start antidiarrheal therapy at the first sign of loose stools, increase fluids, and notify health care provider
• **Thromboembolism:** to report immediately chest pain, worse when breathing deeply or coughing, coughing up blood, dizziness, fainting, tachypnea, rapid heartbeat, irregular heartbeat, shortness of breath, pain, swelling of the extremity with redness and warmth, discoloration including a bluish color
• **Pregnancy/breastfeeding:** not to use in pregnancy, breastfeeding; to use contraception during treatment and for at least 3 wk after last dose

---

⚠ HIGH ALERT

abiraterone (Rx)
(a′bir-a′ter-one)
Zytiga
Func. class.: Antineoplastic
Chem. class.: Androgen inhibitor

ACTION: Converted to abiraterone, which inhibits CYP17, the enzyme required for androgen biosynthesis; androgen-sensitive prostate cancer responds to treatment that decreases androgens

USES: Metastatic, castration-resistant prostate cancer in combination with predniSONE

CONTRAINDICATIONS: Pregnancy, women, children, breastfeeding
Precautions: Adrenal insufficiency, cardiac disease, MI, heart failure, hepatic disease, hypertension, hypokalemia, infection, surgery, ventricular dysrhythmia, stress, trauma

DOSAGE AND ROUTES
• **Adult males:** PO 1000 mg/day with predniSONE 5 mg bid and with GnRH (gonadotropin-releasing hormone analog) or bilateral orchiectomy; with strong CYP3A4 inducers 1000 mg bid
Hepatic dose
• **Adult males (Child-Pugh B, 7-9):** PO 250 mg/day with predniSONE; permanently discontinue if AST/ALT >5 × the upper limit of normal (ULN) or total bilirubin >3 × ULN; Child-Pugh C >10, do not use
Available forms: Tabs 250, 500 mg
Administer:
PO route
• Give whole on empty stomach 2 hr before or 1 hr after meals with full glass of water; do not crush, break, chew
• **Pregnancy:** women who are pregnant or who may become pregnant should not touch tabs without gloves
• Store tabs at room temperature

SIDE EFFECTS
CV: Angina, dysrhythmia exacerbation, atrial flutter/fibrillation/tachycardia, AV block, chest pain, edema, heart failure, MI, hypertension, QT prolongation, sinus tachycardia, supraventricular tachycardia, ventricular tachycardia
ENDO: Hot flashes, adrenocortical insufficiency
GI: Diarrhea, dyspepsia, hepatotoxicity
GU: Increased urinary frequency, nocturia, urinary tract infection

META: Adrenocortical insufficiency, hyperbilirubinemia, hypertriglyceridemia, hypokalemia, hypophosphatemia
MS: Arthralgia, myalgia, fracture
RESP: Cough, upper respiratory infection
SYST: Infection

PHARMACOKINETICS
99% protein binding, converted to abiraterone (active metabolite), half-life 12 hr; excreted 88% (feces), 5% (urine); high-fat food increases effect, give on empty stomach; increased effect in hepatic disease

INTERACTIONS
• **Decrease:** abiraterone effect—CYP3A4 inducers (carBAMazepine, phenytoin, rifAMPin, rifabutin, rifapentine, PHENobarbital); dose may need to be increased
• **Increase:** action of CYP2D6/CYP2C8 substrates—dextromethorphan, thioridazine, pioglitazone; doses of these products should be reduced; avoid concurrent use if possible
Drug/Food
Increase: abiraterone action—must be taken on an empty stomach
Drug/Lab
Increase: ALT, AST, bilirubin, triglycerides, cholesterol, alk phos
Decrease: potassium, phosphate, testosterone, lymphocytes

NURSING CONSIDERATIONS
Assess:
• **Prostate cancer:** monitor prostate-specific antigen (PSA), serum potassium, serum bilirubin baseline and periodically
• **Hepatotoxicity:** monitor liver function tests (AST/ALT) at baseline, every 2 wk for 3 mo, monthly thereafter in patients with no known hepatic disease; interrupt treatment in patients without known hepatic disease at baseline who develop ALT/AST >5 × ULN or total bilirubin >3 × ULN; patients with moderate hepatic disease at baseline, measure ALT, AST, bilirubin before the start of treatment, every wk for 1 mo, every 2 wk for the following 2 mo, monthly thereafter; if elevations in ALT and/or AST >5 × ULN or total bilirubin >3 × ULN occur in patients with moderate hepatic impair-

ment at baseline, discontinue and do NOT restart; measure serum total bilirubin, AST/ALT if hepatotoxicity is suspected; elevations of AST, ALT, bilirubin from baseline should prompt more frequent monitoring

• Monitor B/P, pulse, edema, if hypertensive, control symptoms

• **Musculoskeletal pain, joint swelling, discomfort:** arthritis, arthralgia, joint swelling, and joint stiffness, some severe; muscle discomfort that includes muscle spasms, musculoskeletal pain, myalgia, musculoskeletal discomfort, and musculoskeletal stiffness may be relieved with analgesics

• Signs, symptoms of adrenocorticoid insufficiency (anorexia, nausea, vomiting, fatigue, weight loss); corticosteroids may need to be prescribed during stress, trauma, surgery; assess monthly for hypertension, hypokalemia, fluid retention

• **QT prolongation:** monitor ECG for QT prolongation, ejection fraction in patients with cardiac disease; small increases in the QTc interval such as <10 ms have occurred; monitor for arrhythmia exacerbation such as sinus tachycardia, atrial fibrillation, supraventricular tachycardia (SVT), atrial tachycardia, ventricular tachycardia, atrial flutter, bradycardia, AV block complete, conduction disorder, bradyarrhythmia

Evaluate:

• Therapeutic response: Decreasing spread, progression of prostate cancer

Teach patient/family:

• **Pregnancy:** that women must not come into contact with tabs; to wear gloves if product needs to be handled; that males should wear condoms and use another form of contraception if partner is pregnant during use of product and for 1 wk after discontinuing treatment

• To report chest pain, swelling of joints, burning/pain when urinating

• Not to use with other medications, herbs without prescriber approval

• To take 2 hr before or 1 hr after meals; to swallow tab whole, take with water

• That this product, predniSONE, and a GnRH need to be used together

• Not to stop abruptly without prescriber consent

⚠ **HIGH ALERT**

RARELY USED

acalabrutinib

Calquence

Func. class.: Antineoplastic

USES: For the treatment of mantle cell lymphoma (MCL) in patients who have received at least 1 prior therapy

DOSAGE AND ROUTES

For the treatment of mantle cell lymphoma (MCL) in patients who have received at least 1 prior therapy

• **Adult: PO** 100 mg bid (approximately 12 hr apart) until disease progression

---

acamprosate (Rx)

(a-kam-pro'sate)

Campral ♣

Func. class.: Alcohol deterrent

Chem. class.: Synthetic amino acid neurotransmitter analog

ACTION: Not completely understood; in vitro data suggest it has affinity for type A and type B GABA receptors, lowers neuronal excitability, centrally mediated

USES: Alcohol abstinence management

CONTRAINDICATIONS

Hypersensitivity to this product or sulfites, creatinine clearance ≤30 mL/min

Precautions: Pregnancy, breastfeeding, infants, children, ethanol intoxication, renal impairment, depression, suicidal ideation, driving or operating machinery, geriatric patients

DOSAGE AND ROUTES

• **Adult: PO** 666 mg tid

Renal dosage

• **Adult: PO** CCr 30-50 mL/min 333 mg tid; CCr <30 mL/min do not use

Available forms: Del-rel tabs 333 mg

Administer:
- Without regard to food; do not crush, chew, break del-rel tab
- Use only after alcohol is stopped
- Store at room temperature

SIDE EFFECTS

CNS: Anxiety, depression, dizziness, headache, insomnia, paresthesias, suicidal ideation, tremors, abnormal dreams, chills, drowsiness
CV: Palpitations, hypertension, peripheral edema
EENT: Rhinitis, pharyngitis, abnormal vision
GI: Anorexia, constipation, diarrhea, dry mouth, abdominal pain, flatulence, nausea, vomiting, taste change, weight gain
GU: Impotence
INTEG: Rash, pruritus, increased sweating
MISC: Infection, flulike symptoms
MS: Back pain, myalgias, arthralgia
RESP: Dyspnea, bronchitis

PHARMACOKINETICS
Peak 3-8 hr, half-life 20-33 hr

INTERACTIONS
Drug/Lab
Increase: LFTs, blood glucose, bilirubin, uric acid
Decrease: Hgb/Hct, platelets

NURSING CONSIDERATIONS
Assess:
- **Mental status:** depression, abnormal dreams, suicidal thoughts/behaviors, length of alcohol use, date of discontinuing alcohol use
- **B/P** baseline and periodically
- **Pregnancy/breastfeeding:** use only if benefits outweigh fetal risk; cautious use in breastfeeding, excretion unknown
Evaluate:
- Therapeutic response: continued alcohol abstinence
Teach patient/family:
- To notify prescriber of depression, abnormal thoughts, suicidal thoughts/behaviors
- To take without regard to food; not to break, crush, chew del-rel tabs
- Not to engage in hazardous activities until effect is known; may impair thinking; monitor skills

- Not to use alcohol, to continue treatment for alcohol addiction
- **Pregnancy/breastfeeding:** to notify prescriber if pregnancy is planned or suspected; to use effective contraception; breastfeeding effects are unknown

---

> ## ⚠ HIGH ALERT
>
> ### acarbose (Rx)
> (ay-car′bose)
> Glucobay ✦, Prandase ✦, Precose
> *Func. class.:* Oral antidiabetic
> *Chem. class.:* α-Glucosidase inhibitor

Do not confuse:
Precose/PreCare

ACTION: Delays digestion/absorption of ingested carbohydrates by inhibiting α-glucosidase, results in smaller rise in postprandial blood glucose after meals; does not increase insulin production

USES: Type 2 diabetes mellitus, alone or in combination with a sulfonylurea, metformin, insulin
Unlabeled uses: Adjunct in type 1 diabetes mellitus with insulin

CONTRAINDICATIONS: Breastfeeding, hypersensitivity, diabetic ketoacidosis, cirrhosis, inflammatory bowel disease, ileus, colonic ulceration, partial intestinal obstruction, chronic intestinal disease, serum creatinine >2 mg/dL, CCr <25 mL/min
Precautions: Pregnancy, children, renal/hepatic disease

DOSAGE AND ROUTES
- **Adult: PO** 25 mg tid initially, with 1st bite of meal; maintenance dose may be increased to 50-100 mg tid; dosage adjustment at 4- to 8-wk intervals, individualized
Type 1 diabetes mellitus in those on insulin (unlabeled)
- **Adult: PO** 50 mg tid with meals × 2 wk, then 100 mg tid with meals
Available forms: Tabs 25, 50, 100 mg

Administer:

PO route

- With 1st bite of each meal 3×/day
- Store in a tight container, cool environment

SIDE EFFECTS

GI: *Abdominal pain, diarrhea, flatulence*

PHARMACOKINETICS

Poor systemic absorption, peak 1 hr, duration 2-4 hr, metabolized in GI tract, excreted as intact product in urine, half-life 2 hr

INTERACTIONS

Increase: acetaminophen toxicity—acetaminophen combined with alcohol; avoid concurrent use

Increase or decrease: glycemic control—androgens, lithium, bortezomib, quinolones; check for glucose control

Decrease: effect of digoxin; monitor digoxin levels

Increase: hypoglycemia—sulfonylureas, insulin, MAOIs, salicylates, fibric acid derivatives, bile acid sequestrants, ACE inhibitors, angiotensin II receptor antagonists, β-blockers; check for glucose control

Decrease: effect, increase hyperglycemia—digestive enzymes, intestinal absorbents, thiazide diuretics, loop diuretics, corticosteroids, estrogen, progestins, oral contraceptives, sympathomimetics, isoniazid, phenothiazines, protease inhibitors, atypical antipsychotics, carbonic anhydrase inhibitors, cycloSPORINE, tacrolimus, baclofen

Drug/Herb

Increase: hypoglycemia—chromium, garlic, horse chestnut; check for glucose control

Drug/Lab Test

Increase: ALT, AST

Decrease: calcium, vit B_6, Hgb, Hct

NURSING CONSIDERATIONS

Assess:

- **Hypoglycemia** (weakness, hunger, dizziness, tremors, anxiety, tachycardia, sweating); even though product does not cause hypoglycemia, if patient is on sul-fonylureas or insulin, hypoglycemia may be additive; if hypoglycemia occurs, treat with dextrose or, if severe, with IV glucose or glucagon

- For stress, surgery, or other trauma that may require change in dose

- Monitor AST, ALT q3mo × 1 yr and periodically thereafter; if elevated, dose may need to be reduced or discontinued, usually increased with doses ≥300 mg/day; dose-related elevations may occur and patients are usually asymptomatic; if symptomatic, dosage reduction or withdrawal is needed; A1c q3mo, monitor serum glucose, 1 hr PP throughout treatment

- GI side effects for tolerability/compliance

- **Pregnancy/breastfeeding:** use in pregnancy only if needed; avoid breastfeeding if using acarbose with other antidiabetics

Evaluate:

- Therapeutic response: improved signs/symptoms of diabetes mellitus (decreased polyuria, polydipsia, polyphagia; clear sensorium, absence of dizziness, stable gait)

Teach patient/family:

- The symptoms of hypo/hyperglycemia; what to do about each, that other medications may increase hypoglycemia risk

- That medication must be taken as prescribed; that must be taken with food; explain consequences of discontinuing medication abruptly; that insulin may need to be used for stress, including trauma, surgery, fever

- To avoid medications and herbal supplements unless approved by health care provider

- That diabetes is a lifelong illness; that the diet and exercise regimen must be followed; that this product is not a cure

- To carry emergency ID and a glucose source; to avoid sugar, because sugar is blocked by acarbose

- That blood glucose monitoring is required to assess product effect

- To avoid breastfeeding if using acarbose with other antidiabetics

---

- That GI side effects may occur
- **Pregnancy/breastfeeding:** to notify provider if pregnancy is planned or suspected or if breastfeeding

---

acetaminophen (Rx, OTC) (Paracetamol)

(a-seat-a-mee′noe-fen)

222AF ✤, Abenol ✤, Acephen, Acephen Infant Feverall, ACET ✤, Acetab ✤, Apacet, APAP, Apra, Atasol ✤, Children's FeverAll, Fortolin ✤, Genapap, Infantaire, Mapap, NeoPAP, Novo-Gesic ✤, Pediaphen ✤, Pediatrix ✤, Q-Pap, Q-Pap Children's, Rapid Action Relief ✤, Redutemp, Ridenol, Robigesic ✤, Rounox ✤, Silapap, Taminol ✤, Tempra ✤, T-Painol, Tylenol, ✤ XS pain reliever

Acetaminophen (IV) Ofirmive

Func. class.: Nonopioid analgesic, antipyretic
Chem. class.: Nonsalicylate, paraaminophenol derivative

Do not confuse:
Acephen/Anacin/Aspirin 3/Anacin-3

ACTION: May block pain impulses peripherally that occur in response to inhibition of prostaglandin synthesis; does not possess antiinflammatory properties; antipyretic action results from inhibition of prostaglandins in the CNS (hypothalamic heat-regulating center)

USES: Mild to moderate pain or fever, arthralgia, dental pain, dysmenorrhea, headache, myalgia, osteoarthritis
Unlabeled uses: Migraine

CONTRAINDICATIONS: Hypersensitivity to this product, phenacetin aspartame, saccharin, tartrazine

Precautions: Pregnancy, breastfeeding, geriatric patients, anemia, renal/hepatic disease, chronic alcoholism

Black Box Warning: Hepatotoxicity

DOSAGE AND ROUTES
- **Adult/child >12 yr:** PO/RECT 325-650 mg q4-6hr prn, max 4 g/day; **weight ≥50 kg IV** 1000 mg q6hr or 650 mg q4hr prn, max single dose 1000 mg, min dosing interval 4 hr; **weight <50 kg IV** 15 mg/kg/dose q6hr or 12.5 mg/kg/dose q4hr, max single dose 15 mg/kg, min dosing interval 4 hr, max 75 mg/kg/day from all sources; **EXT REL** 650-1300 mg q8hr as needed, max 4 g/day
- **Child ≥2 yr and <50 kg:** IV 15 mg/kg/dose q6hr or 12.5 mg/kg/dose q4hr, max single dose 15 mg/kg, min dosing interval 4 hr, max 75 mg/kg/day from all sources
Renal dose
- **Adult:** IV CCr <30 mL/min reduce dose and prolong interval, CCr <10 mL/min PO/RECT/IV minimum interval of q8hr
Migraine (unlabeled)
- **Adult and adolescent:** PO/RECT 500-1000 mg, max 1 g/dose or max 4 g/day

Available forms: Rect supp 120, 325, 650 mg; soft chew tabs 80, 160 mg; caps 500 mg; elix 120, 160, 325 mg/5 mL; oral disintegrating tab 80, 160 mg; oral drops 80 mg/0.8 mL, liquid 500 mg/5 mL, 160/5 mL, 1000/30 mL; ext rel 650 mg, 80 mg/mL; tabs 325, 500, 650 mg; sol for inj 1000 mg/100 mL
Administer:
PO route
- Do not confuse 2 × 325 (650 mg), with 650-mg ext rel tab
- Crushed or whole, do not crush ext rel product; chewable tabs may be chewed; give with full glass of water
- With food or milk to decrease gastric symptoms if needed
- Susp after shaken well; check elixir, liquid, suspension concentration carefully; susp and caps are bioequivalent
Rectal route
- Store suppositories <80° F (27° C)

Side effects: *italics* = common; red = life-threatening

Intermittent IV INFUSION route
• No further dilution needed; do not add other medications to vial or infusion device
• For doses equal to single vial, a vented IV set may be used to deliver directly from vial; for doses less than a single vial, withdraw dose and place in an empty sterile syringe, plastic IV container, or glass bottle; infuse over 15 min
• Discard unused portion; if seal is broken, vial penetrated, or drug transferred to another container, give within 6 hr

Y-site: Do not admix

SIDE EFFECTS

CNS: Agitation (child) (IV); headache, fatigue, anxiety (IV)
Resp: Dyspnea (IV), atelectasis (child) (IV)
CV: Hyper- and hypotension (IV)
GI: Nausea, vomiting, abdominal pain; hepatotoxicity, hepatic seizure (overdose), GI bleeding
GU: Renal failure (high, prolonged doses)
HEMA: Leukopenia, neutropenia, hemolytic anemia (long-term use), thrombocytopenia, pancytopenia
INTEG: Rash, urticaria, inj site pain
SYST: Stevens-Johnson syndrome, toxic epidermal necrolysis
TOXICITY: Cyanosis, anemia, neutropenia, jaundice, pancytopenia, CNS stimulation, delirium followed by vascular collapse, seizures, coma, death

PHARMACOKINETICS

85%-90% metabolized by liver, excreted by kidneys; metabolites may be toxic if overdose occurs; widely distributed; crosses placenta in low concentrations; excreted in breast milk; half-life 1-4 hr
PO: Onset 10-30 min, peak $^1/_2$-2 hr, duration 4-6 hr, well absorbed
IV: Onset rapid, peak 30-120 min, duration 3-4 hr
RECT: Onset slow, peak 1-2 hr, duration 4-6 hr, absorption varies

INTERACTIONS

Increase: renal adverse reactions—NSAIDs, salicylates; consider lower dose
Increase: methemoglobinemia—nitric oxide, prilocaine; avoid concurrent use

Increase: hypoprothrombinemia—warfarin, long-term use, high doses of acetaminophen
Increase: hepatotoxicity—barbiturates, alcohol, carBAMazepine, hydantoins, rifAMPin, rifabutin, isoniazid, diflunisal, zidovudine, lamoTRIgine, imatinib, dasatinib, mipomersen; monitor for hepatotoxicity
Decrease: absorption—colestipol, cholestyramine
Decrease: zidovudine, lamoTRIgine effect
Drug/Herb
Increase: hepatotoxicity—St. John's wort, due to acetaminophen metabolism
Drug/Lab Test
Increase: LFTs, potassium, bilirubin, LDH, pro-time
Decrease: Hgb/Hct, WBC, RBC, platelets; albumin, magnesium, phosphate (pediatrics)

NURSING CONSIDERATIONS
Assess:
• **For fever and pain:** Type of pain, location, intensity, duration, aggravating/alleviating factors; assess for diaphoresis, fever, baseline and periodically
• **Hepatic studies:** AST, ALT, bilirubin, creatinine before therapy if long-term therapy is anticipated; may cause hepatic toxicity at doses >4 g/day with chronic use
• **Renal studies:** BUN, urine creatinine, occult blood, albumin, if patient is on long-term therapy; presence of blood or albumin indicates nephritis, I&O ratio; decreasing output may indicate renal failure (long-term therapy)
• **Blood studies:** CBC, PT if patient is on long-term therapy
• **Chronic poisoning:** rapid, weak pulse; dyspnea; cold, clammy extremities; report immediately to prescriber

> **Black Box Warning: Hepatotoxicity:** occurs with high doses (>4 g/day); dark urine; clay-colored stools; yellowing of skin, sclera; itching; abdominal pain; fever; diarrhea if patient is on long-term therapy; may require liver transplant, those malnourished or using alcohol chronically are at higher chance of hepatotoxicity

• **Potentially fatal hypersensitivity, allergic reactions:** rash, urticaria; if these occur, product may have to be discontinued
• Stevens-Johnson syndrome, toxic epidermal necrolysis may occur during beginning treatment or any other dose
• **Pregnancy/breastfeeding:** cautious use in pregnancy, breastfeeding (PO), use only if clearly needed (IV)

Evaluate:
• Therapeutic response: absence of pain using pain scoring; absence of fever

Teach patient/family:

Black Box Warning: **Hepatotoxicity:** not to exceed recommended dosage; the elixir, liquid, suspension come in several concentrations, read label carefully; acute poisoning with liver damage may result; tell parents of children to check products carefully; that acute toxicity includes symptoms of nausea, vomiting, abdominal pain and that prescriber should be notified immediately; that toxicity may occur when used with other combination products

• Not to use with alcohol, herbals, OTC products without approval of prescriber
• **To recognize signs of chronic overdose:** bleeding, bruising, malaise, fever, sore throat
• That those with diabetes may notice blood glucose monitoring changes
• To notify prescriber of pain or fever lasting more than 3 days
• Not to be used in patients <2 yr unless approved by prescriber
• **Hypersensitivity:** to stop product, call prescriber if rash occurs
• **Pregnancy/breastfeeding:** May be used when breastfeeding, short-term

TREATMENT OF OVERDOSE:
Product level, gastric lavage; administer oral acetylcysteine to prevent hepatic damage *(see acetylcysteine monograph)*; monitor for bleeding

---

acetaZOLAMIDE (Rx)
(a-set-a-zole′a-mide)
Acetazolam ✦, Diamox ✦, Novo-Zolamide ✦
Func. class.: Diuretic, carbonic anhydrase inhibitor, antiglaucoma agent, antiepileptic
Chem. class.: Sulfonamide derivative

Do not confuse:
acetaZOLAMIDE/acetoHEXAMIDE
Diamox/Diabinese

ACTION: Inhibits carbonic anhydrase activity in proximal renal tubules to decrease reabsorption of water, sodium, potassium, bicarbonate resulting in increased urine volume and alkalinization of urine; decreases carbonic anhydrase in CNS, increasing seizure threshold; able to decrease secretion of aqueous humor in eye, which lowers intraocular pressure

USES: Open-angle glaucoma, angle-closure glaucoma (preoperatively, if surgery delayed), mixed, tonic-clonic, myoclonic, refractory seizures, epilepsy (petit mal, grand mal, absence), edema in HF, product-induced edema, acute altitude sickness
Unlabeled uses: Urine alkalinization, metabolic alkalosis in mechanical ventilation, decrease CSF production in infants with hydrocephalus, familial periodic paralysis, nystagmus

CONTRAINDICATIONS: Hypersensitivity to sulfonamides, severe renal/hepatic disease, electrolyte imbalances (hyponatremia, hypokalemia), hyperchloremic acidosis, Addison's disease, long-term use for closed-angle glaucoma, adrenocortical insufficiency, metabolic acidosis, acidemia, anuria
Precautions: Pregnancy, breastfeeding, hypercalciuria, respiratory acidosis, pulmonary obstruction/emphysema, COPD

DOSAGE AND ROUTES
Angle-closure glaucoma
• **Adult: PO/IV** 250 mg q4hr or 250 mg bid for short-term therapy

---

Side effects: *italics* = common; red = life-threatening

Chronic open-angle glaucoma
- **Adult:** PO/IV 250 mg 1-4 times per day or 500 mg **EXT REL** bid, max 1 g/day
- **Child (Unlabeled):** PO 8-30 mg/kg/day in divided doses tid or qid, or 300-900 mg/m²/day, max 1 g/day; **IV** 5-10 mg q6hr, max 1 g/day

Edema in heart failure, drug-induced edema
- **Adult:** PO/IV 250-375 mg/day
- **Child (unlabeled):** PO/IV 5 mg/kg/day or 150 mg/m² in AM

Adjunct for epilepsy and myoclonic, refractory, generalized tonic-clonic, absence or mixed seizures
- **Adult:** PO/IV 8-30 mg/kg/day in 1-4 divided doses, usual range 375-1000 mg/day; **EXT REL** not recommended with seizures

Altitude sickness
- **Adult:** PO 125 mg bid, start therapy 24-48 hr before ascent and give for ≥48 hr after arrival at high altitude

Renal dose
- **Adult:** PO/IV CCr 50-80 mL/min give dose ≥q6hr regular release or IV; CCr 10-50 mL/min give dose q12hr; CCr <10 mL/min, avoid use

Urine alkalinization (unlabeled)
- **Adult:** IV 5 mg/kg/dose, repeat 2-3× over 24 hr

Familial periodic paralysis (unlabeled)
- **Adult:** PO 250-375 mg/day in divided doses

Metabolic alkalosis in mechanical ventilation (unlabeled)
- **Adult:** IV 500 mg as a single dose or 250 mg q6hr × 4 doses

Vestibular nystagmus (unlabeled)
- **Adult:** PO 250 mg, increase by 250 mg q3days; max 3 g/day in divided doses

Available forms: Tabs 125, 250 mg; ext rel caps 500 mg; inj 500 mg

Administer:
- In AM to avoid interference with sleep if using product as diuretic
- Potassium replacement if potassium level is <3 mg/dL

PO route
- Do not break, crush, or chew ext rel caps; this product should be used for altitude sickness, glaucoma; store at room temperature
- With food if nausea occurs; absorption may be decreased slightly

IV route
- Reconstitute with 500 mg in ≥5 mL sterile water for inj; **direct IV:** give at 100-150 mg/min
- Store in cool, dark area; use reconstituted solution within 24 hr

SIDE EFFECTS
CNS: Anxiety, *confusion*, seizures, *depression*, dizziness, *drowsiness, fatigue*, headache, *paresthesia*, stimulation
EENT: Myopia, tinnitus
ENDO: *Hyper/hypoglycemia*
GI: *Nausea, vomiting, anorexia, diarrhea*, melena, *weight loss*, hepatic insufficiency, cholestatic jaundice, fulminant hepatic necrosis, *taste alterations*, bleeding
GU: *Frequency, polyuria*, uremia, glucosuria, hematuria, dysuria, crystalluria, renal calculi
HEMA: Aplastic anemia, hemolytic anemia, leukopenia, thrombocytopenia, purpura, pancytopenia
INTEG: *Rash*, pruritus, urticaria, fever, Stevens-Johnson syndrome, photosensitivity, flushing, toxic epidermal necrolysis
META: *Hypokalemia, hyperchloremic acidosis*, hyponatremia, sulfonamide-like reactions, metabolic acidosis, growth inhibition in children, hyperuricemia, hypercalcemia

PHARMACOKINETICS
65% absorbed if fasting (oral), 75% absorbed if given with food; half-life 2½-5½ hr; excreted unchanged by kidneys (80% within 24 hr), crosses placenta
PO: Onset 1-1½ hr, peak 1-4 hr, duration 8-12 hr

PO-EXT REL: Onset 2 hr, peak 3-6 hr, duration 18-24 hr

IV: Onset 2 min, peak 15 min, duration 4-5 hr

INTERACTIONS

Increase: action of—amphetamines, flecainide, phenytoin, procainamide, quiNIDine, anticholinergics, methenamine, mecamylamine, ePHEDrine, memantine, mexiletine, folic acid antagonists; monitor for increased action of each patient

Increase: excretion of lithium, primidone

Increase: alpha/beta blockers, antihypertensives, hypotensive effect; monitor drug levels

Increase: osteomalacia—carBAMazepine, ethotoin

Increase: toxicity—salicylates, cycloSPORINE

Increase: hypokalemia—corticosteroids, amphotericin B, corticotropin, ACTH

Increase: cardiac toxicity if hypokalemia develops—arsenic trioxide, cardiac glycosides, levomethadyl

Increase: renal stone formation, heat stroke—topiramate (avoid concurrent use)

Drug/Lab Test

Increase: glucose, uric acid

Decrease: thyroid iodine uptake, sodium, Hct/Hgb, WBC, platelets

False positive: urinary protein, 17 hydroxysteroid

NURSING CONSIDERATIONS
Assess:

Black Box Warning: Stevens-Johnson syndrome, toxic epidermal necrolysis, blood dyscrasias; discontinue if these occur

• **Edema:** weight daily, I&O daily to determine fluid loss; effect of product may be decreased if used daily; monitor geriatric patients for dehydration
• **Ocular status:** intraocular pressure, ophthalmologic examination
• **B/P** lying, standing; postural hypotension may occur

• Electrolytes: potassium, sodium, chloride; also BUN, blood glucose, CBC, serum creatinine, blood pH, ABGs, LFTs; I&O, platelet count, patient may need to be on a high-potassium diet; identify signs of hypokalemia (vomiting, fatigue, weakness)

• **Seizures:** neurologic status: provide seizure precautions

• **Beers:** avoid in older adults unless safer alternative is not available; may cause ataxia, impaired psychomotor function

• **Pregnancy/breastfeeding:** If pregnancy is planned or suspected or if breastfeeding. Use in pregnancy only if benefits outweigh fetal risk. Women who are pregnant should enroll in the AED Pregnancy Registry (888-233-2334)

Evaluate:

• Therapeutic response: improvement in edema of feet, legs, sacral area daily if medication is being used for HF; decrease in aqueous humor if medication is being used for glaucoma; decreased frequency of seizures, prevention of altitude sickness

Teach patient/family:

• To take exactly as prescribed; if dose is missed, take as soon as remembered; not to double dose; to take with food for GI symptoms; not to crush, chew open capsules

• **Altitude sickness:** to avoid rapid ascent

• **Diabetic:** that drug may alter blood glucose and to monitor blood glucose

• To use sunscreen to prevent photosensitivity, to avoid prolonged sun exposure, phototoxicity may occur

• To avoid hazardous activities if drowsiness occurs

• To report nausea, vertigo, rapid weight gain, change in stools, weakness, numbness, rash, sore throat, bleeding/bruising; Stevens-Johnson syndrome, toxic epidermal necrolysis (blistering, red rash that spreads)

• **Pregnancy/breastfeeding:** to notify prescriber if pregnancy is planned or suspected; to avoid breastfeeding

TREATMENT OF OVERDOSE:
Lavage if taken orally; monitor electrolytes; administer dextrose in saline; monitor hydration, CV, renal status

---

acetylcholine ophthalmic
See Appendix B

---

acetylcysteine (Rx)
(a-se-teel-sis´tay-een)
Acetadote, Cetylev ♥
Func. class.: Mucolytic; antidote—acetaminophen
Chem. class.: Amino acid L-cysteine

ACTION: Decreases viscosity of secretions by breaking disulfide links of mucoproteins; serves as a substrate in place of glutathione, which is necessary to inactivate toxic metabolites with acetaminophen overdose

USES: Acetaminophen toxicity; bronchitis; cystic fibrosis; COPD; atelectasis
Unlabeled uses: Prevention of contrast medium nephrotoxicity

CONTRAINDICATIONS: Hypersensitivity
Precautions: Pregnancy, breastfeeding, hypothyroidism, Addison's disease, CNS depression, brain tumor, asthma, renal/hepatic disease, COPD, psychosis, alcoholism, seizure disorders, bronchospasms, anaphylactoid reactions, fluid restriction, weight <40 kg, increased intracranial pressure, status asthmaticus

DOSAGE AND ROUTES
Acetaminophen toxicity
• **Adult and child: PO** 140 mg/kg, then 70 mg/kg q4hr × 17 doses to total of 1330 mg/kg; ≥ **41-100 kg IV** loading dose 150 mg/kg over 60 min (dilution 150 mg/kg in 200 mL of D_5W); then 50 mg/kg over 4 hr (dilution 50 mg/kg in 500 mL D_5W); then 100 mg/kg over 16 hr (dilution 100 mg/kg in 1000 D_5W)
• **Adult/child 21-40 kg: IV** 150 mg/kg in 100 mL diluent over 1 hr, then 50 mg/kg in 250 mL over 4 hr, then 100 mg/kg in 500 mg over 16 hr
• **Infant/child 5-20 kg: IV** 150 mg/kg in 3 mL/kg diluent over 1 hr, then 50 mg/kg in 7 mL/kg diluent over 4 hr, then 100 mg/kg in 14 mL/kg diluent over 16 hr
Mucolytic
• **Adult and child 1-12 yr: INSTILL** 1-2 mL (10%-20% sol) q6-8hr prn or 3-5 mL (20% sol) or 6-10 mL (10% sol) tid or qid; **NEBULIZER** (face mask, mouthpiece, tracheostomy) 1-10 mL of a 20% sol, or 2-20 mL of a 10% sol, q2-8hr; **NEBULIZER** (tent, croupette) may require large dose, up to 300 mL/treatment
Tracheostomy care
• **Adult/child: INSTILL** 1-2 mL (10%-20% sol) q1-4hr directly into tracheostomy
Diagnostic bronchial lab studies
• **Adult/child: NEBULIZER** 2-3 uses of 1-2 mL of 20% sol or 2-4 mL of 10% sol
Prevention of radiocontrast-induced renal reactions (unlabeled)
• **Adult: PO** 600 mg bid X 2 days before radiocontrast
Available forms: Oral sol 10%, 20%; inj 20% (200 mg/mL); effervescent tab for oral solution 500, 2500 mg
Administer:
PO route
• **Antidotal use:** give within 8 hr for best results; dilute 10% or 20% sol to a 5% sol with diet soda, may use water if giving via gastric tube; dilution of 10% sol 1:1, 20% sol 1:3, store open undiluted solution refrigerated ≤96 hr, repeat dose if vomited within 1 hr
PO route (effervescent tablets for oral solution)
• Dissolve in 100 mL water (50 mg/mL) **1-19 kg;** in 150 mL water **20-59 kg;** 300 mg/mL ≥**60 kg**

Direct intratracheal instill route

• By syringe: 1-2 mL of 10%-20% sol up to q1hr

• Decreased dose to geriatric patients; metabolism may be slowed

• Only if suction machine is available

• Only after patient clears airway by deep breathing, coughing

• Assistance with inhaled dose: bronchodilator if bronchospasm occurs; mechanical suction if cough insufficient to remove excess bronchial secretions

IV route

• **21-hr regimen:** loading dose: dilute 150 mg/kg in 200 mL D_5W; maintenance dose 1: dilute 50 mg/kg in 500 mL D_5W; maintenance dose 2: dilute 100 mg/kg in 1000 mL D_5W; give loading dose over 15 min; give maintenance dose 1 over 4 hr; give maintenance dose 2 over 16 hr, administer sequentially without time between doses

• Store in refrigerator; use within 96 hr of opening

SIDE EFFECTS

CNS: *Dizziness, drowsiness,* fever, chills
CV: Edema, flushing tachycardia
EENT: *Rhinorrhea,* pharyngitis
GI: *Nausea,* stomatitis, vomiting, anorexia
INTEG: Urticaria, rash, clamminess, pruritus
RESP: Bronchospasm, chest tightness, cough, dyspnea
MISC: Anaphylaxis, angioedema, unpleasant odor

PHARMACOKINETICS

IV: Excreted in urine, half-life 5.6 hr (adult), 11 hr (newborn), protein binding 83%, peak up to 60 min (PO), 5-10 min (INH)
Interactions

• Do not use with activated charcoal

NURSING CONSIDERATIONS
Assess:

• **Mucolytic use:** cough—type, frequency, character, including sputum; bronchospasm

• Rate, rhythm of respirations, increased dyspnea; sputum; discontinue if bronchospasm occurs

• VS, cardiac status including checking for dysrhythmias, increased rate, palpitations

• ABGs for increased CO_2 retention in asthma patients

• **Antidotal use:** use within 24 hr of acetaminophen toxicity, give within 10 hr of acetaminophen to minimize hepatotoxicity; monitor LFTs, PT, BUN, creatinine, glucose, electrolytes, acetaminophen levels; inform prescriber if dose is vomited or if vomiting is persistent; 150 mg/kg may be toxic, check acetaminophen level q4hr

• **Hypersensitivity:** anaphylaxis may occur with IV dose; if present, stop infusion, treat, restart; assess for dyspnea, swelling of face, lips, tongue; rash, itching

• Nausea, vomiting, rash; notify prescriber if these occur

• **Pregnancy/breastfeeding:** use only if clearly needed; cautious use in breastfeeding, excretion unknown

Evaluate:

• Therapeutic response: absence of purulent secretions when coughing, clear lung sounds (mucolytic use); absence of hepatic damage with acetaminophen toxicity

Teach patient/family:

• That foul odor and smell may be unpleasant

• To clear airway for inhalation

• To report vomiting because dose may need to be repeated

• **Acetaminophen toxicity:** Explain reason for product, expected result

---

RARELY USED

aclidinium (Rx)
(a′kli-din′ee-um)
Tudorza Pressair
Func. class.: Anticholinergic, bronchodilator
Chem. class.: Synthetic quaternary ammonium compound

USES: Long-term maintenance treatment of bronchospasm in COPD, emphysema, chronic bronchitis, not indicated for initial treatment of acute episodes

CONTRAINDICATIONS: Hypersensitivity

DOSAGE AND ROUTES
• **Adults, including geriatric patients: ORAL INHALATION** 400 mcg (1 actuation) bid; doses should be 12 hr apart

---

acyclovir (Rx)
(ay-sye′kloe-veer)

Avirax ✚, Sitavig, Xerese ✚, Zovirax

Func. class.: Antiviral
Chem. class.: Purine nucleoside analog

Do not confuse:
Zovirax/Zyvox/Valtrex/Zostrix

ACTION: Converted to acyclovir monophosphate by virus-specific thymidine kinase then further converted to acyclovir triphosphate by other cellular enzymes

USES: Mucocutaneous herpes simplex virus, herpes genitalis (HSV-1, HSV-2), varicella infections, herpes zoster, herpes simplex encephalitis
Unlabeled uses: Bell's palsy, prevention of CMV, Epstein-Barr virus, esophagitis, hairy leukoplakia, prevention of herpes labialis, herpes simplex, herpes simplex ocular prophylaxis, keratoconjunctivitis, pharyngitis, pneumonitis, prevention of postherpetic neuralgia, proctitis, stomatitis, tracheobronchitis, varicella prophylaxis

CONTRAINDICATIONS: Hypersensitivity to this product, valACYclovir; milk protein (buccal)
Precautions: Pregnancy, breastfeeding, renal/hepatic/neurologic disease, electrolyte imbalance, dehydration, hypersensitivity to famciclovir, ganciclovir, penciclovir, valGANciclovir, obesity

DOSAGE AND ROUTES
Base dose in obese patients on ideal body weight, not actual body weight
Herpes simplex (recurrent)
• **Adult: PO** 400 mg 3×/day for 5 days or 200 mg 5×/day × 5 days
• **Adult and child >12 yr: IV INFUSION** 5 mg/kg over 1 hr q8hr × 7 days
• **Infant >3 mo/child <12 yr: IV INFUSION** 10 mg/kg q8hr × 7 days; if HIV infected, 5-10 mg/kg q8hr (moderate to severe)
• **Neonate: IV INFUSION** 10 mg/kg q8hr × 10 days, may use higher dose
Genital herpes, initial episodes
• **Adult: PO** 400 mg tid or 200 mg 5×/day × 7-10 days, may extend treatment if healing is not complete after 10 days; **TOP** × 5 days; **IV** 5 mg/kg q8hr or 750 mg/m²/day divided q8hr × 5-7 days
Genital herpes, episodic treatment
• **Adult: PO** 400 mg tid or 800 mg bid × 5 days or 800 mg tid × 2 days; initiate within 1 day of lesion onset
Genital herpes, suppression therapy
• **Adult: PO** 400 mg bid for up to 12 months or 200 mg 3-5 times daily for up to 12 months
Genital herpes, initial limited, mucocutaneous HSV in immunocompromised patients, non–life-threatening
• **Adult/child ≥12 yr: TOP** cover lesions q3hr 6×/day
Herpes simplex encephalitis
• **Adult: IV** 10 mg/kg over 1 hr q8hr × 10 days
• **Child 3 mo-12 yr: IV** 10-15 mg/kg q8hr × 4-21 days
• **Child birth-3 mo: IV** 20 mg/kg q8hr × 21 days
• **Neonates/premature infants: IV** 10 mg/kg q12hr × 14-21 days
Herpes labialis, recurrent
• **Adult/child ≥12 yr: TOP** apply cream 5×/day for 4 days; start as soon as symptoms appear
Herpes labialis, recurrent in immunocompetent patients
• **Adult: Buccal** 50 mg as a single dose in upper gum region within 1 hr after

---

prodromal symptoms and before cold sore formation

Herpes zoster (immunocompetent)
• **Adult:** PO 800 mg q4hr 5×/day while awake × 7-10 days; **IV** 10 mg/kg q8hr × 7 days

Herpes zoster (shingles) immunocompromised patients
• **Adult/adolescent:** PO 800 mg q4hr 5×/day for 7-10 days; **IV** 10-15 mg/kg q8hr × 10-14 days
• **Infant/child <12 yr:** IV 10 mg/kg/dose q8hr × 7-10 days

Herpes zoster (shingles) immunocompetent
• **Adult:** PO 800 mg q4hr 5×/day × 7-10 days; start within 48-72 hr of rash onset

Varicella (chickenpox)
• **Adult/child ≥2 yr:** PO 10 mg/kg/dose (max 800 mg) 4×/day × 5 days

Mucosal/cutaneous herpes simplex infections in immunosuppressed patients
• **Adult and child >12 yr:** IV 5 mg/kg q8hr × 7 days
• **Infant >3 mo/child <12:** IV 10 mg/kg q8hr × 7 days

Renal dose
• **Adult and child:** PO/IV CCr >50 mL/min 100% dose q8hr, CCr 25-50 mL/min 100% dose q12hr, CCr 10-25 mL/min 100% dose q24hr, CCr 0-10 mL/min 50% dose q24hr

Recurrent ocular herpes, prevention (unlabeled)
• **Adult/child ≥12 yr:** PO 600-800 mg every day × 8-12 mo

CMV prophylaxis (unlabeled)
• **Adult:** IV 500 mg/m^2 q8hr

Herpes simplex in pneumonitis/ esophagitis/tracheobronchitis/ proctitis/stomatitis/pharyngitis (unlabeled)
• **Adult and adolescent:** IV 5-10 mg/kg q8hr × 2-7 days or **PO** 200 mg q4hr 5×/day × 7-10 days or 400 mg 3-5×/day × ≥10 days
• **Child 6 mo-12 yr:** IV 1000 mg/day in 3-5 divided doses × 7-14 days

Herpes simplex prophylaxis for chronic suppression therapy (unlabeled)
• **Adult and adolescent:** PO 400 mg bid up to 12 mo

Available forms: Caps 200 mg; tabs 400, 800 mg; powder for inj 500, 1000 mg; sol for inj 50 mg/mL; oral susp 200 mg/5 mL; ointment/cream 5%; buccal tab 50 mg

Administer:
PO route
• Do not break, crush, or chew caps
• May give without regard to meals, with 8 oz of water
• Shake susp before use

Buccal
• Use on the same side as the herpes labialis lesion; after removing tab from blister, place rounded side of tab to the upper gum above incisor tooth; hold in place for 30 sec; once adhered, the tab will dissolve; if tab falls off within 6 hr, reposition the same tab

Topical route
• Use finger cot or glove to cover all lesions completely; do not get in eye; wash hands after use

Intermittent IV INFUSION route
• Increase fluids to 3 L/day to decrease crystalluria; most critical during first 2 hr after IV
• Reconstitute with 10 mL compatible sol/500 mg or 20 mL/1 g of product, concentrations of 50 mg/mL, shake, further dilute in 50-125 mL compatible sol; use within 12 hr; give over at least 1 hr (constant rate) by infusion pump to prevent nephrotoxicity; do not reconstitute with sol containing benzyl alcohol in neonates
• Store at room temperature for up to 12 hr after reconstitution; if refrigerated, sol may show a precipitate that clears at room temperature; yellow discoloration does not affect potency

Y-site compatibilities: Alemtuzumab, alfentanil, allopurinol, amikacin, aminophylline, amphotericin B cholesteryl, amphotericin B liposome, ampicillin, anidulafungin, argatroban, atracurium, bivalirudin, buprenorphine, busulfan, butorphanol, calcium chloride/gluconate, CARBOplatin, cefazolin, cefonicid, cefotaxime, cefoxitin, ceftazidime, ceftizoxime, cefTRIAXone, cefuroxime, chloramphenicol, cholesteryl sulfate complex, cimetidine, clindamycin, dexamethasone sodium phosphate, dimenhyDRINATE, DOXOrubicin, doxycycline, erythromycin, famotidine, filgrastim, fluconazole, gallium, gentamicin, granisetron, heparin, hydrocortisone sodium succinate, HYDROmorphone, imipenem/cilastatin, LORazepam, magnesium sulfate, melphalan, methylPREDNISolone sodium succinate, metoclopramide, metroNIDAZOLE, multivitamin, nafcillin, oxacillin, PACLitaxel, penicillin G potassium, PENTobarbital, perphenazine, piperacillin, potassium chloride, propofol, raNITIdine, remifentanil, sodium bicarbonate, tacrolimus, teniposide, theophylline, thiotepa, ticarcillin, tobramycin, trimethoprimsulfamethoxazole, vancomycin, vasopressin, voriconazole, zidovudine

SIDE EFFECTS

CNS: Tremors, confusion, lethargy, hallucinations, seizures, dizziness, headache, encephalopathic changes
EENT: Gingival hyperplasia
GI: Nausea, vomiting, diarrhea, increased ALT/AST, abdominal pain, colitis
GU: Hematuria, acute renal failure, changes in menses
HEMA: Thrombotic thrombocytopenia purpura, hemolytic uremic syndrome, leukopenia (immunocompromised patients)
INTEG: Rash, urticaria, pruritus, pain or phlebitis at IV site, unusual sweating, alopecia, Stevens-Johnson syndrome
MS: Joint pain
Syst: Angioedema, anaphylaxis

PHARMACOKINETICS

Distributed widely; crosses placenta; CSF concentrations are 50% of plasma; protein binding 9%-33%

PO: Absorbed minimally, onset unknown, peak 1.5-2 hr, half-life 2.5-3.3 hr (adult); 2-3 hr (child); up to 4 hr (neonates)
Buccal: Peak 8 hr
IV: Onset immediate, peak immediate, duration unknown, half-life 20 min-3 hr (terminal); metabolized by liver, excreted by kidneys as unchanged product (95%)

INTERACTIONS

Increase: CNS side effects—zidovudine
Increase: levels, toxicity—probenecid, monitor for toxicity
Increase: nephrotoxicity—aminoglycosides
Increase: concentrations of—entecavir, PEMEtrexed, tenofovir, theophylline
Decrease: action of—hydantoins, valproic acid, monitor drug levels
Drug/Lab Test
Increase: BUN, creatinine
Decrease: WBC

NURSING CONSIDERATIONS
Assess:
• **Infection:** type of lesions, area of body covered, purulent drainage, frequency of lesions
• **Hepatic, renal studies:** AST, ALT; urinalysis, protein, BUN, creatinine, CCr, watch for increasing BUN and serum creatinine or decreased CCr; I&O ratio; report hematuria, oliguria, fatigue, weakness; may indicate nephrotoxicity; check for protein in urine during treatment
• Skin eruptions: rash, urticaria, itching
• Allergies before treatment, reaction to each medication; place allergies on chart in bright red letters
• Neurologic status with herpes encephalitis
• Provide adequate intake of fluids (2 L) to prevent deposits in kidneys, more likely to occur with rapid administration or in dehydration
Evaluate:
• Therapeutic response: absence of itching, painful lesions; crusting and healed lesions; decreased symptoms of chickenpox; healing, decreased pain with herpes zoster

---

Teach patient/family:
• To take as prescribed; if dose is missed, take as soon as remembered up to 1 hr before next dose; do not double dose
• That product may be taken orally before infection occurs; product should be taken when itching or pain occurs, usually before eruptions
• That sexual partners need to be told that patient has herpes because they can become infected; condoms must be worn to prevent reinfections
• Not to touch lesions to avoid spreading infection to new sites, not to use topical products on lesions, spreading may occur
• That product does not cure infection, just controls symptoms and does not prevent infecting others
• That product must be taken in equal intervals around the clock to maintain blood levels for duration of therapy
• That women with genital herpes are more likely to develop cervical cancer; to keep all gynecologic appointments
• **Topical:** Not to use around eyes, to use enough ointment to cover lesions q3hr/6x per day, use finger cot or glove to apply
• **Pregnancy/breastfeeding:** to identify if pregnancy is planned or suspected or if breastfeeding

TREATMENT OF OVERDOSE: Discontinue product; hemodialysis

---

adalimumab (Rx)

(add-a-lim'yu-mab)

Amjevita, Humira, Humira Pen
Func. class.: Antirheumatic agent (disease modifying), immunomodulator, anti-TNF

Chem. class.: Recombinant human IgG1 monoclonal antibody, DMARD

Do not confuse:
Humira/HumuLIN/HumaLOG
Humira Pen/Humapen Memoir

ACTION: A form of human IgG1 monoclonal antibody specific for human tumor necrosis factor (TNF-α); elevated levels of TNF-α are found in patients with rheumatoid arthritis

USES: Moderate to severe active rheumatoid arthritis who are ≥18 years of age and who have not responded to other disease-modifying agents, juvenile rheumatoid arthritis (JRA), psoriatic arthritis, Crohn's disease, moderate to severe plaque psoriasis, ankylosing spondylitis, ulcerative colitis, noninfectious uveitis

CONTRAINDICATIONS: Hypersensitivity, breastfeeding, use of anakinra, abatacept
Precautions: Pregnancy, children, geriatric patients, CNS demyelinating disease, lymphoma, HF, hepatitis B carriers, mannitol hypersensitivity, latex allergy, neoplastic disease, TB

Black Box Warning: Active infections, risk of lymphomas/leukemias

DOSAGE AND ROUTES
Rheumatoid arthritis/ankylosing spondylitis/psoriatic arthritis
• **Adult: SUBCUT** 40 mg every other wk or every wk if not combined with methotrexate
Juvenile rheumatoid arthritis
• **Child ≥2 yr/adolescent ≥30 kg: SUBCUT** 40 mg every other wk
• **Child ≥2 yr/adolescent ≥15 kg to <30 kg: SUBCUT** 20 mg every other wk
• **Child ≥2 yr/adolescent 10-<15 kg: SUBCUT** 10 mg every other wk
Crohn's disease/ulcerative colitis
• **Adult: SUBCUT** 160 mg given as 4 inj on day 1 or 2 inj each on days 1 and 2, then 80 mg at wk 2 and 40 mg every other wk starting at wk 4
Crohn's disease
• **Child >6 yr and ≥40 kg (88 lb): SUBCUT** 160 mg on day 1 (as 4 [40-mg] injections) or 40 mg (as 2 injections)

(80 mg) × 2 days, then 80 mg after 2 wk (day 15), then 40 mg every other week (day 29)

• **Child >6 yr and 17-40 kg (37-88 lb):**
SUBCUT 80 mg day 1 (as 2 [40-mg] injections), then 40 mg after 2 wk (day 15), then 20 mg every other week (day 29)

Plaque psoriasis/noninfectious uveitis

Adult: SUBCUT 80 mg baseline as 2 inj, then 40 mg every other wk starting 1 wk after initial dose (plaque psoriasis)

Available form: Inj 40 mg/0.8 mL; 20 mg/0.4 mL (pediatric)

Administer:

SUBCUT route

• Do not admix with other sol or medications; do not use filter; protect from light; give at 45-degree angle using abdomen, thighs; rotate inj sites; discard unused portions

• Don't inject in bruised, red, tender, abraded areas

SIDE EFFECTS

CNS: *Headache,* Guillain-Barré syndrome, MS

CV: *Hypertension,* HF

EENT: *Sinusitis,* optic neuritis

GI: Abdominal pain, nausea

HEMA: Leukopenia, thrombocytopenia

INTEG: *Rash, inj site reaction*

MISC: Flulike symptoms, increased cancer risk, risk of infection (TB, invasive fungal infections, other opportunistic infections), infections may be fatal; Stevens-Johnson syndrome, anaphylaxis, hyperlipidemia

RESP: *URI,* pulmonary fibrosis, bronchitis

PHARMACOKINETICS

Absorption 65%, distributed to synovial fluid, half-life 2 wk, lower clearance with advancing age (40-75 yr), onset up to 24 wk (inflammation)

INTERACTIONS

Black Box Warning: **Increase:** serious infections—other TNF blockers, rilonacept

Increase: HSTCL-azathioprine, methotrexate

• Do not use with abatacept, anakinra; serious infections may occur

• Do not give concurrently with live virus vaccines; immunizations should be brought up to date before treatment

Drug/Lab Test

Increase: ALT, cholesterol, lipids

NURSING CONSIDERATIONS

Assess:

• **RA:** pain, stiffness, ROM, swelling of joints before, during treatment

• **Crohn's disease/ulcerative colitis:** bowel pattern, cramping, abdominal pain, bleeding

• For inj site pain, swelling, redness—usually occur after 2 inj (4-5 days); use cold compress to relieve pain/swelling

Black Box Warning: **Infections** (fever, flulike symptoms, dyspnea, change in urination, redness/swelling around any wounds), stop treatment if present; some serious infections including sepsis may occur, may be fatal; patients with active infections should not be started on this product

• May reactivate hepatitis B in chronic carriers, may be fatal

Black Box Warning: Latent TB before therapy; treat before starting this product

• **Anaphylaxis, latex allergy:** stop therapy if lupus-like syndrome develops

• **Blood dyscrasias:** CBC, differential periodically

Black Box Warning: **Neoplastic disease (lymphomas/leukemia)** in children, adolescents; hepatosplenic T-cell lymphoma is more likely in adolescent males with Crohn's disease or ulcerative colitis

Evaluate:

• Therapeutic response: decreased inflammation, pain in joints, decreased joint destruction

---

Teach patient/family:

• About self-administration if appropriate: inj should be made in thigh, abdomen, upper arm; rotate sites at least 1 inch from old site; do not inject in areas that are bruised, red, hard, review provided medication guide with patient

• To refrigerate in container that product was received in; to dispose of needles and equipment as instructed

• That if medication is not taken when due, inject dose as soon as remembered and inject next dose as scheduled

• Not to take any live virus vaccines during treatment

• To report signs of infection, allergic reaction, TB, immediately

• To advise all health care professionals of Rx, OTC, herbals, supplements taken

• **Pregnancy/breastfeeding:** To advise health care professional if pregnancy is planned or suspected or if breastfeeding; to register if pregnant at 877-311-8972

• **Prefilled pen use:** Using an alcohol swab, clean area, do not use if solution is cloudy or particulate is present, remove gray cap, the pen is activated, pinch skin and place at 90-degree angle, press button, hold until solution is inserted, remove, dispose of properly

• To do regular skin assessments and report changes to provider

RARELY USED

adefovir (Rx)
(add-ee-foh′veer)
Hepsera
Func. class.: Antiviral
Chem. class.: Nucleoside

ACTION: Inhibits hepatitis B virus DNA polymerase by competing with natural substrates and by causing DNA termination after its incorporation into viral DNA; causes viral DNA death

USES: Chronic hepatitis B

CONTRAINDICATIONS: Hypersensitivity

Precautions: Pregnancy, labor, breastfeeding, children, geriatric patients, dialysis, females, obesity, organ transplant

Black Box Warning: Severe renal disease, impaired hepatic function, lactic acidosis, HIV, hepatitis B exacerbation

DOSAGE AND ROUTES
Chronic hepatitis B
• **Adult/adolescent: PO** 10 mg/day, optimal duration unknown
Renal dose
• **Adult: PO** CCr ≥50 mL/min 10 mg q24hr; CCr 30-49 mL/min 10 mg q48hr; CCr 10-29 mL/min 10 mg q72hr; hemodialysis 10 mg q7days after dialysis

Available forms: Tabs 10 mg

⚠ HIGH ALERT

adenosine (Rx)
(a-den′oh-seen)
Adenocard, Adenoscan ✦
Func. class.: Antidysrhythmic
Chem. class.: Endogenous nucleoside

Do not confuse:
adenosine/adenosine phosphate

ACTION: Slows conduction through AV node, can interrupt reentry pathways through AV node, and can restore normal sinus rhythm in patients with paroxysmal supraventricular tachycardia; decreases cardiac oxygen demand, decreasing hypoxia

USES: PSVT, as a diagnostic aid to assess myocardial perfusion defects in CAD, Wolff-Parkinson-White syndrome
Unlabeled uses: Wide-complex tachycardia diagnosis

CONTRAINDICATIONS: Hypersensitivity, 2nd- or 3rd-degree AV block, sick sinus syndrome, bradycardia
Precautions: Pregnancy, breastfeeding, children, geriatric patients, asthma, atrial flutter, atrial fibrillation, ventricular tachycardia, bronchospastic lung disease,

symptomatic bradycardia, bundle branch block, heart transplant, unstable angina, COPD, hypotension, hypovolemia, vascular heart disease, CV disease

DOSAGE AND ROUTES

Converting paroxysmal supraventricular tachycardia to sinus rhythm (Adenocard)

• **Adult and child >50 kg (110 lb):** IV **BOL** 6 mg; if conversion to normal sinus rhythm does not occur within 1-2 min, give 12 mg by rapid **IV BOL**; may repeat 12-mg dose again in 1-2 min
• **Infant and child <50 kg (110 lb):** IV **BOL** 0.1 mg/kg; if not effective, increase dose by 0.05-0.1 mg/kg q2min to a max of 0.3 mg/kg/dose
• **Neonate:** IV BOL 0.05 mg/kg by rapid IV BOL, may increase by 0.05 mg/kg q2min, max 0.3 mg/kg/dose

Diagnostic Use

• **Adult/child >50 kg:** IV 140 mcg/kg/min x 6 min (0.84 mg/kg total)
Available forms: 3 mg/mL sol for injection

Administer:

IV, direct route

• Warm to room temperature; crystals will dissolve
• Undiluted; give 6 mg or less by rapid inj over 1-2 sec; if using an IV line, use port near insertion site, flush with NS (20 mL), then elevate arm, dose reduction recommended if given by central line
• Store at room temperature; sol should be clear; discard unused product

IV Intermittent Infusion
Diagnostic

• Use 30-mL vial undiluted (3 mg/mL), give at 140 mcg/kg/min over 6 min (total 0.84 mg/kg)
• Thallium-201 should never be given after 3 min of infusion

SIDE EFFECTS

CNS: Light-headedness, dizziness, arm tingling, numbness, headache; seizures, stroke (Adenoscan)
CV: Chest pain, pressure, atrial tachydysrhythmias, sweating, palpitations, hypotension, *facial flushing*, AV block, cardiac arrest, ventricular dysrhythmias, atrial fibrillation
GI: *Nausea,* metallic taste
RESP: *Dyspnea, chest pressure,* hyperventilation, bronchospasm (asthmatics)
EENT: Blurred vision
MS: Back pain

PHARMACOKINETICS

Cleared from plasma in <30 sec, half-life 10 sec, converted to inosine/adenosine monophosphate

INTERACTIONS

Increase: risk for higher degree of heart block—carBAMazepine
Increase: risk for ventricular fibrillation—digoxin, verapamil; monitor ECG
Increase: effects of adenosine—dipyridamole; adenosine dose may need to be reduced
Decrease: activity of adenosine—theophylline or other methylxanthines (caffeine); adenosine dose may need to be increased

Drug/Herb
Increase: adenosine effect—ginger
Decrease: adenosine effect—guarana, green tea

NURSING CONSIDERATIONS
Assess:

• **Cardiopulmonary status:** B/P, pulse, respiration, rhythm, ECG intervals (PR, QRS, QT); check for transient dysrhythmias (PVCs, PACs, sinus tachycardia, AV block)
• **Respiratory status:** rate, rhythm, lung fields for crackles; watch for respiratory depression; bilateral crackles may occur in HF patient; increased respiration, increased pulse, product should be discontinued
• **Pregnancy/breastfeeding:** identify if pregnancy is planned or suspected, or if breastfeeding; use only if benefits outweigh fetal risk; do not breastfeed
• CNS effects: dizziness, confusion, psychosis, paresthesias, seizures; product should be discontinued

Evaluate:
• Therapeutic response: normal sinus rhythm or diagnosis of perfusion defect

Teach patient/family:
• To report facial flushing, dizziness, sweating, palpitations, chest pain; usually transient; chest pressure may occur immediately after administration
• To report IV discomfort
• **Pregnancy/breastfeeding:** to advise prescriber if pregnancy is planned or suspected or if breastfeeding; do not breastfeed

TREATMENT OF OVERDOSE:
Defibrillation, vasopressor for hypotension, theophylline

⚠ HIGH ALERT

ado-trastuzumab (Rx)

(a′doe-tras-tooz′ue-mab)

Kadcyla

Func. class.: Antineoplastic-biologic response modifier

Chem. class.: Signal transduction inhibitors (STIs), humanized anti-HER2 antibody

Do not confuse:
ado-trastuzumab/trastuzumab

ACTION: Humanized ⚠ anti-HER2 monoclonal antibody that is linked to DM1, a small molecule microtubular inhibitor; once the antibody is bound to the HER2 receptor, the complex is internalized and the DM1 is released to bind with tubulin to lead to apoptosis

USES: Breast cancer; metastatic with overexpression of HER2, who previously received trastuzumab and a taxane, separately or in combination

CONTRAINDICATIONS: Hypersensitivity to this product, Chinese hamster ovary cell protein

Black Box Warning: Pregnancy

Precautions: Breastfeeding, children, pulmonary disease, acute bronchospasm, anticoagulant, ⚠ Asian patients, asthma, COPD, extravasation, fever, hepatitis, human anti-human antibody, hypotension, neuropathy, interstitial lung disease/pneumonitis; extravasation; thrombocytopenia

Black Box Warning: Heart failure, hepatotoxicity

DOSAGE AND ROUTES
• **Adult: IV** 3.6 mg/kg over 30-90 min q3wk x14 wk; give first infusion over 90 min; if tolerated, give over 30 min
Dosage adjustments for toxicities
Hepatotoxicity:
• **AST/ALT >5 to ≤20 × ULN:** withhold, resume at a reduced dose when AST/ALT is ≤5 × ULN; first dose reduction: reduce the dose to 3 mg/kg; second dose reduction: reduce the dose to 2.4 mg/kg; requirement for further dose reduction: discontinue **AST/ ALT >20× ULN:** discontinue
• **Total bilirubin >3 to ≤10x ULN:** withhold, resume treatment at a reduced dose when total bilirubin recovers to ≤1.5; first dose reduction: reduce the dose to 3 mg/kg; second dose reduction: reduce the dose to 2.4 mg/kg; requirement for further dose reduction: discontinue treatment
• **Total bilirubin >10x ULN:** permanently discontinue; permanently discontinue treatment in patients with AST/ALT >3x ULN and total bilirubin >2x ULN; permanently discontinue treatment in patients diagnosed with nodular regenerative hyperplasia (NRH)
• **Left ventricular ejection fraction (LVEF):** *LVEF 40%-45% and decrease is <10% from baseline:* continue treatment; repeat LVEF assessment within 3 wk; *LVEF 40%-45% and decrease is ≥10% from baseline:* repeat LVEF assessment within 3 wk; if LVEF remains ≥10% from baseline, discontinue; *LVEF <40%:* withhold; repeat LVEF assessment within 3 wk; if LVEF remains <40%, discontinue; *symptomatic heart failure (HF):* discontinue

---

Thrombocytopenia:

• **Platelet count 25,000/mm³ to <50,000/mm³:** withhold; resume treatment at same dose when platelet count recovers to ≥75,000/mm³

• **Platelet count <25,000/mm³:** withhold; resume treatment at a reduced dose when platelet count recovers to ≥75,000/mm³: first dose reduction: reduce the dose to 3 mg/kg; second dose reduction: reduce the dose to 2.4 mg/kg; requirement for further dose reduction: discontinue

Pulmonary toxicity:

• Permanently discontinue in patients diagnosed with interstitial lung disease or pneumonitis

Peripheral neuropathy:

• Withhold in patients experiencing grade 3 or 4 peripheral neuropathy; resume treatment upon resolution to ≤grade 2

Available forms: Lyophilized powder 100, 160 mg/vial

Administer:

IV route

• Visually inspect for particulate matter and discoloration before use

• Give as (IV) infusion with a 0.2 or 0.22 micron in-line filter; do not administer as an IV push or bolus

• Use cytotoxic handling procedures; do not mix with, or administer as an infusion with, other IV products

Reconstitution:

• Slowly inject 5 mL of sterile water for injection into each 100-mg vial, or 8 mL of sterile water for injection into each 160-mg vial to yield a single-use solution of 20 mg/mL

• Direct the stream of sterile water toward the wall of the vial and not directly at the cake or powder

• Gently swirl the vial to aid in dissolution; do not shake

• After reconstitution, withdraw desired amount from the vial and dilute immediately in 250 mL of 0.9% sodium chloride; do not use dextrose 5% solution; gently invert the bag to mix the solution in order to avoid foaming

• The reconstituted single-use product does not contain a preservative; use the diluted solution immediately or store at 2-8° C (36-46° F) for up to 24 hr after reconstitution; discard any unused drug after 24 hr; do not freeze

IV infusion

• Closely monitor for possible subcutaneous infiltration during drug administration

• **First infusion:** give over 90 min; the infusion rate should be slowed or interrupted if the patient develops an infusion-related reaction; patients should be observed for at least 90 min following the initial dose for fever, chills, or other infusion-related reactions; permanently discontinue for life-threatening infusion-related reactions

• **Subsequent infusions:** administer over 30 min if prior infusions were well tolerated; the infusion rate should be slowed or interrupted if the patient develops an infusion-related reaction; patients should be observed for at least 30 min after the infusion; permanently discontinue for life-threatening infusion-related reactions

SIDE EFFECTS

CNS: Dizziness, insomnia, neuropathy, chills, fatigue, fever, flushing, headache

CV: Hypertension, peripheral edema, left ventricular dysfunction

EENT: Blurred vision, conjunctivitis, stomatitis

GI: Diarrhea, nausea, vomiting, constipation, dyspepsia, hepatotoxicity

HEMA: Anemia, bleeding, thrombocytopenia

INTEG: Rash, infusion-related reactions

MS: Arthralgia, pain

RESP: Cough, dyspnea, pneumonitis, interstitial lung disease

SYST: Anaphylaxis

Other: Elevated LFTs, hand-foot syndrome

PHARMACOKINETICS

93% protein binding, metabolized in the liver by CYP3A4, half-life 4 day

INTERACTIONS
• Do not give with other IV products; do not give with 5% dextrose

Increase: bleeding risk—warfarin, platelet inhibitors, anticoagulants

Increase: ado-trastuzumab toxicity—CYP3A4 inhibitors (clarithromycin, ketoconazole, ritonavir, saquinavir, atazanavir); avoid concurrent use

NURSING CONSIDERATIONS
Assess:
• Pregnancy test, CBC, differential, LFTs

Black Box Warning: **HF, other cardiac symptoms:** dyspnea, coughing; gallop; obtain full cardiac workup including ECG, echo, MUGA; LVEF baseline and q3mo

• Symptoms of infection; may be masked by product
• CNS reaction: LOC, mental status, dizziness, confusion

Black Box Warning: Hypersensitivity reactions, anaphylaxis

Black Box Warning: **Hepatotoxicity:** monitor LFTs, baseline and prior to each dose; fatal liver damage may occur; reduced dose or discontinuing treatment may be required; monitor for infusion reactions during and for 1.5 hrs after conclusion of infusion; slowing infusion may be needed; monitor LFTs, bilirubin baseline and before each dose

• **Infusion reactions that may be fatal:** fever, chills, nausea, vomiting, pain, headache, dizziness, hypotension; discontinue product
• **Pulmonary toxicity:** dyspnea, interstitial pneumonitis, pulmonary hypertension, ARDS; can occur after infusion reaction; those with lung disease may have more severe toxicity, discontinue in those with pneumonitis, interstitial lung disease
• **Bleeding:** monitor for bleeding; grade 3 or 4 bleeding with fatalities has occurred; check platelets baseline and before each dose

Black Box Warning: **Hepatic disease:** may be fatal; monitor LFTs, bilirubin baseline and before each dose

Evaluate:
• Therapeutic response: decrease in size, spread of breast cancer

Teach patient/family:
• Reason for product, expected result
• To take acetaminophen for fever
• To avoid hazardous tasks because confusion, dizziness may occur
• To report signs of infection: sore throat, fever, diarrhea, vomiting; bleeding; decreased heart function/SOB with exertion
• To report weight gain, swelling of the ankles, feet, fatigue, cough, bleeding

Black Box Warning: **Pregnancy/ breastfeeding:** to use effective contraception while taking this product and for additional 7 mo after discontinuing this drug; to notify prescriber if pregnancy is planned or suspected; not to breastfeed; advise patient to enroll in Mother Pregnancy Registry (800-690-6720)

• **Infusion reactions:** to report pain at infusion site

⚠ HIGH ALERT

afatinib (Rx)
(a-fat′i-nib)
Gilotrif, Giotrif ✦

Func. class.: Antineoplastic biologic response modifiers
Chem. class.: Signal transduction inhibitors (STIs), epidermal growth factor receptor, tyrosine kinase inhibitor

Do not confuse:
afatinib/Afinitor/axitinib

ACTION: Selective inhibitor of EGFR (ErbB1), HER2 (ErbB2), and HER4 (ErbB4); irreversible, covalent binding of

---

intracellular tyrosine kinase, inhibiting (and causing regression) tumor growth by decreasing EGFR signal transduction, cell cycle arrest, and inhibition of angiogenesis

USES: Treatment of non–small-cell lung cancer whose tumors have epidermal growth factor receptor Exon 19 deletions or 21 substitution mutations

CONTRAINDICATIONS: Pregnancy, hypersensitivity

Precautions: Contact lenses, dehydration, inflammation, keratitis, ocular disease, pneumonitis, pulmonary disease, renal disease, respiratory distress syndrome, serious rash, skin disease, diarrhea, hepatic disease, ocular disease

DOSAGE AND ROUTES
• **Adult:** PO 40 mg daily, until disease progression or unacceptable toxicity

Dose adjustments for toxicities:
• **Hepatotoxicity:** Hold therapy in patients who develop worsening liver function; when toxicity resolves to grade 1 or less, resume therapy at a reduced dose (10 mg/day less than the dose causing hepatotoxicity); permanently discontinue for severe drug-induced hepatic impairment or if hepatotoxicity persists at a dose of 20 mg/day
• **Grade 2 or higher renal toxicity (CCr >1.5 × ULN):** Hold until the toxicity resolves to grade 1 or less (CCr <1.5 × ULN), then resume at a reduced dose (10 mg/day less than the dose causing nephrotoxicity); permanently discontinue if nephrotoxicity persists at a dose of 20 mg/day
• **Grade 2 diarrhea, lasting 2 or more consecutive days while taking anti-diarrheal medication, or any grade 3 diarrhea:** Hold until the toxicity resolves to grade 1 or less, then resume therapy at a reduced dose (10 mg/day less than the dose causing toxicity); antidiarrheal therapy should continue until no loose bowel movement for 12 hr; permanently discontinue if toxicity persists at a dose of 20 mg/day
• **Grade 2 cutaneous reactions that last more than 7 days or are intolerable:** Hold until the toxicity resolves to grade 1 or less,

then resume at a reduced dose (10 mg/day less than the dose causing toxicity); permanently discontinue for life-threatening bullous, blistering, or exfoliative skin lesions, or if toxicity persists at a dose of 20 mg/day
• **Confirmed interstitial lung disease, persistent ulcerative keratitis, symptomatic left ventricular dysfunction, or any severe/intolerable adverse reaction occurring at a dose of 20 mg/day:** Permanently discontinue
• **Any grade 3 or higher adverse event:** Hold until the toxicity resolves to grade 1 or less, then resume therapy at a reduced dose (10 mg/day less than the dose causing toxicity); permanently discontinue if toxicity persists at a dose of 20 mg/day
• **Permanently discontinue for any severe or intolerable adverse event that occurs at a dose of 20 mg/day.**

Dosage Guidance in Patients on P-glycoprotein (P-gp) inhibitors/inducers
• **P-gp inhibitors:** If use of a P-gp inhibitor is required, reduce the initial daily afatinib dosage to 30 mg/day if not tolerated; resume original dose after discontinuation of the P-gp inhibitor as tolerated
• **P-gp inducers:** If use of a P-gp inducer is required, increase the initial daily afatinib dosage to 50 mg/day as tolerated; resume original dose 2-3 days after discontinuation of the P-gp inducer

Available forms: Tabs 20, 30, 40 mg

Administer:

PO route
• Give on empty stomach 1 hr before, 2 hr after food; give at same time of day
• Do not take a missed dose if within 12 hr of the next dose

SIDE EFFECTS
CNS: Fatigue, fever
CV: Heart failure
EENT: Blurred vision, conjunctivitis
GI: Diarrhea, nausea, vomiting, stomatitis, decreased appetite
HEMA: Anemia, neutropenia, leukopenia, epistaxis
INTEG: Rash, pruritus, acne vulgaris, photosensitivity, nail bed infections
MS: Arthralgia

RESP: Cough, dyspnea, acute respiratory distress syndrome, interstitial lung disease, pneumonitis

Other: Elevated LFTs, infection, hand and foot syndrome, dehydration, renal failure, cystitis, hypokalemia

PHARMACOKINETICS

95% protein binding, half-life 37 hr, primarily excreted as unchanged drug in feces; peak 2-5 hr after dose; time to steady state is approximately 8 days

INTERACTIONS

Increase: afatinib—P-gp inhibitors effect

Drug/Herb

Increase: afatinib concentration—St. John's wort

Drug/Food Test

Increase: afatinib effect—grapefruit juice; avoid use while taking product

NURSING CONSIDERATIONS
Assess:

> **Black Box Warning: Myelosuppression:** anemia, neutropenia; obtain CBC with differential weekly × 1 mo, then monthly as needed; LFTs every mo × 3 mo, then as clinically indicated; hepatic failure may occur

• **Pregnancy/breastfeeding:** do not use in pregnancy, breastfeeding

Evaluate:

• **Therapeutic response:** decrease in progression of disease

Teach patient/family:

• To report adverse reactions, bleeding immediately

• About reason for treatment, expected results

• To use effective contraception during treatment and up to 30 days after discontinuing treatment; not to use product in pregnancy, breastfeeding

• To treat skin rash with topicals and oral antibiotics; use loperamide as prescribed for diarrhea; if any side effect is severe or persistent, contact prescriber

• That complicated dosing changes may occur based on toxicity or drug-drug interaction

• To take on empty stomach 1 hr before or 2 hr after meal; not to take missed dose within 12 hr of next scheduled dose

---

aflibercept (Rx)

(a-fli-ber′sept)

EYLEA

Func. class.: Biologic response modifier; signal transduction inhibitor (STIs) (Ophthalmic)

ACTION: A recombinant fusion protein consisting of portions of human VEGF receptors 1 and 2 extracellular domains fused to human IgG1; acts as a soluble decoy receptor that binds vascular endothelial growth factor-A (VEGF-A) and placental growth factor (PIGF)

USES: For treatment of neovascular (wet) age-related macular degeneration (AMD), macular edema after central retinal vein occlusion, diabetic retinopathy with diabetic macular edema

CONTRAINDICATIONS: Hypersensitivity, ocular/periocular infection, active intraocular inflammation

Precautions: Neonates, infants, children, adolescents, pregnancy, breastfeeding; history of glaucoma, ocular surgery; driving or operating machinery; increased intraocular pressure

DOSAGE AND ROUTES

• **Adult: Intravitreal INJ** 2 mg (0.05 mL) into affected eye(s) q4wk × 12 wk, then 2 mg (0.05 mL) q8wk

Available forms: Sol for inj 2 mg/0.05 mL

Administer:

Intravitreal route

• Visually inspect for particulate matter, discoloration before use; do not use if particulates, cloudiness, discoloration are visible; only for use by physicians trained in administration

• Use each vial for treatment of single eye only; if other eye is being treated, use new vial and change the sterile field, syringe, gloves, drapes, eyelid speculum, filter, injection needles before administering to the other eye

• Immediately after the intravitreal injection, monitor patient for elevation in intraocular pressure (IOP); appropriate monitoring is a check for perfusion of optic nerve head or tonometry; sterile paracentesis needle should be available if required

• Storage: do not freeze, protect from light, refrigerate, store in original package until time of use

SIDE EFFECTS

CV: Arterial thromboembolism, nonfatal stroke, nonfatal myocardial infarction, vascular death

EENT: *Ocular hemorrhage, ocular pain, cataracts, vitreous detachment, vitreous floaters,* conjunctival hyperemia, corneal erosion, detachment of retinal pigment epithelium, injection site pain, foreign body sensation, increased lacrimation, blurred vision, retinal pigment epithelium tear, injection site hemorrhage, blepharedema, corneal edema, increased intraocular pressure/ocular hypertension

SYST: Hypersensitivity

PHARMACOKINETICS

Absorbed into systemic circulation; present in its unbound form and stable inactive form bound with endogenous VEGF; elimination by binding to free endogenous VEGF; metabolism by proteolysis; terminal half-life in plasma 5-6 days

NURSING CONSIDERATIONS
Assess:

• **Infection:** monitor for infection during week after injection to permit early treatment of any ocular infection that may develop; proper aseptic injection technique should be used to minimize infection

• **Increased intraocular pressure:** monitor for acute increases in intraocular pressure within 60 min of injection; sustained increases in intraocular pressure have been reported after repeated intravitreal dosing; monitor intraocular pressure and optic nerve head perfusion, a sterile paracentesis needle should be available

• **Pregnancy/breastfeeding:** use only if benefits outweigh fetal risk, not recommended for breastfeeding

Evaluate:

• Prevention of further vision loss

Teach patient/family:

• To seek immediate care if symptoms of endophthalmitis or retinal detachment develop (ocular pain, hyperemia of the conjunctiva, photophobia, blurry vision)

---

albuterol (Rx)
(al-byoo′ter-ole)

Accuneb, Airomir ✦, ProAir HFA, ProAir RespiClick ✦, Proventil HFA, Ventolin Diskus ✦, Ventolin Nebules ✦, Ventolin HFA, VoSpire ER

Func. class.: Adrenergic β_2-agonist, sympathomimetic, bronchodilator

---

Do not confuse:
albuterol/atenolol/Albutein
Proventil/Prinivil

ACTION: Causes bronchodilation by action on β_2 (pulmonary) receptors by increasing levels of cAMP, which relaxes smooth muscle; produces bronchodilation, CNS or cardiac stimulation as well as increased diuresis and gastric acid secretion; longer acting than isoproterenol

USES: Prevention of exercise-induced asthma, acute bronchospasm, bronchitis, emphysema, bronchiectasis, or other reversible airway obstruction

Unlabeled uses: Hyperkalemia in dialysis patients, COPD, emphysema

CONTRAINDICATIONS: Hypersensitivity to sympathomimetics

Precautions: Pregnancy, breastfeeding, cardiac/renal disease, hyperthyroidism, diabetes mellitus, hypertension, prostatic hypertrophy, angle-closure glaucoma, seizures, exercise-induced bronchospasm (aerosol) in children <12 yr, hypoglycemia, tachydysrhythmias, severe cardiac disease, heart block

---

DOSAGE AND ROUTES
Bronchospasm prophylaxis/treatment

• **Adult and child ≥4 yr: INH** (metered-dose inhaler) 2 puffs (180 mcg) q4-6hr as needed; **>12 yr INH** (powdered inhaler) (ProAir RespiClick) 180 mcg (2 INH) q4-6hr as needed

• **Adult and child ≥13 yr: PO** (ext rel) 4-8 mg q12hr, max 32 mg/day; **PO** (regular release) 2-4 mg tid, max 32 mg/day

• **Child 6-12 yr: PO** (ext rel) 4 mg q12hr, max 24 mg/day; **PO** (regular release) 6-13 yr 2 mg tid-qid, max 24 mg/day

• **Child 2-5 yr: PO** 0.1 mg/kg tid, max 12 mg/day

• **Adult and child ≥15 yr: PO** (syrup) 2-4 mg tid-qid, max 32 mg/day

• **Child 6-14 yr: PO** (syrup) 2 mg tid-qid, max 24 mg/day

• **Child 2-5 yr: PO** (syrup) 0.1 mg/kg tid, max 12 mg/day

Asthma (unlabeled)

• **Child <4 yr: INH** (metered dose inhaler) 180-600 mcg q2 min, max 6 doses; persistent asthma 2 puffs (HFA) q4-6hr

To prevent exercise-induced bronchospasm (not ProAir RespiClick)

• **Adult/child ≥4 yr: INH** 2 puffs before exercise, max 12 puffs/24 hr

• **Adult/child ≥12 yr: INH** (ProAir RespiClick) 2 puffs 15-30 min prior to exercise

Other respiratory conditions

• **Adult and child ≥12 yr: INH** (metered-dose inhaler) 1 puff q4-6hr; **PO** 2-4 mg tid-qid, max 32 mg; **NEB/IPPB** 2.5 mg tid-qid

• **Geriatric: PO** 2 mg tid-qid, may increase gradually to 8 mg tid-qid

• **Child 2-12 yr: INH** (metered-dose inhaler) 0.1 mg/kg tid (max 2.5 mg tid-qid); **NEB/IPPB** 0.1-0.15 mg/kg/dose tid-qid or 1.25 mg tid-qid for child 10-15 kg or 2.5 mg tid-qid for child >15 kg

Hyperkalemia (unlabeled)

• **Adult: ORAL INH** (albuterol nebulizer sol) 10-20 mg over 15 min

Available forms: INH aerosol 108 mcg/actuation; oral syr 2 mg/5 mL; tabs 2, 4 mg; ext rel 4, 8 mg; INH sol 0.63 mg/3 mL, 1.25 mg/3 mL; 0.083%, 0.5%, 0.042%, 0.021%; metered-dose aerosol 90 mcg/actuation

Administer:

• Store in light-resistant container; do not expose to temperatures of more than 86° F (30° C)

PO route

• Do not break, crush, or chew ext rel tabs; give with meals to decrease gastric irritation

• **Oral sol** to children (no alcohol, sugar)

Inhalation route

• For geriatric patients and children, a spacing device is advised

• After shaking metered-dose inhaler, exhale, place mouthpiece in mouth, inhale slowly while depressing inhaler, hold breath, remove, exhale slowly; give INH at least 1 min apart

• **NEB/IPPB** dilute 5 mg/mL sol/2.5 mL 0.9% NaCl for INH; other sol do not require dilution; for neb O_2 flow or compressed air 6-10 L/min, one treatment lasts 10 min; IPPB 5-20 min

ProAir Respistick:

• Before using for the first time, check that the number "200" is showing. The dose counter displays only even numbers; hold the inhaler upright while opening the cap fully; make sure a "click" is heard; do not open the cap unless ready to use; the patient should breathe out through the mouth; then patient should breathe in deeply through the mouth hold breath for about 10 sec; remove check dose counter; make sure the cap closes firmly into place; do not wash or put any part of the inhaler in water; if the mouthpiece needs cleaning, wipe with a dry cloth or tissue; when there are "20" doses left, the counter will change to red; refill

SIDE EFFECTS

CNS: *Tremors, anxiety,* insomnia, headache, stimulation, *restlessness*

CV: Angina, hypo/hypertension, dysrhythmias, chest pain

EENT: Dry nose, irritation of nose and throat

GI: Nausea, vomiting

MISC: Hyperglycemia

RESP: Paradoxical bronchospasm

Side effects: *italics* = common; red = life-threatening

PHARMACOKINETICS

Extensively metabolized in the liver and tissues, crosses placenta, breast milk, blood-brain barrier, half-life 2.7-6 hr, well absorbed

PO: Onset $1/2$ hr, peak 2-3 hr, duration 4-6 hr

PO-ER: Onset $1/2$ hr, peak 2-3 hr, duration 8-12 hr

INH: Onset 5-15 min, peak 1.5-2 hr, duration 2-6 hr, half-life 4 hr

INTERACTIONS

Increase: digoxin level—digoxin
Increase: CNS stimulation—CNS stimulants
Increase: ECG changes/hypokalemia—potassium-losing diuretics
Increase: severe hypotension—oxytocics
Increase: toxicity—theophylline
Increase: action of aerosol bronchodilators
Increase: action of albuterol—tricyclics, MAOIs, other adrenergics; avoid use together
Increase: CV effects—atomoxetine, selegiline
Decrease: albuterol—other β-blockers
Drug/Herb
Increase: stimulation—caffeine (cola nut, green/black tea, guarana, yerba maté, coffee, chocolate)
Drug/Lab Test
Decrease: potassium

NURSING CONSIDERATIONS

Assess:
• **Respiratory function:** vital capacity, pulse oximetry, forced expiratory volume, ABGs, VBGs; lung sounds, heart rate and rhythm, B/P, sputum (baseline and peak); whether patient has received theophylline therapy before giving dose
• Patient's ability to self-medicate
• Trouble breathing with wheezing hold medication, notify prescriber if bronchospasm occurs
• **Pregnancy/breastfeeding:** identify if pregnancy is planned or suspected; use only if necessary; avoid breastfeeding

Evaluate:
• Therapeutic response: absence of dyspnea, wheezing improved airway exchange, improved ABGs, VBGs
Teach patient/family:
• To use exactly as prescribed; to take missed dose when remembered, alter dosing schedule; not to use OTC medications; that excess stimulation may occur, to use this product before other medications, allow 5 min between each
• About use of inhaler: review package insert with patient; use demonstration, return demonstration; shake, prime before 1st use and when not used for >2 wk; release 4 test sprays into air, away from the face; about when empty and when to renew, a bad taste may occur
• To avoid getting aerosol in eyes (blurring of vision may result) or use near flames or sources of heat
• Do not wash inhaler, wipe with dry cloth, to discard product when counter changes to red
• To avoid smoking, smoke-filled rooms, persons with respiratory infections
• That paradoxical bronchospasm may occur; to stop product immediately, call prescriber, usually from first dose of new inhaler
• To limit caffeine products such as chocolate, coffee, tea, colas
• **Pregnancy/breastfeeding:** to advise prescriber if pregnancy is planned or suspected, or if breastfeeding
• To notify health care professional immediately if product does not relieve symptoms, corticosteroids may be needed

TREATMENT OF OVERDOSE: Administer β_1-adrenergic blocker, IV fluids

---

> **⚠ HIGH ALERT**
>
> **RARELY USED**
>
> **alectinib (Rx)**
> [al-ek'ti-nib]
> Alecensa, Alecensaro ✦
> *Func. class.:* Antineoplastics

USES: For the treatment of metastatic, ALK-positive, non–small-cell lung cancer (NSCLC)

CONTRAINDICATIONS: Hypersensitivity

DOSAGE AND ROUTES
• **Adult:** PO 600 mg bid, with food, until disease progression or unacceptable toxicity

---

amlodipine/celecoxib
(am-loe'di-peen sel-e-kox'ib)
Consensi
Func. class.: Antihypertensive/ NSAID
Chem. class.: Calcium channel blocker, dihydropyridine/COX-2 inhibitor

---

ACTION: Amlodipine: inhibits calcium ion influx across cell membrane during cardiac depolarization, results in inhibition of excitation and contraction
Celecoxib: inhibits COX-2 that is needed for prostaglandin synthesis; antiinflammatory, analgesic

USES: Treatment of hypertension and osteoarthritis

CONTRAINDICATIONS: CABG, NSAID/salicylate/sulfonamide hypersensitivity

> **Black Box Warning:** GI bleeding/perforation, thromboembolism

Precautions: Acute bronchospasm, acute MI, alcoholism, anemia, angina, anticoagulant therapy, aortic stenosis, asthma, African-American patients, bone marrow suppression, breastfeeding, cardiac dysrhythmias, CAD, corticosteroid therapy, dehydration, geriatrics, heart failure, hypertension, hypovolemia, immunosuppression, infertility, jaundice, labor/delivery, nasal polyps, pregnancy, renal disease, reproductive risk, stroke, tachycardia, tobacco smoking, urticaria

DOSAGE AND ROUTES
• **Adult:** PO 5 mg/200 mg daily. Initiate with 2.5 mg/200 mg daily with antihypertensive; wait 7-14 days between dosage titration, max 10 mg/200 mg daily
• **Geriatric adult:** PO 2.5 mg/200 mg daily; with antihypertensive, wait 7-14 days between dosage titration, max 10 mg/200 mg daily
Available forms: Tabs 2.5 mg/200 mg, 5 mg/200mg, 10 mg/200 mg

SIDE EFFECTS
CNS: Dizziness, headache, fatigue, insomnia
CV: Peripheral edema, angina, bradycardia, hypotension/hypertension, palpitations, HF, MI, stroke, thrombosis, edema
GI: Gingival hyperplasia, nausea, abdominal pain, diarrhea
INTEG: Flushing
META: Hyperkalemia

PHARMACOKINETICS
Amlodipine: 93% protein binding, extensively metabolized in the liver to inactive compounds, excreted in the urine, half-life 30-50 hr (increased in hepatic disease), peak 6-12 hr
Celecoxib: Widely distributed, 97% protein binding, primarily to albumin, half-life 11.2 hr (increased in hepatic disease), peak 3 hr, delayed peak with high-fat meal

INTERACTIONS
Increase: hypotensive effect—strong CYP3A4 inhibitors (clarithromycin, ketoconazole, itraconazole, ritonavir); alcohol, nitrates, fentanyl, other antihypertensives, alcohol, quinidine
Increase: levels of—CYP2C9 inhibitors; fluconazole
Increase: neurotoxicity—lithium
Increase: levels of—cyclosporine, tacrolimus
Increase: bleeding risk—anticoagulants, salicylates, SNRIs, SSRIs, platelet inhibitors, corticosteroids
Decrease: effect of—ACE inhibitors, thiazides, furosemide
Decrease: hypotensive effect—NSAIDs
Drug/Lab
Increase: AST, ALT, potassium, BUN

Decrease: phosphate

NURSING CONSIDERATIONS

Assess:
• Range of motion, area of pain and inflammation in joints baseline and periodically during treatment
• For allergies to aspirin, sulfonamides, NSAIDs. Patients with these allergies should not receive this product
• For skin rash during treatment, rare but may be fatal; toxic epidermal necrolysis, Stevens-Johnson syndrome may occur during or after treatment
• I&O, daily weight
• Heart failure: increased weight, jugular vein distention, crackles, peripheral edema
• For compliance with amount of refills

Evaluate:
• Therapeutic response: decreased joint pain, tenderness, inflammation; decreased B/P, increased activity tolerance

Teach patient/family:
• To take as prescribed, not to skip or double doses
• How to take B/P, pulse correctly; to contact prescriber if B/P is <50 bpm; instruct caregivers also; to report extra swelling of hands, feet
• To change positions slowly to minimize orthostatic hypotension
• To avoid driving, other hazardous activities until response is known; dizziness may occur
• To obtain good dental care; gingival hyperplasia may occur
• GI toxicity: To report to prescriber abdominal pain, black tarry stools; hypersensitivity: skin rash; or edema, chest pain occur
• Pregnancy/breastfeeding: to notify health care provider if pregnancy is planned or suspected, or if breastfeeding
• To notify all health care providers of all OTC, Rx, herbals, and supplements taken; not to start new products unless approved by prescriber

• To comply with other regimens, including weight loss, exercise

---

RARELY USED

albumin, human 5% (Rx)
(al-byoo′min)
Albumarc, Albuminar-5, Albutein 5%, Buminate 5%, Plasbumin-5
albumin, human 25%
Albuminar-25, Albutein 25%, Buminate 25%, Plasbumin-25
Func. class.: Plasma volume expander

USES: Restores plasma volume after burns, hyperbilirubinemia, shock, hypoproteinemia, prevention of cerebral edema, cardiopulmonary bypass procedures, ARDS, nephrotic syndrome

CONTRAINDICATIONS: Hypersensitivity, HF, severe anemia, renal insufficiency, pulmonary edema

DOSAGE AND ROUTES
Burns
• **Adult:** IV dose to maintain plasma albumin at 3-4 mg/dL
Hypovolemic shock
• **Adult:** IV rapidly give 5% sol, when close to normal, infuse at ≤2-4 mL/min (25% sol ≤1 mL/min)
• **Child:** IV 0.5-1 g/kg/dose 5% sol, may repeat as needed, max 6 g/kg/day
Nephrotic syndrome
• **Adult:** IV 100-200 mL of 25% and loop diuretic × 7-10 days
Hypoproteinemia
• **Adult:** IV 25 g, may repeat in 15-30 min, or 50-75 g of 25% albumin infused at ≤2 mL/min
• **Child and infant:** IV 0.5-1 g/kg/dose over 2-4 hr, may repeat q1-2days
Hyperbilirubinemia/erythroblastosis fetalis
• **Child:** IV 1 g/kg 1-2 hr before transfusion

---

alendronate (Rx)

(al-en-drone′ate)

Binosto, Fosamax, Fosamax plus D

Func. class.: Bone-resorption inhibitor
Chem. class.: Bisphosphonate

Do not confuse:
Fosamax/Flomax

ACTION: Decreases rate of bone resorption and may directly block dissolution of hydroxyapatite crystals of bone; inhibits osteoclast activity

USES: Treatment and prevention of osteoporosis in postmenopausal women, treatment of osteoporosis in men, Paget's disease, treatment of corticosteroid-induced osteoporosis in postmenopausal women not receiving estrogen and in men who are on continuing corticosteroid treatment with low bone mass

Unlabeled uses: Osteogenesis imperfecta, postoperative knee arthroplasty

CONTRAINDICATIONS: Hypersensitivity to bisphosphonates, delayed esophageal emptying, inability to sit or stand for 30 min, hypocalcemia

Precautions: Pregnancy, breastfeeding, children, CCr <35 mL/min, esophageal disease, ulcers, gastritis, poor dental health, increased esophageal cancer risk

DOSAGE AND ROUTES

Osteoporosis in postmenopausal women

• Adult and geriatric: PO 10 mg/day or 70 mg/wk

Paget's disease

• Adult and geriatric: PO 40 mg/day × 6 mo; consider retreatment for relapse

Prevention of osteoporosis in postmenopausal women (excluding Binosto and oral solution)

Adult/postmenopausal female: PO 5 mg/day or 35 mg/wk

Glucocorticoid-induced osteoporosis in those receiving glucocorticosteroids (daily dose $7.5 mg of prednisone)

• Adult: PO 5 mg/day; those not receiving estrogen 10 mg/day

Osteogenesis imperfecta (unlabeled)

• Adult: PO 10 mg/day or 70 mg/wk

• Child/adolescent 2-18 yr and >30 kg (66 lb): PO 10 mg/day

• Child/adolescent 2-18 yr and <30 kg (66 lb): PO 5 mg/day

Postoperative knee arthroplasty (unlabeled)

• Adult: PO 10 mg/day after surgery

Renal dose

• Adult: PO CCr ≤35 mL/min, not recommended

Available forms: Tabs 5, 10, 35, 40, 70 mg; tabs 70 mg with 2800 IU vit D_3, 70 mg with 5600 IU vit D_3; oral sol 70 mg/75 mL; effervescent tab 70 mg

Administer:

• For 6 mo to be effective for Paget's disease

• Store in cool environment, out of direct sunlight

• **Tablet:** take with 8 oz of water 30 min before 1st food, beverage, or medication of the day

• Do not lie down for ≥30 min after dose; do not take at bedtime or before rising

• **Liquid:** use oral syringe or calibrated device; give in AM with ≥2 oz of water ≥30 min before food, beverage, or medication

• **Effervescent tablet:** Dissolve in 4 oz of water, after 5 min, stir and drink

SIDE EFFECTS

Resp: Asthma exacerbation
CV: Atrial fibrillation
Integ: Rash, photosensitivity
CNS: Headache
GI: Abdominal pain, constipation, nausea, vomiting, esophageal ulceration, acid reflux, dyspepsia, esophageal perforation, diarrhea, esophageal cancer
META: Hypophosphatemia, hypocalcemia
MS: Bone pain, osteonecrosis of the jaw, bone fractures

PHARMACOKINETICS

Protein binding 78%, rapidly cleared from circulation, taken up mainly by bones, eliminated primarily through kidneys, bound to bone, half-life >10 yr

INTERACTIONS

Increase: GI adverse reactions—NSAIDs, salicylates, H_2 blockers, proton pump inhibitors, gastric mucosal agents; monitor for GI reactions

Decrease: absorption—antacids, calcium supplements; give alendronate at least 30-60 min before other products

Drug/Food

Decrease: absorption when used with caffeine, orange juice, food; take food at least 30 min after alendronate

Drug/Lab Test

Decrease: calcium, phosphate

NURSING CONSIDERATIONS

Assess:

• Hormonal status of women before treatment, history of fractures

• **For osteoporosis:** bone density test before and during treatment

• **For Paget's disease:** increased skull size, bone pain, headache; decreased vision, hearing; alk phos levels, baseline and periodically, 2× upper limit of normal is indicative of Paget's disease

• **For hypercalcemia:** paresthesia, twitching, laryngospasm; Chvostek's, Trousseau's signs; monitor calcium, vitamin D baseline and during treatment, correct before use

• Dental status: regular dental exams should be performed; dental extractions (cover with antiinfectives before procedure)

• **MS pain:** may occur in a few days or years later, symptoms usually resolve after discontinuing

Evaluate:

• Therapeutic response: increased bone mass, absence of fractures

Teach patient/family:

• To remain upright for 30 min after dose to prevent esophageal irritation; if dose is missed, skip dose, do not double doses or take later in day; to take in AM before food, other meds; to take with 6-8 oz of water only (no mineral water)

• To take calcium, vit D if instructed by health care provider

• To use sunscreen, protective clothing to prevent photosensitivity

• To avoid smoking, alcohol intake, which increase osteoporosis

• To perform weight-bearing exercise to increase bone density

• To maintain good oral hygiene, to use antiinfectives before dental procedures as directed by prescriber

• **Pregnancy/breastfeeding:** to inform prescriber if pregnancy is planned or suspected; that cautious use is advised in breastfeeding

---

alfuzosin (Rx)

(al-fyoo'zoe-sin)

Uroxatral, Xatral ✦

Func. class.: Urinary tract, antispasmodic, α_1-agonist

Chem. class.: Quinazolone

ACTION: Binds to α_{1A}-adrenoceptor subtype located mainly in the prostate, relaxing smooth muscles

USES: Symptoms of benign prostatic hyperplasia

Unlabeled uses: Erectile dysfunction with sildenafil

CONTRAINDICATIONS: Hypersensitivity, moderate to severe hepatic impairment; not indicated for use in women or children, breastfeeding

Precautions: Pregnancy, but not used in females, geriatric patients; CAD, coronary insufficiency, mild hepatic disease, mild/moderate/severe renal disease, history of QT prolongation or coadministration with meds known to prolong QT interval, torsades de pointes, syncope, surgery, prostate cancer, orthostatic hypotension, ocular surgery, dysrhythmias, angina

DOSAGE AND ROUTES

• **Adult: PO EXT REL** 10 mg/day

Available forms: Ext rel tabs 10 mg

Administer:
PO route
• Do not break, crush, chew tabs; give with food; take at same time each day
• Store in tight container in cool environment

SIDE EFFECTS

CNS: *Dizziness, headache,* fatigue, flushing

CV: Postural hypotension (dizziness, lightheadedness, fainting) within a few hours of administration, chest pain, tachycardia, angina

GI: Nausea, abdominal pain, dyspepsia, constipation, diarrhea, liver injury, jaundice

GU: Impotence, priapism

HEMA: Thrombocytopenia

INTEG: Rash, urticaria, angioedema, pruritus, toxic epidermal necrolysis

MISC: Floppy iris syndrome

RESP: Pharyngitis, bronchitis, sinusitis

PHARMACOKINETICS

Peak 8 hr, half-life 10 hr, extensively metabolized in liver by CYP3A4 enzyme, excreted via urine (11% unchanged), protein binding (82%-90%), onset up to 1 hr, peak 8 hr, duration up to 24 hr

INTERACTIONS

• Not to be taken with prazosin, terazosin, doxazosin

Increase: effects of each product—atenolol, cimetidine, diltiazem

Increase: effects of alfuzosin—alcohol

Increase: effects—CYP3A4 inhibitors (ketoconazole, itraconazole, cimetidine and ritonavir); do not use together

Increase: hypotension—β-blockers, phosphodiesterase type 5 inhibitors, nitrates, antihypertensives

NURSING CONSIDERATIONS
Assess:
• **Prostatic hyperplasia:** change in urinary patterns (hesitancy, dribbling, dysuria, urgency), baseline and throughout treatment
• **Serious skin reactions:** Toxic epidermal necrolysis, notify prescriber immediately, stop product

• **Orthostatic hypotension:** Take B/P lying and standing, pulse baseline and frequently, usually occurs within 2-4 hr after beginning dose

Evaluate:
• Therapeutic response: decreased symptoms of benign prostatic hyperplasia

Teach patient/family:
• To take at same time each day with food; not to double doses, take missed doses when remembered
• To inform health care professional of rash, chest pain, dizziness
• That follow-up examinations will be needed
• To inform all health care professionals of use before surgery
• Not to drive or operate machinery; dizziness may occur; take missed doses when remembered
• About orthostatic hypotension; to rise slowly from sitting or lying
• To avoid all OTC products, meds, herbs unless approved by prescriber; not to crush or chew tabs
• To notify prescriber of fainting, dizziness
• That erectile dysfunction is a side effect and is temporary; that priapism has occurred rarely, may cause permanent impotence if not treated properly

---

alirocumab (Rx)
(al′-i-rok′-ue-mab)
Praluent
Func. class.: Antilipemic
Chem. class.: Proprotein convertase subtilisin/kexin type 9 (PCSK9) inhibitor antibody

ACTION: Binds to low-density lipoproteins, a human monoclonal antibody (IgG1)

USES: Heterozygous, familial hypercholesterolemia, atherosclerotic disease

CONTRAINDICATIONS: Hypersensitivity

Precautions: Pregnancy, breastfeeding

Side effects: *italics* = common; red = life-threatening

DOSAGE AND ROUTES
- **Adult: SUBCUT** 75 mg q2wk, may increase to 150 mg q2wk if needed after 4-8 wks or 300 mg q4wk

Available forms: Prefilled pen or prefilled syringe 75 mg/1 mL, 150 mg/1 mL

Administer:
- **SUBCUT route:** If dose is missed, give within 7 days of missed dose; if over 7 days, wait until next scheduled dose
- Visually inspect for particulate matter and discoloration; solution is clear, colorless to pale yellow
- Warm to room temperature for 30-40 min before use. Use as soon as possible after warming
- Do NOT use the prefilled pen or syringe if it has been at room temperature for ≥24 hr
- Give by subcut injection into the thigh, abdomen, or upper arm. Rotate injection site with each injection
- Do NOT inject into areas of active skin disease or injury (sunburn, rash, inflammation, skin infection)
- Do NOT administer with other injectable drugs at the same injection site

SIDE EFFECTS
CNS: Memory impairment, confusion
INTEG: Pruritus, injection-site reaction, vasculitis

PHARMACOKINETICS
Onset 4-8 hr, peak 3-7 days; half-life 17-20 days, distributed to circulation, crosses placenta

INTERACTIONS
None known

NURSING CONSIDERATIONS
Assess:
- **Hypercholesterolemia:** diet history: fat content, lipid levels (triglycerides, LDL, LDL-C 4-8 wk after start or titration, HDL, cholesterol); LFTs at baseline, periodically during treatment
- **Hypersensitivity:** rash, urticaria, itching; may require hospitalization and be severe

Evaluate:
- Therapeutic response: decreased LDL-C

Teach patient/family:

- That compliance is needed, that laboratory testing will be required
- That risk factors should be decreased: high-fat diet, smoking, alcohol consumption, absence of exercise, obesity
- To report confusion, injection-site reactions
- How to self-inject and how to care for equipment; to store in refrigerator, do not freeze; to discard if not refrigerated for >24 hr
- To read the patient information sheet
- To notify all providers that this product is being used
- To notify prescriber if pregnancy is suspected or planned, or if breastfeeding

---

aliskiren (Rx)
(a-lis′kir-en)
Rasilez ♣, Tekturna
Func. class.: Antihypertensive
Chem. class.: Direct renin inhibitor

ACTION: Renin inhibitor that acts on the renin-angiotensin system (RAS)

USES: Hypertension, alone or in combination with other antihypertensives

CONTRAINDICATIONS: Hypersensitivity

Black Box Warning: Pregnancy

Precautions: Breastfeeding, children, geriatric patients, angioedema, aortic/renal artery stenosis, cirrhosis, CAD, dialysis, hyper/hypokalemia, hyponatremia, hypotension, hypovolemia, renal/hepatic disease, surgery, diabetes

DOSAGE AND ROUTES
- **Adult: PO** 150 mg/day, may increase to 300 mg/day if needed, max 300 mg/day

Available forms: Tabs 150, 300 mg

Administer:
- May use with other antihypertensives
- Do not use with a high-fat meal
- Daily with a full glass of water; titrate up to achieve correct dose

---

• Do not discontinue abruptly; correct electrolyte/volume depletion before treatment

• Store in tight container at room temperature

SIDE EFFECTS

CV: Orthostatic hypotension, hypotension
CNS: Headache, dizziness, seizures
GI: *Diarrhea*
GU: Renal stones, increased uric acid
INTEG: Rash
META: Hyperkalemia
MISC: Angioedema, cough

PHARMACOKINETICS

Poorly absorbed, bioavailability 2.5%, peak 1-3 hr, steady state 7-8 days, 91% excreted unchanged in the feces, half-life 24 hr

INTERACTIONS

• Do not use with ACE inhibitors, angiotensin II receptor antagonists in diabetes mellitus

Increase: potassium levels—ACE inhibitors, angiotensin II receptor antagonists, potassium supplements, potassium-sparing diuretics

Increase: hypotension—other antihypertensives, diuretics

Increase: aliskiren levels—atorvastatin, itraconazole, ketoconazole, cycloSPORINE; concurrent use is not recommended

Decrease: levels of warfarin

Drug/Food

Decrease: aliskiren effect—high-fat meal, grapefruit

Drug/Lab Test

Increase: uric acid, BUN, serum creatinine, potassium

NURSING CONSIDERATIONS

Assess:

• Renal studies: uric acid, serum creatinine, BUN may be increased; hyperkalemia may occur; correct salt depletion, hyperkalemia, volume before starting therapy

• Allergic reactions: angioedema may occur (swelling of face; trouble breathing, swallowing)

• Daily dependent edema in feet, legs; weight, B/P, orthostatic hypotension

• **Diabetes:** identify the use of ACE inhibitors, angiotensin II receptor antagonists; if in use, do not use aliskiren

Evaluate:

• Therapeutic response: decrease in B/P

Teach patient/family:

• About the importance of complying with dosage schedule even if feeling better; that if dose is missed, take as soon as possible; that if it is almost time for the next dose, take only that dose; do not double dose; do not take with high-fat meal or grapefruit

• How to take B/P and normal reading for age group

• Not to use OTC products including herbs, supplements unless approved by prescriber

• **To report to prescriber immediately:** dizziness, faintness, chest pain, palpitations, uneven or rapid heartbeat, headache, severe diarrhea, swelling of tongue or lips, trouble breathing, difficulty swallowing, tightening of the throat

• Not to operate machinery or perform hazardous tasks if dizziness occurs

• To rise slowly to avoid faintness

Black Box Warning: **Pregnancy:** To notify if pregnancy is planned or suspected; if pregnant, product will need to be discontinued

---

allopurinol (Rx)

(al-oh-pure′i-nole)
Alloprin ✦, Aloprim ✦, Zyloprim
Func. class.: Antigout drug, antihyperuricemic
Chem. class.: Xanthine oxidase inhibitor

Do not confuse:
Zyloprim/Zovirax/zolpidem

ACTION: Inhibits the enzyme xanthine oxidase, reducing uric acid synthesis

USES: Chronic gout, hyperuricemia associated with malignancies, recurrent calcium oxalate calculi, uric acid calculi

CONTRAINDICATIONS: Hypersensitivity

Side effects: *italics* = common; red = life-threatening

Precautions: Pregnancy, breastfeeding, children, renal/hepatic disease

DOSAGE AND ROUTES
Increased uric acid levels in malignancies
• **Adult: PO** 600-800 mg/day in divided doses for 2-3 days; start up to 1-2 days before chemotherapy; **IV INFUSION** 200-400 mg/m²/day, max 600 mg/day 24-48 hr before chemotherapy, may be divided at 6-, 8-, 12-hr intervals
• **Child 6-10 yr: PO** 300 mg/day, adjust dose after 48 hr
• **Child <6 yr: PO** 150 mg/day, adjust dose after 48 hr
• **Child: IV INFUSION** 200 mg/m²/day, initially as a single dose or divided q6-12hr

Recurrent calculi
• **Adult: PO** 200-300 mg/day in a single dose or divided bid-tid

Uric acid nephropathy prevention
• **Adult and child >10 yr: PO** 600-800 mg/day × 2-3 days

Gout (mild)
• **Adult: PO** 100 mg/day, titrating upward, max 800 mg/day

Gout (moderate to severe)
• **Adult: PO** 400-600 mg/day in a single dose or divided bid-tid, max 800 mg/day, doses >300 mg should be given in divided doses, may start during an acute attack as long as antiinflammatory drugs are being used, do not initiate any new therapy during acute gout flare

Renal dose
• **Adult: PO/IV** CCr 81-100 mL/min 300 mg/day; CCr 61-80 mL/min 250 mg/day; CCr 41-60 mL/min 200 mg/day; CCr 21-40 mL/min 150 mg/day; CCr 10-20 mL/min 100-200 mg/day; CCr 3-9 mL/min 100 mg/day or 100 mg every other day; CCr <3 mL/min 100 mg q24hr or longer or 100 mg every 3rd day

Available forms: Tabs, scored 100, 300 mg; powder for inj 500 mg/vial

Administer:
PO route
• With meals to prevent GI symptoms; may crush, add to foods or fluids

• Begin 1-2 days before antineoplastic therapy

Intermittent IV INFUSION route
• Use in tumor lysis prior to start of chemotherapy (24-48 hr)
• Reconstitute 30-mL vial with 25 mL of sterile water for inj; dilute to desired concentrations (≤6 mg/mL) with 0.9% NaCl for inj or D₅W for inj; begin infusion within 10 hr

Y-site compatibilities: Acyclovir, aminophylline, amphotericin B lipid complex, anidulafungin, argatroban, atenolol, aztreonam, bivalirudin, bleomycin, bumetanide, buprenorphine, butorphanol, calcium gluconate, CARBOplatin, caspofungin, ceFAZolin, cefoTEtan, cefTAZidime, ceftizoxime, cefTRIAXone, cefuroxime, CISplatin, cyclophosphamide, DACTINomycin, DAUNOrubicin citrate liposome, dexamethasone, dexmedetomidine, DOCEtaxel, DOXOrubicin liposomal, enalaprilat, etoposide, famotidine, fenoldopam, filgrastim, fluconazole, fludarabine, fluorouracil, furosemide, gallium, ganciclovir, gatifloxacin, gemcitabine, gemtuzumab, granisetron hydrochloride, heparin, hydrocortisone phosphate, hydrocortisone succinate, HYDROmorphone, ifosfamide, linezolid injection, LORazepam, mannitol, mesna, methotrexate, metroNIDAZOLE, milrinone, mitoXANtrone, morphine, nesiritide, octreotide, oxytocin, PACLitaxel, pamidronate, pantoprazole, PEMEtrexed, piperacillin, piperacillin-tazobactam, plicamycin, potassium chloride, raNITIdine, sodium acetate, sulfamethoxazole-trimethoprim, teniposide, thiotepa, ticarcillin, ticarcillin-clavulanate, tigecycline, tirofiban, vancomycin, vasopressin, vinBLAStine, vinCRIStine, voriconazole, zidovudine, zoledronic acid

SIDE EFFECTS
GI: *Nausea, vomiting, malaise,* diarrhea, hepatitis
INTEG: Rash
CV: Hypo- and hypertension, HF (IV use)
CNS: Drowsiness
GU: Renal failure

Misc: Hypersensitivity, bone marrow depression
MS: Acute gouty attack

PHARMACOKINETICS
Protein binding <1%, half-life 1-2 hr
PO: Peak 1.5 hr; excreted in feces, urine
IV: Peak up to 30 min

INTERACTIONS
Increase: rash—ampicillin, amoxicillin; avoid concurrent use
Increase: action of oral anticoagulants, theophylline
Increase: hypersensitivity, toxicity—ACE inhibitors, thiazides
Increase: bone marrow depression—(mercaptopurine, azaTHIOprine)
Increase: xanthine nephropathy, calculi—rasburicase

NURSING CONSIDERATIONS
Assess:
• **For gout:** joint pain, swelling; may use with NSAIDs for acute gouty attacks; effect may take several wk
• CBC, AST, ALT, BUN, creatinine before starting treatment, periodically
• I&O ratio; increase fluids to 2 L/day to prevent stone formation and toxicity
• For rash, hypersensitivity reactions, discontinue allopurinol immediately, after rash is resolved, treatment may continue at a lower dose
Evaluate:
• Therapeutic response: decreased pain in joints, decreased stone formation in kidneys, decreased uric acid levels
Teach patient/family:
• To take as prescribed; if dose is missed, take as soon as remembered; do not double dose; tabs may be crushed
• To increase fluid intake to 2 L/day
• To report skin rash, stomatitis, malaise, fever, aching; product should be discontinued
• To avoid hazardous activities if drowsiness or dizziness occurs
• To avoid alcohol, caffeine; will increase uric acid levels
• An alkaline diet may be required

• That follow-up examinations and blood work will be needed
• To identify triggers and avoid
• To avoid large doses of vit C; kidney stone formation may occur
• To reduce dairy products, refined sugars, sodium, meat if taking for calcium oxalate stones; to identify triggers and avoid

---

almotriptan (Rx)
(al-moh-trip′tan)
Axert
Func. class.: Antimigraine agent, abortive
Chem. class.: 5-HT$_1$-receptor agonist, triptan

Do not confuse:
Axert/Antivert

ACTION: Binds selectively to the vascular 5-HT$_{1B/1D/1F}$-receptors, exerts antimigraine effect

USES: Acute treatment of migraine with or without aura (adult/adolescent/child ≥12 yr)

CONTRAINDICATIONS: Hypersensitivity, acute MI, angina, CV disease, CAD, stroke, vasospastic angina, ischemic heart disease or risk for, peripheral vascular syndrome, uncontrolled hypertension, basilar or hemiplegic migraine
Precautions: Pregnancy, postmenopausal women, men >40 yr, breastfeeding, children <18 yr, geriatric patients, risk factors for CAD, MI; hypercholesterolemia, obesity, diabetes, impaired renal/hepatic function, sulfonamide hypersensitivity, cardiac dysrhythmias, Raynaud's disease, tobacco smoking, Wolff-Parkinson-White syndrome

DOSAGE AND ROUTES
• **Adult, adolescent, and child ≥12 yr:** PO 6.25 or 12.5 mg; may repeat dose after 2 hr; max 2 doses/24 hr or 4 treatment cycles within any 30-day period
Hepatic/renal dose
• **Adult:** PO (CCr 10-30 mL/min) 6.25 mg initially, max 12.5 mg

---

Available forms: Tabs 6.25, 12.5 mg
Administer:
• Avoid using more than 2×/24 hr; rebound headache may occur
• Swallow tabs whole; do not break, crush, chew tabs, without regard to food

SIDE EFFECTS

CNS: *Dizziness,* headache, seizures, paresthesias
CV: Coronary artery vasospasm, MI, ventricular fibrillation, ventricular tachycardia
GI: Nausea, xerostomia
INTEG: Sweating, rash

PHARMACOKINETICS

Onset of pain relief 2 hr; peak 1-3 hr; duration 3-4 hr; bioavailability 70%; protein binding 35%; metabolized in the liver (metabolite), metabolized by MAO-A, CYP2D6, CYP3A4; excreted in urine (40%), feces (13%); half-life 3-4 hr

INTERACTIONS

Increase: serotonin syndrome—SSRIs, SNRIs, serotonin-receptor agonists, sibutramine
Increase: vasospastic effects—ergot, ergot derivatives, other 5-HT1 agonists; avoid concurrent use
Increase: almotriptan effect—MAOIs; do not use together
Increase: plasma concentration of almotriptan—(CYP3A4 inhibitors) itraconazole, ritonavir, erythromycin, ketoconazole; avoid concurrent use in renal/hepatic disease
Drug/Herb
• Avoid use with feverfew
Increase: serotonin syndrome—St. John's wort

NURSING CONSIDERATIONS
Assess:
• **Migraine:** pain location, aura, duration, intensity, nausea, vomiting; quiet, calm environment with decreased stimulation from noise, bright light, excessive talking
• **Serotonin syndrome:** occurs in those taking SSRIs, SNRIs; agitation, confusion, hallucinations, diaphoresis, hypertension, diarrhea, fever, tremors; usually occurs when dose is increased
• B/P; signs/symptoms of coronary vasospasms
• For stress level, activity, recreation, coping mechanisms
• **Neurologic status:** LOC, blurring vision, nausea, vomiting, tingling, hot sensation, burning, feeling of pressure, numbness, flushing preceding headache
• **Tyramine foods** (pickled products, beer, wine, aged cheese), food additives, preservatives, colorings, artificial sweeteners, chocolate, caffeine, which may precipitate these types of headaches
Evaluate:
• Therapeutic response: decrease in severity of migraine
Teach patient/family:
• To report chest pain, drowsiness, dizziness, tingling, flushing
• To notify prescriber if pregnancy is planned or suspected; to avoid breastfeeding
• That if one dose does not relieve migraine, to take another after 2 hr, max 4 treatment cycles in 30 days; do not take MAOIs for ≥ 24 hr
• That product does not prevent or reduce number of migraine attacks; use to relieve attack only
• **Serotonin syndrome:** To report immediately signs of serotonin syndrome
• To report immediately chest tightness or pain
• Not to drive or operate machinery until reaction is known, drowsiness, dizziness may occur
• To inform all health care professionals of all OTC, Rx, herbals, supplements taken

---

⚠ HIGH ALERT

alogliptin (Rx)
(al′oh-glip′tin)
Nesina
Func. class.: Antidiabetic
Chem. class.: Dipeptidyl peptidase-4 (DPP-4) inhibitor

ACTION: A dipeptidyl-peptidase-IV (DDP-IV) inhibitor for the treatment of type 2 diabetes mellitus (monotherapy or in combination with other antidiabetic agents), potentiates the effects of the incretin hormones by inhibiting their breakdown by DDP-IV

USES: Type 2 diabetes mellitus (T2DM)

CONTRAINDICATIONS: Hypersensitivity, ketoacidosis, type 1 diabetes
Precautions: Pregnancy, breastfeeding, hepatic disease, burns, diarrhea, fever, GI obstruction, hyper/hypoglycemia, hyper/hypothyroidism, hypercortisolism, children, ileus, malnutrition, pancreatitis, surgery, trauma, vomiting, kidney disease, adrenal insufficiency, angioedema

DOSAGE AND ROUTES
• **Adult: PO** 25 mg/day
Renal dose
• **Adult: PO** CCr 30-59 mL/min: 12.5 mg every day; CCr <30 mL/min: 6.25 mg every day; intermittent hemodialysis: 6.25 mg every day; give without regard to the timing of hemodialysis
Available forms: Tabs 6.25, 12.5, 25 mg
Administer:
• Without regard to food

SIDE EFFECTS
CNS: Headache
GI: *Pancreatitis, hepatotoxicity*
CV: Heart failure
SYST: Rash, hypersensitivity, angioedema, Stevens-Johnson syndrome, anaphylaxis

PHARMACOKINETICS
20% protein binding, excreted unchanged (urine), peak 1-2 hr, duration up to 24 hr, effect decreased in liver disease and increased in kidney disease, half-life 21 hr

INTERACTIONS
Increase: hypoglycemia—insulin, androgens, pegvisomant, sulfonylureas; dosage adjustment may be needed

Decrease: hypoglycemia—danazol, thiazides; adjust dose
Drug/Lab Test
Increase: LFTs
Decrease: glucose

NURSING CONSIDERATIONS
Assess:
• **Diabetes:** monitor blood glucose, glycosylated hemoglobin A1c (A1c), LFTs, serum creatinine/BUN baseline and throughout treatment
• **Pancreatitis:** can occur during use; monitor for severe abdominal pain, with or without vomiting
• **Hypersensitivity reactions:** angioedema, Stevens-Johnson syndrome; product should be discontinued
• **HF:** Assess for risk of HF in those with known HF or kidney disease
Evaluate:
• Positive therapeutic response: decrease in polyuria, polydipsia, polyphagia, clear sensorium, absence of dizziness, improvement in A1c
Teach patient/family:
• **Hepatotoxicity:** To report yellowing of skin, eyes, dark urine, clay-colored stools, nausea, vomiting
• That diabetes is a lifelong condition, product does not cure disease
• That all food in diet plan must be eaten to prevent hypoglycemia; to continue with weight control, dietary medical nutrition therapy, physical activity, hygiene
• To carry emergency ID with prescriber, medications, and condition listed
• To test blood glucose using a blood glucose meter, and urine ketones
• To report allergic reactions, nausea, vomiting, abdominal pain, dark urine
• **Hypersensitivity:** To notify health care professional and stop taking product if rash, trouble breathing, swelling of face, lips, tongue occur
• To notify all health care professionals of OTC, Rx, herbs, supplements used
• **Pregnancy/breastfeeding:** To report if pregnancy is planned or suspected, or if breastfeeding

alosetron (Rx)

(ah-loss′a-tron)

Lotronex

Func. class.: Anti-IBS agent
Chem. class.: Serotonin receptor antagonist 5-HT$_3$

Do not confuse:
Lotronex/Lovenox/Protomix

ACTION: A potent and selective antagonist at serotonin 5-HT$_3$ receptors, which are extensively distributed on enteric neurons in GI tract. Antagonism at these receptors in the GI tract modulates the regulation of visceral pain, colonic transit, and GI secretions

USES: Severe, chronic, diarrhea-predominant irritable bowel syndrome (IBS) in women who have failed conventional therapy

CONTRAINDICATIONS: Crohn's disease, severe hepatic disease, diverticulitis, toxic megacolon, GI adhesions/strictures/obstruction/perforation, thrombophlebitis, ulcerative colitis

Black Box Warning: Ischemic colitis, severe constipation

Precautions: Breastfeeding, pregnancy, child <18 yr, mild-moderate hepatic disease

DOSAGE AND ROUTES

• **Adult woman: PO** 0.5 mg bid, may increase to 1 mg bid after 4 wk if well tolerated; if symptoms are not controlled after 4 wk of treatment with 1 mg bid, discontinue

Available forms: Tab 0.5 mg, 1 mg
Administer:

• Without regard to meals with full glass of water

Black Box Warning: Only after "Physician–Patient Agreement Form" is signed and patient receives official Medication Guide

• Store at room temperature, protect from light and moisture

SIDE EFFECTS

CNS: Fatigue, headache
GI: Constipation, abdominal pain, distention, reflux, nausea, obstruction, impaction, ischemic colitis, ileus perforation, small-bowel mesenteric ischemia
GU: Urinary tract infection
MS: Muscle spasm
RESP: Cough, nasopharyngitis, upper respiratory tract infection

PHARMACOKINETICS

Peak 1 hr, half-life 1½ hr, metabolized extensively in the liver, mainly excreted in urine

INTERACTIONS

• Do not use with fluvoxaMINE
Increase: Alosetron metabolism—CYP3A4 inhibitors
Increase: serious adverse reactions—drugs that decrease GI motility, drugs with anticholinergic effect such as TCAs, H^1-blockers, orphenadrine, OLANZapine, maprotiline, disopyramide, cyclobenzaprine, cloZAPine, buPROPion, amoxapine, amantadine
Decrease: Alosetron metabolism—CYP3A4 (clarithromycin, ketoconazole), 1A2, 2C9 inhibitors, hydrALAZINE, procainamide
Drug/Lab Test
Increase: ALT

NURSING CONSIDERATIONS
Assess:

Black Box Warning: **Irritable bowel syndrome:** constipation, diarrhea, abdominal pain, fecal incontinence; discontinue immediately if bloody diarrhea, severe constipation, rectal bleeding, or severe abdominal pain occurs; ischemic colitis has occurred and can be fatal

Black Box Warning: Only clinicians enrolled in the Prometheus Prescribing Program for Lotronex should use this product (888-423-5227)

• Geriatric female patients can experience more severe side effects
Evaluate:
• Therapeutic response: decreasing symptoms of IBS
Teach patient/family:

Black Box Warning: Ischemic colitis: immediately report severe constipation, bloody diarrhea, rectal bleeding, or worsening abdominal pain; stop product, resume only if approved by prescriber

• Not to double doses; if a dose is missed, skip it; do not take with other meds or herbs without prescriber approval
• That product may be taken without regard to food
• That product does not cure disorder, only controls symptoms
• Provide medication guide and clarify, if needed, that improvement in symptoms can take 1-4 wk; symptoms will recur if product is stopped
• That product is used only for women with IBS
• **Pregnancy/breastfeeding:** to report if pregnancy is planned or suspected; product should not be used during pregnancy; effects are unknown; use caution in breastfeeding

---

> ### ⚠ HIGH ALERT
>
> ## ALPRAZolam (Rx)
> (al-pray′zoe-lam)
> Xanax, Xanax XR
> *Func. class.:* Antianxiety
> *Chem. class.:* Benzodiazepine (short/intermediate acting)
>
> **Controlled Substance Schedule IV**

Do not confuse:
ALPRAZolam/LORazepam
Xanax/Zantac

ACTION: Depresses subcortical levels of CNS, including limbic system, reticular formation

USES: Anxiety, panic disorders with or without agoraphobia, anxiety with depressive symptoms
Unlabeled uses: Premenstrual dysphoric disorders, insomnia, PMS, alcohol withdrawal syndrome

CONTRAINDICATIONS: Pregnancy, breastfeeding, hypersensitivity to benzodiazepines, closed-angle glaucoma, psychosis, addiction
Precautions: Geriatric patients, debilitated patients, hepatic disease, obesity, severe pulmonary disease

DOSAGE AND ROUTES
Anxiety disorder
• **Adult:** PO 0.25-0.5 mg tid, may increase q3-4days if needed, max 4 mg/day in divided doses
• **Geriatric:** PO 0.25 mg bid; increase by 0.125 mg as needed
Panic disorder
• **Adult:** PO 0.5 mg tid, may increase up to 1 mg/day q3-4days, max 10 mg/day; **EXT REL** (Xanax XR) give daily in AM, 0.5-1 mg initially, maintenance 3-6 mg/day, max 10 mg/day
Hepatic dose
• Reduce dose by 50%-60%
Premenstrual dysphoric disorders/PMS (unlabeled)
• **Adult:** PO 0.25 mg bid-tid starting on day 16-18 of menses, taper over 2-3 days when menses occurs, max 4 mg/day
Available forms: Tabs 0.25, 0.5, 1, 2 mg; ext rel tabs (Xanax XR) 0.5, 1, 2, 3 mg; orally disintegrating tabs 0.25, 0.5, 1, 2 mg; oral sol 1 mg/mL
Administer:
• Tabs may be crushed, mixed with food, fluids if patient is unable to swallow medication whole; do not break, crush, chew ext rel (XR), give ext rel tab in

---

AM; conversion from regular-release tab to ext rel is at same dose

• With food or milk for GI symptoms; high-fat meal will decrease absorption

• To discontinue, decrease by 0.5 mg q3days

• May divide total daily doses into more times/day if anxiety occurs between doses

• **Orally disintegrating tabs:** place on tongue to dissolve and swallow; protect from moisture, discard unused portion of tab if split

• **Oral solution:** mix with water, juice, applesauce or other soft foods; use calibrated dropper supplied

SIDE EFFECTS

CNS: *Dizziness, drowsiness,* confusion, headache, stimulation, poor coordination, suicide

EENT: *Blurred vision*

GI: Constipation, dry mouth, nausea, vomiting, anorexia, diarrhea, weight gain/loss

GU: Decreased libido

INTEG: Rash, dermatitis

PHARMACOKINETICS

PO: Well absorbed; widely distributed; onset 30 min; peak 1-2 hr; duration 4-6 hr; *oral disintegrating tab* peak 1.5-2 hr; therapeutic response 2-3 days; metabolized by liver (CYP3A4), excreted by kidneys; crosses placenta, breast milk; half-life 12-15 hr, protein binding 80%

INTERACTIONS

Increase: ALPRAZolam action—CYP3A4 inhibitors (cimetidine, disulfiram, erythromycin, FLUoxetine, isoniazid, itraconazole, ketoconazole, metoprolol, propranolol, valproic acid); do not use together

Increase: CNS depression—anticonvulsants, alcohol, antihistamines, sedative/hypnotics, opioids; avoid concurrent use

Decrease: sedation—xanthines

Decrease: ALPRAZolam action—CYP3A4 inducers (barbiturates, carbamazepine rifAMPin), adjust dose as needed

Decrease: action of levodopa

Drug/Herb

Increase: CNS depression—kava, melatonin, St. John's wort, valerian

Drug/Food

Increase: product level—grapefruit juice; avoid concurrent use

Drug/Lab Test

Increase: AST/ALT, alk phos

NURSING CONSIDERATIONS

Assess:

• Mental status: anxiety, mood, sensorium, orientation, affect, sleeping pattern, drowsiness, dizziness, especially in geriatric patients both before and during treatment, suicidal thoughts, behaviors

• Hepatic, blood studies: renal studies, AST, ALT, bilirubin, creatinine, LDH, alk phos, CBC; may cause neutropenia, decreased Hct, increased LFTs

• **Physical dependency, withdrawal symptoms:** anxiety, panic attacks, agitation, seizures, headache, nausea, vomiting, muscle pain, weakness; withdrawal seizures may occur after rapid decrease in dose or abrupt discontinuation; because duration of action is short, considered to be the product of choice for geriatric patients

• **Beers:** avoid in older adults; increased risk of cognitive impairment

Evaluate:

• Therapeutic response: decreased anxiety, restlessness, sleeplessness, panic attacks.

Teach patient/family:

• Not to double doses; to take exactly as prescribed; if dose is missed, take within 1 hr as scheduled; that product may be taken with food

• Not to use for everyday stress or for more than 4 mo unless directed by prescriber; not to take more than prescribed amount; that product may be habit forming; that memory impairment is a result of long-term use

• To avoid OTC preparations unless approved by prescriber, not to use with grapefruit juice

- Not to discontinue medication abruptly after long-term use
- To avoid driving, activities that require alertness because drowsiness may occur
- To avoid alcohol, other psychotropic medications unless directed by prescriber
- To rise slowly or fainting may occur, especially among geriatric patients
- That drowsiness may worsen at beginning of treatment
- **Oral disintegrating tablet:** to place on tongue and allow to dissolve; swallow; if only half tab required, discard other half
- **Oral solution:** to mix with water, juice or other soft foods; to use measuring device supplied
- **Pregnancy/breastfeeding:** If planned or suspected; not to use in pregnancy, to avoid breastfeeding

TREATMENT OF OVERDOSE: Lavage, VS, supportive care, flumazenil

---

RARELY USED

alprostadil (Rx)

(al-pros′ta-dil)

Caverject, Caverject Impulse, Edex, Muse, Prostin VR Pediatric
Func. class.: Hormone

USES: To maintain patent ductus arteriosus (temporary treatment), erectile dysfunction

CONTRAINDICATIONS: Hypersensitivity, respiratory distress syndrome, those at risk for priapism

Black Box Warning: Apnea

DOSAGE AND ROUTES
Patent ductus arteriosus
- **Infant: IV INFUSION** 0.05-0.1 mcg/kg/min until desired response, then reduce to lowest effective amount, max 0.4 mcg/kg/min

Erectile dysfunction of vasculogenic or mixed etiology, psychogenic
- **Men: INTRACAVERNOSAL** 2.5 mcg, may increase by 2.5 mcg, may then increase by 5-10 mcg until adequate response occurs (max 60 mcg/dose); **INTRAURETHRAL** 125-250 mcg, max 2 doses/24 hr, max dose 1000 mcg; administer as needed to achieve erection

---

⚠ HIGH ALERT

alteplase (Rx)

(al-ti-plaze′)

Activase, Activase rt-PA ✤, Cathflo Activase
Func. class.: Thrombolytic enzyme
Chem. class.: Tissue plasminogen activator (TPA)

Do not confuse:
alteplase/Altace
Activase/Cathflo Activase/TNKase

ACTION: Produces fibrin conversion of plasminogen to plasmin; able to bind to fibrin, convert plasminogen in thrombus to plasmin, which leads to local fibrinolysis, limited systemic proteolysis

USES: Lysis of obstructing thrombi associated with acute MI, ischemic conditions that require thrombolysis (i.e., PE, unclotting arteriovenous shunts, acute ischemic CVA), central venous catheter occlusion (Cathflo)
Unlabeled uses: Arterial thromboembolism, deep vein thrombosis (DVT), occlusion prophylaxis, percutaneous coronary intervention (PCI)

CONTRAINDICATIONS: Active internal bleeding, history of CVA, severe uncontrolled hypertension, intracranial/intraspinal surgery/trauma (within 3 mo), aneurysm, brain tumor, platelets <100,000 mm³, bleeding diathesis including INR >1.7 or PR >15 sec, arteriovenous malformation, subarachnoid hemorrhage,

---

Side effects: *italics* = common; red = life-threatening

intracranial hemorrhage, uncontrolled hypertension, seizure at onset of stroke

Precautions: Pregnancy, breastfeeding, children, geriatric patients, neurologic deficits, mitral stenosis, recent GI/GU bleeding, diabetic retinopathy, subacute bacterial endocarditis, arrhythmias, diabetic hemorrhage retinopathy, CVA, recent major surgery, hypertension, acute pericarditis, hemostatic defects, significant hepatic disease, septic thrombophlebitis, occluded AV cannula at seriously infected site

DOSAGE AND ROUTES
MI (standard infusion) (Activase)
• **Adult >65 kg:** 100 mg total given over 3 hr as follows: 60 mg given over 1st hr (6-10 mg bolus over 1-2 min), then 20 mg given over 2nd hr, then 20 mg over 3rd hr
• **Adult <65 kg:** 1.25 mg/kg over 3 hr: 0.75 mg/kg over 1st hr (0.075-0.125 mg/kg given as a bolus over 1st 1-2 min), then 0.25 mg/kg over 2nd hr, then 0.25 mg/kg over 3rd hr, max 100 mg

MI (accelerated infusion) (Activase)
• **Adult ≥67 kg:** 100 mg total dose: give 15-mg IV BOL, then 50 mg over 30 min, then 35 mg over 60 min
• **Adult <67 kg:** 15-mg IV BOL, then 0.75 mg/kg (max 50 mg) over 30 min, then 0.5 mg/kg (max 35 mg) over next 60 min

Pulmonary embolism (Activase)
• **Adult:** IV 100 mg over 2 hr, then heparin

Acute ischemic stroke (Activase)
• **Adult: /child IV** 0.9 mg/kg, max 90 mg; give as **INFUSION** over 1 hr, give 10% of dose **IV BOL** over 1st min

Occluded venous access devices (Cathflo Activase)
• **Adult/child ≥30 kg:** IV 2 mg/2 mL instilled in occluded catheter, may repeat if needed after 2 hr
• **Child 10-29 kg:** IV 110% of lumen volume, max 2 mg/2 mL instilled in occluded catheter, may repeat if needed after 2 hr

Deep venous thrombosis (DVT) (Activase) (unlabeled)
• **Adult:** IV 4 mcg/kg/min as 2-hr infusion, then 1 mcg/kg/min × 33 hr

Percutaneous coronary intervention (PCI) (unlabeled)
• **Adult: INTRACARDIAC** 20 mg over 5 min, then 50 mg over the next 60 min

Occlusion prophylaxis (unlabeled) (Cathflo Activase)
• **Adult/child>30 kg:** IV Do not exceed 2 mg in 2 mL; may use up to 2 doses 120 min apart
• **Adult/child ≤30 kg:** IV 110% lumen volume (max 2 mg/2 mL) in occluded catheter, may repeat after 2 hr

Available forms: Powder for inj 50 mg (29 million international units/vial), 100 mg (58 million international units/vial); Cathflo Activase: lyophilized powder for inj 2 mg

Administer: (Activase)
Intermittent IV INFUSION route
• After reconstituting with provided diluent, add appropriate amount of sterile water for inj (no preservatives) 20-mg vial/20 mL or 50-mg vial/50 mL to make 1 mg/mL, mix by slow inversion or dilute with NaCl, D_5W to a concentration of 0.5 mg/mL; 1.5 to <0.5 mg/mL may result in precipitation of product; use 18G needle; flush line with NaCl after administration, give over 3 hr for MI, 2 hr for PE
• Pressure for 30 sec to minor bleeding sites; 30 min to sites of arterial puncture followed by pressure dressing; inform prescriber if this does not attain hemostasis; apply pressure dressing
• Store powder at room temperature or refrigerate; protect from excessive light
• Heparin therapy after thrombolytic therapy is discontinued, TT, ACT, or APTT less than 2× control (about 3-4 hr); treatment can be initiated before coagulation study results obtained, infusion should be discontinued if pretreatment INR >1.7, PT >15 sec, or elevated APTT is identified
• Use reconstituted IV solution within 8 hr or discard

• Avoid invasive procedures, inj, rectal temperature

• **Cathflo Activase:** Use product after other options used for declotting a line; reconstitute by using 2.2 mL of sterile water provided and injecting in vial, direct flow into powder (1 mg/mL), foam will disappear after standing; swirl, do not shake, sol will be pale yellow or clear, use within 8 hr, instill 2 mL of reconstituted sol into occluded catheter, try to aspirate after ½ hr; if unable to remove, allow 2 hr, a 2nd dose may be used; aspirate 5 mL of blood to remove clot and product, irrigate with normal saline

SIDE EFFECTS
INTEG: Urticaria, rash
SYST: GI, GU, intracranial, retroperitoneal bleeding, anaphylaxis, fever

PHARMACOKINETICS
Cleared by liver, 80% cleared within 10 min of product termination, onset immediate, half-life 35 min, peak 1 hr

INTERACTIONS
Increase: bleeding—anticoagulants, salicylates, dipyridamole, other NSAIDs, abciximab, eptifibatide, tirofiban, clopidogrel, ticlopidine, some cephalosporins, plicamycin, valproic acid; monitor for bleeding
Drug/Herb
Increase: risk for bleeding—feverfew, garlic, ginger, ginkgo, ginseng, green tea
Drug/Lab Test
Increase: PT, APTT, TT

NURSING CONSIDERATIONS
Assess:
• Treatment is not recommended in patients with acute ischemic stroke >3 hr after symptoms onset, with minor neurologic deficit or with rapidly improving symptoms
• VS, B/P, pulse, respirations, neurologic signs, temperature at least q4hr; temperature >104° F (40° C) indicates internal bleeding; monitor rhythm closely; ventricular dysrhythmias may occur with hyperperfusion; monitor heart, breath sounds, neurologic status, peripheral pulses; assess neurologic status, neurologic change may indicate intracranial bleeding
• **For bleeding:** during 1st hour of treatment and 24 hr after procedure: hematuria, hematemesis, bleeding from mucous membranes, epistaxis, ecchymosis; guaiac all body fluids, stools; do not use 150 mg or more total dose because intracranial bleeding may occur; do not use in severe uncontrolled hypertension, aneurysm, head trauma, for MI, pulmonary embolism; obtain noncontrast CT of brain or MRI to take out intracranial hemorrhage prior to systemic use
• **Hypersensitivity:** fever, rash, itching, chills, facial swelling, dyspnea, notify prescriber immediately; stop product, keep resuscitative equipment nearby; mild reaction may be treated with antihistamines
• Previous allergic reactions or streptococcal infection; alteplase may be less effective
• Blood studies (Hct, platelets, PTT, PT, TT, APTT) before starting therapy; PT or APTT must be less than 2× control before starting therapy; TT or PT q3-4hr during treatment
• **MI:** ECG continuously, cardiac enzymes, radionuclide myocardial scanning/coronary angiography; chest pain intensity, character; monitor those with major early infarct signs on CT scan with substantial edema, mass effect, midline shift
• **PE:** pulse, B/P, ABGs, rate/rhythm of respirations
• **Occlusion:** have patient exhale then hold breath when connecting/disconnecting syringe to prevent air embolism
• **Pregnancy/breastfeeding:** usually considered contraindicated in pregnancy except in serious conditions; use cautiously in breastfeeding
Evaluate:

• Therapeutic response: lysis of thrombi, adequate hemodynamic state, absence of HF, cannula/catheter lack of occlusion

Teach patient/family:

• The purpose and expected results of the treatment; to report adverse reactions, bleeding

---

aluminum hydroxide (OTC)

Alugel ♣, AlternaGel, Alu-Cap, Alu-Tab, Amphojel, Basaljel

Func. class.: Antacid, hypophosphatemic

Chem. class.: Aluminum product, phosphate binder

ACTION: Neutralizes gastric acidity; binds phosphates in GI tract; these phosphates are then excreted

USES: Antacid, hyperphosphatemia in chronic renal failure; adjunct in gastric, peptic, duodenal ulcers; hyperacidity, reflux esophagitis, heartburn, stress ulcer prevention in critically ill, GERD

Unlabeled uses: GI bleeding

CONTRAINDICATIONS: Hypersensitivity to product or aluminum products

Precautions: Pregnancy, breastfeeding, geriatric patients, fluid restriction, decreased GI motility, GI obstruction, dehydration, renal disease, sodium-restricted diets, GI bleeding, hypokalemia

DOSAGE AND ROUTES

Antacid

• **Adult: PO** 500-1500 mg 3-6× daily, max 6 doses/day

Hyperphosphatemia

• **Adult: PO** Susp 30-40 mL (regular) or 15-20 mL (concentrated) tid-qid

• **Child: PO** 50-150 mg/kg/day in 4-6 divided doses

Available forms: Susp 320 mg/5 mL, 450 mg/ 5mL, 600 mg/5 mL, 675 mg/5 mL; capsules 475, 500 mg; tablets 300, 500, 600 mg

Administer: 2 tsp (10 mL) will neutralize 20 mEq of acid

PO route

• Give 2 hr before or 6 hr after fluoroquinolones

• **Hyperphosphatemia:** Give with 8 oz water, meals unless contraindicated

• Laxatives or stool softeners if constipation occurs, especially for geriatric patients

• After shaking susp

NG route

• By nasogastric tube if patient unable to swallow

SIDE EFFECTS

GI: *Constipation,* anorexia, fecal impaction

META: *Hypophosphatemia*

PHARMACOKINETICS

PO: Onset 20-40 min, duration 1-3 hr, excreted in feces, onset 20-40 min, peak 30 min, duration 1-3 hr

INTERACTIONS

Decrease: effectiveness of—allopurinol, amprenavir, cephalosporins, corticosteroids, delavirdine, digoxin, fluoroquinolones, gabapentin, gatifloxacin, H$_2$ antagonists, iron salts, isoniazid, ketoconazole, penicillAMINE, phenothiazines, phenytoin, quiNIDine, quinolones, tetracyclines, thyroid hormones, ticlopidine, anticholinergics; separate by at least 4-6 hr

Drug/Food

Decrease: product effect—high-protein meal

NURSING CONSIDERATIONS

Assess:

• **GI pain:** location, intensity, duration, character, aggravating, alleviating factors; monitor for blood in stools, emesis, sputum in ulcer disease

• Phosphate, calcium levels because product is bound in GI system

• **Hypophosphatemia:** anorexia, weakness, fatigue, bone pain, hyporeflexia

---

- Constipation; increase bulk in diet if needed, may use stool softeners or laxatives; record amount and consistency of stools
- **Pregnancy/breastfeeding:** may use occasionally at recommended dose in pregnancy, breastfeeding

Evaluate:
- Therapeutic response: absence of GI pain, decreased acidity, healed ulcers, decreased phosphate levels

Teach patient/family:
- Not to use for prolonged periods for patients with low serum phosphate or patients on low-sodium diets; to shake liquid well
- That stools may appear white or speckled
- To check with prescriber after 2 wk of self-prescribed antacid use
- To separate from other medications by 2 hr
- **Hyperphosphatemia:** to avoid phosphate foods (most dairy products, eggs, fruits, carbonated beverages) during product therapy
- To notify prescriber of black tarry stools, which may indicate bleeding

---

alvimopan (Rx)

(al-vim′oh-pan)

Entereg

Func. class.: Functional GI disorder agent

Chem. class.: Peripheral mu-opioid receptor antagonist

ACTION: A peripherally selective mu-opioid receptor antagonist with activity restricted to the GI tract

USES: Prevention of postoperative ileus
Unlabeled uses: Opiate-agonist–induced constipation

CONTRAINDICATIONS: Those who have taken therapeutic doses of opioids for more than 7 consecutive days immediately before starting alvimopan, end-stage renal disease, Child-Pugh C

Precautions: Risk for MI, surgery for complete GI obstruction, hepatic disease, renal disease, pregnancy, breastfeeding

> Black Box Warning: MI; requires a specialized care setting

DOSAGE AND ROUTES
- **Adult/geriatric patient: PO** 12 mg 30 min-5 hr before surgery; then 12 mg bid beginning the day after surgery; max 7 days or hospital discharge; max 15 doses

Opiate agonist–induced constipation (unlabeled)
- **Adult: PO** 0.5 mg or 1 mg every day

Renal/hepatic dosage
- **Adult: PO** do not use in end-stage renal disease or Child-Pugh Class C

Available forms: Cap 12 mg
Administer:
- Without regard to food

> Black Box Warning: Only in a hospital setting approved for the ENTEREG Access Support and Education (E.A.S.E.) program, MI, max 15 doses inpatient

- Store at room temperature

SIDE EFFECTS
GI: *Constipation, dyspepsia,* flatulence, diarrhea, abdominal pain, cramping
HEMA: *Anemia*
META: Hypokalemia
MISC: Back pain, urinary retention, MI

PHARMACOKINETICS
Half-life 10-17 hr, extended in hepatic/renal disease, protein binding 80%-94%

INTERACTIONS
Increase: Alvimopan concentrations, toxicity —amiodarone, bepridil, cycloSPORINE, diltiaZEM, itraconazole, quiNIDine, quiNINE, spironolactone, verapamil

> Black Box Warning: Do not use if opiate agonists have been used for 7 consecutive days before alvimopan

> Black Box Warning: Do not use concurrently with other opiate antagonists

---

Side effects: *italics* = common; red = life-threatening

NURSING CONSIDERATIONS
Assess:
• Blood studies: Hgb/Hct, potassium; hyperkalemia occurs
• Recent opioid use, do not use within 7 consecutive days

Black Box Warning: Opioid use for chronic pain; MI is more common in this population

Evaluate:
• Therapeutic response: absence of postoperative ileus
Teach patient/family:
• **Pregnancy/breastfeeding:** to notify prescriber if pregnancy is planned or suspected; to avoid breastfeeding
• That product is used for only a limited time (<7 days) in a hospital setting, max 15 doses inpatient
• To report constipation, abdominal pain, cramping, nausea, vomiting, dyskinesia associated with Parkinson's disease

---

amantadine (Rx)
(a-man′ta-deen)
Endantadine ✤, Gocovri, Osmolex ER, Symmetrel ✤
Func. class.: Antiviral, antiparkinsonian agent
Chem. class.: Tricyclic amine

Do not confuse:
amantadine/raNITIdine/rimantidine/amiodarone

ACTION: Prevents uncoating of nucleic acid in viral cell, thereby preventing penetration of virus to host; causes release of DOPamine from neurons

USES: Prophylaxis or treatment of influenza type A, EPS, parkinsonism, Parkinson's disease
Unlabeled uses: Neuroleptic malignant syndrome, MS-associated fatigue

CONTRAINDICATIONS: Hypersensitivity, breastfeeding, children <1, eczematic rash

Precautions: Pregnancy, geriatric patients, epilepsy, HF, orthostatic hypotension, psychiatric disorders, renal/hepatic disease, peripheral edema, CV disease

DOSAGE AND ROUTES
Parkinson's disease
• **Adult:** PO 100 mg bid (monotherapy); after 7 days may increase to 400 mg in divided doses; Osmolex SR: initial dosage 129 mg q day in the AM; may increase q wk, max 322 mg q day in the AM
Influenza type A
• **Adult and child ≥13 yr:** PO 200 mg/day in single dose or divided bid
• **Geriatric:** PO No more than 100 mg/day
• **Child 1-8 yr:** PO 4.4-8.8 mg/kg/day divided bid-tid, max 150 mg/day
Drug-induced EPS
• **Adult:** PO 100 mg bid, up to 300 mg/day in divided doses; **EXT REL** (Gocovri) 137 mg q day at bedtime; after 1 wk, increase to 274 mg q day at bedtime
Renal dose
• **Adult:** PO CCr 30-50 mL/min 200 mg 1st day then 100 mg/day; CCr 15-29 mL/min 100 mg 1st day, then 100 mg on alternate days; CCr 15 mL/min reduce dose and interval to 200 mg q7days
MS-associated fatigue (unlabeled)
• **Adult:** PO 200 mg/day or 100 mg bid
Neuroleptic malignant syndrome (unlabeled)
• **Adult:** PO 100 mg bid × 3 wk
Available forms: Caps 100 mg; oral sol 50 mg/5 mL; tab 100 mg; ext rel (Osmolex ER) 129, 193, 258 mg; ext rel (Gocovri) 68.5, 137 mg
Administer:
• **Prophylaxis:** before exposure to influenza; continue for 10 days after contact; **treatment:** initiate within 24-48 hr of onset of symptoms, continue for 24-48 hr after symptoms disappear
• After meals for better absorption to decrease GI symptoms; at least 4 hr before bedtime to prevent insomnia
• In divided doses to prevent CNS disturbances: headache, dizziness, fatigue, drowsiness
• Store in tight, dry container

SIDE EFFECTS

CNS: *Headache, dizziness,* drowsiness, fatigue, *anxiety,* psychosis, *depression, hallucinations,* tremors, seizures, confusion, *insomnia*

CV: *Orthostatic hypotension,* HF

EENT: Blurred vision

GI: *Nausea, vomiting,* constipation, dry mouth, anorexia

GU: *Frequency, retention*

HEMA: Leukopenia, agranulocytosis

INTEG: Photosensitivity, dermatitis, livedo reticularis

PHARMACOKINETICS

PO: Onset 48 hr, peak 1-4 hr, half-life 24 hr, not metabolized, excreted in urine (90%) unchanged, crosses placenta, excreted in breast milk

INTERACTIONS

Increase: anticholinergic response—atropine, other anticholinergics; reduce dose of anticholinergics

Increase: CNS stimulation—CNS stimulants

Decrease: amantadine effect—metoclopramide, phenothiazines

Decrease: renal excretion of amantadine—triamterene, hydroCHLOROthiazide

Decrease: effect—S/B H1N1 influenza A virus vaccine; avoid use 2 wk before or 48 hr after amantadine

Drug/Lab Test

Increase: BUN, creatinine, alk phos, CK, LDH, bilirubin, AST, ALT, GGT

NURSING CONSIDERATIONS
Assess:

• Mental status: may cause increased psychiatric disorders especially in the elderly

• **HF:** weight gain, jugular venous distention, dyspnea, crackles

• Skin eruptions, photosensitivity after administration of product

• Serum creatinine, BUN in renal impairment

• Reaction to each medication

• Signs of infection

• **Livedo reticularis:** mottling of the skin, usually red; edema; itching in lower extremities, usually in Parkinson's disease

• **Parkinson's disease:** gait, tremors, akinesia, rigidity, may be effective if anticholinergics have not been effective

• **Toxicity:** confusion, behavioral changes, hypotension, seizures

Evaluate:

• Therapeutic response: absence of fever, malaise, cough, dyspnea with infection; tremors, shuffling gait with Parkinson's disease

Teach patient/family:

• To change body position slowly to prevent orthostatic hypotension

• About aspects of product therapy: to report dyspnea, weight gain, dizziness, poor concentration, dysuria, complex sleep behaviors

• To avoid hazardous activities if dizziness, blurred vision occurs

• **Parkinson's disease:** to take product exactly as prescribed; parkinsonian crisis may occur if product is discontinued abruptly; not to double dose; if a dose is missed, not to take within 4 hr of next dose; caps may be opened and mixed with food

• To avoid alcohol

• **Pregnancy/breastfeeding:** Avoid use in pregnancy; identify if pregnancy is suspected; avoid breastfeeding

TREATMENT OF OVERDOSE:
Maintain airway, administer EPINEPHrine, aminophylline, O$_2$, IV corticosteroids, physostigmine

---

ambrisentan (Rx)
(am-bri-sen'tan)

Letairis, Volibris ✦

Func. class.: Antihypertensive

ACTION: Endothelin-A receptor antagonist; endothelin-A is a vasoconstrictor

USES: Pulmonary arterial hypertension, alone or in combination with other antihypertensives in WHO class II (significant exertion), III (mild exertion)

CONTRAINDICATIONS: Breast-feeding, hypersensitivity, idiopathic pulmonary fibrosis (IPF)

Precautions: Children, females, geriatric patients, hepatitis, anemia, heart failure, jaundice, peripheral edema, hepatic disease, pulmonary disease

DOSAGE AND ROUTES
• **Adult: PO** 5 mg/day; may increase q4wk to max 10 mg/day if needed
Hepatic dose
• **Adult: PO** Discontinue if AST/ALT >5× ULN, or if elevations are accompanied by bilirubin >2× ULN, or other signs of liver dysfunction
Available forms: Tabs 5, 10 mg
Administer:
• Do not break, crush, chew tabs
• Daily with a full glass of water without regard to food
• Do not discontinue abruptly

• Store in tight container at room temperature

SIDE EFFECTS
CNS: *Headache,* fever, flushing, fatigue
CV: Orthostatic hypotension, hypotension, *peripheral edema,* palpitations
EENT: Sinusitis, rhinitis
GI: Abdominal pain, constipation, anorexia, hepatotoxicity
GU: Decreased sperm counts
HEMA: *Anemia*
INTEG: Rash, angioedema
RESP: Pharyngitis, dyspnea, pulmonary edema, veno-occlusive disease (VOD)

PHARMACOKINETICS
Rapidly absorbed, peak 2 hr, protein binding 99%, metabolized by CYP3A4, CYP2C19, UGTa, terminal half-life 15 hr, effective half-life 9 hr

INTERACTIONS
• Possibly increase ambrisentan: cimetidine, clopidogrel, efavirenz, felbamate, FLUoxetine, modafinil, OXcarbazepine, ticlopidine
Increase: hypotension—other antihypertensives, diuretics, MAOIs
Increase: ambrisentan—CYP3A4 inhibitors (amprenavir, aprepitant, atazanavir, clarithromycin, conivaptan, cycloSPORINE, dalfopristin, danazol, darunavir, erythromycin, estradiol, imatinib, itraconazole, ketoconazole, nefazodone, nelfinavir, quinupristin, ritonavir, RU-486, saquinavir, tamoxifen, telithromycin, troleandomycin, zafirlukast); CYP2C19/CYP3A4 (chloramphenicol, delavirdine, fluconazole, fluvoxaMINE, isoniazid, voriconazole)
Decrease: ambrisentan—CYP3A4 inducers (carBAMazepine, PHENobarbital, phenytoin, rifampin)
Decrease: ambrisentan absorption—mefloquine, niCARdipine, propafenone, quiNIDine, ranolazine, tacrolimus, testosterone
Drug/Herb
• Need for ambrisentan dosage change: St. John's wort, ephedra (ma huang)
Drug/Food
• Avoid use with grapefruit products
Drug/Lab Test
Increase: LFTs, bilirubin
Decrease: Hct, Hgb

NURSING CONSIDERATIONS
Assess:
• **Pulmonary status:** improvement in breathing, ability to exercise; pulmonary edema that may indicate veno-occlusive disease
• Blood studies: CBC with differential; Hct, Hgb may be decreased
• Liver function tests: AST, ALT, bilirubin

• **Hepatotoxicity:** nausea, vomiting, abdominal pain/cramping, jaundice, anorexia, itching

• **Beers:** use in older adults cautiously; may exacerbate syncope

Evaluate:

• Therapeutic response: decrease in B/P; decreased shortness of breath

Teach patient/family:

• The importance of complying with dosage schedule even if feeling better

• The importance of follow-up with labs

• That sperm count may be decreased

Black Box Warning: To notify if pregnancy is planned or suspected (if pregnant, product will need to be discontinued, pregnancy test done monthly); to use 2 contraception methods while taking this product and for 1 month after concluding therapy

• Not to use OTC products, including herbs, supplements, unless approved by prescriber

• To take tablet whole; not to crush, chew

• **To report to prescriber immediately:** dizziness, faintness, chest pain, palpitations, uneven or rapid heart rate, headache, edema, weight gain

• **To report hepatic dysfunction:** nausea/vomiting, anorexia, fatigue, jaundice, right upper quadrant abdominal pain, itching, fever, malaise

---

amikacin (Rx)

(am-i-kay′sin)

Amikin ✦, Arikayce

Func. class.: Antiinfective

Chem. class.: Aminoglycoside

Do not confuse:

amikacin/Kineret

ACTION: Interferes with protein synthesis in bacterial cells by binding to ribosomal subunits, which causes misreading of genetic code; inaccurate peptide sequence forms in protein chain, thereby causing bacterial death

USES: Severe systemic infections of CNS, respiratory tract, GI tract, urinary tract, bone, skin, soft tissues caused by *Staphylococcus aureus* (MSSA), *Pseudomonas aeruginosa, Escherichia coli, Enterobacter, Acinetobacter, Providencia, Citrobacter, Serratia, Proteus, Klebsiella pneumoniae*

Unlabeled uses: *Mycobacterium avium* complex (MAC) (intrathecal or intraventricular) in combination; actinomycotic mycetoma, febrile neutropenia, cystic fibrosis

CONTRAINDICATIONS: Pregnancy, hypersensitivity to aminoglycosides, sulfites

Precautions: Breastfeeding, neonates, geriatric patients, myasthenia gravis, Parkinson's disease, mild to moderate infections, dehydration

Black Box Warning: Hearing impairment, renal/neuromuscular disease

DOSAGE AND ROUTES

• **Adult/child:** IV INFUSION 15 mg/kg/day in 2-3 divided doses q8-12hr in 100-200 mL D₅W over 30-60 min, max 1.5 g/day; **pulse dosing** (once-daily dosing) may be used with some infections; **IM** 10-15 mg/kg/day in divided doses q8-12hr; or extended-interval dosing as an alternative dosing regimen

• **Neonate:** IV/IM 10 mg/kg initially, then 7.5 mg/kg q8-12hr

Renal dose (extended-interval dosing)

• **Adult:** IV CCr 40-59 mL/min 15 mg/kg q36hr; CCr 20-39 mL/min 15 mg/kg q48hr; <20 mL/min adjust based on serum concentrations and MIC (use traditional dosing)

***Mycobacterium avium* complex (MAC)**

• **Adult and adolescent:** IM/IV 15-20 mg/kg/day or 5× per wk; **Neb (Arikayce)** 590 mg daily in combination

• **Child:** IV 15-30 mg/kg/day divided q12-24hr as part of multiple-drug regimen, max 1.5 g/day

---

Actinomycotic mycetoma (unlabeled)

• **Adult:** IM/IV 15 mg/kg/day in 2 divided doses × 3 wk with co-trimoxazole for 5 wk; repeat cycle once, may be repeated 2×

Available forms: Inj 50, 250 mg/mL; suspension for oral inhalation 590 mg/8.4 mL

Administer:

• Obtain C&S before administration; begin treatment before results are received

IM route

• Inj in large muscle mass; rotate inj sites
• Obtain peak 1 hr after IM, trough before next dose

Inhalation Route (nebulizer)

• Use Lamira Nebulizer System
• May pretreat with short-acting beta-2 antagonists
• Allow to warm to room temperature
• Shake well, pour medication into reservoir
• Press and hold on/off button
• Insert mouthpiece, take slow deep breaths, a beep will be heard when done
• Clean after use

Intermittent IV INFUSION route

• Dilute 500 mg of product/100-200 mL of D₅W, 0.9% NaCl and give over ¹/₂-1 hr; dilute in sufficient volume to allow for infusion over 1-2 hr (infants); flush after administration with D₅W or 0.9% NaCl; sol clear or pale yellow; discard if precipitate or dark color develops
• In children, amount of fluid will depend on ordered dose; in infants, infuse over 1-2 hr
• In evenly spaced doses to maintain blood level, separate from penicillins by at least 1 hr

Y-site compatibilities: Acyclovir, alatrofloxacin, aldesleukin, alemtuzumab, alfentanil, amifostine, aminophylline, amiodarone, amsacrine, anidulafungin, argatroban, ascorbic acid, atracurium, atropine, aztreonam, benztropine, bivalirudin, bumetanide, buprenorphine, butorphanol, calcium chloride/gluconate, CARBOplatin, caspofungin, ceFAZolin, cefepime, cefonicid, cefotaxime, cefoTEtan, cefOXitin, cefTAZidime, ceftizoxime, cefTRIAXone, cefuroxime, chloramphenicol, chlorproMAZINE, cimetidine, cisatracurium, CISplatin, clindamycin, codeine, cyanocobalamin, cyclophosphamide, cycloSPORINE, cytarabine, DACTINomycin, DAPTOmycin, dexamethasone, dexmedetomidine, digoxin, diltiazem, diphenhydrAMINE, DOBUTamine, DOCEtaxel, DOPamine, doripenem, doxacurium, DOXOrubicin, doxycycline, enalaprilat, ePHEDrine, EPINEPHrine, epirubicin, epoetin alfa, eptifibatide, ertapenem, erythromycin, esmolol, etoposide, famotidine, fentaNYL, filgrastim, fluconazole, fludarabine, fluorouracil, foscarnet, furosemide, gemcitabine, gentamicin, glycopyrrolate, granisetron, hydrocortisone, HYDROmorphone, IDArubicin, ifosfamide, IL-2, imipenem/cilastin, isoproterenol, ketorolac, labetalol, levofloxacin, lidocaine, linezolid, LORazepam, magnesium sulfate, mannitol, mechlorethamine, melphalan, meperidine, metaraminol, methotrexate, methoxamine, methyldopate, methylPREDNISolone, metoclopramide, metoprolol, metroNIDAZOLE, midazolam, milrinone, mitoXANTrone, morphine, multivitamins, nafcillin, nalbuphine, naloxone, niCARdipine, nitroglycerin, nitroprusside, norepinephrine, octreotide, ondansetron, oxaliplatin, oxytocin, PACLitaxel, palonosetron, pantoprazole, papaverine, PEMEtrexed, penicillin G, pentazocine, perphenazine, PHENobarbital, phenylephrine, phytonadione, piperacillin/tazobactam, potassium chloride, procainamide, prochlorperazine, promethazine, propranolol, protamine, pyridoxine, quinupristin/dalfopristin, ranitidine, remifentanil, riTUXimab, rocuronium, sargramostim, sodium acetate, sodium bicarbonate, succinylcholine, SUFentanil, tacrolimus, teniposide, theophylline, thiamine, thiotepa, ticarcillin/clavulanate, tigecycline, tirofiban, tobramycin, tolazoline, trimethaphan, urokinase, vancomycin, vasopressin, vecuronium, verapamil, vinCRIStine, vinorelbine, voriconazole, warfarin, zidovudine, zoledronic acid

SIDE EFFECTS
CNS: Dizziness, vertigo
EENT: *Ototoxicity,* deafness
GU: Nephrotoxicity
HEMA: Eosinophilia, anemia
INTEG: *Rash,* burning, urticaria, dermatitis, alopecia
Resp: Apnea
Syst: Hypersensitivity

PHARMACOKINETICS
IM: Onset rapid, peak 1 hr, leads to unpredictable concentrations, IV preferred
IV: Onset immediate, peak 15-30 min, half-life 2 hr, prolonged up to 7 hr in infants; not metabolized; excreted unchanged in urine; crosses placenta; removed by hemodialysis

INTERACTIONS
Increase: masking ototoxicity: dimenhyDRINATE, ethacrynic acid
Increase: neurotoxicity-NSAIDs

Black Box Warning: **Increase:** nephrotoxicity—cephalosporins, acyclovir, vancomycin, amphotericin B, cycloSPORINE, loop diuretics, cidofovir

Black Box Warning: **Increase:** ototoxicity—IV loop diuretics

Black Box Warning: **Increase:** neuromuscular blockade, respiratory depression—anesthetics, nondepolarizing neuromuscular blockers

Decrease: amikacin effect in renal disease-parenteral penicillins, cephalosporins do not combine
Drug/Lab Test
Increase: BUN, creatinine, AST/ALT, alk phos, bilirubin, LDH

NURSING CONSIDERATIONS
Assess:
• Weight before treatment; calculation of dosage is usually based on ideal body weight but may be calculated on actual body weight; in those underweight and not obese, use total body weight (TBW) instead of ideal body weight

• IV site for thrombophlebitis including pain, redness, swelling q30min; change site if needed; apply warm compresses to discontinued site

Black Box Warning: **Nephrotoxicity:** renal impairment; obtain urine for CCr, BUN, serum creatinine; lower dosage should be given with renal impairment; nephrotoxicity may be reversible if product is stopped at 1st sign; I&O ratio; urinalysis daily for proteinuria, cells, casts; report sudden change in urine output

Black Box Warning: **Ototoxicity:** deafness: audiometric testing, ringing, roaring in ears, vertigo; assess hearing before, during, after treatment

• **Dehydration:** high specific gravity, decrease in skin turgor, dry mucous membranes, dark urine, keep well hydrated 2000 mL/day
• **Overgrowth of infection:** increased temperature, malaise, redness, pain, swelling, perineal itching, diarrhea, stomatitis, change in cough, sputum
• **Vestibular dysfunction:** nausea, vomiting, dizziness, headache; product should be discontinued if severe

Black Box Warning: **Neuromuscular blockade;** respiratory paralysis may occur; more common in those receiving anesthetics, neuromuscular blockers; use of calcium salts may be used to reverse effect

Evaluate:
• Therapeutic response: absence of fever, draining wounds; negative C&S after treatment
Teach patient/family:
• To report headache, dizziness, symptoms of overgrowth of infection, renal impairment, symptoms of nephrotoxicity, hepatotoxicity
• **Ototoxicity:** To report loss of hearing; ringing, roaring in ears; feeling of fullness in head

---

Side effects: *italics* = common; red = life-threatening

• **To report hypersensitivity:** rash, itching, trouble breathing, facial edema; notify health care provider
• **Pregnancy/breastfeeding:** tell prescriber if pregnancy is planned or suspected or if breastfeeding; do not use in pregnancy, breastfeeding

TREATMENT OF HYPERSENSITIVITY: Hemodialysis, exchange transfusion in the newborn, monitor serum levels of product, may give ticarcillin or carbenicillin

---

aMILoride (Rx)

(a-mill'oh-ride)
Midamor ♣
Func. class.: Potassium-sparing diuretic
Chem. class.: Pyrazine

Do not confuse:
aMILoride/amLODIPine/amiodarone

ACTION: Inhibits sodium, potassium ion exchange in the distal tubule, cortical collecting duct, resulting in inhibition of sodium reabsorption and decreasing potassium secretion

USES: Edema in HF in combination with other diuretics, for hypertension, adjunct with other diuretics to maintain potassium
Unlabeled uses: Ascites

CONTRAINDICATIONS: Anuria, hypersensitivity, diabetic nephropathy, renal failure

Black Box Warning: Hyperkalemia

Precautions: Pregnancy, breastfeeding, children, geriatric patients, dehydration, diabetes, respiratory acidosis, hyponatremia, impaired renal function

DOSAGE AND ROUTES
• **Adult:** PO 5-10 mg/day in 1-2 divided doses; may be increased to 10-20 mg/day if needed

• **Infant/child (6-20 kg):** PO 0.4-0.625 mg/kg/dose q day, max 20 mg/day, dose daily max 20 mg/day
Renal dose
• **Adult:** PO CCr 10-50 mL/min reduce dose by 50%; CCr <10 mL/min contraindicated

Ascites (unlabeled)
• **Adult:** PO *10 mg/day; max 40 mg
Available forms: Tabs 5 mg
Administer:
• In AM to avoid interference with sleep if using as diuretic; if 2nd daily dose is needed, give in late afternoon
• With food; if nausea occurs, absorption may be decreased slightly

SIDE EFFECTS
CNS: *Headache,* dizziness, weakness, paresthesias, tremors, depression, anxiety, encephalopathy
CV: *Orthostatic hypotension,* dysrhythmias, chest pain
ELECT: Hyperkalemia, dehydration, hyponatremia
GI: *Nausea, diarrhea,* dry mouth, *vomiting, anorexia,* cramps, constipation, abdominal pain, jaundice
INTEG: *Rash, pruritus,* Stevens-Johnson syndrome, toxic epidermal necrolysis
MS: Cramps

PHARMACOKINETICS
Absorption variable 20%-90%; widely distributed; onset 2 hr; peak 6-10 hr; duration 24 hr; excreted in urine, feces; half-life 6-9 hr, crosses placenta

INTERACTIONS

Black Box Warning: **Hyperkalemia:** avoid concurrent use with other potassium-sparing diuretics, potassium products, ACE inhibitors, salt substitutes, cycloSPORINE, tacrolimus; if using together, monitor potassium level

Increase: lithium toxicity: lithium; monitor lithium levels
Increase: action of antihypertensives
Decrease: effect of aMILoride—NSAIDs; avoid concurrent use

Drug/Herb
Increase: effect—hawthorn, horse chestnut
Drug/Food
• Possible hyperkalemia: foods high in potassium, potassium-based salt substitutes
Drug/Lab Test
Increase: LFTs, BUN, potassium, sodium, bilirubin, calcium, cholesterol
Decrease: Potassium, magnesium, sodium
Interference: GTT

NURSING CONSIDERATIONS
Assess:
• Heart rate, B/P lying, standing; postural hypotension may occur
• Electrolytes: potassium, sodium, chloride; glucose (serum), BUN, CBC, serum creatinine, blood pH, ABGs, periodic ECG

Black Box Warning: **Hyperkalemia:** fatigue, weakness, paresthesia, confusion, dyspnea, dysrhythmias, ECG changes; monitor potassium level at baseline and dosage changes, including hyperacute T waves; hyperkalemia is more common in renal disease, geriatric patients, diabetes; if potassium ≥5.5 mEq/L, immediately notify prescriber; discontinue aMILoride 3 days before GTT; hyperkalemia may occur; monitor potassium

• **Fluid volume status:** distended neck veins; crackles in lungs; color, quality, and specific gravity of urine; skin turgor; adequacy of pulse; moist mucous membranes; bilateral lung sounds; peripheral pitting edema; dehydration; symptoms of decreasing output; thirst; hypotension; dry mouth should be reported
• **Hypokalemia:** weakness, polyuria, polydipsia, fatigue, ECG U wave
• **Pregnancy/breastfeeding:** identify if pregnancy is planned or suspected or if breastfeeding; use only if clearly needed
• **Beers:** avoid in older adults; may decrease sodium, increase potassium, decrease creatinine clearance; use with caution; may exacerbate or cause inappropriate antidiuretic hormone secretion/hyponatremia; monitor sodium level carefully
Evaluate:
• Therapeutic response: improvement in edema of feet, legs, sacral area daily if medication is being used for HF; decreased B/P; prevention of hypokalemia (diuretics)
Teach patient/family:
• To take as prescribed; if dose is missed, to take when remembered within 1 hr of next dose; to take with food or milk for GI symptoms; to take early in day to prevent nocturia; to avoid alcohol; not to use other products unless approved by prescriber
• To maintain a weekly record of weight, notify health care professional of weight loss >5 lb
• About adverse reactions: to report muscle cramps, weakness, nausea, dizziness, blurred vision
• **Hyperkalemia:** to avoid potassium-rich foods: oranges, bananas, salt substitutes, dried fruits, salt substitutes, potassium supplements, refer to dietician for assistance, planning
• To rise slowly from sitting to standing to avoid orthostatic hypotension
• To avoid hazardous activities if dizziness occurs
• To continue other medical treatments (exercise, weight loss, relaxation techniques, cessation of smoking)
• To continue taking medication even if feeling better, this product controls symptoms but does not cure condition, to use as directed, not to double or skip doses
• Not to exercise in hot weather or stand for prolonged periods since orthostatic hypotension is enhanced
• How to take own B/P, pulse and record

TREATMENT OF OVERDOSE:
Lavage if taken orally, monitor electrolytes, administer sodium bicarbonate for potassium >6.5 mEq/L, IV glucose, Kayexalate as needed; monitor hydration, CV, renal status

---

Side effects: *italics* = common; red = life-threatening

amino acids (Rx)
(a-mee'noe)

amino acid infusions (crystalline) (Rx)

Aminosyn, Aminosyn II, Aminosyn-PF, Clinisol, FreAmine III, Premasol, Travasol, TrophAmine

amino acid infusions/ dextrose (Rx)

Aminosyn II with dextrose, Clinimix, Amino Acid Infusions/ electrolytes

aminosyn with electrolytes (Rx)

Aminosyn II with electrolytes, FreAmine III with electrolytes, ProcalAmine with electrolytes, Travasol with electrolytes

amino acid infusions/ electrolytes/dextrose (Rx)

Aminosyn II with electrolytes in dextrose

amino acid infusions (hepatic failure) (Rx)

HepatAmine, Hepatasol

amino acid infusions (high metabolic stress) (Rx)

Aminosyn-HBC, FreAmine HBC

amino acid infusions (renal failure) (Rx)

Aminosyn-RF, NephrAmine

Func. class.: Nutritional supplement/ protein

ACTION: Needed for anabolism to maintain structure, decrease catabolism, promote healing

Black Box Warning: Central infusions: administration by central venous catheter should be used only by those familiar with this technique and its complications

USES: Hepatic encephalopathy, cirrhosis, hepatitis, nutritional support in cancer; burn or solid organ transplant patients; to prevent nitrogen loss when adequate nutrition by mouth, gastric, or duodenal tube cannot be obtained

CONTRAINDICATIONS: Hypersensitivity, severe electrolyte imbalances, anuria, severe liver damage, maple syrup urine disease, PKU, azotemia, ✱ genetic disease of amino acid metabolism
Precautions: Pregnancy, breastfeeding, children, renal disease, diabetes mellitus, HF, sulfite sensitivity

DOSAGE AND ROUTES
Nutritional support (cirrhosis, hepatic encephalopathy, hepatitis)
• **Adult: IV** 80-120 g/day amino acids/12-18 g nitrogen of hepatic failure formula
TPN
• **Adult: IV** 1-1.5 g/kg/day
Metabolic stress (severe)
• **Adult: IV** 1.5 g/kg; use formula for high metabolic stress
Renal failure (nutritional support)
• **Adult: IV** Aminosyn-RF 300-600 mL/70% dextrose/day; NephrAmine 250-500 mL/70% dextrose/day; the total daily dosage is calculated based on the daily protein requirements, as well as the patient's metabolic and clinical response. Check product instructions for specific directions
• **Child: IV** 2-3 g/kg/day
Available forms:
Injection: 250, 500, 1000, 2000 mL, containing amino acids in various concentrations; amino acid infusions, crystalline: Aminosyn: 3.5%, 5%, 7%, 8.5%, 10%; Aminosyn II: 3.5%, 5%, 7%, 8.5%, 10%, 15%; Aminosyn-PF: 7%, 10%; Clinisol: 15%; FreAmine III: 8.5%, 10%; Premasol: 6%, 10%; Travasol: 10%; TrophAmine: 6%, 10%
Amino acid infusion/dextrose: Aminosyn II: 3.5% in 5% dextrose, 4.25% in 20% dextrose, 4.25% in 10% dextrose, 4.25% in 25% dextrose; Clinimix: 2.75% in 5% dextrose, 4.25% in 5% dextrose, 4.25%

---

in 10% dextrose, 4.25% in 20% dextrose, 4.25% in 25% dextrose, 5% in 10% dextrose, 5% in 15% dextrose, 5% in 20% dextrose, 5% in 25% dextrose

Amino acid infusions/electrolytes: Aminosyn: 3.5%, 7%, 8.5%; Aminosyn II: 3.5%, 7%, 8.5%; FreAmine III: 3%, 8.5%; ProcalAmine: 3%; Travasol: 3.5%, 5.5%, 8.5%

Amino acid infusions/electrolytes/dextrose: Aminosyn II: 3.5% with electrolytes in 5% dextrose, 3.5% with electrolytes in 25% dextrose, 4.25% with electrolytes in 10% dextrose, 4.25% with electrolytes in 20% dextrose, 4.25% with electrolytes in 25% dextrose; amino acid infusions (hepatic failure): HepatAmine: 8%; Hepatasol: 8%

Amino acid infusions (high metabolic stress): Aminosyn-HBC 7%; Freamine HBC: 6.9%; amino acid infusions (renal failure): Aminosyn-RF: 5.2%; NephrAmine: 5.4%

Administer:

Continuous IV INFUSION route

• Up to 40% protein and dextrose (up to 12.5%) via peripheral vein; stronger sol requires central IV administration

• TPN only mixed with dextrose to promote protein synthesis

• Immediately after mixing under strict aseptic technique, use infusion pump, in-line filter (0.22 µm) unless mixed with fat emulsion and dextrose (3 in 1); use careful monitoring technique; do not speed up infusion; pulmonary edema, glucose overload will result

SIDE EFFECTS

CNS: Dizziness, headache, confusion, loss of concentration, fever
CV: Hypertension, HF/pulmonary edema, flushing, thrombosis
ENDO: Hyperglycemia, rebound hypoglycemia, electrolyte imbalances, hyperosmolar hyperglycemic nonketotic syndrome, alkalosis, hypophosphatemia, hyperammonemia, dehydration, hypocalcemia
GI: Nausea, abdominal pain, cholestasis
GU: Glycosuria osmotic diuresis
INTEG: Extravasation necrosis, phlebitis at inj site

INTERACTIONS

Individual Drugs
Decrease: Protein-sparing effects—tetracycline
Drug/Lab Test
Increase: LFTs, ammonia, glucose
Decrease: Potassium, phosphate, glucose

NURSING CONSIDERATIONS

Assess:
• Electrolytes (potassium, sodium, phosphate, chloride, magnesium, bicarbonate, blood glucose, ammonia, ketones)
• Renal/hepatic studies: BUN, creatinine, ALT, AST, bilirubin
• Weight changes, triglycerides before and after infusion; vit A level with renal disease
• **Inj site for extravasation:** redness along vein, edema at site, necrosis, pain, hard tender area; site should be changed immediately; discontinue infusion, culture tubing and sol
• **Sepsis:** chills, fever, increased temperature, if sepsis is suspected
• **For impending hepatic coma:** asterixis, confusion, uremic fetor, lethargy
• **Hyperammonemia:** nausea, vomiting, malaise, tremors, anorexia, seizures
• Change of dressing and IV tubing every 24-48 hr to prevent infection if chills, fever, other signs of infection occur
Evaluate:
• Therapeutic response: weight gain, decrease in jaundice with liver disorders, increased LOC
Teach patient/family:
• Reason for use of TPN
• To report chills, sweating at once; risk for infection is higher
• About infusion pump, how to care for tubing/site; and blood glucose

---

⚠ HIGH ALERT

amiodarone (Rx)
(a-mee-oh′da-rone)
Nexterone, Pacerone
Func. class.: Antidysrhythmic (class III)
Chem. class.: Iodinated benzofuran derivative

Do not confuse:
amiodarone/amantadine

ACTION: Prolongs duration of action potential and effective refractory period, noncompetitive α- and β-adrenergic inhibition; increases PR and QT intervals, decreases sinus rate, decreases peripheral vascular resistance

USES: Hemodynamically unstable ventricular tachycardia, supraventricular tachycardia, ventricular fibrillation not controlled by 1st-line agents

Unlabeled uses: Atrial fibrillation treatment/prophylaxis, atrial flutter, cardiac arrest, cardiac surgery, CPR, heart failure, PSVT, Wolff-Parkinson-White (WPW) syndrome, supraventricular tachycardia

CONTRAINDICATIONS: Pregnancy, breastfeeding, neonates, infants, severe sinus node dysfunction, hypersensitivity to this product/iodine/benzyl alcohol, cardiogenic shock, 2nd- to 3rd-degree AV block, bradycardia

Precautions: Children, goiter, Hashimoto's thyroiditis, electrolyte imbalances, HF, respiratory disease, torsades de pointes

Black Box Warning: Hepatotoxicity, cardiac arrhythmias, pneumonitis, pulmonary fibrosis; requires an experienced clinician

DOSAGE AND ROUTES
Ventricular dysrhythmias
Adult: PO Loading dose 800-1600 mg/day for 1-3 wk, then 600-800 mg/day for 1 mo, maintenance 400 mg/day; **IV** loading dose (**1st rapid**) 150 mg over the first 10 min, then slow 360 mg over the next 6 hr, **maintenance** 540 mg given over the remaining 18 hr, decrease rate of the slow infusion to 0.5 mg/min
Supraventricular tachycardia
• **Adult:** PO 600-800 mg/day x 1 wk until desired response, then decrease to 400 mg/day x 3 wk, then 200-400 mg/day (maintenance)

• **Child:** PO 10 mg/kg/day x 10 days or until desired response, then decrease to 5 mg/kg/day for several wk, then decrease to 2.5 mg/kg/day or lower (maintenance)
Conversion of atrial fibrillation to sinus rhythm (unlabeled)
• **Adult:** IV 5-7 mg/kg over 30-60 min, then 1.2-1.8 mg/kg **CONT IV INFUSION** or **PO** divided doses
Available forms: Tabs 100, 200, 400 mg; inj 50 mg/mL
Administer:
PO route
• May be used with/without food but be consistent
IV, direct route
• **Peripheral:** max 2 mg/mL for more than 1 hr; preferred through central venous line with in-line filter; concentrations of more than 2 mg/mL should be given by central line
• **Cardiac arrest:** give 300 mg IV bol; diluted to a total volume of 20 mL D₅W; may repeat 150 mg after 3-5 min
Intermittent IV INFUSION route
• **Rapid loading:** add 3 mL (150 mg), 100 mL D₅W (1.5 mg/mL), give over 10 min
• **Slow loading:** add 18 mL (900 mg), 500 mL D₅W (1.8 mg/mL), give over next 6 hr
Continuous IV INFUSION route
• After 24 hr, dilute 50 mL to 1-6 mg/mL, give 1-6 mg/mL at 1 mg/min for the 1st 6 hr, then 0.5 mg/min

Y-site compatibilities: Amikacin, clindamycin, DOBUTamine, DOPamine, doxycycline, erythromycin, esmolol, gentamicin, insulin, isoproterenol, labetalol, lidocaine, metaraminol, metroNIDAZOLE, midazolam, morphine, nitroglycerin, norepinephrine, penicillin G potassium, phenylephrine, potassium chloride, procainamide, tobramycin, vancomycin

SIDE EFFECTS
CNS: *Headache, dizziness,* involuntary movement, *tremors, peripheral neuropathy,* malaise, *fatigue,* ataxia, *paresthesias,* insomnia, confusion, hallucinations

CV: *Hypotension, bradycardia,* HF, dysrhythmias
EENT: *Corneal microdeposits,* dry eyes
ENDO: *Hypo*/hyperthyroidism
GI: *Nausea, vomiting,* diarrhea, abdominal pain, *anorexia, constipation,* hepatotoxicity, pancreatitis
GU: Epididymitis, ED
INTEG: Rash, photosensitivity, blue-gray skin discoloration, alopecia, spontaneous ecchymosis, toxic epidermal necrolysis, urticaria, pancreatitis, phlebitis (IV)
MISC: Flushing, abnormal taste or smell, edema, abnormal salivation
RESP: Pulmonary fibrosis/toxicity, ARDS

PHARMACOKINETICS
PO: Onset 1-3 wk, peak 3-7 hr; **IV:** Onset 2 hr, peak 3-7 hr; half-life 26-107 days, increased in geriatric patients, metabolized by liver (an inhibitor of CYP1A2, CYP3A4, CYP2C8, CYP2C9, CYP2C19, CYP2A6, CYP2B6, CYP2D6, P-glycoprotein), organic cation transporter, excreted by kidneys, 99% protein binding

INTERACTIONS
Increase: QT prolongation—azoles, fluoroquinolones, macrolides, loratadine, trazodone
Increase: amiodarone concentrations, possible serious dysrhythmias—protease inhibitors; reduce dose
Increase: myopathy—HMG-CoA reductase inhibitors; monitor for myopathy
Increase: bradycardia, sinus arrest, AV block—β-blockers, calcium channel blockers; use cautiously
Increase: levels of cycloSPORINE, dextromethorphan, digoxin, disopyramide, flecainide, methotrexate, phenytoin, procainamide, quiNIDine, theophylline, class I antidysrhythmics
Increase: anticoagulant effects—dabigatran, warfarin, dose may need to be decreased (warfarin)
Drug/Herb
• St. John's wort may decrease amiodarone level
Drug/Food

• **Toxicity:** grapefruit juice
Drug/Lab Test
Increase: T_4, ALT, AST, GGT alk phos, cholesterol, lipids, PT, INR
Decrease: T_3

NURSING CONSIDERATIONS
Assess:

Black Box Warning: **Cardiac dysrhythmias:** ECG continuously to determine product effectiveness; measure PR, QRS, QT intervals; check for PVCs, other dysrhythmias, B/P continuously for hypo/hypertension; report dysrhythmias, slowing heart rate; monitor amiodarone level: therapeutic 1-2.5 mcg/mL; toxic >2.5 mcg/mL

Black Box Warning: **Pulmonary toxicity:** dyspnea, fatigue, cough, fever, chest pain; product should be discontinued; for ARDS, pulmonary fibrosis, crackles, tachypnea, increased at higher doses (>400 mg/day), toxicity is common, monitor chest x-ray, pulmonary function tests with diffusion capacity

• **Stevens-Johnson syndrome:** monitor for rash, blistering; discontinue immediately, notify prescriber

Black Box Warning: **Hepatotoxicity:** monitor hepatic enzymes; rarely fatal hepatotoxicity has occurred

• Electrolytes (sodium, potassium, chloride); hepatic studies: AST, ALT, bilirubin, alk phos; for dehydration, hypovolemia; monitor PT, INR if using warfarin
• CNS symptoms: confusion, psychosis, numbness, depression, involuntary movements; product should be discontinued
• **Hypothyroidism:** lethargy; dizziness; constipation; enlarged thyroid gland; edema of extremities; cool, pale skin
• **Hyperthyroidism:** restlessness; tachycardia; eyelid puffiness; weight loss; frequent urination; menstrual irregularities; dyspnea; warm, moist skin; may cause

fatal thyrotoxicosis, cardiac dysrhythmias; may need to discontinue product

• Ophthalmic exams at baseline and periodically (PO); to prevent corneal deposits, use methylcellulose

• Cardiac rate, respirations: rate, rhythm, character, chest pain; start with patient hospitalized and monitored up to 1 wk; for rebound hypertension after 1-2 hr

• **Beers:** Avoid as first-line therapy for atrial fibrillation in older adults unless heart failure or substantial left ventricular hypertrophy is present

Evaluate:

• Therapeutic response: decrease in ventricular tachycardia, supraventricular tachycardia, fibrillation

Teach patient/family:

• To take this product as directed; to avoid missed doses; not to use with grapefruit juice; not to discontinue abruptly, not to use other drugs, herbs without prescriber approval, many interactions

• To use sunscreen or stay out of sun to prevent burns; that dark glasses may be needed for photophobia

• To report side effects immediately; more common at high dose and longer duration

• That skin discoloration is usually reversible

• To report vision changes, weight change, rash, blistering, numbness, temperature intolerance

• **Pregnancy/breastfeeding:** Identify if pregnancy is planned or suspected or if breastfeeding; not to be used in pregnancy, breastfeeding

TREATMENT OF OVERDOSE:

O_2, artificial ventilation, ECG, administer DOPamine for circulatory depression, administer diazepam, thiopental for seizures, isoproterenol

---

amitriptyline (Rx)

(a-mee-trip´ti-leen)

Elavil ♣, Levate ♣

Func. class.: Antidepressant—tricyclic

Chem. class.: Tertiary amine

Do not confuse:

amitriptyline/nortriptyline/aminophylline

ACTION: Blocks reuptake of norepinephrine, serotonin into nerve endings, thereby increasing action of norepinephrine, serotonin in nerve cells

USES: Major depressive disorder

Unlabeled uses: Neuropathic pain, fibromyalgia, anxiety, insomnia

CONTRAINDICATIONS: Hypersensitivity to tricyclics; recovery phase of myocardial infarction

Precautions: Pregnancy, breastfeeding, geriatric patients, seizure disorders, prostatic hypertrophy, schizophrenia, psychosis, severe depression, increased intraocular pressure, closed-angle glaucoma, urinary retention, renal/hepatic/cardiac disease, hyperthyroidism, electroshock therapy, elective surgery

Black Box Warning: Children <12 yr, suicidal patients

DOSAGE AND ROUTES

Depression

• **Adult: PO** Initially, 75 mg/day divided, or 50-100 mg daily at bedtime, max 300 mg/day

• **Geriatric: PO** Initially, 10-25 mg at bedtime; may increase by 10-25 mg weekly, max 150 mg/day

Available forms: Tabs 10, 25, 50, 75, 100, 150 mg

Administer:

• Increase fluids, bulk in diet if constipation, urinary retention occur, especially in geriatric patients

• With food, milk for GI symptoms

• Crushed if patient unable to swallow medication whole, give with food, fluids

• Dosage at bedtime if oversedation occurs during day; may take entire dose at bedtime; geriatric patients may not tolerate once-daily dosing; use tapering when withdrawing product

• Store at room temperature; do not freeze

SIDE EFFECTS

CNS: *Dizziness, drowsiness,* confusion, headache, anxiety, tremors, weakness, *insomnia,* EPS (geriatric patients), seizures, suicidal thoughts, anxiety

CV: *Orthostatic hypotension,* ECG changes, tachycardia, hypertension, palpitations, dysrhythmias, QT prolongation

EENT: *Blurred vision,* tinnitus, mydriasis

GI: *Constipation, dry mouth,* weight gain, nausea, vomiting, paralytic ileus, epigastric distress, hepatitis, diarrhea, constipation

GU: *Urinary retention,* sexual dysfunction

HEMA: Agranulocytosis, thrombocytopenia, eosinophilia, leukopenia, aplastic anemia

INTEG: Rash, urticaria, sweating, photosensitivity

SYST: Hypersensitivity

PHARMACOKINETICS

Onset 45 min; peak 2-12 hr, protein binding >95%; metabolized by liver to nortriptyline; excreted in urine, feces; crosses placenta; excreted in breast milk; half-life 30-46 hr; antidepressant action up to 30 days, peak 2-6 wk, duration up to several weeks

INTERACTIONS

Increase: Hyperpyretic crisis, seizures, hypertensive episode—MAOIs; do not use within 14 days of MAOIs

Increase: risk for agranulocytosis—antithyroid agents

Increase: QT prolongation—procainamide, quiNIDine, amiodarone, tricyclics, class IA, III antidysrhythmics; may need dosage change

Increase: amitriptyline levels, toxicity—carbamazepine, cimetidine, FLUoxetine, phenothiazines, oral contraceptives, antidepressants, carBAMazepine, class IC antidysrhythmics, ritonavir

Increase: effects of direct-acting sympathomimetics (EPINEPHrine), alcohol, barbiturates, benzodiazepines, CNS depressants, opioids, sedative/hypnotics

Increase: serotonin syndrome—linezolid, methylene blue; use cautiously

Increase: hypertensive crisis—clonidine

Drug/Herb

Increase: serotonin syndrome—SAM-e, St. John's wort, yohimbe; avoid concurrent use

Increase: CNS depression—kava, hops, chamomile, lavender, valerian

Drug/Lab Test

Increase: blood glucose, LFTs

Decrease: WBCs, platelets, granulocytes, blood glucose

NURSING CONSIDERATIONS

Assess:

• B/P lying, standing; pulse if systolic B/P drops 20 mm Hg, hold product, notify prescriber; take vital signs more frequently with CV disease; ECG baseline and frequently in cardiac patients; avoid use immediately after MI

• **Blood studies:** CBC, leukocytes, differential, cardiac enzymes if patient is receiving long-term therapy, thyroid function tests

• **Hepatic studies:** AST, ALT, bilirubin

• Weight weekly; appetite may increase with product

• EPS primarily in geriatric patients: rigidity, dystonia, akathisia

• Paralytic ileus, glaucoma exacerbation

Black Box Warning: **Suicidal thinking, behavior:** mood, sensorium, affect, suicidal tendencies; increase in psychiatric symptoms: depression, panic; suicidal tendencies are higher in those ≤24 yr, restrict amount of product available, avoid use in child <12 yr

• Urinary retention, constipation: constipation is most likely to occur in children and geriatric patients

• **Withdrawal symptoms:** headache, nausea, vomiting, muscle pain, weakness; do not usually occur unless product was discontinued abruptly

• **Alcohol consumption:** if alcohol is consumed, hold dose until morning

• **Pain syndromes (unlabeled):** intensity, location, severity; use pain scale; product may be taken for 1-2 mo before effective

• **Sexual dysfunction:** erectile dysfunction, decreased libido

Side effects: *italics* = common; red = life-threatening

• **Beers** Avoid in older adults; highly anticholinergic, sedating, orthostatic hypotension

Evaluate:

• Therapeutic response: decrease in depression, absence of suicidal thoughts

Teach patient/family:

• To take medication as directed (usually at bedtime); not to double dose; that therapeutic effects may take 2-3 wk; not to discontinue medication quickly after long-term use, usually used for at least 3-4 months: may cause nausea, headache, malaise

• To use caution when driving, performing other activities that require alertness because of drowsiness, dizziness, blurred vision; to avoid rising quickly from sitting to standing (especially geriatric patients); how to manage anticholinergic effects

• To avoid alcohol, other CNS depressants

• To wear sunscreen or large hat when outdoors; photosensitivity occurs

• **Pregnancy/breastfeeding:** Identify if pregnancy is planned or suspected or if breastfeeding

---

Black Box Warning: To watch for suicide; advise to watch closely for suicidal thinking, behavior, making a plan or attempts, panic attacks, change in mood

---

• That follow-up examinations will be needed

• That all health care professionals should be notified the product is being used

TREATMENT OF OVERDOSE: ECG monitoring, lavage; administer anticonvulsant, sodium bicarbonate

---

amLODIPine (Rx)

(am-loe'di-peen)

Norvasc

Func. class.: Antianginal, antihypertensive, calcium channel blocker

Chem. class.: Dihydropyridine

Do not confuse:

amLODIPine/aMILoride

ACTION: Inhibits calcium ion influx across cell membrane during cardiac depolarization; produces relaxation of coronary vascular smooth muscle, peripheral vascular smooth muscle; dilates coronary vascular arteries; increases myocardial O_2 delivery in patients with vasospastic angina

USES: Chronic stable angina pectoris, hypertension, variant angina (Prinzmetal's angina)

Unlabeled uses: Hypertension (pediatric patients)

CONTRAINDICATIONS: Hypersensitivity to this product or dihydropyridine, severe aortic stenosis, severe obstructive CAD

Precautions: Pregnancy, breastfeeding, children, geriatric patients, HF, hypotension, hepatic injury, GERD

DOSAGE AND ROUTES

Coronary artery disease

• **Adult:** PO 5-10 mg/day

• **Geriatric:** PO 5 mg/day, max 10 mg/day

Hypertension

• **Adult:** PO 2.5-5 mg/day initially, max 10 mg/day

• **Geriatric:** PO 2.5 mg/day, may increase to 5 mg/day, max 10 mg/day

• **Child 6-17 yr (unlabeled): PO** 2.5-5 mg/day

• **Child 1-5 yr (unlabeled): PO** 0.1 mg/kg/dose daily initially, max 0.6 mg/kg/dose

Hepatic dose

• **Adult: PO** 2.5 mg/day; may increase to 10 mg/day (antihypertensive); 5 mg/day, may increase to 10 mg/day (antianginal)

Available forms: Tabs 2.5, 5, 10 mg

Administer:

• Once a day without regard to meals

SIDE EFFECTS

CNS: *Headache,* fatigue, dizziness, somnolence

CV: *Peripheral edema,* bradycardia, hypotension, angina, edema, palpitations

GI: Nausea, abdominal pain, anorexia, gingival hyperplasia, dyspepsia

INTEG: Rash, pruritus

OTHER: Flushing

PHARMACOKINETICS

Peak 6-12 hr; half-life 30-50 hr; increased in geriatric patients, hepatic disease; metabolized by liver (CYP3A4); excreted in urine (90% as metabolites); protein binding >93%

INTERACTIONS

Increase: a mLODIPine level—strong CPY3A4 inhibitors (clarithromycin, ketoconazole, ritonavir)

Increase: level of cycloSPORINE

Increase: myopathy simvastatin

NURSING CONSIDERATIONS
Assess:

• Cardiac status: B/P, pulse, respirations, ECG; some patients have developed severe angina, acute MI after calcium channel blockers if obstructive CAD is severe

• Fluid volume status, peripheral edema, dyspnea, jugular vein distention, crackles

• **Angina:** intensity, location, duration of pain

• **Pregnancy/breastfeeding:** identify if pregnancy is planned or suspected, or if breastfeeding

Evaluate:

• Therapeutic response: decreased anginal pain, decreased B/P, increased exercise tolerance

Teach patient/family:

• To take product as prescribed, not to double or skip dose, to take even if feeling better

• To avoid hazardous activities until stabilized on product, dizziness is no longer a problem

• To avoid OTC, Rx, herbs, supplements unless directed by prescriber

• To comply in all areas of medical regimen: diet, exercise, stress reduction, product therapy, smoking cessation

• To notify prescriber of irregular heartbeat; shortness of breath; swelling of feet, face, hands; severe dizziness; constipation; nausea; hypotension; if chest pain does not improve, use nitroglycerin when angina is severe

• To use correct technique when monitoring pulse; to contact prescriber if pulse <50 bpm

• To change positions slowly to prevent orthostatic hypotension

• To continue with good oral hygiene to prevent gingival disease

• To use sunscreen, protective clothing to prevent photosensitivity

• To notify all health care providers of use of this product

TREATMENT OF OVERDOSE:

Defibrillation, β-agonists, IV calcium inotropic agents, diuretics, atropine for AV block, vasopressor for hypotension

---

amoxicillin (Rx)
(a-mox-i-sill′in)

Moxatag, Novamoxin ♣

Func. class.: Antiinfective, antiulcer

Chem. class.: Aminopenicillin

ACTION: Interferes with cell wall replication of susceptible organisms; bactericidal: lysis mediated by bacterial cell wall autolysins

USES: Treatment of skin, respiratory, GI, GU infections, otitis media, gonorrhea; for gram-positive cocci *(Staphylococcus aureus, Streptococcus pyogenes, Streptococcus faecalis, Streptococcus pneumoniae)*, gram-negative cocci *(Neisseria gonorrhoeae, Neisseria meningitidis)*, gram-positive bacilli *(Corynebacterium diphtheriae, Listeria monocytogenes)*, gram-negative bacilli *(Haemophilus influenzae, Escherichia coli, Proteus mirabilis, Salmonella)*; gastric ulcer, β-lactase–negative organisms, prophylaxis of bacterial endocarditis; for treatment of ulcers due to *Helicobacter pylori*

Unlabeled uses: Lyme disease, anthrax treatment and prophylaxis, cervicitis, *Chlamydia trachomatis,* dental abscess/infection, dyspepsia, non-gonococcal urethritis, periodontitis, typhoid fever

---

CONTRAINDICATIONS: Hypersensitivity to penicillins

Precautions: Pregnancy, breastfeeding, neonates, hypersensitivity to cephalosporins, carbapenems; severe renal disease, mononucleosis, phenylketonuria, diabetes, geriatric patients, asthma, child, colitis, dialysis, eczema, pseudomembranous colitis, syphilis

DOSAGE AND ROUTES
Tonsillitis and/or pharyngitis (rheumatic fever prophylaxis) secondary to *Streptococcus pyogenes*
• **Adult/adolescent/child ≥12 yr: PO** (Moxatag 775-mg extended-release tablets) 775 mg/day, given within 1 hr of completing a meal, for 10 days
• **Adult: PO** (immediate-release) 1 g/day or 500 mg bid for 10 days
• **Infant/child/adolescent: PO** (immediate-release) 25 mg/kg/dose (max 500 mg/dose) bid for 10 days
Sinusitis
• **Child ≥2 yr/adolescent: PO** (immediate release) **standard-dose therapy,** 45 mg/kg/day divided q12h; **high-dose therapy,** 80-90 mg/kg/day divided q12h (max 2 g/dose)
• **Child <2 yr: PO** Treat with amoxicillin/clavulanate, not amoxicillin alone
Acute otitis media
• **Adult: PO** (immediate-release) 500 mg q12h or 250 mg q8h for mild/moderate infections; 875 mg q12h or 500 mg q8h for severe infections
• **Infant ≥6 mo/child/adolescent: PO** (immediate-release) 80-90 mg/kg/day divided q12h
• **Infant 4-5 mo: PO** (immediate-release) 80-90 mg/kg/day divided q12h for 10 days
• **Infant ≤3 mo: PO** (immediate-release) 30 mg/kg/day divided q12h
Most respiratory Infections
• **Adult: PO** (immediate-release) 500 mg q12h or 250 mg q8h (mild-moderate infections); 875 mg 12 hr or 500 mg q8hr (severe infections)
• **Infant >3 mo/child/adolescent: PO** (immediate-release) 20 mg/kg/day divided q8h (max 250 mg/dose) or 25 mg/kg/day divided q12h (max 500 mg/dose)
• **Neonate/infant ≤3 mo: PO** (immediate-release) 30 mg/kg/day divided q12h
H. pylori
• **Adult: PO** 1000 mg bid with lansoprazole 30 mg bid with clarithromycin 500 mg bid x 14 days or 1000 mg bid with omeprazole 20 mg bid, with clarithromycin 500 mg bid x 14 days or 1000 mg bid with esomeprazole 40 mg daily with clarithromycin 500 mg bid x 10 days; or 1000 mg tid with lansoprazole 30 mg tid x 14 days
Gonorrhea
• **Adult/child ≥ 40 kg: PO** x 3 g single dose
• **Child >2 yr and <40 kg: PO** 50 mg/kg with probenecid 25 mg/kg single dose
Endocarditis prevention
• **Adult: PO** 2 g 60 min prior to procedure
• **Child: PO** 50 mg/kg 60 min prior to procedure, max adult dose
Urinary tract infection (UTI), including cystitis
Mild to moderate infections caused by highly susceptible organisms
• **Adult: PO** (immediate-release) 500 mg q12h or 250 mg q8h
• **Infant >3 mo/child/adolescent: PO** (immediate-release) 20 mg/kg/day divided q8h (max 250 mg/dose) or 25 mg/kg/day divided q12h (max 500 mg/dose)
• **Neonate/infant ≤3 mo: PO** (immediate-release) 30 mg/kg/day divided q12h
Renal disease
• **Adult: PO** CCr 10-30 mL/min 250-500 mg q12h; CCr <10 mL/min 250-500 mg q24hr; do not use 775-, 875-mg strength if CCr <30 mL/min

Available forms: Caps 250, 500 mg; chew tabs 125, 200, 250, 400 mg; tabs, 500, 875 mg; ext rel tab (Moxatag) 775 mg; powder for; susp 125, 200, 250, 400 mg/5 mL; suspension 50 mg/mL

Administer:
PO route
• Identify allergies before use
• **Susp:** shake well before each dose; use calibrated spoon, oral syringe, or measuring cup; may be used alone,

mixed in drinks; use immediately; discard unused portion after 14 days, store in refrigerator

• Give around the clock; caps may be emptied, mixed with liquids if needed without regard to food

• **Ext rel:** do not crush, chew, break; take with food

SIDE EFFECTS

CNS: Seizures, agitation, confusion, dizziness, insomnia

GI: *Nausea, vomiting, diarrhea,* pseudomembranous colitis

HEMA: Anemia, bone marrow depression, granulocytopenia, hemolytic anemia, eosinophilia, thrombocytopenia, agranulocytosis

INTEG: *Urticaria, rash*

SYST: Anaphylaxis, serum sickness, overgrowth of infection, anaphylaxis, hypersensitivity

PHARMACOKINETICS

PO: Peak 1-2 hr, duration 6-8 hr, half-life $1-1^{1}/_{3}$ hr extended in renal disease, metabolized in liver, excreted in urine, crosses placenta, enters breast milk

INTERACTIONS

Increase: rash—allopurinol

Increase: amoxicillin level—probenecid; used for this reason

Increase: anticoagulant action—warfarin

Increase: methotrexate levels—methotrexate; monitor for toxicity

Decrease: contraceptive effect possible—hormonal contraceptives

Drug/Lab Test

Increase: AST/ALT, alk phos, LDH, eosinophils

Decrease: Hgb, WBC, platelets

Interference: urine glucose test (Clinitest, Benedict's reagent)

NURSING CONSIDERATIONS
Assess:

• C&S before product therapy; product may be given as soon as culture is taken

• **CDAD:** bowel pattern before, during treatment; diarrhea, cramping, blood in stool; report to prescriber immediately, product should be discontinued, may occur even weeks after discontinuing product

• Skin eruptions after administration of penicillin to 1 wk after discontinuing product; rash is more common if allopurinol is taken concurrently

• **Pregnancy/breastfeeding:** identify if pregnancy is planned or suspected or if breastfeeding; use only if clearly needed; appears in breast milk, use cautiously in breastfeeding; advise those taking oral contraceptives to use alternative contraceptive since contraceptive may be decreased

• **Anaphylaxis:** rash, itching, dyspnea, facial/laryngeal edema

Evaluate:

• Therapeutic response: absence of infection; prevention of endocarditis, resolution of ulcer symptoms

Teach patient/family:

• That caps may be opened, contents taken with fluids; that chewable form is available; to take as prescribed, not to double dose

• All aspects of product therapy: to complete entire course of medication to ensure organism death; that culture may be taken after completed course of medication

• To report sore throat, fever, fatigue, diarrhea (superinfection or agranulocytopenia), blood in stool, abdominal pain (pseudomembranous colitis)

• That product must be taken in equal intervals around the clock to maintain blood levels; to take without regard to food, that caps may be opened, contents taken with fluids; that chewable form is available; to take as prescribed, not to double dose

• To wear or carry emergency ID if allergic to penicillins

TREATMENT OF ANAPHY-LAXIS: Withdraw product, maintain airway; administer EPINEPHrine, aminophylline, O_2, IV corticosteroids

---

amoxicillin/clavulanate (Rx)

(a-mox-i-sill'in)

Augmentin, Augmentin ES, Augmentin XR, Clavulin ✤

Func. class.: Broad-spectrum antiinfective

Chem. class.: Aminopenicillin β-lactamase inhibitor

ACTION: Bacteriocidal, interferes with cell wall replication of susceptible organisms; lysis mediated by bacterial cell wall autolytic enzymes, combination increases spectrum of activity against β-lactamase–resistant organisms

USES: Lower respiratory tract infections, sinus infections, pneumonia, otitis media, impetigo, skin infection, UTI; effective for *Actinomyces* sp., *Bacillus anthracis*, *Bacteroides* sp., *Bordetella pertussis*, *Borrelia burgdorferi*, *Brucella* sp., *Burkholderia pseudomallei*, *Clostridium perfringens/tetani*, *Corynebacterium diphtheriae*, *Eikenella corrodens*, *Enterobacter* sp., *Enterococcus faecalis*, *Erysipelothrix rhusiopathiae*, *Escherichia coli*, *Eubacterium* sp., *Fusobacterium* sp., *Haemophilus ducreyi/parainfluenzae* (positive/negative beta-lactamase), *Helicobacter pylori*, *Klebsiella* sp., *Lactobacillus* sp., *Listeria monocytogenes*, *Moraxella catarrhalis*, *Neisseria gonorrhoeae/meningitidis*, *Nocardia brasiliensis*, *Peptococcus* sp., *Peptostreptococcus* sp., *Prevotella melaninogenica*, *Propionibacterium* sp., *Shigella* sp., *Staphylococcus aureus (MSSA)/epidermidis/saprophyticus*, *Streptococcus agalactiae (group B streptococci)/dysgalactiae/ pneumoniae/pyogenes (group A streptococci)*, *Treponema pallidum*, *Vibrio cholerae*, *Viridans streptococci*

Unlabeled uses: Actinomycotic mycetoma, chancroid, dental infections, dentoalveolar infection, melioidosis, pericoronitis, SARS

CONTRAINDICATIONS: Hypersensitivity to penicillins, severe renal disease, dialysis

Precautions: Pregnancy, breastfeeding, neonates, children, hypersensitivity to cephalosporins; renal/GI disease, asthma, colitis, diabetes, eczema, leukemia, mononucleosis, viral infections, phenylketonuria

DOSAGE AND ROUTES

Most infections
• **Adult/child >40 kg:** 250 mg q8hr or 500 mg q12hr

Recurrent/persistent otitis media (*Streptococcus pneumoniae*, *Haemophilus*, *Moraxella catarrhalis*)
• **Child ≥3 mo:** PO 90 mg/kg/day (600 mg amoxicillin/42.9 mg clavulanate/5 mL) q12hr × 10 days

Lower respiratory infections, otitis media, sinusitis, skin/skin structure infections, UTIs
• **Adult:** PO 250-500 mg q8hr or 500-875 mg q12hr, depending on severity of infection
• **Child ≤40 kg:** PO 20-90 mg/kg/day in divided doses q8-12hr

Community-acquired pneumonia or acute bacterial sinusitis
• **Adult:** PO 2000 mg/125 mg (Augmentin XR) q12hr × 7-10 days (pneumonia), 10 days (sinusitis)

Renal disease
• **Adult:** PO CCr 10-30 mL/min dose q12hr; CCr <10 mL/min dose q24hr; do not use 875-mg strength or ext rel if CCr <30 mL/min; Augmentin XR is contraindicated with renal disease

Available forms: Tabs 250, 500, 875 mg amoxicillin/125 mg clavulanate; chew tabs 200 mg amoxicillin/28.5 clavulanate, 400 mg amoxacillin/57 mg clavulanate; powder for oral susp 250 mg amoxacillin/28.5 mg clavulanate, 200 amoxacillin mg/28.5 clavulanate mg, 400 amoxacillin mg/57 clavulanate mg,

---

600/42.9 mg/5 mL clavulanate ext rel tabs (XR) 1000 mg amoxicillin/62.5 mg clavulanate; powder for oral susp (ES) 600 mg amoxicillin/42.9 mg clavulanate

Administer:

PO route

• Do not break, crush, chew ext rel product

• Only as directed; two 250-mg tabs not equivalent to one 500-mg tab due to strength of clavulanate

• Shake susp well before each dose; may be used alone, mixed in drinks; use immediately, discard unused portion of susp after 14 days, store in refrigerator

• Give around the clock

• Give with light meal for increased absorption, fewer GI effects, confusion, behavioral changes

SIDE EFFECTS

CNS: Headache, fever, seizures, agitation, insomnia

GI: *Nausea, diarrhea, vomiting,* increased AST/ALT, CDAD

GU: *Vaginitis*

HEMA: Anemia, bone marrow depression, granulocytopenia, leukopenia, eosinophilia, thrombocytopenic purpura

INTEG: *Rash,* urticaria

SYST: Anaphylaxis, respiratory distress, serum sickness

PHARMACOKINETICS

PO: Peak 1-2.5 hr, duration 8–12 hr, half-life 1-1$^1/_3$ hr, metabolized in liver, excreted in urine, crosses placenta, excreted in breast milk, removed by hemodialysis

INTERACTIONS

Increase: amoxicillin levels—probenecid, used for this reason

Increase: anticoagulant effect—warfarin; monitor closely, dose adjustment may be needed

Increase: skin rash—allopurinol

Decrease: contraceptive effect—oral contraceptives

Drug/Food

Decrease: absorption by a high-fat meal

Drug/Lab Test

Increase: AST/ALT, alk phos, LDH

Interference: urine glucose tests (Clinitest, Benedict's reagent, cupric SO_4)

NURSING CONSIDERATIONS

Assess:

• **Infection:** For signs/symptoms of infection (characteristics of wounds, sputum, urine, stool, WBC >10,000/mm³, earache, fever, obtain baseline and during treatment

• **Superinfection:** Perineal itching, fever, malaise, redness, pain, swelling, rash, diarrhea, change in cough sputum; if large doses are given or geriatrics

• Hepatic studies: AST, ALT baseline, periodically in hepatic disease, discontinue if hepatitis occurs

• Blood studies: WBC

• C&S before product therapy; product may be given as soon as culture is taken

• **CDAD:** bowel pattern before, during treatment; diarrhea, cramping, blood in stools; report to prescriber

• **Anaphylaxis:** rash, itching, dyspnea, facial/laryngeal edema; skin eruptions after administration of penicillin to 1 wk after discontinuing product, adrenaline, suction, tracheostomy set, endotracheal intubation equipment on unit

Evaluate:

• Therapeutic response: absence of infection

Teach patient/family:

• To take as prescribed, not to double or skip doses

• All aspects of product therapy: to complete entire course of medication to ensure organism death that culture may be taken after completed course of medication

• That product must be taken in equal intervals around the clock to maintain blood levels

• To report sore throat, fever, fatigue (superinfection or agranulocytosis); diarrhea, cramping, blood in stools (pseudomembranous colitis)

Side effects: *italics* = common; red = life-threatening

• That product must be taken in equal intervals around the clock to maintain blood levels

• To wear or carry emergency ID if allergic to penicillins

• **Pregnancy/breastfeeding:** To notify health care professional if pregnancy is planned or suspected or if breastfeeding; to use another form of contraception if taking oral contraceptives, effect maybe decreased

TREATMENT OF HYPER-SENSITIVITY: Withdraw product, maintain airway, administer EPINEPHrine, aminophylline, O₂, IV corticosteroids for anaphylaxis

---

> **⚠ HIGH ALERT**
>
> **amphotericin B lipid complex (ABLC) (Rx)**
>
> (am-foe-ter′i-sin)
>
> Abelcet
>
> *Func. class.:* Antifungal
> *Chem. class.:* Amphoteric polyene

Do not confuse:
Abelcet/amphotericin B

ACTION: Increases cell membrane permeability in susceptible fungi by binding sterols; alters cell membrane, thereby causing leakage of cell components, cell death

USES: Indicated for the treatment of invasive fungal infections in patients who cannot tolerate or have failed conventional amphotericin B therapy; broad-spectrum activity against many fungal, yeast and mold pathogen infections, including *Aspergillus, Zygomycetes, Fusarium, Cryptococcus,* and many hard-to-treat *Candida* species; *Aspergillus fumigatus, Aspergillus* sp., *Blastomyces dermatitidis, Candida albicans, Candida guilliermondii, Candida* sp., *Candida stellatoidea, Candida tropicalis, Coccidioides immitis, Cryptococcus* sp., *Histoplasma* sp., sporotrichosis

CONTRAINDICATIONS: Hypersensitivity

Precautions: Anemia, breastfeeding, cardiac disease, children, electrolyte imbalance, geriatric patients, hematologic/hepatic/renal disease, hypotension, pregnancy

DOSAGE AND ROUTES
• **Adult: IV** 5 mg/kg/day
Renal dose
• **Adult: IV** CCr <10 mL/min give 5 mg/kg q24-36hr
Available forms: Susp for inj 5 mg/mL
Administer:
• **Do not confuse the four different types; these are not interchangeable:** conventional amphotericin B, amphotericin B cholesteryl, amphotericin B lipid complex, amphotericin B liposome
• May premedicate with acetaminophen, diphenhydrAMINE
• Use only after C&S confirms organism
IV route
• Give product only after C&S confirms organism, product needed to treat condition; make sure product is used for life-threatening infections
• Handle with aseptic technique amphotericin B lipid complex (ABLC) has no preservatives; visually inspect parenteral products for particulate matter and discoloration before use
Filtration and dilution:
• Before dilution, store at 36°-46° F (2°-8° C), protected from moisture and light; do not freeze; the diluted, ready-for-use admixture is stable for up to 48 hours at 36°-46° F (2°-8° C) and an additional 6 hr at room temperature; do not freeze
• Prepare by shaking the vial until no yellow sediment remains
• Transfer the appropriate amount of drug from the required number of vials into one or more sterile syringes using an 18-gauge needle

---

• Attach the provided 5-micron filter needle to the syringe; inject the syringe contents through the filter needle into an IV bag containing the D_5W injection; each filter needle may be used on the contents of no more than four 100-mg vials

• The suspension must be diluted with D_5W injection (1 mg/mL); for pediatric patients and patients with cardiovascular disease, the final concentration may be 2 mg/mL; DO NOT USE SALINE SOLUTIONS OR MIX WITH OTHER DRUGS OR ELECTRO-LYTES

• The diluted ready-for-use admixture is stable for up to 48 hr at 2-8° C (36-46° F) and an additional 6 hr at room temperature; do not freeze

IV INFUSION

• Flush IV line with D_5W injection before use or use a separate IV line; DO NOT USE AN IN-LINE FILTER

• Before infusion, shake the bag until the contents are thoroughly mixed; max rate 2.5 mg/kg/hr; if the infusion time exceeds 2 hr, mix the contents by shaking the infusion bag every 2 hr

Y-site compatibilities: acyclovir, allopurinol, aminocaproic acid, aminophylline, amiodarone, anidulafungin, argatroban, arsenic trioxide, atracurium, azithromycin, aztreonam, bumetanide, buprenorphine, busulfan, butorphanol, CARBOplatin, carmustine, ceFAZolin, cefepime, cefotaxime, cefoTEtan, cefOXitin, cefTAZidime, ceftizoxime, cefTRIAXone, cefuroxime, chloramphenicol, chlorproMAZINE, cimetidine, cisatracurium, clindamycin, cyclophosphamide, cycloSPORINE, cytarabine, DACTINomycin, dexamethasone, digoxin, diphenhydrAMINE, DOCEtaxel, doxacurium, DOXOrubicin liposomal, enalaprilat, EPINEPHrine, eptifibatide, ertapenem, etoposide, famotidine, fentaNYL, fludarabine, fluorouracil, fosphenytoin, furosemide, ganciclovir, granisetron, heparin, hydrocortisone, HYDROmorphone, ifosfamide, insulin, regular ketorolac, lepirudin, lidocaine, linezolid, LORazepam, mannitol, melphalan, meperidine, methotrexate, methylPREDNISolone, metoclopramide, mitoMYcin, mivacurium, nafcillin, nesiritide, nitroglycerin, nitroprusside, octreotide, oxaliplatin, PACLitaxel, pamidronate, pantoprazole, PEMEtrexed, pentazocine, PENTobarbital, PHENobarbital, phentolamine, piperacillin-tazobactam, procainamide, raNITIdine, succinylcholine, SUFentanil, tacrolimus, telavancin, teniposide, theophylline, thiopental, thiotepa, ticarcillin, ticarcillin-clavulanate, trimethobenzamide, verapamil, vinBLAStine, vinCRIStine, zidovudine, zoledronic acid

SIDE EFFECTS

CNS: *Headache, fever, chills,* confusion, anxiety, insomnia

CV: Hypotension, cardiac arrest, chest pain, hypertension, tachycardia, edema

GI: *Nausea, vomiting, anorexia,* diarrhea, cramps, bilirubinemia

GU: Nephrotoxicity

HEMA: Anemia, thrombocytopenia, agranulocytosis, leukopenia

INTEG: *Burning, irritation,* pain, necrosis at inj site with extravasation, rash, pruritus, dermatitis

META: Hyponatremia, hypomagnesemia, hypokalemia

MS: Arthralgia, myalgia, generalized pain, weakness, weight loss

RESP: Dyspnea, wheezing, respiratory failure

SYST: Toxic epidermal necrolysis, exfoliative dermatitis, anaphylaxis, sepsis, infection

PHARMACOKINETICS

IV: half-life 7 days

INTERACTIONS

• Do not use with cidofovir

Increase: nephrotoxicity—other nephrotoxic antibiotics (aminoglycosides, CISplatin, vancomycin, cycloSPORINE, polymyxin B), antineoplastics, pentamidine, salicylates, tacrolimus, tenofovir; use cautiously

Increase: hypokalemia—corticosteroids, digoxin, skeletal muscle relaxants, thiazides, loop diuretics; monitor electrolytes

---

Side effects: *italics* = common; red = life-threatening

Decrease: amphotericin B lipid complex—azole antifungals; may still be used concurrently in serious resistant infections

Drug/Lab Test

Increase: AST/ALT, alk phos, BUN, creatinine, LDH, bilirubin

Decrease: magnesium, potassium, Hgb, WBC, platelets

NURSING CONSIDERATIONS

Assess:

• VS every 15-30 min during first infusion; note changes in pulse, B/P

• Blood studies: CBC, potassium, sodium, calcium, magnesium every 2 wk; BUN, creatinine 2-3 ×/wk

• Weight weekly; if weight increases by more than 2 lb/wk, edema is present; renal damage should be considered

• **For renal toxicity:** increasing BUN, serum creatinine; if BUN is >40 mg/dL or if serum creatinine is >3 mg/dL, product may be discontinued, dosage reduced, I&O ratio; watch for decreasing urinary output, change in specific gravity; discontinue product to prevent permanent damage to renal tubules

• **For hepatotoxicity:** increasing AST, ALT, alk phos, bilirubin

• **For allergic reaction:** dermatitis, rash; product should be discontinued, antihistamines (mild reaction) or EPINEPHrine (severe reaction) should be administered

• **For hypokalemia:** anorexia, drowsiness, weakness, decreased reflexes, dizziness, increased urinary output, increased thirst, paresthesias

• **Infusion reactions:** fever, chills, pain, swelling at site

Evaluate:

• Therapeutic response: resolution of infection, negative C&S for infecting organism

Teach patient/family:

• That long-term therapy may be needed to clear infection (2 wk-3 mo, depending on type of infection), frequent blood draws will be needed

• To notify prescriber of bleeding, bruising, or soft-tissue swelling, neurologic, renal symptoms

• **Pregnancy/breastfeeding:** to advise prescriber if pregnancy is planned or suspected; not to breastfeed

---

⚠ HIGH ALERT

amphotericin B liposomal (LAmB) (Rx)
(am-foe-ter′i-sin)
AmBisome
Func. class.: Antifungal
Chem. class.: Amphoteric polyene

Do not confuse:
AmBisome/amphotericin B

ACTION: Increases cell membrane permeability in susceptible fungi by binding to membrane sterols; alters cell membrane, thereby causing leakage of cell components, cell death

THERAPEUTIC OUTCOME
Resolution of infection

USES: Empirical therapy for presumed fungal infection in febrile neutropenic patients; treatment of cryptococcal meningitis in HIV-infected patients; treatment of *Aspergillus* sp., *Candida* sp., and/or *Cryptococcus* sp. infections refractory to amphotericin B deoxycholate, or in patients where renal impairment or unacceptable toxicity precludes the use of amphotericin B deoxycholate (*Aspergillus flavus, Aspergillus fumigatus, Blastomyces dermatitidis, Candida albicans, Candida krusei, Candida lusitaniae, Candida parapsilosis, Candida tropicalis, Cryptococcus neoformans*); treatment of visceral leishmaniasis

Unlabeled uses: Coccidioidomycosis, histoplasmosis

CONTRAINDICATIONS: Hypersensitivity

Precautions: Anemia, breastfeeding, cardiac disease, children, electrolyte imbalance, geriatric patients, hematologic/hepatic/renal disease, hypotension, pregnancy, severe bone marrow depression

---

DOSAGE AND ROUTES
Systemic fungal infections
• **Adults and children: IV** 3-6 mg/kg/dose q24hr
Esophageal candidiasis (unlabeled) in HIV-infected patients
• **Adults/adolescents: IV** 3-4 mg/kg/dose q24hr for 14 to 21 days
Cryptococcal meningitis in HIV patients
• **Adults/adolescents/children/infants: IV** 6 mg/kg/dose q24hr
Visceral leishmaniasis
• **Adult: IV** 3 mg/kg q24hr on days 1-5, then 3 mg/kg q24hr on days 14, 21 (immunocompetent); 4 mg/kg q24hr on days 1-5, then 4 mg/kg q24hr on days 10, 17, 24, 31, 38 (immunosuppressed)
Severe disseminated (nonmeningeal) or diffuse pulmonary coccidioidomycosis (unlabeled) in HIV-infected patients
• **Adults: IV** 3-5 mg/kg/dose q24hr
Renal dose
• **Adult: IV** CCr <10 mL/min use 3 mg/kg q24hr

Available forms: Powder for inj 50-mg vial

Administer:
• **Do not confuse four different types; these are not interchangeable:** conventional amphotericin B, amphotericin B cholesteryl, amphotericin B lipid complex, amphotericin B liposome
• May premedicate with acetaminophen, diphenhydrAMINE

IV route
• Give after C&S confirms organism, and product needed to treat condition
• Use for life-threatening infections
• Administer by IV infusion only; use aseptic technique as LAmB does not contain any preservatives
• Visually inspect for particulate and discoloration

Reconstitution
• LAmB *must* be reconstituted using sterile water for inj (without a bacteriostatic agent); DO NOT RECONSTITUTE WITH SALINE OR ADD SALINE TO THE RECONSTITUTED SUSPENSION, DO NOT MIX WITH OTHER DRUGS; doing so can cause a precipitate to form
• Reconstitute vials containing 50 mg of LAmB /12 mL of sterile water (4 mg/mL)
• Immediately after the addition of water, SHAKE THE VIAL VIGOROUSLY for 30 sec; the suspension should be yellow and translucent; visually inspect vial for particulate matter and continue shaking until product is completely dispersed
• Store suspension for up to 24 hr refrigerated if using sterile water for inj; do not freeze

Filtration and dilution
• Calculate the amount of reconstituted (4 mg/mL) suspension to be further diluted and withdraw this amount into a sterile syringe
• Attach the provided 5-micron filter to the syringe; inject the syringe contents through the filter into the appropriate amount of D_5W injection; use only one filter per vial
• The suspension must be diluted with D_5W injection (1-2 mg/mL) before administration; for infants and small children, lower concentrations (0.2-0.5 mg/mL) may be appropriate to provide sufficient volume for infusion
• Use injection of LAmB within 6 hr of dilution with D_5W

IV INFUSION
• Flush intravenous line with D_5W injection before infusion; if this cannot be done, then a separate IV line must be used
• An in-line membrane filter may be used provided the mean pore diameter of the filter is not less than 1 micron
• Administer by IV infusion using a controlled infusion device over a period of approximately 120 min; infusion time may be reduced to approximately 60 min in patients who tolerate the infusion; if discomfort occurs during infusion, the duration of infusion may be increased
• Store protected from moisture and light; diluted solution is stable for 24 hr at room temperature

---

Acetaminophen and diphenhydrAMINE
• 30 min before infusion to reduce fever, chills, headache

Y-site compatibilities: Acyclovir, amifostine, aminophylline, anidulafungin, atropine, azithromycin, bivalirudin, bumetanide, buprenorphine, busulfan, butorphanol, CARBOplatin, carmustine, ceFAZolin, ceFOXitin, ceftizoxime, cefTRIAXone, cefuroxime, cimetidine, clindamycin, cyclophosphamide, cytarabine, DACTINomycin, DAPTOmycin, dexamethasone, dexmedetomidine, diphenhydrAMINE, doxacurium, enalaprilat, ePHEDrine, EPINEPHrine, eptifibatide, ertapenem, esmolol, etoposide, famotidine, fenoldopam, fentaNYL, fludarabine, fluorouracil, fosphenytoin, furosemide, granisetron, haloperidol, heparin, hydrocortisone, HYDROmorphone, ifosfamide, isoproterenol, ketorolac, levorphanol, lidocaine, linezolid, mesna, methotrexate, methylPREDNISolone, metoprolol, milrinone, mitoMYcin, nesiritide, nitroglycerin, nitroprusside, octreotide, oxaliplatin, oxytocin, palonosetron, pancuronium, pantoprazole, PEMEtrexed, PENTobarbital, PHENObarbital, phenylephrine, piperacillin/tazobactam, potassium chloride, procainamide, raNITIdine, SUFentanil, tacrolimus, theophylline, thiopental, thiotepa, ticarcillin/clavulanate, tigecycline, trimethoprim-sulfamethoxazole, vasopressin, vinCRIStine, voriconazole, zidovudine

SIDE EFFECTS
CNS: *Headache, fever, chills,* peripheral nerve pain, insomnia
CV: Hypotension, cardiac arrest, tachycardia, edema, flushing
GI: *Nausea, vomiting, anorexia,* diarrhea, cramps, GI hemmorrhage, hyperbilirubinemia
GU: Nephrotoxicity
HEMA: Anemia, thrombocytopenia, agranulocytosis, leukopenia
INTEG: *Burning, irritation,* pain, necrosis at inj site with extravasation, flushing, dermatitis, skin rash (topical route)
MS: Arthralgia, myalgia
RESP: Dyspnea, cough

SYST: Stevens-Johnson syndrome, toxic epidermal necrolysis, exfoliative dermatitis, anaphylaxis

PHARMACOKINETICS
IV: Metabolized in liver; excreted in urine (metabolites), breast milk; protein binding 90%; poorly penetrates CSF, bronchial secretions, aqueous humor, muscle, bone; half-life 4-6 days

INTERACTIONS
Increase: nephrotoxicity—other nephrotoxic antibiotics (aminoglycosides, antineoplastics, CISplatin, vancomycin, cycloSPORINE, polymyxin B)
Increase: hypokalemia—corticosteroids, digoxin, skeletal muscle relaxants, thiazides, loop diuretics
Decrease: amphotericin B liposomal—azole antifungals, may be used concurrently in serious resistant infections

NURSING CONSIDERATIONS
Assess:
• VS every 15-30 min during first infusion; note changes in pulse, B/P
• Blood studies: CBC, potassium, sodium, calcium, magnesium every 2 wk, BUN, creatinine 2-3 ×/wk
• Weight weekly; if weight increases by more than 2 lb/wk, edema is present; renal damage should be considered
• **For renal toxicity:** increasing BUN, serum creatinine; if BUN is >40 mg/dL or if serum creatinine is >3 mg/dL, product may be discontinued, dosage reduced; I&O ratio; watch for decreasing urinary output, change in specific gravity; discontinue product to prevent permanent damage to renal tubules
• **For hepatotoxicity:** increasing AST, ALT, alk phos, bilirubin, monitor LFTs
• **For allergic reaction:** dermatitis, rash; product should be discontinued, antihistamines (mild reaction) or EPINEPHrine (severe reaction) administered
• **For hypokalemia:** anorexia, drowsiness, weakness, decreased reflexes, dizziness, increased urinary output, increased thirst, paresthesias

- **Infusion reaction:** chills, fever, pain, swelling at site

Evaluate:
- Therapeutic response: resolution of infection, negative C&S for infecting organism

Teach patient/family:
- That long-term therapy may be needed to clear infection (2 wk-3 mo, depending on type of infection), that frequent blood draws will be needed
- To notify prescriber of bleeding, bruising, or soft-tissue swelling, renal, neurologic side effects
- **Pregnancy/breastfeeding:** To notify health care professional if pregnancy is planned or suspected, not to breastfeed

ampicillin (Rx)

(am-pi-sill'in)
Func. class.: Antiinfective—broad-spectrum
Chem. class.: Aminopenicillin

ACTION: Interferes with cell wall replication of susceptible organisms; the cell wall, rendered osmotically unstable, swells, bursts from osmotic pressure; lysis mediated by cell wall autolysins

USES: Effective for gram-positive cocci *(Staphylococcus aureus, Streptococcus pyogenes, Streptococcus faecalis, Streptococcus pneumoniae)*, gram-negative cocci *(Neisseria meningitidis)*, gram-negative bacilli *(Haemophilus influenzae, Proteus mirabilis, Salmonella, Shigella, Listeria monocytogenes)*, gram-positive bacilli; meningitis, GI/GU/respiratory infections, endocarditis, septicemia, otitis media, skin infection, bacterial endocarditis

CONTRAINDICATIONS: Hypersensitivity to penicillins, antimicrobial resistance
Precautions: Pregnancy, breastfeeding, neonates, hypersensitivity to cephalosporins, renal disease, mononucleosis

DOSAGE AND ROUTES
Systemic infections
- **Adult and child ≥40 kg:** PO 250-500 mg q6hr; **IV/IM** 2-8 g/day in divided doses q4-6hr
- **Child <40 kg:** PO 50-100 mg/kg/day in divided doses q6-8hr; **IV/IM** 100-150 mg/kg/day in divided doses q6hr

Bacterial meningitis
- **Adult and adolescent:** IM/IV 150-200 mg/kg/day in divided doses q3-4 hr; IDSA dose **IV** 2 g q4hr
- **Infant and child:** IM/IV 150-200 mg/kg/day in divided doses q3-4hr; IDSA dose IV 200-400 mg/kg/day in divided doses q6hr
- **Neonate >7 days and >2000 g:** IM/IV 200 mg/kg/day in divided doses q6hr; IDSA dose **IV** 200 mg/kg/day in divided doses q6-8hr

Prevention of bacterial endocarditis
- **Adult:** IM/IV 2 g 30 min before procedure
- **Child:** IM/IV 50 mg/kg 30 min before procedure, max 2 g

GI/GU infections other than *N. gonorrhoeae*
- **Adult and child >20 kg:** PO 500 mg q6hr, may use larger dose for more serious infections
- **Child <40 kg:** PO 50 mg/kg/day in divided doses q6-8hr

Renal disease
- **Adult and child:** CCr 10-50 mL/min extend to q6-12hr; CCr <10 mL/min extend to q12-16hr

Available forms: Powder for inj 125, 250, 500 mg, 1, 2, 10 g/vial; caps 250, 500 mg; powder for oral susp 125, 250 mg/5 mL

Administer:
- Check allergies before using; obtain C&S before using; begin before results are received

PO route
- Give in even doses around the clock, store caps in tight container, store after reconstituting in refrigerator up to 2 wk, 1 wk room temperature
- Tabs may be crushed or caps opened and mixed with water

• On empty stomach with plenty of water for best absorption (1-2 hr before meals or 2-3 hr after meals)

• Shake susp well before each dose; store after reconstituting in refrigerator up to 2 wk, 1 wk room temperature

IM route

• **Reconstitute** by adding 0.9-1.2 mL/125-mg vial; 0.9-1.9 mL/250-mg vial; 1.2-1.8 mL/500-mg vial; 2.4-7.4 mL/1-g vial; 6.8 mL/2-g vial

IV route

IV direct

• After diluting with sterile water 0.9-1.2 mL/125-mg product, administer over 3-5 min (up to 500 mg), 10-15 min (>500 mg)

Intermittent IV INFUSION route

• May be diluted in 50 mL or more of D_5W, D_5 0.45% NaCl to a concentration of 30 mg/mL or less; IV sol is stable for 1 hr; give at prescribed rate, do not give in same tubing as aminoglycosides, separate by ≥1 hr

Y-site compatibilities: Acyclovir, alemtuzumab, alprostadil, amifostine, aminocaproic acid, anidulafungin, argatroban, atenolol, azithromycin, bivalirudin, bleomycin, CARBOplatin, carmustine, CISplatin, clarithromycin, cyclophosphamide, cytarabine, DACTINomycin, DAPTOmycin, DAUNOrubicin liposome, dexmedetomidine, dexrazoxane, DOCEtaxel, doxacurium, doxapram, DOXOrubicin liposome, eptifibatide, etoposide, etoposide phosphate, filgrastim, fludarabine, fluorouracil, foscarnet, gallium, gatifloxacin, gemcitabine, gemtuzumab, granisetron, hetastarch, ifosfamide, irinotecan, lepirudin, leucovorin, levoFLOXacin, linezolid, mannitol, mechlorethamine, melphalan, methotrexate, metroNIDAZOLE, milrinone, octreotide, ofloxacin, oxaliplatin, PACLitaxel, palonosetron, pamidronate, pancuronium, pantoprazole, PEMEtrexed, penicillin G potassium, perphenazine, potassium acetate, propofol, remifentanil, riTUXimab, rocuronium, sodium acetate, teniposide, thiotepa, tigecycline, tirofiban, TNA, trastuzumab, vecuronium, vinBLAStine, vinCRIStine, vit B/C, voriconazole, zoledronic acid

SIDE EFFECTS

CNS: Seizures (high doses)
GI: *Nausea, vomiting, diarrhea,* CDAD, stomatitis
HEMA: Anemia, bone marrow depression, granulocytopenia, leukopenia, eosinophilia
INTEG: *Rash, urticaria*
MISC: Anaphylaxis, serum sickness

PHARMACOKINETICS

Half-life 50-110 min; excreted in urine, bile, breast milk; crosses placenta; removed by dialysis
PO: Peak 2 hr, duration 6-8 hr
IM: Peak 1 hr, duration 6-8 hr
IV: Peak rapid, duration 6-8 hr

INTERACTIONS

Increase: bleeding—oral anticoagulants, monitor INR/PT
Increase: ampicillin concentrations—probenecid, used for this action
Increase: ampicillin-induced skin rash—allopurinol, monitor for rash
Decrease: ampicillin level—H_2 antagonists, proton pump inhibitors, separate by 2 hr

Drug/Lab Test

Increase: eosinophils, ALT, AST
Decrease: conjugated estrogens during pregnancy, Hgb, WBC, platelets
False positive: urine glucose, direct Coomb's test
Interference: urine glucose (Clinitest, Benedict's reagent, cupric SO_4)

NURSING CONSIDERATIONS

Assess:

• **Infection:** characteristics of wound, sputum; urine, stool, earache, fever WBC baseline, periodically; C&S before product therapy, product may be taken as soon as culture is taken

• Hepatic studies: AST, ALT

• Blood studies: WBC, RBC, Hgb, Hct, bleeding time

• **CDAD:** bowel pattern before/during treatment

• Skin eruptions after administration of penicillin to 1 wk after discontinuing product; identify allergies before using
• Respiratory status: rate, character, wheezing, tightness in chest
• **Anaphylaxis:** rash, itching, dyspnea, facial swelling; stop product, notify prescriber, have emergency equipment available

Evaluate:
• Therapeutic response: absence of fever, draining wounds, resolution of infection

Teach patient/family:
• To take oral ampicillin on empty stomach with full glass of water; to use alternate contraception
• All aspects of product therapy: to complete entire course of medication to ensure organism death (10-14 days); that culture may be taken after completed course of medication
• To report sore throat, fever, fatigue, diarrhea (may indicate superinfection); to report rash, other signs of allergy
• That product must be taken in equal intervals around the clock to maintain blood levels
• To wear or carry emergency ID if allergic to penicillins
• **CDAD:** diarrhea with blood or pus; notify prescriber
• **Pregnancy/breastfeeding:** Identify if pregnancy is planned or suspected or if breastfeeding; to use additional contraception if using oral contraception, effect may be decreased

TREATMENT OF ANAPHYLAXIS: Withdraw product, maintain airway; administer EPINEPHrine, aminophylline, O₂, IV corticosteroids

---

ampicillin, sulbactam (Rx)

Unasyn
Func. class.: Antiinfective—broad-spectrum
Chem. class.: Aminopenicillin with β-lactamase inhibitor

ACTION: Interferes with cell wall replication of susceptible organisms; the cell wall, rendered osmotically unstable, swells, bursts from osmotic pressure; lysis due to cell wall autolytic enzymes; combination extends spectrum of activity by β-lactamase inhibition

USES: Skin infections, intraabdominal infections, cellulitis, diabetic foot ulcer, nosocomial pneumonia, gynecologic infections; *Acinetobacter* sp., *Actinomyces* sp., *Bacillus anthracis, Bacteroides* sp., *Bifidobacterium* sp., *Bordetella pertussis, Borrelia burgdorferi, Brucella* sp., *Clostridium* sp., *Corynebacterium diphtheriae/xerosis, Eikenella corrodens, Enterococcus faecalis, Erysipelothrix rhusiopathiae, Escherichia coli, Eubacterium* sp., *Fusobacterium* sp., *Gardnerella vaginalis, Haemophilus influenzae (beta-lactamase negative/positive), Helicobacter pylori, Klebsiella* sp., *Lactobacillus* sp., *Leptospira* sp., *Listeria monocytogenes, Moraxella catarrhalis, Morganella morganii, Neisseria gonorrhoeae, Pasteurella multocida, Peptococcus* sp., *Peptostreptococcus* sp., *Porphyromonas* sp., *Prevotella* sp., *Propionibacterium* sp., *Proteus mirabilis, Proteus vulgaris, Providencia rettgeri, Providencia stuartii, Salmonella* sp., *Shigella* sp., *Staphylococcus aureus (MSSA)/epidermidis/saprophyticus, Streptococcus agalactiae/dysgalactiae/pneumoniae/pyogenes, Treponema pallidum,* viridans streptococci

CONTRAINDICATIONS: Hypersensitivity to penicillins, sulbactam
Precautions: Pregnancy, breastfeeding, neonates, hypersensitivity to cephalosporins/carbapenems, renal disease, mononucleosis, viral infections, syphilis

DOSAGE AND ROUTES
• **Adult/adolescent/child ≥40 kg: IM/IV** 1.5-3 g q6hr, max 4 g/day sulbactam
• **Child ≤40 kg: IV** 150-300 mg/kg/day divided q6hr

Renal disease
- **Adult ≥40 kg: IM/IV** CCr 15-30 mL/min dose q12hr; CCr 5-15 mL/min dose q24hr

Available forms: Powder for inj 1.5 g (1 g ampicillin, 0.5 g sulbactam), 3 g (2 g ampicillin, 1 g sulbactam), 15 g (10 g ampicillin, 5 g sulbactam)

Administer:

IM route
- Reconstitute by adding 3.2 mL sterile water/1.5-g vial; 6.4 mL/3-g vial, give deep in large muscle, aspirate
- Do not use IM in child

Direct IV route
- After diluting 1.5 g/3.2 mL sterile water for inj or 3 g/6.4 mL (250 mg ampicillin/125 mg sulbactam), allow to stand until foaming stops; may give over 15 min, inject slowly

Intermittent IV INFUSION route
- Dilute further in 50 mL or more of D_5W, NaCl; administer within 1 hr after reconstitution; give over 15-30 min, separate doses from aminoglycosides by ≥1 hr

Y-site compatibilities: Alemtuzumab, amifostine, aminocaproic acid, anidulafungin, argatroban, atenolol, bivalirudin, bleomycin, CARBOplatin, carmustine, cefepime, CISplatin, codeine, cyclophosphamide, cytarabine, DAPTOmycin, DAUNOrubicin liposome, dexmedetomidine, DOCEtaxel, doxacurium, DOXOrubicin liposomal, eptifibatide, etoposide, fenoldopam, filgrastim, fludarabine, fluorouracil, foscarnet, gallium, gatifloxacin, gemcitabine, granisetron, hetastarch, irinotecan, levoFLOXacin, linezolid, methotrexate, metroNIDAZOLE, octreotide, oxaliplatin, PACLitaxel, palonosetron, pamidronate, pancuronium, pantoprazole, PEMEtrexed, remifentanil, riTUXimab, rocuronium, tacrolimus, teniposide, thiotepa, tigecycline, tirofiban, TNA, TPN, trastuzumab, vecuronium, vinCRIStine, voriconazole, zoledronic acid

SIDE EFFECTS

CNS: Coma, seizures (high dose)

GI: *Nausea, vomiting, diarrhea,* abdominal pain, CDAD hepatotoxicity

HEMA: Anemia, bone marrow depression, granulocytopenia, leukopenia, eosinophilia

INTEG: Injection site reactions, rash, urticaria

MISC: Anaphylaxis, serum sickness, Stevens-Johnson syndrome

PHARMACOKINETICS

IV: Peak 5 min, IM 1 hr; half-life 50-110 min (ampicillin) 1-1.4 hr (sulbactam), 10%-50% metabolized in liver, 75%-85% of both products excreted in urine, excreted in breast milk, crosses placenta

INTERACTIONS

Increase: bleeding risk—oral anticoagulants; check INR, PT

Increase: ampicillin-induced skin rash—allopurinol, check for rash

Increase: ampicillin level—probenecid

Increase: methotrexate level—methotrexate

Decrease: contraception effect—oral contraceptives, use additional contraception

Drug/Lab Test

False positive: urine glucose, urine protein

NURSING CONSIDERATIONS

Assess:
- For previous sensitivity to penicillin or cephalosporins, cross-sensitivity is common
- **Infection:** characteristics of wound, sputum; take temperature, WBC count, check allergies before using; C&S before product therapy, product may be given as soon as culture is taken
- **CDAD:** bowel pattern before, during treatment
- Hepatic studies: AST, ALT if on long-term therapy or impaired liver function
- **Anaphylaxis:** skin eruptions after administration of ampicillin to 1 wk after discontinuing product

Evaluate:
• Therapeutic response: absence of fever, draining wounds; negative C&S
Teach patient/family:
• To report superinfection: vaginal itching; loose, foul-smelling stools; black furry tongue
• **CDAD:** to report immediately to health care provider symptoms of fever, diarrhea with pus, blood, mucus; may occur up to 4 wk after treatment
• To wear or carry emergency ID if allergic to penicillin products
• **Pregnancy/breastfeeding:** If pregnancy is planned or suspected; use additional contraception if using oral contraceptives

TREATMENT OF ANAPHY-LAXIS: Withdraw product, maintain airway; administer EPINEPHrine, aminophylline, O_2, IV corticosteroids

---

anakinra (Rx)
(an-ah-kin'rah)
Kineret
Func. class.: Antirheumatic (DMARD), immunomodulator
Chem. class.: Recombinant form of human interleukin-1 receptor antagonist (IL-1Ra)

Do not confuse:
anakinra/amikacin
Kineret/Amikin

ACTION: A form of human interleukin-1 receptor antagonist (IL-1Ra) produced by DNA technology; blocks activity of IL-1, thereby resulting in decreased inflammation, cartilage degradation, bone resorption

USES: Reduction in signs and symptoms of moderate to severe active rheumatic arthritis in patients ≥18 yr who have not responded to other disease-modifying agents, neonatal-onset multisystem inflammatory disease

CONTRAINDICATIONS: Hypersensitivity to *Escherichia coli*–derived proteins, latex; sepsis
Precautions: Pregnancy, breastfeeding, children, geriatric patients, renal impairment, active infections, immunosuppression, neoplastic disease, asthma

DOSAGE AND ROUTES
Rheumatoid arthritis
• **Adult: SUBCUT** 100 mg/day at same time of the day
Neonatal-onset multisystem inflammatory disease
• **Adult/child: SUBCUT** 1-2 mg/kg/day, may increase by 0.5-1 mg to max 8 mg/kg/day
Renal dose
• **Adult: SUBCUT** CCr <30 mL/min 100 mg every other day
Available form: Inj 100 mg/0.67 mL prefilled glass syringe
Administer:
SUBCUT route
• Do not use if cloudy, discolored, if particulate is present; protect from light
• Do not admix with other sol or medications; do not use filter; give at same time each day
• Apply cold compress before, after inj, allow sol to warm to room temperature before use
• Use middle thigh, abdomen (outside 2 inches from navel), upper outer buttocks, upper outer area of arm; rotate sites, give inj at least 1 inch from old site; do not give in skin that is bruised, red, tender, hard; remove needle cover immediately before use, pull gently back on plunger, if no blood appears, inject entire contents of prefilled syringe; discard any unused portion
• Store in refrigerator; do not freeze, shake; protect from light

SIDE EFFECTS
CNS: *Headache, fever*
EENT: *Sinusitis*
GI: *Abdominal pain, nausea, diarrhea, vomiting*
HEMA: Neutropenia

INTEG: Rash, *inj site reaction,* allergic reaction
MISC: Flulike symptoms, infection
MS: *Worsening of RA, arthralgia*
RESP: *URI*

PHARMACOKINETICS
Half-life 4-6 hr; eliminated renally, peak 3-7 hr

INTERACTIONS
Increase: risk for severe infection—etanercept, TNF-blocking agents; do not use together
Decrease: antibody reactions—live virus vaccines; avoid concurrent use

Drug/Lab Test
Increase: eosinophils
Decrease: platelets, WBCs, neutrophils

NURSING CONSIDERATIONS
Assess:
• **Rheumatoid arthritis:** pain, stiffness, ROM, swelling of joints, baseline, periodically during treatment
• For inj site pain, swelling; usually occurs after 2 inj (4-5 days)
• **For infection:** increased WBC, fever, flulike symptoms; stop treatment if present; do not start if patient has active infection; a TB test is required before starting treatment, if TB is present, treat before starting treatment
• CBC with differential, neutrophil counts before treatment, monthly × 3 mo, quarterly for up to 1 yr thereafter
• For allergic reactions (rash, dyspnea); discontinue if severe
• For urinary symptoms: decreasing urinary output
• **Pregnancy/breastfeeding:** identify if pregnancy is planned or suspected, or if breastfeeding; use only if clearly needed
Evaluate:
• Therapeutic response: decreased inflammation, pain in joints
Teach patient/family:
• Not to receive vaccines while taking this product; to update vaccines before treatment
• About self-administration, if appropriate: inj should be made in thigh, abdomen, upper arm; rotate sites at least 1 inch from old site; give at same time of day, store in refrigerator, do not freeze, do not shake
• To notify prescriber of allergic reaction, decreasing urine output, signs/symptoms of infection
• **Pregnancy/breastfeeding:** To notify prescriber if pregnancy is planned, suspected; to avoid breastfeeding

> ### ⚠ HIGH ALERT
>
> ### anastrozole (Rx)
> (an-a-stroh'zole)
> Arimidex
> *Func. class.:* Antineoplastic
> *Chem. class.:* Aromatase inhibitor

ACTION: Highly selective nonsteroidal aromatase inhibitor that lowers serum estradiol concentrations; many breast cancers have strong estrogen receptors

USES: Advanced breast carcinoma in estrogen receptor–positive patients (postmenopausal); patients with advanced disease taking tamoxifen, adjunct therapy
Unlabeled uses: Uterine leiomyomata, endometriosis

CONTRAINDICATIONS: Pregnancy, breastfeeding, hypersensitivity
Precautions: Children, geriatric patients, premenopausal women, osteoporosis, hepatic/cardiac disease

DOSAGE AND ROUTES
• **Adult: PO** 1 mg/day, max 5 yr, may also combine with tamoxifen for up to 10 yr
Available forms: Tabs 1 mg
Administer:
• Give without regard to meals at same time of day
• Store in light-resistant container at room temperature

SIDE EFFECTS
CNS: *Hot flashes, headache, lightheadedness,* depression, dizziness,

confusion, insomnia, anxiety, fatigue, mood changes
CV: Chest pain, *hypertension,* thrombophlebitis, *edema,* angina
GI: *Nausea, vomiting,* altered taste leading to anorexia, diarrhea, constipation, abdominal pain, dry mouth
GU: Vaginal bleeding, vaginal dryness, pelvic pain
INTEG: *Rash,* Stevens-Johnson syndrome, anaphylaxis, angioedema
MISC: Hypercholesterolemia
MS: Bone pain, myalgia, back pain, arthralgia, fractures
RESP: Cough, sinusitis, dyspnea
EENT: Pharyngitis

PHARMACOKINETICS
Peak 4-7 hr; half-life 50 hr; metabolized in liver 85%, excreted in feces, urine, terminal half-life 50 hr

INTERACTIONS
• Do not use with oral contraceptives, estrogen, tamoxifen, androstenedione, DHEA, may decrease the action of anastrozole
Drug/Lab Test
Increase: GGT, AST, ALT, alk phos, cholesterol, LDL

NURSING CONSIDERATIONS
Assess:
• Bone mineral density, cholesterol, lipid panel, periodically
• **Serious skin reactions:** Stevens-Johnson syndrome
Evaluate:
• Therapeutic response: decreased tumor size, spread of malignancy
Teach patient/family:
• To report any complaints, side effects to prescriber
• That vaginal bleeding, pruritus, hot flashes are reversible after discontinuing treatment
• To report continued vaginal bleeding immediately
• That tumor flare—increase in size of tumor, increased bone pain—may occur and will subside rapidly; may take analgesics for pain

• **Pregnancy/breastfeeding:** to tell prescriber if pregnancy is planned or suspected; do not use in pregnancy or breastfeeding during or for 15 days after product is stopped
• To take adequate calcium and vitamin D due to risk for bone loss/fractures

---

antithymocyte
See lymphocyte immune globulin

---

anidulafungin (Rx)
(a-nid-yoo-luh-fun´jin)
Eraxis
Func. class.: Antifungal, systemic
Chem. class.: Echinocandin

ACTION: Inhibits fungal enzyme synthesis; causes direct damage to fungal cell wall

USES: Esophageal candidiasis, *Candida albicans, C. glabrata, C. parapsilosis, C. tropicalis*

CONTRAINDICATIONS: Hypersensitivity to product, other echinocandins
Precautions: Pregnancy, breastfeeding, children, severe hepatic disease

DOSAGE AND ROUTES
Candidemia and other *Candida* infections
• **Adult:** IV 200-mg loading dose on day 1, then 100 mg/day × 14 days or more until last positive culture
Esophageal candidiasis
• **Adult:** IV 200 mg/day × 14-21 days
Available forms: Powder for inj, lyophilized 50 mg/vial for IV use
Administer:

IV route
• Visually inspect prepared infusions for particulate matter and discoloration, do not use if present; give by IV infusion only, after dilution
• **Reconstitution:** Reconstitute each 50-mg or 100-mg vial/15 mL or 30 mL

of sterile water for injection, respectively (3.33 mg/mL)

• **Storage:** Reconstituted solutions are stable for up to 24 hr at room temperature

• **Dilution:** Do not use any other diluents besides D5W or sodium chloride 0.9% (NS)

• **Preparation of the 200-mg loading dose infusion:** Withdraw the contents of either four 50-mg reconstituted vials OR two 100-mg reconstituted vials and add to an IV infusion bag or bottle containing 200 mL of D5W or NS to give a total infusion volume of 260 mL

• **Preparation of the 100-mg daily infusion:** Withdraw the contents of one 100-mg reconstituted vial OR two 50-mg reconstituted vials and add to an IV infusion bag or bottle containing 100 mL of D5W or NS to give a total infusion volume of 130 mL

• **Preparation of a 50-mg daily infusion:** Withdraw the contents of one 50-mg reconstituted vial and add to an IV infusion bag or bottle containing 50 mL of D5W or NS to give a total infusion volume of 65 mL

• **Storage:** Diluted solutions are stable for up to 48 hr at temperatures up to 77° F (25° C) or for 72 hr if stored frozen

Intermittent IV Infusion

• Do not mix or co-infuse with other medications

• Administer as a slow IV infusion at a rate of 1.4 mL/min or 84 mL/h; the minimum duration of infusion is 180 min for the 200-mg dose, 90 min for the 100-mg dose, and 45 min for the 50-mg dose

• Store reconstituted vials at 59°-86° F for up to 24 hr, do not freeze (dehydrated alcohol); store reconstituted vials at 36°-46° F (sterile water) for up to 24 hr, do not freeze

Y-site compatibilities: Acyclovir, alemtuzumab, alfentanil, allopurinol, amifostine, amikacin, aminocaproic acid, aminophylline, amiodarone, amphotericin B lipid complex, amphotericin B liposome, ampicillin, ampicillin sulbactam, argatroban, arsenic trioxide, atenolol, atracurium, azithromycin, aztreonam, bivalirudin, bleomycin, bumetanide, buprenorphine, busulfan, butorphanol, calcium chloride/gluconate, CARBOplatin, carmustine, caspofungin, ceFAZolin, cefepime, cefotaxime, cefoTEtan, cefOXitin, cefTAZidime, ceftizoxime, cefTRIAXone, cefuroxime, chloramphenicol, chlorproMAZINE, cimetidine, ciprofloxacin, cisatracurium, CISplatin, clindamycin, cyclophosphamide, cycloSPORINE, cytarabine, dacarbazine, DACTINomycin, DAUNOrubicin liposome, DAUNOrubicin hydrochloride, dexamethasone, dexmedetomidine, dexrazoxane, digoxin, diltiazem, diphenhydrAMINE, DOBUtamine, DOCEtaxel, dolasetron, DOPamine, doripenem, doxacurium, DOXOrubicin, DOXOrubicin liposomal, doxycycline, droperidol, enalaprilat, ePHEDrine, EPINEPHrine, epiRUBicin, eptifibatide, erythromycin, esmolol, etoposide, etoposide phosphate, famotidine, fenoldopam, fentaNYL, fluconazole, fludarabine, fluorouracil, foscarnet, fosphenytoin, furosemide, gallium nitrate, ganciclovir, gatifloxacin, gemcitabine, gentamicin, glycopyrrolate, granisetron, haloperidol, heparin, hydrALAZINE, hydrocortisone, HYDROmorphone, hydrOXYzine, IDArubicin, ifosfamide, imipenem-cilastatin, inamrinone, insulin (regular), irinotecan, isoproterenol, ketorolac, labetalol, leucovorin, levoFLOXacin, lidocaine, linezolid injection, LORazepam, mannitol, mechlorethamine, melphalan, meperidine, meropenem, mesna, metaraminol, methotrexate, methyldopate, methylPREDNISolone, metoclopramide, metoprolol, metroNIDAZOLE, midazolam, milrinone, mitoMYcin, mitoXANTRONE, mivacurium, morphine, moxifloxacin, mycophenolate mofetil, nafcillin, naloxone, nesiritide, niCARdipine, nitroglycerin, nitroprusside, norepinephrine, octreotide, ondansetron, oxaliplatin, oxytocin, PACLitaxel, palonosetron, pamidronate, pancuronium, pantoprazole, PEMEtrexed, pentamidine, pentazocine, PENTobarbital, PHENobarbital,

phentolamine, phenylephrine, piperacillin/
tazobactam, polymyxin B, potassium ace-
tate/chloride, procainamide, prochlorperazine, promethazine, propranolol,
quiNIDine, quinupristin-dalfopristin,
raNITIdine, remifentanil, rocuronium,
sodium acetate, streptozocin, succinylcholine, SUFentanil, sulfamethoxazole-
trimethoprim, tacrolimus, teniposide,
theophylline, thiopental, thiotepa, ticarcillin, ticarcillin/clavulanate, tirofiban,
tobramycin, topotecan, trimethobenzamide, vancomycin, vasopressin,
vecuronium, verapamil, vinBLAStine,
vinCRIStine, vinorelbine, voriconazole,
zidovudine, zoledronic acid

SIDE EFFECTS
CNS: Dizziness, *headache*, fever,
depression
CV: DVT, hypotension, chest pain, edema
GI: *Nausea, anorexia, vomiting,
diarrhea*
META: Hypokalemia
RESP: Dyspnea, cough
HEMA: Anemia, thrombocytopenia
INTEG: *Rash*, urticaria, itching, flushing
META: Hyperkalemia
GU: UTI
EENT: Oral candidiasis
MS: *Back pain*

PHARMACOKINETICS
Steady state after loading dose, half-life
40-50 hr, protein binding 99%, crosses
placenta, no metabolism

INTERACTIONS
None known
Drug/Lab Test
Increase: amylase, bilirubin, creatinine,
lipase, PT, alk phos, AST, ALT
Decrease: Magnesium, potassium,
glucose

NURSING CONSIDERATIONS
Assess:
• **Infection:** clearing of cultures during
treatment; obtain culture at baseline and
throughout treatment; product may be
started as soon as culture is taken, those

with HIV pharyngeal candidiasis may
need additional antifungals
• Hepatic studies before, during treatment: bilirubin, AST, ALT, alk phos, as
needed; also uric acid
• **GI symptoms:** frequency of stools,
cramping; if severe diarrhea occurs,
electrolytes may need to be given
Evaluate:
• Therapeutic response: decreased symptoms of *Candida* infection, negative culture
Teach patient/family:
• The reason for product, expected result
• **Anaphylaxis:** To report anaphylaxis
symptoms immediately
• **Pregnancy/breastfeeding:** to notify prescriber if pregnancy is suspected, planned;
to use nonhormonal form of contraception
while taking this product; to avoid breastfeeding

RARELY USED

antihemophilic factor Fc fusion protein (Rx)
(an-tee-hee-moe-fil′ik fak′tor)
Eloctate
Func. class.: Hemostatic

USES: Hemophilia A (congenital factor VIII deficiency), control/prevention
of bleeding, perioperative management
of surgical bleeding

DOSAGE AND ROUTES
**Hemophilia A (congenital factor VIII
deficiency)**
• **Adults, adolescents, children, infants,
and neonates:** IV INFUSION Infuse dose
≤10 mL/min; Dose (IU) = body weight
(kg) × desired factor VIII increase (IU/
dL or % of normal) × 0.5 (IU/kg per IU/
dL) *OR* estimated increment of factor
VIII (IU/dL or % of normal) = [total
dose (IU)/body weight (kg)] × 2 (IU/dL
per IU/kg)
Control/prevention of bleeding
• **Adults, adolescents, children, infants,
and neonates:** Dose and duration of

treatment depend on the severity of the factor VIII deficiency, the location and extent of bleeding, and the patient's clinical condition

Perioperative management of surgical bleeding

• **Adults, adolescents, children, infants, and neonates:** Dose and duration of treatment depend on the severity of the factor VIII deficiency, the location and extent of bleeding, and the patient's clinical condition

Routine bleeding prophylaxis to prevent/reduce the frequency of bleeding episodes

• **IV** Initially, 50 IU/kg q4days; adjust dose based on response

> **⚠ HIGH ALERT**
>
> **apalutamide**
> (a′puh-loo′tuh-mide)
> Erleada
> *Func. class.:* Antineoplastic, hormone antagonist
> *Chem. class.:* Anti-androgen

ACTION: An androgen receptor inhibitor that binds directly to the ligand-binding domain of the androgen receptor. It inhibits androgen receptor translocation and DNA binding and impedes androgen receptor–mediated transcription

USES: For the treatment of nonmetastatic castration-resistant prostate cancer

CONTRAINDICATIONS: Pregnancy

Precautions: Bone fractures, breastfeeding, contraception requirements, driving or operating machinery, geriatric patients, infertility, male-mediated teratogenicity, reproductive risk, seizure disorder, seizures

DOSAGE AND ROUTES
Nonmetastatic, castration-resistant prostate cancer

• **Adults: PO** 240 mg q day until disease progression or toxicity; a gonadotropin-releasing hormone (GnRH) analog should be given concurrently or a bilateral orchiectomy should have been performed

Available forms: Tablet 60 mg

SIDE EFFECTS
CNS: Fatigue
CV: Hypertension, peripheral edema, heart failure, MI
GI: Diarrhea, anorexia, nausea, weight loss
GU: Hot flashes
HEMA: Anemia, leukopenia, lymphopenia
INTEG: Rash
META: Hypercholesterolemia, hypertriglyceridemia, hyperkalemia
MS: Arthralgia, bone fractures

PHARMACOKINETICS
96% plasma protein binding, primarily metabolized by CYP2C8 and CYP3A4 to its active metabolite, half-life 3 days, excreted 65% urine (unchanged), 24% feces (unchanged)

INTERACTIONS
Decrease: effects of CYP3A4 substrates—abemaciclib, cyclosporine, tacrolimus, sirolimus, docetaxel, tamoxifen, paclitaxel, cyclophosphamide, doxorubicin, erlotinib, etoposide, ifosfamide, teniposide, vinblastine, vincristine, vindesine, imatinib, irinotecan, sorafenib, sunitinib, vemurafenib, temsirolimus, anastrozole, gefitinib, azole antifungals, macrolides, clarithromycin, erythromycin, telithromycin, dapsone, tricyclic antidepressants, SSRIs, some miscellaneous antidepressants, antipsychotics, opioids, benzodiazepines, some hypnotics, buspirone, statins, calcium channel blockers, class I/III antidysrhythmics, PDE5 inhibitors, sex hormone agonists/antagonists, H1-receptor antagonists, protease inhibitors, non-nucleoside reverse transcriptase inhibitors; avoid concurrent use

NURSING CONSIDERATIONS
Assess
• **Possible bone fractures:** monitor and manage patients at risk for bone fractures; consider the use of bone-targeted agents. Falls and fractures are possible

• **Seizures:** use with caution in those with pre-existing seizure disorders; permanently discontinue if seizure occurs

• **Geriatric patients:** may be at increased risk for related adverse reactions; monitor closely for adverse reactions

• Pregnancy/breastfeeding: contraindicated in pregnancy, as it can cause fetal harm and potential loss of pregnancy; product is not indicated in female patients; male infertility is a possibility

Evaluate:
• Therapeutic response: decrease in prostatic size, decrease in spread of cancer

Teach patient/family
• Male-mediated teratogenicity: that product is not indicated for use in females and is contraindicated during pregnancy; that males with female partners of reproductive potential should avoid pregnancy and use effective contraception during and for at least 3 mo after treatment; that product may impair male fertility

• **Seizures:** about an increase in the risk of seizure and the risk of engaging in any activity where sudden loss of consciousness could cause harm to themselves or others (driving or operating machinery). It is unknown whether antiepileptic medications will prevent seizures

---

⚠ HIGH ALERT

apixaban (Rx)
(a-pix'-a-ban)
Eliquis
Func. class.: Anticoagulant
Chem. class.: Factor Xa inhibitor

ACTION: Inhibits factor Xa and thereby decreases thrombin and clot formation

USES: Deep venous thrombosis (DVT) after hip or knee replacement, to prevent stroke and embolism in atrial fibrillation (nonvalvular)

CONTRAINDICATIONS: Hypersensitivity, active bleeding
Precautions: Breastfeeding, dialysis, hepatic/renal disease, labor, pregnancy, surgery, prosthetic heart valves

> **Black Box Warning:** Abrupt discontinuation, epidural, spinal anesthesia, lumbar puncture

DOSAGE AND ROUTES
DVT or pulmonary embolism (PE)
• **Adult: PO** 10 mg bid × 7 days, then 5 mg bid ≥6 mo, to reduce recurrence >6 mo 2.5 mg bid
Stroke prophylaxis and systemic embolism prophylaxis
• **Adult: PO** 5 mg bid; in those with any 2 of the following—age ≥80 yr, body weight ≤60 kg, or serum creatinine ≥1.5 mg/dL—reduce the dose to 2.5 mg bid. Also decrease the dose to 2.5 mg bid (strong inhibitor of both CYP3A4 and P-glycoprotein)
Reduction in risk of recurrent DVT and/or PE after completion of treatment for acute DVT or PE
• **Adult:** 2.5 mg bid daily after at least 6 mo of treatment for DVT or PE
DVT prophylaxis and PE prophylaxis in patients undergoing knee or hip replacement surgery
• **Adult:** 2.5 mg bid × 12 days after knee replacement surgery or for 35 days after hip replacement surgery. Give initial dose 12-24 hr after surgery
Renal dose:
• No dosage adjustment needed when used for treatment/prevention of venous thromboembolism

---

• **Adult: PO** serum CCr ≥1.5 mg/dL, ≤60 kg, and/or ≥80 yr; if two of these three characteristics are present, then decrease dose to 2.5 mg bid

Hemodialysis end-stage renal disease maintained on hemodialysis

• **Adult: PO** 5 mg bid; reduce to 2.5 mg bid if patient is ≥80 yr or ≤60 kg

Available forms: Tabs 2.5, 5 mg

Administer:

• May be taken without regard to food

• If unable to swallow whole, may crush and suspend the tablet in 60 mL 5% dextrose solution; give immediately via NG

• If a dose is missed, it should be taken as soon as possible on the same day. Twice-daily dosing should be resumed. Do not double the dose to make up for a missed dose.

SIDE EFFECTS

CNS: Syncope, intracranial bleeding
CV: Hypotension
HEMA: Severe bleeding
INTEG: Rash
MISC: Hypersensitivity

PHARMACOKINETICS

Peak 3-4 hr, half-life 12 hr

INTERACTIONS

Increase: bleeding risk—antiplatelets, other anticoagulants, salicylates, NSAIDs, SNRIs, SSRIs, thrombolytics; avoid concurrent use

Increase: apixaban effect—CYP3A4 inhibitors, P-gp; give 2.5 mg apixaban

Decrease: apixaban effect—strong inducers of CYP3A4 and also P-glycoprotein (carBAMazepine, ketoconazole, itraconazole, phenytoin, rifAMPin); use lower dose

Drug/Herb
Decrease: apixaban effect—St. John's wort; avoid concurrent use

Drug/Lab Test
Increase: PT, PTT, INR, coagulation studies

NURSING CONSIDERATIONS

Assess:

• **Bleeding:** bleeding may occur from any body system; may be fatal if severe

Black Box Warning: Neurologic status: monitor for impairment, including numbness, paresthesia, weakness, confusion, back pain, bowel/bladder impairment; notify prescriber immediately

Black Box Warning: Abrupt discontinuation: do not discontinue abruptly; if bleeding occurs, consider using another anticoagulant to prevent thromboembolic events

Black Box Warning: Epidural, spinal anesthesia, lumbar puncture: avoid use in these conditions, risk of hematoma and permanent paralysis, may be increased with use of other anticoagulants, thrombolytics, antiplatelets

• **Hypersensitivity:** rash, itching, chills, fever; report to prescriber

• **Beers:** avoid in older adults; may cause increased risk of bleeding, decreased creatinine clearance

Evaluate:
Therapeutic response: prevention/treatment of DVT, adequate anticoagulation

Teach patient/family:

Black Box Warning: Not to discontinue without prescriber approval; stroke, clots may occur

• **Bleeding:** to report bleeding, bruising, confusion, weakness, numbness of limbs

• To avoid OTC products, supplements, herbs, unless approved by prescriber; serious product interactions may occur

• To carry emergency ID with product taken; to inform all health providers of product use

• To report hypersensitivity reactions: rash, chills, fever, itching

• **Pregnancy/breastfeeding:** To avoid breastfeeding; it is not known if the product appears in breast milk; to notify prescriber if pregnancy is planned or suspected

---

RARELY USED

apomorphine (Rx)
(ah-poe-more'feen)

Apokyn

Func. class.: Antiparkinson agent
Chem. class.: DOPamine agonist,
non-ergot

USES: For use as rescue of "off" episodes associated with advanced Parkinson's disease

CONTRAINDICATIONS: Hypersensitivity to this product, sulfites, or benzyl alcohol, IV use, major psychotic disorder; concurrent treatment with drugs of the 5-HT₃ antagonist class (e.g., ondansetron, granisetron, alosetron)

DOSAGE AND ROUTES
• **Adult: Test dose: SUBCUT** 0.2 mL (2 mg) (test dose) where B/P can be closely monitored (before dose and 20, 40, 60 min after); if tolerated and patient responds, then begin with 0.2 mL (2 mg); may increase by 1 mg every few days, max 0.6 mL (6 mg); if the test dose of 0.2 mL (2 mg) is tolerated but the patient does not respond, give a test dose of 0.4 mL (4 mg) no sooner than 2 hr after the 0.2 mL (2 mg) test dose, where BP can be closely monitored (before dose and 20, 40, and 60 min after the dose); if the 0.4 mL (4 mg) test dose is tolerated, the starting dose should be 0.3 mL (3 mg); may be increased by 1 mg every few days as required, max 0.6 mL (6 mg). If the 0.4 mL (4 mg) test dose is not tolerated, administer a test dose of 0.3 mL (3 mg) no sooner than 2 hr after the 0.4 mL (4 mg) test dose where BP can be closely monitored (before dose and 20, 40, and 60 min after the dose); if the 0.3 mL (3 mg) test dose is not tolerated, begin with 0.2 mL (2 mg); may be increased by 0.1 mL (1 mg) every few days as required, max 0.4 mL (4 mg; outpatient)
• **Usual dosage: SUBCUT** 0.3-0.6 mL (3-6 mg), average frequency three times a day

apraclonidine ophthalmic
See Appendix B

apremilast (Rx)
(a-pre'mi-last)

Otezla

Func. class.: Musculoskeletal agents: disease-modifying antirheumatic drugs (DMARDs)

ACTION: A phosphodiesterase-4 (PDE4) inhibitor specific for cyclic adenosine monophosphate (cAMP). Inhibition of PDE4 results in an increase in intracellular concentration of cAMP, with a partial inhibition of proinflammatory mediators and an increase in the production of some antiinflammatory mediators

USES: Treatment of active psoriatic arthritis; severe plaque psoriasis (in those not a candidate for phototherapy)

CONTRAINDICATIONS: Hypersensitivity
Precautions: Pregnancy, breastfeeding, depression/suicidal, renal disease (CCr <30 mL/min)

DOSAGES AND ROUTES
Active psoriatic arthritis/severe plaque psoriasis
• **Adult: PO** To reduce the risk for gastrointestinal symptoms, titrate to a final dose of 30 mg bid; day 1: 10 mg PO AM; day 2: 10 mg AM and PM; day 3: 10 mg AM and 20 mg PM; day 4: 20 mg AM and PM; day 5: 20 mg AM and 30 mg PM; day 6 and thereafter: 30 mg bid
Renal dose
• **Adult: PO** CCr ≥30 mL/min: no change; CCr <30 mL/min: 30 mg every day. Initially, 10 mg AM days 1-3; 20 mg AM days 4 and 5; 30 mg every day for day 6 and thereafter
Available forms: Tab 30 mg; starter pack

Side effects: *italics* = common; red = life-threatening

Administer:
• Give whole, do not crush, break, or chew; give without regard to meals

SIDE EFFECTS

CNS: *Headache,* depression, suicidal ideation, fatigue, insomnia
GI: Diarrhea, nausea, vomiting, abdominal pain, frequent bowel movements, dyspepsia, weight loss
RESP: URI, pharyngitis, bronchitis
SYST: Hypersensitivity reactions
MS: Back pain

PHARMACOKINETICS
68% protein binding; metabolized by CYP3A4; half-life 6-9 hr; excreted urine 58%, feces 39%; peak 2.5 hr

INTERACTIONS
Decrease: apremilast—CYP3A4 inducers (rifAMPin, isoniazid, pyrazinamide, barbiturates, phenytoin, carBAMazepine, enzalutamide); avoid concurrent use
Drug/Herb
Decrease: apremilast—CYP3A4 inducers (St. John's wort); avoid concurrent use

NURSING CONSIDERATIONS
Assess:
• **Psoriatic arthritis/severe plaque psoriasis:** assess for hypersensitivity reactions
• For depression and suicidal ideation, mood changes
• For renal failure or severe renal impairment (CrCl <30 mL/min), dosage reduction is required
• For significant or unexplained weight loss; report weight loss as therapy may need to be discontinued
• **Pregnancy and breastfeeding:** if pregnancy is planned or suspected; use only if benefits outweigh fetal risk; if used during pregnancy, call 877-311-8972; cautious use in breastfeeding
Evaluate:
• Therapeutic response: resolution of symptoms of psoriatic arthritis or plaque psoriasis
Teach patient/family:
• To report new rash, hypersensitivity reactions; report change in urine output, renal disease history

• To use caution in use in pregnancy and breastfeeding
• To be alert for depression and suicidal ideation, mood changes; if these occur, notify prescriber immediately

---

aprepitant (PO) (Rx)
(ap-re′pi-tant)
Emend
fosaprepitant (IV) (Rx)
Emend
Func. class.: Antiemetic
Chem. class.: Neurokinin antagonist

Do not confuse:
aprepitant/fosaprepitant

ACTION: Selective antagonist of human substance P/neurokinin 1 (NK_1) receptors that decreases emetic reflex

USES: Prevention of nausea/vomiting associated with cancer chemotherapy (highly emetogenic/moderately emetogenic), including high-dose CISplatin; used in combination with other antiemetics; postoperative nausea/vomiting

CONTRAINDICATIONS: Hypersensitivity to this product, polysorbate 80, pimozide
Precautions: Pregnancy, breastfeeding, children, geriatric patients, hepatic disease

DOSAGE AND ROUTES
Prevention of nausea/vomiting after chemotherapy
• **Adult:** PO Day 1 (1 hr before chemotherapy) aprepitant 125 mg with 12 mg dexamethasone PO, with 32 mg ondansetron IV; day 2 aprepitant 80 mg with 8 mg dexamethasone PO; day 3 aprepitant 80 mg with 8 mg dexamethasone PO; day 4 only dexamethasone 8 mg PO; IV INFUSION 150 mg fosaprepitant over 15 min, 30 min before chemotherapy **Child ≥12 yr:** PO caps 125 mg 1 hr prior to chemotherapy; suspension 3 mg/kg 1 hr prior to chemotherapy, max 125 mg

---

Prevention of postoperative nausea/vomiting
• **Adult:** PO 40 mg within 3 hr of induction of anesthesia

Available forms: Caps 40, 80, 125 mg; lyophilized powder for inj, 150 mg; combo pack cap 80-125 mg; powder for oral suspension 125 mg/pouch

Administer:
• Give with dexamethasone and a 5-HT3 antagonist

PO route
• Do not break, crush, or chew
• PO on 3-day schedule, give with full glass of water 1 hr before chemotherapy, with or without food, given with other antiemetics
• Do not open or break capsules
• **Suspension:** Use for children unable to swallow capsules, administer slowly, store at room temperature
• Store at room temperature; keep in original bottles, blisters

Intermittent IV INFUSION route
• **Reconstitution:** use aseptic technique; inject 5 mL 0.9% NaCl into the vial, directing stream to wall of vial to prevent foam; swirl (do not shake)
• Prepare infusion bag 145 mL/150 mg; do not dilute, reconstitute with any divalent cations such as calcium, magnesium, including LR, Hartmann's sol
• Withdraw entire volume from vial, transfer to infusion bag; total volume 115 mL (1 mg/1 mL)
• Gently invert bag 2-3 times; reconstituted sol stable for 24 hr at lower room temperature or <25° C
• Visually inspect for particulates, discoloration
• Infuse over 20-30 min, stable for 24 hr at room temperature, 30 min prior to chemotherapy
• Monitor for IV site reactions

SIDE EFFECTS
CNS: *Headache, dizziness,* insomnia, weakness, headache, fever
CV: Bradycardia, hypo/hypertension
GI: *Diarrhea, constipation,* abdominal pain, *nausea,* vomiting, heartburn
HEMA: Anemia

INTEG: Pruritus, rash, urticaria, injection reaction
MISC: Fatigue, dehydration, fever, alopecia

PHARMACOKINETICS
Absorption 60%-65%, peak 4 hr (PO) infusions end (IV), metabolized in liver by CYP3A4 enzymes to active metabolite, half-life 9-12 hr, 95% protein bound, not excreted in kidneys, crosses blood-brain barrier

INTERACTIONS
Increase: levels of each product—ALPRAZolam, midazolam, triazolam; decrease benzodiazepine dose
Increase: aprepitant action—CYP3A4 inhibitors (ketoconazole, itraconazole, nefazodone, troleandomycin, clarithromycin, ritonavir, nelfinavir, diltiaZEM)
Increase: action of CYP3A4 substrates (pimozide, dexamethasone, methylPREDNISolone, midazolam, ALPRAZolam, triazolam, DOCEtaxel, PACLitaxel, etoposide, irinotecan, imatinib, ifosfamide, vinorelbine, vinBLAStine, vinCRIStine), avoid concurrent use
Decrease: aprepitant action—CYP3A4 inducers (rifAMPin, carBAMazepine, phenytoin)
Decrease: action of CYP2C9 substrates (warfarin, phenytoin), hormonal contraceptives
Decrease: action of both products—PARoxetine
Drug/Food
Decrease: effect—grapefruit juice
Drug/Lab
Increase: AST/ALT, alkaline phosphatase
Decrease: Hgb, WBC

NURSING CONSIDERATIONS
Assess:
• **For hypersensitivity reactions:** pruritus, rash, urticaria, anaphylaxis
• CV status: hypo/hypertension, bradycardia, tachycardia, DVT
• For absence of nausea, vomiting during chemotherapy
• CBC, LFTs, creatinine baseline and periodically

Side effects: *italics* = common; red = life-threatening

Evaluate:

• Therapeutic response: absence of nausea, vomiting during cancer chemotherapy, or post-op

Teach patient/family:

• To take only as prescribed; to take first dose 1 hr before chemotherapy or within 3 hr of surgery to prevent nausea, vomiting

• To report all medications and herbals to prescriber before taking this medication

• That those patients also taking warfarin should have clotting monitored closely during 2-wk period after administration of aprepitant

• **Pregnancy/breastfeeding:** to use nonhormonal form of contraception while taking this agent and for 1 mo thereafter; oral contraceptive effect may be decreased; to avoid breastfeeding

---

arformoterol (Rx)

(ar-for-moe′ter-ole)

Brovana

Func. class.: Long-acting adrenergic β₂-agonist, sympathomimetic, bronchodilator

Do not confuse:

Brovana/Boniva

ACTION: Causes bronchodilation by action on β₂ (pulmonary) receptors by increasing levels of cAMP, which relaxes smooth muscle; produces bronchodilation and CNS, cardiac stimulation, as well as increased diuresis and gastric acid secretion; longer acting than isoproterenol

USES: Maintenance bronchospasm prevention in COPD, including chronic bronchitis, emphysema

CONTRAINDICATIONS: Hypersensitivity to sympathomimetics, product, racemic formoterol; tachydysrhythmias, severe cardiac disease, heart block, children, monotherapy in asthma

Precautions: Pregnancy, breastfeeding, cardiac disorders, hyperthyroidism, diabetes mellitus, hypertension, prostatic hypertrophy, angle-closure glaucoma, seizures, hypoglycemia

Black Box Warning: Asthma-related death

DOSAGE AND ROUTES

COPD

• **Adult:** NEB 15 mcg, bid, AM, PM

Available forms: Inh sol 15 mcg/2 mL

Administer:

• By nebulization only; no dilution needed; give over 5-10 min; sol should be colorless

• Store in refrigerator; if stored at room temperature, discard after 6 wk or if past expiration date, whichever is sooner

SIDE EFFECTS

CNS: *Tremors, paralysis*

CV: Chest pain AV block, heart failure, prolonged QT, supraventricular tachycardia

EENT: Sinusitis

GI: Diarrhea, constipation

MISC: Bad taste/smell changes, hypokalemia, anaphylaxis, *hypoglycemia, flu-like symptoms*

MS: Muscle cramps, back pain

RESP: Dyspnea, bronchospasm

PHARMACOKINETICS

Onset 10-20 min: peak 1-1$^1/_2$ hr; duration 4-6 hr; half-life (COPD) 26 hr; extensively metabolized by direct conjugation by CYP2D6, CYP2C19; crosses placenta; protein binding 52%-65%; excreted in urine 63%, feces 11%

INTERACTIONS

Increase: QT prolongation—Class IA/III antidysrhythmics, MAOIs, tricyclics

Increase: hyperkalemia—theophylline

Increase: ECG changes/hypokalemia—potassium-losing diuretics

Increase: action of nebulized bronchodilators

Increase: action of arformoterol—tricyclics, MAOIs, other adrenergics; do not use together

---

Decrease: arformoterol action, increased asthma-related death—other β-blockers; avoid concurrent use

Drug/Herb

Increase: stimulation—caffeine (cola nut, green/black tea, guarana, yerba maté, coffee, chocolate)

NURSING CONSIDERATIONS
Assess:

Black Box Warning: **Asthma-related death:** Respiratory function: vital capacity, forced expiratory volume, ABGs; lung sounds, heart rate, rhythm, B/P, sputum (baseline, peak); actively deteriorating COPD and asthma-related death may occur; a rescue inhaler should be readily available

- Whether patient has received theophylline therapy, other bronchodilators before giving dose
- Patient's ability to self-medicate
- For evidence of allergic reactions
- **For paradoxical bronchospasm:** hold medication, notify prescriber if bronchospasm occurs

Evaluate:

- Therapeutic response: absence of dyspnea, wheezing after 1 hr, improved airway exchange, improved ABGs

Teach patient/family:

Black Box Warning: **Asthma-related death:** to use exactly as prescribed; that death has resulted from asthma with products similar to this one; to have a rescue inhaler always

- How to self-medicate
- Not to use OTC medications because excess stimulation may occur
- That an opened unit-dose vial should be used right away, store vials in refrigerator
- To notify prescriber if more frequent use is needed
- **Pregnancy/breastfeeding:** use only if benefits outweigh fetal risk; cautious use in breastfeeding

⚠ **HIGH ALERT**

argatroban (Rx)
(are-ga-troe′ban)
Func. class.: Anticoagulant
Chem. class.: Direct thrombin inhibitor

Do not confuse:
argatroban/Aggrastat

ACTION: Direct inhibitor of thrombin; it reversibly binds to thrombin active site

USES: Anticoagulation prevention/treatment of thrombosis in heparin-induced thrombocytopenia; adjunct to percutaneous coronary intervention (PCI) in those with history of HIT, deep vein thrombosis, pulmonary embolism

CONTRAINDICATIONS: Hypersensitivity, overt major bleeding
Precautions: Pregnancy, breastfeeding, children, intracranial bleeding, renal function impairment, hepatic disease, severe hypertension, after lumbar puncture, spinal anesthesia, major surgery/trauma, congenital/acquired bleeding, GI ulcers, abrupt discontinuation

DOSAGE AND ROUTES
Prevention/treatment of thrombosis (heparin-induced thrombocytopenia)
- **Adult:** CONT IV INFUSION 2 mcg/kg/min; adjust dose until steady-state aPTT is 1.5-3 × initial baseline, max 100 sec, max dose 10 mcg/kg/min
- **Infant/child/adolescent (unlabeled):** CONT IV INFUSION 0.75 mcg/kg/min, monitor aPTT q2hr until stable, then at least daily

Hepatic dose
- **Adult:** CONT INFUSION 0.5 mcg/kg/min; adjust rate based on aPTT

Percutaneous coronary intervention (PCI) in HIT
- **Adult:** IV INFUSION 25 mcg/kg/min and bolus of 350 mcg/kg given over 3-5 min, check ACT 5-10 min after bolus completed, proceed if ACT >300 sec; if ACT <300 sec, give another 150 mcg/kg BOL,

increase infusion rate to 30 mcg/kg/min, recheck ACT in 5-10 min; if ACT >450 sec, decrease infusion rate to 15 mcg/kg/min, recheck ACT in 5-10 min; when ACT is therapeutic, continue for duration of procedure

DIC (unlabeled)
• **Adult: CONT IV** 0.7 mcg/kg/min
Available forms: Inj 100 mg/mL (2.5 mL; must dilute 100-fold), 50 mg/50 mL, 125 mg/125 mL
Administer:
• Avoid all IM inj that may cause bleeding

IV, direct route
• **For PCI:** 350 mg/kg bol and continuous infusion of 25 mcg/kg/min; check ACT 5-10 min after bolus
Intermittent IV INFUSION route
• **Dilute** in 0.9% NaCl, D$_5$W, LR to a final concentrations of 1 mg/mL; **dilute** each 2.5-mL vial 100-fold by mixing with 250 mL of diluent, mix by repeated inversion of the diluent bag for 1 min; may briefly be slightly hazy
• Dosage adjustment may be made after review of aPTT, max 10 mcg/kg/min

SIDE EFFECTS
CNS: *Fever,* intracranial bleeding, headache
CV: Atrial fibrillation, coronary thrombosis, MI, myocardial ischemia, coronary occlusion, ventricular tachycardia, bradycardia, *chest pain, hypotension*
GI: *Nausea, vomiting, abdominal pain, diarrhea,* GI bleeding
HEMA: Bleeding
SYST: Anaphylaxis

PHARMACOKINETICS
Metabolized in liver, distributed to extracellular fluid, 54% plasma protein binding, half-life 39-51 min, excreted in feces, peak 1-2 hr (anticoagulant action)

INTERACTIONS
Increase: bleeding risk—antiplatelets, NSAIDs, salicylates, dipyridamole, clopidogrel, ticlopidine, heparin, warfarin, glycoprotein IIb/IIIa antagonists (abciximab, tirofiban, eptifibatide),

thrombolytics (alteplase, reteplase, urokinase, tenecteplase), other anticoagulants; avoid using concurrently
Drug/Herb
Increase: bleeding risk—ginger, garlic, ginkgo, horse chestnut
Drug/Lab
Decrease: Hgb/Hct

NURSING CONSIDERATIONS
Assess:
• Obtain baseline aPTT before treatment, do not start if aPTT ratio ≥2.5, then aPTT 4 hr after initiation of treatment and at least daily thereafter; if aPTT is above target, stop infusion for 2 hr, then restart at 50%, take aPTT in 4 hr; if below target, increase infusion rate of 0.21 mg/kg/hr without checking for coagulation abnormalities
• **Bleeding:** gums; petechiae; ecchymosis; black, tarry stools; hematuria/epistaxis; decreased B/P, Hct; vaginal bleeding, possible hemorrhage
• **Anaphylaxis:** dyspnea, rash during treatment
• Fever, skin rash, urticaria
• **Pregnancy/breastfeeding:** if pregnancy is planned or suspected; if pregnant, use only if benefits outweigh fetal risk; do not breastfeed, excretion unknown
Evaluate:
• Therapeutic response: prevention of thrombosis
Teach patient/family:
• Reason for product, expected results
• To use a soft-bristle toothbrush to avoid bleeding gums; avoid contact sports; use electric razor; avoid IM inj
• To report any signs of bleeding: gums, under skin, urine, stool; trouble breathing, wheezing, skin rash
• **Pregnancy/breastfeeding:** to notify prescriber if planning to become pregnant, breastfeeding
• Not to use OTC meds, herbal products unless approved by prescriber

---

• To notify prescriber of hepatic/GI disease, recent surgery, injury

---

ARIPiprazole (Rx)

(a-rip-ip-pra′zol)

Abilify, Abilify Discmelt, Abilify Maintena, Aristada

Func. class.: Antipsychotic

Chem. class.: Quinolinone

Do not confuse:

aripiprazole/rabeprazole

ACTION: Exact mechanism unknown; may be mediated through both DOPamine type 2 (D_2, D_3) and serotonin type 2 ($5-HT_{1A}$, $5-HT_{2A}$) antagonism, DOPamine System Stabilizer

USES: Schizophrenia and bipolar disorder (adults and adolescents), mania, major depressive disorder, short-term mania or mixed episodes of bipolar disorder; irritability in patients with autism

CONTRAINDICATIONS: Breastfeeding, hypersensitivity, seizure disorders **Precautions:** Pregnancy, geriatric patients, renal/hepatic/cardiac disease, neutropenia

Black Box Warning: Children with depression; suicidal ideation; dementia

DOSAGE AND ROUTES

Major depressive disorder

• **Adult: PO** 2-5 mg/day as an adjunct to other antidepressant treatment; adjust by 5 mg at ≥1 wk (range, 2-15 mg/day)

Schizophrenia

• **Adult: PO** 10-15 mg/day; if needed, dosage may be increased to 30 mg/day after 2 wk; maintenance 15 mg/day; periodically reassess; **IM/ext rel** (monthly inj susp) 400 mg monthly

• **Adolescent 13-17 yr: PO** 2 mg/day, may increase to 5 mg after 2 days, then 10 mg after 2 more days, max 30 mg/day

Bipolar disorder

• **Adult: PO** 15 mg/day, may increase to 30 mg if needed (monotherapy); adjunctive to lithium or valproate **PO** 10-15 mg daily, may increase to 30 mg if needed

• **Child >10 yr, adolescent: PO** 2 mg, titrate to 5 mg/day after 2 days to target of 10 mg/day after another 2 days

Agitation with bipolar disorder/ schizophrenia

• **Adult: IM** 9.75 mg as a single dose, may start with a lower dose, max 30 mg/day

Irritability associated with autism

• **Child ≥6 yr, adolescent: PO** 2 mg/day, increase to 5 mg/day after 1 wk, may increase to 10-15 mg/day if needed; dose changes should not occur more frequently than q1wk

Tourette's syndrome

• **Child 6-18 yr ≥50 kg: PO** 2 mg/day × 2 days, then increase to 5 mg/day, target 10 mg/day on day 8

• **Child 6-18 yr <50 kg: PO** 2 mg/day, increase to 5 mg/day after 2 days; may increase to 10 mg/day; adjust dose ≥1 wk

Potential CYP2D6 inhibitor, strong CYP3A4 inhibitors

• **Adult: PO** reduce to 50% of usual dose; increase dose when CYP2D6, CYP3A4 inhibitors withdrawn

Combination of strong CYP3A4/ CYP2D6 inhibitors

• **Adult: PO** reduce to 25% of usual dose

Available forms: Tabs 2, 5, 10, 15, 20, 30 mg; inj 9.75 mg/1.3 mL; orally disintegrating tab 10, 15 mg; oral sol 1 mg/mL; susp for inj 441 mg/1.6 mL, 662 mg/2.4 mL, 882 mg/3.2 mL

Administer:

PO route

• Store in tight, light-resistant container

• May be given without regard to meals

• **Orally disintegrating tabs:** do not open blister until ready to use, do not push tab through foil; place on tongue, allow to dissolve, swallow, do not divide

• **Oral liquid:** use calibrated measuring device

• **Oral solution:** can be substituted for tablet mg per mg, up to 25-mg dose. Patients

---

receiving 30-mg tablets should receive 25 mg, immediate release of solution

IM (Ext Rel) route

• Give IM only; inject slowly, deeply into muscle mass; discard unused portion; do not give IV or subcut
• Available as ready to use
• Ext rel monthly (Abilify Maintena)

SIDE EFFECTS

CNS: *Drowsiness, insomnia, agitation, anxiety, headache,* seizures, neuroleptic malignant syndrome, *light-headedness, akathisia, tremor,* suicidal ideation, tardive dyskinesia, EPS

CV: Orthostatic hypotension, tachycardia, chest pain, hypertension, peripheral edema

EENT: *Blurred vision, rhinitis*

GI: *Constipation, nausea, vomiting, weight gain*

INTEG: *Rash, dry skin, sweating*

META: Hyperglycemia

MS: Myalgia

RESP: *Cough,* dyspnea, hypercholesterolemia

Hema: Agranulocytosis, anemia, leukemia

SYST: Death among geriatric patients with dementia, hypersensitivity

PHARMACOKINETICS

PO: Absorption 87%; extensively metabolized by liver to a major active metabolite by CYP3A4/CYP2D6; plasma protein binding >99%; half-life 75 hr; excretion via urine 25%, feces 55%; clearance decreased in geriatric patients

INTERACTIONS

Increase: effects of ARIPiprazole—CYP3A4 inhibitors (ketoconazole, erythromycin), CYP2D6 inhibitors (quiNIDine, FLUoxetine, PARoxetine); reduce dose of ARIPiprazole

Increase: sedation—other CNS depressants, alcohol

Increase: EPS—other antipsychotics, lithium

Decrease: ARIPiprazole level—famotidine, valproate

Decrease: effects of ARIPiprazole—CYP3A4 inducers (carBAMazepine);

dose of ARIPiprazole may need to be increased

Increase: antihypertensive effect—antihypertensives; monitor B/P

Drug/Herb

Decrease: ARIPiprazole effect—St. John's wort

Drug/Lab

False positive: amphetamine drug screen

NURSING CONSIDERATIONS

Assess:

> **Black Box Warning:** Mental status before initial administration; children/young adults may exhibit suicidal thoughts/behaviors; therefore smallest amount of product should be given; elderly patients with dementia-related psychosis are at increased risk of death

• AIMS assessment, neurologic function, LFTs, weight, lipid profile, blood glucose monthly
• Affect, orientation, LOC, reflexes, gait, coordination, sleep pattern disturbances
• B/P standing and lying; also pulse, respirations; take q4hr during initial treatment; establish baseline before starting treatment; report drops of 30 mm Hg; watch for ECG changes
• Dizziness, faintness, palpitations, tachycardia on rising
• EPS, including akathisia (inability to sit still, no pattern to movements), tardive dyskinesia (bizarre movements of the jaw, mouth, tongue, extremities), pseudoparkinsonism (rigidity, tremors, pill rolling, shuffling gait)
• **Neuroleptic malignant syndrome:** hyperthermia, increased CPK, altered mental status, muscle rigidity; notify prescriber immediately
• **Beers:** avoid in older adults, high risk of delirium, CVA; may use in schizophrenia, bipolar disorder, or short-term as antiemetic in chemotherapy

Evaluate:

• Therapeutic response: decrease in emotional excitement, hallucinations, delusions, paranoia; reorganization of patterns of thought, speech

Teach patient/family:

- That orthostatic hypotension may occur; to rise from sitting or lying position gradually
- To avoid hot tubs, hot showers, tub baths; hypotension may occur
- To avoid abrupt withdrawal of this product; EPS may result; product should be withdrawn slowly
- To avoid OTC preparations (cough, hay fever, cold) unless approved by prescriber because serious product interactions may occur; to avoid use with alcohol, CNS depressants because increased drowsiness may occur
- To avoid hazardous activities if drowsy, dizzy
- About compliance with product regimen
- To report impaired vision, tremors, muscle twitching
- That examinations and blood work will be needed during treatment
- That weight gain may occur, to notify health care professional of large weight gain
- That heat stroke may occur in hot weather; to take extra precautions to stay cool

Black Box Warning: To report suicidal thoughts/behaviors, dementia immediately

- **Pregnancy/breastfeeding:** Identify if pregnancy is planned or suspected; pregnant patient should be enrolled in the National Pregnancy Registry for Atypical Antipsychotics 866-961-2388; avoid breastfeeding; use only if benefits outweigh fetal risk

TREATMENT OF OVERDOSE: Lavage if orally ingested; provide airway; *do not induce vomiting*

RARELY USED

armodafinil (Rx)
(ar-moe-daf′in-il)
Nuvigil
Controlled Substance Schedule IV

USES: Narcolepsy, obstructive sleep apnea/hypoapnea syndrome, circadian rhythm disruption (shift-work sleep problems)

CONTRAINDICATIONS: Hypersensitivity to this product or modafinil

DOSAGE AND ROUTES
Narcolepsy, obstructive sleep apnea/hypoapnea syndrome
- **Adult and adolescent ≥17 yr: PO** 150-250 mg in AM
Circadian rhythm disruption (shift-work sleep problems)
- **Adult and adolescent ≥17 yr: PO** 150 mg at start of shift

---

asenapine (Rx)
(a-sen′a-peen)
Saphris
Func. class.: Antipsychotic, atypical; DOPamine-serotonin antagonist
Chem. class.: Dibenzapine

ACTION: Unknown; may be mediated through both DOPamine type 2 (D2) and serotonin type 2 (5-HT2A) antagonism

USES: Bipolar 1 disorder, schizophrenia

CONTRAINDICATIONS: Breastfeeding, hypersensitivity
Precautions: Pregnancy, children, geriatric patients, cardiac/renal/hepatic disease, breast cancer, Parkinson's disease, dementia, seizure disorder, CNS depression, agranulocytosis, QT prolongation, torsades de pointes, suicidal ideation, substance abuse, diabetes mellitus

Black Box Warning: Increased mortality in elderly patients with dementia-related psychosis

DOSAGE AND ROUTES
Schizophrenia
• **Adult: SL** 5 mg bid, may increase to 10 mg BID after 1 wk, max 20 mg/day
Acute mania/mixed episodes (bipolar 1 disorder, monotherapy)
• **Adult: SL** 10 mg bid, may decrease to 5 mg bid as needed, max 20 mg/day; with lithium or valproate 5 mg bid, may increase to 10 mg bid
• **Child 10-17 yr: SL** 2.5 mg bid, may increase after 3 days to 5 mg bid, then after 3 more days 10 mg bid can be tolerated
Available forms: SL tab 2.5, 5, 10 mg
Administer:
• Anticholinergic agent to be used for EPS
• Store in tight, light-resistant container
• **SL tab:** remove tab; place tab under tongue; after it dissolves, swallow; advise patient not to chew, crush, swallow tabs, not to eat, drink for 10 min

SIDE EFFECTS
CNS: *EPS, pseudoparkinsonism, akathisia, dystonia, tardive dyskinesia; drowsiness, insomnia, agitation, anxiety, headache,* seizures, neuroleptic malignant syndrome, dizziness, suicidal ideation
CV: Orthostatic hypotension, tachycardia; QT prolongation
ENDO: Hyperglycemia
GI: *Nausea,* vomiting, oral hypoesthesia/paresthesia, (SL)
HEMA: Agranulocytosis, anemia, leukopenia
INTEG: Serious allergic reactions (anaphylaxis, angioedema)

PHARMACOKINETICS
Extensively metabolized by liver by CYP3A4/UGTA14, protein binding 95%, peak 0.5-1.5 hr, half-life 24 hr, excreted urine 50%, feces 40% (metabolites)

INTERACTIONS
Increase: sedation—other CNS depressants, alcohol

Increase: EPS—CYP2D6 inhibitors/substrates (SSRIs)
Increase: serotonin syndrome—SSRIs
Increase: Seizure risk—buPROPion
Increase: EPS—other antipsychotics
Increase: asenapine excretion—carBAMazepine
Increase: QT prolongation—class IA/III antidysrhythmics, some phenothiazines, β-agonists, local anesthetics, tricyclics, haloperidol, methadone, chloroquine, clarithromycin, droperidol, erythromycin, pentamidine; avoid concurrent use
Decrease: asenapine action—CYP2D6 inducers (carBAMazepine, barbiturates, phenytoins, rifAMPin)
Drug/Herb
Increase: CNS depression—kava
Increase: EPS—betel palm, kava
Drug/Lab Test
Increase: prolactin levels, glucose, cholesterol, LFTs, lipids, triglycerides
Decrease: sodium

NURSING CONSIDERATIONS
Assess:

> Black Box Warning: Mental status before initial administration; watch for suicidal thoughts and behaviors; dementia and death may occur among elderly patients

• Affect, orientation, LOC, reflexes, gait, coordination, sleep pattern disturbances
• B/P standing and lying; also pulse, respirations; take these during initial treatment; establish baseline before starting treatment; report drops of 30 mm Hg; watch for ECG changes; QT prolongation may occur
• Dizziness, faintness, palpitations, tachycardia on rising
• **EPS,** including akathisia, tardive dyskinesia (bizarre movements of the jaw, mouth, tongue, extremities), pseudoparkinsonism (rigidity, tremors, pill rolling, shuffling gait)
• **Neuroleptic malignant syndrome:** hyperthermia, increased CPK, altered mental status, muscle rigidity

• Weight, thyroid function studies, serum prolactin, lipid profile, serum electrolytes, creatinine, pregnancy test, neurologic function, LFTs, glycosylated hemoglobin A1c, CBC, blood glucose, AIMS assessment baseline and periodically

• Supervised ambulation until patient stabilized on medication; do not involve patient in strenuous exercise program because fainting is possible; patient should not stand still for a long time

• **Beers:** avoid use in older adults; high risk of delirium, CVA, worsening parkinsonian symptoms, increased CNS effects; may use in schizophrenia, bipolar disorder, or as antiemetic in chemotherapy

Evaluate:

• Therapeutic response: decrease in emotional excitement, hallucinations, delusions, paranoia; reorganization of patterns of thought, speech

Teach patient/family:

• That orthostatic hypotension may occur; to rise from sitting or lying position gradually

• To avoid hot tubs, hot showers, tub baths; hypotension may occur

• To avoid abrupt withdrawal of this product; EPS may result; product should be withdrawn slowly

• To avoid OTC preparations (cough, hay fever, cold) unless approved by prescriber; serious product interactions may occur; to avoid use of alcohol; increased drowsiness may occur

• To avoid hazardous activities if drowsy, dizzy

• About compliance with product regimen

• That heat stroke may occur in hot weather; to take extra precautions to stay cool

• To notify provider if history of diabetes in patient or family; if so, blood sugar should be checked before starting this product

Black Box Warning: To report suicidal thoughts/behaviors, dementia immediately

• **Pregnancy/breastfeeding:** use only if benefits outweigh fetal risk; identify if pregnancy is planned or suspected; if pregnant, register at National Pregnancy Registry for Atypical Antipsychotics (866-961-2388)

TREATMENT OF OVERDOSE: Lavage if orally ingested; provide airway; *do not induce vomiting*

⚠ HIGH ALERT

RARELY USED

asparaginase *Erwinia chrysanthemi* (Rx)

Erwinaze
Func. class.: Antineoplastic, natural and semisynthetic

USES: Treatment of acute lymphocytic leukemia (ALL) in combination with other chemotherapeutic agents in patients who have developed hypersensitivity to *Escherichia coli*–derived asparaginase

CONTRAINDICATIONS: Hypersensitivity, breastfeeding, history of serious pancreatitis, bleeding, or serious thrombosis with prior L-asparaginase therapy

DOSAGE AND ROUTES

• **Adult, adolescent, child ≥2 yr (substitute for pegaspargase):** IM 25,000 IU/m^2 3×/wk (Monday/Wednesday/Friday) × 6 doses for each planned dose of pegaspargase within a treatment

• **Adult (substitute for L-asparaginase E. coli):** IM 25,000 IU/m^2 for each scheduled dose of native *E. coli* asparaginase within a treatment

> ## ⚠ HIGH ALERT
>
> ## aspirin (acetylsalicylic acid, ASA) (OTC)
> (as′pir-in)
> Acuprin, Asaphen ✦, Asatab ✦, A.S.A. Ascriptin Enteric, Aspergum, Aspir-Low, Aspir-trin, Bayer Aspirin, Easprin, Ecotrin, Entrophen ✦, Halfprin, Lowprin ✦, Novasen ✦, Rivasa ✦, Sloprin, St. Joseph Adult, Zorprin
> *Func. class.:* Nonopioid analgesic, nonsteroidal antiinflammatory, antipyretic, antiplatelet
> *Chem. class.:* Salicylate

Do not confuse:
Aspirin/Anacin Adult Low/Anacin-3

ACTION: Blocks pain impulses by blocking COX-1 in CNS, reduces inflammation by inhibition of prostaglandin synthesis; antipyretic action results from vasodilation of peripheral vessels; decreases platelet aggregation

USES: Mild to moderate pain or fever, including rheumatoid arthritis (RA), osteoarthritis, thromboembolic disorders; TIAs, rheumatic fever, post-MI, prophylaxis of MI, ischemic stroke, angina, acute MI, Kawasaki disease
Unlabeled uses: Colorectal cancer prophylaxis

CONTRAINDICATIONS: Pregnancy, breastfeeding, children <12 yr, children with flulike symptoms, hypersensitivity to salicylates, tartrazine (FD&C yellow dye #5), GI bleeding, bleeding disorders, vit K deficiency, peptic ulcer, acute bronchospasm, agranulocytosis, increased intracranial pressure, intracranial bleeding, nasal polyps, urticaria
Precautions: Abrupt discontinuation, acetaminophen/NSAIDs hypersensitivity, acid/base imbalance, alcoholism, ascites, asthma, bone marrow suppression in elderly patients, dehydration, G6PD deficiency, gout, heart failure, anemia, renal/hepatic disease, pre/postoperatively, gastritis

DOSAGE AND ROUTES
Pain/fever
• **Adult:** PO/RECT 325-1000 mg q4hr prn, max 4 g/day
• **Child 2-11 yr:** PO 10-15 mg/kg/dose q4hr, max 4 g/day
RA, osteoarthritis, other inflammatory conditions
• **Adult:** PO 2.4 g/day in divided doses q4-6hr, maintenance 3.6-5.4 g/day; **ext rel** 650 mg q8hr or 800 mg q12hr; target salicylate level 150-300 mcg/mL
Juvenile RA
• **Child:** PO/RECT 90-130 mg/kg/day in divided doses, target salicylate level 150-300 mcg/mL
Thromboembolic disorders
• **Adult:** PO 325-650 mg/day or bid
Transient ischemic attacks
• **Adult:** PO 50-325 mg/day (grade 1A)
Evolving MI with ST segment elevation (STEMI)
• **Adult:** PO 160-325 mg nonenteric, chewed and swallowed immediately, maintenance 75-162 mg daily
MI, stroke prophylaxis
• **Adult:** PO 50-325 mg/day
Prevention of recurrent MI/antiplatelet
• **Adult:** PO 80-325 mg/day
CABG
• **Adult:** PO 325 mg/day starting 6 hr postprocedure, continue for 1 yr
PTCA
• **Adult:** PO 325 mg 2 hr before surgery, then 160-325 mg daily
Kawasaki disease
• **Child:** PO 80-100 mg/kg/day in 4 divided doses, maintenance 3-5 mg/kg/day
Available forms: Tabs 81, 162.5, 325, 500, 650, 975 mg; chewable tabs 81 mg; supp 60, 120, 125, 130, 150 ✦, 160 ✦, 195, 200, 300, 600 mg; chewing gum 227

---

mg; enteric-coated tabs 81, 325, 500, 975 mg; del rel tabs 325, 500, 600 ♣, 650, 975 mg; 640, 650, 1200 mg

Administer:

PO route

• Do not break, crush, or chew enteric product

• Crushed or whole (regular PO product), chewable tablets may be chewed

• With food or milk to decrease gastric symptoms; separate by 2 hr from enteric products

• With 8 oz of water; sit upright for $1/2$ hr after dose to facilitate product passing into stomach

Rectal route

• Place suppository in refrigerator for at least 30 minutes before removing wrapper

SIDE EFFECTS

CNS: Confusion, seizures, headache, intracranial hemorrhage

CV: Tachycardia, hypotension, dysrhythmias

EENT: Tinnitus, hearing loss

ENDO: Hypoglycemia, hypokalemia

GI: *Nausea, vomiting,* GI bleeding, pancreatitis, hepatotoxicity

HEMA: Thrombocytopenia, leukopenia, DIC, increased PT, aPTT, bleeding time

INTEG: *Rash,* urticaria, bruising

SYST: Reye's syndrome (children), anaphylaxis, laryngeal edema, angioedema

PHARMACOKINETICS

Enteric metabolized by liver; inactive metabolites excreted by kidneys; crosses placenta; excreted in breast milk; half-life 15-20 min, up to 30 hr in large dose; rectal products may be erratic; protein binding 90%

PO: Onset 15-30 min, peak 1-2 hr, duration 4-6 hr, well absorbed

PO: Enteric coated: onset 10-30 min, duration 2-4 hr

RECT: Onset slow, duration 4-6 hr

INTERACTIONS

Increase: gastric ulcer risk—corticosteroids, antiinflammatories, NSAIDs, alcohol

Increase: bleeding—alcohol, plicamycin, cefamandole, thrombolytics, ticlopidine, clopidogrel, tirofiban, eptifibatide, anticoagulants; monitor for bleeding

Increase: effects of insulin, methotrexate, thrombolytic agents, penicillins, phenytoin, valproic acid, oral hypoglycemics, sulfonamides; monitor for increased effects of each product

Increase: salicylate levels—urinary acidifiers, ammonium chloride, nizatidine

Increase: hypotension—nitroglycerin

Decrease: effects of aspirin—antacids (high doses), urinary alkalizers, corticosteroids; monitor for decreased effects

Decrease: antihypertensive effect—ACE inhibitors, monitor B/P

Decrease: effects of probenecid, spironolactone, sulfinpyrazone, sulfonylamides, NSAIDs, β-blockers, loop diuretics

Drug/Herb

Increase: risk of bleeding—feverfew, garlic, ginger, ginkgo, ginseng *(Panax),* horse chestnut

Drug/Food

Increase: risk of bleeding—fish oil (omega-3 fatty acids)

• Foods that acidify urine may increase aspirin level

Drug/Lab Test

Increase: coagulation studies, LFTs, serum uric acid, amylase, CO_2, urinary protein

Decrease: serum potassium, cholesterol

Interference: VMA, 5-HIAA, xylose tolerance test, TSH, pregnancy test

NURSING CONSIDERATIONS

Assess:

• **Pain:** character, location, intensity; ROM before and 1 hr after administration

• **Fever:** temperature before and 1 hr after administration

• Hepatic studies: AST, ALT, bilirubin, creatinine if patient is receiving long-term therapy

• Renal studies: BUN, urine creatinine; I&O ratio; decreasing output may indicate renal failure (long-term therapy)

- Blood studies: CBC, Hct, Hgb, PT if patient is receiving long-term therapy
- **Hepatotoxicity:** dark urine, clay-colored stools, yellowing of skin, sclera, itching, abdominal pain, fever, diarrhea if patient is receiving long-term therapy
- **Allergic reactions:** rash, urticaria; if these occur, product may have to be discontinued; patients with asthma, nasal polyps, allergies: severe allergic reaction may occur
- **Ototoxicity:** tinnitus, ringing, roaring in ears; audiometric testing needed before, after long-term therapy
- **Salicylate level:** therapeutic level 150-300 mcg/mL for chronic inflammation
- **Beers:** avoid chronic use in older adults; GI bleeding may occur
- **Pregnancy/breastfeeding:** do not use in 1st trimester; may cause fetal harm; use only if benefits outweigh fetal risks (2nd/3rd trimester); avoid breastfeeding

Evaluate:
- Therapeutic response: decreased pain, inflammation, fever

Teach patient/family:
- To report any symptoms of hepatotoxicity, renal toxicity, visual changes, ototoxicity, allergic reactions, bleeding (long-term therapy)
- To avoid if allergic to tartrazine
- Not to exceed recommended dosage; acute poisoning may result
- To read labels on other OTC products because many contain aspirin, salicylates
- That the therapeutic response takes 2 wk (arthritis)
- To report tinnitus, confusion, diarrhea, sweating, hyperventilation
- To avoid alcohol ingestion; GI bleeding may occur
- That patients who have allergies, nasal polyps, asthma may develop allergic reactions
- To discard tabs if vinegar-like smell is detected
- That medication is not to be given to children or teens with flulike symptoms or chickenpox, because Reye's syndrome may develop

- To take with a full glass of water
- Not to use in children with flulike symptoms or chickenpox, risk of Reye's syndrome
- **Pregnancy/breastfeeding:** to inform prescriber if pregnancy is planned or suspected; avoid breastfeeding

TREATMENT OF OVERDOSE: Lavage, monitor electrolytes, VS

atazanavir (Rx)
(at-a-za-na′veer)

Reyataz

Func. class.: Antiretroviral
Chem. class.: Protease inhibitor

ACTION: Inhibits human immunodeficiency virus (HIV-1) protease, which prevents maturation of the infectious virus

USES: HIV-1 infection in combination with other antiretroviral agents

CONTRAINDICATIONS: Hypersensitivity, Child-Pugh Class C
Precautions: Pregnancy, breastfeeding, children, geriatric patients, hepatic disease, alcoholism, drug resistance, AV block, diabetes, dialysis, geriatric patients, females, hemophilia, hypercholesterolemia, immune reconstitution syndrome, lactic acidosis, pancreatitis, cholelithiasis, serious rash

DOSAGE AND ROUTES
Antiretroviral-naive patients
- **Adult: PO** 400 mg/day (unable to take ritonavir); 300 mg with ritonavir 100 mg/day
- **Child ≥6 yr/adolescent ≥40 kg: PO** 300 mg with ritonavir 100 mg daily
- **Child ≥6 yr/adolescent 20 to <40 kg: PO** 200 mg with ritonavir 100 mg daily
- **Child ≥6 yr/adolescent 15 to <20 kg: PO** 150 mg with ritonavir 100 mg daily
Antiretroviral-experienced patients
- **Adult: PO** 300 mg with ritonavir 100 mg daily

- **Pregnant adults/adolescents (2nd/3rd trimester) with H$_2$ blocker or tenofovir:** PO 400 mg with ritonavir 100 mg daily
- **Child ≥6 yr/adolescent ≥40 kg:** PO 300 mg with ritonavir 100 mg daily
- **Child ≥6 yr/adolescent 20 to <40 kg:** PO 200 mg with ritonavir 100 mg daily
- **Children and adolescents ≥25 kg:** PO (oral powder) 300 mg q24hr with ritonavir 100 mg q24hr
- **Children 15 to 24 kg:** PO (oral powder) 250 mg q24hr with ritonavir 80 mg q24hr
- **Infants and children ≥3 mo and 5 to 14 kg:** PO (oral powder) 200 mg q24hr with ritonavir 80 mg q24hr

Hepatic dose
- **Adult:** PO Child-Pugh B: 300 mg/day; Child-Pugh C: do not use

Renal dose
- **Adult:** PO Therapy-naive and HD: 300 mg q day; with ritonavir: 100 mg q day; therapy experienced and HD: do not use

Available forms: Caps 100, 150, 200, 300 mg; oral powder 50 mg/packet

Administer:
- **Capsules:** With food; 2 hr before or 1 hr after antacid or didanosine; swallow cap whole, do not open
- **Oral Powder:** Use with food or beverage; mix 1 tablespoon of food with powder, feed, then add another tablespoon of food to container, mix, and feed; or mix with 30 mL of liquid, give, then add another 15 mL of liquid to cup to remove residual, give; use within 1 hr of mixing

SIDE EFFECTS

CNS: Headache, depression, dizziness, insomnia, peripheral neuropathy

CV: Increased PR interval

GI: Vomiting, *diarrhea, abdominal pain, nausea,* hepatotoxicity, cholelithiasis

INTEG: *Rash,* Stevens-Johnson syndrome, *photosensitivity,* DRESS

MISC: Fatigue, fever, arthralgia, back pain, cough, lipodystrophy, pain, gynecomastia, nephrolithiasis; lactic acidosis, hyperbilirubinemia (pregnancy, females, obesity), immune reconstitution syndrome

PHARMACOKINETICS

Rapidly absorbed, absorption increased with food, peak $2^1/_2$ hr, 86% protein bound, extensively metabolized in liver by CYP3A4, 27% excreted unchanged in urine/feces (minimal), half-life 7 hr

INTERACTIONS

Increase: levels, toxicity of immunosuppressants (cycloSPORINE, sirolimus, tacrolimus), sildenafil, antifungals (itraconazole, ketoconazole, voriconazole), tricyclic antidepressants, warfarin, calcium channel blockers, clarithromycin, clorazepate, diazePAM, irinotecan, HMG-CoA reductase inhibitors, antidysrhythmics, midazolam, triazolam, ergots, pimozide, other protease inhibitors; monitor for toxicity (amprenavir, darunavir, fosamprenavir, indinavir, nelfinavir, ritonavir, saquinavir)

Increase: effects of estrogens, oral contraceptives (unboosted), decreased (boosted with ritonavir)

Increase: atazanavir levels—CYP3A4 substrates, CYP3A4 inhibitors

Increase: hyperbilirubinemia—indinavir

Decrease: telaprevir level when used with atazanavir and ritonavir

Increase: QT prolongation—salmeterol, clarithromycin, romiDEPsin, ranolazine; dose reduction of each of these products may be needed

Increase: effect of alfuzosin, ARIPiprazole, benzodiazepine, brentuximab, cabazitaxel, carBAMazepine, cilostazol, colchicine, corticosteroids, eletriptan, eplerenone, crizotinib, DOCEtaxel, ixabepilone, iloperidone, lurasidone, maraviroc, muscarinic receptor antagonists, nilotinib, opioids, vinca alkaloids (vinCRIStine, vinBLAStine), vilazodone, vasopressin antagonists, dasatinib, lapatinib, SORAfenib, traZODone, risperIDONE, raltegravir, QUEtiapine

Decrease: atazanavir levels—CYP3A4 inducers, rifAMPin, antacids, didanosine, efavirenz, proton pump inhibitors, H$_2$-receptor antagonists; give atazanavir 2 hr before or 1 hr after these products

---

Drug/Herb

Decrease: atazanavir levels—St. John's wort; avoid concurrent use

Increase: myopathy, rhabdomyolysis—red yeast rice

Drug/Lab Test

Increase: AST, ALT, total bilirubin, amylase, lipase, CK

Decrease: Hgb, neutrophils, platelets

Drug/Food

• Increased drug bioavailability (to be taken with food)

NURSING CONSIDERATIONS
Assess:

• **For hepatic failure; hepatic studies:** ALT, AST, bilirubin; do not use in Child-Pugh C

• For lactic acidosis, hyperbilirubinemia (females, pregnancy, obesity); if pregnant, call Antiretroviral Pregnancy Registry 800-258-4263; do not breastfeed; use additional contraception when boosted with ritonavir

• PR interval in those taking calcium channel blockers, digoxin

• For signs of infection, anemia, nephrolithiasis

• Bowel pattern before, during treatment; if severe abdominal pain with bleeding occurs, product should be discontinued; monitor hydration

• Viral load, CD4 count throughout treatment

• **Serious rash (Stevens-Johnson syndrome, DRESS):** most rashes last 1-4 wk; if serious, discontinue product

• **Immune reconstitution syndrome:** time of onset is variable when given with combination antiretroviral therapy

Evaluate:

• Therapeutic response: increasing CD4 counts; decreased viral load, resolution of symptoms of HIV-1 infection

Teach patient/family:

• To take as prescribed with other antiretrovirals as prescribed; if dose is missed, to take as soon as remembered up to 1 hr before next dose; not to double dose or share with others

• That product must be taken daily to maintain blood levels for duration of therapy

• To report yellowing of skin, sclera

• To notify prescriber if diarrhea, nausea, vomiting, rash occurs; dizziness, light-headedness may occur; ECG may be altered

• That product interacts with many products, including St. John's wort; to advise prescriber of all products, herbal products used

• That redistribution of body fat may occur, the effect is not known

• That product does not cure HIV-1 infection, prevent transmission to others; only controls symptoms

• That, if taking phosphodiesterase type 5 inhibitor with atazanavir, there may be increased risk of phosphodiesterase type 5 inhibitor–associated adverse events (hypotension, prolonged penile erection); to notify physician promptly of these symptoms

• **Pregnancy/breastfeeding:** that registration with Antiretroviral Pregnancy Registry is strongly encouraged for pregnant patients; to notify prescriber if pregnancy is planned or suspected; to use additional contraception when boosted with ritonavir

---

> ## ⚠ HIGH ALERT
>
> ## atazanavir/cobicistat (Rx)
> (at-a-za-na′veer / koe-bik′-i-stat)
> Evotaz
> *Func. class.:* Antiretroviral
> *Chem. class.:* Protease inhibitor

ACTION: Inhibits HIV-1 protease, which prevents maturation of the infectious virus; it combines a protease inhibitor with an enhancer

USES: HIV-1 infection in combination with other antiretroviral agents

CONTRAINDICATIONS: Hypersensitivity, Child-Pugh Class C

Precautions: Pregnancy, breastfeeding, children, geriatric patients, hepatic disease, alcoholism, drug resistance, AV block, diabetes, dialysis, female patients, hemophilia, hypercholesterolemia, immune reconstitution syndrome, lactic acidosis, pancreatitis, cholelithiasis, serious rash

DOSAGE AND ROUTES
• **Adult:** PO 300 mg/150 mg daily in both treatment-naive and treatment-experienced patients
• **Adolescent (unlabeled):** PO 300 mg/150 mg daily in combination with other antiretroviral agents as part of an alternative initial regimen (treatment-naive)
Renal dose
• Adult: PO CCr <70 mL/min; if receiving tenofovir, should not use
Available forms: Tab 300 mg/150 mg
Administer:
• Antiretroviral drug resistance testing (preferably genotypic testing) is recommended before initiation of therapy in antiretroviral treatment-naive patients and before changing therapy for treatment failure
• With food

SIDE EFFECTS
CNS: Headache, depression, dizziness, insomnia, peripheral neurologic symptoms
CV: Increased PR interval
EENT: Yellowing of sclera
GI: Vomiting, *diarrhea, abdominal pain, nausea,* hepatotoxicity, cholelithiasis
INTEG: Rash, Stevens-Johnson syndrome, photosensitivity, DRESS
MISC: Fatigue, fever, arthralgia, back pain, cough, lipodystrophy, pain, gynecomastia, nephrolithiasis; lactic acidosis, hyperbilirubinemia (pregnancy, female patients, obesity)

PHARMACOKINETICS
Rapidly absorbed, absorption increased with food, peak 2.5 hr, 86% protein bound, extensively metabolized in liver by CYP3A4, 27% excreted unchanged in urine/feces (minimal), half-life 7 hr

INTERACTIONS
Increase: levels, toxicity of immunosuppressants (cycloSPORINE, sirolimus, tacrolimus), sildenafil, tricyclic antidepressants, warfarin, calcium channel blockers, clarithromycin, clorazepate, diazePAM, irinotecan, HMG-CoA reductase inhibitors, antidysrhythmics, midazolam, triazolam, ergots, pimozide, other protease inhibitors
Increase: effects of estrogens
Increase: atazanavir levels—CYP3A4 substrates, CYP3A4 inhibitors
Increase: hyperbilirubinemia—indinavir
Decrease: telaprevir level when used with atazanavir and ritonavir
Decrease: atazanavir levels—CYP3A4 inducers, rifAMPin, antacids, didanosine, efavirenz, proton pump inhibitors, H$_2$-receptor antagonists
Decrease: effects of oral contraceptives
Drug/Herb
Decrease: atazanavir levels—St. John's wort; avoid concurrent use
Increase: myopathy, rhabdomyolysis—red yeast rice
Drug/Lab Test
Increase: AST, ALT, total bilirubin, amylase, lipase, CK
Decrease: Hgb, neutrophils, platelets
Drug/Food
• Increased drug bioavailability (to be taken with food)

NURSING CONSIDERATIONS
Assess:
• For hepatic failure; hepatic studies: ALT, AST, bilirubin
• Immune reconstitution syndrome: when given with combination antiretroviral therapy
• For lactic acidosis, hyperbilirubinemia (female patients, pregnancy, obesity); if pregnant, call Antiretroviral Pregnancy Registry 800-258-4263
• PR interval in those taking calcium channel blockers, digoxin
• For signs of infection, anemia, nephrolithiasis

• Bowel pattern before, during treatment; if severe abdominal pain with bleeding occurs, product should be discontinued; monitor hydration

• Viral load, CD4 count throughout treatment

• **Serious rash (Stevens-Johnson syndrome, DRESS):** most rashes last 1-4 wk; if serious, discontinue product

• **Immune reconstitution syndrome:** time of onset is variable

• **Pregnancy/breastfeeding:** use only if benefits outweigh fetal risk; do not breastfeed

Evaluate:

• Therapeutic response: increasing CD4 counts; decreased viral load, resolution of symptoms of HIV-1 infection

Teach patient/family:

• To take as prescribed with other antiretrovirals as prescribed; if dose is missed, to take as soon as remembered up to 1 hr before next dose; not to double dose, share with others

• That product must be taken daily to maintain blood levels for duration of therapy

• To report yellowing of skin, sclera

• To notify prescriber if diarrhea, nausea, vomiting, or rash occurs; dizziness, light-headedness may occur; ECG may be altered

• That product interacts with many products, including St. John's wort; to advise prescriber of all products, herbal products used

• That redistribution of body fat may occur; the effect is not known

• That product does not cure HIV-1 infection or prevent transmission to others; only controls symptoms

• That if taking phosphodiesterase type 5 inhibitor with atazanavir, there may be increased risk of phosphodiesterase type 5 inhibitor–associated adverse events (hypotension, prolonged penile erection); to notify physician promptly of these symptoms

---

⚠ HIGH ALERT

atenolol (Rx)

(a-ten′oh-lole)

Tenormin

Func. class.: Antihypertensive, antianginal

Chem. class.: β-Blocker, β₁-, β₂-blocker (high doses)

Do not confuse:
atenolol/albuterol
Tenormin/thiamine/Imuran

ACTION: Competitively blocks stimulation of β-adrenergic receptor within vascular smooth muscle; produces negative chronotropic activity (decreases rate of SA node discharge, increases recovery time), slows conduction of AV node, decreases heart rate, negative inotropic activity decreases O_2 consumption in myocardium; decreases action of renin-aldosterone-angiotensin system at high doses, inhibits β₂ receptors in bronchial system at higher doses

USES: Hypertension, angina pectoris; suspected or known MI (IV use); MI prophylaxis

Unlabeled uses: Migraine prophylaxis, supraventricular tachycardia prophylaxis (PSVT), unstable angina, alcohol withdrawal, lithium-induced tremor

CONTRAINDICATIONS: Pregnancy, hypersensitivity to β-blockers, cardiogenic shock, 2nd- or 3rd-degree heart block, sinus bradycardia, cardiac failure

Precautions: Breastfeeding, major surgery, diabetes mellitus, thyroid/renal disease, HF, COPD, asthma, well-compensated heart failure, dialysis, myasthenia gravis, Raynaud's disease, pulmonary edema

Black Box Warning: Abrupt discontinuation

DOSAGE AND ROUTES
Hypertension
• **Adult:** PO 25-50 mg/day, increasing q1-2wk to 100 mg/day; may increase to 200 mg/day for angina, up to 100 mg/day for hypertension

• **Child:** PO 0.8-1 mg/kg/dose initially; range, 0.8-1.5 mg/kg/day; max 2 mg/kg/day

• **Geriatric:** PO 25 mg/day initially
Angina
• **Adult:** PO 50 mg/day, then 100 mg/day as needed after 7 days, max 200 mg/day
MI
• **Adult:** PO 100 mg/day in 1-2 divided doses; may need for 1-3 yr after MI
Renal disease
• **Adult:** PO CCr 15-35 mL/min, max 50 mg/day; CCr <15 mL/min, max 25 mg/day; hemodialysis 25-50 mg after dialysis
PSVT prophylaxis (unlabeled)
• **Child:** PO 0.3-1.3 mg/kg/day
Cardiac risk reduction during surgery (unlabeled)
• **Adult:** PO 50 mg, start before planned procedure, titrate to heart rate, continue 7-30 days after procedure
Unstable angina (unlabeled)
• **Adult:** PO 50-200 mg/day
Ethanol withdrawal prevention (unlabeled)
• **Adult:** PO 50-100 mg/day
Migraine prophylaxis (unlabeled)
• **Adult:** PO 50-150 mg/day, titrate to response
Lithium-induced tremor (unlabeled)
• **Adult:** PO 50 mg/day
Available forms: Tabs 25, 50, 100 mg
Administer:
PO route
• Before meals, at bedtime; tab may be crushed, swallowed whole, same time of day
• Reduced dosage with renal dysfunction
• Store protected from light, moisture; place in cool environment

SIDE EFFECTS
CNS: *Insomnia, fatigue, dizziness, mental changes,* memory loss, depression, lethargy, drowsiness, strange dreams

CV: Profound hypotension, bradycardia, HF

ENDO: Hypo- and hyperglycemia

GI: *Nausea, diarrhea,* vomiting, constipation

GU: Impotence, decreased libido, urinary frequency

INTEG: Rash

RESP: Bronchospasm, dyspnea, wheezing, pulmonary edema

PHARMACOKINETICS
PO: Peak 2-4 hr; onset 1 hr; duration 24 hr; half-life 6-7 hr; excreted unchanged in urine, feces (50%); protein binding 5%-15%

INTERACTIONS
• Mutual inhibition: sympathomimetics (cough, cold preparations)

Increase: hypotension, bradycardia—reserpine, hydrALAZINE, methyldopa, prazosin, anticholinergics, digoxin, diltiaZEM, verapamil, cardiac glycosides, calcium channel blockers, antihypertensives; monitor and adjust dose if needed

Increase: hypoglycemia—insulins, oral antidiabetics

Increase: hypertension—amphetamines, ePHEDrine, pseudoephedrine

Increase: toxicity risk—dolasetron; lidocaine (IV)

Decrease: atenolol effect—salicylates, rifamycins, penicillins, NSAIDs, calcium carbonate, aluminum antacids

Drug/Herb

Increase: atenolol effect—hawthorn

Decrease: atenolol effect—ephedra (ma huang)

Drug/Lab Test

Increase: BUN, potassium, triglycerides, uric acid, ANA titer, platelets, alkaline phosphatase, creatinine, LDH, AST/ALT

Decrease: glucose

NURSING CONSIDERATIONS
Assess:
• I&O, weight daily; watch for HF (rales/crackles, jugular vein distention, weight gain, edema)
• **Hypertension:** B/P, pulse q4hr; note rate, rhythm, quality; apical/radial pulse

---

before administration; notify prescriber of any significant changes (<50 bpm); ECG
• **Hypoglycemia:** may be masked in diabetes mellitus (tachycardia, sweating)

Black Box Warning: Taper gradually, do not discontinue abruptly, may precipitate angina, MI

• If pregnancy is planned or suspected; do not use in pregnancy, breastfeeding
Evaluate:
• Therapeutic response: decreased B/P after 1-2 wk, increased activity tolerance, decreased anginal pain
Teach patient/family:

Black Box Warning: Not to discontinue product abruptly, taper over 2 wk (angina); to take at same time each day as directed

• Not to use OTC products unless directed by prescriber
• To report bradycardia, dizziness, confusion, depression, fever
• To take pulse at home; advise when to notify prescriber (heart rate <50 bpm)
• To limit alcohol, smoking, sodium intake
• To comply with weight control, dietary adjustments, modified exercise program
• To carry emergency ID to identify product, allergies, conditions being treated
• To avoid hazardous activities if dizziness is present
• To change position slowly, to limit orthostatic hypotension
• That product may mask symptoms of hypoglycemia in diabetic patients
• **Pregnancy/breastfeeding:** if pregnancy is planned or suspected; do not use in pregnancy, breastfeeding; to use contraception while taking this product; to avoid breastfeeding

TREATMENT OF OVERDOSE:
Lavage, IV atropine for bradycardia, IV theophylline for bronchospasm, dextrose for hypoglycemia, digoxin, O_2, diuretic for cardiac failure, hemodialysis

⚠ HIGH ALERT

RARELY USED

atezolizumab (Rx)
(a-te-zoe-liz' ue-mab)
Tecentriq ✦
Func. class.: Antineoplastic

USES: Treatment of locally advanced or metastatic urothelial carcinoma, including bladder cancer and other urinary system cancers, in patients who progress during or following platinum-containing chemotherapy for advanced disease, or within 12 months of neoadjuvant or adjuvant platinum-containing chemotherapy

CONTRAINDICATIONS: Hypersensitivity

DOSAGE AND ROUTES
• **Adult:** IV 1200 mg over 60 min q3wks until disease progression or unacceptable toxicity. If the first infusion is tolerated, infusions may be given over 30 min

atomoxetine (Rx)
(at-o-mox'eh-teen)
Strattera
Func. class.: Psychotherapeutic—miscellaneous
Chem. class.: Selective norepinephrine reuptake inhibitor

Do not confuse:
atomoxetine/atorvastatin

ACTION: Selective norepinephrine reuptake inhibitor; may inhibit the presynaptic norepinephrine transporter

USES: Attention-deficit/hyperactivity disorder
Unlabeled uses: Nocturnal enuresis

CONTRAINDICATIONS: Hypersensitivity, closed-angle glaucoma, MAOI therapy, history of pheochromocytoma

Precautions: Pregnancy, breastfeeding, hepatic disease, angioedema, bipolar disorder, dysrhythmias, CAD, hypo/hypertension, arteriosclerosis, cardiac disease, cardiomyopathy, heart failure, jaundice

> Black Box Warning: Children <6 yr, suicidal ideation

DOSAGE AND ROUTES
ADHD
• **Child >6 yr and ≤70 kg: PO** 0.5 mg/kg/day, increase after 3 days to target daily dose of 1.2 mg/kg in AM or evenly divided doses AM, late afternoon; max 1.4 mg/kg/day or 100 mg/day, whichever is less

• **Adult and child >6 yr and >70 kg: PO** 40 mg/day, increase after 3 days to target daily dose of 80 mg in AM or evenly divided doses AM, late afternoon; max 100 mg/day

Initial dose titration with strong CYP2D6 inhibitors
• **Adult and child >6 yr weighing >70 kg: PO** 40 mg/day each AM or 2 evenly divided doses, titrate to target of 80 mg/day if symptoms do not improve after 4 wk and dose is well tolerated

Hepatic dose
• Adult/Child PO Child-Pugh B: reduce dose by 50%; Child-Pugh C: reduce dose by 75%

Nocturnal enuresis (unlabeled)
• **Child: PO** 1.5 mg/kg divided bid × 12 wk

Available forms: Caps 10, 18, 25, 40, 60, 80, 100 mg

Administer:
• Whole; do not break, crush, chew
• Gum, hard candy, frequent sips of water for dry mouth
• Without regard to food

SIDE EFFECTS
CNS: *Insomnia,* dizziness, irritability, crying, mood swings, fatigue, lethargy, paresthesia, suicidal ideation

CV: *Palpitations,* hot flushes, tachycardia, increased B/P, palpitations, orthostatic hypotension, QT prolongation

GI: Dyspepsia, nausea, anorexia, dry mouth, weight loss, vomiting, diarrhea, constipation, hepatotoxicity

GU: Urinary hesitancy, retention, dysmenorrhea, erectile disturbance, ejaculation failure, impotence, prostatitis

INTEG: Sweating, rash

MISC: Rhabdomyolysis, angioneurotic edema, anaphylaxis

PHARMACOKINETICS
Peak 1-2 hr duration up to 24 hr, metabolized by liver, some are poor metabolizers ⚛, excreted by kidneys, 98% protein binding, half-life 5 hr

INTERACTIONS
Increase: hypertensive crisis—MAOIs or within 14 days of MAOIs, vasopressors

Increase: cardiovascular effects of albuterol, pressor agents

Increase: effects of atomoxetine—CYP2D6 inhibitors (amiodarone, cimetidine [weak], clomiPRAMINE, delavirdine, gefitinib, imatinib, propafenone, quiNIDine [potent], ritonavir, citalopram, escitalopram, FLUoxetine, sertraline, PARoxetine, thioridazine, venlafaxine)

NURSING CONSIDERATIONS
Assess:

> Black Box Warning: **Mental status:** mood, sensorium, affect, stimulation, memory loss, confusion, insomnia, aggressiveness, suicidal ideation in children/young adults, to notify prescriber immediately

• VS, B/P; check patients with cardiac disease more often for increased B/P
• **Hepatic injury:** may cause liver failure: monitor LFT; assess for jaundice, pruritus, flulike symptoms, upper right quadrant pain
• **Priapism:** monitor for urinary function (hesitancy, retention), sexual changes
• Appetite, sleep, speech patterns
• **ADHD:** For increased attention span, decreased hyperactivity with ADHD, growth

---

rate, weight; therapy may need to be discontinued

Evaluate:

• Therapeutic response: decreased hyperactivity (ADHD), improved attention

Teach patient/family:

• To avoid OTC preparations, other medications, herbs, supplements unless approved by prescriber; no tapering needed when discontinuing product

• To avoid alcohol ingestion

• To avoid hazardous activities until stabilized on medication

• To get needed rest; patients will feel more tired at end of day; not to take dose late in day, insomnia may occur

Black Box Warning: To report suicidal ideation

• To notify prescriber immediately if erection >4 hr

• To report immediately fainting, chest pain, difficulty breathing

• **Pregnancy/breastfeeding:** to notify prescriber if pregnancy is planned or suspected, or if breastfeeding; avoid in pregnancy or breastfeeding

atorvastatin (Rx)

(a-tore′va-stat-in)

Lipitor

Func. class.: Antilipidemic

Chem. class.: HMG-CoA reductase inhibitor (statin)

Do not confuse:

atorvastatin/atomoxetine

Lipitor/Loniten/ZyrTEC

ACTION: Inhibits HMG-CoA reductase enzyme, which reduces cholesterol synthesis; high doses lead to plaque regression

USES: As adjunct for primary hypercholesterolemia (types Ia, Ib), dysbetalipoproteinemia, elevated triglyceride levels, prevention of CV disease by reduction of heart risk in those with mildly elevated cholesterol

CONTRAINDICATIONS: Pregnancy, breastfeeding, hypersensitivity, active hepatic disease

Precautions: Previous hepatic disease, alcoholism, severe acute infections, trauma, severe metabolic disorders, electrolyte imbalance

DOSAGE AND ROUTES

• **Adult: PO** 10-20 mg/day, usual range 10-80 mg/day, dosage adjustments may be made in 2- to 4-wk intervals, max 80 mg/day; patients who require >45% reduction in LDL may be started at 40 mg/day; concurrent use with clarithromycin, itraconazole, saquinavir/ritonavir, derunavir, fosamprenivir, fosamprenavir/ritonavir max 20 mg/day

• **Child 10-17 yr: PO** 10 mg daily, adjust q4wk, max 20 mg/day

Available forms: Tabs 10, 20, 40, 80 mg

Administer:

• Total daily dose at any time of day without regard to meals

• Store in cool environment in tight container protected from light

SIDE EFFECTS

CNS: Headache, asthenia, insomnia

EENT: Lens opacities

GI: *Abdominal cramps, constipation, diarrhea, flatus, heartburn,* dyspepsia, liver dysfunction, pancreatitis, nausea, increased serum transaminase

GU: Impotence, UTI

INTEG: Rash

MISC: Hypersensitivity; gynecomastia (child)

MS: Arthralgia, myalgia, rhabdomyolysis, myositis

Resp: Pharyngitis, sinusitis

PHARMACOKINETICS

Peak 1-2 hr, metabolized in liver, highly protein-bound, excreted primarily in urine, half-life 14 hr, protein binding 98%

INTERACTIONS

Increase: rhabdomyolysis—azole antifungals, cycloSPORINE, erythromycin, niacin, gemfibrozil, clofibrate, amiodarone, boceprevir, nelfinavir, gemfibrozil, lopinavir/ritonavir, macrolides, tacrolimus, telaprevim; use lower dose

Increase: serum level of digoxin

Increase: toxicity, decreased metabolism of HMG-CoA: colchicine, diltiazem, fibric acid derivatives, protease inhibitors

Increase: levels of oral contraceptives

Increase: levels of atorvastatin, myopathy—CYP3A4 inhibitors

Increase: effects of warfarin

Decrease: atorvastatin levels—colestipol, antacids, cholestyramine

Drug/Herb

Decrease: effect—St. John's wort

Drug/Food

• Possible toxicity when used with grapefruit juice (large amounts); oat bran may reduce effectiveness

Drug/Lab Test

Increase: ALT, AST, CK

NURSING CONSIDERATIONS

Assess:

• **Hypercholesterolemia:** diet, obtain diet history including fat, cholesterol in diet; cholesterol triglyceride levels periodically during treatment; check lipid panel 6-12 wk after changing dose

• Hepatic studies q1-2mo, at initiation, 6, 12 wk after initiation or change in dose, periodically thereafter; AST, ALT, LFTs may be increased

• Bowel status: constipation, stool softeners may be needed; if severe, add fiber, water to diet

• **Rhabdomyolysis:** for muscle pain, tenderness, obtain CPK baseline; if markedly increased, product may need to be discontinued; many drug interactions may increase possibility for rhabdomyolysis

• **Pregnancy/breastfeeding:** do not breastfeed or use in pregnancy

Evaluate:

• Therapeutic response: decrease in LDL, total cholesterol, triglycerides, CAD; increase in HDL:LDL ratio

Teach patient/family:

• That compliance is needed for positive results to occur, not to skip or double doses

• That blood work and eye exam will be necessary during treatment

• To report blurred vision, severe GI symptoms, headache, muscle pain, and weakness; to avoid alcohol

• That previously prescribed regimen will continue: low-cholesterol diet, exercise program, smoking cessation

• **Pregnancy/breastfeeding:** identify if pregnancy is planned or suspected, or if breastfeeding

---

atovaquone (Rx)

(a-toe′va-kwon′)

Mepron

Func. class.: Antiprotozoal

Chem. class.: Analog of ubiquinone

ACTION: Interferes with DNA/RNA synthesis in protozoa

USES: *Pneumocystis jiroveci* infections in patients intolerant of trimethoprim-sulfamethoxazole; prophylaxis

CONTRAINDICATIONS: Hypersensitivity or history of developing life-threatening allergic reactions to any component of the formulation, benzyl alcohol sensitivity

Precautions: Pregnancy, breastfeeding, neonates, hepatic disease, GI disease, respiratory insufficiency

DOSAGE AND ROUTES

Acute, mild, moderate

***Pneumocystis jiroveci* pneumonia**

• **Adult and adolescent 13-16 yr: PO** 750 mg with food bid for 21 days

***Pneumocystis jiroveci* pneumonia, prophylaxis**

• **Adult and adolescent >13 yr: PO** 1500 mg/day with meal

Available forms: Susp 750 mg/5 mL

Administer:

• If vomiting occurs after ingestion, notify prescribe

• With high-fat food to increase absorption of product and higher plasma concentrations
• Oral susp; shake gently before using
• All contents of foil pouch, pour in spoon or directly into mouth

SIDE EFFECTS

CNS: *Dizziness, headache, anxiety, insomnia,* asthenia, fever
CV: Hypotension
GI: *Nausea, vomiting, diarrhea,* anorexia, increased AST/ALT, acute pancreatitis, constipation, abdominal pain
HEMA: Anemia, neutropenia
INTEG: Pruritus, urticaria, *rash*
META: Hypoglycemia, hyponatremia
OTHER: Cough, dyspnea

PHARMACOKINETICS

Excreted unchanged in feces (94%), protein binding (99%), half-life 2-3 days, peak 1-8 hr

INTERACTIONS

Increase: level of—zidovudine; monitor for toxicity
Decrease: effect of atovaquone—metoclopramide, rifAMPin, rifabutin, tetracycline; avoid concurrent use
Drug/Food
• Increased absorption with food
Drug/Lab Test
Increase: AST, ALT, alk phos
Decrease: glucose, neutrophils, Hgb, sodium

NURSING CONSIDERATIONS

Assess:
• **Infection:** WBC, vital signs; sputum baseline, periodically; obtain specimens needed before giving 1st dose
• Bowel pattern before, during treatment
• Respiratory status: rate, character, wheezing, dyspnea; risk for respiratory infection
• Allergies before treatment, reaction to each medication
Evaluate:
• Therapeutic response: C&S negative
• Decreased infection signs/symptoms

Teach patient/family:
• To take with food to increase plasma concentrations
• **Pregnancy/breastfeeding:** identify if pregnancy is planned or suspected; use cautiously in breastfeeding
• To take product as prescribed, not to skip or double dose

---

atovaquone/proguanil (Rx)

(a-toe′va-kwon)
Malarone, Malarone Pediatric
Func. class.: Antimalarial
Chem. class.: Aromatic diamide derivative

ACTION: The constituents of Malarone, atovaquone, and proguanil hydrochloride interfere with 2 different pathways involved in DNA/RNA synthesis in protozoa

USES: Malaria, malaria prophylaxis

CONTRAINDICATIONS: Hypersensitivity to this product, malaria prophylaxis in patients with severe renal impairment
Precautions: Pregnancy, breastfeeding, children, hepatic/GI/renal disease

DOSAGE AND ROUTES
Treatment of acute, uncomplicated *P. falciparum* malaria
Malarone adult-strength tabs
• **Adult/adolescent/child >40 kg: PO** 4 adult-strength tabs every day as a single dose × 3 consecutive days
• **Child 31-40 kg: PO** 3 adult-strength tabs every day as a single dose × 3 consecutive days
• **Child 21-30 kg: PO** 2 adult-strength tabs every day as a single dose × 3 consecutive days
• **Infant/child 11-20 kg: PO** 1 adult-strength tab every day × 3 consecutive days
Malarone Pediatric tabs
• **Infant/child 11-20 kg: PO** 4 pediatric tabs every day × 3 consecutive days

---

- **Infant/child 9-10 kg:** PO 3 pediatric tabs every day × 3 consecutive days
- **Infant/child 5-8 kg:** PO 2 pediatric tabs every day × 3 consecutive days

***P. falciparum* malaria prophylaxis, including chloroquine resistance areas**

Malarone adult-strength tabs

- **Adult/adolescent/child >40 kg:** PO 1 adult-strength tab every day; begin prophylaxis 1-2 days before entering the endemic area; continue daily during the stay and for 7 days after leaving the area

Malarone Pediatric tabs

- **Child 31-40 kg:** PO 3 pediatric tabs every day; begin prophylaxis 1-2 days before entering the endemic area; continue daily during the stay and for 7 days after leaving the area
- **Child 21-30 kg:** PO 2 pediatric tabs every day; begin prophylaxis 1-2 days before entering the endemic area; continue daily during the stay and for 7 days after leaving the area
- **Infant/child 11-20 kg:** PO 1 pediatric tab every day; begin prophylaxis 1-2 days before entering the endemic area; continue daily during the stay and for 7 days after leaving the area

Renal dose

- **Adult:** PO CCr <30 mL/min, do not use for prophylaxis

Available forms: Tabs (adult) 250 mg atovaquone/proguanil 100 mg; tabs (pediatric) 62.5 atovaquone/proguanil 25 mg

Administer:

- Give with food or with milk or milk-based drink (nutritional supplement shake) to enhance oral absorption of atovaquone; food with high fat content is desired
- Give dose at the same time each day; administer a repeat dose if vomiting occurs within 1 hr after dosing
- Tabs may be crushed and mixed with condensed milk for children unable to swallow whole tablets

SIDE EFFECTS

CNS: *Dizziness, headache, anxiety, insomnia,* asthenia, fever
CV: Hypotension
GI: *Nausea, vomiting, diarrhea,* anorexia, increased AST/ALT, acute pancreatitis, constipation, abdominal pain
INTEG: Pruritus
OTHER: Cough, dyspnea

PHARMACOKINETICS

Atovaquone excreted unchanged in feces (94%), highly protein-bound (99%), proguanil 75% protein-bound, 40%-60% excreted in urine, hepatic metabolism; half-life 2-3 days

INTERACTIONS

Increase: level of warfarin; monitor INR
Decrease: effect of atovaquone—rifAMPin, rifabutin, tetracycline, metoclopramide; avoid using concurrently

Drug/Lab
Increase: AST, ALT, alk phos
Decrease: glucose, neutrophils, Hgb

NURSING CONSIDERATIONS
Assess:

- **Malaria:** identify when the patient will be entering an area with malaria
- Bowel pattern before, during treatment
- Respiratory status: rate, character, wheezing, dyspnea; risk for respiratory infection
- Allergies before treatment, reaction to each medication
- CBC, LFTs, serum amylase, creatinine/BUN, sodium; increases in LFTs can persist for 4 wk after discontinuation of treatment
- **Pregnancy/breastfeeding:** identify if pregnancy is planned or suspected; avoid in breastfeeding if possible

Evaluate:

- Therapeutic response: resolution/prevention of malaria

Teach patient/family:

- To take with food to increase plasma concentrations, at same time of day
- To take whole course of treatment

• That product may be crushed and mixed with fluid if unable to swallow

> **⚠ HIGH ALERT**
>
> **RARELY USED**

atracurium (Rx)
(a-tra-kyoor'ee-um)
Func. class.: Neuromuscular blocker (nondepolarizing)

USES: Facilitation of endotracheal intubation, skeletal muscle relaxation during mechanical ventilation, surgery, or general anesthesia

CONTRAINDICATIONS: Hypersensitivity

Black Box Warning: Respiratory insufficiency

DOSAGE AND ROUTES
• **Adult and child >2 yr:** IV BOL 0.4-0.5 mg/kg, then 0.08-0.1 mg/kg 20-45 min after 1st dose if needed for prolonged procedures; give smaller doses with halothane
• **Child 1 mo-2 yr:** IV BOL 0.3-0.4 mg/kg

atropine (Rx)
(a'troe-peen)
Atro-Pen
Func. class.: Antidysrhythmic, anticholinergic parasympatholytic, antimuscarinic
Chem. class.: Belladonna alkaloid

ACTION: Blocks acetylcholine at parasympathetic neuroeffector sites; increases cardiac output, heart rate by blocking vagal stimulation in heart; dries secretions by blocking vagus

USES: Bradycardia <40-50 bpm, bradydysrhythmia, reversal of anticholinesterase agents, insecticide poisoning, blocking cardiac vagal reflexes, decreasing secretions before surgery, antispasmodic with GU, biliary surgery, bronchodilator, AV heart block
Unlabeled uses: Cardiac arrest, CPR, pulseless electrical activity, ventricular asystole, asthma, irinotecan-induced diarrhea, rapid-sequence intubation

CONTRAINDICATIONS: Hypersensitivity to belladonna alkaloids, closed-angle glaucoma, GI obstructions, myasthenia gravis, thyrotoxicosis, ulcerative colitis, prostatic hypertrophy, tachycardia/tachydysrhythmias, asthma, acute hemorrhage, severe hepatic disease, myocardial ischemia, paralytic ileus
Precautions: Pregnancy, breastfeeding, children <6 yr, geriatric patients, renal disease, HF, hyperthyroidism, COPD, hypertension, intraabdominal infection, Down syndrome, spastic paralysis, gastric ulcer

DOSAGE AND ROUTES
Bradycardia/bradydysrhythmia
• **Adult:** IV BOL 0.5-1 mg given q3-5 min, max 2 mg
• **Child:** IV BOL 0.02 mg/kg, may repeat ×1; min dose 0.1 mg to avoid paradoxical reaction, max single dose 0.5 mg, max total dose 1 mg; endotracheal IV dose dilute before use
Organophosphate poisoning
• **Adult and child:** IM/IV 1-2 mg q20-30min until muscarinic symptoms disappear; may need 6 mg every hr
• **Adult and child >90 lb, usually >10 yr:** AtroPen 2 mg
• **Child 40-90 lb, usually 4-10 yr:** Atro-Pen 1 mg
• **Child 15-40 lb:** AtroPen 0.5 mg
• **Infant <15 lb:** IM/IV 0.05 mg/kg q5-20min as needed
Presurgery
• **Adult and child >20 kg:** SUBCUT/IM/IV 0.4-0.6 mg 30-60 min before anesthesia

---

- **Child <20 kg: IM/SUBCUT** 0.01 mg/kg up to 0.4 mg, $\frac{1}{2}$-1 hr preop, max 0.6 mg/dose

Available forms: Inj 0.05, 0.1, 0.4, 0.8, 1 mg/mL; AtroPen 0.25, 0.5, 1, 2/0.7 mL mg inj prefilled autoinjectors

Administer:

IM route

- Atropine flush may occur in children and is not harmful, usually 15-20 min after use

AtroPen

- Use no more than 3 AtroPen inj unless under the supervision of trained medical provider
- Use as soon as symptoms appear (tearing, wheezing, muscle fasciculations, excessive oral secretions), may use through clothing

IV route

- Undiluted or diluted with 10 mL sterile water; give at 0.6 mg/min through Y-tube or 3-way stopcock; do not add to IV sol; may cause paradoxical bradycardia for 2 min

Y-site compatibilities: Amrinone, etomidate, famotidine, heparin, hydrocortisone, meropenem, nafcillin, potassium chloride, SUFentanil, vit B/C

Endotracheal Route

- Dilute with 5-10 mL of 0.9% NaCl, inject into endotracheal tube, then positive pressure ventilation

SIDE EFFECTS

CNS: Headache, dizziness, involuntary movement, confusion, flushing, drowsiness

CV: *Tachycardia, bradycardia*

EENT: Blurred vision, photophobia, dry eyes

GI: Dry mouth, constipation

Resp: Tachypnea, pulmonary edema

GU: Retention, hesitancy, impotence

INTEG: Flushing, decreased sweating

PHARMACOKINETICS

Half-life 4-5 hr, excreted by kidneys unchanged (50%), metabolized in liver, crosses placenta, excreted in breast milk

IM/SUBCUT: Onset 15-50 min, peak 30 min, duration 4-6 hr, well absorbed

IV: Peak 2-4 min, duration 4-6 hr

INTERACTIONS

Increase: mucosal lesions—potassium chloride tab; avoid concurrent use

Increase: anticholinergic effects—tricyclics, amantadine, antiparkinson agents, phenothiazines, antidysrhythmics

Increase: altered response—β blockers

Decrease: absorption—ketoconazole, levodopa

Decrease: effect of atropine—antacids

NURSING CONSIDERATIONS

Assess:

- I&O ratio; check for urinary retention, daily output
- VS during treatment, ECG for ectopic ventricular beats, PVC, tachycardia in cardiac patients
- For bowel sounds, constipation, abdominal distension, if constipation occurs add fluids, bulk in diet
- **Beers:** avoid in older adults; highly anticholinergic, high risk of delirium, in men decreased urinary flow

Evaluate:

- Therapeutic response: decreased dysrhythmias, increased heart rate, secretions; GI, GU spasms; bronchodilation

Teach patient/family:

- To report blurred vision, chest pain, allergic reactions, constipation, urinary retention; to use sunglasses to protect the eyes
- Not to perform strenuous activity in high temperatures; heat stroke may result
- To take as prescribed; not to skip or double doses
- Not to operate machinery if drowsiness occurs
- Not to take OTC products, herbals, supplements without approval of prescriber
- Not to freeze or expose to light (AtroPen)
- To use sunglasses for photophobia

• **Pregnancy/breastfeeding:** identify if pregnant or if breastfeeding; use only if benefits outweigh fetal risk

TREATMENT OF OVERDOSE: O_2, artificial ventilation, ECG; administer DOPamine for circulatory depression; administer diazePAM or thiopental for seizures; assess need for antidysrhythmics

---

atropine ophthalmic
See Appendix B

---

avanafil (Rx)
(a-van′a-fil)
Stendra
Func. class.: Impotence agent
Chem. class.: Phosphodiesterase type 5 inhibitor

ACTION: Inhibits phosphodiesterase type 5 (PDE5); enhances erectile function by increasing the amount of cGMP, causing smooth muscle relaxation and increasing blood flow to the corpus cavernosum

USES: Treatment of erectile dysfunction

CONTRAINDICATIONS: Hypersensitivity, severe renal/hepatic disease, current nitrates/nitrites, patients <18 yr
Precautions: Pregnancy, although not indicated for women, anatomic penile deformities, sickle cell anemia, leukemia, multiple myeloma, renal/hepatic/CV disease, bleeding disorders, active peptic ulcer, prolonged erection, aortic stenosis, HIV, stroke, geriatric patients, tinnitus, MI, visual disturbances, retinitis pigmentosa

DOSAGE AND ROUTES
Erectile dysfunction
• **Adult:** PO 100 mg 30 min before sexual activity, dose may be reduced to 50 mg or increased to 200 mg; usual max dose frequency is 1 time/day
Dosage adjustments
Potent CYP3A4 inhibitors/nitrates
• Do not use
Moderate CYP3A4 inhibitors/ α-blockers
• Max 50 mg/day
Hepatic dosage/severe renal disease
Child-Pugh C: Not recommended
Available forms: Tabs 50, 100, 200 mg
Administer:
PO route
• May be taken 30 min before sexual activity on an as-needed basis, but no more than once per day
• May be used without regard to meals
• Product should not be used with nitrates or strong CYP3A4 inhibitors

SIDE EFFECTS
CNS: *Headache, flushing, dizziness*
EENT: Nasal congestion, nasopharyngitis, sudden hearing/vision loss
GI: Nausea, diarrhea, constipation
MS: Back pain, arthralgia
Resp: URI, bronchitis

PHARMACOKINETICS
99% protein binding, metabolized by CYP3A4, excreted as metabolites, urine 62%, feces 21%; half-life 5 hr, peak 30-45 min

INTERACTIONS
• Do not use with nitrates/nitrites because of unsafe drop in B/P, which could result in MI, stroke
• Do not use with strong CYP3A4 inhibitors (ketoconazole, ritonavir, atazanavir, clarithromycin, indinavir, itraconazole, nefazodone, nelfinavir, saquinavir, telithromycin, isoniazid, boceprevir, delavirdine, telaprevir, tipranavir)
• Avoid use with other phosphodiesterase-type inhibitors (vardenafil, sildenafil, tadalafil)
Increase: Avanafil level—moderate CYP3A4 inhibitors (erythromycin, amprenavir, aprepitant, diltiaZEM,

fluconazole, fosamprenavir, verapamil, amiodarone, crizotinib, darunavir, dasatinib, dronedarone, imatinib, lapatinib, ticagrelor, voriconazole); lower avanafil dose

Decrease: B/P—alcohol, α-blockers, amLODIPine, antihypertensives

Drug/Food

Increase: Avanafil effect—grapefruit juice; do not use together

NURSING CONSIDERATIONS
Assess:

• **Erectile dysfunction:** assess for underlying cause before treatment; use of organic nitrates that should not be used with this product; any loss of vision/hearing while taking this product; hypersensitivity reactions

• **Hepatic/renal disease:** avoid use in Child-Pugh C

• **Pregnancy/breastfeeding:** not indicated for women

Evaluate:

• Therapeutic response: ability to engage in sexual intercourse

Teach patient/family:

• Sexual dysfunction: may be taken 30 min before sexual activity on an as-needed basis, but no more than once per day

• May be used without regard to meals

• That product should not be used with nitrates/nitrites or strong CYP3A4 inhibitors

• That product does not protect against sexually transmitted disease, including HIV

• That product has no effect in the absence of sexual stimulation; to seek help if erection lasts >4 hr

• To tell prescriber about all medication, vitamins, herbs being taken, especially ritonavir, indinavir, ketoconazole, itraconazole, erythromycin, nitrates, α-blockers

• Not to drink large amounts of alcohol

• To notify prescriber immediately and to stop taking product if vision or hearing loss occurs, if erection lasts >4 hr, or if chest pain occurs

---

⚠ HIGH ALERT   A

avelumab
(a vel′ue mab)

Bavencio

Func. class.: Antineoplastic monoclonal antibody

Chem. class.: Human IgG1 monoclonal antibody

ACTION: A human IgG1 monoclonal antibody that binds to the programmed death ligand found on T cells and blocks the interaction on receptors on the tumor cell

USES: For the treatment of Merkel cell carcinoma, urothelial carcinoma

CONTRAINDICATIONS: Pregnancy, hypersensitivity

Precautions: Adrenal insufficiency, autoimmune disease, breastfeeding, colitis, Crohn's disease, contraception requirements, diabetes mellitus, diarrhea, hepatic disease, hepatitis, hyperglycemia, infertility, infection, infusion-related reactions, organ transplant, pulmonary disease, pneumonitis, reproductive risk, thyroid disease

DOSAGE AND ROUTES
Metastatic Merkel cell carcinoma

• **Adult/adolescent/child ≥12 yr:** IV 800 mg over 60 min q2wk until disease progression. Give antihistamine (diphenhydramine) and acetaminophen 30-60 min before first 4 infusions; premedication may be administered before subsequent doses as necessary

Locally advanced or metastatic urothelial carcinoma

• **Adult:** IV 10 mg/kg over 60 min q2wk until disease progression or unacceptable toxicity. Give antihistamine (diphenhydramine) and acetaminophen 30-60 min before first 4 infusions; premedication may be administered before subsequent doses as necessary

---

Side effects: *italics* = common; red = life-threatening

Available forms: Sol for injection 200 mg/10 mL

Administer:

Management of treatment-related toxicity/immune-mediated reactions

Colitis

• **Grade 2 or 3 toxicity:** Hold and give corticosteroids (prednisone 1-2 mg/kg/day or equivalent, then taper); resume therapy when adverse event recovers to grade ≤1 after corticosteroid taper; permanently discontinue if grade 3 toxicity recurs

• **Grade 4 toxicity:** Permanently discontinue; give corticosteroids (prednisone 1-2 mg/kg/day or equivalent, then taper)

Endocrinopathies:

• Including hyperglycemia, hypothyroidism, hyperthyroidism, adrenal insufficiency

• **Grade 3 or 4 toxicity:** Hold, give corticosteroids, and manage the endocrinopathy with insulin or antihyperglycemics for hyperglycemia, or with hormone replacement therapy for hypothyroidism; resume when adverse event recovers to grade ≤1 after corticosteroid taper

Hepatitis

• **Grade 2 toxicity** (AST or ALT level of 3-5× the upper limit of normal [ULN] or total bilirubin level of 1.5-3× ULN): Hold, give corticosteroids (prednisone 1-2 mg/kg/day or equivalent initially, then taper); resume when adverse event recovers to grade ≤1 after corticosteroid taper

• **Grade 3 or 4 toxicity** (AST or ALT level >5× ULN or total bilirubin level >3× ULN): Permanently discontinue; give corticosteroids (prednisone 1-2 mg/kg/day or equivalent initially, then taper)

Nephritis

• **Grade 2 or 3 toxicity** (serum creatinine [SCr] level 1.5-6× ULN): Hold, give corticosteroids (prednisone 1-2 mg/kg/day or equivalent initially, then taper); resume therapy when adverse event recovers to grade ≤1 after corticosteroid taper

• **Grade 4 toxicity** (SCr level >6× ULN): Permanently discontinue, give corticosteroids (prednisone 1-2 mg/kg/day or equivalent initially, then taper)

Pneumonitis

• **Grade 2 toxicity:** Hold, give corticosteroids (prednisone 1-2 mg/kg/day or equivalent initially, then taper); resume when adverse event recovers to grade ≤1 after corticosteroid taper; permanently discontinue if grade 2 toxicity recurs

• **Grade 3 or 4 toxicity:** Permanently discontinue; give corticosteroids (prednisone 1-2 mg/kg/day or equivalent initially, then taper)

IV route

• Visually inspect for particulate matter and discoloration before use

• **Dilution:** Add required amount/volume of drug to a 250-mL bag of 0.9% sodium chloride injection or 0.45% sodium chloride injection; mix by gentle inversion

• Discard any unused drug left in vial

• **Storage following dilution:** Store at room temperature (up to 25° C or 77° F) for up to 4 hr or refrigerated (2-8° C; 36-46° F) for up to 24 hr from the time of dilution. Do not freeze or shake; protect from light. If refrigerated, allow the diluted solution to warm to room temperature before use

Intermittent IV Infusion:

• Administer diluted solution IV over 60 min

• Use a sterile, nonpyrogenic, low-protein binding 0.2-micron in-line filter

• Do not administer other drugs through the same infusion line

• Follow cytotoxic handling procedures

SIDE EFFECTS

CNS: Fatigue, chills, fever, dizziness, headache, flushing

CV: Peripheral edema, hypertension

GI: Nausea, vomiting, diarrhea, constipation, abdominal pain, anorexia

HEMA: Anemia, thrombocytopenia, lymphopenia

INTEG: Urticaria, rash

MS: Back pain, arthralgia, myalgia

PHARMACOKINETICS

Half-life 6.1 days, steady state 4-6 wk

INTERACTIONS

• None known

NURSING CONSIDERATIONS
Assess:
• Serious infection: some may be fatal. Monitor patients for signs and symptoms of infection; hold therapy for grade ≥3 infection. Serious *Pneumocystis jiroveci* pneumonia (PJP) has occurred; consider PJP prophylaxis in at-risk patients before starting treatment, hold if PJP is suspected. If PJP diagnosis is confirmed, treat infection until resolution, then resume at previous dose and give PJP prophylaxis for the duration of therapy
• Myelosuppression: assess for anemia, thrombocytopenia, neutropenia; obtain CBC at least weekly during treatment
• Pregnancy/breastfeeding: product can cause fetal harm; females of reproductive potential should avoid becoming pregnant while taking this product; do not breastfeed during treatment and for at least 1 mo after last dose

Evaluate
• Therapeutic response: improving blood counts

Teach patient/family
• To report adverse reactions immediately; to report diarrhea, flulike symptoms
• About reason for treatment, expected results
• Pregnancy/breastfeeding: to notify provider if pregnancy is planned or suspected; not to use during pregnancy and to use effective contraception during treatment and for at least 1 mo after last dose of drug; not to breastfeed during treatment or for at least 1 mo after last dose

---

axicabtagene ciloleucel
(ax-i-cab' tay-jeen-sye-lo' loo-sel)
Yescarta
Func. class.: Antineoplastic, cellular immunotherapies
Chem. class.: Chimeric antigen receptor (CAR) T-cell therapy

ACTION: A chimeric antigen receptor (CAR) T-cell therapy that works by redirecting T cells to target an antigen on B cells in patients with hematologic malignancies

USES: For the treatment of non-Hodgkin's lymphoma

CONTRAINDICATIONS: Hypersensitivity
Precautions: Neurotoxicity, allergic reactions, anemia, neutropenia, thrombocytopenia, secondary malignancy, hypogammaglobulinemia, B-cell aplasia, pregnancy, breastfeeding, hepatitis B, vaccinations, infection

> **Black Box Warning:** Cytokine release syndrome

DOSAGE AND ROUTES
Large B-cell lymphoma
• **Adult:** IV 2×10^6 CAR-positive viable T cells per kg of body weight (max dose of 2×10^8 CAR-positive viable T cells) as a single IV dose
Therapeutic drug monitoring: management of treatment-related toxicity
Cytokine release syndrome (CRS) (without concurrent neurologic toxicity):
• For grade ≥2 toxicity: give tocilizumab 8 mg/kg **IV** over 1 hr (max 800 mg); repeat tocilizumab 8 mg/kg **IV** q8hr as needed if IV fluids or supplemental oxygen is ineffective. Max 3 doses/24 hr, or max 4 doses
• **Grade 2 toxicity (oxygen requirement <40% FiO₂, hypotension responsive to fluids or a low dose of 1 vasopressor agent, or grade 2 organ toxicity):** no improvement within 24 hr after starting tocilizumab, start methylPREDNISolone 1 mg/kg **IV** bid or dexamethasone 10 mg **IV** q6hr; continue corticosteroids until toxicity resolves to grade ≤1, then taper over 3 days
• **Grade 3 toxicity (oxygen requirement of ≥40% FiO₂, hypotension requiring high-dose or multiple vasopressor**

agents, grade 3 organ toxicity, or grade 4 transaminitis): start methylPREDNISolone 1 mg/kg **IV** bid or dexamethasone 10 mg **IV** q6hr; continue corticosteroids until toxicity resolves to grade ≤1, then taper over 3 days

• **Grade 4 toxicity (i.e., requirements for ventilator support, continuous venovenous hemodialysis (CVVHD), or grade 4 organ toxicity (excluding transaminitis):** give methylPREDNISolone 1,000 mg **IV**/day for 3 days. If condition improves, begin methylPREDNISolone 1 mg/kg **IV** bid or dexamethasone 10 mg **IV** q6hr. Continue corticosteroids until toxicity resolves to grade ≤1, then taper over 3 days

Neurologic toxicity (without concurrent CRS):

• Consider seizure prophylaxis with a nonsedating antiseizure medication

• **Grade 2 toxicity:** start dexamethasone 10 mg **IV** q6hr until toxicity resolves to grade ≤1, then taper over 3 days

• **Grade 3 toxicity:** start dexamethasone 10 mg **IV** q6hr until toxicity resolves to grade ≤1, then taper over 3 days

• **Grade 4 toxicity:** give methylPREDNISolone 1,000 mg **IV** daily for 3 days. If condition improves, begin dexamethasone 10 mg **IV** q6hr. Continue corticosteroids until toxicity resolves to grade ≤1, then taper over 3 days

Neurologic toxicity (with concurrent CRS):

• May use seizure prophylaxis with a nonsedating antiseizure medication. For grade ≥2 CRS, give tocilizumab 8 mg/kg **IV** over 1 hr (max dose, 800 mg); may repeat tocilizumab 8 mg/kg **IV** q8hr as needed, max 3 doses/24 hr or max 4 doses

• **Grade 2 neurotoxicity:** if no improvement in 24 hr after starting tocilizumab, start dexamethasone 10 mg **IV** q6hr (if not already taking other corticosteroids); continue corticosteroids until toxicity resolves to grade ≤1, then taper over 3 days

• **Grade 3 neurotoxicity:** give dexamethasone 10 mg **IV** q6hr; start with the first dose of tocilizumab. Continue corticosteroids until toxicity resolves to grade ≤1, then taper over 3 days

• **Grade 4 neurotoxicity:** give methylPREDNISolone 1,000 mg **IV** daily for 3 days; start with the first dose of tocilizumab. If condition improves, start dexamethasone 10 mg **IV** q6hr. Continue corticosteroids until toxicity resolves to grade ≤1, then taper over 3 days

Administer

IV route

• Premedicate patients with acetaminophen 650 mg and diphenhydramine 12.5 mg IV or PO 1 hr before use

• Confirm that tocilizumab is available at the facility before the infusion

• Visually inspect infusion bag for any breaks or cracks before thawing. Do not infuse if bag is compromised; follow local guidelines or call Kite Pharma at 1-844-454-5483

• For autologous and IV use

• Each dose contains a max of 2×10^8 CAR-positive viable T cells suspended in a single patient-specific infusion bag; the total infusion bag volume is about 68 mL

• Ensure that tocilizumab and emergency equipment are available before use

• Coordinate the timing of the product's thaw and infusion; confirm infusion time in advance, and adjust the start time for thaw so that the patient will be ready

• Premedicate with acetaminophen and diphenhydrAMINE approximately 1 hr before infusion; avoid corticosteroids use except for life-threatening emergency

Preparation:

• Match patient's identity with the patient identifiers on the cassette; do not remove product bag from the cassette if the patient-specific label does not match the intended recipient

• Remove the product bag from the cassette; verify that the patient information on the cassette label matches the bag label

• Put the infusion bag inside a second, sterile bag to protect against leaks and port contamination

• Thaw the infusion bag at 37° C using a water bath or dry thaw method; once there is no visible ice, gently mix the contents of the bag

- Do not wash, spin down, and/or resuspend in new media before use
- **Storage:** after thawing, may store at room temperature (20-25° C) ≤3 hr

IV infusion

- Confirm patient's identity with the patient identifiers on the infusion bag
- Prime the tubing with normal saline before use; do not use a leukocyte-depleting filter
- Give as an IV infusion within 30 min via gravity or a peristaltic pump until infusion bag is empty
- Gently agitate during infusion to prevent cell clumping
- Rinse tubing with normal saline at the same infusion rate to ensure that all product is given

SIDE EFFECTS

GI: Abdominal pain, nausea, vomiting, anorexia, constipation, diarrhea, weight loss

CNS: Confusion, chills, delirium, dizziness, drowsiness, fatigue, fever, hallucinations, irritability, malaise, neurotoxicity, paranoia, tremor, weakness

HEMA: Anemia, leukopenia, lymphopenia, neutropenia, thrombocytopenia, thromboembolism, thrombosis

CV: Atrial fibrillation/flutter, AV block, bundle branch block, orthostatic hypotension, QT prolongation, sinus tachycardia, supraventricular tachycardia, ventricular tachycardia, hypotension

META: Hypokalemia, hyponatremia, hypophosphatemia, hyperuricemia

PHARMACOKINETICS

Peak 7-14 days; return to baseline within 28 days

INTERACTIONS

- None known

NURSING CONSIDERATIONS

Assess

- Allergic reactions, anaphylaxis: premedicate with acetaminophen and diphenhydrAMINE before use. Use with caution in those with DMSO or aminoglycoside hypersensitivity

- **Cytopenias (anemia, neutropenia, and thrombocytopenia):** monitor complete blood counts regularly until recovery
- Secondary malignancy: lifelong monitoring for the development of secondary malignancies is recommended. Report cases of secondary malignancy to Kite at 1-844-454-5483; instructions will be provided regarding patient sample collection for testing
- **Hypogammaglobulinemia and B-cell aplasia:** monitor immunoglobulin levels after therapy; provide infection precautions, antibiotic therapy, and immunoglobulin replacement as required
- **Hepatitis B virus (HBV) reactivation:** may cause hepatitis B exacerbation, fulminant hepatitis, hepatic failure, and death; may occur with drugs directed against B cells. Screen all patients for HBV, hepatitis C virus, and HIV before cell collection (leukapheresis)
- Serious infections (bacterial, fungal, viral): may be life-threatening or fatal. Monitor for infection before and after use; use anti-infective therapy as needed. Febrile neutropenia has also been reported; it may occur concurrently with cytokine release syndrome; assess for infection and give broad-spectrum antibiotics, fluids as needed
- Patients should avoid cell, organ, tissue, and blood donation

Black Box Warning: **Cytokine release syndrome (CRS)** may be fatal or life-threatening. Do not use in active infection or inflammatory disorders. Confirm that 2 tocilizumab doses are available before infusion. Observe for CRS q day for ≥7 days in a certified facility following the infusion; continue monitoring for ≥4 wk after infusion. Assess for fever, hypoxia, and hypotension. Treat severe or life-threatening CRS with tocilizumab or tocilizumab and corticosteroids. Those with mild symptoms (fever, nausea, fatigue, headache, myalgia, and malaise) may require symptomatic treatment only. Monitor patients with grade ≥2 CRS (hypotension, not responsive to fluids, or hypoxia requiring supplemental oxygenation) with continuous cardiac telemetry and pulse oximetry. Possible ECG to assess cardiac function

---

Side effects: *italics* = common; red = life-threatening

• **Severe neurotoxicity** (encephalopathy, seizures, cerebral edema), may be fatal, usually occurs within 8 wk. Assess for neurotoxicity daily ≥7 days in a certified health care facility after infusion and for ≥4 wk after infusion. Monitor those with grade ≥2 neurotoxicity with continuous cardiac telemetry and pulse oximetry. Nonsedating antiseizure medicines (levETIRAcetam) may be required for seizure prophylaxis

• **Pregnancy/breastfeeding:** should be avoided; there are no available studies; test for pregnancy before starting treatment; use contraception during treatment, but the recommended length of time for using contraception after treatment is unknown; avoid breastfeeding, excretion unknown

Evaluate:

• Therapeutic response: prevention of spread of cancer

Teach patient/family:

• To avoid driving, operating machinery, or performing other dangerous duties for 8 wk after treatment; mental status changes, seizures may occur or change in consciousness or coordination

• Not to donate blood, organs, tissues

• To report to health care provider any symptoms of fever, fast heartbeat, confusion, or inability to speak

• To avoid vaccinations (live virus) during and for 6 wk after treatment

---

⚠ HIGH ALERT

axitinib (Rx)

Inlyta

Func. class.: Antineoplastics, biologic response modifiers, signal transduction inhibitors (STIs)

Chem. class.: Tyrosine kinase inhibitor

ACTION: Inhibits receptor tyrosine kinases including vascular endothelial growth factor receptor 1 (VEGFR-1), VEGFR-2, and VEGFR-3; inhibits tumor growth and phosphorylation of VEGFR-2 and VEGF-mediated endothelial cell proliferation

USES: Treatment of advanced renal cell cancer after failure of 1 prior systemic therapy

CONTRAINDICATIONS: Pregnancy, breastfeeding

Precautions: Risk for or history of thromboembolic disease, recent bleeding, untreated brain metastasis, recent GI bleeding, GI perforation, fistula, surgery, moderate hepatic disease, uncontrolled hypertension, hyper/hypothyroidism, proteinuria, infertility, end-stage renal disease (CrCl <15 mL/min); not intended for use in adolescents, children, infants, neonates

DOSAGE AND ROUTES

• **Adult: PO** 5 mg bid (at 12-hr intervals), may increase to 7 mg bid and then to 10 mg bid in intervals of 6 wk; in those not receiving antihypertensives who tolerate the lower dosage for at least 2 consecutive wk with no more than grade 2 adverse reactions; reduce to 3 mg bid if a dose reduction is needed; if further reduction is necessary, reduce to 2 mg bid

• **Adult receiving a strong CYP3A4/5 inhibitor:** Reduce dose by ½, adjust as needed

Available forms: Tabs 1, 5 mg

Administer:

• Use safe handling precautions

• Give with or without food; swallow tablet whole with a glass of water

• If patient vomits or misses a dose, an additional dose should not be taken; the next dose should be taken at the usual time

• Store at room temperature

SIDE EFFECTS

CNS: Dizziness, headache, reversible posterior leukoencephalopathy syndrome (RPLS), fatigue

CV: Hypertension, arterial thromboembolic events (ATE), venous thromboembolic events (VTE)

ENDO: Hypothyroidism, hyperthyroidism

GI: Lower GI bleeding/perforation/fistula, abdominal pain, constipation, diarrhea, dysgeusia, dyspepsia, dysphonia, hemorrhoids, nausea, mucosal inflammation, stomatitis, vomiting, increased ALT/AST

GU: Proteinuria
HEMA: Bleeding, intracranial bleeding, anemia, polycythemia, decreased/increased hemoglobin, lymphopenia, thrombocytopenia, neutropenia
INTEG: Palmar-plantar erythrodysesthesia (hand and foot syndrome), rash, dry skin, pruritus, alopecia, erythema
MISC: Weight loss, dehydration, metabolic and electrolyte laboratory abnormalities
MS: Asthenia, arthralgia, musculoskeletal pain, myalgia
RESP: Cough, dyspnea

PHARMACOKINETICS

Absorption: bioavailability 58%; distribution: protein binding >99%; metabolized in liver by CYP3A4/5, CYP1A2, CYP2C19, and UGT1A1; metabolites are carboxylic acid, sulfoxide, and N-glucuronide; excretion 41% in feces and 23% in urine, 12% unchanged; half-life: 2.5-6.1 hr; steady state 2-3 days; onset unknown, peak 2.5-4.1 hr, increased in moderate hepatic disease; duration unknown

INTERACTIONS

Increase: effect of axitinib—CYP3A4/5 inhibitors, strong/moderate (ketoconazole, boceprevir, chloramphenicol, conivaptan, delavirdine, fosamprenavir, imatinib, indinavir, isoniazid, itraconazole, dalfopristin, quinupristin, posaconazole, ritonavir, telithromycin, tipranavir [boosted with ritonavir], darunavir [boosted with ritonavir], aldesleukin [IL-2], amiodarone, aprepitant, fosaprepitant, atazanavir, bromocriptine, clarithromycin, crizotinib, danazol, diltiaZEM, dronedarone, erythromycin, fluvoxaMINE, lanreotide, lapatinib, miconazole, miFEPRIStone, nefazodone, nelfinavir, niCARdipine, octreotide, pantoprazole, saquinavir, tamoxifen, verapamil, voriconazole, grapefruit juice); avoid using together, or reduce axitinib
Decrease: effect of axitinib—CYP3A4/5 inducers, strong/moderate (rifAMPin, carBAMazepine, dexamethasone, phenytoin, PHENobarbital, rifabutin, rifapentine, St. John's wort, ethanol, bexarotene, bosentan, efavirenz, etravirine, griseofulvin, metyraPONE, modafinil, nafcillin, nevirapine, OXcarbazepine, vemurafenib, pioglitazone, topiramate); avoid using together
Increase or decrease: effect of axitinib—CYP3A4/5 inhibitors and inducers (quiNINE)

Drug/Lab Test
Increase: creatinine, lipase, amylase, potassium
Decrease: bicarbonate, calcium, albumin, glucose, phosphate, sodium
Increase or decrease: sodium, glucose

Drug/Food
Increase: drug effect—grapefruit or grapefruit juice

Drug/Herb
Decrease: effect of axitinib—St. John's wort

NURSING CONSIDERATIONS

Assess:
• **Bleeding:** monitor for GI bleeding or perforation; temporarily discontinue therapy if a patient develops any bleeding that requires treatment
• **Surgery:** discontinue ≥24 hr before surgery; may be resumed after adequate wound healing
• **Hepatic/renal disease:** dosage should be reduced in patients with moderate (Child-Pugh Class B) hepatic disease; monitor liver function tests (ALT, AST, bilirubin) before and periodically during therapy; monitor CCr before and during treatment
• **Hypertension:** B/P should be well controlled before starting treatment; monitor patients for hypertension and administer antihypertensive therapy as needed before and during therapy; dose should be reduced for persistent hypertension; therapy should be discontinued if B/P remains elevated after a dosage reduction or if there is evidence of hypertensive crisis; after discontinuation, monitor B/P for hypotension in those receiving antihypertensives
• **Hyper/hypothyroidism:** monitor thyroid function tests before and periodically during therapy; thyroid disease should be treated with thyroid medications
• Monitor for proteinuria before and periodically during therapy; product

---

may need to be decreased or discontinued if moderate to severe proteinuria occurs

• **Pregnancy/breastfeeding:** determine if the patient is pregnant or breastfeeding before using this product; may also cause infertility; do not use in pregnancy or breastfeeding

Evaluate:

• Therapeutic response: decreased spread of malignancy

Teach patient/family:

• That product will be discontinued ≥24 hr before surgery; may be resumed after adequate wound healing

• **Pregnancy/breastfeeding:** to use contraception during treatment or to avoid use of this product; to notify prescriber if pregnancy is planned or suspected; not to breastfeed

• To notify prescriber of bleeding that is severe or that requires treatment

• That laboratory testing will be required before and periodically during product use

• How to monitor B/P and that B/P products should be continued as directed by prescriber

---

> **⚠ HIGH ALERT**
>
> ## azaCITIDine (Rx)
>
> (a-za-sie-ti′deen)
>
> Vidaza
>
> *Func. class.:* Antineoplastic
> *Chem. class.:* Pyrimidine nucleoside analogue

Do not confuse:
azaCITIDine/azaTHIOprine

ACTION: Cytotoxic by producing damage to double-strand DNA during DNA synthesis

USES: Myelodysplastic syndrome (MDS)

Unlabeled uses: Acute myelogenous leukemia (AML), chronic myelogenous leukemia (CML)

CONTRAINDICATIONS: Pregnancy, hypersensitivity to product or mannitol, advanced malignant hepatic tumors

Precautions: Breastfeeding, children, geriatric patients, renal/hepatic disease, baseline albumin <30 g/L; a man should not father a child while taking product

DOSAGE AND ROUTES

• **Adult: SUBCUT/IV** 75 mg/m²/day × 7 days q4wk, dose may be increased to 100 mg/m² if no response seen after 2 treatment cycles; minimum treatment, 4 cycles

Available forms: Powder for inj 100 mg

Administer:

• Use cytotoxic handling procedures

SUBCUT route

• **Reconstitute** with 4 mL sterile water for inj (25 mg/mL), inject diluents slowly into vial, invert vial 2-3 times, gently rotate; sol will be cloudy, use immediately; divide doses >4 mL into 2 syringes; invert contents 2-3 times, gently roll syringe between the palms for 30 sec immediately before administration, rotate inj site

Intermittent IV INFUSION route

• **Reconstitute** each vial with 10 mL sterile water for inj, shake well until all solids are dissolved, withdraw sol (10 mg/mL), inject in 50-100 NS or LR infusion, run over 10-40 min

SIDE EFFECTS

CNS: *Anxiety, depression, dizziness, fatigue, headache, fever, insomnia*

CV: Cardiac murmur, hypotension, tachycardia, peripheral edema, *chest pain*

GI: *Diarrhea, nausea, vomiting,* anorexia, *constipation,* abdominal pain, distention, tenderness, hemorrhoids, mouth hemorrhage, tongue ulceration, stomatitis, dyspepsia, hepatotoxicity, hepatic coma

GU: Renal failure, renal tubular acidosis, dysuria, UTI

HEMA: Leukopenia, anemia, thrombocytopenia, neutropenia, febrile neutropenia, ecchymosis, petechiae

INTEG: *Irritation at site, rash,* sweating, pyrexia, pruritus

META: Hypokalemia

MS: Weakness, arthralgia, muscle cramps, myalgia, back pain
RESP: Cough, *dyspnea, pharyngitis,* pleural effusion

PHARMACOKINETICS
Rapidly absorbed, peak $1/2$ hr, metabolized in the liver, half-life 4 hr, excreted in urine

INTERACTIONS
Increase: bone marrow suppression—other antineoplastics
Increase: bleeding—anticoagulants
Drug/Lab
Increase: BUN, creatinine
Decrease: WBC, platelets, neutrophils, potassium

NURSING CONSIDERATIONS
Assess:
• For CNS symptoms: fever, headache, chills, dizziness
• **Bone marrow suppression/hematologic response:** CBC with differential, baseline WBC ≥3000/mm^3, absolute neutrophil count (ANC) ≥1500/mm^3, platelets >75,000/mm^3, adjust dose based on nadir; ANC <500/mm^3, platelets <25,000/mm^3, give 50% dose next course; ANC 500-1500/mm^3, platelets 25,000-50,000/mm^3, give 67% next course; bruising, bleeding, blood in stools, urine, sputum, emesis; myelodysplastic syndrome (MDS), splenomegaly
• Buccal cavity q8hr for dryness, sores, or ulceration, white patches, oral pain, bleeding, dysphagia
• **Myelodysplastic syndrome:** severe anemia, cytopenias, splenomegaly
• Blood studies: BUN, bicarbonate, creatine, LFTs
• Increased fluid intake to 2-3 L/day to prevent dehydration unless contraindicated
• Rinsing of mouth tid-qid with water, club soda; brushing of teeth bid-tid with soft brush or cotton-tipped applicator for stomatitis; use unwaxed dental floss
Evaluate:
• Therapeutic response: improvement in blood counts with refractory anemia, or refractory anemia with excess blasts

Teach patient/family:
• To avoid crowds, persons with known infections; not to receive immunizations
• To avoid foods with citric acid or hot or rough texture if stomatitis is present; to drink adequate fluids
• To report stomatitis; any bleeding, white spots, ulcerations in mouth; to examine mouth daily, report symptoms, infection site reactions, pruritus, fever
• **Pregnancy/breastfeeding:** to use contraception during and for several months after therapy; not to breastfeed; not to father a child while receiving product

---

azaTHIOprine (Rx)
(ay-za-thye'oh-preen)
Azasan, Imuran ✦
Func. class.: Immunosuppressant
Chem. class.: Purine antagonist

Do not confuse:
azaTHIOprine/azaCITIDine

ACTION: Produces immunosuppression by inhibiting purine synthesis in cells

USES: Renal transplants to prevent graft rejection, refractory rheumatoid arthritis
Unlabeled uses: Chronic ulcerative colitis, Crohn's disease, autoimmune hepatitis, dermatomyositis, thrombocytopenic purpura, lupus nephritis, polymyositis, pulmonary fibrosis, systemic lupus erythematosus (SLE), Wegener's granulomatosis, vasculitis, atopic dermatitis

CONTRAINDICATIONS: Pregnancy, hypersensitivity, breastfeeding
Precautions: Severe renal/hepatic disease, geriatric patients, ✦ thiopurine methyltransferase deficiency, infection, bone marrow suppression; must be used by an experienced clinician

Black Box Warning: Neoplastic disease

DOSAGE AND ROUTES
Immunosuppression in kidney transplantation
• **Adult and child: PO/IV** 3-5 mg/kg/day, then maintenance **(PO)** of ≥1-3 mg/kg/day
Renal dose
• **Adult: PO** Give lower dose in tubular necrosis in immediate postcadaveric transplant period
Refractory rheumatoid arthritis
• **Adult: PO** 1 mg/kg/day, may increase dose after 2 mo by 0.5 mg/kg/day and then q4wk, max 2.5 mg/kg/day
Lupus nephritis/SLE/Wegener's granulomatosis/idiopathic pulmonary fibrosis/multiple sclerosis (unlabeled)
• **Adult: PO** 2-3 mg/kg/day
Atopic dermatitis (unlabeled)
• **Adult/adolescent ≥16 yr: PO** 2.5 mg/kg/day
Crohn's disease, ulcerative colitis (unlabeled)
• **Adult/child: PO** 50 mg/day; may increase by 25 mg/day q1-2wk up to 2-3 mg/kg/day, if tolerated
Available forms: Tabs 50, 75, 100 mg; powder for injection 50 mg ✦, 100 mg/vial
Administer:
• For several days before transplant surgery
• All medications PO if possible; avoid IM inj because bleeding may occur
PO route
• With meals to reduce GI upset
IV route
• Prepare in biologic cabinet with gown, gloves, mask
Direct IV
• **Dilute** to 10 mg/mL with 0.9% NaCl, 0.45% NaCl, D₅W, **give** over 5 min
Intermittent IV INFUSION route
• **Reconstitute** 100 mg/10 mL of sterile water for inj; rotate to dissolve; **further dilute** with 50 mL or more saline or glucose in saline, **give** over ¹/₂-1 hr

Y-site compatibilities: Alfentanil, atracurium, atropine, benztropine, calcium gluconate, cycloSPORINE, enalaprilat, epoetin alfa, erythromycin, fentaNYL, fluconazole, folic acid, furosemide, glycopyrrolate, heparin, insulin, mannitol, mechlorethamine, metoprolol, naloxone, nitroglycerin, oxytocin, penicillin G, potassium chloride, propranolol, protamine, SUFentanil, trimethaphan, vasopressin

SIDE EFFECTS
CNS: Progressive multifocal leukoencephalopathy
EENT: Retinopathy
Resp: Pulmonary edema
GI: *Nausea, vomiting,* stomatitis, esophagitis, pancreatitis, hepatotoxicity, jaundice, hepatic veno-occlusive disease
HEMA: Leukopenia, thrombocytopenia, anemia, pancytopenia, bleeding
INTEG: Rash, alopecia
MISC: Serum sickness, Raynaud's symptoms, secondary malignancy, infection, chills, fever
MS: Arthralgia, muscle wasting

PHARMACOKINETICS
Metabolized in liver, excreted in urine (active metabolite), crosses placenta, half-life 3 hr

INTERACTIONS
Increase: leukopenia—ACE inhibitors, sulfamethoxazole-trimethoprim; monitor for increased leukopenia
Increase: myelosuppression—cycloSPORINE, antineoplastics; monitor for increased myelosuppression
Increase: action of azaTHIOprine—allopurinol; decrease dose of allopurinol, or avoid using
Decrease: immune response—vaccines, toxoids
Drug/herb
Decrease: product's effect—cat's-claw, echinacea; avoid concurrent use
Drug/Lab Test
Increase: LFTs
Decrease: uric acid
Interference: CBC, differential count

NURSING CONSIDERATIONS
Assess:
• **For infection:** increased temperature, WBC; sputum, urine, vital signs baseline and during treatment

• I&O, weight daily, report decreasing urine output; toxicity may occur

• **Bone marrow suppression:** severe leukopenia, pancytopenia, thrombocytopenia; Hgb, WBC, platelets during treatment monthly; if leukocytes are <3000/mm³ or platelets <100,000/mm³, product should be discontinued, CBC

• **Hepatotoxicity:** if dark urine, jaundice, itching, light-colored stools, increased LFTs, product should be discontinued; hepatic studies: alk phos, AST, ALT, bilirubin

• **Arthritis:** pain, ROM, swelling, mobility before, during treatment

Evaluate:

• Therapeutic response: absence of graft rejection, immunosuppression in autoimmune disorders

Teach patient/family:

• To take as prescribed; not to miss doses; if dose is missed on daily regimen, to skip dose; if taking multiple doses/day, to take as soon as remembered

• That therapeutic response may take 3-4 mo with RA; to continue with prescribed exercise, rest, other medications

• To report fever, rash, severe diarrhea, chills, sore throat, fatigue because serious infections may occur; report unusual bleeding, bruising; signs/symptoms of renal/hepatic toxicity

• To avoid vaccinations, bring up to date before use

• To avoid crowds to reduce risk for infection

• That treatment is ongoing to prevent transplant rejection

• To avoid use with OTC, herbals, supplements unless approved by prescriber

• **RA:** Advise patient to continue with other prescribed treatment, other medications, physical therapy

---

RARELY USED

azelaic acid (Rx)
(aze-eh-lay′ik)
Azelex, Finacea
Func. class.: Antiacne agent
Chem. class.: Dicarboxylic acid

USES: Mild to moderate inflammatory acne vulgaris, rosacea

CONTRAINDICATIONS: Hypersensitivity

DOSAGE AND ROUTES
Adult/child ≥12 yr: Apply a thin film and massage into affected areas bid AM and PM
Available forms: Cream 20%, gel 15%

---

azelastine (ophthalmic) (Rx)
(ah-zell′ah-steen)
Optivar
Func. class.: Antihistamine (ophthalmic)
Chem. class.: H₁ receptor antagonist

ACTION: Decreases the allergic response by inhibiting histamine release

USES: Pruritus from allergic conjunctivitis

CONTRAINDICATIONS: Hypersensitivity
Precautions: Pregnancy, breastfeeding, child <3 yr

DOSAGE AND ROUTES
• **Adult/child ≥3 yr: OPHTH** 1 drop into each affected eye bid
Available forms: Ophthalmic sol: 0.05%
Administer:
• Tip of dropper should not touch the eye
• Store upright and tightly closed at room temperature

SIDE EFFECTS
CNS: Headache
EENT: *Eye burning/stinging/irritation,* blurred vision, rhinitis, bitter taste
INTEG: Pruritus
RESP: Asthma, dyspnea, wheezing

PHARMACOKINETICS
Onset 3 min, duration 8 hr, half-life 22 hr, protein binding 88%

Side effects: *italics* = common; red = life-threatening

NURSING CONSIDERATIONS
Assess:
• Eyes: for itching, redness, use of soft or hard contact lenses
Evaluate:
• Therapeutic response: absence of redness, itching in the eyes
Teach patient/family:
• To use in the eyes only; not to touch dropper to eye/eyelid
• Not to wear contact lenses if eyes are red and itching
• To wait at least 10 min before inserting contact lenses; soft contact lenses can absorb preservative

---

azelastine nasal agent
See Appendix B

---

azilsartan (Rx)
(a-zill-sar'tain)
Edarbi
Func. class.: Antihypertensive
Chem. class.: Angiotensin II receptor antagonist

ACTION: Antagonizes angiotensin II at the AT_1 receptor in tissues such as vascular smooth muscle and the adrenal gland

USES: Hypertension, alone or in combination with other antihypertensives

CONTRAINDICATIONS

Black Box Warning: Pregnancy

Precautions: Pregnancy 1st trimester, breastfeeding, children, geriatric patients, angioedema, ⟐ African descent, renal disease, renal artery stenosis, heart failure, hypovolemia

DOSAGE AND ROUTES
• **Adult: PO** 80 mg/day, may give an initial dose of 40 mg/day in patients receiving high-dose diuretic therapy

Available forms: Tabs 40, 80 mg
Administer:
• May administer without regard to food
• Use original package to protect from light and moisture, heat

SIDE EFFECTS
CNS: Dizziness, fatigue, insomnia, headache, depression
CV: Hypotension, orthostatic hypotension
GI: Nausea, diarrhea, vomiting, abdominal pain
INTEG: Angioedema, rash, pruritus
MS: Muscle cramps, arthralgia, myalgia
Meta: Hyperkalemia

PHARMACOKINETICS
Protein binding >99% to serum albumin; metabolized by CYP2C9; half-life 11 hr; elimination 55% in feces, 42% in urine; hydrolyzed to the active metabolite, in GI tract during absorption, rapidly absorbed, peak 1.5-3 hr; absolute bioavailability (60%) not affected by food

INTERACTIONS
Increase: hypotensive effect—other antihypertensives, other angiotensin receptor antagonists, MAOIs; monitor B/P
Increase: hypoglycemia—antidiabetics; reduce antidiabetic dose if needed
Increase: level of digoxin
Increase: hyperkalemia—diuretics; potassium sparing, potassium salt substitute, potassium products; monitor potassium levels
Increase: renal failure risk—cycloSPORINE, diuretics, NSAIDs in those with poor renal function; monitor closely
Increase: lithium toxicity—lithium; reduce lithium dose if needed
Drug/Herb
Increase: antihypertensive effect—hawthorn
Decrease: antihypertensive effect—ephedra

NURSING CONSIDERATIONS
Assess:
• **Angioedema:** Assess for facial swelling, difficulty breathing; discontinued product, notify prescriber immediately

---

more effective against gram-negative organisms

USES: Mild to moderate infections of the upper respiratory tract, lower respiratory tract; uncomplicated skin and skin structure infections caused by *Bacillus anthracis, Bacteroides bivius, Bordetella pertussis, Borrelia burgdorferi, Campylobacter jejuni, CDC coryneform group G, Chlamydia trachomatis, Chlamydophila pneumoniae, Clostridium perfringens, Gardnerella vaginalis, Haemophilus ducreyi, influenzae* (beta-lactamase negative/positive), *Helicobacter pylori, Klebsiella granulomatis, Legionella pneumophila, Moraxella catarrhalis, Mycobacterium avium-intracellulare, Mycoplasma genitalium/hominis/pneumoniae, Neisseria gonorrhoeae, Peptostreptococcus* sp., *Prevotella bivia, Rickettsia tsutsugamushi, Salmonella typhi, Staphylococcus aureus (MSSA)/epidermidis, Streptococcus* sp., *Toxoplasma gondii, Treponema pallidum, Ureaplasma urealyticum, Vibrio cholerae, Viridans streptococci;* **PO:** acute pharyngitis/tonsillitis (group A streptococcal); acute skin/soft-tissue infections; community-acquired pneumonia; **Ophthalmic:** bacterial conjunctivitis
Unlabeled uses: Babesiosis, cholera, cystic fibrosis, dental abscess/infection, endocarditis prophylaxis, granuloma inguinale, Legionnaire's disease, Lyme disease, lymphogranuloma venereum, MAC, periodontitis, pertussis, prostatitis, shigellosis, syphilis, toxoplasmosis, typhoid fever

CONTRAINDICATIONS: Hypersensitivity to azithromycin, erythromycin, any macrolide, hepatitis, jaundice
Precautions: Pregnancy, breastfeeding; geriatric patients; renal/hepatic/cardiac disease; <6 mo for otitis media; <2 yr for pharyngitis, tonsillitis, QT prolongation, ulcerative colitis, torsades de pointes, sunlight exposure, sodium restriction, myasthenia gravis, pseudomembranous colitis, contact lenses, hypokalemia, hypomagnesemia

---

• Response and adverse reactions especially in renal disease
• **HF:** Daily weight, for fluid overload, dyspnea, jugular venous distension, edema, crackles
• Renal function studies; BUN, creatinine, electrolytes (potassium)
• B/P, pulse when beginning therapy and periodically thereafter; note rhythm, rate, quality; obtain electrolytes before beginning therapy
Evaluate:
• Therapeutic response: decreased B/P
Teach patient/family:
• To comply with dosage schedule even if feeling better

• That diarrhea, dehydration, excessive perspiration, vomiting may lead to fall in B/P; to consult prescriber if these occur
• To rise slowly from lying or sitting to minimize orthostatic hypotension; that product may cause dizziness
• To avoid OTC medications unless approved by prescriber; to inform all health care providers of product use
• To use proper technique for obtaining B/P

---

azithromycin (Rx)

(ay-zi-thro-my'sin)

AzaSite, Zithromax, Zmax
Func. class.: Antiinfective
Chem. class.: Macrolide

Do not confuse:
azithromycin/erythromycin
Zithromax/Zinacef

ACTION: Binds to 50S ribosomal subunits of susceptible bacteria and suppresses protein synthesis; much greater spectrum of activity than erythromycin;

DOSAGE AND ROUTES
Most infections
- **Adult: PO** 500 mg on day 1, then 250 mg/day on days 2-5 for a total dose of 1.5 g or 500 mg a day × 3 days
- **Child 2-15 yr: PO** 10 mg/kg on day 1, then 5 mg/kg × 4 days

Disseminated MAC infections
- **Adult: PO** 600 mg/day with ethambutol 15 mg/kg/day;

MAC in HIV:
PO 1.2 g q1wk, alone or with rifabutin

Cervicitis, chlamydia, chancroid, nongonococcal urethritis, syphilis
- **Adult: PO** 1 g single dose

Gonorrhea
- **Adult: PO** 1 g single dose with ceftriaxine 250 mg IM

Lower respiratory tract infections
- **Adult: PO** 500 mg day 1, then 250 mg × 4 days
- **Child: PO** 5-12 mg/kg/day × 5 days

Bacterial conjunctivitis
- **Adult/child ≥1 yr: Ophthalmic** Instill 1 drop in affected eye bid × 2 days, then 1 drop in eye daily × 5 days

Legionnaire's disease/early Lyme disease (unlabeled)
- **Adult: PO** 500 mg/day × 5-7 days

Traveler's diarrhea
- **Adult: PO** 1000 mg as a single dose

Pertussis (unlabeled)
- **Adult: PO** 500 mg on day 1, then 250 mg/day for 2-5 days
- **Infant ≥6 mo and child: PO** 10 mg/kg/day (max 500 mg) on day 1, then 5 mg/kg/day (max 250 mg) on days 2-5
- **Infant <6 mo: PO** 10 mg/kg/day × 5 days

Available forms: Tabs 250, 500, 600 mg; powder for inj 500 mg; susp 100, 200 mg/5 mL, 1 g single-dose powder for susp; ext rel powder for susp 2 (ZMAX); ophthalmic drops 1% solution

Administer:
Ophthalmic route
- Store in refrigerator
- Do not touch dropper to eye

PO route
- **Susp** 1 hr before meal or 2 hr after meal; reconstitute 1 g packet for susp with 60 mL water, mix, rinse glass with more water and have patient drink to consume all medication; packets not for pediatric use
- Store at room temperature

Intermittent IV INFUSION route
- **Reconstitute** 500 mg of product with 4.8 mL sterile water for inj (100 mg/mL); shake, **dilute** with 250 or 500 mL 0.9% NaCl, 0.45% NaCl, or LR to 1-2 mg/mL; diluted sol stable for 24 hr or 7 days if refrigerated
- **Give** 1 mg/mL sol over 3 hr or 2 mg/mL sol over 1 hr; never give IM or as bolus
- Reconstituted product is stable for 24 hr at room temperature or 7 days refrigerated

Y-site compatibilities: Acyclovir, alatrofloxacin, alemtuzumab, alfentanil, aminocaproic acid, aminophylline, amphotericin B liposome/lipid complex, ampicillin, ampicillin-sulbactam, anidulafungin, atenolol, bivalirudin, bleomycin, bumetanide, buprenorphine, butorphanol, calcium chloride/gluconate, CARBOplatin, carmustine, ceFAZolin, cefepime, cefoTEtan, cefOXitin, ceftaroline, cefTAZidime, ceftizoxime, cimetidine, cisatracurium, CISplatin, cyclophosphamide, cycloSPORINE, cytarabine, DAPTOmycin, DAUNOrubicin liposome, dexamethasone, dexmedetomidine, dexrazoxane, digoxin, diltiaZEM, diphenhydrAMINE, DOBUTamine, DOCEtaxel, dolasetron, doripenem, doxacurium, DOXOrubicin liposomal, doxycycline, droperidol, enalaprilat, EPINEPHrine, epiRUBicin, eptifibatide, ertapenem, esmolol, etoposide, etoposide phosphate, fenoldopam, fluconazole, fluorouracil, foscarnet, fosphenytoin, gallium, ganciclovir, gatifloxacin, gemcitabine, granisetron, haloperidol, heparin, hydrocortisone phosphate/succinate, HYDROmorphone, hydrOXYzine, IDArubicin, ifosfamide, inamrinone, irinotecan, isoproterenol, labetalol, lepirudin, magnesium sulfate, mannitol, meperidine, meropenem, mesna, mechlorethamine, methohexital, methotrexate, methylPREDNISolone, metoclopramide, metroNIDAZOLE, milrinone, minocycline, mivacurium, nalbuphine, naloxone, nesiritide, nitroglycerin, nitroprusside, octreotide, ofloxacin, ondansetron, oxaliplatin, oxytocin, PACLitaxel, palonosetron, pamidronate, pantoprazole, PEMEtrexed, PENTobarbital, phenylephrine, piperacillin, potassium acetate/phosphates, procainamide, prochlorperazine, promethazine, propranolol, raNITIdine, remifentanil, rocuronium, sodium acetate, succinylcholine, SUFentanil, sulfamethoxazole-trimethoprim, tacrolimus, telavancin, teniposide, thiotepa, ticarcillin, tigecycline, tirofiban, TPN, trimethobenzamide, vancomycin, vasopressin, vecuronium, verapamil, vinCRIStine, voriconazole, zidovudine, zoledronic acid

SIDE EFFECTS

CNS: Dizziness, headache, seizures, fatigue
CV: Palpitations, chest pain, QT prolongation, torsades de pointes (rare)
EENT: Hearing loss, tinnitus
GI: *Nausea, diarrhea,* hepatotoxicity, abdominal pain, stomatitis, heartburn, dyspepsia, flatulence, melena, cholestatic jaundice, CDAD
GU: Vaginitis, nephritis
HEMA: Anemia, leukopenia, thrombocytopenia
INTEG: Rash, urticaria, pruritus, photosensitivity, pain at inj site
SYST: Angioedema, Stevens-Johnson syndrome, toxic epidermal necrolysis

PHARMACOKINETICS

PO: Peak 2-4 hr, duration 24 hr
IV: Peak end of infusion; duration 24 hr; half-life 11-57 hr; excreted in bile, feces, urine primarily as unchanged product; may be inhibitor of P-glycoprotein

INTERACTIONS

Increase: ergot toxicity—ergotamine
Increase: dysrhythmias—pimozide; fatal reaction, do not use concurrently
Increase: QT prolongation—amiodarone, quiNIDine, nilotinib, droperidol, methadone, propafenone, fluoroquinolones, lithium, paliperidone
Increase: effects of oral anticoagulants, digoxin, theophylline, methylPREDNISolone,

cycloSPORINE, bromocriptine, disopyramide, triazolam, carBAMazepine, phenytoin, tacrolimus, nelfinavir
Decrease: clearance of triazolam
Decrease: absorption of azithromycin—aluminum, magnesium antacids, separate by ≥2 hr
Drug/Lab Test
Increase: CPK, ALT, AST, bilirubin, BUN, creatinine, alk phos, potassium, blood glucose
Drug/Food
Decrease: absorption—food (susp)
Decrease: blood glucose, potassium, sodium

NURSING CONSIDERATIONS

Assess:
• I&O ratio; report hematuria, oliguria with renal disease
• Hepatic studies: AST, ALT, CBC with differential
• Renal studies: urinalysis, protein, blood
• C&S before product therapy; product may be taken as soon as culture is taken; C&S may be repeated after treatment
• **QT prolongation, torsades de pointes:** assess for patients with serious bradycardia, ongoing proarrhythmic conditions, or elderly; more common in these patients
• **Serious skin reactions:** Stevens-Johnson syndrome, toxic epidermal necrolysis, angioedema; discontinue if rash develops, treat symptomatically
• **Superinfection:** sore throat, mouth, tongue; fever, fatigue, diarrhea, anogenital pruritus
• **CDAD:** diarrhea, abdominal pain, fever, fatigue, anorexia; obtain CBC, serum albumin
• Bowel pattern before, during treatment
• Respiratory status: rate, character; wheezing, tightness in chest: discontinue product
• Cardiovascular death has occurred in those with serious bradycardia or ongoing hypokalemia, hypomagnesemia; avoid use

• **Pregnancy/breastfeeding:** use only if clearly needed; cautious use in breastfeeding, excreted in breast milk

Evaluate:

• Therapeutic response: C&S negative for infection; decreased signs of infection

Teach patient/family:

• To report sore throat, fever, fatigue, severe diarrhea, anal/genital itching (may indicate superinfection)

• Not to take aluminum-magnesium–containing antacids simultaneously with this product (PO)

• To notify nurse of diarrhea, dark urine, pale stools; yellow discoloration of eyes, skin; severe abdominal pain

• To complete dosage regimen

• To take ZMAX 1 hr before or 2 hr after a meal; shake well before use

• To use protective clothing or stay out of the sun, photosensitivity may occur

TREATMENT OF HYPERSENSITIVITY: Withdraw product, maintain airway; administer EPINEPHrine, aminophylline, O_2, IV corticosteroids

---

azithromycin ophthalmic

See Appendix B

RARELY USED

aztreonam (Rx)

(az-tree′oh-nam)

Azactam, Cayston

Func. class.: Antibiotic—miscellaneous

USES: Urinary tract infection; septicemia; skin, muscle, bone infection; lower respiratory tract, intraabdominal infections; other infections caused by gram-negative organisms

CONTRAINDICATIONS: Hypersensitivity to product, severe renal disease

DOSAGE AND ROUTES
Urinary tract infections

• **Adult: IM/IV** 500 mg-1 g q8-12hr

Systemic infections

• **Adult: IM/IV** 1-2 g q8-12hr

• **Child: IM/IV** 90-120 mg/kg/day in divided doses q6-8hr; max 8 g/day **IV**

Severe systemic infections

• **Adult: IM/IV** 2 g q6-8hr; max 8 g/day; continue treatment for 48 hr after negative culture or until patient is asymptomatic

Cystic fibrosis with *Pseudomonas aeruginosa*

• **Adult, adolescent, child ≥7 yr: NEB** 75 mg tid × 28 days, then 28 days off; give q4hr or more; give bronchodilator before aztreonam

---

B

bacitracin topical
See Appendix B

baclofen (Rx)
(bak'loe-fen)

Gablofen, Lioresal Intrathecal

Func. class.: Skeletal muscle relaxant, central acting

Chem. class.: GABA chlorophenyl derivative

Do not confuse:

Lioresal/Lotensin

baclofen/Bactroban/bacitracin

ACTION: Inhibits synaptic responses in CNS by stimulating GABAb receptor subtype, which decreases neurotransmitter function; decreases frequency, severity of muscle spasms

USES: Spasticity with spinal cord injury, multiple sclerosis

Unlabeled uses: Neuropathic pain, trigeminal neuralgia

CONTRAINDICATIONS: Hypersensitivity, epidural, IM, IV, subcut administration

Precautions: Pregnancy, breastfeeding, geriatric patients, peptic ulcer disease, renal/hepatic disease, stroke, seizure disorder, diabetes mellitus, psychosis, abrupt discontinuation (intrathecal), CNS depressants, especially opiates

DOSAGE AND ROUTES
Spasticity in multiple sclerosis/spinal cord injury
• **Adult/child ≥12 yr: PO** 5 mg tid × 3 days, then 10 mg tid × 3 days, then 15 mg tid × 3 days, then 20 mg tid × 3 days, then titrated to response, max 80 mg/day (20 mg qid); **INTRATHECAL** use implantable intrathecal infusion pump; use screening trial of 3 separate bolus doses if needed 24 hr apart (50 mcg, 75 mcg, 100 mcg)

• **Child <8 yr:** As above; max 60 mg/day

• **Child >2-7 yr: PO** 10-15 mg/day divided q8hr; titrate q3days by 5-15 mg/day to max 40 mg/day

• **Child: INTRATHECAL** initial test dose same as adult; for small children, initial dose of 25 mcg/dose may be used; 25-1200 mcg/day infusion titrated to response in screening phase

Neuropathic pain including trigeminal neuralgia (unlabeled)
• **Adult: PO** 10 mg tid, may increase by 10 mg every other day; max 80 mg/day

Available forms: Tabs 5, 10, 20 mg; IT inj 10,000 mcg/20 mL, 20,000 mcg/20 mL, 40,000 mcg/20 mL; 50 mcg/mL, 0.5 mg/mL, 10 mg/20 mL, 10 mg/5 mL, 40 mg/20 mL

Administer:
PO route

• With meals for GI symptoms

• Store in a tight container at room temperature

IT route

For screening, dilute to a concentration of 50 mcg/mL with NaCl for inj (preservative free); give test dose over 1 min; watch for decreasing muscle tone, frequency of spasm; if inadequate, use 2 more test doses q24hr, those with inadequate response should not receive chronic IT therapy; **maintenance infusion** via implantable pump of 500-2000 mcg/mL because individual titration is required

• Do not give IT dose by inj, IV, IM, SUBCUT, epidural

> **Black Box Warning:** Do not discontinue abruptly; may be fatal

SIDE EFFECTS
CNS: *Dizziness, weakness, fatigue, drowsiness,* headache, *disorientation,* insomnia, paresthesias, tremors; seizures (IT)

CV: Hypotension, bradycardia, flushing, edema

EENT: Nasal congestion, blurred vision, tinnitus

GI: *Nausea,* constipation, dry mouth, anorexia, weight gain

GU: Urinary frequency, hematuria

INTEG: Rash, pruritus

RESP: Dyspnea

MISC: Hypersensitivity, sweating, hyperglycemia

PHARMACOKINETICS

IT: Peak 2-3 hr, duration >8 hr, half-life $2^{1}/_{2}$-4 hr, partially metabolized in liver, excreted in urine (unchanged), protein binding 30%; CSF levels with plasma levels 100 × that of the oral route

INTERACTIONS

Increase: CNS depression—alcohol, tricyclics, opiates, barbiturates, sedatives, hypnotics, MAOIs, antihistamines; increases CNS depression; avoid concurrent use

> **Black Box Warning:** Increased respiratory depression, death—opiates; avoid concurrent use; limit quantity provided

Increase: hypotension—antihypertensives
Drug/Herb
Increase: CNS depression—kava, valerian, chamomile
Drug/Lab Test
Increase: AST, ALT, alk phos, blood glucose

NURSING CONSIDERATIONS
Assess:

• **MS:** Assess for spasms, spasticity, improvement should occur

• **Abrupt discontinuation;** serious adverse reactions may occur (intrathecal)

• **Intrathecal:** Have emergency equipment nearby; assess test dose and titration; if no response, check pump, catheter for proper functioning

• B/P, weight, blood glucose, hepatic function periodically

• **Seizures (IT):** for increased seizure activity with seizure disorders; product decreases seizure threshold; EEG in epileptic patients

• **Withdrawal symptoms:** agitation, tachycardia, insomnia, hyperpyrexia

• **Allergic reactions:** rash, fever, respiratory distress

• Severe weakness, numbness in extremities

• **CNS depression:** dizziness, drowsiness

Evaluate:

• Therapeutic response: decreased pain, spasticity, ability to perform ADLs

Teach patient/family:

• **Black Box Warning: IT:** Not to discontinue medication quickly; hallucinations, spasticity, tachycardia will occur; product should be tapered off over 1-2 wk, especially intrathecal form

• Not to take with alcohol, other CNS depressants

• To avoid hazardous activities if drowsiness, dizziness occurs; to rise slowly to prevent orthostatic hypotension

• To avoid using OTC medications; not to take cough preparations, antihistamines unless directed by prescriber; to take PO with food or milk

• To notify prescriber if nausea, headache, tinnitus, insomnia, confusion, constipation, inadequate or painful urination continues

• **MS:** may require 1-2 mo for full response

• **Pregnancy/breastfeeding:** to notify prescriber if pregnancy is planned or suspected; avoid breastfeeding

TREATMENT OF OVERDOSE:
Induce emesis in conscious patient, dialysis, physostigmine to reduce life-threatening CNS side effects

---

baloxavir marboxil
(ba lox'a'veer mar box'el)
Xofluza
Func. class.: Antiviral—influenza

ACTION: Baloxavir, the active metabolite of baloxavir marboxil, is responsible for the drug's antiviral activity; inhibits the activity of polymerase acidic

(PA) protein, an influenza virus–specific enzyme

USES: Treatment of uncomplicated influenza A virus or influenza B virus infection

CONTRAINDICATIONS: Hypersensitivity

Precautions: Bacterial infections, child <12 yr

DOSAGE AND ROUTES
• **Adult/adolescent/child >12 yr ≥80 kg: PO** 80 mg single dose; **40-79 kg:** 40 mg single dose

Available forms: Tabs 20 mg, 40 mg

Administer:
• Begin treatment within 48 hr of symptom onset
• Administer with or without food
• Avoid with dairy products, calcium-fortified beverages, laxatives, antacids, or oral supplements (calcium, iron, magnesium, selenium, zincs)

SIDE EFFECTS
CNS: Headache
GI: *Diarrhea, nausea*
RESP: Bronchitis, nasopharyngitis

PHARMACOKINETICS
Plasma protein binding >92%, metabolic pathway by UGT1A3, CYP3A4, excretion urine 14.7%, feces 80%

INTERACTIONS
• Avoid use with laxatives, antacids, oral supplements (calcium, iron, magnesium, selenium, zinc), dairy products
• Avoid use with live attenuated influenza vaccines

NURSING CONSIDERATIONS
Assess:
• **Flu-like symptoms:** duration, onset, specific symptoms (fever, cough, muscle aches and pains)
• **Pregnancy/breastfeeding:** no adverse effects in animals regarding pregnancy and breastfeeding; influenza may pose health hazard to mother and fetus

Evaluate:
• **Therapeutic response:** relief of symptoms of influenza A or B

Teach patient/family:
• **Pregnancy/lactation:** to notify health care provider if pregnancy is planned or suspected, or if breastfeeding
• To avoid use with laxatives, antacids, oral supplements (calcium, iron, magnesium, selenium, zinc), dairy products
• To avoid use with live attenuated influenza vaccines

---

baricitinib
(bar i sye′ ti nib)
Olumiant
Func. class.: Antirheumatic, antiinflammatory
Chem. class.: JAK inhibitor

ACTION: An oral Janus kinase (JAK) inhibitor. Janus kinases are enzymes that transmit signals arising from cytokine or growth factor receptor interactions

USES: Treatment of moderately to severely active rheumatoid arthritis in patients who have had an inadequate response to 1 or more tumor necrosis factor (TNF) antagonists

CONTRAINDICATIONS: Hypersensitivity

Precautions: Vaccinations, lipid elevations, anemia, lymphopenia, neutropenia, GI perforation, viral reactivation, TB

> **Black Box Warning:** Hepatitis exacerbation, hepatotoxicity, lactic acidosis, HIV

DOSAGE AND ROUTES
• **Adult: PO** 2 mg daily; may give with or without methotrexate or other nonbiologic disease-modifying antirheumatic drugs (DMARDs)

Available forms: Tabs 2 mg

Administer:
• Without regard to food

SIDE EFFECTS

EENT: Rhinitis, sinusitis
GI: Nausea, GI perforation, hepatotoxicity
INTEG: Skin cancer
RESP: Pulmonary embolism
SYST: Infection, new primary malignancy

PHARMACOKINETICS

Protein binding 45%-50%, metabolized by CYP3A4, excreted 75% urine, 20% feces, half-life 24 hr

INTERACTIONS

Increase: effect of product—strong OAT3 inhibitors (probenecid)

NURSING CONSIDERATIONS

Assess:
• For pain, swelling in joints, ADLs, aggravating factors
• CBC with differential, hemoglobin/hematocrit, LFTs, serum cholesterol profile, serum creatinine/BUN, tuberculin skin test baseline and periodically
• For new primary malignancies, skin cancer screening exam
• **Pregnancy/breastfeeding:** do not use in pregnancy, breastfeeding

Evaluate:
• Therapeutic response: decreased pain, swelling of joints; slowing of destruction of joints; increased physical function

Teach patient/family:
• About the potential benefits and risk of this product
• **Infections:** that infections are more common; to report any symptoms of infection to health care provider
• **New malignancies:** that product may increase the risk of new cancers, including lymphoma; to notify health care provider
• **Thrombosis:** that DVT and PE may occur; to report any symptoms to health care provider
• That lab work will be needed on a continuing basis
• **Pregnancy/breastfeeding:** not to breastfeed during therapy

---

⚠ HIGH ALERT

basiliximab (Rx)

(bas-ih-liks'ih-mab)

Simulect

Func. class.: Immunosuppressant
Chem. class.: Murine/human monoclonal antibody (interleukin-2) receptor antagonist

ACTION: Binds to and blocks the IL-2 receptor, which is selectively expressed on the surface of activated T lymphocytes; impairs the immune system to antigenic challenges

USES: Acute allograft rejection in renal transplant patients when used with cycloSPORINE and corticosteroids
Unlabeled uses: Liver transplant rejection prophylaxis

CONTRAINDICATIONS: Mannitol, murine protein hypersensitivity
Precautions: Pregnancy, children, geriatric patients, human anti-murine antibody, infections, breastfeeding, neoplastic disease, vaccination

Black Box Warning: Requires a specialized care setting and experienced clinician

DOSAGE AND ROUTES

For acute kidney transplant rejection prophylaxis

• **Adults, adolescents, and children ≥35 kg: IV** 20 mg within 2 hr before transplantation, then 20 mg IV 4 days after surgery
• **Children and adolescents <35 kg: IV** 10 mg within 2 hr before transplantation, then 10 mg IV 4 days after transplantation

For acute liver transplant rejection prophylaxis (unlabeled)

• **Adults: IV** 20 mg within 2 hr of graft reperfusion, then 20 mg IV 4 days after transplantation

---

Available forms: Powder for inj 10, 20 mg/vial

Administer:

IV direct route

• May give undiluted by bolus at 4 mg/mL given over 30 min by central or peripheral IV line

Intermittent IV INFUSION route

• **Reconstitute** 10-mg vial/2.5 mL or 20-mg vial in 5 mL sterile water for inj; shake gently to dissolve; **dilute** reconstituted sol in 25 mL (10-mg vial) or 50 mL (20-mg vial) with 0.9% NaCl or D_5W; gently invert bag, do not shake; **give** over $^1/_2$ hr, do not admix, usually given with corticosteroids and other immunosuppressants

• Store reconstituted sol refrigerated for up to 24 hr or at room temperature for 4 hr

SIDE EFFECTS

CNS: Pyrexia, chills, tremors, headache, insomnia, weakness, dizziness, psychiatric/behavioral changes (child)

CV: Chest pain, angina, cardiac failure, Hypotension, hypertension, edema

GI: Vomiting, nausea, diarrhea, constipation, abdominal pain, GI bleeding, gingival hyperplasia, stomatitis, weight gain

INTEG: Acne, pruritus, impaired wound healing

META: Hypercholesterolemia, hyperuricemia, hypokalemia, hypocalcemia, hypophosphatemia

MISC: Infection, moniliasis, anaphylaxis, allergic reaction

MS: Arthralgia, myalgia

RESP: Cough

PHARMACOKINETICS

Peak $^1/_2$ hr (adults); half-life 7 days (adult), $9^1/_2$ days (children)

INTERACTIONS

Increase: immunosuppression—other immunosuppressants

• Do not use with or within 2 wk of live virus vaccines

Drug/Herb

Decrease: immunosuppression—echinacea, melatonin, St. John's wort, turmeric

Drug/Lab Test

Increase: cholesterol, BUN, uric acid, creatinine, calcium blood glucose, Hgb, Hct

Decrease: Hgb, Hct, platelets, magnesium, phosphate, potassium, glucose

NURSING CONSIDERATIONS

Assess:

For infection: increased temperature, WBC, sputum, urine; may be fatal (bacterial, protozoal, fungal)

• Blood studies: Hgb, WBC, platelets baseline; electrolytes, B/P, edema assessment

• Hepatic studies: alk phos, AST, ALT, bilirubin

• **Anaphylaxis, hypersensitivity:** dyspnea, wheezing, rash, pruritus, hypotension, tachycardia; if severe hypersensitivity reactions occur, product should not be used again

Evaluate:

• Therapeutic response: absence of graft rejection

Teach patient/family:

• To avoid crowds, persons with known upper respiratory tract infections

• To report fever, chills, sore throat, fatigue; serious infection may occur

• Advise patient not to receive any live virus vaccines within 2 wk of this product

• Reason for product, expected result

• Not to drive or engage in hazardous activities, dizziness may occur

• **Pregnancy/breastfeeding:** If pregnancy is planned or suspected; to use contraception during treatment

• To report GI symptoms, bleeding, allergic reactions

---

beclomethasone, inhalation (Rx)

(be-kloe-meth'a-sone)

QVAR, RediHaler

beclamethasone nasal (Rx)

Beconase AQ, QNASL, Rivanage AQ

Func. class.: Antiasthmatic

Chem. class.: Corticosteroid

Side effects: *italics* = common; red = life-threatening

Do not confuse:
beclomethasone/betamethasone

ACTION: Prevents inflammation by suppression of the migration of polymorphonuclear leukocytes, fibroblasts and the reversal of increased capillary permeability and lysosomal stabilization; does not suppress hypothalamus and pituitary function

USES: Chronic asthma, allergic/vasomotor rhinitis, nasal polyps

CONTRAINDICATIONS: Hypersensitivity, status asthmaticus (primary treatment)
Precautions: Pregnancy, breastfeeding, children <12 yr, nasal disease/surgery, nonasthmatic bronchial disease; bacterial, fungal, viral infections of mouth, throat, lungs; HPA suppression, osteoporosis, Cushing's syndrome, diabetes mellitus, measles, cataracts, corticosteroid hypersensitivity, glaucoma, herpes infection

DOSAGE AND ROUTES
• **Adult and child >12 yr: INH** 40-80 mcg bid (alone) or 40-160 mcg bid (previous inhaled corticosteroids); max 320 mcg bid; **Nasal:** 1-2 sprays in each nostril bid
• **Child 5-11 yr: INH** 40 mcg bid; max 80 mcg bid; **Nasal** 1-2 sprays in each nostril bid
Available forms: Oral inh 40, 80, 250 ♣ mcg/metered spray
Administer:
• **Oral inhalation:** no shaking, spacer, or priming needed
• **Nasal:** Shake, invert, tilt head backward, insert nozzle into nostril, compress activator, inhale through nose, exhale through mouth

SIDE EFFECTS
CNS: *Headache,* psychiatric/behavioral changes (child)
EENT: *Hoarseness, candidal infection of oral cavity, sore throat,* loss of taste/smell, dysgeusia, pharyngitis, rhinitis, sinusitis, cataracts, fungal infections, epistaxis

ENDO: HPA suppression
GI: Dry mouth, dyspepsia
MISC: Angioedema, adrenal insufficiency, facial edema, Churg-Strauss syndrome (rare)
RESP: Bronchospasm, wheezing, cough
Nasal
CNS: Headache, dizziness
EENT: Nasal burning/irritation, sneezing
GI: Dry mouth, esophageal candidiasis
Resp: Cough

PHARMACOKINETICS
INH: Onset 1-4 wk; excreted in feces, urine (metabolites); half-life 2.8 hr; crosses placenta; metabolized in lungs, liver (by CYP3A)

NURSING CONSIDERATIONS
Assess:
• **Bronchospasm:** use short-acting bronchodilator
• **Fungal infections:** assess mucous membranes often for infection
• Adrenal function periodically for HPA axis suppression during prolonged therapy; monitor growth/development
• Provide gum, rinsing of mouth for dry mouth
• **Beers:** avoid in older adults; high risk of delirium
Evaluate:
• Therapeutic response: decreased dyspnea, wheezing, dry crackles; nasal polyps are reduced
Teach patient/family:
• To take as prescribed, not to double or skip doses
• To gargle/rinse mouth after each use to prevent oral fungal infections
• To notify prescriber if therapeutic response decreases; dosage adjustment may be needed
• Proper administration technique and cleaning technique
• About all aspects of product usage, including cushingoid symptoms
• About **adrenal insufficiency symptoms:** nausea, anorexia, fatigue, dizziness, dyspnea, weakness, joint pain, depression

• To check growth in child on long-term therapy

• To taper PO products before starting inhalation products

• That peak response may take up to 1 mo

• To carry medical alert ID with corticosteroid user listed

• **Allergic reaction:** To inform health care professional of rash, itching, swelling of face, lips, trouble breathing

• **Pregnancy/breastfeeding:** To notify prescriber if pregnancy is planned or suspected; may breastfeed

---

bedaquiline (Rx)

(bed-ak'-wi-leen)

Sirturo

Func. class.: Antiinfective/antituberculotic

Chem. class.: Diarylquinoline

ACTION: Inhibits an enzyme that binds to adenosine 5'-triphosphate (ATP) synthase and prevents ATP synthase from using the energy from hydrogen and/or sodium

USES: For use as part of a combination regimen to treat pulmonary multidrug-resistant tuberculosis infection (MDR-TB) when other effective treatment regimens are not available

CONTRAINDICATIONS: Hypersensitivity

Precautions: Alcoholism, bradycardia, breastfeeding, arrhythmias, cardiac disease, children, coronary artery disease, diabetes mellitus, females, geriatric patients, heart failure, hepatic disease, hypertension, hypocalcemia, hypokalemia, hypomagnesemia, malnutrition, MI, pregnancy, syncope, thyroid disease

Black Box Warning: QT prolongation, increased mortality risk

DOSAGE AND ROUTES

• **Adults: PO** 400 mg daily × 2 wk, then reduce dose to 200 mg 3×/wk with food (≥48 hr between doses). Total duration is 24 wk

Available forms: Tabs 100 mg

Administer:

• If a dose is missed during the first 2 wk of treatment, instruct patient not to make up the missed dose but to continue with the usual dosing schedule. If a dose is missed during treatment wk 3-24, the missed dose should be taken as soon as possible and then resume 3×/wk regimen

• Give in combination with at least 3 other drugs proven to be or at least 4 other drugs suspected of being effective against the patient's *Mycobacterium tuberculosis* isolate

• Give with food. Swallow tablets whole with water; do not break, crush, chew

• Store at room temperature in light-resistant container

SIDE EFFECTS

CNS: *Headache*

CV: QTc prolongation, chest pain

GI: Nausea, anorexia

MISC: Arthralgia, rash, hemoptysis

PHARMACOKINETICS

Half-life 5 mo, peak 5 hr

INTERACTIONS

Increase: QT prolongation—other drugs that prolong QT (class IA/III antidysrhythmics, some phenothiazines, beta agonists, local anesthetics, tricyclics, haloperidol, chloroquine, droperidol; CYP3A4 inhibitors (amiodarone, clarithromycin, erythromycin); CYP3A4 substrates (methadone, pimozide, QUEtiapine, quiNIDine, risperiDONE, ziprasidone); ECG should be taken often, if possible; avoid concurrent use

Increase: adverse reactions—lopinavir/ritonavir; avoid concurrent use if possible

Increase: bedaquiline effect—strong CYP3A4 inhibitors; avoid use over 14 days

---

Side effects: *italics* = common; red = life-threatening

Decrease: bedaquiline effect—strong CYP3A4 inducers; avoid concurrent use

Drug/Lab Test

Increase: hepatic enzymes

NURSING CONSIDERATIONS

Assess

• **Acute TB:** chest x-ray, sputum culture, blood culture

• **Pregnancy/breastfeeding:** identify if pregnancy is planned or suspected; avoid use unless benefits outweigh risk; avoid breastfeeding

Black Box Warning: **Increased mortality risk:** use only when other treatments cannot be used

• **Liver function:** monitor LFTs baseline and monthly if needed, repeat if >3 × ULN, test for viral hepatitis before use; monitor for dark urine, anorexia, jaundice, nausea, fatigue, hepatomegaly, abdominal tenderness

Black Box Warning: **QT prolongation:** monitor ECG baseline, at 2, 12, and 24 wk or more often if QT prolongation is suspected; close monitoring of the ECG is needed in those with QT-prolonging risk factors; if prolongation of the QT interval is detected, electrolyte monitoring and frequent ECG (to ensure QTc interval return to baseline) are recommended; those developing a clinically significant ventricular arrhythmia or a QTcF interval >500 ms (confirmed by repeat ECG) should discontinue this product and all other QT-prolonging products

• Monitor calcium, magnesium, potassium at baseline, and periodically correct imbalances

Evaluate:

• Positive therapeutic outcome: negative culture

Teach patient/family:

• The importance of compliance with the entire course of therapy, that tabs should be swallowed whole, taken with water and food, and used as part of a multidrug regimen (DOT)

• To report symptoms of TB exacerbation or infection, hemoptysis, respiratory symptoms

• **Pregnancy/breastfeeding:** To avoid breastfeeding and to notify prescriber if pregnancy is planned or suspected

• To avoid the use of alcohol and all medications, herbs unless approved by prescriber; to continue with other prescribed TB regimen

• That scheduled appointments must be kept because relapse may occur

---

belatacept (Rx) REMS

(bel-a-ta′sept)

Nulojix

Func. class.: Immunosuppressant

Chem. class.: Fusion protein

ACTION: Activated T-lymphocytes are the mediators of immunologic rejection. This product is a selective T-cell costimulation blocker; blocks the CD28 mediated costimulation of T-lymphocytes by binding to CD80 and CD86 on antigen-presenting cells; inhibits T-lymphocyte proliferation and the production of the cytokines.

USES: Kidney transplant rejection prophylaxis given with basiliximab induction, mycophenolate mofetil, corticosteroids

CONTRAINDICATIONS: Hypersensitivity, Epstein-Barr virus (EBV) seronegative, EBV status unknown

Precautions: Breastfeeding, child/infant/neonate, pregnancy, diabetes mellitus, progressive multifocal leukoencephalopathy, immunosuppression, sunlight exposure, TB

Black Box Warning: Infection, organ transplant, requires an experienced clinician and specialized care setting, secondary malignancy, posttransplant lymphoproliferation disorder (PLD), immunosuppression

---

DOSAGE AND ROUTES

• **Adult:** IV *Initial:* 10 mg/kg rounded to the nearest 12.5-mg increment; give over 30 min the day of transplantation (day 1) but before transplantation, on day 5 approximately 96 hours after the day 1 dose, at the end of wk 2, at the end of wk 4, at the end of wk 8, and at the end of wk 12; *maintenance* 5 mg/kg rounded to the nearest 12.5-mg increment; give over 30 min at the end of wk 16 and q4wk ± 3 days thereafter; doses should be calculated on actual body weight on the transplantation day unless the patient's weight varies by >10%

Available forms: Powder for inj 250 mg

Administer:

Black Box Warning: Only providers skilled in the use of immunosuppressants and the management of transplants should use these products

IV route

• Visually inspect for particulate matter, discoloration; discard if present
• Calculate the number of vials required
• Reconstitute each vial/10.5 mL of either sterile water for injection, 0.9% sodium chloride, D5W, using the silicone-free disposable syringe provided and an 18-21G needle; if you need additional silicone-free disposable syringes, call 1-888-685-6549; if the powder is accidentally reconstituted using a different syringe than the one provided, the sol may develop a few translucent particles; discard any sol prepared using siliconized syringes
• Inject the diluent into the vial and direct the stream to the glass wall; to minimize foaming, rotate and invert with gentle swirling; do not shake when reconstituted (25 mg/mL), product should be clear to slightly opalescent and colorless to pale yellow; do not use if opaque particles, discoloration, or other foreign particles are present

• Calculate the total volume of the reconstituted 25 mg/mL sol required; further dilute this volume with a volume of infusion fluid equal to the volume of the reconstituted drug sol required; use either NS or D5W if drug was reconstituted with SWFI; use NS if drug was reconstituted with NS; use D5W if drug was reconstituted with D5W; with the same silicone-free disposable syringe; final concentrations in infusion container should range from 2-10 mg/mL; but total infusion volumes ranging from 50-250 mL may be used; discard any unused sol; after reconstitution, immediately transfer the reconstituted sol from the vial to the infusion bag or bottle; complete within 24 hr
• Give over 30 min; use an infusion set and a sterile, nonpyrogenic, low–protein-binding filter (0.2-1.2 mm); use a separate line
• Store refrigerated, protected from light ≤24 hr; max 4 hr of the total 24 hr can be at room temperature and room light

SIDE EFFECTS

CV: Hypo/hypertension
CNS: Progressive multifocal leukoencephalopathy (PML), headache, fever
GI: Abdominal pain, constipation, diarrhea, nausea, vomiting
GU: Proteinuria
HEMA: Anemia, neutropenia, leukopenia
INTEG: Infusion reaction
META: Hyperglycemia, hyper/hypokalemia
SYST: Secondary malignancy, posttransplant lymphoproliferation disorder, wound dehiscence

PHARMACOKINETICS

Half-life, 6.1-15.1 days steady state by wk 8 after transplantation and by mo 6 during maintenance phase, peak infusion end

INTERACTIONS

• **Increase:** effect, toxicity—mycophenolic acid
• Do not use 30 days before or with this product: live virus vaccines

Side effects: *italics* = common; red = life-threatening

NURSING CONSIDERATIONS
Assess:

Black Box Warning: **Transplant rejection:** flulike symptoms, decreasing urinary output, malaise; some may experience pain in area (rare; monitor BUN/creatinine)

Black Box Warning: **Infection:** monitor for fever, chills, increased WBC, wound dehiscences; immunosuppression occurs

Black Box Warning: **Posttransplant lymphoproliferation disorder:** may lead to secondary malignancy (lymphoma) or infectious mononucleosis–like lesions (mood change, confusion, memory loss, change in gait, talking); may be treated with antivirals or immunosuppressant; product may need to be discontinued

• **Progressive multifocal leukoencephalopathy (PML):** apathy, confusion, ataxia may occur during treatment
• **Pregnancy/breastfeeding:** use only if benefits outweigh risk to the fetus; pregnant females should enroll in the National Transplant Pregnancy Registry by calling 1-877-955-6877; use adequate contraception during treatment and for 4 mo after last dose; discontinue breastfeeding or product; excretion in breast milk is unknown
Evaluate:
• Therapeutic response: absence of renal transplant rejection
Teach patient/family:
• Reason for product and expected result; use REMS guidelines
• To avoid exposure to sunlight, tanning beds; risk of secondary malignancy, including skin cancer
• To avoid crowds, persons with known infections
• That repeated lab test will be needed
• To avoid with vaccines; to inform providers of all OTC, prescription medications, herbs, supplements
• That immunosuppressants will be needed for life to prevent rejection; to call provider immediately if symptoms of rejection/infection arise

---

belimumab (Rx)
(be-lim′ue-mab)
Benlysta
Func. class.: Immunosuppressant, monoclonal antibody
Chem. class.: Disease-modifying antirheumatic drugs (DMARDs)

ACTION: Inhibits B-lymphocyte stimulator (BLyS), needed for B-cell survival; normally, soluble BLyS binds to its receptors on B cells and allows B-cell survival; binds BLyS and prevents binding to its receptors on B cells

USES: Active, autoantibody-positive, systemic lupus erythematosus (SLE) in combination with standard therapy

CONTRAINDICATIONS: Hypersensitivity
Precautions: Pregnancy, breastfeeding, children/infants, geriatric patients, ✧◐✦ patients of African descent, depression, immunosuppression, infection, suicidal ideation, vaccination, secondary malignancy, cardiac disease; requires experienced clinician

DOSAGE AND ROUTES
• **Adult: IV** 10 mg/kg over 1 hr q2wk for the first 3 doses, then q4wk; **SUBCUT** 200 mg weekly
• **Child/adolescent 5-17 yr:** 10 mg/kg/dose over 1 hr q2wk × 3 doses, then q4wk
Available forms: Powder for inj 120, 400 mg; autoinjector 200 mg/mL, prefilled syringe sol 200 mg/mL
Administer:
• Only health care providers prepared to manage anaphylaxis should administer this product; may give premedication for prophylaxis against infusion and hypersensitivity reactions (antihistamine, antipyretic)

Intermittent IV INFUSION route

• Visually inspect for particulate matter and discoloration whenever sol and container permit

• **Give** as IV infusion only; do not give IV bolus or push; give over 1 hr and slow or stop if infusion reactions occur

• Do not give with any other agents in the same IV line

• Allow to stand at room temperature for 10-15 min before using

• **Reconstitute** with the appropriate amount of sterile water for injection (80 mg/mL); add 1.5 mL of sterile water (120 mg/vial) or 4.8 mL of sterile water (400 mg/vial)

• Direct the stream of sterile water toward the side of the vial to minimize foaming; gently swirl for 60 sec, allow to sit during reconstitution, gently swirl for 60 sec q5min until powder is dissolved; do not shake; reconstitution is complete in 10-30 min

• If a mechanical reconstitution device (swirler) is used, max 500 rpm swirled for ≤30 min

• Sol should be opalescent and colorless to pale yellow and without particles; small air bubbles are expected; protect from sunlight

• **Dilution:** dilute only in normal saline for injection, 0.45% NaCl, lactated Ringer's; dilute reconstituted sol with enough compatible solution to 250 mL; from a 250-mL infusion bag or bottle of compatible solution, withdraw and discard a volume equal to the volume of the reconstituted sol required for dose; add the required volume of the reconstituted sol to the infusion bag/bottle; gently invert to mix

• Discard any unused sol

• Store in refrigerator or at room temperature; total time from reconstitution to completion of infusion max 8 hr

SUBCUT route

Use of the prefilled syringe or autoinjector:

• Allow 30 min to reach room temperature. Do not warm in any other way

• Inspect for particulate matter and discoloration; product should be clear to opalescent and colorless to pale yellow. It is normal to see 1 or more air bubbles in the solution

• Do not use the autoinjector or prefilled syringe if dropped on a hard surface

Storage of unopened prefilled syringes or autoinjectors:

• Protect from light and store refrigerated at 2° C-8° C (36° F-46° F) until time of use. Do not freeze. Do not shake. Avoid exposure to heat

Administration:

• Subcut administration sites include the abdomen and thigh. Do not inject within 2 inches of the umbilicus. Do not administer where skin is tender, bruised, erythematous, or hard

• For the prefilled syringe, insert the entire needle into the pinched area of the skin at a slight 45-degree angle. Push the plunger all the way down until all of the solution is injected. While keeping your hold on the syringe, slowly move your thumb back, allowing the plunger to rise up. The needle will automatically rise up into the needle guard

• For the autoinjector, position autoinjector straight over inj site at 90-degree angle. Make sure the gold needle guard is flat on the skin. To start injection, firmly press autoinjector all the way down onto inj site and hold in place. A "click" will be heard at the start of injection. Continue to hold autoinjector down until you see that the purple indicator has stopped moving. A second "click" may be heard

• Rotate inj site with each dose

• **Missed dose:** if a dose is missed, administer as soon as possible. Do not give 2 doses on same day

SIDE EFFECTS

CNS: Headache, dizziness, *depression*, fever, *insomnia, migraine*, suicidal ideation, progressive multifocal leukoencephalopathy

GU: UTI

CV: Bradycardia

GI: *Nausea, diarrhea*

MISC: Rash, allergic reactions, myalgia

SYST: Anaphylaxis, angioedema, antibody formation, secondary malignancy, infection, influenza, infusion reactions

INTERACTIONS

• Don't use with cyclophosphamide (IV)

Side effects: *italics* = common; red = life-threatening

• Don't use with live virus vaccines within 30 days of belimumab; response to vaccine will be decreased

Drug/herb

• Decrease belimumab effect—echinacea

Drug/Lab Test

Decrease: leukocytes

PHARMACOKINETICS
Half-life 19.4 days

NURSING CONSIDERATIONS
Assess:

• **SLE improvement:** monitor for decreasing fever, malaise, fatigue, joint pain, myalgias

• **Progressive multifocal leukoencephalopathy:** apathy, confusion, ataxia, cognitive problems

• **Suicidal ideation:** more common in those with preexisting depression

• **Infection:** determine if a chronic or acute infection is present, may be fatal; do not begin therapy if any products are being used for a chronic infection; leukopenia may occur and susceptibility to infections is increased

• **Anaphylaxis** (angioedema, rash, pruritus, wheezing), infusion site reactions: if these occur, stop infusion

• **African descent patients:** use cautiously in these patients; may not respond to this product

• **Pregnancy/breastfeeding:** determine if pregnant or if pregnancy is planned or suspected; if pregnant, enroll in registry; do not breastfeed; contraception is required during and for 4 mo after conclusion of therapy

Evaluate:

• Positive response: decreasing symptoms of SLE; decreasing fatigue, fever, malaise

Teach patient/family:

• To seek treatment immediately for serious hypersensitive reactions

• Not to receive live vaccinations during treatment; bring up to date before treatment

• That compliance is required

• **Infection:** To report fever, shortness of breath, diarrhea, urinary frequency/burning, sweating, chills; to avoid others with known infections

• To report history of cancer in patient or family

• Subcut injection technique, must give at same time of day every wk

• To take as prescribed, not to double or skip doses; if dose is missed, then take as soon as remembered, then resume correct schedule, provide "Medication Guide" and go over with patient

---

> **⚠ HIGH ALERT**
>
> **belinostat (Rx)**
> (beh-lih'noh-stat')
> **Beleodaq**
> *Func. class.:* Antineoplastic-biologic response modifier
> *Chem. class.:* Histone deacetylase inhibitors

Do not confuse:
belinostat/beractant

ACTION: A class I and II inhibitor of the histone deacetylase (HDAC) enzymes. Overexpression of 🔬 HDACs is present in some cancer cells. HDAC inhibitors have been shown to activate differentiation, inhibit the cell cycle, and induce apoptosis

USES: For the treatment of relapsed or refractory peripheral T-cell lymphoma (PTCL)

CONTRAINDICATIONS: Hypersensitivity, pregnancy

Precautions: Hematologic toxicity (thrombocytopenia, leukopenia, neutropenia, lymphopenia, anemia), serious infections (pneumonia, sepsis), fatal hepatic toxicity, tumor lysis syndrome (TLS), breastfeeding

DOSAGE AND ROUTES

• **Adult:** IV 1000 mg/m^2 over 30 min on days 1-5 q21 days. Reduce the dose to 750 mg/m^2 in those who are 🔬 homozygous for the UGT1A1∗28 allele. Cycles should be repeated until disease progression or unacceptable toxicity

Available forms: Powder for inj 500 mg (single-use vial)

Administer:

Intermittent IV route

• Reconstitution: Add 9 mL of sterile water for injection/500 mg, swirl until there are no visible particles in the solution (50 mg/mL); stable at room temperature for up to 12 hr

• Withdraw the appropriate amount from the reconstituted vial and further dilute in 250 mL 0.9% sodium chloride for injection, the final solution is stable at room temperature for up to 36 hr, including infusion time; use a 0.22-micron in-line filter; give over 30 min; if pain occurs at infusion site, run over 45 min

Dose adjustments due to treatment-related toxicity

Hematologic toxicities:

• Do not begin the next cycle of treatment until the absolute neutrophil count (ANC) is ≥1000/mm^3 and platelet count ≥50,000/mm^3

• ANC nadir ≥500/mm^3 *and* platelet count nadir ≥25,000/mm^3: no dose adjustment

• ANC nadir <500/mm^3 (any platelet count): begin next cycle of treatment at a reduced dose of 750 mg/m^2. For the second occurrence of an ANC nadir <500/mm^3, reduce the dose of the next cycle to 500 mg/m^2; if the ANC nadir is <500/mm^3 after 2 dose reductions, discontinue therapy

• Platelet nadir <25,000/mm^3 (any ANC): begin next cycle of treatment at a reduced dose of 750 mg/m^2. For the second occurrence of a platelet nadir <25,000/mm^3, reduce the dose of the next cycle to 500 mg/m^2. If the platelet nadir is <25,000/mm^3 after 2 dose reductions, discontinue therapy

Nonhematologic toxicities:

• Grade 3 or 4 nausea, vomiting, or diarrhea for >7 days with supportive management, or other grade 3 or 4 toxicity of any duration: hold treatment. When toxicity resolves to grade ≤2, restart the next cycle at a reduced dose of 750 mg/m^2.

For the second occurrence of grade 3 or 4 toxicity (for a duration >7 days with supportive management for GI toxicities), resume therapy at 500 mg/m^2 upon resolution to grade ≤2. If the grade 3 or 4 toxicity recurs after 2 dose reductions, discontinue therapy

SIDE EFFECTS

CNS: Fatigue, headache, dizziness, fever, chills

CV: Hypotension, QT prolongation

GI: *Constipation, anorexia, abdominal pain, nausea, vomiting, diarrhea,* hepatotoxicity

HEMA: Anemia, thrombocytopenia, neutropenia

RESP: Dyspnea, cough

INTEG: Injection-site reactions, rash, phlebitis,

MISC: Hypokalemia

SYST: Multi-organ failure, tumor lysis syndrome (TLS), serious infections

PHARMACOKINETICS

Half-life of 1.1 hr; 92.9%-95.8% protein bound, 80%-90% metabolized by hepatic UGT1A1; metabolized in the liver, 40% excreted renally, primarily as metabolites

INTERACTIONS

Increase: belinostat—strong UGT1A1 inhibitors (atazanavir, indinavir); avoid concurrent use if possible

Drug/Lab

Increase: creatinine, LDH

Decrease: platelets, neutrophils, RBC

NURSING CONSIDERATIONS

Assess:

• **Hematologic toxicity (thrombocytopenia, leukopenia, neutropenia, lymphopenia, anemia):** monitor CBC before starting therapy and then every week. Dose modifications may be necessary in patients with bone marrow suppression and should be determined by the ANC and platelet count nadirs of the previous cycle of therapy. Platelet counts should be ≥50,000/mm^3 and ANC >1000/mm^3 before starting each cycle

• **Serious infections (pneumonia, sepsis):** may be fatal. Do not use in those with an active infection. Use caution in patients with a history of extensive or intensive chemotherapy, as they may be at higher risk of life-threatening infections; monitor for dyspnea, cough, characteristics of sputum

• **Fatal hepatic toxicity:** monitor LFTs before the start of each cycle. Those with signs of hepatic disease may require dose modification or discontinuation

• **Tumor lysis syndrome (TLS):** those with high tumor burden or advanced stage disease are at greater risk for development of TLS; consider tumor lysis prophylaxis with antihyperuricemic agents and hydration beginning 12-24 hr before treatment; for TLS treatment, administer aggressive IV hydration, antihyperuricemic agents, correct electrolyte abnormalities, and monitor renal function

• **Pregnancy/breastfeeding:** consider discontinuing breastfeeding; identify whether the patient is pregnant before using; do not use if pregnant

• **Renal studies:** monitor BUN/creatinine periodically; if renal disease is present, use cautiously

Evaluate:

• Therapeutic response: prevention of spread of disease

Teach patient/family:

• To avoid use in breastfeeding; not to use in pregnancy; that fertility may be impaired

• To report infusion-site reactions, rash, severe constipation or diarrhea, abdominal pain, nausea, vomiting

• **Bleeding:** to report increased bruising, bleeding, melanotic or dark tarry stools

• **Tumor lysis syndrome:** to report fatigue, dark urine, nausea, weakness, confusion, change in heart rate

• **Infection:** to report sore throat, cough, trouble breathing

• **Hepatic toxicity:** to report dark urine, anorexia, yellow skin/eyes, itching, abdominal pain

• **Child ≥6 yr:** CCr< 30 mL/min do not use

• That compliance is needed with product and lab testing

---

benazepril (Rx)
(ben-aze'uh-pril)
Lotensin
Func. class.: Antihypertensive
Chem. class.: Angiotensin-converting enzyme (ACE) inhibitor

Do not confuse:
benazepril/Benadryl
Lotensin/lovastatin

ACTION: Selectively suppresses renin-angiotensin-aldosterone system; inhibits ACE, thus preventing conversion of angiotensin I to angiotensin II

USES: Hypertension, alone or in combination with thiazide diuretics
Unlabeled uses: HF, diabetic nephropathy, proteinuria, renal impairment

CONTRAINDICATIONS: Breastfeeding, children, hypersensitivity to ACE inhibitors, hereditary angioedema

Black Box Warning: Pregnancy

Precautions: Geriatric patients, impaired renal/hepatic function, dialysis patients, hypovolemia, blood dyscrasias, HF, asthma, bilateral renal artery stenosis

DOSAGE AND ROUTES

Hypertension
• **Adult:** PO 10 mg/day initially, then 20-40 mg/day divided bid or daily (without a diuretic); reduce initial dose to 5 mg **PO** daily (with a diuretic); max 80 mg/day
• **Child ≥6 yr:** **PO** 0.2 mg/kg/day, max 40 mg/day
Renal dose
• **Adult:** PO CCr <30 mL/min or CCr >3 mg/dL, use 5 mg daily, max 40 mg/day
• **Child ≥6 yr:** PO CCr <30 mL/min, do not use

Renal impairment due to diabetic nephropathy (unlabeled)
• **Adult: PO** 5-10 mg/day
Heart failure (unlabeled)
• **Adult: PO** 2-20 mg/day
Available forms: Tabs 5, 10, 20, 40 mg
Administer:
• May give without regard to food
• Do not discontinue product abruptly
• Store in a tight container at 86° F (30° C) or less

SIDE EFFECTS
CNS: Insomnia, headache, dizziness, fatigue
CV: Hypotension, postural hypotension
GI: Nausea, constipation, vomiting, diarrhea
GU: Increased BUN, creatinine, decreased libido, impotence, renal insufficiency
HEMA: Agranulocytosis
INTEG: Rash, flushing, sweating
META: Hyperkalemia
MISC: Angioedema, Stevens-Johnson syndrome, hypersensitivity, dry cough

PHARMACOKINETICS
Peak 1-2 hr fasting, 2-4 hr after food; protein binding 89%-95%; half-life 10-11 hr; metabolized by liver (metabolites); excreted in urine 33%

INTERACTIONS
Increase: hypotension—phenothiazines, nitrates, acute alcohol ingestion, diuretics, other antihypertensives; may need to reduce dose, monitor B/P
Increase: hyperkalemia—potassium-sparing diuretics, potassium supplements; monitor potassium, BUN, creatinine
Increase: hypotension, hyperkalemia in diabetes, renal disease—aliskiren; do not use in diabetes, avoid use in GFR <60 mL/min
Increase: myelosuppression—azaTHIOprine
Increase: serum levels of lithium, digoxin; may cause toxicity; monitor lithium or digoxin levels
Decrease: hypotensive effects—NSAIDs, COX-2 inhibitors; monitor B/P
Drug/Herb
Increase: antihypertensive effect—hawthorn

Decrease: antihypertensive effect—ephedra (ma huang); avoid concurrent use
Drug/Lab Test
Increase: AST, ALT, alk phos, bilirubin, uric acid, blood glucose, potassium, BUN, creatinine

NURSING CONSIDERATIONS
Assess:
• **Hypertension:** B/P, pulse at baseline, periodically; orthostatic hypotension, syncope when used with diuretic; notify prescriber of changes; monitor compliance
• **Renal studies:** protein, BUN, creatinine; increased levels may indicate nephrotic syndrome; monitor urine for protein; LFTs, uric acid, glucose may be increased; diuretic should be discontinued 3 days before initiation of benazepril; if hypertension is not controlled, a diuretic can be added; measure B/P at peak 2-4 hr and trough (before next dose); ᴬᵂᵃˣ this product is less effective in patients of African descent; CBC, ALT/AST alkaline phosphatase
• Potassium levels, although hyperkalemia rarely occurs
• **Allergic reactions:** rash, fever, pruritus, urticaria; product should be discontinued if antihistamines fail to help; Stevens-Johnson syndrome; angioedema is more common in patients of African descent
• **Renal symptoms:** polyuria, oliguria, frequency, dysuria
• **HF (unlabeled):** edema in feet, legs daily; weight daily
Evaluate:
• Therapeutic response: decrease in B/P; decreased HF (unlabeled)
Teach patient/family:
• Not to use OTC products (cough, cold, allergy) unless directed by prescriber; not to use salt substitutes that contain potassium without consulting prescriber
• The importance of complying with dosage schedule, even if feeling better

Black Box Warning: To notify prescriber of pregnancy; product will need to be discontinued immediately

• To rise slowly to sitting or standing position to minimize orthostatic hypotension

• To notify prescriber of mouth sores, sore throat, fever, swelling of hands or feet, irregular heartbeat, chest pain, bruising, bleeding, swelling of face, tongue, lips, difficulty breathing, signs of infection, cough

• To report excessive perspiration, dehydration, vomiting, diarrhea; may lead to fall in B/P; to use caution in hot weather, strenuous exercise; to consume adequate fluids

• That product may cause dizziness, fainting, light-headedness; that this may occur during first few days of therapy

• That product may cause skin rash or impaired perspiration

• **Diabetes:** blood glucose, glucose may be decreased, especially during early treatment

• **Hypertension:** How to take B/P, and normal readings for age group

TREATMENT OF OVERDOSE: 0.9% NaCl IV infusion, hemodialysis

⚠ HIGH ALERT

bendamustine (Rx)
(ben-da-muss′teen)
Bendeka, Treanda
Func. class.: Antineoplastic alkylating agent
Chem. class.: Mechlorethamine derivative

ACTION: Cross-linking DNA that causes single-strand and double-strand breaks, inhibits several mitotic checkpoints, combines alkylating and antimetabolite properties

USES: Chronic lymphocytic leukemia, non-Hodgkin's lymphoma

CONTRAINDICATIONS: Pregnancy, fetal harm may occur; breastfeeding, children, hepatic disease, renal impairment, hypersensitivity to product or mannitol

Precautions: Hyperuricemia, infusion-related reactions, myelosuppression, infection, skin reactions

DOSAGE AND ROUTES
Chronic lymphocytic leukemia (CLL)
• **Adult: IV INFUSION** 100 mg/m² over 30 min (Treanda) or 10 min (Bendeka) on days 1, 2 q28days up to 6 cycles
Non-Hodgkin's lymphoma
• **Adult: IV INFUSION** 120 mg/m² over 60 min (Treanda) or 10 min (Bendeka) on days 1, 2 q21days up to 8 cycles
Mantle cell lymphoma (unlabeled)
• **Adult: IV INFUSION** 90 mg/m² on days 1, 2 with rituximab on day 1 q28days for 6 cycles
Renal/hepatic dose
• **Adult: IV INFUSION** CCr <40 mL/min, do not use; AST or ALT 2.5-10 × ULN or bilirubin 1.5-3 × ULN, do not use
Available forms: Powder for inj 25, 100 mg; sol for inj 100 mg/4 mL
Administer:
• Allopurinol for 1-2 wk to those at high risk for tumor lysis syndrome; usually develops in first treatment cycle
• Blood transfusions; RBC colony-stimulating factors to counter anemia unless cure is the intent
• Antiemetic 30-60 min before giving product to prevent vomiting
• All medications PO; if possible, avoid IM inj if platelets are <100,000/mm³
Intermittent IV INFUSION route (Treanda)
• Prepare in biologic cabinet wearing gown, gloves, mask; avoid contact with skin, can cause burning, stain the skin brown; use cytotoxic handling procedures
• Before dilution, Treanda injection 45 mg/0.5 mL or 180 mg/2 mL solution cannot be used with any closed-system transfer devices (CSTD), adapters, or syringes that contain polycarbonate or acrylonitrile-butadiene-styrene (ABS)
• After **reconstituting** 100 mg product/20 mL or 25 mg/5 mL sterile water for inj (5 mg/mL), sol should be clear,

colorless to pale yellow, completely dissolve in 5 min; if particulate is present, do not use

• Within 30 min of reconstitution, withdraw volume needed and **further dilute** in 500 mL NS or D2.5/0.45%NS to a final concentration of 0.2-0.6 mg/mL; doses of ≤100 mg/m^2, **give** over 30 min; doses of >100 mg/m^2, **give** over 60 min

• Monitor for infusion reactions; may use antihistamines or corticosteroids for grade 1, 2 reactions; if grade 3 or 4 occurs, discontinue if needed

• Store reconstituted sol in refrigerator for 24 hr or at room temperature for 3 hr; protect from light; store vials at room temperature

Intermittent IV INFUSION route (Bendeka)
• Allow to reach room temperature before use

• Withdraw necessary volume from vial and immediately add to 50 mL bag of NS, dextrose 2.5%/sodium chloride 0.45%, or D$_5$W

• Mix thoroughly; final concentration should be 1.85 to 5.6 mg/mL

SIDE EFFECTS

CNS: Asthenia, *fatigue,* fever, *headache,* chills, hypertension
CV: Hypertension, hypertensive crisis, peripheral edema
GI: *Nausea, vomiting, diarrhea,* hyperbilirubinemia, *constipation,* stomatitis, *anorexia,* weight loss
GU: Renal failure
HEMA: Thrombocytopenia, leukopenia, anemia, lymphocytopenia, neutropenia, secondary malignancy
INTEG: *Bulbous rash, pruritus,* extravasation
META: Hyperuricemia
SYST: Anaphylaxis, infection, dehydration, severe skin toxicities, tumor lysis syndrome, Stevens-Johnson syndrome, toxic epidermal necrolysis, tumor lysis syndrome

PHARMACOKINETICS

95% protein binding, metabolized by hydrolysis via CYP450 1A2, 2 metabolites are produced, half-life 40 min, 90% excreted unchanged (feces)

INTERACTIONS

Increase: agranulocytosis risk—cloZAPine (do not use concurrently)
Increase: bleeding risk—aspirin, anticoagulants, NSAIDs, platelet inhibitors, thrombolytics
Increase: myelosuppression—myelosuppressive agents
Increase: toxicity—other antineoplastics, radiation
Increase: adverse reactions, decreased antibody reaction—live vaccines
Increase: bendamustine—CYP1A2 inhibitors (atazanavir, cimetidine, ciprofloxacin, enoxacin, ethyl estradiol, fluvoxaMINE, mexiletine, norfloxacin, tacrine, thiabendazole, zileuton)
Decrease: bendamustine—CYP1A2 inducers (barbiturates, carBAMazepine, rifampin)
Drug/Lab Test
Increase: LFTs

NURSING CONSIDERATIONS
Assess:
• **Blood dyscrasias:** CBC with differential, platelet count weekly; withhold product if ANC is <1000 or if platelet count is <75,000; notify prescriber of results

• Hepatic studies: AST, ALT, bilirubin
• Renal studies: BUN, serum uric acid, urine CCr before, during therapy; I&O ratio; report fall in urine output of 30 or 40 mL/hr; electrolytes
• Monitor for cold, cough, fever (may indicate beginning infection)
• For malignancy regression
• Bleeding: hematuria, guaiac, bruising, petechiae, mucosa, orifices q8hr
• **Serious skin toxicities:** toxic epidermal necrolysis, Stevens-Johnson syndrome; product should be discontinued
• **Tumor lysis syndrome:** monitor uric acid, potassium; may occur during 1st treatment cycle; use allopurinol for patients at high risk for this condition, usually during the 1st 2 wk; provide adequate hydration
• **Pregnancy/breastfeeding:** fetal toxicity, not to be used in pregnancy; discontinue breastfeeding or product

---

Side effects: *italics* = common; red = life-threatening

Evaluate:
• Therapeutic response: improvement in blood counts, morphology

Teach patient/family:
• To avoid hazardous activity that requires mental alertness
• To avoid crowds, persons with upper respiratory infections
• To report immediately fever, sore throat, flulike symptoms; indicates infection
• To report immediately allergic reaction, facial swelling, difficulty breathing, itchy rash
• Not to breastfeed; males should also use contraception during therapy and for 3 mo after therapy ends
• To avoid use of aspirin, ibuprofen, razors, commercial mouthwash
• To report signs of anemia (fatigue, irritability, SOB, faintness)
• To report signs of infection, myelosuppression, skin toxicities, diarrhea, nausea, vomiting

---

benzocaine topical
See Appendix B

RARELY USED

benzonatate (Rx)
(ben-zoe′na-tate)
Tessalon Perles, Zonatuss
Func. class.: Antitussive, nonopioid

USES: Nonproductive cough

CONTRAINDICATIONS: Hypersensitivity

DOSAGE AND ROUTES
• **Adult and child >10 yr: PO** 100-200 mg up to tid; max 600 mg/day

---

benztropine (Rx)
(benz′troe-peen)
Cogentin
Func. class.: Anticholinergic, antiparkinson agent
Chem. class.: Tertiary amine

Do not confuse:
benztropine/bromocriptine

ACTION: Blockade of central acetylcholine receptors, balances cholinergic activity

USES: Parkinson's symptoms, EPS associated with neuroleptic products, acute dystonic reactions

CONTRAINDICATIONS: Children <3 yr, hypersensitivity, closed-angle glaucoma, dementia, tardive dyskinesia

Precautions: Pregnancy, breastfeeding, geriatric patients, tachycardia, renal/hepatic disease, substance abuse history, dysrhythmias, hypo/hypertension, myasthenia gravis, GI/GU obstruction, peptic ulcer, megacolon, prostate hypertrophy, psychosis

DOSAGE AND ROUTES
Drug-induced EPS (not tardive dyskinesia)
• **Adult: IM/IV/PO** 1-4 mg daily/bid; give **PO** dose as soon as possible
• **Child >3 yr: IM/IV/PO** 0.02-0.05 mg/kg/dose 1-2×/day

Parkinson's symptoms
• **Adult: PO/IM** 0.5-1 mg at bedtime; increase by 0.5 mg q5-6days titrated to patient response, max 6 mg/day

Acute dystonic reactions
• **Adult: IM/IV** 1-2 mg, may increase to 1-2 mg bid **(PO)**

Postencephalitic parkinsonism
• **Adult: PO/IM/IV**
2 mg/day in 1 dose or divided, max 6 mg/day

Available forms: Tabs 0.5, 1, 2 mg; inj 1 mg/mL

Administer:
PO route
• With or after meals to prevent GI upset; may give with fluids other than water
• At bedtime to avoid daytime drowsiness with parkinsonism
• Store at room temperature

IM route
• Inject deeply in muscle; use filtered needle to remove solution from ampule

IV, direct route
• Use in emergencies, not used often; rate 1 mg/min

Y-site compatibilities: Alfentanil, amikacin, aminophylline, ascorbic acid injection, atracurium, atropine, azaTHIOprine, aztreonam, bumetanide, buprenorphine, butorphanol, calcium chloride, gluconate, ceFAZolin, cefotaxime, cefoTEtan, cefOXitin, cefTAZidime, ceftizoxime, cefTRIAXone, cefuroxime, chlorproMAZINE, cimetidine, clindamycin, cyanocobalamin, cycloSPORINE, dexamethasone, digoxin, diphenhydrAMINE, DOBUTamine, DOPamine, doxycycline, enalaprilat, ePHEDrine, epinephrine, epoetin alfa, erythromycin lactobionate, esmolol, famotidine, fentaNYL, fluconazole, folic acid (as sodium salt), gentamicin, glycopyrrolate, heparin, hydrocortisone sodium succinate, hydrOXYzine, imipenem-cilastatin, inamrinone, insulin (regular), isoproterenol, ketorolac, labetalol, lactated Ringer's, lidocaine, magnesium sulfate, mannitol, meperidine, metaraminol, methyldopate, methylPREDNISolone, metoclopramide, metoprolol, midazolam, minocycline, morphine, multiple vitamins injection, nafcillin, nalbuphine, naloxone, netilmicin, nitroglycerin, nitroprusside, norepinephrine, ondansetron, oxacillin, oxytocin, papaverine, penicillin G potassium/sodium, pentamidine, pentazocine, PHENobarbital, phentolamine, phenylephrine, phytonadione, piperacillin, polymyxin B, potassium chloride, procainamide, prochlorperazine, promethazine, propranolol, protamine, pyridoxine, quiNIDine, ranitidine, Ringer's injection, sodium bicarbonate, succinylcholine, SUFentanil, tacrolimus, theophylline, thiamine, ticarcillin, ticarcillin-clavulanate, tobramycin, tolazoline, urokinase, vancomycin, vasopressin, verapamil

SIDE EFFECTS

CNS: Hallucinations, depression, dizziness, memory loss; *confusion;* delirium (geriatric headache, sedation)
CV: Palpitations, tachycardia, hypotension, bradycardia
EENT: Blurred vision, photophobia
GI: *Dry mouth, constipation,* nausea
GU: Urinary hesitancy/retention
INTEG: Rash
MISC: Decreased sweating

PHARMACOKINETICS

PO: Onset 1 hr, peak 7 hr, duration 24 hr
IM/IV: Onset 15 min, duration 6-10 hr

INTERACTIONS

Increase: anticholinergic effect— antihistamines, phenothiazines, tricyclics, disopyramide, quiNIDine; reduce dose
Decrease: absorption—antidiarrheals, antacids
Decrease: anticholinergic effect of—cholinergics; monitor response
Drug/Herb
Increase: anticholinergic action—jimsonweed, *Scopola*

NURSING CONSIDERATIONS

Assess:
• **Parkinsonism:** EPS, shuffling gait, muscle rigidity, involuntary movements, loss of balance, tardive dyskinesia; may exacerbate symptoms
• I&O ratio; commonly causes decreased urinary output; urinary hesitancy, retention; palpate bladder if retention occurs
• Constipation: increase fluids, bulk, exercise if this occurs
• Mental status: affect, mood, CNS depression, worsening of mental symptoms during early therapy
• Use caution during hot weather; product may increase susceptibility to heat stroke by decreasing sweating
• With benztropine "buzz" or "high," patients may imitate EPS
• Hard candy, gum, frequent drinks to relieve dry mouth
• **Withdrawal symptoms:** do not discontinue abruptly; taper
• **Beers:** Avoid in older adults; high risk of delirium, CNS effects, decreased urinary flow
Evaluate:
• Therapeutic response: absence of involuntary movements after 2 days of treatment

---

Side effects: *italics* = common; red = life-threatening

Teach patient/family:

• To report urinary hesitancy/retention, dysuria

• That tabs may be crushed, mixed with food; may take whole dose at bedtime if approved by prescriber

• Not to discontinue product abruptly; to taper off over 1 wk or withdrawal symptoms may occur (EPS, tremors, insomnia, tachycardia, restlessness); to take as directed; not to double dose

• To avoid driving, other hazardous activities; drowsiness/dizziness may occur

• To avoid OTC medications: cough, cold preparations with alcohol, antihistamines, antacids, antidiarrheals within 2 hr unless directed by prescriber

• To change positions slowly to prevent orthostatic hypotension

• To use good oral hygiene, frequent sips of water, sugarless gum for dry mouth

• To avoid strenuous exercise or activities in hot weather; overheating may occur

• That routine exams will be needed

• To separate antacids by 2 hr of this product

---

bepotastine (Rx)

(beh-pot'uh-steen)

Bepreve

Func. class.: Antihistamine (ophthalmic)

Chem. class.: Histamine-1 receptor antagonist

ACTION: A topically active, direct H_1-receptor antagonist and mast cell stabilizer; by reducing these inflammatory mediators, relieves the ocular pruritus associated with allergic conjunctivitis

USES: Ocular pruritus associated with signs/symptoms of allergic conjunctivitis

CONTRAINDICATIONS: Hypersensitivity

Precautions: Pregnancy, breastfeeding, children, contact lenses

DOSAGE AND ROUTES

• **Adult/child ≥2 yr: OPHTH** Instill 1 drop in affected eye bid, max 2 drops/day in each eye

Available forms: Ophthalmic solution 1.5%

Administer:

Ophthalmic route

• For topical ophthalmic use only

• Wash hands before and after use; tilt the head back slightly and pull the lower eyelid down with the index finger; squeeze the prescribed number of drops into the conjunctival sac and gently close eyes for 1-2 min; do not blink

• Do not touch the tip of the dropper to the eye, fingertips, or other surface

• Wait ≥10 min after instilling the ophthalmic solution before inserting contact lenses; contact lenses should not be worn if eye is red; the preservative in this product may be absorbed by soft contact lenses

• Do not share ophthalmic drops with others

SIDE EFFECTS

CNS: Headache

EENT: Taste change, ocular irritation, pharyngitis

SYST: Hypersensitivity

NURSING CONSIDERATIONS

Assess:

• Eyes for itching, redness, use of soft or hard contact lenses

Evaluate:

• Therapeutic response: absence of redness, itching in the eyes

Teach patient/family:

Ophthalmic route

• Product is for topical ophthalmic use only

• Wash hands before and after use; tilt the head back slightly and pull the lower eyelid down with the index finger; squeeze the prescribed number of drops into the conjunctival sac and gently close eyes for 1-2 min; do not blink

• Do not touch the tip of the dropper to the eye, fingertips, or other surface

---

- Do not share ophthalmic drops with others
- Remove **contact lenses** before use because the preservative, benzalkonium chloride, may be absorbed by soft contact lenses; product should not be used to treat contact lens–related irritation; wait ≥10 min after instilling the ophthalmic solution before inserting contact lenses; contact lenses should not be worn if eye is red

---

**betamethasone
(augmented) topical**
See Appendix B

**betamethasone (topical)
(Rx)**
(bay-ta-meth´a-sone)
**betamethasone
augmented
dipropionate (Rx)**

**betamethasone
dipropionate (Rx)**
Diprolene, Diprolene AF, Sernivo
betamethasone valerate
Beta-Val, Dermabet, Luxiq, Valnac
Func. class.: Corticosteroid, topical

ACTION: Crosses cell membrane to attach to receptors to decrease inflammation, itching; inhibits multiple inflammatory cytokines

USES: Inflammation/itching corticosteroid-responsive dermatoses on the skin/scalp

CONTRAINDICATIONS: Hypersensitivity, use of some preparations on face, axilla, groin
Precautions: Pregnancy, skin infections

DOSAGE AND ROUTES
- **Adult: TOP** 1-2 times/day (dipropionate) or **1**-3 times/day (valerate); or apply spray 0.05% bid up to 4 wk (plaque psoriasis, mild to moderate)

Available forms: dipropionate: gel, lotion, ointment, cream, spray 0.05%; **valerate:** cream, lotion, ointment 0.1%, foam 0.12%

SIDE EFFECTS
INTEG: Burning, folliculitis, pruritus, dermatitis, maceration, erythema
MISC: Hyperglycemia, glycosuria, Cushing syndrome, HPA axis suppression

PHARMACOKINETICS
Unknown

NURSING CONSIDERATIONS
Assess:
- **Skin reactions:** - burning, pruritus, folliculitis, dermatitis
- **HPA axis suppression:** usually rare with topical products
Evaluate:
- Decreased itching, inflammation on the skin, scalp
Teach patient/family:
Topical route:
- That betamethasone valerate may be used with occlusive dressings for psoriasis or recalcitrant conditions; not to use dipropionate with occlusive dressings
Cream/ointment/lotion:
- To apply sparingly in a thin film, using gloves, and to rub gently into the cleansed, slightly moist affected area
- Not to use on broken, wet skin, area of infection, face, or groin, axilla
Gel:
- To apply sparingly in a thin film, using gloves, and to rub gently into the cleansed, slightly moist affected area
Scalp foam:
- To invert can and dispense a small amount of foam onto a saucer or other cool surface; not to dispense directly onto hands; to pick up small amounts of foam with fingers and gently massage into affected area until foam disappears; repeat until entire affected scalp area is treated
- That treatment should be limited to 2 wk

Side effects: *italics* = common; red = life-threatening

⚠ HIGH ALERT

betaxolol (Rx)
(beh-tax'oh-lol)

Betoptic-S, Kerlone
Func. class.: Antiglaucoma
Chem. class.: β-Blocker

ACTION: Can decrease aqueous humor and increase outflows, resulting in reduction of intraocular pressure; PO reduces B/P, heart rate, cardiac output by beta-1 receptor blockade

USES: Treatment of chronic open-angle glaucoma and ocular hypertension; **PO** for hypertension

CONTRAINDICATIONS: Hypersensitivity, AV block, heart failure, bradycardia, sick sinus syndrome
Precautions: Abrupt discontinuation, children, pregnancy, breastfeeding, asthma, COPD, depression, diabetes mellitus, myasthenia gravis, hyperthyroidism, pulmonary disease, angle-closure glaucoma

DOSAGE AND ROUTES
Chronic open-angle glaucoma
• **Adult:** Instill 1-2 drops in the affected eye(s) bid
Hypertension
• **Adult:** PO 10 mg/day, may increase to 20 mg after 1-2 wk; may be used with or without diuretics
Geriatric
• **PO** Initially, 5 mg/day, may increase 5 mg/day q2wk, max 20 mg/day
Angina pectoris, chronic (unlabeled)
• **Adult:** PO 5-80 mg/day
Cardiac dysrhythmia (unlabeled)
• **Adult:** PO 20 mg/day started 2 days before CABG and continuing for no less than 10 days postop
Available forms: Ophthalmic sol 0.5%, ophthalmic susp 0.25%, tabs 10, 20 mg
Administer:
Ophthalmic

• Do not touch dropper to eye; shake suspension; press on lacrimal sac after use
PO route
• May be used without regard to food

SIDE EFFECTS
CNS: Insomnia, headache, dizziness
CV: Palpitations, heart block, heart failure
EENT: Eye stinging/burning, tearing, photophobia
MISC: Bronchospasm, asthma

PHARMACOKINETICS
Ophthalmic: Onset 30 min, peak 2 hr, duration ≥12 hr
PO: Peak 3 hr

INTERACTIONS
Increase: bradycardia—digoxin; may need to decrease dose
Increase: antihypertensive effect, negative inotropic effect, bradycardia—calcium channel blockers, other beta blockers; monitor B/P, other cardiac parameters
Increase: hyperglycemia/hypoglycemia—insulins, antidiabetics; adjust dose if needed

NURSING CONSIDERATIONS
Assess:
• **Systemic absorption:** when used in the eye, systemic absorption is common, with the same adverse reactions and interactions as other forms
• Glaucoma: monitor intraocular pressure
• **HPA axis suppression:** usually rare with topical products
• Monitor serum creatinine, BUN, baseline and periodically
• **Pregnancy/breastfeeding:** use only if benefits outweigh risks to fetus; use caution in breastfeeding
Evaluate:
• Decreasing intraocular pressure
Teach patient/family:
Ophthalmic route
• That strength is expressed in betaxolol base
• That ophthalmic product is for ophthalmic use only; shake the ophthalmic suspension well before use

---

• Not to touch the tip of the dropper to the eye, fingertips, or other surface to prevent contamination

• To wash hands before and after use; tilt the head back slightly and pull the lower eyelid down with the index finger to form a pouch; squeeze the prescribed number of drops into the pouch; close eyes to spread drops; to avoid excessive systemic absorption, apply finger pressure on the lacrimal sac for 1-2 min following use

• That if more than one topical ophthalmic drug product is being used, the drugs should be administered at least 5 min apart

• To avoid contamination or the spread of infection, do not use dropper for more than one person

• To report symptoms of heart failure

PO route

• Not to perform hazardous tasks until response is known

---

bethanechol (Rx)

(be-than′e-kole)

Urecholine, Duvoid, Myotonachol ✦

Func. class.: Urinary tract stimulant, cholinergic

Chem. class.: Synthetic choline ester

ACTION: Stimulates muscarinic ACH receptors directly; mimics effects of parasympathetic nervous system stimulation; stimulates gastric motility, micturition; increases lower esophageal sphincter pressure

USES: Urinary retention (postoperative, postpartum), neurogenic atony of bladder with retention

Unlabeled uses: Ileus, GERD, anticholinergic syndrome

CONTRAINDICATIONS: Hypersensitivity, severe bradycardia, asthma, severe hypotension, hyperthyroidism, peptic ulcer, parkinsonism, seizure disorders, CAD, COPD, coronary occlusion, mechanical obstruction, peritonitis, recent urinary/GI surgery, GI/GU obstruction

Precautions: Pregnancy, breastfeeding, children <8 yr, hypertension

DOSAGE AND ROUTES

• **Adult: PO** 10-50 mg bid-qid

• **Child (unlabeled): PO** 0.5 mg/kg/day in 3-4 divided doses

Ileus (unlabeled)

• **Adult: PO** 10-20 mg tid-qid before meals

Available forms: Tabs 5, 10, 25, 50 mg

Administer:

• To avoid nausea, vomiting, take on an empty stomach

• Only after all other cholinergics have been discontinued; cholinergic effects at higher doses may be cumulative

• Store at room temperature

SIDE EFFECTS

CNS: Dizziness, headache, malaise

CV: Hypotension, bradycardia, reflex tachycardia, cardiac arrest, circulatory collapse

EENT: Miosis, increased salivation, lacrimation, blurred vision

GI: *Nausea, bloody diarrhea, belching, vomiting, cramps, fecal incontinence*

GU: Urgency

INTEG: Rash, urticaria, flushing, increased sweating

RESP: Acute asthma, dyspnea, bronchoconstriction

PHARMACOKINETICS

PO: Onset 30-90 min, duration 6 hr

INTERACTIONS

Increase: severe hypotension—ganglionic blockers; avoid concurrent use

Increase: action or toxicity—cholinergic agonists, anticholinesterase agents; avoid concurrent use

Decrease: action of anticholinergics, procainamide, quiNIDine, belladonna; monitor for adequate effect

Drug/Lab Test

Increase: AST, lipase/amylase, bilirubin

NURSING CONSIDERATIONS

Assess:

Side effects: *italics* = common; red = life-threatening

- **Urinary patterns:** retention, urgency
- **B/P, pulse:** observe after parenteral dose for 1 hr; may need to use atropine subcut 0.6 mg or IV push slowly for bronchoconstriction
- **I&O ratio:** check for urinary retention, urge incontinence
- **Toxicity:** bradycardia, hypotension, bronchospasm, headache, dizziness, seizures, respiratory depression; product should be discontinued if toxicity occurs
- **Orthostatic hypotension:** monitor frequently, monitor ambulation to prevent falling
- **Pregnancy/breastfeeding:** use only if clearly needed; discontinue breastfeeding or product

Evaluate:
- Therapeutic response: absence of urinary retention, abdominal distention

Teach patient/family:
- To take product exactly as prescribed; 1 hr before meals or 2 hr after meals to avoid nausea
- To make position changes slowly; orthostatic hypotension may occur
- To avoid driving, hazardous activities until effects are known

TREATMENT OF OVERDOSE: Administer atropine 0.6-1.2 mg IV or IM (adult)

---

betrixaban (Rx)
(be-trix′-a-ban)

Bevyxxa
Func. class.: Antithrombotic agents
Chem. class.: Synthetic, selective factor Xa inhibitor

ACTION: Inhibits factor Xa; neutralization of factor Xa interrupts blood coagulation and thrombin formation

USES: Prevention/treatment of deep venous thrombosis, PE in at-risk, acutely ill, hospitalized medical patients

CONTRAINDICATIONS: Hypersensitivity, active major bleeding

Precautions: Pregnancy, breastfeeding, children, geriatric patients, hepatic disease, renal disease

Black Box Warning: Spinal/epidural anesthesia, lumbar puncture

DOSAGE AND ROUTES

For venous thromboembolism prophylaxis (i.e., deep venous thrombosis [DVT] prophylaxis, pulmonary embolism prophylaxis) in at-risk, acutely ill, hospitalized medical patients
- **Adult: PO** 160 mg once, followed by 80 mg/day for 35-42 days

Available Forms: Capsules 40, 80 mg
Administer:
- Give with food
- If a dose is missed, take as soon as remembered on the same day; do not double

PHARMACOKINETICS
Protein binding 60%, half-life 19-27 hr; excreted in urine 11%, feces 85%; affected cytochrome P450 isoenzymes and drug transporters: P-gp; betrixaban is a substrate of P-glycoprotein (P-gp)

INTERACTIONS
Increase: bleeding risk—salicylates, NSAIDs, abciximab, eptifibatide, tirofiban, clopidogrel, dipyridamole, quiNIDine, valproic acid

Drug/Herb
Increase: bleeding risk—feverfew, garlic, ginger, ginkgo, ginseng, green tea, horse chestnut, kava

NURSING CONSIDERATIONS
Assess:

Black Box Warning: Monitor patients who have received epidural/spinal anesthesia or lumbar puncture for neurologic impairment, including spinal hematoma; may lead to permanent disability or paralysis

- **Hepatic impairment:** avoid use
- **Renal impairment:** dose reduction is required

• For bleeding: gums, petechiae, ecchymosis, black tarry stools, hematuria; decreased Hct; notify prescriber

• For risk of hemorrhage if coadministering with other products that may cause bleeding

• For hypersensitivity: rash, fever, chills; notify prescriber

• **Pregnancy/breastfeeding:** consider risks of bleeding and stroke; use only if benefits outweigh risks; consider potential adverse effects before breastfeeding

• **Beers:** avoid in older adults; increased risk of bleeding, lower creatinine clearance

Evaluate:

• Therapeutic response: prevention of DVT

Teach patient/family:

• To use soft-bristle toothbrush to avoid bleeding gums; to use electric razor

• To report any signs of bleeding: gums, under skin, urine, stools; bleeding risk may continue up to 72 hr after stopping therapy

• To avoid OTC products containing aspirin, NSAIDs

• To take with food

⚠ HIGH ALERT

bevacizumab (Rx)

(beh-va-kiz'you-mab)

Avastin

Func. class.: Antineoplastic—miscellaneous

Chem. class.: Monoclonal antibody

Do not confuse:
Avastin/Astelin

ACTION: Monoclonal antibody selectively binds to and inhibits activity of human vascular endothelial growth factor (VEGF) to reduce microvascular growth and metastatic disease progression

USES: Non–small-cell lung cancer (NSCLC), metastatic carcinoma of the colon or rectum, renal cell carcinoma, glioblastoma

Unlabeled uses: Adjunctive for ovarian cancer; (wet) macular degeneration

CONTRAINDICATIONS: Hypersensitivity, serious bleeding, hypertensive crisis, recent surgery

Precautions: Pregnancy, breastfeeding, children, geriatric patients, HF, blood dyscrasias, CV disease, hypertension, surgery, thromboembolic disease, hamster protein/murine hypersensitivity

> Black Box Warning: GI perforation, wound dehiscence, bleeding

DOSAGE AND ROUTES
Non–small-cell lung cancer

• **Adult: IV** 15 mg/kg over 60-90 min with CARBOplatin and paclitaxel q3wk

Metastatic colorectal cancer

• **Adult: IV** in combination with (5-FU) 5 mg/kg q 14 days over 90 min, **INFUSION** over 22 hr on day 1. On day 2, repeat leucovorin 200 mg/m² **IV** over 2 hr followed by 5-FU 400 mg/m² **IV BOL**, then 5-FU 600 mg/m² **CONT IV INFUSION** over 22 hr. The order of administration is bevacizumab, followed by oxaliplatin and leucovorin, followed by 5-FU. This 2-day regimen (FOLFOX4-bevacizumab) is repeated q2wk until disease progression or unacceptable toxicity

First-line treatment of metastatic colorectal cancer in combination with capecitabine and oxaliplatin (unlabeled)

• **Adult: IV** 7.5 mg/kg **IV** on day 1 in combination with oxaliplatin (130 mg/m² **IV** on day 1) and capecitabine (1000 mg/m² **PO** bid on days 1 through 14), repeated q3wk

First-line or second-line treatment of metastatic colorectal cancer in combination with 5-fluorouracil, leucovorin, and irinotecan

• **Adult: IV** 5 mg/kg over 30-90 min q2wk. On days 1, 8, 15, and 22, give irinotecan 125 mg/m² **IV** over 90 min, followed by leucovorin 20 mg/m² **IV BOL** and then 5-FU 500 mg/m² **IV BOL**; repeat every 6 wk (IFL). On bevacizumab treatment days, give bevacizumab concomitantly (but in separate bags) with or without irinotecan. The sequence of administration is irinotecan, concomitantly with or without bevacizumab, followed by leucovorin, then 5-FU

Platinum-resistant epithelial ovarian, fallopian tube, or primary peritoneal cancer

• **Adult: IV** 10 mg/kg q2wk in combination with paclitaxel (80 mg/m² **IV** on days 1, 8, 15, and 22 every 4 wk), until disease progression or unacceptable toxicity

Recurrent platinum-resistant epithelial ovarian, fallopian tube, or primary peritoneal cancer

• **Adult: IV** 10 mg/kg q2wk in combination with pegylated liposomal doxorubicin (PLD, 40 mg/m² **IV** on day 1 q4wk), until disease progression or unacceptable toxicity

Recurrent platinum-resistant epithelial ovarian, fallopian tube, or primary peritoneal cancer

• **Adult: IV** 10 mg/kg q2wk in combination with topotecan (4 mg/m² **IV** on days 1, 8, and 15 q4wk), until disease progression or unacceptable toxicity

Neovascular (wet) age-related macular degeneration (AMD) (unlabeled)

• **Adult/geriatric patients: INTRAVITREAL INJ** 1.25 mg (0.05 mL) monthly into affected eye. Before injection, prepare the eye with a local anesthetic and povidone iodine and/or a broad-spectrum antibiotic. After injection, monitor patient for elevation in intraocular pressure and for endophthalmitis. Treatment continues monthly until macular edema, subretinal fluid, and/or pigment epithelial detachment is resolved

Cervical cancer

• **Adult: IV** 15 mg/kg q3wk

Renal cell carcinoma

• **Adult: IV** 10 mg/kg q2wk

Glioblastoma

• **Adult: IV** 10 mg/kg q2wk

Available forms: Sol for inj 25 mg/mL

Administer:
Intermittent IV INFUSION route

• Do not give by IV bolus, IV push; do not shake vial, do not admix

• Withdraw amount of product to be given, dilute in 100 mL 0.9% NaCl, discard any unused portion

> Black Box Warning: **Wound dehiscence:** discontinue 28 days prior to elective surgery, do not give for ≥28 days after surgery; make sure wound is healed before giving product

• Give as IV infusion over 90 min for 1st dose and 60 min thereafter if well tolerated; subsequent infusion may be given over 30 min; do not admix with dextrose

SIDE EFFECTS

CNS: *Asthenia, dizziness,* abnormal gait, syncope, headache, confusion
CV: Deep vein thrombosis, arterial thrombosis, hypo/hypertension, heart failure
GI: Nausea, vomiting, *anorexia, diarrhea,* constipation, *abdominal pain,* colitis, taste change, dyspepsia, stomatitis, GI hemorrhage/perforation
GU: Proteinuria, vaginal hemorrhage
HEMA: Leukopenia, neutropenia, thrombocytopenia
META: Bilirubinemia, hypokalemia
MISC: Exfoliative dermatitis, *alopecia*
RESP: Dyspnea, upper respiratory tract infection, hemoptysis
INTEG: Skin discoloration, infusion reactions, dry skin, skin ulcer, palmar-plantar erythrodysesthesia

PHARMACOKINETICS

Half-life 20 days, steady state 100 days

INTERACTIONS

• Avoid concurrent use with SUNItinib; microangiopathic hemolytic anemia may occur
Increase: CV toxicity antineoplastics
Increase: osteonecrosis of the jaw—biophosphates
Decrease: immune response to live virus vaccines

Drug/Lab
Increase: bilirubin
Decrease: neutrophil, platelets, WBC, potassium

NURSING CONSIDERATIONS
Assess:
• B/P; take frequently if hypertension develops, discontinue if hypertensive crisis occurs
• For symptoms of infection; may be masked by product
• **CNS reaction:** dizziness, confusion
• **HF:** crackles, jugular venous distention, dyspnea during treatment
• **GU status(proteinuria):** nephrotic syndrome may occur; monitor urinalysis for increasing protein level; product should be held if protein ≥2 g/24 hr; resume when <2 g/24 hr

Black Box Warning: **Wound dehiscence:** hold for ≥28 days until incision is healed, discontinue 28 days prior to elective surgery

Black Box Warning: **GI perforation** (constipation, fever, abdominal pain, nausea, vomiting), **serious bleeding** (bleeding from any orifice, stroke, deep vein thrombosis), **nephrotic syndrome, hypertensive crisis;** product should be discontinued permanently; surgery should be postponed

• **Thromboembolic events:** monitor for stroke, TIA, MI; usually occurs in geriatric patients who used this product previously
• **Fistulas:** may occur within 6 mo of beginning treatment, may be fatal
• **Pregnancy/breastfeeding:** drug may lead to fetal harm; do not use in pregnancy, do not breastfeed during and for 6 months after last dose; use contraception during and for 6 months after last dose
• **Reversible posterior leukoencephalopathy syndrome (RPLS):** discontinue if this disorder develops (headache, vision changes, seizures, altered mental status); MRI may be ordered, occurs 16 hr-1 yr after beginning treatment

Evaluate:
• Therapeutic response: decrease in size of tumors
Teach patient/family:
• To avoid hazardous tasks because confusion, dizziness may occur
• To report signs of infection: sore throat, fever, diarrhea, vomiting

Black Box Warning: **Hemorrhage/ bleeding:** to report bleeding, changes in urinary patterns, edema, abdominal pain

• To avoid live virus vaccines
• About the need to discontinue product a month before surgery and not to restart until wound is healed
• **Pregnancy/breastfeeding:** that fetal harm may occur, not to breastfeed, not to become pregnant while taking this product or for 6 months after discontinuing treatment; discuss possible infertility with patient

---

bezlotoxumab
(bez′ loe-tox′ ue-mab)
Zinplava
Func. class.: Antidiarrheal
Chem class.: Monoclonal antibody

ACTION: Binds to *Clostridium difficile* toxin B

USES: For *Clostridium difficile* infection (CDI) in patients who are receiving antibacterial treatment of CDI and are at a high risk for CDI recurrence

CONTRAINDICATIONS: Hypersensitivity

Precautions: Breastfeeding, pregnancy, heart failure

DOSAGE AND ROUTES
• **Adult:** IV 10 mg/kg as a single dose
Available forms: Sol for inj 25 mg/mL

Side effects: *italics* = common; red = life-threatening

Administer:

Intermittent IV infusion route

• Give by IV infusion, visually inspect parenteral products for particulate matter and discoloration prior to use

• **Dilution of vials:** Do not shake; withdraw the required volume from the vial based on the patient's weight and transfer into an IV bag of either 0.9% NaCl or D₅W injection (1-10 mg/mL). Mix the diluted solution by gentle inversion, do not shake

• Infuse the diluted solution IV over 60 min using a sterile, nonpyrogenic, low–protein-binding 0.2-0.5 micron in-line or add-on filter; give via a central line or a peripheral catheter; do not give IV push or bolus; do not coadminister other drugs simultaneously through the same infusion line

• **Storage:** Diluted solution may be stored at room temperature for 16 hr or refrigerated at 2-8°C (36-46°F) up to 24 hr; if refrigerated, allow the solution to come to room temperature before use; do not freeze

SIDE EFFECTS

CNS: Fever, headache
CV: Heart failure, hypertension
MISC: Infusion-related reactions

PHARMACOKINETICS

Eliminated by catabolism, half-life 19 days

INTERACTIONS

None known

NURSING CONSIDERATIONS

Assess:

• **CDI:** diarrhea that is watery or bloody, fever, abdominal cramping/pain, pus or mucus in the stools, dehydration

• **Heart failure:** monitor for heart failure during administration, death has occurred; causes of death included infections, cardiac failure, and respiratory failure in those with existing heart failure

• **Pregnancy/breastfeeding:** pregnant or breastfeeding; report if pregnancy is planned or suspected or if breastfeeding

Evaluate:

• Therapeutic response: no recurrence of CDI when used with antibiotic therapy

Teach patient/family:

• Reason for product and expected result

• **CDI:** to report immediately diarrhea that is watery or bloody, fever, abdominal cramping/pain, pus or mucus in the stools, dehydration

• **Infusion-related reactions:** to report immediately infusion-related reactions, redness, swelling; if these occur, infusion should be discontinued

---

bictegravir/emtricitabine/tenofovir alafenamide

Biktarvy

Func. class.: HIV antivirals
Chem. class.: Integrase strand transfer inhibitor (INSTI); nucleoside and nucleotide reverse transcriptase inhibitor (NRTI) combinations

---

ACTION: A three-drug combination of bictegravir (BIC), an HIV-1 integrase strand transfer inhibitor (INSTI), and emtricitabine (FTC) and tenofovir alafenamide (TAF), both HIV-1 nucleoside analog reverse transcriptase inhibitors (NRTIs)

USES: Complete regimen for the treatment of HIV-1 infection in adults who have no antiretroviral treatment history or to replace the current antiretroviral regimen in those who are virologically suppressed (HIV-1 RNA <50 copies per mL)

CONTRAINDICATIONS: Do not use with dofetilide, rifampin; hypersensitivity

---

Precautions: Alcoholism, breastfeeding, Graves' disease, pregnancy, hepatic impairment, HIV resistance, immune reconstitution syndrome, infection resistance, osteoporosis, renal impairment, lactic acidosis/severe hepatomegaly with steatosis, suicidal ideation

Black Box Warning: Hepatitis B and HIV coinfection, hepatitis B exacerbation

DOSAGE AND ROUTES
- **Adult:** 1 tablet daily

Available forms: Tabs 50 mg bictegravir, 200 mg emtricitabine, 25 mg tenofovir alafenamide

Administer:
- With or without food
- Do not use 2 hr before or after dairy products or antacids that contain aluminum, magnesium, or calcium

SIDE EFFECTS
CNS: Fatigue, abnormal dreams, headache, depression, suicidal ideation
GI: Nausea, vomiting, diarrhea

PHARMACOKINETICS
Bictegravir: Protein binding >99%, elimination via metabolism, mediated by CYP3A and UGT1A1 enzymes; excreted in feces (60.3%), urine (35%), half-life 17.3 hr
Emtricitabine: Protein binding <4%, excreted in urine (70%), feces (13.7%), half-life 10 hr
Tenofovir AF: Protein binding 80%, elimination via metabolism (more than 80% of dose), excreted in feces (31.7%), elimination of metabolite via kidneys (70%-80%) by a combination of glomerular filtration and active tubular secretion, half-life 0.51 hr; metabolite half-life of 150-180 hr
Affected cytochrome P450 isoenzymes and drug transporters: CYP3A4, UGT1A1, OCT2, MATE1, P-gp, BCRP, OATP1B1, OATP1B3

INTERACTIONS
- Do not use with other antiretrovirals for HIV, rifampin

Increase: effect of metformin
Increase: effect of this HIV combination product—OCT2 and MATE1 (dofetilide); CYP3A4 inhibitors, UGT1A1 inhibitors
Decrease: concentration of this HIV combination product—carbamazepine, oxcarbazepine, phenobarbital, phenytoin; use alternative anticonvulsants
Decrease: concentration of this HIV combination product—products that inhibit P-gp and BCRP

Drug/Herb
Avoid use with St. John's wort

NURSING CONSIDERATIONS
Assess:
- **HIV:** symptoms and change in severity; opportunistic infections may occur with HIV; assess for these infections throughout therapy
- **Osteoporosis and bone mineral loss:** assess those who have had prior fractures, osteoporosis, or mineral bone loss
- **Hepatitis B infection:** before use test for hepatitis B virus infection; monitor hepatitis B serology, plasma hepatitis C RNA
- **Lab testing:** before use and periodically during treatment, assess serum creatinine, estimated creatinine clearance, urine glucose, urine protein, serum phosphorus in those with chronic kidney disease
- Monitor blood glucose, CBC with differential, CD4+ T-cell count, LFTs, plasma HIV RNA, pregnancy testing (if applicable), serum bilirubin (total and direct), serum cholesterol, BUN, serum lipid profile, urinalysis
- **Pregnancy/breastfeeding:** for pregnant women, therapy should begin immediately after HIV diagnosis, as early maternal viral suppression is associated with lower risk of perinatal transmission. Therapy may be initiated before drug

resistance testing results are available; modify based on the assay results
• **Depression and suicidal ideation:** although rare, has occurred in those with depression before treatment
Evaluate:
• Therapeutic response: improving signs and symptoms of HIV, improving CD4+ counts, plasma HIV RNA with only moderate side effects

TEACH PATIENT/FAMILY
• To take as directed, not to skip or double doses; if missed, to take when remembered; not to share with others
• That product is not a cure; that patient is still infective and may transmit infection to others via sexual contact, blood transfusions, or sharing needles; to practice safe sex, as using a condom will prevent transmission from person to person; not to donate blood
• That lab testing will be required periodically during treatment
• **Immune reconstitution syndrome:** that patients may develop an inflammatory response to opportunistic infections (such as *Mycobacterium avium* infection, cytomegalovirus, *Pneumocystis jirovecii* pneumonia [PCP], or TB), autoimmune disorders (Graves' disease, polymyositis, and Guillain-Barré syndrome); response may occur during or many months after starting treatment
• **Pregnancy/breastfeeding:** to notify health care provider if pregnancy is planned or suspected; if pregnant, to enroll in the Antiretroviral Pregnancy Registry (800-258-4263); to avoid breastfeeding
• **Lactic acidosis/hepatomegaly with stenosis:** to report immediately nausea, vomiting, abdominal pain, severe weakness
• To inform all health care providers of OTC, Rx, herbal products, supplements taken; not to start or stop without consent of prescriber; to avoid St. John's wort
• Not to use antacids, dairy products 2 hr before or after this product

---

bimatoprost (ophthalmic/topical) (Rx)
(by-mat′oh-prost)
Latisse, Lumigan
Func. class.: Antiglaucoma agent
Chem. class.: Prostaglandin agonist

Do not confuse:
bimatoprost/travoprost

ACTION
Latisse
Promotion of eyelash growth, thickness, and darkness: unknown; possible increase in the percent of hairs and an increase in the duration of the hair-growth (anagen) phase

Lumigan
Reduction of intraocular pressure (IOP) in patients with ocular hypertension or open-angle glaucoma; selectively mimics endogenous prostamides to produce ocular hypotension

USES: Increased intraocular pressure in those with open-angle glaucoma/ocular hypertension (Lumigan); eyelash hypotrichosis (Latisse)

CONTRAINDICATIONS: Hypersensitivity to this product, benzalkonium chloride
Precautions: Children, intraocular inflammation, closed-angle glaucoma, macular edema, contact lenses, ocular infection, surgery, trauma; corneal abrasion, iritis, urethritis

DOSAGE AND ROUTES
Increased intraocular pressure/ocular hypertension (Lumigan)
• **Adult: OPHTH** Instill 1 drop in each affected eye (conjunctival sac) every night
Eyelash hypotrichosis (Latisse)
• **Adult: Apply** 1 drop to skin of upper eyelid margin at base of eyelashes every night using a new supplied disposable sterile applicator
Available forms: Ophthalmic solution 0.01%; topical solution 0.03%

SIDE EFFECTS

EENT: *Conjunctival hyperemia, growth of eyelashes (hypertrichosis), ocular pigment changes, ocular pruritus,* xerophthalmia, visual disturbance, ocular irritation/burning, foreign body sensation, ocular pain, blepharitis, cataracts, superficial punctate keratitis

INTEG: Hyperpigmentation of the periocular skin, eyelash darkening, lacrimation, photophobia, conjunctivitis, asthenopia, iritis, macular edema

MISC: Influenza, upper respiratory tract infections, asthenia, headache, hirsutism

PHARMACOKINETICS

Ophthalmic: Onset 4 hr, peak 8-12 hr; half-life 45 min

INTERACTIONS

Decrease: Intraocular pressure–latanoprost, travoprost (no longer available in the U.S.)

Drug/Lab Test
Increase: LFTs

NURSING CONSIDERATIONS

Assess:

• **Intraocular pressure:** in those with ongoing increased IOP or those using latanoprost, travoprost (no longer available in the U.S.)

Evaluate:

• Decreasing IOP or increased growth of eyelashes

Teach patient/family:

Ophthalmic route (Lumigan):

• To wash hands before and after use; remove contact lenses before use and reinsert 15 min after use; Lumigan contains benzalkonium chloride, which can be absorbed by soft contact lenses

• To tilt the head back slightly and pull the lower eyelid down with the index finger to form a pouch; squeeze the prescribed number of drops into the pouch and gently close the eyes for 1-2 min; do not blink; to avoid contamination, do not touch the tip of the dropper to the eye, fingertips, or other surface

• That the solution may be used concomitantly with other topical ophthalmic drug products to lower IOP; if more than one topical ophthalmic drug is being used, the drugs should be administered at least 5 min apart

Topical route (Latisse):

• To ensure the patient's face is clean and makeup is removed before using Latisse; the disposable sterile applicator is the only applicator that should be used; each applicator should be used for 1 eye only; dispose of the applicator after each use; after applying 1 drop of solution to the applicator, apply evenly along the skin of the upper eyelid margin at the base of the eyelashes; blot excess solution runoff outside the upper eyelid margin with a tissue or other absorbent eyelash line

---

RARELY USED

binimetinib
(bih′-nee-meh′-tih-nib)
Mektovi
Func. class.: Antineoplastic

USES: Treatment of unresectable/metastatic melanoma (BRAF V600E or V600K mutations) with encorafenib

CONTRAINDICATIONS: Hypersensitivity

DOSAGE AND ROUTES

• **Adult: PO** 45 mg bid with encorafenib **PO** 450 mg daily until disease progression

---

bisacodyl (Rx, OTC)

(bis-a-koe′dill)
Bisac-EVAC ✦, Bisacolax, Bisacolax, Correctol, Carter's Little Pills ✦, Codulax ✦, Dacodyl, Doxidan, Dulcolax, Ex-Lax Ultra, Femilax, Fleet, Soflax-Ex ✦
Func. class.: Laxative, stimulant
Chem. class.: Diphenylmethane

Do not confuse:
Dulcolax (bisacodyl)/Dulcolax (docusate)

ACTION: Acts directly on intestine by increasing peristalsis; thought to irritate colonic intramural plexus

USES: Short-term treatment of constipation; bowel or rectal preparation for surgery, examination

CONTRAINDICATIONS: Hypersensitivity, abdominal pain, nausea, vomiting, appendicitis, acute surgical abdomen, ulcerated hemorrhoids, acute hepatitis, fecal impaction, intestinal/biliary tract obstruction
Precautions: Pregnancy, breastfeeding, rectal fissures, severe CV disease

DOSAGE AND ROUTES
• **Adult and child ≥12 yr: PO** 5-15 mg in PM or AM; may use up to 30 mg for bowel or rectal preparation; **RECT** 10 mg as a single dose; 30-mL enema
• **Child 3-11 yr: PO** 5-10 mg as a single dose; **RECT** 5-10 mg as a single dose
Available forms: Tabs del rel 5, 10 mg; enteric-coated tabs 5 mg; supp 5, 10 mg; rectal solution 10 mg/30 mL
Administer:
PO route
• Swallow tabs whole with full glass of water; do not break, crush, chew tabs
• Alone only with water for better absorption; do not take within 1 hr of other products or within 1 hr of antacids, milk, H₂ antagonists; do not take enteric product with proton-pump inhibitors
• In AM or PM
Rectal route
• Insert high in rectum

SIDE EFFECTS
CNS: Muscle weakness
GI: *Nausea, anorexia, cramps,* diarrhea, rectal burning (suppositories)
META: Protein-losing enteropathy (extended use), hypokalemia (extended use), tetany

PHARMACOKINETICS
Small amounts absorbed/metabolized by liver; excreted in urine, bile, feces, breast milk
PO: Onset 6-10 hr
RECT: Onset 15-60 min

INTERACTIONS
Increase: gastric irritation—antacids, milk, H₂ blockers, gastric acid pump inhibitors
Drug/Food
• Increase irritation—dairy products, separate by 2 hr
Drug/Lab
Increase: Sodium phosphate
Decrease: Calcium, magnesium
Drug/Herb
Increase: laxative action—flexibility of the valley, pheasant's eye, senna, squill

NURSING CONSIDERATIONS
Assess:
• Blood, urine electrolytes if product is used often by patient
• I&O ratio to identify fluid loss
• Cause of constipation; identify whether fluids, bulk, exercise missing from lifestyle; determine use of constipating products
• **GI symptoms:** cramping, rectal bleeding, nausea, if these symptoms occur, product should be discontinued
• Multiple products/routes may be used for bowel prep
Evaluate:
• Therapeutic response: decrease in constipation, removal of stool from colon
Teach patient/family:
• Not to use laxatives for long-term therapy because bowel tone will be lost; 1-wk use is usually sufficient
• That normal bowel movements do not always occur daily
• Not to use in presence of abdominal pain, nausea, vomiting
• To notify prescriber if constipation is unrelieved or if symptoms of electrolyte imbalance occur: muscle cramps, pain, weakness, dizziness

---

• To take with a full glass of water; if using with dairy products (separate by 2 hr); to separate from other foods by 1 hr
• Identify bulk, water, constipating products, exercise in patient's life

---

bismuth subsalicylate (OTC)

(bis'muth sub-sal-iss'uh-late)

Bismatrol, Bismed ✤, Bismylate ✤, Kaopectate, Kao-Tin, Peptic Relief, Pepto-Bismol, Pink Bismuth, Stomak-care ✤, Kaopectolin, K-Pek, Maalox Total Stomach Relief, Stomach Relief

Func. class.: Antidiarrheal, weak antacid
Chem. class.: Salicylate

Do not confuse:
Kaopectate/Kayexalate

ACTION: Inhibits the prostaglandin synthesis responsible for GI hypermotility, intestinal inflammation; stimulates absorption of fluid and electrolytes; binds toxins produced by *Escherichia coli*

USES: Diarrhea (cause undetermined), prevention of diarrhea when traveling; may be included to treat *Helicobacter pylori*, heartburn, indigestion, nausea
Unlabeled uses: Traveler's diarrhea, gastric/duodenal ulcer, *H. pylori* eradication

CONTRAINDICATIONS: Children <3 yr, children with chickenpox, history of GI bleeding, flulike symptoms, hypersensitivity to product or salicylates, PUD
Precautions: Pregnancy, breastfeeding, geriatric patients, gout, diabetes mellitus, bleeding disorders, previous hypersensitivity to NSAIDs, *Clostridium difficile*–associated diarrhea when used with anti-infectives for *H. pylori*

DOSAGE AND ROUTES
Antidiarrheal/gastric distress
• **Adult/adolescent:** PO 524 mg (2 tabs or 30 mL) q30-60min as needed, max 8 doses/day; or 1050 mg (30 mL) qhr as needed, max 4 doses/day
Antiulcer (unlabeled)
• **Adult/adolescent: PO** • 525 mg qid, max 4.2 g/24 hr; given with metroNIDAZOLE or tetracycline and acid-suppressive therapy × 14 days
Traveler's diarrhea (unlabeled)
• **Adult: PO** • 30 mL q30min (8×/day regular strength, 4×/day max strength)
Available forms: Tabs 262 mg; chewable tabs 262 mg; liquid 262 mg/15 mL, 525 mg/15 mL
Administer:
• Increase fluids to rehydrate patient
• **Susp:** shake liquid before using; use measuring cup, syringe
• Tabs can be chewed, dissolved in mouth; caplets to be swallowed whole with water

SIDE EFFECTS
CNS: Confusion, twitching, neurotoxicity (high doses)
EENT: Hearing loss, tinnitus, metallic taste, blue gums, black tongue
GI: Increased fecal impaction (high doses), dark stools, constipation, diarrhea, nausea
HEMA: Increased bleeding time
MISC: Reye's syndrome

PHARMACOKINETICS
PO: Onset 1 hr, peak 2 hr, duration 4 hr

INTERACTIONS
Increase: toxicity—salicylates, methotrexate
Increase: effect of anticoagulants (PO), antidiabetics (PO)
Decrease: absorption of tetracycline, quinolones, phenytoin; separate for ≥2 hr
Drug/Lab Test
Interference: radiographic studies of GI system

NURSING CONSIDERATIONS
Assess:
• **Diarrhea:** bowel pattern before product therapy, after treatment
• **Pregnancy/breastfeeding:** avoid in pregnancy; do not breastfeed

---

• Electrolytes K, Na, Cl if diarrhea is severe or continues long term; assess skin turgor, other signs of dehydration

Evaluate:

• Therapeutic response: decreased diarrhea, absence of diarrhea when traveling; resolution of ulcers

Teach patient/family:

• To chew, dissolve tablets in mouth; not to swallow whole; to shake liquid before using, maintain hydration

• To avoid other salicylates unless directed by prescriber; not to give to children, possibility of Reye's syndrome

• That stools may turn black; that tongue may darken; that impaction may occur in debilitated patients

• To stop use if symptoms do not improve within 2 days or become worse, or if diarrhea is accompanied by high fever

• To separate quinolones, phenytoin, tetracyclines by ≥2 hr

⚠ HIGH ALERT

bisoprolol (Rx)

(bis-oh′pro-lole)

Func. class.: Antihypertensive
Chem. class.: β₁-blocker

ACTION: Blocks stimulation of β₁-adrenergic receptors within cardiac muscle (decreases rate of SA node discharge, increases recovery time), slows conduction of AV node, decreases heart rate, which decreases O_2 consumption in myocardium; decreases renin-angiotensin-aldosterone system

USES: Mild to moderate hypertension

CONTRAINDICATIONS: Hypersensitivity to β-blockers, cardiogenic shock, heart block (2nd, 3rd degree), sinus bradycardia, acute cardiac failure

Precautions: Pregnancy, breastfeeding, children, major surgery, diabetes mellitus, HF, thyroid/renal/hepatic disease, COPD, asthma, well-compensated heart failure, aortic or mitral valve disease, peripheral vascular disease, myasthenia gravis, abrupt discontinuation

DOSAGE AND ROUTES

• **Adult: PO** 5 mg/day; reduce to 2.5 mg in bronchospastic disease; may increase to 20 mg/day if necessary; max 20 mg/day

Renal/hepatic dose

• **Adult: PO** CCr <40 mL/min 2.5 mg, titrate upward

Available forms: Tabs 5, 10 mg

Administer:

• Take apical pulse before each dose, if <50 bpm withhold

• Tab may be crushed, swallowed whole; may give without regard to meals

• Store protected from light, moisture; place in cool environment

SIDE EFFECTS

CNS: Insomnia, fatigue, dizziness

CV: Bradycardia, HF, postural hypotension, peripheral edema, cold extremities

EENT: Blurred vision, dry mouth

ENDO: Hypoglycemia

GI: Nausea, diarrhea, vomiting, constipation

INTEG: Rash

RESP: Dyspnea, cough

GU: Erectile dysfunction, decreased libido, urinary frequency

PHARMACOKINETICS

Peak 2-4 hr, half-life 9-12 hr, 50% excreted unchanged in urine, protein binding 30%-36%, metabolized in liver to inactive metabolites

INTERACTIONS

Increase: myocardial depression—calcium channel blockers, phenytoin (IV) verapamil

Increase: antihypertensive effect—ACE inhibitors, α-blockers, calcium channel blockers, diuretics, nitrates

Increase: bradycardia—digoxin, amiodarone clonidine, diltiazem, verapamil

Increase: antidiabetic effect—antidiabetics; may mask hypoglycemic symptoms

Drug/Herb

Increase: β-blocking effect—hawthorn

Decrease: β-blocking effect—ephedra

Drug/Lab Test
Increase: AST, ALT, blood glucose, BUN, uric acid, potassium

NURSING CONSIDERATIONS
Assess:
• **Hypertension:** B/P, pulse during beginning treatment, periodically thereafter; pulse: note rate, rhythm, quality; apical/radial pulse before administration; notify prescriber of any significant changes (pulse <50 bpm); monitor ECG baseline and periodically
• Baselines of renal, hepatic studies before therapy begins
• **Heart failure:** I&O, weight daily; increased weight, jugular venous distention, dyspnea, crackles, edema in feet, legs daily
• Skin turgor, dryness of mucous membranes for hydration status, especially for geriatric patients
Evaluate:
• Therapeutic response: decreased B/P after 1-2 wk
Teach patient/family:
• Not to discontinue product abruptly, taper over 1 wk; may cause precipitate angina, rebound hypertension; evaluate noncompliance
• Not to use OTC products that contain α-adrenergic stimulants (e.g., nasal decongestants, OTC cold preparations) unless directed by prescriber
• To report slow heart rate, dizziness, confusion, depression, fever, cold extremities
• To take pulse at home; advise when to notify prescriber
• To avoid alcohol, smoking; to limit sodium intake
• To comply with weight control, dietary adjustments, modified exercise program
• To carry emergency ID to identify product, allergies
• To avoid hazardous activities if dizziness is present
• **To report symptoms of heart failure:** difficulty breathing especially on exertion or when lying down, night cough, swelling of extremities

• That if diabetic, product may mask signs of hypoglycemia or alter blood glucose levels
Pregnancy/breastfeeding: To notify health care professional if pregnancy is planned or suspected

TREATMENT OF OVERDOSE:
Lavage, IV atropine for bradycardia; IV theophylline for bronchospasm; digoxin, O_2, diuretic for cardiac failure; hemodialysis, IV glucose for hypoglycemia; IV diazepam or phenytoin for seizures

---

⚠ HIGH ALERT

bivalirudin (Rx)
(bye-val-i-rue'din)
Angiomax
Func. class.: Anticoagulant
Chem. class.: Thrombin inhibitor

ACTION: Direct inhibitor of thrombin that is highly specific; able to inhibit free and clot-bound thrombin

USES: Unstable angina in patients undergoing percutaneous transluminal coronary angioplasty (PTCA), used with aspirin; heparin-induced thrombocytopenia, with/without thrombosis syndrome, PCI with IIb/IIIa

CONTRAINDICATIONS: Hypersensitivity, active bleeding, cerebral aneurysm, intracranial hemorrhage, recent surgery, CVA
Precautions: Pregnancy, breastfeeding, children, geriatric patients, renal function impairment, hepatic disease, asthma, blood dyscrasias, thrombocytopenia, GI ulcers, hypertension, inflammatory bowel disease, vitamin K deficiency, asthma

DOSAGE AND ROUTES
Unstable angina in those undergoing PTCA
• **Adult:** IV **BOL** 0.75 mg/kg, then **IV INFUSION** 1.75 mg/kg/hr for 4 hr; another **IV INFUSION** may be used at

---

Side effects: *italics* = common; red = life-threatening

0.2 mg/kg/hr for ≤20 hr; this product is intended to be used with aspirin (325 mg/day) adjusted to body weight

HIT/HITTS

Adult: IV Bolus 0.75 mg/kg, then continuous infusion 1.75 mg/kg/hr for duration of procedure

DVT prophylaxis (major hip or knee surgery)

Adult: SUBCUT 1 mg/kg q8hr up to 14 days

Renal dose

• **Adult:** IV CCr ≥30 mL/min no adjustment; CCr 10-29 mL/min consider reducing to 1 mL/kg/hr

Available forms: Inj, lyophilized 250 mg/vial

Administer:

• Before PTCA; give with aspirin (325 mg)

• Store reconstituted vials in refrigerator for up to 24 hr; store diluted concentrations at room temperature for 24 hr

IV, direct route

• Dilute by adding 5 mL of sterile water for inj/250 mg bivalirudin, swirl until dissolved, further dilute in 50 mL of D₅W or 0.9% NaCl (5 mg/mL), give by bolus inj 0.75 mg/kg, then intermittent infusion

Continuous IV INFUSION route

• To each 250-mg vial add 5 mL of sterile water for inj, swirl until dissolved, further dilute in 500 mL D₅W or 0.9% NaCl (0.5 mg/mL); give infusion after bolus dose at a rate of 1.75 mg/kg/hr; may give an additional infusion at 0.2 mg/kg/hr

• Do not mix other IV medications with bivalirudin or provide via the same IV line as bivalirudin

Y-site compatibilities: Abciximab, acyclovir, alfentanil, allopurinol, amifostine, amikacin, aminocaproic acid, aminophylline, amphotericin B liposome, ampicillin, ampicillin-sulbactam, anidulafungin, argatroban, arsenic trioxide, atenolol, atracurium, atropine, azithromycin, aztreonam, bleomycin, bumetanide, buprenorphine, busulfan, butorphanol, calcium chloride/gluconate, capreomycin, CARBOplatin, carmustine, ceFAZolin, cefepime, cefotaxime, cefoTEtan, cefOXitin, cefTAZidime, ceftizoxime, cefTRIAXone, cefuroxime, chloramphenicol, cimetidine, ciprofloxacin, cisatracurium, CISplatin, clindamycin, cyclophosphamide, cycloSPORINE, cytarabine, dacarbazine, DACTINomycin, DAPTOmycin, DAUNOrubicin, DAUNOrubicin liposome, dexamethasone, dexmedetomidine, dexrazoxane, digoxin, diltiazem, diphenhydrAMINE, DOCEtaxel, dolasetron, DOPamine, DOXOrubicin, DOXOrubicin liposomal, doxycycline, droperidol, enalaprilat, ePHEDrine, EPINEPHrine, epirubicin, epoprostenol, eptifibatide, ertapenem, erythromycin, foscarnet, fosphenytoin, furosemide, gallium, ganciclovir, gatifloxacin, gemcitabine, gentamicin, glycopyrrolate, granisetron, haloperidol, heparin, hydrALAZINE, hydrocortisone, HYDROmorphone, hydrOXYzine, IDArubicin, ifosfamide, imipenem-cilastatin, inamrinone, insulin (regular), irinotecan, isoproterenol, ketorolac, labetalol, leucovorin, levofloxacin, lidocaine, linezolid, LORazepam, magnesium, mannitol, mechlorethamine, melphalan, meperidine, meropenem, mesna, methohexital, methotrexate, methyldopa, methylPREDNISolone, metoclopramide, metoprolol, metroNIDAZOLE, midazolam, milrinone, mitoMYcin, mitoXANtrone, mivacurium, morphine, moxifloxacin, mycophenolate mofetil, nafcillin, nalbuphine, naloxone, nesiritide, niCARdipine, nitroglycerin, nitroprusside, norepinephrine, octreotide, ofloxacin, ondansetron, oxaliplatin, oxytocin, PACLitaxel, palonosetron, pamidronate, pancuronium, PEMEtrexed, PENTobarbital, PHENobarbital, phenylephrine, piperacillin, piperacillin-tazobactam, polymyxin B, potassium acetate/chloride/phosphates, procainamide, promethazine, propranolol, ranitidine, remifentanil, rocuronium, sodium acetate/bicarbonate/phosphates, streptozocin, succinylcholine, SUFentanil, sulfamethoxazole-trimethoprim, tacrolimus, teniposide, theophylline, thiopental, thiotepa, ticarcillin, ticarcillin-clavulanate, tigecycline, tirofiban, tobramycin, topotecan, vasopressin, vecuronium, verapamil, vinBLAStine, vinCRIStine, vinorelbine, voriconazole, warfarin, zidovudine, zoledronic acid

SIDE EFFECTS

CNS: *Headache, insomnia, anxiety, nervousness*
CV: *Hypo/hypertension, bradycardia,* ventricular fibrillation
GI: *Nausea, vomiting, abdominal pain, dyspepsia*
HEMA: Hemorrhage, thrombocytopenia
MISC: Pain at inj site, pelvic pain, urinary retention, fever, anaphylaxis, infection
MS: *Back pain*
GU: Urinary retention, renal failure, oliguria

PHARMACOKINETICS

Excreted in urine, half-life 25 min, duration 1 hr, no protein binding

INTERACTIONS

Increase: bleeding risk—abciximab, anticoagulants, aspirin, thrombolytics, cephalosporins, use together cautiously
Drug/Herb
Increase: bleeding risk—angelica, chamomile, devil's claw, dong quai, garlic, ginger, ginkgo, ginseng, horse chestnut, licorice, saw palmetto; avoid concurrent use

NURSING CONSIDERATIONS
Assess:
• **Bleeding:** check arterial and venous sites, IM inj sites, catheters; all punctures should be minimized; fall in B/P or Hct may indicate hemorrhage; hematoma, hemorrhage at puncture site are more common in the elderly; monitor coagulation studies, Hct before use ; baseline and periodic ACT, aPTT, PT, INR, TT, platelets, Hgb, Hct
• CV status: B/P; watch for hypo/hypertension, bradycardia
• Neurologic status: any focal or generalized deficits should be reported immediately

• **PCI use:** possible thrombosis, stenosis, unplanned stent, prolonged ischemia, decreased reflow
• **Renal function:** dosage reductions may be required
Evaluate:
• Therapeutic response: anticoagulation with PTCA; resolution of heparin-induced thrombocytopenia, thrombosis syndrome
Teach patient/family:
• About the reason for the product and expected results
• To report black, tarry stools; blood in urine; difficulty breathing
• Not to use any OTC, herbal products unless approved by prescriber
• Not to use hard-bristle toothbrush or regular razor to avoid any injury; hemorrhage may result
• **Pregnancy/breastfeeding:** Report if pregnancy is planned or suspected or if breastfeeding

⚠ HIGH ALERT

bleemycin (Rx)
(blee-oh-mye′sin)
Blenoxane
Func. class.: Antineoplastic, antibiotic
Chem. class.: Glycopeptide

ACTION: Inhibits synthesis of DNA, RNA, protein; derived from *Streptomyces verticillus;* phase specific to the G_2 and M phases; a nonvesicant, sclerosing agent

USES: Cancer of head, neck, penis, cervix, vulva of squamous cell origin; Hodgkin's/non-Hodgkin's disease; testicular carcinoma; as a sclerosing agent for malignant pleural effusion

CONTRAINDICATIONS: Pregnancy, breastfeeding, hypersensitivity
Precautions: Patients >70 yr old, renal/hepatic disease, respiratory disease, max lifetime dose 400 units, fever

Black Box Warning: Pulmonary fibrosis; requires specialized care setting, experienced clinician

Side effects: *italics* = common; red = life-threatening

DOSAGE AND ROUTES

Test dose
• Adult/child (unlabeled): IM/IV/SUB-CUT ≤2 units for first 2 doses followed by 24 hr of observation

Non-Hodgkin's lymphoma, testicular cancer, squamous cell carcinoma
• Adult/child: SUBCUT/IV/IM 0.25-0.5 unit/kg 1-2×/wk or 10-20 units/m², then 1 unit/day or 5 units/wk; max total dose of 400 units during lifetime

Hodgkin's lymphoma
• Adult/adolescent ≥15 yr: IV IM 5-20 units/m² may be given in combination, use 2 units or less for first 2 doses (anaphylaxis is common)

Malignant pleural effusion
• Adult: BOL INTRAPLEURAL 60 units as a single dose

Testicular cancer
• Adult: IV 10-20 units/m² 1-2 times per wk

Renal dose
• Adult/child: CCr 40-50 mL/min reduce dose by 30%; CCr 30-39 mL/min reduce dose by 40%; CCr 20-29 mL/min reduce dose by 45%; CCr 10-19 mL/min reduce dose by 55%; CCr 5-10 mL/min reduce dose by 60%

Available forms: Powder for inj, 15, 30 units/vial

Administer:
• Antiemetic 30-60 min before giving product to prevent vomiting
• Topical or systemic analgesics for pain of stomatitis as ordered; antihistamines and antipyretics for fever, chills
• May be given IM, subcut, IV, intrapleurally, intralesionally, intraarterially

IM/SUBCUT route
• After reconstituting 15 units/1-5 mL or 30 units/2-10 mL of 0.9% NaCl or bacteriostatic water for inj, max concentrations 5 units/mL, rotate inj sites; do not use products that contain benzyl alcohol when giving to neonates or that contain dextrose because of loss of potency

IV route
• Use cytotoxic handling procedures
• After reconstituting 15- or 30-unit vial with 5 or 10 mL of NS, respectively, inject slowly over 10 min or, after further dilution with 50-100 mL 0.9% NaCl, give at prescribed rate
• For patients with lymphoma, give 2 test doses of 2-5 units before initial dose; monitor for anaphylaxis
• Store for 2 wk after reconstituting if refrigerated or for 24 hr at room temperature; discard unused portions

Y-site compatibilities: Acyclovir, alfentanil, allopurinol, amifostine, amikacin, aminocaproic acid, aminophylline, amiodarone, ampicillin, ampicillin-sulbactam, anidulafungin, atenolol, atracurium, azithromycin, aztreonam, bivalirudin, bumetanide, buprenorphine, busulfan, butorphanol, calcium chloride/gluconate, CARBOplatin, carmustine, caspofungin, ceFAZolin, cefepime, cefotaxime, cefoTEtan, cefOXitin, cefTAZidime, ceftizoxime, cefTRIAXone, cefuroxime, chloramphenicol, chlorproMAZINE, cimetidine, ciprofloxacin, cisatracurium, CISplatin, clindamycin, codeine, cyclophosphamide, cycloSPORINE, cytarabine, dacarbazine, DACTINomycin, DAPTOmycin, DAUNOrubicin, dexamethasone, dexmedetomidine, dexrazoxane, digoxin, diltiazem, diphenhydrAMINE, DOBUTamine, DOCEtaxel, DOPamine, doxacurium, DOXOrubicin, DOXOrubicin liposomal, doxycycline, droperidol, enalaprilat, ePHEDrine, EPINEPHrine, epirubicin, ertapenem, erythromycin, esmolol, etoposide, famotidine, fenoldopam, fentaNYL, filgrastim, fluconazole, fludarabine, fluorouracil, foscarnet, fosphenytoin, furosemide, ganciclovir, gatifloxacin, gemcitabine, gentamicin, glycopyrrolate, granisetron, haloperidol, heparin, hydrALAZINE, hydrocortisone sodium succinate, HYDROmorphone, hydrOXYzine, IDArubicin, ifosfamide, imipenem-cilastatin, inamrinone, insulin (regular), irinotecan, isoproterenol, ketorolac, labetalol, leucovorin, levofloxacin, levorphanol, lidocaine, linezolid, LORazepam, magnesium sulfate, mannitol, mechlorethamine, melphalan, meperidine, meropenem, mesna, metaraminol, methohexital, methotrexate, methyldopate, methylPREDNISolone, metoclopramide, metoprolol, metroNIDAZOLE, midazolam, milrinone, minocycline, mitoMYcin, mitoXANtrone, mivacurium, morphine, nafcillin, nalbuphine, naloxone, nesiritide, niCARdipine, nitroglycerin, nitroprusside, norepinephrine, octreotide, ondansetron, oxaliplatin, palonosetron, pamidronate, pancuronium, pantoprazole, PEMEtrexed, pentamidine, pentazocine, PENTobarbital, PHENobarbital, phenylephrine, piperacillin, piperacillin-tazobactam, polymyxin B, potassium chloride, potassium phosphates, procainamide, prochlorperazine, promethazine, propranolol, quiNIDine, ranitidine, remifentanil, riTUXimab, rocuronium, sargramostim, sodium acetate, sodium bicarbonate, sodium phosphates, succinylcholine, SUFentanil, sulfamethoxazole-trimethoprim, tacrolimus, teniposide, theophylline, thiopental, thiotepa, ticarcillin, ticarcillin-clavulanate, tirofiban, tobramycin, tolazoline, trastuzumab, trimethobenzamide, vancomycin, vasopressin, vecuronium, verapamil, vinBLAStine, vinCRIStine, vinorelbine, voriconazole, zidovudine

SIDE EFFECTS

CNS: Pain at tumor site, headache, confusion, *fever*, chills, malaise
CV: Hypotension, peripheral vasoconstriction
GI: *Nausea, vomiting, anorexia, stomatitis, weight loss*
GU: Hemolytic-uremic syndrome
INTEG: *Rash, alopecia,* hyperpigmentation
RESP: Fibrosis, pneumonitis, wheezing, pulmonary toxicity
SYST: Anaphylaxis

PHARMACOKINETICS

Half-life 2-4 hr; when CCr is >35 mL/min, half-life is increased with lower clearance; metabolized in liver; 70% excreted in urine (unchanged) **IV, IM, subcut:** Peak 30-60 min

INTERACTIONS

• Avoid live virus vaccines concurrently; adverse reactions may occur
Increase: bleomycin toxicity-cisplatin
Increase: oxygen requirements—anesthesia
Decrease: serum phenytoin levels—phenytoin, fosphenytoin; check drug level periodically
Drug/Lab Test
Increase: uric acid

NURSING CONSIDERATIONS
Assess:
• IM test dose of 1-2 units in patients with lymphoma before 1st 2 doses
• CBC, differential baseline and periodically, thrombocytopenia, leukopenia may occur (nadir 12 days)

Black Box Warning: Pulmonary toxicity/fibrosis: risk increases >70 yr; pulmonary function tests; chest x-ray before, during therapy, should be obtained q2wk during treatment; pulmonary diffusion capacity for carbon monoxide (DLCO) monthly, if <40% of pretreatment value, stop treatment; treat pulmonary infection before treatment; dyspnea, crackles, unproductive cough, chest pain, tachypnea, fatigue, increased pulse, pallor, lethargy, more common in the elderly, radiation therapy, pulmonary disease; usually occurs with cumulative doses >400 units

• Temperature; fever may indicate beginning infection
• Renal status: serum creatinine/BUN; CBC
• Effects of alopecia, skin color alterations on body image; discuss feelings about body changes
• Buccal cavity q8hr for dryness, sores, ulceration, white patches, oral pain, bleeding, dysphagia
• Local irritation, pain, burning, discoloration at inj site
• **Anaphylaxis:** rash, pruritus, urticaria, purpuric skin lesions, itching, flushing,

wheezing, hypotension; have emergency equipment available

Black Box Warning: Idiosyncratic reaction: severe reaction in those with lymphoma, hypotension, mental confusion, fever, chills, wheezing in lymphoma

Black Box Warning: Requires a specialized care setting and experienced clinician due to severe reactions

• Rinsing of mouth tid-qid with water, club soda; brushing of teeth with soft brush or cotton-tipped applicators for stomatitis; use unwaxed dental floss
• **Pregnancy/breastfeeding:** do not use in pregnancy/breastfeeding
Evaluate:
• Therapeutic response: decrease in size of tumor
Teach patient/family:
• To report any changes in breathing, coughing, fever
• That hair may be lost during treatment and that wig or hairpiece may make patient feel better; that new hair may be different in color, texture
• To report any bleeding, white spots, ulcerations in mouth; to examine mouth daily and report symptoms; to report decreased urination
• That continuing exams and lab work will be needed
• **Skin toxicity:** To report rash, color changes, sensitivity, irritation
• **Stomatitis:** Teach patient that mouth ulcerations, redness may occur, use soft toothbrush
• **Pregnancy/breastfeeding:** to use contraception during treatment; to avoid breastfeeding
• Not to receive vaccines during treatment

RARELY USED

boceprevir
(boe-se′pre-vir)
Victrelis
Func. class.: Antiviral, antihepatitis agents

ACTION: Prevents hepatitis C viral (HCV) replication by blocking the activity of HCV NS3/4A serine protease. Hepatitis C virus NS3/4A serine protease is an enzyme responsible for the conversion of HCV-encoded polyproteins to mature/functioning viral proteins

USES: Hepatitis C infection in combination with peginterferon alfa and ribavirin with compensated liver function

CONTRAINDICATIONS: Pregnancy, male partners of women who are pregnant
Precautions: Breastfeeding, neonates, infants, children, adolescents <18 years of age, anemia, neutropenia, thrombocytopenia, HIV, hepatitis B, decompensated hepatic disease, in liver or other organ transplants, hypersensitivity

DOSAGE AND ROUTES
Chronic hepatitis C infection (genotype 1) compensated liver disease (without cirrhosis, previously untreated with interferon and ribavirin therapy/partial responders/relapsers/null responders)
• **Adults:** PO Before starting therapy peginterferon alfa and ribavirin must be given 4 wk, then add boceprevir 800 mg (four 200-mg caps) **PO** tid (7-9 hr); treatment length is determined by HCV RNA concentrations at treatment wk 4, 8, 12, and 24; if patient has undetectable HCV RNA concentrations at wk 8 and 24, discontinue all 3 medications at wk 28 (previously untreated); 36 wk (partial responders/relapsers); if HCV RNA is detectable at wk 8 but undetectable at wk 24, continue the 3-drug regimen through wk 36, then give only peginterferon alfa and ribavirin through treatment wk 48; if the patient has a poor response to peginterferon alfa and ribavirin during the initial 4 wk, continue treatment with all 3 medications for a total of 48 wk; discontinue the 3-drug regimen if the HCV RNA concentrations >100 international units/

mL at treatment wk 12 or a detectable HCA RNA concentration at treatment wk 24

Chronic hepatitis C infection (genotype 1) compensated liver disease with cirrhosis

• **Adults:** PO Before starting therapy with boceprevir, peginterferon alfa and ribavirin must be given 4 wk; then add boceprevir 800 mg (four 200-mg caps) **PO** tid (7-9 hr) to peginterferon alfa and ribavirin for an additional 44 wk (48 wk total)

Available forms: Caps 200 mg

Administer:

• Only use in combination with peginterferon alfa and ribavirin; never give as monotherapy

• Discontinue in hepatitis C virus (HCV) if RNA concentrations ≥100 international units/mL at wk 12 or a confirmed detectable HCV RNA concentration at wk 24

• Any contraindication to peginterferon alfa or ribavirin also applies to boceprevir

• Give with food

SIDE EFFECTS

When used in combination with peginterferon/ribavirin

CNS: *Fatigue, chills, asthenia,* insomnia, irritability, dizziness

GI: Nausea, vomiting, diarrhea, dysgeusia, decreased appetite, xerostomia

HEMA: Anemia (Hgb <10 g/dL), neutropenia, thrombocytopenia

INTEG: *Alopecia, rash,* xerosis

MISC: *Arthralgia, exertional dyspnea,* drug rash with eosinophilia and systemic symptoms (DRESS) syndrome, exfoliative dermatitis, Stevens-Johnson syndrome, toxic epidermal necrolysis

INTERACTIONS

Increase: life-threatening reactions of each product: alfuzosin, ergots (dihydroergotamine, ergotamine, ergonovine, methylergonovine), cisapride, pimozide, lovastatin, simvastatin, ezetimibe, niacin with simvastatin and boceprevir; triazolam, oral midazolam; sildenafil, tadalafil (pulmonary arterial hypertension); do not use concurrently

Increase: adverse reactions of each product—phosphodiesterase type 5 (PDE5) inhibitors (for erectile dysfunction), acetaminophen, alfentanil, aliskiren, almotriptan, alosetron, ALPRAZolam, aminophylline, amiodarone, amitriptyline, amLODIPine, ARIPiprazole, astemizole, atorvastatin, bepridil, boceprevir, bosentan, budesonide, bupivacaine, buprenorphine, busPIRone, carvedilol, cevimeline, chloroquine, cilostazol, cinacalcet, citalopram, clarithromycin, clomiPRAMINE, clonazePAM, clopidogrel, cloZAPine, colchicine, cyclobenzaprine, cycloSPORINE, dapsone, DAUNOrubicin, desipramine, desloratadine, dexamethasone, dexlansoprazole, dextromethorphan, diazepam, diclofenac, digoxin, diltiazem, disopyramide, disulfiram, DOCEtaxel, dolasetron, donepezil, DOXOrubicin, droperidol, dutasteride, ebastine, eletriptan, eplerenone, erlotinib, erythromycin, estazolam, eszopiclone, ethosuximide, etoposide, exemestane, felodipine, fentaNYL, fexofenadine, finasteride, flecainide, flunitrazepam, flurazepam, galantamine, gefitinib, glyburide, granisetron, halofantrine, haloperidol, HYDROcodone, ifosfamide, imipramine, indiplon, irinotecan, isradipine, itraconazole, ivermectin, ixabepilone, ketoconazole, lansoprazole, lidocaine, loperamide, loratadine, losartan, maraviroc, mefloquine, meloxicam, mirtazapine, mitoMYcin, montelukast, morphine, nateglinide, niCARdipine, NIFEdipine, nisoldipine, nortriptyline, omeprazole, ondansetron, oxybutynin, oxyCODONE, PACLitaxel, palonosetron, paricalcitol, plicamycin, posaconazole, prasugrel, praziquantel, propafenone, quazepam, QUEtiapine, quinacrine, quiNIDine, ramelteon, repaglinide, rifabutin, risperiDONE, ropivacaine, salmeterol, selegiline, sertraline, sibutramine, silodosin, sirolimus, sitaxentan, solifenacin, SUFentanil, SUNItinib, systemic corticosteroids, tacrolimus, telithromycin, teniposide, terfenadine, testosterone, theophylline, tiaGABine, tinidazole, tolterodine, tolvaptan, traMADol, traZODone, vardenafil, venlafaxine, verapamil, vinBLAStine, vinCRIStine, voricon-

---

Side effects: *italics* = common; red = life-threatening

azole, warfarin, and others; use cautiously, may need to reduce dose

Increase: hyperkalemia—drospirenone
Decrease: estrogen levels—ethinyl estradiol
Decrease: boceprevir effect—CYP3A4 inhibitors (phenytoin, carBAMazepine, PHENobarbital, rifampin)
Decrease: effect of—methadone
Possible treatment failure: efavirenz, ritonavir, atazanavir, lopinavir with ritonavir
Drug/Herb

• Do not use with St. John's wort
Drug/Lab Test
Decrease: Hgb, platelets

NURSING CONSIDERATIONS
Assess:

• **Pregnancy:** obtain a pregnancy test before, monthly during, and for 6 mo after treatment is completed; those who are not willing to practice strict contraception should not receive treatment; report any cases of prenatal ribavirin exposure to the Ribavirin Pregnancy Registry at 800-593-2214

• **Anemia:** monitor Hgb, CBC with differential before, at treatment wk 2, 8, 12, and as needed. If Hgb is <10 g/dL, decrease ribavirin dosage; if Hgb is <8.5 g/dL, discontinuation of therapy is recommended; dosage should not be altered based on adverse reactions; anemia may be managed through ribavirin dose modifications; never alter the dose of boceprevir; if anemia persists despite a reduction in ribavirin dose, consider discontinuing boceprevir; if management of anemia requires permanent discontinuation of ribavirin, treatment with boceprevir MUST also be permanently discontinued; once boceprevir has been discontinued, it must not be restarted; monitor CBC with differential at treatment wk 4, 8, 12, and at other treatment points as needed

• Serious skin disorders (DRESS, Stevens-Johnson syndrome, toxic epidermal necrolysis, exfoliative dermatitis): These reactions may be due to combination use with peginterferon alfa, ribavirin; if serious skin reactions occur, discontinue all 3 products

Teach patient/family:

• To take with food to increase absorption; do not start new meds/herbs without prescriber's approval

• To use precautions to prevent transmission of hepatitis C

• To inform prescriber of all medications, herbs, supplements used

• **Pregnancy/breastfeeding:** To use 2 forms of effective contraception (intrauterine devices and barrier methods) during treatment and for 6 mo after treatment; to avoid breastfeeding

---

⚠ HIGH ALERT

bortezomib (Rx)
(bor-tez′oh-mib)
Velcade
Func. class.: Antineoplastic—miscellaneous
Chem. class.: Proteasome inhibitor

ACTION: Reversible inhibitor of chymotrypsin-like activity; causes delay in tumor growth by disrupting normal homeostatic mechanisms

USES: Multiple myeloma previously untreated or when at least 2 other treatments have failed; mantle cell lymphoma in patients who have received ≥1 prior therapy
Unlabeled uses: Non-Hodgkin's lymphoma (NHL)

CONTRAINDICATIONS: Pregnancy, breastfeeding; hypersensitivity to product, boron, mannitol
Precautions: Children, geriatric patients, peripheral neuropathy, cardiac/hepatic disease, hypotension, tumor lysis syndrome, thrombocytopenia, infection, diabetes mellitus, bone marrow suppression, intracranial bleeding, injection site irritation

DOSAGE AND ROUTES
Multiple myeloma (previously untreated)

• **Adult:** IV BOL/SUBCUT • Give for nine 6-wk cycles; cycles 1-4, 1.3 mg/m^2/dose given on days 1, 4, 8, 11, then a

---

10-day rest period (days 12-21), then give again on days 22, 25, 29, 32, then a 10-day rest period (days 33-42); given with melphalan (9 mg/m²/day on days 1-4) and predniSONE (60 mg/m²/day on days 1-4); during cycles 5-9, give bortezomib 1.3 mg/m²/dose on days 1, 8, 22, 29 with melphalan (9 mg/m²/day on days 1-4) and predniSONE (60 mg/m²/day on days 1-4); this 6-wk cycle is considered 1 course; at least 72 hr should elapse between consecutive doses

Mantle cell lymphoma in combination

• **Adult:** IV BOL/SUBCUT 1.3 mg/m²/dose on days 1, 4, 8, 11 followed by a 10-day rest period (days 12-21); ×6 (3-wk) cycles with rituximab 375 mg/m², cyclophosphamide 750 mg/m², doxorubicin 50 mg/m² all on day 1, and prednisone 100 mg/m² daily on days 1-5, give bortezomib before rituximab

Relapsed multiple myeloma or mantle cell lymphoma

• **Adult:** IV BOL/SUBCUT 1.3 mg/m²/2 × per wk on days 1, 4, 8, 11 followed by a 10-day rest period

Hepatic dose

• **Adult:** IV bilirubin >1.5 × ULN, reduce to 0.7 mg/m² during cycle 1; consider dose escalation to 1 mg/m² or further reduction to 0.5 mg/m² during next cycles based on tolerability

Available forms: Lyophilized powder for inj 3.5 mg

Administer:

IV bolus route

• **Reconstitute** each vial with 3.5 mL of 0.9% NaCl (1 mg/mL); sol should be clear/colorless; **inj** as bolus over 3-5 sec

• Store unopened product at room temperature, protect from light

• Wear protective clothing during handling, preparation; avoid contact with skin

• Check for extravasation at inj site

SUBCUT route

• Only Velcade can be given subcut

• Reconstitute with 1.4 mL of NS to a final concentration of 2.5 mg/mL; if inj site reaction occurs, reconstitute vial with 3.5 mL of NS to a final concentration of 1 mg/ mL or consider IV administration; use within 8 hr

• Administer calculated dose into the thigh or abdomen; rotate sites with each inj; inject at least 1 inch from old sites

• Space apart consecutive doses by at least 72 hr. Consider subcut in patients with preexisting peripheral neuropathy or at high risk for the condition

SIDE EFFECTS

CNS: Posterior reversible encephalopathy syndrome (PRESS), progressive multifocal leukoencephalopathy (PML), dizziness, headache, *peripheral neuropathy,* fever, headache, *fatigue, malaise, weakness*

CV: *Hypotension,* edema

GI: Abdominal pain, *constipation, diarrhea, nausea, vomiting,* anorexia, hepatotoxicity

HEMA: *Anemia,* neutropenia, thrombocytopenia

MISC: Tumor lysis syndrome

RESP: Cough, pneumonia, dyspnea

PHARMACOKINETICS

Half-life 9-15 hr, protein binding 83%, metabolized by CYP450 enzymes (3A4, 2D6, 2C19, 2C9, 1A2)

INTERACTIONS

Increase: risk for bleeding—anticoagulants, NSAIDs, platelet inhibitors, salicylates, thrombolytics

Increase: peripheral neuropathy—amiodarone, antivirals (amprenavir, atazanavir, didanosine, lamiVUDine, 3TC, ritonavir, stavudine, zidovudine), chloramphenicol, CISplatin, colchicine, cycloSPORINE, dapsone, disulfiram, DOCEtaxel, gold salts, HMG-CoA reductase inhibitors, iodoquinol, INH, metroNIDAZOLE, nitrofurantoin, oxaliplatin, PACLitaxel, penicillamine, phenytoin, sulfaSALAzine, thalidomide, vinBLAStine, vinCRIStine, zalcitabine ddc, isoniazid, statins, others

Decrease: effect of norethindrone, estradiol, combination oral contraceptives; another nonhormonal contraceptive should be used

Drug/Herb

Increase: toxicity or decrease efficacy—St. John's wort

Drug/Lab
Increase: LFTs, glucose
Decrease: Platelets

NURSING CONSIDERATIONS
Assess:
• VS baseline and frequently, hypotension may occur, patient who are dehydrated are at greater risk
• GI toxicity: nausea, vomiting, diarrhea, constipation, may require antiemetics, antidiarrheals
• **Thrombocytopenia, neutropenia:** CBC baseline and periodically, platelets before each dose, dose adjustment may be required (nadir 11 platelets)
• **Fatal pulmonary toxicity:** assess for risk factors or new or worsening pulmonary symptoms
• **Fatal pulmonary toxicity:** assess for risk factors or new or worsening pulmonary symptoms
• **Tumor lysis syndrome:** usually in patients with a high tumor burden (hyperkalemia, hyperuricemia, hyperphosphatemia, renal failure)
• **PRES:** Headache, malaise, confusion, seizures, blindness, hypertension, usually occurs within a few hours up to 1 yr after starting treatment, most symptoms do not need treatment, MRI confirms
• **PML:** For new infections of the brain
Evaluate:
• Therapeutic response: improvement of multiple myeloma symptoms
Teach patient/family:
• To monitor blood glucose levels if diabetic
• To contact prescriber about new or worsening peripheral neuropathy, severe vomiting, diarrhea, easy bruising, bleeding, infection
• To avoid driving, operating machinery until effect is known
• To avoid using other medications unless approved by prescriber
• About bleeding risk; to report bruising, bleeding
• To immediately report headache, confusion, lethargy (PRES)

• **Pregnancy/breastfeeding:** To use contraception while taking this product; to avoid breastfeeding

---

bosentan (Rx) REMS
(boh′sen-tan)
Tracleer
Func. class.: Vasodilator
Chem. class.: Endothelin receptor antagonist

Do not confuse:
Tracleer/ Tricor

ACTION: Peripheral vasodilation occurs via the antagonism of the effect of endothelin on endothelium and vascular smooth muscle

USES: Pulmonary arterial hypertension with WHO class III, IV symptoms
Unlabeled uses: Septic shock to improve microcirculatory blood flow, functional class II pulmonary arterial hypertension

CONTRAINDICATIONS: Hypersensitivity, CVA, CAD

Black Box Warning: Pregnancy

Precautions: Breastfeeding, children, geriatric patients, mitral stenosis, anemia, edema, jaundice, hypovolemia, hypotension

Black Box Warning: Hepatic disease, requires an experienced clinician, contraceptive requirements, pregnancy testing

DOSAGE AND ROUTES
Pulmonary hypertension (pulmonary arterial hypertension WHO Group 1)
• **Adults/adolescents >40 kg: PO** tab 62.5 mg bid × 4 wk, then increase to 125 mg bid
• **Adults/adolescents ≤40 kg: PO** tab 62.5 mg bid
• **Children 21-40 kg (unlabeled): PO** tab 62.5 mg bid
• **Infants/children 10-20 kg (unlabeled): PO** 31.25 mg q day for 4 wk

---

• **Infants <10 kg (unlabeled):** PO 2 mg/kg/dose bid, initiate at half of maintenance dose and increase to target dosage after 4 wk
• **Children 3-12 yr and 25-40 kg:** PO tab for susp 64 mg bid
• **Children 3-12 yr and 17-24 kg:** PO tab for susp 48 mg bid
• **Children 3-12 yr and 9-16 kg:** PO tab for susp 32 mg bid
• **Children 3-12 yr and 4-8 kg:** PO tab for susp 16 mg bid

Persistent pulmonary hypertension of the newborn (PPHN) (unlabeled)
• **Premature and term neonates ≥34 wk gestation:** PO 1 mg/kg/dose bid
Hepatic dose
• **Adult:** PO baseline AST/ALT <3 × ULN no dosage change, monitor LFTs monthly, reduce or interrupt if elevated; AST/ALT >3 and ≤5 × ULN repeat test, if confirmed reduce to 62.5 mg bid or interrupt; monitor LFTs q2wk, if interrupted, restart when LFTs <3 × ULN, check LFTs within 3 days; increase in AST/ALT >5 and ≤5 × ULN; during treatment repeat test to confirm, discontinue, monitor LFTs q2wk until LFTs <3 × ULN, restart at starting dose; AST/ALT >8 × ULN **discontinue permanently**
Available forms: Tabs 62.5, 125 mg; tab for oral suspension 32 mg
Administer:
• Give without regard to meals
• Only available through the TAP program; 866-228-3546
• Do not stop product abruptly; taper
• Store at room temperature

SIDE EFFECTS
CNS: Headache, flushing, fatigue, fever
CV: Hypotension, chest pain, palpitations, edema of lower limbs, fluid retention
GI: Abnormal hepatic function, diarrhea, dyspepsia, hepatotoxicity
HEMA: Anemia, leukopenia, neutropenia, lymphopenia, thrombocytopenia
INTEG: Pruritus, anaphylaxis, rash, Stevens-Johnson syndrome, toxic epidermal necrolysis
MISC: Oligospermia, tumor lysis syndrome, respiratory infection, arthralgia
SYST: Secondary malignancy

PHARMACOKINETICS
Metabolized by inducer of CYP2C9, CYP3A4, possibly CYP2C19; metabolized by the liver; terminal half-life 5 hr; steady state 3-5 days

INTERACTIONS
• Do not coadminister cycloSPORINE with bosentan; bosentan is increased, cycloSPORINE is decreased
• Do not coadminister glyBURIDE with bosentan; glyBURIDE is decreased significantly, bosentan is also decreased, hepatic enzymes may be increased
Increase: bosentan effects—CYP2C9, CYP3A4 inhibitors
Increase: bosentan level—ketoconazole
Decrease: effects of warfarin, hormonal contraceptives, statins
Drug/Lab Test

Black Box Warning: **Increase:** ALT, AST

Decrease: Hgb, Hct

NURSING CONSIDERATIONS
Assess:
• **Serious skin toxicities:** angioedema occurring 8-21 days after initiating therapy
• B/P, pulse during treatment until stable
• Blood studies: Hct, Hgb after 1 mo, 3 mo, then every 3 mo; may be decreased
• **Pulmonary hypertension/HF:** fluid retention, weight gain, increased leg edema; may occur within weeks

Black Box Warning: **Hepatic toxicity:** vomiting, jaundice; product should be discontinued; hepatic studies: AST, ALT, bilirubin; hepatic enzymes may increase; if ALT/AST >3 × and ≤5 × ULN, decrease dose or interrupt treatment and monitor AST/ALT q2wk; if bilirubin >2 × ULN or signs of hepatitis or hepatic disease are present, stop treatment

Black Box Warning: **Experienced clinician:** must be enrolled in the Tracleer REMS program (1-866-228-3546) and comply with requirements

Black Box Warning: **Pregnancy:** perform pregnancy testing prior to and during treatment in all female patients of childbearing potential, do not use unless a negative serum or urine pregnancy test is confirmed during the first 5 days of a normal menstrual period and at least 11 days after the last unprotected sex then monthly; do not use hormonal contraceptive as sole method

• **Beers:** use with caution in older adults; syncope may be exacerbated
Evaluate:
• Therapeutic response: decrease in pulmonary hypertension
Teach patient/family:
• To report jaundice, dark urine, joint pain, fatigue, malaise, bruising, easy bleeding, fluid retention

Black Box Warning: Patient must use nonhormonal contraception during and ≥1 mo after conclusion of treatment

• That lab work will be required periodically
• To take without regard to food; not to take new meds/herbs without prescriber approval; to take in AM or PM

⚠ HIGH ALERT

RARELY USED

bosutinib (Rx)
(boe-sue′ti-nib)
Bosulif
Func. class.: Antineoplastic biologic response modifiers
Chem. class.: Signal transduction inhibitors (STIs), tyrosine kinase inhibitor

---

USES: Treatment of CML (chronic accelerator phase); Philadelphia chromosome–positive patients in blast-cell crisis

CONTRAINDICATIONS: Pregnancy, hypersensitivity

DOSAGE AND ROUTES
• **Adult:** PO 400 mg daily with food, may increase to 600 mg/day in those who have not developed grade 3 toxicity or in patients who do not reach complete hematological response by wk 8 or complete cytogenic response (CCyR) by wk 12
Hepatic dosage
• **Adult:** PO Any baseline hepatic impairment: start at 200 mg/day; liver transaminase >5 × ULN, hold dose until levels are ≤2.5 × ULN, then resume at 400 mg/day; liver transaminase level ≥3 × ULN and bilirubin >2 × ULN and alk phos <2 × ULN, discontinue

---

⚠ HIGH ALERT

brentuximab vedotin (Rx)
(bren-tuk′see-mab)
Adcetris
Func. class.: Antineoplastic
Chem. class.: Monoclonal antibody

ACTION: The anticancer activity is due to the binding of the ⍉ꞏ ADC to CD30-expressing cells, followed by the internalization and transportation of the ADC-CD30 complex to lysosomes and the release of MMAE via selective proteolytic cleavage; MMAE binds to tubulin and disrupts the microtubule network within the cell, inducing cell cycle arrest and apoptotic death of the cells

USES: Hodgkin's disease after failure of autologous stem cell transplant (ASCT) or after failure of at least 2 prior multiagent chemotherapy regimens in patients who are not ASCT candidates; non-Hodgkin's lymphoma (NHL); systemic anaplastic large cell lymphoma (sALCL) after failure of at least 1 prior multiagent chemotherapy regimen

CONTRAINDICATIONS: Hypersensitivity, pregnancy

Precautions: Breastfeeding, children, infants, neonates, neutropenia, peripheral neuropathy, tumor lysis syndrome (TLS)

Black Box Warning: Progressive multifocal leukoencephalopathy

DOSAGE AND ROUTES
• **Adult: IV** 1.8 mg/kg q3wk until disease progression or unacceptable toxicity

Renal dose
• **Adult:** IV CCr <30 mL/min, avoid use
Hepatic dose
• **Adult:** IV (Child-Pugh A) 1.2 mg/kg q3wk; (Child-Pugh B or C avoid use)
Available forms: Powder for inj 50 mg/vial
Administer:
Intermittent IV INFUSION route
• Visually inspect for particulate matter and discoloration whenever sol and container permit
• Only as an IV infusion, do not give as an IV push or bolus
• Use cytotoxic handling procedures
• Do not mix, or administer as an infusion, with other IV products
• Calculate the dose (mg) and the number of vials required. For patients weighing >100 kg, use 100 kg to calculate the dose; reconstitute each 50-mg vial per 10.5 mL of sterile water for inj (5 mg/mL)
• Direct the stream of sterile water toward the wall of the vial and not directly at the cake or powder; gently swirl the vial to aid in dissolution, do not shake
• Discard any unused portion left in the vial
• After reconstitution, dilute immediately with ≥100 mL of 0.9% sodium chloride, 5% dextrose, or lactated Ringer's solution to a final concentration (0.4 mg/mL-1.8 mg/mL)
• Infuse over 30 min
• Use the diluted sol immediately or store in refrigerator for ≤24 hr after reconstitution; do not freeze

SIDE EFFECTS
CNS: Headache, dizziness, *fever*, peripheral neuropathy, anxiety, chills, *fatigue*, insomnia, night sweats, progressive multifocal leukoencephalopathy
CV: Peripheral edema
GI: *Abdominal pain, nausea, vomiting,* constipation, *diarrhea*, weight loss, GI hemorrhage/perforation/obstruction
INTEG: *Rash,* pruritus, alopecia, xerosis
RESP: Pneumothorax, pneumonitis dyspnea, *cough*
SYST: Anaphylaxis, tumor lysis syndrome, Stevens-Johnson syndrome, infusion reactions, toxic epidermal necrolysis
HEMA: Anemia, neutropenia, thrombocytopenia, lymphadenopathy

PHARMACOKINETICS
Protein binding is 68%-82%, only a small amount is metabolized; potent inhibitors or inducers of CYP3A4 may alter action; terminal half-life is 4-6 days; 3 components are released

INTERACTIONS
Increase: brentuximab action—CYP3A4 inhibitors, P-gb inhibitors, ketoconazole, boceprevir, delavirdine, isoniazid, indinavir, itraconazole, dalfopristin, quinupristin, telithromycin, tipranavir, rifampin, ritonavir
Increase: Toxicity of live virus vaccines
Increase: Pulmonary toxicity—bleomycin; do not use together
Decrease: brentuximab action—CYP3A4 inducers
Drug/Herb
Increase: brentuximab component action—St. John's wort
Drug/Lab
Decrease: WBC, platelets, RBCs

NURSING CONSIDERATIONS
Assess:
• **Pulmonary toxicity**: cough, trouble breathing, report immediately
• **Infection**: report immediately, fever, chills
• **Tumor lysis syndrome (TLS):** assess for hyperkalemia, hypophosphatemia, hypocalcemia; may develop renal failure;

---

may use allopurinol or rasburicase to prevent TLS; monitor serum BUN/creatinine

• **Pregnancy:** determine if pregnancy is planned or suspected; do not use in pregnancy/breastfeeding; reliable contraception should be used

Black Box Warning: **Peripheral neuropathy, progressive multifocal leukoencephalopathy:** assess for weakness or paralysis, vision loss, impaired speech, and cognitive deterioration; often fatal

• Monitor CBC and differential, LFTs, serum bilirubin (direct and indirect), electrolytes, uric acid, neurologic function

• **Bone marrow suppression:** monitor CBC before each dose

• **GI toxicity:** monitor for changes in bowel habits, bowel obstruction, constipation, pancreatitis

• **Anaphylaxis:** monitor for symptoms; high risk during administration

• **Stevens-Johnson syndrome:** monitor and report skin reactions or rash; discontinue if toxic epidermal necrolysis or Stevens-Johnson syndrome occurs

Evaluate:

• Decreasing symptoms of Hodgkin's disease (decreased lymph nodes, night sweats, weight loss, splenomegaly, hepatomegaly)

Teach patient/family:

• To report immediately weakness, change in vision, impaired speech, peripheral neuropathy, neutropenia if severe, rash, change in bowel habits

• To use reliable contraception; not to breastfeed

• **Hepatotoxicity:** AST/ALT, bilirubin baseline and periodically, if elevated product may need to be discontinued or decreased

• **Pulmonary toxicity:** dyspnea, cough if these occur product may need to be discontinued

• **Infusion site reactions:** check site frequently, if reaction occurs (redness, swelling at site) stop infusion, give antihistamines

brexpiprazole
brex-pip′-ra-zole

Rexulti

Func. class.: Antipsychotic, atypical

ACTION: May exert its effects through a combination of partial agonist activity at dopaminergic D-2 receptors, serotonergic 5-HT1A receptors, antagonist activity at serotonergic 5-HT2A receptors

USES: Adjunctive treatment of major depressive disorder, schizophrenia

CONTRAINDICATIONS: Hypersensitivity

Precautions: Elderly patients, dementia-related psychosis, suicidal ideation, stroke, neuroleptic malignant syndrome, tardive dyskinesia, leukopenia, neutropenia, agranulocytosis, orthostatic hypotension, seizures, cognitive impairment

DOSAGE AND ROUTES

Schizophrenia

• **Adult: PO** Initially, 1 mg daily on Days 1-4; increase to 2 mg daily on Days 5-7, then increase to 4 mg daily on Day 8 based on response and tolerability. Recommended dose range 2-4 mg/day (max: 4 mg/day)

Adjunctive treatment of major depressive disorder

• **Adult: PO** Initially, 0.5 to 1 mg daily; after titration to 1 mg/day, increase to target dose of 2 mg/day; titrate dosage at weekly intervals based on response and tolerability

Hepatic dose

• **Adult: PO** Mild hepatic impairment: no change; moderate to severe hepatic impairment (Child-Pugh score ≥7): max 2 mg/day for major depressive disorder, 3 mg/day for schizophrenia

Renal dose

• **Adult: PO** CCr ≥60 mL/min: no change; CCr <60 mL/min, including end-stage renal disease (ESRD): max 2 mg/day for major depression, 3 mg/day for schizophrenia

Available forms: Tabs 0.25, 0.50, 1, 2, 3, 4 mg

Administer:

• Initiate treatment at low end of dosage range in geriatric adults

• Periodically reassess for need of continued maintenance therapy

• Without regard to food

SIDE EFFECTS

CNS: Akathisia, fatigue, drowsiness, dizziness, tremor, sedation, insomnia, EPS

EENT: Blurred vision, dry mouth, nasopharyngitis

GI: Constipation, diarrhea, nausea, flatulence, abdominal cramping/pain

GU: UTI

MISC: Weight gain, myalgia

PHARMACOKINETICS

Half-life 91 hr, peak 4 hr

INTERACTIONS

Increase: temperature—anticholinergics

Increase: CNS depression—other CNS depressants

Increase: brexpiprazole effect—strong CYP2D6 inhibitors, strong CYP3A4 inhibitors

Drug/Herb:

Decrease: brexpiprazole effect—St. John's wort; may need to increase product dose

Drug/Food:

Increase: brexpiprazole effect—grapefruit juice; avoid using together

NURSING CONSIDERATIONS

Assess:

• **Hypersensitivity:** rash, facial swelling, urticaria, and anaphylaxis have been observed; discontinue immediately

Black Box Warning: Suicidal ideation: provide close supervision and control; give the smallest quantity consistent with good management to reduce the risk of overdose. In those who exhibit changes in symptoms, worsening of depression, suicidality, or other unusual changes in mood or behavior, a decision should be made to change or discontinue treatment. If discontinuing, taper as rapidly as possible, but with recognition that abrupt discontinuation of drug can also cause adverse symptoms. Children and young adults <24 yr are at increased risk

• **Tardive dyskinesia:** periodic evaluation for movement disorders (AIMS) is recommended. If signs and symptoms of tardive dyskinesia appear, consider discontinuation

• **Seizure disorder:** use cautiously in patients with history of seizure disorder, or with conditions that may lower the seizure threshold. Conditions that lower the seizure threshold may be more prevalent in patients 65 yr or older

• **Orthostatic hypotension:** dizziness, light-headedness, tachycardia, and occasionally syncope. Risks are generally greatest at beginning of treatment and during dose escalation. Patients at higher risk include those with dehydration, hypovolemia, treatment with antihypertensive medications, history of cardiac disease (HF, MI, CAD, ischemia, or conduction abnormalities), history of cerebrovascular disease, and patients who are antipsychotic-naive. Monitor orthostatic vital signs, such as pulse and BP. Complete fall risk assessments in at-risk patients on long-term antipsychotic therapy

• **Hematologic disease:** those with a history of clinically significant low WBC count or drug-induced leukopenia/neutropenia should have frequent CBC assessments in first few months of treatment. Consider discontinuing drug if a clinically significant decline in WBC occurs in the absence of an identifiable cause. Monitor patients

with neutropenia for fever, infection. Discontinue in patients with ANC <1000/mm^3
• **Pregnancy/breastfeeding:** no well-controlled studies; use only when benefits outweigh fetal risks. Neonates exposed to antipsychotics in the third trimester of pregnancy are at risk for extrapyramidal and/or withdrawal symptoms after delivery. Enroll patient in National Pregnancy Registry for Psychiatric Medications, 1-866-961-2388. Consider benefits of breastfeeding, risk of potential infant drug exposure, and risk of untreated or inadequately treated condition. If a breastfeeding infant experiences an adverse effect related to a maternally ingested drug, providers are encouraged to report the adverse effect to the FDA
Teach patient/family:
• To use caution when driving or operating machinery or performing other tasks that require mental alertness until the effects are known
• To avoid ethanol ingestion during treatment. Somnolence could lead to falls with the potential for fractures and other injuries

---

⚠ HIGH ALERT
RARELY USED

brigatinib
(bri-ga′-ti-nib)
Alunbrig
Func. class.: Antineoplastic

USES: Advanced ALK-positive metastatic non–small-cell lung cancer who have progressed on or are intolerant to crizotinib

DOSAGE AND ROUTES
• **Adult: PO** 90 mg/day × 7 days; if tolerated during the first 7 days, increase to 180 mg/day. Continue until disease progression or unacceptable toxicity

---

brimonidine (ophthalmic) (Rx)
(bri-moe′ni-deen)
Alphagan P, Qoliana
Func. class.: Antiglaucoma
Chem. class.: Selective α-2 agonist

Do not confuse:
brimonidine/bimatoprost

ACTION: Select α-agonist that decreases aqueous humor and increases outflows

USES: Treatment of chronic open-angle glaucoma and ocular hypertension

CONTRAINDICATIONS: Hypersensitivity, AV block, heart failure, bradycardia, sick sinus syndrome, within 14 days of MAOI therapy
Precautions: Breastfeeding, depression, cerebrovascular disease, hepatic/renal impairment, Raynaud's phenomenon, orthostatic hypotension, thromboangiitis obliterans

DOSAGE AND ROUTES
• **Adult/child >2 yr:** Instill 1 drop in the affected eye(s) tid
Available forms: Ophthalmic solution 0.1%, 0.15%, 0.2%

SIDE EFFECTS
RESP: Cough, dyspnea, bronchitis, pharyngitis
CNS: Headache, dizziness, somnolence
CV: Hyper/hypotension, hypercholesterolemia
EENT: Eye stinging/burning, tearing, photophobia, change in vision, sinus infection, blurred vision, pruritus, photophobia, eyelid erythema, ocular pain, nasal dryness

PHARMACOKINETICS
Peak $^1/_2$-2 hr, half-life 2 hr

INTERACTIONS

Increase: intraocular pressure reduction—apraclonidine, dorzolamide, pilocarpine, timolol

Increase: effects of—CNS depressants

Decrease: B/P—β-blockers, antihypertensives

Decrease: brimonidine effect—tricyclic antidepressants, may cause HTN crisis MAOIs, linezolid

NURSING CONSIDERATIONS
Assess:
• Glaucoma: monitor intraocular pressure

Evaluate:
• Decreasing intraocular pressure

Teach patient/family:
• That drug is for ophthalmic use only
• Not to touch the tip of the dropper to the eye, fingertips, or other surface to prevent contamination
• Not to use alcohol
• To wait 15 min before inserting soft contact lenses
• To avoid hazardous activities until response is known
• To wash hands before and after use; to tilt the head back slightly and pull the lower eyelid down with the index finger to form a pouch; to squeeze the prescribed number of drops into the pouch, then close eyes to spread drops; to apply finger pressure on the lacrimal sac for 1-2 min following use to avoid excessive systemic absorption
• That if more than one topical ophthalmic drug product is being used, the drugs should be administered at least 10 min apart
• To avoid contamination or the spread of infection by not using dropper for more than one person

---

brinzolamide ophthalmic
See Appendix B

---

brivaracetam
(briv-a- ra′ se-tam)
Briviact
Func. class.: Anticonvulsant

Controlled Substance V

B

ACTION: The exact mechanism is not known, may occur in modulation of synaptic vesicle proteins; additional anticonvulsant activity may be related to the modulation of voltage-dependent sodium channels

USES: For the adjunctive treatment of partial seizures

CONTRAINDICATIONS: Hypersensitivity

Precautions: Abrupt discontinuation, breastfeeding, depression, driving or operating machinery, geriatric patients, hepatic disease, pregnancy, suicidal ideation

DOSAGE AND ROUTES
• **Adult/adolescent ≥16: PO/IV** • 50 mg bid. Adjust dose to 25 mg bid or 100 mg bid based on clinical response; max 100 mg bid. Use **IV** when **PO** is temporarily not feasible
• **Child/adolescent 4-15 yr and >50 kg: PO** 25-50 mg bid
• **Child/adolescent 4-15 yr and 20-49 kg: PO** 0.5-1 mg/kg/dose bid
• **Child/adolescent 4-12 yr and 11-19 kg: PO** 0.5-2.5 mg/kg/dose, max 5 mg/kg/day

Available forms:
• Tabs 10, 25, 50, 75, 100; oral solution 10 mg/mL; sol for inj 50 mg/5 mL (10 mg/mL)

Administer:
• May be administered without regard to meals
• To discontinue, gradually reduce the dose to minimize the risk for increased seizure frequency and status epilepticus

Tablets:
• Swallow tablets whole; do not crush or chew

Oral solution:
• No dilution is necessary
• Measure and administer oral solution using a calibrated measuring device
• A nasogastric tube or gastrostomy tube may be used for administration
• **Storage:** discard any unused solution 5 months after first opening the bottle

IV infusion
• Visually inspect parenteral products for particulate matter and discoloration prior to use; do not use if discoloration or particulate matter is present; injection is a clear, colorless solution
• May be given IV without further dilution or may be mixed with a diluent, including 0.9% NaCl injection, LR injection, or D_5 injection
• Infuse over 2 to 15 min
• **Storage:** after dilution, the solution may be stored ≤4 hr at room temperature and may be stored in polyvinyl chloride (PVC) bags; discard any unused injection vial contents; for single dose only

SIDE EFFECTS

CNS: Dizziness, drowsiness, ataxia, euphoria, fatigue, irritability, depression, emotional lability, hallucinations, psychosis, suicidal ideation

GI: Constipation, nausea, vomiting

HEMA: Leukopenia

INTEG: Angioedema

RESP: Bronchospasm

PHARMACOKINETICS

Protein binding 20%, primarily metabolized by hydrolysis to form a hydroxy metabolite, metabolized by CYP2C19, excreted in urine, feces <1%, half-life 9 hr, all forms may be used interchangeably, peak 1 hr without food, high-fat meal slows absorption

INTERACTIONS

Increase: sedation—TCAs, antihistamines, benzodiazepines, other CNS depressants
Increase: possible toxicity—carBAMazepine

Decrease: brivaracetam absorption—sevelamer

Drug/Lab Test:
Increase: LFTs
Decrease: Hct/Hgb, WBC, RBC

NURSING CONSIDERATIONS

Assess:
• Seizures: type, location, duration, character; provide seizure precautions
• Renal studies: urinalysis, BUN, urine creatinine q3mo
• Blood studies: CBC, LFTs
• Mental status: mood, sensorium, affect, behavioral changes, suicidal thoughts/behaviors; if mental status changes, notify prescriber
• Assistance with ambulation during early part of treatment; dizziness, drowsiness occurs
• **Pregnancy/breastfeeding:** use only if benefits outweigh fetal risk; pregnant patients should be registered at the North American Antiepileptic Drug Pregnancy Registry (1-888-233-2334); discontinue breastfeeding or product; excretion is unknown

Evaluate:
• Therapeutic response: decreased seizure activity

Teach patient/family:
• To carry emergency ID stating patient's name, medications taken, condition, prescriber's name and phone number
• How to use oral solution, use calibrated device to measure
• To notify prescriber if pregnancy is planned or suspected
• To avoid driving, other activities requiring alertness until response is known; drowsiness occurs during beginning therapy
• Not to discontinue quickly after long-term use; withdrawal seizure may occur; date bottle, throw away oral solution after 5 mo
• Not to breastfeed; to notify prescriber immediately if pregnancy is planned

---

• To report immediately suicidal thoughts/behaviors, psychotic symptoms (hallucination, delusions, or unusual behaviors)

brodalumab (Rx)

(broe-dal´-ue-mab)

Siliq

Func. class.: Immunosuppressive
Chem. class.: Recombinant human IgG2 monoclonal antibody

ACTION: Human IgG2 monoclonal antibody that binds to interleukin-17 receptor A (IL-17RA) and prevents IL-17 cytokines from activating the receptor

USES: For the treatment of moderate to severe plaque psoriasis in adult patients who are candidates for phototherapy or systemic therapy and who have failed to respond or have lost response to other systemic therapies

CONTRAINDICATIONS: Hypersensitivity, Crohn's disease
Precautions: Pregnancy, breastfeeding, children, depression, geriatric patients, immunosuppression, infection, suicidal ideation, vaccination

DOSAGE AND ROUTES

• **Adult: SUBCUT** • 210 mg at weeks 0, 1, and 2, then 210 mg q2wk; discontinue if inadequate response after 12-16 wk
• **Available forms:** Prefilled syringe 210 mg/1.5 mL

Administer:
SUBCUT route

• Due to suicidal ideation/behavior, the drug is available only through a restricted program (Siliq Risk Evaluation and Mitigation Strategy [REMS] Program). Prescribers must be certified in the program. Patients must sign a patient-prescriber agreement form. For information, visit the Siliq REMS website or cell 1-855-511-6135

• Remove prefilled syringe from refrigerator and allow to reach room temperature (about 30 min) without removing the needle cap; once brought to room temperature, do not return to the refrigerator. If needed, the prefilled syringe may be stored at room temperature for up to 14 days. Any prefilled syringe that has been stored at room temperature for more than 14 days must be discarded.
• Do not shake. Do not use the prefilled syringe if it has been dropped on a hard surface. Use a new syringe and call 1-800-321-4576
• Visually inspect for particulate matter and discoloration; the solution should be clear to slightly opalescent, colorless to slightly yellow, and may contain a few small translucent particles. Do not use if discolored, cloudy, or if foreign particulate matter is present
• Only an individual trained in subcut drug delivery should administer the injection. A patient who is properly trained in injection technique may self-inject using the prefilled syringe or vial if appropriate. The first injection needs to be under the supervision of a qualified health care professional
• Use front part of the middle thigh, the gluteal or abdominal region, and the outer area of the upper arm. Rotate injection sites. Do not use where skin is tender, bruised, red, hard, thick, scaly, or affected by psoriasis
• Gently pinch the cleaned area of skin, and insert needle at about a 45-degree angle subcut, using a quick dart-like motion. Push plunger slowly and evenly to deliver dose, remove the needle, and release pinched skin. Do not rub injection site; slight bleeding may occur
• Each single-use prefilled syringe contains 210 mg/1.5 mL of product. Inject the entire 1.5 mL contents of the syringe. No preservatives are present; discard unused portion
• Protect from light, do not freeze

SIDE EFFECTS
CNS: Headache, fatigue, suicidal ideation

Side effects: *italics* = common; red = life-threatening

EENT: Sinusitis
GI: Nausea, diarrhea
MS: Arthralgia
INTEG: Erythema, pruritus
HEMA: Bleeding, neutropenia
MISC: Infection, injection site reactions, antibody formation, pharyngitis, TB

PHARMACOKINETICS
Peak 3 days

INTERACTIONS
• **Increase:** altered effect of each product—CYP450 enzymes (carbamazepine, cyclosporine, ethosuximide, fosphenytoin, phenytoin, tacrolimus, theophylline, aminophylline, warfarin); monitor if products are initiated or discontinued; dose adjustments may be needed
• Do not give concurrently with live virus vaccines; bring immunizations up-to-date before treatment

NURSING CONSIDERATIONS
Assess:
• For injection site pain, swelling, redness; use cold compress to relieve pain/swelling
• **Infection:** fever, flulike symptoms, dyspnea, change in urination, redness/swelling around any wounds; stop treatment if present; serious infections including sepsis may occur, may be fatal; patients with active infections should not be started on this product
• **TB:** test for TB before starting product; do not use in active TB; for latent TB, give antituberculosis therapy before use of product; monitor closely for signs and symptoms of active tuberculosis infection during and after treatment
• **Pregnancy/breastfeeding:** no data for use in pregnancy, breastfeeding; excretion in breast milk unknown

Black Box Warning: **Suicidal ideation:** there is an increased incidence of suicidal ideation and behavior among recipients with a history of suicidality or depression; assess risks and benefits of treatment when considering use in those with a history of depression or psychosis

Evaluate:
• Therapeutic response: decrease in lesions
Teach patient/family:
• About self-administration if appropriate: injection should be made in thigh, abdomen, upper arm; rotate sites at least 1 inch from old site; do not inject in areas that are bruised, red, hard
• That if medication is not taken when due, to inject dose as soon as remembered and inject the next dose as scheduled
• Not to take any live virus vaccines during treatment
• To report signs of infection (fever, sweats, or chills, muscle aches, weight loss, cough, warm, red, or painful skin or sores on the body different from psoriasis, diarrhea or stomach pain, shortness of breath, blood in phlegm [mucus], burning in urination or urinating more often than normal); allergic reactions (itching, rash)
• To tell provider of all prescription and OTC medication, herbals, and supplements currently taken

Black Box Warning: **Suicidal ideation:** to seek medical attention for suicidal ideation, new onset or worsening depression, anxiety, or other mood changes

bromfenac (ophthalmic) (Rx)
(brom′fen-ak)
BromSite, Prolensa, Xibrom
Func. class.: Antiinflammatory (ophthalmic)
Chem. class.: Nonsteroidal antiinflammatory drug

ACTION: The mechanism of action is thought to be ability to block prostaglandin synthesis by inhibiting cyclooxygenase 1 and 2. In studies performed in animal eyes, prostaglandins have been shown to produce disruption of the blood–aqueous humor barrier, vasodilation, increased vascular permeability, leukocytosis, and increased intraocular pressure

USES: To reduce pain and inflammation after cataract surgery

CONTRAINDICATIONS: Hypersensitivity to this product, sulfites, NSAIDs, salicylates

Precautions: Bleeding disorders, complicated ocular surgery, corneal denervation, diabetes mellitus, rheumatoid arthritis, dry eye syndrome, pregnancy, breastfeeding

Do not administer while wearing contact lenses

DOSAGE AND ROUTES
• **Adult:** Instill 1 drop into affected eye twice daily (0.07%), q day (0.09%) beginning 24 hr before cataract surgery, continued on the day of surgery and through the first 14 days of the postoperative period

Available forms: Ophthalmic solution 0.07%, 0.09%

Administer:
• Apply topically to the eye
• Remove contact lenses before instilling solution; contact lenses should not be worn during use of this product
• Instruct patient on proper instillation of eye solution
• Do not touch the tip of the dropper to the eye, fingertips, or other surface
• Do not share bottle with other patients
• If more than one ophthalmic medication is being used, the medications should be administered at least 5 min apart

SIDE EFFECTS
CNS: Headache
EENT: Abnormal sensation in eye, conjunctival hyperemia, ocular irritation, ocular pain, ocular pruritus, conjunctival hyperemia, iritis, keratitis

PHARMACOKINETICS
Unknown

INTERACTIONS
Increase: corneal erosion, poor healing—topical corticosteroids

Increase: bleeding—anticoagulants
Increase: intraocular pressure—latanoprost
Drug/Lab
Increase: bleeding time

NURSING CONSIDERATIONS
Assess:
• Eyes for pain, inflammation, burning, redness after cataract surgery
• Identify if patient is using topical corticosteroids, anticoagulants; use cautiously in those using these products
• **Pregnancy/breastfeeding:** use if benefits outweigh fetal risks; avoid in 3rd trimester; cautious use in breastfeeding
Evaluate:
• Decreased pain and inflammation after cataract surgery
Teach patient/family:
• To apply topically to the eye
• To remove contact lenses before instilling solution; contact lenses should not be worn during use of this product; reinsert after 10 min (Prolensa)
• Proper instillation of eye solution
• Not to touch the tip of the dropper to the eye, fingertips, or other surface
• Not to share bottle with other patients
• That if more than one ophthalmic medication is being used, the medications should be administered at least 5 min apart

---

⚠ HIGH ALERT

bromocriptine (Rx)
(broe-moe-krip′teen)
Cycloset, Parlodel
Func. class.: Antiparkinson agent
Chem. class.: Dopamine receptor agonist

Do not confuse:
Parlodel/ pindolol/ Provera
bromocriptine/ benztropine /brimonidine

ACTION: Inhibits prolactin release by activating postsynaptic dopamine receptors; activation of striatal dopamine receptors may be reason for improvement in Parkinson's disease

USES: Parkinson's disease, amenorrhea/galactorrhea caused by hyperprolactinemia, infertility, acromegaly, pituitary adenomas, adjunct for type 2 diabetes
Unlabeled uses: Neuroleptic malignant syndrome, alcoholism, premenstrual syndrome, mastalgia, cocaine withdrawal

CONTRAINDICATIONS: Basilar migraine, hemiplegic migraine, breastfeeding, uncontrolled hypertension, severe peripheral vascular disease; hypersensitivity to ergot, bromocriptine; preeclampsia/eclampsia
Precautions: Pregnancy, breastfeeding, children, renal/hepatic disease, pituitary tumors, peptic ulcer disease, sulfite hypersensitivity, pulmonary fibrosis, dementia, GI bleeding, bipolar disorder, abrupt discontinuation, acute MI, angina, type 1 diabetes mellitus

DOSAGE AND ROUTES
Parkinson's disease (not Cycloset)
• **Adult:** PO 1.25 mg bid with meals; may increase q2-4wk by 2.5 mg/day, max 100 mg/day; levodopa should be continued while bromocriptine is being instituted
Hyperprolactinemia (not Cycloset)
• **Adult:** PO 1.25-2.5 mg with meals; may increase by 2.5 mg q3-7days, usual range 2.5-15 mg/day, max 30 mg/day
Acromegaly (not Cycloset)
• **Adult:** PO 1.25-2.5 mg at bedtime; may increase by 1.25-2.5 mg q3-7days; usual range 20-30 mg/day, max 100 mg/day
Pituitary adenoma (not Cycloset)
• **Adult/adolescent ≥16 yr:** PO 1.25 mg bid-tid; may increase over several wk to 10-20 mg/day
Type 2 diabetes (Cycloset only)
• **Adult:** PO (initially) 0.8 mg daily in AM within 2 hr of waking; titrate by 0.8 mg/day no more than weekly to max 1.6-4.8 mg/day
Female infertility (in vitro fertilization)
• **Adult female:** PO 1.25 mg/day on days 4-6 of follicular phase, then 2.5 mg/day

until 3 days after onset of menstruation as part of standard protocol
Available forms: Caps 5 mg; tabs 2.5 mg (Parodel), 0.8 mg (Cycloset)
Administer:
• With meal to prevent GI symptoms; Cycloset: give with food in AM within 2 hr of waking
• At bedtime so that dizziness, orthostatic hypotension do not occur
• Store at room temperature in tight, light-resistant container

SIDE EFFECTS
CNS: *Headache,* depression, restlessness, anxiety, nervousness, confusion, seizures, *hallucinations,* dizziness, fatigue, drowsiness, abnormal involuntary movements, psychosis, weakness
CV: Orthostatic hypotension, decreased B/P, palpitations, extrasystole, shock, dysrhythmias, bradycardia, MI
EENT: Blurred vision, diplopia, burning eyes, nasal congestion
GI: *Nausea, vomiting, anorexia,* cramps, constipation, diarrhea, dry mouth, GI hemorrhage
GU: Frequency, retention, incontinence, diuresis
INTEG: *Rash on face, arms;* alopecia; coolness, pallor of fingers, toes; peripheral edema
META: Hypoglycemia

PHARMACOKINETICS
Peak 1-3 hr, duration 4-8 hr, 90%-96% protein bound, half-life 3 hr, metabolized by liver (inactive metabolites), 85%-98% of dose excreted in feces, >90% of absorbed dose undergoes 1st-pass metabolism

INTERACTIONS
• Disulfiram-like reaction: alcohol
Increase: action of antihypertensives, levodopa, chloramphenicol, probenecid, salicylates, sulfonamides; dose of both products may need to be adjusted
Decrease: action of bromocriptine—phenothiazines, oral contraceptives, progestins, estrogens, haloperidol, loxapine, methyldopa, metoclopramide, MAOIs, reserpine; dose may need to be decreased

---

Decrease/increase: effect of Cycloset—CYP3A4 inhibitors/inducers; use cautiously
Decrease: effect of Cycloset—butyrophenones, metoclopramide, phenothiazine, thioxanthenes; avoid concurrent use
Drug/Lab Test
Increase: growth hormone, AST, ALT, CK, BUN, uric acid, alk phos

NURSING CONSIDERATIONS
Assess:
• B/P; establish baseline, compare with other readings; this product decreases B/P and causes orthostatic hypotension; obtain chest X-ray baseline
• **Parkinson's symptoms:** pill rolling, shuffling gait, restlessness, tremors, postural instability before and during treatment
• **Neuroleptic malignant syndrome:** decrease in temperature and sweating, lower pulse rate, and lessening of seizures indicates resolution of symptoms
• Change in size of soft-tissue volume with acromegaly
• **CNS symptoms:** CNS depression, hallucinations, vertigo; report symptoms immediately
• **Pregnancy:** fertility may occur before onset of menses after pregnancy; use pregnancy testing q4wk or if menstruation does not occur
Evaluate:
• Therapeutic response (Parkinson's disease): decreased dyskinesia, drooling, spasm, rigidity
Teach patient/family:
• That tabs may be crushed, mixed with food; Cycloset to be taken within 2 hr of rising; that 8 wk are needed for full effect
• To change position slowly to prevent orthostatic hypotension
• To use contraceptives during treatment with this product; that pregnancy may occur; to use methods other than oral contraceptives/subdermal implants
• That therapeutic effect for Parkinson's disease may take 2 mo, titrate slowly
• To avoid hazardous activity if dizziness occurs

• To report symptoms of MI immediately
• To take with food, avoid alcohol

---

budesonide (Rx)
(byoo-des'oh-nide)
Inhaation
Pulmicort Respules, Pulmicort Flexhaler
Nasal
Rhinocort Allergy
Systemic
Entocort EC, Uceris
Func. class.: Glucocorticoid
Chem. class.: Nonhalogenated

ACTION: Prevents inflammation by depressing migration of polymorphonuclear leukocytes and fibroblasts, reversal of increased capillary permeability, and lysosomal stabilization; does not suppress hypothalamus or pituitary function

USES: Rhinitis; prophylaxis for asthma; Crohn's disease, ulcerative colitis, nasal polyps
Unlabeled uses: Microscopic colitis, laryngotracheobronchitis (croup)

CONTRAINDICATIONS: Hypersensitivity, status asthmaticus, acute bronchospasm
Precautions: Pregnancy, breastfeeding; children; TB; fungal, bacterial, systemic viral infections; ocular herpes simplex; nasal septal ulcers; hepatic disease, diabetes, GI disease, increased intraocular pressure

DOSAGE AND ROUTES
Rhinitis
• **Adult and child >12 yr:** SPRAY/INH 2 sprays in each nostril AM, PM or 4 sprays in each nostril AM
Asthma
• **Adult:** INH 360 mcg bid, max 720 mcg bid
• **Child 1-8 yr previously taking bronchodilator alone:** NEB (Respules) 0.5 mg daily or 0.25 mg bid; susp via jet nebulizer, max 0.5 mg daily; previously

Side effects: italics = common; red = life-threatening

using inhaled corticosteroid 0.5 mg daily or 0.25 mg bid susp via jet nebulizer, max 0.5 mg bid

Crohn's disease/ulcerative colitis (Uceris)
• **Adult:** PO 9 mg/day AM × 8 wk

Laryngotracheobronchitis (croup) (unlabeled)
• **Infant ≥3 mo-child ≤5 yr:** NEB (Pulmicort Respules INH susp) 2 mg inhaled as a single dose

Available forms: Dry powder for INH 90, 100 ✦, 180, 200, 400 ✦; 32 mcg/actuation (Rhinocort Aqua) nasal spray; susp for INH 0.5 mg/2 mL, 0.25 mg/2 mL.; cap 3 mg; ext rel tab (Uceris) 9 mg, rectal foam 2 mg/actuation

Administer:

PO route (Crohn's disease/ulcerative colitis)
• Swallow caps whole; do not break, crush, chew; take in AM
• May repeat 8-wk course if needed; may taper to 6 mg/day for 2 wk before cessation
• Store at 59° F-86° F (15° C-30° C); keep away from heat, open flame

Rectal foam route
• Product is flammable, may use before bedtime, applicators are single use only

Inhalation route
• Prime inhaler before initial use only. Do not shake; do not use with spacer. After inhalation, rinse and spit with water

Nasal route
• Shake gently before use
• Prime by actuating 8 times before initial use
• Reprime if not used for 2 consecutive days. If not used for 14 days, rinse the applicator and reprime until a fine mist appears

SIDE EFFECTS

CNS: *Headache,* insomnia, hypertonia, syncope, dizziness, drowsiness
CV: Chest pain, hypertension, sinus tachycardia, palpitation
EENT: *Sinusitis, pharyngitis,* rhinitis, oral candidiasis

ENDO: Adrenal insufficiency, growth suppression in children
GI: Dry mouth, dyspepsia, nausea, vomiting, abdominal pain
MISC: Ecchymosis, fever, *hypersensitivity,* flulike symptoms, epistaxis, dysuria
MS: Back pain, myalgias, fractures
RESP: Nasal irritation, cough, nasal bleeding, *respiratory infections,* bronchospasm

PHARMACOKINETICS

Peak: Respules 4-6 wk, Rhinocort Aqua 2 wk, half-life 2-3.6 hr
Onset: Respules 2-8 days, Rhinocort Aqua 10 hr
Enters breast milk

INTERACTIONS

Increase: budesonide effect—CYP3A inhibitors; dose adjustment may be needed
• Avoid concurrent use of varicella live vaccine in pediatric patients

NURSING CONSIDERATIONS
Assess:
• Respiratory status: rate, rhythm, increase in bronchial secretions, wheezing, chest tightness; provide fluids to 2 L/day to decrease thickness of secretions; check for oral candidiasis
• **Bronchospasm:** stop treatment, give bronchodilator
• **Crohn's disease/ulcerative colitis:** assess for improvement in symptoms, decreased stools, abdominal cramps, urgency
• **HPA axis suppression:** do not stop abruptly, taper
• Viral infections: corticosteroid use can mask infections
• Increased intraocular pressure: discontinue use if this occurs
• **Beers:** avoid in older adults; high risk of delirium
• **Pregnancy/breastfeeding:** fetal harm appears remote; excreted in breast milk; consider risk factors in continuing breastfeeding

Evaluate:
• Therapeutic response: absence of asthma, rhinitis

Teach patient/family:

• To notify prescriber of pharyngitis, nasal bleeding, oral candidiasis

• Not to exceed recommended dose because adrenal suppression may occur

• To carry emergency ID that identifies steroid use

• To read and follow package directions

• To prevent exposure to infections (especially viral)

• To use good oral hygiene if using nebulizer or inhaler

• To avoid breastfeeding

• That burning or stinging may occur with first few doses of inhalation use

• That product is not a bronchodilator and not to be used for asthma; to use regularly

• How to use as described in "administer"

• To notify prescriber if symptoms persist after wks, that results usually take 2 wk

• To notify prescriber if exposure to measles, chickenpox occurs

---

bumetanide (Rx)

(byoo-met′a-nide)

Burinex ✦

Func. class.: Loop diuretic, antihypertensive

Chem. class.: Sulfonamide derivative

ACTION: Acts on ascending loop of Henle by inhibiting reabsorption of chloride, sodium

USES: Edema in heart failure, renal disease

CONTRAINDICATIONS: Hypersensitivity to sulfonamides, anuria, hepatic coma

Black Box Warning: Fluid and electrolyte depletion

Precautions: Pregnancy, breastfeeding, neonates, ascites, severe renal disease, hepatic cirrhosis, blood dyscrasias, ototoxicity, hyperuricemia, hypokalemia, hyperglycemia, oliguria, hypomagnesemia, hypovolemia

Black Box Warning: Dehydration

DOSAGE AND ROUTES

• **Adult and adolescent:** PO 0.5-2 mg/day; **IV/IM** 0.5-1 mg; may give 2nd or 3rd dose at 2-3 hr intervals, not to exceed 10 mg/day

• **Child and infant:** PO/IM/IV 0.015-0.1 mg/kg dose q6-24hr, max 10 mg/day

• **Neonates:** PO/IM/IV 0.01-0.05 kg/dose q12-24hr

Available forms: Tabs 0.5, 1, 2, 5 ✦ mg; inj 0.25 mg/mL

PO route

• Use in AM to prevent nocturia

• Without regard to food

IV, direct route

• Direct IV undiluted slowly over 1-2 min through Y-tube, 3-way stopcock, or hep-lock

Intermittent IV INFUSION route

• Dilute in LR, D₅W, 0.9% NaCl (rarely given by this method), give over 12 hr with renal disease; give at 4 mg/min or less, use infusion pump

Y-site compatibilities: Acyclovir, alfentanil, allopurinol, amifostine, amikacin, aminocaproic acid, aminophylline, amiodarone, amoxicillin, amphotericin B lipid complex (Abelcet), amphotericin B liposome (AmBisome), anidulafungin, ascorbic acid injection, atenolol, atracurium, atropine, aztreonam, benztropine, bivalirudin, bleomycin, buprenorphine, butorphanol, calcium chloride/gluconate, CARBOplatin, caspofungin, cefamandole, ceFAZolin, cefepime, cefmetazole, cefonicid, cefotaxime, cefoTEtan, cefOXitin, cefTAZidime, ceftizoxime, ceftobiprole, cefTRIAXone, cefuroxime, cephapirin, chloramphenicol, cimetidine, cisatracurium, CISplatin, cladribine, clarithromycin, clindamycin, codeine, cyanocobalamin, cyclophosphamide, cycloSPORINE, cytarabine,

---

DACTINomycin, DAPTOmycin, dexamethasone, dexmedetomidine, digoxin, diltiazem, diphenhydrAMINE, DOBUTamine, DOCEtaxel, DOPamine, doripenem, doxacurium, DOXOrubicin, doxycycline, enalaprilat, ePHEDrine, EPINEPHrine, epirubicin, epoetin alfa, eptifibatide, ertapenem, erythromycin, esmolol, etoposide, famotidine, fentaNYL, filgrastim, fluconazole, fludarabine, fluorouracil, folic acid, furosemide, gatifloxacin, gemcitabine, gentamicin, glycopyrrolate, granisetron, heparin, hydrocortisone sodium succinate, HYDROmorphone, hydrOXYzine, IDArubicin, ifosfamide, imipenem-cilastatin, indomethacin, insulin (regular), irinotecan, isoproterenol, ketorolac, labetalol, levofloxacin, lidocaine, linezolid, LORazepam, magnesium sulfate, mannitol, mechlorethamine, melphalan, meperidine, metaraminol, methotrexate, methoxamine, methyldopate, methylPREDNISolone, metoclopramide, metoprolol, metroNIDAZOLE, mezlocillin, micafungin, miconazole, milrinone, mitoXANtrone, morphine, moxalactam, multiple vitamins injection, mycophenolate, nafcillin, nalbuphine, naloxone, netilmicin, nitroglycerin, nitroprusside, norepinephrine, octreotide, ondansetron, oxacillin, oxaliplatin, oxytocin, palonosetron, pamidronate, pancuronium, pantoprazole, PEMEtrexed, penicillin G potassium/sodium, pentazocine, PENTobarbital, PHENobarbital, phenylephrine, phytonadione, piperacillin, piperacillin-tazobactam, polymyxin B, potassium chloride, procainamide, promethazine, propofol, propranolol, protamine, pyridoxine, quiNIDine, ranitidine, remifentanil, rifampin, ritodrine, riTUXimab, rocuronium, sodium acetate, sodium bicarbonate, succinylcholine, SUFentanil, tacrolimus, teniposide, theophylline, thiamine, thiotepa, ticarcillin, ticarcillin-clavulanate, tigecycline, tirofiban, TNA, tobramycin, tolazoline, TPN, traMADol, trastuzumab, trimetaphan, urokinase, vancomycin, vasopressin, vecuronium, verapamil, vinCRIStine, vinorelbine, voriconazole

SIDE EFFECTS

CNS: *Headache,* fatigue, weakness, *dizziness, encephalopathy*

CV: *Hypotension,* ECG changes, dehydration

EENT: *Loss of hearing*

ELECT: *Hypokalemia, hypochloremic alkalosis, hypomagnesemia, hyperuricemia, hypocalcemia, hyponatremia*

ENDO: *Hyperglycemia*

GI: Dry mouth, upset stomach, vomiting, diarrhea, nausea

GU: *Polyuria,* glycosuria,

INTEG: *Rash, pruritus*

MS: *Myalgia, arthralgia*

PHARMACOKINETICS

Excreted by kidneys (50% unchanged), feces (20%); crosses placenta; excreted in breast milk; protein binding >72%; half-life 1-1$\frac{1}{2}$ hr

PO: Onset $\frac{1}{2}$-1 hr, peak 1-2 hr, duration 3-6 hr

IM: Onset 40 min, peak 1-2 hr, duration 4-6 hr

IV: Onset 5 min, peak 15-30 min, duration 3-6 hr

INTERACTIONS

Increase: ototoxicity—aminoglycosides, avoid concurrent use

Increase: hypokalemia—corticosteroids, diuretics, laxatives (stimulants); monitor closely

Increase: toxicity—lithium, digoxin

Increase: hypotension, antihypertensives, nitrates

Decrease: diuretic effect—NSAIDs, other diuretics

Decrease: antidiabetic effects—antidiabetics

Drug/Herb

Increase: effect—hawthorn, horse chestnut

Decrease: effect of bumetanide—ginseng, ephedra

Drug/Lab

Increase: glucose

Decrease: chloride, potassium, sodium, calcium, phosphorus

NURSING CONSIDERATIONS
Assess

• For tinnitus, hearing loss, ear pain; obtain audiometric testing for long-term IV treatment

Black Box Warning: **Dehydration:** weight, I&O daily to determine fluid loss; if urinary output decreases or azotemia occurs, product should be discontinued; safest dosage schedule is alternate days

• B/P lying, standing; postural hypotension may occur

Black Box Warning: **Fluid and electrolyte depletion:** potassium, sodium, calcium; include BUN, blood glucose, CBC, serum creatinine, blood pH, ABGs, uric acid, calcium, magnesium; severe electrolyte depletion should be corrected before starting treatment

• Blood glucose if patient is diabetic; blood uric acid levels in those with gout
• Improvement in edema of feet, legs, sacral area daily if medication is being used for HF
• Signs of metabolic alkalosis: drowsiness, restlessness
• **Hypokalemia:** postural hypotension, malaise, fatigue, tachycardia, leg cramps, weakness
• Rashes, temperature elevation daily
• Confusion, especially in geriatric patients; take safety precautions if needed
• **Digoxin toxicity** in patients taking digoxin products: anorexia, nausea, vomiting, confusion, paresthesia, muscle cramps; **lithium toxicity** in those taking lithium
• **Beers:** Use cautiously in older adults; may cause or exacerbate syndrome of inappropriate antidiuretic hormone secretion

Evaluate:
• Therapeutic response: decreased edema, B/P

Teach patient/family:
• To increase fluid intake to 2-3 L/day unless contraindicated; to take potassium supplement; to rise slowly from lying or sitting position

• To recognize adverse reactions: muscle cramps, weakness, nausea, dizziness, edema, weight gain
• To take with food, milk for GI symptoms; to avoid alcohol
• To take early in day to prevent nocturia; if another dose is needed, take after noon, not to double or miss dose
• To take B/P, pulse, weight weekly
• That orthostatic hypotension may occur, to avoid rising rapidly
• To continue other medical regimens
• **Pregnancy/breastfeeding:** To report if pregnancy is planned or suspected or if breastfeeding
• That continuing exams and blood work will be needed
• To notify other health care professionals of condition being treated, medications taken

TREATMENT OF OVERDOSE:
Lavage if taken orally; monitor electrolytes; administer dextrose in saline; monitor hydration, CV, renal status

---

⚠ HIGH ALERT

buprenorphine (Rx)
REMS
(byoo-pre-nor′feen)
Belbuca, Buprenex, Butrans, Probuphine, Sublocade
Func. class.: Opioid analgesic, partial agonist
Chem. class.: Thebaine derivative

Controlled Substance Schedule III

ACTION: Depresses pain impulse transmission at the spinal cord level by interacting with opioid receptors, partial agonist at μ-opioid receptor

USES: Moderate to severe pain, opiate agonist withdrawal/dependence
Unlabeled uses: Cocaine withdrawal

CONTRAINDICATIONS: Hypersensitivity, ileus, status asthmaticus

Black Box Warning: Respiratory depression

Precautions: Pregnancy, breastfeeding, substance abuse/alcoholism, increased intracranial pressure, MI (acute), severe heart disease, respiratory depression, renal/hepatic/pulmonary disease, hypothyroidism, Addison's disease, QT prolongation, accidental exposure, neonatal opioid withdrawal syndrome

Black Box Warning: Potential for overdose/poisoning, substance abuse, IM, coadministration with other CNS depressants, implant insertion and removal

DOSAGE AND ROUTES
• **Adult: IM/IV** 0.3 mg q4-6hr as needed: **TD** each patch is worn for 7 days (moderate-severe pain); **opioid-naive patients** (those taking <30 mg of oral morphine or equivalent before beginning treatment with TD buprenorphine), 5 mcg/hr q7days, overestimating dose can be fatal; **conversion from other opiate agonist therapy,** titrate from other opioids for up to 7 days to no more than 30 mg oral morphine or equivalent before beginning TD therapy, begin with 5 mcg/hr q7days; for those with daily dose of 30-80 mg oral morphine or equivalent, start with 10 mcg/hr q7days; for those taking >80 mg oral morphine or equivalent, start with 20 mcg/hr q7days
• **Geriatric/debilitated patients: IM/IV** 0.15 mg slowly
• **Child 2-12 yr: IM/IV** 2-6 mcg/kg q4-8hr
Hepatic dose
Adult TD (mild-moderate): 5 mcg/hr system initially
Buccal (severe hepatic disease): decrease dose by 50%, titrate upward by 75 mcg q12hr ≥q4days
Available forms: Inj 0.3 mg/mL (1-mL vials); SL tab 2, 8 mg as base; TD system 5, 7.5, 10, 15, 20 mcg/hr (weekly);

dissolving film (buccal) 75, 150, 300, 450, 600, 750, 900 mcg; sol for inj, ext rel 100 mg/0.5 mL, 300 mg/1.5 mL; SD implant 74.2 mg/implant
Administer:
SL route
• Do not chew; dissolve under tongue, use 2 or more at same time
Transdermal route (REMS)
• Apply to clean, dry, intact skin; each patch should be worn for 7 days, do not exceed dose, Qtc prolongation may occur; do not apply direct heat source to patch, will increase absorption of product, may use first-aid tape if edge of patch is not adhering
• Apply to upper outer arm, upper chest/back, or side of chest
Subcut route (ext-rel injection— Sublocade)
• Inject only in abdominal region. DO NOT use IM/IV
• Visually inspect for particulate matter, discoloration before use; product is clear, colorless to yellow to amber solution
• Give monthly with a minimum of 26 days between doses
• Use only the syringe and safety needle included. Do not attach the needle until time of use
• Do not inject into an area where skin is irritated, reddened, bruised, infected, or scarred
• Do not rub area after injection
• To avoid irritation, rotate inj site with each injection
• Inj site should be examined for infection, evidence of tampering, or attempts to remove the depot
• **Storage:** store unopened prefilled syringes in the refrigerator in original packaging; do not freeze. Once outside the refrigerator this product may be stored in original packaging at room temperature for up to 7 days before administration. Discard injection if left at room temperature for longer than 7 days
Subdermal route (Probuphine)
• Inserted in inner side of upper arm
• Maintenance dose must be 8 mg/day or less

- Use guideline from manufacturer
- Available from REMS program 1-844-859-6341, health care professional must complete training program
- Inserts are removed after 6 mo, if other insert is not used, use transmucosal

IM route
- In deep muscle mass

IV, direct route
- Give undiluted over ≥2 min, titrate to patient response; rapid injection will increase side effects
- With antiemetic if nausea, vomiting occur
- When pain is beginning to return; determine dosage interval by patient response

Y-site compatibilities: Acyclovir, alfentanil, allopurinol, amifostine, amikacin, aminocaproic acid, amphotericin B liposome (AmBisome), anidulafungin, ascorbic acid injection, atenolol, atracurium, atropine, aztreonam, benztropine, bivalirudin, bleomycin, bumetanide, butorphanol, calcium chloride/gluconate, CARBOplatin, cefamandole, ceFAZolin, cefepime, cefotaxime, cefoTEtan, cefOXitin, cefTAZidime, ceftizoxime, cefTRIAXone, cefuroxime, chloramphenicol, chlorproMAZINE, cimetidine, cisatracurium, CISplatin, cladribine, clindamycin, cyanocobalamin, cyclophosphamide, cycloSPORINE, cytarabine, D₅W-dextrose 5%, DACTINomycin, DAPTOmycin, dexamethasone, dexmedetomidine, digoxin, diltiazem, diphenhydrAMINE, DOBUTamine, DOCEtaxel, DOPamine, doxacurium, DOXOrubicin HCl, doxycycline, enalaprilat, ePHEDrine, EPINEPHrine, epirubicin, epoetin alfa, eptifibatide, ertapenem, erythromycin, esmolol, etoposide, famotidine, fenoldopam, fentaNYL, filgrastim, fluconazole, fludarabine, gatifloxacin, gemcitabine, gentamicin, glycopyrrolate, granisetron, heparin, hydrocortisone, hydrOXYzine, IDArubicin, ifosfamide, imipenem-cilastatin, inamrinone, insulin (regular), irinotecan, isoproterenol, ketorolac, labetalol, lactated Ringer's injection, levofloxacin, lidocaine, linezolid, LORazepam, magnesium sulfate, mannitol, mechlorethamine, melphalan, meperidine, metaraminol, methicillin, methotrexate, methoxamine, methyldopate, methylPREDNISolone, metoclopramide, metoprolol, metroNIDAZOLE, mezlocillin, miconazole, midazolam, milrinone, minocycline, mitoXANtrone, morphine, moxalactam, multiple vitamins injection, mycophenolate mofetil, nafcillin, nalbuphine, naloxone, nesiritide, netilmicin, nitroglycerin, nitroprusside, norepinephrine, octreotide, ondansetron, oxacillin, oxaliplatin, oxytocin, palonosetron, pamidronate, pancuronium, papaverine, PEMEtrexed, penicillin G potassium/sodium, pentamidine, pentazocine, phenylephrine, phytonadione, piperacillin, piperacillin-tazobactam, polymyxin B, potassium chloride, procainamide, prochlorperazine, promethazine, propofol, propranolol, protamine, pyridoxine, quiNIDine, ranitidine, remifentanil, Ringer's injection, riTUXimab, rocuronium, sodium acetate, succinylcholine, SUFentanil, tacrolimus, teniposide, theophylline, thiamine, thiotepa, ticarcillin, ticarcillin-clavulanate, tigecycline, tirofiban, TNA (3-in-1), tobramycin, tolazoline, TPN, trastuzumab, trimetaphan, urokinase, vancomycin, vasopressin, vecuronium, verapamil, vinCRIStine, vinorelbine, voriconazole

SIDE EFFECTS
CNS: *Drowsiness, dizziness, confusion, headache, sedation, euphoria, hallucinations, strange dreams*
CV: Palpitations, QT prolongation, hypo/hypertension
EENT: Tinnitus, blurred vision, *miosis,* diplopia
GI: *Nausea,* vomiting, anorexia, constipation, dry mouth, hepatotoxicity
GU: Urinary retention
INTEG: *Rash,* diaphoresis, pruritus
RESP: Respiratory depression, bronchospasm
Misc: Anaphylaxis, angioedema, dependency

Side effects: *italics* = common; red = life-threatening

PHARMACOKINETICS

Metabolized in liver by CYP3A4, excreted by kidneys and in feces, crosses placenta, excreted in breast milk, half-life $2^1/_2$-$3^1/_2$ hr, 96% bound to plasma proteins

IM: Onset 15 min, peak 1 hr, duration 6-10 hr

SL: Onset, peak, duration unknown, half-life 37 hr

IV: Onset 1 min, peak 5 min, duration 6 hr, half-life 2.2 hr

TD: Half-life 26 hr

Epidural: Duration dose dependent

INTERACTIONS

Increase: effect with other CNS depressants—alcohol, opioids, sedative/hypnotics, antipsychotics, skeletal muscle relaxants, MAOIs

Increase: buprenorphine effect—CYP3A4 inhibitors (erythromycin, indinavir, ketoconazole, ritonavir, saquinavir)

Increase: QT prolongation—class IA, III antidysrhythmics

Increase: serotonin syndrome 5-HT3 antagonists, linezolid, methylene blue, MAOIs, SSRIs, SNRIs, tricyclics

Decrease: buprenorphine effect—CYP3A4 inducers (carBAMazepine, PHENobarbital, phenytoin, rifampin)

Drug/Herb

Increase: CNS depression—chamomile, kava, St. John's wort

NURSING CONSIDERATIONS

Assess:

• **Pain:** intensity, location, type before treatment, after 5, 15, 30 min (IV); need for pain medication, tolerance

> **Black Box Warning: Accidental exposure:** keep away from children and pets; may be fatal

• I&O ratio; check for decreasing output; may indicate urinary retention
• Bowel pattern; severe constipation can occur

• CNS changes, dizziness, drowsiness, hallucinations, euphoria, LOC, pupil reaction; withdrawal in opioid-dependent persons
• Allergic reactions: rash, urticaria

> **Black Box Warning: Respiratory dysfunction:** respiratory depression, character, rate, rhythm; notify prescriber if respirations are <12/min, may be fatal

> **Black Box Warning: Potential for overdose** may occur from chewing, swallowing, snorting, or injecting extracted product from TD formulation

• **QT prolongation:** in those taking class Ia, III antidysrhythmics; patients with hypokalemia, cardiac instability (TD), max TD 20 mcg/hr q7day
• **Beers:** avoid in older adults unless safer alternatives are not available, may cause impaired psychomotor function, syncope
• **Pregnancy/breastfeeding:** avoid use in pregnancy and breastfeeding; in those using product and breastfeeding, watch infant for decreased respiration, lethargy, decreased heart rate

Evaluate:

• Therapeutic response: decrease in pain, decreased withdrawal symptoms

Teach patient/family:

• To report any symptoms of CNS changes, allergic reactions

> **Black Box Warning:** That psychologic dependence leading to substance abuse may result when used for extended periods; that long-term use is not recommended

• That product can cause serious breathing problems; call provider right away if feeling faint, dizzy or if breathing gets much slower than normal
• To avoid hazardous activities such as driving unless reaction is known
• Do not start new meds/herbs without prescriber approval; do not double, skip doses

• Start stool softener/laxatives to lessen constipation

• **SL route:** to place under tongue and allow to dissolve

• **Transdermal route:** how to apply and dispose of patch; not to use a heating pad or other heat source; do not cut

TREATMENT OF OVERDOSE: Naloxone 0.4 mg ampule diluted in 10 mL 0.9% NaCl given by direct IV push 0.02 mg q2min (adult)

---

buPROPion (Rx)

(byoo-proe′pee-on)

Aplenzin, Forfivo XL, Wellbutrin SR, Wellbutrin XL, Zyban

Func. class.: Antidepressant—miscellaneous smoking deterrent

Chem. class.: Aminoketone

Do not confuse:
buPROPion/busPIRone

ACTION: Inhibits reuptake of DOPamine, norepinephrine, serotonin

USES: Depression (Wellbutrin), smoking cessation (Zyban); seasonal affective disorder, substance abuse, glaucoma, smoking, cardiac disease, heart failure

Unlabeled uses: ADHD (SR); increase libido in women

CONTRAINDICATIONS: Hypersensitivity, head trauma, stroke, intracranial mass, eating disorders, seizure disorders

Precautions: Pregnancy, breastfeeding, geriatric patients, renal/hepatic disease, recent MI, cranial trauma, seizure disorder, substance abuse, glaucoma, smoking, cardiac disease, heart failure, head trauma, stroke, intracranial mass, Tourette's syndrome, tics, tobacco smoking, abrupt discontinuation

Black Box Warning: Children <18 yr, suicidal thinking/behavior (young adults)

DOSAGE AND ROUTES
Depression

• **Adult: PO** 100 mg bid initially, then increase after 3 days to 100 mg tid if needed, max 150 mg single dose; **ER/SR** initially 150 mg AM, increase to 300 mg/day if initial dose is tolerated, after no less than 4 days; after several wk, titrate to 200 mg bid; Aplenzin 174 mg q AM, may increase to 348 mg q AM on day 4, may increase to 522 mg after several weeks if needed; Forfivo XL (not for initial treatment) 450 mg daily after titration with another product (300 mg/day × ≥2 wk)

• **Geriatric: PO** 50-100 mg/day, may increase by 50-100 mg q3-4days

Smoking cessation (Zyban)

• **Adult: SR** 150 mg daily × 3 days, then 150 mg bid for remainder of treatment

Seasonal affective disorder

• **Adult: PO** (Wellbutrin XL) 150 mg as a single dose in the AM, after 1 wk may be increased to 300 mg/day; (Aplenzin) 174 mg daily in AM, after 7 days may increase to 348 mg daily

Hepatic dose
Adult: PO (moderate-severe) Aplenzin max 174 mg every other day

ADHD (unlabeled) (Wellbutrin)

• **Adult: PO** 100 mg bid, after ≥3 days titrate to 100 mg tid; **SR** 300 mg/day, 200 mg 8 AM, 100 mg 4 PM

Available forms: Tabs 75, 100 mg; sus rel tabs (SR) 100, 150, 200; ext rel tab (XL) 100, 150, 300, 450 mg; (SR-12 hr, XL-24 hr); tab ext rel (Aplenzin) 174, 348, 522 mg

Administer:
PO route

• When switching to Aplenzin from Wellbutrin, Wellbutrin SR or XL, use these equivalents: 174 mg buPROPion HBr = 150 mg buPROPion HCl; 348 mg buPROPion HBr = 300 mg buPROPion HCl; 522 mg buPROPion HBr = 450 mg buPROPion HCl

• **Wellbutrin immediate rel**, separate by ≥6 hr, give in 3 divided doses; **Wellbutrin SR**, if multiple doses are used, separate by ≥8 hr; **Wellbutrin XL,** give daily in AM; **Zyban SR,** give in 2 divided doses, ≥8 hr apart; **Aplenzin ER,** give daily in AM, a larger dose of Aplenzin is needed because these products are not equivalent

• Do not break, crush, chew sus rel, ext rel tab

• At evenly spaced times to prevent seizures; seizure risk increases with high doses

• Increase fluids, bulk in diet if constipation occurs

• With food, milk for GI symptoms

• Sugarless gum, hard candy, frequent sips of water for dry mouth

• Avoid giving at night to prevent insomnia

SIDE EFFECTS

CNS: *Headache, agitation, dizziness, akinesia, confusion,* seizures, delusions, *insomnia, sedation, tremors,* suicidal/homicidal ideation, flushing
CV: *Dysrhythmias, hypertension,* palpitations, *tachycardia,* hypotension, chest pain, chills
EENT: *Blurred vision, auditory disturbance*
GI: *Nausea, vomiting,* anorexia, diarrhea, *dry mouth,* increased appetite, *constipation,* altered taste
GU: Impotence, urinary frequency, retention
INTEG: *Rash,* pruritus, *sweating*
MISC: *Hot flashes*

PHARMACOKINETICS

Onset 1-4 wk, half-life 14 hr (immediate release), extensively metabolized by liver, some conversion to active metabolites, protein binding 84%, excreted in urine and feces

INTERACTIONS

• Do not use within 14 days of MAOIs
Increase: adverse reactions: amantadine, haloperidol seizures—levodopa, MAOIs, phenothiazines, antidepressants, benzodiazepines, alcohol, theophylline, systemic steroids
Increase: action of citalopram
Decrease: effect of tamoxifen
Decrease: buPROPion effect—carBAMazepine, cimetidine, PHENobarbital,

phenytoin or other products (CYP2D6); CYP2B6 inducers
Drug/Herb
Increase: CNS depression—kava, valerian
Drug/Lab Test
Positive: urine drug screen for amphetamine possible

NURSING CONSIDERATIONS
Assess:
• **Smoking:** For smoking cessation after 7-12 wk; if progress has not been made, product should be discontinued
• For increased risk of seizures; if patient has excessively used CNS depressants and OTC stimulants, dosage of buPROPion should not be exceeded
• Monitor weight regularly

> Black Box Warning: **Mental status:** mood, sensorium, affect, suicidal /homicidal tendencies, increase in psychiatric symptoms

• **Beers:** avoid in older adults; lowers seizure threshold, may be acceptable for those with well-controlled seizures for which other treatment has been ineffective
Evaluate:
• Therapeutic response: decreased depression, ability to perform daily activities, ability to sleep throughout the night, smoking cessation
Teach patient/family:
• That therapeutic effects may take 2-4 wk; not to increase dose without prescriber's approval; that treatment for smoking cessation lasts 7-12 wk
• To use caution when driving, performing other activities that require alertness; sedation, blurred vision may occur
• To avoid alcohol, other CNS depressants; alcohol may increase risk of seizures
• That ext rel shell may be seen in stools
• That exams and lab work will be needed
• To notify health care professionals of all Rx, herbals, supplements taken, not

to start new product unless discussed before use
• Not to use with nicotine patches unless directed by prescriber; may increase B/P
• To notify prescriber immediately if urinary retention occurs
• That risk of seizures increases when dose is exceeded, if patient has seizure disorder

Black Box Warning: That suicidal/homicidal ideas, behaviors, hostility, depression may occur in children or young adults, to report immediately

• **Pregnancy/breastfeeding:** To notify prescriber if pregnancy is suspected, planned, or if breastfeeding

TREATMENT OF OVERDOSE: ECG monitoring; lavage; administer anticonvulsant

---

burosumab

(bur- oh' sue-mab)

Crysvita

Func. class.: Fibroblast growth factor blocking antibody

USES: X-linked hypophosphatemia (XLH) in adult and pediatric patients 1 year of age and older

CONTRAINDICATIONS: Use with oral phosphate or active vit D analogs; serum phosphorus is within or above the normal range for age; severe renal impairment or end-stage renal disease

DOSAGE AND ROUTES
•**Adult: SUBCUT** 1 mg/kg body weight rounded to nearest 10 mg (max 90 mg) q4wk
• **Child: SUBCUT** 0.8 mg/kg body weight rounded to nearest 10 mg (max 90 mg) q2wk. Dose may be increased up to approximately 2 mg/kg (max 90 mg) q2wk to achieve normal serum phosphorus

---

⚠ HIGH ALERT

busPIRone (Rx)

(byoo-spye'rone)

Buspirex ✚, Bustab ✚

Func. class.: Antianxiety, sedative
Chem. class.: Azaspirodecanedione

Do not confuse:
busPIRone/buPROPion

ACTION: Acts by inhibiting the action of serotonin (5-HT); has shown little potential for abuse; a good choice with substance abuse

USES: Generalized anxiety disorders

CONTRAINDICATIONS: Children <18 yr, hypersensitivity, MAOIs
Precautions: Pregnancy, breastfeeding, geriatric patients, impaired hepatic/renal function

DOSAGE AND ROUTES
• **Adult: PO** 7.5 mg bid; may increase by 5 mg/day q2-3 days, max 60 mg/day
Hepatic/renal dose
• **Adult: PO** reduce by 25%-50% for mild-moderate hepatic disease; do not use for severe hepatic disease; CCr 11-70 mL/min reduce by 25%-50%; CCr <10 mL/min do not use
Available forms: Tabs 5, 7.5, 10, 15, 30 mg
Administer:
• With food, milk for GI symptoms; avoid grapefruit juice; give drug at same time of day, with/without food consistently
• Crushed if patient unable to swallow medication whole
• Sugarless gum, hard candy, frequent sips of water for dry mouth

SIDE EFFECTS
CNS: *Dizziness, headache, stimulation, insomnia, nervousness, numbness, paresthesia, incoordination*

CV: *Tachycardia, palpitations,* hypo/hypertension, chest pain

EENT: *Sore throat, tinnitus, blurred vision, nasal congestion;* red, change in taste, smell

GI: *Nausea, dry mouth, diarrhea, constipation,* increased appetite

GU: Frequency, hesitancy, change in libido

INTEG: *Rash,* edema, pruritus, alopecia, dry skin

MISC: *Sweating,* fatigue, fever

MS: *Pain, weakness,* muscle cramps, myalgia

RESP: Hyperventilation, chest congestion, shortness of breath

PHARMACOKINETICS

Peak 40-90 min, half-life 2-4 hr, rapidly absorbed, metabolized by liver (CYP3A4), excreted in feces, protein binding 86%

INTERACTIONS

Increase: busPIRone—CYP3A4 inhibitors (erythromycin, itraconazole, nefazodone, ketoconazole, ritonavir, verapamil, diltiazem, several other protease inhibitors)

Increase: B/P—procarbazine, MAOIs; do not use together

Increase: CNS depression—psychotropic products, alcohol (avoid use)

Increase: serotonin syndrome—SSRIs, SNRIs, serotonin receptor agonists

Decrease: busPIRone effects—rifampin

Decrease: busPIRone action—CYP3A4 inducers (rifampin, phenytoin, PHENobarbital, carBAMazepine, dexamethasone)

Drug/Herb

Increase: CNS depression—chamomile, kava, valerian

Drug/Food

Increase: peak concentration of busPIRone—grapefruit juice

NURSING CONSIDERATIONS
Assess:

• B/P lying, standing; pulse; if systolic B/P drops 20 mm Hg, hold product, notify prescriber

• CNS reactions because some may be unpredictable

• Mental status: mood, sensorium, affect, sleeping pattern, drowsiness, dizziness; withdrawal symptoms when dose reduced, product discontinued

• Safety measures if drowsiness, dizziness occurs

• **Beers:** avoid in older adults with delirium or at high risk for delirium

Evaluate:

• Therapeutic response: decreased anxiety, restlessness, sleeplessness

Teach patient/family:

• That product may be taken consistently with/without food

• To avoid OTC products, alcohol ingestion, other psychotropic medications unless approved by prescriber; to avoid large amounts of grapefruit juice

• To avoid activities that require alertness because drowsiness may occur

• Not to discontinue medication abruptly after long-term use; if dose is missed, do not double

• To rise slowly because fainting may occur, especially among geriatric patients

• That drowsiness may worsen at beginning of treatment; that 2 wk of therapy may be required before therapeutic effects occur, max effect 3-6 wk

• **Serotonin syndrome:** to report immediately (fever, tremor, sweating, diarrhea, delirium)

• **Pregnancy/breastfeeding:** report if pregnancy is planned or suspected or if breastfeeding

---

⚠ HIGH ALERT

busulfan (Rx)

(byoo-sul'fan)

Busulfex, Myleran

Func. class.: Antineoplastic alkylating agent

Chem. class.: Bifunctional alkylating agent

Do not confuse:
Myleran/Leukeran/Alkeran

ACTION: Changes essential cellular ions to covalent bonding with resultant alkylation; this interferes with the normal biological function of DNA; activity is not phase-specific; action is due to myelosuppression

USES: Chronic myelocytic leukemia, bone marrow ablation, stem cell transplant preparation with CML

CONTRAINDICATIONS: Pregnancy, breastfeeding, blastic phase of chronic myelocytic leukemia, hypersensitivity

Precautions: Women of childbearing age, leukopenia, anemia, hepatotoxicity, renal toxicity, seizures, tumor lysis syndrome, hyperkalemia, hyperphosphatemia, hypocalcemia, hyperuricemia, radiation, chemotherapy, male-mediated teratogenicity, veno-occlusive disease (VOD), sinusoidal obstruction syndrome, head trauma

> Black Box Warning: Thrombocytopenia, neutropenia, new primary malignancy, bone marrow suppression

DOSAGE AND ROUTES
Chronic myelocytic leukemia
• **Adult:** PO 4-8 mg/day or 1.8-4 mg/m²/day initially, reduce dose if WBC reaches 30,000-40,000/mm³, discontinue if WBC ≤20,000/mm³, maintenance 1-3 mg/day
• **Child:** PO 0.06-0.12 mg/kg/day or 1.8-4.6 mg/m²/day; reduce if WBC reaches 30,000-40,000/mm³, discontinue if WBC ≤20,000/mm³

Allogenic hematopoietic stem cell transplantation
• **Adult:** IV 0.8 mg/kg over 2 hr, q6hr × 4 days (total 16 doses); give cyclophosphamide IV 60 mg/kg over 1 hr daily for 2 days starting after 16th dose of busulfan; PO (unlabeled) 1 mg/kg q6hr × 16 doses
• **Adolescent and child >12 kg (unlabeled):** IV 0.8 mg/kg over 2 hr q6hr × 16 doses (4 days), then high-dose cyclophosphamide 50 mg/kg/day × 4 days

• **Infant/child ≤12 kg (unlabeled):** IV 1.1 mg/kg over 2 hr q6hr × 16 doses (4 days), then high-dose cyclophosphamide 50 mg/kg/day × 4 days
Available forms: Tabs 2 mg; inj 6 mg/mL
Administer:
• Store in tight container
PO route
• Give at same time daily on empty stomach
Intermittent IV INFUSION route
• Prepare in biologic cabinet while wearing gloves, gown, mask; **dilute** with 10 times volume of product with D₅W, 0.9% NaCl (0.5 mg/mL); when withdrawing product, use needle with 5-micron filter provided, remove amount needed, remove filter, and **inject** product into diluent; always add product to diluent (not vice versa); stable for 8 hr at room temperature (using D₅W) or 12 hr refrigerated; **give** by central venous catheter over 2 hr q6hr × 4 days, use infusion pump, do not admix
• Give antiemetics before IV route on schedule
• In those with history of seizures, give phenytoin before IV drug to prevent seizures (using 0.9% NaCl)

Y-site compatibilities: Acyclovir, amphotericin B lipid complex, amphotericin B liposome, anidulafungin, atenolol, bivalirudin, bleomycin, caspofungin, codeine, DAPTOmycin, dexmedetomidine, diltiazem, DOCEtaxel, ertapenem, fenoldopam, gatifloxacin, granisetron, HYDROmorphone, levofloxacin, linezolid, LORazepam, meperidine, metroNIDAZOLE, milrinone, nesiritide, octreotide acetate, ondansetron, palonosetron, pancuronium, piperacillin-tazobactam, riTUXimab, sodium acetate, tacrolimus, tigecycline, tirofiban, trastuzumab, vasopressin

SIDE EFFECTS
CV: *Hypotension*, thrombosis, *chest pain*, tachycardia, atrial fibrillation, heart block, pericardial effusion, cardiac tamponade (high dose with cyclophosphamide)
GI: *Anorexia, constipation, diarrhea, dry mouth, nausea, vomiting*

Side effects: *italics* = common; red = life-threatening

CNS: *Depression, dizziness, insomnia, headache*
EENT: Blurred vision
GU: Impotence, sterility, amenorrhea, gynecomastia, renal toxicity, hyperuremia, adrenal insufficiency–like syndrome
HEMA: Thrombocytopenia, leukopenia, pancytopenia, severe bone marrow depression
INTEG: Dermatitis, hyperpigmentation, alopecia
OTHER: Chromosomal aberrations, graft-versus-host disease (GVHD), sinusoidal obstruction syndrome, veno-occlusive disease (VOD), new primary malignancy
RESP: Alveolar hemorrhage, atelectasis, cough, hemoptysis, hypoxia, irreversible pulmonary fibrosis, pleural effusion, pneumonia, pneumonitis, pulmonary fibrosis, sinusitis

PHARMACOKINETICS
Well absorbed orally, excreted in urine, crosses placenta, excreted in breast milk, half-life 2.5 hr

INTERACTIONS
Increase: cardiac tamponade—cyclophosphamide
Increase: toxicity—other antineoplastics, radiation
Increase: risk for bleeding—anticoagulants, salicylates
Increase: antibody response—live virus vaccines
Decrease: busulfan level—phenytoin
Decrease: busulfan clearance—acetaminophen, itraconazole
Drug/Lab Test
False positive: breast, bladder, cervix, lung cytology tests

NURSING CONSIDERATIONS
Assess:

Black Box Warning: **Bone marrow suppression,** CBC, differential, platelet count weekly; withhold product if WBC is <15,000/mm³ or platelet count is <150,000/mm³; notify prescriber of results; institute thrombocytopenia precautions; levels for withholding product will be different for children; bone marrow status before chemotherapy; seizure history; bone marrow suppression may be prolonged (up to 2 mo)

• **Pulmonary fibrosis:** pulmonary function tests, chest x-ray films before, during therapy; chest film should be obtained q2wk during treatment; pulmonary fibrosis may occur up to 10 yr after treatment with busulfan

Black Box Warning: **New primary malignancy:** monitor for new malignancies

Black Box Warning: **Hepatotoxicity, including sinusoidal obstruction syndrome (SOS):** some have been fatal; monitor LFTs, including bilirubin, alkaline phosphatase prior to and daily through day 28; use cautiously with a preexisting hepatic disease; those with busulfan >1500 micromoles × min, prior radiation, 3 or more cycles of chemotherapy, prior stem cell transplantation, or those receiving multiple alkylating agents may be at greater risk

• Renal studies: BUN, serum uric acid, urine CCr before, during therapy; monitor ALT, alk phos, bilirubin, uric acid before and during treatment; I&O ratio; report fall in urine output of <30 mL/hr; hyperuricemia
• For **secondary malignancy** within 5-8 yr of chronic oral therapy; long-term follow-up may be required
• Monitor for cold, fever, sore throat (may indicate beginning infection)
• Bleeding: hematuria, guaiac, bruising, petechiae; mucosa, orifices q8hr; no rectal temperatures
• Dyspnea, crackles, nonproductive cough, chest pain, tachypnea
• Inflammation of mucosa, breaks in skin; use viscous xylocaine for oral pain
• Comprehensive oral hygiene
• Strict medical asepsis, protective isolation if WBC levels low
• Increased fluid intake to 2-3 L/day to prevent urate deposits, calculi formation
• **Pregnancy/breastfeeding:** do not use in pregnancy, breastfeeding
Evaluate:
• Therapeutic response: decreased exacerbations of chronic myelocytic leukemia

---

Teach patient/family:

• To avoid use of products that contain aspirin, ibuprofen; razors; commercial mouthwash

• To use effective contraception during and for at least 3 mo after treatment; to avoid breastfeeding; may cause infertility, discuss family planning before initiating therapy

• To report signs of **anemia** (fatigue, headache, irritability, faintness, shortness of breath); symptoms of **infection;** jaundice; persistent cough, congestion, skin pigmentation, darkening of skin; sudden weakness, weight loss (may resemble adrenal insufficiency)

• To report symptoms of bleeding (hematuria, tarry stools)

• To avoid vaccinations, crowds, persons with known infections

• That impotence, amenorrhea can occur; that these are reversible after discontinuing treatment

---

butoconazole vaginal antifungal
See Appendix B

⚠ HIGH ALERT

butorphanol (Rx)
(byoo-tor′fa-nole)
Stadol ✦
Func. class.: Opioid analgesic
Chem. class.: Mixed opioid antagonist, partial agonist

Controlled Substance Schedule IV

ACTION: Depresses pain impulse transmission at the spinal cord level by interacting with opioid receptors

USES: Moderate to severe pain, general anesthesia induction/maintenance, headache, migraine, preanesthesia
Unlabeled uses: Pruritus

CONTRAINDICATIONS: Hypersensitivity to product, preservative; addiction (opioid)

Precautions: Pregnancy, breastfeeding, children <18 yr, addictive personality, increased intracranial pressure, renal/hepatic disease, ileus, COPD, potential for overdose

Black Box Warning: Coadministration with other CNS depressants, respiratory depression, accidental exposure (intranasal), neonatal opioid withdrawal syndrome, substance abuse

DOSAGE AND ROUTES
Moderate-severe pain

• **Adult: IM** 1-4 mg q3-4hr prn; **IV** 0.5-2 mg q3-4hr prn; **INTRANASAL** 1 spray in 1 nostril, may give another dose 1-1$^1/_2$ hr later; repeat if needed 3-4 hr after last dose

• **Geriatric: IV** $^1/_2$ adult dose at 2× the interval; **INTRANASAL** if no relief after 90-120 min, may repeat with 1 spray

Anesthesia—maintenance in balanced anesthesia; anesthetic adjunct

• **Adult: IV** Initially, 2 mg shortly before anesthesia induction. Maintenance, 0.5-1 mg **IV** during anesthesia, up to 0.06 mg/kg; usual total dose, 4-12.5 mg (approximately 0.06 to 0.18 mg/kg)

Atrial cardioversion—pain

• **Adult: INTRANASAL** 1 mg 30 min before internal atrial defibrillation shock

Renal/hepatic dose

• **Adult: INTRANASAL** max 1 mg followed by 1 mg after 90-120 min; IM/IV give 50% of dose (0.5 mg IV, 1 mg IM), do not repeat within 6 hr

Opioid-induced pruritus (unlabeled)

• **Adult: INTRANASAL** 1 mg (1 spray) in each nostril q4-6hr

Intractable pruritus with inflammatory skin or systemic disease (unlabeled)

• **Adult: INTRANASAL** 1-4 mg/day
Available forms: Inj 1, 2 mg/mL; nasal spray 10 mg/mL
Administer:
• With antiemetic if nausea, vomiting occur

Side effects: *italics* = common; red = life-threatening

- When pain is beginning to return; determine dosage interval according to patient response
- Store in light-resistant container at room temperature

Nasal route

- Prime before first use, point sprayer away from the face, pump activator 7 × until a fine, wide spray occurs; if not used for 48 hr, reprime by pumping 1-2 ×
- If more than 1 spray is needed, use other nostril
- Do not share with others
- Nasal congestion/irritation may occur

IM route

- Deeply in large muscle mass

IV direct route

- Undiluted at a rate of <2 mg/>3-5 min, titrate to patient response; inject directly in vein or tubing of free-flowing compatible IV infusion

Y-site compatibilities: Acyclovir, alfentanil, allopurinol, amifostine, amikacin, aminocaproic acid, aminophylline, amphotericin B liposome (AmBisome), anidulafungin, ascorbic acid injection, atenolol, atracurium, atropine, aztreonam, benztropine, bivalirudin, bleomycin, bumetanide, buprenorphine, calcium chloride/gluconate, CARBOplatin, caspofungin, cefamandole, ceFAZolin, cefepime, cefotaxime, cefoTEtan, cefOXitin, cefTAZidime, ceftizoxime, cefTRIAXone, cefuroxime, cephalothin, chlorproMAZINE, cimetidine, cisatracurium, CISplatin, cladribine, clindamycin, cyanocobalamin, cyclophosphamide, cycloSPORINE, cytarabine, DACTINomycin, DAPTOmycin, dexamethasone phosphate, dexmedetomidine, digoxin, diltiazem, diphenhydrAMINE, DOBUTamine, DOCEtaxel, DOPamine, doxacurium, DOXOrubicin, DOXOrubicin liposomal, doxycycline, enalaprilat, ePHEDrine, EPINEPHrine, epirubicin, epoetin alfa, eptifibatide, ertapenem, erythromycin, esmolol, etoposide, famotidine, fenoldopam, fentaNYL, filgrastim, fluconazole, fludarabine, fluorouracil, gatifloxacin, gemcitabine, gentamicin, glycopyrrolate, granisetron, heparin, hydrocortisone, hydrOXYzine, IDArubicin, ifosfamide, imipenem-cilastatin, irinotecan, isoproterenol, ketorolac, labetalol, lactated Ringer's injection, levofloxacin, lidocaine, linezolid injection, LORazepam, magnesium, mannitol, mechlorethamine, melphalan, meperidine, metaraminol, methicillin, methotrexate, methoxamine, methyldopate, methylPREDNISolone, metoclopramide, metoprolol, metroNIDAZOLE, mezlocillin, milrinone, minocycline, mitoXANtrone, morphine, multiple vitamins injection, mycophenolate mofetil, nafcillin, nalbuphine, naloxone, nesiritide, netilmicin, niCARdipine, nitroglycerin, nitroprusside, norepinephrine, octreotide, ondansetron, oxacillin, oxaliplatin, oxytocin, palonosetron, pamidronate, pancuronium, papaverine, PEMEtrexed, penicillin G potassium/sodium, pentazocine, PHENobarbital, phenylephrine, phytonadione, piperacillin, piperacillin-tazobactam, polymyxin B, potassium chloride, procainamide, prochlorperazine, promethazine, propofol, propranolol, protamine, pyridoxine, quiNIDine, ranitidine, remifentanil, Ringer's injection, riTUXimab, rocuronium, sargramostim, sodium acetate, succinylcholine, SUFentanil, tacrolimus, teniposide, theophylline, thiamine, thiotepa, ticarcillin, ticarcillin-clavulanate, tigecycline, tirofiban, TNA, tobramycin, tolazoline, TPN, trastuzumab, urokinase, vancomycin, vasopressin, vecuronium, verapamil, vinCRIStine, vinorelbine, voriconazole

SIDE EFFECTS

CNS: *Drowsiness, dizziness, confusion, headache, sedation, euphoria, weakness, hallucinations,* insomnia (nasal)

CV: Palpitations, bradycardia, hypotension

EENT: Tinnitus, blurred vision, miosis, diplopia, nasal congestion, unpleasant taste

GI: *Nausea, vomiting, anorexia, constipation, cramps*

GU: Urinary retention

INTEG: Rash, urticaria, bruising, flushing, diaphoresis, pruritus
RESP: Respiratory depression

PHARMACOKINETICS
Metabolized by liver, excreted by kidneys, crosses placenta, excreted in breast milk, half-life 2-9 hr, protein binding 80%
IM: Onset 5-15 min, peak 30-60 min, duration 3-4 hr
INTRANASAL: Onset within 15 min, peak 1-2 hr, duration 4-5 hr
IV: Onset 1 min, peak 4-5 min, duration 2-4 hr

INTERACTIONS
Black Box Warning: **Increase:** CNS effects—alcohol, opioids, sedative/hypnotics, antipsychotics, skeletal muscle relaxants, other CNS depressants, MAOIs

NURSING CONSIDERATIONS
Assess:
• For decreasing output; may indicate urinary retention
• For withdrawal symptoms in opioid-dependent patients; PE, vascular occlusion, abscesses, ulcerations
• CNS changes: dizziness, drowsiness, hallucinations, euphoria, LOC, pupil reaction
• Allergic reactions: rash, urticaria

Black Box Warning: **Respiratory dysfunction:** respiratory depression, character, rate, rhythm; notify prescriber if respirations are <10/min

Black Box Warning: **Neonatal opioid withdrawal:** if mother used this product for prolonged periods during pregnancy, monitor neonate for withdrawal

Black Box Warning: **Substance abuse:** identify if there has been substance abuse (including alcoholism) in the past or present; addiction is more common in these patients

Black Box Warning: **Accidental exposure (intranasal):** keep out of reach of children

Black Box Warning: Avoid with benzodiazepines

• Need for pain medication, physical dependence
• Safety measures: night-light, call bell within easy reach, assistance with ambulation, especially for geriatric patients
• **Pregnancy/breastfeeding:** use only if benefits outweigh risks; usually compatible with breastfeeding
Evaluate:
• Therapeutic response: decrease in pain
Teach patient/family:

Black Box Warning: To report any symptoms of CNS changes

• That physical dependency may result when used for extended periods
• That withdrawal symptoms may occur: nausea, vomiting, cramps, fever, faintness, anorexia
• How to use nasal product
• To avoid hazardous activities

TREATMENT OF OVERDOSE:
Naloxone 0.4-2 mg IV, O$_2$, IV fluids, vasopressors

RARELY USED

C1 esterase inhibitor subcutaneous, human
Haegarda

USES: Acute attacks of hereditary angioedema

CONTRAINDICATIONS: Leporine protein hypersensitivity

DOSAGE AND ROUTES
• **Adult/adolescent ≥84 kg: IV** Inject 4200 units (2 vials) as a slow intravenous injection over approximately 5 min; may give second dose
• **Adult/adolescent <84 kg: IV** Inject 50 units per kg body weight up to 4200 units as a slow intravenous injection over approximately 5 min; may give second dose

---

cabozantinib
(ka-boe-zanʹti-nib)
Cabometyx, Cometriq ✦
Func. class.: Antineoplastic, biologic response modifier, signal transduction inhibitor
Chem. class.: Multi-tyrosine kinase inhibitor

ACTION: Blocks abnormal tyrosine kinase proteins ⚠ (RET, MET, VEGFR-1, VEGFR-2, VEGFR-3, KIT, TRKB, FLT-3, AXL, TIE-2, ROS1, TYRO3, and MER); inhibits these receptor tyrosine kinases (RTK) that are responsible for the control of cell migration, metabolism, proliferation, and differentiation

USES: In patients with progressive, metastatic medullary thyroid cancer, advanced renal cell cancer (RCC) who have received prior anti-angiogenic therapy

CONTRAINDICATIONS: Hypersensitivity, pregnancy

Black Box Warning: Bleeding, fistula, GI perforation

Precautions: Breastfeeding, contraception requirements, dental disease, dental work, diarrhea, encephalopathy, GI bleeding, hypertension, infertility, MI, proteinuria, reproductive risk, skin disease, surgery, thromboembolic disease, wound dehiscence

DOSAGE AND ROUTES
Progressive, metastatic medullary thyroid cancer (capsules only; do not substitute with tablets):
• **Adult: PO** 140 mg daily on an empty stomach until disease progression or unacceptable toxicity occurs
Advanced renal cell cancer (RCC) in patients who have received prior anti-angiogenic therapy (tablets only; do not substitute with capsules):
• **Adult: PO** 60 mg daily on an empty stomach until disease progression or unacceptable toxicity
Hepatic dose
Cometriq capsules:
• Mild or moderate hepatic impairment (Child-Pugh class A or B): reduce the starting dose to 80 mg qday; severe hepatic impairment (Child-Pugh class C): do not use
Cabometyx tablets:
• Mild or moderate hepatic impairment (Child-Pugh class A or B): reduce the starting dose to 40 mg qday; severe hepatic impairment (Child-Pugh class C): do not use
Available forms: Caps 60, 100, 140 mg; tabs 20, 40, 60 mg

Administer:
• Do not substitute tablets with capsules
• Take on an empty stomach; do not eat for at least 2 hr before and at least 1 hr after taking, swallow capsules and tablets whole; do not open or crush
• Do not take with grapefruit juice or nutritional supplements that are known to inhibit CYP450
• Do not take a missed dose within 12 hr of the next dose. If the next dose is in 12 hr or more, take the missed dose; if the next dose is in <12 hr, skip the missed dose and take the next dose at the scheduled time

Dosage adjustments due to treatment-related toxicity
Cometriq capsules:

• Serious arterial thromboembolic event (MI, cerebral infarction); development of visceral perforation or fistula formation; severe hemorrhage; malignant hypertension, hypertensive crisis, or persistent severe hypertension despite optimal management; nephrotic syndrome; osteonecrosis of the jaw; reversible posterior leukoencephalopathy syndrome (RPLS): Permanently discontinue.

• Palmar-plantar erythrodysesthesia (hand and foot syndrome) (intolerable grade 2, or grade 3): Hold, when toxicity resolves to grade 1 or less, reduce the daily dose by 40 mg; if the patient was previously receiving 60 mg/day, resume therapy at this dosage if tolerated, otherwise discontinue therapy

• Wound dehiscence or healing complications: Hold

• Grade 4 hematologic toxicity, any other grade 3 or higher nonhematologic toxicity, or intolerable grade 2 toxicity: Hold, when toxicity resolves to grade 1 or less, reduce the daily dose by 40 mg. If the patient was previously receiving 60 mg/day, resume therapy at this dosage if tolerated, otherwise discontinue therapy

Cabometyx tablets:

• Arterial thromboembolic event (e.g., myocardial infarction, cerebral infarction); development of unmanageable fistula or GI perforation; severe hemorrhage; hypertensive crisis or severe hypertension despite optimal management; nephrotic syndrome; reversible posterior leukoencephalopathy syndrome (RPLS): Permanently discontinue

• Palmar-plantar erythrodysesthesia (hand and foot syndrome) (intolerable grade 2, or grade 3): Hold; when toxicity improves to grade 1 or less, reduce the daily dose by 20 mg; if the patient was previously receiving 20 mg/day, resume therapy at this dose if tolerated, otherwise discontinue therapy.

• Any other grade 4 toxicity or grade 3/intolerable grade 2 toxicities that cannot be managed with a dose reduction or supportive care (hematologic or nonhematologic): Hold; when toxicity improves to grade 1 or less, reduce the daily dose by 20 mg; if the patient was previously receiving 20 mg/day, resume therapy at this dose if tolerated, otherwise discontinue therapy

Dosage guidance in patients on strong CYP3A4 inducers/inhibitors
Cometriq capsules:

• **Strong CYP3A4 inhibitors:** avoid concomitant use if possible. If a strong CYP3A4 inhibitor is required, reduce the daily dose by 40 mg; resume the prior dose after 2 to 3 days if the strong CYP3A4 inhibitor is discontinued

• **Strong CYP3A4 inducers:** avoid chronic concomitant use if possible. If a strong CYP3A4 inducer is required, increase the daily dose by 40 mg as tolerated. Max 180 mg/day. Resume the prior dose after 2 to 3 days if the strong CYP3A4 inducer is discontinued.

Cabometyx tablets:

• **Strong CYP3A4 inhibitors:** Reduce the daily dose by 20 mg; resume the prior dose after 2 to 3 days if the strong CYP3A4 inhibitor is discontinued.

• **Strong CYP3A4 inducers:** Increase the daily dose by 20 mg as tolerated. Max 80 mg/day. Resume the prior dose after 2 to 3 days if the strong CYP3A4 inducer is discontinued.

SIDE EFFECTS
RESP: Cough, dyspnea
CNS: Dizziness, headache, fatigue
CV: Hypertension, hypertriglyceridemia
EENT: Rash, erythema, hair discoloration, oral ulceration, stomatitis
META: Hyperbilirubinemia, hyperglycemia, hypocalcemia, hypokalemia, hypoalbuminemia, hypomagnesemia, hyponatremia, hypophosphatemia
MISC: Arthralgia, asthenia, dysgeusia, hand and foot syndrome, hypothyroidism, dysphonia
GI: Anorexia, nausea, vomiting, weight loss, abdominal pain, diarrhea, constipation, dyspepsia
HEMA: Thrombocytopenia, lymphopenia, neutropenia, anemia

Side effects: *italics* = common; red = life-threatening

PHARMACOKINETICS
• Protein binding ≥99.7%, half-life 55 hr, excretion 54% feces (43% as unchanged drug), 21% urine, peak 2-5 hr
• Affected cytochrome P450 isoenzymes and drug transporters: CYP1A1, CYP2C8, CYP2C9, CYP2C19, CYP3A4, P-gp, MRP2
• Metabolized in the liver and is a substrate of CYP3A4

INTERACTIONS
• **Increase:** GI bleeding—warfarin, NSAIDs
• **Increase:** cabozantinib effects—CYP3A4 inhibitors (amprenavir, bocenavir, delavirdine, ketoconazole, indinavir, itraconazole, dalfopristin/quinupristin, ritonavir, tipranavir, fluconazole, isoniazid, miconazole)
• **Decrease:** cabozantinib effects—CYP3A4 inducers (rifampin, rifapentine, rifabutin, primadone, phenytoin, phenobarbital, nevirapine, nafcillin, modafinil, griseofulvin, etravirine, efavirenz, barbiturates, bexarotene, bosentan, carbamazepine, enzalutamide, dexamethasone)

Drug/Food
Increase: cabozantinib effects—grapefruit juice
Drug/Herb
Decrease: cabozantinib effects—St. John's wort
Drug/Smoking
Decrease: cabozantinib effects—smoking, dose may need to be increased
Drug/Lab
Increase: INR, PT, AST, ALT, bilirubin

NURSING CONSIDERATIONS
Assess:

> Black Box Warning: **GI perforation/ bleeding:** some cases have been fatal, usually occurs in those using NSAIDs, taxanes, or those with diverticulitis or peptic ulcer disease, discontinue if these occur

• **Serious arterial and venous thromboembolic disease:** some have been fatal, permanently discontinue if myocardial infarction or any other arterial thromboembolic complication occurs

• **Wound dehiscence:** temporary suspension of therapy is recommended at least 28 days before scheduled surgery, including dental surgery. Resume therapy based on clinical judgment of adequate wound healing. Hold therapy in those who develop wound dehiscence or wound healing complications requiring medical intervention

• **Hypertension:** monitor BP prior to and regularly during treatment, hold in those hypertensive patients not adequately controlled with medical management; resume therapy at a reduced dose. Permanently discontinue if patients develop malignant hypertension, hypertensive crisis, or persistent uncontrolled hypertension despite optimal management

• **Dental disease:** an oral examination should be performed prior to starting therapy to evaluate for dental disease; good oral hygiene practices should be encouraged. Temporary suspension of therapy is recommended at least 28 days before invasive dental work or surgery. Resume therapy based on clinical judgment of adequate wound healing. Osteonecrosis of the jaw (ONJ) has been reported; permanently discontinue capsules (Cometriq) in those who develop ONJ

• **Palmar-plantar erythrodysesthesia (hand and foot syndrome):** hold in those who develop intolerable grade 2 or grade 3 or 4 hand and foot syndrome, resume at a reduced dose when toxicity has improved to grade 1

• **Proteinuria:** monitor urine protein regularly; permanently discontinue in those who develop nephrotic syndrome

• **Severe diarrhea:** those with preexisting diarrhea should be treated prior to receiving this product; hold (Cabometyx) therapy for intolerable grade 2 diarrhea, or for grade 3 or higher diarrhea that cannot be managed with standard antidiarrheal treatments until improvement to grade 1 or less; a dose reduction may be necessary. Those with severe diarrhea should also be given fluid and electrolyte replacement if they become dehydrated

---

• **Reversible posterior leukoencephalopathy syndrome (RPLS):** assess for seizures, headache, visual disturbances, confusion, and altered mental status. Discontinue if RPLS is suspected or diagnosed; this syndrome may be confirmed on magnetic resonance imaging

• **Pregnancy/breastfeeding:** assess if pregnancy is planned or suspected. Females of reproductive potential should avoid becoming pregnant during treatment; women who become pregnant while receiving product should be apprised of the potential hazard to the fetus.

• Counsel patients about the reproductive risk and contraception requirements during treatment. Females and men with female partners who are able to become pregnant should avoid pregnancy and use effective contraception during and for ≥4 mo after the last dose. Females of reproductive potential should undergo pregnancy testing prior to initiation; do not breastfeed

Evaluate:

• **Therapeutic response:** decreased spread of cancer

Teach Patient/Family:

• To report adverse reactions immediately, SOB, severe abdominal pain, persistent diarrhea, severe hypertension, bleeding

• About reason for treatment, expected results

• To use reliable contraception during treatment and for ≥4 mo after treatment

---

⚠ **HIGH ALERT**

RARELY USED

calcitonin (salmon) (Rx)
Miacalcin, Calcimar ✦, Caltine ✦

Func. class.: Parathyroid agents (calcium regulator)
Chem. class.: Polypeptide hormone

Do not confuse:
Calcitonin/calcitriol/calcifediol/calcium
Fortical/Foradil

ACTION: Decreases bone resorption, blood calcium levels; increases deposits of calcium in bones; opposes parathyroid hormone

USES: Paget's disease, postmenopausal osteoporosis, hypercalcemia

CONTRAINDICATIONS: Hypersensitivity to this product, fish
Precautions: Pregnancy, breastfeeding, children, hypotension, hypocalcemia, secondary malignancy

DOSAGE AND ROUTES
Postmenopausal osteoporosis
• **Adult:** SUBCUT/IM 100 units every other day; **INTRANASAL** 200 units (1 spray) daily, alternating nostrils daily
Paget's disease
• **Adult:** SUBCUT/IM 100 units/day; maintenance 50 units daily, every other day, or 3 × per wk
Hypercalcemia
• **Adult:** SUBCUT/IM 4 units/kg q12hr, increase to 8 units/kg q12hr if response is unsatisfactory, may increase to 8 units/kg q6hr if needed after 2 more days
Available forms: Inj 200 units/mL; nasal spray 200 units/actuation
Administer:
• Store at <77° F (25° C); protect from light
SUBCUT route
• Rotate inj sites; use within 2 hr of reconstitution; **give** at bedtime to minimize nausea, vomiting
IM route
• After test dose of 10 units/mL, 0.1 mL intradermally; watch for 15 min; **give** only with EPINEPHrine, emergency meds available
• IM inj slowly into deep muscle mass; rotate sites; preferred route if volume is >2 mL; use within 2 hr of reconstitution
Nasal route
• Prime pump before first dose
• Use at bedtime; alternate nostrils daily, prime to get full spray before first dose, store in refrigerator
• Allow to come to room temperature before using
• Discard after 30 days

Side effects: *italics* = common; red = life-threatening

SIDE EFFECTS
CNS: Headache, (nasal)
EENT: Eye pain (nasal)
GI: Nausea, diarrhea, vomiting, anorexia, (IM/SUBCUT)
GU: Nocturia, frequency
INTEG: Rash, flushing, reaction at inj site
MS: Backache, myalgia, arthralgia
RESP: Dyspnea, flulike symptoms, bronchospasm
SYST: Anaphylaxis, infection

PHARMACOKINETICS
IM/SUBCUT: Onset 15 min, peak 2 hr, duration 6-8 hr, metabolized by kidneys, excreted as inactive metabolites via kidneys

INTERACTIONS
Decrease: lithium effect; monitor lithium level
Decrease: effect of nasal spray—bisphosphonates (Paget's disease); monitor for adequate effect

NURSING CONSIDERATIONS
Assess:
• Anaphylaxis, hypersensitivity reaction (rash, fever, inability to breathe); emergency equipment should be nearby
• GI symptoms, polyuria, flushing, head swelling, tingling, headache; may indicate hypercalcemia
• Nutritional status; diet for sources of vit D (milk, some seafood), calcium (dairy products, dark green vegetables), phosphates
• **Postmenopausal osteoporosis:** vit D (50-135 international units/dL), alk phos baseline, q3-6mo; monitor urine hydroxyproline with Paget's disease, biochemical markers of bone formation/absorption, radiologic evidence of fracture; bone density
• **Toxicity (can occur rapidly),** increased drug level; have parenteral calcium on hand if calcium level drops too low; check for tetany (irritability, paresthesia, nervousness, muscle twitching, seizures, tetanic spasms)
Evaluate:
• Therapeutic response: calcium levels 9-10 mg/dL, decreasing symptoms of Paget's disease

Teach patient/family:
SUBCUT route/IM route
• About the method of inj if patient will be responsible for self-medication; to rotate sites, not to inject into broken, irritated skin; provide written instructions
• To report difficulty swallowing, any changes in side effects to prescriber immediately
• To report immediately signs/symptoms of hypocalcemia: tetany, seizures
• **Pregnancy/breastfeeding:** to advise prescriber if pregnancy is planned or suspected; or if breastfeeding
• **Postmenopausal osteoporosis:** to take vitamin D and calcium differential; that nausea, vomiting, and facial flushing occur often
Nasal route
• To use alternating nostrils; to use after allowing to warm to room temperature; to prime to get full spray; to discard after 30 days

---

calcitriol vitamin D$_3$ (Rx)
(kal-sih-try'ole)
Calcijex ✚, Rocaltrol, SilKis ✚
Func. class.: Parathyroid agent (calcium regulator)
Chem. class.: Vit D hormone

Do not confuse:
calcitriol/Calciferol/calcitonin/calcium

ACTION: Increases intestinal absorption of calcium; provides calcium for bones; increases renal tubular reabsorption of phosphate

USES: Hypocalcemia with chronic renal disease, hyperparathyroidism, pseudohypoparathyroidism, psoriasis, renal osteodystrophy

CONTRAINDICATIONS: Hypersensitivity, hyperphosphatemia, hypercalcemia, vit D toxicity
Precautions: Pregnancy, breastfeeding, renal calculi, CV disease

---

DOSAGE AND ROUTES
Hypocalcemia
• **Adult and child ≥6 yr: PO** 0.25 mcg/day; **IV** 0.5 mcg (0.01 mcg/kg) 3 × per wk, may increase by 0.25-0.5 mcg/dose q2-4wk

• **Child 1-5 yr: PO** 0.25-2 mcg/day; **IV** 0.01-0.05 mcg/kg 3 × per wk
Hypoparathyroidism
• **Adult and child ≥6 yr: PO** 0.25 mcg/day, may increase q2-4wk, maintenance 0.5-2 mcg/day

• **Child 1-5 yr: PO** 0.25-0.75 mcg daily

• **Child <1 yr: PO** 0.04-0.08 mcg/kg/day

Available forms: Caps 0.25, 0.5 mcg; inj 1 mcg/mL; oral sol 1 mcg/mL, 2 mcg/mL; top 3 mcg/g
Administer:
PO route
• Do not break, crush, chew caps
• Give without regard to meals
• Store protected from light, heat, moisture
Topical route
• Rub into skin
IV route
• **Hypocalcemia:** Give by direct IV over 1 min through catheter at hemodialysis conclusion

SIDE EFFECTS
CNS: Drowsiness, headache, vertigo
CV: Hypertension, *dysrhythmias*, edema
EENT: Blurred vision, photophobia, rhinorrhea
ENDO: Hypercalcemia
GI: Nausea, vomiting, jaundice, anorexia, dry mouth, constipation, cramps, metallic taste, *pancreatitis*
GU: Polyuria
MS: Myalgia, arthralgia, weakness
SYST: *Anaphylaxis*
INTEG: Pain at injection site, rash, pruritus

PHARMACOKINETICS
PO: Absorbed readily from GI tract, peak 10-12 hr, duration 3-5 days, half-life hr, undergoes hepatic recycling, excreted in bile

INTERACTIONS
Increase: hypercalcemia—thiazide diuretics, calcium supplements

Increase: cardiac dysrhythmias—cardiac glycosides, verapamil; use cautiously
Increase: hypermagnesemia—magnesium antacids/supplements
Increase: toxicity—other vit D products
Increase: metabolism of vit D—phenytoin
Decrease: absorption of calcitriol—cholestyramine, mineral oil, fat-soluble vitamins; avoid concurrent use
Drug/Food
• Large amounts of high-calcium foods may cause hypercalcemia
Drug/Lab Test
Increase: AST/ALT, BUN, creatinine
False increase: Cholesterol
Interference: Alk phos, electrolytes

NURSING CONSIDERATIONS
Assess:
• **Vitamin D deficiency:** Baseline and periodically
• May increase calcium; should be kept at 9-10 mg/dL, vit D 50-135 units/dL, phosphate 70 mg/dL; toxic reactions may occur rapidly
• Serum calcium, phosphate 2 × per wk during beginning treatment; serum calcium magnesium, alkaline phosphatase and intact PTH ≤ monthly
• **Hypercalcemia:** dry mouth, metallic taste, polyuria, bone pain, muscle weakness, headache, fatigue, change in level of consciousness, dysrhythmias, increased respirations, anorexia, nausea, vomiting, cramps, constipation; **Hypocalcemia:** paresthesia, twitching, Chvostek's sign, Trousseau's sign
• Nutritional status, diet for sources of vit D (milk, some seafood); calcium (dairy products, dark green vegetables), phosphates (dairy products) must be avoided
• Restrict sodium, potassium if required; restriction of fluids if required for chronic renal failure
• Height, weight in children, baseline and periodically if on long-term high-dose therapy
Evaluate:
• **Therapeutic response:** calcium 9-10 mg/dL; decreasing symptoms of hypocalcemia, hypoparathyroidism

---

Side effects: *italics* = common; red = life-threatening

Teach patient/family:

• **About symptoms of hypercalcemia:** renal stones, nausea, vomiting, anorexia, lethargy, thirst, bone or flank pain, confusion

• To follow prescribed diet, usually; to avoid products with sodium: cured meats, dairy products, cold cuts, olives, beets, pickles, soups, meat tenderizers with chronic renal failure; products with potassium: oranges, bananas, dried fruit, peas, dark green leafy vegetables, milk, melons, beans

• To avoid OTC products that contain calcium, potassium, sodium with chronic renal failure, to take as prescribed, not to double or skip doses

• To monitor weight weekly; to maintain fluid intake

• To continue with exams and lab work

• To avoid large doses of vitamins or supplements

• **Pregnancy/breastfeeding:** identify if pregnancy is planned or suspected or if breastfeeding; do not breastfeed

TREATMENT OF OVERDOSE: Discontinue treatment, diuretics, hemodialysis

---

calcium carbonate (OTC)

Alka-Mints, Apo-Cal ✦, Calcarb, Calci-Chew, Calci-Mix, Calcite ✦, Calsan ✦, Caltrate ✦, Maalox Antacid, Os-Cal, Rolaids Extra Strength Softchew, Tums, Tums E-X

calcium acetate (OTC)

(kal'see-um ass'e-tate)

Eliphos, PhosLo, Phoslyra, Calphron

Func. class.: Antacid, calcium supplement

Chem. class.: Calcium product

Do not confuse:
Os-Cal/Asacol
calcium/calcitriol/calcitonin

ACTION: Neutralizes gastric acidity

USES: Antacid, calcium supplement

CONTRAINDICATIONS: Hypersensitivity, hypercalcemia

Precautions: Pregnancy, breastfeeding, geriatric patients, fluid restriction, decreased GI motility, GI obstruction, dehydration, renal disease, hyperparathyroidism, bone tumors

DOSAGE AND ROUTES

Hypocalcemia prevention, osteoporosis

• **Adult yr:** PO 1-2 g

• **Adult 19-50 yr:** PO 1000 mg/day elemental calcium (2500 mg/day calcium carbonate)

Chronic hypocalcemia

• **Adult:** PO 2-4 g/day elemental calcium (5-10 g/day calcium carbonate) in 3-4 divided doses

• **Child:** PO 45-65 mg/kg/day elemental calcium (112.5-162.5 mg/kg/day calcium carbonate) in 4 divided doses

• **Neonate:** PO 50-150 mg/kg/day elemental calcium (125-375 mg/kg/day in 4-6 divided doses, max 1 g/day)

Supplementation

• **Child:** PO 45-65 mg/kg/day

Hyperphosphatemia (Acetate)

• **Adult:** PO 1334 mg with meals

Heartburn, dyspepsia, hyperacidity (OTC)

• **Adult:** PO 1-2 tabs q2hr, max 9 tabs/24 hr (Alka-Mints); chew 2-4 tab q1hr prn, max 16 tabs (Tums regular strength); chew 2-4 tab q1hr prn, max 10 tabs (Tums E-X)

Available forms: Calcium carbonate: chewable tabs 350, 420, 450, 500, 750, 1000, 1250 mg; **tabs** 500, 600, 650, 667, 1000, 1250, 1500 mg; **gum** 300, 450, 500 mg; **susp** 1250 mg/5 mL; **caps** 1250 mg; **powder** 6.5 g/packet; **calcium acetate: tabs** 667 mg (169 mg elemental Ca), **gelcaps:** 667 mg (169 mg elemental calcium); caps 500 mg (125 mg elemental Ca)

Administer:

PO route

• 1 g calcium carbonate = 400 mg elemental calcium = 10 mmol calcium = 20 mEq calcium

---

- Do not give enteric-coated within 1 hr of calcium carbonate
- **For ulcer treatment** (adjunct): give 1 and 3 hr after meals and at bedtime
- **For a phosphate binder:** give 1 hr after each meal or snack and at bedtime
- **For supplement:** give 1-1$\frac{1}{2}$ hr after meals; avoid oxalic acid foods (spinach, rhubarb), phytic acid (brans, cereals) or phosphorus (milk, dairy), may decrease calcium absorption
- **Suspension:** shake well; use calibrated measuring device
- Laxatives or stool softeners if constipation occurs

SIDE EFFECTS

GI: *Constipation,* anorexia, nausea, vomiting, diarrhea
GU: Calculi, hypercalciuria

PHARMACOKINETICS

$\frac{1}{3}$ of dose absorbed by small intestine, excreted in feces and urine, crosses placenta, must have adequate vit D for absorption

INTERACTIONS

Increase: digoxin toxicity—hypercalcemia
Increase: plasma levels of quiNIDine, amphetamines
Increase: hypercalcemia—thiazide diuretics, calcium supplements
Decrease: levels of salicylates, calcium channel blockers, ketoconazole, iron salts, tetracyclines, fluoroquinolones, phenytoin, etidronate, risedronate, atenolol PO
Drug/Food
Decrease: calcium supplement effect—cereal, spinach
Drug/Lab Test
Decrease: phosphates
False increase: chloride
False positive: benzodiazepines
False decrease: magnesium, oxalate, lipase

NURSING CONSIDERATIONS
Assess:
- Calcium (serum, urine), serum calcium should be 8.5-10.5 mg/dL, correct or use ionized calcium in low albumin or acid/base disorders, monitor weekly if used to treat electrolyte imbalances or use a daily supplement; urine calcium should be 150 mg/day, monitor weekly; serum phosphate
- **Milk-alkali syndrome:** nausea, vomiting, disorientation, headache
- Constipation; increase bulk in the diet if needed
- **Hypercalcemia:** headache, nausea, vomiting, confusion
- **Hypocalcemia:** paresthesia, twitching, colic, dysrhythmias, Chvostek's sign, Trousseau's sign
- Those taking digoxin for toxicity; monitor frequently
- Antacid—for abdominal pain, heartburn, indigestion before, after administration
Evaluate:
- Therapeutic response: absence of pain, decreased acidity; decreased hyperphosphatemia with renal failure
Teach patient/family:
- To increase fluids to 2 L unless contraindicated; to add bulk to diet for constipation; to notify prescriber of constipation
- Not to switch antacids unless directed by prescriber; not to use as antacid for >2 wk without approval by prescriber
- That therapeutic dose recommendations are figured as elemental calcium
- To avoid excessive use of alcohol, caffeine, tobacco
- To avoid spinach, cereals, dairy products in large amounts, other foods high in oxalates before taking the product; may interfere with absorption of calcium

CALCIUM SALTS

calcium acetate
Eliphos, PhosLo, Phoslyra
calcium chloride (Rx)
calcium citrate (OTC)
Cal-Citrate, Citracal
Calcium glubionate
calcionate
calcium gluceptate (Rx)
calcium gluconate (Rx)
Kalcinate
calcium lactate (Rx)
Cal-Lac
Tri calcium phosphate (OTC)
Posture

Func. class.: Electrolyte replacement—calcium product

ACTION: Calcium needed for maintenance of nervous, muscular, skeletal function; enzyme reactions; normal cardiac contractility; coagulation of blood; affects secretory activity of endocrine, exocrine glands

USES: Prevention and treatment of hypocalcemia, hypermagnesemia, hypoparathyroidism, neonatal tetany, cardiac toxicity caused by hyperkalemia, lead colic, hyperphosphatemia, vit D deficiency, osteoporosis prophylaxis, calcium antagonist toxicity (calcium channel blocker toxicity)
Unlabeled uses: Electrolyte abnormalities in cardiac arrest, CPR

CONTRAINDICATIONS: Hypercalcemia, digoxin toxicity, ventricular fibrillation, renal calculi
Precautions: Pregnancy, breastfeeding, children, respiratory/renal disease, cor pulmonale, digitalized patient, respiratory failure, diarrhea, dehydration

DOSAGE AND ROUTES
Acute hypocalcemia
• **Adult:** IV 7-14 mEq **For tetany** 4.5-16 mEq
• **Child/infant:** IV 1-7 mEq **For tetany** 0.5-0.7 mEq/kg tid-qid
For nutritional supplementation
PO (any oral calcium salt; dosage expressed as elemental calcium)
• **Adult:** PO 1-2 g mg/day
• **Child:** PO 45-65 mg/kg/day

Available forms: Calcium chloride: injection 10% (1.36 mEq); **calcium citrate:** tabs 250 mg; **calcium glubionate:** syrup 1.8 g/5 mL; **calcium gluconate:** tabs 500, 650, 975, 1 g; injection 10% (0.45 mEq); **calcium lactate:** tabs 325, 500, 650 mg; **tricalcium phosphate:** tabs 600 mg
Administer:
PO route (only acetate, carbonate, citrate, glubionate, lactate, phosphate)
• Give in 3-4 divided doses with or 1 hr after meals, follow with full glass of water; if using as phosphate binder in renal dialysis, do not follow with water, do not give oral medications within 1 hr of oral calcium; **chew tab:** chew thoroughly; **effervescent tab:** dissolve in full glass of water; **oral powder:** mix and give with food; **oral solution:** give before meals; **oral suspension:** shake well
• Store at room temperature
IM route
• **Glycerophosphate,** lactate may be given IM
IV route
• Warm to room temperature
• Undiluted or diluted with equal amounts of NS to a 5% sol for inj, give 0.5-1 mL/min, give slowly, rapid administration may cause cardiac arrest
• Through small-bore needle into large vein, do not use scalp vein; if extravasation occurs, necrosis will result (IV)
• Remain recumbent ½ hr after IV dose, drop in B/P may result

Calcium chloride
Y-site compatibilities: Acyclovir, alemtuzumab, alfentanil, amikacin, aminocaproic

acid, aminophylline, amiodarone, anidulafungin, argatroban, arsenic trioxide, ascorbic acid injection, asparaginase, atenolol, atracurium, atropine, azithromycin, aztreonam, benztropine, bivalirudin, bleomycin, bumetanide, buprenorphine, butorphanol, calcium gluconate, CARBOplatin, carmustine, caspofungin acetate, cefotaxime, cefoTEtan, cefOXitin, ceftaroline, ceftizoxime, chloramphenicol, chlorothiazide, chlorpheniramine, chlorproMAZINE, cimetidine, CISplatin, clindamycin, cloxacillin, colistimethate, cyanocobalamin, cyclophosphamide, cycloSPORINE, cytarabine, DACTINomycin, DAPTOmycin, DAUNOrubicin, dexmedetomidine, dexrazoxane, digoxin, diltiaZEM, diphenhydrAMINE, DOBUTamine, DOCEtaxel, dolasetron, DOPamine, doxacurium, doxapram, DOXOrubicin, doxycycline, edetate calcium disodium, enalaprilat, ePHEDrine, EPINEPHrine, epiRUBicin, epoetin alfa, eptifibatide, ergonovine, ertapenem, erythromycin, esmolol, etoposide, etoposide phosphate, famotidine, fenoldopam, fentaNYL, fluconazole, fludarabine, furosemide, gallamine, gallium, ganciclovir, gatifloxacin, gemcitabine, gentamicin, glycopyrrolate, granisetron, heparin sodium, HYDROmorphone, hydrOXYzine, IDArubicin, ifosfamide, inamrinone, insulin (regular), irinotecan, isoproterenol, kanamycin, labetalol, lactated Ringer's, lepirudin, leucovorin, lidocaine, lincomycin, linezolid, LORazepam, mannitol, meperidine, mephentermine, mesna, methohexital, methotrexate, methyldopate, metoclopramide, metoprolol, metroNIDAZOLE, micafungin, midazolam, milrinone, minocycline, mitoMYcin, mitoXANTRONE, mivacurium, morphine, moxifloxacin, multiple vitamins injection, mycophenolate mofetil, nafcillin, nalbuphine, nalorphine, naloxone, nesiritide, niCARdipine, nitroglycerin, nitroprusside, norepinephrine, octreotide, ondansetron, oxytocin, PACLitaxel (solvent/surfactant), pancuronium, papaverine, penicillin G potassium/sodium, pentazocine, PENTobarbital, PHENobarbital, phentolamine, phenylephrine, phytonadione, piperacillin, piperacillin-tazobactam, polymyxin B, potassium, potassium chloride, procainamide, prochlorperazine, promazine, promethazine, propranolol, protamine, pyridoxine, quinupristin-dalfopristin, raNITIdine, Ringer's injection, rocuronium, streptomycin, succinylcholine, SUFentanil, tacrolimus, teniposide, theophylline, thiamine, thiotepa, ticarcillin-clavulanate, tigecycline, tirofiban, TNA (3-in-1), tobramycin, tolazoline, topotecan, trimetaphan, tubocurarine, urokinase, vancomycin, vasopressin, vecuronium, verapamil, vinBLAStine, vinCRIStine, vinorelbine, voriconazole

Calcium gluconate

Y-site compatibilities: Acyclovir, aldesleukin, alemtuzumab, alfentanil, allopurinol, amifostine, amikacin, aminocaproic acid, aminophylline, amiodarone, anidulafungin, argatroban, arsenic trioxide, ascorbic acid injection, asparaginase, atenolol, atracurium, atropine, azaTHIOprine, azithromycin, aztreonam, benztropine, bivalirudin, bleomycin, bumetanide, buprenorphine, butorphanol, calcium chloride, CARBOplatin, carmustine, caspofungin, ceFAZolin, cefepime, cefoperazone, cefotaxime, cefoTEtan, cefOXitin, ceftaroline, cefTAZidime, ceftizoxime, cefuroxime, chloramphenicol sodium succinate, chlorothiazide, chlorpheniramine, chlorproMAZINE, cimetidine, ciprofloxacin, cisatracurium, CISplatin, cladribine, clindamycin, cloxacillin, codeine, colistimethate, cyanocobalamin, cyclophosphamide, cycloSPORINE, cytarabine, DACTINomycin, DAPTOmycin, DAUNOrubicin liposome, DAUNOrubicin, dexmedetomidine, dexrazoxane, digoxin, diltiaZEM, dimenhyDRINATE, diphenhydrAMINE, DOBUTamine, DOCEtaxel, dolasetron, DOPamine, doripenem, doxacurium, doxapram, DOXOrubicin, DOXOrubicin liposomal, doxycycline, edetate calcium disodium, enalaprilat, ePHEDrine, EPINEPHrine, epiRUBicin, epoetin alfa, eptifibatide, ergonovine, ertapenem, erythromycin, esmolol, etoposide, etoposide phosphate, famotidine, fenoldopam, fentaNYL, filgrastim, fludarabine, fluorouracil, folic acid (as sodium salt), furosemide, gallamine, gallium, ganciclovir, gatifloxacin, gemcitabine, gentamicin, glycopyrrolate, granisetron, heparin sodium, HYDROmorphone, hydrOXYzine, IDArubicin, ifosfamide, insulin (regular), irinotecan, isoproterenol, kanamycin, ketamine, labetalol, lactated Ringer's injection, lepirudin, leucovorin, levoFLOXacin, lidocaine, lincomycin, linezolid, LORazepam, magnesium sulfate, mannitol, melphalan, meperidine, mephentermine, mesna, methohexital, methotrexate, methyldopa, metoclopramide, metoprolol, metroNIDAZOLE, micafungin, midazolam, milrinone, mitoMYcin, mitoXANTRONE, mivacurium, morphine, moxifloxacin, multiple vitamins injection, nafcillin, nalbuphine, nalorphine, naloxone, nesiritide, netilmicin, niCARdipine, nitroglycerin, nitroprusside, norepinephrine, octreotide, ondansetron, oritavancin, oxaliplatin, oxytocin, PACLitaxel (solvent/surfactant), palonosetron, pancuronium, papaverine, penicillin G potassium/sodium, pentamidine, pentazocine, PENTobarbital, PHENobarbital, phentolamine, phenylephrine, phytonadione, piperacillin, polymyxin B, potassium acetate/chloride, procainamide, prochlorperazine, promazine, promethazine, propofol, propranolol, protamine, pyridoxine, quiNIDine, raNITIdine, remifentanil, Ringer's, riTUXimab, rocuronium, sargramostim, sodium acetate, streptomycin, succinylcholine, SUFentanil, tacrolimus, telavancin, teniposide, theophylline, thiamine, thiotepa, ticarcillin, ticarcillin-clavulanate, tigecycline, tirofiban, TNA (3-in-1), tobramycin, tolazoline, TPN (2-in-1), trastuzumab, trimetaphan, tubocurarine, urokinase, vancomycin, vasopressin, vecuronium, verapamil, vinBLAStine, vinCRIStine, vinorelbine, vitamin B complex with C, voriconazole

SIDE EFFECTS

CV: Hypotension, bradycardia, dysrhythmias; cardiac arrest (IV)
GI: Vomiting, nausea, constipation
GU: Hypercalciuria, renal calculi
META: Hypercalcemia
INTEG: Pain, burning at IV site, severe venous thrombosis, necrosis, extravasation

PHARMACOKINETICS

Crosses placenta, enters breast milk, excreted via urine and feces, half-life unknown, protein binding 40%-50%
PO: Onset, peak, duration unknown, absorption from GI tract
IV: Onset immediate, duration ½-2 hr

INTERACTIONS

Increase: milk-alkali syndrome—antacids
Increase: dysrhythmias—digoxin glycosides
Increase: toxicity—verapamil, diltiaZEM
Increase: hypercalcemia—thiazide diuretics
Decrease: absorption of fluoroquinolones, tetracyclines, iron salts, phenytoin, thyroid hormones when calcium is taken PO
Decrease: effects of atenolol—verapamil
Drug/Herb
Increase: action/side effects—lily of the valley, pheasant's eye, shark cartilage, squill
Drug/Food
Decrease: calcium absorption—cereal, spinach
Drug/Lab Test
Increase: calcium

NURSING CONSIDERATIONS
Assess:
• **ECG** for decreased QT and T wave inversion: hypercalcemia, product should be reduced or discontinued, consider cardiac monitoring
• Calcium levels during treatment (8.5-11.5 g/dL is normal level); urine calcium if hypercalciuria occurs
• Cardiac status: rate, rhythm, CVP (PWP, PAWP if being monitored directly)
• **Hypocalcemia:** muscle twitching, paresthesia, dysrhythmias, laryngospasm
• **Digoxin therapy:** monitor frequently; an increase in calcium increases digoxin toxicity risk
• Store at room temperature
Evaluate:
• Therapeutic response: decreased twitching, paresthesias, muscle spasms; absence of tremors, seizures, dysrhythmias, dyspnea, laryngospasm; negative Chvostek's sign, negative Trousseau's sign

Teach patient/family:
• To increase fluids to 2 L unless contraindicated; to add bulk to diet for constipation; to notify prescriber of constipation
• Not to switch antacids unless directed by prescriber; not to use as antacid for >2 wk without approval by prescriber
• That therapeutic dose recommendations are figured as elemental calcium
• To avoid excessive use of alcohol, caffeine, tobacco

---

canagliflozin

(kan′a-gli-floe′zin)

Invokana

Func. class.: Oral antidiabetic

Chem. class.: Sodium-glucose co-transporter 2 (SGLT 2) inhibitor

---

ACTION: Blocks glucose reabsorption by the kidney, increases glucose excretion, lowers blood glucose concentrations by inhibiting proximal renal tubular sodium glucose transporter 2 (SGLT2)

USES: Type 2 diabetes mellitus, with diet and exercise; may use in combination

CONTRAINDICATIONS: Dialysis, renal failure, hypersensitivity, breastfeeding, diabetic ketoacidosis
Precautions: Pregnancy, children, renal/hepatic disease, hypothyroidism, hyperglycemia, hypotension, pituitary insufficiency, type 1 diabetes mellitus, malnutrition, fever, dehydration, adrenal insufficiency, geriatric patients

Black Box Warning: Lower limb amputation

DOSAGE AND ROUTES
• **Adult:** PO eGFR ≥60 mL/min/1.73 m² 100 mg/day, may increase to 300 mg/day
Renal dose
• **Adult:** PO eGFR 45-59 mL/min/1.73 m², max 100 mg/day; <45 mL/min/1.73 m² do not use

Available forms: Tabs 100, 300 mg
Administer:
PO route
• Once daily with first meal of the day
• Correct volume depletion before use
• Adjust dose in times of stress, surgery, trauma
• Store at room temperature

SIDE EFFECTS
CV: Hypotension, orthostatic hypotension
GU: *Cystitis, candidiasis, urinary frequency, polydipsia, polyuria,* renal impairment
INTEG: *Photosensitivity, rash, pruritus*
META: *Hypercholesterolemia, lipidemia, hypoglycemia,* hyperkalemia, *hypermagnesemia, hyperphosphatemia,* hypersensitivity, *ketoacidosis*
MISC: Bone fractures

PHARMACOKINETICS
99% protein binding, metabolized by UGT1A9, UGT2B4, excreted 33% in urine, peak 1-2 hr, half-life 10.6-13 hr depending on dose

INTERACTIONS
• Do not use gatifloxacin
Increase: hypoglycemia—sulfonylureas, insulin, MAOIs, salicylates, fibric acid derivatives, bile acid sequestrants, ACE inhibitors, angiotensin II receptor antagonists, beta blockers, SSRIs; monitor for hypoglycemia
Increase: hyperkalemia—potassium-sparing diuretics
Increase or decrease: glycemic control—androgens, lithium, bortezomib, quinolones; monitor for glycemic control
Decrease: effect hyperglycemia—digestive enzymes, intestinal absorbents, thiazide diuretics, loop diuretics, corticosteroids, estrogen, progestins, oral contraceptives, sympathomimetics, isoniazid, phenothiazines; protease inhibitors, atypical antipsychotics, carbonic anhydrase inhibitors, cycloSPORINE, tacrolimus, baclofen, UGT inducers (PHENobarbital, phenytoin, rifAMPin, ritonavir); dose may need to be increased based on eGFR

Drug/Lab

Increase: urine glucose, potassium, lipids, cholesterol, magnesium phosphate, uric acid, serum creatinine

Decrease: serum glucose, eGFR

NURSING CONSIDERATIONS
Assess:

• Hypoglycemia (weakness, hunger, dizziness, tremors, anxiety, tachycardia, sweating), hyperglycemia; even though product does not cause hypoglycemia, if patient is on sulfonylureas or insulin, hypoglycemia may be additive; if hypoglycemia occurs, treat with dextrose, or, if severe, with IV glucagon

• **Ketoacidosis:** monitor for increased ketone levels; may occur with any glucose level, more common in those with severe illnesses

• **Volume depletion:** monitor for orthostatic hypotension, weakness, dizziness; may occur after beginning treatment; correct volume depletion before starting treatment

• For stress, surgery, or other trauma that may require a change in dose

• A1c q3mo; monitor serum glucose 1 hr PP throughout treatment; serum cholesterol, serum creatinine/BUN, serum electrolytes

• **Bone fractures:** monitor bone density, other conditions that may lead to bone fractures; fractures may occur within 3 mo of starting therapy

• **Renal impairment:** monitor more frequently in those with renal disease; increased creatinine, eGFR may be decreased BUN may occur

Black Box Warning: **Lower limb amputation:** Increased risk of amputation; monitor wound and feet closely for complications

• **Pregnancy/breastfeeding:** identify whether pregnancy is planned or suspected or if breastfeeding

Evaluate:

• Therapeutic response: improved signs/symptoms of diabetes mellitus (decreased polyuria, polydipsia, polyphagia); clear sensorium, absence of dizziness, stable gait

Teach patient/family:

• The symptoms of hypo/hyperglycemia, what to do about each

• That medication must be taken as prescribed; explain consequences of discontinuing medication abruptly; that insulin may need to be used for stress, including trauma, fever, surgery, to take as soon as remembered if dose is missed unless close to next dose, then skip and take at next scheduled dose, do not double

• To avoid OTC medications and herbal supplements unless discussed with health care professional

• That diabetes is a lifelong illness; that the diet and exercise regimen must be followed; that this product is not a cure

• To carry emergency ID and glucose source

• That blood glucose monitoring is required to assess product effect

• **Hypersensitivity:** to notify prescriber immediately of itching, hives, rash, swelling of face/lips

Black Box Warning: **Lower limb amputation risk:** Inspect feet; monitor for new ulcerations, wounds; educate about foot care

• Ketoacidosis: to notify prescriber immediately of nausea, vomiting, lack of appetite, sleepiness, difficulty breathing

• **Yeast infections (women/men):** That yeast infections can occur with this product (women, vaginal; men, penile); to report discharge, itching, swelling

• **Pregnancy/breastfeeding:** Not to breastfeed; to advise prescriber if pregnancy is planned or suspected

---

candesartan (Rx)

(can-deh-sartan)

Atacand

Func. class.: Antihypertensive

Chem. class.: Angiotensin II receptor (type AT$_1$) antagonist

Do not confuse:

Atacand/antacid

ACTION: Blocks the vasoconstrictor and aldosterone-secreting effects of angiotensin II; selectively blocks the binding of angiotensin II to the AT_1 receptor found in tissues

USES: Hypertension, alone or in combination; diabetic nephropathy in hypertension and type 2 diabetes

CONTRAINDICATIONS: Hypersensitivity

Black Box Warning: Pregnancy

Precautions: breastfeeding, children, geriatric patients, hypersensitivity to ACE inhibitors, volume depletion, renal/hepatic impairment, renal artery stenosis, hypotension, electrolyte abnormalities

DOSAGE AND ROUTES
Hypertension
• **Adult:** PO single agent 16 mg/day initially in patients who are not volume depleted, range 8-32 mg/day, with diuretic or volume depletion 8-32 mg/day as single dose or divided bid
• **Adolescent and child ≥6 yr and weight >50 kg:** PO 8-16 mg/day or divided bid, adjust to B/P; usual range 4-32 mg/day, max 32 mg/day
• **Child ≥6 yr, weight <50 kg:** PO 2-16 mg/day divided 1-2 doses, max 16 mg/day
• **Child ≥1 yr and <6 yr:** PO 0.2 mg/kg/day in 1 dose or in 2 divided doses, adjust to B/P, max 0.4 mg/kg/day
Heart failure
• **Adult:** PO 4 mg/day, may be doubled ≥2 wk, target dose 32 mg/day
Renal/hepatic disease
• **Adult:** PO ≤8 mg/day for severe renal disease/moderate hepatic disease; adjust dose as needed
Available forms: Tabs 4, 8, 16, 32 mg
Administer:
• Without regard to meals
• Oral liquid (compounded): shake well, do not freeze

SIDE EFFECTS
CNS: *Dizziness,* fatigue, headache, syncope, insomnia

CV: Chest pain, peripheral edema, hypotension, palpitations
EENT: Sinusitis, rhinitis, pharyngitis
GI: *Diarrhea,* nausea, abdominal pain, vomiting
GU: Renal dysfunction
MS: Arthralgia, back pain, myalgia
SYST: Angioedema, hypersensitivity reactions

PHARMACOKINETICS
Peak 3-4 hr, protein binding 90%, half-life 9-12 hr, duration 24 hr, extensively metabolized, excreted in urine (33%) and feces (67%)

INTERACTIONS
Increase: lithium level—lithium
Increase: hyperkalemia—potassium, potassium-sparing diuretics, ACE inhibitors
Increase: hypotension—ACE inhibitors, β-blockers, calcium channel blockers, α-blockers, MAOIs, diuretics
Decrease: hypotensive effect—COX-2 inhibitors, NSAIDs
Drug/Herb
Increase: antihypertensive effect—hawthorn
Decrease: antihypertensive effect—ephedra
Drug/Lab
Increase: albumin, ALT/AST, potassium

NURSING CONSIDERATIONS
Assess
• **Hypotension:** B/P, pulse; note rate, rhythm, quality; notify prescriber of significant changes
• **Electrolytes:** potassium, sodium, calcium; baselines of renal/hepatic studies before therapy begins
• **Hydration:** Skin turgor, dryness of mucous membranes, correct volume depletion
• **Blood studies:** BUN, creatinine, LFTs baseline, all may be increased
• **Serious hypersensitivity reaction:** angioedema, anaphylaxis: facial swelling, difficulty breathing (rare)
• **Hyperkalemia:** more common with other diuretics
• Response and adverse reactions, especially with renal disease; diuretic may be added

---

Side effects: *italics* = common; red = life-threatening

• **Heart failure:** monitor for jugular venous distention, weight, peripheral edema, dyspnea, crackles

Black Box Warning: Pregnancy/breastfeeding: This product can cause fetal death when given during pregnancy; do not breastfeed

Evaluate:
• Therapeutic response: decreased B/P, decreased heart failure–related complications, death

Teach patient/family:
• To notify prescriber of mouth sores, fever, swelling of hands or feet, irregular heartbeat, chest pain
• That excessive perspiration, dehydration, vomiting, diarrhea may lead to fall in B/P; to consult prescriber if these occur
• To avoid all OTC medications unless approved by prescriber; to inform all health care providers of medication use, full effect 4 wk, onset 2 wk; that product may be taken with or without meals; to store at room temperature, to comply with dosage schedule, even if feeling better
• To use proper technique for obtaining B/P; to understand acceptable parameters; to rise slowly to sitting or standing position to minimize orthostatic hypotension; that product may cause dizziness, fainting, light-headedness
• To continue to follow other requirements, no smoking, lose weight, exercise
• To limit potassium foods or salt substitutes/supplements containing potassium unless discussed with health care professional

---

cangrelor (Rx)

(kan′grel-or)

Kengreal

Func. class.: Platelet aggregation inhibitor

Chem. class.: ADP receptor antagonist

ACTION: A direct competitive inhibitor of a platelet receptor, prevents further signaling and platelet activation, results in inhibition of platelet activation and aggregation, does not require hepatic conversion to an active metabolite

USES: For use as an adjunct to percutaneous coronary intervention (PCI) for myocardial infarction prophylaxis, repeat coronary revascularization, and stent thrombosis in patients who have not been treated with a P2Y12 platelet inhibitor and are not being given a glycoprotein IIb/IIIa inhibitor

CONTRAINDICATIONS: Hypersensitivity, active bleeding

Precautions: Pregnancy, breastfeeding, children, increased bleeding risk, neutropenia, agranulocytosis, renal disease

DOSAGE AND ROUTES
• **Adult: IV BOLUS** 30 mcg/kg as a single, then follow immediately by 4 mcg/kg/min continuous IV infusion; the bolus should be given before PCI and maintenance infusion should be continued for ≥2 hr or for the duration of PCI, whichever is longer; use ticagrelor, prasugrel, or clopidogrel to maintain platelet inhibition

Available forms: Powder for injection 50 mg

Administer:
• Visually inspect parenteral products for particulate matter and discoloration before use, use IV only
• **Reconstitution:** Reconstitute by adding 5 mL sterile water for inj to a 50-mg vial, swirl until dissolved, do not shake, allow foam to settle, solution should be clear and colorless to pale yellow, withdraw contents of one reconstituted 50-mg vial and add to one 250-mL bag of 0.9% sodium chloride injection or dextrose 5% injection resulting in a final infusion concentration of 200 mcg/mL; usually, one bag should be sufficient for most patients for ≥2 hr of dosing; those weighing >100 kg will require a minimum of 2 bags
• Use diluted product immediately. When stored at room temperature, diluted product stable for ≤12 hr in dextrose 5% injec-

tion and 24 hr in 0.9% sodium chloride injection, use a dedicated line
• Bolus injection should be administered rapidly (<1 min). The bolus volume may be withdrawn from the diluted infusion bag and given by IV push or using an infusion pump
• Ensure the bolus dose is completely administered before start of PCI
• Start the continuous IV infusion immediately after administration of the bolus; use infusion pump for the continuous IV infusion

SIDE EFFECTS
CNS: Intracranial bleeding
GI: GI bleeding
GU: Hematuria
HEMA: Bleeding
RESP: Wheezing, dyspnea, bronchospasm
SYST: Anaphylaxis, angioedema

PHARMACOKINETICS
Half-life 3-6 min; plasma protein binding 97%; effect on platelets 2 min, excreted in urine

INTERACTIONS
Do not give clopidogrel or prasugrel until infusion is discontinued

NURSING CONSIDERATIONS
Assess:
• **Bleeding:** intracranial, retroperitoneal, other frank bleeding, after completion of infusion, platelet inhibition decreases rapidly within 1 hr; monitor Hct/Hgb
• **Hypersensitivity:** identify if patient has a known cangrelor hypersensitivity
• **Severe renal impairment:** decreased renal function may occur in those with severe renal impairment creatinine clearance >30 mL/min); however, no dosage change is required
• **Pregnancy/breastfeeding:** identify whether the patient is pregnant or breastfeeding; it is not known whether product is excreted in breast milk, no well-controlled studies
Evaluate:
• Therapeutic response: platelet inhibition during PCI

Teach patient/family:
• Use and expected results
• **Pregnancy/breastfeeding:** to inform prescriber if pregnancy is planned or suspected, or if breastfeeding
• **Bleeding:** to report bleeding immediately (blood in stools, urine, gums, bruising)
• **Hypersensitivity:** to report immediately any difficulty breathing, hives, swelling of face, lips, mouth

---

cannabidiol
(ka-na'bi-dye-ole)
Epidiolex
Func. class.: Anticonvulsant
Chem. class.: Cannabinoid

ACTION: Appears to bind to cannabinoid receptors. It may be effective in epilepsy by modulation of the endocannabinoid system

USES: Seizures associated with Lennox-Gastaut syndrome or Dravet syndrome

CONTRAINDICATIONS: Hypersensitivity to this product or sesame seed oil
Precautions: Abrupt discontinuation, breastfeeding, depression, driving or operating machinery, hepatic disease, pregnancy, suicidal ideation

DOSAGE AND ROUTES
• **Adult/adolescent/child ≥2 yr: PO** Initially, 2.5 mg/kg bid; after 1 wk may increase to 5 mg/kg bid, may increase weekly by 2.5 mg/kg bid, max 10 mg/kg bid
Available forms: Solution 100 mg/mL
Administer
• Consistently either with or without food
• Use the adapter and oral dosing syringes provided
• **Storage**: Discard any unused solution remaining 12 wk after first opening the bottle

SIDE EFFECTS
CNS: Drowsiness, dizziness, fatigue, insomnia, irritability, agitation, lethargy, suicidal ideation

---

GI: Anorexia, nausea, diarrhea, weight loss, hepatic dysfunction
HEMA: Anemia
INTEG: Angioedema, erythema
MISC: Infection

PHARMACOKINETICS
Protein binding >94%, metabolized by the liver primarily and the gut by CYP2C19, CYP3A4, UGT1A7, UGT1A9, and UGT2B7, half-life 56 to 61 hr, excreted in feces

Affected cytochrome P450 isoenzymes and drug transporters: CYP1A2, CYP2B6, CYP2C8, CYP2C9, CYP2C19, CYP3A4, UGT1A9, and UGT2B7

INTERACTIONS
Increase: cannabinoid effects—moderate or strong inhibitors of CYP3A4 or CYP2C19; consider dose reduction of cannabidiol
Decrease: cannabinoid effects—strong inducer of CYP3A4 or CYP2C19; consider dose increase of cannabidiol
• Consider a dose reduction of substrates of UGT1A9, UGT2B7, CYP2C8, CYP2C9, and CYP2C19 (clobazam)
• Substrates of CYP1A2 and CYP2B6 may also require dose adjustment

NURSING CONSIDERATIONS
Assess:
• **Seizures:** location, frequency, duration of seizures, with or without aura; EEG will be monitored baseline and periodically
• Suicidal ideation: for changes in behavior, worsening depression, suicidal thoughts, mental status; report these immediately
• **Hepatic dysfunction:** nausea, vomiting, abdominal pain, fatigue, anorexia, jaundice, dark urine; obtain liver function tests baseline and periodically
Evaluate:
• Therapeutic response: decrease in amount and severity of seizures
Teach patient/family:
• How to use the adapter and oral dosing syringes provided; provide instructions for use

• To take consistently either with or without food
• To discard any unused oral solution after 12 wk of first opening the bottle; to take as directed, not to miss or double doses
• That lab work will be necessary before and during treatment
• **Hepatic dysfunction:** to contact health care provider promptly if nausea, vomiting, abdominal pain, fatigue, anorexia, jaundice, or dark urine occurs
• To avoid operating hazardous machinery, driving until response is known; dizziness, drowsiness may occur; to get clearance from prescriber when seizures are controlled
• Suicidal thinking and behavior: that product may increase the risk of suicidal thoughts and behavior; to be alert for worsening depression, changes in mood/behavior, suicidal thoughts or behavior, or thoughts of self-harm; to report any of these behaviors immediately to health care provider
• Not to discontinue abruptly without consulting health care provider; gradually withdraw to reduce possibility for increase in seizures
• **Pregnancy/breastfeeding:** to notify health care provider if pregnancy is planned or suspected; that those who are pregnant and taking this product should register with the North American Antiepileptic Drug (NAAED) Pregnancy Registry, 888-233-2334 or www.aedpregnancyregistry.org; that patients must register themselves
• That a positive cannabis drug screen may occur
• To notify all health care providers of product use
• To carry identification with medications taken, condition being treated, and emergency contacts
• To notify all health care providers of OTC, Rx, herbals, supplements taken and to avoid using new products without approval of health care provider

---

> **⚠ HIGH ALERT**

capecitabine (Rx)

(cap-eh-sit′ah-been)

Xeloda

Func. class.: Antineoplastic, antimetabolite

Chem. class.: Fluoropyrimidine carbamate

Do not confuse:

Xeloda/Xenical

ACTION: Competes with physiologic substrate of DNA synthesis, thereby interfering with cell replication in the S phase of cell cycle (before mitosis); also interferes with RNA and protein synthesis; product is converted to 5-FU

USES: PACLitaxel- and anthracycline-resistant metastatic breast, colorectal cancer when 5-FU monotherapy is preferred; treatment of colorectal cancer patients who have undergone complete resection of their primary tumors

CONTRAINDICATIONS: Pregnancy, hypersensitivity to 5-FU, infants, severe renal impairment (CCr <30 mL/min)

Precautions: Breastfeeding, children, infections, radiation therapy, anticoagulation, geriatric patients, renal/hepatic/cardiac disease, ⬥ DPD deficiency

Black Box Warning: Anticoagulant therapy

DOSAGE AND ROUTES

• **Adult:** PO 2500 mg/m^2/day divided q12hr after a meal × 2 wk, repeat q3wk; Dukes C colon cancer 8 cycles (24 wk), max 5600 mg/day

Renal dose

• **Adult:** PO CCr 30-50 mL/min, decrease initial dose to 75% of usual dose; CCr <30 mL/min, contraindicated

Available forms: Tabs 150, 500 mg

SIDE EFFECTS

CNS: Dizziness, *headache, paresthesia, fatigue,* insomnia

CV: Venous thrombosis, edema, chest pain

GI: *Nausea, vomiting, anorexia, diarrhea, stomatitis, abdominal pain, constipation, dyspepsia,* hyperbilirubinemia

HEMA: Neutropenia, lymphopenia, thrombocytopenia, anemia

INTEG: *Dermatitis,* nail disorders, alopecia, rash

OTHER: *Eye irritation, edema,* limb pain, *pyrexia,* dehydration, renal impairment, Stevens-Johnson syndrome

RESP: *Cough, dyspnea,* pulmonary embolism

PHARMACOKINETICS

Readily absorbed, peak 1^1/$_2$ hr, food decreases absorption, extensively metabolized in the liver, elimination half-life 45 min

INTERACTIONS

Increase: toxicity—leucovorin; monitor for toxicity

Increase: capecitabine levels—antacids (aluminum, magnesium)

Increase: phenytoin level—phenytoin; monitor phenytoin level

Black Box Warning: **Increase:** bleeding risk—anticoagulants, NSAIDs, salicylates, platelet inhibitors, thrombolytics; monitor PT and INR

Drug/Food

Increase: absorption; give within 30 min of a meal

Drug/Lab Test

Increase: bilirubin

Decrease: Hgb/Hct/RBC, neutrophils, platelets, WBC

NURSING CONSIDERATIONS

Assess:

• **Bone marrow suppression,** CBC (RBC, Hct, Hgb), differential, platelet count weekly; withhold product if WBC is <1000/mm^3, platelet count is <50,000/mm^3, or RBC, Hct, Hgb low; notify prescriber of

these results; frequently monitor INR in those receiving warfarin concurrently
• Renal studies: BUN, serum uric acid, urine CCr, electrolytes before, during therapy
• Infection: Monitor temperature q4hr; fever may indicate beginning infection; no rectal temperatures
• Hepatic studies before, during therapy: bilirubin, ALT, AST, alk phos as needed or monthly

Black Box Warning: Bleeding: hematuria, heme-positive stools, bruising or petechiae of mucosa or orifices q8hr; monitor INR and PT in those taking coumarin-derivative anticoagulants; adjustment of dose may be needed

• Dyspnea, crackles, unproductive cough, chest pain, tachypnea, fatigue, increased pulse, pallor, lethargy; personality changes with high doses
• **Hand and foot syndrome/Stevens-Johnson syndrome:** paresthesia, tingling, painful/painless swelling, blistering, erythema with severe pain of hands or feet, toxicity is divided into grade 1, 2, 3; if grade 2 or 3 product should be discontinued until grade 1
• **GI toxicity:** severe diarrhea (multiple times/day or at night), nausea, vomiting, stomatitis, fever; adjust dose, stop treatment if severe
• Buccal cavity q8hr for dryness, sores, ulceration, white patches, oral pain, bleeding, dysphagia
• Fluid, electrolytes may need to be given; elderly patients are at greater risk of GI symptoms
• Rinsing of mouth tid-qid with water, club soda; brushing of teeth bid-tid with soft brush or cotton-tipped applicators for stomatitis; use unwaxed dental floss
Evaluate:
• Therapeutic response: decreased tumor size, spread of malignancy
Teach patient/family:
• To avoid foods with citric acid, hot temperature, or rough texture if stomatitis is present; to take with water within 30 min of end of meal; not to take if dose is missed

• How to take (on for 14 days then 7 days off, then start a new cycle); do not crush, cut
• Not to double dose if dose is missed
• To immediately report severe diarrhea, vomiting, stomatitis, fever of more than 100° F (37.8° C), hand and foot syndrome, anorexia; stop taking product
• **To report signs of infection:** increased temperature, sore throat, flulike symptoms, to avoid crowds, persons with known infections; signs of **anemia:** fatigue, headache, faintness, shortness of breath, irritability; **bleeding;** to avoid use of razors, commercial mouthwash
• OTC antidiarrheals for mild diarrhea (4-6 stools/day or diarrhea at night)
• **Pregnancy/breastfeeding:** To notify prescriber if pregnancy is planned or suspected; to avoid pregnancy while taking this product, use adequate contraception during and for 6 mo after last dose; males should use contraception during and for 3 mo after last dose if partner is of child-bearing potential; not to breastfeed
• That continuing exams and blood work will be needed

---

captopril (Rx)
(kap′toe-pril)
Func. class.: Antihypertensive
Chem. class.: Angiotensin-converting enzyme (ACE) inhibitor

Do not confuse:
captopril/carvedilol

ACTION: Selectively suppresses renin-angiotensin-aldosterone system; inhibits ACE; prevents conversion of angiotensin I to angiotensin II

USES: Hypertension, HF, left ventricular dysfunction after MI, diabetic nephropathy, proteinuria
Unlabeled uses: Acute MI, hypertensive emergency/urgency, scleroderma renal crisis (SRC)

CONTRAINDICATIONS: Breastfeeding, children, hypersensitivity, heart block, potassium-sparing diuretics, bilateral renal artery stenosis, ACE inhibitors, ACE inhibitor–induced angioedema

Precautions: Dialysis patients, hypovolemia, leukemia, scleroderma, SLE, blood dyscrasias, HF, diabetes mellitus, thyroid/renal/hepatic disease, ⚫ African descent, pregnancy 1st trimester, collagen vascular disease, hyperkalemia, hyponatremia

DOSAGE AND ROUTES
Hypertension
• **Adult:** PO initial dose: 12.5-25 mg bid-tid; may increase to 50 mg bid-tid at 1-2 wk intervals; usual range: 25-150 mg bid-tid; max 450 mg/day
• **Child (unlabeled):** PO 0.3-0.5 mg/kg/dose, may titrate up to 6 mg/kg/day in 2-4 divided doses
• **Infant (unlabeled):** PO 0.15-0.3 mg/kg/dose initially, max 6 mg/kg/day
• **Neonate (unlabeled):** PO 0.01-0.1 mg/kg/dose, may increase as needed
Heart failure
• **Adult:** PO 25 mg bid; may increase to 50 mg tid; after 14 days, may increase to 150 mg tid if needed
• **Adolescent (unlabeled):** PO 6.25-12.5 mg q8-12hr titrated up to max 50-75 mg/dose
• **Child (unlabeled):** PO 0.1-2 mg/kg/dose q6-12hr, max 6 mg/kg/day
• **Infant (unlabeled):** PO 0.15-0.3 mg/kg/dose, max 6 mg/kg/day in 1-4 divided doses
• **Neonate (unlabeled):** PO 0.05-0.1 mg/kg q8-24hr titrate to 0.5 mg/kg q6-24hr, max 2 mg/kg/day
Diabetic nephropathy
• **Adult:** PO 25 mg tid
Renal dose
• **Adult:** PO CCr 10-50 mL/min, decrease dose by 25%; CCr <10 mL/min, decrease dose by 50%
Acute MI (unlabeled) or post-MI
• **Adult:** PO 6.25-12.5 mg tid, increase to 25 mg tid gradually

Hypertensive emergency/urgency (unlabeled)
• **Adult:** PO 25 mg, may repeat q30min
Available forms: Tabs 12.5, 25, 50, 100 mg
Administer:
• Store in tight container at 86° F (30° C) or less
• 1 hr before or 2 hr after meals
• Correct volume depletion before starting treatment
• **Oral sol:** may crush 25-mg tab, dissolve in 50-100 mL water; give within ½ hr; make sure tab completely dissolved

SIDE EFFECTS
CNS: Fever, chills, dizziness, drowsiness, fatigue, headache, insomnia, weakness
CV: *Hypotension,* postural hypotension, *tachycardia,* angina
GI: Loss of taste, increased LFTs
GU: Impotence, dysuria, nocturia, proteinuria, nephrotic syndrome, acute reversible renal failure, polyuria, oliguria, urinary frequency
HEMA: Neutropenia, agranulocytosis, pancytopenia, thrombocytopenia, anemia
INTEG: Rash, pruritus
MISC: Angioedema, hyperkalemia
RESP: Bronchospasm, *dyspnea, cough*

PHARMACOKINETICS
Peak 1 hr; duration 2-6 hr; half-life <2 hr, increased in renal disease; metabolized by liver (metabolites); excreted in urine; crosses placenta; excreted in breast milk, small amounts; protein binding 25%-30%

INTERACTIONS
• Do not use with potassium-sparing diuretics, sympathomimetics, potassium supplements
Increase: possible toxicity—lithium, digoxin; monitor individual drug levels
Increase: hyperkalemia—aliskiren
Increase: hypoglycemia—insulin, oral antidiabetics; monitor blood glucose
Increase: hypotension—diuretics, other antihypertensives, acute alcohol ingestion, MAOIs

Decrease: captopril effect—antacids, COX-2 inhibitors, NSAIDs, salicylates

Drug/Herb

Increase: antihypertensive effect—hawthorn

Decrease: antihypertensive effect—ephedra

Drug/Food

Decrease: absorption of captopril

Drug/Lab Test

Increase: AST, ALT, alk phos, bilirubin, uric acid, potassium

Decrease: platelets, WBC, RBC, Hgb/Hct

False positive: urine acetone

Positive: ANA titer

NURSING CONSIDERATIONS

Assess:

• **Blood dyscrasias:** blood studies: decreased platelets; CBC with differential at baseline, q2wk and periodically during 1 yr; if neutrophils <1000/mm^3, discontinue treatment (recommended with collagen-vascular or renal disease)

• **Hypertension:** B/P, pulse rates at baseline, frequently; notify prescriber of significant changes

• **Heart failure:** dyspnea, jugular venous distention, weight gain, edema, rales/crackles in lungs, increased B/P

• Renal studies: protein, BUN, creatinine electrolytes, watch for raised levels, if increased dose may need to be reduced

• **Angioedema/allergic reaction:** rash, fever, pruritus, urticaria; discontinue product if antihistamines fail to help; swelling of lips, mouth, face, difficulty breathing/swallowing (angioedema), provide supportive care, discontinue product

• Monitor AST, ALT alkaline phosphatase, glucose, urine protein bilirubin, uric acid baseline and periodically

• **Cough:** monitor for development of dry cough unexplained by other illness; notify prescriber

Black Box Warning: **Pregnancy/breastfeeding:** Discontinue ACE inhibitors when pregnancy is detected; monitor fetal development regularly; do not breastfeed

Evaluate:

• Therapeutic response: decrease in B/P with hypertension; decreased edema, moist crackles (HF); decreased diabetic nephropathy symptoms

Teach patient/family:

• To take 1 hr before or 2 hr after meals; not to discontinue product abruptly; if dose is missed, take as soon as remembered but not if almost time for next dose; not to double doses, advise patient to tell all persons associated with care that product is being used

• Not to use OTC products (cough, cold, or allergy) unless directed by prescriber; to avoid salt substitutes, high-potassium or high-sodium foods

• To adhere to dosage schedule, even if feeling better

• To rise slowly to sitting or standing position to minimize orthostatic hypotension

• To notify prescriber of fever, swelling of hands or feet, irregular heartbeat, chest pain, signs of angioedema, rash, hoarseness, difficulty breathing

• **Infection:** to report fever, sore throat, flulike symptoms, other signs of infection

• That excessive perspiration, dehydration, vomiting, diarrhea may lead to fall in B/P; to consult prescriber if these occur

• That dizziness, fainting, light-headedness may occur during first few days of therapy; to avoid activities that require concentration

• How to take B/P and when to notify prescriber

• **Diabetes:** to monitor blood glucose often, hypoglycemia

Black Box Warning: **Pregnancy/breastfeeding:** to notify if pregnancy is planned or suspected; not to breastfeed, contraception should be used, if pregnancy occurs, discontinue medication

TREATMENT OF OVERDOSE:
0.9% NaCl IV/INFUSION; hemodialysis

---

carbachol ophthalmic
See Appendix B

carBAMazepine (Rx)

(kar-ba-maz'e-peen)

Carbatrol ♣, Carnexiv, Epitol, Equetro, Mazepine ♣, TEGretol ♣, TEGretol-XR

Func. class.: Anticonvulsant
Chem. class.: Iminostilbene derivative

Do not confuse:

carBAMazepine/OXcarbazepine
TEGretol/Tegrotol XR/Tequin/TRENtal

ACTION: Exact mechanism unknown; appears to decrease polysynaptic responses and block posttetanic potentiation

USES: Tonic-clonic, complex-partial, mixed seizures; trigeminal neuralgia; bipolar disorder
Unlabeled uses: Neurogenic pain

CONTRAINDICATIONS: Pregnancy, hypersensitivity to carBAMazepine or tricyclics, MAOI therapy, bone marrow suppression
Precautions: Breastfeeding, children <6 yr, glaucoma, AV or bundle branch block, cardiac/renal/hepatic disease, psychosis, alcoholism, hepatic porphyria

Black Box Warning: Hematologic disease, ⏣ Asian patients or those with positive HLA-B 1502 or HLA-A 3101 alleles, agranulocytosis, leukopenia, neutropenia, thrombocytopenia

DOSAGE AND ROUTES—NTI
Seizures
• **Adult and child >12 yr:** PO 200 mg bid, may be increased by 200 mg/day in weekly intervals, give in divided doses q6-8hr; maintenance 800-1200 mg/day, max 1600 mg/day (adult); max child 12-15 yr 1000 mg/day; max child >15 yr 1200 mg/day; **EXT REL** give bid; rectal administration of **ORAL SUSP** 200 mg/10 mL or 6 mg/kg as a single dose
• **Child 6-12 yr:** PO tabs 100 mg bid or ext rel 50 mg qid; may increase by <100 mg weekly; max 1000 mg/day, usual dose 15-30 mg/kg/day
• **Child <6 yr:** PO 10-20 mg/kg/day in 2-3 divided doses or 4 divided doses (susp), may increase every wk, do not use ext rel, max 35 mg/kg/day
Trigeminal neuralgia
• **Adult:** PO 100 mg bid with meals; may increase 100 mg q12hr until pain subsides, max 1200 mg/day; maintenance 200-400 mg bid
Diabetic neuropathy (unlabeled)
• **Adult:** PO 100 mg bid or 50 mg qid, titrate to 600-800 mg/day
Bipolar disorder
• **Adult:** PO (Equetro only) 200 mg bid, increase by 200 mg/day until response, max 1600 mg/day
Available forms: Chewable tabs 100, 200 mg; tabs 200 mg; ext rel tabs (XR) 100, 200, 400 mg; oral susp 100 mg/5 mL; ext rel caps 100, 200, 300 mg
Administer:
PO route
• When converting from tabs to oral susp, give same amount/day, or regular release to extended release same amount
• Do not crush, chew ext rel tab; ext rel cap may be opened and beads sprinkled over food; patient should chew chewable tab, not swallow it whole
• With food, milk to decrease GI symptoms
Susp: Turn off NG/enteral feeding 15 min before and hold for 15 min after
• Mix an equal amount of water, D$_5$W, 0.9% NaCl when giving by NG tube; flush tube with 15-30 mL, do not give at same time as other liquid products or diluents
• Shake oral susp before use
• Store at room temperature

SIDE EFFECTS
CNS: *Drowsiness,* dizziness, fatigue, headache, suicidal thoughts/behaviors
CV: Hypertension, AV block, hypotension
EENT: Dry mouth, blurred vision, diplopia, nystagmus

Side effects: *italics* = common; red = life-threatening

ENDO: SIADH (geriatric patients)
GI: *Nausea,* anorexia, increased hepatic enzymes, pancreatitis, hepatotoxicity
GU: retention, increased BUN, renal dysfunction
HEMA: Thrombocytopenia, leukopenia, agranulocytosis, aplastic anemia, eosinophilia, lymphadenopathy
INTEG: *Rash,* Stevens-Johnson syndrome, urticaria, photosensitivity, toxic epidermal necrolysis, DRESS, alopecia, pruritus
RESP: Pulmonary hypersensitivity (fever, dyspnea, pneumonitis)

PHARMACOKINETICS

Onset slow; peak 4-5 hr (PO), 1.5 hr (susp) metabolized by liver; excreted in urine, feces; crosses placenta, blood-brain barrier; excreted in breast milk; half-life 6-12 hr; protein binding 76%; metabolized by CYP3A4

INTERACTIONS

• **Increase:** CNS toxicity—lithium; avoid concurrent use
• **Fatal reaction:** MAOIs; do not use within 14 days of beginning carBAMazepine
• Do not use with: NNRTIs (nonnucleoside reverse transcriptase inhibitors), nefazodone

Increase: carBAMazepine levels—CYP3A inhibitors (cimetidine, clarithromycin, danazol, diltiaZEM, erythromycin, FLUoxetine, fluvoxaMINE, isoniazid, valproic acid, verapamil, voriconazole), SSRIs, tricyclics; adjust dose if needed, or do not use together
Increase: effects of desmopressin, lithium, lypressin, vasopressin
Decrease: carBAMazepine effect—CYP1A2, CYP2C9 substrates
Decrease: effect of CYP3A inducers
Decrease: effects of benzodiazepines, doxycycline, felbamate, haloperidol, oral contraceptives, PHENobarbital, phenytoin, primidone, theophylline, thyroid hormones, warfarin; adjust dose as needed
Decrease: carBAMazepine levels—CYP3A4 inducers (CISplatin, darunavir, delavirdine, DOXOrubicin, felbamate, nefazodone, OXcarbazepine, PHENobarbital, phenytoin, primidone, rifAMPin, theophylline); monitor carBAMazepine effectiveness

Drug/Herb
Decrease: carBAMazepine metabolism, increased levels—echinacea
Decrease: anticonvulsant effect—St. John's wort

Drug/Food
Increase: peak concentration of carBAMazepine—grapefruit juice; avoid use

Drug/Lab Test
Decrease: serum calcium, sodium
Increase: cholesterol

NURSING CONSIDERATIONS
Assess:

> Black Box Warning: ✒ Asian patients for serious skin reaction; genetic test for ✒ HLA-B1502 allele before administration; these patients may develop toxic epidermal necrolysis, Stevens-Johnson syndrome, DRESS; may be fatal

• **Seizures:** character, location, duration, intensity, frequency, presence of aura, in mixed seizure disorder, worsening of symptoms may occur
• **Trigeminal neuralgia:** facial pain, including location, duration, intensity, character, activity that stimulates pain
• Renal studies: urinalysis, BUN, urine creatinine q3mo
• **Bipolar disorder:** assess for symptoms at baseline and during treatment
• **DRESS:** fever, lymphadenopathy with multiorgan involvement, including liver, kidney, cardiac; discontinue carBAMazepine

> Black Box Warning: **Bone marrow depression:** blood studies: CBC reticulocyte counts every wk for 4 wk, then q3-6mo if on long-term therapy; if myelosuppression occurs, product should be discontinued; blood dyscrasias: fever, sore throat, bruising, rash, jaundice, agranulocytosis, and aplastic anemia may occur

• Blood studies: ALT, AST, bilirubin; serum calcium, may be decreased and lead to osteoporosis; cholesterol periodically

• Drug levels during initial treatment or when changing dose; should remain at 4-12 mcg/mL; anorexia may indicate increased blood levels

• **Mental status:** mood, sensorium, affect, behavioral changes, **suicidal thoughts/behaviors;** if mental status changes, notify prescriber

• **Eye problems:** need for ophthalmic examinations before, during, after treatment (slit lamp, funduscopy, tonometry)

• **Allergic reaction:** purpura, red, raised rash; if these occur, product should be discontinued; increased risk if past hypersensitivity to hydantoins

• *Toxicity:* bone marrow depression, nausea, vomiting, ataxia, diplopia, CV collapse

• Hard candy, gum, frequent rinsing for dry mouth

• **Beers:** Avoid use in older adults unless safer alternative is unavailable; ataxia, impaired psychomotor function may occur

Evaluate:

• Therapeutic response: decreased seizure activity; document on patient's chart

Teach patient/family:

• To carry emergency ID stating patient's name, products taken, condition, prescriber's name, and phone number

• To avoid driving, other activities that require alertness usually for the first 3 days of treatment; dizziness, drowsiness may occur

• Not to discontinue medication quickly after long-term use; seizures may occur

• To immediately report chills, rash, light-colored stools, dark urine, yellowing of skin and eyes, abdominal pain, sore throat, mouth ulcers, bruising, blurred vision, dizziness, skin rash, fever

• That urine may turn pink to brown

• Not to use with grapefruit juice; to take on an empty stomach; that toxicity may occur

• **Pregnancy/breastfeeding:** to notify health care provider if pregnancy is planned or suspected; not to breastfeed; that if pregnant, patient should register with American Antiepileptic Drug Pregnancy Registry, 888-233-2334, to use nonhormonal contraceptive

• That ophthalmic examinations will be needed; to report changes in vision

TREATMENT OF OVERDOSE: Lavage, VS

⚠ HIGH ALERT

CARBOplatin (Rx)

(kar-boe-pla′-tin)

Func. class.: Antineoplastic alkylating agent

Chem. class.: Platinum coordination compound

Do not confuse:
CARBOplatin/CISplatin

ACTION: Produces interstrand DNA cross-links and, to a lesser extent, DNA-protein cross-links; activity is not cell-cycle–phase specific

USES: Advanced ovarian cancer in combination with other agents; palliative treatment of ovarian carcinoma recurrent after treatment with other antineoplastic agents

CONTRAINDICATIONS: Pregnancy, breastfeeding, hypersensitivity, significant bleeding, aluminum products used to prepare or administer CARBOplatin

Black Box Warning: Severe bone marrow depression, platinum compound hypersensitivity (anaphylaxis)

Precautions: Geriatric patients, radiation therapy within 1 mo, other cancer chemotherapy within 1 mo, renal/hepatic disease, hearing impairment, infection

Black Box Warning: Anemia, chemotherapy-induced nausea/vomiting; requires a specialized care setting and an experienced clinician

DOSAGE AND ROUTES

• **Adult: IV INFUSION** 300 mg/m² on day 1 with cyclophosphamide, 600 mg/

Side effects: *italics* = common; red = life-threatening

m^2 **IV** on day 1, repeat q4wk × 6 cycles; refractory tumors 360 mg/m^2 single dose, may repeat q4wk as needed

Renal Dose

Adult: (single agent) IV INF CCr 41–59 mL/min 250mg/m2; CCr 16–40mL/min 200mg mg/m2; do not use if CCr < 15 mL/min

Available forms: Sol for injection 10 mg/mL

Administer:

Black Box Warning: Give antiemetic 30-60 min before product and prn for vomiting

IV route

• Do not use needles or IV administration sets that contain aluminum; may cause precipitate or loss of potency
• Use cytotoxic handling procedures
• Store protected from light at room temperature; reconstituted vials stable for 24 hr at room temperature, solutions further diluted in D$_5$W or NS are stable for 8 hr at room temperature. Paraplatin multidose (10 mg/mL) vials stable for up to 14 days after entry into vial
• Reconstitute CARBOplatin 50, 150, or 450 mg with 5, 15, or 45 mL, respectively, of sterile water for inj, D$_5$W, or NaCl (10 mg/mL); then further **dilute** with the same sol to 0.5-4 mg/mL; **give** over 15 min-1 hr (intermittent INFUSION)
• **Continuous IV INFUSION** give over 24 hr; max dose based on (GFR=125 mg/mL)

Solution compatibilities: D$_5$/0.2% NaCl, D$_5$/0.45% NaCl, D$_5$/0.9% NaCl, 0.9% NaCl, D$_5$W, sterile water for inj

Y-site compatibilities: Acyclovir, alfentanil, allopurinol, amifostine, amikacin, aminocaproic acid, aminophylline, amiodarone, amphotericin B lipid complex, amphotericin B liposome, ampicillin, ampicillin-sulbactam, anidulafungin, atenolol, atracurium, azithromycin, aztreonam, bivalirudin, bleomycin, bumetanide, buprenorphine, butorphanol, calcium chloride/gluconate, caspofungin, ceFAZolin, cefepime, cefotaxime, cefoTEtan, cefOXitin, cefTAZidime, ceftizoxime, cefTRIAXone, cefuroxime, cimetidine, ciprofloxacin, cisatracurium, CISplatin, cladribine, clindamycin, codeine, cyclophosphamide, cycloSPORINE, cytarabine, DAPTOmycin, DAUNOrubicin, dexamethasone, dexmedetomidine, dexrazoxane, digoxin, diltiaZEM, diphenhydrAMINE, DOBUTamine, DOCEtaxel, DOPamine, doripenem, doxacurium, DOXOrubicin, DOXOrubicin liposomal, doxycycline, droperidol, enalaprilat, ePHEDrine, EPINEPHrine, epiRUBicin, ertapenem, erythromycin, esmolol, etoposide, famotidine, fenoldopam, fentaNYL, filgrastim, fluconazole, fludarabine, fluorouracil, foscarnet, fosphenytoin, furosemide, ganciclovir, gatifloxacin, gemcitabine, gentamicin, granisetron, haloperidol, heparin, hydrocortisone, HYDROmorphone, hydrOXYzine, IDArubicin, ifosfamide, imipenem-cilastatin, inamrinone, insulin (regular), irinotecan, isoproterenol, ketorolac, labetalol, levoFLOXacin, levorphanol, lidocaine, linezolid injection, LORazepam, magnesium sulfate, mannitol, melphalan, meperidine, meropenem, mesna, methohexital, methotrexate, methylPREDNISolone, metoclopramide, metoprolol, metroNIDAZOLE, micafungin, midazolam, milrinone, minocycline, mitoXANTRONE, mivacurium, morphine, nafcillin, nalbuphine, naloxone, nesiritide, niCARdipine, nitroglycerin, nitroprusside, norepinephrine, octreotide, ofloxacin, ondansetron, oxaliplatin, PACLitaxel, palonosetron, pamidronate, pancuronium, pantoprazole, PEMEtrexed, pentamidine, PENTobarbital, PHENobarbital, phenylephrine, piperacillin, piperacillin-tazobactam, potassium chloride, potassium phosphates, prochlorperazine, promethazine, propofol, propranolol, raNITIdine, remifentanil, riTUXimab, rocuronium, sargramostim, sodium acetate, sodium bicarbonate, sodium phosphates, succinylcholine, SUFentanil, sulfamethoxazole-trimethoprim, tacrolimus, teniposide, theophylline, thiotepa, ticarcillin, ticarcillin-clavulanate, tigecycline, tirofiban, TNA, tobramycin, topotecan, TPN, trastuzumab, trimethobenzamide, vancomycin, vasopressin, vecuronium, verapamil, vinBLAStine, vinCRIStine, vinorelbine, voriconazole, zidovudine

SIDE EFFECTS

CNS: Central neurotoxicity, *peripheral neuropathy,* dizziness, confusion
CV: Cardiac abnormalities (fatal CV events), stroke, HF, embolism
EENT: Tinnitus, hearing loss
GU: Nephrotoxicity
GI: *Severe nausea, vomiting,* diarrhea, weight loss, mucositis, anorexia, constipation, taste change
HEMA: Thrombocytopenia, leukopenia, neutropenia, anemia
INTEG: Dermatitis, rash
META: Hypomagnesemia, hypocalcemia, hypokalemia, hyponatremia, hyperuricemia
SYST: Anaphylaxis, hypersensitivity

PHARMACOKINETICS

Initial half-life 2-6 hr, postdistribution half-life $2\frac{1}{2}$-6 hr, not bound to plasma proteins, excreted by the kidneys

INTERACTIONS

• Do not use with or within 3 mo of live virus vaccines
Increase: nephrotoxicity or ototoxicity—aminoglycosides, amphotericin B
Increase: toxicity—radiation, bone marrow suppressants; monitor for blood counts often
Increase: myelosuppression—myelosuppressives
Decrease: phenytoin levels; monitor levels
Drug/Lab Test
Increase: AST, BUN, alk phos, bilirubin, creatinine
Decrease: platelets, neutrophils, WBC, RBC, Hgb/Hct, calcium, potassium, magnesium, phosphate

NURSING CONSIDERATIONS
Assess:

Black Box Warning: To be used only in a specialized care setting by a person experienced in the use of chemotherapeutic products

Black Box Warning: **Bone marrow depression:** CBC, differential, platelet count weekly; withhold product if neutrophil count is <2000/mm³ or platelet count is <100,000/mm³; notify prescriber of results; calcium, magnesium, phosphate, potassium, sodium, uric acid, CCr, bilirubin; CCr <60 mL/min may be responsible for increased bone marrow suppression; assess frequently for infection and treat active infection before use

Black Box Warning: **Nausea/vomiting:** may occur a few hr after administration; antiemetics are used, give fluids, food as tolerated

• Renal studies: BUN, creatinine, serum uric acid; urine CCr before, during therapy; I&O ratio; report fall in urine output to <30 mL/hr
• Hepatic studies before, during therapy (bilirubin, AST, ALT, LDH) as needed or monthly; jaundice of skin, sclera; dark urine, clay-colored stools, itchy skin, abdominal pain, fever, diarrhea

Black Box Warning: **Anaphylaxis:** hypotension, rash, pruritus, wheezing, tachycardia may occur within a few minutes of use; notify prescriber after discontinuing product; resuscitation equipment, corticosteroids, EPINEPHrine should be available

• **Peripheral neuropathy:** may be increased in geriatric patients
• **Beers:** Use with caution in older adults; may exacerbate or cause syndrome of inappropriate antidiuretic hormone secretion or hyponatremia
Evaluate:
• Therapeutic response: decreasing size of tumor, spread of malignancy
Teach patient/family:
• To report ringing/roaring in the ears; numbness, tingling in face, extremities; weight gain
• **Pregnancy/breastfeeding:** that impotence or amenorrhea can occur; that this is reversible after treatment is

discontinued; to notify prescriber if pregnancy is suspected or planned; that contraception should be used if patient is fertile; not to breastfeed during treatment
• To avoid OTC products with aspirin, NSAIDs, alcohol; not to receive live virus vaccines during treatment or for 3 mo after completion of treatment
• To notify prescriber immediately of fever, fatigue, sore throat, bleeding, bruising, chills, back pain, dyspnea, tingling in extremities, blood in stools, urine, emesis
• To avoid crowds, persons with known infections; to avoid the use of razors, stiff-bristle toothbrushes

---

⚠ HIGH ALERT

RARELY USED

carfilzomib

(car-fil′zoe-mib)

Kyprolis

Func. class.: Antineoplastic biologic response modifiers

Chem. class.: Signal transduction inhibitors (STIs)

ACTION: Antiproliferative and proapoptotic activity

USES: Multiple myeloma in those who have received ≥2 therapies (including bortezomib and immunomodulatory agents)

CONTRAINDICATIONS: Pregnancy, hypersensitivity

DOSAGE AND ROUTES

• **Adult:** IV 20 mg/m^2 over 2-10 min on days 1, 2, 8, 9, 15, 16, then 12-day rest (days 17-28), then may increase to 27 mg/m^2 on days 1, 2, 8, 9, 15, 16 repeated every 28 days
• Refer to package insert for dosage adjustments for treatment-related toxicity

---

RARELY USED

carglumic acid

(kar-gloo′mik)

Carbaglu

Func. class.: Antihyperammonemic agent

USES: Acute or chronic hyperammonemia in persons with *N*-acetylglutamate synthetase deficiency

DOSAGE AND ROUTES

• **Adult/child:** PO 100-250 mg/kg/day (rounded to the nearest 100 mg) initially, divided bid-qid, given immediately before meals, titrate to ammonia level; usual maintenance dose <100 mg/kg/day

---

carisoprodol (Rx)

(kar-eye-soe-proe′dole)

Soma

Func. class.: Skeletal muscle relaxant, central acting

Chem. class.: Meprobamate congener

Controlled Substance Schedule IV

Do not confuse:
Soma/Soma Compound

ACTION: Depresses CNS by blocking interneuronal activity in descending reticular formation, spinal cord, thereby producing sedation and possibly altering pain perception

USES: Relieving pain, stiffness with musculoskeletal disorders

CONTRAINDICATIONS: Hypersensitivity to these products or carbamates, intermittent porphyria
Precautions: Pregnancy, breastfeeding, geriatric patients, ⚛ Asian patients, renal/hepatic disease, substance abuse,

---

seizure disorder, CNS depression, abrupt discontinuation

DOSAGE AND ROUTES
• **Adult/adolescent ≥16 yr: PO** 250-350 mg qid, max 3 wk of use
Available forms: Tabs 250, 350 mg
Administer:
• With meals for GI symptoms
• For short term (2-3 wk), potential for habituation
• Store in tight container at room temperature

SIDE EFFECTS
CNS: *Dizziness, weakness, drowsiness,* headache, insomnia, irritability
CV: Postural hypotension, tachycardia
GI: *Nausea,* vomiting, hiccups, epigastric discomfort
HEMA: Eosinophilia, leukopenia
INTEG: Rash, facial flushing, erythema multiforme
RESP: Asthmatic attacks
SYST: Angioedema, anaphylaxis

PHARMACOKINETICS
PO: Onset ½ hr; peak 4 hr; duration 4-6 hr; extensively metabolized by liver, substrate of CYP2C19 ⟳, some Asians, blacks, whites are poor metabolizers; excreted in urine; crosses placenta; excreted in breast milk (large amounts); half-life 8 hr

INTERACTIONS
• Do not use together with meprobamate
Increase: CNS depression—alcohol, tricyclics, opioids, barbiturates, sedatives, hypnotics; avoid concurrent use
Increase: carisoprodol metabolite, decreasing carisoprodol effect—CYP2C19 inhibitors (FLUoxetine, fluvoxaMINE, isoniazid, modafinil)
Decrease: carisoprodol metabolism, increasing carisoprodol effect—CYP219 inducers (rifAMPin)
Drug/Herb
Increase: CNS depression—kava, valerian
Increase: metabolism of carisoprodol—St. John's wort
Drug/Lab Test

Increase: eosinophils
Increase: RBC, WBC, platelets

NURSING CONSIDERATIONS
Assess:
• **Pain,** stiffness, mobility, activities of daily living at baseline and throughout treatment
• **Idiosyncratic reaction:** (weakness, dizziness, blurred vision, confusion, euphoria), anaphylaxis within a few minutes or hours of 1st to 4th dose, withhold and notify prescriber, usually seen in poor CYP2C19 metabolizers
• **Allergic reactions:** rash, fever, respiratory distress, anaphylaxis, angioedema
• **CNS depression:** dizziness, drowsiness, psychiatric symptoms, abuse potential
• **Abrupt discontinuation:** withdrawal reactions do occur but may be mild, dependence may occur
• **Beers:** avoid in older adults; may cause sedation, anticholinergic effects; may decrease urinary flow, cause retention (men)
Evaluate:
• Therapeutic response: decreased pain, spasticity; increased ROM
Teach patient/family:
• There is a hight incidence of dependence when using this product
• To avoid hazardous activities if drowsiness, dizziness occur; not to drive while taking product; to avoid rapid position changes, postural hypotension occurs, not to use for >2-3 wk
• To avoid using OTC medications (cough preparations, antihistamines) unless directed by prescriber; not to take with alcohol, other CNS depressants; that there is a high incidence of dependence when using this product
• **Idiosyncratic reaction:** to report weakness, dizziness, blurred vision, confusion, euphoria; if these occur, to withhold product and call prescriber
• **To report allergic reaction immediately:** rash, swelling of tongue/lips, hives, dyspnea
• To take with food or milk for GI symptoms

• **Pregnancy/breastfeeding:** If pregnancy is planned or suspected or if breastfeeding

TREATMENT OF OVERDOSE: Dialysis, lavage

⚠ HIGH ALERT

carmustine (Rx)
(kar-mus'teen)
BiCNU, Gliadel
Func. class.: Antineoplastic alkylating agent
Chem. class.: Nitrosourea

ACTION: Alkylates DNA, RNA; able to inhibit enzymes that allow for the synthesis of amino acids in proteins; activity is not cell-cycle–phase specific

USES: Brain tumors such as glioblastoma, medulloblastoma, brain stem glioma, astrocytoma, ependymoma, metastatic brain tumors; multiple myeloma (with predniSONE), non-Hodgkin's disease, Hodgkin's disease, other lymphomas; GI, breast, bronchogenic, renal carcinomas; wafer, as adjunct to surgery/radiation for patients newly diagnosed with high-grade malignant glioma
Unlabeled uses: Ablation, mycosis fungoides, stem cell transplant preparation

CONTRAINDICATIONS: Pregnancy, breastfeeding, hypersensitivity, leukopenia, thrombocytopenia
Precautions: Dental disease, extravasation, females, infection, secondary malignancy, thrombocytopenia, renal disease

Black Box Warning: Bone marrow suppression, pulmonary fibrosis, bleeding, infection

DOSAGE AND ROUTES
Brain tumors, Hodgkin's disease, malignant lymphoma, multiple myeloma
• **Adult: IV** 75-100 mg/m² over 1-2 hr × 2 days or 150-200 mg/m² × 1 dose

q6-8wk or 40-75 mg/m²/day × 5 days q6wk **INTRACAVITARY** up to 8 wafers inserted into resection cavity
• **Child (unlabeled): IV** 200-250 mg/m² as a single dose q4-6wk
Stem cell transplant/bone marrow ablation (unlabeled)
• **Adult: IV** 450-600 mg/m² as a single dose or 2 divided doses q12hr at a rate of no more than 3 mg/m²/min
Available forms: Powder for inj 100 mg; wafer 7.7 mg (intracavitary)
Administer:
• Store reconstituted sol in refrigerator for 24 hr or at room temperature for 8 hr; protect from light
• Blood transfusions, RBC colony-stimulating factors to counter anemia
• Antiemetic, serotonin antagonists, dexamethasone
• All medications PO, if possible; avoid IM inj if platelets are <100,000/mm³

Black Box Warning: Carmustine should not be given until platelets >100,000/mm³ and WBC >4000/mm²

Wafer route
• Use cytotoxic handling procedures
• If wafers are broken into several pieces, they should not be used
• Foil pouches may be kept at room temperature for 6 hr if unopened
Intermittent IV INFUSION route
• Use cytotoxic handling procedures; do not use if an oil film appears on vial (decomposition)
• Do not use with PVC IV tubing, do not admix
• After **diluting** 100 mg product/3 mL ethyl alcohol (provided), **further dilute** with 100-500 mL 0.9% NaCl or D₅W, **give** over 1 hr or more, reduce rate if discomfort is felt; use only glass containers, protect from light
• **Flush** IV line after carmustine with 10 mL 0.9% NaCl to prevent irritation at site

Y-site compatibilities: Amifostine, amphotericin B lipid complex, amphotericin B liposome, anidulafungin, aztreonam, bivalirudin, bleomycin, caspofungin, cefepime, codeine, DAPTOmycin, dexmedetomidine, DOCEtaxel, ertapenem, etoposide, fenoldopam, filgrastim, fludarabine, gemcitabine, granisetron, levoFLOXacin, melphalan, meperidine, mitoXANTRONE, nesiritide, octreotide, ondansetron, PACLitaxel, palonosetron, pamidronate, pantoprazole, PEMEtrexed, piperacillin-tazobactam, riTUXimab, sargramostim, sodium acetate, tacrolimus, teniposide, thiotepa, tigecycline, tirofiban, trastuzumab, vinCRIStine, vinorelbine, voriconazole

SIDE EFFECTS

GI: *Nausea, vomiting, anorexia, stomatitis,* hepatotoxicity

GU: *Azotemia,* renal failure

HEMA: Thrombocytopenia, leukopenia, myelosuppression, anemia

INTEG: Pain, burning, hyperpigmentation at inj site, alopecia

RESP: Fibrosis, pulmonary infiltrate

SYST: Secondary malignant neoplastic disease

PHARMACOKINETICS

Degraded within 15 min; crosses blood-brain barrier; 70% excreted in urine within 96 hr; 10% excreted as CO_2, fate of 20% is unknown

INTERACTIONS

Increase: bleeding risk—aspirin, anticoagulants, platelets inhibitors

Increase: myelosuppression—myelosuppressive agents, cimetidine

Increase: toxicity—other antineoplastics, radiation, cimetidine

Increase: adverse reactions, decreased antibody reaction—live vaccines

Decrease: effects of digoxin, phenytoins

Drug/Lab Test

Increase: bilirubin, prolactin, uric acid, LFTs

Decrease: platelets, WBC, neutrophils, Hct

NURSING CONSIDERATIONS

Assess:

Black Box Warning: **Bone marrow suppression:** CBC, differential, platelet count weekly; withhold product if WBC is <4000 or platelet count is <100,000; notify prescriber of results

• Hepatic studies: AST, ALT, bilirubin; monitor regularly; hepatotoxicity occurs rarely

• **Pregnancy/breastfeeding:** identify if pregnancy is planned or suspected, or if breastfeeding; do not use in pregnancy, breastfeeding; contraception should be used

Black Box Warning: **Pulmonary fibrosis/infiltrate:** pulmonary function tests, chest x-ray films before, during therapy; chest film should be obtained q2wk during treatment; monitor for dyspnea, cough, pulmonary fibrosis; infiltrate occurs after high doses or several low-dose courses (>1400 mg/m^2 cumulative dose), may occur months or years after treatment

Black Box Warning: Only to be used by an experienced clinician in cases of cancer, immune suppression

• Renal studies: BUN, serum uric acid, urine CCr before, during therapy; I&O ratio; report fall in urine output of 30 mL/hr, may use allopurinol for hyperuricemia with increased fluids

• Monitor for cold, cough, fever (may indicate beginning infection)

• **Bleeding:** hematuria, guaiac, bruising, petechiae, mucosa, orifices q8hr

• Rinsing of mouth tid-qid with water or club soda; use of sponge brush for stomatitis

• Warm compresses at inj site for inflammation; reduce flow rate if patient complains of burning at infusion site

Evaluate:

• Therapeutic response: decreasing size of tumor, spread of malignancy

Teach patient/family:

Black Box Warning: To report any changes in breathing or coughing; to avoid smoking

• To avoid foods with citric acid, hot temperature, or rough texture if stomatitis is present; to report any bleeding, white spots, ulceration in mouth to prescriber; to examine mouth daily

---

Side effects: *italics* = common; red = life-threatening

• To avoid aspirin, ibuprofen, razors, commercial mouthwash
• To report signs of anemia (fatigue, irritability, shortness of breath, faintness); to report signs of infection (sore throat, fever); pulmonary toxicity can occur up to 15 yr after treatment
• **Pregnancy/breastfeeding:** to use contraception during treatment; not to breastfeed
• Not to receive live vaccines during treatment
• That infusion can be painful to veins and that product contains ethanol
• To report chest pain

---

carteolol (ophthalmic)

(kar·tee-oh-lol)
Func. class.: Antiglaucoma
Chem. class.: β-Blocker

ACTION: May decrease aqueous humor and increase outflows

USES: Treatment of chronic open-angle glaucoma and ocular hypertension

CONTRAINDICATIONS: Hypersensitivity, AV block, heart failure, bradycardia, sick sinus syndrome
Precautions: Abrupt discontinuation, children, pregnancy, breastfeeding, COPD, depression, diabetes mellitus, myasthenia gravis, hyperthyroidism, pulmonary disease, angle-closure glaucoma

DOSAGE AND ROUTES
• **Adult:** Instill 1 drop in the affected eye(s) bid
Available forms: Ophthalmic solution 1%
Administer:
• For ophthalmic use only
• Do not touch the tip of the dropper to the eye, fingertips, or other surface to prevent contamination
• Wash hands before and after use; tilt head back slightly and pull the lower eyelid down with the index finger; squeeze the prescribed number of drops into the pouch; close eyes to spread; to

avoid excessive systemic absorption, apply finger pressure on the lacrimal sac for 1-2 min after use
• If more than one topical ophthalmic drug product is being used, the drugs should be administered at least 5 min apart
• Decreased intraocular pressure can take several weeks; monitor IOP after 1 mo

SIDE EFFECTS
CNS: Insomnia, headache, dizziness
CV: Palpitations
EENT: Eye stinging/burning, tearing, photophobia, sinusitis

INTERACTIONS
Increase: β-blocking effect—oral β-blockers
Increase: intraocular pressure reduction—topical miotics, dipivefrin, EPINEPHrine, carbonic anhydrase inhibitors; this may be beneficial
Increase: B/P, severe—when abruptly stopping cloNIDine
Increase: depression of AV nodal conduction, bradycardia, or hypotension—adenosine, cardiac glycosides, disopyramide, other antiarrhythmics, class 1C antiarrhythmic drugs (flecainide, propafenone, moricizine, encainide, quiNIDine, or drugs that significantly depress AV nodal conduction)
Increase: AV block nodal conduction, induce AV block—high doses of procainamide
Increase: antihypertensive effect—other antihypertensives

NURSING CONSIDERATIONS
Assess:
• **Systemic absorption:** when used in the eye, systemic absorption is common with the same adverse reactions and interactions
• Glaucoma: monitor intraocular pressure
Evaluate:
• Decreasing intraocular pressure
Teach patient/family:
• For ophthalmic use only

• Not to touch the tip of the dropper to the eye, fingertips, or other surface to prevent contamination

• To wash hands before and after use; tilt the head back slightly and pull the lower eyelid down with the index finger to form a pouch; squeeze the prescribed number of drops into the pouch; close eyes to spread drops; to avoid excessive systemic absorption, apply finger pressure on the lacrimal sac for 1-2 min following use

• If more than one topical ophthalmic drug product is being used, the drugs should be administered at least 5 min apart

---

⚠ HIGH ALERT

carvedilol (Rx)

(kar-ved′i-lole)

Coreg, Coreg CR

Func. class.: Antihypertensive, α-/β-adrenergic blocker

Do not confuse:
carvedilol/captopril

ACTION: A mixture of nonselective α-/β-adrenergic blocking activity; decreases cardiac output, exercise-induced tachycardia, reflex orthostatic tachycardia; causes vasodilation, reduction in peripheral vascular resistance

USES: Essential hypertension alone or in combination with other antihypertensives, HF, LV dysfunction after MI, cardiomyopathy
Unlabeled uses: Angina, pediatric patients, atrial fibrillation/flutter

CONTRAINDICATIONS: Hypersensitivity, asthma, class IV decompensated cardiac failure, 2nd- or 3rd-degree heart block, cardiogenic shock, severe bradycardia, pulmonary edema, severe hepatic disease, sick sinus symptoms
Precautions: Pregnancy, breastfeeding, children, geriatric patients, cardiac failure, hepatic injury, peripheral vascular disease, anesthesia, major surgery, diabetes mellitus, thyrotoxicosis, emphysema, chronic bronchitis, renal disease, abrupt discontinuation

DOSAGE AND ROUTES
Hypertension
• **Adult:** PO 6.25 mg bid × 7-14 days; may increase to 25 mg bid; max 50 mg/day; **EXT REL** cap 20 mg/day, may double after 7-14 days to 40 mg/day, max 80 mg/day

Heart failure
• **Adult:** PO 3.125 mg bid × 2 wk; may increase to give 6.25 mg bid × 2 wk, then double q2wk to max dose of 25 mg bid <85 kg or 50 mg bid >85 kg; **EXT REL** caps (Coreg CR) 10 mg/day × 2 wk, increase to 20, 40, 80 mg/day over successive intervals of 2 wk

Postmyocardial infarction
• **Adult:** PO 6.25 mg bid × 2 wk; titrate upward as tolerated q2wk; may increase to 12.5 mg bid, then titrate to 25 mg bid; **PO EXT REL** 20 mg daily; titrate upward after 3-10 days, increase to 40 mg daily; max 80 mg/day

Available forms: Tabs 3.125, 6.25, 12.5, 25 mg; ext rel cap 10, 20, 40, 80 mg
Administer:
• With food to minimize orthostatic hypotension; regular tabs may be crushed or swallowed whole; give ext rel every AM with food; do not break, crush, chew ext rel cap; separate alcohol (including OTC products that contain ethanol) by ≥2 hr; caps may be opened and sprinkled over applesauce

• Take apical pulse before use; notify prescriber if <50 bpm and hold dose

• Conversion from immediate release to extended release: 3.125 mg bid is 10 mg qd; 6.25 mg bid is 20 mg qd; 12.5 mg bid is 40 mg qd; 25 mg bid is 80 mg qd

• Do not discontinue before surgery

SIDE EFFECTS
CNS: *Dizziness, fatigue, weakness,* somnolence, insomnia, ataxia, drowsiness, memory loss, paresthesia, vertigo, depression
CV: Bradycardia, *postural hypotension,* HF, pulmonary edema

GI: *Diarrhea,* abdominal pain, constipation, nausea, vomiting
GU: Decreased libido, *impotence*
INTEG: Rash, Stevens-Johnson syndrome, toxic epidermal necrolysis
MISC: Pruritus, *hyperglycemia,* weight gain, anaphylaxis, angioedema, lupus-like syndrome
RESP: Dyspnea, bronchospasm
EENT: Blurred vision, floppy iris syndrome, dry eyes

PHARMACOKINETICS
Peak 1-2 hr; duration 7-9 hr; ext rel onset 30 min, peak 5 hr, readily and extensively absorbed PO; >98% protein binding; extensively metabolized (CYP2D6, CYP2C9) by liver; excreted through bile into feces; half-life 7-10 hr with increases in geriatric patients, hepatic disease; ✱ some individuals may be poor metabolizers

INTERACTIONS
Increase: conduction disturbances—calcium channel blockers
Increase: carvedilol level—CYP2D6 inhibitors (FLUoxetine, quiNIDine)
Increase: bradycardia, hypotension—levodopa, MAOIs
Increase: hypoglycemia—antidiabetic agents, monitor blood glucose level, dosage of antidiabetics may need to be decreased
Increase: concentrations of digoxin, cycloSPORINE, CYP2D6 inhibitors (FLUoxetine, quiNIDine)
Increase: toxicity of carvedilol—cimetidine, other antihypertensives, nitrates, acute alcohol ingestion; monitor for toxicity
Decrease: heart rate, B/P—cloNIDine; monitor B/P, pulse frequently
Decrease: carvedilol levels—rifAMPin, NSAIDs, thyroid medications; monitor B/P
Drug/Herb
Increase: antihypertensive effect—hawthorn
Decrease: antihypertensive effect—ephedra (ma huang)

Drug/Lab Test
Increase: blood glucose, BUN, potassium, triglycerides, uric acid, bilirubin, cholesterol, creatinine, LFTs, ANA titer
Decrease: sodium, HDL

NURSING CONSIDERATIONS
Assess:
• **Hypertension:** B/P when beginning treatment, periodically thereafter; pulse: note rate, rhythm, quality; apical/radial pulse before administration; in those with lower heart rate (<55 bpm) dose may need to be lowered; notify prescriber of significant changes; identify orthostatic hypotension when patient rises
• **Heart failure:** edema in feet, legs daily; fluid overload: dyspnea, weight gain, jugular venous distention, fatigue, crackles, monitor I&O
Evaluate:
• Therapeutic response: decreased B/P with hypertension; decreased anginal pain
Teach patient/family:
• To comply with dosage schedule even if feeling better; that improvement may take several weeks; not to crush, chew caps
• To rise slowly to sitting or standing position to minimize orthostatic hypotension
• To report slow pulse, dizziness, confusion, depression, fever, weight gain, SOB, cold extremities, rash, sore throat, bleeding, bruising
• To weigh, take pulse, B/P at home; to advise if weight gain of >2 lb/day or 5 lb/wk and when to notify prescriber
• Not to discontinue product abruptly; to taper over 1-2 wk; life-threatening dysrhythmias may occur
• To avoid hazardous activities until stabilized on medication; dizziness may occur
• To carry emergency ID with product name, prescriber information at all times
• To inform all health care providers of products, supplements taken; to avoid all OTC medications unless approved by prescriber

---

• That product may mask hypoglycemia, thyroid symptoms

• **Pregnancy/breastfeeding:** to notify provider if pregnancy is planned or suspected; to avoid breastfeeding

caspofungin (Rx)

(cas-po-fun′gin)

Cancidas

Func. class.: Antifungal, systemic
Chem. class.: Echinocandin

ACTION: Inhibits an essential component in fungal cell walls; causes direct damage to fungal cell wall

USES: Treatment of invasive aspergillosis and candidemia that has not responded to other treatment, including peritonitis, intraabdominal abscesses; susceptible species: *Aspergillus flavus, A. fumigatus, A. terreus, Candida albicans, C. glabrata, C. krusei, C. lusitaniae, C. parapsilosis, C. tropicalis,* esophageal candidiasis; empirical therapy for presumed fungal infection in febrile, neutropenic patients

Unlabeled uses: *Aspergillus niger,* fungal infections in premature neonates, neonates, infants, children <2 yr

CONTRAINDICATIONS:

Hypersensitivity

Precautions: Pregnancy, breastfeeding, children, geriatric patients, severe hepatic disease

DOSAGE AND ROUTES

• **Adult:** IV loading dose 70 mg on day 1, then 50 mg/day maintenance dose, depending on condition; max 70 mg/day

• **Adolescent/child/infant ≥3 mo:** IV INFUSION 70 mg/m^2 loading dose, then 50 mg/m^2/day; max 70 mg/m^2

• **Neonate and infant <3 mo (unlabeled):** IV 25 mg/m^2/day

Esophageal candidiasis

• **Adult:** IV 50 mg × 7-14 days over 1 hr

Hepatic dose

• **Adult:** IV (Child-Pugh 7-9, class B) loading dose 70 mg, then 35 mg/day

• **Child 3 mo-17 yr:** IV 70 mg/m^2 loading dose, then 50 mg/m^2 daily; max 70 mg/m^2

Available forms: Powder for inj 50, 70 mg

Administer:

• Do not mix or confuse with other medications; do not use dextrose-containing products to dilute; do not give as bolus

• Store at room temperature for up to 24 hr or refrigerated for 48 hr; store reconstituted sol at room temperature for 1 hr before preparation of sol for administration

Intermittent IV INFUSION route

• Allow to warm to room temperature

• May administer loading dose on day 1

• **Reconstitute** 50-mg vial or 70-mg vial with 10.8 mL 0.9% NaCl, sterile water for inj, or bacteriostatic water for inj (5 mg/mL or 7 mg/mL), respectively; **swirl** to dissolve, withdraw 10 mL reconstituted sol, and **further dilute** with 250 mL 0.9% NaCl, 0.45% NaCl, 0.225% NaCl, RL; **run** over 1 hr or more

SIDE EFFECTS

CNS: Dizziness, *headache,* fever, chills
CV: Sinus tachycardia, hypertension
GI: Abdominal pain, *nausea, anorexia, vomiting, diarrhea, increased AST/ALT, alk phos*
GU: Renal failure
HEMA: Thrombophlebitis, vasculitis, anemia
INTEG: *Rash, pruritus, inj site pain*
META: Hypokalemia
MS: Myalgia
RESP: Acute respiratory distress syndrome (ARDS), pleural effusions
SYST: Anaphylaxis, histamine-related reactions, Stevens-Johnson syndrome

PHARMACOKINETICS

Metabolized in liver to inactive metabolites; excretion in feces, urine; phase II terminal half-life 9-11 hr; phase III terminal half-life 40-50 hr; protein binding 97%

INTERACTIONS

Increase: caspofungin levels, hepatic toxicity—cycloSPORINE; avoid concurrent use

Side effects: *italics* = common; red = life-threatening

Decrease: levels of tacrolimus, sirolimus
Decrease: caspofungin levels—carBAMazepine, dexamethasone, efavirenz, nelfinavir, nevirapine, phenytoin, rifAMPin; caspofungin dose may need to be increased
Drug/Lab Test
Increase: AST, ALT, RBC, eosinophils, glucose, bilirubin, alk phos, serum creatinine
Decrease: Hct/Hgb, WBC, potassium, magnesium

NURSING CONSIDERATIONS
Assess:
• **Infection:** clearing of cultures during treatment; obtain culture at baseline, throughout treatment; product may be started as soon as culture is taken (esophageal candidiasis); monitor cultures during hematopoietic stem cell transplantation (HSCT) for prevention of *Candida* infections
• Blood studies before, during treatment: bilirubin, AST, ALT, alk phos, as needed; obtain baseline renal studies; CBC with differential, serum potassium
• **Hypersensitivity:** rash, pruritus, facial swelling; also for phlebitis; anaphylaxis (rare)
• GI symptoms: frequency of stools, cramping; if severe diarrhea occurs, electrolytes may need to be given
• **Pregnancy/breastfeeding:** no well-controlled studies; use in pregnancy only if benefits outweigh fetal risk; excreted in breast milk, use cautiously in breastfeeding
Evaluate:
• Therapeutic response: decreased symptoms of *Candida, Aspergillus* infections
Teach patient/family:
• **Pregnancy/breastfeeding:** to notify prescriber if pregnancy is suspected or planned; to use cautiously in breastfeeding
• To inform prescriber of renal/hepatic disease
• To report bleeding, facial swelling, wheezing, difficulty breathing, itching, rash, hives, increasing warmth, flushing; anaphylaxis can occur

---

cefaclor
See cephalosporins—2nd generation
cefadroxil
See cephalosporins—1st generation
ceFAZolin
See cephalosporins—1st generation
cefdinir
See cephalosporins—3rd generation
cefditoren pivoxil
See cephalosporins—3rd generation
cefepime
See cephalosporins—3rd generation
cefixime
See cephalosporins—3rd generation
cefotaxime
See cephalosporins—3rd generation
cefoTEtan
See cephalosporins—2nd generation
cefOXitin
See cephalosporins—2nd generation
cefpodoxime
See cephalosporins—3rd generation
cefprozil
See cephalosporins—2nd generation
cefTAZidime
See cephalosporins—3rd generation
ceftibuten
See cephalosporins—3rd generation
ceftizoxime
See cephalosporins—3rd generation
cefTRIAXone
See cephalosporins—3rd generation
cefuroxime
See cephalosporins—2nd generation

---

ceftaroline (Rx)
(sef-tar′oh-leen)
Teflaro
Func. class.: Antiinfective-cephalosporin derivative (5th generation)

ACTION: Cephalosporin action: Inhibits cell wall synthesis through binding to essential penicillin-binding protein (PBP)

USES: Acute bacterial skin/skin structure infections (ABSSI), bacterial community-acquired pneumonia

CONTRAINDICATIONS: Cephalosporin hypersensitivity

Precautions: Child/infant/neonate, breastfeeding, elderly patients, antimicrobial resistance, carbapenem/penicillin hypersensitivity, coagulopathy, colitis, dialysis, diarrhea, GI disease, hypoprothrombinemia, IBS, pregnancy, pseudomembranous colitis, renal disease, ulcerative colitis, viral infection, vit K deficiency

DOSAGE AND ROUTES
• **Adult: IV** 600 mg q12hr × 5-14 days (skin/skin-structure infections) or × 5-7 days (bacterial community-acquired pneumonia)
• **Child 2-17 yr and >33 kg: IV** 400 mg q8hr or 600 mg q12hr; **2-17 yr and <33 kg;** 12 mg/kg q8hr
• **Child 2 mo to <2 yr: IV** 8 mg/kg q8hr
Renal dose
• **Adult: IV** CCr >30-≤50 mL/min, 400 mg q12hr; CCr ≥15-≤30 mL/min, 300 mg q12hr; CCr <15 mL/min, 200 mg q12hr, includes hemodialysis
Available forms: Powder for inj 400 mg, 600 mg/vial
Administer:
• Obtain culture specimen before use, first dose may be given before results are received
• Identify allergies before use; identify reactions to penicillins, cephalosporins, carbapenems
Intermittent IV INFUSION route
• Visually inspect for particulate matter, discoloration
• **Reconstitute:** add 20 mg of sterile water to 400- or 600-mg vial (20 mg/mL for 400 mg; 30 mg/mL for 600 mg), mix gently until dissolved; **dilute** in 250 mL of 0.9% NaCl, 0.45% NaCl, LR, D₅W, dextrose 2.5%, **give** over 1 hr, do not admix, use within 6 hr at room temperature or 24 hr refrigerated

SIDE EFFECTS
CNS: Dizziness, seizures
GI: Diarrhea, nausea, vomiting, *Clostridium difficile*-associated diarrhea (CDAD)
HEMA: Aplastic anemia
INTEG: Rash, anaphylaxis
GU: Renal failure
META: Hypokalemia, hyperkalemia, hyperglycemia
MISC: Injection site reactions

PHARMACOKINETICS
Protein binding 20%; excreted in urine 88%, feces 6%; half-life 1.6 hr; not hepatically metabolized

INTERACTIONS
Increase: prothrombin time risk—anticoagulants
Drug/Lab Test
Increase: LFTs, glucose, potassium
Decrease: potassium, eosinophils, platelets

NURSING CONSIDERATIONS
Assess:
• **Infection:** vital signs, sputum, WBC before, during therapy, obtain culture and sensitivity, should be done before starting treatment, may start medication before results are obtained
• **Hypersensitivity:** before use, obtain a history of hypersensitivity reactions to cephalosporins, carbapenems, penicillins; cross-sensitivity may occur
• **Hemolytic anemia (rare):** discontinue product, obtain direct Coomb's test, result will be positive
• **Anaphylaxis (rare):** rash, pruritus, laryngeal edema, dyspnea, wheezing; discontinue product, notify health care provider immediately, keep emergency equipment nearby
• **CDAD:** diarrhea, abdominal pain, fever, bloody stools; report immediately if these occur; may occur several weeks after terminating therapy
• Monitor BUN, creatinine baseline, periodically; elderly and those with renal disease are at greater risk of renal dysfunction
Evaluate:
• Therapeutic response: negative C&S, resolution of symptoms of infection

Side effects: *italics* = common; red = life-threatening

Teach patient/family:
• About the reason for treatment and expected result
• To immediately report rash, itching, difficulty breathing, bloody diarrhea, fever, abdominal pain
• **Pregnancy/breastfeeding:** if pregnancy is planned or suspected, or if breastfeeding

---

⚠ HIGH ALERT

celecoxib (Rx)
(sel-eh-cox′ib)
CeleBREX
Func. class.: Nonsteroidal antiinflammatory, antirheumatic
Chem. class.: COX-2 inhibitor

Do not confuse:
CeleBREX/CeleXA/Cerebyx

ACTION: Inhibits prostaglandin synthesis by selectively inhibiting cyclooxygenase-2 (COX-2), an enzyme needed for biosynthesis

USES: Acute, chronic rheumatoid arthritis, osteoarthritis, acute pain, primary dysmenorrhea, ankylosing spondylitis, juvenile rheumatoid arthritis (JRA)
Unlabeled uses: Acute gout

CONTRAINDICATIONS: Pregnancy; hypersensitivity to salicylates, iodides, other NSAIDs, sulfonamides; for perioperative pain in CABG
Precautions: Breastfeeding, children <18 yr, geriatric patients, bleeding, GI/renal/hepatic/cardiac disorders, PVD, hypertension, severe dehydration, asthma, sulfa allergy, peptic ulcer disease, MI, stroke

> **Black Box Warning:** GI bleeding/perforation, thromboembolism

DOSAGE AND ROUTES
Acute pain/primary dysmenorrhea
• **Adult: PO** 400 mg initially, then 200 mg if needed on 1st day, then 200 mg bid as needed on subsequent days; start with ½ dose for poor CYP2C9 metabolizers
Osteoarthritis
• **Adult: PO** 200 mg/day as a single dose or 100 mg bid
Rheumatoid arthritis
• **Adult: PO** 100-200 mg bid; start with ½ dose for poor CYP2C9 metabolizers
Ankylosing spondylitis
• **Adult: PO** 200 mg/day or in divided doses (bid)
Juvenile rheumatoid arthritis (JRA)
• **Adolescent/child ≥2 yr (>25 kg): PO** 100 mg bid
• **Child ≥2 yr (10-25 kg): PO** 50 mg bid
Hepatic disease
• **Adult: PO** (Child-Pugh B) reduce dose by 50%; (Child-Pugh C) do not use
Acute gout (unlabeled)
• **Adult: PO** 800 once, then 400 mg on day 1, then 400 mg bid × 1 wk
Available forms: Caps 50, 100, 200, 400 mg
Administer:
• Do not break, crush, chew, or dissolve caps; give with a full glass of water to enhance absorption; caps may be opened into applesauce or soft food, ingest immediately with water
• With food, milk to decrease gastric symptoms (with higher doses [400 mg bid]); do not increase dose

SIDE EFFECTS
CNS: *Fatigue, nervousness,* insomnia, headache
CV: Stroke, MI, HF, hypertension, fluid retention
GI: Nausea, anorexia, dry mouth, GI bleeding/ulceration
INTEG: Serious (sometimes fatal) Stevens-Johnson syndrome, toxic epidermal necrolysis, exfoliative dermatitis, rash

PHARMACOKINETICS
Well absorbed, crosses placenta, metabolized by CYP2C9 in liver, ✪ some patients may be poor metabolizers; very little excreted by kidneys/in feces, peak 3 hr, half-life 11 hr, protein binding ~97%

INTERACTIONS

Increase: bleeding risk—anticoagulants, SNRIs, SSRIs, antiplatelets, thrombolytics, salicylates, alcohol

Increase: adverse reactions—glucocorticoids, NSAIDs, aspirin

Increase: toxicity—lithium

Increase: celecoxib blood level—CYP2C9 inhibitors (fluconazole)

Decrease: effect of aspirin, ACE inhibitors, thiazide diuretics, furosemide

Drug/Lab Test

Increase: ALT, AST, BUN, cholesterol, glucose, potassium, sodium

Decrease: glucose, sodium, WBC, platelets

NURSING CONSIDERATIONS

Assess

• **Pain** of rheumatoid arthritis, osteoarthritis; check ROM, inflammation of joints, characteristics of pain, baseline and periodically

Black Box Warning: For cardiac disease that may be worse after taking product; MI, stroke; do not use with coronary artery bypass graft (CABG)

• CBC during therapy; watch for decreasing platelets; if low, therapy may need to be discontinued, restarted after hematologic recovery; LFTs; serum creatinine/BUN

• **For blood dyscrasias (thrombocytopenia):** bruising, fatigue, bleeding, poor healing

Black Box Warning: GI toxicity: black, tarry stools; abdominal pain; monitor stool guaiac

• **Serious skin disorders:** Stevens-Johnson syndrome, toxic epidermal necrolysis; may be fatal, treat symptomatically; may reoccur after therapy is discontinued; if severe, may require discontinuing

• **Beers:** Avoid use in older adults; may increase risk of kidney injury, exacerbate heart failure, increase fluid retention

Evaluate:

• Therapeutic response: decreased pain, inflammation in arthritic conditions; decreased number of polyps

Teach patient/family:

Black Box Warning: Not to exceed recommended dose; to notify prescriber immediately of chest pain, skin eruptions; to stop product if these occur

• To check with prescriber to determine when product should be discontinued before surgery

• That product must be continued for prescribed time to be effective; to avoid other NSAIDs, aspirin, sulfonamides

Black Box Warning: To notify prescriber immediately of GI symptoms: black, tarry stools; cramping or rash; edema of extremities; weight gain or hepatotoxicity: nausea, pruritus, yellowing skin, eyes, lethargy; itching upper abdominal pain

• To report bleeding, bruising, fatigue, malaise because blood abnormalities do occur

• **Pregnancy/breastfeeding:** to report if pregnancy is planned or suspected; avoid use in breastfeeding; not to use during pregnancy, breastfeeding; those who are pregnant should register at the Organization of Teratology of Information Specialists Autoimmune Diseases in Pregnancy Study, 877-311-8972

---

cemiplimab
(seh-mip' lih-mab)

Libtayo

Func. class.: Antineoplastic—monoclonal antibody

Chem. class.: Death receptor-1 (PD-1)/PD-L1

ACTION: Binds to the programmed death receptor-1 (PD-1) found on T cells. Blocking the PD-1/PD-L1 pathway improves the antitumor immune response by reducing immunosuppressive signals between immune cells and tumor cells and causes inhibition of T-cell proliferation and cytokine production

---

Side effects: *italics* = common; red = life-threatening

USES: Squamous cell skin carcinoma in patients who are not candidates for curative surgery/radiation

CONTRAINDICATIONS: Hypersensitivity, pregnancy, breastfeeding
Precautions: Adrenal insufficiency, autoimmune disease, colitis, contraception requirements, Crohn's disease, hepatitis, hyperthyroidism, immune-mediated reactions, infusion-related reactions, organ transplant, pneumonitis, pregnancy testing, renal impairment, reproductive risk, serious rash, type 1 diabetes mellitus, ulcerative colitis

DOSAGE AND ROUTES
• **Adult:** IV 350 mg over 30 min q3wk until disease progression
Administer
IV INFUSION route
• Visually inspect for particulate matter and discoloration before use; product is clear to slightly opalescent, colorless to pale yellow and may contain trace amounts of translucent to white particles
• Do not shake vial
Dilution:
• Withdraw the required amount/volume, dilute in 0.9% sodium chloride injection or 5% dextrose injection to a final concentration between 1 and 20 mg/mL; mix by gentle inversion, do not shake
• Discard any unused portion
• **Storage following dilution:** store at room temperature (up to 25° C or 77° F) for up to 8 hr or refrigerated (2-8° C; 36-46° F) for up to 24 hr from time of dilution. Do not freeze
Administration:
• If refrigerated, allow to warm to room temperature
• Give diluted solution over 30 min through a sterile, in-line or add-on 0.2- to 0.5-micron filter

SIDE EFFECTS
CNS: Fatigue, asthenia
EENT: Immune-mediated optic nephritis
ENDO: Immune-mediated hypophysitis, immune-mediated hypothyroidism/hyperthyroidism, immune-mediated type 1 diabetes mellitus
GI: Anorexia, nausea, vomiting, abdominal pain, constipation, diarrhea, immune-mediated colitis, immune-mediated hepatitis
GU: Immune-mediated nephritis
HEMA: Anemia
INTEG: Rash, pruritus, infusion-related reactions
MS: Immune-mediated rhabdomyolysis, back pain, myalgia, MS pain
RESP: Immune-mediated pneumonitis

PHARMACOKINETICS
Half-life 19 days

NURSING CONSIDERATIONS
Assess:
• *Immune-mediated pneumonitis:* short-ness of breath, chest pain, new or worsening cough periodically; if present, obtain x-ray; withhold product until grade ≤1; usually treated with corticosteroids
• *Immune-mediated colitis:* severe diarrhea or abdominal pain, blood or mucus in stool. If present, therapy may need to be interrupted or discontinued based on severity; corticosteroids may be used; permanently discontinue if grade 4 toxicity
• *Immune-mediated hepatitis:* jaundice of skin/eyes, severe nausea/vomiting; obtain liver function tests before starting and periodically during therapy; if hepatitis occurs, therapy may need to be interrupted or discontinued based on severity of the toxicity; corticosteroids may be given
• *Infusion-related reactions:* fever, pruritus, wheezing, rigors; if severe grade 3 or 4, discontinue permanently
• *Immune-mediated dermatologic reactions:* erythema multiforme, Stevens-Johnson syndrome, toxic epidermal necrolysis have occurred with similar products; interrupt or discontinue therapy in patients who develop severe skin toxicity; provide corticosteroids followed by a 1-mo taper, starting when the toxicity resolves to grade ≤1

• *Immune-mediated hypophysitis:* continual headache, weakness, fatigue, blurred vision, dizziness; provide corticosteroids for grade 2; if severe (grade 3), withhold or discontinue product until toxicity resolves to grade ≤1; permanently discontinue for grade 4

• *Immune-mediated nephritis:* monitor serum creatinine and BUN baseline and periodically; corticosteroids may be used for grade ≥2 nephritis; withhold for grade 2, resume when recovery is grade ≤1; discontinue for grade 4

• *Pregnancy/breastfeeding:* product should not be used in pregnancy or breastfeeding; perform pregnancy test in all women of childbearing potential

• Blood glucose baseline and periodically; may cause hyperglycemia

• Thyroid function test baseline and periodically; may cause hypo/hyperthyroidism; corticosteroids may be used for grade 3 hypothyroidism; withhold product for severe grade 3, permanently discontinue for grade 4

EVALUATE:
• Therapeutic response: decreased spread of skin cancer

Teach patient/family
• That product treats a type of skin cancer by working with your immune system
• To notify prescriber immediately of new or worsening cough, shortness of breath, chest pain, diarrhea, stools that are black, tarry, sticky, or have blood or mucus, abdominal pain, yellowing of skin/eyes, severe nausea/vomiting, bleeding or bruising more easily, unusual headaches, rapid heartbeat, increased sweating, extreme tiredness, weight gain/weight loss, dizziness/fainting, feeling hungrier or thirstier than usual, hair loss, feeling cold, constipation, skin rash with blisters

• Pregnancy/breastfeeding: to inform health care provider if pregnancy is planned or suspected. That product should not be used in pregnancy or breastfeeding. That a pregnancy test is required before treatment begins and that a nonhormonal form of contraception will be needed to prevent pregnancy during

treatment and for 4 mo after treatment ends. Not to breastfeed during treatment or for 4 mo after last dose

• To inform health care provider of all Rx, OTC, vitamins, and herbal products taken and not to take others without prescriber's approval

• That blood work and regular exams will be needed throughout treatment

---

cephalexin
See cephalosporins—1st generation

CEPHALOSPORINS— 1ST GENERATION

cefadroxil (Rx)
(sef-a-drox′ill)
Duricef ✦
ceFAZolin (Rx)
(sef-a′zoe-lin)
Ancef ✦, Kefzol ✦
cephalexin (Rx)
(sef-a-lex′in)
Keflex
Func. class.: Antiinfective
Chem. class.: Cephalosporin (1st generation)

ACTION: Inhibits bacterial cell wall synthesis; renders cell wall osmotically unstable, leads to cell death; lysis mediated by cell wall autolytic enzymes

USES: **cefadroxil:** Gram-negative bacilli: *Escherichia coli, Proteus mirabilis, Klebsiella* (UTI only); gram-positive organisms: *Streptococcus pneumoniae, Streptococcus pyogenes, Staphylococcus aureus;* upper, lower respiratory tract, urinary tract, skin infections; otitis media; tonsillitis; UTIs
ceFAZolin: Gram-negative bacilli: *Haemophilus influenzae, Escherichia coli, Proteus mirabilis, Klebsiella pneumoniae;* gram-positive organisms:

Side effects: *italics* = common; red = life-threatening

Staphylococcus aureus/epidermidis; upper, lower respiratory tract, urinary tract, skin infections; bone, joint, biliary, genital infections; endocarditis, surgical prophylaxis, septicemia; *Streptococcus sp.*

cephalexin: Gram-negative bacilli: *Haemophilus influenzae, Escherichia coli, Proteus mirabilis, Klebsiella pneumoniae;* gram-positive organisms: *Streptococcus pneumoniae, Streptococcus pyogenes, Streptococcus agalactiae, Staphylococcus aureus;* upper, lower respiratory tract, urinary tract, skin, bone infections; otitis media

CONTRAINDICATIONS: Hypersensitivity to cephalosporins, infants <1 mo

Precautions: Pregnancy, breastfeeding, hypersensitivity to penicillins, renal disease

DOSAGE AND ROUTES
cefadroxil
• **Adult:** PO 1-2 g/day or divided q12hr; loading dose of 1 g initially
• **Child:** PO 30 mg/kg/day in divided doses bid, max 2 g/day
Catheter-related bloodstream infections
• **Adult:** IV 2 g q8h
Renal dose
• **Adult:** PO CCr 25-50 mL/min, 1 g, then 500 mg q12hr; CCr 10-24 mL/min, 1 g, then 500 mg q24hr; CCr <10 mL/min, 1 g, then 500 mg q36hr
Available forms: Caps 500 mg; tabs 1 g; oral susp 250, 500 mg/5 mL
ceFAZolin
Surgical prophylaxis
• **Adult:** IM/IV 1 g 30-60 min before surgery, then 0.5-1 g q6-8hr × 24 hr
Life-threatening infections
• **Adult:** IM/IV 1-2 g q6-8hr; max 12 g/day
• **Child >1 mo:** IM/IV 75-100 mg/kg/day in 3-4 divided doses; max 6 g/day
Mild/moderate infections
• **Adult:** IM/IV 250 mg-1 g q8hr, max 12 g/day
• **Child >1 mo:** IM/IV 50 mg/kg in 3-4 equal doses, max 6 g/day, or 2 g as a single dose

Renal dose
• **Adult: IM/IV** after loading dose, CCr 35-54 mL/min, dose q8hr; CCr 10-34 mL/min, 50% of dose q12hr; CCr <10 mL/min, 50% of dose q18-24hr
• **Child: IM/IV** CCr >70 mL/min, no dosage adjustment; CCr 40-70 mL/min after loading dose, reduce dose to 7.5-30 mg/kg q12hr; CCr 20-39 mL/min, give 3.125-12.5 mg/kg after loading dose q12hr; CCr 5-19 mL/min, 2.5-10 mg/kg after loading dose q24hr
Available forms: Powder for Inj 500 mg, 1, 10, 20 g/vial; premixed infusion 500 mg, 1 g/50 mL, 500 mg/50-mL vial
cephalexin
Moderate infections
• **Adult:** PO 250-500 mg q6hr, max 4 g/day
• **Child:** PO 25-100 mg/kg/day in 4 equal doses, max 4 g/day
Moderate skin infections
• **Adult:** PO 500 mg q12hr
Endocarditis prophylaxis
• **Adult:** PO 2 g 1 hr before procedure
Severe infections
• **Adult:** PO 500 mg-1 g q6hr, max 4 g
• **Child:** PO 50-100 mg/kg/day in 4 equal doses, max 4 g/day
Otitis media
• **Child:** PO 18.75-25 mg/kg q6hr, max 4 g/day
Community-acquired pneumonia (unlabeled)
• **Child: >3 mo:** PO 75-100 mg/kg/day divided in 3 or 4 doses × 10 days
Renal dose
• **Adult:** PO CCr 10-40 mL/min, 250-500 mg then 250-500 mg q8-12hr; CCr <10 mL/min, 250-500 mg, then 250 mg q12-24hr
Available forms: Caps 250, 500, 750 mg; tabs 250, 500 mg 1g; oral suspension 125, 250 mg/5 mL
Administer:
cefadroxil
• For prescribed time to ensure organism death, prevent superinfection
• With food if needed for GI symptoms
• Shake susp, refrigerate, discard after 2 wk
• Identify allergies before use
• After C&S specimen is obtained

---

ceFAZolin

- Obtain C&S specimen before use
- Identify allergies before use

IV route

- Check for irritation, extravasation often; dilute in 2 mL/500 mg or 2.5 mL/1 g sterile water for inj, inject over 3-5 min; may be further diluted with 50-100 mL of NS, D₅W sol, run over 10 min-1 hr by Y-tube or 3-way stopcock
- After C&S completed

Y-site compatibilities: Acyclovir, alfentanil, allopurinol, alprostadil, amifostine, amikacin, aminocaproic acid, aminophylline, amphotericin B liposome, anidulafungin, ascorbic acid injection, atenolol, atracurium, atropine, aztreonam, benztropine, bivalirudin, bleomycin, bumetanide, buprenorphine, butorphanol, calcium gluconate, CARBOplatin, cefamandole, cefmetazole, cefonicid, cefoTEtan, cefOXitin, cefpirome, cefTAZidime, ceftizoxime, cefTRIAXone, cefuroxime, chloramphenicol, cimetidine, CISplatin, clindamycin, codeine, cyanocobalamin, cyclophosphamide, cycloSPORINE, cytarabine, DACTINomycin, DAPTOmycin, dexamethasone, dexmedetomidine, digoxin, diltiaZEM, DOCEtaxel, doxacurium, doxapram, DOXOrubicin liposomal, enalaprilat, ePHEDrine, EPINEPHrine, epirubicin, epoetin alfa, eptifibatide, esmolol, etoposide, fenoldopam, fentaNYL, filgrastim, fluconazole, fludarabine, fluorouracil, folic acid (as sodium salt), foscarnet, furosemide, gallium, gatifloxacin, gemcitabine, gentamicin, glycopyrrolate, granisetron, heparin, hydrocortisone, hydrOXYzine, IDArubicin, ifosfamide, imipenem-cilastatin, indomethacin, insulin (regular), irinotecan, isoproterenol, ketorolac, lidocaine, linezolid, LORazepam, LR's injection, mannitol, mechlorethamine, melphalan, meperidine, methotrexate, methyldopate, methylPREDNISolone, metoclopramide, metoprolol, metroNIDAZOLE, miconazole, midazolam, milrinone, morphine, moxalactam, multiple vitamins injection, nafcillin, nalbuphine, naloxone, nesiritide, niCARdipine, nitroglycerin, nitroprusside, norepinephrine, octreotide, ondansetron, oxacillin, oxaliplatin, oxytocin, PACLitaxel, palonosetron, pamidronate, pancuronium, pantoprazole, penicillin G potassium/sodium, peritoneal dialysis solution, perphenazine, PHENobarbital, phenylephrine, phytonadione, piperacillin, Plasma-Lyte M in dextrose 5%, polymyxin B, potassium chloride, procainamide, propofol, propranolol, raNITIdine, remifentanil, Ringer's injection, ritodrine, riTUXimab, sargramostim, sodium acetate, sodium bicarbonate, succinylcholine, SUFentanil, tacrolimus, teniposide, tenoxicam, theophylline, thiamine, thiotepa, ticarcillin, ticarcillin-clavulanate, tigecycline, tirofiban, TNA, tolazoline, trastuzumab, trimetaphan, urokinase, vasopressin, vecuronium, verapamil, vinCRIStine, vitamin B complex with C, voriconazole, warfarin, zoledronic acid

cephalexin

- Shake susp, refrigerate, discard after 2 wk; use calibrated oral syringe, spoon, or measuring cup
- With food if needed for GI symptoms
- After C&S specimen is obtained
- Identify allergies before use

SIDE EFFECTS

CNS: Headache, dizziness, weakness, paresthesia, fever, chills, confusion, fatigue, hallucinations, seizures (with high doses)

GI: Nausea, vomiting, *diarrhea, anorexia,* abdominal pain, *Clostridium difficile-associated diarrhea (CDAD)*

GU: Vaginitis, pruritus, candidiasis

HEMA: Thrombocytopenia, anemia, neutropenia, eosinophilia, hemolytic anemia

INTEG: Rash, urticaria, dermatitis, injection site reactions

SYST: Anaphylaxis, serum sickness, superinfection, Stevens-Johnson syndrome

PHARMACOKINETICS

cefadroxil: Peak 1-1$^1/_2$ hr, duration 12-24 hr, half-life 1-2 hr, 20% bound by plasma proteins, crosses placenta, excreted in breast milk

ceFAZolin

IV: Onset 10 min, peak infusions end, duration 6-12 hr, eliminated unchanged in urine, 75%-85% protein bound

IM: Peak 1-2 hr, duration 6-12 hr, half-life 1$^1/_2$-2 hr

cephalexin: Peak 1 hr, duration 6-12 hr, half-life 30-72 min, 5%-15% bound by plasma proteins, 80%-100% eliminated unchanged in urine, crosses placenta, excreted in breast milk

INTERACTIONS

Increase: toxicity—aminoglycosides, loop diuretics, probenecid

Drug/Lab Test

Increase: AST, ALT, alk phos, LDH, BUN, creatinine, bilirubin

False positive: urinary protein, direct Coombs' test, urine glucose

Interference: cross-matching

NURSING CONSIDERATIONS

Assess:

• **Infection:** characteristics of wounds, sputum, urine, stools, WBC >10,000/mm^3, earache, fever; obtain baseline and periodically during treatment; obtain C&S before treatment starts, may start treatment before results are received

• Cross-sensitivity to penicillin and other cephalosporins; hypersensitivity reaction may occur

• **Nephrotoxicity:** increased BUN, creatinine; urine output: if decreasing, notify prescriber

• Blood studies: AST, ALT, CBC, Hct, bilirubin, LDH, alk phos, Coombs' test monthly if patient is on long-term therapy

• **CDAD:** bowel pattern daily; if severe diarrhea occurs, product should be discontinued

• **Anaphylaxis:** rash, urticaria, pruritus, chills, fever, joint pain; angioedema; may occur a few days after therapy begins; discontinue product, notify prescriber immediately, keep emergency equipment nearby

• **Stevens-Johnson syndrome, toxic epidermal necrolysis:** painful, red rash; flulike symptoms, discontinue product, do not restart

• **Overgrowth of infection:** perineal itching, fever, malaise, redness, pain, swelling, drainage, rash, diarrhea, change in cough, sputum

Evaluate:

• Therapeutic response: decreased symptoms of infection, negative C&S

Teach patient/family:

• To take all medication prescribed for length of time ordered; take missed dose as soon as remembered, unless close to next dose; do not double dose; use calibrated device for syrup, liquid, suspension

• To report vaginal itching; loose, foul-smelling stools; furry tongue occurs; may indicate superinfection

• To report immediately rash, flulike symptoms, blisters, stop product

• Diarrhea with mucus, blood (may indicate **CDAD**)

TREATMENT OF ANAPHYLAXIS: EPINEPHrine, antihistamines; resuscitate if needed

CEPHALOSPORINS— 2ND GENERATION

cefaclor (Rx)
(sef'a-klor)
Ceclor ✦
cefoTEtan (Rx)
(sef'oh-tee-tan)
Cefotan
cefOXitin (Rx)
(se-fox'i-tin)
Mefoxin
cefprozil (Rx)
(sef-proe'zill)
Cefzil
cefuroxime (Rx)
(sef-yoor-ox'eem)
Ceftin, Kefurox ✦, Zinacef
Func. class.: Antiinfective
Chem. class.: Cephalosporin (2nd generation)

Do not confuse:
cefaclor/cephalexin
Cefotan/Ceftin
cefprozil/ceFAZolin/cefuroxime
Cefzil/Ceftin

ACTION: Inhibits bacterial cell wall synthesis, renders cell wall osmotically unstable, leads to cell death by binding to cell wall membrane

USES: cefaclor: Gram-negative bacilli: *Haemophilus influenzae, Escherichia coli, Proteus mirabilis, Klebsiella;* gram-positive organisms: *Streptococcus pneumoniae, Streptococcus pyogenes, Staphylococcus aureus;* respiratory tract, urinary tract, skin, infections; otitis media
cefoTEtan: Gram-negative organisms: *Haemophilus influenzae, Escherichia coli, Enterobacter aerogenes, Proteus mirabilis, Klebsiella, Citrobacter, Salmonella, Shigella, Acinetobacter, Bacteroides fragilis, Neisseria, Serratia;* gram-positive organisms: *Streptococcus pneumoniae, Streptococcus pyogenes,*

Staphylococcus aureus; lower, serious respiratory tract, urinary tract, skin, bone, joint, gynecologic, gonococcal, intraabdominal infections
cefOXitin: Gram-negative bacilli: *Haemophilus influenzae, Escherichia coli, Proteus, Klebsiella, Bacteroides fragilis, Neisseria gonorrhoeae;* gram-positive organisms: *Streptococcus pneumoniae, Streptococcus pyogenes, Staphylococcus aureus;* anaerobes including *Clostridium;* lower respiratory tract, urinary tract, skin, bone, gynecologic, gonococcal infections; septicemia, peritonitis
cefprozil: Pharyngitis/tonsillitis; otitis media; secondary bacterial infection of acute bronchitis; acute bacterial exacerbation of chronic bronchitis; uncomplicated skin and skin-structure infections; acute sinusitis
cefuroxime: Gram-negative bacilli: *Haemophilus influenzae, Escherichia coli, Neisseria, Proteus mirabilis, Klebsiella;* gram-positive organisms: *Streptococcus pneumoniae, Streptococcus pyogenes, Staphylococcus aureus;* serious lower respiratory tract, urinary tract, skin, bone, joint, gonococcal infections; septicemia, meningitis, surgery prophylaxis

CONTRAINDICATIONS: Hypersensitivity to cephalosporins or related antibiotics; seizures
Precautions: Pregnancy, breastfeeding, children, GI/renal disease, diabetes mellitus, coagulopathy, pseudomembranous colitis

DOSAGE AND ROUTES
cefaclor
• **Adult:** PO 250-500 mg q8hr; ext rel 500 mg q12hr; max 1.5 g/day (cap, oral susp); 1 g/day (ext rel)
• **Child >1 mo:** PO 20-40 mg/kg/day in divided doses q8hr or total daily dose may be divided and given q12hr, max 1 g/day
Available forms: Caps 250, 500 mg; oral susp 125, 250, 375 mg/5 mL; ext rel tab 375, 500 mg

---

Side effects: *italics* = common; red = life-threatening

cefoTEtan
- **Adult:** IM/IV 1-3 g q12hr × 5-10 days

Renal dose
- **Adult:** IM/IV CCr 30-50 mL/min 1-2 g, then 1-2 g q8-12hr; CCr 10-29 mL/min 1-2 g, then 1-2 g q12-24hr; CCr 5-9 mL/min 1-2 g, then 0.5-1 g q12-24hr; CCr<5 mL/min 1-2 g, then 0.5-1 g q24-48hr

Perioperative prophylaxis
- **Adult:** IV 1-2 g ½-1 hr before surgery

Available forms: Inj 1, 2, 10 g; premixed 1 g/50 mL D₅W, 2 g/50 mL D₅W

cefOXitin
- **Adult:** IM/IV 1-2 g q6-8hr
- **Child/infant >3 mo:** IV/IM 13.3-26.7 mg/kg q4hr or 20-40 mg/kg q6hr

Renal dose
- **Adult:** IM/IV after loading dose, CCr 30-50 mL/min, 1-2 g q8-12hr; CCr 10-29 mL/min, 1-2 g q12-24hr; CCr <10 mL/min, 0.5-1 g q12-24hr

Severe infections
- **Adult:** IM/IV 2 g q4hr
- **Child ≥3 mo:** IM/IV 80-160 mg/kg/day divided q4-6hr; max 12 g/day

Available forms: Powder for inj 1, 2, 10 g; premixed 1 g/50 mL D⁵W, 2 g/50 mL D₅W

cefprozil

Upper respiratory infections
- **Adult:** PO 500 mg q24hr × 10 days

Otitis media
- **Child 6 mo-12 yr:** PO 15 mg/kg q12hr × 10 days

Lower respiratory infections
- **Adult:** PO 500 mg q12hr × 10 days

Skin/skin-structure infections
- **Adult:** PO 250-500 mg q12hr × 10 days

Renal dose
- **Adult:** PO CCr <30 mL/min, 50% of dose

Available forms: Tabs 250, 500 mg; susp 125, 250 mg/5 mL

cefuroxime
- **Adult/child:** PO 250 mg q12hr; may increase to 500 mg q12hr for serious infections
- **Adult:** IM/IV 750 mg-1.5 g q8hr for 5-10 days

Urinary tract infections
- **Adult:** PO 125 mg q12hr; may increase to 250 mg q12hr if needed

Otitis media
- **Child <2 yr:** PO 125 mg bid
- **Child >2 yr:** PO 250 mg bid

Surgical prophylaxis
- **Adult:** IV 1.5 g ½-1 hr before surgery

Severe infections
- **Adult:** IM/IV 1.5 g q6hr; may give up to 3 g q8hr for bacterial meningitis
- **Child >3 mo:** IM/IV 50-100 mg/kg/day or IM in divided doses q6-8hr

Uncomplicated gonorrhea
- **Adult:** IM 1.5 g as single dose in 2 separate sites with oral probenecid

Renal dose
- Dosage reduction indicated with severe renal impairment (CCr <20 mL/min)

Available forms: Tabs 250, 500 mg; solution for inj 1.5 g/50 mL, 750 mg/50 mL; susp 125, 250 mg/5 mL

Administer:
- Do not break, crush, or chew ext rel tabs or caps
- On an empty stomach 1 hr before or 2 hr after a meal

cefaclor
- Identify allergies before use
- Obtain C&S specimen before use
- Shake susp, refrigerate, discard after 2 wk
- For 10-14 days to ensure organism death, prevent superinfection
- With food if needed for GI symptoms
- After C&S completed
- Swallow ext rel whole

cefoTEtan
- Identify allergies before use
- Obtain C&S specimen before use

Direct IV route
- IV direct after diluting 1 g/10 mL sterile water for inj, give over 3-5 min

Intermittent IV infusion route
- May be diluted further with 50-100 mL NS or D₅W; shake; run over ½-1 hr by Y-tube or 3-way stopcock; discontinue primary infusion during administration
- May be stored 96 hr refrigerated or 24 hr at room temperature

Y-site compatibilities: Allopurinol, amifostine, aztreonam, diltiazem, famotidine, filgrastim, fluconazole, fludarabine, heparin, insulin (regular), melphalan, meperidine, morphine, PACLitaxel, remifentanil, sargramostim, tacrolimus, teniposide, theophylline, thiotepa

cefOXitin
IV route
Direct IV route
• After diluting 1 g/10 mL or more D_5W, NS, give over 3-5 min
intermittent IV infusion route may be diluted further with 50-100 mL NS or D_5W; run over ½-1 hr by Y-tube or 3-way stopcock; discontinue primary infusion during administration
continuous infusion route give by cont infusion at prescribed rate; may store 96 hr refrigerated or 24 hr at room temperature
• After C&S completed

Y-site compatibilities: Acyclovir, amifostine, amphotericin B cholesteryl sulfate complex, aztreonam, cyclophosphamide, diltiazem, DOXOrubicin liposome, famotidine, fluconazole, foscarnet, HYDROmorphone, magnesium sulfate, meperidine, morphine, ondansetron, perphenazine, remifentanil, teniposide, thiotepa

cefprozil
PO route
• Without regard to meals
• Identify allergies before use
• Obtain C&S specimen before use
• Refrigerate/shake susp before use; discard after 14 days

cefuroxime
PO route
• Identify allergies before use
• Obtain C&S specimen before use
• With food if needed for GI symptoms
Y-site compatibilities: Acyclovir, allopurinol, amifostine, atracurium, aztreonam, cyclophosphamide, diltiazem, famotidine, fludarabine, foscarnet, HYDROmorphone, melphalan, meperidine, morphine, ondansetron, pancuronium, perphenazine, remifentanil, sargramostim, tacrolimus, teniposide, thiotepa, vecuronium

SIDE EFFECTS
CNS: Dizziness, headache, seizures
GI: *Diarrhea,* nausea, vomiting, anorexia, CDAD
HEMA: Leukopenia, thrombocytopenia, agranulocytosis, neutropenia, eosinophilia, hemolytic anemia
INTEG: Rash, urticaria, dermatitis, Stevens-Johnson syndrome, IV site reactions
SYST: Anaphylaxis, serum sickness, superinfection

PHARMACOKINETICS
cefaclor
PO: Peak ½-1 hr, half-life 36-54 min, 25% bound by plasma proteins, 60%-85% eliminated unchanged in urine, crosses placenta, excreted in breast milk (low concentrations)
cefoTEtan
IM/IV: Peak 1½-3 hr, half-life hr, 75%-90% proteins binding, 50%-80% eliminated unchanged in urine, crosses placenta, excreted in breast milk
cefOXitin
Half-life ½-1 hr; 65%-80% protein binding 90%-100%; eliminated unchanged in urine; crosses placenta, blood-brain barrier; eliminated in breast milk; not metabolized
IM: Peak 15-30 min
IV: Infusion's end, duration 6-8 hr
cefprozil
PO: Peak 1.5 hr, protein binding 36%, half-life 1.3 hr (normal renal function), 2 hr (hepatic disease), 5½-6 hr (end-stage renal disease), extensively metabolized to an active metabolite, eliminated in urine 60%
cefuroxime
Peak **PO** 2 hr, **IM** 45 min, **IV** 2-3 min, 66% excreted unchanged in urine, half-life 1-2 hr in normal renal function

INTERACTIONS
Increase: effect/toxicity—aminoglycosides, probenecid
Increase: bleeding risk (cefoTEtan)—anticoagulants, thrombolytics, NSAIDs, antiplatelets

C

Decrease: absorption of cephalosporin
—antacids
Drug/Lab Test
False increase: creatinine (serum urine),
urinary 17-KS
False positive: urinary protein, direct
Coombs' test, urine glucose testing
(Clinitest)
Interference: cross-matching

NURSING CONSIDERATIONS
Assess:
• I&O ratio
• Blood studies: AST, ALT, CBC, Hct, bilirubin, LDH, alk phos, Coombs' test
monthly if patient is on long-term therapy
• Electrolytes: potassium, sodium, chlorine monthly if patient is on long-term
therapy
• *Clostridium difficile–associated diarrhea (CDAD):* bowel pattern daily; if
severe diarrhea occurs, product should be
discontinued
• **Anaphylaxis:** rash, flushing, urticaria,
pruritus, dyspnea; discontinue product,
notify prescriber, have emergency equipment available; cross-sensitivity may occur with penicillins or other beta-lactam
antibiotics
• **Bleeding:** ecchymosis, bleeding gums,
hematuria, stool guaiac daily
• **Overgrowth of infection:** perineal
itching, fever, malaise, redness, pain,
swelling, drainage, rash, diarrhea, change
in cough, sputum
Evaluate:
• Therapeutic response: negative C&S,
decreased symptoms of infections
Teach patient/family:
• To complete full course of product
therapy; to take missed dose as soon as
remembered unless close to next dose,
do not double dose; to use calibrated
device for syrup, liquid suspension
• To report diarrhea with mucus, blood
CDAD; symptoms of hypersensitivity

TREATMENT OF ANAPHY-
LAXIS: EPINEPHrine, antihistamines;
resuscitate if needed

CEPHALOSPORINS— 3RD/4TH GENERATION

cefdinir (Rx)
(sef′dih-ner)
cefditoren (Rx)
(sef-dit′oh-ren)
Spectracef
cefepime (Rx) (4th generation)
(sef′e-peem)
Maxipime
cefixime (Rx)
(sef-icks′ime)
Suprax
cefotaxime (Rx)
(sef-oh-taks′eem)
Claforan
cefpodoxime (Rx)
(sef-poe-docks′eem)
cefTAZidime (Rx)
(sef′tay-zi-deem)
Fortaz, Tazicef
ceftibuten (Rx)
(sef-ti-byoo′tin)
Cedax
cefTRIAXone (Rx)
(sef-try-ax′one)
Func. class.: Broad-spectrum antiinfective
Chem. class.: Cephalosporin (3rd
generation)

Do not confuse:
cefTAZidime/ceftizoxime

ACTION: Inhibits bacterial cell wall
synthesis, renders cell wall osmotically
unstable, leads to cell death

USES:
cefdinir: Community-acquired pneumonia, otitis media, sinusitis, pharyngitis,
skin and skin-structure infections, acute
exacerbations of chronic bronchitis,

---

pneumonia, tonsillitis, *Citrobacter diversus, Escherichia coli, Klebsiella pneumoniae, Proteus mirabilis, Staphylococcus epidermidis, Streptococcus agalactiae* (group B), viridans streptococci alpha, *Haemophilus influenzae, Haemophilus parainfluenzae, Moraxella catarrhalis;* gram-positive organisms: *Streptococcus pneumoniae, Streptococcus pyogenes, Staphylococcus aureus* (MSSA)

cefditoren pivoxil: Acute bacterial exacerbations of chronic bronchitis caused by *Haemophilus influenzae, Haemophilus parainfluenzae, Streptococcus pneumoniae, Moraxella catarrhalis*; pharyngitis/tonsillitis caused by *Streptococcus pyogenes;* uncomplicated skin and skin-structure infections caused by *Staphylococcus aureus, Streptococcus pyogenes;* community-acquired pneumonia, viridans streptococci

cefixime: Uncomplicated UTI *(Escherichia coli, Proteus mirabilis),* pharyngitis and tonsillitis *(Streptococcus pyogenes),* otitis media *(Haemophilus influenzae), Moraxella catarrhalis,* acute bronchitis and acute exacerbations of chronic bronchitis *(Streptococcus pneumoniae, H. influenzae),* uncomplicated gonorrhea

cefotaxime: *Haemophilus influenzae, Haemophilus parainfluenzae, Escherichia coli, Enterococcus faecalis, Neisseria gonorrhoeae, Neisseria meningitidis, Proteus mirabilis, Klebsiella, Citrobacter, Serratia, Salmonella, Shigella, Pseudomonas; Streptococcus pneumoniae, Streptococcus pyogenes, Staphylococcus aureus;* serious lower respiratory tract, urinary tract, skin, bone, gonococcal infections; bacteremia, septicemia, meningitis, skin, skin-structure infections; CNS infections; perioperative prophylaxis, intraabdominal infections, PID, UTI, ventriculitis

cefpodoxime: *Bacteroides, Neisseria gonorrhoeae, Haemophilus influenzae, Escherichia coli, Proteus mirabilis, Klebsiella;* gram-positive organisms: *Streptococcus pneumoniae, Streptococcus pyogenes, Staphylococcus aureus;* upper and lower respiratory tract, urinary tract, skin infections; otitis media; sexually transmitted diseases

cefTAZidime: *Haemophilus influenzae, Escherichia coli, Enterobacter aerogenes, Pseudomonas aeruginosa, Proteus mirabilis, Klebsiella, Citrobacter, Enterobacter, Salmonella, Shigella, Acinetobacter, Bacteroides fragilis, Neisseria, Serratia; Streptococcus pneumoniae, Streptococcus pyogenes, Staphylococcus aureus;* serious lower respiratory tract, urinary tract, skin, gynecologic, bone, joint, intraabdominal infections; septicemia, meningitis

ceftibuten: Pharyngitis/tonsillitis, otitis media, secondary bacterial infection of acute bronchitis

cefTRIAXone: Gram-negative bacilli: *Haemophilus influenzae, Escherichia coli, Enterobacter aerogenes, Proteus mirabilis, Klebsiella, Citrobacter, Enterobacter, Salmonella, Shigella, Acinetobacter, Bacteroides fragilis, Neisseria, Serratia;* gram-positive organisms: *Streptococcus pneumoniae, Streptococcus pyogenes, Staphylococcus aureus;* serious lower respiratory tract, urinary tract, skin, gonococcal, intraabdominal infections; septicemia, meningitis, bone, joint infections; otitis media; PID

CONTRAINDICATIONS: Hypersensitivity to cephalosporins, infants <1 mo

Precautions: Pregnancy, breastfeeding, children, hypersensitivity to penicillins, GI/renal disease, geriatric patients, pseudomembranous colitis, viral infection, vit K deficiencies, diabetes

DOSAGE AND ROUTES
cefdinir

Uncomplicated skin and skin-structure infections/community-acquired pneumonia
• **Adult and child ≥13 yr: PO** 300 mg q12hr × 10 days or 600 mg q24hr
• **Child 6 mo-12 yr: PO** 7 mg/kg q12hr or 14 mg/kg q24hr × 10 days

---

Acute exacerbations of chronic bronchitis/acute maxillary sinusitis
- Adult and child ≥13 yr: **PO** 300 mg q12hr or 600 mg q24hr × 10 days

Pharyngitis/tonsillitis
- Adult and child ≥13 yr: **PO** 300 mg q12hr or 600 mg q24hr × 10 days
- Child 6 mo-12 yr: **PO** 7 mg/kg q12hr × 5-10 days or 14 mg/kg q24hr × 10 days

Renal dose
- Adult/child >13 yr: **PO** CCr <30 mL/min, 300 mg/day (adult); 7 mg/kg/day (child 6 mo-12 yr)

Available forms: Caps 300 mg; susp 125 mg, 250 mg/5 mL

cefditoren
- Adult: **PO** 200-400 mg bid × 10-14 days

Renal dose
- Adult: **PO** CCr 30-49 mL/min, max 200 mg bid; CCr <30 mL/min, max 200 mg daily

Available forms: Tabs 200, 400 mg

cefepime

Febrile neutropenia
- Adult/adolescent >16 yr/child ≥40 kg: **IV** 2 g q8hr × 7 days or until neutropenia resolves
- Infant ≥2 mo/child/adolescent ≤16 yr and ≤40 kg: **IV** 50 mg/kg/dose q8hr × 7 days or until neutropenia resolves

Urinary tract infections (mild to moderate)
- Adult: **IV/IM** 0.5-1 g q12hr × 7-10 days

Urinary tract infections (severe)
- Adult/adolescent >16 yr/child ≥40 kg: **IV** 2 g q12hr × 10 days

Pneumonia (moderate to severe)
- Adult: **IV** 1-2 g q12hr × 10 days

Available forms: Powder for inj 500 mg, 1, 2 g; 1 g/50 mL, 2 g/100 mL

cefixime
- Adult/adolescent/child >12 yr old >45 kg: **PO** 400 mg/day
- Child ≤45 kg/infant ≥6 mo: **PO** 8 mg/kg/day

Renal dose
- Adult: **PO** CCr 21-59 mL/min, give 65% of dose; CCr <20 mL/min, give 50% of dose

Available forms: Powder for oral susp 100 mg/5 mL, 200 mg/5 mL, 500 mg/mL; chew tabs 100, 200 mg, cap 400 mg

cefotaxime
- Adult/adolescent/child ≥50 kg: **IV/IM** (uncomplicated infections) 1 g q12hr, (moderate-severe infection) 1-2 g q8hr, (severe infections) 2 g q6-8hr, (life-threatening infections) 2 g q4hr, max 12 g/day
- Adolescent/child <50 kg and infants: **IV/IM** 50-180 mg/kg/day divided q6-8hr, max 2 g/dose; (severe infections) 200-225 mg/kg/day divided q4-6hr, max 12 g
- Neonate >7 days: **IV/IM** 50 mg/kg/dose q8-12hr

Uncomplicated gonorrhea
- Adult: **IM** 500 mg as a single dose

Renal dose
- Adult: **IM** CCr <20 mL/min 50% dose reduction

Available forms: Powder for inj 500 mg, 1, 2, 10 g; inj 1, 2 g premixed frozen

cefpodoxime

Pneumonia
- Adult >12 yr: **PO** 200 mg q12hr × 14 days

Skin and skin structure
- Adult >13 yr: **PO** 400 mg q12hr × 7-14 days

Pharyngitis and tonsillitis
- Adult >13 yr: **PO** 100 mg q12hr × 5-10 days
- Child 5 mo-12 yr: **PO** 5 mg/kg q12hr (max 100 mg/dose or 200 mg/day) × 5-10 days

Uncomplicated UTI
- Adult >13 yr: **PO** 100 mg q12hr × 7 days; dosing interval increased with severe renal impairment

Acute otitis media
- Child 5 mo-12 yr: **PO** 5 mg/kg q12hr × 5 days

Available forms: Tabs 100, 200 mg; granules for susp 50 mg, 100 mg/5 mL

cefTAZidime
- Adult: **IV/IM** 1-2 g q8hr
- Child: **IV/IM** 30-50 mg/kg q8hr, max 6 g/day
- Neonate: **IV/IM** 30-50 mg/kg q8-12hr

Renal dose
- **Adult:** IM/IV CCr 31-50 mL/min 1 g q12hr; CCr 16-30 mL/min 1 g q24hr; CCr 6-15 mL/min 1 g loading dose, then 0.5 g q24hr; CCr <5 mL/min 1 g loading dose, then 0.5 g q48hr

Available forms: Inj, 500 mg, 1, 2, 6 g/ vial

ceftibuten
- **Adult:** PO 400 mg/day × 10 days
- **Child 6 mo-12 yr:** PO 9 mg/kg/day × 10 days

Renal dose
- **Adult:** PO CCr 30-49 mL/min, give 200 mg q24hr; CCr 5-29 mL/min, give 100 mg q24hr

Available forms: Caps 400 mg; susp 90 mg, 180 mg/5 mL

cefTRIAXone
- **Adult:** IM/IV 1-2 g/day, max 4 g/24 hr
- **Child:** IM/IV 50-75 mg/kg/day in equal doses q12-24hr

Uncomplicated gonorrhea
- **Adult:** 250 mg **IM** as single dose
- Reduce dosage in severe renal impairment (CCr <10 mL/min)

Available forms: Inj 250, 500 mg, 1, 2, 10 g

Administer
cefdinir
- Oral susp after adding 39 mL water to the 60-mL bottle or 65 mL water to the 120-mL bottle; discard unused portion after 10 days; give without regard to food, do not give within 2 hr of antacids, iron supplements
- After C&S completed

cefditoren
- For 10-14 days to ensure organism death, prevent superinfection
- With food; do not give with antacids
- After C&S completed

cefepime
Intermittent IV INFUSION route
- IV after diluting in 50-100 mL or more D₅, NS; give over 30 min
- For 7-10 days to ensure organism death, prevent superinfection

Y-site compatibilities: DOXOrubicin liposome

cefixime
- For 10-14 days to ensure organism death, prevent superinfection
- Without regard to food
- Chew tabs before swallowing

cefotaxime
IV route
- IV after **diluting** 1 g/10 mL D₅W, NS, sterile water for inj, **give** over 3-5 min by Y-tube or 3-way stopcock; may be **diluted further** with 50-100 mL NS or D₅W; **run** over ½-1 hr; discontinue primary infusion during administration; may be **diluted** in larger vol of sol, given as a cont infusion
- For 10-14 days to ensure organism death, prevent superinfection
- Thaw frozen container at room temperature or refrigeration; do not force thaw by immersion or microwave; visually inspect container for leaks

Y-site compatibilities: Acyclovir, alfentanil, alprostadil, amifostine, amikacin, aminocaproic acid, aminophylline, anidulafungin, ascorbic acid injection, atenolol, atracurium, atropine, aztreonam, benztropine, bivalirudin, bleomycin, bumetanide, buprenorphine, butorphanol, caffeine, calcium chloride/gluconate, CARBOplatin, cefamandole, cefmetazole, cefonicid, cefoperazone, cefoTEtan, cefOXitin, cefTAZidime (ʟ-arginine), cefTRIAXone sodium, cefuroxime, cimetidine, CISplatin, clindamycin, codeine, cyanocobalamin, cyclophosphamide, cycloSPORINE, cytarabine, DACTINomycin, DAPTOmycin, dexamethasone, dexmedetomidine, digoxin, diltiaZEM, DOCEtaxel, DOPamine, doxacurium, doxycycline, enalaprilat, ePHEDrine, EPINEPHrine, epiRUBicin, epoetin alfa, eptifibatide, erythromycin, esmolol, etoposide, famotidine, fenoldopam, fentaNYL, fludarabine, fluorouracil, folic acid, furosemide, gatifloxacin, gentamicin, glycopyrrolate, granisetron, heparin, hydrocortisone, HYDROmorphone, ifosfamide, imipenem-cilastatin, insulin (regular), isoproterenol, ketorolac, lidocaine, linezolid, LORazepam, LR, magnesium sulfate, mannitol, mechlorethamine, melphalan, meperidine, metaraminol, methicillin, methotrexate, methoxamine, methyldopate, metoclopramide, metoprolol, metroNIDAZOLE, mezlocillin, miconazole, midazolam, milrinone, minocycline, mitoXANTRONE, morphine, moxalactam, multiple vitamins, mycophenolate, nafcillin, nalbuphine, naloxone, nesiritide, netilmicin, nitroglycerin, nitroprusside, norepinephrine, normal saline, octreotide, ofloxacin, ondansetron, ornidazole, oxacillin, oxaliplatin, oxytocin, PACLitaxel, palonosetron, pamidronate, pancuronium, pantoprazole, papaverine, pefloxacin, PEMEtrexed, penicillin G potassium/sodium, pentamidine, pentazocine, PENTobarbital, peritoneal dialysis solution, perphenazine, PHENobarbital, phenylephrine, phenytoin, phytonadione, piperacillin, polymyxin B, potassium chloride, procainamide, prochlorperazine, promethazine, propofol, propranolol, protamine, pyridoxine, quiNIDine, quinupristin, raNITIdine, remifentanil, Ringer's injection, ritodrine, riTUXimab, rocuronium, sargramostim, sodium acetate/bicarbonate, sodium fusidate, sodium lactate, succinylcholine, SUFentanil, sulfamethoxazole-trimethoprim, tacrolimus, teniposide, theophylline, thiamine, thiotepa, ticarcillin, ticarcillin-clavulanate, tigecycline, tirofiban, TNA, tobramycin, tolazoline, TPN, trastuzumab, trimetaphan, urokinase, vancomycin, vasopressin, vecuronium, verapamil, vinorelbine, voriconazole

cefpodoxime

- Do not break, crush, or chew tabs due to taste
- For 10-14 days to ensure organism death, prevent superinfection
- With food for better absorption; do not give within 2 hr of antacids, H$_2$-receptor antagonists
- Shake susp well, refrigerate, discard after 2 wk

cefTAZidime

IM route

- **Fortaz, Tazidime vials:** reconstitute 500 mg or 1 g with 1.5 or 3 mL, respectively, of sterile or bacteriostatic water for inj or 0.5%-1% lidocaine (approx 280 mg/mL)
- **Tazicef vials:** reconstitute 1 g/3 mL sterile water for inj (approx 280 mg/mL)
- **Ceptaz vials:** reconstitute 1 g/3 mL sterile or bacteriostatic water for inj or 0.5%-1% lidocaine (approx 250 mg/mL)
- **Withdraw** dose while making sure needle remains in vial; **ensure** no CO$_2$ bubbles present; **inject** deeply in large muscle mass, **aspirate** before injection

IV route

- Visually inspect for particulate matter, discoloration, if possible
- **Fortaz, Tazicef, Tazidime packs:** reconstitute 1 or 2 g/100 mL sterile water for inj or other compatible IV sol (10 or 20 mg/mL, respectively); reconstitution is done in two stages: first, **inject** 10 mL of the diluent into the pack and **shake** well to dissolve and become clear; CO$_2$ pressure inside container will occur, **insert** vent needle to release pressure; **add** remaining diluents, **remove** vent needle
- **Fortaz, Tazicef, Tazidime vials:** reconstitute 500 mg, 1 g, 2 g with 5, 10, 10 mL, respectively, of sterile water for inj or other compatible IV solution (100, 95-100, or 170-180 mg/mL, respectively); **shake** well to dissolve
- **Fortaz, Tazidime ADD-Vantage vials (for IV only):** reconstitute 1 or 2 g with NS, ½ NS, D$_5$W in either 50- or 100-mL flexible diluent container; to release CO$_2$ pressure, **insert** vent needle after dissolving, **remove** vent before using
- **Ceptaz packs:** reconstitute 1 or 2 g/100 mL sterile water for inj or compatible IV sol (10 or 20 mg/mL, respectively); reconstitution is done in two stages: first, **inject** 10 mL of the diluent into the pack and **shake** well to dissolve, **add** the remaining diluent, **insert** vent needle before giving
- **Ceptaz vials:** reconstitute 1 or 2 g/10 mL of sterile water for inj or compatible IV sol (90-95, or 170-180 mg/mL, respectively)
- **Ceptaz ADD-Vantage vials (for IV only):** reconstitute 1 or 2 g with NS, ½ NS, or D$_5$W in either 50- or 100-mL diluent container

Direct Intermittent IV INFUSION route
• Vials: **withdraw** dose while making sure needle remains in sol; make sure there are no CO_2 bubbles in syringe before inj; **inject** directly over 3-5 min or slowly into tubing of a free-flowing compatible IV solution

Intermittent IV INFUSION route
• Vials: **withdraw** dose while making sure needle opening remains in sol; make sure there are no CO_2 bubbles in syringe before inj; infusion packs and ADD-Vantage systems ready for infusion after reconstitution, **infuse** over 15-30 min

Y-site compatibilities: Acyclovir, alfentanil, allopurinol, amifostine, amikacin, aminocaproic acid, aminophylline, amphotericin B lipid complex, anakinra, anidulafungin, atenolol, atropine sulfate, aztreonam, benztropine, bivalirudin, bleomycin, bumetanide, buprenorphine, butorphanol, calcium gluconate, CARBOplatin, cefamandole, ceFAZolin, cefonicid, cefoperazone, cefoTEtan, cefOXitin, cefTAZidime, ceftizoxime, cefTRIAXone, cefuroxime, cephalothin, cephapirin, cimetidine, ciprofloxacin, CISplatin, clindamycin, codeine, cyanocobalamin, cyclophosphamide, cycloSPORINE, cytarabine, DACTINomycin, DAPTOmycin, dexamethasone, dexmedetomidine, digoxin, diltiaZEM, DOCEtaxel, DOPamine, doxacurium, doxapram, enalaprilat, ePHEDrine, EPINEPHrine, epoetin alfa, eptifibatide, esmolol, etoposide, famotidine, fenoldopam, fentaNYL, filgrastim, fludarabine, fluorouracil, folic acid, foscarnet, furosemide, gallium, gatifloxacin, gemcitabine, gentamicin, glycopyrrolate, granisetron, heparin, HYDROmorphone, ifosfamide, imipenemcilastatin, indomethacin, insulin (regular), irinotecan, isepamicin, isoproterenol, isosorbide, ketamine, ketorolac, labetalol, levoFLOXacin, lidocaine, linezolid, LORazepam, LR, magnesium sulfate, mannitol, mechlorethamine, melphalan, meperidine, metaraminol, methicillin, methotrexate, methoxamine, methyldopate, methylPREDNISolone, metoclopramide, metoprolol, metroNIDAZOLE, miconazole, milrinone, morphine, moxalactam, multiple vitamins inj, nafcillin, nalbuphine, PACLitaxel, raNITIdine, remifentanil, tacrolimus, teniposide, theophylline, thiotepa, vinorelbine, zidovudine

ceftibuten
• For 10 days to ensure organism death, prevent superinfection
• On empty stomach

cefTRIAXone
• For 10-14 days to ensure organism death, prevent superinfection
• **IM** inj deeply in large muscle mass

IV route
• **IV** after **reconstituting** 250 mg/2.4 mL, 500 mg/4.8 mL, 1 g/9.6 mL, 2 g/19.2 mL D_5W, water for inj, 0.9% NaCl; **further dilute** with 50-100 mL (40 mg/mL) NS, D_5W, $D_{10}W$; shake; **run** over ½ hr
• Do not mix with calcium salts

Y-site compatibilities: Acetaminophen, acyclovir, alfentanil, allopurinol, amifostine, amikacin, aminocaproic acid, aminophylline, amiodarone, amphotericin B liposome, anidulafungin, argatroban, atenolol, atracurium, atropine, aztreonam, benztropine, bivalirudin, bleomycin, bumetanide, buprenorphine, butorphanol, CARBOplatin, cefamandole, ceFAZolin, cefmetazole, cefonicid, cefoperazone, cefoTAXime, cefoTEtan, cefOXitin, cefTAZidime, ceftizoxime, cefuroxime, cephalothin, cephapirin, cimetidine, cisatracurium, CISplatin, codeine, cyanocobalamin, cyclophosphamide, cycloSPORINE, cytarabine, DACTINomycin, DAPTOmycin, dexamethasone, dexmedetomidine, digoxin, diltiaZEM, DOCEtaxel, DOPamine, doxacurium, DOXOrubicin liposomal, doxycycline, drotrecogin alfa, enalaprilat, ePHEDrine, EPINEPHrine, epoetin alfa, eptifibatide, erythromycin, esmolol, etoposide, fenoldopam, fludarabine, fluorouracil, folic acid, foscarnet, furosemide, gallium, gatifloxacin, gemcitabine, gentamicin, glycopyrrolate, granisetron, heparin, hydrocortisone, HYDROmorphone, ifosfamide, indomethacin, insulin (regular), isoproterenol, ketorolac, lansoprazole, levoFLOXacin, lidocaine, linezolid, LORazepam, mannitol, mechlorethamine, melphalan, meperidine, metARAMinol, methicillin, methotrexate, methoxamine, methyldopa, methylPREDNISolone, metoclopramide, metoprolol, metroNIDAZOLE, mezlocillin, miconazole, midazolam, milrinone, morphine, moxalactam, multiple vitamins injection, nafcillin, nalbuphine, naloxone, nesiritide, netilmicin, nitroglycerin, nitroprusside, norepinephrine, octreotide, oxacillin, oxaliplatin, oxytocin, PACLitaxel, palonosetron, pamidronate, pancuronium, pantoprazole, PEMEtrexed, penicillin G potassium/sodium, PHENobarbital, phenylephrine, phytonadione, piperacillin, polymyxin B, potassium chloride, procainamide, propofol, propranolol, pyridoxine, raNITIdine, remifentanil, ritodrine, riTUXimab, rocuronium, sargramostim, sodium acetate/bicarbonate, succinylcholine, SUFentanil, tacrolimus, teniposide, theophylline, thiamine, thiotepa, ticarcillin, ticarcillin-clavulanate, tigecycline, tirofiban, tolazoline, trastuzumab, trimetaphan, urokinase, vasopressin, vecuronium, verapamil, vinCRIStine, voriconazole, warfarin, zidovudine

SIDE EFFECTS

CNS: Headache, dizziness, seizures
GI: *Nausea, vomiting, diarrhea, anorexia,* abdominal pain, CDAD; cholestasis (cefotaxime)
GU: renal failure
HEMA: Thrombocytopenia, agranulocytosis, neutropenia, lymphocytosis, eosinophilia, pancytopenia, hemolytic anemia
INTEG: Rash, urticaria, dermatitis, injection site reaction
MS: Arthralgia (cefditoren)
SYST: Anaphylaxis, serum sickness, Stevens-Johnson syndrome, toxic epidermal necrolysis

PHARMACOKINETICS

cefdinir
Unchanged in urine; crosses placenta, blood-brain barrier; eliminated in breast milk, not metabolized; 60%-70% protein binding, half-life 1.7 hr

cefditoren
Well absorbed when broken down (prodrug), wide distribution, half-life 100 min, onset rapid, peak 1.5-3 hr, duration 12 hr, 88% protein binding

cefepime
Peak 79 min; half-life 2 hr; 20% bound by plasma proteins; 90% excreted unchanged in urine; crosses placenta, blood-brain barrier; excreted in breast milk, not metabolized

cefixime
PO: Peak 2-8 hr, half-life 3-4 hr, 65%-70% protein binding, 50% eliminated unchanged in urine, crosses placenta, excreted in breast milk

cefotaxime
Half-life 1 hr, 35%-65% is bound by plasma proteins, 40%-65% is eliminated unchanged in urine in 24 hr, 25% metabolized in the liver to active metabolites, excreted in breast milk (small amounts)
IM: Onset 30 min
IV: Onset 5 min

cefpodoxime
Half-life 1-1.5 hr, 13%-38% bound by plasma proteins, 30% eliminated unchanged in urine in 8 hr, crosses placenta, excreted in breast milk

cefTAZidime
IM/IV: Half-life 1½-2 hr, 10% bound by plasma proteins, 80% eliminated unchanged in urine, crosses placenta, excreted in breast milk

ceftibuten
PO: Peak 2-3 hr; plasma protein binding 65%, elimination half-life 2 hr, extensively metabolized to an active metabolite
IM: Peak 1 hr
IV: Onset 5 min

cefTRIAXone
Half-life 6-9 hr, 58%-96% eliminated unchanged in urine, crosses placenta, excreted in breast milk
IM: Peak $1\frac{1}{2}$-4 hr
IV: Peak 30 min

INTERACTIONS

Many products should not be used with calcium salts (mixed or administered) or H_2 blocker antacids (PO)
Increase: bleeding—anticoagulants, thrombolytics, NSAIDs (ceftriaxone)
Increase: toxicity—aminoglycosides, furosemide loop diuretics, probenecid

Decrease: absorption of cefdinir—iron
Drug/Food
Decrease: absorption—iron-rich cereal, infant formula
Drug/Lab Test
Increase: ALT, AST, alk phos, LDH, bilirubin, BUN, creatinine
False increase: creatinine (serum urine), urinary 17-KS
False positive: urinary protein, direct Coombs' test, urine glucose
Interference: cross-matching

NURSING CONSIDERATIONS
Assess:
• **Infection:** characteristics of wounds, sputum, urine, stool, WBC >10,000/mm³, fever; obtain baseline and periodically during treatment
• Cross-sensitivity to penicillin, other cephalosporins; hypersensitivity reaction may occur
• Obtain C&S prior to treatment, may start treatment before results are received
• Blood studies: AST, ALT, CBC, Hct, bilirubin, LDH, alk phos, Coombs' test monthly if patient is on long-term therapy
• Electrolytes: potassium, sodium, chloride monthly if patient is on long-term therapy
• **CDAD:** bowel pattern daily; if severe diarrhea occurs, product should be discontinued
• IV site for extravasation, phlebitis
• **Anaphylaxis:** rash, urticaria, pruritus, chills, fever, joint pain, angioedema; may occur a few days after therapy begins
• **Serious skin disorders:** Rash, blisters; toxic epidermal necrolysis, Stevens-Johnson syndrome may occur
• **Overgrowth of infection:** perineal itching, fever, malaise, redness, pain, swelling, drainage, rash, diarrhea, change in cough, sputum
Evaluate:
• Therapeutic response: decreased symptoms of infection; negative C&S
Teach patient/family:
• If diabetic, to check blood glucose
• To report sore throat, bruising, bleeding, joint pain, may indicate **blood dyscrasias (rare);** diarrhea with mucus, blood, may indicate **CDAD**

• To complete full course of treatment, to take missed dose as soon as remembered unless close to next dose, do not double dose; to use calibrated device for suspension

TREATMENT OF ANAPHYLAXIS: EPINEPHrine, antihistamines; resuscitate if needed

---

⚠ HIGH ALERT

ceritinib (Rx)
(cerr-ah-tin′ib)
Zykadia
Func. class.: Antineoplastic—miscellaneous
Chem. class.: Protein-tyrosine kinase inhibitor

ACTION: A tyrosine kinase inhibitor targeting ▶ anaplastic lymphoma kinase (ALK); also targets insulin-like growth factor 1 (IFG-1) receptor, insulin receptor (InsR), ROS1

USES: ▶ Anaplastic lymphoma kinase (ALK)–positive metastatic non–small-cell lung cancer (NSCLC) in patients who have progressed on or are intolerant to crizotinib

CONTRAINDICATIONS: Pregnancy, hypersensitivity, QT prolongation
Precautions: Breastfeeding, children, geriatric patients, cardiac/hepatic disease, GI bleeding, bone marrow suppression, infection, diarrhea, hyperglycemia, diabetes mellitus, nausea/vomiting, pancreatitis, pneumonitis, QT prolongation, torsades de pointes, bradycardia, cardiac arrhythmias, electrolyte imbalances, corticosteroid therapy

DOSAGE AND ROUTES
• **Adult: PO** 450 mg daily on an empty stomach until disease progression or unacceptable toxicity. Decrease dose by ⅓, round to nearest 150 mg strong 3A4 inhibitors or inducers

---

Side effects: *italics* = common; red = life-threatening

Available forms: Caps 150 mg
Administer:
Dosage adjustments due to treatment-related toxicity

• **Any grade interstitial lung disease (ILD) or pneumonitis:** Permanently discontinue

• **Strong CYP3A4 inhibitors:** Close monitoring of the QT interval is recommended. If the strong CYP3A4 inhibitor is discontinued, resume the previous dosage

• Take on an empty stomach. Do not give within 2 hr of a meal; swallow tablets whole; do not crush or dissolve; if a dose is missed, make it up unless the next dose is due within 12 hr. Do not take 2 doses at the same time if missed; if vomiting occurs, do not give an additional dose. Take the next dose at the next scheduled time

SIDE EFFECTS

CNS: Weakness, fatigue, paresthesias
CV: QT prolongation, torsades de pointes, bradycardia
GI: *Nausea,* hepatotoxicity, vomiting, *anorexia,* pancreatitis, GERD, *abdominal pain,* diarrhea, constipation
INTEG: *Rash*
META: Hyperglycemia, hyperphosphatemia, hyperamylasemia
MISC: Renal failure
RESP: Cough, dyspnea, pneumonitis

PHARMACOKINETICS

Protein binding 97%; metabolized by CYP3A4; peak 4-6 hr; half-life 41 hr, excretion 68% feces

INTERACTIONS

Increase: QT prolongation—drugs that increase QT prolongation
Increase: blood levels, toxicity of—CYP3A4, CYP2C of substrates (alfentanil, cycloSPORINE, ergots, fentaNYL, phenytoin, tirolimus, tacrolimus)
Increase: ceritinib concentrations—CYP3A4 inhibitors (ketoconazole, itraconazole, erythromycin, clarithromycin); avoid concurrent use
Increase: bradycardia—β-blockers, avoid using concurrently
Increase: plasma concentrations of calcium channel blockers, ergots

Increase: of warfarin; avoid use with warfarin; use low-molecular-weight anticoagulants instead
Decrease: ceritinib concentrations—CYP3A4 inducers (dexamethasone, phenytoin, carBAMazepine, rifAMPin, PHENobarbital); avoid concurrent use

Drug/Food
Increase effect, toxicity—grapefruit, grapefruit juice
Drug/Herb
Decrease: ceritinib concentration—St. John's wort
Drug/Lab Test
Increase: bilirubin, amylase, LFTs

NURSING CONSIDERATIONS
Assess:

• **Hepatotoxicity:** pruritus, jaundice, nausea/vomiting, upper quadrant pain, dark urine

• **Bradycardia:** monitor pulse; avoid use with other agents that may lower pulse

• **Bradycardia:** Symptomatic but not life-threatening: Hold and evaluate other medications that may cause bradycardia. When asymptomatic or heart rate ≥60 bpm, resume with an adjusted dose, do not resume in those unable to tolerate 300 mg daily; life-threatening: discontinue product

• **QT prolongation:** assess for a history of cardiac arrhythmias, congestive heart failure, bradycardia, electrolyte imbalance, or congenital long QT syndrome; correct electrolyte abnormalities before starting product; monitor ECG baseline and periodically; **QTc prolongation**

• *QTc >500 msec on at least 2 separate ECGs*: Hold. When QTc returns to <481 msec (or baseline if >481 msec), resume with a 150-mg dose reduction. Do not resume in those unable to tolerate 300 mg daily. Any occurrence of QTc prolongation in combination with torsades de pointes or polymorphic ventricular tachycardia or signs/symptoms of serious arrhythmia: permanently discontinue

• **Hyperglycemia:** monitor for hyperglycemia, may be 6-8–fold in diabetic patients; if hyperglycemia continues even with antidiabetic, withhold product until controlled, restart with 150 mg

• **Persistent hyperglycemia >250 mg/ dL despite optimal antihyperglycemic therapy:** hold dose; when hyperglycemia is controlled, resume with a 150-mg dose reduction. Do not resume in those unable to tolerate 300 mg daily. If blood sugars cannot be controlled medically, discontinue

• **Pancreatitis:** monitor for nausea, vomiting, severe abdominal pain; monitor serum lipase baseline and periodically; if lipase or amylase >2× upper limit of normal (ULN), withhold product; when lipase, amylase <1.5 × ULN, start with 150 mg

Evaluate:

• Therapeutic response: decrease in progression of lung cancer

Teach patient/family:

• To report adverse reactions immediately: abdominal pain, nausea, vomiting, increased blood glucose in diabetic patients

• About reason for treatment, expected results, to avoid grapefruit juice

• To avoid OTC products unless approved by prescriber, to take as directed, not to double or miss doses

• **Pregnancy/breastfeeding:** to notify prescriber if pregnancy is planned or suspected; not to use in pregnancy

---

cephradine
See cephalosporins—1st generation

RARELY USED

cerliponase alfa
(ser-LIP-oh-nase-AL-fa)
Brineura
Func. class.: Alimentary tract and metabolism agents; lysosomal storage disorder agents

---

USES: Late infantile neuronal ceroid lipofuscinosis type 2

DOSAGE AND ROUTES

• **Adolescent/child 3-17 yr:** IV 300 mg every other wk. Give first at an infusion rate of 2.5 mL/hr, then with the required infusion of intraventricular electrolytes at the same infusion rate of 2.5 mL/hr (complete infusion time is 4.5 hr). Pretreatment with antihistamines with or without antipyretics or corticosteroids is recommended 30-60 min before the start of the infusion

---

⚠ HIGH ALERT

certolizumab (Rx)
(ser'tue-liz'oo-mab)
Cimzia
Func. class.: GI antiinflammatory antirheumatic
Chem. class.: Antitissue necrosis factor (anti-TNF) agent

ACTION: Monoclonal antibody that neutralizes the activity of tumor necrosis factor α (TNF-α) found in Crohn's disease; decreases infiltration of inflammatory cells

USES: Crohn's disease (moderate to severe) that has not responded to conventional therapy, rheumatoid arthritis (moderate to severe), psoriatic arthritis, ankylosing spondylitis
Unlabeled uses: Moderate to severe chronic plaque psoriasis, fistulizing Crohn's disease

CONTRAINDICATIONS: Influenza, IV administration, sepsis, hypersensitivity
Precautions: Pregnancy, breastfeeding, children, geriatric patients, AIDS, coagulopathy, diabetes, fungal infection, heart failure, hepatitis, human antichimeric antibody, immunosuppression, leukopenia, MS, cancer, neurologic/renal disease, surgery, thrombocytopenia, TB, vaccinations

---

Side effects: *italics* = common; red = life-threatening

Black Box Warning: Infection, neoplastic disease in children

DOSAGE AND ROUTES
Crohn's disease (moderate to severe)
• **Adult: SUBCUT** 400 mg given as 2 inj at wk 0, 2, 4; if clinical response occurs, give 400 mg q4wk
Rheumatoid arthritis (moderate to severe)/ankylosing spondylitis/psoriatic arthritis
• **Adult: SUBCUT** 400 mg (as 2 inj of 200 mg) once, then repeat at wks 2 and 4; maintenance, 200 mg q2wk or 400 mg q4wk
Available forms: Solution for inj 200 mg/mL; prefilled syringe 400-mg kit
Administer:
SUBCUT route
• **TB testing:** required before use, should be done baseline, periodically, use in TB or active infection is contraindicated
• Give by subcut inj only
• Reconstitution: allow to warm to room temperature; add 1 mL sterile water for inj to each vial; 2 vials will be needed for patients with Crohn's disease
• Gently swirl; do not shake; full reconstitution may take up to 30 min; reconstituted product may remain at room temperature for up to 2 hr or refrigerated up to 24 hr
• If reconstituted product has been refrigerated, allow to warm to room temperature
• Use 2 syringes and two 20G needles
• Withdraw reconstituted sol from each vial into separate syringes; each will contain 200 mg; switch 20G to 23G needle; inject into 2 separate sites in abdomen or thigh
• Store in refrigerator; do not freeze

SIDE EFFECTS
CNS: Anxiety, bipolar disorder, suicidal ideation
CV: Heart failure, MI, cardiac dysrhythmia, angina, stroke, thrombophlebitis, hypertension

GI: Abdominal pain
HEMA: Anemia, pancytopenia
INTEG: *Rash, urticaria,* angioedema
MISC: Anaphylaxis, antibody formation, arthralgia, bleeding, infection, lupuslike symptoms, lymphadenopathy, malignancies, serum sickness
RESP: upper respiratory tract infection, cough

PHARMACOKINETICS
Peak 54-171 hr, terminal half-life 14 days

INTERACTIONS
• Do not administer live vaccines, toxoids concurrently
Increase: possible infections—abatacept, adalimumab, anakinra, etanercept, immunosuppressive agents, inFLIXimab, rilonacept; do not use concurrently
Increase: immunosuppressant toxicity—pimecrolimus, tofacitinib, tocilzumab

NURSING CONSIDERATIONS
Assess:
• Antinuclear antibody test (ANA), hepatitis B serology, CBC with differential, blood dyscrasias
• **Rheumatoid arthritis/ankylosing spondylitis:** pain, range of motion baseline and during treatment
• **Crohn's disease:** nausea, vomiting, abdominal pain, hepatitis, increased LFTs
• CV status: B/P, pulse, chest pain
• **Allergic reaction, anaphylaxis:** rash, dermatitis, urticaria, dyspnea, hypotension, fever, chills; discontinue if severe; administer EPINEPHrine, corticosteroids, antihistamines; assess for allergies to murine proteins before starting therapy

Black Box Warning: Fungal infection: fever, weight loss, diaphoresis, fatigue, dyspnea; discontinue if infection occurs; do not administer to patients with active infection

Black Box Warning: Identify TB, risk for HBV before beginning treatment; TB test should be obtained; if present, TB should be treated before certolizumab treatment

---

Hepatitis B virus: Carriers of HBV should be monitored; those at risk for HBV should be evaluated before use

Black Box Warning: Do not use in children; lymphoma may occur

Evaluate:
• Therapeutic response: absence of fever, mucus in stools; decreased inflammation in joints, ability to move without pain

Teach patient/family:
• Those pregnant should enroll in the Mother to Baby Autoimmune Disease Study, 877-311-8972; not to breastfeed while taking this product
• To notify prescriber of GI symptoms, hypersensitivity reactions, infections, fluid retention; redness, pain, swelling at inj site
• Not to operate machinery, drive if dizziness, vertigo occur
• Not to receive live virus vaccines while taking this product
• How to inject medications if given prefilled syringes for home use
• To discuss with provider all OTC, Rx, herbals, supplements taken
• Anaphylaxis, angioedema, hypersensitivity • To report immediately rash, itching, swollen lips, tongue, face
• To discuss possible secondary malignancy

---

cetirizine (Rx, OTC)
(se-teer'i-zeen)
Aller Relief ✸, Reactine ✸,
Rhinaris Relief ✸, ZyrTEC
Func. class.: Antihistamine (2nd generation, peripherally selective)
Chem. class.: Piperazine, H_1-histamine antagonist

Do not confuse:
cetirizine/sertraline/stavudine
ZyrTEC/Xanax/Zantac/Zocor/ZyPREXA/
Zerit

ACTION: Acts on blood vessels, GI, respiratory system by competing with histamine for H_1-receptor site; decreases allergic response by blocking pharmacologic effects of histamine; minimal anticholinergic, sedative action

USES: Rhinitis, allergy symptoms, chronic idiopathic urticaria
Unlabeled uses: Asthma, atopic dermatitis

CONTRAINDICATIONS: Breastfeeding, newborn or premature infants, hypersensitivity to this product or hydrOXYzine, severe hepatic disease
Precautions: Pregnancy, children, geriatric patients, respiratory disease, angle-closure glaucoma, prostatic hypertrophy, bladder neck obstruction, asthma

DOSAGE AND ROUTES
• **Adult and child ≥6 yr:** PO 5-10 mg/day
• **Child 2-5 yr:** PO 2.5 mg/day, may increase to 5 mg/day or 2.5 mg bid
• **Child 1-2 yr:** PO 2.5 mg/day, may increase to 2.5 mg q12hr
• **Geriatric:** PO 5 mg/day, may increase to 10 mg/day
Renal dose/hemodialysis dose
• **Adult:** PO CCr 11-31 mL/min, 5 mg/day
Hepatic dose
• **Adult:** PO 5 mg daily
• **Child 6-11 yr:** PO 2.5 mg daily
Available forms: Tabs 5, 10 mg; syr 5 mg/5 mL; chew tabs 5, 10 mg; oral disintegrating tab 10 mg
Administer:
• Without regard to meals
• Store in tight, light-resistant container
• **Chew tabs:** chew before swallowing; may use with or without water
• **Syrup:** use calibrated measuring device

SIDE EFFECTS
CNS: *Headache, drowsiness,* sedation, *fatigue*
EENT: Pharyngitis, dry mouth
INTEG: Rash, eczema
RESP: Pharyngitis

PHARMACOKINETICS
Absorption rapid; onset ½ hr; peak 1-2 hr; duration 24 hr; protein binding

---

93%; half-life 8.3 hr, decreased in children, increased in renal/hepatic disease

INTERACTIONS

Increase: CNS depression—alcohol, opiates, sedative/hypnotics, other CNS depressants

Increase: anticholinergic/sedative effect—MAOIs

Drug/Lab Test

False negative: skin allergy tests

NURSING CONSIDERATIONS

Assess:

• **Allergy symptoms:** pruritus, urticaria, watering eyes at baseline and during treatment

• Respiratory status: rate, rhythm, increase in bronchial secretions, wheezing, chest tightness

Evaluate:

• Therapeutic response: absence of running or congested nose, rashes

Teach patient/family:

• About all aspects of product use; to notify prescriber if confusion, sedation, or hypotension occurs

• To avoid driving, other hazardous activity if drowsiness occurs; to take at night as drowsiness may occur, especially in children

• To avoid alcohol, other CNS depressants, OTC antihistamines

• To avoid exposure to sunlight; burns may occur

• To use sugarless gum, candy, frequent sips of water to minimize dry mouth

TREATMENT OF OVERDOSE:

Administer diazePAM, vasopressors, phenytoin IV

> ⚠ **HIGH ALERT**
>
> **RARELY USED**
>
> ## cetrorelix (Rx)
> (set-roe-ree'lix)
> Cetrotide
> *Func. class.:* Gonadotropin-releasing hormone antagonist
> *Chem. class.:* Synthetic decapeptide

USES: For inhibition of premature LH surges in women undergoing controlled ovarian hyperstimulation

CONTRAINDICATIONS: Pregnancy, breastfeeding, hypersensitivity, latex allergy, renal disease, KRA5 mutation

DOSAGE AND ROUTES

Single-dose regimen

• **Adult:** SUBCUT 3 mg when serum estradiol level at appropriate stimulation response, usually on stimulation day 7; if hCG not given within 4 days after inj of 3 mg cetrorelix, give 0.25 mg daily until day of hCG administration

Multiple-dose regimen

• **Adult:** SUBCUT 0.25 mg given on stimulation day 5 (either morning or evening) or 6 (morning) and continued daily until day hCG is given

BPH (unlabeled)

• **Adult (male):** SUBCUT 5 mg bid × 2 days, then 1 mg/day

Endometriosis (unlabeled)

• **Adult (female):** SUBCUT 3 mg weekly

> ⚠ **HIGH ALERT**
>
> ## cetuximab (Rx)
> (se-tux'i-mab)
> Erbitux
> *Func. class.:* Antineoplastic—miscellaneous, monoclonal antibody
> *Chem. class.:* Epidermal growth factor receptor inhibitor

ACTION: Not fully understood; binds to 🔟 K-RAS wild-type epidermal growth factor receptors (EGFRs); inhibits phosphorylation and activation of receptor-associated kinase, thereby resulting in inhibition of cell growth

USES: Alone or in combination with irinotecan for 🔟 K-RAS wild-type EGFRs expressing metastatic colorectal carcinoma, head/neck cancer

---

Unlabeled uses: Front-line use for non–small-cell lung cancer in combination with CISplatin and vinorelbine

CONTRAINDICATIONS:
Hypersensitivity to this product, murine proteins, ✱ɴᴀ RAS-mutant metastatic colorectal cancer or unknown RAS mutation
Precautions: Pregnancy, breastfeeding, children, geriatric patients; CV/renal/hepatic disease; ocular or pulmonary disorders, arrhythmias, CAD, radiation/platinum-based therapy, respiratory arrest

> Black Box Warning: Infusion-related reactions, cardiac arrest

DOSAGE AND ROUTES
• **Adult: IV INFUSION** 400 mg/m^2 loading dose given over 120 min, max infusion rate 5 mL/min; weekly maintenance dose (all other infusion) is 250 mg/m^2 given over 60 min, max infusion rate 5 mL/min (10 mg/min); premedicate with an H$_1$-antagonist (diphenhydrAMINE 50 mg IV); dosage adjustments made for infusion reactions or dermatologic toxicity; other protocols used
Available forms: Sol for inj 2 mg/mL
Administer:
• Premedicate with diphenhydramine 50 mg 30-60 min before first dose; use during infusion for reactions
Intermittent IV INFUSION route
• Use cytoxic handling procedures
• By IV infusion only; do not give by IV push or bolus; do not shake or dilute
• Do not dilute with other products
• Store refrigerated at 36° F-46° F, discard unused portions
• **Infusion pump:** draw up volume of vial using appropriate syringe/needle (vented spike or other appropriate transfer device); fill Erbitux into sterile evacuated container/bag, repeat until calculated volume put into the container; use new needle for each vial; give through in-line filter (low protein binding 0.22 micrometer); affix infusion line and prime before starting infusion, max rate 5 mL/min; flush line at end of infusion with 0.9% NaCl; use a low–protein-binding 0.22-micrometer in-line filter.
• **Syringe pump:** draw up volume of vial using appropriate syringe/needle (vented spike); place syringe into syringe driver of syringe pump and set rate; use in-line filter (low protein binding 0.22-micrometer); connect infusion line, start infusion after priming; repeat until calculated volume given
• Use new needle and filter for each vial, max 5 mL/min rate; use 0.9% NaCl to flush line after infusion
• Do not piggyback to patient infusion line
• Observe patient for adverse reactions for 1 hr after infusion

> Black Box Warning: Infusion reactions (bronchospasm, stridor, urticaria, hypotension, MI): if mild (grade 1 or 2), reduce all doses by 50%; if severe (grade 3 or 4), permanently discontinue; monitor for at least 1 hr after completion of therapy; reactions usually occur during first dose; have emergency equipment nearby

SIDE EFFECTS
CNS: *Headache, insomnia, depression,* aseptic meningitis
CV: Cardiac arrest
GI: *Nausea, diarrhea, vomiting, anorexia, mouth ulceration, dehydration, constipation, abdominal pain*
HEMA: Leukopenia, anemia, neutropenia
INTEG: Rash, pruritus, acne, toxic epidermal necrolysis, angioedema, acute infusion reactions, other skin toxicities
MISC: *Conjunctivitis* hypomagnesemia
RESP: Interstitial lung disease, *cough, dyspnea,* pulmonary embolus, respiratory arrest
SYST: Anaphylaxis, sepsis, infection, mucosal inflammation, Stevens-Johnson syndrome, toxic epidermal necrolysis

PHARMACOKINETICS
Half-life 114 hr, steady state by 3rd wkly infusion

Side effects: *italics* = common; red = life-threatening

INTERACTIONS
Drug/Lab Test
Increase: LFTs

NURSING CONSIDERATIONS
Assess:
• **Pulmonary changes:** lung sounds, cough, dyspnea; interstitial lung disease may occur, may be fatal; discontinue therapy if confirmed

Black Box Warning: Cardiac arrest: monitor electrolytes; in those undergoing radiation therapy, electrolytes may be decreased; monitor cardiac patients who receive this product and radiation therapy or platinum-based therapy with 5-FU (head, neck cancer)

• **Serious hypersensitivity reactions:** toxic epidermal necrosis, angioedema, anaphylaxis, Stevens-Johnson syndrome
• Monitor serum calcium, magnesium, potassium during and for 8 wk after treatment; low levels may occur from a few days to several months after treatment
• GI symptoms: frequency of stools, dehydration, abdominal pain, stomatitis
• **K-RAS mutations** with metastatic colorectal carcinoma; if K-RAS mutation on codon 12 or 13 detected, patient should not receive anti-EGFR antibody therapy
Evaluate:
• Therapeutic response: decreased growth, spread of EGFR-expressing metastatic colorectal, head/neck carcinoma
Teach patient/family:
• **To report adverse reactions immediately:** shortness of breath, severe abdominal pain, skin eruptions
• About the reason for treatment, expected results
• To use contraception (both female and male) during treatment and for 6 mo after treatment; not to breastfeed during treatment and for 2 mo after treatment
• To wear sunscreen and hats to limit sun exposure; sun exposure can exacerbate any skin reactions

• To avoid crowds, persons with known infections

---

chlordiazePOXIDE (Rx)
(klor-dye-az-e-pox′ide)
Librium ✦, Solium ✦
Func. class.: Antianxiety
Chem. class.: Benzodiazepine, long-acting

Controlled Substance Schedule IV

Do not confuse:
Librium/Librax

ACTION: Potentiates the actions of GABA, especially in the limbic system, reticular formation

USES: Short-term management of anxiety, acute alcohol withdrawal, preoperatively for relaxation

CONTRAINDICATIONS: Pregnancy, breastfeeding, children <6 yr, hypersensitivity to benzodiazepines, closed-angle glaucoma, psychosis
Precautions: Geriatric patients, debilitated, renal/hepatic disease, suicidal ideation, abrupt discontinuation, respiratory depression, Parkinson's disease, myasthenia gravis

DOSAGE AND ROUTES
Mild anxiety
• **Adult: PO** 5-10 mg tid-qid
• **Geriatric: PO** 5 mg bid initially, increase as needed
• **Child >6 yr: PO** 5 mg bid-qid, max 10 mg bid-tid
Severe anxiety
• **Adult: PO** 25-50 mg tid-qid
Preoperatively
• **Adult: PO** 5-10 mg tid-qid on day before surgery
Alcohol withdrawal
• **Adult: PO** 50-100 mg q4-6hr prn, max 300 mg/day
Renal disease
• **Adult: PO** CCr <10 mL/min, give 50% dose

Available forms: Caps 5, 10, 25 mg
Administer:
PO route
• With food or milk for GI symptoms

SIDE EFFECTS

CNS: *Dizziness, drowsiness,* confusion, headache, anxiety, tremors, stimulation, fatigue, depression, insomnia, hallucinations
CV: *Orthostatic hypotension,* edema, ECG changes, tachycardia, hypotension
EENT: *Blurred vision,* tinnitus, mydriasis
GI: Constipation, dry mouth, nausea, vomiting, anorexia, diarrhea
GU: Irregular periods, decreased libido
HEMA: Agranulocytosis
INTEG: Rash, dermatitis, itching

PHARMACOKINETICS

PO: Onset 30 min, peak within 2 hr, duration 4-6 hr, metabolized by liver, excreted by kidneys, crosses placenta, excreted in breast milk, half-life 5-30 hr (increased in geriatric patients)

INTERACTIONS

Increase: CNS depression—CNS depressants, alcohol
Increase: chlordiazePOXIDE—cimetidine, disulfiram, FLUoxetine, isoniazid, ketoconazole, metoprolol, oral contraceptives, propranolol, valproic acid
Decrease: action of levodopa
Decrease: action of chlordiazePOXIDE—CYP3A4 inhibitors (protease inhibitors, barbiturates, rifamycins)
Drug/Lab Test
Increase: LFTs
False increase: 17-OHCS
False positive: pregnancy test (some methods)

NURSING CONSIDERATIONS

Assess:
• B/P (lying, standing), pulse; if systolic B/P drops 20 mm Hg, hold product, notify prescriber
• Hepatic studies: AST, ALT, bilirubin, creatinine, LDH, alk phos during long-term therapy

• For ataxia, oversedation of geriatric patients, debilitated patients; provide assistance with ambulation during beginning therapy
• Physical dependency, withdrawal symptoms: headache, nausea, vomiting, muscle pain, weakness after long-term use.
• Need for assistance with ambulation during beginning therapy because drowsiness, dizziness occur
• Check to confirm that PO medication has been swallowed if patient is depressed, suicidal
• Sugarless gum, hard candy, frequent sips of water for dry mouth
• **Pregnancy/breastfeeding:** do not use in pregnancy or breastfeeding
Evaluate:
• Therapeutic response: decreased anxiety, restlessness, sleeplessness
Teach patient/family:
• That product may be taken with food
• Not to use product for everyday stress or use for more than 4 mo unless directed by prescriber, tolerance occurs
• Not to take more than prescribed amount; may be habit forming
• To avoid OTC preparations unless approved by prescriber
• To avoid driving, activities that require alertness because drowsiness may occur
• To avoid alcohol ingestion, other psychotropic medications unless directed by prescriber
• Not to discontinue medication abruptly after long-term use because this may precipitate seizures
• To rise slowly because fainting may occur, especially among geriatric patients
• That drowsiness may be worse at beginning of treatment
• To notify prescriber if pregnancy is suspected or planned; not to use in pregnancy or breastfeeding
• To immediately report suicidal thoughts/behaviors

TREATMENT OF OVERDOSE:
Lavage, VS, supportive care, give flumazenil

chloroquine (Rx)

(klor'oh-kwin)

Aralen ✚

Func. class.: Antimalarial
Chem. class.: Synthetic 4-amino-quinoline derivative

ACTION: Inhibits parasite replication, transcription of DNA to RNA by forming complexes with DNA of parasite

USES: Malaria of *Plasmodium vivax, P. malariae, P. ovale, P. falciparum* (some strains); amebiasis
Unlabeled uses: Discoid lupus erythematosus, polymorphous light eruption, rheumatoid arthritis, ulcerative colitis

CONTRAINDICATIONS: Hypersensitivity, retinal field changes
Precautions: Pregnancy, breastfeeding, children, blood dyscrasias, severe GI/neurologic/cardiac disease, alcoholism, hepatic disease, ✚ G6PD deficiency, psoriasis, eczema, seizures, preexisting auditory damage, torsades de pointes, infection

DOSAGE AND ROUTES
Acute malaria attacks
• **Adult: PO** 1000 mg (600-mg base), then 500 mg (300-mg base) in 6-8 hr, 500 mg (300-mg base) daily × 2 days for a total of 2.5 g (1.5-g base) in 3 days
• **Adult/adolescent of low body weight, child/infant: PO** 16.5 mg (10-mg base)/kg, max 600-mg base, then 8.3 mg (5-mg base)/kg, max 300-mg base 6 hr after 1st dose, then 8.3 mg (5-mg base)/kg, max 300-mg base 24 hr after 1st dose, then 8.3 mg (5-mg base)/kg, max 300-mg base 36 hr after 1st dose
Malaria prophylaxis (in areas with chloroquine-sensitive *P. falciparum*)
• **Adult: PO** 500 mg (300-mg base) weekly on same day of each wk starting 2 wk before travel and for 8 wk after leaving
Extraintestinal amebiasis
• **Adult: PO** 1 g (600-mg base) daily × 2 days, then 500 mg (300-mg base) for ≥2-3 wk

• **Child (unlabeled): PO** 16.6 mg (10-mg base)/kg (max 300-mg base) daily × 2-3 wk
Rheumatoid arthritis/discoid lupus erythematosus (unlabeled)
• **Adult: PO** 250 mg (150-mg base) daily
Available forms: Tabs 250 mg (150-mg base), 500 mg (300-mg base) phosphate
Administer:
• Product in mg or base; they are different
PO route
• Before or after meals at same time each day to maintain product level
• Store in tight, light-resistant container at room temperature; keep inj in cool environment

SIDE EFFECTS
CNS: Headache, stimulation, fatigue, seizures, psychosis, hallucinations, insomnia
CV: Hypotension, heart block, asystole with syncope, ECG changes, cardiomyopathy
EENT: *Blurred vision, corneal changes, retinal changes, difficulty focusing,* tinnitus, vertigo, deafness, photophobia, corneal edema
GI: *Nausea, vomiting, anorexia,* diarrhea, cramps
HEMA: Thrombocytopenia, agranulocytosis, hemolytic anemia, leukopenia
INTEG: Pruritus, pigmentary changes, skin eruptions, lichen-planus–like eruptions, eczema, exfoliative dermatitis

PHARMACOKINETICS
Metabolized in liver; excreted in urine, feces, breast milk; crosses placenta
PO: Peak 1-3 hr, half-life 3-5 days

INTERACTIONS
• Reduced oral clearance and metabolism of chloroquine, cimetidine
Increase: QT prolongation, torsades de pointes—class IA, III antidysrhythmics
Increase: effects—2D6 inhibitors (amiodarone, chlorpheniramine, FLUoxetine, haloperidol, ritonavir, PARoxetine, terbinafine, ticlopidine); CYP3A4 inhibitors (diltiaZEM, verapamil, itraconazole, ketoconazole, erythromycin, doxycycline, clarithromycin)

Decrease: action of chloroquine—magnesium, aluminum compounds, kaolin; do not use concurrently

Decrease: effects of ampicillin, rabies vaccine (ID)

Drug/Lab Test

Decrease: Hgb, platelets, WBC

NURSING CONSIDERATIONS
Assess:

• **Infection:** resistance is common; not to be used for *P. falciparum* acquired in areas of resistance or where prophylaxis has failed

• Ophthalmic test if long-term treatment or dosage of >150 mg/day, baseline and periodically

• Screen for G6PD deficiency; identify risk of hemolysis

• Blood studies: CBC, as blood dyscrasias occur

• **ECG** during therapy; watch for depression of T waves, widening of QRS complex

• **Allergic reactions:** pruritus, rash, urticaria

• **Blood dyscrasias:** malaise, fever, bruising, bleeding (rare)

• **For ototoxicity** (tinnitus, vertigo, change in hearing); audiometric testing should be done before, after treatment

• **For toxicity:** blurring vision; difficulty focusing; headache; dizziness; decreased knee, ankle reflexes; seizures; CV collapse; product should be discontinued immediately and IV fluids given

Evaluate:

• Therapeutic response: decreased symptoms of infection

Teach patient/family:

• To take with meals or immediately after meals

• To use sunglasses in bright sunlight to decrease photophobia

• That urine may turn rust or brown color

• To report hearing, visual problems; fever, fatigue, bruising, bleeding (may indicate blood dyscrasias)

• To keep away from pets, children; overdose is fatal

• **Pregnancy/breastfeeding:** to avoid use in pregnancy unless suppression of malaria is needed and benefits outweigh fetal risk; do not use in breastfeeding

TREATMENT OF OVERDOSE:
• Administer barbiturate (ultrashort-acting), vasopressor; tracheostomy may be necessary.

---

chlorproMAZINE (Rx)
(klor-proe′ma-zeen)
Func. class.: Antipsychotic/antiemetic
Chem. class.: Phenothiazine-aliphatic

Do not confuse:
chlorproMAZINE/chlorproPAMIDE/prochlorperazine

ACTION: Depresses cerebral cortex, hypothalamus, limbic system, which control activity, aggression; blocks neurotransmission produced by DOPamine at synapse; exhibits a strong α-adrenergic, anticholinergic blocking action; mechanism for antipsychotic effects is unclear

USES: Psychotic disorders, mania, schizophrenia, anxiety, intractable hiccups in adults, nausea, vomiting; preoperatively for relaxation; acute intermittent porphyria, behavioral problems in children, nonpsychotic, demented patients, Tourette's syndrome

Unlabeled uses: Vascular headache, agitation, dementia, neonatal abstinence syndrome

CONTRAINDICATIONS: Children <6 mo, hypersensitivity, circulatory collapse, liver damage, cerebral arteriosclerosis, coronary disease, coma

Precautions: Pregnancy, breastfeeding, geriatric patients, seizure disorders, hypertension, hepatic/cardiac disease, prostatic enlargement, Parkinson's disease, pulmonary disease, severe hypo/hypertension, blood dyscrasias, brain damage, bone marrow depression, alcohol/barbiturate withdrawal, closed-angle glaucoma

Black Box Warning: Dementia; increased mortality in geriatric patients with dementia-related psychosis

---

DOSAGE AND ROUTES
Psychosis
- **Adult: PO** 10-50 mg q1-4hr initially then increase up to 2 g/day if necessary; **IM** 10-50 mg q1-4hr, usual dose 300-800 mg/day
- **Geriatric: PO** 10-25 mg daily-bid, increase by 10-25 mg/day q4-7days, max 800 mg/day
- **Child >6 mo: PO** 0.55 mg/kg q4-6hr; **IM** 0.5 mg/kg q6-8hr

Nausea and vomiting
- **Adult: PO** 10-25 mg q4-6hr prn; **IM** 12.5-25 mg q3hr prn, then 25-50 mg q6-8 hr prn if no hypotension, max 400 mg/day; **IV** 25-50 mg daily-qid
- **Child ≥6 mo: PO** 0.55 mg/kg q4-6hr; **IM** q6-8hr; **IM** ≤5 yr or ≤22.7 kg, 40 mg; max **IM** 5-10 yr or 22.7-45.5 kg, 75 mg

Intractable hiccups/acute intermittent porphyria
- **Adult: PO** 25-50 mg tid-qid; **IM** 25-50 mg (only if **PO** dose does not work); **IV** 25-50 mg in 500-1000 mL NS(only for severe hiccups)

Available forms: Tabs 10, 25, 50, 100, 200 mg; inj 25 mg/mL

Administer:
Anticholinergic agent for EPS if ordered
PO route
- With full glass of water, milk or with food to decrease GI upset
- Periodically attempt dosage reduction in those with behavioral problems
- Store in tight, light-resistant container

Syrup:
- Use calibrated measuring device, do not spill on skin or clothes

IM route
- Use gloves to prepare product; if product touches skin, wash with soap and water to prevent contact dermatitis
- IM, inject in deep muscle mass with patient recumbent, do not give SUBCUT, no dilution needed; if irritation occurs, may dilute in NS or procaine 2%
- Avoid skin contact with injection solution—may cause contact dermatitis

IV route (surgery only)
Direct IV: After **diluting** 1 mg/1 mL with NS, **give** 1 mg or less/2 min or more with patient recumbent, never give undiluted

Intermittent IV INFUSION: Dilute 25-50 mg/500-1000 NS or other compatible large IV sol, **give** over ½ hour, protect from light

Y-site compatibilities: Alfentanil, amikacin, amphotericin B lipid complex, amsacrine, anidulafungin, ascorbic acid injection, atenolol, atracurium, atropine, benztropine, bleomycin sulfate, buprenorphine, butorphanol, calcium chloride/gluconate, caspofungin, cimetidine, cisatracurium, CISplatin, cladribine, codeine, cyanocobalamin, cyclophosphamide, cycloSPORINE, cytarabine, DACTINomycin, DAPTOmycin, dexmedetomidine, digoxin, diltiaZEM, diphenhydrAMINE, DOBUTamine, DOCEtaxel, DOPamine, doxacurium, DOXOrubicin, DOXORUBicin liposomal, doxycycline, enalaprilat, ePHEDrine, EPINEPHrine, epiRUBicin, erythromycin, esmolol, etoposide, famotidine, fenoldopam, fentaNYL, filgrastim, fluconazole, gatifloxacin, gemcitabine, gentamicin, glycopyrrolate, granisetron, hydrocortisone, HYDROmorphone, hydrOXYzine, IDArubicin, ifosfamide, isoproterenol, labetalol, levoFLOXacin, lidocaine, LORazepam, LR, magnesium sulfate, mannitol, mechlorethamine, meperidine, methicillin, methoxamine, methyldopate, methylPREDNISolone, metoclopramide, metoprolol, metroNIDAZOLE, miconazole, midazolam, milrinone, minocycline, mitoXANTRONE, morphine, multiple vitamins injection, mycophenolate mofetil, nafcillin, nalbuphine, naloxone, netilmicin, nitroglycerin, norepinephrine, octreotide, ondansetron, oxacillin, oxaliplatin, palonosetron, pamidronate, pancuronium, papaverine, penicillin G potassium, pentamidine, pentazocine, phytonadione, polymyxin B, potassium chloride, procainamide, prochlorperazine, promethazine, propofol, propranolol, protamine sulfate, pyridoxine, quiNIDine, quinupristin-dalfopristin, raNITIdine, Ringer's injection, ritodrine, riTUXimab, rocuronium, sodium acetate, succinylcholine, SUFentanil, tacrolimus, teniposide, theophylline, thiamine, thiotepa, tirofiban, TNA, tolazoline, TPN, trimetaphan, vancomycin, vasopressin, vecuronium, verapamil, vinCRIStine, vinorelbine, vitamin B complex with C, voriconazole, zoledronic acid

SIDE EFFECTS

CNS: *EPS: pseudoparkinsonism, akathisia, dystonia, tardive dyskinesia,* seizures, *headache,* neuroleptic malignant syndrome, dizziness

CV: *Orthostatic hypotension,* hypertension, cardiac arrest, ECG changes, tachycardia

EENT: Blurred vision, glaucoma, dry eyes

ENDO: SIADH

GI: *Dry mouth, nausea, vomiting, anorexia, constipation,* diarrhea, cholestatic jaundice, weight gain

GU: Urinary retention, enuresis, impotence, amenorrhea, gynecomastia, breast engorgement

HEMA: Anemia, leukopenia, leukocytosis, agranulocytosis

INTEG: *Rash,* photosensitivity, dermatitis

RESP: Laryngospasm, dyspnea, respiratory depression

SYST: Death in geriatric patients with dementia

PHARMACOKINETICS

Metabolized by liver, excreted in urine (metabolites), crosses placenta, enters breast milk, 95% bound to plasma proteins, elimination half-life 23-37 hr

PO: Absorption variable, widely distributed, onset erratic 30-60 min, duration 4-6 hr

PO-ER: Onset 30-60 min, peak unknown, duration 10-12 hr

IM: Well absorbed, peak 15-20 min, duration 4-8 hr

IV: Onset 5 min, peak 10 min, duration unknown

INTERACTIONS

Increase: CNS depression—other CNS depressants, alcohol, barbiturate anesthetics, antihistamines, sedatives/hypnotics, antidepressants

Increase: toxicity—EPINEPHrine

Increase: agranulocystosis—antithyroid agents

Increase: effects of both products—β-adrenergic blockers, alcohol

Increase: anticholinergic effects—anticholinergics, antidepressants, antiparkinsonian agents, MAOIs

Increase: valproic acid level

Decrease: seizure threshold—anticonvulsants

Decrease: absorption—aluminum hydroxide, magnesium hydroxide antacids, cimetidine

Decrease: antiparkinson activity—levodopa, bromocriptine

Decrease: serum chlorproMAZINE—lithium, barbiturates

Decrease: anticoagulant effect—warfarin

Drug/Herb:

Increase: CNS depression—kava, chamomile, hops, valerian

Increase: anticholinergic effect—jimson weed, scopolia

Drug/Lab Test

Increase: hepatic studies

Decrease: WBC, platelets, Hgb/Hct

False positive: pregnancy tests, PKU

False negative: urinary steroids, 17-OHCS

NURSING CONSIDERATIONS
Assess:

Black Box Warning: **Beers:** avoid in older adults except in schizophrenia, bipolar disorder, or short-term use as antiemetic in chemotherapy; increased risk for stroke and greater rate of cognitive decline and mortality in dementia

• Mental status: AIMS assessment, orientation, mood, behavior, presence and type of hallucinations before initial administration and monthly

• Any potentially reversible causes of behavioral problems in geriatric patients before and during therapy

• I&O ratio; palpate bladder if low urinary output occurs, especially in geriatric patients

• Monitor B/P, pulse, lying, sitting

• Bilirubin, CBC, LFTs, ocular exam; agranulocytosis, glaucoma, cholestatic jaundice may occur

• Respirations q4hr during initial treatment; establish baseline before starting treatment; report drops of 30 mm Hg; obtain baseline ECG; Q-wave and T-wave changes

- Dizziness, faintness, palpitations, tachycardia on rising
- **Neuroleptic malignant syndrome:** hyperpyrexia, muscle rigidity, increased CPK, altered mental status, for acute dystonia (check chewing, swallowing, eyes, pill rolling)
- **Extrapyramidal symptoms:** akathisia (inability to sit still, no pattern to movements), tardive dyskinesia (bizarre movements of the jaw, mouth, tongue, extremities), pseudoparkinsonism (rigidity, tremors, pill rolling, shuffling gait)
- Constipation, urinary retention daily; increase bulk, water in diet
- Supervised ambulation until stabilized on medication; do not involve in strenuous exercise program because fainting is possible; patient should not stand still for long periods
- Increased fluids, roughage to prevent constipation
- Candy, gum, sips of water for dry mouth
- **Pregnancy/breastfeeding:** no well-controlled studies; use in pregnancy only if benefits outweigh fetal risk; excreted in breast milk, discontinue breastfeeding or product

Evaluate:

- Therapeutic response: decrease in emotional excitement, hallucinations, delusions, paranoia; reorganization of patterns of thought, speech; increase in target behaviors

Teach patient/family:

- To use good oral hygiene; to use frequent rinsing of mouth, sugarless gum, candy, ice chips for dry mouth
- To avoid hazardous activities until product response is determined
- That orthostatic hypotension occurs often; to rise gradually from sitting or lying position
- To remain lying down for at least 30 min after IM inj
- To avoid hot tubs, hot showers, tub baths because hypotension may occur; that during hot weather, heat stroke may occur; to take extra precautions to stay cool

- To avoid abrupt withdrawal of product or EPS may result; product should be withdrawn slowly
- To avoid OTC preparations (cough, hay fever, cold) unless approved by prescriber since serious product interactions may occur; avoid use with alcohol, increased drowsiness may occur
- To use a sunscreen and sunglasses to prevent burns and photophobia
- To take antacids 2 hr before or after this product
- To report sore throat, malaise, fever, bleeding, mouth sores; CBC should be drawn and product discontinued
- To employ contraceptive measures
- That urine may turn pink or reddish brown

TREATMENT OF OVERDOSE: Lavage if orally ingested; provide airway; *do not induce vomiting or use EPINEPHrine*

---

cholestyramine (Rx)
(koe-less-tir′a-meen)
Prevalite
Func. class.: Antilipemic
Chem. class.: Bile acid sequestrant

Do not confuse:
Questran/Quarzan

ACTION: Adsorbs, combines with bile acids to form insoluble complex that is excreted through feces; loss of bile acids lowers LDL, cholesterol levels

USES: Primary hypercholesterolemia (esp. type IIa/IIb hyperlipoproteinemia), pruritus associated with biliary obstruction
Unlabeled uses: Diarrhea caused by excess bile acid, thyroid storm

CONTRAINDICATIONS: Hypersensitivity; complete biliary obstruction; hyperlipidemia III, IV, V
Precautions: Pregnancy, breastfeeding, children, PKU, renal disease, coagulopathy

---

DOSAGE AND ROUTES
• **Adult:** PO 4 g/day or bid, max 24 g/day
• **Child:** PO 240 mg/kg/day in 3 divided doses with food or drink, max 8 g/day titrated up over several weeks to decrease GI effects
Available forms: Powder for susp 4 g cholestyramine/packet or scoop; tab 1 g
Administer:
• Product daily or bid; give all other medications 1 hr before or 4-6 hr after cholestyramine to avoid poor absorption
• Product mixed with applesauce or stirred into beverage (2-6 oz), let stand for 2 min; do not take dry, avoid inhaling powder, avoid GI tube administration, take with food
• Supplemental doses of vit A, D, K if levels are low
• Doses are expressed in anhydrous cholestyramine resin; amount of resin varies with each product

SIDE EFFECTS
CNS: Headache, dizziness, drowsiness, vertigo, tinnitus, anxiety
GI: *Constipation, abdominal pain, nausea,* fecal impaction, hemorrhoids, flatulence, vomiting, steatorrhea, peptic ulcer
HEMA: Bleeding, increased PT
INTEG: Rash, irritation of perianal area, tongue, skin
META: Decreased vit A, D, K, red cell folate content; hyperchloremic acidosis
MS: Muscle, joint pain

PHARMACOKINETICS
PO: Excreted in feces, LDL lowered within 4-7 days, serum cholesterol lowered within 1 mo, duration 2-4 wk

INTERACTIONS
Decrease: absorption of warfarin, thiazides, cardiac glycosides, propranolol, corticosteroids, iron, thyroid hormones, acetaminophen, amiodarone, penicillin G, tetracyclines, clofibrate, gemfibrozil, oral vancomycin, glipiZIDE, vit A, D, E, K
Drug/Lab Test
Increase: AST, ALT, alk phos
Decrease: sodium, potassium

NURSING CONSIDERATIONS
Assess:
• Cardiac glycoside level if both products administered, may need to adjust dose of cardiac glycoside if this product is increased or decreased
• For signs of vit A, D, K deficiency
• **Hypercholesterolemia:** fasting LDL, HDL, total cholesterol, triglyceride levels, electrolytes if receiving extended therapy; diet history
• **Pruritus:** for signs of itching
• Bowel pattern daily; increase bulk, water in diet for constipation; diarrhea may also occur
• **Pregnancy/breastfeeding:** no well-controlled studies; may decrease vitamin absorption (fat-soluble); use only if benefits outweigh fetal risks; cautious use in breastfeeding, vitamins may be decreased
Evaluate:
• Therapeutic response: decreased LDL, cholesterol level (hyperlipidemia); diarrhea, pruritus (excess bile acids)
Teach patient/family:
• **About the symptoms of hypoprothrombinemia:** bleeding mucous membranes, dark tarry stools, hematuria, petechiae; report immediately
• To take with food, never use dry
• That PKU patients should avoid Questran Light (contains aspartame and phenylalanine)
• About the importance of compliance
• That risk factors should be decreased: high-fat diet, smoking, alcohol consumption, absence of exercise
• That GI side effects will resolve with continued use

---

cidofovir (Rx)
(si-doh-foh'veer)
Vistide
Func. class.: Antiviral
Chem. class.: Nucleotide analog

ACTION: Suppresses cytomegalovirus (CMV) replication by selective inhibition of viral DNA synthesis

---

USES: CMV retinitis in patients with HIV; used with probenecid

Unlabeled uses: Adenovirus, condylomata acuminata, eczema vaccination, Epstein-Barr virus, generalized vaccinia, herpes genitalis/simplex, HPV, molluscum contagiosum, vaccinia necrosum, vaccinia, varicella-zoster, variola

CONTRAINDICATIONS: Hypersensitivity to this product, probenecid, sulfa products; direct intraocular injection; proteinuria, renal disease/failure

Precautions: Pregnancy, breastfeeding, children <6 mo, geriatric patients, preexisting cytopenias, renal function impairment, platelet count <25,000/mm^3, dehydration

> **Black Box Warning:** Neutropenia, infertility, secondary malignancy, pregnancy, nephrotoxicity

DOSAGE AND ROUTES

• **Adult: IV INFUSION** Induction: 5 mg/kg over 1 hr q wk × 2 wks; maintenance: 5 mg/kg over 1 hr every other wk, give with probenecid

Renal dose

• **Adult: IV** CCr ≤55 mL/min, do not use; SCr increase of 0.3-0.4 mg/dL above baseline, decrease dose to 3 mg/kg; CCr increase of ≥0.5 mg/dL above baseline or ≥2+ proteinuria, discontinue

Available forms: Inj 75 mg/mL

Administer:

> **Black Box Warning:** Use cytotoxic handling procedures

• Allow to warm to room temperature
• If product comes in contact with skin, wash with soap and water immediately
• If zidovudine is used, reduce dose to 50% on cidofovir treatment days

Intermittent IV INFUSION route

• **Dilute** in 100 mL 0.9% saline sol before administration; **give** probenecid PO 2 g 3 hr before the cidofovir infusion and 1 g at 2 and 8 hr after ending the cidofovir infusion; **give** 1 L of 0.9% saline sol IV with each INFUSION of cidofovir, give saline INFUSION over 1-2 hr period immediately before cidofovir; patient should be given a 2nd L if the patient can tolerate the fluid load (2nd L given at time of cidofovir or immediately afterward, should be given over 1-3 hr)

• **Give** slowly; do not give by bolus IV, SUBCUT inj
• Use diluted sol within 24 hr, do not freeze; do not use sol with particulate matter or discoloration
• Do not admix

SIDE EFFECTS

CNS: *Fever, chills,* coma, confusion, abnormal thoughts, *dizziness,* bizarre dreams, *headache,* psychosis, tremors, somnolence, paresthesia, *amnesia, anxiety, insomnia,* seizures

CV: Dysrhythmias, hypo/hypertension

EENT: Retinal detachment with CMV retinitis

GI: Abnormal LFTs, *nausea, vomiting, anorexia, diarrhea,* abdominal pain, hemorrhage

GU: Hematuria, increased creatinine, BUN, nephrotoxicity

HEMA: Granulocytopenia, thrombocytopenia, irreversible neutropenia, anemia, eosinophilia

INTEG: *Rash, alopecia, pruritus, acne,* urticaria, pain at inj site, phlebitis

RESP: Dyspnea

PHARMACOKINETICS

Terminal half-life 2.6 hr

INTERACTIONS

> **Black Box Warning: Nephrotoxicity:** amphotericin B, foscarnet, aminoglycosides, pentamidine IV, NSAIDs, salicylates; wait 7 days after use to begin cidofovir

Drug/Lab

Increase: ALT, AST, alk phos, glucose, cholesterol, BUN, creatinine, urine protein

Decrease: neutrophils, platelets, calcium, potassium

NURSING CONSIDERATIONS
Assess:
• Culture before treatment is initiated; cultures of blood, urine, and throat may all be taken; CMV not confirmed by this method; diagnosis made by ophthalmic exam

Black Box Warning: Renal, hepatic, increased hemopoietic studies, BUN; serum creatinine, AST, ALT, creatinine, CCr, A-G ratio, baseline and drip treatment, blood counts should be done q2wk; watch for decreasing granulocytes, Hgb; if low, therapy may have to be discontinued and restarted after hematologic recovery; blood transfusions may be required, renal failure can occur also, Fanconi syndrome

• For GI symptoms: severe nausea, vomiting, diarrhea; severe symptoms may necessitate discontinuing product
• Electrolytes and minerals: calcium, phosphorus, magnesium, sodium, potassium; watch closely for tetany during 1st administration

Black Box Warning: **Blood dyscrasias** (anemia, granulocytopenia); bruising, fatigue, bleeding, poor healing; leukopenia, neutropenia, thrombocytopenia: WBCs, platelets q2days during 2×/day dosing and every wk thereafter; check for leukopenias with daily WBC count in patients with prior leukopenia, with other nucleoside analogs, or for whom leukopenia counts are <1000 cells/mm^3 at start of treatment

• Allergic reactions: flushing, rash, urticaria, pruritus
• Monitor serum creatinine or CCr at least q2wk; give only to those with creatinine levels ≤1.5 mg/dL, CCr >55 mL/min, urine protein <100 mg/dL

Black Box Warning: **Pregnancy/breastfeeding:** may cause fetal harm; use only if benefits outweigh fetal risk; do not use in breastfeeding

Evaluate:
• Therapeutic response: decreased symptoms of CMV
Teach patient/family:
• To notify prescriber if sore throat, swollen lymph nodes, malaise, fever occur; may indicate other infections
• To report perioral tingling, numbness in extremities, paresthesias; report rash immediately, mental/vision changes, urinary problems, abnormal bleeding
• That serious product interactions may occur if OTC products are ingested; check with prescriber
• That product is not a cure but will control symptoms
• That regular ophthalmic exams, renal studies must be continued
• That major toxicities may necessitate discontinuing product
• To use contraception during treatment, that infertility may occur, and that men should use barrier contraception for 90 days after treatment

TREATMENT OF OVERDOSE:
Discontinue product; use hemodialysis; increase hydration

▲ HIGH ALERT

cilostazol (Rx)
(sih-los′tah-zol)
Func. class.: Platelet aggregation inhibitor
Chem. class.: Quinolinone derivative

ACTION: Multifactorial effects (antithrombotic, antiplatelet vasodilation)

USES: Intermittent claudication associated with PVD

CONTRAINDICATIONS: Hypersensitivity, acute MI, active bleeding conditions, hemostatic conditions

Black Box Warning: HF

Precautions: Pregnancy, breastfeeding, children, geriatric patients, previous

---

hepatic disease, cardiac/renal disease, increased bleeding risk, low platelet count, platelet dysfunction, smoking

DOSAGE AND ROUTES
• **Adult: PO** 100 mg bid or 50 mg bid if using products that inhibit CYP3A4 and CYP2C19
Available forms: Tabs 50, 100 mg
Administer:
• Give bid 30 min before or 2 hr after meals with a full glass of water; do not give with grapefruit juice

SIDE EFFECTS
CNS: *Dizziness, headache*
CV: *Palpitations, tachycardia,* postural hypotension, chest pain
GI: *Nausea,* vomiting, *diarrhea,* GI discomfort, colitis, cholelithiasis, ulcer, esophagitis, gastritis, anorexia, *flatulence, dyspepsia*
INTEG: *Rash,* Stevens-Johnson syndrome
RESP: *Cough, pharyngitis, rhinitis*

PHARMACOKINETICS
95%-98% protein binding; metabolism: hepatic extensively by CYP3A4, 2C19 enzymes (active metabolite); excreted in urine (74%), feces (20%); half-life 11-13 hr

INTERACTIONS
Increase: bleeding tendencies—anticoagulants, NSAIDs, thrombolytics, abciximab, eptifibatide, tirofiban, ticlopidine
Increase: cilostazol levels—CYP3A4, CYP2C19 inhibitors; diltiazem, erythromycin, clarithromycin, verapamil, protease inhibitors, omeprazole; exercise caution when coadministering with fluvoxaMINE, FLUoxetine, ketoconazole, isoniazid, gemfibrozil, omeprazole, itraconazole, voriconazole, fluconazole; reduce dose to 50 mg bid
Decrease: cilostazol levels—CYP3A4 inducers

Black Box Warning: **Decrease:** survival rates—when used with phosphodiesterase III inhibitors (milrinone) in those with heart failure class III, IV

Drug/Herb
Decrease: action—chamomile, coenzyme Q10, feverfew, garlic, ginger, ginkgo biloba, flax, goldenseal, St. John's wort
Drug/Food
• Do not use with grapefruit juice; toxicity may occur
Increase: cilostazol action—fatty meal; avoid giving with food

NURSING CONSIDERATIONS
Assess:

Black Box Warning: For underlying CV disease because CV risk is great; for CV lesions with repeated oral administration; do not administer to patients with HF of any severity; for severe headache, signs of toxicity

• Blood studies: CBC q2wk, Hct, Hgb, PT
• **Beers:** avoid in older adults; may promote fluid retention and/or exacerbate heart failure
Evaluate:
• Therapeutic response: improved walking distance, duration; decreased pain
Teach patient/family:
• To avoid hazardous activities until effect is known; dizziness may occur
• To report any unusual bleeding
• To report side effects such as diarrhea, skin rashes, subcutaneous bleeding
• That effects may take 2-4 wk; treatment of up to 12 wk may be required for necessary effect
• That reading the patient package insert is necessary
• That it is best to discontinue tobacco use, not to use grapefruit juice
• That there are many drug and herb interactions; to obtain approval from prescriber before use

cimetidine (OTC, Rx)
(sye-met′i-deen)
Tagamet, Tagamet HB
Func. class.: H$_2$-histamine receptor antagonist
Chem. class.: Imidazole derivative

ACTION: Inhibits histamine at H_2-receptor site in the gastric parietal cells, which inhibits gastric acid secretion

USES: Short-term treatment of duodenal and gastric ulcers and maintenance; management of GERD (PO) and Zollinger-Ellison syndrome; prevention of upper GI bleeding; prevent, relieve heartburn, acid indigestion

CONTRAINDICATIONS: Hypersensitivity to this product, H_2 blockers, benzyl alcohol
Precautions: Pregnancy, breastfeeding, children <16 yr, geriatric patients, organic brain syndrome, renal/hepatic disease

DOSAGE AND ROUTES
Short-term treatment of active ulcers
• **Adult/adolescents ≥16 yr: PO** 300 mg qid × 8-12 wk or 400 mg bid × 8 wk
• **Child: PO** 20-40 mg/kg/day, divided q6hr
Prophylaxis of duodenal ulcer
• **Adult and child >16 yr: PO** 400 mg at bedtime or 300 mg bid
GERD
• **Adult: PO** 800-1600 mg/day in divided doses × up to 12 wk
Hypersecretory conditions (Zollinger-Ellison syndrome)
• **Adult: PO** 300-600 mg q6hr; may increase to 12 g/day if needed; OTC use ≤200 mg daily or bid, max 2×/wk
Heartburn
• **Adult/child ≥12 yr: PO** 200 mg up to bid, may use before eating, max 400 mg/day, max daily use up to 2 wk
Renal disease
• **Adult: PO** CCr <30 mL/min, 300 mg q12hr
Available forms: Tabs 100, 200, 300, 400, 800 mg
Administer:
PO route
• With meals for prolonged product effect; antacids 1 hr before or 1 hr after cimetidine

SIDE EFFECTS
CNS: *Confusion, headache,* depression, dizziness, psychosis

CV: Bradycardia, tachycardia, dysrhythmias
GI: *Diarrhea,* abdominal cramps
GU: Gynecomastia, galactorrhea, impotence, increase in BUN, creatinine
INTEG: Urticaria, rash
RESP: Pneumonia

PHARMACOKINETICS
Half-life $1^1/_2$-2 hr; 30%-40% metabolized by liver, excreted in urine (unchanged), crosses placenta, enters breast milk
PO: Onset 30 min, peak 45-90 min; duration 4-5 hr, well absorbed

INTERACTIONS
Increase: toxicity due to CYP450 pathway—benzodiazepines, β-blockers, calcium channel blockers, carBAMazepine, chloroquine, lidocaine, metroNIDAZOLE, moricizine, phenytoin, quiNIDine, quiNINE, sulfonylureas, theophylline, tricyclics, valproic acid, warfarin
Increase: bone marrow suppression—carmustine
Decrease: absorption of cimetidine—antacids, sucralfate
Decrease: absorption—ketoconazole, itraconazole
Drug/Lab Test
Increase: alk phos, AST, creatinine, prolactin
False positive: gastroccult, hemoccult tests
False negative: TB skin tests

NURSING CONSIDERATIONS
Assess:
• **Ulcer symptoms:** epigastric pain, duration, intensity; aggravating, ameliorating factors; blood in stools; emesis
• **Beers:** avoid in older adults with delirium or at high risk for delirium, adverse CNS reactions
Evaluate:
• Therapeutic response: decreased pain in abdomen; healing of ulcers; absence of gastroesophageal reflux; gastric pH of 5
Teach patient/family:
• That gynecomastia, impotence may occur, are reversible

Side effects: *italics* = common; red = life-threatening

• To avoid driving, other hazardous activities until stabilized on this medication; drowsiness or dizziness may occur
• To avoid OTC preparations: aspirin; cough, cold preparations; condition may worsen; OTC therapy is used for short term (2 wk)
• Not to smoke because smoking decreases effectiveness of product
• That product must be taken exactly as prescribed and continued for prescribed time to be effective; not to double dose; if taking OTC, not to take maximum dose >2 wk unless directed by prescriber
• To report diarrhea, black tarry stools, sore throat, rash, dizziness, confusion, delirium to prescriber
• To use increased fluids, bulk in diet to decrease constipation
• **Pregnancy/breastfeeding:** to report if pregnancy is planned or suspected or if breastfeeding, avoid breastfeeding

cinacalcet (Rx)
(sin-a-kal′set)
Sensipar
Func. class.: Calcium receptor agonist
Chem. class.: Polypeptide hormone

ACTION: Directly lowers PTH levels by increasing sensitivity of calcium-sensing receptors to extracellular calcium

USES: Hypercalcemia with parathyroid carcinoma, secondary hyperparathyroidism with chronic kidney disease for patient on dialysis, primary hyperparathyroidism

CONTRAINDICATIONS: Hypersensitivity, hypocalcemia
Precautions: Pregnancy, breastfeeding, children, seizure disorders, hepatic disease

DOSAGE AND ROUTES
Parathyroid carcinoma
• Adult: PO 30 mg bid, titrate q2-4wk, with sequential doses of 30 mg bid, 60 mg bid, 90 mg bid, 90 mg tid-qid to normalize calcium levels

Secondary hyperparathyroidism
• Adult: PO 30 mg/day, titrate no more frequently than q2-4wk with sequential doses of 30, 60, 90, 120, 180 mg/day
Available forms: Tabs 30, 60, 90 mg
Administer:
• Swallow tabs whole; do not break, crush, or chew; use with food or right after a meal
• Can be used alone or in combination with vit D sterols, phosphate binders
• Storage at <77° F (25° C)
Chronic kidney disease: Titrate q2-4wk to target iPTH consistent with National Kidney Foundation–Kidney Disease Outcomes Quality Initiative (NKF-K/DOQI) for chronic kidney disease patient on dialysis of 150-300 pg/mL; if iPTH <150-300 pg/mL, reduce dose of cinacalcet and/or vit D sterols or discontinue treatment

SIDE EFFECTS
CNS: Dizziness, asthenia, seizures, paresthesia, fatigue, headache
CV: Dysrhythmia hypotension
GI: Nausea, diarrhea, vomiting, anorexia, constipation
MISC: Infection, dehydration, hypercalcemia, anemia, hypocalcemia
MS: Myalgia, bone fractures binding

PHARMACOKINETICS
93%-97% plasma; proteins metabolized by CYP3A4, 2D6, 1A2; half-life 30-40 hr; renal excretion of metabolites (80% renal, 15% in feces)

INTERACTIONS
Increase: cinacalcet levels—CYP3A4 inhibitors (ketoconazole, erythromycin, itraconazole), dose may need to be reduced
Increase: levels of CYP2D6 inhibitors (flecainide, vinBLAStine, thioridazine, tricyclics)
Drug/Food
Increase: action by high-fat meal

NURSING CONSIDERATIONS
Assess:
• **Hypocalcemia:** cramping, seizures, tetany, myalgia, paresthesia; calcium, phosphorous within 1 wk and iPTH 1-4 wk after initiation or dosage adjustment

when maintenance established; measure calcium, phosphorus monthly; iPTH q1-3mo, target range 150-300 pg/mL for iPTH level; biochemical markers of bone formation/resorption; radiologic evidence of fracture; serum testosterone

• **Renal disease (without dialysis):** these patients should not receive treatment with this product; high risk of hypocalcemia

• Liver studies in those with liver disease

• If calcium <8.4 mg/dL, do not start therapy; if calcium is 7.5-8.4 mg/dL, give calcium-containing phosphate binders, vitamin D sterols to increase calcium; if calcium <7.5 mg/dL or if symptoms of hypocalcemia continue and vitamin D cannot be increased, withhold product until calcium reaches 8.0 mg/dL, symptoms resolve, start product at next lowest dose

• **Pregnancy/breastfeeding:** no well-controlled studies, use only if benefits outweigh fetal risk; those who are pregnant should enroll in Amgen's Pregnancy Surveillance Program (1-800-772-6436); discontinue breastfeeding or product, it is unknown if excreted in breast milk

Evaluate:

• Therapeutic response: calcium levels 9-10 mg/dL, decreasing symptoms of hypercalcemia

Teach patient/family:

• To take with food or shortly after a meal; to take tabs whole, not to take any other meds, supplements without prescriber approval

• **Hypocalcemia:** to report cramping, seizures, muscle pain, tingling, tetany immediately

• To continue exams and lab work

---

ciprofloxacin (Rx)

(sip-ro-floks′a-sin)

Cipro, Cipro XR

Func. class.: Antiinfective—broad spectrum

Chem. class.: Fluoroquinolone

Do not confuse:
ciprofloxacin/cephalexin

ACTION: Interferes with conversion of intermediate DNA fragments into high-molecular-weight DNA in bacteria; DNA gyrase inhibitor

USES: Infection caused by susceptible *Escherichia coli, Enterobacter cloacae, Proteus mirabilis, Klebsiella pneumoniae, Proteus vulgaris, Citrobacter freundii, Serratia marcescens, Pseudomonas aeruginosa, Staphylococcus aureus, Staphylococcus epidermidis, Enterobacter, Campylobacter jejuni, Salmonella, Streptococcus pyogenes, Bacillus anthracias;* chronic bacterial prostatitis, acute sinusitis, postexposure inhalation anthrax, infectious diarrhea, typhoid fever, complicated intraabdominal infections, nosocomial pneumonia, urinary tract infections, plague

CONTRAINDICATIONS: Hypersensitivity to quinolones

Precautions: Pregnancy, breastfeeding, children, geriatric patients, renal disease, seizure disorder, stroke, CV disease, hepatic disease, QT prolongation, hypokalemia, colitis

> **Black Box Warning:** Tendon pain/rupture, tendinitis, myasthenia gravis, nephrotoxicity

DOSAGE AND ROUTES
Uncomplicated urinary tract infections

• **Adult:** PO 250 mg q12hr × 3 days or **XL** 500 mg q24hr × 3 days

Complicated/severe urinary tract infections

• **Adult:** PO 500 mg q12hr or **XL** 1000 mg q24hr × 7-14 days; **IV** 400 mg q12hr

• **Child/adolescent:** PO 10-20 mg/kg/dose q12hr × 10-21 days; not first choice in pediatric patients due to high incidence of adverse reactions

Respiratory, bone, skin, joint infections (mild-moderate)

• **Adult:** PO 500-750 mg q12hr × 7-14 days; **IV** 400 mg q12hr

---

Nosocomial pneumonia
- **Adult: IV** 400 mg q8hr × 10-14 days

Intraabdominal infections, complicated
- **Adult: PO** 500 mg q12hr × 7-14 days; **IV** 400 mg q12hr × 7-14 days, usually given with metroNIDAZOLE

Acute sinusitis, mild/moderate
- **Adult: PO** 500 mg q12hr × 10 days; **IV** 400 mg q12hr × 10 days

Inhalational anthrax (postexposure)
- **Adult: PO** 500 mg q12hr × 60 days; **IV** 400 mg q12hr × 60 days
- **Child: PO** 15 mg/kg/dose q12hr × 60 days, max 500 mg/dose; **IV** 10 mg/kg q12hr, max 400 mg/dose

Infectious diarrhea
- **Adult: PO** 500-750 mg q12hr × 5-7 days

Chronic bacterial prostatitis
- **Adult: PO** 500 mg q12hr × 28 days; **IV** 400 mg q12hr × 28 days

Renal disease
- **Adult:** CCr 30-50 mL/min, **PO** 250-500 mg q12hr; CCr 5-29 mL/min, **PO** 250-500 mg q18hr, **IV** 200-400 mg q18-24hr

Available forms: Tabs 100, 250, 750 mg; ext rel tabs (XR) 500, 1000 mg; inj 200 mg/100 mL D_5W, 400 mg/200 mL D_5W; inj 200, 400 mg; oral susp 250 mg, 500 mg/5 mL

Administer:
- Obtain C&S before use, may give first dose before results are received
- Use caution when giving with antidysrhythmics IA, III

PO route
- Do not break, crush, chew XR (ext rel) product, use adequate fluids to prevent crystalluria
- 2 hr before or 6 hr after antacids, zinc, iron, calcium
- Do not give oral susp by GI tube

IV route
- Over 1 hr as an infusion, comes in premixed plastic infusion container or diluted 20- or 40-mL vial to a final concentration of 0.5-2 mg/mL of NS or D_5W; give through Y-tube or 3-way stopcock, diluted vials can be stored for 14 days at room temperature or refrigerator; do not freeze

Y-site compatibilities: Amifostine, anakinra, anidulafungin, argatroban, arsenic, atenolol, aztreonam, bivalirudin, bleomycin, calcium gluconate, CARBOplatin, caspofungin, cefTAZidime, cisatracurium, CISplatin, clarithromycin, codeine, cytarabine, DACTINomycin, DAPTOmycin, dexmedetomidine, digoxin, diltiaZEM, diphenhydrAMINE, DOBUTamine, DOCEtaxel, doripenem, DOPamine, doxacurium, DOXOrubicin, epiRUBicin, eptifibatide, ertapenem, etoposide, fenoldopam, fludarabine, gallium, gemcitabine, gentamicin, granisetron, HYDROmorphone, hydrOXYzine, IDArubicin, ifosfamide, irinotecan, lidocaine, linezolid, LORazepam, LR, mechlorethamine, meperidine, methotrexate, metoclopramide, metroNIDAZOLE, midazolam, midodrine, milrinone, mitoXANTRONE, mycophenolate, nesiritide, octreotide, ondansetron, oxaliplatin, oxytocin, PACLitaxel, palonosetron, pamidronate, pancuronium, piperacillin, potassium acetate/chloride, promethazine, raNITIdine, remifentanil, rocuronium, sodium chloride, tacrolimus, teniposide, thiotepa, tigecycline, tirofiban, TNA, tobramycin, trastuzumab, vasopressin, vecuronium, verapamil, vinCRIStine, vinorelbine, voriconazole

SIDE EFFECTS

CNS: *Headache*, dizziness, fatigue, insomnia, depression, *restlessness,* seizures, suicidal ideation, pseudotumor cerebri, confusion, hallucinations

GI: *Nausea, diarrhea,* increased ALT/AST, flatulence, *vomiting,* abdominal pain, pancreatitis, hepatotoxicity, CDAD

GU: Vaginitis

INTEG: *Rash,* pruritus, urticaria, photosensitivity, toxic epidermal necrolysis, injection site reactions

MISC: Anaphylaxis, Stevens-Johnson syndrome, QT prolongation, pseudotumor cerebri

MS: Arthralgia, tendon rupture

META: Hypo- and hyperglycemia

PHARMACOKINETICS

PO: Peak 1-2 hr; half-life 4 hr; excreted in urine as active product, metabolites 35%-40%, 20%-40% protein binding

INTERACTIONS

Increase: nephrotoxicity—cycloSPORINE
Increase: ciprofloxacin levels—probenecid; monitor for toxicity
Increase: levels of theophylline, warfarin; monitor blood levels, reduce dose
Increase: hypoglycemia risk—antidiabetics
Increase: QT prolongation—astemizole, droperidol, class IA/III antidysrhythmics, tricyclics, tetracyclines, local anesthetics, phenothiazines, haloperidol, risperiDONE, sertindole, ziprasidone, alfuzosin, arsenic trioxide, β-agonists, chloroquine, cloZAPine, cyclobenzaprine, dasatinib, dolasetron, droperidol, flecainide, halogenated anesthetics, lapatinib, levomethadyl, macrolides, methadone, octreotide, ondansetron, paliperidone, palonosetron, pentamidine, propafenone, ranolazine, SUNItinib, tacrolimus, terfenadine, vardenafil, vorinostat; less likely than other quinolones
Decrease: ciprofloxacin absorption—antacids that contain magnesium, aluminum; zinc, iron, sucralfate, enteral feedings, calcium, sevelamer

Drug/Food
Increase: effect of caffeine
Decrease: absorption—dairy products, food

Drug/Lab Test
Increase: AST, ALT, BUN, creatinine, LDH, bilirubin, alk phos, glucose, proteinuria, albuminuria
Decrease: WBC, glucose

NURSING CONSIDERATIONS
Assess:
• **Infection:** WBC, temperature before treatment, periodically
• **QT prolongation:** monitor for changes in QTc if taking other products that increase QT

• **CNS symptoms:** headache, dizziness, fatigue, insomnia, depression, seizures
• Renal, hepatic studies: BUN, creatinine, AST, ALT
• I&O ratio, urine pH <5.5 is ideal, to prevent crystalluria

• **Anaphylaxis:** fever, flushing, rash, urticaria, pruritus, dyspnea; discontinue immediately, have emergency equipment nearby
• **Pseudotumor cerebri:** may occur at excessive doses
• **Hepatotoxicity:** report immediately dark urine, jaundice, pruritus, clay-colored stools
• Limited intake of alkaline foods, products: milk, dairy products, alkaline antacids, sodium bicarbonate; caffeine intake if excessive cardiac or CNS stimulation
• Increase fluids to 3 L/day to avoid crystallization in kidneys
• *Clostridium difficile*–associated diarrhea (CDAD): monitor for diarrhea, abdominal pain, cramps, fever, bloody stools; usually occurs several weeks after completion of therapy; report to prescriber immediately
• **Pregnancy/breastfeeding:** no well-controlled studies; use in pregnancy only if benefits outweigh fetal risk; excreted in breast milk, discontinue breastfeeding or discontinue product
Evaluate:
• Therapeutic response: decreased pain, frequency, urgency, C&S; absence of infection
Teach patient/family:
• Not to take any products that contain magnesium, calcium (such as antacids), iron, aluminum with this product or 2 hr before, 6 hr after product; to drink fluids to prevent crystals in urine; not to crush, chew the extended-release product

---

Side effects: *italics* = common; red = life-threatening

Black Box Warning: To report tendon pain, chest pain, palpitations

• To complete full course of product therapy; not to double or miss doses
• To notify prescriber if rash occurs; discontinue product
• To notify prescriber if pregnancy is planned or suspected; not to breastfeed
• **Suicidal thoughts/behaviors:** To report immediately, suicidal thoughts, behaviors
• To contact prescriber if taking theophylline, warfarin
• That extended-release and regular-release products are not interchangeable
• Not to add or stop products without prescriber's approval
• To use calibrated measuring device for suspension

---

ciprofloxacin (ophthalmic)

(sip-roe-flox′a-sin)

Ciloxan

Func. class.: Ophthalmic antiinfective
Chem. class.: Fluoroquinolone

Do not confuse:
ciprofloxacin/gatifloxacin/levoFLOXAcin/moxifloxacin/ofloxacin

ACTION: Inhibits DNA gyrase, thereby decreasing bacterial replication

USES: Corneal ulcers, bacterial conjunctivitis

CONTRAINDICATIONS: Hypersensitivity to this product or fluoroquinolones
Precautions: Pregnancy, breastfeeding

DOSAGE AND ROUTES
Bacterial conjunctivitis
• **Adult/adolescent/child ≥1 yr: Ophthalmic (sol):** 1-2 drops in affected eye(s) every 2 hr while awake × 2 days, then every 4 hr while awake for the next 5 days

• **Adult/adolescent/child ≥2 yr: Ophthalmic (ointment):** $^1/_2$-inch ribbon to conjunctival sac tid × 2 days, then $^1/_2$ inch bid for next 5 days
Ophthalmic infection associated with corneal ulcer
• **Adult/adolescent/child ≥1 yr: Ophthalmic (sol):** 2 drops in affected eye(s) every 15 min × 6 hr, then every 30 min for the remainder of the first day; for the second day, 2 drops every hr; for days 3-14, 2 drops every 4 hr
Available forms: Ophthalmic ointment, solution 0.3%
Administer:
• Commercially available ophthalmic solutions are not for injection subconjunctivally or into the anterior chamber of the eye
Ophthalmic route
• Apply topically to the eye, taking care to avoid contamination
• Do not touch the tip of the dropper to the eye, fingertips, or other surface
• Apply pressure to lacrimal sac for 1 min after instillation
• Avoid wearing contact lens(es) while treating eye infection
• Protect from light, store at room temperature

SIDE EFFECTS
EENT: Burning, hypersensitivity, pruritus, precipitate in those with corneal ulcers, lid margin crusting

NURSING CONSIDERATIONS
Assess:
• **Allergic reaction:** assess for hypersensitivity; discontinue product
Evaluate:
• Therapeutic response: decreased ophthalmic infection
Teach patient/family:
Ophthalmic route:
• To apply topically to the eye, taking care to avoid contamination; for ophthalmic use only
• Not to touch the tip of the dropper to the eye, fingertips, or other surface
• To apply pressure to lacrimal sac for 1 min after instillation

---

• To avoid wearing contact lens(es) while treating eye infection

---

⚠ HIGH ALERT

cisatracurium
(sis-ah-trah-kyoo′ree-um)

Nimbex

Func. class.: Skeletal muscle relaxant
Chem. class.: Nondepolarizing neuromuscular blocker

ACTION: Antagonizes acetylcholine by binding to cholinergic receptors on the motor end plate, resulting in neuromuscular blockade

USES: To maintain neuromuscular blockade during mechanical ventilation and as an adjunct to general anesthesia

CONTRAINDICATIONS: Hypersensitivity
Precautions: Pregnancy, breastfeeding, children, benzyl alcohol hypersensitivity, electrolyte imbalances, long-term use in ICU, trauma, or burns, dehydration, metabolic alkalosis, respiratory acidosis, myopathy, myasthenia gravis

DOSAGE AND ROUTES
Endotracheal intubation
• **Adult/adolescent (healthy):** IV 0.15-0.2 mg/kg, one time
• **Adult with myasthenia gravis:** IV use peripheral nerve stimulator monitoring and an initial dose ≤0.02 mg/kg
• **Child 2-12 yr:** IV 0.1-0.15 mg/kg over 5-10 sec during either halothane or opioid anesthesia
• **Infant/child ≤23 mo:** IV 0.15 mg/kg over 5-10 sec during either halothane or opioid anesthesia
To maintain neuromuscular blockade during prolonged surgical procedures:
• **Adult/adolescent/child ≥2 yr (healthy):** IV Maintenance dose 0.03 mg/kg; maintenance dosing is generally required

40-50 min after an initial dose of 0.15 mg/kg IV or 50-60 min after an initial dose of 0.2 mg/kg; the need for maintenance doses should be determined by clinical criteria
Available forms: Injection solution 2, 10 mg/mL
Administer:
IV route
• Visually inspect for particulate matter and discoloration before use
• Only experienced clinicians, familiar with the use of neuromuscular blocking drugs, should administer or supervise the use of this product
• Use by rapid IV injection or by continuous IV infusion
IV INFUSION route
• Inject IV over 5-10 sec
Continuous IV INFUSION route
• Dilute with NS, D₅W, or D₅NS (0.1-0.4 mg/mL); adjust the rate of infusion according to peripheral nerve stimulation
• The amount of infusion sol required per minute depends on the concentration of cisatracurium in the infusion sol, the desired dose of cisatracurium, and the patient's weight
• Store Nimbex injection diluted to 0.1 mg/mL either under refrigeration or at room temperature for 24 hr; dilutions to 0.1 mg/mL or 0.2 mg/mL in D₅W/LR injection may be stored under refrigeration for 24 hr
• Not an analgesic, treat pain with other agents

SIDE EFFECTS
CV: Bradycardia, *flushing*, hypotension
RESP: Apnea, bronchospasm, prolonged neuromuscular block

PHARMACOKINETICS
Onset 2 min, peak 3-5 min, duration 25-44 min, half-life 22-30 min

INTERACTIONS
Increase: neuromuscular blockade—aminoglycosides, clindamycin, lithium, local anesthetics, magnesium salts, colistin, colistimethate, procainamide, quiNIDine, tetracyclines, bacitracin, capreomycin, polymyxin B, vancomycin; amphotericin B,

CISplatin, corticosteroids, loop/thiazide diuretics (if hypokalemia is present)
Decrease: neuromuscular blockade—carBAMazepine, phenytoin; dose of cisatracurium may need to be increased

NURSING CONSIDERATIONS
Assess:
• **Neuromuscular function:** use nerve stimulator to monitor neuromuscular function; if no response, stop until response; not to be used for rapid-sequence endotracheal intubation
• **Sedation/pain:** those undergoing neuromuscular blockage (paralytics) must receive treatment with sedative and pain control before and during therapy
• **Electrolytes:** electrolytes and acid-base balance may be altered
• **Malignant hyperthermia:** those with a family history of malignant hyperthermia should not receive this product or it should be used cautiously
• **Pregnancy/breastfeeding:** no well-controlled studies; use in pregnancy only if benefits outweigh fetal risk; use caution in breastfeeding; excretion is unknown
Evaluate:
• Maintenance of neuromuscular blockade
Teach patient/family:
• Reason for product and expected results

⚠ HIGH ALERT

CISplatin (Rx) ✦
(sis′pla-tin)
Func. class.: Antineoplastic alkylating agent
Chem. class.: Platinum complex

Do not confuse:
CISplatin/CARBOplatin

ACTION: Alkylates DNA, RNA; inhibits enzymes that allow for the synthesis of amino acids in proteins; activity not cell cycle–phase specific

USES: Advanced bladder cancer; adjunct in metastatic testicular cancer; adjunct in metastatic ovarian cancer, head and neck, lung cancer

CONTRAINDICATIONS: Pregnancy, breastfeeding

Black Box Warning: Bone marrow suppression, platinum compound hypersensitivity

Precautions: Geriatric patients, vaccination, infections, extravasation, peripheral neuropathy, radiation therapy

Black Box Warning: Chemotherapy-induced nausea/vomiting, children, nephrotoxicity, ototoxicity; requires a specialized care setting and an experienced clinician

DOSAGE AND ROUTES
Dosage protocols may vary
Metastatic testicular cancer
• **Adult:** IV 20 mg/m^2/day × 5 days, repeat q3wk for 2 cycles or more, depending on response
Advanced bladder cancer
• **Adult:** IV 50-70 mg/m^2 q3-4wk
Metastatic ovarian cancer
• **Adult:** IV 100 mg/m^2 q4wk or 75-100 mg/m^2 q3wk with cyclophosphamide
Hodgkin's/non-Hodgkin's lymphoma (unlabeled)
• **Adult/child:** IV INFUSION 100 mg/m^2 24 hr continuous infusion day 1 of 4-day regimen with cytarabine/dexamethasone q3-4wk
Gastric cancer (unlabeled)
• **Adult:** IV 75 mg/m^2 on day 1 with DOCEtaxel 75 mg/m^2 and fluorouracil 750 mg/m^2 on days 1-5, q21days
Available forms: Inj 0.5 ✦, 1 mg/mL
Administer:
IV route
• Do not use aluminum equipment during any preparation or administration, will form precipitate; do not refrigerate unopened powder or solution; protect from sunlight

---

- Prepare in biologic cabinet using gown, gloves, mask; do not allow product to come in contact with skin; use soap and water if contact occurs; use cytotoxic handling procedures
- Hydrate patient with 1-2 L 0.9% NaCl over 8-12 hr before treatment
- EPINEPHrine, antihistamines, corticosteroids for hypersensitivity reaction
- Antiemetic 30-60 min before product and prn; allopurinol to maintain uric acid levels, alkalinization of urine; diuretic (furosemide 40 mg IV) or mannitol after INFUSION

Intermittent IV INFUSION route

- Check solution for particulate and color, do not use if present or if discolored
- **Dilute** 10 mg/10 mL or 50 mg/50 mL sterile water for inj, withdraw prescribed dose; **dilute** ½ dose with 1000 mL $D_5$0.2NaCl, $D_5$0.45NaCl with 37.5 g mannitol; IV INFUSION is **given** over 3-4 hr; use a 0.45-µm filter; total dose 2 L over 6-8 hr; check site for irritation, phlebitis

Continuous IV INFUSION route

- **Give** over 24 hr × 5 days

Y-site compatibilities: Acyclovir, alfentanil, allopurinol, amikacin, aminophylline, amiodarone, ampicillin, ampicillin-sulbactam, anidulafungin, atenolol, atracurium, azithromycin, aztreonam, bivalirudin, bleomycin, bumetanide, buprenorphine, butorphanol, calcium chloride/gluconate, carmustine, caspofungin, ceFAZolin, cefoperazone, cefotaxime, cefoTEtan, cefOXitin, cefTAZidime, ceftizoxime, cefTRIAXone, cefuroxime, chlorproMAZINE, cimetidine, ciprofloxacin, cisatracurium, cladribine, clindamycin, codeine, cyclophosphamide, cycloSPORINE, cytarabine, DACTINomycin, DAPTOmycin, DAUNOrubicin, dexamethasone, dexmedetomidine, dexrazoxane, digoxin, diltiaZEM, diphenhydrAMINE, DOBUTamine, DOCEtaxel, DOPamine, doripenem, doxacurium, DOXOrubicin, DOXOrubicin liposomal, doxycycline, droperidol, enalaprilat, ePHEDrine, EPINEPHrine, epiRUBicin, ertapenem, erythromycin, esmolol, etoposide, famotidine, fenoldopam, fentaNYL, filgrastim, fluconazole, fludarabine, fluorouracil, foscarnet, fosphenytoin, furosemide, ganciclovir, gatifloxacin, gemcitabine, gentamicin, glycopyrrolate, granisetron, haloperidol, heparin, hydrocortisone, HYDROmorphone, IDArubicin, ifosfamide, imipenem-cilastatin, inamrinone, indomethacin, irinotecan, isoproterenol, ketorolac, labetalol, leucovorin, levoFLOXacin, levorphanol, lidocaine, linezolid, LORazepam, magnesium sulfate, mannitol, melphalan, meperidine, meropenem, methohexital, methotrexate, methylPREDNISolone, metoclopramide, metoprolol, metroNIDAZOLE, midazolam, milrinone, minocycline, mitoMYcin, mitoXANTRONE, mivacurium, nafcillin, naloxone, nesiritide, niCARdipine, nitroglycerin, nitroprusside, norepinephrine, octreotide, ofloxacin, ondansetron, oxaliplatin, PACLitaxel, palonosetron, pamidronate, pancuronium, PEMEtrexed, pentamidine, pentazocine, PENTobarbital, PHENobarbital, phenylephrine, phenytoin, piperacillin, polymyxin B, potassium chloride/phosphates, procainamide, prochlorperazine, promethazine, propofol, propranolol, quiNIDine, quinupristin-dalfopristin, raNITIdine, remifentanil, riTUXimab, sargramostim, sodium acetate/bicarbonate/phosphates, succinylcholine, SUFentanil, sulfamethoxazole-trimethoprim, tacrolimus, teniposide, theophylline, thiopental, ticarcillin, ticarcillin-clavulanate, tigecycline, tirofiban, TNA, tobramycin, topotecan, trastuzumab, vancomycin, vasopressin, vecuronium, verapamil, vinBLAStine, vinCRIStine, vinorelbine, voriconazole, zidovudine, zoledronic acid

SIDE EFFECTS

CNS: Seizures, *peripheral neuropathy*
EENT: *Tinnitus, hearing loss, vestibular toxicity,* blurred vision, altered color perception
GI: *Severe nausea, vomiting, diarrhea, weight loss,* hepatotoxicity
GU: Renal tubular damage, *renal insufficiency,* sterility

HEMA: Thrombocytopenia, leukopenia, pancytopenia, *anemia*
INTEG: *Alopecia,* dermatitis
META: *Hypomagnesemia, hypocalcemia, hypokalemia*
RESP: Fibrosis
SYST: Anaphylaxis

PHARMACOKINETICS
Absorption complete, metabolized in liver, excreted in urine, half-life 30-90 min accumulates in body tissues for several months, enters breast milk

INTERACTIONS
Increase: bleeding risk—aspirin, NSAIDs, alcohol
Increase: myelosuppression—myelosuppressive agents, radiation
Increase: nephrotoxicity—aminoglycosides, loop diuretics, salicylates
Decrease: effects of phenytoin
Decrease: antibody response—live virus vaccines
Decrease: potassium, magnesium levels—loop diuretics
Drug/Lab Test
Increase: uric acid, BUN, creatinine
Decrease: CCr, calcium, phosphate, potassium, magnesium
Positive: Coombs' test

NURSING CONSIDERATIONS
Assess:

> Black Box Warning: **Bone marrow depression:** CBC, differential, platelet count weekly; withhold product if WBC is <4000 or platelet count is <100,000; notify prescriber of results

> Black Box Warning: **Renal toxicity:** BUN, creatinine, serum uric acid, urine CCr before, electrolytes during therapy; dose should not be given if BUN <25 mg/dL; creatinine <1.5 mg/dL; I&O ratio; report fall in urine output of <30 mL/hr; toxicity is cumulative; withhold until renal function returns to normal

> Black Box Warning: **Anaphylaxis:** wheezing, tachycardia, facial swelling, fainting; discontinue product, report to prescriber; resuscitation equipment should be nearby, may occur within minutes; often EPINEPHrine, corticosteroids, antihistamines may alleviate symptoms

• **Infection:** monitor temperature; may indicate beginning infection; report signs of infection, cough, sore throat, fever
• **Hepatotoxicity:** report jaundice, dark urine, clay-colored stools, pruritus, abdominal pain
• Hepatic studies before, during therapy (bilirubin, AST, ALT, LDH) as needed
• **Bleeding:** hematuria, guaiac, bruising, petechiae, mucosa, or orifices q8hr; obtain prescription for viscous lidocaine (Xylocaine)

> Black Box Warning: **Ototoxicity:** more common in genetic variants TPMT 3B and 3C in children; use audiometric testing baseline and before each dose; tinnitus or loss of high-frequency sounds is usually first indication of ototoxicity

• Effects of alopecia on body image; discuss feelings about body changes
• Comprehensive oral hygiene
• **RPLS:** Headache, change in eyesight, confusion, seizures, increased B/P, usually occurs a few hours up to a year after treatment starts, discontinue treatment
• **Hyperuricemia in lymphoma:** increase fluid intake to 2-3 L/day to prevent urate deposits, calculi formation, promote elimination of product; usually occurs between 3-5 days after a dose, may use allopurinol
Evaluate:
• Therapeutic response: decreased tumor size, spread of malignancy
Teach patient/family:
• **To report signs of infection:** increased temperature, sore throat, flulike symptoms
• **To report signs of anemia:** fatigue, headache, faintness, SOB, irritability
• To report bleeding, bruising, petechiae; to avoid use of razors, commercial mouthwash; to avoid aspirin, ibuprofen, NSAIDs, alcohol; may cause GI bleeding
• That impotence or amenorrhea can occur but is reversible after discontinuing treatment

• To maintain adequate fluids; to report decreased urine output, flank pain

• That hair may be lost during treatment; a wig or hairpiece may make patient feel better; that new hair may be different in color, texture

• To report numbness, tingling in face or extremities; poor hearing; joint pain, swelling

• Not to receive vaccinations during treatment

• **Pregnancy/breastfeeding:** to use contraception during treatment and for 4 mo after treatment; that product may cause infertility; not to breastfeed

Black Box Warning: **Ototoxicity:** to report loss of hearing, ringing, or roaring in the ears

---

citalopram (Rx)

(sigh-tal'oh-pram)

CeleXA

Func. class.: Antidepressant
Chem. class.: Selective serotonin reuptake inhibitor (SSRI)

Do not confuse:
CeleXA/CeleBREX/Cerebyx/ZyPREXA

ACTION: Inhibits CNS neuron uptake of serotonin but not of norepinephrine; weak inhibitor of CYP450 enzyme system, thus making it more appealing than other products

USES: Major depressive disorder
Unlabeled uses: Obsessive-compulsive disorder in adolescents

CONTRAINDICATIONS: Hypersensitivity

Precautions: Pregnancy, breastfeeding, geriatric patients, renal/hepatic disease, seizure disorder, hypersensitivity to escitalopram, bradycardia, recent MI, abrupt discontinuation, QT prolongation

Black Box Warning: Children, suicidal ideation

DOSAGE AND ROUTES
Depression
• **Adult: PO** 20 mg/day AM or PM, may increase if needed to 40 mg/day after 1 wk; maintenance: after 6-8 wk of initial treatment, continue for 24 wk (32 wk total), reevaluate long-term usefulness (max 40 mg/day); poor metabolizers of CYP2C19 or use of CYP2C19 inhibitors max 20 mg/day

Hepatic dose/geriatric
• **Adult: PO** 20 mg/day

OCD (unlabeled)
• **Adult: PO** 20-40 mg/day
Available forms: Tabs 10, 20, 40 mg; oral sol 10 mg/5 mL
Administer:
• With food or milk for GI symptoms
• Crushed if patient is unable to swallow medication whole
• Dosages at bedtime if oversedation occurs during the day; may take entire dose at bedtime
• Do not give within 14 days of MAOIs
• Store at room temperature; do not freeze

SIDE EFFECTS
CNS: *Headache, insomnia, drowsiness, anxiety, tremor, dizziness, fatigue, sedation, poor concentration,* seizures, suicidal attempts, neuroleptic malignant–like syndrome reactions
CV: Tachycardia, QT prolongation, orthostatic hypotension, torsades de pointes
EENT: Visual changes
GI: *Nausea, diarrhea, dry mouth, anorexia, dyspepsia, vomiting, flatulence, decreased appetite*
GU: *Dysmenorrhea, decreased libido,* amenorrhea, impotence
INTEG: *Sweating, rash, pruritus,* photosensitivity
MS: Arthritis, myalgia
RESP: *Infection, cough, dyspnea*
SYST: Hyponatremia (geriatric patients), serotonin syndrome

PHARMACOKINETICS
Metabolized in liver by CYP3A4, CYP2C19, some individuals are poor metabolizers; excreted in urine; steady state 1 wk; peak 4 hr; half-life 35 hr

Side effects: *italics* = common; red = life-threatening

INTERACTIONS

• **Fatal reactions:** do not use within 14 days of MAOIs

Increase: QTc interval—dofetilide, halofantrine, probucol, pimozide, quinolones, ziprasidone; do not use together

Increase: serotonin syndrome—serotonin receptor agonists, SSRIs, traMADol, lithium, MAOIs, traZODone, SNRIs (venlafaxine, DULoxetine), linezolid, methylene blue, tricyclics, fentaNYL, busPIRone, triptans

Increase: bleeding risk—NSAIDs, salicylates, thrombolytics, anticoagulants, antiplatelets

Increase: CNS effects—barbiturates, sedative/hypnotics, other CNS depressants

Increase: citalopram levels—macrolides, azole antifungals

Increase: plasma levels of β-blockers

Decrease: citalopram levels—carBAMazepine, cloNIDine

Drug/Herb

Increase: serotonin syndrome—St. John's wort, SAM-e; fatal reaction may occur; do not use concurrently

Increase: CNS stimulation—yohimbe

Drug/Lab Test

Increase: serum bilirubin, blood glucose, alk phos

Decrease: VMA, 5-HIAA

False increase: urinary catecholamines

NURSING CONSIDERATIONS

Assess:

> **Black Box Warning: Suicide:** mood, sensorium, affect, suicidal tendencies, increase in psychiatric symptoms, depression, panic; risk for suicide is greater in children and those ≤24 yr; these patients should be evaluated weekly × 4 wk and then q3wk × 4 wk, give only a small amount of product

• **Serotonin syndrome:** increased heart rate, sweating, dilated pupils, tremors, twitching, hyperthermia, agitation, hyperreflexia, nausea, vomiting, diarrhea, coma, hallucinations; may be worse in those taking SSRIs, SNRIs, triptans

• **QT prolongation:** Flattening T-wave, bundle branch block, AV block

• B/P lying, standing, pulse q4hr; if systolic B/P drops 20 mm Hg, hold product, notify prescriber; take vital signs q4hr in patients with CV disease

• Weight weekly; appetite may decrease or increase with product

• **Torsades de pointes, QT prolongation:** is dose-dependent; ECG for flattening of T wave, bundle branch, AV block, dysrhythmias in cardiac patients

• Alcohol consumption; if alcohol is consumed, hold dose until AM

• **Sexual dysfunction:** erectile dysfunction, decreased libido

• **Beers:** avoid in older adults unless safer alternative is unavailable; may cause ataxia, impaired psychomotor function

• **Pregnancy/breastfeeding:** no well-controlled studies; use in pregnancy only if benefits outweigh fetal risk; excreted in breast milk, discontinue breastfeeding or discontinue product

Evaluate:

• Therapeutic response: decreased depression

Teach patient/family:

• That therapeutic effect may take 4-6 wk; that patient may have increased anxiety 1st 5-7 days of therapy; not to discontinue abruptly

• To use caution when driving, performing other activities that require alertness because of drowsiness, dizziness, blurred vision; to report signs, symptoms of bleeding

• To use sunscreen, protective clothing to prevent photosensitivity

• To avoid alcohol, other CNS depressants

> **Black Box Warning: Suicide:** That suicidal ideas, behavior may occur in children or young adults, to watch closely for suicidal thoughts, behaviors, notify prescriber immediately

• **About the effects of serotonin syndrome:** nausea/vomiting, tremors; if symptoms occur, to discontinue immediately, notify prescriber

---

clarithromycin (Rx)

(klare-ith'row-my-sin)

Biaxin, Biaxin XL

Func. class.: Antiinfective
Chem. class.: Macrolide

ACTION: Binds to 50S ribosomal subunits of susceptible bacteria and suppresses protein synthesis

USES: Mild to moderate infections of the upper and lower respiratory tract, uncomplicated skin and skin structure infections caused by *Streptococcus pneumoniae, Mycoplasma pneumoniae, Legionella pneumophila, Moraxella catarrhalis, Neisseria gonorrhoeae, Corynebacterium diphtheriae, Listeria monocytogenes, Haemophilus influenzae, Streptococcus pyogenes, Staphylococcus aureus, Mycobacterium avium* complex (MAC); complex infection in AIDS patients; *Mycobacterium avium intracellulare, Helicobacter pylori* in combination with omeprazole, *H. parainfluenzae*
Unlabeled uses: Endocarditis prophylaxis, dyspepsia, gastric ulcer, Legionnaire's disease, pertussis, SARS

CONTRAINDICATIONS: Hypersensitivity to this product or macrolide antibiotics, torsades de pointes, QT prolongation
Precautions: Pregnancy, breastfeeding, geriatric patients, renal/hepatic disease, heart disease

DOSAGE AND ROUTES
Acute exacerbation of chronic bronchitis
• **Adult: PO** 250-500 mg q12hr × 7-14 days or 1000 mg/day × 7 days (XL)
Pharyngitis/tonsillitis
• **Adult: PO** 250 mg q12hr × 10 days
Community-acquired pneumonia
• **Adult: PO** 250 mg q12hr × 7-14 days or 1000 mg/day × 7 days (XL)
Endocarditis prophylaxis
• **Adult: PO** 500 mg 1 hr before procedure

• **Child: PO** 15 mg/kg 1 hr prior to procedure
MAC prophylaxis/treatment
• **Adult: PO** 500 mg bid; will require an additional antiinfective for active infection
H. pylori infection
• **Adult: PO** 500 mg with 30 mg lansoprazole and 1 g amoxicillin together q12hr × 10-14 days or 500 mg with omeprazole 20 mg and 1 g amoxicillin together q12hr × 10 days or 500 mg q8hr and omeprazole 40 mg daily × 14 days, continue omeprazole for 14 more days
Acute maxillary sinusitis
• **Adult: PO** 500 mg q12hr × 14 days
Most infections
• **Child: PO** 7.5 mg/kg q12hr × 10 days, max 500 mg/dose for MAC
Renal dose
• **Adult/child: PO** CCr 30-60 mL/min decrease dose by 50% if using with ritonavir; <30 mL/min, reduce dose by 50%, if used with ritonavir reduce by 75%

Available forms: Tabs 250, 500 mg; oral susp 125 mg/5 mL, 250 mg/5 mL; ext rel tab (XL) 500 mg
Administer:
• Do not break, crush, or chew ext rel
• Adequate intake of fluids (2 L) during diarrhea episodes
• q12hr to maintain serum levels
• Store at room temperature
• **Susp:** Shake well, store at room temperature, discard after 2 wk
• **Ext Rel:** Give with food

SIDE EFFECTS
CV: Ventricular dysrhythmias, QT prolongation, torsades de pointes
GI: *Nausea, vomiting, diarrhea,* hepatotoxicity, *abdominal pain,* anorexia, *abnormal taste,* CDAD, pancreatitis
INTEG: Rash, urticaria, pruritus, Stevens-Johnson syndrome, toxic epidermal necrolysis, angioedema
MISC: *Headache,* hearing loss

PHARMACOKINETICS
Regular release: peak 2-2.5 hr; duration 12 hr; ext release: peak 5-7 hr; half-life 5-7 hr; metabolized by liver; excreted in

---

Side effects: *italics* = common; red = life-threatening

bile, feces; possible inhibition of P-glycoprotein, protein binding 70%

INTERACTIONS

Increase: levels, toxicity—ALPRAZolam, benzodiazepines, busPIRone, carBAMazepine, cycloSPORINE, digoxin, disopyramide, ergots, felodipine, fluconazole, omeprazole, tacrolimus, theophylline, antidiabetics, midazolam, triazolam

Increase: atorvastatin, pravastatin

Increase: myopathy, rhabdomyolysis risk—lovastatin, simvastatin; do not use concurrently

Increase: action, risk for toxicity—all products metabolized by CYP3A enzyme system

Increase: levels of sildenafil, tadalafil, vardenafil

Increase: effect of calcium channel blockers

Increase: QT prolongation—class IA, III antidysrhythmics, quinidines, procainamide, dofetilide, sotalol, amiodarone or other products that prolong QT

Increase or decrease action: zidovudine

Drug/Food
• Do not use with grapefruit juice

Drug/Herb
Decrease: clarithromycin effect—St. John's wort

Drug/Lab Test
Increase: AST, ALT, BUN, creatinine, LDH, total bilirubin, INR, PT

NURSING CONSIDERATIONS
Assess:
• **Infection:** wound characteristics, urine, stool, sputum, WBC, temperature; C&S before product therapy; product may be given as soon as culture is taken; C&S may be repeated after treatment
• **Bleeding:** check INR if anticoagulants are taken
• **Hypersensitivity:** allergies before treatment, reaction to each medication
• **Heart failure:** increased risk of heart-related disease and death in some patients; use caution in those with increased CV risk, and weigh benefits and risk

• **QT prolongation, ventricular dysrhythmias:** monitor ECG, cardiac status in those with underlying cardiac abnormalities
• *Clostridium difficile*–associated diarrhea (CDAD): monitor for diarrhea, cramping, blood in stools, fever; report immediately to prescriber; may start up to several weeks after conclusion of treatment
• **Serious skin reaction:** Stevens-Johnson syndrome, toxic epidermal necrolysis; product should be discontinued immediately; may occur after therapy is concluded
• **Pregnancy/breastfeeding:** no well-controlled studies; use in pregnancy only if benefits outweigh fetal risk; excreted in breast milk, use caution in breastfeeding

Evaluate:
• Therapeutic response: C&S negative for infection, prevention of endocarditis

Teach patient/family:
• To take with full glass of water; may give with food to decrease GI symptoms; to take ext rel with food
• To report sore throat, fever, fatigue; may indicate superinfection
• To notify prescriber of diarrhea, dark urine, pale stools, yellow discoloration of eyes or skin, severe abdominal pain
• To take at evenly spaced intervals; to complete dosage regimen; to notify prescribers of all products used
• To notify prescriber if pregnancy is suspected or planned or if breastfeeding

TREATMENT OF HYPERSENSITIVITY: Withdraw product, maintain airway, administer EPINEPHrine, aminophylline, O_2, IV corticosteroids

---

clevidipine (Rx)
(klev-id'i-peen)

Cleviprex

Func. class.: Calcium channel blocker (L-type)

Chem. class.: Dihydropyridine

ACTION: L-type calcium channels mediate the influx of calcium during depolarization in arterial smooth muscle;

reduces mean arterial B/P by decreasing systemic vascular resistance

USES: Reduction of B/P when oral therapy is not feasible

CONTRAINDICATIONS: Hypersensitivity to this product, eggs, soya lecithin; defective lipid metabolism; severe aortic stenosis, pancreatitis

Precautions: Pregnancy, labor, breastfeeding, children <18 yr, heart failure, hyperlipidemia, chronic hypertension, pheochromocytoma

DOSAGE AND ROUTES
• **Adult:** CONT IV 1-2 mg/hr; dose may be doubled q90sec initially; as B/P reaches goal, adjust dose less frequently (q5-10min) with smaller increases in dose; most patients require 4-6 mg/hr, max 32 mg/hr; no more than 1000 mL should be infused per 24-hr period due to lipid load restrictions

Available forms: Single-dose vial 50, 100 mL (0.5 mg/mL)

Administer:

Intermittent IV INFUSION route
• Do not give through same line as other medications; do not dilute, do not filter
• Gently invert several times before use; do not use if discolored or if particulate matter is present
• Give through central or peripheral line at 1-2 mg/hr; use infusion device
• Store vials in refrigerator; do not freeze; leave vials in carton until use; product is photosensitive, but protection from light during administration is not required

Solution compatibilities: water for injection, 0.9% NaCl, D₅W/0.9% NaCl, D₅/LR, LR, 10% amino acid

SIDE EFFECTS
CNS: Headache
CV: Reflex tachycardia, hypotension, rebound hypertension, atrial fibrillation
GI: Nausea, vomiting
MS: Arthralgia
GU: Acute renal failure

PHARMACOKINETICS
Onset 2-4 min; half-life initially 1 min, terminal 15 min; metabolized via esterases in blood, extravascular tissues; excreted in urine 63%-74%, feces 7%-22%; protein binding >99%

NURSING CONSIDERATIONS
Assess:
• **Cardiac status:** B/P, pulse, respiration, ECG; some patients have developed severe angina, acute MI after calcium channel blockers if obstructive CAD is severe; if not transitioned to oral antihypertensive therapies after clevidipine infusion, patients should be monitored ≥8 hr for rebound hypertension; monitor for rebound hypertension after product stoppage
• **Pregnancy/breastfeeding:** no well-controlled studies; use in pregnancy only if benefits outweigh fetal risk; excretion is unknown, use cautiously in breastfeeding

Evaluate:
• Therapeutic response: decreased B/P

Teach patient/family:
• To notify prescriber immediately if neurologic symptoms, visual changes, or symptoms of HF occur
• To inform the patient of reason for product, expected result
• To continue follow-up for hypertension in patients with hypertension
• To notify prescriber if pregnancy is planned or suspected, or if breastfeeding

---

clindamycin (Rx)
(klin-da-myˈsin)
Cleocin, Cleocin T, Clinda-Derm, Clinda-T ✿, Clindagel, Clindesse, Clindets, Dalacin T ✿, Evolin, Dalacin C ✿
Func. class.: Antiinfective—miscellaneous
Chem. class.: Lincomycin derivative

ACTION: Binds to 50S subunit of bacterial ribosomes, suppresses protein synthesis

USES: Skin, skin structure, respiratory tract infections; septicemia; intra-abdominal infections; endocarditis prophylaxis; infections caused by staphylococci, streptococci, *Rickettsia, Fusobacterium, Actinomyces, Peptococcus, Bacteroides, Pneumocystis jiroveci*

Unlabeled uses: *Pneumocystis jiroveci* pneumonia (PCP)

CONTRAINDICATIONS: Hypersensitivity to this product or lincomycin, tartrazine dye; ulcerative colitis/enteritis

> Black Box Warning: Pseudomembranous colitis

Precautions: Pregnancy, breastfeeding, GI/hepatic disease, asthma, allergy, diarrhea

DOSAGE AND ROUTES
Most infections
• **Adult: PO** 150-450 mg q6hr, max 2700 mg/day; **IM/IV** 1.2-2.7 g/day in 2-4 divided doses, max 4800 mg/day severe infections
• **Child >1 mo: PO** 8-25 mg/kg/day in divided doses q6-8hr; **IM/IV** 20-40 mg/kg/day in 3-4 equal divided doses q6-8hr
• **Neonate: IM/IV** 15-20 mg/kg/day divided doses q6-8hr

PID
• **Adult: IV** 900 mg q8hr plus gentamicin

Bacterial endocarditis prophylaxis
• **Adult: PO/IV** 600 mg 1 hr (PO), 30 min (IV) before procedure

Bacterial vaginosis
• **Adult/adolescent:** **Vaginal:** (Cleocin, Clindamax) 1 applicator (5 g) at bedtime × 3-7 day; (Clindesse) 1 applicator (5 g) single dose or 1 suppository (100 mg) at bedtime × 3 nights

***P. jiroveci* pneumonia (unlabeled)**
• **Adult: PO** 1200-1800 mg/day in divided doses with 15-30 mg primaquine/day × 21 days

Available forms: caps 75, 150, 300 mg; oral sol 75 mg/5 mL; inj 150, 300, 600 mg base/16 mL; 900 mg base/mL; inj infusion in D_5 300 mg, 600 mg, 900 mg/16 mL

Administer:
• In equal intervals around the clock to maintain blood levels
• Obtain C&S before use, may start product before results are received

PO route
• Do not break, crush, chew caps
• Orally with at least 8 oz of water

Oral solution
• Do not refrigerate reconstituted product; store at room temperature ≤2 wk
• Reconstitute granules with most of 75 mL of water, shake well, add remaining water, shake well (75 mg/5 mL)

Vaginal route
• Use applicator supplied
• Partner is not treated

Topical route
• Do not get in eyes, mouth cuts

IM route
• IM deep inj; rotate sites; do not give >600 mg in single IM inj

IV route
• Visually inspect parenteral products for particulate matter and discoloration before use
• **Vials:** dilute 300 and 600 mg doses with 50 mL of a compatible diluent; dilute 900-mg doses with 50-100 mL of a compatible diluent; dilute 1200-mg doses with 100 mL of a compatible diluent, final concentration max 18 mg/mL
• **ADD-vantage vials:** dilute 600- and 900-mg ADD-vantage containers with 50 or 100 mL, respectively, of NS or D_5W
• **Storage:** when diluted in D_5W, NS, or LR, solutions with concentrations of 6, 9, or 12 mg/mL are stable for 16 days at room temperature or 32 days under refrigeration when stored in glass bottles or minibags; when diluted in D_5W, solutions with a concentration of 18 mg/mL are stable for 16 days at room temperature

Intermittent IV infusion route
• Infuse over at least 10-60 min, infusion rates max 30 mg/min and ≤1.2 g should be infused in a 1-hr period
• Infuse 300-mg doses over 10 min; 600-mg doses over 20 min, 900-mg doses over 30 min, and 1200-mg doses over 40 min

Continuous IV infusion route

• Give first dose rapidly, then follow with continuous infusion

• Rate is based on desired serum clindamycin levels

• To maintain serum concentrations above 4 mcg/mL, use a rapid infusion rate of 10 mg/min for 30 min and a maintenance rate of 0.75 mg/min; to maintain serum concentrations above 5 mcg/mL, use a rapid infusion rate of 15 mg/min for 30 min and a maintenance rate of 1 mg/min; to maintain serum concentrations above 5 mcg/mL, use a rapid infusion rate of 20 mg/min for 30 min and a maintenance rate of 1.25 mg/min

Y-site compatibilities: Acyclovir, alfentanil, amifostine, amikacin, aminocaproic acid, aminophylline, amiodarone, amphotericin B cholesteryl, amphotericin B lipid complex, amsacrine, anakinra, anidulafungin, ascorbic acid injection, atenolol, atracurium, atropine, aztreonam, benztropine, bivalirudin, bleomycin, bumetanide, buprenorphine, butorphanol, calcium chloride/gluconate, CARBOplatin, cefamandole, ceFAZolin, cefmetazole, cefonicid, cefoperazone, cefotaxime, cefoTEtan, cefOXitin, cefpirome, cefTAZidime, ceftizoxime, ceftobiprole, cefuroxime, cephalothin, cephapirin, chloramphenicol, cimetidine, cisatracurium, CISplatin, codeine, cyanocobalamin, cyclophosphamide, cycloSPORINE, cytarabine, DACTINomycin, DAPTOmycin, dexamethasone, dexmedetomidine, digoxin, diltiaZEM, diphenhydrAMINE, DOCEtaxel, DOPamine, doxacurium, DOXORUBicin, DOXOrubicin liposomal, doxycycline, enalaprilat, ePHEDrine, EPINEPHrine, epirubicin, epoetin alfa, eptifibatide, esmolol, etoposide, famotidine, fenoldopam, fentaNYL, fludarabine, fluorouracil, folic acid, foscarnet, furosemide, gatifloxacin, gemcitabine, gemtuzumab, gentamicin, glycopyrrolate, granisetron, heparin, hydrocortisone, HYDROmorphone, ifosfamide, imipenem-cilastatin, indomethacin, insulin (regular), irinotecan, isoproterenol, ketorolac, levoFLOXacin, lidocaine, linezolid, LORazepam, LR, magnesium sulfate, mannitol, mechlorethamine, melphalan, meperidine, metaraminol, methicillin, methotrexate, methoxamine, methyldopate, methylPREDNISolone, metoclopramide, metoprolol, metroNIDAZOLE, mezlocillin, miconazole, milrinone, morphine, moxalactam, multiple vitamins injection, nafcillin, nalbuphine, naloxone, nesiritide, netilmicin, niCARdipine, nitroglycerin, nitroprusside, norepinephrine, octreotide, ondansetron, oxacillin, oxaliplatin, oxytocin, PACLitaxel, palonosetron, pamidronate, pancuronium, pantoprazole, PEMEtrexed, penicillin G potassium/sodium, pentazocine, perphenazine, PHENobarbital, phenylephrine, phytonadione, piperacillin, piperacillin-tazobactam, potassium chloride, procainamide, propofol, propranolol, protamine, pyridoxine, raNITIdine, remifentanil, Ringer's, ritodrine, riTUXimab, rocuronium, sargramostim, sodium acetate/bicarbonate, succinylcholine, SUFentanil, tacrolimus, teniposide, theophylline, thiamine, thiotepa, ticarcillin, ticarcillin-clavulanate, tigecycline, tirofiban, TNA, tobramycin, tolazoline, TPN, trimetaphan, urokinase, vancomycin, vasopressin, vecuronium, verapamil, vinCRIStine, vinorelbine, vitamin B complex/C, voriconazole, zidovudine, zoledronic acid

SIDE EFFECTS

GI: *Nausea, vomiting, abdominal pain, diarrhea*, CDAD, anorexia

CV: Dysrrhythmias, hypotension

INTEG: Rash, urticaria, pruritus, abscess at inj site

SYST: Stevens-Johnson syndrome, exfoliative dermatitis

Misc: Candidiasis

PHARMACOKINETICS

PO: Peak 45 min, duration 6-8 hr

IM: Peak 3 hr (adult), 1 hr (child); duration 8-12 hr; half-life 2½ hr; metabolized in liver by CYP3A4; excreted in urine, bile, feces as inactive metabolites; crosses placenta; excreted in breast milk, protein binding 94%

INTERACTIONS

• May block clindamycin effect: erythromycin; avoid using together

Increase: neuromuscular blockade—neuromuscular blockers

Decrease: absorption—kaolin/pectin

Drug/Lab Test

Increase: alk phos, bilirubin, CPK, AST, ALT

NURSING CONSIDERATIONS
Assess:

• **Infection:** C&S before product therapy; product may be given as soon as culture is taken; monitor appearances of wounds, sputum, stools, urine baseline and periodically

> **Black Box Warning: CDAD:** bowel pattern before, during treatment; if severe diarrhea occurs, product should be discontinued; may occur several wk after therapy is terminated; use this product in serious infections only

• **Monitor blood studies:** CBC

• **Serious skin reactions:** Stevens-Johnson syndrome, exfoliative dermatitis (monitor for rash); discontinue at first appearance of rash, may occur after conclusion of therapy

• **Pregnancy/breastfeeding:** no well-controlled studies; use in pregnancy only if benefits outweigh fetal risk; excreted in breast milk, not recommended if breastfeeding

Evaluate:

• Therapeutic response: negative C&S

Teach patient/family:

• To take oral product with full glass of water; that antiperistaltic products may worsen diarrhea

• About all aspects of product therapy; to complete entire course of medication to ensure organism death (10-14 days); culture may be taken after medication course completed

• To report sore throat, fever, fatigue; may indicate **superinfection**

• To take with food to reduce GI symptoms

> **Black Box Warning:** • To notify nurse or prescriber of diarrhea with pus, mucus, rash

TREATMENT OF HYPER-SENSITIVITY:

• Withdraw product; maintain airway; administer EPINEPHrine, O_2, IV corticosteroids

---

clindamycin (topical, vaginal)

(klin-da-mye′sin)

Cleocin, Cleocin-T, Clindacin-P, Clindagel, ClindaMax, Clindasol ✦, Clinda-T ✦, Clindesse, Clindets, Dalacin ✦, Evoclin

Func. class.: Topical antiinfective
Chem. class.: Lincosamide derivative

ACTION: Antibacterial activity results from inhibition of protein synthesis; bacteriostatic

USES: For the treatment of acne vulgaris; treatment of bacterial vaginosis and anaerobic bacteria

CONTRAINDICATIONS: Hypersensitivity to this product or lincomycin, history of antibiotic-associated colitis or ulcerative colitis

Precautions: Breastfeeding, children <12 yr

DOSAGE AND ROUTES
Acne vulgaris

• **Adult/adolescent: TOP** (gel, lotion, solution) Apply a thin film of 1% to affected areas bid; **TOP (foam)** Apply 1% topical foam to affected areas once daily; if there is no improvement after 6-8 weeks or if the condition worsens, discontinue treatment; **TOP** (medicated pledgets) Use a pledget to apply a thin film to the affected area bid

Bacterial vaginosis and anaerobic bacteria

Nonpregnant adult/adolescent/postmenarchal females: Intravaginal cream: one applicatorful (100 mg clindamycin/5 g cream) intravaginally, preferably at bedtime, for 3 or 7 consecutive days in

---

nonpregnant women and for 7 consecutive days in pregnant women; Clindesse is administered as a single dose at any time of the day

• **Intravaginal ovules/suppositories:** one ovule (100 mg clindamycin) inserted intravaginally at bedtime for 3 days

Available forms: Topical gel, foam, lotion, pledget, solution 1%; vaginal cream 2%, vaginal suppositories 100 mg

Administer:

Topical route:

• Improvement occurs after 6 wk but can require 8-12 wk

• Topical skin products are not for intravaginal therapy and are for external use only; do not use skin products near the eyes, nose, or mouth

• Wash hands before and after use; wash affected area and gently pat dry

Cream/ointment/lotion: Shake well before use (lotion); apply a thin film to the cleansed affected area; massage gently into affected areas

Foam formulations: Do not dispense foam directly onto hands or face; the warmth of the skin will cause the foam to melt; instead, dispense desired amount directly into the cap or onto a cool surface; if the can feels warm or the foam seems runny, run the can under cold water; to apply, pick up small amounts of the foam with the fingertips and gently massage into the affected areas

Solution formulations: Shake well before use; apply a thin film to the cleansed affected area; massage gently into affected areas; if using a solution-soaked pledget, patient may use more than 1 pledget per application as needed to treat affected areas, but each pledget should be used only once and then discarded

Intravaginal route: Only use dosage formulations specified for intravaginal use; intravaginal dosage forms are not for topical therapy; do not ingest

Suppository: Unwrap vaginal ovule (suppository) before insertion; use applicator(s) supplied by the manufacturer

Cream: Use applicator(s) supplied by the manufacturer

SIDE EFFECTS

GU: Colitis, diarrhea, overgrowth, vaginitis, *vaginal moniliasis*, UTI

INTEG: Redness, burning, dermatitis, rash, pruritus

NURSING CONSIDERATIONS

Assess:

• Contact prescriber immediately if severe diarrhea, stomach cramps/pain, or bloody stools occur

Infection: Assess for number of lesions, severity in acne, itching in vaginosis

Evaluate:

• Decreased lesions in acne, infection in vaginosis

Teach patient/family:

Topical route

• That improvement occurs after 6 wk but can require 8-12 wk

• That topical skin products are not for intravaginal therapy and are for external use only; not to use skin products near the eyes, nose, or mouth

• To wash hands before and after use; to wash affected area and gently pat dry

• **Cream/ointment/lotion:** to shake well before use; **lotion:** to apply a thin film to the cleansed affected area and massage gently into affected area

• **Foam formulations:** not to dispense foam directly onto hands or face; pick up small amounts of the foam with the fingertips and gently massage into the affected areas

• **Solution formulations:** to shake well before use; to apply a thin film to the cleansed affected area and massage gently into affected areas; if using a solution-soaked pledget, patient may use more than one pledget per application as needed to treat affected areas, but each pledget should be used only once and then discarded

Intravaginal route

• To use only dosage formulations specified for intravaginal use; not to ingest

• **Suppository:** to unwrap vaginal ovule (suppository) before insertion; to use applicator(s) supplied by the manufacturer

• **Cream:** to use applicator(s) supplied by the manufacturer

clobetasol

(kloe-bay′ta-sol)

Clobex, Cormax, Olux, Olux-E, Temovate, Temovate-E

Func. class.: Corticosteroid, topical

ACTION: Crosses cell membrane to attach to receptors to decrease inflammation, itching

USES: Inflammation/itching in corticosteroid-responsive dermatoses on the skin/scalp

Unlabeled uses: aphthous ulcer, hemangioma, vulvar lichen sclerosus

CONTRAINDICATIONS: Hypersensitivity, use of some preparations on face, axilla, groin; monotherapy for primary bacterial infections

Precautions: Pregnancy, breastfeeding, children <12 yr

DOSAGE AND ROUTES

• **Adult: TOP** Apply to infected areas bid (shampoo: daily up to 4×/wk)

Available forms: Gel, lotion, ointment, cream, shampoo, solution, spray, foam 0.05%

Administer

Topical route

• Do not use with occlusive dressings

• Treatment should be limited to 2 wk

• **Cream/ointment/lotion:** using gloves, apply sparingly in a thin film and rub gently into the cleansed, slightly moist affected area

• **Gel:** using gloves, apply sparingly in a thin film and rub gently into the cleansed, slightly moist affected area

• **Scalp foam:** invert can and dispense a small amount of foam onto a saucer or other cool surface; do not dispense directly onto hands; pick up small amounts of foam with fingers and gently massage into affected area until foam disappears; repeat until entire affected scalp area is treated

• **Shampoo:** apply onto dry scalp in thin film, leave lather on scalp for 15 min, rinse off

SIDE EFFECTS

GU: Glycosuria

INTEG: Burning, folliculitis, pruritus, dermatitis, irritation, erythema, hypertrichosis, acne

MISC: Hyperglycemia, HPA axis suppression

NURSING CONSIDERATIONS

Assess:

• Skin reactions: burning, pruritus, folliculitis, dermatitis

• **Beers:** avoid in older adults with delirium or with high risk for delirium; may induce or worsen delirium

Evaluate:

• Therapeutic response: decrease in itching, inflammation on the skin, scalp

Teach patient/family:

Topical route

• Not to use with occlusive dressings

• That treatment should be limited to 2 wk

• **Cream/ointment/lotion:** to apply sparingly in a thin film and rub gently into the cleansed affected area

• **Gel:** to apply sparingly in a thin film and rub gently into the cleansed, slightly moist affected area

• **Scalp foam:** to invert can and dispense a small amount of foam onto a saucer or other cool surface; not to dispense directly onto hands; to pick up small amounts of foam with fingers and gently massage into affected area until foam disappears; repeat until entire affected scalp area is treated

clomiPHENE (Rx)

(kloe′mi-feen)

Clomid

Func. class.: Ovulation stimulant

Chem. class.: Selective estrogen receptor modulator (SERM)

Do not confuse:

clomiPHENE/clomiPRAMINE

ACTION: Increases LH, FSH release from the pituitary, which increases the maturation of the ovarian follicle, ovulation, and the development of the corpus luteum

USES: Female infertility (ovulatory failure)

CONTRAINDICATIONS: Pregnancy, hypersensitivity, hepatic disease, undiagnosed uterine bleeding, uncontrolled thyroid or adrenal dysfunction, intracranial lesion, ovarian cysts, endometrial carcinoma

Precautions: Hypertension, depression, seizures, diabetes mellitus, abnormal ovarian enlargement, ovarian hyperstimulation

DOSAGE AND ROUTES

• **Adult: PO** 50 mg/day × 5 days or 50 mg/day beginning on day 5 of menstrual cycle, may increase to 100 mg daily × 5 days with next cycle; may be repeated until conception occurs or max 6 cycles of therapy

Available forms: Tabs 50 mg

Administer:

• After discontinuing estrogen therapy

• At same time daily to maintain product level, without regard to food

• Avoid heat, moisture, light; store at room temperature

SIDE EFFECTS

CNS: *Headache, depression,* restlessness, anxiety, nervousness, fatigue, insomnia, dizziness, flushing

CV: Vasomotor flushing, phlebitis, deep venous thrombosis

EENT: Blurred vision, diplopia, photophobia

GI: *Nausea, vomiting, constipation,* abdominal pain, bloating, hepatitis

GU: Polyuria, urinary frequency, birth defects, spontaneous abortions, multiple ovulation, breast pain, oliguria, abnormal uterine bleeding, ovarian cyst, hypertrophy of ovary, hot flashes

INTEG: *Rash, dermatitis,* urticaria, alopecia

PHARMACOKINETICS

Metabolized in liver, excreted in feces

INTERACTIONS

Drug/Herb

Decrease: clomiPHENE effect—DHEA, black cohosh, chaste tree fruit

Drug/Food

Decrease: clomiPHENE effect—soy

Drug/Lab Test

Increase: LFTs

NURSING CONSIDERATIONS

Assess:

• Verify infertility workup, pelvic exam

• LFTs before therapy: AST, ALT, alk phos

• Serum progesterone, urinary excretion of pregnanediol to identify occurrence of ovulation

• Ovarian size, cervical condition by pelvic examination

• Rule out endometrial carcinoma in women >35 yr by endometrial biopsy

• **Pregnancy/breastfeeding:** do not use in pregnancy or breastfeeding

Evaluate:

• Therapeutic response: fertility

Teach patient/family:

• That multiple births are common

• To notify prescriber immediately if low abdominal pain occurs; may indicate ovarian cyst, cyst rupture, ovarian hyperstimulation syndrome (OHSS) symptoms (abdominal bloating, nausea, diarrhea, weight gain, vomiting, dark urine)

• To notify prescriber of photophobia, blurred vision, diplopia, abnormal bleeding

• That if dose is missed, to double it next time; if more than one dose is missed, to call prescriber

• That response usually occurs 4-10 days after last day of treatment

• About the method for taking, recording basal body temperature to determine whether ovulation has occurred

• If ovulation can be determined (there is a slight decrease in temperature then a sharp increase with ovulation), to attempt coitus 3 days before and every other day until after ovulation

• To notify prescriber immediately if pregnancy is suspected

clomiPRAMINE (Rx)

(kloe-mip'ra-meen)

Anafranil

Func. class.: Antidepressant, tricyclic
Chem. class.: Tertiary amine

Do not confuse:
clomiPRAMINE/clomiPHENE

ACTION: Potentiates serotonin and norepinephrine; moderate anticholinergic effect

USES: Obsessive-compulsive disorder
Unlabeled uses: Autism, depression, premature ejaculation

CONTRAINDICATIONS: Hypersensitivity to this product, carBAMazepine, tricyclics, immediate post-MI, MAOI therapy
Precautions: Pregnancy, breastfeeding, geriatric patients, seizures, cardiac disease, glaucoma, prostatic hypertrophy, urinary retention

Black Box Warning: Children, suicidal ideation

DOSAGE AND ROUTES
Obsessive-compulsive disorder
• **Adult:** PO 25 mg at bedtime, increase gradually over 4 wk to 75-250 mg/day in divided doses
• **Child 10-18 yr:** PO 25 mg/day, gradually increase over 2 wk; max 3 mg/kg/day or 200 mg/day, whichever is smaller
Autism (unlabeled)
• **Adult:** PO 25 mg/day, may increase to 75-100 mg/day, max 250 mg/day
• **Child:** PO 25 mg/day, may increase if needed
Premature ejaculation (unlabeled)
• **Adult:** PO 25-50 mg/day
Depression (unlabeled)
• **Adult:** PO 25 mg at bedtime and increase gradually over 4 wk to 75-250 mg/day in divided doses
• **Child 10-18 yr:** PO 25-50 mg/day gradually increased; max 3 mg/kg/day or 200 mg/day, whichever is smaller
Available forms: Caps 25, 50, 75 mg

Administer:
• Do not break, crush, or chew caps
• Increased fluids, bulk in diet for constipation, especially for geriatric patients
• Without regard to food; during initial dosing and titration give with meals
• After titration, may be given as a single dose at bedtime to reduce daytime sedation
• Store in tight container, at room temperature; do not freeze

SIDE EFFECTS
CNS: *Dizziness, tremors, mania,* seizures, aggressiveness, EPS, drowsiness, headache, neuroleptic malignant syndrome, insomnia, agitation, anxiety, impaired memory
CV: Hypotension, tachycardia, cardiac arrest, hypertension, palpitations
EENT: Blurred vision, altered taste, tinnitus, increased intraocular pressure
ENDO: Galactorrhea, hyperprolactinemia
GI: *Constipation, dry mouth, nausea, dyspepsia,* weight gain, hepatic toxicity
GU: *Delayed ejaculation, anorgasmia,* urinary retention, decreased libido
HEMA: Agranulocytosis, neutropenia, pancytopenia
INTEG: Diaphoresis, photosensitivity, abnormal skin odor, flushing, rash, pruritus
META: Hyponatremia
RESP: Pharyngitis, rhinitis, bronchospasm
SYST: Suicide in children, adolescents

PHARMACOKINETICS
Onset ≥ 2 wk (depression), 4-10 wk (OCD); peak 2-6 hr; extensively bound to tissue and plasma proteins; demethylated in liver; active metabolites excreted in urine (50%-60%), feces (24%-32%); half-life 32 hr; steady state 1-2 wk

INTERACTIONS
Increase: hypertensive crisis, seizures, hypertensive episode—MAOIs
Increase: serotonin syndrome—SSRIs, SNRIs, linezolid, methylene blue IV
Increase: clomiPRAMINE levels—cimetidine, FLUoxetine, fluvoxaMINE, sertraline; do not use together

Increase: hypertensive effect—cloNI-Dine, EPINEPHrine, norepinephrine
Increase: clomiPRAMINE level—CYP1A2, CYP2D6
Increase: CNS depression—alcohol, CNS depressants, general anesthetics
Increase: QT prolongation—other tricyclics, phenothiazines, quinolones, antidysrhythmics, droperidol, mefloquine, mesoridazine, moxifloxacin, pentamidine, pimozide, tacrolimus, ziprasidone
Decrease: effect of cloNIDine, levodopa, skeletal muscle relaxants, haloperidol, opiates
Decrease: clomiPRAMINE levels—barbiturates, carBAMazepine, phenytoin

Drug/Herb
Increase: serotonin syndrome—St. John's wort; do not use concurrently
Increase: CNS depression—hops, kava, valerian

Drug/Lab Test
Increase: prolactin, TBG, AST, ALT, blood glucose
Decrease: serum thyroid hormone (T_3, T_4)

NURSING CONSIDERATIONS
Assess:
• B/P lying, standing; pulse q4hr; if systolic B/P drops 20 mm Hg, withhold product, notify prescriber; take VS q4hr in patients with CV disease
• **Serotonin syndrome:** hyperpyrexia, rigidity, irregular pulse, diaphoresis
• **ECG** for flattening of T wave, QTc prolongation, bundle branch block, AV block, dysrhythmias in cardiac patients, may lead to cardiac collapse
• Blood studies: CBC, leukocytes, differential, cardiac enzymes if patient is receiving long-term therapy and signs of blood dyscrasias
• Hepatic studies: AST, ALT, bilirubin

Black Box Warning: Mental status: mood, sensorium, affect, suicidal tendencies; increase in psychiatric symptoms: depression, panic, frequency of obsessive-compulsive behaviors; watch closely for evidence of suicidal thoughts in children, adolescents; seizure disorders

• **Beers:** avoid in older adults with or at high risk for delirium or orthostatic hypotension
• **Pregnancy/breastfeeding:** no well-controlled studies; use in pregnancy only if benefits outweigh fetal risk; excreted in breast milk, discontinue breastfeeding or discontinue product
• Urinary retention, constipation; constipation more likely in children
• **Withdrawal symptoms:** headache, nausea, vomiting, muscle pain, weakness; not usual unless product discontinued abruptly
• Alcohol consumption; if alcohol is consumed, withhold dose until AM
• Assistance with ambulation during beginning therapy since drowsiness, dizziness occurs
• Gum, hard candy, or frequent sips of water for dry mouth

Evaluate:
• Therapeutic response: decreased anxiety, depression

Teach patient/family:
• That the effects may take 4-6 wk to appear
• About risk for seizures
• To use caution when driving, performing other activities that require alertness because drowsiness, dizziness, blurred vision may occur
• To avoid alcohol, other CNS depressants
• Not to discontinue medication quickly after long-term use because this may cause nausea, headache, malaise

Black Box Warning: That suicidal thoughts/behaviors may occur in children, young adults; report immediately

• To wear sunscreen, protective clothing to prevent photosensitivity
• To notify prescriber if pregnancy is planned, suspected
• That men may experience a high incidence of sexual dysfunction
• **Serotonin syndrome:** to report immediately sweating, diarrhea, twitching
• **Abrupt discontinuation:** not to stop abruptly

Side effects: *italics* = common; red = life-threatening

TREATMENT OF OVERDOSE:

ECG monitoring; induce emesis; lavage, anticonvulsant; diazePAM IV

⚠ HIGH ALERT

clonazePAM (Rx)

(kloe-na′zi-pam)

KlonoPIN, Rivotril ✤

Func. class.: Anticonvulsant

Chem. class.: Benzodiazepine derivative

Controlled Substance Schedule IV

Do not confuse:

clonazePAM/LORazepam/cloNIDine
KlonoPIN/cloNIDine

ACTION: Inhibits spike, wave formation during absence seizures (petit mal); decreases amplitude, frequency, duration, spread of discharge during minor motor seizures

USES: Absence, atypical absence, akinetic, myoclonic seizures; Lennox-Gastaut syndrome, panic disorder

Unlabeled uses: Insomnia, restless legs syndrome, acute mania, neuralgia

CONTRAINDICATIONS: Pregnancy, hypersensitivity to benzodiazepines, acute closed-angle glaucoma, psychosis, severe hepatic disease

Precautions: Breastfeeding, geriatric patients, open-angle glaucoma, chronic respiratory disease, renal/hepatic disease

Black Box Warning: Coadministration with other CNS depressants, especially opiates

DOSAGE AND ROUTES

Lennox-Gastaut syndrome/atypical absence seizures/akinetic and myclonic seizures

• **Adult:** PO up to 1.5 mg/day in 3 divided doses; may be increased 0.5-1 mg q3days until desired response, max 20 mg/day

• **Geriatric:** PO 0.25 daily-bid initially, increase by 0.25/day q7-14days as needed

• **Child ≤10 yr or ≤30 kg:** PO initial 0.01-0.03 mg/kg/day in divided doses q8hr, max 0.05 mg/kg/day; may be increased 0.25-0.5 mg q3days until desired response, max 0.1-0.2 mg/kg/day

Panic disorder

• **Adult:** PO 0.25 mg bid, increase to 1 mg daily after 3 days, max 4 mg/day

Restless legs syndrome (RLS) (unlabeled)

• **Adult:** PO 0.5 mg tid or 0.5 mg in the evening and 30 min before bedtime

Insomnia/anxiety (unlabeled)

• **Adult:** PO 0.125-0.25 mg at bedtime, titrate up q3-4days as needed

Available forms: Tabs 0.5, 1, 2 mg; orally disintegrating tabs 0.125, 0.25, 0.5, 1, 2 mg

Administer:

PO route

• With food, milk for GI symptoms

• **Orally disintegrating tablets:** open pouch by peeling back foil on blister pack (do not push tab through foil), place on tongue, allow to dissolve; may be swallowed with/without water

• Store at room temperature

SIDE EFFECTS

CNS: *Drowsiness,* dizziness, confusion, behavioral changes, tremors, insomnia, headache, suicidal tendencies, slurred speech, fatigue

CV: Palpitations, bradycardia

EENT: *Nystagmus, diplopia*

GI: *Nausea, constipation,* anorexia, diarrhea

GU: Dysuria, enuresis, nocturia, retention, libido changes

HEMA: Anemia, thrombocytopenia, leukopenia

INTEG: Rash

RESP: Congestion, respiratory depression

PHARMACOKINETICS

PO: Peak 1-2 hr, metabolized by liver, excreted in urine, half-life 18-50 hr, duration 6-12 hr, protein binding 85%

INTERACTIONS

Increase: clonazePAM effects—CYP3A4 inhibitors (azoles, cimetidine, clarithromycin, diltiazem, erythromycin, FLUoxetine), oral contraceptives; adjust dosage

Black Box Warning: **Increase:** CNS depression—alcohol, barbiturates, opiates, antidepressants, other anticonvulsants, general anesthetics, hypnotics, sedatives

Decrease: clonazePAM effect—CYP3A4 inducers (carBAMazepine, PHENobarbital, phenytoin); monitor effect
Drug/Herb

Black Box Warning: **Increase:** CNS depression—kava, chamomile, valerian

Increase: clonazePAM effect—ginkgo, melatonin
Decrease: clonazePAM effect—ginseng, St. John's wort
Drug/Lab Test
Increase: AST, alk phos, bilirubin
Decrease: platelets, WBC

NURSING CONSIDERATIONS
Assess:
• **Seizures:** monitor duration, type, intensity, with/without aura
• Blood studies: RBC, Hct, Hgb, reticulocyte counts periodically
• Hepatic studies: ALT, AST, bilirubin, creatinine
• **Abrupt discontinuation:** do not discontinue abruptly; seizures may increase
• Signs of physical withdrawal if medication suddenly discontinued
• **Mental status:** mood, sensorium, affect, oversedation, behavioral changes, **suicidal thoughts/behaviors;** if mental status changes, notify prescriber
• **Allergic reaction:** red, raised rash; product should be discontinued
• **Blood dyscrasias:** fever, sore throat, bruising, rash, jaundice
• **Toxicity:** bone marrow depression, nausea, vomiting, ataxia, diplopia, CV collapse; drug levels during initial treatment (therapeutic 20-80 ng/mL)

Black Box Warning: **Coadministration with other CNS depressants, especially opioids:** increased risk of sedation causing death with benzodiazepines and opioids

• **Beers:** may be appropriate in older adults for seizure disorders, rapid eye movement sleep disorder, benzodiazepine/ethanol withdrawal; avoid in those with delirium or at high risk of delirium
Evaluate:
• Therapeutic response: decreased seizure activity
Teach patient/family:
• To carry emergency ID bracelet stating name, products taken, condition, prescriber's name, phone number
• About potential drug tolerance, withdrawal symptoms
• To continue with follow-up exams, lab work

Black Box Warning: **Coadministration with other CNS depressants, especially opioids:** to avoid driving, other activities that require alertness

• To take as prescribed, not to skip or take double doses, provide "Medication Guide"
• To avoid driving and other hazardous activities until response is known
• **ODT:** open when ready to use, peel foil back with dry hands, place on tongue to dissolve
• To avoid alcohol, other CNS depressants; increased sedation may occur
• Not to discontinue medication quickly after long-term use; to taper off over several wk
• **Pregnancy/breastfeeding:** to notify prescriber if pregnancy is planned or suspected or if breastfeeding, to register with North American Antiepileptic Drug Pregnancy Registry, 1-888-233-2334, if pregnant, not to use during pregnancy/breastfeeding
• To notify prescriber of yellowing of skin/eyes, clay-colored stools, bleeding,

fever, extreme fatigue, sore throat, suicidal thoughts/behaviors

TREATMENT OF OVERDOSE:
Lavage, flumazenil, monitor electrolytes, VS, administer vasopressors, sodium bicarbonate

cloNIDine (Rx)

(klon'i-deen)

Catapres, Catapres-TTS, Duraclon, Kapvay, Dixant ✦

Func. class.: Antihypertensive
Chem. class.: Central α-adrenergic agonist

Do not confuse:
cloNIDine/KlonoPIN/clonazePAM

ACTION: Inhibits sympathetic vasomotor center in CNS, which reduces impulses in sympathetic nervous system; blood pressure, pulse rate, cardiac output are decreased; prevents pain signal transmission in CNS by α-adrenergic receptor stimulation of the spinal cord

USES: Mild to moderate hypertension, used alone or in combination; severe pain in cancer patients (epidural), attention-deficit/hyperactivity disorder (ADHD)
Unlabeled uses: Diabetic neuropathy, opioid withdrawal

CONTRAINDICATIONS: Hypersensitivity; (epidural) bleeding disorders, anticoagulants
Precautions: Pregnancy, breastfeeding, children <12 yr (transdermal), geriatric patients, noncompliant patients, MI (recent), diabetes mellitus, chronic renal failure, Raynaud's disease, thyroid disease, depression, COPD, asthma, pheochromocytoma

Black Box Warning: Labor (epidermal cloNIDIne)

DOSAGE AND ROUTES
Hypertension
• **Adult:** PO 0.1 mg bid then increase by 0.1-0.2 mg/day at weekly intervals until desired response; max 2.4 mg; range 0.2-0.6 mg/day in divided doses or **TRANSDERMAL** q7days, start 0.1 mg and adjust q1-2wk
• **Geriatric:** PO 0.1 mg at bedtime; may increase gradually
• **Child:** PO 5-10 mcg/kg/day in divided doses q8-12hr, max 0.9 mg/day
Severe pain
• **Adult:** CONT EPIDURAL INFUSION 30 mcg/hr
• **Child:** CONT EPIDURAL INFUSION 0.5 mcg/kg/hr, then titrate to response
ADHD
• **Adolescent/child ≥6 yr:** PO 0.05 mg/kg/day in 3-4 divided doses, may increase by 0.1 mg/day weekly up to 0.4 mg/day; ext rel 0.1 mg at bedtime, increase dose by 0.1 mg/day up to 0.4 mg/day

Available forms: Tabs 0.025 ✦, 0.1, 0.2, 0.3 mg; transdermal 2.5, 5, 7.5 mg delivering 0.1, 0.2, 0.3 mg/24 hr, respectively; inj 100, 500 mcg/mL; ext rel tab 0.1 mg (Kapvay)
Administer:
• Store patches in cool environment, tablets in tight container
PO route
• Give last dose at bedtime
• Do not crush, cut, chew, or break ext rel tabs; Kapvay is not interchangeable with other products
Transdermal route
• Once weekly; apply to site without hair; best absorption over chest or upper arm; rotate sites with each application; clean site before application; apply firmly, especially around edges; may secure with adhesive tape if loose; fold sticky sides together and discard
• Should be removed before MRI
Epidural route
• Used for severe cancer pain
• May be used with opiates

• Use only if familiar with epidural infusion devices
• Dilute 500 mcg/mL with 0.9% NaCl (100 mcg/mL)

Black Box Warning: Do not use for labor

SIDE EFFECTS
CNS: *Drowsiness,* nightmares, anxiety, depression, hallucinations, syncope, dizziness
CV: *Orthostatic hypotension,* HF, ECG abnormalities, sinus tachycardia
EENT: Taste change, dry eyes
ENDO: Hyperglycemia
GI: *Nausea, vomiting,* constipation, *dry mouth*
GU: Impotence, urinary retention, decreased libido
INTEG: *Rash,* pruritus, excoriation (transdermal patches)
MISC: Withdrawal symptoms

PHARMACOKINETICS
PO: Onset ½ to 1 hr, peak 2-4 hr, duration 8-12 hr, half-life 6-12 hr
TRANSDERMAL: Onset 3 days; duration 1 wk; metabolized by liver (metabolites); excreted in urine (45% unchanged, inactive metabolites), feces; crosses blood-brain barrier; excreted in breast milk

INTERACTIONS
• **Increase:** bradycardia, verapamil, diltiaZEM
• **Life-threatening elevations of B/P:** tricyclics, β-blockers
Increase: CNS depression—opiates, sedatives, hypnotics, anesthetics, alcohol
Increase: hypotensive effects—diuretics, other antihypertensive nitrates
Increase: bradycardia—amphetamines, beta blockers, digoxin, diltiazem, MAO inhibitors, verapamil
Decrease: hypotensive effects—tricyclics, MAOIs, appetite suppressants, amphetamines, prazosin, antipsychotics
Decrease: effect of levodopa
Drug/Herb
Increase: antihypertensive effect—hawthorn

Decrease: antihypertensive effect—ephedra, ginseng
Drug/Lab Test
Increase: blood glucose
Decrease: VMA, urinary catecholamines, aldosterone
Positive: Coombs' test

NURSING CONSIDERATIONS
Assess:
• **Hypertension:** B/P, pulse; report significant changes
• **Allergic reaction:** rash, fever, pruritus, urticaria; product should be discontinued if antihistamines fail to help
• **HF:** edema, dyspnea, wet crackles, B/P, more common in geriatric patients
• **ADHD:** B/P, pulse, palpitations, syncope
• **Beers:** avoid as first-line in older adults; high risk of CNS effects, bradycardia, orthostatic hypotension

Black Box Warning: **Pregnancy/breastfeeding:** do not use for labor/epidural; excreted in breast milk, discontinue breastfeeding or product

Evaluate:
• Therapeutic response: decrease in B/P with hypertension, decrease in withdrawal symptoms (opioid), decrease in pain
Teach patient/family:
• To avoid hazardous activities and driving until response is known, product may cause drowsiness
• To notify all health care providers of medication use
• Not to discontinue product abruptly or withdrawal symptoms may occur: anxiety, increased B/P, headache, insomnia, increased pulse, tremors, nausea, sweating; to comply with dosage schedule even if feeling better
• Not to use OTC (cough, cold, or allergy), alcohol, or CNS depressant products unless directed by prescriber
• To rise slowly to sitting or standing position to minimize orthostatic hypotension, especially among geriatric patients

Side effects: *italics* = common; red = life-threatening

• To notify prescriber of mouth sores, sore throat, fever, swelling of hands or feet, irregular heartbeat, chest pain, signs of **angioedema**

• About excessive perspiration, dehydration, vomiting; diarrhea may lead to fall in B/P; consult prescriber if these occur; that product may cause dizziness, fainting; that light-headedness may occur during first few days of therapy

• That product may cause dry mouth; to use hard candy, saliva product, sugarless gum, or frequent rinsing of mouth

• Not to skip or stop product unless directed by prescriber; tolerance may develop with long-term use

• **Transdermal:** how to use patch; that patch comes in two parts: product patch and overlay to keep patch in place; not to trim or cut; that response may take 2-3 days, if switching from tabs to patch, to taper tabs to avoid withdrawal; to remove for MRI; can use during bathing, swimming

TREATMENT OF OVERDOSE:
Supportive treatment; administer tolazoline, atropine, DOPamine prn

---

⚠ HIGH ALERT

clopidogrel (Rx)
(klo-pid′oh-grel)

Plavix
Func. class.: Platelet aggregation inhibitor
Chem. class.: Thienopyridine derivative

Do not confuse:
Plavix/Paxil

ACTION: Inhibits ADP-induced platelet aggregation

USES: Reducing the risk of stroke, MI, vascular death, peripheral arterial disease in high-risk patients, acute coronary syndrome, transient ischemic attack (TIA), unstable angina

Unlabeled uses: Cardiac surgery (infant and child), Kawasaki disease

CONTRAINDICATIONS: Hypersensitivity, active bleeding
Precautions: Pregnancy, breastfeeding, children, previous hepatic disease, increased bleeding risk, neutropenia, agranulocytosis, renal disease, ✖️Ⓖ Asian/black/Caucasian patients

Black Box Warning: ✖️Ⓖ CYP2C19 allele (poor metabolizers)

DOSAGE AND ROUTES
Recent MI, stroke, peripheral arterial disease, TIA
• **Adult:** PO 75 mg/day with/without aspirin
Acute MI (ST-segment elevation, MI)
• **Adult:** PO 75 mg/day with aspirin 75-325 mg/day; with or without loading dose or thrombolytics; those >75 yr no loading dose should be given; continue this product for 2 wk to <1 yr with aspirin 81 mg indefinitely
Acute coronary syndrome
• **Adult:** PO loading dose 300 mg, then 75 mg/day with aspirin
Cardiac surgery/other cardiac conditions (unlabeled)
• **Child ≤2 yr/infant/neonate:** PO 0.2 mg/kg/day for platelet inhibition
Available forms: Tabs 75, 300 mg
Administer:
• Without regard to food
• Should be discontinued 5 days before elective surgery if an antiplatelet action is not desired

SIDE EFFECTS
CNS: Headache, dizziness, depression
CV: Edema, hypertension, chest pain
GI: Diarrhea, constipation, GI discomfort
HEMA: Bleeding (major/minor from any site), neutropenia, aplastic anemia, agranulocytosis, thrombotic thrombocytopenic purpura
INTEG: Rash, pruritus, anaphylaxis
MISC: Fatigue, intracranial hemorrhage, toxic epidermal necrolysis, Stevens-Johnson syndrome, flulike syndrome

MS: Arthralgia
RESP: Bronchospasm

PHARMACOKINETICS
Rapidly absorbed; metabolized by liver (CYP3A4, CYP2B6, CYP1A2, CYP2C8); excreted in urine, feces; half-life 6 hr; protein binding 95%; effect on platelets after 3-7 days

INTERACTIONS

Black Box Warning: Avoid use with CYP2C19 inhibitors (omeprazole, esomeprazole)

Increase: bleeding risk—anticoagulants, aspirin, NSAIDs, abciximab, eptifibatide, tirofiban, thrombolytics, ticlopidine, SSRIs, treprostinil, rifampin, SNRIs, prasugrel
Increase: action of some NSAIDs, phenytoin, TOLBUTamide, tamoxifen, torsemide, fluvastatin, warfarin
Decrease: clopidogrel effect—proton pump inhibitor (PPIs)
Decrease: CYP3A4 inhibitors/substrates—atorvastatin, simvastatin, cerivastatin
Drug/Herb
Increase: clopidogrel effect—feverfew, fish oil, omega-3 fatty acid, garlic, ginger, ginkgo biloba, green tea, horse chestnut
Decrease: clopidogrel effect—bilberry, saw palmetto
Drug/Lab Test
Increase: AST, ALT, bilirubin, uric acid, total cholesterol, nonprotein nitrogen (NPN)

NURSING CONSIDERATIONS
Assess:
• Thrombotic/thrombocytic purpura: fever, thrombocytopenia, hemolytic anemia, neurologic changes, treat immediately

Black Box Warning: CYP2C19 allele (poor metabolizers): consider using another antiplatelet product; higher CV reaction occurs after acute coronary syndrome or PCI; tests are available to determine CYP2C19 allele

• Hepatic studies: AST, ALT, bilirubin, creatinine (long-term therapy)
• Blood studies: CBC, differential, Hct, Hgb, PT, cholesterol (long-term therapy); thrombocytopenia, neutropenia are rare
• **Hypersensitivity:** rash, angioedema may occur
Evaluate:
• Therapeutic response: absence of stroke, MI
Teach patient/family:
• That blood work will be necessary during treatment (CBC, liver function tests)
• To report any unusual bruising, bleeding to prescriber; that it may take longer to stop bleeding
• To take without regard to food
• To tell all health care providers that clopidogrel is being used; may be held for 5 days before surgery, restart as soon as possible
• **Hypersensitivity:** To report immediately rash, pruritus
• **Pregnancy/breastfeeding:** to notify provider if pregnancy is planned or suspected or if breastfeeding; do not breastfeed, use cautiously in pregnancy

---

clotrimazole (topical, vaginal, oral)
(kloe-trim′a-zole)
Cruex, Gyne-Lotrimin, Lotrimin, Lotrimin AF, MyCelex, MyCelex-7, Trivagizole 3, Desenex
Func. class.: Topical antifungal
Chem. class.: Imidazole derivative

Do not confuse:
clotrimazole/miconazole/clobetasol

ACTION: Antifungal activity results from altering cell wall permeability

USES: Vulvovaginal, oropharyngeal candidiasis; topical fungal infections

CONTRAINDICATIONS: Hypersensitivity, ophthalmic use
Precautions: Hepatic impairment (oral)

DOSAGE AND ROUTES
Tinea corporis, cruris, pedis, versicolor; candidiasis
• **Adult/child ≥2 yr: TOP** Apply to affected area and rub into area AM/PM × 2-4 wk
Vulvovaginal candidiasis
• **Adult/child ≥12 yr: VAG CREAM** 1 applicator at bedtime × 3 days (2%) or 7 days (1%)
Oropharyngeal candidiasis
• **Adult/child ≥3 yr: LOZENGE** 1 PO dissolved 5×/day × 2 wk or adults 1 lozenge dissolved tid (prevention)
Available forms: Topical cream, solution, 1%; vaginal cream 1%, 2%; lozenges, troches 10 mg
Administer:
Topical route
• Topical skin products are not for intravaginal therapy and are for external use only; do not use skin products near the eyes, nose, or mouth
• Wash hands before and after use; wash affected area and gently pat dry
• **Cream/solution:** apply to the cleansed affected area; massage gently into affected areas
PO route
• **Troches:** allow to dissolve; do not chew or swallow whole
Intravaginal route
• Only use dosage formulations specified for intravaginal use; intravaginal dosage forms are not for topical therapy; do not ingest
• **Cream:** use applicator(s) supplied by the manufacturer

SIDE EFFECTS
GI: Nausea, vomiting
GU: Vaginal burning, irritation
INTEG: Burning, peeling, rash, pruritus

PHARMACOKINETICS
PO duration 3 hr

INTERACTIONS
Drug/Lab Test
Increase: LFTs

NURSING CONSIDERATIONS
Assess:
• **Allergic reaction:** assess for hypersensitivity; product might need to be discontinued
• **Infection:** assess for severity of infection, itching
• Hepatic function studies periodically if using oral troches
Evaluate:
• Decreased infection, itching
Teach patient/family:
Topical route:
• That topical skin products are not for intravaginal therapy and are for external use only; do not use skin products near the eyes, nose, or mouth; do not use occlusive dressings
• To wash hands before and after use; wash affected area and gently pat dry
• **Cream:** to shake well before use; apply a thin film to the cleansed affected area; massage gently into affected areas
PO route:
• **Troches:** allow to dissolve; do not chew or swallow whole
• **Cream:** to use applicator(s) supplied by the manufacturer

---

cloZAPine (Rx)
(kloz′a-peen)
Clozaril, FazaClo, Versacloz
Func. class.: Antipsychotic
Chem. class.: Tricyclic dibenzodiazepine derivative

Do not confuse:
Clozaril/Colazal
cloZAPine/cloNIDine/clofazimine/clonazePAM/KlonoPIN

ACTION: Interferes with DOPamine receptor binding with lack of EPS; also acts as an adrenergic, cholinergic, histaminergic, serotonergic antagonist

USES: Management of psychotic symptoms for schizophrenic patients for

---

whom other antipsychotics have failed; recurrent suicidal behavior

CONTRAINDICATIONS: Hypersensitivity, severe granulocytopenia (WBC <3500 before therapy), coma, ileus
Precautions: Pregnancy, breastfeeding, children <16 yr, geriatric patients; CV, pulmonary, cardiac, renal, hepatic disease; seizures, prostatic enlargement, closed-angle glaucoma, stroke

Black Box Warning: Bone marrow suppression, hypotension, myocarditis, orthostatic hypotension, geriatric patients with dementia-related psychosis, seizures, syncope

DOSAGE AND ROUTES
• **Adult:** PO 12.5 mg daily or bid; may increase by 25-50 mg/day; over 2 wk; dose >500 mg requires 3 divided doses; do not increase dose more than 2×/wk; max 900 mg/day; if dose is to be discontinued, taper over 1-2 wk
Available forms: Tabs 25, 50, 100, 200 mg; orally disintegrating tabs 12.5, 25, 100, 150, 200 mg; oral suspension 50 mg/mL
Administer:
• May be taken with or without food
• Patient-specific registration required before administration (clozapine REMS program); if WBC <3500 cells/mm³ or ANC <2000 cells/mm³, therapy should not be started; may only dispense the 7-, 14-, 28-day supply upon receipt of lab report that is appropriate
• Check to confirm PO medication swallowed; monitor for hoarding or giving of medication to other patients, if hospitalized; avoid giving patient >7 days' worth of medication if outpatient
• Store in tight, light-resistant container
• **Orally disintegrating tab:** do not push through foil; leave in foil blister until ready to take, peel back foil, place tab in mouth; allow to dissolve, swallow; water is not needed
• **Oral suspension:** shake before using; use oral syringe and syringe adapter

SIDE EFFECTS
CNS: Neuroleptic malignant syndrome, *sedation, dizziness, headache,* seizures, *insomnia,* dystonia
CV: *Tachycardia, hypo/hypertension,* orthostatic hypotension
EENT: *Blurred vision*
GI: *Drooling or excessive salivation, constipation, nausea, abdominal discomfort, vomiting,* anorexia, *dry mouth, dyspepsia,* hepatotoxicity
GU: *Urinary abnormalities,* incontinence
HEMA: Leukopenia, agranulocytosis
RESP: Dyspnea, pulmonary embolism
SYST: Death among geriatric patients with dementia, aggravation of diabetes mellitus

PHARMACOKINETICS
Bioavailability 27%-47%; 97% protein bound; completely metabolized by liver enzymes involved in metabolism CYP1A2, 2D6, 3A4; excreted in urine (50%), feces (30%) (metabolites); half-life 8-12 hr

INTERACTIONS
Increase: CNS depression—CNS depressants, psychoactives, alcohol, antihistamines, opioids, sedative/hypnotics
Increase: cloZAPine level—caffeine, citalopram, FLUoxetine, sertraline, ritonavir, risperiDONE, CYP1A2 inhibitors (fluvoxaMINE), CYP3A4 inhibitors (ketoconazole, erythromycin), CYP2D6 inhibitors
Increase: plasma concentration—warfarin, digoxin, other highly protein-bound products
Increase: QT prolongation—β blockers, class IA/III antidysrhythmias, and other drugs that increase QT
Increase: hypotension, respiratory, cardiac arrest, collapse—benzodiazepines
Increase: bone marrow suppression—antineoplastics, radiation therapy
Increase: seizures—lithium
Decrease: cloZAPine level—CYP1A2 inducers (carBAMazepine, omeprazole, rifAMPin); PHENobarbital; CYP3A4 inducers
Drug/Herb
Decrease: clozapine action—St. John's wort

Side effects: *italics* = common; red = life-threatening

Drug/Lab Test
Increase: cholesterol, blood glucose, triglycerides
Decrease: WBC, ANC

NURSING CONSIDERATIONS
Assess:

Black Box Warning: **Myocarditis:** if suspected, discontinue use; myocarditis usually occurs during 1st month of treatment; dyspnea, fever, palpitations, ECG changes

Black Box Warning: **Seizures:** usually occur with higher doses >600 mg/day or dosage change >100 mg/day; do not use in uncontrolled seizure disorder; use cautiously in those with a predisposition to seizures

• AIMS assessment, blood glucose, CBC differential, glycosylated hemoglobin A1c, LFTs, neurologic function, pregnancy test, serum creatinine, electrolytes, lipid profile, prolactin, thyroid function tests, weight

Black Box Warning: **Bone marrow depression:** bilirubin, CBC, LFTs monthly; discontinue treatment if WBC <3000-3500/mm³ or ANC <1500/mm³; test weekly; may resume when normal; if WBC <2000/mm³ or ANC <1000/mm³, discontinue; if agranulocytosis develops, never restart product

• Affect, orientation, LOC, reflexes, gait, coordination, sleep pattern disturbances

Black Box Warning: **Hypotension, bradycardia, syncope:** B/P standing and lying; take pulse, respirations q4hr during initial treatment; establish baseline before starting treatment; report drops of 30 mm Hg; dizziness, faintness, palpitations, tachycardia on rising

• **Extrapyramidal symptoms:** including akathisia (inability to sit still, no pattern to movements), tardive dyskinesia (bizarre movements of the jaw, mouth, tongue, extremities), pseudoparkinsonism (rigidity, tremors, pill rolling, shuffling gait)

• **Neuroleptic malignant syndrome:** tachycardia, seizures, fever, dyspnea, diaphoresis, increased/decreased B/P; notify prescriber immediately
• **Beers:** avoid in older adults except for schizophrenia, bipolar disorder; increased risk of stroke and cognitive decline
• **Pregnancy/breastfeeding:** no well-controlled studies; use in pregnancy only if benefits outweigh fetal risk; excreted in breast milk; discontinue breastfeeding or discontinue product; EPS may be present in neonates exposed to this product during 3rd trimester
Evaluate:
• Therapeutic response: decrease in emotional excitement, hallucinations, delusions, paranoia, reorganization of patterns of thought, speech
Teach patient/family:
• About symptoms of agranulocytosis and need for blood tests weekly for 6 mo, then q2wk; to report flulike symptoms
• That orthostatic hypotension often occurs; to rise gradually from sitting or lying position; to avoid hot tubs, hot showers, tub baths; hypotension may occur
• To avoid abrupt withdrawal of this product because EPS may result; that product should be withdrawn over 1-2 wk
• To avoid OTC preparations (cough, hay fever, cold) unless approved by prescriber because serious product interactions may occur; to avoid use with alcohol or CNS depressants, increased drowsiness may occur
• About compliance with product regimen

Black Box Warning: To report sore throat, malaise, fever, bleeding, mouth sores; if these occur, CBC should be drawn and product discontinued

• That heat stroke may occur in hot weather; to take extra precautions to stay cool
• To avoid driving, other hazardous activities; seizures may occur
• To notify prescriber if pregnant or if pregnancy is intended; not to breastfeed

TREATMENT OF OVERDOSE:
Lavage; provide an airway; do not induce vomiting

RARELY USED

cobicistat/darunavir/ emtricitabine/tenofovir

Symtuza
Func. class.: Antiviral-HIV protease inhibitor/nucleotide reverse transcriptase inhibitor (NRTI) combination

USES: Human immunodeficiency virus (HIV) infection in treatment-naive adults/virologically suppressed adults on an antiretroviral regimen ≥6 mo and who are without resistance-associated substitutions to darunavir or tenofovir

CONTRAINDICATIONS: Hypersensitivity

Black Box Warning: Hepatitis B exacerbation

DOSAGE AND ROUTES
• **Adult/adolescent: PO** 1 tablet (800 mg darunavir; 150 mg cobicistat; 200 mg emtricitabine; 10 mg tenofovir alafenamide) daily with food

---

⚠ HIGH ALERT

RARELY USED

cobimetinib

(koe-bi-me′ ti-nib)
Cotellic
Func. class.: Antineoplastic

USES: Orphan drug. For the treatment of unresectable or metastatic melanoma in patients with a BRAF V600E or V600K mutation, in combination with vemurafenib

CONTRAINDICATIONS: Hypersensitivity

DOSAGE AND ROUTES
• **Adult: PO** 60 mg (three 20-mg tablets) q day × 21 days, in combination with vemurafenib 960 mg bid × 28 days; repeat cycle q28days until disease progression or unacceptable toxicity

---

⚠ HIGH ALERT

codeine (Rx)

(koe′deen)
Func. class.: Opiate analgesic, antitussive
Chem. class.: Opiate, phenathrene derivative

Controlled Substance Schedule II, III, IV, V (depends on content)

Do not confuse:
codeine/Iodine/iodine

ACTION: Depresses pain impulse transmission at the spinal cord level by interacting with opioid receptors; decreases cough reflex, GI motility

USES: Mild to moderate pain
Unlabeled uses: Diarrhea

CONTRAINDICATIONS: Breastfeeding, hypersensitivity to opiates, respiratory depression, increased intracranial pressure, seizure disorders, severe respiratory disorders

Black Box Warning: Children recovering from tonsillectomy/adenoidectomy who are ultrarapid metabolizers

Precautions: Pregnancy, geriatric patients, cardiac dysrhythmias, prostatic hypertrophy, bowel impaction

DOSAGE AND ROUTES
Pain
• **Adult: PO** 15-60 mg q4hr prn
• **Child 6-17 yr: PO** 3 mg/kg/day in divided doses q4hr prn

Side effects: *italics* = common; red = life-threatening

Renal disease
- **Adult:** PO CCr 10-50 mL/min, 75% of dose; CCr <10 mL/min, 50% of dose

Diarrhea (unlabeled)
- **Adult:** PO 30 mg; may repeat qid prn

Arthralgia/bone pain/back pain/dental pain/headache/migraine/myalgia (unlabeled)
- **Adult:** PO 15-60 mg q4-6hr
- **Child ≥3 yr:** PO 0.5-1 mg/kg or 15 mg/m^2 (max 60 mg/dose) q4-6hr

Available forms: Tabs 15, 30 mg; inj 15, 30, 60 mg/mL; oral sol 10 mg/5 mL ✦, 25 mg/5 mL ✦

Administer:
- Discontinue gradually after long-term use, use stool softener, laxative for constipation
- Store in light-resistant container at room temperature

SIDE EFFECTS

CNS: *Drowsiness, sedation,* dizziness, dependency, headache, confusion
CV: Bradycardia, palpitations, orthostatic hypotension
GI: *Nausea, vomiting, anorexia, constipation,* dry mouth
GU: Urinary retention
INTEG: Flushing, rash, sweating
RESP: Respiratory depression

PHARMACOKINETICS

Bioavailability 60%-90%; peak ½-1 hr; duration 4-6 hr; metabolized by liver (CYP3A4 to morphine); excreted by kidneys, in breast milk; crosses placenta; half-life 3 hr; protein binding 7%; ⟡ altered codeine metabolism occurs in different ethnic groups
PO: Onset 30-60 min

INTERACTIONS

Increase: CNS depression—alcohol, antihistamines, antidepressants, opiates, sedative/hypnotics, antipsychotics, skeletal muscle relaxants; monitor response
Increase: toxicity—MAOIs; use cautiously

Drug/Herb
Increase: CNS depression—chamomile, kava, valerian

Drug/Lab Test
Increase: lipase, amylase
Decrease: opioid effect—opioid antagonists

NURSING CONSIDERATIONS
Assess:
- **Pain:** intensity, type, location, aggravating, alleviating factors; need for pain medication, tolerance; use pain scoring
- I&O ratio; check for decreasing output; may indicate urinary retention, especially among geriatric patients
- GI function: nausea, vomiting, constipation
- **Cough:** type, duration, ability to raise secretion for productive cough; do not use to suppress productive cough
- CNS changes, dizziness, drowsiness, hallucinations, euphoria, LOC, pupil reaction
- Allergic reactions: rash, urticaria
- B/P, pulse respirations baseline and periodically

> **Black Box Warning:** Children (tonsillectomy/adenoidectomy and are ultrarapid metabolizers): deaths have occurred; use is contraindicated

- **Respiratory dysfunction:** respiratory depression, character, rate, rhythm; notify prescriber if respirations are <10/min, shallow; obstructive sleep apnea (children) (tonsillectomy/adenoidectomy)
- **Beers:** avoid in older adults unless safer alternative is unavailable; may cause ataxia, impaired psychomotor function

Evaluate:
- Therapeutic response: decrease in pain, absence of grimacing, decreased cough, decreased diarrhea

Teach patient/family:
- To report any symptoms of CNS changes, allergic reactions
- That physical dependency may result after extended periods, product should be used short term
- To change position slowly; orthostatic hypotension may occur

- To avoid hazardous activities if drowsiness or dizziness occurs
- To avoid alcohol, other CNS depressants unless directed by prescriber
- To increase fiber, water in diet to help avoid constipation
- **Pregnancy/breastfeeding:** to notify prescriber if pregnancy is planned or suspected; infants born to those using opioids are at risk of neonatal opiate withdrawal; not to breastfeed

TREATMENT OF OVERDOSE: Naloxone 0.4-mg ampule diluted in 10 mL 0.9% NaCl and given by direct IV push, 0.02 mg q2min (adult)

colchicine (Rx)
(kol′chih-seen)
Colcigel, Colcrys, Mitagere
Func. class.: Antigout agent
Chem. class.: Alkaloid

Do not confuse:
colchicine/Cortrosyn

ACTION: Inhibits microtubule formation of lactic acid in leukocytes, which decreases phagocytosis and inflammation in joints

USES: Gout, gouty arthritis (prevention, treatment); to arrest the progression of neurologic disability in those with MS, Mediterranean fever

CONTRAINDICATIONS: Serious GI, severe cardiac/renal/hepatic disorders, hypersensitivity
Precautions: Pregnancy (PO), breastfeeding, children, geriatric patients, blood dyscrasias, hepatic disease

DOSAGE AND ROUTES
Gout prevention
- **Adult: PO** 0.6-1.2 mg/day in 1-2 divided doses, depending on severity
Gout treatment
- **Adult: PO** 1.2 mg initially, then 0.6 mg 1 hr later (1.8 mg); *for those on strong CYP3A4 inhibitor* (during past 14 days), 0.6 mg initially, then 0.3 mg 1 hr later

Mediterranean fever
- **Adult on no interacting products: PO** 1.2-2.4 mg/day in 1-2 divided doses; **strong CYP3A4 inhibitors; P-glycoprotein inhibitors within 14 days:** max 0.6 mg/day in 1-2 divided doses; **moderate CYP3A4 inhibitors within 14 days:** max 1.2 mg/day in 1-2 divided doses
- **Adolescent: PO** 1.2-2.4 mg/day in 1-2 divided doses, titrate by 0.3 mg/day
- **Child >6-12 yr: PO** 0.9-1.8 mg/day in 1-2 divided doses
- **Child 4-6 yr: PO** 0.3-1.8 mg/day in 1-2 divided doses
Renal dose
- **Adult: PO** CCr <30 mL/min, for acute gout, do not repeat course for 2 wk; for familial Mediterranean fever, 0.3 mg daily, increase cautiously
Available forms: Tabs 0.6 mg; caps 0.6 mg; topical gel 4×
Administer:
PO route
- Without regard to food
- Cumulative doses ≤4 mg, renal patients ≤2 mg

SIDE EFFECTS
GI: *Nausea, vomiting, anorexia,* cramps
HEMA: Agranulocytosis, thrombocytopenia, aplastic anemia, pancytopenia
MISC: Alopecia, peripheral neuritis

PHARMACOKINETICS
PO: Peak ½-2 hr, half-life 30 hr, deacetylates in liver, excreted in feces (metabolites/active product)

INTERACTIONS
Increase: colchicine level/toxicity—moderate/strong CYP3A4 inhibitors (atazanavir, clarithromycin, indinavir, itraconazole, ketoconazole, ritonavir, nefazodone, nelfinavir, saquinavir, telithromycin), P-glycoprotein inhibitors; reduce dose
Increase: GI effects—NSAIDs, ethanol
Increase: bone marrow depression—radiation, bone marrow depressants, cycloSPORINE
Increase: rhabdomyolysis HMG-CoA reductase inhibitors—digoxin

Side effects: *italics* = common; red = life-threatening

Decrease: action of vit B_{12}; may cause reversible malabsorption

Drug/Food

Increase: colchicine level—grapefruit juice

Drug/Lab Test

Increase: alk phos, AST

Decrease: platelets, WBC, granulocytes

False positive: urine Hgb

Interference: urinary 17-hydroxycorticosteroids

NURSING CONSIDERATIONS
Assess:

• **Gout:** relief of pain, uric acid levels decreasing; monitor response to treatment q1hr

• **Familial Mediterranean fever:** chest pain, fever, joint pain, red lesions baseline and during treatment

• I&O ratio; observe for decrease in urinary output

• CBC, platelets, reticulocytes before, during therapy (q3mo); may cause aplastic anemia, agranulocytosis, decreased platelets in those on long-term therapy

• **Toxicity:** weakness, abdominal pain, nausea, vomiting, diarrhea; product should be discontinued, report symptoms immediately

• **Beers:** reduce dose in older adults; monitor for adverse reactions

• **Pregnancy/breastfeeding:** no well-controlled studies; use in pregnancy only if benefits outweigh fetal risk; neonatal codeine withdrawal may occur; don't use in labor (premature infant); excreted in breast milk, avoid breastfeeding

Evaluate:

• Therapeutic response: decreased stone formation, decreased pain in kidney region, absence of hematuria, decreased pain in joints, reduced familial Mediterranean fever episodes

Teach patient/family:

• To avoid alcohol, OTC preparations that contain alcohol

• To report any pain, redness, hard areas, usually in legs; rash, sore throat, fever, bleeding, bruising, weakness, numbness, tingling, nausea, vomiting, abdominal pain, muscle pain, weakness

• To avoid grapefruit and juice, may increase colchicine level

• About the importance of complying with medical regimen (diet, weight loss, product therapy); about the possibility of bone marrow depression occurring; not to double or skip doses, during acute attacks other products may be needed

• To advise all providers of product use; that surgery may increase the possibility of acute gout symptoms

TREATMENT OF OVERDOSE: D/C medication; may need opioids to treat diarrhea

---

colesevelam (Rx)
(koe-leh-seve′eh-lam)
WelChol, Lodalis ✦
Func. class.: Antilipemic
Chem. class.: Bile acid sequestrant

ACTION: Adsorbs, combines with bile acids to form insoluble complex excreted through feces; loss of bile acids lowers cholesterol levels

USES: Elevated LDL cholesterol, alone or in combination with HMG-COA reductase inhibitor; type 2 diabetes (adjunct)

CONTRAINDICATIONS: Hypersensitivity, bowel disease, primary biliary cirrhosis, triglycerides >500 mg/dL, bowel obstruction, pancreatitis, biliary obstruction, dysphagia, fat-soluble vitamin deficiency

Precautions: Pregnancy, breastfeeding, children

DOSAGE AND ROUTES
Hyperlipidemia

• **Adult: PO** three 625-mg tabs bid with meals or 6 tabs daily with meal; may increase to 7 tabs if needed (monotherapy); 3 tabs bid with meals or 6 tabs daily with meal given with an HMG-CoA reductase inhibitor (combination)

Type 2 diabetes
• **Adult and geriatric: PO** Approx 3.8 g (6 tabs)/day or approx 1.9 g (3 tabs) bid
Heterozygous familial hypercholesterolemia
• **Females (postmenarchal and >10 yr) and males ≥10 yr: PO** 1.875-g packet bid or 3.75-g packet daily dissolved in 4-8 oz of water with meal
Available forms: Tabs 625 mg; granules for oral susp 3.75 g/packet
Administer:
• Swallow tabs whole; do not break, crush, or chew
• Give product daily or bid with meals; give all other medications 4 hr before colesevelam; with liquid to avoid poor absorption
• **Granules for oral susp:** empty contents of packet into a cup/glass, add $^1/_2$-1 cup (4-8 oz) of water, fruit juice, diet soda; stir well before drinking

SIDE EFFECTS
GI: *Constipation, nausea,* flatulence

PHARMACOKINETICS
Excreted in feces, peak response 2 wk

INTERACTIONS
Decrease: absorption of—diltiaZEM, gemfibrozil, mycophenolate, phenytoin, propranolol, warfarin, thiazides, digoxin, penicillin G, tetracyclines, corticosteroids, iron, thyroid, fat-soluble vitamins, glyBURIDE, fluoroquinolones
Decrease: action of—oral contraceptives, give ≥4 hr prior to colesevelam
Drug/Lab Test
Increase: LFTs

NURSING CONSIDERATIONS
Assess:
• Cardiac glycoside level if used with an HMG-CoA
• **Hypercholesterolemia:** fasting LDL, HDL, total cholesterol, triglyceride levels baseline and q4-6wk after initiation of treatment and periodically, electrolytes if on extended therapy; monitor BUN/creatinine, take diet history
• Bowel pattern daily; increase bulk, water in diet for constipation

• **Diabetes:** hypoglycemia (weakness, hunger, dizziness, diaphoresis) can result from use of this product, monitor blood glucose, A1C
Evaluate:
• Therapeutic response: decreased total cholesterol level, LDL cholesterol, apolipoproteins
Teach patient/family:
• About the importance of compliance; timing of dose 4 hr after other meds
• **Hypercholesterolemia:** That risk factors should be decreased: high-fat diet, smoking, alcohol consumption, absence of exercise
• To take with meal and fluids
• To discuss with health care professional all OTC, herbals, supplements, to use oral contraceptive at least 4 hr before this product
• Diabetes: to monitor glucose
• **Pregnancy/breastfeeding:** to notify prescriber if pregnancy is planned or suspected or if breastfeeding; that insulin may be used in diabetes during pregnancy; to use another form of contraception other than oral contraceptives

---

conivaptan (Rx)
(kon-ih-vap′tan)
Vaprisol
Func. class.: Vasopressin receptor antagonist

ACTION: Dual arginine vasopressin (AVP) antagonist with affinity for V_{1A}, V_2 receptors; level of AVP in circulating blood is critical for regulation of water, electrolyte balance and is usually elevated in euvolemic/hypervolemic hyponatremia

USES: Euvolemia hyponatremia in hospitalized patients; not indicated for HF, hypervolemic hyponatremia
Unlabeled uses: Increased intracranial pressure

CONTRAINDICATIONS: Hypersensitivity, hypovolemia

Side effects: *italics* = common; red = life-threatening

Precautions: Pregnancy, breastfeeding, orthostatic disease, renal disease, heart failure, rapid correction of serum sodium

DOSAGE AND ROUTES
• **Adult: IV INFUSION** loading dose 20 mg given over 30 min then **CONT IV** over 24 hr; after 1 day, give for an additional 1-3 days as a **CONT INFUSION** of 20 mg/day total; can be titrated up to 40 mg/day if serum sodium is not rising at desired rate; max time 4 days
Hepatic/renal dose
• **Adult: IV** Child-Pugh A-C or CCr 30-60 mL/min: give IV loading dose over 10 min then **CONT IV INFUSION** 10 mg over 24 hr × 2-4 days

Available forms: Injection (premixed) 0.2 mg/mL in 100 mL D$_5$W
Administer:
Intermittent IV Infusion
• Premixed, do not need dilution (0.2 mg/mL)
Continuous IV INFUSION route
• Give over 24 hr; or give 40 mg 24 hr

SIDE EFFECTS
CNS: Headache, confusion, insomnia
CV: Hypo/hypertension, *orthostatic hypotension*
GI: Nausea, vomiting, constipation, dry mouth
GU: Hematuria, infertility (women), polyuria
INTEG: Erythema, inj site reaction
META: Dehydration, hypokalemia, hypomagnesemia, hyponatremia
MISC: Oral candidiasis

PHARMACOKINETICS
Protein binding 99%, metabolized by CYP3A4, half-life 5 hr

INTERACTIONS
Increase: effect of—CYP3A4 substrates (alfuzosin, ARIPiprazole, bexarotene, bortezomib, bosentan, bupivacaine, buprenorphine, carBAMazepine, cevimeline, cilostazol, cinacalcet, clopidogrel, colchicine, cyclobenzaprine, dapsone, darifenacin, disopyramide, DOCEtaxel, donepezil, DOXOrubicin, dutasteride, eletriptan, eplerenone, ergots, erlotinib, eszopiclone, ethinyl estradiol, ethosuximide, etoposide, fentaNYL, galantamine, gefitinib, ifosfamide, irinotecan, lidocaine, loperamide, loratadine, mefloquine, methadone, modafinil, PACLitaxel, paricalcitrol, pimozide, praziquantel, quiNIDine, quiNINE, ramelteon, repaglinide, rifabutin, sibutramine, sildenafil, sirolimus, SUFentanil, SUNItinib, tacrolimus, tamoxifen, teniposide, testosterone, tiaGABine, tinidazole, trimetrexate, vardenafil, vinca alkaloids, ziprasidone, zolpidem, zonisamide); do not use concurrently

NURSING CONSIDERATIONS
Assess:
• Renal, hepatic function
• **Sodium levels/volume status:** monitor serum sodium levels q2-3hr until stable; overly rapid correction of sodium concentration (>12 mEq/L per 24 hr) may result in osmotic demyelination syndrome
• Neurologic status: confusion, headache
• **Injection site reactions:** redness, inflammation, pain, if these occur product needs to be discontinued
• CV status: atrial fibrillation, hypo/hypertension, orthostatic hypotension; monitor B/P, pulse baseline and periodically
• Monitor other electrolytes (magnesium and potassium)
• **Pregnancy/breastfeeding:** no well-controlled studies; use in pregnancy only if benefits outweigh fetal risk, may cause fetal harm; discontinue breastfeeding or discontinue product; excretion is unknown
Evaluate:
• Therapeutic response: correction of serum sodium levels
Teach patient/family:
• To report neurologic changes: headache, insomnia, confusion
• About administration procedure and expected results
• To report inj site pain, redness, swelling

CONTRACEPTIVES, HORMONAL

Monophasic, Oral

ethinyl estradiol/ desogestrel (Rx)

Apri-28, Desogen, EnsKyce, Isibloom, Kalliga, Reclipsen, Solia, Emoquette

ethinyl estradiol/ drospirenone (Rx)

Beyaz, Gianvi, Loryna, Nikki, Safyral, Syeda, Vestura, Yaela, Zarah, Yasmin, Yaz, Ocella

ethinyl estradiol/ ethynodiol (Rx)

Kelnor, Zovia 1/35, Zovia 1/50

ethinyl estradiol/ levonorgestrel (Rx)

Aviane-28, Altavera, Aubra, Chateal, Falmina, Kurvelo, Marlissa, Vienva, Lessina, Levora, Lutera, Sronyx

ethinyl estradiol/ norethindrone (Rx)

Alyacen 1/35, Brevicon, Briellyn, Cyclafem 1/35, Dasetta, Generess Fe, Larin 1/20, Larin Fe 1.5/30, Junel 1/20, Junel 1.5/30, Loestrin 1.5/30, Loestrin 1/20, Necon 0.5/35, Norinyl 1+35, Nortrel 1/35, Nortrel 7/7/7

ethinyl estradiol/ norgestimate (Rx)

Estarylla, Mono-Linyah, MonoNessa, Ortho-Cyclen, Previfem, Sprintec

ethinyl estradiol/ norgestrel (Rx)

Cryselle, Elinest, Lo/Ovral, Low-Ogestrel, Ogestrel

mestranol/ norethindrone (Rx)

Necon 1/50, Norinyl 1+50

Biphasic, Oral

ethinyl estradiol/ norethindrone (Rx)

Ortho-Novum 10/11

Triphasic, Oral

ethinyl estradiol/ desogestrel (Rx)

Azurette, Bekyree, Cyclessa, Kariva, Kimidess, Pimtrea, Viorele

ethinyl estradiol/ norethindrone (Rx)

Nortrel 7/7/7, Ortho-Novum 7/7/7, Tri-Norinyl

ethinyl estradiol/ norgestimate (Rx)

Ortho Tri-Cyclen, Ortho Tri-Cyclen Lo, Tri-Estarylla, Tri-Linyah

ethinyl estradiol/ levonorgestrel (Rx)

Enpresse, Levonest, Myzilra, Tri-Levlen, Triphasil

Four phasic oral estradiol, Valeriate/dienogest, Natazia

Four phasic oral

Estradiol/valerate/ dienogest Natazia

Extended Cycle, Oral

ethinyl estradiol/ levonorgestrel (Rx)

Seasonale

Progestin, Oral

norethindrone (Rx)

Errin, Jencycla, Nor-QD, Nora-BE, Ortho-Micronar, Camila, Jolivette

---

Side effects: *italics* = common; red = life-threatening

Progressive Estrogen, Oral

ethinyl estradiol/ norethindrone acetate (Rx)

Estrostep, Estrostep Fe

Emergency

levonorgestrel (Rx)

Fallback Solo, Plan BUlipristal, Ella, Logilia

medroxyPROGESTER-one (Rx)

Depo-SubQ, Depo-Provera, Provera 104

Intrauterine

levonorgestrel (Rx)

Mirena, Skyla

Implant

etonogestrel (Rx)

Implanon, Nexplanon

Vaginal Ring

ethinyl estradiol/ etonogestrel (Rx)

NuvaRing

Transdermal

ethinyl estradiol/ norelgestromin (Rx)

Xulane

ACTION: Prevents ovulation by suppressing FSH and LH; *monophasic:* estrogen/progestin (fixed dose) used during a 21-day cycle; ovulation is inhibited by suppression of FSH and LH; thickness of cervical mucus and endometrial lining prevents pregnancy; *biphasic:* ovulation is inhibited by suppression of FSH and LH; alteration of cervical mucus, endometrial lining prevents pregnancy; *triphasic:* ovulation is inhibited by suppression of FSH and LH; change of cervical mucus, endometrial lining prevents pregnancy; variable doses of estrogen/ progestin combinations may be similar to natural hormonal fluctuations; *extended cycle:* estrogen/progestin continuous for 84 days, off for 7 days, results in 4 menstrual periods/yr; *progressive estrogen:* constant progestin with 3 progressive doses of estrogen; *progestin-only pill, implant, intrauterine:* change of cervical mucus and endometrial lining prevents pregnancy; ovulation may be suppressed

USES: To prevent pregnancy, regulation of menstrual cycle, treatment of acne in women >14 yr for whom other treatment has failed, emergency contraception; *injection:* inhibits gonadotropin secretion, ovulation, follicular maturation; *emergency:* inhibits ovulation and fertilization, decreases transport of sperm and egg from fallopian tube to uterus; *vaginal ring, transdermal:* inhibits ovulation, prevents sperm entry into uterus; *antiacne:* may decrease sex hormone binding globulin, results in decreased testosterone

CONTRAINDICATIONS: Pregnancy, breastfeeding, women ≥40 yr, reproductive cancer, thrombophlebitis, MI, hepatic tumors, hepatic disease, CAD, CVA, breast cancer, jaundice, stroke, vaginal bleeding

Precautions: Depression, hypertension, renal disease, seizure disorders, lupus erythematosus, rheumatic disease, migraine headache, amenorrhea, irregular menses, gallbladder disease, diabetes mellitus, heavy smoking, acute mononucleosis, sickle cell disease

Black Box Warning: Tobacco smoking

DOSAGE AND ROUTES
Monophasic

• **Adult: PO** Take first tab on Sunday after start of menses × 21 days; skip 7 days, then repeat cycle; may contain 7 placebo tabs when 1 tab is taken daily

Biphasic
• **Adult: PO** Take 10 days of small progestin, then large progestin; estrogen is the same during cycle; skip 7 days, then repeat cycle; may contain 7 placebo tabs when 1 tab is taken daily

Triphasic
• **Adult: PO** Estrogen dose remains constant; progestin changes throughout 21-day cycle; some products contain 28 tabs per month

Extended cycle
• **Adult: PO** Start taking on 1st day of menses; continue for 84 days of active tab, then 7 days of placebo; repeat cycle

Progestin
• **Adult: PO** Start on 1st day of menses, then daily and continuously

Progressive estrogen
• **Adult: PO** Progestin dose remains constant; estrogen increases q7days throughout 21-day cycle; may include 7 placebo tabs for 28-day cycle

Emergency
• **Adult/adolescent: PO** Give within 72 hr of intercourse, repeat 12 hr later; **Plan B** 1 tab, then 1 tab 12 hr later; **Preven** 2 tab, then 2 tab 12 hr later; **Ovral** 2 white tabs; **Lo/Ovral (unlabeled)** 4 white tabs; **Levlen, Nordette** 4 orange tabs; **Triphasil, Tri-Levlen** 4 yellow tabs

Injectable
• **Adult: IM (Depo-Provera)** 150 mg within 5 days of start of menses or within 5 days postpartum (must not be breastfeeding); if breastfeeding, give 6 wk postpartum, repeat q3mo

Intrauterine
• **Adult: INTRAUTERINE** To be inserted using the levonorgestrel-releasing intrauterine system (LRIS) by those trained in procedure; inserted into uterine cavity within 7 days of the onset of menstruation; use should not exceed 5 yr per implant

Vaginal ring
• **Adult: VAG** Insert 1 ring on or before day 5 of cycle; leave in place 3 wk; remove for 1 wk, then repeat

Transdermal
• **Adult: TD** Apply patch within 7 days of menses; change weekly × 3 wk; no patch wk 4; repeat cycle

Implant
• **Adult: SUBDERMAL** In inner side of upper arm on days 1-5 of menses, replace q3yr

Acne
• **Adult: PO (Ortho Tri-Cyclen)** Take daily × 21 days, off 7 days

Administer:
• PO with food for GI symptoms; give at same time each day
• Subdermal implant of 6 caps effective for 5 yr, then should be removed
• IM inj deep in large muscle mass after shaking suspension; ensure patient not pregnant if inj are 2 wk or more apart

SIDE EFFECTS

CNS: Depression, fatigue, dizziness, nervousness, anxiety, headache
CV: Increased BP, cerebral hemorrhage, thrombosis, pulmonary embolism, fluid retention, edema, MI
EENT: Optic neuritis, retinal thrombosis, cataracts
ENDO: Decreased glucose tolerance, increased TBG, PBI, T_4, T_3, temporary infertility
GI: *Nausea*, vomiting, cramps, diarrhea, bloating, constipation, change in appetite, cholestatic jaundice, weight change
GU: Breakthrough bleeding, amenorrhea, spotting, dysmenorrhea, galactorrhea, endocervical hyperplasia, vaginitis, cystitis-like syndrome, breast changes
HEMA: Increased fibrinogen, clotting factor
INTEG: *Chloasma, melasma,* acne, rash, urticaria, erythema, pruritus, hirsutism, alopecia, photosensitivity

PHARMACOKINETICS
Excreted in breast milk

INTERACTIONS
Decrease: oral contraceptives' effectiveness—anticonvulsants, rifAMPin, analgesics, antibiotics, antihistamines, griseofulvin

Decrease: oral anticoagulants' action
Drug/Herb
• Altered action: black cohosh
Decrease: oral contraceptives' effect—
saw palmetto, St. John's wort
Drug/Food
Increase: peak level—grapefruit juice
Drug/Lab Test
Increase: PT; clotting factors VII, VIII, IX, X; TBG, PBI, T_4, platelet aggregability, BSP, triglycerides, bilirubin, AST, ALT
Decrease: T_3, antithrombin III, folate, metyrapone test, GTT, 17-OHCS

NURSING CONSIDERATIONS
Assess:
• Glucose, thyroid function, LFTs, BP
• Reproductive changes: changes in breasts, tumors; positive Pap smear; product should be discontinued
Evaluate:
• Therapeutic response: absence of pregnancy, endometriosis, hypermenorrhea
Teach patient/family:
• To use sunscreen or avoid sunlight; photosensitivity can occur
• To take at same time each day to ensure equal product level
• To report GI symptoms that occur after 4 mo
• **Pregnancy/breastfeeding:** to use another birth control method during 1st 3 weeks of oral contraceptive use; to avoid use in breastfeeding; many antibiotics interfere with oral contraceptives
• To take another tablet as soon as possible if one is missed
• That, after product is discontinued, pregnancy may not occur for several months
• To report abdominal pain, change in vision, shortness of breath, change in menstrual flow, spotting, breakthrough bleeding, breast lumps, swelling, headache, severe leg pain
• That continuing medical care is needed: Pap smear and gynecologic examinations q6mo
• To notify health care providers and dentists of oral contraceptive use; many antibiotics interfere with oral contraceptive effect

Black Box Warning: Do not smoke; increased risk of CV side effects

---

⚠ HIGH ALERT

copanlisib
(koh-pan´-lih-sib)
Aliqopa
Func. class.: Antineoplastic biologic response modifiers
Chem. class.: Tyrosine kinase inhibitor

ACTION: Inhibits tyrosine kinase created in patients with non-Hodgkin's lymphoma; induces tumor cell death by apoptosis and by inhibiting the proliferation of primary malignant B-cell lines.

USES: For the treatment of non-Hodgkin's lymphoma

CONTRAINDICATIONS: Pregnancy, hypersensitivity
Precautions: Breastfeeding, contraception requirements, children, diabetes mellitus, diarrhea, geriatric patients, hepatic/pulmonary disease, hyperglycemia, hypertension, infertility, male-mediated teratogenicity, neutropenia, pneumonitis, bone marrow suppression, infection, reproductive risk, serious rash, thrombocytopenia

DOSAGE AND ROUTES
Relapsed follicular lymphoma
• **Adult:** IV 60 mg over 1 hr on days 1, 8, and 15 repeated q28days until disease progression
Dosage adjustment for related toxicities
Infection:
• **Grade ≥3 toxicity:** hold until infection resolves
• **Suspected** *Pneumocystis jirovecii* **pneumonia (PJP) infection (any grade):** hold; if PJP diagnosis is confirmed, treat infection until resolution and

then resume product at previous dose. PJP prophylaxis is recommended for the duration of therapy

Hyperglycemia:

• **Predose fasting blood glucose of ≥160 mg/dL or a random/nonfasting blood glucose of ≥200 mg/dL:** hold until fasting glucose is ≤160 mg/dL or a random/nonfasting blood glucose is ≤200 mg/dL

• **Pre- or postdose blood glucose of ≥500 mg/dL (first occurrence):** hold until fasting glucose is ≤160 mg/dL or a random/nonfasting blood glucose is ≤200 mg/dL; resume product at 45 mg

• **Pre- or postdose blood glucose of ≥500 mg/dL (subsequent occurrences):** hold product until fasting glucose is ≤160 mg/dL or a random/nonfasting blood glucose is ≤200 mg/dL; resume at 30 mg. Discontinue if hyperglycemia persists at the 30-mg dose

Hypertension:

• **Predose systolic B/P of ≥150 mm Hg or predose diastolic B/P of ≥90 mm Hg:** hold until B/P is <150/90 mm Hg based on 2 consecutive measurements (taken at least 15 min apart)

• **Postdose B/P of ≥150/90 mm Hg (non–life-threatening):** continue product at the previous dose if antihypertensive treatment is not required. Consider a dose reduction (from 60 mg to 45 mg or from 45 mg to 30 mg) if antihypertensive treatment is required. Discontinue if hypertension persists despite antihypertensive treatment

• **Postdose B/P (life-threatening):** discontinue

Noninfectious pneumonitis:

• **Grade 2 toxicity:** hold and treat with systemic corticosteroids. Resume at 45 mg when toxicity recovers to grade ≤1. Discontinue if grade 2 toxicity recurs

• **Grade ≥3 toxicity:** discontinue

Neutropenia:

• **Absolute neutrophil count (ANC) 0.5-1 × 10^3 cells/mm³:** continue at previous dose and monitor ANC at least weekly

• **ANC <0.5 × 10^3 cells/mm³:** hold, monitor ANC at least weekly until ANC is

≥0.5 × 10^3 cells/mm³; resume at previous dose. Reduce to 45 mg if an ANC of <0.5 × 10^3 cells/mm³ recurs

Thrombocytopenia:

• **Platelet count <25 × 10^9 cells/L:** hold, resume at a reduced dose (from 60 mg to 45 mg or from 45 mg to 30 mg) if platelet count recovers to ≥75 × 10^9 cells/L within 21 days. Discontinue if platelet count does not recover to 75 × 10^9 cells/L within 21 days

Severe cutaneous reactions:

• **Grade 3 toxicity:** hold until toxicity resolves. Resume at a reduced dose (from 60 mg to 45 mg or from 45 mg to 30 mg)

• **Life-threatening (grade 4) toxicity:** discontinue

Other severe and non–life-threatening toxicities:

• **Grade 3 toxicity:** hold until toxicity resolves. Resume at reduced dose (from 60 mg to 45 mg or from 45 mg to 30 mg)

• **Grade 4 or life-threatening toxicity:** discontinue

Available forms: Powder for injection 60 mg

Administer:

IV route

• Visually inspect for particulate matter and discoloration before use

Reconstitution

• Add 4.4 mL of sterile 0.9% NaCl injection to the 60-mg lyophilized powder vial (15 mg/mL)

• Gently shake and then allow to stand for 1 min, letting bubbles rise to the surface; repeat if needed; solution will be colorless to slightly yellowish

• **Storage of reconstituted vial:** if not diluted immediately, store refrigerated at 2-8° C (36-46° F) for up to 24 hr before use; protect from direct sunlight

Dilution

• Into an infusion bag containing 100 mL of sterile 0.9% sodium chloride injection, add the appropriate volume (based on the desired dose) from the reconstituted vial as follows: **60-mg dose:** 4 mL; **45-mg dose:** 3 mL; **30-mg dose:** 2 mL

• Invert the infusion bag to mix

• Discard any unused contents from the reconstituted vial

• **Storage of diluted admixture:** if not used immediately, store refrigerated at 2-8° C (36-46° F) for up to 24 hr (from vial reconstitution) before use; protect from direct sunlight

Intermittent IV INFUSION route

• Allow the diluted admixture in the infusion bag to warm to room temperature (if stored in refrigerator) before use

• Give over 1 hr

• Do not mix or inject product with other drugs or diluents

• Follow cytotoxic handling procedures

SIDE EFFECTS

CNS: Fatigue
GI: Nausea, vomiting, diarrhea, stomatitis
HEMA: *Anemia*, neutropenia, thrombocytopenia, bleeding, lymphopenia
INTEG:
• Rash, exfoliative dermatitis
MISC:
• Hypertriglyceridemia, hyperuricemia

PHARMACOKINETICS

Protein binding 84.2%; avoid use with strong CYP3A inhibitors or inducers; this product is a substrate of the P-glycoprotein (P-gp) and breast cancer resistance protein (BCRP) transporters and a multidrug and toxin extrusion member 2 (MATE2)-K inhibitor

INTERACTIONS

Increase: copanlisib concentrations—CYP3A4 inhibitors (ketoconazole, itraconazole, erythromycin, clarithromycin), P-gb inhibitors
Increase: plasma concentrations of simvastatin, calcium channel blockers, ergots
Decrease: copanlisib concentrations—CYP3A4 inducers (dexamethasone, phenytoin, carBAMazepine, rifAMPin, PHENobarbital), antacids, proton pump inhibitors

Drug/Food
Increase: copanlisib effect—grapefruit juice; avoid use while taking product
Drug/Herb
Decrease: copanlisib concentration—St. John's wort

Drug/Lab Test
Increase: uric acid, blood glucose, triglycerides
Decrease: phosphate

NURSING CONSIDERATIONS

Assess:

• **Serious infection:** some may be fatal. Monitor patients for signs and symptoms of infection; hold therapy for grade ≥3 infection. Serious *Pneumocystis jirovecii* pneumonia (PJP) has occurred; consider PJP prophylaxis in at-risk patients before starting treatment, hold if PJP is suspected. If PJP diagnosis is confirmed, treat infection until resolution; then resume at previous dose and give PJP prophylaxis for the duration of therapy

• **Myelosuppression:** anemia, thrombocytopenia, neutropenia; obtain a CBC at least weekly during treatment

• **Pregnancy/breastfeeding:** product can cause fetal harm; females of reproductive potential should avoid becoming pregnant while taking this product; malformations may occur; do not breastfeed during and for at least 1 mo after last dose; men with female partners of reproductive potential should avoid fathering a child and use effective contraception during and for at least 1 mo after therapy

• **Severe hyperglycemia:** elevated HbA1c and infusion-related hyperglycemia have occurred; monitor blood glucose levels before and after infusion; product interruption, dose reduction, or discontinuation may be needed. Blood glucose levels typically peak at 5-8 hr postinfusion and then decline to baseline levels in most patients. Use with caution in patients with diabetes mellitus. Initiate product after these patients have achieved optimal blood glucose control; monitor blood glucose levels closely in these patients

• **Severe hypertension and infusion-related hypertension:** use with caution in those with preexisting hypertension; monitor B/P before and after infusion; optimal B/P control should be achieved before each dose. Therapy interruption, dose reduction, or therapy discontinuation may be necessary in patients who develop hypertension. A mean increase in systolic (+16.8 mm Hg) and diastolic (+7.8 mm Hg) B/P was observed at 2 hr postinfusion on day 1 of cycle 1; B/P may remain elevated for 6-8 hr after start of infusion

Evaluate: Therapeutic response: improving blood counts

Teach patient/family

• To report adverse reactions immediately, bleeding; to report diarrhea, hepatic, hematologic symptoms/toxicity, flulike symptoms, rash

• About reason for treatment, expected results

• **Pregnancy/breastfeeding:** to notify provider if pregnancy is planned or suspected; to use effective contraception during treatment and up to 30 days after discontinuing treatment; not to use during pregnancy, breastfeeding; that men with female partners of reproductive potential should be cautioned to avoid fathering a child and to use effective contraception during and for at least 1 mo after therapy

---

crisaborole

(kris′a-bor-ole)

Eucrisa

Func. class.: Dermatologic agent
Chem. class.: Phosphodiesterase 4 enzyme inhibitor

ACTION: Increases intracellular cyclic adenosine monophosphate (cAMP) levels in the skin

USES: Mild to moderate atopic dermatitis

CONTRAINDICATIONS: Hypersensitivity
Precautions: Children, pregnancy, breastfeeding

DOSAGE AND ROUTES

• **Adult/child ≥2 yr: TOP** Apply ointment bid in a thin film to cover area
Available forms: Topical ointment 2%
Administer:
Topical route:
• For external use only; store at room temperature
• Tube should be tightly closed
• Apply only to affected areas

SIDE EFFECTS

INTEG: Burning, stinging, application site pain

PHARMACOKINETICS

97% protein bound, excreted renally

INTERACTIONS

• None known

NURSING CONSIDERATIONS

Assess:
• **Contact dermatitis**: for redness, itching, inflammation; assess if these symptoms are relieved after application
• **Hypersensitivity**: for pruritus, inflammation, rash; if present, product should be discontinued
• **Pregnancy/breastfeeding:** no adverse reactions in animal studies, no human studies available; consider benefits to mother and infant if breastfeeding; product is systemically absorbed
Evaluate:
• Therapeutic response: decreasing redness, itching, inflammation
Teach patient/family:
• **Contact dermatitis:** to identify whether symptoms are relieved after application; to apply a thin film and wash hands after use; to use externally only
• **Hypersensitivity:** to report immediately itching, inflammation, rash; if present, product should be discontinued
• **Pregnancy/breastfeeding:** to advise prescriber if pregnant or planning to get pregnant, or if breastfeeding; effects are unknown

> ### ⚠ HIGH ALERT

crizotinib
(kriz-oh′ti-nib)

XALKORI

Func. class.: Antineoplastic
Chem. class.: Signal transduction inhibitors (STIs)

ACTION: Inhibits 🐱 receptor tyrosine kinases (anaplastic lymphoma kinase [ALK]), hepatocyte growth factor receptor (HGFR, c-Met), recepteur d'origine nantais (RON)

USES: 🐱 Locally advanced or metastatic non–small-cell lung cancer (NSCLC) that is anaplastic lymphoma kinase (ALK)-positive as detected by an FDA-approved test

CONTRAINDICATIONS: Pregnancy, breastfeeding, hypersensitivity, concurrent use of strong CYP3A4 inducers/inhibitors
Precautions: Neonates, infants, children, adolescents, pneumonitis, severe hepatic disease, congenital long QT syndrome, severe renal impairment, endstage renal disease, vision disorders

DOSAGE AND ROUTES
• **Adult:** PO 250 mg bid; continue as long as beneficial
Available forms: Cap 200, 250 mg
Administer:
• May be taken orally with or without food
• Have the patient swallow capsule whole; do not crush or chew
• If a dose is missed, it can be taken up to 6 hr before the next dose is due to maintain the twice-daily regimen; do not take both doses at the same time
• Store at room temperature

SIDE EFFECTS
CNS: Dizziness, peripheral neuropathy, headache, insomnia

CV: QT prolongation, disseminated intravascular coagulation (DIC), septic shock, bradycardia
EENT: *Diplopia, blurred vision,* reduced *visual acuity*
GI: *Nausea, diarrhea, vomiting, constipation,* decreased appetite, dysgeusia, abdominal pain, stomatitis, hepatotoxicity, epigastric discomfort/pain, esophagitis
HEMA: Grade 3/4 neutropenia, thrombocytopenia, lymphopenia
MISC: Fatigue, fever, *edema*, chest pain
RESP: Severe, life-threatening pneumonitis, dyspnea

PHARMACOKINETICS
Protein binding 91%; distribution into the tissues and plasma; metabolized by the CYP3A4/5; primary metabolic pathways are oxidation to metabolites; terminal half-life 42 hr; excreted 63% feces, 22% urine; unchanged drug 53% feces, 2.3% urine; absolute bioavailability is 43%; peak is 4-6 hr; steady state is reached within 15 days; 🐱 dosage adjustments may need to be made in hepatic/renal disease and Asian patients

INTERACTIONS
Increase: CYP2B6 substrates (prasugrel, selegiline, cyclophosphamide)
Increase: CYP3A4 inhibitors (ketoconazole, atazanavir, indinavir, itraconazole, nefazodone, nelfinavir, ritonavir, voriconazole, boceprevir, delavirdine, isoniazid, dalfopristin-quinupristin, tipranavir)
Decrease: CYP3A4 inducers (rifAMPin, carBAMazepine, PHENobarbital, phenytoin, rifabutin); antacids, H₂ blockers, proton pump inhibitors (PPIs)
Increase: action of—midazolam
• Avoid use with CYP3A4 substrates (alfentanil, cycloSPORINE, ergotamine, dihydroergotamine fentaNYL, sirolimus, colchicine)
Increase: QT prolongation, torsades de pointes—arsenic trioxide, certain phenothiazines (chlorproMAZINE, mesoridazine, thioridazine), grepafloxacin, pentamidine, probucol, sparfloxacin, troleandomycin,

class IA antiarrhythmics (disopyramide, procainamide, quiNIDine), class III antiarrhythmics (amiodarone, dofetilide, ibutilide, sotalol), clarithromycin, ziprasidone, pimozide, haloperidol, halofantrine, quiNIDine, chloroquine, dronedarone, droperidol, erythromycin, methadone, posaconazole, propafenone, saquinavir, abarelix, amoxapine, apomorphine, asenapine, β-agonists, ofloxacin, eriBULin, ezogabine, flecainide, gatifloxacin, gemifloxacin, halogenated anesthetics, iloperidone, levoFLOXacin, local anesthetics, magnesium sulfate, potassium sulfate, sodium, maprotiline, moxifloxacin, nilotinib, norfloxacin, ciprofloxacin, OLANZapine, paliperidone, some phenothiazines (fluPHENAZine, perphenazine, prochlorperazine, trifluoperazine), telavancin, tetrabenazine, tricyclic antidepressants, venlafaxine, vorinostat, citalopram, alfuzosin, cloZAPine, cyclobenzaprine, dolasetron, palonosetron, QUEtiapine, rilpivirine, SUNItinib, tacrolimus, vardenafil, indacaterol, dasatinib, fluconazole, lapatinib, lopinavir/ritonavir, mefloquine, octreotide, ondansetron, ranolazine, risperiDONE, telithromycin, vemurafenib

Drug/Herb

Do not use with St. John's wort

Drug/Food

Do not use with grapefruit juice or grapefruit

NURSING CONSIDERATIONS
Assess:

• **Severe, life-threatening, or fatal treatment-related pneumonitis:** all cases occurred within 2 mo of treatment initiation; monitor for pulmonary symptoms that may indicate pneumonitis, other causes of pneumonitis should be excluded; permanently discontinue in patients with treatment-related pneumonitis

• **Hepatic disease:** liver function test (LFT) abnormalities, altered bilirubin levels may occur during treatment; monitor LFTs and bilirubin levels before treatment, then monthly; more frequent testing is needed in those presenting with grade 2 or greater toxicities; laboratory alterations should be managed with dose reduction, treatment interruption, or discontinuation

• **QT prolongation;** monitor ECG and electrolytes in patients with congestive heart failure, bradycardia, electrolyte imbalance (hypokalemia, hypomagnesemia), or in patients taking concomitant medications known to prolong the QT interval; treatment interruption, dosage adjustment, treatment discontinuation may be needed in patients who develop QT prolongation

• **For grade 1-2 QTc prolongation:** no dosage adjustment necessary; for grade 3 QTc prolongation: interrupt treatment until toxicity resolves to grade ≤1; when resuming treatment, reduce dosage to 200 mg PO bid; in case of recurrence, interrupt treatment until toxicity resolves to grade ≤1 and when resuming treatment, reduce dosage to 250 mg PO daily; permanently discontinue in case of further recurrence; for grade 4 QTc prolongation: permanently discontinue

• **Vision disorders,** generally start within 2 wk of the start of therapy; ophthalmological evaluation should be considered, particularly if patients experience photopsia or new or increased vitreous floaters; caution should be used when driving or operating machinery by patients who experience vision disorders

• **Pregnancy/breastfeeding:** identify if pregnancy is planned or suspected; do not breastfeed

• CBC with differential; BUN/creatinine

• **Hematologic toxicities: Grade 3:** Interrupt treatment until toxicity resolves to grade ≤2, then continue with the same dosage schedule; in case of recurrence after a grade 4 event with dose reduction, interrupt treatment until toxicity resolves to grade ≤2; when resuming treatment, reduce dosage to 250 mg PO daily; grade 4: interrupt treatment until toxicity resolves to grade ≤2; when resuming treatment, reduce dosage to 200 mg PO bid; in case of grade 4 recurrence, permanently discontinue treatment

Evaluate:

• Decreasing spread of malignancy

Teach patient/family:

• That missed doses can be taken up to 6 hr before the next dose is due to maintain the twice-daily regimen; do not double or skip doses

• To use reliable contraception; both women and men of childbearing age should use adequate contraceptive methods during therapy and for at least 90 days after completing treatment
• To report immediately shortness of breath, cough, fatigue, visual changes
• Not to take with grapefruit juice or grapefruit
• To avoid activities requiring mental alertness until effects are known
• To report signs of QT prolongation (abnormal heartbeats, dizziness, syncope)
• To swallow caps whole and avoid contact with broken cap
• To report immediately nausea, vomiting, abdominal pain, yellowing of skin, eyes, dark urine, itching

---

crofelemer
(kroe-fel′e-mer)
Mytesi
Func. class.: Antidiarrheal
Chem. class.: Red sap of *Croton lechleri* plant

ACTION: Blocks chloride channel and high-volume water loss in diarrhea

USES: Noninfectious diarrhea in those with HIV/AIDS using antiretrovirals

CONTRAINDICATIONS: Hypersensitivity
Precautions: Pregnancy, ✖️ breastfeeding, black patients, children/adolescents, GI disease, infection, malabsorption syndrome, pancreatitis

DOSAGE AND ROUTES
• **Adult: PO** 125 mg bid
Available forms: Delayed rel tabs 125 mg
Administer:
• Do not break, crush, or chew
• Without regard to meals

SIDE EFFECTS
CNS: Dizziness, depression
GI: Nausea, constipation, abdominal pain, anorexia, flatulence

INTEG: Acne vulgaris, contact dermatitis
MISC: Arthralgia, cough, increased urinary frequency

INTERACTIONS
Increase: serious constipation, bowel obstruction—alosetron (IBS)
Increase: constipation—may occur with antimuscarinics, opiate agonists

NURSING CONSIDERATIONS
Assess:
• Stools: volume, color, characteristic, frequency; bowel pattern before protein rebound constipation
• Electrolytes (K, Na, Cl), hydration status
• Monitor effect in black patients; may be less effective
Evaluate: Therapeutic response: decreased diarrhea
Teach patient/family:
• To avoid OTC products unless directed by prescriber
• If drowsiness occurs, not to operate machinery

RARELY USED

crotamiton
(kroe-tam′-ih-tuhn)
Eurax
Func. class.: Scabicide/pediculicide

USES: Scabies, lice

CONTRAINDICATIONS: Hypersensitivity; raw, inflamed skin

DOSAGE AND ROUTES
• **Adult: TOP** After routine bath, apply over the entire body from the chin to the soles; do not apply to the face or head; repeat in 24 hr; patient may take a cleansing bath 48 hr after the second dose
Treatment of pruritus
• **Adult: TOP** Apply topically by massaging gently into affected area until medication is completely absorbed; repeat if needed
Available forms: Lotion, cream 10%

---

cyanocobalamin
(vit B₁₂) (otc, Rx)
(sye-an-oh-koe-bal′a-min)
Nascobal, Rubramin PC
hydroxocobalamin
(otc, Rx)
CytoKit ✦

Func. class.: Vit B₁₂, water-soluble vitamin

ACTION: Needed for adequate nerve functioning, protein and carbohydrate metabolism, normal growth, RBC development, cell reproduction

USES: Vit B₁₂ deficiency, pernicious anemia, vit B₁₂ malabsorption syndrome, Schilling test, increased requirements with pregnancy, thyrotoxicosis, hemolytic anemia, hemorrhage, renal/hepatic disease, nutritional supplementation

CONTRAINDICATIONS: Hypersensitivity to this product, cobalt, benzyl alcohol, optic nerve atrophy
Precautions: Pregnancy, breastfeeding, children, renal/hepatic disease, folic acid/iron deficiency anemia, infection

DOSAGE AND ROUTES
cyanocobalamin
• **Adult:** PO Up to 1000 mcg/day **SUBCUT/IM** 30-100 mcg/day × 1 wk, then 100-200 mcg/mo
Schilling test
• **Adult/child:** IM 1000 mcg in 1 dose
• **Child:** PO Up to 1000 mcg/day **SUBCUT/IM** 30-50 mcg/day × 2 wk, then 100 mcg/mo; **NASAL** 500 mcg weekly

hydroxocobalamin
• **Adult:** SUBCUT/IM 30-50 mcg/day × 5-10 days, then 100-200 mcg/mo
• **Child:** SUBCUT/IM 30-50 mcg/day × 5-10 days, then 30-50 mcg/mo
Available forms: *Cyanocobalamin:* tabs 50, 100, 250, 500, 1000, 5000 mcg; ext rel tabs 1000 mcg; lozenges 100, 250, 500 mcg; nasal 500 mcg/spray; inj 100, 1000 mcg/mL;

hydroxocobalamin: inj 1000 mcg/mL, powder for inj 5 g/vial
Administer:
PO route
• With fruit juice to disguise taste; immediately after mixing
• With meals if possible for better absorption; large doses should not be used because most is excreted
• Protect from light, heat
IM route
• By IM inj for pernicious anemia for life unless contraindicated
Intranasal route
• Avoid use within 1 hr of hot fluids, food, no priming needed
IV route
• IV route not recommended but may be admixed in TPN solution

Additive compatibilities: Ascorbic acid, chloramphenicol, hydrocortisone, vit B/C
Solution compatibilities: Dextrose/Ringer's or LR combinations, dextrose/saline combinations, D₅W, D₁₀W, 0.45% NaCl, Ringer's or LR sol
Y-site compatibilities: Alfentanil, amikacin, aminophylline, ascorbic acid, atracurium, atropine, azaTHIOprine, aztreonam, benztropine, bretylium, bumetanide, buprenorphine, butorphanol, calcium chloride/gluconate, ceFAZolin, cefmetazole, cefonicid, cefotaxime, cefoTEtan, cefOXitin, cefTAZidime, ceftizoxime, cefTRIAXone, cefuroxime, chloramphenicol, chlorproMAZINE, cimetidine, clindamycin, dexamethasone, digoxin, diphenhydrAMINE, DOBUTamine, DOPamine, doxycycline, enalaprilat, ePHEDrine, EPINEPHrine, epoetin alfa, erythromycin, esmolol, famotidine, fentaNYL, fluconazole, folic acid, furosemide, ganciclovir, gentamicin, glycopyrrolate, heparin, hydrocortisone, hydrOXYzine, imipenem-cilastatin, indomethacin, insulin (regular), isoproterenol hydrochloride, ketorolac, labetalol, lidocaine, magnesium, mannitol, meperidine, methoxamine, methyldopate, methylPREDNISolone, metoclopramide, metoprolol, miconazole, midazolam, minocycline, morphine, moxalactam, multiple vitamins

Side effects: *italics* = common; red = life-threatening

injection, nafcillin, nalbuphine, naloxone, netilmicin, nitroglycerin, nitroprusside, norepinephrine, ondansetron, oxacillin, oxytocin, papaverine, penicillin G potassium/sodium, pentamidine, pentazocine, PENTobarbital, PHENobarbital, phentolamine, phenylephrine, phytonadione, piperacillin, polymyxin B, potassium chloride, procainamide, prochlorperazine, promethazine, propranolol, protamine, pyridoxine, quiNIDine, raNITIdine, ritodrine, sodium bicarbonate, succinylcholine, SUFentanil, theophylline, thiamine, ticarcillin, ticarcillin-clavulanate, tobramycin, tolazoline, trimetaphan, urokinase, vancomycin, vasopressin, verapamil, vitamin B complex with C

SIDE EFFECTS

CNS: Flushing, optic nerve atrophy
CV: HF, peripheral vascular thrombosis, pulmonary edema
GI: *Diarrhea*
INTEG: Itching, rash, pain at inj site
META: Hypokalemia
SYST: Anaphylactic shock

PHARMACOKINETICS

Gastric intrinsic factor must be present for absorption to occur; stored in liver, kidneys, stomach; 50%-90% excreted in urine; crosses placenta; excreted in breast milk

INTERACTIONS

Increase: absorption—predniSONE
Decrease: absorption—aminoglycosides, anticonvulsants, colchicine, chloramphenicol, aminosalicylic acid, potassium preparations, cimetidine
Drug/Herb
Decrease: vit B_{12} absorption—goldenseal
Drug/Lab Test
False positive: intrinsic factor

NURSING CONSIDERATIONS
Assess:
• For vit B_{12} deficiency: red, beefy tongue; psychosis; pallor; neuropathy, ataxia, positive Romberg
• GI function: diarrhea, constipation

• Potassium levels during beginning treatment in megaloblastic anemia; q6mo in pernicious anemia; folic acid, plasma vit B_{12} (after 1 wk), reticulocyte counts
• Nutritional status: egg yolks, fish, organ meats, dairy products, clams, oysters: good sources of vit B_{12}
• For pulmonary edema, worsening of HF in cardiac patients

Evaluate:
• Therapeutic response: decreased anorexia, dyspnea on exertion, palpitations, paresthesias, psychosis, visual disturbances

Teach patient/family:
• That treatment must continue for life for pernicious anemia
• To eat a well-balanced diet
• To avoid contact with persons with infection; that infections are common

TREATMENT OF OVERDOSE:
Discontinue product

---

cyclobenzaprine (Rx)
(sye-kloe-ben′za-preen)
Amrix
Func. class.: Skeletal muscle relaxant, central acting
Chem. class.: Tricyclic amine salt

ACTION: Reduces tonic muscle activity at the brain stem; may be related to antidepressant effects

USES: Adjunct for relief of muscle spasm and pain in musculoskeletal conditions
Unlabeled uses: Fibromyalgia

CONTRAINDICATIONS: Acute recovery phase of MI, dysrhythmias, heart block, HF, hypersensitivity, intermittent porphyria, thyroid disease, QT prolongation, within 14 days of MAOIs
Precautions: Pregnancy, breastfeeding, geriatric patients, renal/hepatic disease, addictive personality, CV disease, child <15 yr

---

DOSAGE AND ROUTES
Muscloskeletal disorders
• **Adult/adolescent ≥15 yr: PO** 5 mg tid × 1 wk, max 30 mg/day × 3 wk
• **Adult: EXT REL** 15 mg/day, max 30 mg/day × 3 wk
• **Geriatric: PO** 5 mg tid
Hepatic dose
• **Adult (mild hepatic disease): PO** 5 mg, titrate slowly
Fibromyalgia (unlabeled)
• **Adult: PO** 10 mg at bedtime, titrated up
Available forms: Tabs 5, 7.5, 10 mg; ext rel tab 15, 30 mg
Administer:
• Without regard to meals, give with food for GI symptoms
• Do not crush, break, chew ext rel cap
• Store in tight container at room temperature

SIDE EFFECTS
CNS: *Dizziness, weakness, drowsiness,* headache, insomnia, confusion, nervousness, fatigue
CV: Postural hypotension, dysrhythmias
EENT: Diplopia, temporary loss of vision, blurred vision, dry mouth
GI: *Nausea,* dry mouth, constipation
GU: Urinary retention
INTEG: Rash

PHARMACOKINETICS
PO: Onset 1 hr, peak 3-8 hr, duration 12-24 hr, half-life 1-3 days, 32 hr ext rel, metabolized by liver, excreted in urine, crosses placenta, excreted in breast milk

INTERACTIONS
• Do not use within 14 days of MAOIs, traMADol
Increase: QT interval—Class IA/III antidysrhythmics and other products that increase QT interval
Increase: serotonin syndrome—SSRIs, SNRIs, tricyclics, triptans, fentaNYL, busPIRone, traMADol
Increase: CNS depression—alcohol, tricyclics, opiates, barbiturates, sedatives, hypnotics
Drug/Herb
Increase: CNS depression—kava, chamomile, hops, valerian

NURSING CONSIDERATIONS
Assess:
• **Serotonin syndrome:** If using with SSRIs, SNRIs, monitor closely; if syndrome occurs, discontinue both products immediately, hallucinations, nausea, vomiting, diarrhea, tachycardia, hyperthermia
• **Pain:** location, duration, mobility, stiffness at baseline, periodically
• **Allergic reactions:** rash, fever, respiratory distress
• Severe weakness, numbness in extremities
• Assistance with ambulation if dizziness, drowsiness occur, especially for geriatric patients
• **Beers:** avoid use in older adults; anticholinergic effects
• **Pregnancy/breastfeeding:** no well-controlled studies; use only if clearly needed; use cautiously in breastfeeding
Evaluate:
• Therapeutic response: decreased pain, spasticity; relief of muscle spasms of acute, painful musculoskeletal conditions generally short term; long-term therapy seldom warranted
Teach patient/family:
• Not to discontinue medication abruptly; that insomnia, nausea, headache, spasticity, tachycardia will occur; that product should be tapered off over 1-2 wk
• Not to take with alcohol, other CNS depressants or MAOIs
• To avoid hazardous activities if drowsiness, dizziness occur
• To avoid using OTC medication (cough preparations, antihistamines) unless directed by prescriber
• To use gum, frequent sips of water for dry mouth
• To notify prescriber of serotonin syndrome
• To report feeling of fullness of bladder, inability to void adequate amounts
• To use fluids, bulk in diet to prevent constipation

TREATMENT OF OVERDOSE:
Use anticonvulsants if indicated; monitor cardiac function

Side effects: *italics* = common; red = life-threatening

cyclopentolate ophthalmic
See Appendix B

⚠ HIGH ALERT

cyclophosphamide (Rx)
(sye-kloe-foss′fa-mide)
Procytox ✦
Func. class.: Antineoplastic alkylating agent
Chem. class.: Nitrogen mustard

Do not confuse:
cyclophosphamide/cycloSPORINE

ACTION: Alkylates DNA; is responsible for cross-linking DNA strands; activity is not cell-cycle–phase specific

USES: Hodgkin's disease, lymphomas, leukemia; cancer of female reproductive tract, breast, multiple myeloma; neuroblastoma; retinoblastoma; Ewing's sarcoma; nephrotic syndrome

CONTRAINDICATIONS: Pregnancy, hypersensitivity, prostatic hypertrophy, bladder neck obstruction
Precautions: Radiation therapy, cardiac disease, anemia, dysrhythmias, child, dental disease/work, dialysis, geriatric patients, heart failure, hematuria, infections, leukopenia QT prolongation, secondary malignancy surgery, tumor lysis syndrome, vaccinations, breastfeeding, severely depressed bone marrow function

DOSAGE AND ROUTES
Acute lymphocytic leukemia (ALL)
• **Adult/adolescent/child:** IV Total doses of IV 300-1500 mg/m^2 have been incorporated into induction, intensification, consolidation regimens, possibly using vinCRIStine, predniSONE, or others; PO 1-5 mg/kg/day depending on response

Neuroblastoma
• **Adult/child:** IV For induction, 40-50 mg/kg in divided doses over 2-5 days or 10-15 mg/kg q7-10days, 3-5 mg/kg 2×/wk or 1-5 mg/kg daily
• **Child and infant:** PO 150 mg/m^2/day, days 1-7 with DOXOrubicin (IV 35 mg/m^2 on day 8) q21days × 5 cycles
• **Child:** IV 70 mg/kg/day with hydration on days 1, 2 with DOXOrubicin and vinCRIStine q21days for courses 1, 2, 4, 6 alternating with CISplatin and etoposide q21days for courses 3, 5, 7

Breast cancer
• **Adult:** PO 100-200 mg/m^2/day or 2 mg/kg/day × 4-14 days; IV 500-1000 mg/m^2 on day 1 in combination with fluorouracil and methotrexate or DOXOrubicin or DOXOrubicin alone, also cyclophosphamide 600 mg/m^2; may be given dose-dense on day 1 of q14days with DOXOrubicin (60 mg/m^2) with growth-factor support

Operable node-positive breast cancer IV (TAC regimen)
• **Adult:** IV 500 mg/m^2 with DOXOrubicin (50 mg/m^2 IV), then DOCEtaxel (75 mg/m^2) IV given 1 hr later q3wk × 6 cycles

Nephrotic syndrome
• **Child:** PO 2.5-3 mg/kg daily × 60-90 days
Available forms: Powder for inj ✦ 200, 500 mg, 1, 2 g/vials; caps 25, 50 mg
Administer:
• Use cytotoxic handling procedures
• In AM so product can be eliminated before bedtime
• Fluids IV or PO before chemotherapy to hydrate patient
• Antacid before oral agent; give after evening meal, before bedtime
• Antiemetic 30-60 min before product and prn
• Allopurinol or sodium bicarbonate to maintain uric acid levels, alkalinization of urine
PO route
• Take on empty stomach; do not crush, break, chew caps; wash hands immediately if in contact with caps

---

• May be taken as a single dose or divided doses

• Take in AM or afternoon, avoid evening

• Store in tight container at room temperature

Direct IV route

• Reconstitute with NS only 100 mg/5mL, swirl, inject slowly

Intermittent IV INFUSION route

• Use cytotoxic handling procedures

• IV after diluting 100 mg/5 mL, 0.9% NaCl of sterile water or bacteriostatic water; shake; let stand until clear; may be further diluted in ≤250 mL D$_5$/NS, 0.45% NaCl; give 100 mg or less/min (2 mg/mL)

• Use 21, 23, 25G needle; check site for irritation, phlebitis

Y-site compatibilities: Acyclovir, alfentanil, allopurinol, amifostine, amikacin, aminocaproic acid, aminophylline, amiodarone, amphotericin B lipid complex, amphotericin B liposome, ampicillin, ampicillin-sulbactam, anidulafungin, atenolol, atracurium, azlocillin, aztreonam, bivalirudin, bleomycin, bumetanide, buprenorphine, butorphanol, calcium chloride/gluconate, CARBOplatin, caspofungin, cefamandole, ceFAZolin, cefepime, cefoperazone, cefotaxime, cefoTEtan, cefOXitin, cefTAZidime, ceftizoxime, cefTRIAXone, cefuroxime, chloramphenicol, chlorproMAZINE, cimetidine, ciprofloxacin, cisatracurium, CISplatin, cladribine, clindamycin, codeine, cycloSPORINE, cytarabine, DACTINomycin, DAPTOmycin, DAUNOrubicin, dexamethasone, dexmedetomidine, dexrazoxane, digoxin, diltiaZEM, diphenhydrAMINE, DOBUTamine, DOCEtaxel, dolasetron, DOPamine, doripenem, doxacurium, DOXOrubicin, DOXOrubicin liposomal, doxycycline, droperidol, enalaprilat, ePHEDrine, EPINEPHrine, epiRUBicin, ertapenem, erythromycin, esmolol, etoposide, famotidine, fenoldopam, fentaNYL, filgrastim, fluconazole, fludarabine, fluorouracil, foscarnet, fosphenytoin, furosemide, gallium, ganciclovir, gatifloxacin, gemcitabine, gentamicin, granisetron, haloperidol, heparin, hydrocortisone, HYDROmorphone, hydrOXYzine, IDArubicin, imipenem-cilastatin, inamrinone, insulin (regular), irinotecan, isoproterenol, kanamycin, ketorolac, labetalol, leucovorin, levoFLOXacin, levorphanol, lidocaine, linezolid, LORazepam, magnesium sulfate, mannitol, melphalan, meperidine, meropenem, mesna, methohexital, methotrexate, methylPREDNISolone, metoclopramide, metoprolol, metroNIDAZOLE, midazolam, milrinone, minocycline, mitoMYcin, mitoXANTRONE, mivacurium, morphine, nafcillin, nalbuphine, naloxone, nesiritide, nitroglycerin, nitroprusside, norepinephrine, octreotide, ondansetron, oxacillin, oxaliplatin, PACLitaxel, palonosetron, pamidronate, pancuronium, pantoprazole, PEMEtrexed, penicillin G potassium, pentamidine, PENTobarbital, PHENobarbital, phenylephrine, piperacillin, piperacillin-tazobactam, potassium chloride/phosphates, procainamide, prochlorperazine, promethazine, propofol, propranolol, quinupristin-dalfopristin, raNITIdine, rapacuronium, remifentanil, riTUXimab, rocuronium, sargramostim, sodium acetate/bicarbonate/phosphates, succinylcholine, SUFentanil, sulfamethoxazole-trimethoprim, tacrolimus, teniposide, theophylline, thiopental, thiotepa, ticarcillin, ticarcillin-clavulanate, tigecycline, tirofiban, TNA, tobramycin, topotecan, TPN, trastuzumab, vancomycin, vasopressin, vecuronium, verapamil, vinBLAStine, vinCRIStine, vinorelbine, voriconazole, zidovudine, zoledronic acid

SIDE EFFECTS

CV: Cardiotoxicity (high doses), myocardial fibrosis, hypotension

ENDO: SIADH, gonadal suppression

GI: *Nausea, vomiting, weight loss,* anorexia

GU: Hemorrhagic cystitis, *hematuria*

HEMA: Thrombocytopenia, leukopenia, myelosuppression

INTEG: *Alopecia*

META: Hyperuricemia

MISC: Secondary neoplasms

RESP: Pulmonary fibrosis, interstitial pneumonia

Side effects: *italics* = common; red = life-threatening

PHARMACOKINETICS

Metabolized by liver, excreted in urine, half-life $4-6\frac{1}{2}$ hr, 50% bound to plasma proteins

INTERACTIONS

Increase: neuromuscular blockade—succinylcholine

Increase: action of warfarin

Increase: bone marrow depression—other antineoplastics, radiation, allopurinol, thiazides

Decrease: digoxin levels—digoxin

Decrease: cyclophosphamide effect

Decrease: antibody response—live virus vaccines

Drug/Herb

Increase: toxicity—St. John's wort

Drug/Lab Test

Increase: uric acid

False positive: Pap smear

False negative: PPD, mumps, *Candida*, *Trichophyton*, Pap smear

NURSING CONSIDERATIONS
Assess:

• **Hemorrhagic cystitis; renal studies:** BUN, serum uric acid, urine CCr before, during therapy; I&O ratio; report fall in urine output <30 mL/hr; provide increased fluid intake to 3 L/day (adults)

• **Bone marrow depression:** CBC, differential, platelet count baseline, weekly; withhold product if WBC is <2500 or platelet count is <75,000; notify prescriber of results. Assess for hematuria, guaiac, bruising or petechiae, mucosa or orifices q8hr

• **Pulmonary fibrosis/interstitial pneumonia:** pulmonary function tests, chest x-ray films before, during therapy; chest film should be obtained q2wk during treatment; monitor for dyspnea, rales/crackles, edema

• **Hepatotoxicity:** hepatic studies before, during therapy (bilirubin, AST, ALT, LDH), as needed; jaundice of skin, sclera; dark urine, clay-colored stools; itchy skin; abdominal pain; fever; diarrhea

• Unproductive cough, chest pain, tachypnea

• Buccal cavity q8hr for dryness, sores or ulceration, white patches, oral pain, bleeding, dysphagia; obtain prescription for viscous lidocaine (Xylocaine); provide rinsing of mouth tid-qid with water, club soda; brushing of teeth bid-tid with soft brush or cotton-tipped applicators for stomatitis; use unwaxed dental floss

• Increase fluid intake to 2-3 L/day to prevent urate deposits, calculi formation, reduce incidence of hemorrhagic cystitis

• Warm compresses at inj site for inflammation

• **Beers:** avoid in older adults; delirium, dementia may occur; avoid in men due to decrease in urine flow, retention

Evaluate:

• Therapeutic response: decreased tumor size, spread of malignancy; nephrotic syndrome

Teach patient/family:

• To take adequate fluids (3 L/day, adults) to eliminate product

• That amenorrhea can occur and may last up to 1 yr after therapy but is reversible after stopping treatment

• To report any changes in breathing or coughing

• To avoid foods with citric acid, hot temperature, or rough texture; that skin, fingernails may become darker

• **To report signs of infection:** increased temperature, sore throat, flulike symptoms

• **To report signs of anemia:** fatigue, headache, faintness, SOB, irritability

• To report bleeding (bruising, hematuria, petechiae); to avoid the use of razors, commercial mouthwash

• To avoid the use of aspirin products, ibuprofen

• To avoid vaccinations during therapy

• About proper handling and disposal of chemotherapy drugs

• **Pregnancy/breastfeeding:** to use reliable contraception during treatment and for 1 yr after treatment (women); men should use condoms during and for 4 mo following treatment; not to breastfeed

cycloSPORINE (Rx)

(sye'kloe-spor-een)

Gengraf, Neoral, SandIMMUNE

Func. class.: Immunosuppressant, antirheumatic (DMARD)

Chem. class.: Fungus-derived peptide

Do not confuse:

cycloSPORINE/cycloSERINE/ cyclophosphamide

ACTION: Produces immunosuppression by inhibiting T-lymphocytes

USES: Organ transplants (liver, kidney, heart) to prevent rejection (GVHD), rheumatoid arthritis, psoriasis

Unlabeled uses: Recalcitrant ulcerative colitis, aplastic anemia, Crohn's disease, thrombocytopenia purpura, lupus, nephritis, myasthenia gravis, psoriatic arthritis, atopic dermatitis

CONTRAINDICATIONS: Breastfeeding, hypersensitivity to polyoxyethylated castor oil (inj only); psoriasis or RA in renal disease (Neoral/Gengraf); Gengraf/Neoral used with PUVA/UVB, methotrexate, coal tar; ocular infections

Black Box Warning: Uncontrolled malignant hypertension

Precautions: Pregnancy, geriatric patients, severe hepatic disease

Black Box Warning: Immunosuppression, nephrotoxicity, skin cancer; requires a specialized care setting and experienced clinician; infections; new primary malignancy (lymphoma, skin cancer)

DOSAGE AND ROUTES—NTI
Prevention of transplant rejection (nonmodified) (Sandimmune)

• **Adult/child:** PO 15 mg/kg 4-12 hr before surgery, daily for 2 wk, reduce dosage by 2.5 mg/kg/wk to 5-10 mg/kg/day; **IV** 5-6 mg/kg 4-12 hr before surgery, daily, switch to **PO** form as soon as possible

Prevention of transplant rejection (modified) (Neoral)

• **Adult/child:** PO 4-12 mg/kg/day divided q12hr, depends on organ transplanted

Rheumatoid arthritis (Neoral/Gengraf)

• **Adult:** PO 2.5 mg/kg/day divided bid, may increase 0.5-0.75 mg/kg/day after 8-12 wk, max 4 mg/kg/day

Psoriasis (Neoral/Gengraf)

• **Adult:** PO 2.5 mg/kg/day divided bid, × 4 wk, then increase by 0.5 mg/kg/day q2wk, max 4 mg/kg/day

Autoimmune diseases (Sandimmune)

• **Adult/child:** PO 1-3 mg/kg/day

Atopic dermatitis (unlabeled)

• **Adult/adolescent/child ≥2 yr:** PO 5 mg/kg/day

Crohn's disease that is resistant to/ intolerant of corticosteroids (unlabeled)

• **Adult:** PO 2.5-15 mg/kg/day (non-modified)

Available forms: Oral sol 100 mg/mL; soft gel cap 25, 50, 100 mg; inj 50 mg/mL

Administer:

PO route

• Some brands are not interchangeable

• Do not break, crush, or chew caps

• Use pipette provided to draw up oral sol; may mix with milk or juice; wipe pipette, do not wash (Neoral)

• For several days before transplant surgery; give at same time of day

• With corticosteroids

• With meals for GI upset or in chocolate milk, milk, or orange juice (SandIMMUNE)

Rheumatoid arthritis

• Give Neoral or Gengraf 2.5 mg/kg/day divided bid; may use with salicylates, NSAIDs, PO corticosteroids

• Always give the daily dose of Neoral/Gengraf in 2 divided doses on consistent schedule

• Give initial SandIMMUNE PO dose 4-12 hr before transplantation as a single dose of 15 mg/kg, continue the single daily dose for 1-2 wk, then taper 5%/wk to a maintenance dose of 5-10 mg/kg/day

Side effects: *italics* = common; red = life-threatening

Intermittent IV INFUSION route
• After diluting each 50 mg/20-100 mL of 0.9% NaCl or D$_5$W (2.5 mg/mL), run over 2-6 hr, use an infusion pump

Continuous IV INFUSION route
• May run over 24 hr
• **For SandIMMUNE parenteral,** give $1/3$ of PO dose, initial dose 4-12 hr before transplantation as a single IV dose 5-6 mg/kg/day, continue the single daily dose until PO can be used

Y-site compatibilities: Abciximab, alatrofloxacin, alfentanil, amikacin, aminocaproic acid, aminophylline, amphotericin B lipid complex, anidulafungin, argatroban, ascorbic acid injection, atenolol, atracurium, atropine, azaTHIOprine, aztreonam, benztropine, bivalirudin, bleomycin, bretylium, bumetanide, buprenorphine, butorphanol, calcium chloride/gluconate, CARBOplatin, carmustine, caspofungin, ceFAZolin, cefmetazole, cefonicid, cefotaxime, cefoTEtan, cefOXitin, cefTAZidime, ceftizoxime, cefTRIAXone, cefuroxime, chloramphenicol, chlorproMAZINE, cimetidine, ciprofloxacin, CISplatin, clindamycin, codeine, cyanocobalamin, cyclophosphamide, cytarabine, DACTINomycin, DAPTOmycin, DAUNOrubicin, dexamethasone, dexmedetomidine, digoxin, diltiaZEM, diphenhydrAMINE, DOBUTamine, DOCEtaxel, DOPamine, doripenem, doxacurium, DOXOrubicin, doxycycline, enalaprilat, ePHEDrine, EPINEPHrine, epiRUBicin, epoetin alfa, eptifibatide, ertapenem, erythromycin, esmolol, etoposide, famotidine, fenoldopam, fentaNYL, fluconazole, fludarabine, fluorouracil, folic acid, furosemide, gallium, ganciclovir, gatifloxacin, gemcitabine, gentamicin, glycopyrrolate, granisetron, heparin, hydrocortisone, HYDROmorphone, hydrOXYzine, ifosfamide, imipenem-cilastatin, indomethacin, irinotecan, isoproterenol, ketorolac, labetalol, lansoprazole, levoFLOXacin, lidocaine, linezolid, LORazepam, mannitol, mechlorethamine, meperidine, meropenem, methotrexate, methyldopate, methylPREDNISolone, metoclopramide, metoprolol, metroNIDAZOLE, micafungin, miconazole, midazolam, milrinone, minocycline, mitoXANTRONE, morphine, multiple vitamins injection, nafcillin, naloxone, nesiritide, netilmicin, nitroglycerin, nitroprusside, norepinephrine, octreotide, ondansetron, oxacillin, oxaliplatin, oxytocin, PACLitaxel, palonosetron, pamidronate, pancuronium, pantoprazole, papaverine, PEMEtrexed, penicillin G potassium/sodium, pentamidine, pentazocine, phentolamine, phenylephrine, phytonadione, piperacillin, piperacillin-tazobactam, polymyxin B, potassium acetate/chloride, procainamide, prochlorperazine, promethazine, propofol, propranolol, protamine, pyridoxine, quiNIDine, quinupristin-dalfopristin, raNITIdine, ritodrine, sargramostim, sodium acetate/bicarbonate, succinylcholine, SUFentanil, tacrolimus, teniposide, theophylline, thiamine, thiotepa, ticarcillin, ticarcillin-clavulanate, tigecycline, tirofiban, tobramycin, trimetaphan, urokinase, vancomycin, vasopressin, vecuronium, verapamil, vinCRIStine, vinorelbine, zoledronic acid

SIDE EFFECTS

CNS: *Tremors, headache,* seizures, progressive multifocal leukoencephalopathy, confusion, migraine, paresthesia
GI: Nausea, vomiting, diarrhea, *oral candida, gum hyperplasia,* hepatotoxicity, pancreatitis
GU: Nephrotoxicity
INTEG: Rash, acne, *hirsutism*
META: Hyperkalemia, hypomagnesemia, hyperlipidemia, hyperuricemia
MISC: *Infection,* gingival hyperplasia, hypersensitivity, malignancy

PHARMACOKINETICS

Peak 4 hr; highly protein bound; half-life (biphasic) 1.2 hr, 25 hr; metabolized in liver; excreted in feces, 6% in urine; crosses placenta; excreted in breast milk

---

INTERACTIONS

Increase: action, toxicity of cycloSPORINE—allopurinol, amiodarone, amphotericin B, androgens, azole antifungals, β-blockers, bromocriptine, calcium channel blockers, carvedilol, cimetidine, colchicine, corticosteroids, fluoroquinolones, foscarnet, imipenem-cilastatin, macrolides, metoclopramide, oral contraceptives, NSAIDs, melphalan, SSRIs

Increase: effects of aliskiren, digoxin, etoposide, HMG-CoA reductase inhibitors, methotrexate, potassium-sparing diuretics, sirolimus, tacrolimus

Increase: action, toxicity of—digoxin, colchicine

Increase: hyperkalemia—potassium-sparing diuretics, potassium supplements, ACE inhibitors

Increase: renal dysfunction—aminoglycosides, ciprofloxacin, NSAIDs, fibric acid derivatives, vancomycin, melphalan, ketoconazole

Decrease: cycloSPORINE action—anticonvulsants, nafcillin, orlistat, PHENobarbital, phenytoin, rifamycins, sulfamethoxazole-trimethoprim, terbinafine, ticlopidine

Decrease: antibody reaction—live virus vaccines

Drug/Herb

Decrease: immunosuppression—echinacea, melatonin; do not use together

Decrease: cycloSPORINE levels—St. John's wort; do not use together

Drug/Food

• Slowed metabolism of product—grapefruit juice, food

NURSING CONSIDERATIONS
Assess:

Black Box Warning: **Nephrotoxicity:** BUN, creatinine at least monthly during treatment, 3 mo after treatment; nephrotoxicity increases with increasing doses and duration of treatment

• Product blood level during treatment 12 hr after dose, toxic >400 ng/mL
• Hepatic studies: alk phos, AST, ALT, bilirubin; **hepatotoxicity:** dark urine, jaundice, itching, light-colored stools; product should be discontinued

• Serum lipids, magnesium, potassium, cycloSPORINE blood concentrations, therapeutic cycloSPORINE range: 100-400 mg/mL

• **Posterior reversible encephalopathy:** impaired cognition, seizures, visual changes including blindness, loss of motor function, movement disorders, and psychiatric changes; dosage reduction or discontinuation may be needed in severe cases

• **Progressive multifocal leukoencephalopathy (PML):** apathy, confusion, cognitive changes; may be fatal, withhold dose, notify prescriber immediately

• **Immunosuppression/infection:** bacterial, viral, protozoal, and fungal infections are common; assess for signs of infection often

• **Nephrotoxicity:** Increased with increased doses and duration

• **Psoriasis:** Lesions baseline and during treatment

• **RA:** Pain, ROM, ADLs baseline and during treatment

Black Box Warning: **Requires a specialized care setting and experienced clinician:** product must be given in a facility equipped with adequate laboratory and supportive medical services

Black Box Warning: **New primary malignancy:** lymphoma, skin cancer; increased risk in psoriasis with use of PUVA or UVB therapy, methotrexate, other immunosuppressives, coal tar or radiation; these patients may be at increased risk of skin cancer also

Evaluate:

• Therapeutic response: absence of rejection; decreased pain in rheumatoid arthritis, decreased lesions in psoriasis

Teach patient/family:

• To report fever, chills, sore throat, fatigue since serious infections may occur; tremors, bleeding gums, increased B/P

• To take at same time of day, every day; not to skip doses or double dose; not to use with grapefruit juice or receive vaccines; that there are many drug interactions; not to add new products without approval of prescriber

• That treatment is lifelong to prevent rejection; to identify signs of rejection
• To report severe diarrhea because drug loss and rejection may result
• **About the signs of nephrotoxicity:** increased B/P, tremors of the hands, changes in gums, increased hair on body, face
• To continue with all lab work and follow-up appointments
• That types of products are not interchangeable
• Not to wash syringe/container with water; variation in dose may result
• To notify prescriber of all medications, herbal products, supplements that are taken
• **Pregnancy/breastfeeding:** to use contraceptive measures during treatment, for 12 wk after ending therapy; to notify prescriber if pregnancy is planned or suspected; no well-controlled studies; use only if benefits outweigh risks; discontinue breastfeeding or product

---

⚠ HIGH ALERT

cytarabine (Rx)
(sye-tare′a-been)
Cytosar ✦
cytarabine liposomal (Rx)
DepoCyt
Func. class.: Antineoplastic, antimetabolite
Chem. class.: Pyrimidine nucleoside analog

Do not confuse:
Cytosar/Cytoxan/Cytovene

ACTION: Competes with physiologic substrate of DNA synthesis, thus interfering with cell replication in the S phase of the cell cycle (before mitosis)

USES: Acute myelocytic leukemia, acute nonlymphocytic leukemia, chronic myelocytic leukemia; lymphomatous meningitis (intrathecal/intraventricular) **Unlabeled uses:** Hodgkin's/non-Hodgkin's lymphoma, malignant meningitis, mantle cell lymphoma

CONTRAINDICATIONS: Pregnancy, hypersensitivity
Precautions: Breastfeeding, children, renal/hepatic disease, tumor lysis syndrome, infection, hyperkalemia, hyperphosphatemia, hyperuricemia, hypocalcemia

DOSAGE AND ROUTES
Regimens will vary
Acute myelogenous leukemia (AML)
• Adult: **CONT IV INFUSION** 100 mg/m^2/day × 7 days q2wk as single agent or 2-6 mg/kg/day (100-200 mg/m^2/day) as a single dose or 2-3 divided doses for 5-10 days until remission, used in combination; maintenance 70-200 mg/m^2/day for 2-5 days monthly; **SUBCUT/IM** maintenance 100 mg/m^2/day × 5 days q28days
Meningeal leukemia
• Adult/child: **INTRATHECAL** For induction 50 mg (liposomal) q14days × 2 doses (wk 1, 3); consolidation 50 mg (liposomal) q14days × 3 doses (wk 5, 7, 9), then another dose at wk 13; maintenance 50 mg (liposomal) q28days (wk 17, 21, 25, 29)
Refractory acute Hodgkin's/ refractory non-Hodgkin's lymphoma (unlabeled)
• Adult/child: **IV** 2 g/m^2/day; on day 5 q21days, with etoposide, methylPREDNISolone, and CISplatin

---

Carcinomatous meningitis (liposomal)

• **Adult:** **IT** 50 mg over 1-5 min q14days, during induction and consolidation wk 1, 3, 5, 7, 9, give another 50 mg **IT** wk 13; maintenance 50 mg q28days on wk 17, 21, 25, 29, use with dexamethasone 4 mg **PO/IV** × 5 days on each day of cytarabine

Renal dose

• **Adult:** **IV** CCr ≤60 mL/min, serum creatinine 1.5-1.9 mg/dL or increase of 0.5-1.2 mg/dL from baseline during treatment: reduce to 1 g/m²/dose; serum creatinine ≥2 mg/dL or change from baseline serum creatinine was 1.2 mg/dL: reduce to 100 mg/m²/day

Available forms: Solution for injection 20 mg/mL, 100 mg/mL; liposomal intrathecal injection 10 mg/mL

Administer:

• Antiemetic 30-60 min before product and prn

• Allopurinol to maintain uric acid levels and alkalinization of the urine

IT route

• Use preservative-free NS, add 5 mL/100-mg vial or 10 mL/500-mg vial; use immediately, discard unused product

IV route

• Use cytotoxic handling precautions

Direct IV route

• Give undiluted, give by direct IV over 1-3 min through free-flowing tubing (IV)

Intermittent IV INFUSION route

• Dilute in 50-100 mL NS or D₅W, given over 30 min to 24 hr, depending on dose

Continuous IV INFUSION route

• May also be given by continuous infusion

Y-site compatibilities: Acyclovir, alfentanil, amifostine, amikacin, aminocaproic acid, aminophylline, amphotericin B lipid complex, amphotericin B liposome, ampicillin, ampicillin-sulbactam, amsacrine, anidulafungin, atenolol, atracurium, azithromycin, aztreonam, bivalirudin, bleomycin, bumetanide, buprenorphine, butorphanol, calcium chloride/gluconate, CARBOplatin, ceFAZolin, cefepime, cefotaxime, cefoTEtan, cefOXitin, cefTAZidime, ceftizoxime, cefTRIAXone, cefuroxime, chlorproMAZINE, cimetidine, ciprofloxacin, cisatracurium, CISplatin, cladribine, clindamycin, codeine, cyclophosphamide, cycloSPORINE, DAUNOrubicin, dexamethasone, dexmedetomidine, dexrazoxane, digoxin, diltiaZEM, diphenhydrAMINE, DOBUTamine, DOCEtaxel, dolasetron, DOPamine, doxacurium, DOXOrubicin, DOXOrubicin liposomal, doxycycline, droperidol, enalaprilat, ePHEDrine, EPINEPHrine, ertapenem, erythromycin, esmolol, etoposide, famotidine, fenoldopam, fentaNYL, filgrastim, fluconazole, fludarabine, foscarnet, fosphenytoin, furosemide, gatifloxacin, gemcitabine, gemtuzumab, gentamicin, granisetron, haloperidol, heparin, hydrocortisone, HYDROmorphone, hydrOXYzine, IDArubicin, ifosfamide, imipenemcilastatin, inamrinone, insulin (regular), irinotecan, isoproterenol, ketorolac, labetalol, leucovorin, levoFLOXacin, levorphanol, lidocaine, linezolid, LORazepam, magnesium sulfate, mannitol, melphalan, meperidine, meropenem, mesna, methohexital, methotrexate, methylPREDNISolone, metoclopramide, metoprolol, metroNIDAZOLE, midazolam, milrinone, minocycline, mitoXANTRONE, mivacurium, morphine, nalbuphine, naloxone, nesiritide, niCARdipine, nitroglycerin, nitroprusside, norepinephrine, octreotide, ofloxacin, ondansetron, oxaliplatin, PACLitaxel, palonosetron, pamidronate, pancuronium, pantoprazole, PEMEtrexed, pentamidine, PENTobarbital, PHENobarbital, phenylephrine, piperacillin, piperacillin-tazobactam, potassium chloride/phosphates, procainamide, prochlorperazine, promethazine, propofol, propranolol, quinupristin-dalfopristin, raNITIdine, rapacuronium, remifentanil, riTUXimab, rocuronium, sargramostim, sodium acetate/bicarbonate/phosphates, succinylcholine, SUFentanil, sulfamethoxazole-trimethoprim, tacrolimus, teniposide, theophylline, thiopental, thiotepa, ticarcillin, ticarcillin-clavulanate, tigecycline, tirofiban, TNA, tobramycin, trastuzumab, trimethobenzamide, vanco-mycin, vasopressin, vecuronium, verap-amil, vinCRIStine, vinorelbine, voricon-azole, zidovudine, zoledronic acid

SIDE EFFECTS
CNS: Dizziness, headache, confusion, drowsiness, chemical arachnoiditis (IT)
CV: Edema
EENT: Conjunctivitis, visual changes
GI: *Nausea, vomiting, anorexia, diarrhea, stomatitis,* hepatotoxicity, abdominal pain, GI ulceration (high dose)
GU: Urinary retention, renal dysfunction
HEMA: Thrombophlebitis, bleeding, thrombocytopenia, leukopenia, myelosuppression, anemia
INTEG: *Rash*
META: Hyperuricemia
RESP: Dyspnea, pulmonary edema (high doses)
SYST: Anaphylaxis, tumor lysis syndrome
Cytarabine syndrome: *Fever,* myalgia, bone pain, chest pain, *rash,* conjunctivitis, malaise (6-12 hr after administration)

PHARMACOKINETICS
INTRATHECAL: Half-life 100-236 hr; metabolized in liver; excreted in urine (primarily inactive metabolite); crosses blood-brain barrier, placenta
IV/SUBCUT: Distribution half-life 10 min, elimination half-life 1-3 hr

INTERACTIONS
• Do not use with live virus vaccines
• Do not use within 24 hr of chemotherapy—sargramostim, GM-CSF, filgrastim, G-CSF
Increase: toxicity—immunosuppressants, methotrexate, flucytosine, radiation, or other antineoplastics
Increase: bleeding risk—anticoagulants, platelet inhibitors, salicylates, thrombolytics, NSAIDs
Decrease: effects of oral digoxin, gentamicin

NURSING CONSIDERATIONS
Assess:

Black Box Warning: **Bone marrow suppression:** CBC (RBC, Hct, Hgb), differential, platelet count weekly; withhold product if WBC is <1000/mm^3, platelet count is <50,000/mm^3, or RBC, Hct, Hgb are low; notify prescriber of these results; assess for bleeding: hematuria, hemepositive stools, bruising or petechiae, mucosa, or orifices q8hr

• Renal studies: BUN, serum uric acid, urine CCr, electrolytes before and during therapy
• I&O ratio; report fall in urine output to <30 mL/hr
• Monitor temperature; fever may indicate beginning infection; no rectal temperatures

Black Box Warning: **Hepatotoxicity:** hepatic studies before and during therapy: bilirubin, ALT, AST, alk phos, as needed or monthly; check for jaundice of skin, sclera; dark urine; clay-colored stools; pruritus; abdominal pain; fever; diarrhea

• Serum uric acid during therapy
• **For anaphylaxis:** rash, pruritus, facial swelling, dyspnea; resuscitation equipment should be nearby

Black Box Warning: **Chemical arachnoiditis (IT):** headache, nausea, vomiting, fever; neck rigidity/pain, meningism, CSF pleocytosis; may be decreased by dexamethasone

• **Cytarabine syndrome** 6-12 hr after infusion: fever, myalgia, bone pain, chest pain, rash, conjunctivitis, malaise; corticosteroids may be ordered
• Dyspnea, crackles, unproductive cough, chest pain, tachypnea, fatigue, increased pulse, pallor, lethargy; personality changes, with high doses; pulmonary edema may be fatal (rare)
• Buccal cavity q8hr for dryness, sores or ulceration, white patches, oral pain, bleeding, dysphagia
• Local irritation, pain, burning, discoloration at inj site
• GI symptoms: frequency of stools, cramping; antispasmodic may be used
• Increased fluid intake to 2-3 L/day to prevent urate deposits and calculi formation unless contraindicated

• Rinsing of mouth tid-qid with water, club soda; brushing of teeth bid-tid with soft brush or cotton-tipped applicators for stomatitis; use unwaxed dental floss

Evaluate:

• Therapeutic response: improvement of hematologic parameters, decrease in size, spread of tumor

Teach patient/family:

• To report any coughing, chest pain, changes in breathing; may indicate beginning pneumonia, pulmonary edema

• **Stomatitis:** To avoid foods with citric acid, hot temperature, or rough texture if stomatitis is present; use sponge brush and rinse with water after each meal; to report stomatitis: any bleeding, white spots, ulcerations in mouth; to examine mouth daily, report any symptoms

• To report signs of infection: increased temperature, sore throat, flulike symptoms; to avoid crowds, persons with infections

• To report signs of **anemia:** fatigue, headache, faintness, SOB, irritability

• To report bleeding; to avoid use of razors, commercial mouthwash, salicylates, NSAIDs, anticoagulants

• To use thrombocytopenia precautions

• To take fluids to 3 L/day to prevent renal damage

• To avoid receiving vaccines during treatment

• That fever, headache, nausea, vomiting are likely to occur

• **Pregnancy/breastfeeding:** to use reliable contraception during treatment and for 4 mo thereafter; not to breastfeed

dabigatran
(da-bye-gat′ran)

Pradaxa

Func. class.: Anticoagulant

Chem. class.: Thrombin inhibitor

ACTION: Direct thrombin inhibitor that inhibits both free and clot-bound thrombin; prevents thrombin-induced platelet aggregation and thrombus formation by preventing conversion of fibrinogen to fibrin

USES: Stroke/systemic embolism prophylaxis with nonvalvular atrial fibrillation, DVT, pulmonary embolism in hip replacement

CONTRAINDICATIONS: Hypersensitivity, active bleeding, prosthetic heart valves, use with PgP inducers

Precautions: Pregnancy, labor, obstetric delivery, breastfeeding, children, geriatric patients, abrupt discontinuation, anticoagulant therapy, renal disease, surgery

Black Box Warning: Abrupt discontinuation, epidural/spinal anesthesia, lumbar puncture

DOSAGE AND ROUTES
Stroke prophylaxis, atrial fibrillation, and DVT/PE prophylaxis
• **Adult: PO** 150 mg bid

For conversion from an alternative anticoagulant to dabigatran
• When converting from warfarin to dabigatran, discontinue warfarin and initiate dabigatran therapy when the INR is <2.0; when converting from a parenteral anticoagulant to dabigatran, initiate dabigatran 0-2 hr before the time of the next scheduled anticoagulant dose or at the time of discontinuation of a continuously administered anticoagulant (e.g., intravenous unfractionated heparin)

For conversion from dabigatran to warfarin
• **Adult:** CCr >50 mL/min, start warfarin 3 days before discontinuing dabigatran; CCr 31-50 mL/min, start warfarin 2 days before discontinuing dabigatran; CCr 15-30 mL/min, start warfarin 1 day before discontinuing dabigatran

For conversion from dabigatran to parenteral anticoagulants
• **Adult: PO** discontinue dabigatran; start parenteral anticoagulant 12 hr (CCr ≥30 mL/min) or 24 hr (CCr <30 mL/min) after the last dabigatran dose

Deep venous thrombus (DVT)/ pulmonary embolism (PE) prophylaxis
• **Adult: PO** 220 mg or 150 mg/day × 28-35 days, starting with $^1/_2$ dose 1-4 hr after surgery (knee replacement); 110 mg on first day 1-4 hr after surgery, hemostasis achieved, then 220 mg daily × 28-35 days; those previously treated 150 mg bid (hip replacement)

DVT/PE/treated with a parenteral anticoagulant × 5-10 days
• **Adult: PO** 150 mg bid

Renal dose
• **Adult: PO** CCr 15-30 mL/min, 75 mg bid (for reduction in stroke risk and systemic embolism in nonvalvular atrial fibrillation)

Available forms: Caps 75, 110, 150 mg

Administer:
• Before surgery, discontinue product; restart after surgery is completed
• Do not crush, break, chew, or empty contents of capsule
• Without regard to food
• Store in original package at room temperature until time of use; discard after 30 days; protect from moisture

SIDE EFFECTS
GI: Abdominal pain, dyspepsia, esophagitis, gastritis, diarrhea

HEMA: Bleeding (any site)

SYST: Anaphylaxis (rare), angioedema

PHARMACOKINETICS
Protein binding 35%, half-life 12-17 hr (extended in renal disease), peak 1 hr, high-fat meal delays peak

INTERACTIONS
Increase: bleeding risk—amiodarone, other anticoagulants, clopidogrel, ketoconazole, quiNIDine, thrombolytics, verapamil

Pgp inhibitors: dose should be reduced to 150 mg/day (75 mg bid) in those with CCr 30-50 mL/min

Decrease: dabigatran effect—rifampin; avoid concurrent use

Decrease: dabigatran effect—P-glycoprotein inducers (carBAMazepine, rifampin, tipranavir)

Drug/Herb

Decrease: dabigatran—St. John's wort

Drug/Lab Test

Increase: thrombin time, aPTT

NURSING CONSIDERATIONS

Assess:

• **Stroke:** facial palsy, weakness, headache, blurred vision, speaking difficulty

• **DVT/PE** Pain in calf, swelling, or behind knee, trouble breathing, chest pain, lightheadedness

• **Bleeding:** blood in urine or emesis, dark tarry stools, lower back pain; caution with arterial/venous punctures, catheters, NG tubes; monitor vital signs frequently; elderly patients more prone to serious bleeding, monitor aPTT, ecarin clotting time baseline and during treatment

Black Box Warning: **Premature discontinuation: risk of thrombosis/MI/emboli:** swelling, pain, redness, difficulty breathing, chest pain, tachypnea, cough, coughing up blood, cyanosis

• **Postthrombotic syndrome:** pain, heaviness, itching/tingling, swelling, varicose veins, brownish/reddish skin discoloration, ulcers; use of ambulation, compression stockings, adequate anticoagulation can prevent this syndrome

• **Surgery:** discontinue 24-48 hr before surgery in those with CCr ≥50 mL/min, 72-96 hr in those with CCr <50 mL/min; longer times may be needed in major surgery; restart after surgery, spinal epidural catheter

Black Box Warning: **Epidural/spinal anesthesia, lumbar puncture:** risk of hematoma that may cause permanent paralysis; indwelling epidural catheters and products that cause coagulation changes (NSAIDs, anticoagulants) may increase the risk of paralysis

Black Box Warning: Do not discontinue abruptly

• **Pregnancy/breastfeeding:** no well-controlled studies; bleeding may occur if used during pregnancy; discontinue breastfeeding or product, unknown if excreted in breast milk

Evaluate:

• Therapeutic response: decreased thrombus formation/extension, absence of emboli, postthrombotic effects

Teach patient/family:

• About the purpose and expected results of this product; to take at same time of day; not to skip or double doses; if dose is missed, to take as soon as remembered if on the same day; do not administer if <6 hr before next dose; to store in original container, protect from moisture

• To take without regard to food; to swallow cap whole, not to open; to take with a full glass of water

• To notify all providers that this product is being used; to check with prescriber about when to discontinue

• **Bleeding:** to report any bleeding or bruising, including blood in stool, emesis, urine; nosebleeds

Black Box Warning: **Neurological changes:** to notify prescriber immediately of bowel or bladder changes, numbness in lower extremities, midline back pain

• Not to use any other OTC products, herbs without prescriber approval

• That lab tests may be required during treatment

---

dabrafenib

(da-braf'e-nib)

Tafinlar

Func. class.: Antineoplastic

Chem. class.: Signal transduction inhibitor, kinase inhibitor

---

Side effects: *italics* = common; red = life-threatening

ACTION: Inhibits kinase, inhibitor against mutated forms ⁿᴼᴱᴷ of BRAF kinases in melanoma cells

USES: ⁿᴼᴱᴷ Unresectable or metastatic BRAF V600E-mutated malignant melanoma, or V600K-mutated melanoma in combination with tramatinib

CONTRAINDICATIONS: Pregnancy, hypersensitivity

Precautions: Breastfeeding, children, infection, dehydration, diabetes mellitus, fever, G6PD deficiency, hemolytic anemia, hyperglycemia, hypotension, infertility, iritis, renal failure, secondary malignancy

DOSAGE AND ROUTES
• **Adult: PO** 150 mg q12hr until disease progression; avoid strong CYP3A4/CYP2C8 inhibitors or inducers

Available forms: Caps 50, 75 mg

Administer:

PO route
• Obtain testing for genetic evidence of BRAF V60E or K
• Swallow whole, do not open, crush, chew caps
• If dose is missed, take within 6 hr of missed dose; if >6 hr have passed, skip dose
• Space doses q12hr
• Take at least 1 hr before or 2 hr after a meal

SIDE EFFECTS
CNS: Headache, fever, fatigue
GI: Pancreatitis
INTEG: Rash, alopecia
MISC: Myalgia
OTHER: Hyperglycemia, hypophosphatemia, hyponatremia, secondary malignancy, hand/foot syndrome
CV: Cardiomyopathy, HF, thromboembolism
EENT: Uveitis, retinal detachment

PHARMACOKINETICS
Protein binding 99.7%, half-life 8 hr (dabrafenib), 10 hr, 21-22 hr metabolites, excreted 71% (feces), 23% (urine)

INTERACTIONS
Altered: dabrafenib concentrations—CYP3A4 inhibitors (ketoconazole, itraconazole, erythromycin, clarithromycin)
Decrease: dabrafenib concentrations—CYP3A4 inducers (dexamethasone, phenytoin, carBAMazepine, rifampin, PHENobarbital), antacids, proton pump inhibitors
Decrease: effect of CYP3A4, CYP2C9 substrates

Drug/Herb
Decrease: dabrafenib concentrations—St. John's wort

Drug/Food Test
Increase: dabrafenib effect—grapefruit juice; avoid use while taking product

NURSING CONSIDERATIONS
Assess:
• **Secondary malignancy:** has been reported with monotherapy; cutaneous squamous cell carcinoma (cuSCC), keratoacanthoma, and new primary malignant melanomas are increased when used in combination with trametinib, usually within 9 wk (cutaneous squamous cell carcinoma); basal cell carcinoma (4-36 wk). Perform a dermatologic evaluation before therapy, q2mo while on therapy, and for up to 6 mo after discontinuing therapy
• **Serious fever and febrile reaction:** hypotension, rigors/chills, dehydration, renal failure may occur; the incidence and severity of fever are higher when given with trametinib. Interruption of therapy, a dose reduction, or permanent therapy discontinuation may be needed. Monitor for signs and symptoms of infection. If a severe fever or febrile reaction occurs, monitor renal function (BUN/serum creatinine) during and after the event and give antipyretic agents when therapy is resumed. In those who develop a febrile reaction that does not resolve within 3 days of onset, give corticosteroids (predniSONE 10 mg/day **PO**) for at least 5 days; ensure that there is no evidence of active infection before starting corticosteroids

- **Hyperglycemia:** Monitor serum glucose levels at baseline and as clinically indicated
- **Uveitis, iritis, and iridocyclitis:** steroid and mydriatic ophthalmic drops may provide symptomatic relief for these conditions. Monitor for visual signs and symptoms of uveitis (blurred vision, photophobia, and eye pain). Continue at the same dose in iritis. Hold for mild or moderate uveitis that does not respond to ocular therapy, severe uveitis, or iridocyclitis; initiate treatment as indicated. Permanently discontinue in those who develop persistent grade 2 or higher uveitis that lasts longer than 6 wk
- **Bleeding:** major intracranial bleeding/ GI bleeding can occur when used in combination with trametinib. Monitor for signs of bleeding (frank blood, blood in stools, urine, vomit); evaluate any unexplained fall in hematocrit, hypotension, grade 3 bleeding hold product, grade 4 discontinue
- **Cardiomyopathy:** a decrease in left ventricular ejection fraction (LVEF) of 10% or greater from baseline and below the lower limit of normal (LLN) may occur and was higher when given in combination with trametinib. Obtain an echocardiogram or multigated acquisition (MUGA) scan prior to starting combination therapy, 1 mo after starting dabrafenib, and then q2-3mo during treatment. Hold dabrafenib for symptomatic congestive heart failure or LVEF below the LLN with an absolute decrease of greater than 20% from baseline. Resume dabrafenib at the same dose if LVEF improves to the institutional LLN and an absolute decrease of 10% or less from baseline
- **Palmar-plantar erythrodysesthesia syndrome (hand and foot syndrome):** may occur when given in combination with trametinib, usually within 37 days; hospitalization may be required due to a secondary infection of the skin. Interruption of therapy, a dose reduction, or permanent therapy discontinuation may be needed in those who develop severe skin toxicity

Evaluate:
- Therapeutic response: decrease in melanoma progression

Teach patient/family:
- To notify prescriber of new lesions
- To notify providers of all OTC, Rx, herbal products taken
- To take as prescribed 1 hr prior to or 2 hr after meals, to take a missed dose at least 6 hr before next dose
- To report adverse reactions immediately
- About reason for treatment, expected results
- Advise patients to report symptoms of severe hyperglycemia (excessive thirst, increased urinary frequency)
- Advise that other malignancies are possible
- **Pregnancy:** to use effective nonhormonal contraception during treatment and for at least 30 days after discontinuing treatment; not to breastfeed

---

⚠ HIGH ALERT

dacarbazine (Rx)
(da-kar′ba-zeen)
Func. class.: Antineoplastic alkylating agent
Chem. class.: Cytotoxic triazine

ACTION: Alkylates DNA, RNA; inhibits DNA, RNA synthesis; also responsible for breakage, cross-linking of DNA strands; activity is not cell-cycle–phase specific

USES: Hodgkin's disease, malignant melanoma
Unlabeled uses: Metastatic soft-tissue sarcoma in combination with other agents

CONTRAINDICATIONS: Breastfeeding, hypersensitivity
Precautions: Renal disease, infection

Black Box Warning: Pregnancy 1st trimester, radiation therapy, hepatic disease, bone marrow suppression, secondary malignancy, requires an experienced clinician

---

DOSAGE AND ROUTES
Metastatic malignant melanoma
- **Adult: IV** 2-4.5 mg/kg/day × 10 days or 100-250 mg/m^2/day × 5 days; repeat q3-4wk depending on response

Hodgkin's lymphoma
- **Adult: IV** 150 mg/m^2/day × 5 days with other agents, repeat q4wk; or 375 mg/m^2 on days 1 and 15 when given in combination, repeat q28days

Soft-tissue sarcoma (unlabeled)
- **Adult/child: IV** 250-300 mg/m^2/day as continuous infusion × 3 days q21-28days

Available forms: Powder for inj 100, 200, 500 mg vials

Administer:
- Antiemetic 30-60 min before giving product to prevent vomiting, nausea; vomiting may subside after several doses, nausea/vomiting may be severe and last several hours
- Antibiotics for prophylaxis of infection

IV route
- Use cytotoxic handling precautions
- Clarify all orders, double-check original order; may be fatal if wrong dose is given

Direct IV route
- After diluting 100 mg/9.9 or 200 mg/19.7 mL of sterile water for inj (10 mg/mL), give by direct IV over 2-3 min through Y-tube or 3-way stopcock

Intermittent IV INFUSION route
- May be further diluted in 50-250 mL D$_5$W or NS for inj, given as an infusion over $^1/_2$-1 hr
- Watch for extravasation; stop infusion, apply ice to area
- Store in light-resistant container in a dry area

Y-site compatibilities: Amifostine, anidulafungin, atenolol, aztreonam, bivalirudin, bleomycin, caspofungin, DAPTOmycin, dexmedetomidine, DOCEtaxel, DOXOrubicin, ertapenem, etoposide, fenoldopam, filgrastim, fludarabine, gemtuzumab, granisetron, levofloxacin, mechlorethamine, melphalan, nesiritide, octreotide, ondansetron, oxaliplatin, PACLitaxel, palonosetron, pamidronate, quinupristin-dalfopristin, sargramostim, teniposide, thiotepa, tigecycline, tirofiban, vinorelbine, voriconazole, zoledronic acid

SIDE EFFECTS
GI: *Nausea, anorexia, vomiting,* hepatotoxicity, diarrhea
HEMA: Thrombocytopenia, leukopenia, anemia
INTEG: *Alopecia,* dermatitis, pain at inj site, photosensitivity; severe sun reactions (high doses)
MISC: Flulike symptoms, malaise, fever, myalgia, hypotension
SYST: Anaphylaxis

PHARMACOKINETICS
Metabolized by liver; excreted in urine; half-life 5 hr, 5% protein bound

INTERACTIONS

Black Box Warning: **Toxicity, bone marrow suppression:** bone marrow suppressants, radiation, other antineoplastics

Increase: adverse reaction, decrease antibody reaction—live virus vaccines
Decrease: dacarbazine effect—phenytoin, PHENobarbital
Drug/Lab Test
Increase: BUN, AST, ALT
Decrease: platelets, WBC, RBC

NURSING CONSIDERATIONS
Assess:

Black Box Warning: **Bone marrow suppression:** monitor CBC, differential, platelet count weekly; notify prescriber of results

- Monitor temperature, may indicate beginning infection, I&O, for nausea, appetite

Black Box Warning: **Secondary malignancy:** assess for secondary malignancy that may occur with this product

- **Bleeding:** hematuria, guaiac, bruising, petechiae of mucosa or orifices q8hr
- Effects of alopecia on body image; discuss feelings about body changes

Black Box Warning: **Hepatotoxicity:** assess for jaundice of skin, sclera; dark urine; clay-colored stools; itchy skin; abdominal pain; fever; diarrhea; monitor hepatic studies before, during therapy (bilirubin, AST, ALT, LDH) as needed or monthly

• Inflammation of mucosa, breaks in skin
• IV site for irritation, redness, pain; if infiltration occurs, use hot packs at site
• **Hypersensitivity reactions, anaphylaxis:** discontinue product, administer meds for anaphylaxis
• Increased fluid intake to 2-3 L/day to prevent urate deposits, calculi formation

Black Box Warning: Product must be administered by those experienced in the use of cancer chemotherapy

Evaluate:
• Therapeutic response: decreased tumor size, spread of malignancy
Teach patient/family:
• That patient should avoid prolonged exposure to sun, wear sunscreen
• That hair may be lost during treatment; that a wig or hairpiece may make the patient feel better; that new hair may be different in color, texture
• To report signs of **infection:** fever, sore throat, flulike symptoms
• To report signs of **anemia:** fatigue, headache, faintness, SOB, irritability
• To report bleeding; to avoid use of razors, commercial mouthwash
• To avoid aspirin products or ibuprofen

Black Box Warning: **Pregnancy:** to notify prescriber if pregnancy is planned or suspected; to use reliable contraceptives during and for several mo after therapy; not to breastfeed

daclatasvir
(dak-lat′-as-vir)
Daklinza
Func. class.: Antiviral, antihepatitis C agent
Chem. class.: Hepatitis C virus NS5A replication inhibitor

ACTION: Active against chronic infections caused by ℞ genotype 3 hepatitis C virus (HCV); prevents viral RNA replication by impairing protein function

USES: Chronic hepatitis C, genotype 3 with complicated liver disease

CONTRAINDICATIONS: Hypersensitivity
Precautions: Pregnancy, breastfeeding, antimicrobial resistance, hepatic disease, hepatitis C with HIV coinfection, liver transplant

Black Box Warning: Hepatitis B exacerbation

DOSAGE AND ROUTES
HCV genotype 1 or 3
• **Adult: PO** 60 mg daily x 12 wk in combination with sofosbuvir
Adults without cirrhosis or who have compensated (Child-Pugh A) cirrhosis
• **Adult: PO** 60 mg once daily in combination with sofosbuvir
Adults receiving strong CYP3A inhibitors who do not have cirrhosis or who have compensated (Child-Pugh A) cirrhosis
• **Adult: PO** 30 mg once daily in combination with sofosbuvir
Adults receiving moderate CYP3A inducers who do not have cirrhosis or who have compensated (Child-Pugh A) cirrhosis
• **Adult: PO** 90 mg once daily in combination with sofosbuvir

SIDE EFFECTS
CNS: *Headache, fatigue*
GI: Diarrhea, nausea
MISC: HBV reactivation

PHARMACOKINETICS
Peak 2 hr, excreted feces 88%, protein binding; half-life 12-15 hr, metabolized in the liver by CYP3A4, affected by P-glycoprotein (P-gp), organic anion transporting polypeptides (OATP1B1 and OATP1B3), breast cancer resistance protein (BCRP)

Side effects: *italics* = common; red = life-threatening

INTERACTIONS

• Do not use with potent CYP3A4 inducers

Increase: each product—P-glycoprotein (P-gp) substrates

Increase: bradycardia—amiodarone; avoid concurrent use

Increase: HMG-COA reductase inhibitors effect

Increase: daclatasvir effect—potent CYP3A4 inhibitors (clarithromycin, indinavir, ketoconazole, voriconazole); reduce dose of daclatasvir

Decrease: daclatasvir effect—moderate CYP3A4 inducers (carBAMazepine, rifampin); increase dose of daclatasvir

Drug/Lab Test

Increase: lipase

Drug/Herb

Decrease: daclatasvir effect—St. John's wort

NURSING CONSIDERATIONS

Assess:

• **Liver transplant/cirrhosis:** may have lower sustained virologic response rates in cirrhosis, and use in prior liver transplant is unknown

• **HIV/hepatitis C coinfection:** all patients with HIV infection should be tested for hepatitis C, with continued annual screening for persons considered at high risk for acquiring hepatitis C. If hepatitis C and HIV coinfection is identified, treating both viral infections concurrently

• **Strong CYP3A4 inducers:** do not use concurrently; may lead to treatment failure; review patient's medication profile for potential drug interactions before starting treatment

Black Box Warning: **Hepatitis B exacerbation:** baseline HBV DNA concentration should be obtained before starting treatment; monitor HBsAg, HBV DNA, hepatic enzymes, bilirubin

• **Bradycardia:** <60 bpm, pulse, dizziness, confusion, memory problems, retake, then notify prescriber

• **Hepatitis C:** monitor plasma hepatitis C RNA and plasma HIV RNA baseline and during treatment, HBsAq and anti-HBC

NS5A resistance testing in type 1a with cirrhosis

• **Pregnancy/breastfeeding:** no well-controlled studies; use only if benefits outweigh fetal risk; use caution in breastfeeding, excretion is unknown

Evaluate:

• Therapeutic response: decreased symptoms of chronic hepatitis C

Teach patient/family:

• That optimal duration of treatment is 12 wk; that product is not a cure; that transmission may still occur and that drug must be taken with sofosbuvir, not to stop or double doses

• To avoid use with other medications, herbs, supplements unless approved by prescriber

• Not to stop abruptly unless directed; worsening of hepatitis may occur

• **Pregnancy/breastfeeding:** To notify prescriber if pregnancy is planned or suspected or if breastfeeding

---

dalbavancin
(dal-ba-van'sin)

Dalvance

Func. class.: Antiinfective

Chem. class.: Glycopeptide

ACTION: Binds to the bacterial cell walls, inhibiting their synthesis

USES: Treatment of acute bacterial skin and skin structure infections due to gram-positive organisms (cellulitis, major abscess, wound infections); *Staphylococcus aureus, Streptococcus agalactiae, S. anginosus, S. pyogenes*

CONTRAINDICATIONS: Hypersensitivity

Precautions: Antimicrobial resistance, breastfeeding, colitis, diarrhea, GI disease, inflammatory bowel disease, infusion-related reactions, pregnancy, pseudomembranous colitis, ulcerative colitis, vancomycin hypersensitivity, viral infection

---

DOSAGE AND ROUTES
• **Adult:** IV 1500 mg once or 1000 mg once, then 500 mg **IV** 1 wk later
Renal dose
• **Adult:** IV CCr <30 mL/min 1125 mg as a single dose or 750 mg once then 375 mg one week later
Available forms: Powder for injection 500 mg/vial
Administer:
IV INFUSION route
• Visually inspect parenteral products for particulate matter and discoloration
• **Reconstitution:** Reconstitute each 500 mg/25 mL sterile water for injection; to avoid foaming, alternate between gentle swirling and inversion until completely dissolved, do not shake; further dilution is required
• **Storage:** Refrigerate or store at room temperature. Do not freeze. The total time from reconstitution to dilution to use should not exceed 48 hr
• **Dilution:** Transfer the dose of reconstituted solution from the vial(s) to an IV bag or bottle containing D$_5$W (1-5 mg/mL), discard unused product
Intermittent IV INFUSION
• Give over 30 min, do not infuse with other medications or electrolytes, saline-based infusion solutions may cause precipitation and should not be used; if a common IV line is being used to administer other drugs, the line should be flushed before and after each dose

SIDE EFFECTS
CNS: Dizziness, headache, flushing
GI: Nausea, CDAD, abdominal pain, diarrhea
SYST: Red man syndrome, hypersensitivity reactions
INTEG: Rash, urticaria, infusion-related reactions, pruritus

PHARMACOKINETICS
Protein binding 93%, primarily to albumin, excreted in feces and urine, metabolism decreased in renal disease, half-life 8 days, peak infusions end

INTERACTIONS
None known

NURSING CONSIDERATIONS
Assess:
• BUN/creatinine; lower dose may be required in severe renal disease
• **CDAD:** bowel pattern daily; if severe diarrhea occurs, product should be discontinued
• **Infection:** B/P, pulse, temperature, characteristics of urine, stools, sputum baseline and during treatment
• IV site for infusion-site reactions
• **Anaphylaxis:** rash, urticaria, pruritus, wheezing; may occur a few days after administration
• **Red man–like syndrome:** flushing, rash over upper torso and neck; may occur after a few minutes of infusion; may be treated with antihistamines and a slower infusion
Evaluate:
• Therapeutic response: decreased symptoms of infection, negative C&S
Teach patient/family:
• To report sore throat, bruising, bleeding, joint pain **(blood dyscrasias)**; diarrhea with mucus, blood **(pseudomembranous colitis)**; rash, pruritus, wheezing **(hypersensitivity reactions)**
• **Pregnancy/breastfeeding:** To use non-hormonal contraceptive if on long-term therapy to notify health care professional if pregnancy is planned or suspected or if breastfeeding
• To notify prescriber of all OTC, prescription medications, and herbals used

---

dalfampridine (Rx)
(dal-fam′pri-deen)
Ampyra, Fampyra ✦
Func. class.: Neurological agent—multiple sclerosis
Chem. class.: Broad-spectrum potassium channel blocker

ACTION: Mechanism of action is not fully understood; a broad-spectrum potassium channel blocker that inhibits potassium channels and increased action potential conduction in demyelinated axons

Side effects: *italics* = common; red = life-threatening

USES: For improved walking in patients with multiple sclerosis

CONTRAINDICATIONS: Renal failure (CCr <50 mL/min), seizures
Precautions: Pregnancy, breastfeeding, geriatric patients, renal disease

DOSAGE AND ROUTES
• **Adult: PO** 10 mg q12hr
Renal dose
• **Adult: PO** CCr 51-80 mL/min, no dosage adjustment needed but seizure risk unknown; CCr ≤50 mL/min, do not use
Available forms: Ext rel tab 10 mg
Administer:
• Do not break, crush, or chew; give without regard to meals
• Do not give closer together than q12hr; seizures may occur
• Do not double doses; if a dose is missed, skip it

SIDE EFFECTS
CNS: Seizures, paresthesias, headache, dizziness, asthenia, insomnia
GI: Nausea, constipation, dyspepsia
GU: Urinary tract infection
MS: Back pain
SYST: Anaphylaxis

PHARMACOKINETICS
Bioavailability 96%; peak 3-4 hr (fasting), longer if taken with food; largely unbound to plasma proteins; 96% recovered in urine, half-life 5-6 hr

INTERACTIONS
• None known

NURSING CONSIDERATIONS
Assess:
• **Multiple sclerosis:** improved walking, including speed baseline and during treatment
• **Seizures:** more common in those with previous seizure disorder; risk increases with higher doses, discontinue, if seizures occur
• **Anaphylaxis:** wheezing, rash, pruritus, angioedema
Evaluate:
• Therapeutic response: ability to walk at improved speed in multiple sclerosis

Teach patient/family:
• To take as directed, not to double or skip doses, to take 12 hr apart, provide "Medication Guide"
• Expected results; side effects, including seizures
• To notify prescriber of all OTC, prescription medications, herbals, supplements taken
• **Anaphylaxis:** to notify prescriber immediately of wheezing, throat tightening, rash, swelling of face, lips
• **Seizures:** to notify prescriber immediately
• **Urinary tract infection:** to report burning, stinging on urination
• **Pregnancy/breastfeeding:** to notify prescriber if pregnancy is planned or suspected; not to breastfeed

---

⚠ HIGH ALERT

dalteparin (Rx)
(dahl′ta-pear-in)
Fragmin
Func. class.: Anticoagulant
Chem. class.: Low-molecular-weight heparin

ACTION: Inhibits factor Xa/IIa (thrombin), resulting in anticoagulation

USES: Unstable angina/non–Q-wave MI; prevention/treatment of deep venous thrombosis in abdominal surgery, hip replacement, or in those with restricted mobility during acute illness, pulmonary embolism
Unlabeled uses: VTE prophylaxis in gynecologic surgery

CONTRAINDICATIONS: Hypersensitivity to this product, heparin, or pork products; active major bleeding, hemophilia, leukemia with bleeding, thrombocytopenic purpura, cerebrovascular hemorrhage, cerebral aneurysm; those undergoing regional anesthesia for unstable angina, non–Q-wave MI, dalteparin-induced thrombocytopenia
Precautions: Hypersensitivity to benzyl alcohol, pregnancy, breastfeeding, children, recent childbirth, geriatric patients; hepatic

---

disease; severe renal disease; blood dyscrasias; bacterial endocarditis; acute nephritis; uncontrolled hypertension; recent brain, spine, eye surgery; congenital or acquired disorders; severe cardiac disease; peptic ulcer disease; hemorrhagic stroke; history of HIT; pericarditis; pericardial effusion; recent lumbar puncture; vasculitis; other diseases in which bleeding is possible

Black Box Warning: Epidural/spinal anesthesia, lumbar puncture

DOSAGE AND ROUTES
DVT/pulmonary embolism (cancer-associated venous thrombosis)
• **Adult: SUBCUT** 200 units/kg daily during 1st mo (max single dose 18,000 units), then 150 units/kg daily for mo 2-6 (max single dose 18,000 units), use prefilled syringe that is closest to calculated dose; if platelets are 50,000-100,000/mm^3, reduce dose by 2500 units until platelets ≥100,000 mm^3; if platelets <50,000/mm^3, discontinue until >50,000/mm^3

Hip replacement surgery/DVT prophylaxis
• **Adult: SUBCUT** 2500 units 2 hr before surgery and 2nd dose in the evening on the day of surgery (4-8 hr postop), then 5000 units **SUBCUT** 1st postop day and daily × 5-10 days

Unstable angina/non–Q-wave MI
• **Adult: SUBCUT** 120 units/kg q12hr × 5-8 days, max 10,000 units q12hr × 5-8 days with concurrent aspirin; continue until stable

DVT, prophylaxis for abdominal surgery
• **Adult: SUBCUT** 2500 units 1-2 hr before surgery; repeat daily × 5-10 days; for high-risk patients, >3400 units should be used

DVT prophylaxis in medical patients with severely restricted mobility due to acute illness
Adult: SUBCUT 5000 units q day × 12-14 days

Renal dose
• Adult: SUBCUT cancer patient with CCr <30 mL/min, monitor and adjust based on anti-factor Xa during extended treatment

VTE prophylaxis in gynecologic surgery (unlabeled)
• **Adults: SUBCUT** 2500 units daily starting 1-2 hr prior to surgery then daily

Available forms: Prefilled syringes, 2500, 5000 units/0.2 mL; 7500 units/0.3 mL; 10,000, 12,500, 15,000, 18,000, 25,000 units/mL

Administer:
• Cannot be used interchangeably (unit for unit) with unfractionated heparin or other LMWHs
• Do not give IM or IV product route; approved is SUBCUT only; do not mix with other inj or sol
• Have patient sit or lie down; SUBCUT inj may be 2 inches from umbilicus in a U-shape, upper outer side of thigh, or upper outer quadrangle of the buttocks; rotate inj sites
• Change inj site daily; use at same time of day

SIDE EFFECTS
CNS: Intracranial bleeding
HEMA: Thrombocytopenia, DIC
INTEG: Skin necrosis, inj site reaction
SYST: Hypersensitivity, hemorrhage, anaphylaxis

PHARMACOKINETICS
87% absorbed, excreted by kidneys, elimination half-life 2-2.3 hr, peak 2-4 hr, onset 1-2 hr, duration up to 24 hr

INTERACTIONS
Increase: bleeding risk—aspirin, oral anticoagulants, platelet inhibitors, NSAIDs, salicylates, thrombolytics, some cephalosporins

Drug/Herb
Increase: bleeding risk— angelica, capsicum, chamomile, dandelion, dan shen, feverfew, garlic, ginger, ginkgo, horse chestnut

Drug/Lab Test
Increase: AST, ALT
Decrease: platelets

NURSING CONSIDERATIONS
Assess:

• **Blood studies** (Hct/Hgb, CBC, platelets, anti-Xa,) during treatment because bleeding can occur

• **Bleeding:** bleeding gums, petechiae, ecchymosis, black tarry stools, hematuria, epistaxis; decrease in Hct, B/P may indicate bleeding, possible hemorrhage; notify prescriber immediately; product should be discontinued

Black Box Warning: **Epidural/spinal anesthesia:** neurologic impairment may occur frequently when neuraxial anesthesia has been used; spinal/epidural hematomas may occur, with paralysis; numbness in lower extremities; bowel, bladder changes; back pain; notify prescriber immediately; those at greatest risk are those taking products that cause increased bleeding risk

• **Hypersensitivity:** fever, skin rash, urticaria; notify prescriber immediately

• Needed dosage change q1-2wk; dose may need to be decreased if bleeding occurs

• **Pregnancy/breastfeeding:** no well-controlled studies; use only if clearly needed; LMWH does not cross placenta; benefits and risk must be weighed with provider; if used, discontinue 24 hr before induction or cesarean delivery; use of multidose vials containing benzyl alcohol is contraindicated; use caution in breastfeeding

Evaluate:

• Therapeutic response: absence of DVT/PE, prevention of complication (unstable angina, non-Q-wave MI)

Teach patient/family:

• To avoid OTC preparations that contain aspirin, other anticoagulants unless approved by prescriber; serious product interactions may occur

• To use soft-bristle toothbrush to avoid bleeding gums; to avoid contact sports; to use electric razor; to avoid IM inj

• **Bleeding:** To report any signs of bleeding (gums, under skin, urine, stools), unusual bruising

TREATMENT OF OVERDOSE:
Protamine sulfate 1% given IV; 1 mg protamine/100 anti-Xa international units of dalteparin given

---

⚠ HIGH ALERT

dantrolene (Rx)
(dan'troe-leen)
Dantrium, Revonto, Ryanodex
Func. class.: Skeletal muscle relaxant, direct acting
Chem. class.: Hydantoin

Do not confuse:
Dantrium/danazol

ACTION: Interferes with intracellular release of calcium from the sarcoplasmic reticulum necessary to initiate contraction; slows catabolism in malignant hyperthermia

USES: Spasticity in multiple sclerosis, stroke, spinal cord injury, cerebral palsy, malignant hyperthermia
Unlabeled uses: Neuroleptic malignant syndrome

CONTRAINDICATIONS: Hypersensitivity, hepatic disease, hepatitis
Precautions: Pregnancy, breastfeeding, geriatric patients, peptic ulcer disease, cardiac/renal/hepatic disease, stroke, seizure disorder, diabetes mellitus, ALS, COPD, MS, mannitol/gelatin hypersensitivity, labor, lactase deficiency, extravasation

Black Box Warning: Hepatotoxicity

DOSAGE AND ROUTES
Spasticity

• **Adult:** PO 25 mg/day × 7 days; may increase to 25-100 mg bid-qid, max 400 mg/day, may be increased q7days as needed

• **Child:** PO 0.5 mg/kg/day given in divided doses bid, may be increased q7days as needed, max 400 mg/day

Prevention of malignant hyperthermia

• **Adult/child:** PO 4-8 mg/kg/day in 3-4 divided doses × 1-3 days before procedure, give last dose 4 hr preop; **IV** 2.5 mg/kg before anesthesia

---

Malignant hyperthermia
• **Adult/child:** IV 1-2.5 mg/kg, may repeat to total dose of 10 mg/kg; **PO** 4-8 mg/kg/day in 4 divided doses × 1-3 days
Neuroleptic malignant syndrome (unlabeled)
• **Adult:** PO 100-300 mg/day in divided doses; IV 1.25-1.5 mg/kg
Available forms: Caps 25, 50, 100 mg; powder for inj 20 mg/vial, 250 mg/vial
Administer:
• Avoid use with other CNS depressants
PO route
• Do not crush or chew caps
• Caps may be opened, mixed with juice, and swallowed
• With meals for GI symptoms
IV direct route (Revonto)
• **Dantrium:** IV after reconstituting each 20 mg/60 mL sterile water for inj without bacteriostatic agent (333 mcg/mL); shake until clear; give by rapid IV push through Y-tube or 3-way stopcock; follow with prescribed doses immediately; may also give by intermittent infusion over 1 hr before anesthesia
• Considered incompatible in sol or syringe; compatibility unknown
• Store in tight container at room temperature; protect diluted sol from light, use reconstituted sol within 6 hr

IV, direct route (Ryanodex) (malignant hyperthermia)
• Reconstitute vial (250 mg) with 5 mL sterile water for inj without a bacteriostatic agent and shake vial
• Do not dilute or transfer reconstituted solution
• Administer into IV catheter with continuous sodium chloride 0.9% IV or dextrose 5% injection or into an indwelling catheter after ensuring its patency, and flush the line after administration

SIDE EFFECTS
CNS: *Dizziness, weakness, drowsiness,* headache, insomnia, seizures, flushing
CV: Hypotension
EENT: Blurred vision, mydriasis, excessive lacrimation

GI: *Nausea,* constipation, vomiting, increased AST, alk phos, anorexia, hepatitis, dyspepsia, hepatotoxicity
GU: Urinary frequency, nocturia, impotence, crystalluria
HEMA: Eosinophilia, aplastic anemia, leukopenia, thrombocytopenia
INTEG: Rash, pruritus, extravasation (tissue necrosis), phlebitis
RESP: Pleural effusion, pulmonary edema, respiratory depression, dyspnea
SYST: Anaphlaxis

PHARMACOKINETICS
PO: Peak 5 hr, highly protein bound, half-life 8.7-11 hr, metabolized in liver, excreted in urine (metabolites), absorption poor (35%)

INTERACTIONS
Increase: dysrhythmias—verapamil
Increase: hepatotoxicity—estrogens, other hepatotoxics
Increase: CNS depression—alcohol, tricyclics, opiates, barbiturates, sedatives, hypnotics, antihistamines, tramadol

NURSING CONSIDERATIONS
Assess:
• **Spasticity:** muscle, nervous system status baseline and during treatment, identify improvement
• **Malignant hyperthermia:** patient/family reactions to anesthesia, monitor ECG, B/P, I&O
• **Respiratory status:** dyspnea, trouble breathing
• **Seizures:** increased seizure activity, ECG in epilepsy patient; poor seizure control has occurred
• I&O ratio; check for urinary retention, frequency, hesitancy, especially geriatric patients

Black Box Warning: **Hepatotoxicity:** hepatic function by frequent determination of AST, ALT, bilirubin, alk phos, GGTP; renal function studies, BUN, creatinine, CBC, use lowest dose possible; check for jaundice, dark urine, diarrhea, weakness; product should be discontinued, occurs with oral form

- **Allergic reactions:** rash, fever, respiratory distress
- Severe weakness, numbness in extremities; prescriber should be notified and product discontinued
- Tolerance: increased need/more frequent requests for medication, increased pain
- CNS depression: dizziness, drowsiness, insomnia, psychiatric symptoms
- **Pregnancy/breastfeeding:** no well-controlled studies; avoid use in pregnancy, breastfeeding

Evaluate:
- Therapeutic response: decreased pain, spasticity

Teach patient/family:
- Not to discontinue medication quickly because hallucinations, spasticity, tachycardia will occur; product should be tapered off over 1-2 wk; to notify prescriber of abdominal pain, jaundiced sclera, clay-colored stools, change in color of urine
- That if improvement does not occur within 6 wk, prescriber may discontinue product
- To avoid hazardous activities if drowsiness, dizziness occurs
- To report severe weakness, seizures, signs of liver insufficiency
- To avoid using OTC medications: cough preparations, antihistamines, other CNS depressants, alcohol unless directed by prescriber
- To take with meals
- **Malignant hyperthermia:** to carry a medical ID stating condition, products used

---

⚠ HIGH ALERT

dapagliflozin
(dap'a-gli-floe'zin)

Farxiga

Func. class.: Oral antidiabetic
Chem. class.: Sodium-glucose co-transporter 2 (SGLT 2) inhibitor

Do not confuse:
Farxiga/Fetzima

ACTION:
Blocks reabsorption of glucose by the kidney, increases glucose excretion, lowers blood glucose concentrations

USES: Type 2 diabetes mellitus, with diet and exercise

CONTRAINDICATIONS: Dialysis, renal failure, hypersensitivity, breastfeeding, diabetic ketoacidosis
Precautions: Pregnancy, children, renal/hepatic disease, hypothyroidism, hyperglycemia, hypotension, bladder cancer, hypercholesterolemia, pituitary insufficiency, type 1 diabetes mellitus, malnutrition, fever, dehydration, adrenal insufficiency, geriatrics, genital fungal infections, hypoglycemia

DOSAGE AND ROUTES
- **Adult: PO** 5 mg in AM; may increase to 10 mg daily if needed

Renal dose
- **Adult:** PO eGFR ≥60 mL/min/1.73 m² no change, eGFR <60 mL/min, do not use

Available forms: Tabs 5, 10 mg
Administer:

PO route
- Once daily in AM without regard to food
- Store at room temperature

SIDE EFFECTS
GI: Pancreatitis, constipation, nausea
GU: Cystitis, candidiasis, urinary frequency, polydipsia, polyuria, increased serum creatinine; renal impairment/failure; infections
INTEG: Photosensitivity, rash, pruritus
META: Hypercholesterolemia, lipidemia, hypoglycemia, hyperkalemia, hypomagnesemia, hypo/hyperphosphatemia
MISC: Bone fractures, hypotension; dehydration; orthostatic hypotension; hypersensitivity; new bladder cancer

PHARMACOKINETICS
91% protein binding, primary excretion in urine, half-life 12.9 hr; primarily metabolized by O-glucuronidation by UGT1A9; minor CYP3A4; Cmax is less than 2 hr

---

INTERACTIONS

• Do not use gatifloxacin

Increase: hypoglycemia—sulfonylureas, insulin, MAOIs, salicylates, fibric acid derivatives, bile acid sequestrates, ACE inhibitors, angiotensin II receptor antagonists, beta blockers; adjust antidiabetics

Increase or decrease: glycemic control—androgens, lithium, bortezomib, quinolones

Decrease: effect, hyperglycemia—digestive enzymes, intestinal absorbents, thiazide diuretics, loop diuretics, corticosteroids, estrogen, progestins, oral contraceptives, sympathomimetics, isoniazid, phenothiazines, protease inhibitors, atypical antipsychotics, carbonic anhydrase inhibitors, cycloSPORINE, tacrolimus, baclofen

Drug/Lab Test

Increase: Hct, LDL

Decrease: eGFR

NURSING CONSIDERATIONS

Assess:

• **Hypoglycemia** (weakness, hunger, dizziness, tremors, anxiety, tachycardia, sweating) when used with other agents even though product does not cause hypoglycemia; if patient is on sulfonylureas or insulin, hypoglycemia may be additive; if hypoglycemia occurs, treat with dextrose or, if severe, with IV glucagon; monitor HbA1c, lipid panel, blood glucose, BUN, creatinine; if renal function is reduced, discontinue; monitor volume status, B/P, usually in those with eGFR <60 mL/min/1.73m^2; more frequent in those with poor renal function

• **Pregnancy/breastfeeding:** avoid use in pregnancy; do not breastfeed

• Renal function: baseline and periodically; discontinue if renal function is reduced; assess for signs of urinary tract infections (serious)

• **Bone fracture risk:** avoid use in those at increased risk of fractures; renal impairment increases fracture risk

• **Mycotic infections:** increased risk of mycotic infections, especially genital; caution in those with previous infections or in uncircumcised males

• Hypersensitivity: discontinue immediately

• Ketoacidosis: increased urine/serum ketone levels, may occur without increased glucose levels, may occur more frequently in those with reduced intake of food, fluids, or in serious conditions

Evaluate:

• Therapeutic response: improved signs/symptoms of diabetes mellitus (decreased polyuria, polydipsia, polyphagia); clear sensorium, absence of dizziness, stable gait; HbA1c WNL

Teach patient/family:

• The symptoms of hypo/hyperglycemia, what to do about each

• That medication must be taken as prescribed; explain consequences of discontinuing medication abruptly; that insulin may need to be used for stress, including trauma, fever, surgery

• To avoid OTC medications and herbal supplements unless approved by health care provider

• That diabetes is a lifelong illness; that the diet and exercise regimen must be followed; that this product is not a cure

• To carry emergency ID and glucose source

• That blood glucose monitoring and periodic lab tests are required to assess product effect

• That GI side effects may occur

• That there is a risk of renal impairment, dehydration, and bladder cancer

• To report immediately fever, itching, change in urine output, light-headedness or feeling faint, other signs of urinary tract infection

• To ensure adequate fluid intake to avoid dehydration and/or hypotension; to report symptoms to provider

---

- **Ketoacidosis:** to report immediately confusion, abdominal pain, fatigue, trouble breathing, nausea, vomiting, food intolerance

---

> **⚠ HIGH ALERT**

dapagliflozin/saxagliptin

(dap′a-gli-floe′zin/sax-a-glip′tin)

Qtern

Func. class.: Oral antidiabetic

Chem. class.: Sodium-glucose cotransporter 2 (SGLT2) inhibitor/dipeptidyl peptidase-4 (DPP-4) inhibitor antidiabetics

ACTION: Blocks reabsorption of glucose by the kidney, increases glucose excretion, lowers blood glucose concentrations

USES: Type 2 diabetes mellitus, with diet and exercise

CONTRAINDICATIONS: Dialysis, renal failure, hypersensitivity, breastfeeding, diabetic ketoacidosis

Precautions: Pregnancy, children, renal/hepatic disease, hypothyroidism, hyperglycemia, hypotension, bladder cancer, hypercholesterolemia, pituitary insufficiency, type 1 diabetes mellitus, malnutrition, fever, dehydration, adrenal insufficiency, geriatrics, genital fungal infections, hypoglycemia

DOSAGE AND ROUTES

For the treatment of type 2 diabetes mellitus in combination with diet and exercise

- **Adult: PO** 10 mg dapagliflozin and 5 mg saxagliptin once daily, taken in the morning, with or without food

Renal dose

- **Adult: PO** eGFR 60 mL/min/1.73 m^2 or more: no change; eGFR <60 mL/min/1.73 m^2: do not start in these patients. In patients currently taking the product, discontinue when eGFR is persistently <60 mL/min/1.73 m^2; eGFR <45 mL/min/1.73 m^2: do not use

Available forms: Tabs 10 mg, 5 mg

Administer:

- Do not cut, split, crush; swallow whole
- Give q day in the morning, with or without food

SIDE EFFECTS

CNS: Dizziness, fatigue

GI: Abdominal pain, pancreatitis, constipation, nausea

GU: Cystitis, candidiasis, urinary frequency, polydipsia, polyuria, increased serum creatinine, renal impairment/failure, infections

INTEG: Photosensitivity, rash, pruritus

META: Hypercholesterolemia, lipidemia, hypoglycemia, hyperkalemia, hypomagnesemia, hypo/hyperphosphatemia

MISC: Bone fractures, hypotension, dehydration, orthostatic hypotension, hypersensitivity, bladder cancer

PHARMACOKINETICS

91% protein binding, primary excretion in urine, half-life 12.9 hr; primarily metabolized by O-glucuronidation by UGT1A9, minor CYP3A4; Cmax is <2 hr

INTERACTIONS

Increase: hypoglycemia—sulfonylureas, insulin, MAOIs, salicylates, fibric acid derivatives, bile acid sequestrates, ACE inhibitors, angiotensin II receptor antagonists, beta blockers

Increase or decrease glycemic control: androgens, lithium, bortezomib, quinolones

Decrease: effect, hyperglycemia—digestive enzymes, intestinal absorbents, thiazide diuretics, loop diuretics, corticosteroids, estrogens, progestins, hormonal contraceptives, sympathomimetics, isoniazid, phenothiazines, protease inhibitors, atypical antipsychotics, carbonic anhydrase inhibitors, cyclosporine, tacrolimus, baclofen

Drug/Lab Test

Increase: Hct, LDL

NURSING CONSIDERATIONS

Assess:

- **Hypoglycemia** (weakness, hunger, dizziness, tremors, anxiety, tachycardia):

---

even though product does not cause hypoglycemia, if patient is on sulfonylureas or insulin, hypoglycemia may be additive; if hypoglycemia occurs, treat with dextrose or IV glucagon, monitor HbA1c, lipid panel, blood glucose, BUN, creatinine; if renal function is decreased, discontinue

• **Renal function:** baseline and periodically; discontinue if renal function is reduced; monitor for signs of infection (urinary infections)

• **Hypersensitivity:** discontinue immediately

• **Hypotension:** monitor volume status, B/P, usually in those with eGFR <60 mL/min/1.73m^2; more frequent in those with poor renal function

Evaluate:

• Therapeutic response: improved signs/symptoms of diabetes mellitus (decreased polyuria, polydipsia, polyphagia); clear sensorium, absence of dizziness, stable gait; HbA1c WNL

Teach patient/family:

• The symptoms of hypoglycemia/hyperglycemia and what to do about each

• That medication must be taken as prescribed; explain consequences of discontinuing abruptly, that insulin may be needed in times of stress, trauma, surgery, fever

• To report immediately fever, itching, change in urine output, light-headedness, or feeling faint

• To avoid OTC medications and herbal supplements unless approved by health provider

• That diabetes is a lifelong illness; that the diet and exercise regimen must be followed; that this product is not a cure

• To carry emergency ID and glucose source

• That blood glucose monitoring and periodic lab tests are required to assess product effect

• That there is a risk of renal impairment, dehydration, and bladder cancer

v• To use adequate fluids to decrease hypotension

• **Ketoacidosis:** to report immediately confusion, abdominal pain, fatigue, trouble breathing

DAPTOmycin (Rx)

(dap'toe-mye-sin)

Cubicin Cubicin RF

Func. class.: Antiinfective—miscellaneous

Chem. class.: Lipopeptides

D

ACTION: A new class of antiinfective; it binds to the bacterial membrane and results in a rapid depolarization of the membrane potential, thereby leading to inhibition of DNA, RNA, and protein synthesis

USES: Bacteremia, endocarditis, UTI, complicated skin, skin-structure infections caused by *Staphylococcus aureus* (MRSA, MSSA) including methicillin-resistant strains, *Streptococcus agalactiae, Streptococcus dysgalactiae, Enterococcus faecalis* (vancomycin-susceptible strains), *Streptococcus pyogenes* (group A beta hemolytic), *Staphylococcus aureus, Staphylococcus epidermidis, Corynebacterium jeikeium, Staphylococcus haemolyticus*

CONTRAINDICATIONS: Hypersensitivity

Precautions: Pregnancy, breastfeeding, children, geriatric patients, GI/renal disease, myopathy, ulcerative/pseudomembranous colitis, rhabdomyolysis, eosinophilic pneumonia

DOSAGE AND ROUTES

Complicated skin and skin structure infections

• **Adult:** IV INFUSION 4 mg/kg over ½ hr diluted in 0.9% NaCl, give q24hr × 7-14 days; some indications may use up to 6 mg/kg

• **Adolescent/child/infant ≥5 mo (unlabeled):** IV 4-6 mg/kg/day

***Staphylococcus aureus* bacteremia, right-sided infective endocarditis**

• **Adult:** IV INFUSION 6 mg/kg daily × 2-6 wk, up to 8-10 mg/kg daily; treatment failures should use another agent

• **Child 12-17 yr:** IV INFUSION 5 mg/kg/dose q24hr for up to 14 days

• **Child 7-11 yr:** IV INFUSION 7 mg/kg/dose q24hr up to 14 days

Side effects: *italics* = common; red = life-threatening

- **Child 2-6 yr: IV INFUSION** 9 g/kg/dose q24hr up to 14 days

Renal dose

- **Adult: IV INFUSION** CCr <30 mL/min, hemodialysis, CAPD 4 mg/kg q48hr, 6 mg/kg q48hr (bacteremia)

Available forms: Lyophilized powder for inj 500 mg/vial

Administer:

Intermittent IV infusion route

- Obtain culture and sensitivity; can begin treatment before results
- After reconstitution with 10 mL 0.9% NaCl (500 mg/10 mL), further dilution is needed with 0.9 NaCl; infuse over $1/2$ hr or give reconstituted sol (50 mg/mL) by

Direct IV route

- inj over 2 min; do not use dextrose-containing solutions
- Refrigerate vials, for single use only, discard unused portion; prepared solutions are stable for 12 hr at room temperature or 48 hr refrigerated

Cubin RF:

Direct IV Route (Push)

- Reconstitute 500mg/10mL (50mg/mL) sterile water for injection or bacteriostatic water for injection, us ≤ 21 G needle, swirl, give over 2 mins

Intermittent IV Infusion Route

- Further dilute in 50 mL 0.9% NaCl give over 30 mins; child ≥7 yrs give over 30 mins at 1.67 mL/min

Y-site compatibilities: Alfentanil, amifostine, amikacin, aminocaproic acid, aminophylline, amiodarone, amphotericin B liposome, ampicillin, ampicillin-sulbactam, argatroban, arsenic trioxide, atenolol, atracurium, azithromycin, aztreonam, bivalirudin, bleomycin, bumetanide, buprenorphine, busulfan, butorphanol, calcium chloride/gluconate, CARBOplatin, carmustine, caspofungin, ceFAZolin, cefepime, cefotaxime, cefoTEtan, cefOXitin, cefTAZidime, ceftizoxime, cefTRIAXone, cefuroxime, chloramphenicol, chlorproMAZINE, cimetidine, ciprofloxacin, cisatracurium, CISplatin, clindamycin, cyclophosphamide, cycloSPORINE, dacarbazine, DACTINomycin, DAUNOrubicin, dexamethasone, dexmedetomidine, dexrazoxane, diazepam, digoxin, diltiazem, diphenhydrAMINE, DOBUTamine, DOCEtaxel, DOPamine, doripenem, doxacurium, DOXOrubicin, DOXOrubicin liposomal, doxycycline, droperidol, enalaprilat, ePHEDrine, EPINEPHrine, epirubicin, eptifibatide, ertapenem, erythromycin, esmolol, etoposide, famotidine, fenoldopam, fentaNYL, fluconazole, fludarabine, fluorouracil, foscarnet, fosphenytoin, furosemide, ganciclovir, gentamicin, glycopyrrolate, granisetron, haloperidol, heparin, hydrALAZINE, hydrocortisone, HYDROmorphone, hydrOXYzine, IDArubicin, ifosfamide, inamrinone, insulin (regular), irinotecan, isoproterenol, ketorolac, labetalol, lepirudin, leucovorin, levofloxacin, lidocaine, linezolid, LORazepam, magnesium sulfate, mannitol, mechlorethamine, melphalan, meperidine, meropenem, mesna, metaraminol, methyldopate, methylPREDNISolone, metoclopramide, metoprolol, midazolam, milrinone, mitoXANtrone, mivacurium, morphine, moxifloxacin, mycophenolate mofetil, nafcillin, nalbuphine, naloxone, niCARDipine, nitroprusside, norepinephrine, octreotide, ondansetron, oxaliplatin, oxytocin, PACLitaxel, palonosetron, pamidronate, pancuronium, PEMEtrexed, pentamidine, PHENobarbital, phenylephrine, piperacillin-tazobactam, polymyxin B, potassium acetate/chloride/phosphates, procainamide, prochlorperazine, promethazine, propranolol, quinupristin-dalfopristin, ranitidine, rocuronium, sodium acetate/bicarbonate/citrate/phosphates, succinylcholine, sulfamethoxazole-trimethoprim, tacrolimus, teniposide, theophylline, thiotepa, ticarcillin, ticarcillin-clavulanate, tigecycline, tirofiban, tobramycin, topotecan, trimethobenzamide, vasopressin, vecuronium, verapamil, vinBLAStine, vinCRIStine, vinorelbine, voriconazole, zidovudine, zoledronic acid

SIDE EFFECTS

CNS: Headache, insomnia, dizziness

CV: Hypo/hypertension

GI: Nausea, constipation, diarrhea, vomiting, dyspepsia, CDAD, abdominal pain

GU: Nephrotoxicity

HEMA: Anemia

INTEG: Rash, pruritus, injection site reactions

MS: Rhabdomyolysis
RESP: Cough, eosinophilic pneumonia, dyspnea
SYST: Anaphylaxis, DRESS, Stevens-Johnson syndrome, **angioedema**

PHARMACOKINETICS
Site of metabolism unknown, protein binding 92%, terminal half-life 8.1 hr, 78% excreted unchanged (urine), excreted in breast milk, peak infusions end, duration 24 hr

INTERACTIONS
• May alter anticoagulant levels—warfarin; monitor PT, INR
Increase: tobramycin levels
Increase: daptomycin action—tobramycin
Increase: myopathy—HMG-CoA reductase inhibitors
Drug/Lab Test
Increase: CPK, AST, ALT, BUN, creatinine, albumin, LDH
Increase/Decrease: glucose
Decrease: alkaline phosphatase, magnesium, phosphate, bicarbonate

NURSING CONSIDERATIONS
Assess:
• **Eosinophilic pneumonia:** dyspnea, fever, cough, shortness of breath; if left untreated, can lead to respiratory failure and death
• **DRESS:** swelling, rash, fever, may lead to organ involvement, discontinue product
• **Nephrotoxicity:** any patient with compromised renal system; toxicity may occur; BUN, creatinine
• **Rhabdomyolysis:** check for myopathy, CPK >1000 U/L (>5 × ULN), discontinue product, muscle pain, weakness; caution if concomitant HMG-CoA reductase inhibitor therapy, consider discontinuation of therapy
• **Bowel function:** diarrhea, fever, abdominal pain; report to prescriber; CDAD may occur
• **I&O ratio:** report hematuria, oliguria; nephrotoxicity may occur
• **B/P** during administration; hypotension/hypertension may occur
• Signs of infection
• **Pregnancy/breastfeeding:** identify whether pregnancy is planned or suspected; avoid use in pregnancy or breastfeeding, lack of controlled studies

Evaluate:
• Therapeutic response: negative culture, resolution of infection
Teach patient/family:
• About allergies before treatment, reaction to each medication
• To report sore throat, fever, fatigue; could indicate superinfection; diarrhea; muscle weakness, pain, shortness of breath
• To avoid driving, hazardous activities until response is known; may cause dizziness
• To avoid breastfeeding, use in pregnancy

⚠ HIGH ALERT
RARELY USED

daratumumab
(dar′ a- toom-ue-mab)
Darzalex
Func. class.: Antineoplastic

USES: For the treatment of multiple myeloma in patients who have received at least 3 prior lines of therapy including a proteasome inhibitor (PI) and an immunomodulatory agent or who are double-refractory to a PI and an immunomodulatory agent

CONTRAINDICATIONS: Hypersensitivity

DOSAGE AND ROUTES
• **Adult: IV** 16 mg/kg (actual body weight) wkly on wk 1 to 8 (8 doses), 16 mg/kg q other week on wk 9 to 24 (8 doses), and then 16 mg/kg q4weeks starting on wk 25 until disease progression; premedicate 1-3 hr before infusion with corticosteroid, oral antipyretic, oral or IV antihistamine

⚠ HIGH ALERT

darbepoetin alfa (Rx)
(dar′bee-poh′eh-tin)
Aranesp
Func. class.: Hematopoietic agent
Chem. class.: Recombinant human erythropoietin

ACTION: Stimulates erythropoiesis by the same mechanism as endogenous

Side effects: *italics* = common; red = life-threatening

erythropoietin; in response to hypoxia, erythropoietin is produced in the kidney and released into the bloodstream, where it interacts with progenitor stem cells to increase red-cell production

USES: Anemia associated with chronic renal failure in patients on and not on dialysis, and anemia in nonmyeloid malignancies for patients receiving coadministered chemotherapy

CONTRAINDICATIONS: Hypersensitivity to hamster protein products, human albumin, polysorbate 80; uncontrolled hypertension; red-cell aplasia
Precautions: Pregnancy, breastfeeding, children, seizure disorder, porphyria, hypertension, sickle cell disease; vit B_{12}, folate deficiency; chronic renal failure, dialysis; latex hypersensitivity, CABG, angina, anemia

> Black Box Warning: Hgb >11 g/dL, neoplastic disease, MI, stroke, thromboembolic disease

DOSAGE AND ROUTES
Correction of anemia in chronic renal failure
• **Adult:** SUBCUT/IV 0.45 mcg/kg as a single inj; every wk, titrate, max target Hgb of 11 g/dL
Anemia due to chemotherapy
• **Adult:** SUBCUT 2.25 mcg/kg/wk or 500 mcg q3wk
Epoetin alfa to darbepoetin conversion
• **Adult:** SUBCUT/IV (epoetin alfa <2500 units/wk) 6.25 mcg/wk; (epoetin alfa 2500-4999 units/wk) 12.5 mcg/wk; (epoetin alfa 5000-10,999 units/wk) 25 mcg/wk; (epoetin alfa 11,000-17,999 units/wk) 40 mcg/wk; (epoetin alfa 18,000-33,999 units/wk) 60 mcg/wk; (epoetin alfa 34,000-89,999 units/wk) 100 mcg/wk; (epoetin alfa >90,000 units/wk) 200 mcg/wk
Available forms: Sol for inj 25, 40, 60, 100, 150, 200, 300, 500 mcg/mL
Administer:
• Transfusions may still be required for anemia, use iron supplements with this product

SUBCUT route
• May be used without diluting into vein
• Do not give intradermally
IV route
• Without shaking; check for discoloration, particulate matter, do not use if present; do not dilute, do not mix with other products or sol, discard unused portion, do not pool unused portions
• IV given direct undiluted or bolus into IV tubing or venous line after completion of dialysis; watch for clotting of line
• Adjust dosage every mo or more
• Store refrigerated, do not freeze; protect from light

SIDE EFFECTS
CNS: Seizures, headache, dizziness, stroke
CV: *Hypo/hypertension,* cardiac arrest, *angina pectoris,* HF, acute MI, dysrhythmias, chest pain, edema
GI: *Diarrhea, vomiting, nausea, abdominal pain, constipation*
HEMA: Red-cell aplasia
MISC: *Infection, fatigue, fever*
MS: *Bone pain, myalgia, limb pain, back pain, arthralgia*
RESP: *Dyspnea, cough, bronchitis*
SYST: Allergic reactions, anaphylaxis

PHARMACOKINETICS
IV: Onset of increased reticulocyte count 2-6 wk; distributed to vascular space; absorption slow and rate limiting; terminal half-life 49 hr (SUBCUT), 21 hr (IV); peak concentrations at 34 hr; increased Hgb levels not generally observed until 2-6 wk after treatment initiated

INTERACTIONS
Increase: darbepoetin alfa effect—androgens
Drug/Lab Test
Increase: WBC, platelets, Hgb
Decrease: bleeding time

NURSING CONSIDERATIONS
Assess:
• Symptoms of anemia: fatigue, dyspnea, pallor
• **Serious allergic reactions:** rash, urticaria; if anaphylaxis occurs, stop product, administer emergency treatment (rare)

Black Box Warning: Increased risk of death if hemoglobin >11 g/dL: monitor Hgb prior to and weekly × 4 wk or after change in dose and then often after target range has been reached; a rise >1g/dL over 2 wk may increase risks; reduce dose, keep Hgb <10 g/dL in chronic kidney disease

Black Box Warning: Renal studies: urinalysis, protein, blood, BUN, creatinine, electrolytes; monitor dialysis shunts; during dialysis, heparin may need to be increased; those with renal dysfunction may be at greater risk of death. Keep Hgb <10 g/dL in chronic kidney disease

Black Box Warning: Blood studies: ferritin, transferrin monthly; transferrin saturation ≥20%, ferritin ≥100 ng/mL; Hgb 2×/wk until stabilized in target range (30%-33%), then at regular intervals; those with endogenous erythropoietin levels of <500 units/L respond to this agent; iron stores should be corrected before beginning therapy; if there is lack of response, obtain folic acid, iron, B$_{12}$ levels

Black Box Warning: Neoplastic disease: breast, non–small-cell lung, head and neck, lymphoid, or cervical cancers, increased tumor progression; use lowest dose to avoid RBC transfusion

• B/P: check for rising B/P as Hgb rises; antihypertensives may be needed

Black Box Warning: CV status: hypertension may occur rapidly, leading to **hypertensive encephalopathy;** Hgb >11 g/dL may lead to stroke, MI, death; do not administer

• I&O; report drop in output to <50 mL/hr
• **Seizures:** if Hgb is increased by 1 g/dL within 2 wk, institute seizure precautions, decrease dose
• CNS symptoms: sweating, pain in long bones
• **Dialysis patients:** thrill, bruit of shunts; monitor for circulation impairment
• **Pregnancy/breastfeeding:** Those who become pregnant should register with

Amgen's Pregnancy Surveillance Program 800–772–6436, may cause fetal harm

Evaluate:
• Therapeutic response: increase in reticulocyte count, Hgb/Hct; increased appetite, enhanced sense of well-being

Teach patient/family:
• To avoid driving or hazardous activity during beginning of treatment
• To monitor B/P, Hgb, max Hgb 11 g/dL
• To take iron supplements, vit B$_{12}$, folic acid as directed

Black Box Warning: To report to prescriber any chest pain, SOB, swelling/pain in legs, confusion, inability to speak; to comply with treatment regimen

• That menses and fertility may return; to use contraception
• About home administration procedures, if appropriate
• **Seizures:** discuss injury prevention in those who are prone to seizures may occur if Hgb is increased too rapidly, to report immediately if seizures occur
• **Chronic renal failure:** that product does not cure condition, that other treatment regimens should be followed

darifenacin
(da-ree-fen'ah-sin)
Enablex
Func. class.: Antispasmodic/GU anticholinergic

Do not confuse:
Enablex/Effexor XR

ACTION: Bladder smooth muscle relaxation by decreasing the action of muscarinic receptors, thereby relieving overactive bladder

USES: Urge incontinence, frequency, urgency in overactive bladder

CONTRAINDICATIONS: Hypersensitivity, urinary retention, narrow-angle glaucoma (uncontrolled)
Precautions: Severe hepatic disease (Child-Pugh C), GI/GU obstruction,

controlled narrow-angle glaucoma, ulcerative colitis, myasthenia gravis, moderate hepatic disease (Child-Pugh B), elderly

DOSAGE AND ROUTES
• **Adult: PO** 7.5 mg/day, initially; may increase to 15 mg/day after 14 days if needed
With CYP3A4 inhibitor ✖️☞
• **Adult: PO** max 7.5 mg/day
Hepatic dosage
• **Adult: PO** (Child-Pugh B) max 7.5 mg/day; do not use in severe hepatic disease
Available forms: Tabs, ext rel 7.5, 15 mg
Administer:
• Without regard to meals, do not crush, break, chew extended-release tabs
• Store at room temperature

SIDE EFFECTS
CNS: Dizziness, headache, confusion, hallucinations, drowsiness
EENT: Blurred vision
GI: Constipation, dry mouth, nausea, dyspepsia
INTEG: Rash, pruritus, skin drying
MISC: Angioedema

PHARMACOKINETICS
Peak 7 hr, half-life 12-19 hr, extensively metabolized by CYP2D6, less metabolism ✖️☞ in poor metabolizers; some metabolism by CYP3A4, protein binding 98%, duration 24 hr

INTERACTIONS
Increase: level of—digoxin
Increase: anticholinergic effect—anticholinergics
Increase: darifenacin level—CYP3A4 and CYP2D6 inhibitors (ketoconazole, itraconazole, ritonavir)
Increase: levels of—drugs metabolized by CYP2D6 (flecainide, tricyclics)

NURSING CONSIDERATIONS
Assess:
• **Urinary function:** urgency, frequency, retention, incontinence in bladder outflow obstruction

• **Bowel pattern:** constipation, abdominal pain, increase fluids, bulk in diet if constipation occurs
• **Pregnancy/breastfeeding:** no well-controlled studies; use only if benefit outweighs fetal risk; caution use in breastfeeding, excretion is unknown
Evaluate:
• Therapeutic response: decreasing urgency, frequency of urination
Teach patient/family:
• To take without regard to meals; not to crush, break, chew extended-release tabs, not to use other products unless approved by prescriber
• Not to double or skip doses, provide "Patient Information" and ask to read
• To discuss with provider all OTC, Rx, herbals, supplements used
• To store at room temperature
• To avoid breastfeeding; to notify prescriber if pregnancy is planned or suspected
• About anticholinergic symptoms (dry mouth, constipation, dry eyes, heat prostration); not to become overheated
• To avoid hazardous activities until reaction is known; dizziness, blurred vision can occur
• **Angioedema:** to report facial swelling, difficulty swallowing, or large tongue

---

darunavir/cobicistat (Rx)
(da-roon′a-veer/koe-bik′i-stat)
Prezcobix
Func. class.: Antiretroviral
Chem. class.: Protease inhibitor

Do not confuse:
Prezcobix/Prezistra

ACTION: Inhibits HIV-1 protease, which prevents maturation of the infectious virus; combines a protease inhibitor with an enhancer

USES: HIV-1 infection in combination with other antiretroviral agents

CONTRAINDICATIONS: Hypersensitivity, Child-Pugh Class C

Precautions: Pregnancy, breastfeeding, children, geriatric patients, hepatic disease, alcoholism, drug resistance, AV block, diabetes, dialysis, elderly, females, hemophilia, hypercholesterolemia, immune reconstitution syndrome, lactic acidosis, pancreatitis, cholelithiasis, serious rash

DOSAGE AND ROUTES

• **Adult: PO** 800 mg/150 mg daily in treatment-naive and treatment-experienced adults with no darunavir-resistance–associated substitutions (V11I, V32I, L33F, I47V, I50V, I54L, I54M, T74P, L76V, I84V, L89V)

• **Adolescent (unlabeled): PO** 800 mg/150 mg daily in combination with other antiretroviral agents for treatment-naive adolescents with no darunavir-resistance–associated substitutions (V11I, V32I, L33F, I47V, I50V, I54L, I54M, T74P, L76V, I84V, L89V)

Hepatic dose

• Do not use in severe hepatic disease

Available forms: Tabs 800 mg/150 mg

Administer:

• With food

• Antiretroviral drug resistance testing (preferably genotypic testing) is recommended before initiation of therapy in antiretroviral treatment-naive patients and before changing therapy for treatment failure

SIDE EFFECTS

CNS: Headache, depression, dizziness, insomnia, peripheral neurologic symptoms

CV: Increased PR interval

EENT: Yellowing of sclera

GI: Vomiting, *diarrhea, abdominal pain, nausea,* hepatotoxicity, cholelithiasis

INTEG: *Rash,* Stevens-Johnson syndrome, *photosensitivity,* DRESS

MISC: Fatigue, fever, arthralgia, back pain, cough, lipodystrophy, pain, gynecomastia, nephrolithiasis; lactic acidosis, hyperbilirubinemia (pregnancy, female patients, obesity)

PHARMACOKINETICS

Rapidly absorbed, absorption increased with food, peak 2.5 hr, 86% protein bound, extensively metabolized in liver by CYP3A4, 27% excreted unchanged in urine/feces (minimal), half-life 7 hr

INTERACTIONS

Increase: levels, toxicity of immunosuppressants (cycloSPORINE, sirolimus, tacrolimus, sildenafil), tricyclic antidepressants, warfarin, calcium channel blockers, clarithromycin, clorazepate, diazePAM, irinotecan, HMG-CoA reductase inhibitors, antidysrhythmics, midazolam, triazolam, ergots, pimozide, other protease inhibitors

Increase: effects of estrogens with ritonavir

Increase: atazanavir levels—CYP3A4 substrates, CYP3A4 inhibitors

Increase: hyperbilirubinemia—indinavir

Decrease: telaprevir level when used with atazanavir and ritonavir

Decrease: atazanavir levels—CYP3A4 inducers, rifampin, antacids, didanosine, efavirenz, proton pump inhibitors, H$_2$-receptor antagonists

Decrease: oral contraceptives

Drug/Herb

Decrease: atazanavir levels—St. John's wort; avoid concurrent use

Increase: myopathy, rhabdomyolysis—red yeast rice

Drug/Lab Test

Increase: AST, ALT, total bilirubin, amylase, lipase, CK

Decrease: Hgb, neutrophils, platelets

Drug/Food

• Increased drug bioavailability (to be taken with food)

NURSING CONSIDERATIONS

Assess:

• **For hepatic failure:** hepatic studies—ALT, AST, bilirubin

• **Immune reconstitution syndrome:** when given with combination antiretroviral therapy, time of onset is variable

• **For lactic acidosis, hyperbilirubinemia** (female patients, pregnancy, obesity);

D

---

if pregnant, call Antiretroviral Pregnancy Registry, 1-800-258-4263

• PR interval in those taking calcium channel blockers, digoxin

• For signs of infection, anemia, nephrolithiasis

• Bowel pattern before, during treatment; if severe abdominal pain with bleeding occurs, product should be discontinued; monitor hydration

• Viral load, CD4 count throughout treatment

• **Serious rash (Stevens-Johnson syndrome, DRESS):** most rashes last 1-4 wk; if serious, discontinue product

• **Pregnancy/breastfeeding:** no well-controlled studies; use only if benefit outweighs fetal risk; if pregnant, call Antiretroviral Pregnancy Registry, 800-258-4263; avoid use in breastfeeding

Evaluate:

• Therapeutic response: increasing CD4 counts; decreased viral load, resolution of symptoms of HIV-1 infection

Teach patient/family:

• To take as prescribed with other antiretrovirals as prescribed; if dose is missed, to take as soon as remembered up to 1 hr before next dose; not to double dose, share with others

• That product must be taken daily to maintain blood levels for duration of therapy

• To report yellowing of skin, sclera

• To notify prescriber if diarrhea, nausea, vomiting, or rash occurs; dizziness, light-headedness may occur; ECG may be altered

• That product interacts with many products, including St. John's wort; to advise prescriber of all products, herbal products used

• That redistribution of body fat may occur, the effect is not known

• That product does not cure HIV-1 infection, prevent transmission to others; only controls symptoms

• That, if taking phosphodiesterase type 5 inhibitor with atazanavir, there may be increased risk of phosphodiesterase type 5 inhibitor–associated adverse events (hypotension, prolonged penile erection); to notify physician promptly of these symptoms

---

RARELY USED

dasatinib (Rx)

(da-si′ti-nib)

Sprycel

Func. class.: Antineoplastic—miscellaneous

Chem. class.: Protein-tyrosine kinase inhibitor

USES: Treatment of accelerated, chronic blast phase CML or acute lymphoblastic leukemia (ALL); chronic phase CML with resistance or intolerance to prior therapy; Philadelphia chromosome–positive CML in chronic phase

CONTRAINDICATIONS: Pregnancy, hypersensitivity

DOSAGE AND ROUTES

Accelerated or myeloid/lymphoid blast phase CML with resistance/intolerance to prior therapy

• **Adult:** PO 140 mg daily titrated up to 180 mg daily in those resistant to therapy

Chronic phase CML with resistance/intolerance to prior therapy

• **Adult:** PO 100 mg daily either AM or PM

Dosage reduction for those taking a strong CYP3A4 inhibitor

• **Adult:** PO 20-40 mg daily

⚠ HIGH ALERT

DAUNOrubicin (Rx)

(daw-noe-roo′bi-sin)

Cerubidine ✦

Func. class.: Antineoplastic, antibiotic

Chem. class.: Anthracycline glycoside

Do not confuse:
DAUNOrubicin/DOXOrubicin

ACTION: Inhibits DNA synthesis, primarily; derived from *Streptomyces coeruleorubidus;* replication is decreased by

---

binding to DNA, binds DNA causing confirmational changes; a vesicant

USES: Acute lymphocytic leukemia (ALL), acute myelogenous leukemia (AML)

CONTRAINDICATIONS: Pregnancy, breastfeeding, hypersensitivity, systemic infections, cardiac disease, bone marrow depression

Black Box Warning: IM/SUBCUT use

Precautions: Tumor lysis syndrome, MI, infection, thrombocytopenia, renal/hepatic disease; gout

Black Box Warning: Bone marrow suppression, cardiac disease, extravasation, renal failure, hepatic disease; requires a specialized care setting and an experienced clinician

DOSAGE AND ROUTES
• **Adult <60 yr: IV** 45 mg/m^2/day × 3 day, 1st cycle, then 2 days 2nd cycle
Adult <60 yr: IV 45 mg/m^2/day × 3 day, 1st cycle, then 2 days 2nd cycle
• **Adult ≥60 yr: IV** 30 mg/m^2/day × 3 days, then 2 days of subsequent courses in combination, max 400-600 mg/m^2 total cumulative dose
• **Child ≥2 yr: IV** 25 mg/m^2/day depending on cycle weekly in combination; **<2 yr or BSA <0.5 m^2** determine on mg/kg basis
Available forms: Inj 20 mg powder/vial
Administer:
• Antiemetic 30-60 min before giving product to prevent vomiting

Black Box Warning: To be used in a care setting with emergency equipment available; to be used by a clinician knowledgeable in cytotoxic therapy; do not give by IM/subcut injection

IV route
• Use cytotoxic handling precautions
• After diluting 20 mg/4 mL sterile water for inj (5 mg/mL), rotate, further dilute in 10-15 mL 0.9% NaCl; give over 3-5 min by direct IV through Y-tube or 3-way stop-cock of infusion of D$_5$W or 0.9% NaCl; or dilute in 50 mL 0.9% NaCl and give over 10-15 min; or dilute in 100 mL and give over 30 min, may use premix vial 5 mg/mL
• Apply ice compress after stopping infusion for extravasation

Y-site compatibilities: Amifostine, anidulafungin, atenolol, bivalirudin, bleomycin, CARBOplatin, caspofungin, CISplatin, codeine, cyclophosphamide, cytarabine, DACTINomycin, DAPTOmycin, dexmedetomidine, etoposide, fenoldopam, filgrastim, gemcitabine, gemtuzumab, granisetron, melphalan, meperidine, methotrexate, nesiritide, octreotide, ondansetron, oxaliplatin, PACLitaxel, palonosetron, quinupristin-dalfopristin, riTUXimab, sodium acetate/bicarbonate, teniposide, thiotepa, tigecycline, trastuzumab, vinCRIStine, vinorelbine, voriconazole, zoledronic acid

SIDE EFFECTS
CNS: Fever, chills
CV: HF, peripheral edema, cardiotoxicity, dysrhhthmias, tachycardia
GI: *Nausea, vomiting, anorexia, mucositis,* hepatotoxicity
GU: Impotence, sterility, red/orange urine
HEMA: Thrombocytopenia, leukopenia, anemia
INTEG: *Rash,* extravasation, dermatitis, alopecia, thrombophlebitis at inj site
SYST: Anaphylaxis, tumor lysis syndrome, secondary malignancies

PHARMACOKINETICS
Half-life $18^1/_2$ hr, metabolized by liver; crosses placenta; excreted in breast milk, (40–50%), bile

INTERACTIONS
Increase: QT prolongation, torsades de pointes—arsenic trioxide, chloroquine, clarithromycin, class IA, class III antidysrhythmics, dasatinib, dolasetron, droperidol, erythromycin, flecainide, haloperidol, methadone, ondansetron, palonosetron, pentamidine, some phenothiazines,

---

propafenone, risperiDONE, sparfloxacin; tricyclic antidepressants (high doses); vorinostat, ziprasidone

Increase: toxicity—other antineoplastics, radiation, cyclophosphamide

Decrease: DAUNOrubicin effects—hematopoietic progenitor cells given within 24 hr

Decrease: antibody reaction—live virus vaccines

Drug/Lab Test

Increase: uric acid

NURSING CONSIDERATIONS
Assess:

Black Box Warning: **Bone marrow suppression:** CBC, differential, platelet count weekly, leukocyte nadir within 2 wk after administration, recovery within 3 wk; do not administer if absolute granulocyte count is <750/mm³ (liposome)

Black Box Warning: **Acute renal failure, uric acid nephropathy:** renal studies: BUN, urine CCr, electrolytes, uric acid baseline before each dose; I&O ratio; report fall in urine output to <30 mL/hr; provide aggressive alkalinization of urine and use of allopurinol; can prevent urate nephropathy

Black Box Warning: **Hepatotoxicity:** monitor hepatic studies baseline before each dose: bilirubin, AST, ALT, alk phos; check for jaundice of skin, sclera; dark urine, clay-colored stools; itchy skin, abdominal pain, fever; diarrhea

Black Box Warning: **Cardiac toxicity:** chest x-ray, echocardiography, radionuclide angiography, MUGA, ECG; watch for ST-T wave changes, low QRS and QT prolongation, possible dysrhythmias (sinus tachycardia, heart block, PVCs); watch for HF (jugular vein distention, weight gain, edema, crackles), may occur after 2-6 mo of treatment, cumulative dose (400-550 mg/m²), or 450 mg/m² if used in combination with radiation, cyclophosphamide

• Bleeding: hematuria, guaiac stools, bruising, petechiae, mucosa, or orifices q8hr

• Effects of alopecia on body image; discuss feelings about body changes

• Buccal cavity for dryness, sores, ulceration, white patches, oral pain, bleeding, dysphagia, rinse mouth tidqid with water, club soda; brush teeth bid-qid with soft brush or cottontipped applicators for stomatitis; use unwaxed dental floss

• **Tumor lysis syndrome:** hyperkalemia, hyperphosphatemia, hyperuricemia, hypocalcemia

Black Box Warning: **Extravasation:** swelling, pain, decreased blood return; if extravasation occurs, stop infusion, remove tubing, attempt to aspirate the drug before removing the needle, elevate area, treat with ice pack

• GI symptoms: frequency of stools, cramping

• Increase fluid intake to 2-3 L/day to prevent urate and calculi formation

Evaluate:

• Therapeutic response: decreased tumor size, spread of malignancy

Teach patient/family:

• To report signs of infection, bleeding, bruising, SOB, swelling, change in heart rate

• That hair may be lost during treatment; that wig or hairpiece may make patient feel better; that new hair may be different in color, texture

• To avoid foods with citric acid, hot temperature, or rough texture if stomatitis is present

• To report any bleeding, white spots, ulcerations in mouth; to examine mouth daily

• That urine and other body fluids may be red-orange for 48 hr

• To avoid vaccines, aspirin, while taking this product

• To avoid crowds, those with known infections

• Not to use during pregnancy while taking product and for 4 mo thereafter; not to breastfeed

---

⚠ HIGH ALERT

RARELY USED

daunorubicin/ cytarabine

(daw-noe-roo'bi-sin/sye-tare'a-been)

Vyxeos

Func. class.: Antineoplastic

USES: For the treatment of newly diagnosed therapy-related AML or AML with myelodysplasia-related changes

DOSAGE AND ROUTES

• **Adult:** IV **First induction,** 44 mg/m² daunorubicin liposomal and 100 mg/m² cytarabine liposomal over 90 min on days 1, 3, and 5; patients who do not achieve a response may receive a second induction. **Second induction** (given 2-5 wk after first induction cycle), 44 mg/m² daunorubicin liposomal and 100 mg/m² cytarabine liposomal on days 1 and 3. **Consolidation therapy** (given 5-8 wk after start of the last induction), 29 mg/m² daunorubicin liposomal and 65 mg/m² cytarabine liposomal on days 1 and 3. Patients without disease progression or unacceptable toxicity should receive a second cycle of consolidation therapy given 5-8 wk after the start of the previous consolidation

---

RARELY USED

deferasirox (Rx)

(def-a'sir-ox)

Exjade, Jadence ✦, Jadenu, Jadenu Sprinkle

Func. class.: Heavy-metal chelating agent

USES: Chronic iron overload, transfusion hemosiderosis

CONTRAINDICATIONS: Breastfeeding, children, hypersensitivity, severe renal/hepatic disease, GI hemorrhage

> **Black Box Warning:** Renal failure, GI bleeding/perforation, hepatotoxicity, nephrotoxicity

DOSAGE AND ROUTES

• **Adult and child >2 yr:** PO 20-30 mg/kg/day; oral dispersion tablet is dissolved in water <1 g in 3.5 oz; >1 g in 7 oz or more; give on empty stomach at least 30 min before meals

---

⚠ HIGH ALERT

degarelix

(day-gah-rel'iks)

Firmagon

Func. class.: Antineoplastic
Chem. class.: GnRH-receptor antagonist

ACTION: Reduces release of gonadotropins and testicular steroidogenesis by reversibly binding to GnRH receptors

USES: Advanced prostate cancer

CONTRAINDICATIONS: Hypersensitivity, QT prolongation, osteoporosis, severe hepatic/renal disease, pregnancy, breastfeeding
Precautions: CV disease, electrolyte abnormalities, geriatric patients

DOSAGE AND ROUTES

• **Adult (male):** SUBCUT 240 mg given as two 120-mg injections (40 mg/mL concentrations); maintenance 80 mg (20 mg/mL concentration) every 28 days, starting 28 days after first dose
Available forms: Injection 80, 120 mg vial
Administer:
• Do not give IV, subcut only
General reconstitution information:
• Use double gloves, gown, aseptic technique during preparation and administration
• Keep vials vertical at all times; do *not* shake the vials; give reconstituted drug

---

Side effects: *italics* = common; red = life-threatening

within 1 hr after addition of sterile water for injection

Reconstitution of 120-mg vial (240-mg dose *only*):

• For a 240-mg dose, use two 120-mg vials; repeat for each 120-mg vial: draw up 3 mL of sterile water for injection with a 2-inch, 21-G needle; do not use bacteriostatic water for injection; inject the sterile water slowly into vial containing 120 mg; to maintain sterility, do not remove the syringe or the needle from the vial; keep the vial in an upright position and swirl gently; avoid shaking; reconstitution can take up to 15 min; tilt the vial slightly and withdraw 3 mL (40 mg/mL); avoid turning the vial upside down; repeat with a new vial, needle, and syringe for the second 120-mg dose (total dose = 240 mg)

Reconstitution of 80-mg vial:

• Draw up 4.2 mL of sterile water for injection with a 2-inch, 21-G needle; do not use bacteriostatic water for injection; inject the sterile water slowly into vial containing 80 mg; do not remove the syringe or the needle from the vial; swirl gently; avoid shaking; reconstitution can take up to 15 min; withdraw 4 mL (20 mg/mL); avoid turning upside down during withdrawal

Subcut injection:

• Exchange the reconstitution needle with a 1.25-inch, 27-G needle; remove air bubbles; give in the abdominal region; rotate injection site periodically; use area not exposed to pressure; grasp the skin of abdomen, elevate the subcutaneous tissue, and insert the needle deeply at an angle ≥45 degrees; aspirate before injection; inject the dose subcut; when giving the loading dose of two 120-mg doses, the second dose should be injected at a different site

SIDE EFFECTS

CNS: Chills, dizziness, fatigue, fever, headache, insomnia

CV: Increased QT prolongation, hypotension, hot flashes, hypertension

GI: Diarrhea, constipation, nausea

GU: ED, UTI, gynecomastia, testicular atrophy

INTEG: Injection site reactions, pain at site, redness, swelling

MS: Back pain, decreased bone density

SYST: Hypersensitivity, anaphylaxis, angioedema

PHARMACOKINETICS

Peak 2 days, duration 50 days, half-life 53 days

INTERACTIONS

Increase: QT prolongation—Class IA/III antidysrhythmics, methyldopa, metoclopramide, reserpine

Drug/Lab Test

Increase: PSA, LFTs

Decrease: bone density test

NURSING CONSIDERATIONS

Assess:

• HbA1c, lipids, B/P prior to initiation and 3-6 mo after

• **QT prolongation:** more common in those taking Class IA/III antidysrhythmics, heart failure, congenital long QT syndrome; monitor cardiac status at baseline and often thereafter, include ECG periodically

• **Anaphylaxis, angioedema (rash, trouble breathing):** discontinue treatment and do not restart in serious reactions; assess for rash, dyspnea, wheezing, facial swelling

• Liver function studies, PSA, GGT that may be elevated; bone density that may be decreased; electrolytes; if PSA is elevated, monitor testosterone levels

• **Pregnancy:** identify if pregnancy is planned or suspected or if breastfeeding; do not use in pregnancy or breastfeeding

Evaluate:

• Therapeutic response: decreasing spread, size of tumor

Teach patient/family:

• To notify all prescribers of cardiac disease or use of all cardiac products, irregular pulse, heartbeat

• Injection technique if patient/family will be giving product (provide patient information)

• **Pregnancy:** to notify prescriber if pregnancy is planned or suspected; do not breastfeed

RARELY USED

delafloxacin
(dela-flox´-a-sin)
Baxdela
Func. class.: Antiinfective

USES: For the treatment of acute bacterial skin and skin structure infections

DOSAGE AND ROUTES
• **Adult: PO** 450 mg q12hr × 5-14 days
• **Adult: IV** 300 mg q12hr × 5-14 days

⚠ HIGH ALERT

delavirdine (Rx)
(de-la-veer´deen)
Rescriptor
Func. class.: Antiretroviral
Chem. class.: Nonnucleoside reverse transcriptase inhibitor (NNRTI)

ACTION: Binds directly to reverse transcriptase; blocks RNA-, DNA-dependent polymerase activities, causing a disruption of the enzyme's site

USES: HIV-1 in combination with at least 2 other antiretrovirals

CONTRAINDICATIONS: Hypersensitivity
Precautions: Pregnancy, breastfeeding, children, hepatic disease, achlorhydria, antimicrobial resistance, exfoliative dermatitis, hepatitis, immune reconstitution syndrome

DOSAGE AND ROUTES
• **Adult and adolescent ≥16 yr: PO** 400 mg tid, max 1200 mg/day
Available forms: Tabs 100, 200 mg
Administer:

• 100-mg tab: dispersion by adding 4 tab/3-4 oz water, let stand, stir, swallow, rinse glass, swallow; use only 100-mg tabs for dispersion; 200-mg tab take as intact tab
• Do not give within 1 hr of antacids or didanosine
• Always use as combination therapy; this product is not recommended for initial treatment; due to inferior virologic effect, it is no longer listed as part of any preferred regimens

SIDE EFFECTS
CNS: Headache, fatigue, anxiety, insomnia, fever
GI: Diarrhea, abdominal pain, nausea, anorexia, vomiting, dyspepsia, hepatotoxicity
GU: Nephrotoxicity
HEMA: Neutropenia, leukopenia, thrombocytopenia, anemia, granulocytopenia
INTEG: Rash, pruritus
MISC: Cough
MS: Pain, myalgia, rhabdomyolysis
SYST: Stevens-Johnson syndrome, immune reconstitution syndrome (combination therapy)

PHARMOCOKINETICS
98% protein bound, half-life 5.8 hr, peak 1 hr, duration 8 hr, extensively metabolized by CYP3A4, excreted in urine, feces

INTERACTIONS
Do not coadminister with nevirapine, efavirenz, rilpivirine; combined use not beneficial
Increase: serious life-threatening adverse reactions—amphetamines, ergots, benzodiazepines, calcium channel blockers, sedative/hypnotics, antidysrhythmics, sildenafil, pimozide, ALPRAZolam, astemizole, midazolam, opiates, triazolam
Increase: levels of ALPRAZolam, clarithromycin, dapsone, ergots, felodipine, midazolam, NIFEdipine, indinavir, saquinavir, lovastatin, simvastatin, atorvastatin, other CYP3A4, 2D6 inhibitors
Increase: delavirdine levels—FLUoxetine, ketoconazole
Increase: levels of both products—quiNIDine, warfarin, clarithromycin

Decrease: delavirdine levels—antacids, anticonvulsants, rifamycins, protease inhibitors, didanosine, H₂ blockers, PPIs

Decrease: action of oral contraceptives, didanosine

Drug/Herb

Decrease: delavirdine level—St. John's wort; avoid use

Drug/Lab Test

Increase: ALT/AST, alkaline phosphatase, bilirubin, creatinine, CK, lipase, GGT, eosinophils, PT, PTT

Decrease: RBCs, WBCs, platelets, granulocytes

NURSING CONSIDERATIONS

Assess:

• **HIV:** obtain hepatitis B virus (HBV) screening to ensure proper treatment; if coinfected, use a fully suppressive antiretroviral regimen with products against both; CBC, blood chemistry, plasma HIV RNA, absolute CD41/CD81/cell counts/%, serum β₂ microglobulin, serum ICD124 antigen levels

• **Immune reconstitution syndrome:** when treated with combination therapy; development of opportunistic infections (*Mycobacterium avium complex [MAC]*, cytomegalovirus [CMV], *Pneumocystis carinii* pneumonia [PCP], TB)

• Signs of infection, anemia

• Hepatic studies: ALT, AST; renal studies

• Bowel pattern before, during treatment; if severe abdominal pain with bleeding occurs, product should be discontinued; monitor hydration

• Allergies before treatment, reaction to each medication; place allergies on chart

• Plasma delavirdine concentrations (trough 10 micromolar)

• **Toxicity:** severe nausea/vomiting, maculopapular rash

• **Serious skin reactions:** Stevens-Johnson syndrome; rash may occur within 1-3 wk of beginning treatment; if rash is not severe, manage with diphenhydrAMINE, hydrOXYzine, topical corticosteroids

Evaluate:

• Therapeutic response: increased CD4 cell count, decreased viral load, improvement in symptoms of HIV

Teach patient/family:

• To take as prescribed; if dose is missed, to take as soon as remembered up to 1 hr before next dose; not to double dose; do not take antacids concurrently, separate by 1 hr

• That tabs may be dissolved in ¹/₂ cup of water (100 mg only); to stir; when dissolved, drink right away; to rinse cup with water and drink to get all medication

• To make sure health care provider knows about all medications being taken

• That if severe rash, mouth sores, swelling, aching muscles/joints, or eye redness occur, to notify health care provider

• **Pregnancy/breastfeeding:** identify if pregnancy is planned or suspected; if pregnant, use in pregnancy only if benefits outweigh fetal risk; that patient should register with the Antiretroviral Pregnancy Registry (800-258-4263); not to breastfeed

• That this product is not a cure, only controls symptoms

---

denosumab (Rx)

(den-oh′sue-mab)

Prolia, Xgeva

Func. class.: Bone resorption inhibitor

Chem. class.: Monoclonal antibody, bone resorption

ACTION: Neutralizes activity of receptor activator nuclear factor kappa-B ligand (RANKL) by binding to it and blocking its interaction with cell-surface receptors; use of a RANKL inhibitor may reduce bone turnover and decrease tumor burden

USES: **Prolia:** Osteoporosis in postmenopausal women or men at high risk for fractures; increase bone mass in men who are receiving androgen deprivation therapy for prostate cancer and women receiving aromatase inhibitor therapy for breast cancer at high risk for fractures; **Xgeva:** prevention of skeletal-related events in bone metastases from solid tumors

CONTRAINDICATIONS: Hypersensitivity, hypocalcemia, pregnancy

Precautions: Breastfeeding, child/infant/neonate, anemia, coagulopathy, diabetes mellitus, dialysis, eczema, hypoparathyroidism, immunosuppression, latex hypersensitivity, malabsorption syndrome, neoplastic disease, pancreatitis, parathyroid disease, dental/renal/thyroid disease, TB, vit D deficiency

DOSAGE AND ROUTES
Postmenopausal osteoporosis (Prolia)
• **Adult female:** SUBCUT 60 mg q6mo
Bone metastases from solid tumors (Xgeva)
• **Adult:** SUBCUT 120 mg q4wk, max 120 mg q4wk
Giant cell tumor (bone) (Xgeva)
• **Adult:** SUBCUT 120 mg, then 120 mg q4wk on day 1, 8, 15
Hypercalcemia of malignancy (Xgeva)
• **Adult:** SUBCUT 120 mg q4wk, another dose of 120 mg given on day 8 and 15 of first month of treatment
Available forms: Sol for inj 60 mg/mL (Prolia); 120 mg/1.7 mL (Xgeva)
Administer:
SUBCUT route
• Give acetaminophen before and for 72 hr after to decrease pain
• Do not use if particulate matter or discoloration is present; sol is clear and colorless to slightly yellow with small white/opalescent particles; remove from refrigerator and allow to warm to room temperature (15-30 min)
• **Use of prefilled syringe with needle safety guard:** leave green guard in original position until after use; remove and discard needle cap immediately before inj; give by subcut inj in upper arm/thigh or abdomen; after inj, point needle away from people and slide green guard over needle
• **Use of single-use vials:** use 27-G needle; give in upper arm/thigh or abdomen; do not reinsert needle in vial; discard supplies as appropriate
• Store and use out of direct sunlight/heat; do not freeze; use within 14 days after removal from refrigerator; store unopened containers in refrigerator

SIDE EFFECTS
CNS: Headache, vertigo, fatigue, insomnia
CV: Angina, atrial fibrillation
GI: Abdominal pain, constipation, *diarrhea,* flatulence, GERD, *vomiting, nausea,* pancreatitis
GU: Cystitis
HEMA: Anemia
INTEG: Dermatitis, pruritus
META: Hypercholesterolemia, hypocalcemia, hypophosphatemia
MS: Back, bone pain; MS pain, myalgia, osteonecrosis of the jaw
RESP: Cough, *dyspnea*
SYST: Infection, secondary malignancy, anaphylaxis

PHARMACOKINETICS
Half-life 25.4 days, bioavailability 62%, max serum concentrations 3-21 days

INTERACTIONS
Increase: infection, possible—immunosuppressives (except cytarabine liposomal), corticosteroids
Drug/Lab Test
Increase: cholesterol
Decrease: calcium, phosphate

NURSING CONSIDERATIONS
Assess:
• **Acute phase reaction:** fever, myalgia, headache, flulike symptoms for 72 hr after inj; usually resolves after 72 hr
• **Blood tests:** serum calcium, creatinine, BUN, magnesium, phosphate; provide adequate calcium, vitamin D, magnesium
• **Hypocalcemia (may be fatal):** paresthesia, twitching, laryngospasm, Chvostek's and Trouseau's signs; preexisting hypocalcemia should be corrected before treatment; patient with vit D deficiency may require higher doses of vit D
• **Hypercalcemia:** nausea, vomiting, anorexia, weakness, thirst, constipation, dysrhythmias
• **Dental status:** correct dental complications before product use; good oral hygiene should be maintained; if dental work is to be performed, antiinfectives

---

should be given to prevent osteonecrosis of the jaw

• **Infection:** do not start treatment in patients with active infections; infections should be resolved first

• **Pregnancy:** identify whether pregnancy is planned or suspected; women who become pregnant should enroll in Amgen's Pregnancy Surveillance Program (1-800-772-6436); do not use in pregnancy, breastfeeding

Evaluate:

• Therapeutic response: increased/maintained bone density, decreased calcium levels

Teach patient/family:

• To report hypercalcemic relapse: nausea, vomiting, bone pain, thirst

• To notify prescriber immediately if rash, infection, cramps, twitching occur

• To continue with dietary recommendations, including additional Ca 1000 mg/day and vit D ≥400 units (Prolia product labeling)

• That product must be continued or fractures may occur

• To use acetaminophen before and for 72 hr after inj to lessen bone pain

• About the purpose of this product and its expected results

• To avoid OTC, Rx medications and herbs and supplements unless approved by prescriber

• To exercise regularly, stop smoking, and avoid alcohol to maintain bone health

• To inform all health care providers of product use; to avoid dental procedures/surgery if possible; to practice good oral hygiene

• That lab tests and follow-up exams will be required

• **Pregnancy/breastfeeding:** not to use during pregnancy and breastfeeding; to notify prescriber if pregnancy is planned, suspected; to use contraception during and for (Xgeva) 5 mo after completion of therapy; that males

should use contraception if partner is pregnant

RARELY USED

deoxycholic acid
(dee-ox′-i-koe′-lik as′-id)
Kybella ✿
Func. class.: Lypolytic

USES: For the improvement in the appearance of moderate to severe convexity or fullness associated with submental fat

CONTRAINDICATIONS: Infection

DOSAGE AND ROUTES

• **Adult: SUBCUT** 0.2 mL per injection site. A single treatment session consists of up to a maximum of 50 injections (10 mL total dose), with each injection spaced 1 cm apart. Up to 6 single treatments may be given at intervals of no less than 1 mo. Injections are made into the subcutaneous fat of the submental region, between the dermis and the platysma. Do not inject into the platysma

---

desipramine (Rx)
(dess-ip′ra-meen)
Norpramin
Func. class.: Antidepressant, tricyclic
Chem. class.: Dibenzazepine, secondary amine

Do not confuse:
desipramine/disopyramide

ACTION: Blocks reuptake of norepinephrine, serotonin into nerve endings, thereby increasing action of norepinephrine, serotonin in nerve cells

USES: Depression
Unlabeled uses: Chronic pain, insomnia, anxiety

CONTRAINDICATIONS: Hypersensitivity to tricyclics, carBAMazepine, closed-angle glaucoma, acute MI, MAOIs

---

Precautions: Pregnancy, breastfeeding, geriatric patients, severe depression, increased intraocular pressure, seizure disorder, CV disease, urinary retention, cardiac dysrhythmias, cardiac conduction disturbances, family history of sudden death, prostatic hypertrophy, thyroid disease

Black Box Warning: Children <18 yr, suicidal patients

DOSAGE AND ROUTES
• **Adult:** PO 50-75 mg/day in 1-4 divided doses; titrate by 25-50 mg weekly up to 300 mg/day in single or divided doses (inpatient), 200 mg/day (outpatient)
• **Geriatric:** PO 25 mg/day at bedtime, titrate weekly; may increase to 150 mg/day
• **Adolescent:** PO 25-50 mg/day in divided doses; max 100 mg/day
• **Child 6-12 yr:** PO 1-3 mg/kg/day in divided doses; max 5 mg/kg/day
Available forms: Tabs 10, 25, 50, 75, 100, 150 mg
Administer:
• Increased fluids, bulk in diet for constipation, especially in geriatric patients; with food or milk for GI symptoms; crushed if patient is unable to swallow medication whole; without regard for food
• Dosage at bedtime if oversedation occurs during day; may take entire dose at bedtime; geriatric patients may not tolerate once-daily dosing

SIDE EFFECTS
CNS: *Dizziness, drowsiness,* confusion, headache, fatigue, anxiety, tremors, stimulation, weakness, insomnia, nightmares, EPS (geriatric patients), increased psychiatric symptoms, paresthenia, suicidal ideation, impaired memory, seizures, serotonin syndrome
CV: *Orthostatic hypotension,* ECG changes, *tachycardia, hypertension,* palpitations
EENT: *Blurred vision,* tinnitus, mydriasis, ophthalmoplegia
ENDO: SIADH
GI: *Diarrhea, dry mouth,* nausea, vomiting, paralytic ileus, increased appetite, cramps, epigastric distress, jaundice, hepatitis, stomatitis, constipation, weight gain
GU: *Retention,* dereased libido
HEMA: Agranulocytosis, thrombocytopenia, eosinophilia, leukopenia
INTEG: Rash, urticaria, sweating, pruritus, photosensitivity

PHARMACOKINETICS
Well absorbed, widely distributed, protein binding 92%, extensively metabolized in the liver ⟩⟩ (CYP2D6) to active metabolite of imipramine; ⟩⟩ some patients are poor metabolizers; half-life 15-60 hr

INTERACTIONS
Increase: serotonin syndrome, neuroleptic malignant syndrome—SSRIs, SNRIs, serotonin-receptor agonists, other tricyclic antidepressants
Increase: CNS depression—alcohol, barbiturates, opioids, CNS depressants, skeletal muscle relaxants
Increase: desipramine level—cimetidine, diltiazem, fluvoxaMINE, FLUoxetine, PARoxetine, sertraline, verapamil
Increase: life-threatening B/P elevations—cloNIDine; do not use concurrently
Increase: hypertension—EPINEPHrine, norepinephrine
Increase: hyperpyrexia, seizures, excitation; do not use within 14 days of MAOIs
Increase: QT interval—tricyclics, SUNItinib, vorinostat, ziprasidone, gatifloxacin, levoFLOXacin, moxifloxacin, sparfloxacin, class IA/III antidysrhythmics, linezolid, methylene blue
Drug/Herb
Increase: serotonin syndrome—St. John's wort, SAM-e, yohimbe; avoid concurrent use
Increase: CNS depression—kava, valerian
Drug/Lab Test
Increase: serum bilirubin, blood glucose, alk phos, LFTs

NURSING CONSIDERATIONS
Assess:
• **Pain:** characteristics, including locations, intensity, alleviating factors, prior to and periodically

---

• B/P (lying, standing), pulse; if systolic B/P drops 20 mm Hg, hold product, notify prescriber; take VS, ECG in cardiac patients
• Hepatic studies: AST, ALT, bilirubin; thyroid function studies; monitor blood glucose and cholesterol in those who are overweight
• Weight weekly, BMI initially and periodically; appetite may increase with product
• **EPS** primarily in geriatric patients: rigidity, dystonia, akathisia
• **Seizure activity** in those with a history of seizures; may be prior to cardiac events

Black Box Warning: **Depression:** monitor mental status: mood, sensorium, affect, **suicidal tendencies,** increase in psychiatric symptoms (depression, panic); this product is not indicated for children; monitor mental status baseline and during first few months of treatment

• Urinary retention, constipation; constipation most likely in children
• **Withdrawal symptoms:** headache, nausea, vomiting, muscle pain, weakness; not usual unless product discontinued abruptly
• **Beers:** avoid in older adults with delirium or at high risk for delirium; assess for confusion; highly anticholinergic
• **Pregnancy/breastfeeding:** no well-controlled studies, use only if benefit outweighs fetal risk; avoid breastfeeding, excretion is unknown
Evaluate:
• Therapeutic response: decreased depression
Teach patient/family:
• That therapeutic effects may take 2-3 wk

Black Box Warning: That suicidal thoughts/behaviors may occur; to notify prescriber immediately

• To use caution when driving, performing other activities requiring alertness because of drowsiness, dizziness, blurred vision
• To avoid alcohol, other CNS depressants

• Not to discontinue medication abruptly after long-term use because this may cause nausea, headache, malaise
• To wear sunscreen or large hat because photosensitivity occurs

TREATMENT OF OVERDOSE: ECG monitoring; lavage; administer anticonvulsant

---

desloratadine (Rx)
(des′lor-at′ah-deen)
Clarinex, Clarinex RediTabs
Func. class.: Antihistamine, 2nd generation
Chem. class.: Selective histamine (H_1)-receptor antagonist

ACTION: Binds to peripheral histamine receptors, thus providing antihistamine action without sedation

USES: Seasonal/perennial allergic rhinitis, chronic idiopathic urticaria, pruritus

CONTRAINDICATIONS: Hypersensitivity, infants/neonates
Precautions: Pregnancy, breastfeeding, child, asthma, renal/hepatic impairment, phenylketonuria

DOSAGE AND ROUTES
• **Adult and child ≥12 yr: PO** 5 mg/day
• **Child 6-11 yr: PO** 2.5 mg/day
• **Child 2-5 yr: PO** 1.25 mg/day
• **Child 6-11 mo: PO** 1 mg/day (urticaria only)
Hepatic/renal dose
• Adult: PO 5 mg every other day
Available forms: Tabs 5 mg; orally disintegrating tabs 2.5, 5 mg (RediTabs); syr 0.5 mg/mL
Administer:
• Without regard to meals
• Do not remove RediTabs from blister until ready to use
• RediTabs directly on tongue; may take with or without water

---

• Use calibrated device for syrup

SIDE EFFECTS
CNS: Sedation (more common with increased doses), headache, psychomotor hyperactivity, *seizures*, fatigue, dizziness
GI: *Hepatitis*, nausea, dry mouth
MISC: Flulike symptoms, pharyngitis, myalgias

PHARMACOKINETICS
Onset antihistamine effect 1 hr, peak 1½ hr, elimination half-life 8½-28 hr, metabolized in liver to active metabolites, excreted in urine

INTERACTIONS
Increase: CNS depression (rare)—alcohol, opiates, sedative/hypnotics, H_1 blockers, antipsychotics, tricyclic antidepressants, anxiolytics
Increase: desloratadine—nilotinib, etravirine

NURSING CONSIDERATIONS
Assess:
• **Allergy:** hives, rash, rhinitis; monitor respiratory status; stop product 4 days before antigen skin test
• **Pregnancy/breastfeeding:** identify whether pregnancy is planned or suspected; use only if benefits outweigh fetal risk; avoid breastfeeding, excretion unknown
Evaluate:
• Therapeutic response: absence of running or congested nose, other allergy symptoms
Teach patient/family:
• To avoid driving, other hazardous activities if drowsiness occurs; to use caution until product's effects are known
• That product may cause photosensitivity; to use sunscreen or stay out of the sun to prevent burns
• Not to exceed max dose, to take without regard to meals
• To use RediTab by removing from pack and allowing to dissolve on tongue, without regard to water

---

desmopressin (Rx)
(des-moe-press'in)
DDAVP, DDAVP Melt ✦, DDAVP Rhinal Tube ✦, DDAVP Rhinyle Drops ✦, Noctiva, Nocdurna ✦, Stimate
Func. class.: Pituitary hormone
Chem. class.: Synthetic antidiuretic hormone

D

ACTION: Promotes reabsorption of water by action on renal tubular epithelium; causes smooth muscle constriction, increase in plasma factor VIII levels, which increases platelet aggregation, thereby resulting in vasopressor effect; similar to vasopressin

USES: Hemophilia A, von Willebrand's disease type 1, nonnephrogenic diabetes insipidus, symptoms of polyuria/polydipsia caused by pituitary dysfunction, nocturnal enuresis, nocturia
Unlabeled uses: Uremic bleeding

CONTRAINDICATIONS: Hypersensitivity, nephrogenic diabetes insipidus, severe renal disease

> **Black Box Warning:** Hyponatremia

Precautions: Pregnancy, breastfeeding, coronary artery disease, hypertension, cystic fibrosis, thrombus, electrolyte imbalances, male infertility

DOSAGE AND ROUTES
Primary nocturnal enuresis
• **Adult/child ≥6 yr: PO** 20 mcg at bedtime, max 0.6 mg at bedtime; **INTRANASAL** 0.2 mL at bedtime, half in each nostril
Diabetes insipidus
• **Adult: INTRANASAL** 10-40 mcg in divided doses (1-4 sprays with pump); **PO** Initially 0.05 mg bid, adjust based on diurnal pattern of response; usual range (0.1-1.2 mg)/day in 2-3 divided doses

---

IV/SUBCUT 2-4 mcg/day or **SUBCUT** in 2 divided doses

• **Child 3 mo to 12 yr: INTRANASAL** 5-30 mcg/day in divided doses

Hemophilia/von Willebrand's disease

• **Adult/child >3 mo: IV** 0.3 mcg/kg in 0.9% NaCl over 15-30 min; may repeat if needed

• **Adult/child >11 mo: NASAL SPRAY** 300 mcg (1 spray in each nostril); give 2 hr prior to surgery

Antihemorrhagic

• **Adult/child >3 mo: IV/SUBCUT** 0.2-0.4 mcg/kg/dose

• **Adult/child <50 kg: INTRANASAL** 1 spray in 1 nostril

• **Adult/child >50 kg: INTRANASAL** 1 spray in each nostril

Nocturia

• **Adult 50-64 yr: INTRANASAL** 1 spray in 1 nostril 30 min before going to bed (not at increased risk for hyponatremia)

Uremic bleeding (unlabeled)

• **Adult: SUBCUT/IV** 0.3-0.4 mcg/kg as a single inj

Available forms: Inj 4 mcg/mL, rhinal tube delivery 2.5 mg/vial (0.1 mg/mL); tabs 0.1, 0.2 mg; nasal spray pump (DDAVP) 10 mcg/spray (0.1 mg/mL); nasal spray (Stimate) 1.5 mg/mL (150 mcg/dose); tablet 0.1, 0.2 mg

Administer:

PO route

• Store at room temperature

Nasal route

• DDAVP and Stimate are not interchangeable

• Prime before 1st dose (press down 4 times), pump stays primed for 1 wk; to reprime, press down 1 time

• **Nocturia:** do not shake bottle, prime by pumping 5 times into the air away from the face; if not used for >3 days, reprime with 2 actuations, have patient blow nose, tilt head back slightly, close nostril, inhale while pumping 1 time, wipe applicator and replace cap

Direct IV route

• Undiluted over 1 min for diabetes insipidus

Intermittent IV INFUSION route

• Diluted single dose/50 mL of 0.9% NaCl (adult and child >10 kg), single dose/10 mL as IV infusion over 15-30 min for von Willebrand's disease or hemophilia A

• Store in refrigerator

SIDE EFFECTS

CNS: Drowsiness, headache, lethargy, flushing, seizures

CV: Increased B/P, palpitations, tachycardia

EENT: Nasal irritation, congestion, rhinitis

GI: Nausea, heartburn, cramps

GU: Vulval pain

META: Hyponatremia, hyponatremia-induced seizures

SYST: Anaphylaxis (IV)

PHARMACOKINETICS

PO: Onset 1 hr, peak 4-7 hr

INTRANASAL: Onset 1 hr; peak 1-4 hr; duration 8-20 hr

IV: Onset 1 min, peak $1/2$ hr, duration >3 hr

INTERACTIONS

Increase: antidiuretic action—carBAMazepine, chlorproPAMIDE, clofibrate, SSRIs, lamotrigine

Increase: pressor effect—pressor products

Decrease: antidiuretic action—lithium, alcohol, demeclocycline, heparin, large doses of EPINEPHrine

NURSING CONSIDERATIONS

Assess:

• Pulse, B/P when giving IV or SUBCUT

• I&O ratio, weight daily; check for edema in extremities; if water retention severe, diuretic may be prescribed

• **Water intoxication:** lethargy, behavioral changes, disorientation, neuromuscular excitability

• **Intranasal use:** nausea, congestion, cramps, headache; usually decreased with decreased dose; for nasal mucosa changes: congestion, edema, discharge, scarring (nasal route)

• For severe allergic reaction, including anaphylaxis (IV route); notify prescriber, discontinue use

• **Nocturnal enuresis:** identify how often enuresis is occurring; avoid use in those prone to water intoxication or sodium depletion

• **Diabetes insipidus:** urine volume/osmolality and plasma osmolality; monitor for dry skin, poor turgor, thirst (dehydration)

• **Hemophilia/von Willebrand's disease:** factor VIII coagulant activity, bleeding time before using for hemostasis; assess for bleeding, frank and occult

• **Pregnancy/breastfeeding:** no well-controlled studies; use only if benefit outweighs fetal risk; use caution in breastfeeding, excretion is unknown

• **Beers:** avoid for treatment of nocturia or nocturnal polyuria; high risk of hyponatremia

Evaluate:

• Therapeutic response: absence of severe thirst, decreased urine output, decreased osmolality

Teach patient/family:

• About the proper technique for nasal instillation: to insert tube into nostril to instill product, clear nasal passage before use

• To avoid OTC products (cough, hay fever) because these preparations may contain EPINEPHrine, decrease product response; not to use with alcohol because adverse reactions may occur

• To wear emergency ID specifying therapy

• That, if dose is missed, to take when remembered up to 1 hr before next dose; not to double dose; to avoid fluids from 1 hr to up to 8 hr after PO dose

• To report upper respiratory infection, nasal congestion to prescriber

• How to use subcut, rotate sites

---

desonide topical
See Appendix B

---

desoximetasone
(dess-ox'ee-met'ah-sone)
Topicort, Topicort Spray
Func. class.: Corticosteroid, topical

ACTION: Crosses cell membrane to attach to receptors to decrease inflammation, itching; inhibits multiple inflammatory cytokines

USES: Inflammation/itching of corticosteroid-responsive dermatoses on the skin; spray—plaque psoriasis

CONTRAINDICATIONS: Hypersensitivity, use of some preparations on face, axilla, groin, intertriginous areas; monotherapy in primary bacterial infection, TB
Precautions: Pregnancy, breastfeeding, children, skin infections, Cushing's syndrome

DOSAGE AND ROUTES

• **Adult/child >10 yr:** Apply to affected areas 2 times/day
Available forms: Cream 0.05%, 0.25%; ointment 0.05%, 0.25%; gel 0.05%; spray 0.25%
Administer:
Topical route

• Do not use with occlusive dressings

• **Cream/ointment/lotion:** apply sparingly in a thin film and rub gently into the cleansed affected area

• **Gel:** apply sparingly in a thin film and rub gently into the cleansed affected area

• **Spray:** discard after 30 days; keep away from heat/flame; store at room temperature

SIDE EFFECTS
INTEG: Burning, folliculitis, pruritus, dermatitis, maceration
MISC: Hyperglycemia, glycosuria, systemic absorption, hypothalamic-pituitary-adrenal (HPA) axis suppression, Cushing's syndrome

NURSING CONSIDERATIONS
Assess:

• Skin reactions: burning, pruritus, folliculitis, dermatitis

• **Systemic absorption:** HPA suppression and possible adrenocortical insufficiency after stopping treatment

---

• **Pregnancy/breastfeeding:** if pregnancy is planned or suspected; no well-controlled studies; use only if benefit outweighs fetal risk; caution use in breastfeeding; do not apply to breast
Evaluate:
• Decrease in itching, inflammation on the skin
Teach patient/family:
Topical route
• Not to use with occlusive dressings
• **Cream/ointment/lotion:** apply sparingly in a thin film and rub gently into the cleansed affected area
• **Gel:** apply sparingly in a thin film and rub gently into the cleansed affected area
• **Spray:** discard after 30 days; keep away from heat/flame; store at room temperature

---

desvenlafaxine

Khedezla, Pristiq
Func. class.: Antidepressant
Chem. class.: Serotonin-receptor norepinephrine reuptake inhibitor (SNRI)

Do not confuse:
Pristiq/Prilosec

ACTION: May work by blocking the central presynaptic reuptake of 5-HT and NE, resulting in an increased sustained level of these neurotransmitters

USES: Major depressive disorder
Unlabeled uses: Vasomotor symptoms (hot flashes) associated with menopause

CONTRAINDICATIONS: Hypersensitivity to this product or venlafaxine, MAOI therapy
Precautions: CNS depression, abrupt discontinuation, hypertension, hepatic/renal disease, hyponatremia, geriatric patients, pregnancy, labor and delivery, breastfeeding, angina, bleeding, cardiac dysrhythmias, MI, stroke, mania, hypovolemia, dehydration, increased intraocular pressure

Black Box Warning: Children, suicidal ideation

DOSAGE AND ROUTES
Major depressive disorder
• **Adult: PO** Initially, 50 mg/day; max 400 mg/day with adjustments as needed
Reduction of hot flash frequency/severity in women with natural or medically induced menopause (unlabeled)
• **Adult: PO** 100-150 mg/day, max 200 mg/day
Renal/hepatic dose
• **Adult: PO** CCr 30-50 mL/min 50 mg daily; CCr <30 mL/min or end-stage renal disease 50 mg every other day; moderate to severe hepatic disease, max 100 mg/day

Available forms: Extended release tabs 25, 50, 100 mg
Administer:
• Without regard to food; food may minimize GI symptoms
• Extended release tab: do not crush, break, or chew
• Store at room temperature

SIDE EFFECTS
CNS: *Dizziness,* drowsiness, *headache,* tremor, paresthesias, asthenia, suicidal thoughts/behaviors, seizures, fatigue, chills, yawning, hot flashes, flushing, *irritability, insomnia, anxiety, abnormal dreams, fatigue*
CV: Palpitations, sinus tachycardia, increased blood pressure, orthostatic hypotension
EENT: Blurred vision, mydriasis, tinnitus, bruxism
GI: *Nausea,* xerostomia, *diarrhea,* constipation, vomiting, anorexia, weight loss, dysgeusia, hypercholesterolemia, hypertriglyceridemia
GU: Urinary retention/hesitancy, orgasm dysfunction, decreased libido, impotence, proteinuria
HEMA: Impaired platelet aggregation
INTEG: Photosensitivity, hyperhidrosis, diaphoresis, rash

SYST: Serotonin syndrome, neuroleptic malignant syndrome–like symptoms, toxic epidermal necrolysis, Stevens-Johnson syndrome, erythema multiforme, angioedema; neonatal abstinence syndrome (fetal exposure)

PHARMACOKINETICS

Protein binding 30%, elimination half-life 11 hr; elimination half-life is increased (hepatic/renal disease)

INTERACTIONS

Increase: serotonin syndrome, neuroleptic malignant syndrome–like reactions—SSRIs, other SNRIs, serotonin receptor agonists (almotriptan, eletriptan, frovatriptan, naratriptan, rizatriptan, SUMAtriptan, ZOLMitriptan), tricyclics, traZODone, sibutramine, ergots, lithium, nefazodone, meperidine, phentermine, MAOIs, dextromethorphan, linezolid, promethazine, methylphenidate, dexmethylphenidate, mirtazapine, pentazocine, tryptophan, methylene blue IV; do not administer concurrently

Increase: bleeding risk—salicylates, thrombolytics, NSAIDs, platelet inhibitors, anticoagulants

Increase: CNS depression—alcohol, opioids, antihistamines, sedatives/hypnotics

Increase: hallucinations, delusions, disorientation—zolpidem

Drug/Herb

Increase: desvenlafaxine action—kava, valerian

Drug/Lab Test

Increase: cholesterol, triglycerides

False positive: amphetamine, phencyclidine

Decrease: sodium

NURSING CONSIDERATIONS

Assess:

Black Box Warning: Suicidal thoughts/behaviors: mental status and mood; identify suicidal ideation

• **Serious skin reactions:** assess during and after treatment; discontinue product immediately if rash develops

• **Serotonin syndrome, neuroleptic malignant syndrome–like symptoms:** assess for nausea/vomiting, sedation, dizziness, diaphoresis (sweating), facial flush, hallucinations, mental status changes, myoclonia, restlessness, shivering, elevated blood pressure, hyperthermia, muscle rigidity, autonomic instability, mental status changes; if serotonin syndrome occurs, discontinue desvenlafaxine and any other serotonergic agents

• Monitor B/P baseline and periodically during treatment, lipid levels, signs of glaucoma

• Appetite and nutritional intake; weight loss is common, change diet as needed to support weight

• **Pregnancy/breastfeeding:** no well-controlled studies; use only if benefit outweighs fetal risk; discontinue breastfeeding or product, excreted in breast milk

Evaluate:

• Decreased depression, increased sense of well-being, renewed interest in activities

Teach patient/family:

• To take as directed, not to double or skip doses; if a dose is missed, take as soon as remembered unless close to next dose; do not discontinue abruptly, decrease gradually

Black Box Warning: To report immediately suicidal thoughts/behaviors; have family members look for symptoms of suicidal ideation

• Not to operate machinery or engage in hazardous activities until reaction is known, may cause dizziness, drowsiness

• To avoid all other products unless approved by prescriber

• To report if pregnancy is planned or suspected or if breastfeeding

• **Serious skin reactions:** to report immediately allergic reactions, including rash, hives, difficulty breathing, or swelling of face, lips

• **Serotonin syndrome, neuroleptic malignant syndrome:** to report immediately nausea/vomiting, sedation, dizziness, sweating, facial flush

• That continuing follow-up exams will be needed; that low sodium levels may occur, to watch for headache, confusion, weakness

---

RARELY USED

deutetrabenazine
(du-tet-ra-BEN-a-zeen)
Austedo

USES: For the treatment of chorea associated with Huntington's disease and tardive dyskinesia

CONTRAINDICATIONS
Hypersensitivity, hepatic disease, MAOIs

Black Box Warning: Suicidal ideation

DOSAGE AND ROUTES
• **Adult (treatment naïve; not switching from tetrabenazine): PO** Initially, 6 mg/day; increase at weekly intervals by increments of 6 mg/day to a max of 48 mg/day
• **Adult (switching from tetrabenazine): PO** Discontinue tetrabenazine and start deutetrabenazine the next day. Use 6 mg/day for patients taking tetrabenazine 12.5 mg/day

dexamethasone (Rx)
(dex-ah-meth'a-sone)
Dexasone ✦
dexamethasone sodium phosphate (Rx)
Func. class.: Corticosteroid, synthetic
Chem. class.: Glucocorticoid, long acting

ACTION: Decreases inflammation by suppression of migration of polymorphonuclear leukocytes, fibroblasts, reversal of increased capillary permeability and lysosomal stabilization, suppresses normal immune response, no mineralocorticoid effects

USES: Inflammation, allergies, neoplasms, cerebral edema, septic shock, collagen disorders, dexamethasone suppression test for Cushing syndrome, adrenocortical insufficiency, TB, meningitis, acute exacerbations of MS

CONTRAINDICATIONS: Hypersensitivity to corticosteroids, sulfites, or benzyl alcohol; fungal infections, abrupt discontinuation, coagulopathy, ulcerative colitis, seizure disorders
Precautions: Pregnancy, breastfeeding, diabetes mellitus, osteoporosis, seizure disorders, ulcerative colitis, HF, myasthenia gravis, renal disease, peptic ulcer, esophagitis, recent MI, hypertension, TB, active hepatitis, psychosis, sulfite hypersensitivity, thromboembolic disorders

DOSAGE AND ROUTES
Inflammatory condition/neoplasias
• **Adult: PO** 0.75-9 mg/day in divided doses q6-12hr or phosphate **IM** 0.5-9 mg/day divided q6-12hr
• **Child: PO** 0.024-0.34 mg/kg/day in divided doses q6-12hr
Anaphylactic shock
• **Adult: IV** (phosphate) single dose 1-6 mg/kg or **IV** 40 mg q2-6hr as needed up to 72 hr
Airway edema/extubation
• **Adult: PO/IM/IV** 0.5-2 mg/kg/day divided q6hr; use 24 hr before extubation and use for 24 hr after extubation
Chemotherapy-induced vomiting
• **Adult: PO/IV** 10-20 mg 15-30 min before chemotherapy or 10 mg q12hr on each treatment day
• **Child: IV** 5-20 mg 15-30 min before chemotherapy
Cerebral edema
• **Adult: IV** (phosphate) 10 mg, then 4-6 mg **IM** q6hr × 2-4 days, then taper over 1 wk
• **Child:** loading dose 1-2 mg/kg **(PO/IM/IV)**, then 1-1.5 mg/kg/day, max 16 mg/day divided q4-6hr for 2-4 days, then taper down weekly
Palliative management of recurrent or inoperable brain tumors
• **Adult: IM/IV** 2 mg bid-tid (maintenance)
Adrenocortical insufficiency
• **Adult: PO** 0.75-9 mg/day in divided doses

- **Child: PO** 0.03-0.3 mg/kg/day in 2-4 divided doses

Suppression test for Cushing's syndrome

- **Adult: PO** 1 mg at 11 PM or 0.5 mg q6hr × 48 hr

Available forms: Tabs 0.5, 0.75, 1, 1.5, 2, 4, 6 mg; oral sol 0.5 mg/5 mL; elixir 0.5 mg/5 mL, oral concentrate 1 mg/mL; injection 4 mg/mL, 10 mg/mL

Administer:

PO route

- Titrated dose; use lowest effective dose
- With food or milk to decrease GI symptoms, give once daily in AM for less toxicity, fewer adverse reactions

IM route

- IM inj deeply in large muscle mass; rotate sites; avoid deltoid; use 21-G needle
- In 1 dose in AM to prevent adrenal suppression; avoid SUBCUT administration, may damage tissue

Intra-articular/intralesional route

- Use rarely as injections may damage joints

Continuous IV infusion

- Change IV solution q24hr

Direct IV route (sodium phosphate)

- Undiluted direct over ≤1 min

Intermittent IV INFUSION route

- Diluted with 0.9% NaCl or D₅W, give as IV infusion at prescribed rate

Y-site compatibilities: Acetaminophen, acyclovir, alfentanil, allopurinol, amifostine, amikacin, aminocaproic acid, aminophylline, amphotericin B cholesteryl, amphotericin B lipid complex, amphotericin B liposome, amsacrine, anidulafungin, argatroban, ascorbic acid injection, atenolol, atracurium, atropine, aztreonam, benztropine, bivalirudin, bleomycin, bumetanide, buprenorphine, butorphanol, caffeine, CARBOplatin, carmustine, ceFAZolin, cefepime, cefmetazole, cefonicid, cefotaxime, cefoTEtan, cefOXitin, cefpirome, ceftaroline, cefTAZidime, ceftizoxime, cefTRIAXone, chloramphenicol, cimetidine, cisatracurium, CISplatin, cladribine, clindamycin, codeine, cyanocobalamin, cyclophosphamide, cycloSPORINE, cytarabine, DACTINomycin,

DAPTOmycin, DAUNOrubicin, dexmedetomidine, digoxin, diltiazem, DOCEtaxel, DOPamine, doripenem, doxacurium, DOXOrubicin, DOXOrubicin liposomal, enalaprilat, ePHEDrine, EPINEPHrine, epoetin alfa, eptifibatide, ertapenem, etoposide, etoposide phosphate, famotidine, fentaNYL, filgrastim, fluconazole, fludarabine, fluorouracil, folic acid, fosaprepitant, foscarnet, furosemide, ganciclovir, gatifloxacin, gemcitabine, glycopyrrolate, granisetron, heparin, hydrocortisone, HYDROmorphone, ifosfamide, imipenem-cilastatin, indomethacin, insulin (regular), irinotecan, isoproterenol, ketorolac, lansoprazole, leucovorin, levofloxacin, lidocaine, linezolid, liposome, LORazepam, LR, mannitol, mechlorethamine, melphalan, meropenem, metaraminol, methadone, methicillin, methoxamine, methyldopate, methylPREDNISolone, metoclopramide, metoprolol, metroNIDAZOLE, mezlocillin, miconazole, milrinone, morphine, multiple vitamins injection, nafcillin, nalbuphine, naloxone, nitroglycerin, nitroprusside, norepinephrine, octreotide, ondansetron, oxacillin, oxaliplatin, oxyCODONE, oxytocin, PACLitaxel, palonosetron, pamidronate, pancuronium, PEMEtrexed, penicillin G potassium/sodium, PENTobarbital, PHENobarbital, phenylephrine, phytonadione, piperacillin, piperacillin-tazobactam, potassium chloride, procainamide, propofol, propranolol, pyridoxine, ranitidine, remifentanil, Ringer's, ritodrine, riTUXimab, sargramostim, sodium acetate/bicarbonate, succinylcholine, SUFentanil, tacrolimus, telavancin, teniposide, theophylline, thiamine, thiotepa, ticarcillin, ticarcillin-clavulanate, tigecycline, tirofiban, TNA, tolazoline, topotecan, trastuzumab, urokinase, vancomycin, vasopressin, vecuronium, verapamil, vinCRIStine, vinorelbine, vitamin B complex/C, voriconazole, zidovudine, zoledronic acid

SIDE EFFECTS

CNS: *Depression,* headache, mood changes, euphoria
CV: *Hypertension*

EENT: Increased intraocular pressure, cataracts

ENDO: HPA suppression, hyperglycemia, sodium, fluid retention, pheochromocytoma

GI: *Nausea,* peptic ulceration, vomiting

INTEG: Acne, poor wound healing, ecchymosis, petechiae, hirsutism

META: Hypokalemia, fluid retention, hypokalemic alkalosis

MS: Fractures, osteoporosis, weakness, arthralgia, myopathy

PHARMACOKINETICS

Half-life 1-2 days

PO: Onset 1 hr, peak 1-2 hr, duration $2^1/_2$ days

IM: Onset 1 hr, peak 1 hr, duration 2 days-3 wk

IV: Onset 1 hr, peak 1 hr, duration varies

INTERACTIONS

Increase: toxicity—cycloSPORINE

Increase: side effects—alcohol, salicylates, amphotericin B, digoxin, cycloSPORINE, diuretics, NSAIDs

Increase: dexamethasone action—salicylates, estrogens, hormonal contraceptives, ketoconazole, macrolide antiinfectives, NSAIDs

Increase: tendinitis, tendon rupture risk—quinolones

Decrease effect of—antidiabetics, insulin

Decrease: dexamethasone action—cholestyramine, colestipol, barbiturates, rifampin, phenytoin, theophylline, antacids, bosentan, carBAMazepine

Decrease: anticoagulant effect—anticonvulsants, antidiabetics, ambenonium, neostigmine, isoniazid, toxoids, vaccines, anticholinesterases, salicylates, somatrem

Decrease: potassium levels—thiazide/loop diuretics, amphotericin B

Drug/Lab Test

Increase: cholesterol, sodium, blood glucose

Decrease: calcium, potassium, T_4, T_3, thyroid ^{131}I uptake test

False negative: skin allergy tests

NURSING CONSIDERATIONS
Assess:

• Potassium, blood, urine glucose while receiving long-term therapy; hypo/hyperglycemia, Weight daily; notify prescriber of weekly gain >5 lb, B/P, pulse; notify prescriber of chest pain

• I&O ratio; be alert for decreasing urinary output, increasing edema

• **Cerebral edema:** LOC, and headache, baseline and periodically

• **Adrenal insufficiency:** weight loss, nausea, vomiting, anorexia, confusion, decreased B/P, baseline and periodically

• **Epidural injections (unlabeled):** may cause rare events (vision loss, paralysis, stroke, death)

• **Cushingoid symptoms:** assess for buffalo hump, moon face, increased B/P; monitor plasma cortisol levels during long-term therapy (normal: 138-635 nmol/L SI units when drawn at 8 AM); prolonged use can cause cushingoid symptoms

• **Infection:** fever, WBC even after withdrawal of medication; product masks infection

• **Potassium depletion:** paresthesias, fatigue, nausea, vomiting, depression, polyuria, dysrhythmias, weakness

• **Edema,** hypertension, cardiac symptoms

• **Mental status:** affect, mood, behavioral changes, aggression

• **Abrupt withdrawal:** acute adrenal insufficiency and death may occur following abrupt discontinuation of systemic therapy; withdraw gradually

• **Pregnancy/breastfeeding:** no well-controlled studies; use only if benefit outweighs fetal risk; discontinue breastfeeding or product

Evaluate:

• Therapeutic response: decreased inflammation

Teach patient/family:

• To carry medical alert ID as corticosteroid user at all times

• To contact prescriber if surgery, trauma, stress occurs because dose may need to be adjusted

---

• To notify prescriber if therapeutic response decreases because dosage adjustment may be needed
• To take with food or milk
• That bruising may occur easily
• That if on long-term therapy, a high-protein diet may be needed
• Not to discontinue abruptly because **adrenal crisis** can result
• **About symptoms of adrenal insufficiency:** nausea, anorexia, fatigue, dizziness, dyspnea, weakness, joint pain, hypertension
• To avoid OTC products: salicylates, alcohol in cough products, cold preparations unless directed by prescriber
• About all aspects of product usage, including cushingoid symptoms; to notify health care provider of infection
• To avoid exposure to chickenpox or measles, persons with infection

dexamethasone (ophthalmic)
(dex-a-meth′a-sone)
Maxidex
Func. class.: Ophthalmic antiinflammatory
Chem. class.: Corticosteroid

Do not confuse:
dexamethasone/desoximetasone

ACTION: Exact mechanism of antiinflammatory action unknown; inhibits multiple inflammatory cytokines; decreases inflammation, collagen deposits, capillary dilation, edema

USES: Treatment of corticosteroid-responsive ophthalmic disorders

CONTRAINDICATIONS: Hypersensitivity to this product or sulfites, ocular TB, acute herpes simplex (superficial), fungal/viral infections of the eye, posterior lens capsule rupture
Precautions: Corneal infected abrasions, glaucoma, pregnancy, breastfeeding, migration of intravitreal implant risk, children

DOSAGE AND ROUTES
Corticosteroid-responsive ophthalmic disorders
• **Adult:** Instill 1 or 2 drops of 0.1% ophthalmic sol or susp every hr during the day and every 2 hr at night; reduce application to every 4 hr after response occurs
Available forms: Ophthalmic solution, suspension 0.1%
Administer:
• For ophthalmic use only
• Instruct patient on proper instillation of eye ointment or solution; do not touch the tip of the dropper to the eye, fingertips, or other surface; wait ≥15 min before inserting soft contact lens

SIDE EFFECTS
EENT: Burning, stinging, poor vision, corneal ulcerations, increased IOP, optic nerve damage

NURSING CONSIDERATIONS
Assess:
• **Corneal effects:** ulcerations, infections can worsen with this product
Evaluate:
• Decreased corneal inflammation
Teach patient/family:
• How to use products
• Not to share with others or use for other conditions
• To notify prescriber immediately if vision changes or if condition worsens
• To take as prescribed

dexlansoprazole (Rx)
(dex-lan-so-prey′zole)
Dexilant
Func. class.: Antiulcer, proton pump inhibitor
Chem. class.: Benzimidazole

ACTION: Suppresses gastric secretion by inhibiting hydrogen/potassium ATPase enzyme system in gastric parietal cell; characterized as gastric acid pump inhibitor because it blocks final step of acid production

USES: Gastroesophageal reflux disease (GERD), severe erosive esophagitis, heartburn

CONTRAINDICATIONS: Hypersensitivity

Precautions: Pregnancy, breastfeeding, children, proton-pump hypersensitivity, gastric cancer, hepatic disease, vit B_{12} deficiency, colitis

DOSAGE AND ROUTES
Erosive esophagitis
• **Adult:** PO 60 mg daily for up to 8 wk; maintenance: **PO** 30 mg daily for up to 6 mo
GERD
• **Adult:** PO 30 mg daily × 4 wk
Hepatic disease
• **Adult:** PO (Child-Pugh B): max 30 mg/day
Available forms: Del rel caps 30, 60 mg
Administer:
• Swallow caps whole; do not crush, chew caps; caps may be opened, contents sprinkled on food, use immediately; do not chew contents of capsule; give without regard to food

SIDE EFFECTS
CNS: Headache, dizziness, confusion, agitation, amnesia, depression, anxiety, seizures, insomnia, migraine
CV: Chest pain, angina, bradycardia, palpitations, CVA, hypertension, MI
EENT: Tinnitus
GI: Diarrhea, abdominal pain, vomiting, nausea, constipation, flatulence, colitis, dysgeusia, pseudomembranous colitis
HEMA: Anemia, neutropenia, thrombocytopenia, pernicious anemia, thrombosis
INTEG: Rash, urticaria, pruritus
META: Gout
MS: Arthralgia, mylagia
RESP: Upper respiratory infections, cough, epistaxis, dyspnea, pneumonia
SYST: Anaphylaxis, Stevens-Johnson syndrome, toxic epidermal necrolysis, exfoliative dermatitis

PHARMACOKINETICS
Absorption 57%-64%; half-life 1-2 hr; protein binding 96.1%-98.8%; extensively metabolized in liver 🦎 by CYP2C19/CYP3A4; excreted in urine, feces; clearance decreased in geriatric patients, renal/hepatic impairment; peak 4 hr

INTERACTIONS
Increase: dexlansoprazole effect—CYP2C19, 3A4 inhibitors (fluvoxaMINE, voriconazole)
Decrease: dexlansoprazole absorption —sucralfate
Decrease: absorption of ketoconazole, itraconazole, iron, delavirdine, ampicillin, calcium carbonate
Drug/Herb
Decrease: dexlansoprazole effect—St. John's wort
Drug/Lab Test
Increase: LFTs, bilirubin, creatinine, glucose, lipids
Decrease: platelets, magnesium

NURSING CONSIDERATIONS
Assess:
• **CDAD (rare):** diarrhea, abdominal cramps, fever; report to prescriber promptly
• **Hepatotoxicity (rare):** hepatitis, jaundice; monitor hepatic studies (AST, ALT, alk phos) if hepatic adverse reactions occur
• **Hypomagnesemia:** usually 3 mo to 1 yr after beginning therapy; monitor magnesium level, assess for irregular heartbeats, muscle spasms; in children, fatigue, upset stomach, dizziness; magnesium supplement may be used
• **Anaphylaxis (rare), serious skin disorders:** require emergency intervention
• **Beers:** avoid scheduled use >8 wk in older adults who are at high risk for erosive esophagitis, pathologic hypersecretory conditions
• **Pregnancy/breastfeeding:** no well-controlled studies; use only if benefit outweighs fetal risk; avoid breastfeeding, excretion is unknown

---

Evaluate:

• Therapeutic response: absence of epigastric pain, swelling, fullness; healing of erosive esophagitis

Teach patient/family:

• **CDAD:** to report to prescriber at once abdominal cramps, bloody diarrhea, fever
• That diabetic patient should know that hypoglycemia may occur
• To avoid hazardous activities; dizziness may occur
• To avoid alcohol, salicylates, ibuprofen; may cause GI irritation
• To report allergic reactions, symptoms of low magnesium levels
• To notify prescriber if pregnancy is planned or suspected; not to breastfeed
• To swallow cap whole, not to chew, crush; to report all products being used to prescriber

dexmethylphenidate (Rx)

(dex′meth-ul-fen′ih-dayt)

Focalin, Focalin XR

Func. class.: Central nervous system (CNS) stimulant, psychostimulant
Controlled Substance Schedule II

Do not confuse:

dexmethylphenidate/methylphenidate

ACTION: Increases release of norepinephrine and DOPamine into the extraneuronal space; also blocks the reuptake of norepinephrine and DOPamine into the presynaptic neuron; mode of action for treating attention-deficit/hyperactivity disorder (ADHD) is unknown

USES: ADHD

CONTRAINDICATIONS: Hypersensitivity to methylphenidate, anxiety, history of Gilles de la Tourette's syndrome, tics, glaucoma, concurrent treatment with MAOIs or within 14 days of discontinuing treatment with MAOIs

Precautions: Pregnancy, hypertension, depression, seizures, CV disorders, breastfeeding, child <6 yr, geriatric patients, psychosis, thyrotoxicosis

Black Box Warning: Substance abuse, alcoholism

DOSAGE AND ROUTES

• **Adult/adolescent/child >6 yr: PO** 2.5 mg bid with doses at least 4 hr apart, gradually increase to a maximum of 20 mg/day (10 mg bid); for those taking methylphenidate, use ¹/₂ of methylphenidate dose initially, then increase as needed to a max of 20 mg/day
• **Adolescent/child ≥6 yr: EXT REL** 5 mg/day, may adjust to 20 mg/day in 5-mg increments, max 30 mg/day
• **Adult: PO EXT REL** 10 mg/day, may adjust to 20 mg/day in 10-mg increments, max 40 mg/day

Available forms: Tabs 2.5, 5, 10 mg; ext rel caps 5, 10, 15, 20, 25, 30, 35, 40 mg

Administer:

• Twice daily at least 4 hr apart; ext rel once a day; in the morning, ext rel cap may be opened and contents sprinkled onto applesauce and consumed without chewing
• Without regard to meals
• Do not break, crush, or chew ext rel product
• Med guide should be provided by dispenser

SIDE EFFECTS

CNS: Dizziness, headache, drowsiness, nervousness, insomnia, toxic psychosis, neuroleptic malignant syndrome (rare), Tourette's syndrome

CV: Palpitations, B/P changes, angina, dysrhythmias, tachycardia, MI, stroke

GI: *Nausea, anorexia,* abnormal hepatic function, hepatic coma, *abdominal pain*

HEMA: Leukopenia, anemia, thrombocytopenic purpura

INTEG: Exfoliative dermatitis, urticaria, rash, erythema multiforme

MISC: *Fever,* arthralgia, scalp hair loss, rhabdomyolysis

PHARMACOKINETICS

Readily absorbed, elimination half-life 2.2 hr, metabolized by liver, excreted by kidneys

PO: Peak 1¹/₂ hr, onset ¹/₂-1 hr
PO-ER: Onset unknown, peak 4 hr

Side effects: *italics* = common; red = life-threatening

INTERACTIONS

Increase: hypertensive crisis—MAOIs or within 14 days of MAOIs, vasopressors

Increase: sympathomimetic effect—decongestants, vasoconstrictors

Increase: effects of anticonvulsants, tricyclics, SSRIs, coumarin

Decrease: effects of antihypertensives

Drug/Herb

• Synergistic effect—melatonin

NURSING CONSIDERATIONS

Assess:

Black Box Warning: Substance abuse, past or current; psychotic episodes may occur, especially with parenteral abuse; avoid use in a history of substance abuse or alcoholism as dependence may occur

• **Toxicity:** rhabdomyolysis, headache, flushing, vomiting, agitation, tachycardia, tremor, euphoria, hallucinations, hyperreflexia

• VS, B/P; may reverse antihypertensives; check patients with cardiac disease more often for increased B/P

• CBC, differential platelet counts during long-term therapy, urinalysis; with diabetes: blood glucose, urine glucose; insulin changes may have to be made because eating will decrease

• Height, growth rate q3mo in children; growth rate may be decreased; weight loss, anorexia may occur

• Mental status: mood, sensorium, affect, stimulation, insomnia, aggressiveness, hostility

• **Withdrawal symptoms:** headache, nausea, vomiting, muscle pain, weakness

• Appetite, sleep, speech patterns

• For attention span, decreased hyperactivity in persons with ADHD

• **Pregnancy/breastfeeding:** no well-controlled studies; use only if benefit outweighs fetal risk; avoid breastfeeding, excretion is unknown

Evaluate:

• Therapeutic response: decreased hyperactivity or ability to stay awake

Teach patient/family:

• To decrease caffeine consumption (coffee, tea, cola, chocolate); may increase irritability, stimulation

• To take early in day to prevent insomnia; not to take more than prescribed, dependence may occur

• To avoid OTC preparations unless approved by prescriber; to avoid alcohol ingestion

• To taper off product over several wk to avoid depression, increased sleeping, lethargy

• To report weight loss; anorexia may occur

• To avoid hazardous activities until stabilized on medication

• To get needed rest; patients will feel more tired at end of day

• To notify all health care workers, including school nurse, of medication and schedule

• About information, instructions provided in patient information section

• To notify prescriber if pregnancy is planned or suspected; to avoid breastfeeding

• **To report toxicity immediately:** vomiting, agitation, tremor, hyperreflexia, euphoria, confusion, hallucinations, flushing, headache, tachycardia, rhabdomyolysis

TREATMENT OF OVERDOSE:
Administer fluids; hemodialysis: or peritoneal dialysis; antihypertensive for increased B/P; administer short-acting barbiturate before lavage

---

dextroamphetamine (Rx)

(dex-troe-am-fet′a-meen)

Dexedrine, ProCentra, Zenzedi

Func. class.: Cerebral stimulant

Chem. class.: Amphetamine

Controlled Substance Schedule II

ACTION: Increases release of norepinephrine, DOPamine in cerebral cortex to reticular activating system

USES: Narcolepsy, attention-deficit/hyperactivity disorder (ADHD)

Unlabeled uses: Obesity

CONTRAINDICATIONS: Hypersensitivity to sympathomimetic amines, hyperthyroidism, glaucoma, severe arteriosclerosis

Black Box Warning: Substance abuse

Precautions: Pregnancy, breastfeeding, children <3 yr, depression, Gilles de la Tourette's disorder, cardiomyopathy, bipolar disorder, abrupt discontinuation, acute MI; benzyl alcohol, salicylate hypersensitivity; hypercortisolism, obesity, psychosis, seizure disorder, hypertension, anxiety, anorexia nervosa, tartrazine dye hypersensitivity

Black Box Warning: Symptomatic cardiac disease

DOSAGE AND ROUTES
Narcolepsy
• **Adult:** PO 5 mg bid, titrate daily dose by no more than 10 mg/wk, max 60 mg/day
• **Child 6-12 yr:** PO 5 mg/day, titrate daily dose by no more than 5 mg/day at weekly intervals, max 60 mg/day
ADHD
• **Adult:** PO 5-60 mg/day daily or divided bid, max 40 mg/day
• **Child 3-5 yr:** PO 2.5 mg/day increasing by 2.5 mg/day at weekly intervals, max 40 mg/day
• **Child >6-12 yr:** PO 5 mg daily-bid increasing by 5 mg/day at weekly intervals
Obesity, exogenous (unlabeled)
• **Adult and adolescent:** PO 5-30 mg/dose given 30-60 min before meals, use for 3-6 wk only
Available forms: Tabs 2.5, 5, 7.5, 10, 15, 20, 30 mg; oral sol 5 mg/5 mL; caps: ext rel 5, 10, 15 mg
Administer:
• At least 6 hr before bedtime to avoid sleeplessness
• Use calibrated measuring device for oral sol
• Store all forms at room temperature

SIDE EFFECTS
CNS: *Hyperactivity, insomnia, restlessness, talkativeness,* dizziness, headache, chills, stimulation, dysphoria, irritability, aggressiveness, tremor, dependence, addiction
CV: *Palpitations, tachycardia,* hypertension, decrease in heart rate, dysrhythmias
GI: *Anorexia,* dry mouth, diarrhea, constipation, weight loss, metallic taste
GU: Impotence, change in libido
INTEG: Urticaria
MISC: Rhabdomyolysis

PHARMACOKINETICS
Onset 30-60 min, peak 2 hr, duration 4 hr; ext rel onset 1 hr, peak 2 hr, duration 8 hr; metabolized by liver; urine excretion pH dependent; crosses placenta, breast milk; half-life 6-8 hr (child), 10-12 hr (adult)

INTERACTIONS
• Hypertensive crisis: MAOIs or within 14 days of MAOIs
Increase: serotonin syndrome, neuroleptic malignant syndrome: SSRIs, SNRIs, serotonin-receptor agonists; do not use concurrently
Increase: dextroamphetamine effect—acetaZOLAMIDE, antacids, sodium bicarbonate
Increase: CNS effect—haloperidol, tricyclics, phenothiazines
Decrease: absorption of barbiturates, phenytoin
Decrease: dextroamphetamine effect—ascorbic acid, ammonium chloride
Decrease: effect of adrenergic blockers, antidiabetics, antihypertensives, antihistamines
Drug/Herb
• Serotonin syndrome—St. John's wort
Decrease: stimulant effect—eucalyptus
Drug/Food
Increase: amine effect—caffeine (cola, coffee, tea [green/black])
Decrease: effect—fruit juice (oral solution)
Drug/Lab Test
Increase: plasma corticosteroids, urinary steroids

Side effects: *italics* = common; red = life-threatening

NURSING CONSIDERATIONS
Assess:

Black Box Warning: **Cardiac disease:** VS, B/P; product may reverse antihypertensives; check patients with cardiac disease often

Black Box Warning: **Substance abuse:** use for prolonged periods may lead to dependence; sudden death or serious CV events can occur from misuse; chronic intoxication (insomnia, irritability, personality changes)

• CBC, urinalysis; with diabetes: blood glucose, urine glucose; insulin changes may be required because eating will decrease
• Height, growth rate in children (growth rate may be decreased), weight
• **Toxicity:** symptoms may vary in children; anxiety, headache, flushing, vomiting, rhabdomyolysis, tremor, hyperreflexia, confusion, euphoria, tachycardia
• **ADHD:** change in behavior, growth retardation in children
• Mental status: mood, sensorium, affect, stimulation, insomnia, irritability
• Tolerance or dependency: increased amount may be used to get same effect; will develop after long-term use
• **Pregnancy/breastfeeding:** no well-controlled studies; use only if benefit outweighs fetal risk; avoid breastfeeding, excreted in breast milk
Evaluate:
• Therapeutic response: increased CNS stimulation, decreased drowsiness
Teach patient/family:
• To take before meals (obesity)
• To decrease caffeine consumption (coffee, tea, cola, chocolate); may increase irritability, stimulation
• To avoid OTC preparations unless approved by prescriber; to avoid alcohol ingestion; to avoid fruit juice at same time as solution, effect is decreased
• To tell parents that change in behavior may occur in beginning treatment, irritability, hostility

• **Seizures:** that those with a seizure disorder may have decreased seizure threshold
• To taper product over several wk; depression, increased sleeping, lethargy may occur
• To avoid hazardous activities until stabilized on medication
• To get needed rest; patient will feel more tired at end of day

TREATMENT OF OVERDOSE: Administer fluids, hemodialysis; antihypertensive for increased B/P, ammonium chloride for increased excretion

---

dextromethorphan (OTC)
(dex-troe-meth-or′fan)
Balminil ✦, Benylin DM ✦, Bronchophan Forte DM ✦, Buckley's Mixture, Delsym 12-Hour, ElixSure Cough, Koffex ✦, Robitussin, Robitussin Cough with honey, Robitussin Long Acting Strength, Scot-Tussin Diabetes CF, Triaminic Long Acting Cough, Vicks Formula 44, Wal-Tussin
Func. class.: Antitussive, nonopioid
Chem. class.: Levorphanol derivative

ACTION: Depresses cough center in medulla by direct effect

USES: Nonproductive cough caused by colds or inhaled irritants

CONTRAINDICATIONS: Hypersensitivity, MAOIs, SSRIs
Precautions: Pregnancy, fever, hepatic disease, asthma/emphysema, chronic cough, child <4 yr, breastfeeding

DOSAGE AND ROUTES
• **Adult/child ≥12 yr: PO** 10-20 mg q4hr or 30 mg q6-8hr, max 120 mg/day; **SUS REL LIQ** 60 mg q12hr, max 120 mg/day

---

- **Child 6-11 yr: PO** 5-10 mg q4hr; **SUS REL LIQ** 30 mg bid, **LOZ** 5-10 mg q1-4hr; max 60 mg/day
- **Child 4-5 yr: PO** 2.5-7.5 mg q4-8hr, max 30 mg/day; **SUS REL LIQ** 15 mg bid

Available forms: Liq 7.5, 15 mg/5 mL; syr 10 mg/5 mL, 15 mg/5 mL, 30 mg/15 mL; gel caps 15 mg; caps 15 mg; ext rel susp: 30 mg/5 mL

Administer:
- **Chew tabs:** chew well; **syrup:** use calibrated measuring device; **ext rel susp:** shake well, use calibrated measuring device
- Decreased dose for geriatric patients; metabolism may be slowed

SIDE EFFECTS
CNS: *Dizziness,* sedation, confusion, ataxia, fatigue
GI: *Nausea*

PHARMACOKINETICS
PO: Onset 15-30 min, duration 3-6 hr
SUS: Duration 12 hr, terminal half-life 11 hr, metabolized by the liver, excreted via kidneys

INTERACTIONS
- Do not give with MAOIs or within 2 wk of MAOIs; avoid furazolidone, linezolid, procarbazine (MAOI activity)
Increase: CNS depression—alcohol, antidepressants, antihistamines, opioids, sedative/hypnotics
Increase: adverse reactions—amiodarone, quiNIDine, serotonin receptor agonist, sibutramine, SSRI

NURSING CONSIDERATIONS
Assess:
- **Cough:** type, frequency, character, lung sounds, sputum
- Increase fluids to liquefy secretions, unless contraindicated
- **Pregnancy/breastfeeding:** no well-controlled studies; use only if benefit outweighs fetal risk; avoid breastfeeding
Evaluate:
- Therapeutic response: absence of cough
Teach patient/family:

- To avoid driving, other hazardous activities until stabilized on medication
- To avoid smoking, smoke-filled rooms, perfumes, dust, environmental pollutants, cleaners that increase cough
- To avoid alcohol, CNS depressants
- To notify prescriber if cough persists over a few days
- Not to use if breastfeeding, or in child <4 yr

> **⚠ HIGH ALERT**

diazepam (Rx)
(dye-az′-e-pam)
Diastat, Valium
Func. class.: Antianxiety, anticonvulsant, skeletal muscle relaxant, central acting
Chem. class.: Benzodiazepine, long-acting

Controlled Substance Schedule IV

Do not confuse:
diazepam/Ditropan/LORazepam

ACTION: Potentiates the actions of GABA, especially in the limbic system, reticular formation; enhances presympathetic inhibition, inhibits spinal polysynaptic afferent paths

USES: Anxiety, acute alcohol withdrawal, adjunct for seizure disorders; preoperatively as a relaxant for skeletal muscle relaxation; rectally for acute repetitive seizures

CONTRAINDICATIONS: Pregnancy, hypersensitivity to benzodiazepines, closed-angle glaucoma, coma, myasthenia gravis, ethanol intoxication, hepatic disease, sleep apnea
Precautions: Breastfeeding, children <6 mo, geriatric patients, debilitation, renal disease, asthma, bipolar disorder, COPD, CNS depression, labor, Parkinson's disease, neutropenia, psychosis, seizures, substance abuse, smoking

Black Box Warning: Coadministration with other CNS depressants, respiratory depression

---

Side effects: *italics* = common; red = life-threatening

DOSAGE AND ROUTES

Anxiety/seizure disorders

- **Adult: PO** 2-10 mg bid-qid; **IM/IV** 2-5 mg q3-4hr
- **Geriatric: PO** 2-2.5 mg daily-bid, increase slowly as needed
- **Child >6 mo: PO** 1-2.5 mg tid/qid; **IM/IV** 0.04-0.3 mg/kg/dose q2-4hr, max 0.6 mg/kg in an 8-hr period

Precardioversion

- **Adult: IV** 5-15 mg 5-10 min precardioversion

Preendoscopy

- **Adult: IV** 2.5-20 mg; **IM** 5-10 mg $^1/_2$ hr preendoscopy

Muscle relaxation

- **Adult: PO** 2-10 mg tid-qid or **EXT REL** 15-30 mg/day; **IV/IM** 5-10 mg, repeat in 2-4 hr

Tetanic muscle spasms

- **Child >5 yr: IM/IV** 5-10 mg q3-4hr prn
- **Infant >30 days: IM/IV** 1-2 mg q3-4hr prn

Status epilepticus

- **Adult: IV/IM** 5-10 mg, 2 mg/min, may repeat q10-15min, max 30 mg; may repeat in 2-4 hr if seizures reappear
- **Child >5 yr: IM** 1 mg q2-5min; **IV** 1 mg slowly
- **Child 1 mo-5 yr: IV** 0.2-0.5 mg slowly; **IM** 0.2-0.5 mg slowly q2-5min up to 5 mg, may repeat in 2-4 hr prn

Seizures other than status epilepticus

- **Adult: RECT** 0.2 mg/kg, may repeat in 4-12 hr
- **Child 6-11 yr: RECT** 0.3 mg/kg, may repeat in 4-12 hr
- **Child 2-5 yr: RECT** 0.5 mg/kg, may repeat in 4-12 hr

Alcohol withdrawal

- **Adult: IV** 10 mg initially, then 5-10 mg q3-4hr prn

Psychoneurotic reactions

- **Adult: IM/IV** 2-10 mg, may repeat in 3-4 hr

Available forms: Tabs 2, 5, 10 mg; inj 5 mg/mL; oral sol 5 mg/5 mL, rectal 2.5 (pediatric), 10, 20 mg, twin packs; ext rel cap 15 mg, rectal gel

Administer:

PO route

- With food or milk for GI symptoms; crushed if patient is unable to swallow medication whole
- Reduce opioid dose by $^1/_3$ if given concomitantly with diazepam
- **Concentrate:** use calibrated dropper only; mix with water, juice, pudding, applesauce; to be consumed immediately

Rectal route

- Do not use more than 5×/mo or for an episode q5days (Diastat)

IM route

- Painful, use deltoid if used this route

Direct IV route

- Have emergency equipment nearby
- Observe for several hours after IV; if used in combination with opioids, decrease opioid dose
- Into large vein; give IV 5 mg or less/1 min or total dose over 3 min or more (children, infants); continuous infusion is not recommended; inject as close to vein insertion as possible; do not dilute or mix with other products

SIDE EFFECTS

CNS: *Dizziness, drowsiness,* headache, hangover, slurred speech, paradoxical excitation

CV: Hypotension

EENT: *Blurred vision*

GI: Constipation, nausea, vomiting, diarrhea, weight gain

INTEG: Rash, dermatitis, itching, phlebitis (IV), venous thrombosis

RESP: Respiratory depression

MISC: Psychological/physical dependency, tolerance

PHARMACOKINETICS

Metabolized by liver via ⚕ CYP2C19, CYP3A4; 15%-20% of ⚕ Asian patients and up to 5% of Caucasians and black patients are poor metabolizers; excreted by kidneys; crosses placenta; excreted in breast milk; crosses the blood-brain barrier; half-life 1-12 days; more reliable by mouth; 99% protein binding

PO: Rapidly absorbed, onset $^1/_2$ hr, peak 2 hr, duration up to 24 hr

IM: Onset 15-30 min, duration 1-1$^1/_2$ hr, absorption slow and erratic

RECT: Peak 1.5 hr

IV: Onset immediate, duration 15 min-1 hr

INTERACTIONS

Increase: diazepam effect—amiodarone, protease inhibitors, diltiazem, cimetidine, clarithromycin, dalfopristin-quinupristin, delavirdine, disulfiram, efavirenz, erythromycin, fluconazole, fluvoxaMINE, imatinib, itraconazole, ketoconazole, IV miconazole, nefazodone, niCARdipine, ranolazine, troleandomycin, valproic acid, verapamil, voriconazole, zafirlukast, zileuton; monitor for increased sedation

Increase: toxicity—barbiturates, SSRIs, cimetidine, CNS depressants, valproic acid, CYP3A4 inhibitors

Increase: CNS depression—CNS depressants, alcohol; monitor for increased sedation

Decrease: diazepam metabolism—oral contraceptives, valproic acid, disulfiram, isoniazid, propranolol

Decrease: diazepam effect—CYP3A4 inducers (rifampin, barbiturates, carBAMazepine, ethotoin, phenytoin, fosphenytoin), smoking

Drug/Herb

Increase: CNS depression—kava, chamomile, valerian

Drug/Lab Test

Increase: AST/ALT, alk phos

NURSING CONSIDERATIONS

Assess:

• B/P (lying, standing), pulse; if systolic B/P drops 20 mm Hg, hold product, notify prescriber

• Blood studies: CBC during long-term therapy; blood dyscrasias (rare); hepatic studies: AST, ALT, bilirubin, creatinine, LDH, alk phos

• **IV site:** frequently, watch for phlebitis

• **Degree of anxiety:** what precipitates anxiety and whether product controls symptoms

• **Alcohol withdrawal symptoms,** including hallucinations (visual, auditory), delirium, irritability, agitation, fine to coarse tremors

• Seizure control and type, duration, intensity of seizures

• For muscle spasms; pain relief

> **Black Box Warning:** Avoid coadministration with other CNS depressants; do not use with opioids

> **Black Box Warning: Respiratory depression:** monitor for respiratory depression, respirations q5-15 min if given IV

• IV site for thrombosis or phlebitis, which may occur rapidly

• Mental status: mood, sensorium, affect, sleeping pattern, drowsiness, dizziness, suicidal tendencies

• **Physical dependency, withdrawal symptoms:** headache, nausea, vomiting, muscle pain, weakness after long-term, high-dose use

• **Beers:** avoid use in older adults; may be appropriate for seizures, sleep disorders, benzodiazepine/ethanol withdrawal, severe anxiety disorders

• **Pregnancy/breastfeeding:** use in pregnancy not recommended; do not breastfeed, excretion in breast milk

Evaluate:

• Therapeutic response: decreased anxiety, restlessness, insomnia

Teach patient/family:

• That product may be taken with food

• That product not to be used for everyday stress or for >4 mo unless directed by prescriber; to take no more than prescribed amount; that product may be habit forming, review package insert with patient

• To avoid OTC preparations unless approved by prescriber

• To avoid driving, activities that require alertness; drowsiness may occur

• To avoid alcohol, other psychotropic medications unless directed by prescriber; that smoking may decrease diazepam effect by increasing diazepam metabolism

• Not to discontinue medication abruptly after long-term use; to gradually taper

• To rise slowly or fainting may occur, especially in geriatric patients

• That drowsiness may worsen at beginning of treatment

• To notify prescriber if pregnancy is planned or suspected; to avoid breastfeeding

TREATMENT OF OVERDOSE: Lavage, VS, supportive care, flumazenil

dibucaine topical
See Appendix B

diclofenac epolamine (Rx)
(dye-kloe'fen-ak)

Flector

diclofenac potassium (Rx)
Cambia, Zipsor

diclofenac sodium (Rx)
Dyloject, PENNSAID, Solaraze Topical Gel, Voltaren, Voltaren Topical Gel, Voltaren XR, Zorvolex

Func. class.: Nonsteroidal antiinflammatory products (NSAIDs), nonopioid analgesic

Chem. class.: Phenylacetic acid

Do not confuse:
Cataflam/Catapres

ACTION: Inhibits COX-1, COX-2 by blocking arachidonate, resulting in analgesic, antiinflammatory, antipyretic effects

USES: Acute, chronic RA; osteoarthritis; ankylosing spondylitis; analgesia; primary dysmenorrhea; patch: mild to moderate pain

Unlabeled uses: Arthralgia, headache, migraine, bone pain, myalgia

CONTRAINDICATIONS: Hypersensitivity to aspirin, iodides, other NSAIDs, bovine protein, asthma, serious CV disease; eczema, exfoliative dermatitis, skin abrasions (gel, patch); treatment of perioperative pain in CABG surgery

Precautions: Pregnancy, breastfeeding, children, bleeding disorders, GI disorders, cardiac disorders, hypersensitivity to other antiinflammatory agents, CCr <30 mL/min, accidental exposure, acute bronchospasm, hypersensitivity to benzyl alcohol

Black Box Warning: GI bleeding/perforation, MI, stroke

DOSAGE AND ROUTES
Osteoarthritis
• **Adult:** PO (Cataflam) 50 mg bid-tid, max 150 mg/day; **DEL REL** (Voltaren) 50 mg bid-tid or 75 mg bid, max 150 mg/day; **EXT REL** (Voltaren-XR) 100 mg daily, max 150 mg/day; **TOP GEL** 1% (Voltaren gel) 4 g for each of lower extremities qid, max 16 g/day; 2 g for each of upper extremities qid, max 8 g/day; **TOP SOL** (Pennsaid) apply 40 drops to each affected knee qid; apply 10 drops at a time, spread over entire knee

Rheumatoid arthritis
• **Adult:** PO (Cataflam) 50 mg tid-qid, max 200 mg/day; **DEL REL** (Voltaren) 50 mg tid-qid or 75 mg bid, max 200 mg/day; **EXT REL** (Voltaren-XR) 100 mg daily, may increase to 200 mg/day, max 200 mg/day

Ankylosing spondylitis
• **Adult:** PO DEL REL (Voltaren) 25 mg qid and 25 mg at bedtime, max 125 mg/day

Acute migraine with/without aura
• **Adult:** PO (powder for oral sol) (Cambia) 50 mg as a single dose, mix contents of packet in 1-2 oz water

Mild to moderate pain
• **Adult:** PO (Zipsor) 25 mg qid

Dysmenorrhea or nonrheumatic inflammatory conditions
• **Adult:** PO (Cataflam) 50 mg tid or 100 mg initially, then 50 mg tid, max 200 mg 1st day, then 150 mg/day, immediate release only

Pain of strains/sprains
* **Adult:** **TOP PATCH** (Flector) apply patch to area bid

Actinic keratosis
* **Adult:** **TOP GEL** (Solaraze) apply to area bid

Hepatic dose
* **Adult:** PO max 18 mg tid

Renal dose
* **Avoid:** Use of topical gel, patch, sol, potassium oral tab for advanced renal disease

Available forms: **Epolamine:** topical patch 1.3%; **potassium:** tabs 50 mg; tabs liquid filled 25 mg; oral powder for sol 50 mg; **sodium:** delayed rel tabs (enteric-coated) 25, 50, 75 mg; Pennsaid: ext rel tabs, 100 mg

Administer:

PO route
* Do not break, crush, or chew enteric products
* Take with a full glass of water to enhance absorption, remain upright for $1/2$ hr; if dose is missed, take as soon as remembered within 2 hr if taking 1-2×/day; do not double doses
* Allow 6 hr between use with another NSAID
* Store at room temperature

Powder:
* Mix powder in 30-60 mL water only
* Mix solution; have patient drink immediately
* Powder (Cambia) and Zorvolex may be less effective if taken with food; Zorvolex capsules are not interchangeable with other formulations of oral product

Topical patch route (Flector)
* Wash hands before handling patch
* Remove and release liner before administration
* Use only on normal, intact skin
* Remove before bath, shower, swimming, do not use heat or occlusive dressings
* Discard removed patch in trash away from children, pets
* Store at room temperature

Topical gel route
* Apply to intact skin; do not use heat or occlusive dressings

* Use only for osteoarthritis, mild to moderate pain
* Store at room temperature, avoid heat, do not freeze

Topical solution route
* Apply to clean, dry skin
* Wait until dry before applying clothing, other creams/lotions
* Wait $\geq$30 min after use before bathing, swimming
* Store at room temperature

SIDE EFFECTS

CNS: *Dizziness, headache*
CV: HF, MI, stroke, edema
EENT: Tinnitus
GI: Nausea, anorexia, vomiting, diarrhea, constipation, flatulence, GI bleeding, hepatotoxicity
GU: Nephrotoxicity: hematuria
HEMA: Anemia
INTEG: Rash, pruritus, photosensitivity
SYST: Anaphylaxis, Stevens-Johnson syndrome, exfoliative dermatitis, toxic epidermal necrolysis

PHARMACOKINETICS

PO: Peak 2-3 hr; **TOP Patch:** peak 12 hr; elimination half-life 1-2 hr, patch 12 hr, 99% bound to plasma proteins, metabolized in liver to metabolite, excreted in urine

INTERACTIONS

* Need for dosage adjustment: antidiabetics
Increase: hyperkalemia—potassium-sparing diuretics
Increase: anticoagulant effect—anticoagulants, NSAIDs, platelet inhibitors, salicylates, thrombolytics, SSRIs
Increase: toxicity—phenytoin, lithium, cycloSPORINE, methotrexate, digoxin, lithium, cidofovir
Increase: GI side effects—aspirin, other NSAIDs, bisphosphonates, corticosteroids
Decrease: antihypertensive effect—β-blockers, diuretics, ACE inhibitors
Decrease: effect of diuretics

Drug/Herb
Increase: bleeding risk—garlic, ginger, ginkgo; monitor for bleeding

NURSING CONSIDERATIONS
Assess:

• **CABG:** do not use oral, top, gel, patch in perioperative pain in coronary artery bypass graft surgery for 10-14 days

Black Box Warning: Stroke/MI: may increase HF and hypertension; increased CV thrombotic events, which may be fatal; those with CV disease may be at greater risk

• **Pain:** location, character, aggravating/alleviating factors, ROM before and 1 hr after dose
• **Actinic keratosis:** check lesions prior to use and periodically
• LFTs (may be elevated), uric acid (may be decreased—serum; increased—urine) periodically; also BUN, creatinine, electrolytes (may be elevated)
• **Serious skin disorders/anaphylaxis:** if rash develops, discontinue immediately, may be fatal; patients with asthma, aspirin hypersensitivity, nasal polyps may develop hypersensitivity
• **Beers:** avoid chronic use in older adults unless other alternatives are ineffective; increased risk of GI bleeding
• **Pregnancy/breastfeeding:** use only if benefit outweighs fetal risks <30 wk, do not use after 30 wk; discontinue breastfeeding, excretion is unknown

Evaluate:
• Therapeutic response: decreased inflammation in joints, after cataract surgery

Teach patient/family:
• That product must be continued for prescribed time to be effective; to contact prescriber before surgery regarding when to discontinue this product
• To report bleeding, bruising, fatigue, malaise; **blood dyscrasias** do occur
• To notify prescriber immediately, stop product if rash occurs
• To avoid aspirin, alcoholic beverages, NSAIDs, or other OTC medications unless approved by prescriber
• To take with food, milk, or antacids to avoid GI upset; to swallow whole

• To use caution when driving; drowsiness, dizziness may occur
• To report **hepatotoxicity:** flulike symptoms, nausea, vomiting, jaundice, pruritus, lethargy
• To use sunscreen to prevent photosensitivity
• To notify all providers of product use
• To notify prescriber if pregnancy is planned or suspected
• **Stroke/MI:** to notify prescriber immediately, seek medical attention if chest pain, slurred speech, weakness, shortness of breath occur
• **Gel:** to use dosing card to measure; not to apply where cosmetics, sunscreen have been applied
• **Transdermal:** not to use in water (swimming/bathing); to use only on intact skin; not to cover with occlusive dressing; to apply adhesive tape or mesh sleeve if patch begins to peel off

---

diclofenac ophthalmic
See Appendix B

RARELY USED

dicyclomine (Rx)
(dye-sye′kloe-meen)
Bentyl, Bentylol ♦, Formulex ♦, Lomine ♦
Func. class.: Gastrointestinal anticholinergic, antispasmodic

USES: IBS

CONTRAINDICATIONS: Hypersensitivity to anticholinergics, closed-angle glaucoma, GI obstruction, myasthenia gravis, paralytic ileus, GI atony, toxic megacolon, dementia

DOSAGE AND ROUTES
• **Adult:** PO 10-20 mg tid-qid, max 160 mg/day; IM 10-20 mg q6hr; max 1-2 days
• **Child >2 yr:** PO 10 mg tid-qid
• **Child 6 mo-2 yr:** PO 5 mg tid-qid

---

didanosine (Rx)

(dye-dan'oh-seen)

ddI, Videx Pediatric Powder, Videx EC

Func. class.: Antiretroviral
Chem. class.: Nucleoside reverse transcriptase inhibitor (NRTI)

ACTION: Nucleoside analog incorporating into cellular DNA by viral reverse transcriptase, thereby terminating the cellular DNA chain

USES: HIV-1 infection in combination with at least 2 other antiretrovirals
Unlabeled uses: HIV prophylaxis

CONTRAINDICATIONS: Hypersensitivity, lactic acidosis, pancreatitis, phenylketonuria
Precautions: Pregnancy, breastfeeding, children, renal disease, sodium-restricted diets, elevated amylase, preexisting peripheral neuropathy, hyperuricemia, gout, HF, noncirrhotic portal hypertension

Black Box Warning: Hepatic disease, lactic acidosis, pancreatitis

DOSAGE AND ROUTES

• **Adult/adolescent/child ≥6 yr and ≥60 kg:** PO EXT REL CAP 400 mg/day; if used with tenofovir, reduce to 250 mg/day
• **Adult/adolescent/child ≥6 yr and 25 kg to <60 kg:** PO EXT REL CAP 250 mg/day; if used with tenofovir, reduce to 200 mg/day
• **Adolescent 20 kg to <25 kg:** PO EXT REL CAP 200 mg/day
• **Adult ≥60 kg:** PO ORAL SOL 200 mg bid or 400 mg/day; if used with tenofovir, reduce to 250 mg/day
• **Adult <60 kg:** PO ORAL SOL 125 mg bid or 250 mg/day; if used with tenofovir, reduce to 200 mg/day
• **Adolescent/child/infant >8 mo:** PO ORAL SOL 120 mg/m² every 12 hr, max adult dosing
• **Infant <8 mo/neonate ≥2 wk:** PO ORAL SOL 100 mg/m² every 12 hr for up to 3 months

Renal dose
• **Adult:** PO CrCl ≥60 mL/min: No change
• **Adult/adolescent ≥60 kg:** PO CCr 30-59 mL/min: reduce oral sol to 100 mg every 12 hr or 200 mg every 24 hr; reduce EXT-REL caps to 200 mg/day; CCr 10-29 mL/min: reduce oral sol to 150 mg every 24 hr; reduce EXT-REL caps to 125 mg/day; CCr <10 mL/min: reduce oral sol to 100 mg every 24 hr; reduce EXT-REL caps to 125 mg/day
• **Adult/adolescent <60 kg:** PO CCr 30-59 mL/min: reduce oral sol to 75 mg every 12 hr or to 150 mg every 24 hr; reduce EXT-REL caps to 125 mg/day; CCr 10-29 mL/min: reduce oral sol to 100 mg every 24 hr; reduce EXT-REL caps to 125 mg/day; CCr <10 mL/min: reduce oral sol to 75 mg every 24 hr; EXT-REL caps are not recommended

Intermittent hemodialysis/continuous ambulatory peritoneal dialysis
• **Adult/adolescent >60 kg:** Give 100 mg **ORAL SOL** or 125 mg **DEL REL CAPS** every 24 hr
• **Adult/adolescent <60 kg:** Give 75 mg **ORAL SOL** every 24 hr, **DEL REL CAPS** are not recommended

Available forms: Powder for oral sol 10 mg/mL; del rel caps 125, 200, 250, 400 mg

Administer:
• Pediatric powder for oral sol after preparation by pharmacist; dilution required using purified USP water, then antacid (10 mg/mL), refrigerate, shake before use
• On an empty stomach ≥30 min before or 2 hr after meals
• Adjust dose with renal impairment
• Store tabs, caps in tightly closed bottle at room temperature; store oral sol after dissolving at room temperature ≤4 hr

SIDE EFFECTS

CNS: Peripheral neuropathy, seizures, confusion, *anxiety,* hypertonia, abnormal thinking, asthenia, *insomnia,* CNS depression, pain, dizziness, chills, fever
CV: Hypertension, vasodilation, dysrhythmia, syncope, HF, palpitation

---

Side effects: *italics* = common; red = life-threatening

D

EENT: Ear pain, otitis, photophobia, visual impairment, retinal depigmentation, optic neuritis

GI: Pancreatitis, *diarrhea, nausea,* vomiting, *abdominal pain,* constipation, stomatitis, dyspepsia, liver abnormalities, flatulence, taste perversion, dry mouth, oral thrush, melena, increased ALT/AST, alk phos, amylase, hepatic failure, noncirrhotic portal hypertension

GU: Increased bilirubin, uric acid

HEMA: Leukopenia, granulocytopenia, thrombocytopenia, anemia

INTEG: *Rash, pruritus,* alopecia, ecchymosis, hemorrhage, petechiae, sweating

MS: Myalgia, arthritis, myopathy, muscular atrophy

RESP: Cough, pneumonia, dyspnea, asthma, epistaxis, hypoventilation, sinusitis

SYST: Lactic acidosis, anaphylaxis

PHARMACOKINETICS

PO: Peak 0.67 hr, del rel 2 hr; elimination half-life 48 min; extensive metabolism; administration within 5 min of food will decrease absorption (50%); excreted in urine, feces

INTERACTIONS

Increase: didanosine level—allopurinol, tenofovir

Increase: side effects from magnesium, aluminum antacids

Increase: pancreatitis risk—stavudine

Decrease: absorption—ketoconazole, dapsone

Decrease: concentrations of fluoroquinolones, other antiretrovirals, itraconazole, tetracyclines

> Black Box Warning: **Increase:** fatal lactic acidosis—stavudine, tenofovir, other antiretrovirals; do not use together

• **Do not use with these products PO:** gatifloxacin, gemifloxacin, levoFLOXacin, moxifloxacin, norfloxacin

Drug/Food
• Any food decreases rate of absorption 50%; do not use with food
• Do not use with acidic juices

NURSING CONSIDERATIONS
Assess:

> Black Box Warning: **Pancreatitis:** do not use in those with symptoms of pancreatitis; may be dose related in advanced HIV, alcoholism, history of pancreatitis

• **Peripheral neuropathy:** tingling or pain in hands and feet, distal numbness; onset usually occurs 2-6 mo after beginning treatment; may persist if product not discontinued

> Black Box Warning: **Lactic acidosis, severe hepatomegaly, pancreatitis:** abdominal pain, nausea, vomiting, elevated hepatic enzymes; product should be discontinued because condition can be fatal

• Children by dilated retinal exam q6mo to rule out retinal depigmentation
• CBC, differential, platelet count monthly; notify prescriber of results; alk phos, monitor amylase; viral load, CD4 count
• Renal studies: BUN, serum uric acid, urine CCr before, during therapy
• Temperature may indicate beginning infection
• Hepatic studies before, during therapy (bilirubin, AST, ALT) as needed, monthly
• Cleanup of powdered products; use wet mop or damp sponge
• **Pregnancy/breastfeeding:** identify if pregnancy is planned or suspected; product is not recommended in initial treatment due to toxicity; do not breastfeed; enroll in the Antiretroviral Pregnancy Registry (800-258-4263)

Evaluate:
• Therapeutic response: absence of infection; symptoms of HIV

Teach patient/family:

> Black Box Warning: **Pancreatitis:** to report immediately abdominal pain, diarrhea, nausea, vomiting

• To report numbness, tingling in extremities
• To take on an empty stomach; not to take dapsone at same time as ddI; not to

mix powder with fruit juice; to chew tab or crush and dissolve in water; to drink powder immediately after mixing

• To report signs of **infection**: increased temperature, sore throat, flulike symptoms; other infections and complications may still occur

• To report signs of **anemia**: fatigue, headache, faintness, SOB, irritability

• To report **bleeding**; to avoid use of razors, commercial mouthwash

• That hair may be lost during therapy (rare); that a wig or hairpiece may make patient feel better

• That product does not cure symptoms, only controls them; that infection of others may occur via sex or blood

---

difluprednate (ophthalmic)

(die-flu′pred-nate)

Durezol

Func. class.: Ophthalmic antiinflammatory

Chem. class.: Corticosteroid

ACTION: Exact mechanism of antiinflammatory action unknown; inhibits multiple inflammatory cytokines; decreases release of arachidonic acid, which increases in inflammation

USES: For the treatment of postoperative ocular pain and postoperative ocular inflammation; for the treatment of endogenous anterior uveitis

CONTRAINDICATIONS: Hypersensitivity to this product, glycerin, polysorbate, ocular TB, acute herpes simplex (superficial), fungal/viral infections of the eye

Precautions: Pregnancy, breastfeeding, children, corneal infected abrasions, glaucoma

DOSAGE AND ROUTES
Postoperative ocular pain, postoperative ocular inflammation

• **Adult/geriatric/adolescents/children/infants:** OPHTH Instill 1 drop into the conjunctival sac of the affected eye(s) qid beginning 24 hr after surgery; continue giving 4 ×/day for the first 2 wk of the postoperative period, then administer bid × 1 wk; at the end of the third wk, taper dosage based on response

Endogenous anterior uveitis

• **Adult:** OPHTH Instill 1 drop into the conjunctival sac of the affected eye(s) qid × 14 days, followed by tapering based on response

Available forms: Ophthalmic emulsion 0.05%

Administer:

• Apply topically to the eye, shake well before use

• Do not touch the tip of the dropper to the eye, fingertips, or other surface

• Instruct patient on proper instillation of eye sol

• When using this product, the patient should not wear contact lenses

SIDE EFFECTS

EENT: Burning, stinging, poor vision, corneal ulcerations, increased IOP, optic nerve damage

NURSING CONSIDERATIONS
Assess:

• **Corneal effects:** ulcerations; infections can worsen with this product; monitor IOP used intraocularly over 10 days

Evaluate:

• Therapeutic response: decreased corneal inflammation

Teach patient/family:

• How to use product

• Not to share with others or use for other conditions

• To notify prescriber immediately if vision changes or if condition worsens

• To take as prescribed

⚠ HIGH ALERT

digoxin (Rx) NTI

(di-jox′in)

Toloxin ✦, Digitek, Lanoxin

Func. class.: Cardiac glycoside, inotropic, antidysrhythmic

Chem. class.: Digoxin preparation

Do not confuse:
Lanoxin/Lasix/Lonox/Lomotil/Xanax/
naloxone

ACTION: Inhibits the sodium-potassium ATPase pump, which makes more calcium available for contractile proteins, thereby resulting in increased cardiac output (positive inotropic effect); increases force of contractions; decreases heart rate (negative chronotropic effect); decreases AV conduction speed

USES: Heart failure, atrial fibrillation/flutter
Unlabeled uses: Paroxysmal supraventricular tachycardia (PSVT) treatment/prophylaxis

CONTRAINDICATIONS: Hypersensitivity to digoxin, ventricular fibrillation, ventricular tachycardia
Precautions: Pregnancy, breastfeeding, geriatric patients, renal disease, acute MI, AV block, severe respiratory disease, hypothyroidism, sinus nodal disease, hypokalemia, carotid sinus syndrome, 2nd- or 3rd-degree heart block, electrolyte disturbances, hypertension, cor pulmonale, Wolff-Parkinson-White syndrome

DOSAGE AND ROUTES—NTI
Loading dose, IV route
• **Adult/adolescent/child >10 yr: IV** 8-12 mcg/kg, divided into ≥3 doses, with the first dose equaling one-half the total, give subsequent doses every 6-8 hr
• **Child 5-10 yr: IV** 15-30 mcg/kg divided into ≥3 doses, with the first dose equaling one-half the total, give subsequent doses every 6-8 hr
• **Child 2-4 yr: IV** 25-35 mcg/kg, divided into ≥3 doses, with the first dose equaling one-half the total, give subsequent doses every 6-8 hr
• **Infant/child <2 yr: IV** 30-50 mcg/kg, divided into ≥3 doses, with the first dose equaling one-half the total, give subsequent doses every 6-8 hr
• **Full-term neonate: IV** 20-30 mcg/kg, divided into ≥3 doses, with the first dose

equaling one-half the total, give subsequent doses every 6-8 hr
• **Premature neonate: IV** 15-25 mcg/kg, divided into ≥3 doses, with the first dose equaling one-half the total, give subsequent doses every 6-8 hr
Loading dose, PO (tablets)
• **Adult/adolescent/child >10 yr: PO** Total dosage of 10-15 mcg/kg in 3 divided doses, give one-half the total loading dose initially, then one-fourth the loading dose every 4-8 hr × 2 doses
• **Child 5-10 yr: PO** Total dosage of 20-45 mcg/kg in 3 divided doses, give one-half the total loading dose initially, then one-fourth the loading dose every 4-8 hr × 2 doses
Loading dose, PO (elixir)
• **Adult/adolescent/child >10 yr: PO** Total dosage of 10-15 mcg/kg, give one-half the total loading dose initially, then additional fractions of the planned total dose at 4-8 hr
• **Child 5-10 yr: PO** Total dosage of 20-35 mcg/kg, give one-half the total loading dose initially, then additional fractions of the planned total dose at 4-8 hr
• **Child 2-4 yr: PO** Total dosage of 30-45 mcg/kg, give one-half the total loading dose initially, then additional fractions of the planned total dose at 4-8 hr
• **Infant/child <2 yr: PO** Total dosage of 35-60 mcg/kg, give one-half the total loading dose initially, then additional fractions of the planned total dose at 4-8 hr
• **Full-term neonate: PO** Total dosage of 25-35 mcg/kg, give one-half the total loading dose initially, then additional fractions of the planned total dose at 4-8 hr
• **Premature neonate: PO** Total dosage of 20-30 mcg/kg, give one-half the total loading dose initially, then additional fractions of the planned total dose at 4-8 hr
Available forms: Elix 0.05 mg/mL; tabs 0.0625, 0.125, 0.1875, 0.25, 0.5 mg; inj 0.5 ✦, 0.25 mg/mL; pediatric inj 0.1 mg/mL
Administer:
PO route
• Bioavailability varies among different oral dosage forms of digoxin and among different brands of the same dosage form;

changing from one preparation to another might require dosage adjustments

- **All dosage forms:** may be administered without regard to meals
- **Tab:** may be crushed and administered with food or fluids
- **Pediatric elixir:** administer using a calibrated measuring device

Injectable

- When changing from PO to IM/IV, use 20%-25% less
- IV is preferred over IM because it is less painful and more rapid action
- PO should replace parenteral therapy as soon as possible
- Visually inspect parenteral products for particulate matter and discoloration before use

IM route

- Do not administer >2 mL at any one IM injection site
- Inject deeply into gluteal muscle, then massage area

IV route

- Monitor ECG during and for 6 hr after IV use; watch for dysrhythmias or bradycardia; notify prescriber
- May be given undiluted or each 1 mL may be diluted in 4 mL of sterile water for injection, NS, D$_5$W, or LR; diluent volumes <4 mL will cause precipitation; use diluted solutions immediately
- Inject over ≥5 min in Y-site or 3-way stopcock; in patients with pulmonary edema, administer over 10-15 min; to avoid inadvertent overdosage, do not flush the syringe following administration
- Check for potency and check site for redness, inflammation, infiltration; tissue sloughing can occur

Y-site compatibilities: Acyclovir, alfentanil, amikacin, aminocaproic acid, aminophylline, amphotericin B lipid complex, anidulafungin, ascorbic acid injection, atenolol, atracurium, atropine, aztreonam, benztropine, bivalirudin, bleomycin, bumetanide, buprenorphine, butorphanol, calcium chloride/gluconate, CARBOplatin, ceFAZolin, cefonicid, cefotaxime, cefoTEtan, cefOXitin, cefTAZidime, ceftizoxime, cefTRIAXone, cefuroxime, chloramphenicol, chlorproMAZINE, cimetidine, ciprofloxacin, cisatracurium, CISplatin, clindamycin, codeine, cyanocobalamin, cyclophosphamide, cycloSPORINE, cytarabine, DACTINomycin, DAPTOmycin, dexamethasone, dexmedetomidine, diltiazem, diphenhydrAMINE, DOBUTamine, DOCEtaxel, DOPamine, doripenem, doxacurium, doxycycline, enalaprilat, ePHEDrine, EPINEPHrine, epirubicin, epoetin alfa, eptifibatide, ertapenem, erythromycin, esmolol, etoposide, famotidine, fenoldopam, fentaNYL, fludarabine, fluorouracil, folic acid, furosemide, ganciclovir, gatifloxacin, gemcitabine, gentamicin, glycopyrrolate, granisetron, heparin, hydrocortisone, HYDROmorphone, hydrOXYzine, ifosfamide, imipenem-cilastatin, indomethacin, irinotecan, isoproterenol, ketorolac, labetalol, levofloxacin, lidocaine, linezolid, LORazepam, LR, magnesium sulfate, mannitol, mechlorethamine, meperidine, meropenem, methicillin, methotrexate, methyldopate, methylPREDNISolone, metoclopramide, metoprolol, metroNIDAZOLE, mezlocillin, miconazole, midazolam, milrinone, morphine, multiple vitamins injection, mycophenolate mofetil, nafcillin, nalbuphine, naloxone, nesiritide, metilmicin, nitroglycerin, nitroprusside, norepinephrine, octreotide, ondansetron, oxacillin, oxaliplatin, oxytocin, palonosetron, pamidronate, pancuronium, pantoprazole, papaverine, PEMEtrexed, penicillin G potassium/sodium, pentazocine, PENTObarbital, PHENobarbital, phenylephrine, phytonadione, piperacillin, piperacillin-tazobactam, polymyxin B, potassium chloride, procainamide, prochlorperazine, promethazine, propranolol, protamine, pyridoxine, quiNIDine, ranitidine, remifentanil, Ringer's, ritodrine, riTUXimab, rocuronium, sodium acetate/bicarbonate, succinylcholine, SUFentanil, tacrolimus, teniposide, theophylline, thiamine, thiotepa, ticarcillin, ticarcillin-clavulanate, tigecycline, tirofiban, TNA, tobramycin, tolazoline, TPN, trastuzumab, trimetaphan, urokinase, vancomycin, vasopressin, vecuronium, verapamil, vinCRIStine, vinorelbine, vitamin B complex, voriconazole, zoledronic acid

SIDE EFFECTS

CNS: *Headache,* drowsiness, apathy, confusion, disorientation, fatigue, depression, hallucinations
CV: Dysrhythmias, *hypotension,* bradycardia, AV block
EENT: Blurred vision, yellow-green halos, photophobia, diplopia
GI: Nausea, vomiting, anorexia, abdominal pain, diarrhea

PHARMACOKINETICS

Half-life 30-40 hr, excreted in urine, protein binding 20%-30%
PO: Onset $1/2$-2 hr, peak 2-6 hr, duration 3-4 days
IV: Onset 5-30 min, peak 1-4 hr, duration variable

INTERACTIONS

Increase: toxicity—azole antifungals, macrolides, tetracyclines, ritonavir; monitor for toxicity
Increase: hypercalcemia, hypomagnesemia, digoxin toxicity—thiazides, parenteral calcium; monitor electrolytes
Increase: hypokalemia, digoxin toxicity—diuretics, amphotericin B, carbenicillin, ticarcillin, corticosteroids
Increase: digoxin levels—propantheline, quiNIDine, verapamil, amiodarone, anticholinergics, diltiazem, NIFEdipine, indomethacin
Increase: bradycardia—β-adrenergic blockers, antidysrhythmics
Increase: cardiac dysrhythmia risk—sympathomimetics
Decrease: digoxin absorption—antacids, kaolin/pectin, cholestyramine, metoclopramide
Decrease: digoxin level—thyroid agents, cholestyramine, colestipol, metoclopramide, aMILoride
Drug/Food
Decrease: digoxin effect—food, separate by ≥1 hr
Decrease: GI absorption—flaxseed, psyllium

Drug/Herb
Increase: cardiac effects—foxglove, goldenseal, hawthorn, rue
Decrease: product effect—St. John's wort
Drug/Lab Test
Increase: CPK

NURSING CONSIDERATIONS
Assess:
• Apical pulse for 1 min before giving product; if pulse <60 in adult or <90 in infant, take again in 1 hr; if <60 in adult, call prescriber; note rate, rhythm, character; monitor ECG continuously during parenteral loading dose; monitor I&O, daily weight; check for edema
• Electrolytes: potassium, sodium, chloride, magnesium, calcium; renal function studies: BUN, creatinine; blood studies: ALT, AST, bilirubin, Hct, Hgb before initiating treatment and periodically thereafter; monitor for decrease or increase in potassium
• Monitor product levels; therapeutic level 0.5-2 ng/mL, draw ≥6-8 hr after last dose, optimally 12-24 hr after a dose
• **Beers:** avoid dosage >0.125 mg/dL in atrial fibrillation, heart failure in older adults; decreased renal clearance may lead to toxicity
• **Pregnancy/breastfeeding:** no well-controlled studies; use only if clearly needed; excreted in breast milk (small amounts), may breastfeed
Evaluate:
• Therapeutic response: decrease in heart failure, dysrhythmias; serum digoxin level (0.5-2 ng/mL)
Teach patient/family:
• Not to stop product abruptly; about all aspects of product; to take exactly as ordered; how to monitor heart rate
• To avoid OTC medications, herbal remedies because many adverse product interactions may occur; not to take antacid within 2 hr of this product
• To notify prescriber of loss of appetite, lower stomach pain, diarrhea, weakness, drowsiness, headache, blurred or yellow vision, rash, depression, toxicity
• About the toxic symptoms of this product; when to notify prescriber

---

- To maintain a sodium-restricted diet as ordered
- To use one brand consistently, to keep in original container
- To notify prescriber if pregnancy is planned or suspected
- To carry ID stating condition treated, products taken
- How to take pulse, when to notify prescriber

TREATMENT OF OVERDOSE: Discontinue product; give potassium; monitor ECG; give adrenergic-blocking agent, digoxin immune FAB

RARELY USED

digoxin immune FAB (ovine) (Rx)
(di-jox'in im-myoon' FAB)

DigiFab
Func. class.: Antidote—digoxin specific

USES: Life-threatening digoxin toxicity

CONTRAINDICATIONS: Mild digoxin toxicity, hypersensitivity to this product, papain or ovine protein

DOSAGE AND ROUTES
1 (40 mg) DigiFab binds 0.5 mg digoxin
Digoxin toxicity (known amount) (tabs, oral sol, IM)
- **Adult and child:** IV dose (mg) = dose ingested (mg) × 0.8/1000 × 38- or 40-mg vial
Toxicity (known amount) (cap, IV)
- **Adult and child:** IV dose = dose ingested (mg)/0.5 × 38- or 40-mg vial
Toxicity (known amount) by serum digoxin concentrations (SDCs)
- **Adult and child:** IV SDC (ng/mL) × kg of weight/100 × 38- or 40-mg vial
Digoxin toxicity (unknown amount)
- **Adult and child >20 kg:** IV 228 mg (6 vials)
- **Infant and child <20 kg:** IV 38 mg (1 vial)

Acute ingestion
- **Adult:** IV 380 mg (10 vials)
Life-threatening ingestion
- **Adult:** IV 760 mg (20 vials)
Skin test
- **Adult:** ID 0.1 mL of 1:100 dilution, check after 20 min

⚠ HIGH ALERT

diltiazem (Rx)
(dil-tye'a-zem)

Cardizem, Cardizem CD, Cardizem LA, Cartia XT, Taztia XT, Tiazac, Tiazac XC ✤
Func. class.: Calcium channel blocker, antiarrhythmic class IV, antihypertensive
Chem. class.: Benzothiazepine

Do not confuse:
Cardizem/Cardene
Tiazac/Ziac

ACTION: Inhibits calcium ion influx across cell membrane during cardiac depolarization; produces relaxation of coronary vascular smooth muscle, dilates coronary arteries, slows SA/AV node conduction times, dilates peripheral arteries

USES: **PO** angina pectoris due to coronary artery spasm, hypertension, improvement in exercise tolerance (chronic stable angina), **IV** atrial fibrillation, flutter, paroxysmal supraventricular tachycardia
Unlabeled uses: Unstable angina, proteinuria, cardiomyopathy, diabetic neuropathy

CONTRAINDICATIONS: Sick sinus syndrome, AV heart block, hypotension <90 mm Hg systolic, acute MI, pulmonary congestion, cardiogenic shock
Precautions: Pregnancy, breastfeeding, children, geriatric patients, HF, aortic stenosis, bradycardia, GERD, hepatic disease, hiatal hernia, ventricular dysfunction

---

Side effects: *italics* = common; red = life-threatening

DOSAGE AND ROUTES
Prinzmetal's or variant angina, chronic stable angina
• **Adult:** PO 30 mg qid, increasing dose gradually to 180-360 mg/day in divided doses or **EXT REL** (LA, CD, XT, XR products) 180-360 mg, max 480-540 mg/day, depending on brand

Atrial fibrillation/flutter, paroxysmal supraventricular tachycardia
• **Adult:** IV BOL 0.25 mg/kg over 2 min initially, then 0.35 mg/kg may be given after 15 min; if no response, may give **CONT INFUSION** 5-15 mg/hr for up to 24 hr

Hypertension
• **Adult:** PO 30 mg tid, increase to max 480 mg/day; **EXT REL** 120-240 mg q day, max 540 mg/day; **SUS REL** 60 mg bid, max 360 mg/day

Rapid ventricular rate secondary to dysrhythmias (unlabeled)
• **Adolescent/child/infant >7 mo:** IV BOL 0.25 mg/kg over 5 min, then **CONT IV INFUSION** 0.11 mg/kg/hr

Available forms: Tabs 30, 60, 90, 120 mg; ext rel tabs 120, 180, 240, 300, 360, 420 mg; ext rel caps 60, 90, 120, 180, 240, 300, 360, 420 mg; inj 5 mg/mL (5, 10 mL); powder for inj 100 mg

Administer:
PO route
• Not all products are interchangeable
• Store at room temperature
• **Cardizem LA** ext rel tab 24 hr: give daily, either AM or PM, without regard to meals
• **Dilacor XR/Diltia XT** ext rel cap 24 hr: give daily; take on empty stomach; swallow whole; do not cut, crush, chew, open
• **Tiazac, Tiztia XT:** give daily without regard to meals
• **Conventional regular-rel tab:** give before meals, at bedtime
• **Cardizem CD or equivalent (Cartia XT):** generic ext rel cap 24 hr: give daily, without regard to meals
• May crush, sprinkle regular tab on applesauce for administration

Direct IV route
• IV undiluted over 2 min
Continuous IV INFUSION route
• Diluted 125 mg/100 mL, 250 mg/250 mL of D$_5$W, 0.9% NaCl, D$_5$/0.45% NaCl, give 10 mg/hr, may increase by 5 mg/hr to 15 mg/hr, continue infusion up to 24 hr max

Y-site compatibilities: Albumin, amikacin, amphotericin B, aztreonam, bumetanide, ceFAZolin, cefotaxime, cefoTEtan, cefOXitin, cefTAZidime, cefTRIAXone, cefuroxime, cimetidine, ciprofloxacin, clindamycin, digoxin, DOBUTamine, DOPamine, doxycycline, EPINEPHrine, erythromycin, esmolol, fentaNYL, fluconazole, gentamicin, hetastarch, HYDROmorphone, imipenem-cilastatin, labetalol, lidocaine, LORazepam, meperidine, metoclopramide, metroNIDAZOLE, midazolam, milrinone, morphine, multivitamins, niCARdipine, nitroglycerin, norepinephrine, oxacillin, penicillin G potassium, pentamidine, piperacillin, potassium chloride, potassium phosphates, ranitidine, sodium nitroprusside, theophylline, ticarcillin, ticarcillin/clavulanate, tobramycin, trimethoprim-sulfamethoxazole, vancomycin, vecuronium

SIDE EFFECTS
CNS: Tremor, paresthesia
CV: Dysrhythmia, *edema,* HF, bradycardia, hypotension, palpitations
GI: *Nausea,* vomiting, diarrhea, *constipation*
GU: Nocturia, polyuria, sexual dysfunction, dysuria
INTEG: *Rash,* flushing, photosensitivity, burning, pruritus, Stevens-Johnson syndrome, sweating
RESP: Rhinitis, dyspnea, pharyngitis, cough
EENT: Blurred vision, epistaxis, tinnitus
Endo: Hyperglycemia, gynecomastia
HEMA: Anemia, leukopenia, thrombocytopenia
MS: Stiffness, muscle cramps
MISC: Gingival hyperplasia

PHARMACOKINETICS
Onset 30-60 min; peak 2-3 hr immediate rel, 10-14 hr ext rel, 11-18 hr sus rel;

half-life $3^1/_2$-9 hr; metabolized by liver; excreted in urine (96% as metabolites)

INTERACTIONS

Increase: effect, toxicity—theophylline, lithium

Increase: effects of β-blockers, digoxin, lithium, carBAMazepine, cycloSPORINE, anesthetics, HMG-CoA reductase inhibitors, benzodiazepines, methylPREDNISolone; monitor for increased action of each product

Increase: AV node slowing—cimetidine, ranitidine; monitor closely

Decrease: antihypertensive effect—NSAIDs, phenobarbital, phenytoin

Drug/Food

Increase: diltiazem effect—grapefruit juice; avoid use

NURSING CONSIDERATIONS

Assess:

• **HF:** dyspnea, weight gain, edema, jugular venous distention, rales; monitor I&O ratios daily, weight

• **Angina:** location, duration, alleviating factors, activity when pain starts

• **Dysrhythmias:** cardiac status: B/P, pulse, respiration, ECG and intervals PR, QRS, QT; if systolic B/P <90 mm Hg or HR <50 bpm, hold dose, notify prescriber; monitor B/P, ECG continuously if using IV; report bradycardia, have emergency equipment nearby

• Monitor if refills are being purchased

• Monitor digoxin levels if taking both products, digoxin toxicity is more common

• Potassium baseline and periodically; LFTs, renal studies

• Stevens-Johnson syndrome: assess for rash, fever, fatigue, mouth blistering; discontinue product immediately if severe

• **Beers:** avoid extended-release capsule in older adults; promotes fluid retention, exacerbates heart failure

• **Pregnancy/breastfeeding:** identify whether pregnancy is planned or suspected or if breastfeeding; no well-controlled studies; use only if benefit outweighs fetal risk; discontinue breastfeeding or product, excreted in breast milk

Evaluate:

• Therapeutic response: decreased anginal pain, decreased B/P, increased exercise tolerance

Teach patient/family:

• How to take pulse, B/P before taking product; that a record or graph should be kept

• To avoid hazardous activities until stabilized on product, dizziness is no longer a problem

• To limit caffeine consumption; to avoid grapefruit juice

• To discuss OTC, Rx, herbals, supplements with provider

• About the importance of complying with all areas of medical regimen: diet, exercise, stress reduction, product therapy

• To report dizziness, SOB, palpitations, rash, nausea, headache, swelling of face, hands

• Not to discontinue abruptly

• To use sunscreen, protective clothing to prevent photosensitivity

• To rise or change positions slowly, orthostatic hypotension may occur

• **Angina:** To discuss other therapy, including nitrates, β-blockers and when to take

• To use good oral hygiene and teeth cleaning, gingival hyperplasia occurs

• **Pregnancy:** to avoid pregnancy and breastfeeding

TREATMENT OF OVERDOSE:

Atropine for AV block, vasopressor for hypotension

---

dimenhyDRINATE (OTC, Rx)

(dye-men-hye′dri-nate)

Dramamine, Driminate, Gravol ✤, Dinate ✤, Nauseatol ✤

TripTone, Wal-Dram

Func. class.: Antiemetic, antihistamine, anticholinergic

Chem. class.: H₁-receptor antagonist, ethanolamine derivative

---

Do not confuse:
dimenhyDRINATE/diphenhydrAMINE

ACTION: Competes with histamine for
H_1 receptors in GI tract, blood vessels,
respiratory tract; central anticholinergic
activity, which results in decreased vestibular stimulation and blockade of chemoreceptor trigger zone

USES: Motion sickness, nausea, vomiting, vertigo
Unlabeled uses: Hyperemesis gravidarum, Ménière's syndrome

CONTRAINDICATIONS: Hyper-
sensitivity, infants, neonates, tartrazine
dye hypersensitivity
Precautions: Pregnancy, breastfeeding,
children, geriatric patients, cardiac dysrhythmias, asthma, prostatic hypertrophy,
bladder-neck obstruction, closed-angle
glaucoma, stenosing peptic ulcer, pyloro-
duodenal obstruction

DOSAGE AND ROUTES
• **Adult: PO** 50-100 mg q4hr; **IM/IV** 50
mg q4hr as needed (Canada only)
• **Child 6-12 yr: PO** 25-50 mg q6-8hr
prn, max 150 mg/day
• **Child 2-5 yr: PO** 12.5-25 mg q6-8hr,
max 75 mg/day
Available forms: Tabs 50 mg; inj 50
mg/mL ✿; elixir 15 mg/5 mL ✿; chew
tabs 50 mg
Administer:
• IM inj in large muscle mass; aspirate
to avoid IV administration (Canada only)
• Tablets may be swallowed whole,
chewed, or allowed to dissolve
IV route (Canada only)
• After diluting 50 mg/10 mL of NaCl inj,
give ≤50 mg over 2 min

SIDE EFFECTS
CNS: *Drowsiness,* restlessness, headache, dizziness, insomnia, confusion,
nervousness, tingling, vertigo
CV: Hypertension, *hypotension,*
palpitation
EENT: *Dry mouth,* blurred vision, diplopia, nasal congestion, photosensitivity,
xerostomia

GI: Nausea, anorexia, vomiting,
constipation
INTEG: Rash, urticaria, fever, chills,
flushing
MISC: Anaphylaxis

PHARMACOKINETICS
PO/IM: Onset 15-30 min, duration
4-6 hr

INTERACTIONS
Increase: effect—alcohol, anticholiner-
gics, tricyclics, MAOIs, opiates, sedative/
hypnotics, other CNS depressants
Drug/Lab Test
False negative: Allergy skin testing

NURSING CONSIDERATIONS
Assess:
• VS, B/P; check patients with cardiac
disease more often
• **Signs of toxicity** of other products or
masking of symptoms of disease: brain
tumor, intestinal obstruction
• Observe for drowsiness, dizziness
• **Beers:** avoid use in older adults;
highly anticholinergic
• **Pregnancy/breastfeeding:** no well-
controlled studies; use only if benefit
outweighs fetal risk; avoid breastfeeding,
excreted in breast milk
Evaluate:
• Therapeutic response: absence of
nausea, vomiting, or vertigo
Teach patient/family:
• To avoid hazardous activities, activities
requiring alertness because dizziness
may occur; to request assistance with
ambulation
• To avoid alcohol, other CNS depressants

---

dimethyl fumarate (Rx)
(dahy-meth'ul fyoo' muh-reyt)
Tecfidera
Func. class.: Immunomodulator

ACTION: Has beneficial effects on
inflammation and oxidative stress.
Induces an antioxidant effect–related
neuronal death, and damage to myelin in

the CNS may also improve mitochondrial function.

USES: Relapsing multiple sclerosis

CONTRAINDICATIONS: Hypersensitivity

Precautions: Pregnancy, breastfeeding, immunosuppression, infertility, male-mediated teratogenicity

DOSAGE AND ROUTES
• **Adult: PO** 120 mg bid × 7 days, may increase to 240 mg bid for maintenance
Available forms: Caps, del rel 120, 240 mg
Administer:
• Do not break, crush, or chew, do not open cap; give without regard to meals, use with food may decrease flushing

SIDE EFFECTS
CNS: *Flushing*, progressive multifocal leukoencephalopathy
GI: *Nausea*, dyspepsia, *abdominal pain*, *diarrhea*, vomiting
GU: Albuminuria
INTEG: Rash, pruritus
HEMA: Lymphopenia, leukopenia
SYST: Anaphylaxis, angioedema

PHARMACOKINETICS
Half-life 1 hr, peak 2½ hr

INTERACTIONS
None known

NURSING CONSIDERATIONS
Assess:
• **Multiple sclerosis:** monitor for improved number and severity of spasms, chronic pain, fatigue and weakness, balance and dizziness
• CBC with differential baseline and every 6 months thereafter; leukopenia and lymphopenia may occur
• **Anaphylaxis:** usually during first dose, but may occur any time during treatment; monitor for difficulty breathing, urticaria, and swelling of the throat and tongue
• **Progressive multifocal leukoencephalopathy:** ataxia, vision changes, weakness, trouble using arms/legs, confusion; discontinue at first sign of PML

• **Pregnancy:** identify if pregnancy is planned or suspected, or if breastfeeding; use only if benefit outweighs fetal risk; cautious use in breastfeeding, excretion is unknown; if pregnant, register by calling 866-810-1462 or by visiting www.tecfiderapregnancyregistry.com
Evaluate:
• Therapeutic response: improved symptoms of multiple sclerosis
Teach patient/family:
• To notify prescriber if pregnancy is planned or suspected; not to breastfeed
• Expected results; side effects
• **Anaphylaxis:** to discontinue the drug and seek immediate medical treatment if patient experiences difficulty breathing, urticaria, or swelling of the throat/tongue
• **Progressive multifocal leukoencephalopathy:** to notify prescriber immediately of vision changes, confusion, ataxia, weakness, trouble using arms/legs

dinoprostone (Rx)
(dye-noe-prost′one)
Cervidil, Prepidil, Prostin E-2
Func. class.: Oxytocic, abortifacient
Chem. class.: Prostaglandin E_2

Do not confuse:
Prepidil/bepridil

ACTION: Stimulates uterine contractions, causing abortion; acts within 30 hr for complete abortion

USES: Abortion during 2nd trimester, benign hydatidiform mole, expulsion of uterine contents in fetal deaths to 28 wk, missed abortion, to efface and dilate the cervix in pregnancy at term

CONTRAINDICATIONS: Hypersensitivity, C-section, surgery, fetal distress, multiparity, vaginal bleeding, cephalopelvic disproportion
Precautions: Pregnancy, cardiac disease, asthma, anemia, jaundice, diabetes mellitus, seizure disorders, hypertension, glaucoma, uterine fibrosis, cervical stenosis, pelvic surgery, pelvic inflammatory disease, respiratory disease

Black Box Warning: Requires a specialized setting and an experienced clinician

DOSAGE AND ROUTES
Abortifacient
• **Adult: VAG SUPP** 20 mg, repeat q3-5hr until abortion occurs, max dose is 240 mg
Cervical ripening
• **Adult: GEL** 0.5 mg vag gel placed in cervical canal, may repeat after 6 hr, max 1.5 mg/24 hr; vag insert 10 mg high in vagina, remove at onset of active labor or within 12 hr

Available forms: VAG SUPP 20 mg; endocervical gel 0.5 mg/3 g (prefilled syringe); vag insert 10 mg

Administer:
By gel
• Antiemetic/antidiarrheal before administration of this product
• Keep patient supine for 15-30 min after administration. Use after warming to room temperature. Remove seal from end of syringe, remove protective end cap, and insert into plunger stopper assembly; make sure patient is in dorsal position; **insert.** Must be kept frozen until use; warm to room temperature before use

Suppository
• Keep patient supine for 10 min after insertion; continuous administration for >2 days is not recommended

SIDE EFFECTS
CNS: *Headache,* dizziness, chills, fever, flushing, drowsiness
CV: Hypotension, dysrhythmias, DIC
EENT: Blurred vision
FETAL: Bradycardia (i.e., deceleration)
GI: *Nausea, vomiting, diarrhea*
GU: Vaginitis, vaginal pain, vulvitis, vaginismus
INTEG: Rash, skin color changes
MS: *Leg cramps, joint swelling,* weakness
GEL: Uterine contractile abnormality, GI side effects, back pain, fever, amniotic fluid embolism
INSERT: Uterine hyperstimulation, fever, nausea, vomiting, diarrhea, abdominal pain, amniotic fluid embolism

SUPPOSITORY: Uterine rupture, anaphylaxis
SYST: Anaphylactoid syndrome of pregnancy

INTERACTIONS
Increase: effect—other oxytocics

PHARMACOKINETICS
Metabolized in spleen, kidney, lungs; excreted in urine
GEL: Onset 10 min, peak 30-45 min
SUPP: Onset 10 min, duration 2-3 hr

NURSING CONSIDERATIONS
Assess:

Black Box Warning: **Specialized setting, specialized clinician:** use only with emergency equipment nearby, by a clinician experienced when used in pregnancy termination; complete abortion should result within 17 hr; use only in 12-20 wk or up to 28 wk for removal of remaining material after miscarriage

• **Cervical ripening:** dilation, effacement of cervix and uterine contraction, fetal heart tones; check for contractions over 1 min
• **Abortifacient:** monitor contractions for frequency, duration, force
• **Anaphylaxis:** monitor for rash, wheezing
• B/P baseline and during treatment for fever that occurs $1/2$ hr after suppository insertion (abortion)
• **Vaginal discharge:** check for itching, irritation, amount; indicates vaginal infection
Evaluate:
• Therapeutic response: expulsion of fetus
Teach patient/family:
• **Cervical ripening:** To remain supine for 10-15 min after insertion of vaginal suppository, 15-30 min after vaginal gel, 2 hr after vaginal insert (make sure it remains in place)
• To report excessive cramping, bleeding, chills, fever

• About some methods of pain, comfort control
• To avoid intercourse, tub baths, douches, tampon use for at least 2 wk

diphenhydrAMINE (OTC, Rx)

(dye-fen-hye′dra-meen)

Allerdryl ♣, AllerMax ♣, Banophen, Benadryl, Benadryl Allergy, Benadryl Allergy Dye Free, Diphedryl, Diphenhist, Silphen, Sominex, Unisom ♣, Benylin ♣, Calmex ♣, Dormex ♣, Dormiphen ♣

Func. class.: Antihistamine (1st generation, nonselective)

Chem. class.: Ethanolamine derivative, H_1-receptor antagonist

Do not confuse:

diphenhydrAMINE/ dicyclomine/dimenhy-DRINATE

ACTION: Acts on blood vessels, GI, respiratory system by competing with histamine for H_1-receptor site; decreases allergic response by blocking histamine

USES: Allergy symptoms, rhinitis, motion sickness, antiparkinsonism, nighttime sedation, infant colic, nonproductive cough, insomnia in children

CONTRAINDICATIONS: Hypersensitivity to H_1-receptor antagonist, neonates

Precautions: Pregnancy, breastfeeding, children <6 yr, increased intraocular pressure, cardiac/renal disease, hypertension, bronchial asthma, seizure disorder, stenosed peptic ulcers, hyperthyroidism, prostatic hypertrophy, bladder neck obstruction

DOSAGE AND ROUTES
Antihistamine/antiemetic/antivertigenia
• **Adult/child >12 yr: PO** 25-50 mg q4-6hr, max 300 mg/day; **IM/IV** 10-50 mg, max 300 mg/day

• **Child 6-12 yr: PO/IM/IV** 5 mg/kg/day in 4 divided doses, max 300 mg/day
Nighttime sleep aid
• **Adult and child ≥12 yr: PO** 25-50 mg at bedtime
Antitussive (syrup only)
• **Adult and child >12 yr: PO** 25 mg q4hr, max 150 mg/24 hr
• **Child 6-12 yr: PO** 12.5 mg q4hr, max 75 mg/24 hr
Motion sickness
• **Adult: IM/IV** 10-50 mg, max 25 mg/min; doses up to 100 mg/dose may be used; **PO** 25-50 mg q4-6hr

Available forms: Caps 25, 50 mg; tabs 25, 50 mg; chew tabs 12.5, 25 mg; elix 12.5 mg/5 mL; syr 12.5 mg/5 mL; inj 50 mg/mL; orally disintegrating tabs 12.5 mg; orally disintegrating strips 12.5, 25 mg

Administer:

• Avoid use in children <6 yr; death has occurred; overdose has occurred with topical gel taken orally (adult/child)
• With meals for GI symptoms; absorption rate may slightly decrease
• At bedtime only if using for sleep aid
IM route
• Deep IM in large muscle; rotate site
Direct IV route
• Undiluted; give 25 mg/min or less
Intermittent IV INFUSION route
• Dilute with 0.9% NaCl, 0.45% NaCl, D_5W, 0.9% NaCl, $D_{10}W$, LR, Ringer's

Y-site compatibilities: Acetaminophen, aldesleukin, alfentanil hydrochloride, amifostine, amikacin sulfate, aminocaproic acid, amphotericin B lipid complex (Abelcet), amphotericin B liposome (AmBisome), amsacrine, anidulafungin, argatroban, ascorbic acid injection, atenolol, atracurium besylate, atropine sulfate, azithromycin, benztropine mesylate, bivalirudin, bleomycin, bumetanide, buprenorphine, butorphanol, calcium chloride/gluconate, CARBOplatin, caspofungin, cefTAZidime, ceftizoxime, chlorproMAZINE, cimetidine, ciprofloxacin, cisatracurium, CISplatin, cladribine, clindamycin, codeine, cyanocobalamin, cyclophosphamide, cycloSPORINE, cytarabine,

D

Side effects: *italics* = common; red = life-threatening

DACTINomycin, DAPTOmycin, digoxin, diltiazem, DOBUTamine, DOCEtaxel, DOPamine, doripenem, doxacurium, DOXOrubicin, DOXOrubicin liposomal, doxycycline, enalaprilat, ePHEDrine, EPINEPHrine, epirubicin, epoetin alfa, eptifibatide, ertapenem, erythromycin, esmolol, etoposide, famotidine, fenoldopam, fentaNYL, filgrastim, fluconazole, fludarabine, folic acid, gallium, gatifloxacin, gemcitabine, gemtuzumab, gentamicin, glycopyrrolate, granisetron, HYDROmorphone, hydrOXYzine, IDArubicin, ifosfamide, imipenem-cilastatin, irinotecan, isoproterenol, labetalol, levofloxacin, lidocaine, linezolid, LORazepam, LR, magnesium sulfate, mannitol, mechlorethamine, melphalan, meperidine, meropenem, metaraminol, methadone, methicillin, methotrexate, methoxamine, methyldopate, metoclopramide, metoprolol, metroNIDAZOLE, miconazole, midazolam, minocycline, mitoXANtrone, morphine, multiple vitamins injection, mycophenolate, nalbuphine, naloxone, nesiritide, netilmicin, nitroglycerin, norepinephrine, octreotide, ondansetron, oxaliplatin, oxytocin, PACLitaxel, palonosetron, pamidronate, pancuronium, papaverine, PEMEtrexed, penicillin G potassium/sodium, pentamidine, pentazocine, phenylephrine, phytonadione, piperacillin, piperacillin-tazobactam, polymyxin B, potassium chloride, procainamide, prochlorperazine, promethazine, propofol, propranolol, protamine, pyridoxine, quiNIDine, quinupristin-dalfopristin, ranitidine, remifentanil, Ringer's, ritodrine, riTUXimab, rocuronium, sargramostim, sodium acetate, succinylcholine, SUFentanil, tacrolimus, teniposide, theophylline, thiamine, thiotepa, ticarcillin, ticarcillin-clavulanate, tigecycline, tirofiban, TNA, tobramycin, tolazoline, TPN, trastuzumab, trimetaphan, urokinase, vancomycin, vasopressin, vecuronium, verapamil, vinCRIStine, vinorelbine, vitamin B complex/C, voriconazole, zoledronic acid

SIDE EFFECTS

CNS: *Dizziness, drowsiness,* confusion, headache, seizures
CV: Hypotension, palpitations
EENT: Blurred vision, tinnitus, nasal stuffiness
GI: Nausea, anorexia, diarrhea
GU: *Retention,* dysuria, frequency
HEMA: Thrombocytopenia, agranulocytosis, hemolytic anemia
INTEG: Photosensitivity, rash
MISC: Anaphylaxis
RESP: Increased thick secretions, wheezing, chest tightness

PHARMACOKINETICS

Metabolized in liver, excreted by kidneys, crosses placenta, excreted in breast milk, half-life 2-4 hr
PO: Peak 2-4 hr, duration 4-8 hr
IM: Onset $1/2$ hr, peak 2-4 hr, duration 4-8 hr
IV: Onset immediate, duration 4-8 hr

INTERACTIONS

Increase: CNS depression—barbiturates, opiates, hypnotics, tricyclics, alcohol
Increase: diphenhydrAMINE effect—MAOIs
Drug/Herb
Increase: CNS depression—chamomile, kava, valerian
Drug/Lab Test
False negative: skin allergy tests

NURSING CONSIDERATIONS
Assess:
• Urinary retention, frequency, dysuria; product should be discontinued
• CBC during long-term therapy; blood dyscrasias may occur
• Respiratory status: rate, rhythm, increase in bronchial secretions, wheezing, chest tightness
• **EPS:** If using for dystonic reactions, assess type of involuntary movement and evaluate response to medication
• **Cough:** Characteristics (type, frequency, thickness of secretions); evaluate response to this medication, increase fluids to 2L/day unless contraindicated
• Anaphylaxis: Used for this rash, throat tightness, have emergency equipment nearby
• Store in tight container at room temperature

• **Pregnancy/breastfeeding:** no well-controlled studies; use only if benefit outweighs fetal risk; avoid breastfeeding, excreted in breast milk

Evaluate:

• Therapeutic response: absence of running or congested nose or rashes, improved sleep

Teach patient/family:

• About all aspects of product use; to notify prescriber of confusion, sedation, hypotension

• To avoid driving, other hazardous activity if drowsiness occurs

• That photosensitivity may occur use sunscreen, protective clothing

• To avoid concurrent use of alcohol, other CNS depressants

• To use hard candy, gum, frequent rinsing of mouth for dryness

• Product should be discontinued 4 days before skin allergy tests

• Not to use in child <4 yr, deaths have occurred; do not use in any child for sleep

• **Pregnancy/breastfeeding:** To report if pregnancy is planned or suspected or if breastfeeding, avoid if breastfeeding

TREATMENT OF OVERDOSE: Administer diazepam, vasopressors, phenytoin IV

RARELY USED

diphenoxylate/atropine (Rx)

(dye-fen-ox'ee-late/a'troe-peen)

Lomotil, Lonox

difenoxin/atropine (Rx)

(dye-fen-ox'in/a'troe-peen)

Motofen

Func. class.: Antidiarrheal
Chem. class.: Phenylpiperidine derivative opiate agonist

Controlled Substance Schedule V

diphenoxylate/atropine

Controlled Substance Schedule **IV:**

difenoxin/atropine

USES: Acute nonspecific and acute exacerbations of chronic functional diarrhea

CONTRAINDICATIONS: Children <2 yr, hypersensitivity, pseudomembranous colitis, severe electrolyte imbalances, diarrhea associated with organisms that penetrate intestinal mucosa

DOSAGE AND ROUTES

Diphenoxylate/atropine

• **Adult: PO** 5 mg qid titrated to patient response needed, max 8 tabs/day

• **Child 2-12 yr: PO** (liquid only) 0.3-0.4 mg/kg/day in 4 divided doses

Difenoxin/atropine

• **Adult: PO** 2 tabs, then 1 tab after each loose stool or q3-4hr prn, max 8 tabs/day

---

dipyridamole (Rx)

(dye-peer-id'a-mole)

Persantine ✤

Func. class.: Coronary vasodilator, antiplatelet agent
Chem. class.: Nonnitrate

ACTION: Inhibits adenosine uptake, which produces coronary vasodilation; increases oxygen saturation in coronary tissues, coronary blood flow; acts on small resistance vessels with little effect on vascular resistance; may increase development of collateral circulation; decreases platelet aggregation by the inhibition of phosphodiesterase (an enzyme)

USES: Prevention of transient ischemic attacks, inhibition of platelet adhesion to prevent myocardial reinfarction, thromboembolism, with warfarin in prosthetic heart valves, prevention of coronary bypass graft occlusion with aspirin; IV form used to evaluate CAD; used as alternative to exercise with thallium myocardial perfusion imaging to evaluate CAD

Unlabeled uses: Cardiomyopathy, MI prophylaxis, proteinuria, TIA, valvular heart disease

---

Side effects: *italics* = common; red = life-threatening

CONTRAINDICATIONS: Hypersensitivity

Precautions: Pregnancy, breastfeeding, hypotension, unstable angina, asthma, hepatic disease, labor

DOSAGE AND ROUTES
Inhibition of platelet adhesion
• **Adult: PO** 75-100 mg qid in combination with warfarin, 75 mg qid with aspirin
Thallium myocardial perfusion imaging
• **Adult: IV** 570 mcg/kg, max 60 mg/day
TIA with aspirin (unlabeled)
• **Adult: PO** 225-400 mg/day max 400 mg/day

Available forms: Tabs 25, 50, 75 mg; inj 10 mg/2 mL

Administer:
PO route
• On empty stomach: 1 hr before meals or 2 hr after; give with 8 oz water for better absorption
• Store at room temperature
IV route
• IV after diluting to at least 1:2 ratio using D_5W, 0.45% NaCl, or 0.9% NaCl to a total vol of 20-50 mL; give over 4 min; do not give undiluted
• Inject thallium 201 within 5 min after product infusion
• Do not admix

SIDE EFFECTS
CNS: *Headache, dizziness, weakness, fainting, syncope;* IV: transient cerebral ischemia, weakness
CV: *Postural hypotension;* IV: MI
GI: *Nausea, vomiting,* anorexia, diarrhea
INTEG: *Rash,* flushing

PHARMACOKINETICS
PO: Peak 75 min; **IV** peak 2 min, therapeutic response may take several mo, metabolized in liver, excreted in bile, undergoes enterohepatic recirculation, protein binding 91%-99%, terminal half-life 12 hr

INTERACTIONS
• Prevention of coronary vasodilation: theophylline, other xanthines; do not use

together, causes a false-negative thallium imaging result
Increase: digoxin effect—digoxin
Increase: bleeding risk—NSAIDs, cefoTEtan, valproic acid, salicylates, sulfinpyrazole, anticoagulants, thrombolytics; monitor for bleeding
Increase: adenosine effects—adenosine
Increase: myasthenia gravis effects—cholinesterase inhibitors

NURSING CONSIDERATIONS
Assess:
• B/P, pulse during treatment until stable; take B/P lying, standing; orthostatic hypotension is common
• Cardiac status: chest pain; what aggravates, ameliorates condition
• **Pregnancy/breastfeeding:** no well-controlled studies, use only if clearly needed; cautious use in breastfeeding, excreted in breast milk
Evaluate:
• Therapeutic response: decreased platelet adhesion
Teach patient/family:
• That medication is not a cure; may have to be taken continuously in evenly spaced doses only as directed
• To avoid hazardous activities until stabilized on medication; dizziness may occur
• To rise slowly from sitting or lying to prevent orthostatic hypotension
• Not to use alcohol or OTC medications unless approved by prescriber
• About cardiac stress testing, expectations

⚠ HIGH ALERT

DOBUTamine (Rx)
(doe-byoo′ta-meen)
Func. class.: Adrenergic direct-acting β_1-agonist, cardiac stimulant
Chem. class.: Catecholamine

Do not confuse:
DOBUTamine/DOPamine

ACTION: Causes increased contractility, increased cardiac output without marked increase in heart rate by acting on β_1-receptors in heart; minor α and β_2 effects

USES: Cardiac decompensation due to organic heart disease or cardiac surgery
Unlabeled uses: Cardiogenic shock in children; congenital heart disease in children undergoing cardiac catheterization

CONTRAINDICATIONS: Hypersensitivity, idiopathic hypertrophic subaortic stenosis
Precautions: Pregnancy, breastfeeding, children, hypertension, CAD, MI, hypovolemia, dysrhythmias, sulfite hypersensitivity, renal failure, geriatric patients

DOSAGE AND ROUTES
• **Adult and child:** IV INFUSION 0.5-1 mcg/kg/min; titrate to 2-20 mcg/kg/min, may increase to 40 mcg/kg/min if needed
Available forms: Inj 12.5 mg/mL; premixed infusion 250 mg/mL, 500 mg/500 mL, 500 mg/250 mL, 1000 mg/250 mL
Administer:
Injectable
• Visually inspect parenteral products for particulate matter and discoloration before administration whenever solution and container permit
• Store reconstituted sol for 24 hr if refrigerated
IV route
Note: Infusions lasting up to 72 hr have been given without development of tolerance; however, beta-receptor desensitization can occur with prolonged infusion of any beta-adrenergic agonist, including DOBUTamine, or as a consequence of sympathetic compensatory mechanisms associated with advanced congestive heart failure, resulting in alterations in DOBUTamine pharmacodynamics
• Must be diluted before administration
• Infuse into a large vein
Dilution
• Concentrate for injection must be diluted with ≥50 mL of a compatible IV solution (strongly alkaline [e.g., sodium bicarbonate] solutions are incompatible); a common dilution is 500 mg (40 mL) in 210 mL D₅W or NS (withdraw 40 mL from

a 250-mL bag) to produce a final concentration of 2000 mcg/mL; or 1000 mg (80 mL) in 170 mL D₅W or NS (withdraw 80 mL from a 250-mL bag) to produce a final concentration of 4000 mcg/mL; max 5000 mcg/mL and should be adjusted according to the patient's fluid requirements
Infusion
• Continuous: Use a controlled-infusion device
• Premixed bags in D₅W solutions can be a pink color that increases with time; this color change is due to slight oxidation of the drug, but there is no significant loss of potency
• Do not give DOBUTamine simultaneously with solutions containing sodium bicarbonate or strong alkaline solutions (incompatible)
• Infusion should be started at a low rate and titrated frequently to reach the optimal dosage; dosage titration is guided by the patient's response, including systemic blood pressure, urine flow, frequency of ectopic activity, heart rate, and measurements of cardiac output, central venous pressure, and/or pulmonary capillary wedge pressure

Y-site compatibilities: Alfentanil, alprostadil, amifostine, amikacin, aminocaproic acid, amiodarone, anidulafungin, argatroban, ascorbic acid injection, atenolol, atracurium, atropine, aztreonam, benztropine, bleomycin, bumetanide, buprenorphine, butorphanol, calcium chloride/gluconate, CARBOplatin, caspofungin, chlorproMAZINE, cimetidine, ciprofloxacin, cisatracurium, CISplatin, cladribine, clarithromycin, cloNIDine, codeine, cyanocobalamin, cyclophosphamide, cycloSPORINE, cytarabine, DACTINomycin, DAPTOmycin, dexmedetomidine, digoxin, diltiazem, diphenhydrAMINE, DOCEtaxel, DOPamine, doripenem, doxacurium, DOXOrubicin, DOXOrubicin liposomal, doxycycline, enalaprilat, ePHEDrine, EPINEPHrine, epirubicin, epoetin alfa, eptifibatide, erythromycin, esmolol, etoposide, famotidine, fenoldopam, fentaNYL, fluconazole, fludarabine, gatifloxacin, gemcitabine, gentamicin, glycopyrrolate, granisetron, HYDROmorphone, hydrOXYzine, IDArubicin, ifosfamide, irinotecan, isoproterenol, labetalol, levofloxacin, lidocaine, linezolid, LORazepam, LR, magnesium sulfate, mannitol, mechlorethamine, meperidine, meropenem, metaraminol, methoxamine, methyldopate, methylPREDNISolone, metoclopramide, metoprolol, metroNIDAZOLE, miconazole, milrinone, minocycline, mitoXANtrone, morphine, multiple vitamins injection, mycophenolate mofetil, nafcillin, nalbuphine, naloxone, netilmicin, niCARdipine, nitroglycerin, norepinephrine, octreotide, ondansetron, oxaliplatin, oxytocin, PACLitaxel, palonosetron, pamidronate, pancuronium, papaverine, pentamidine, pentazocine, phenylephrine, polymyxin B, potassium chloride, procainamide, prochlorperazine, promethazine, propofol, propranolol, protamine, pyridoxine, quiNIDine, ranitidine, remifentanil, Ringer's, ritodrine, riTUXimab, rocuronium, sodium acetate, succinylcholine, SUFentanil, tacrolimus, temocillin, teniposide, theophylline, thiamine, thiotepa, tigecycline, tirofiban, TNA, tobramycin, tolazoline, TPN, trastuzumab, trimetaphan, urokinase, vancomycin, vasopressin, vecuronium, verapamil, vinCRIStine, vinorelbine, voriconazole, zidovudine, zoledronic acid

SIDE EFFECTS

CNS: *Anxiety,* headache, dizziness, fatigue
CV: Palpitations, tachycardia, hypo/hypertension, PVCs, angina
ENDO: Hypokalemia
GI: Heartburn, nausea, vomiting
MS: Muscle cramps (leg)
RESP: Dyspnea

PHARMACOKINETICS

IV: Onset 1-2 min, peak 10 min, half-life 2 min, metabolized in liver (inactive metabolites), excreted in urine

INTERACTIONS

Increase: severe hypertension— guanethidine
Increase: dysrhythmias—general anesthetics
Increase: pressor effect, dysrhythmias— atomoxetine, COMT inhibitors, tricyclics, MAOIs, oxytocics
Decrease: DOBUTamine action—other β-blockers

NURSING CONSIDERATIONS
Assess:
• **Hypovolemia:** if present, correct first; administer any cardiac glycoside before DOBUTamine
• **Oxygenation/perfusion deficit:** check B/P, chest pain, dizziness, loss of consciousness
• **Heart failure:** S$_3$ gallop, dyspnea, neck venous distention, bibasilar crackles in patients with HF, cardiomyopathy; palpate peripheral pulses, report if extremities become cold or mottled or if peripheral pulses decrease
• **ECG** during administration continuously; if B/P increases, product is decreased; CVP or PCWP, cardiac output during infusion; report changes, may induce ectopic rhythms
• Serum electrolytes, urine output; correct before use
• **Sulfite sensitivity,** which may be life threatening
• **Pregnancy/breastfeeding:** no well-controlled studies; use only if benefit outweighs fetal risk; cautious use in breastfeeding, excretion is unknown
Evaluate:
• Therapeutic response: increased B/P with stabilization, increased urine output
Teach patient/family:
• About the reason for product administration
• To report shortness of breath, chest pain, numbness of extremities, headache, IV site discomfort, exercise intolerance, inability to complete ADLs

TREATMENT OF OVERDOSE:
Administer a β$_1$-adrenergic blocker; reduce IV or discontinue, ensure

oxygenation/ventilation; for severe tachy-dysrhythmias (ventricular), give lido-caine or propranolol

A HIGH ALERT

DOCEtaxel (Rx)
(doe-se-tax'el)

Docefrez, Taxotere

Func. class.: Antineoplastic—miscel-laneous

Chem. class.: Taxane

Do not confuse:
Taxotere/Taxol

ACTION: Inhibits reorganization of microtubule network needed for inter-phase and mitotic cellular functions; also causes abnormal bundles of microtubules during cell cycle and multiple esters of microtubules during mitosis

USES: Locally advanced or metastatic breast cancer, non–small-cell lung can-cer, androgen-independent metastatic prostate cancer, postsurgery operable node-positive breast cancer, induction treatment of locally advanced squamous cell of the head and neck, gastric adenocarcinoma

Unlabeled uses: Malignant melanoma, ovarian cancer, front-line use with beva-cizumab for metastatic breast cancer, adjuvant treatment of breast cancer with CARBOplatin and trastuzumab

CONTRAINDICATIONS: Preg-nancy, breastfeeding, hypersensitivity to this product, bilirubin exceeding upper normal limit

Black Box Warning: Other products with polysorbate 80, neutropenia of <1500/mm^3

Precautions: Children, cardiovascular disease, pulmonary disorders, bone mar-row depression, herpes zoster, pleural effusion

Black Box Warning: Edema, hepatic dis-ease, lung cancer, taxane hypersensitivity

DOSAGE AND ROUTES:
• Other regimens are used
• **Adult:** IV 60-100 mg/m^2 given over 1 hr q3wk; if neutrophil count is <500 cells/mm^3 for >1 wk, reduce dose by 25%

Operable node-positive breast cancer, adjuvant
• **Adult:** IV (TAC regimen) 75 mg/m^2 1 hr after DOXOrubicin 50 mg/m^2 and cyclophosphamide 500 mg/m^2 q3wk × 6 cycles

Locally advanced or metastatic non–small-cell lung cancer after failure of CISplatin chemotherapy
• **Adult:** IV 75 mg/m^2 over 1 hr q3wk; if neutrophil count is <500 cells/mm^3 for >1 wk, reduce dose to 55 mg/m^2; if pa-tient develops grade 3 peripheral neu-ropathy, stop product

Androgen-independent metastatic prostate cancer
• **Adult:** IV 75 mg/m^2 given over 1 hr q3wk with 5 mg predniSONE **PO** bid continuously; give dexamethasone 8 mg **PO** at 12 hr, 3 hr, and 1 hr prior to DOCEtaxel; if neutrophil count is <500 cells/mm^3 for more than 1 wk or other toxicities occur, reduce dose to 60 mg/m^2

Squamous cell of head and neck
• **Adult:** IV 75 mg/m^2 over 1 hr, then CISplatin 100 mg/m^2 over 1 hr on day 1, then 5FU 1000 mg/m^2/day **CONT INFU-SION** × 5 days, repeat cycle q3wk

Available forms: Inj 10 mg/mL, 20 mg/0.5 mL, 20 mg/mL, 80 mg/2 mL, 80 mg/4 mL; 20, 80 mg powder for injection/vial

Administer:
• Premedicate with dexamethasone 8 mg **PO** bid × 3 days starting 1 day before treatment
• Antiemetic 30-60 min before product and prn

Side effects: *italics* = common; red = life-threatening

• Confirmation that dexamethasone was given 8 mg bid x 3 days starting 1 day before infusion; for prostate cancer give 8 mg 12 hr, 3 hr, and 1 hr prior to infusion
• Store prepared sol up to 27 hr in refrigerator

Intermittent IV INFUSION route
• Use cytotoxic handling procedures
• Use non-PVC bag and use non-DEHP tubing
• Double-check all orders and products; errors can be fatal
• Solution is yellow to brown, do not use if particulate is present
• Allow vials to warm to room temperature; withdraw all diluent, inject in vial of DOCEtaxel; rotate gently to mix; allow to stand to decrease foaming, then withdraw the required amount (10 mg/mL), inject in 250 mL of 0.9% NaCl, D₅W; mix gently; give over 1 hr

Y-site compatibilities: Acyclovir, alfentanil, allopurinol, amifostine, amikacin, aminocaproic acid, aminophylline, amiodarone, amphotericin B lipid complex, ampicillin, ampicillin-sulbactam, anidulafungin, atenolol, atracurium, azithromycin, aztreonam, bivalirudin, bleomycin, bumetanide, buprenorphine, busulfan, butorphanol, calcium chloride/gluconate, CARBOplatin, carmustine, caspofungin, ceFAZolin, cefepime, cefonicid, cefotaxime, cefoTEtan, cefOXitin, cefTAZidime, ceftizoxime, cefTRIAXone, cefuroxime, chloramphenicol, chlorproMAZINE, cimetidine, ciprofloxacin, cisatracurium, CISplatin, clindamycin, codeine, cyclophosphamide, cycloSPORINE, cytarabine, dacarbazine, DACTINomycin, DAPTOmycin, dexamethasone, dexmedetomidine, dexrazoxane, diazepam, digoxin, diltiazem, diphenhydrAMINE, DOBUTamine, DOPamine, doripenem, doxacurium, DOXOrubicin HCl, doxycycline, droperidol, enalaprilat, ePHEDrine, EPINEPHrine, epirubicin, ertapenem, erythromycin, esmolol, etoposide, famotidine, fenoldopam, fentaNYL, fluconazole, fludarabine, fluorouracil, foscarnet, fosphenytoin, furosemide, ganciclovir, gatifloxacin, gemcitabine, gentamicin, glycopyr-rolate, granisetron, haloperidol, heparin, hydrALAZINE, hydrocortisone, HYDROmorphone, hydrOXYzine, ifosfamide, imipenem-cilastatin, inamrinone, insulin (regular), irinotecan, isoproterenol, ketorolac, labetalol, leucovorin, levofloxacin, levorphanol, lidocaine, linezolid, LORazepam, LR, magnesium sulfate, mannitol, meperidine, meropenem, mesna, methotrexate, methyldopate, metoclopramide, metoprolol, metroNIDAZOLE, midazolam, milrinone, minocycline, mitoXANtrone, mivacurium, morphine, nafcillin, naloxone, nesiritide, netilmicin, niCARdipine, nitroglycerin, nitroprusside, norepinephrine, octreotide, ofloxacin, ondansetron, oxaliplatin, palonosetron, pamidronate, pancuronium, pantoprazole, PEMEtrexed, pentamidine, pentazocine, PENTobarbital, PHENobarbital, phenylephrine, piperacillin, piperacillin-tazobactam, polymyxin B, potassium chloride/phosphates, procainamide, prochlorperazine, promethazine, propranolol, quiNIDine, quinupristin-dalfopristin, ranitidine, remifentanil, riTUXimab, rocuronium, sodium acetate/bicarbonate/phosphates, succinylcholine, SUFentanil, sulfamethoxazole-trimethoprim, tacrolimus, teniposide, theophylline, thiopental, thiotepa, ticarcillin, ticarcillin-clavulanate, tigecycline, tirofiban, tobramycin, tolazoline, trastuzumab, trimethobenzamide, vancomycin, vasopressin, vecuronium, verapamil, vinCRIStine, vinorelbine, voriconazole, zidovudine, zoledronic acid

SIDE EFFECTS
EENT: Altered hearing, cystoid macular edema
CNS: Seizures, fatigue, weakness
CV: *Fluid retention, peripheral edema*
GI: *Nausea, vomiting, diarrhea,* hepatotoxicity, stomatitis
HEMA: Leukopenia, thrombocytopenia, anemia
INTEG: *Alopecia,* nail changes, rash, skin eruptions
MISC: Secondary malignancy, Stevens-Johnson syndrome
MS: *Arthralgia, myalgia,* back pain, weakness

NEURO: *Peripheral neuropathy*
RESP: Dyspnea, pulmonary edema, fibrosis, embolism, acute respiratory distress syndrome, interstitial lung disease
SYST: Hypersensitivity reactions

PHARMACOKINETICS
Metabolized in liver, excreted in feces, half-life 11.1 hr, peak 5-9 days, duration 1 wk

INTERACTIONS
Increase: Docetaxel effect—CYP3A inhibitors: anastrozole (high doses), aprepitant, fosaprepitant, clarithromycin, conivaptan, delavirdine, efavirenz (induces or inhibits), erythromycin, fluconazole, FLUoxetine, fluvoxaMINE, imatinib, itraconazole, ketoconazole, nefazodone, voriconazole, and others
Increase: Modified effect of docetaxel CYP3A inducers: barbiturates, bosentan, carBAMazepine, nevirapine, phenytoin, fosphenytoin, rifabutin, rifampin, rifapentine
Increase: myelosuppression—other antineoplastics, radiation
Decrease: immune response—live virus vaccines

NURSING CONSIDERATIONS
Assess:

Black Box Warning: **Neutropenia:** CBC, differential, platelet count before treatment and weekly; withhold product if WBC is <1500/mm³ or platelet count is <100,000/mm³; notify prescriber, nadir 8 days

Black Box Warning: DOCEtaxel, polysorbate 80 hypersensitivity: contraindicated; some products may contain polysorbate 80

Black Box Warning: **Edema:** oral corticosteroids should be given as premedication; assess for fluid retention; may be severe, is usually dose related

Black Box Warning: **Lung cancer:** increased mortality in those with increased LFTs and a history of platinum-based products

Black Box Warning: **Hepatic disease:** hepatic studies before each cycle (bilirubin, AST, ALT, LDH); check for jaundiced skin and sclera, dark urine, clay-colored stools, itchy skin, abdominal pain, fever, diarrhea, if LFTs are >5x upper limit discontinue

- **CNS changes:** confusion, paresthesias, peripheral neuropathy, dysesthesia, pain, weakness; if severe, product should be discontinued or pyridoxine used
- VS during 1st hr of infusion, check IV site for signs of infiltration

Black Box Warning: **Hypersensitivity reactions, anaphylaxis,** including hypotension, dyspnea, angioedema, generalized urticaria; discontinue infusion immediately, usually during first or second dose; mild reactions can be treated by slowing infusion, treating symptomatically; do not retreat in those with severe reactions

- **Bone marrow depression/bleeding:** hematuria, guaiac, bruising or petechiae, mucosa or orifices q8hr; obtain prescription for viscous lidocaine (Xylocaine); avoid invasive procedures, avoid IM injections, rectal temps if platelets are low
- Effects of alopecia on body image; discuss feelings about body changes

Evaluate:
- Therapeutic response: decreased tumor size, spread of malignancy

Teach patient/family:
- To report signs of infection: fever, sore throat, flulike symptoms
- To report signs of anemia: fatigue, headache, faintness, SOB, irritability
- To report bleeding; to avoid use of razors, commercial mouthwash
- To avoid use of aspirin, ibuprofen, alcohol
- That hair may be lost during treatment; that a wig or hairpiece may make patient feel better; that new hair may be different in color and texture
- That pain in muscles and joints 2-5 days after infusion is common

• To avoid receiving vaccinations while taking product

• **Pregnancy/breastfeeding:** to use barrier contraception during and for several mo after treatment; to avoid breastfeeding

---

docosanol topical
See Appendix B

---

docusate calcium (OTC)
(dok'yoo-sate cal'see-um)
Kaopectate Stool Softener, Kao-Tin
docusate sodium (OTC)
Colace, Correctol, Diocto, Docu DOK, Doculace, Dulcolax, Dulcolax stool softener, Enemeez, Fleet Pedialax, Fleet Sof-Lax, Phillips Liquid-Gels, Selex ✦, Silace, Soflax ✦
Func. class.: Laxative, emollient; stool softener
Chem. class.: Anionic surfactant

Do not confuse:
Colace/Cozaar
Dulcolax (docusate)/Dulcolax (bisacodyl)

ACTION: Increases water, fat penetration in intestine; allows for easier passage of stool

USES: Prevention of dry, hard stools

CONTRAINDICATIONS: Hypersensitivity, obstruction, fecal impaction, nausea/vomiting
Precautions: Pregnancy, breastfeeding

DOSAGE AND ROUTES
• **Adult:** PO 50-400 mg/day in divided doses (sodium) or 240 mg q day (calcium); **Rectal ENEMA** 4 mL
• **Child >12 yr:** ENEMA 2 mL
• **Child 6-12 yr:** PO 40-150 mg/day (sodium) in divided doses
• **Child 3-6 yr:** PO 20-60 mg/day (sodium) in divided doses

• **Child <3 yr:** PO 10-40 mg/day (sodium) in divided doses
• **Infant:** PO 5 mg/kg/day in divided doses
Available forms: *Calcium:* 240 mg; *sodium:* caps 50, 100, 250 mg; tabs 100 mg; syr 20 mg/5 mL; liquid 50 mg/5 mL, enema 283 mg/5mL
Administer:
• Swallow tabs whole; do not break, crush, or chew
• Oral sol: diluted in milk, fruit juice to decrease bitter taste
• In morning or evening (oral dose)
• Store in cool environment; do not freeze

SIDE EFFECTS
EENT: Bitter taste, throat irritation
GI: Nausea, anorexia, cramps, diarrhea
INTEG: Rash

PHARMACOKINETICS
Onset 12-72 hr (PO), 2-15 min (rectal)

INTERACTIONS
• **Toxicity:** mineral oil
Drug/Herb
Increase: laxative action—flax, senna

NURSING CONSIDERATIONS
Assess:
• **Cause of constipation;** identify whether fluids, bulk, or exercise is missing from lifestyle; constipating products
• Cramping, rectal bleeding, nausea, vomiting; if these occur, product should be discontinued
• **Pregnancy/breastfeeding:** low risk of fetal harm in pregnancy, breastfeeding
Evaluate:
• Therapeutic response: decrease in constipation
Teach patient/family:
• That normal bowel movements do not always occur daily
• Not to use in presence of abdominal pain, nausea, vomiting
• To notify prescriber if constipation is unrelieved or if symptoms of electrolyte imbalance occur: muscle cramps, pain, weakness, dizziness, excessive thirst

• That product may take up to 3 days to soften stools
• To take oral preparations with a full glass of water (unless on fluid restrictions) and to increase fluid intake

⚠ HIGH ALERT

dofetilide (Rx)

Tikosyn
Func. class.: Antidysrhythmic (Class III)

ACTION: Blocks cardiac ion channel carrying the rapid component of delayed potassium current; no effect on sodium channels

USES: Atrial fibrillation, flutter, maintenance of normal sinus rhythm

CONTRAINDICATIONS: Children, hypersensitivity, digoxin toxicity, aortic stenosis, pulmonary hypertension, severe renal disease, QT prolongation, torsades de pointes, renal failure
Precautions: Pregnancy, breastfeeding, AV block, bradycardia, electrolyte imbalance, renal disease

Black Box Warning: Arrhythmias, ventricular arrhythmias/tachycardia; requires an experienced clinician in specialized care setting

DOSAGE AND ROUTES

Adult: PO 500 mcg bid initially; maintenance 250 mcg bid, max 500 mcg bid; adjust dose based on QT and renal function
Renal dose
• **Adult: PO** CCr >60 mL/min, 500 mcg bid; CCr 40-60 mL/min, 250 mcg bid; CCr 20-39 mL/min, 125 mcg bid; CCr <20 mL/min, do not use
Available forms: Caps 125, 250, 500 mcg
Administer:
• Physician and pharmacy must be registered to use product
• With patient hospitalized for ≥3 days

Black Box Warning: **Step 1: Assess cardiac conduction:** Before first dose, the QTc interval must be determined using an average of 5-10 beats; if the QTc interval is >440 msec (or >500 msec in ventricular conduction abnormalities), do not use; if baseline heart rate is <60 bpm, then the QT interval should be used

Black Box Warning: **Step 2: Assess renal function:** Before first dose, determine renal function using the Cockcroft-Gault equation, use actual body weight to calculate creatinine clearance

Black Box Warning: **Step 3: Adjust starting dose according to renal function:** Refer to the renal dose section above to determine the appropriate initial dosage

Black Box Warning: **Step 4: ECG monitoring:** Begin continuous ECG monitoring starting with the first dose

Black Box Warning: **Step 5: Dosage adjustments:** Approximately 2-3 hr after the first dose, determine the QTc interval; if the QTc interval has increased by >15% (compared to baseline), or if the QTc interval is >500 msec (>550 msec in patients with ventricular conduction abnormalities), the initial dosage should be reduced by half as follows:
• Decrease an initial dose of 500 mcg bid to 250 mcg bid
• Decrease an initial dose of 250 mcg bid to 125 mcg bid
• Decrease an initial dose of 125 mcg bid to 125 mcg/day

Black Box Warning: **Step 6: Reassess QTc interval:** Reassess the QTc interval 2-3 hr after each subsequent dose; if the QTc interval lengthens to >500 msec (or >550 msec in patients with ventricular conduction abnormalities), discontinue

Black Box Warning: **Step 7: ECG monitoring:** Monitor continuous ECG for a minimum of 3 days or for 12 hr after conversion to normal sinus rhythm, whichever is greater

D

SIDE EFFECTS

CNS: *Dizziness,* headache, stroke
CV: QT prolongation, torsades de pointes, ventricular dysrhythmias, chest pain
GI: *Nausea,* diarrhea

PHARMACOKINETICS

Well absorbed, max plasma concentrations 2-3 hr, steady state 2-3 days, half-life 10 hr, metabolized by liver, excreted by kidneys, peak 3 hr, duration up to 24 hr

INTERACTIONS

• Do not use with cimetidine, ketoconazole, verapamil, prochlorperazine, trimethoprim-sulfamethoxazole, megestrol, hydroCHLOROthiazide

Increase: QT prolongation, torsades de pointes—class IA/III antidysrhythmics, arsenic trioxide, chloroquine, clarithromycin, droperidol, erythromycin, halofantrine, haloperidol, methadone, pentamidine, some phenothiazines, ziprasidone, ciprofloxacin

Increase: hypokalemia—potassium-depleting diuretics

Increase: toxicity—aMILoride metFORMIN, entecavir, lamiVUDine, memantine, triamterene, procainamide, trospium

Increase: dofetilide levels—antiretroviral protease inhibitors

Increase: dysrhythmias—CYP3A4 inhibitors (SSRIs, macrolides, azoles, protease inhibitors, amiodarone, diltiazem, quinine)

Drug/Food
• Do not use with grapefruit juice

NURSING CONSIDERATIONS
Assess:
• AF patients should receive anticoagulation prior to cardioversion

Black Box Warning: Dysrhythmias: 3 days of continuous ECG monitoring, monitoring of CCr are required when starting or restarting medication; have cardiac resuscitation equipment nearby

• Cardiac status: rate, rhythm, character, continuously; B/P
• **Severe renal impairment CCr <20 mL/min:** do not use for mild to moderate renal disease; monitor BUN/creatinine; adjust dose based on creatinine clearance
• **Pregnancy/breastfeeding:** no well-controlled studies; use only if benefit outweighs fetal risk; avoid breastfeeding, excretion is unknown

Evaluate:
• Therapeutic response: control of atrial fibrillation, normal sinus rhythm

Teach patient/family:
• To make position changes slowly; orthostatic hypotension may occur
• To notify prescriber if fast heartbeats with fainting or dizziness occur
• To notify all prescribers of all medications, supplements taken
• That if dose is missed, not to double; to take next dose at usual time
• To avoid breastfeeding

---

dolasetron (Rx)
(do-la'se-tron)
Anzemet
Func. class.: Antiemetic
Chem. class.: 5-HT3 receptor antagonist

Do not confuse:
Anzemet/Avandamet

ACTION: Prevents nausea, vomiting by blocking serotonin peripherally, centrally, and in the small intestine

USES: Prevention of chemotherapy-induced and postoperative nausea, vomiting

CONTRAINDICATIONS: Hypersensitivity
Precautions: Pregnancy, breastfeeding, children, geriatric patients, hypokalemia, electrolyte imbalances; granisetron/ondansetron/palonosetron hypersensitivity, QT prolongation

DOSAGE AND ROUTES
Prevention of cancer chemotherapy nausea/vomiting
• **Adult:** PO 100 mg 1 hr prior to chemotherapy

• **Child 2-16 yr:** PO 1-8 mg/kg given1 hr prior to chemotherapy
Available forms: Tabs 50, 100 mg; inj
Administer:
PO route
• Do not mix product for oral administration in apple or apple-grape juice until immediately before administration; diluted product can be kept for 2 hr at room temperature
• Store at room temperature 48 hr after dilution

SIDE EFFECTS

CNS: *Headache,* dizziness, fatigue, drowsiness, serotonin syndrome
CV: Dysrhythmias, ECG changes, hypo/hypertension, tachycardia, bradycardia; ventricular tachycardia/fibrillation, QT prolongation, torsades de pointes, cardiac arrest (IV)
GI: *Diarrhea,* constipation, increased AST/ALT, abdominal pain, anorexia
GU: Urinary retention, oliguria
MISC: Rash, bronchospasm

PHARMACOKINETICS
Well absorbed, metabolized to active metabolite, half-life of active metabolite 8 hr, max concentrations after 1 hr

INTERACTIONS
Increase: dysrhythmias—antidysrhythmics
Increase: dolasetron levels—cimetidine
Increase: QT prolongation—thiazide/loop diuretics, antidysrhythmics (class IA, III), arsenic trioxide, chloroquine, clarithromycin, droperidol, erythromycin, halofantrine, haloperidol, methadone, pentamidine, some phenothiazines, ziprasidone; occurs at higher dose of dolasetron
Decrease: dolasetron levels—rifampin

NURSING CONSIDERATIONS
Assess:
• **Hypersensitivity reaction:** rash, bronchospasm
• Nausea, vomiting, before and after use
• **Cardiac conduction conditions:** monitor ECG, electrolyte imbalances, dysrhythmias, heart rate

• **QT prolongation:** QRS, PR prolongation; do not use in those with congenital long QT syndrome, hypokalemia, hypomagnesemia, complete heart block (unless a pacemaker is in place), correct electrolytes before use, monitor ECG in elderly patients, renal cardiac disease
• **Serotonin syndrome:** usually when combined with SSRIs, SNRIs, MAOIs
• **Pregnancy/breastfeeding:** no well-controlled studies; use only if clearly needed, cautious use in breastfeeding, excretion is unknown
Evaluate:
• Therapeutic response: absence of nausea, vomiting during cancer chemotherapy
Teach patient/family:
• To report diarrhea, constipation, nausea, vomiting, rash, or changes in respirations, heart rate, nausea, vomiting
• May cause headache; use analgesic

⚠ HIGH ALERT

dolutegravir
(dole-oo-teg′ra-vir)
Tivicay

ACTION: Inhibits catalytic activity of HIV integrase, which is an HIV-encoded enzyme needed for replication

USES: HIV in combination with other antiretrovirals

CONTRAINDICATIONS: Breastfeeding, hypersensitivity
Precautions: Pregnancy, children, geriatric patients, hepatic disease, immune reconstitution syndrome, hepatitis, antimicrobial resistance, lactase deficiency

DOSAGE AND ROUTES
• **Adult and child ≥12 yr and ≥40 kg (treatment naïve or treatment experienced but integrase strand transfer inhibitor naïve):** PO 50 mg daily; if given with efavirenz, fosamprenavir/ritonavir, tipranavir/ritonavir, or rifampin, give 50 mg bid

Child 30-39 kg: PO 35 mg/day; if using efavirenz, fosamprenavir/ritonavir, tipranavir/ritonavir, rifampin

Available forms: Tabs 10, 25, 50 mg

Administer:

• May give without regard to meals, with 8 oz of water

• Store at room temperature

• Give 2 hr before or 6 hr after cation-containing antacids or laxatives, sucralfate, oral iron, oral calcium, or buffered products

SIDE EFFECTS

CNS: Fatigue, headache, insomnia

GI: Nausea, vomiting, diarrhea, hepatotoxicity

INTEG: Rash, pruritus

META: Hyperglycemia

SYST: Immune reconstitution syndrome

GU: Renal dysfunction

PHARMACOKINETICS

Peak 2-3 hr, steady state 5 days, half-life 14 hr, 98% protein binding, metabolized in the liver, excreted in feces 53%, urine 31%

INTERACTIONS

Decrease: effect of dolutegravir—antacids, laxatives/sucralfate, oral iron, oral calcium, buffered products

Decrease: levels—rifampin efavirenz, tenofovir, tipranavir/ritonavir

Drug/Herb

• Avoid concurrent use with St. John's wort

NURSING CONSIDERATIONS

Assess:

• HIV infection: CD4, T-cell count, plasma HIV RNA, viral load; resistance testing before treatment, at treatment failure

• Drug resistance testing before use in treatment naïve patients

• Immune reconstitution syndrome, usually during initial phase of treatment; may need antiinfective before starting

• Monitor total HDL/LDL cholesterol baseline and periodically; all may be elevated

• **Pregnancy/breastfeeding:** all HIV-positive women should receive antiretroviral therapy, report pregnancy to the Antiretroviral Pregnancy Registry, 1-800-258-4263; avoid breastfeeding, excretion unknown; glucose screening should be performed at 24-48 wk gestation, confirm gestation age in each trimester by ultrasound

Evaluate:

• Therapeutic response: improvement in cell counts, T-cell counts

Teach patient/family:

• To take as prescribed; if dose is missed, to take as soon as remembered up to 1 hr before next dose; not to double dose; not to share with others

• That sexual partners need to be told that patient has HIV; that product does not cure infection, just controls symptoms, does not prevent infecting others

• To report sore throat, fever, fatigue (may indicate superinfection)

• That continued follow-up and lab work will be needed

• That fat accumulation/redistribution may occur

• To notify prescriber if pregnancy is planned or suspected; to avoid breastfeeding and to continue follow-up exams and lab work

---

RARELY USED

dolutegravir/rilpivirine

(doe-loo-teg′-ra-vir/ril-pi-vir′-een)

Juluca

Func. class.: Antiviral

USES: For the treatment of HIV-1 infection in adults

DOSAGE AND ROUTES

• **Adult:** PO 1 tablet (dolutegravir 50 mg; rilpivirine 25 mg) plus an additional 25-mg tablet of rilpivirine (total daily rilpivirine dose of 50 mg) daily with a meal. When rifabutin coadministration is stopped, reduce rilpivirine dose to 25 mg daily with a meal

Human immunodeficiency virus (HIV) infection without concurrent rifabutin

---

• **Adult:** PO 1 tablet (dolutegravir 50 mg; rilpivirine 25 mg) daily with a meal

donepezil (Rx)

(don-ep-ee'zill)

Aricept

Func. class.: Anti-Alzheimer's agent

Chem. class.: Reversible cholinesterase inhibitor

Do not confuse:

Aricept/Aciphex/Azilect

ACTION: Elevates acetylcholine concentrations (cerebral cortex) by slowing degradation of acetylcholine released in cholinergic neurons; does not alter underlying dementia

USES: Mild to severe dementia with Alzheimer's disease

CONTRAINDICATIONS: Hypersensitivity to this product or piperidine derivatives

Precautions: Pregnancy, breastfeeding, children, sick sinus syndrome, history of ulcers, GI bleeding, hepatic disease, bladder obstruction, asthma, seizures, COPD, abrupt discontinuation, AV block, GI obstruction, Parkinson's disease, surgery

DOSAGE AND ROUTES

• **Adult:** PO 5 mg/day at bedtime; may increase to 10 mg/day after 4-6 wk, may increase to 23 mg/day after 3 mo of 10 mg/day (moderate to severe); 5 mg daily may be increased by 10 mg daily after 4-6 wk; after 3 mo may increase to 23 mg daily (severe)

Available forms: 5, 23, 10 mg

Administer:

• Give between meals, may give with meals for GI symptoms

SIDE EFFECTS

CNS: Dizziness, *insomnia, headache,* fatigue, abnormal dreams, syncope, seizures, drowsiness, agitation, depression, confusion, hallucinations

CV: Atrial fibrillation, hypo/hypertension

GI: *Nausea, vomiting,* anorexia, *diarrhea,* abdominal pain, weight gain

GU: Urinary frequency

INTEG: Rash, flushing, diaphoresis, bruising

MS: Cramps, arthritis, arthralgia, back pain

PHARMACOKINETICS

Well absorbed PO; metabolized by CYP2D6, CYP3A4; half-life 10 hr single dose, 70 hr multiple doses; protein binding 96%

INTERACTIONS

Increase: donepezil effects—CYP2D6, CYP3A4 inhibitors

Increase: synergistic effect—succinylcholine, cholinesterase inhibitors, cholinergic agonists

Increase: GI bleeding—NSAIDs

Decrease: donepezil effects—CYP2D6, CYP3A4 inducers

Decrease: action of anticholinergics

Increase: QT prolongation—dofetilide, dronedarone, grepafloxacin, mesoridazine, pimozide, probucol, sparfloxacin, ziprasidone; do not use concurrently

Decrease: donepezil effect—carBAMazepine, dexamethasone, phenytoin, PHENobarbital, rifampin

Drug/Herb

Decrease: donepezil—St. John's wort

Drug/Lab

Increase: CK

NURSING CONSIDERATIONS

Assess:

• **Alzheimer's disease:** ADLs, memory, language, confusion baseline and during treatment

• B/P: hypo/hypertension, heart rate, ECG, QT

• Mental status: affect, mood, behavioral changes, depression, complete neurologic status

• GI status: nausea, vomiting, anorexia, diarrhea; monitor weight, active/occult GI bleeding

• GU status: urinary frequency, incontinence, I&O

• **Beers:** avoid use in older adults; increases risk of hypotension/bradycardia

---

Side effects: *italics* = common; red = life-threatening

• **Pregnancy/breastfeeding:** no well-controlled studies; use only if benefit outweighs fetal risk; avoid breastfeeding, excretion is unknown

Evaluate:

• Therapeutic response: decrease in confusion, improved mood, memory

Teach patient/family:

• To report side effects: twitching, nausea, vomiting, sweating, dizziness; indicates cholinergic crisis or overdose

• That continuing follow-up will be needed

• To use product exactly as prescribed, not to use with other products unless approved by prescriber

• To notify prescriber of nausea, vomiting, diarrhea (dose increase or beginning treatment), or rash

• Not to increase or abruptly decrease dose; serious side effects may result

• That product is not a cure, relieves symptoms

• To report if pregnancy is planned or suspected; to avoid breastfeeding

---

⚠ HIGH ALERT

DOPamine (Rx)

(dope' a-meen)

Func. class.: Adrenergic
Chem. class.: Catecholamine

Do not confuse:
DOPamine/DOBUTamine

ACTION: Causes increased cardiac output; acts on β_1- and α-receptors, causing vasoconstriction in blood vessels; low dose causes renal and mesenteric vasodilation; β_1 stimulation produces inotropic effects with increased cardiac output

USES: Shock, increased perfusion, hypotension, cardiogenic/septic shock

Unlabeled uses: Bradycardia, cardiac arrest, CPR, acute renal failure, cirrhosis, barbiturate intoxication

CONTRAINDICATIONS: Hypersensitivity, ventricular fibrillation, tachy-dysrhythmias, pheochromocytoma, hypovolemia

Precautions: Pregnancy, breastfeeding, geriatric patients, arterial embolism, peripheral vascular disease, sulfite hypersensitivity, acute MI

Black Box Warning: Extravasation

DOSAGE AND ROUTES

• **Adult:** IV INFUSION 2-5 mcg/kg/min, titrate upward in 5-10 mcg/kg/min increments, max 50 mcg/kg/min; titrate to patient's response

• **Child:** IV 1-5 mcg/kg/min initially; usual dosage range, 2-20 mcg/kg/min

HF

• **Adult:** IV 3-10 mcg/kg/min

Bradycardia (unlabeled)

• **Adult:** IV 2-10 mcg/kg/min, titrate as needed

Available forms: Inj 40 mg, 80 mg, 160 mg/mL; concentrations for IV infusion 0.8, 1.6, 3.2 mg/mL in 250, 500 mL D_5W

Administer:

• Correct volume depletion before use

• Store reconstituted sol for up to 24 hr if refrigerated

• Do not use discolored sol; protect from light

IV route

• IV after diluting 200-400 mg/250-500 mL of D_5W, $D_5$0.45%NaCl, $D_5$0.9%NaCl, D_5LR, LR; use large vein

• After reconstituting, use infusion pump; give at rate of 0.5-5 mcg/kg/min, increase by 1-4 mcg/kg/min at 10-30 min intervals until desired response, titrate as needed, decrease infusion gradually

---

Black Box Warning: Extravasation: if extravasation occurs, stop infusion; may inject area with phentolamine 10 mg/15 mL of NS

Y-site compatibilities: Alfentanil, alprostadil, amifostine, amikacin, aminocaproic acid, aminophylline, amiodarone, anidulafungin, argatroban, ascorbic acid injection, atenolol, atracurium, atropine, aztreonam, benztropine, bivalirudin, bleomycin, bumetanide, buprenorphine, butorphanol,

---

calcium chloride/gluconate, CARBOplatin, caspofungin, cefmetazole, cefonicid, cefotaxime, cefoTEtan, cefOXitin, cefTAZidime, ceftizoxime, cefTRIAXone, cefuroxime, chlorproMAZINE, cimetidine, ciprofloxacin, cisatracurium, CISplatin, cladribine, clarithromycin, clindamycin, cloNIDine, codeine, cyanocobalamin, cyclophosphamide, cycloSPORINE, cytarabine, DACTINomycin, DAPTOmycin, dexamethasone, dexmedetomidine, digoxin, diltiazem, diphenhydrAMINE, DOBUTamine, DOCEtaxel, doripenem, doxacurium, DOXOrubicin, DOXOrubicin liposomal, doxycycline, droperidol, enalaprilat, ePHEDrine, EPINEPHrine, epirubicin, epoetin alfa, eptifibatide, ertapenem, erythromycin, esmolol, etoposide, famotidine, fenoldopam, fentaNYL, fluconazole, fludarabine, fluorouracil, folic acid, foscarnet, gatifloxacin, gemcitabine, gemtuzumab, gentamicin, glycopyrrolate, granisetron, heparin, hydrocortisone, HYDROmorphone, hydrOXYzine, IDArubicin, ifosfamide, imipenem-cilastatin, irinotecan, isoproterenol, ketorolac, labetalol, levofloxacin, lidocaine, linezolid, LORazepam, LR, magnesium sulfate, mannitol, mechlorethamine, meperidine, methicillin, methyldopate, methylPREDNISolone, metoclopramide, metoprolol, metroNIDAZOLE, micafungin, miconazole, midazolam, milrinone, minocycline, mitoXANtrone, morphine, multiple vitamins injection, mycophenolate, nafcillin, nalbuphine, naloxone, netilmicin, niCARdipine, nitroglycerin, nitroprusside, norepinephrine, octreotide, ondansetron, oxacillin, oxaliplatin, oxytocin, PACLitaxel, palonosetron, pamidronate, pancuronium, pantoprazole, papaverine, PEMEtrexed, penicillin G potassium/sodium, pentamidine, pentazocine, PENTobarbital, PHENobarbital, phenylephrine, phytonadione, piperacillin, piperacillin-tazobactam, polymyxin B, potassium chloride, procainamide, prochlorperazine, promethazine, propofol, propranolol, protamine, pyridoxine, quiNIDine, ranitidine, remifentanil, Ringer's, ritodrine, riTUXimab, rocuronium, sargramostim, sodium acetate, succinylcholine, SUFentanil, tacrolimus, temocillin, teniposide, theophylline, thiamine, thiotepa, ticarcillin, ticarcillin-clavulanate, tigecycline, tirofiban, TNA, tobramycin, tolazoline, TPN, trastuzumab, trimetaphan, urokinase, vancomycin, vasopressin, vecuronium, verapamil, vinCRIStine, vinorelbine, vitamin B complex/C, voriconazole, warfarin, zidovudine, zoledronic acid

SIDE EFFECTS
CNS: *Headache*, anxiety
CV: *Palpitations, angina*, wide QRS complex, peripheral vasoconstriction, hypotension
GI: *Nausea, vomiting, diarrhea*
INTEG: Necrosis, tissue sloughing with extravasation
RESP: Dyspnea

PHARMACOKINETICS
IV: Onset 5 min; duration <10 min; metabolized in liver, kidney, plasma; excreted in urine (metabolites); half-life 2 min

INTERACTIONS
• Do not use within 2 wk of MAOIs; hypertensive crisis may result
Increase: bradycardia, hypotension—phenytoin
Increase: dysrhythmias—general anesthetics
Increase: severe hypertension—ergots
Increase: B/P—oxytocics
Increase: pressor effect—tricyclics, MAOIs
Decrease: DOPamine action—β-/α-blockers
Drug/Lab Test
Increase: urinary catecholamine, serum glucose

NURSING CONSIDERATIONS
Assess:
• Hypovolemia; if present, correct first
• **Oxygenation/perfusion deficit:** check B/P, chest pain, dizziness, loss of consciousness
• **Heart failure:** S_3 gallop, dyspnea, neck venous distention, bibasilar crackles in patients with HF, cardiomyopathy, palpate peripheral pulses

---

Side effects: *italics* = common; red = life-threatening

• I&O ratio: if urine output decreases without decrease in B/P, product may need to be reduced
• **ECG** during administration continuously; if B/P increases, product should be decreased; PCWP, CVP during infusion
• B/P, pulse q5min
• Paresthesias and coldness of extremities; peripheral blood flow may decrease
• **Pregnancy/breastfeeding:** no well-controlled studies; use only if benefit outweighs fetal risk, may cause toxicity; avoid use in breastfeeding, excretion is unknown

Evaluate:
• Therapeutic response: increased B/P with stabilization; increased urine output

Teach patient/family:
• About the reason for product administration
• To report immediately chest pain, shortness of breath, numbness/tingling of extremities
• To report immediately pain, burning, redness at IV site

TREATMENT OF OVERDOSE: Discontinue IV, may give a short-acting α-adrenergic blocker

---

doravirine
(dor′a-vir′een)

Pifeltro

Func. class.: Antiviral
Chem. class.: Nonnucleoside reverse transcriptase inhibitor (NNRTI)

ACTION: Binds directly to a site on reverse transcriptase that is distinct from where NRTIs bind, causing disruption of the enzyme's active site, blocking RNA-dependent and DNA-dependent DNA polymerase

USES: Human immunodeficiency virus (HIV) infection in antiretroviral-naive adults in combination with other antiretrovirals

CONTRAINDICATIONS: Hypersensitivity

DOSAGE AND ROUTES
• **Adult: PO** 100 mg daily; when given with rifabutin 100 mg q12hr
Available forms: Tabs 100 mg

SIDE EFFECTS
CNS: Dizziness, malaise, headache, fatigue, nightmares, abnormal dreams, insomnia, depression, suicidal ideation
GI: Nausea, vomiting, diarrhea
INTEG: Rash
META: Hypertriglyceridemia, hypercholesterolemia, hyperbilirubinemia
MISC: Immune reconstitution syndrome

PHARMACOKINETICS
76% protein binding, metabolized by CYP3A4 enzymes, half-life 15 hr, peak 2 hr, high-fat meal increases exposure

INTERACTIONS
Decrease: doravirine effects—mitotane, enzalutamide, carbamazepine, oxcarbazepine, phenobarbital, phenytoin, rifampin, rifapentine; do not use together, a 4-wk cessation period is needed before using doravirine
Decrease: doravirine effects—efavirenz, etravirine, nevirapine; concurrent use is not recommended

Drug/Herb
Decrease: doravirine effects—St. John's wort; do not use together, a 4-wk cessation period is needed before using doravirine

NURSING CONSIDERATIONS
Assess:
• **HIV:** symptoms of HIV, either increasing or lessening
• **Suicidal ideation:** assess for depression, suicidal thought, behaviors; monitor mental status frequently for mood, orientation, behavior, abnormal dreams
• Monitor bilirubin, blood glucose, CBC with differential, CD4+ T cell count, hepatitis B serology, LFTs, plasma hepatitis C RNA, plasma HIV

RNA, pregnancy testing, serum bilirubin (total and direct), serum cholesterol, serum creatinine, serum lipid profile, urinalysis

• **Immune reconstitution syndrome:** assess for this condition in patients treated with combination antiretroviral therapy; monitor for inflammatory response to opportunistic infections (progressive multifocal leukoencephalopathy [PML], *Mycobacterium avium* complex [MAC], cytomegalovirus [CMV], *Pneumocystis* pneumonia, or tuberculosis)

Evaluate:

• Therapeutic response: decreased viral load and improving CD4 counts; decreased symptoms of HIV

Teach patient/family

• To take only as prescribed, not to double or skip doses, not to stop taking unless discussed with prescriber, not to share with others; to read the "patient information" sheet

• That regular exams and blood work will be needed

• **Pregnancy/breastfeeding:** to report whether pregnancy is planned or suspected, or if breastfeeding; to avoid breastfeeding; to register with the Antiretroviral Pregnancy Registry at 1-800-258-4263 if pregnant and using this product

• To notify health care provider of all OTC, Rx, herbal, or supplement products taken; not to change products without discussing with prescriber

• That this product does not cure HIV, but controls the symptoms; that product does not prevent transmission to others through sexual contact, sharing needles, or blood contamination; to use a condom during sexual contact; not to share needles or donate blood

• **Suicidal thoughts/behaviors:** to report immediately depression, thought of suicide, hopelessness

doravirine/lamivudine/tenofovir

(dor' a-vir' een lam-i-voo'deen ten-oh-foh'veer)

Delstrigo

Func. class.: Antiretroviral

Chem. class.: Nonnucleoside reverse transcriptase inhibitor (NNRTI), nucleoside reverse transcriptase inhibitor (NRTI)

ACTION: Doravirine is a nonnucleoside reverse transcriptase inhibitor (NNRTI), lamivudine is a nucleoside reverse transcriptase inhibitor (NRTI), and tenofovir is a nucleotide reverse transcriptase inhibitor. Combination therapy targets different points in the life cycle of HIV, reducing viral capacity to mutate to drug-resistant strains

USES: Human immunodeficiency virus (HIV) infection in antiretroviral-naive adults

CONTRAINDICATIONS: Hypersensitivity

Precautions: Alcoholism, autoimmune disorders, bipolar disease, breastfeeding, children, depression, driving or operating hazardous machinery, geriatric patients, Graves' disease, Guillain-Barré syndrome, hepatic disease, hepatitis B and HIV coinfection, hepatitis C and HIV coinfection, HIV resistance, immune reconstitution syndrome, pregnancy, psychosis, substance abuse

Black Box Warning: Hepatitis B exacerbation

DOSAGE AND ROUTES

• **Adult:** PO 1 tablet (doravirine 100 mg; lamivudine 300 mg; tenofovir disoproxil fumarate 300 mg) daily

Concurrent treatment with rifabutin

• **Adult:** PO 1 tablet (doravirine 100 mg; lamivudine 300 mg; tenofovir disoproxil fumarate 300 mg) daily, then 12 hr later, give an additional 100 mg of doravirine by mouth each day of rifabutin concurrent therapy

Available forms: Tabs 100 mg-300 mg

SIDE EFFECTS

CNS: Dizziness, malaise, headache, fatigue, nightmares, abnormal dreams, insomnia, depression, suicidal ideation
GI: Nausea, vomiting, diarrhea
INTEG: Rash
META: Hypertriglyceridemia, hypercholesterolemia, hyperbilirubinemia
MISC: Immune reconstitution syndrome

PHARMACOKINETICS

Doravirine: protein binding 76%, extensive metabolism in the liver by CYP3A enzymes, 6% excreted in the urine unchanged, half-life 15 hr
Lamivudine: protein binding <36%, minimally metabolized, 71% eliminated unchanged in urine by glomerular filtration and active organic cationic secretion, half-life 5-7 hr
Tenofovir: protein binding negligible, intracellularly undergoes phosphorylation to an active metabolite, tenofovir diphosphate (PMPApp), half-life 17 hr, 70%-80% excreted unchanged in urine, eliminated by glomerular filtration and active renal tubular secretion; affected isoenzymes and transporters: CYP3A, P-gp, BRCP

INTERACTIONS

• **Decrease:** doravirine combination product effects—mitotane, enzalutamide, carbamazepine, oxcarbazepine, phenobarbital, phenytoin, rifampin, rifapentine; do not use together; a 4-wk cessation period is needed before using doravirine
• **Decrease:** doravirine combination product effects—efavirenz, etravirine, nevirapine; concurrent use is not recommended

Drug/Herb
• **Decrease:** doravirine combination product effects—St. John's wort; do not use together; a 4-wk cessation period is needed before using doravirine

NURSING CONSIDERATIONS
Assess
• **HIV:** symptoms of HIV, either increasing or lessening
• **Suicidal ideation:** assess for depression, suicidal thought, behaviors; monitor mental status frequently for mood, orientation, behavior, abnormal dreams
• Monitor blood glucose, CBC with differential, CD4+ T-cell count, hepatitis B serology, LFTs, plasma hepatitis C RNA, plasma HIV RNA, pregnancy testing, serum bilirubin (total and direct), serum cholesterol, serum creatinine, serum lipid profile, urinalysis
• **Immune reconstitution syndrome:** assess for this condition in patients treated with combination antiretroviral therapy; monitor for inflammatory response to opportunistic infections (progressive multifocal leukoencephalopathy [PML], *Mycobacterium avium* complex [MAC], cytomegalovirus [CMV], *Pneumocystis* pneumonia, or tuberculosis)

> **Black Box Warning: Hepatitis B exacerbation:** monitor hepatic studies, AST/ALT, bilirubin; amylase, lipase, triglycerides periodically during treatment

Evaluate:
• Therapeutic response: decreased viral load and improving CD4 counts; decreased symptoms of HIV

Teach patient/family
• To take only as prescribed, not to double or skip doses, not to stop taking unless discussed with prescriber, not to share with others; to read the "patient information" sheet
• That regular exams and blood work will be needed
• **Pregnancy/breastfeeding:** to report if pregnancy is planned or suspected or if breastfeeding; the patient should avoid breastfeeding; register patient with Antiretroviral Pregnancy Registry at 1-800-258-4263 if pregnant and using this product
• To notify health care providers of all products taken, OTC, Rx, herbals, sup-

plements; not to change products without discussing with prescribers

• That this product does not cure HIV, but controls the symptoms, does not prevent transmission to others through sexual contact, sharing needles or blood contamination; to use a condom during sexual contact, not to share needles or donate blood

• **Suicidal thoughts/behaviors:** to report immediately depression, thought of suicide; hopelessness

doripenem (Rx)

(dore-i-pen′em)

Doribax

Func. class.: Antiinfective—miscellaneous

Chem. class.: Carbapenem

Do not confuse:

Doribax/Zovirax

ACTION: Bactericidal; interferes with cell-wall replication of susceptible organisms; osmotically unstable cell-wall swells, bursts from osmotic pressure

USES: Serious infections caused by *Acinetobacter baumannii, Bacteroides caccae, Bacteroides fragilis, Bacteroides thetaiotaomicron, Bacteroides uniformis, Bacteroides vulgatus, Citrobacter freundii, Escherichia coli, Klebsiella pneumoniae, Peptostreptococcus micros, Proteus mirabilis, Pseudomonas aeruginosa, Serratia marcescens, Staphylococcus aureus, Streptococcus constellatus, Streptococcus intermedius*; complicated urinary tract infections, pyelonephritis, complicated intraabdominal infections

CONTRAINDICATIONS: Hypersensitivity to carbapenems (meropenem, doripenem, imipenem), penicillin, β-lactam; viral infection

Precautions: Pregnancy, breastfeeding, geriatric patients, renal disease, seizure disorder, pseudomembranous colitis, nebulizer or inhalation use, hypersensitivity to cephalosporins, children/adolescents

DOSAGE AND ROUTES

• **Adult:** IV 500 mg q8hr × 5-14 days; if improvement occurs after 3 days, switch to appropriate oral product

Renal dose

• **Adult:** IV CCr 30-50 mL/min, 250 mg over 1 hr, q8hr; CCr >10 to <30 mL/min, 250 mg over 1 hr q12hr; CCr ≤10 mL/min, no data

Available forms: Powder for inj 250, 500 mg

Administer:

IV route

• Visually inspect parenteral products for particulate matter and discoloration before use, diluted range in color from clear, colorless solutions to solutions that are clear and slightly yellow

• **Reconstitution:** no bacteriostatic preservative is present; observe aseptic technique while preparing the infusion

• **500-mg dose using the 500-mg vial:** reconstitute the vial with 10 mL of sterile water for injection or sodium chloride 0.9% (normal saline); gently shake (50 mg/mL); *the reconstituted suspension is not for direct injection; further dilution is required;* using a syringe with a 21-G needle, withdraw the suspension and add it to an infusion bag containing 100 mL of NS or D$_5$W; gently shake until clear; final concentration: 4.5 mg/mL

• **250-mg dose using the 500-mg vial:** reconstitute the vial with 10 mL of sterile water for injection or sodium chloride 0.9% (normal saline); gently shake (50 mg/mL); *the reconstituted suspension is not for direct injection; further dilution is required;* using a syringe with a 21-G needle, withdraw 5 mL (250 mg) and add it to an infusion bag containing 100 mL of normal saline or D$_5$W; gently shake until clear; remove 55 mL of this solution and discard; the remaining infusion sol contains 250 mg (4.5 mg/mL)

• **250-mg dose using the 250-mg vial:** reconstitute the vial with 10 mL of sterile water for injection or sodium chloride 0.9% (normal saline); gently shake (25 mg/mL); *the reconstituted suspension is not for direct injection; further dilution is required;* using a syringe with a 21-G needle, withdraw the contents of the vial and add it to an infusion bag containing 50 or 100 mL of normal saline or D₅W; gently shake until clear; final concentrations 4.2 mg/mL (50-mL infusion bag) or 2.3 mg/mL (100-mL infusion bag)

• **Storage:** reconstituted suspensions may be held in vial for up to 1 hr before transfer and dilution in the infusion bag; including storage and infusion time, diluted infusion sols are stable for up to 12 hr (NS) or 4 hr (D₅W) at controlled room temperature; diluted infusion sols are stable for up to 72 hr (NS) or 24 hr (D₅W) refrigerated; do not freeze reconstituted solutions

• If Baxter Minibag Plus infusion bags are to be used, consult the instructions provided by the infusion bag manufacturer

Intermittent IV INFUSION route

• After C&S is taken

• Do not mix with or physically add to solutions containing other drugs; infuse over 1 hr

Y-site compatibilities: Acyclovir, amikacin, aminophylline, amiodarone, anidulafungin, atropine, azithromycin, bumetanide, calcium gluconate, CARBOplatin, caspofungin, ceftaroline, ceftobiprole, cimetidine, ciprofloxacin, CISplatin, cyclophosphamide, cycloSPORINE, DAPTOmycin, dexamethasone, digoxin, diltiazem, diphenhydrAMINE, DOBUTamine, DOCEtaxel, DOPamine, DOXOrubicin, enalaprilat, esmolol, esomeprazole, etoposide, famotidine, fentaNYL, fluconazole, fluorouracil, foscarnet, furosemide, gemcitabine, gentamicin, granisetron, heparin, hydrocortisone, HYDROmorphone, ifosfamide, insulin (regular), labetalol, levofloxacin, linezolid, LORazepam, magnesium sulfate, mannitol, meperidine, methotrexate, methylPREDNISolone, metoclopramide, metroNIDAZOLE, micafungin, midazolam, milrinone, morphine, moxifloxacin, norepinephrine, ondansetron, PACLitaxel, pantoprazole, PHENobarbital, phenylephrine, potassium chloride, ranitidine, sodium bicarbonate/

phosphates, tacrolimus, telavancin, tigecycline, tobramycin, vancomycin, voriconazole, zidovudine

Solution compatibilities: D₅W, 0.9% NaCl, sterile water for inj

SIDE EFFECTS

CNS: Seizures, headache

GI: *Diarrhea, nausea,* vomiting, pseudomembranous colitis, hepatitis

GU: Renal impairments/failure

HEMA: Neutropenia, leukopenia, anemia

INTEG: *Rash,* urticaria, phlebitis, erythema at inj site, Stevens-Johnson syndrome, toxic epidermal necrolysis, pruritus

RESP: Pneumonitis (inhalation)

SYST: Anaphylaxis, Stevens-Johnson syndrome, toxic epidermal necrolysis

PHARMACOKINETICS

IV: Distributed to most body fluids/tissue, excreted mainly unchanged in urine, 70% recovered in 48 hr, half-life 1 hr, half-life extended in renal disease

INTERACTIONS

Increase: doripenem plasma levels—probenecid

Decrease: effect of valproic acid, divalproex sodium

Drug/Lab Test

Increase: AST, ALT, LDH, BUN, alk phos, bilirubin, creatinine

False positive: direct Coombs' test

NURSING CONSIDERATIONS

Assess:

• For sensitivity to carbapenem antibiotics, penicillins, cephalosporins, other beta lactams

• Renal disease: lower dose may be required

• **Pseudomembranous colitis:** bowel pattern daily, diarrhea, abdominal cramps, fever; if severe diarrhea occurs, product should be discontinued

• **Infection:** temperature; sputum; characteristics of wound before, during, and after treatment

• **Allergic reactions, anaphylaxis:** rash, urticaria, pruritus; may occur a few days after therapy begins; discontinue,

notify prescriber, have emergency equipment nearby
• **Overgrowth of infection:** perineal itching, fever, malaise, redness, pain, swelling, drainage, rash, diarrhea, change in cough, sputum
• **Pregnancy/breastfeeding:** use only if clearly needed, likely safe in breastfeeding

Evaluate:
• Therapeutic response: negative C&S; absence of symptoms and signs of infection

Teach patient/family:
• To report severe diarrhea with abdominal cramping, fever; may indicate pseudomembranous colitis
• To report sore throat, bruising, bleeding, joint pain; may indicate blood dyscrasias (rare)
• To report overgrowth of infection: black, furry tongue; vaginal itching; foul-smelling stools
• That product is probably safe in breastfeeding

TREATMENT OF HYPERSENSITIVITY: EPINEPHrine, antihistamines; resuscitate if needed (anaphylaxis)

---

dorzolamide (ophthalmic)

(dor-zole'ah-mide)

Trusopt

Func. class.: Antiglaucoma
Chem. class.: Carbonic anhydrase inhibitor

ACTION: Decreases aqueous humor secretion by decreasing bicarbonate, thus decreasing IOP

USES: For the treatment of elevated intraocular pressure in patients with ocular hypertension or open-angle glaucoma

CONTRAINDICATIONS: Hypersensitivity

Precautions: Hypersensitivity to sulfonamides, hepatic/renal disease, angle-closure glaucoma, electrolyte disturbances

DOSAGE AND ROUTES
• **Adult/adolescent/child/infant/neonate ≥1 wk: Ophthalmic** Instill 1 drop of a 2% solution into the affected eye(s) tid
Available forms: Ophthalmic solution 2%

Administer:
• Wash hands before and after use, tilt the head back slightly and pull the lower eyelid down with the index finger to form a pouch, squeeze the prescribed number of drops into the pouch and gently close eyes for 1-2 min; do not blink
• Care should be taken to avoid contamination; do not touch the tip of the dropper to the eye, fingertips, or other surface
• The sol may be used concomitantly with other topical ophthalmic drug products to lower IOP; if more than one topical ophthalmic drug is being used, administer ≥10 min apart

SIDE EFFECTS
CNS: Headache
EENT: Blurred vision, tearing, allergy, burning/stinging, photophobia
GI: Bitter taste

PHARMACOKINETICS
Onset 1-2 hr, peak 3 hr, duration 8 hr, half-life 4 mo

INTERACTIONS
Increase: effects—carbonic anhydrase inhibitors (PO)

NURSING CONSIDERATIONS
Assess:
• Hypersensitivity
• Monitor IOP during treatment

Evaluate:
• Decreasing IOP

Teach patient/family:
• How to use product
• Not to share with others or use for other conditions
• To notify prescriber immediately if vision changes or if condition worsens
• To take as prescribed

---

doxazosin (Rx)

(dox-ay′zoe-sin)

Cardura, Cardura XL

Func. class.: Peripheral α$_1$-adrenergic receptor blocker

Chem. class.: Quinazoline

Do not confuse:

Cardura/Coumadin/Cardene/Ridaura

ACTION: Dilates peripheral blood vessels, lowers peripheral resistance; reduction in B/P results from peripheral α$_1$-adrenergic receptors being blocked

USES: Hypertension, urinary outflow obstruction, symptoms of benign prostatic hyperplasia

CONTRAINDICATIONS: Hypersensitivity to quinazolines

Precautions: Pregnancy, breastfeeding, children, hepatic disease, geriatric patients

DOSAGE AND ROUTES
BPH

• **Adult: PO** 1 mg/day at bedtime; increase in stepwise manner to 2, 4, 8 mg/day as needed at 1-2 wk intervals, max 8 mg; ext rel tab (Cardura XL) 4 mg daily with breakfast, adjust dose q3-4wk, up to 8 mg daily

Hypertension

• **Adult: PO** 1 mg/day at bedtime, increasing gradually up to 16 mg/day if required; usual range 4-16 mg/day

• **Geriatric: PO** 0.5 mg nightly, gradually increase

Available forms: Tabs 1, 2, 4, 8 mg; ext rel tabs 4, 8 mg

Administer:

• Store in tight container at room temperature

• **Tabs:** may be broken, crushed, or chewed; if chewed, will be bitter; do not break, crush, chew XL tabs

• **Immediate release tab:** without regard to meals; **ext rel tabs:** give with breakfast; when switching from immediate release to ext rel, the final evening dose of immediate release should not be taken

SIDE EFFECTS

CNS: *Dizziness, headache,* drowsiness, anxiety, depression, *vertigo,* weakness, fatigue

CV: Palpitations, *orthostatic hypotension,* tachycardia, *edema,* dysrhythmias, chest pain

EENT: Epistaxis, tinnitus, dry mouth, red sclera, pharyngitis, rhinitis, blurred vision

GI: *Nausea,* vomiting, diarrhea, constipation, abdominal pain, hepatitis

GU: Priapism, impotence, decreased libido

RESP: Dyspnea

PHARMACOKINETICS

PO: Onset 2 hr, peak 2-3 hr, duration up to 24 hr, half-life 22 hr, metabolized in liver, excreted via bile/feces (<63%) and in urine (9%), extensively protein bound (98%)

INTERACTIONS

Increase: hypotensive effects—alcohol, other antihypertensives, nitrates, PDE-5 inhibitors

Decrease: hypotensive effects—NSAIDs, estrogens, sympathomimetics

NURSING CONSIDERATIONS
Assess:

• **Hypertension:** B/P (lying, standing), pulse 2-6 hr after each dose, with each increase; postural effects may occur, crackles, dyspnea, orthopnea with increased B/P; increased pulse; jugular venous distention during beginning treatment

• **BPH:** urinary pattern changes (hesitancy, dribbling, incomplete bladder emptying, dysuria, urgency, nocturia, urgency incontinence, intermittency) before and during treatment

• I&O, weight daily; edema in feet, legs daily

• **Pregnancy/breastfeeding:** no well-controlled studies; use only if clearly needed; use caution in breastfeeding

Evaluate:

• Therapeutic response: decreased B/P; decreased symptoms of BPH

Teach patient/family:

• That fainting occasionally occurs after 1st dose; not to drive, operate machinery

---

for 4 hr after 1st dose, after dosage increase; to take 1st dose at bedtime; may take 1-2 wk to respond with BPH
• To rise slowly from sitting position
• To comply with hypertension regimen: low-sodium diet, exercise, weight reduction, stress management; not to smoke
• How to take B/P, to check at least once/wk
• For male to notify prescriber of erection >4 hr or priapism
• To notify all health care providers of all Rx and OTC medications and herbal supplements; not to add any products unless approved by prescriber
• To avoid hazardous activities until response is known; dizziness or drowsiness may occur
• To continue to take product even if feeling better; to take at same time each day, not to double doses

TREATMENT OF OVERDOSE:
Administer volume expanders or vasopressors; discontinue product; place patient in supine position

---

⚠ HIGH ALERT

doxepin (Rx)
(dox′e-pin)
Prudoxin Cream, Silenor, Zonalon Topical Cream, Sinequan ✿
Func. class.: Antidepressant, tricyclic, antihistamine (topical)
Chem. class.: Dibenzoxepine, tertiary amine

Do not confuse:
Sinequan/Seroquel/Saquinavir/Singulair/Zonegran

ACTION: Blocks reuptake of norepinephrine, serotonin into nerve endings, increasing action of norepinephrine, serotonin in nerve cells

USES: Major depression, anxiety; *topical:* lichen simplex, atopic dermatitis, eczema, insomnia, migraine prophylaxis
Unlabeled uses: Topical pruritus

CONTRAINDICATIONS: Hypersensitivity to tricyclics, urinary retention, closed-angle glaucoma, prostatic hypertrophy, acute recovery from MI
Precautions: Pregnancy, breastfeeding, geriatric patients, seizures

Black Box Warning: Children, suicidal patients

D

DOSAGE AND ROUTES
Depression/anxiety
• **Adult: PO** 50-75 mg/day, may increase to 300 mg/day for severely ill; give in divided doses if >150 mg/day
• **Geriatric: PO** 25-50 mg at bedtime, increase weekly by 25-50 mg to desired dose, max 150 mg/day
Pruritus
• **Adult: PO** 10 mg at bedtime, may increase to 25 mg at bedtime; **TOP** apply thin film qid at least 3 hr apart
Insomnia (Silenor)
• **Adult: PO** 6 mg 30 min before bedtime, 3 mg may be sufficient, max 6 mg/night
Available forms: Caps 10, 25, 50, 75, 100, 150 mg; oral concentrations 10 mg/mL; cream 5%; tabs (Silenor) 3, 6 mg
Administer:
• **Oral concentrations:** should be diluted with 120 mL water, milk, or orange, grapefruit, tomato, prune, or pineapple juice; do not mix with grape juice
• Increased fluids, bulk in diet for constipation
• With food, milk for GI symptoms; do not give with carbonated beverages
• Dosage at bedtime to avoid oversedation during day; may take entire dose at bedtime; geriatric patients may not tolerate daily dosing
• Gum, hard candy, or frequent sips of water for dry mouth
• Store in tight container protected from direct sunlight
• **Topical:** by applying to affected area, rub slightly; do not use occlusive dressings

SIDE EFFECTS
CNS: *Dizziness, drowsiness,* confusion, headache, anxiety, tremors, stimulation, weakness, insomnia, nightmares, EPS

Side effects: *italics* = common; red = life-threatening

(geriatric patients), increased psychiatric symptoms, paresthesia, suicidal ideation

CV: *Orthostatic hypotension, ECG changes, tachycardia,* hypertension, palpitations, dysrhythmias

EENT: *Blurred vision,* tinnitus, mydriasis, ophthalmoplegia, glossitis

GI: *Diarrhea, dry mouth,* nausea, vomiting, paralytic ileus, increased appetite, cramps, epigastric distress, jaundice, hepatitis, stomatitis, constipation

GU: *Urinary retention,* acute renal failure

HEMA: Agranulocytosis, thrombocytopenia, eosinophilia, leukopenia, pancytopenia, purpuric disorder

INTEG: Rash, urticaria, sweating, pruritus, photosensitivity

PHARMACOKINETICS

PO: Peak 2 hr, metabolized in liver by CYP2C19/CYP2D6, which exert genetic polymorphism; Asians, black patients may be poor metabolizers; excreted by kidneys, crosses placenta, excreted in breast milk, half-life 8-24 hr

INTERACTIONS

Increase: hyperpyretic crisis, seizures, hypertensive episode—MAOIs

Increase: hypertensive action—EPINEPHRine, norepinephrine

Increase: hypertensive crisis—cloNIDine; do not use together

Increase: doxepin effect—cimetidine, FLUoxetine, fluvoxaMINE, PARoxetine, sertraline

Increase: CNS depression—barbiturates, benzodiazepines, sedative/hypnotics, alcohol, other CNS depressants

Increase: QT interval—class IC/III antiarrhythmics (propafenone, flecainide), quinolones

Increase: serotonin syndrome, toxicity—SSRIs, SNRIs, serotonin-receptor agonists, triptans

Increase: anticholinergic effects—anticholinergics

Drug/Herb

• **Serotonin syndrome:** St. John's wort; avoid using together

Drug/Lab Test

Increase: serum bilirubin, blood glucose, alk phos, LFTs

NURSING CONSIDERATIONS
Assess:

• B/P (lying, standing), pulse q4hr; if systolic B/P drops 20 mm Hg, hold product, notify prescriber; VS q4hr in patients with CV disease

• Blood studies: CBC, leukocytes, differential, cardiac enzymes if patient is receiving long-term therapy

• Hepatic studies: AST, ALT, bilirubin

• Weight weekly; appetite may increase with product

• **ECG** for flattening of T wave, bundle branch block, AV block, dysrhythmias in cardiac patients; product should be discontinued gradually several days before surgery

• **EPS** primarily in geriatric patients: rigidity, dystonia, akathisia

• **Depression:** mood, sensorium, affect, suicidal tendencies, increase in psychiatric symptoms; assess often during initial treatment; restrict the amount of the product given to the patient

• **Chronic pain:** location, severity, type before and during treatment, alleviating/aggravating factors

• **Sexual dysfunction:** decreased libido and erectile dysfunction may occur

• Urinary retention, constipation; constipation most likely in children, geriatric patients

• **Withdrawal symptoms:** headache, nausea, vomiting, muscle pain, weakness; not usual unless product is discontinued abruptly

• Alcohol consumption; if alcohol is consumed, hold dose until morning

• Assistance with ambulation during beginning therapy because drowsiness/dizziness occurs; safety measures primarily for geriatric patients

• **Serotonin syndrome:** nausea, vomiting, diarrhea, agitation, hallucinations, hyperthermia, incoordination; may occur when used with other products known to cause serotonin syndrome

• **Beers:** avoid use in older adults; highly anticholinergic, sedating; causes orthostatic hypotension, may cause delirium

- **Pregnancy/breastfeeding:** no well-controlled studies; use only if benefit outweighs fetal risk; use caution in breastfeeding, excreted in breast milk

Evaluate:
- Therapeutic response: decreased anxiety, depression

Teach patient/family:
- That therapeutic effect (depression) may take 2-3 wk, antianxiety effects sooner
- To use caution when driving, during other activities requiring alertness because of drowsiness, dizziness, blurred vision
- To avoid alcohol, other CNS depressants; may potentiate effects; not to take other products unless approved by prescriber
- Not to discontinue medication abruptly after long-term use; may cause nausea, headache, malaise
- To wear sunscreen or large hat; photosensitivity occurs
- That clinical worsening and suicide may occur, usually in children, young adults ≤24 yr
- To immediately report urinary retention

TREATMENT OF OVERDOSE:
ECG monitoring; lavage, administer anticonvulsant, sodium bicarbonate

---

⚠ HIGH ALERT

DOXOrubicin
(dox-oh-roo'bi-sin)
Adriamycin ✹, Caelyx ✹, Myocet ✹
Func. class.: Antineoplastic, antibiotic
Chem. class.: Anthracycline glycoside

Do not confuse:
DOXOrubicin/DOXOrubicin liposomal/DAUNOrubicin

ACTION: Inhibits DNA synthesis primarily; replication is decreased by binding to DNA, which causes strand splitting; active throughout entire cell cycle; a vesicant

USES: Wilms' tumor; bladder, breast, lung, ovarian, stomach, thyroid cancer; Hodgkin's/non-Hodgkin's disease; acute lymphoblastic leukemia; myeloblastic leukemia; neuroblastomas; soft tissue/bone sarcomas

CONTRAINDICATIONS: Pregnancy, breastfeeding, hypersensitivity, systemic infections, cardiac disorders, severe myelosuppression, lifetime dose of 550 mg/m², hepatic disease
Precautions: Accidental exposure, cardiac disease, dental work, electrolyte imbalance, infection, hyperuricemia

> **Black Box Warning:** Bone marrow suppression, extravasation, heart failure, secondary malignancy; requires an experienced clinician, IM/SUBCUT use

DOSAGE AND ROUTES
- **Adult: IV** 60-75 mg/m² every 3 wk, or 25-30 mg/m² q day × 2-3 days, repeat q3-4 wk or 20 mg/m²/wk, or may be used in combination with other antineoplastics with 40-75 mg/m² every 21-28 days, max cumulative dose 550 mg/m² or 450 mg/m² if prior DAUNOrubicin, cyclophosphamide, mediastinal XRT
- **Child: IV** 30 mg/m²/day × 3 days q4wk

Hepatic dose
- **Adult: IV** Bilirubin 1.2-3 mg/dL, give 50% of dose; bilirubin 3.1-5 mg/dL, give 25% of dose

Renal dose
- **Adult: IV** CCr <10 mL/min give 75% of dose

Available forms: Powder for inj 10, 20, 50 mg/vial; solution for injection 2 mg/mL

Administer:
IV route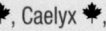
- Give antiemetic 30-60 min before product to prevent vomiting
- Give allopurinol or sodium bicarbonate to maintain uric acid levels, alkalization of urine
- Use cytotoxic handling procedures: inspect for particulate and discoloration before use

> **Black Box Warning:** Do not give IM, subcut

Side effects: *italics* = common; red = life-threatening

> **Black Box Warning:** If extravasation occurs, stop infusion and complete via another vein, preferably in another limb, use dexrazoxane topically

- Aluminum needles may be used during administration; avoid aluminum during storage
- Rapid injection can cause facial flushing or erythema along the vein

Reconstitution:

- To avoid risks with reconstitution, the commercially available injection may be used; there are still risks involved in handling the injection
- Do not use diluents containing preservatives to reconstitute powder for injection
- Reconstitute 10, 20, 50, 100 mg of DOXOrubicin with 5, 10, 25, 50 mL, respectively, of nonbacteriostatic NS injection (2 mg/mL), shake until completely dissolved; use reconstituted solution within 24 hr; do not expose to sunlight

- **IV injection**

Inject reconstituted solution over >3-5 min via Y-site or 3-way stopcock into a free-flowing IV infusion of NS or D$_5$W; a butterfly needle inserted into a large vein is preferred

- Increase fluid intake to 2-3 L/day to prevent urate, calculi formation
- Store at room temperature for 24 hr after reconstituting

Y-site compatibilities: Alemtuzumab, alfentanil, amifostine, amikacin, anidulafungin, argatroban, aztreonam, bivalirudin, bleomycin, bumetanide, buprenorphine, butorphanol, calcium chloride/gluconate, CARBOplatin, carmustine, caspofungin, ceftizoxime, chlorproMAZINE, cimetidine, ciprofloxacin, CISplatin, cladribine, clindamycin, cyclophosphamide, cycloSPORINE, cytarabine, DACTINomycin, DAPTOmycin, dexamethasone, diltiazem, diphenhydrAMINE, DOBUTamine, DOCEtaxel, dolasetron, DOPamine, doripenem, doxycycline, droperidol, enalaprilat, ePHEDrine, EPINEPHrine, erythromycin, esmolol, etoposide, etoposide phosphate, famotidine, fenoldopam, fentaNYL, filgrastim, fluconazole, fludarabine, gemcitabine, gentamicin, granisetron, haloperidol, hydrocortisone, HYDROmorphone, ifosfamide, imipenem cilastatin, inamrinone, isoproterenol, ketorolac, labetalol, leucovorin, levorphanol, lidocaine, linezolid, LORazepam, mannitol, mechlorethamine, melphalan, meperidine, mesna, methotrexate, metoclopramide, metoprolol, metroNIDAZOLE, midazolam, milrinone, mitoMYcin, morphine, nalbuphine, naloxone, nesiritide, niCARDipine, nitroglycerin, nitroprusside, octreotide, ofloxacin, ondansetron, oxaliplatin, PACLitaxel, palonosetron, pancuronium, phenylephrine, potassium chloride, procainamide, prochlorperazine, promethazine, propranolol, quinupristin-dalfopristin, ranitidine, sargramostim, sodium acetate, tacrolimus, teniposide, theophylline, thiotepa, ticarcillin/clavulanate, tigecycline, tirofiban, tobramycin, topotecan, trastuzumab, trimethobenzamide, vancomycin, vasopressin, vecuronium, verapamil, vinBLAStine, vinCRIStine, vinorelbine, zidovudine, zoledronic acid

SIDE EFFECTS

CV: Increased B/P, sinus tachycardia, PVCs, chest pain, bradycardia, extrasystoles, irreversible cardiomyopathy, acute left ventricular failure

GI: *Nausea, vomiting,* anorexia, *mucositis,* hepatotoxicity

GU: Impotence, sterility, amenorrhea, gynecomastia, hyperuricemia, urine discoloration

HEMA: Thrombocytopenia, leukopenia, anemia

RESP: Recall pneumonitis

INTEG: *Rash,* necrosis at inj site, dermatitis, reversible *alopecia,* cellulitis, thrombophlebitis at inj site, radiation recall

SYST: Anaphylaxis, secondary malignancy

PHARMACOKINETICS

Half-life 30 min, terminal 16.5 hr; metabolized by liver; crosses placenta; excreted in urine, bile, breast milk

INTERACTIONS

Increase: life-threatening dysrhythmias—posaconazole, fluconazole; do not use together

Increase: QT prolongation—other drugs that increase QT prolongation

Increase: neutropenia, thrombocytopenia—progesterone

Increase: cardiomyopathy—calcium-channel blockers

Increase: toxicity—other antineoplastics, cycloSPORINE, radiation, mercaptopurine

Increase: hemorrhagic cystitis risk, cardiac toxicity—cyclophosphamide

Increase: effect of phenytoin, fosphenytoin

Increase: DOXOrubicin effect—streptozocin

Decrease: DOXOrubicin effect—PHENobarbital

Decrease: antibody response—live virus vaccine

Decrease: clearance of DOXOrubicin—PACLitaxel

Drug/Lab Test

Increase: uric acid

NURSING CONSIDERATIONS
Assess:

Black Box Warning: **Bone marrow depression:** CBC, differential, platelet count weekly; withhold or reduce dose of product if WBC is <1500/mm^3 or platelet count is <50,000/mm^3; notify prescriber of these results

• **Renal studies:** BUN, serum uric acid, urine CCr, electrolytes before, during therapy
• **I&O ratio:** report fall in urine output to <30 mL/hr
• **Monitor temperature:** fever might indicate beginning infection
• **Hepatotoxicity:** hepatic studies before, during therapy: bilirubin, AST, ALT, alk phos as needed or monthly; check for jaundice of skin and sclera, dark urine, clay-colored stools, itchy skin, abdominal pain, fever, diarrhea

Black Box Warning: **Dysrhythmias:** ECG; watch for ST-T wave changes, low QRS and T, possible dysrhythmias (sinus tachycardia, heart block, PVCs), ejection fraction before treatment, signs of irreversible cardiomyopathy, can occur up to 6 mo after treatment begins

• Bleeding: hematuria, guaiac, bruising, petechiae of mucosa or orifices every 8 hr
• Effects of alopecia on body image; discuss feelings about body changes; almost total alopecia is expected
• Buccal cavity every 8 hr for dryness, sores, ulceration, white patches, oral pain, bleeding, dysphagia
• Alkalosis if severe vomiting is present

Black Box Warning: **Secondary malignancy:** assess for AML and MDS, which may occur

Black Box Warning: **Extravasation:** local irritation, pain, burning at inj site; a vesicant; if extravasation occurs, stop drug, restart at another site, apply ice, elevate extremity to reduce swelling; if resolution does not occur, surgical debridement may be required

• GI symptoms: frequency of stools, cramping
• Rinsing of mouth tid-qid with water, club soda; brushing of teeth bid-tid with soft brush or cotton-tipped applicators for stomatitis; use unwaxed dental floss

Evaluate:
• Therapeutic response: decreased tumor size, spread of malignancy

Teach patient/family:
• To add 2-3 L of fluids unless contraindicated before and for 24-48 hr after to decrease possible hemorrhagic cystitis
• To report any complaints, side effects to nurse or prescriber
• That hair may be lost during treatment; that wig or hairpiece might make patient feel better; that new hair might be different in color, texture

---

- That continuing follow-up and lab work will be needed
- To notify health care professional of trouble breathing, swelling of hands, feet, increase in weight, change in heart rate
- That body fluids should not be handled unless protective equipment is used
- To discuss OTC, Rx, herbals, supplements with health care professional
- To avoid foods with citric acid, hot temperature, or rough texture
- To report any bleeding, white spots, ulcerations in mouth to prescriber; to examine mouth daily
- That urine, other body fluids may be red-orange for 48 hr
- To avoid crowds and persons with infections when granulocyte count is low
- To avoid vaccinations
- **Pregnancy/breastfeeding:** that barrier contraceptive measures are recommended during therapy and for 4 mo after ending therapy; to avoid breastfeeding

---

⚠ HIGH ALERT

DOXOrubicin liposomal

(dox-oh-roo′bi-sin)

Doxil, Lipodox
Func. class.: Antineoplastic, antibiotic
Chem. class.: Anthracycline glycoside

Do not confuse:
DOXOrubicin/DOXOrubicin liposomal/ DAUNOrubicin

ACTION: Inhibits DNA synthesis primarily; replication is decreased by binding to DNA, which causes strand splitting; active throughout entire cell cycle; a vesicant

USES: AIDS-related Kaposi's sarcoma, multiple myeloma, metastatic ovarian carcinoma

CONTRAINDICATIONS: Pregnancy, breastfeeding, hypersensitivity
Precautions: Children, infection, leukopenia, stomatitis, thrombocytopenia, systemic infections, cardiac disorders

Black Box Warning: Cardiotoxicity, infusion reactions, myelosuppression, hepatic disease

DOSAGE AND ROUTES

Max lifetime cumulative dose 550 mg/m^2; 400 mg/m^2 for those who have received other cardiotoxics or mediastinal radiation
Kaposi's sarcoma
- **Adult: IV** 20 mg/m^2 every 3 wk
Multiple myeloma
- **Adult: IV** 30 mg/m^2 IV infusion on day 4 every 3 wk plus bortezomib 1.3 mg/m^2/ dose IV bolus on days 1, 4, 8, 11 of each cycle; give DOXOrubicin liposomal after bortezomib receipt on day 4; administer up to 8 treatment cycles or until disease progression or unacceptable toxicity occurs
Ovarian cancer
- **Adult: IV** 50 mg/m^2 q4wk
Hematologic toxicity in patients with ovarian cancer or HIV-related Kaposi's sarcoma
Grade 1 (ANC of 1500-1900/mm^3, platelets ≥75,000/mm^3): No dose reduction; **Grade 2 (ANC of 1000-1499/mm^3, platelets ≥50,000/mm^3 and <75,000/mm^3:** Wait until ANC ≥1500 cells/mm^3 and platelets ≥75,000 cells/mm^3; redose with no dose reduction; **Grade 3 (ANC of 500-999/mm^3, platelets ≥25,000/mm^3 and <50,000/mm^3):** Wait until ANC ≥1500 cells/mm^3 and platelets ≥75,000 cells/mm^3; redose with no dose reduction; **Grade 4 (ANC <500/mm^3, platelets <25,000/mm^3):** Wait until ANC ≥1500 cells/mm^3 and platelets ≥75,000 cells/mm^3; reduce dose by 25% or continue with full dose with colony-stimulating factor
Available forms: Liposomal dispersion for inj: 2 mg/mL
Administer:
- Prepared liposomal DOXOrubicin is a translucent, red liposomal dispersion; visually inspect for particulate matter and discoloration before use
- Pegylated liposomal DOXOrubicin (Doxil) is for IV INFUSION use only and should not be given IM/subcut; give under the supervision of a physician who is experienced in cancer chemotherapy

Black Box Warning: Care should be taken to avoid extravasation because the drug is irritating to extravascular tissue

• Premedication with antiemetics is recommended

IV route

• **Reconstitution (Doxil):** dilute the appropriate dose, not to exceed 90 mg/250 mL D$_5$W; do not mix with any other diluent, drugs, or bacteriostatic agent; use aseptic technique; product contains no preservative or bacteriostatic agent; diluted solution must be refrigerated and used within 24 hr

• **IV INFUSION (Doxil):** do not administer as a bolus injection or an undiluted solution; rapid injection can increase the risk of an infusion-related reaction

Black Box Warning: Care should be taken to avoid extravasation because the drug is irritating to extravascular tissue

• An acute infusion reaction can occur during the first infusion and is usually resolved by slowing the rate of infusion; most patients can tolerate subsequent infusion

• **Rate:** infuse at an initial rate of 1 mg/min; if no infusion-related action, the rate can be increased to complete the infusion over 1 hr; do not filter

• Give antiemetic 30-60 min before product to prevent vomiting

• Use allopurinol or sodium bicarbonate to maintain uric acid levels, alkalinization of urine

• Avoid mixing with other products

• Increase fluid intake to 2-3 L/day to prevent urate, calculi formation

• Store refrigerated for 24 hr after reconstituting

SIDE EFFECTS

CNS: Paresthesias, headache, depression, insomnia, fatigue, fever

CV: Chest pain, decreased B/P, cardiomyopathy, heart failure, dysrhythmias, tachycardia

EENT: Optic neuritis, rhinitis, pharyngitis, stomatitis

GI: *Nausea, vomiting,* anorexia, *mucositis,* hepatotoxicity, abdominal pain

HEMA: Thrombocytopenia, leukopenia, anemia, secondary malignancy

INTEG: *Rash,* necrosis at inj site, dermatitis, *reversible alopecia,* exfoliative dermatitis, palmar-plantar erythrodysesthesia, thrombophlebitis at inj site

RESP: Dyspnea, cough, respiratory infections

PHARMACOKINETICS

Half-life 55 hr; metabolized by liver; crosses placenta; excreted in urine, bile, breast milk

INTERACTIONS

Increase: life-threatening dysrhythmias—posaconazole, fluconazole; do not use together

Increase: QT prolongation—other drugs that increase QT prolongation

Increase: neutropenia, thrombocytopenia—progesterone

Increase: cardiomyopathy—calcium channel blockers

Increase: toxicity—other antineoplastics, cycloSPORINE, radiation, mercaptopurine

Increase: hemorrhagic cystitis risk, cardiac toxicity—cyclophosphamide

Increase: effect of—phenytoin, fosphenytoin

Increase: DOXOrubicin effect—streptozocin

Decrease: DOXOrubicin effect—PHENobarbital

Decrease: antibody response—live virus vaccine

Decrease: antineoplastic effect—hematopoietic progenitor cell; do not use 24 hr before or after treatment

Decrease: clearance of DOXOrubicin—PACLitaxel

Drug/Lab Test

Increase: uric acid

NURSING CONSIDERATIONS

Assess:

Black Box Warning: **Bone marrow depression:** CBC, differential, platelet count weekly; withhold product if WBC is <4000/mm^3 or platelet count is <75,000/mm^3; notify prescriber of these results

• Renal studies: BUN, serum uric acid, urine CCr, electrolytes before, during therapy
• I&O ratio: report fall in urine output to <30 mL/hr
• **Hepatotoxicity:** Hepatic studies before, during therapy: bilirubin, AST, ALT, alk phos as needed or monthly; check for jaundice of skin and sclera, dark urine, clay-colored stools, itchy skin, abdominal pain, fever, diarrhea

Black Box Warning: Dysrhythmias: ECG: watch for ST-T wave changes, low QRS and T, possible dysrhythmias (sinus tachycardia, heart block, PVCs), ejection fraction before treatment, signs of irreversible cardiomyopathy, can occur up to 6 mo after treatment begins

• Bleeding: hematuria, guaiac, bruising, petechiae of mucosa or orifices every 8 hr
• Effects of alopecia on body image; discuss feelings about body changes; almost total alopecia is expected
• Buccal cavity every 8 hr for dryness, sores, ulceration, white patches, oral pain, bleeding, dysphagia
• **Secondary malignancy:** assess for acute myelogenous leukemia and oral cancer

Black Box Warning: Extravasation: local irritation, pain, burning at inj site; a vesicant; if extravasation occurs, stop drug, restart at another site, apply ice, elevate extremity to reduce swelling; if resolution does not occur, surgical debridement may be required

• GI symptoms: frequency of stools, cramping
• Rinsing of mouth tid-qid with water, club soda; brushing of teeth bid-tid with soft brush or cotton-tipped applicators for stomatitis; use unwaxed dental floss
Evaluate:
• Therapeutic response: decreased tumor size, spread of malignancy

Teach patient/family:
• To add 2-3 L of fluids unless contraindicated before and for 24-48 hr after to decrease possible **hemorrhagic cystitis**
• To report any complaints, side effects to nurse or prescriber
• That hair may be lost during treatment; that wig or hairpiece might make patient feel better; that new hair may be different in color, texture
• To avoid foods with citric acid, hot temperature, or rough texture
• To report any bleeding, white spots, ulcerations in mouth to prescriber; to examine mouth daily
• That urine, other body fluids may be red-orange for 48 hr
• To avoid crowds and persons with infections when granulocyte count is low
• To avoid vaccinations because reactions can occur; to avoid alcohol
• **Pregnancy/breastfeeding:** that barrier contraceptive measures are recommended during therapy and for 4 mo after therapy ends; to avoid breastfeeding

doxycycline (Rx)

(dox-i-sye′kleen)
Acticlate ♥, Apprilon ♥, Atridox ♥, Adoxa, ♥, Doryx, Doxy, Doxycin ♥, Monodox, Oracea, Periostat, Vibramycin, Vibra-Tabs
Func. class.: Antiinfective
Chem. class.: Tetracycline

Do not confuse:
doxycycline/doxepin/dicyclomine

ACTION: Inhibits protein synthesis, phosphorylation in microorganisms by binding to 30S ribosomal subunits; bacteriostatic

USES: *Acinetobacter* sp., *Actinomyces israelii, Bacillus anthracis, Bacteroides* sp., *Balantidium coli, Bartonella bacilliformis, Borrelia recurrentis, Brucella* sp., *Campylobacter fetus, Chlamydia psittaci, Chlamydia trachomatis, Clostridium* sp., *Entamoeba histolytica, Enterobacter aerogenes, Enterococcus* sp., *Escherichia coli, Francisella tularensis, Fusobacterium fusiforme, Haemophilus ducreyi, Haemophilus influenzae* (beta-lactamase negative), *Haemophilus influenzae* (beta-lactamase positive), *Klebsiella granulomatis, Klebsiella* sp., *Leptospira* sp., *Listeria monocytogenes, Mycoplasma pneumoniae, Neisseria gonorrhoeae, Neisseria meningitidis, Orientia tsutsugamushi, Plasmodium falciparum, Propionibacterium acnes, Rickettsia akari, Rickettsia prowazekii, Rickettsia rickettsii, Shigella* sp., *Staphylococcus aureus* (MSSA), *Streptococcus pneumoniae, Streptococcus pyogenes* (group A beta-hemolytic streptococci), *Streptococcus* sp., *Treponema pallidum, Treponema pertenue, Ureaplasma urealyticum, Vibrio cholerae,* viridans streptococci, *Yersinia pestis;* syphilis, gonorrhea, lymphogranuloma venereum, uncommon gram-negative/gram-positive organisms, malaria prophylaxis

Unlabeled uses: Enterocolitis, biliary tract, intraabdominal infections; epididymitis *(Chlamydia trachomatis);* chronic prostatitis *(Ureaplasma urealyticum);* traveler's diarrhea (enterotoxigenic *Escherichia coli);* Legionnaire's disease *(Legionella pneumophila);* Lyme disease *(Borrelia burgdorferi),* Lyme disease (erythema migrans); Lyme arthritis; Lyme carditis; pleural effusion; malaria (chloroquine-resistant *Plasmodium falciparum);* pelvic inflammatory disease (PID), tubo-ovarian abscess in combination; acute dental infection, dentoalveolar infection, endodontic infection; aggressive juvenile periodontitis, plaque prophylaxis *(Yersinia pestis);* tularemia prophylaxis *(Francisella tularensis);* Bancroft's filariasis (elephantiasis) *(Wuchereria bancrofti);* melioidosis due to *Burkholderia pseudomallei;* leptospirosis *(Leptospira* sp); infection prophylaxis for gynecologic procedures/surgical infection prophylaxis hysterosalpingogram or chromotubation/induced abortion/dilation and evacuation; methicillin-resistant *Staphylococcus aureus* (MRSA)-associated bone and joint infections

CONTRAINDICATIONS: Pregnancy, children <8 yr, hypersensitivity to tetracyclines, esophageal ulceration
Precautions: Breastfeeding, hepatic disease, pseudomembranous colitis, ulcerative colitis, sulfite hypersensitivity, excessive sunlight

DOSAGE AND ROUTES
Most infections
• **Adult: PO/IV** 100 mg q12hr on day 1, then 100 mg/day; **IV** 200 mg in 1-2 infusions on day 1, then 100-200 mg/day
• **Child >8 yr, ≥45 kg: PO** 100 mg q12hr on day 1, then 100 mg daily; severe infections 100 mg q12hr; **IV** 200 mg on day 1, then 100-200 mg daily, give 200 mg dose as 1 or 2 infusions
• **Child >8 yr, ≤45 kg: PO** 2.2 mg/kg q12hr on day 1, then 2.2 mg/kg daily, severe infections 2.2 mg/kg q12hr; **IV** 4.4 mg/kg divided on day 1, then 2.2-4.4 mg/kg daily in 1 to 2 divided doses
Gonorrhea in patients allergic to penicillin
• **Adult: PO** 100 mg q12hr × 7 days or 300 mg followed 1 hr later by another 300 mg
Malaria prophylaxis
• **Adult: PO** 100 mg/day 1-2 days before travel, daily during travel, and for 4 wk after return
• **Adolescent/child ≥8 yr, <45 kg: PO** 2 mg/kg/day (up to 100 mg/day) begin 1-2 days before travel, continue for 4 wk after return
C. trachomatis
• **Adult: PO** 100 mg bid × 7 days
Syphilis (early)
• **Adult: PO** 100 mg bid × 14 days
Anthrax, postexposure
• **Adult and child >8 yr and ≥45 kg: IV** 100 mg q12hr; change to **PO** when able × 60 days
• **Adolescent/child ≥8 yr and <45 kg: PO** 2.2 mg/kg q12hr × 60 days; **IV** 100

mg q12hr, change to **PO** when able ×
60 days

Lyme disease

- **Adult/adolescent/child ≥8 yr: PO**
100 mg bid × 10-21 days

Periodontitis

- **Adult:** 20 mg bid after scaling and root
planing for ≤9 mo; give close to mealtime AM or PM

Pleural effusion (unlabeled)

- **Adult: INTRACAVITARY** 500 mg diluted with 250 mL 0.9% NaCl given by
chest tube lavage and drainage

Available forms: cap 40 mg; susp 50
mg/5 mL; cap 20, 50, 100 mg; del rel tabs
75, 100, 150 mg; del rel cap 75, 100 mg;
inj 42.5, 100, 200 mg; tabs 20, 100 mg;
caps 50, 100, 150 mg; tabs 50, 75, 100
mg; oral susp 25 mg/5 mL

Administer:

PO route

- Do not break, crush, or chew caps;
may crush tabs and mix with food
- On empty stomach or with full glass of
water 2 hr before or after meals; avoid
dairy products, antacids, laxatives, iron-
containing products; if these must be
taken, give 2 hr before or after product;
avoid giving oral products within 1 hr of
bedtime, esophageal ulceration may occur
- **Delayed-release cap:** Swallow whole
or open and sprinkle on applesauce
- **Susp:** Shake well, use calibrated device, may give with food/milk for GI irritation, store at room temperature, discard after 14 days

Intermittent IV INFUSION route

- After diluting 100 mg or less/10 mL or
200 mg/20 mL of sterile water or NS for
inj, each 100 mg must be further diluted
with 100-1000 mL of NaCl, D_5W, Ringer's, LR, D_5LR, Normosol-M, Normosol-R
in D_5W; run 100 mg or less over 1-4 hr;
infusion must be completed in 6 hr when
diluted in LR sol or 12 hr with other sol;
protect from light, heat
- Avoid rapid use, extravasation
- Store in tight, light-resistant container
at room temperature; IV stable for 12 hr
at room temperature, 72 hr refrigerated;
discard if precipitate forms

Y-site compatibilities: Acyclovir, alemtuzumab, alfentanil, amifostine, amikacin,
aminophylline, amiodarone, anidulafungin, ascorbic acid, atracurium, atropine,
aztreonam, bivalirudin, bumetanide,
buprenorphine, butorphanol, calcium
chloride/gluconate, CARBOplatin, caspofungin, cefonicid, cefotaxime, cefTRI-
AXone, chlorproMAZINE, cimetidine,
cisatracurium, CISplatin, clindamycin,
codeine, cyanocobalamin, cyclophosphamide, cycloSPORINE, cytarabine,
DACTINomycin, DAPTOmycin, dexmedetomidine, digoxin, diltiazem, diphenhydrAMINE, DOBUTamine, DOCEtaxel,
DOPamine, doxacurium, DOXOrubicin,
enalaprilat, ePHEDrine, EPINEPHrine,
epirubicin, epoetin alfa, eptifibatide,
ertapenem, esmolol, etoposide, etoposide phosphate, famotidine, fenoldopam,
fentaNYL, filgrastim, fluconazole, fludarabine, gemcitabine, gemtuzumab, gentamicin, glycopyrrolate, granisetron,
HYDROmorphone, IDArubicin, ifosfamide, imipenem/cilastatin, insulin, isoproterenol, labetalol, levofloxacin, lidocaine, linezolid, LORazepam, magnesium
sulfate, mannitol, mechlorethamine,
melphalan, meperidine, methyldopate,
metoclopramide, metoprolol, metro-
NIDAZOLE, miconazole, midazolam,
milrinone, mitoXANtrone, morphine,
multivitamins, nalbuphine, naloxone,
nesiritide, netilmicin, nitroglycerin,
nitroprusside, norepinephrine, octreotide, ondansetron, oxaliplatin, oxytocin,
PACLitaxel, pancuronium, pantoprazole,
papaverine, pentamidine, pentazocine,
perphenazine, phentolamine, phenylephrine, phytonadione, potassium chloride,
procainamide, prochlorperazine, promethazine, propofol, propranolol, protamine, pyridoxine, quinupristin/dalfo-
pristin, ranitidine, remifentanil,
ritodrine, riTUXimab, rocuronium, sargramostim, sodium acetate, succinylcholine,
SUFentanil, tacrolimus, telavancin, teniposide, theophylline, thiamine, thiotepa,
tirofiban, tobramycin, tolazoline, TPN (2 in
1), trastuzumab, trimetaphan, urokinase,
vancomycin, vasopressin, vecuronium,

verapamil, vinCRIStine, vinorelbine, voriconazole, zoledronic acid

SIDE EFFECTS

CNS: Fever, headache
CV: Pericarditis
EENT: Dysphagia, glossitis, decreased calcification of deciduous teeth, oral candidiasis, tooth discoloration
GI: *Nausea, abdominal pain, vomiting, diarrhea,* anorexia, enterocolitis, hepatotoxicity, flatulence, abdominal cramps, gastric burning, stomatitis
GU: *Increased BUN*
HEMA: Eosinophilia, neutropenia, thrombocytopenia, hemolytic anemia
INTEG: *Rash, urticaria, photosensitivity, increased pigmentation,* exfoliative dermatitis, pruritus, phlebitis, injection site reaction
MS: Bone growth retardation (<8 yr old), muscle, joint pain
RESP: Cough
SYST: Stevens-Johnson syndrome, angioedema, anaphylaxis, toxic epidermal necrolysis

PHARMACOKINETICS

PO: Well absorbed, widely distributed; peak $1\frac{1}{2}$-4 hr; half-life 1 day; excreted in urine, feces, bile; 90% protein bound; crosses placenta; enters breast milk

INTERACTIONS

Increase: effect of—anticoagulants, digoxin, methotrexate
Decrease: doxycycline effect—antacids, $NaHCO_3$, dairy products, alkali products, iron, kaolin/pectin, barbiturates, carBAMazepine, phenytoin, cimetidine sucralfate, cholestyramine, colestipol, rifampin, bismuth; iron, magnesium, zinc, calcium, aluminum salts, sevelamer
Decrease: effects—penicillins, oral contraceptives, digoxin

Drug/Lab Test
Increase: BUN, alk phos, bilirubin, amylase, ALT, AST, eosinophils, WBC
Decrease: Hgb
False increase: urinary catecholamines

NURSING CONSIDERATIONS
Assess:

doxylamine/pyridoxine   **439**

- I&O ratio
- Blood studies: PT, CBC, AST, ALT, BUN, creatinine
- Signs of infection
- **Allergic reactions:** rash, itching, pruritus, angioedema
- Nausea, vomiting, diarrhea; administer antiemetic, antacids as ordered
- **Overgrowth of infection:** fever, malaise, redness, pain, swelling, drainage, perineal itching, diarrhea, changes in cough or sputum
- IV site for phlebitis/thrombosis; product is highly irritating
- After C&S is obtained, do not wait for results
- **Pregnancy/breastfeeding:** no well-controlled studies; may affect skeletal development, do not use in 2nd half of pregnancy unless benefit outweighs fetal risk; discontinue breastfeeding or product, excreted in small amounts in breast milk

Evaluate:
- Therapeutic response: decreased temperature, absence of lesions, negative C&S

Teach patient/family:
- To avoid sun because burns may occur; that sunscreen does not seem to decrease photosensitivity
- That all prescribed medication must be taken to prevent superinfection; not to use outdated products because Fanconi syndrome may occur (reversible nephrotoxicity)
- That if children ≤8 yr old are undergoing tooth development, teeth may be permanently discolored
- Not to use with antacids, iron products, H_2 blockers, sevelamer, calcium (milk), magnesium, zinc
- To take with full glass of water; if nausea occurs, take with food

---

RARELY USED

doxylamine/pyridoxine
(docks-ill'ah-meen/peer-reh-dock'seen)
Diclegis
Func. class.: Antiemetic

Side effects: *italics* = common; red = life-threatening

USES: Nausea and vomiting of pregnancy in women who do not respond to other treatment

CONTRAINDICATIONS: Hypersensitivity

DOSAGE AND ROUTES

• **Adult pregnant females: PO** 2 tabs (on an empty stomach) at bedtime, on day 1; if dose controls symptoms the next day, continue regimen. If symptoms persist on the afternoon of day 2, continue 2 tabs at bedtime, then take 3 tabs starting on day 3 (1 tab in AM and 2 tabs at bedtime); if symptoms are controlled, continue regimen. If symptoms persist, on day 4, take 4 tabs (1 tab in AM, 1 tab midafternoon, and 2 tabs at bedtime); max 4 tabs/day. Use only as needed

---

⚠ HIGH ALERT

dronedarone (Rx)

(drone′da′rone)

Multaq

Func. class.: Antidysrhythmic (class III)

Chem. class.: Iodinated benzofuran derivative

ACTION: Prolongs duration of action potential and effective refractory period, noncompetitive α- and β-adrenergic inhibition; increases PR and QT intervals, decreases sinus rate, decreases peripheral vascular resistance

USES: Atrial fibrillation, atrial flutter

CONTRAINDICATIONS: Pregnancy, breastfeeding; 2nd-, 3rd-degree AV block; bradycardia, severe sinus node dysfunction, hypersensitivity, heart failure, hepatic disease, QT prolongation, aminodarone-induced lung/liver toxicity

Black Box Warning: NYHA Class IV heart failure or Class II-III with recent decompensation requiring hospitalization, permanent atrial fibrillation (cannot restore sinus rhythm)

Precautions: Children, geriatric patients, ✱☞ Asian patients, females, electrolyte imbalances, atrial fibrillation/flutter

DOSAGE AND ROUTES

• **Adult: PO** 400 mg bid; discontinue class I, III antidysrhythmics or strong CYP3A4 inhibitors before beginning treatment; max 800 mg/day

Available forms: Tabs 400 mg
Administer:
PO route
• Give bid with morning, evening meals
• Give MedGuide; should be dispensed with each prescription, refill

SIDE EFFECTS

CNS: Weakness
CV: *Bradycardia,* heart failure, QT prolongation, torsades de pointes, atrial flutter
GI: Nausea, vomiting, diarrhea, abdominal pain, severe hepatic injury, hepatic failure
INTEG: Rash, photosensitivity, anaphylaxis, angioedema
RESP: Interstitial pneumonitis, pulmonary fibrosis

PHARMACOKINETICS

Peak 3-6 hr, half-life 13-19 hr, metabolized by liver, by CYP3A excreted in feces (84%), via kidneys (6%), protein binding >98%

INTERACTIONS

Increase: dronedarone levels—CYP3A inhibitors/2D6 inhibitors
Decrease: dronedarone levels—3A/2D6 inducers
Increase: bradycardia—β-blockers, calcium channel blockers
Increase: levels of cycloSPORINE, dextromethorphan, digoxin, disopyramide, flecainide, methotrexate, phenytoin, procainamide, quiNIDine, theophylline
Increase: anticoagulant effects—dabigatran, warfarin

Drug/Herb

Increase: anticoagulant effect—yohimbine

Decrease: dronedarone effect—St. John's wort

Drug/Food:

Increase: dronedarone effect—grapefruit; avoid use

Drug/Lab Test

Increase: T4, creatinine, LFTs, bilirubin

Decrease: potassium, magnesium

NURSING CONSIDERATIONS
Assess:

Black Box Warning: NYHA Class IV heart failure or symptomatic heart failure with recent decomposition requiring hospitalization doubles risk of death

• **ECG** to determine product effectiveness; measure PR, QRS, QT intervals; check for PVCs, other dysrhythmias, B/P continuously for hypo/hypertension; report dysrhythmias, slowing heart rate

• Serum creatinine, potassium, magnesium

• I&O ratio; electrolytes (potassium, creatinine, magnesium)

• Dehydration or hypovolemia

• Rebound hypertension after 1-2 hr

• Cardiac rate; respiration: rate, rhythm, character; chest pain; start with patient hospitalized and monitored up to 1 wk

• **Pregnancy/breastfeeding:** do not use in pregnancy, breastfeeding

Evaluate:

• Therapeutic response: maintenance of normal heart rhythm following atrial fibrillation, flutter

Teach patient/family:

• To take this product as directed in AM, PM with meals; to avoid missed doses; not to use with grapefruit juice, to avoid all other products without approval of provider

• To immediately report weight gain, edema, difficulty breathing, fatigue, peripheral edema

• **Pregnancy/breastfeeding:** to use effective contraception during treatment; not to breastfeed

TREATMENT OF OVERDOSE: O_2, artificial ventilation, ECG, administer DOPamine for circulatory depression

---

droxidopa
(drox'-i-doe'-pa)
Northera
Func. class.: Cardiovascular agent-vasopressor

ACTION: A synthetic amino acid precursor of norepinephrine. It is used to increase blood pressure with symptomatic neurogenic orthostatic hypotension (NOH) caused by primary autonomic failure (e.g., Parkinson's disease, multiple system atrophy, and pure autonomic failure), dopamine β-hydroxylase deficiency, or nondiabetic autonomic neuropathy

USES: To increase blood pressure

CONTRAINDICATIONS: Hypersensitivity

Precautions: Angina, breastfeeding, cardiac arrhythmias, cardiac disease, children, coronary artery disease, heart disease, hyperthermia, infants, mental status changes, myocardial infarction, neonates, pregnancy, salicylate/tartrazine dye hypersensitivity

Black Box Warning: Supine hypertension

DOSAGE AND ROUTES
• **Adult: PO** 100 mg tid: upon arising in the morning, at midday, and in the late afternoon at least 3 hr before bedtime; titrate to response, by 100 mg tid q24-48hr up to a dose of 600 mg **PO** tid, max 1800 mg/day

Available forms: Caps 100, 200, 300 mg

Administer:

Black Box Warning: Give tid at the following times: upon arising in the morning, at midday, and in the late afternoon at least 3 hr before bedtime (to reduce the potential for supine hypertension during sleep)

• Use without regard to food, but should be taken consistently in regard to food to ensure consistent absorption
• Swallow capsules whole

SIDE EFFECTS

CNS: Headache, dizziness, fatigue
CV: Supine hypertension, arrhythmia exacerbation, chest pain
MISC: Urinary tract infection, neuroleptic malignant syndrome

PHARMACOKINETICS
Peak 3-4 hr

INTERACTIONS
Increase: droxidopa effects—carbidopa, serotonin receptor agonists, sympathomimetics
Increase: hypertensive crisis—MAOIs

NURSING CONSIDERATIONS
Assess:

Black Box Warning: **Supine hypertension:** monitor supine B/P before and at every dosage increase; assess response periodically. Advise to elevate the head of the bed when resting or sleeping to lessen the risk for supine hypertension. B/P should be monitored in supine position and in the recommended head-elevated sleeping position. Reduce or discontinue if supine hypertension persists

• **Neuroleptic malignant syndrome:** hyperthermia, severe extrapyramidal dysfunction, alterations in consciousness, mental status changes, and autonomic instability (tachycardia, blood pressure fluctuations, diaphoresis). In those with Parkinson's disease, this condition may occur with abrupt reduction of products with dopaminergic properties
• **Arrhythmia exacerbation:** exacerbation of existing ischemic cardiac disease (coronary artery disease, angina, myocardial infarction, HF); consider the potential risk before initiating therapy; if chest pain occurs during use, assess cardiac status
• **Pregnancy/breastfeeding:** no well-controlled studies in pregnancy, breastfeeding

Evaluate:
• **Therapeutic response:** increased B/P
Teach patient/family:

Black Box Warning: Instruct patients to rest and sleep in an upper-body-elevated position and to monitor blood pressure (to reduce the potential for supine hypertension); to take ≥3 hr prior to bedtime

• To take consistently with or without food
• Not to double doses

⚠ HIGH ALERT

dulaglutide (Rx)
(doo-la-gloo'-tide)
Trulicity
Func. class.: Antidiabetic
Chem. class.: Incretin mimetic

ACTION: Binds and activates known human glucagon-like peptide-1 (GLP-1) receptor agonist, mimics natural physiology for self-regulating glycemic control

USES: Type 2 diabetes mellitus, once-weekly dosing

CONTRAINDICATIONS: Hypersensitivity

Black Box Warning: Medullary thyroid carcinoma, multiple endocrine neoplasia syndrome type 2 (MEN-2), thyroid cancer

Precautions: Pregnancy, breastfeeding, children, geriatric patients, severe renal/hepatic/GI disease, pancreatitis, vit D deficiency, burns, colitis, diarrhea, fever, GI bleeding/perforation/obstruction, ileus, infection, pseudomembranous colitis, thyroid disease, trauma, surgery, type 1 diabetes mellitus, tobacco smoking, vomiting

DOSAGE AND ROUTES
• **Adult:** SUBCUT 0.75 mg weekly, may increase to 1.5 mg weekly
Available forms: Solution for SUBCUT injection 0.75 mg/0.5 mL, 1.5 mg/0.5 mL

(single-use pen); 1.5 mg/0.5 mL (single-dose prefilled syringe)

Administer:

SUBCUT route

• Do not use as first-line therapy for those who have inadequate glycemic control on diet and exercise

• Administer the dose at any time of day, with or without meals

• If a dose is missed, take as soon as remembered, as long as the next dose is due at least 3 days later; if it is more than 3 days after the missed dose, wait until the next regularly scheduled dose

• Give SUBCUT only, do not give IV or IM, inject into the thigh, abdomen, or upper arm, rotate sites with each injection to prevent lipodystrophy

• Properly dispose of the pen or syringe

• Store in refrigerator for unopened pen; may store at room temperature after opening for up to 30 days, do not freeze

• When using concomitantly with insulin, give as separate injections. Never mix them together. The two injections may be injected in the same body region, but not adjacent to each other

Prefilled pen administration: Part of pen is glass; if dropped on a hard surface, do not use. Uncap the pen after checking that it is locked, place base flat, and firmly unlock by turning the lock ring, press and hold green button, click will be heard, continue holding until another click is heard. Injection is complete when the gray plunger is visible. Remove the pen and dispose of the used pen

SIDE EFFECTS

CNS: Fatigue
ENDO: Hypoglycemia
GI: Nausea, vomiting, diarrhea, anorexia, gastroesophageal reflux, pancreatitis, flatulence, abdominal pain, constipation
SYST: Secondary malignancy
INTEG: Injection-site reactions, rash, urticaria

PHARMACOKINETICS

Peak 24-72 hr, half-life 5 days, metabolized by catabolism

INTERACTIONS

Increase: hypoglycemia—ACE inhibitors, disopyramide, sulfonylureas, androgens, fibric acid derivatives, alcohol
Increase: hyperglycemia—phenothiazines, corticosteroids, anabolic steroids
Decrease: effect of dulaglutide—niacin, dextrothyroxine, thiazide diuretics, triamterene, estrogens, progestins, oral contraceptives, MAOIs

NURSING CONSIDERATIONS

Assess:

• Fasting blood glucose, A1c levels (check twice a yr or quarterly in those with therapy changes or uncontrolled disease), postprandial glucose during treatment to determine diabetes control

• **Pancreatitis:** severe abdominal pain, with or without vomiting; product should be discontinued

• Hypo/hyperglycemic reaction that can occur soon after meals; for severe hypoglycemia, give IV $D_{50}W$, then IV dextrose solution

• Nausea, vomiting, diarrhea, ability to tolerate product, may cause dehydration

• **Pregnancy/breastfeeding:** no well-controlled studies; use only if benefit outweighs fetal risk; avoid breastfeeding, excretion is unknown

Evaluate:

• Therapeutic response: decrease in polyuria, polydipsia, polyphagia, clear sensorium, improving A1c, weight; absence of dizziness, stable gait

Teach patient/family:

• About the symptoms of hypo/hyperglycemia, what to do about each; to have glucagon emergency kit available; to carry a glucose source (candy, sugar cube) to treat hypoglycemia

---

DULoxetine (Rx)

(du-lox'uh-teen)
Cymbalta
Func. class.: Antidepressant
Chem. class.: Serotonin-norepineph-rine reuptake inhibitor (SNRI)

Do not confuse:
Cymbalta/Symbyax
duloxetine/fluoxetine

ACTION: May potentiate serotonergic, noradrenergic activity in the CNS; in studies, DULoxetine is a potent inhibitor of neuronal serotonin and norepinephrine reuptake

USES: Major depressive disorder (MDD), neuropathic pain associated with diabetic neuropathy, generalized anxiety disorder, fibromyalgia, chronic low back pain, osteoarthritis pain
Unlabeled uses: Stress, urinary incontinence

CONTRAINDICATIONS: Alcohol intoxication, alcoholism, closed-angle glaucoma, hepatic disease, hepatitis, jaundice, hypersensitivity
Precautions: Pregnancy, breastfeeding, geriatric patients, mania, hypertension, renal/cardiac disease, seizures, increased intraocular pressure, anorexia nervosa, bleeding, dehydration, diabetes, hyponatremia, hypotension, hypovolemia, orthostatic hypotension, abrupt product withdrawal

> Black Box Warning: Children, suicidal ideation

DOSAGE AND ROUTES NTI
Depression
• **Adult: PO** 40-60 mg/day as single dose or 2 divided doses
Diabetic neuropathy
• **Adult: PO** 60 mg/day
Generalized anxiety disorder
• **Adult: PO** 60 mg/day, may start with 30 mg/day × 1 wk, then increase to 60 mg/day; maintenance 60-120 mg/day
Fibromyalgia
• **Adult: PO** 30 mg/day × 1 wk, then 60 mg/day
Musculoskeletal pain
• **Adult: PO** 60 mg/day or 30 mg/day × 1 wk, then 60 mg/day
Renal dose
• **Adult: PO** Start with 20 mg, gradually increase; avoid use in severe renal disease

Available forms: Caps 20, 30, 40, 60 mg
Administer:
• Swallow cap whole; do not break, crush, or chew; do not sprinkle on food or mix with liquid
• Without regard to food
• Store in tight container at room temperature; do not freeze

SIDE EFFECTS
CNS: Insomnia, anxiety, dizziness, tremor, somnolence, fatigue, decreased appetite, decreased weight, agitation, diaphoresis, hallucinations, neuroleptic malignant–like syndrome reaction, aggression, seizures, *headache,* abnormal dreams, flushing, hot flashes, chills
CV: Thrombophlebitis, peripheral edema, hypertension, palpitations, supraventricular dysrhythmia, orthostatic hypotension
EENT: *Abnormal vision*
ENDO: Hypo/hyperglycemia, SIADH
GI: Constipation, diarrhea, dysphagia, *nausea,* vomiting, anorexia, dry mouth, colitis, gastritis, abdominal pain, hepatic failure
GU: Abnormal ejaculation, urinary hesitation/retention/frequency, ejaculation delayed, erectile dysfunction, gynecologic bleeding
INTEG: Photosensitivity, bruising, sweating, Stevens-Johnson syndrome
MS: Gait disturbance, muscle spasm, restless legs syndrome, myalgia
SYST: Anaphylaxis, angioedema, serotonin syndrome, Stevens-Johnson syndrome

PHARMACOKINETICS
Well absorbed; extensively metabolized ☞ (CYP2D6, CYP1A2) in the liver to an active metabolite; 70% of product recovered in urine, 20% in feces; 90% protein binding; elimination half-life 9.2-19.1 hr

INTERACTIONS
• Do not use with linezolid or methylene blue IV
• **Narrow therapeutic index:** CYP2D6 extensively metabolized products (flecainide, phenothiazines, propafenone, tricyclics, thioridazine)

• Hyperthermia, rigidity, rapid fluctuations of vital signs, mental status changes, neuroleptic malignant syndrome—MAOIs; coadministration contraindicated within 14 days of MAOI use

Increase: CNS depression—opioids, antihistamines, sedative/hypnotics

Increase: serotonin syndrome, neuroleptic malignant syndrome—SSRIs, serotonin-receptor agonists

Increase: bleeding risk—anticoagulants, antiplatelets, salicylates, NSAIDs

Increase: action of DULoxetine—CYP1A2 inhibitors (fluvoxamine, quinolone anti-infectives); CYP2D6 inhibitors (FLUoxetine, quiNIDine, PARoxetine)

Drug/Herb

Increase: serotonin syndrome—St. John's wort; avoid using together

Increase: CNS depression—kava, valerian

Drug/Lab Test

Increase: ALT, bilirubin—alcohol

Increase: blood glucose

NURSING CONSIDERATIONS
Assess:

Black Box Warning: **Depression:** mood, sensorium, affect, **suicidal tendencies,** increase in psychiatric symptoms, depression, panic; monitor children weekly face to face during first 4 wk, or dosage change, then every other wk for next 4 wk, then at 12 wk

• B/P lying, standing; pulse q4hr; if systolic B/P drops 20 mm Hg, hold product, notify prescriber; take VS q4hr in patients with CV disease

• **Hypo/hyperglycemia:** assess for each during treatment and before dosing

• Hepatic studies: AST, ALT, bilirubin

• Weight weekly; weight loss or gain; appetite may increase; peripheral edema may occur

• **Withdrawal symptoms:** headache, nausea, vomiting, muscle pain, weakness; not common unless product is discontinued abruptly

• Malignant neuroleptic–like syndrome reaction

• **Serotonin syndrome:** nausea/vomiting, dizziness, facial flush, shivering, sweating

• **Sexual dysfunction:** ejaculation dysfunction, erectile dysfunction, decreased libido, orgasm dysfunction

• Assistance with ambulation during beginning therapy; drowsiness, dizziness occur

• **Beers:** use with caution in older adults; may exacerbate or cause SIADH

• **Pregnancy/breastfeeding:** no well-controlled studies; use only if benefit outweighs fetal risk, complications in late 3rd trimester have occurred; pregnancy should be registered with the Cymbalta Pregnancy Registry, 1-866-814-6975; excreted in breast milk

Evaluate:

• Therapeutic response: decreased depression

Teach patient/family:

• To use sugarless gum, hard candy, frequent sips of water for dry mouth

• To report urinary retention; about signs and symptoms of bleeding (GI bleeding, nosebleed, ecchymoses, bruising)

• To use with caution when driving, performing other activities requiring alertness because of drowsiness, dizziness, blurred vision

• To avoid alcohol ingestion, MAOIs, other CNS depressants

• To notify prescriber of nausea, vomiting, dizziness, facial flushing, shivering, sweating, confusion, hallucinations, incoordination; may indicate serotonin syndrome

• Not to discontinue medication quickly after long-term use; may cause nausea, headache, malaise; taper

Black Box Warning: That clinical worsening and suicide risk may occur

• To wear sunscreen or large hat; photosensitivity may occur

• To notify prescriber if pregnancy is planned or suspected, or if breastfeeding

• Improvement may occur in 4-8 wk or in up to 12 wk (geriatric patients)

RARELY USED

dupilumab
(doo-pil′-ue-mab)
Dupixent
Func. class.: Dermatologicals

USES: Moderate to severe atopic dermatitis in patients whose disease is not adequately controlled with topical therapies or when those therapies are not advised

DOSAGE AND ROUTES
• **Adult: SUBCUT** Initially, 600 mg (administered as two 300-mg injections), then 300 mg every other week

---

⚠ HIGH ALERT

durvalumab
(dur-val′-yoo-mab)
Imfinzi
Func. class.: Antineoplastic monoclonal antibodies

ACTION: A human IgG1 kappa (IgG1k) monoclonal antibody, produced in Chinese hamster ovary; inhibits programmed death ligand interactions

USES: For the treatment of advanced or metastatic urothelial carcinoma
Unlabeled uses: For the consolidation treatment of locally advanced or unresectable non–small-cell lung cancer (NSCLC) after treatment with and response to platinum-based chemoradiotherapy

CONTRAINDICATIONS: Pregnancy, hypersensitivity
Precautions: Adrenal insufficiency, aseptic meningitis, autoimmune disease, breastfeeding, colitis, contraception requirements, Crohn's disease, diabetes mellitus, diarrhea, hemolytic anemia, hepatic disease, hepatitis, hypophysitis, hypopituitarism, IBS, infusion-related reactions, keratitis, myocarditis, organ transplant, pneumonitis, pulmonary disease, reproductive risk, serious rash, SLE, thyroid disease, ulcerative colitis, uveitis

DOSAGE AND ROUTES
Locally advanced or metastatic urothelial carcinoma
• **Adult: IV** 10 mg/kg over 60 min q2wk until disease progression or unacceptable toxicity

Consolidation treatment of locally advanced or unresectable non–small-cell lung cancer (NSCLC) (unlabeled)
• **Adult: IV** 10 mg/kg, beginning 1-42 days after the last radiation dose, q2wk until disease progression or unacceptable toxicity, for up to 12 mo

Management of immune-mediated toxicities
Adrenal insufficiency
• **Grade 2 to 4:** hold until patient is stable and start corticosteroids (1-2 mg/kg/day of prednisone or equivalent). Begin hormone replacement therapy as needed. When adrenal insufficiency improves to grade ≤1, begin a steroid taper over at least 1 mo
Colitis or diarrhea
• **Grade 2:** hold and start corticosteroids (1-2 mg/kg/day of prednisone or equivalent). If there is worsening or no improvement, increase corticosteroids and/or other systemic immunosuppressants. When colitis improves to grade ≤1, begin a steroid taper over at least 1 mo. Treatment may be resumed without a dose reduction when colitis is grade ≤1 and the corticosteroid dose has been reduced to <10 mg of prednisone or equivalent per day
• **Grade 3 or 4:** permanently discontinue and start corticosteroids (1-2 mg/kg/day of prednisone or equivalent). If there is worsening or no improvement, consider increasing the dose of corticosteroids and/or other systemic immunosuppressants. When colitis improves to

---

grade ≤1, begin a steroid taper over at least 1 mo

Diabetes, type 1:

• **Grade 2 to 4:** hold until patient is stable and start insulin as needed

Hypophysitis

• **Grade 2 to 4:** hold until patient is stable and start corticosteroids (1-2 mg/kg/day of prednisone or equivalent). Begin hormone replacement therapy as needed. When hypophysitis improves to grade ≤1, begin a steroid taper over at least 1 mo

Infection

• **Grade 3 or 4:** hold and initiate symptomatic management; treat with anti-infectives for suspected or confirmed infections

Infusion-related reactions

• **Grade 1 or 2:** interrupt or slow the rate of the infusion. Consider premedications before subsequent dosing

• **Grade 3 or 4:** permanently discontinue

Pneumonitis/interstitial lung disease (ILD)

• **Grade 2:** hold and start corticosteroids (1-2 mg/kg/day of prednisone or equivalent). If there is worsening or no improvement, increase the dose of corticosteroids, other systemic immunosuppressants. When pneumonitis improves to grade ≤1, begin a steroid taper over at least 1 mo. Treatment may be resumed without a dose reduction when pneumonitis is grade ≤1 and the corticosteroid dose has been reduced to <10 mg of prednisone or equivalent per day.

• **Grade 3 or 4:** permanently discontinue and start corticosteroids (1-4 mg/kg/day of prednisone or equivalent). If there is worsening or no improvement, consider increasing dose of corticosteroids and/or other systemic immunosuppressants. When pneumonitis improves to grade ≤1, begin a steroid taper over at least 1 mo

Rash

• **Grade 2 for >1 wk or Grade 3:** hold and start corticosteroids (1-2 mg/kg/day of prednisone or equivalent). If there is worsening or no improvement, consider

increasing the dose of corticosteroids and/or other systemic immunosuppressants. When the rash improves to grade ≤1, begin a steroid taper over at least 1 mo. Treatment may be resumed without a dose reduction when the rash is grade ≤1 and the corticosteroid dose has been reduced to <10 mg of prednisone or equivalent per day

• **Grade 4:** permanently discontinue and start corticosteroids (1-2 mg/kg/day of prednisone or equivalent). If there is worsening or no improvement, consider increasing the dose of corticosteroids and/or other systemic immunosuppressants. When the rash improves to grade ≤1, begin a steroid taper over at least 1 mo

Thyroid disorders

• **Hypothyroidism, grade 2 to 4:** initiate thyroid hormone replacement as needed

• **Hyperthyroidism, grade 2 to 4:** hold until patient is clinically stable. Manage patient symptomatically as clinically indicated

Other immune-mediated toxicities:

• **Grade 3:** hold and begin symptomatic management of the toxicity. Based on severity of the reaction, may use corticosteroids. If there is worsening or no improvement, consider increasing dose of corticosteroids and/or other systemic immunosuppressants. When toxicity improves to grade ≤1, begin a steroid taper over at least 1 mo. Treatment may be resumed without a dose reduction when toxicity is grade ≤1 and the corticosteroid dose has been reduced to <10 mg of prednisone or equivalent per day

• **Grade 4:** permanently discontinue and start symptomatic treatment and corticosteroids (1-4 mg/kg/day of prednisone or equivalent). If there is worsening or no improvement, consider increasing the dose of corticosteroids and/or other systemic immunosuppressants. When toxicity improves to grade ≤1, begin a steroid taper over at least 1 mo

Patients with hepatic impairment dosing

- **Mild hepatic impairment:** no change
- **Moderate (bilirubin 1.5-3× the upper limit of normal [ULN] and any AST) or severe (bilirubin >3× ULN and any AST):** specific guidelines unknown

Management of immune-mediated hepatitis

- **ALT/AST 3.1-5× ULN or total bilirubin 1.6-3× ULN (grade 2):** hold and start treatment with corticosteroids (1-2 mg/kg/day of prednisone or equivalent). If there is worsening or no improvement, consider increasing the dose of corticosteroids, other systemic immunosuppressants. When hepatitis improves to grade ≤1, begin a steroid taper over at least 1 mo
- **ALT/AST ≤8× ULN or total bilirubin ≤5× ULN (grade 3a):** hold and start corticosteroids (1-2 mg/kg/day prednisone or equivalent). If there is worsening or no improvement, increase corticosteroids, systemic immunosuppressants. When hepatitis improves to grade ≤1, begin a steroid taper over at least 1 mo
- **ALT/AST >8× ULN or total bilirubin >5× ULN (grade 3b):** permanently discontinue and start corticosteroids (1-2 mg/kg/day of prednisone or equivalent). If there is worsening or no improvement, increase dose of corticosteroids, systemic immunosuppressants. When hepatitis improves to grade ≤1, begin a steroid taper over at least 1 mo
- **Concurrent ALT/AST >3× ULN and total bilirubin >2× ULN with no other cause:** permanently discontinue and start corticosteroids (1-2 mg/kg/day of prednisone or equivalent). If there is worsening or no improvement, consider increasing the dose of corticosteroids, systemic immunosuppressants. When hepatitis improves to grade ≤1, begin a steroid taper over at least 1 mo

Renal dose

- **Mild to moderate renal impairment (CCr ≥30 mL/min):** no change
- **Severe renal impairment (CCr 15-29 mL/min):** unknown

Available forms: Powder for inj 120 mg/2.4 mL, 500 mg/10 mL

Administer:

IV route

- Follow cytotoxic handling procedures
- Visually inspect for particulate matter and discoloration, product should be clear to opalescent, colorless to slightly yellow, free from particles. Discard if solution is cloudy or discolored or if particles are observed
- Do not shake

Preparation:

- Withdraw the required volume of drug and transfer into an intravenous container containing 0.9% sodium chloride injection or 5% dextrose injection to prepare an infusion with a final concentration ranging from 1 mg/mL to 15 mg/mL
- Mix diluted solution by gentle inversion. Do not shake
- Discard partially used or empty vials of durvalumab

Storage of diluted solution:

- Does not contain a preservative; give immediately after preparation
- If storage of diluted solution is necessary, the total time from vial puncture to the start of administration should be <24 hr if refrigerated (2-8° C; 36-46° F), or <4 hr at room temperature (up to 25° C; up to 77° F). Do not freeze

IV Infusion:

- Give diluted over 60 min through an IV line using a low protein-binding 0.2- or 0.22-micron in-line filter
- Do not admix or give other products through the same line

SIDE EFFECTS

CNS: Fatigue, fever

GI: Nausea, diarrhea, constipation, anorexia, abdominal pain, colitis

HEMA: Anemia, hemolytic anemia, lymphopenia

RESP: Cough, dyspnea

META: Hyponatremia, hyperbilirubinemia, hypercalcemia, hypermagnesium, hypoalbuminemia

ENDO: Hyperglycemia, hyperthyroidism, hypothyroidism

MISC: Infection, peripheral edema, musculoskeletal pain, rash, antibody formation, aseptic meningitis, dehydration, infusion reactions, keratitis, myocarditis, uveitis

PHARMACOKINETICS
Steady state 16 wk, half-life 17 days

INTERACTIONS
• None known

Drug/Lab Test
Increase: LFTs, blood glucose, serum creatinine/BUN, thyroid function tests
Decrease: thyroid function tests

NURSING CONSIDERATIONS
Assess:
• Monitor baseline and periodically blood glucose, LFTs, serum creatinine/BUN
• **Serious infection:** may be fatal; monitor for signs and symptoms of infection; use prophylactic anti-infectives as appropriate.
• **Pregnancy/breastfeeding:** product can cause fetal harm; females of reproductive potential should avoid becoming pregnant during and for 3 mo after final dose; obtain a pregnancy test before starting product; do not breastfeed during and for at least 3 mo after last dose
• **Immune-mediated pneumonitis or interstitial lung disease (ILD):** may be fatal; monitor for signs or symptoms (new or worsening chest pain or shortness of breath) of pneumonitis. If pneumonitis is suspected, obtain a chest x-ray; an interruption or discontinuation of therapy and treatment with high-dose corticosteroids (followed by a steroid taper) may be necessary. The median time to onset of immune-mediated pneumonitis was 55.5 days (range, 24 to 423 days)
• **Immune-mediated hepatitis:** may be fatal; monitor for abnormal liver tests before each cycle of treatment; interruption or discontinuation of therapy may be needed with high-dose corticosteroids (followed by a steroid taper). The median time to onset of immune-mediated hepatitis was 51.5 days (range, 15 to 312 days)
• **Diarrhea and immune-mediated colitis:** monitor for signs and symptoms of colitis (diarrhea or severe abdominal pain). Treatment with antidiarrheal agents

and high-dose corticosteroids (followed by a steroid taper), along with an interruption or discontinuation of therapy, may be necessary. The median time to onset of immune-mediated colitis was 73 days (range, 13 to 345 days). Use with caution in those with inflammatory bowel disease such as ulcerative colitis or Crohn's disease
• **Thyroid disease/disorders (hypothyroidism/hyperthyroidism):** monitor thyroid function tests (TFTs) at baseline and periodically during treatment. Asymptomatic patients with abnormal TFTs can receive treatment; manage these patients with hormone replacement and symptomatic management as needed. The median time to onset of hypothyroidism was 42 days (range, 15 to 239 days), and the median time to first onset of hyperthyroidism was 43 days (range, 14-71 days)
• **Immune-mediated adrenal insufficiency and hypophysitis/hypopituitarism:** monitor for signs and symptoms of adrenal insufficiency (hypotension, decreased cortisol level, fatigue, weakness, and weight loss) and hypophysitis (decreased pituitary hormone levels, pituitary gland inflammation, severe intractable headache, and vision impairment) during and after treatment. An interruption of therapy, treatment with high-dose corticosteroids, and hormone replacement may be necessary
• **Immune-mediated nephritis:** monitor renal function at baseline and before each cycle of treatment. No initial dose adjustment is recommended in patients with renal dysfunction; use with caution in patients with renal disease or renal impairment. If immune-mediated nephritis occurs, an interruption or discontinuation of therapy may be needed with treatment with high-dose corticosteroids
• **Immune-mediated reactions (aseptic meningitis, hemolytic anemia, immune thrombocytopenic purpura, myocarditis, myositis) and ocular inflammatory toxicity (uveitis and keratitis):** monitor for signs and symptoms of immune-mediated reactions; confirm etiology or exclude other causes. Therapy may need to

be temporarily withheld or permanently discontinued; administer corticosteroids as needed

• **Severe infusion-related reactions:** monitor signs and symptoms of an infusion-related reaction. Interrupt or slow the rate of infusion in those with mild or moderate infusion reactions. Permanently discontinue in those with grade 3 or 4 infusion reactions

Evaluate:

• Therapeutic response: lack of disease progression

Teach patient/family:

• To report adverse reactions immediately; to report diarrhea, hepatic, flu-like symptoms, cough, trouble breathing, rash

• About reason for treatment, expected results

• **Pregnancy/breastfeeding:** to notify provider if pregnancy is planned or suspected; to use effective contraception during treatment and for 3 mo after discontinuing treatment; do not breastfeed during or for 3 mo after final dose

---

dutasteride (Rx)

(doo-tass′ter-ide)

Avodart

Func. class.: Androgen inhibitor

Chem. class.: Synthetic 5α-reductase inhibitor, 4-azasteroid compound

---

ACTION: Inhibits both type 1 and type 2 forms of a steroid enzyme that converts testosterone to 5α-dihydrotestosterone (DHT), which is responsible for the initial growth of prostatic tissue

USES: Treatment of benign prostatic hyperplasia (BPH) in men with an enlarged prostate gland; may be used in combination with tamsulosin

CONTRAINDICATIONS: Pregnancy, breastfeeding, women, children, hypersensitivity

Precautions: Hepatic disease

DOSAGE AND ROUTES

Benign prostatic hyperplasia (BPH)

• **Adult:** PO 0.5 mg/day; may use without tamsulosin

Available form: Caps 0.5 mg

Administer:

• Swallow caps whole; do not break, crush, chew

• Without regard to meals

SIDE EFFECTS

GU: Decreased libido, impotence, gynecomastia, ejaculation disorders (rare), mastalgia, teratogenesis

INTEG: Serious skin infections

PHARMACOKINETICS

Peak 2-3 hr, protein binding 99%, metabolized in liver by CYP3A4, excreted in feces, half-life 5 wk at steady state

INTERACTIONS

Increase: dutasteride concentrations—ritonavir, ketoconazole, verapamil, diltiazem, cimetidine, ciprofloxacin, antiretroviral protease inhibitors, or other products metabolized by CYP3A4

Drug/Lab Test

Decrease: PSA

NURSING CONSIDERATIONS

Assess:

• **For decreasing symptoms of BPH:** decreasing urinary retention, frequency, urgency, nocturia

• PSA levels; urinary obstruction; determine the absence of urinary or prostate cancer before starting treatment

• Blood studies: ALT, AST, bilirubin, CBC with differential, serum creatinine, serum electrolytes

Evaluate:

• Therapeutic response: decreasing symptoms of BPH; decreased urinary retention, frequency, urgency, nocturia

Teach patient/family:

• To read patient information leaflet before starting therapy; to reread it upon prescription renewal

• To notify prescriber if therapeutic response decreases, if edema occurs

• Not to discontinue product abruptly

• About changes in sex characteristics, gynecomastia, breast hardness; that decreased libido decreases after 6 months

• That men taking dutasteride should not donate blood for at least 6 mo after last dose to prevent blood administration to pregnant female

• That caps should not be handled by a woman who is pregnant or who may become pregnant because product can be absorbed through skin

• That ejaculate volume may decrease during treatment; that product rarely interferes with sexual function

• That product should not be used or handled by breastfeeding women

• To swallow whole; do not crush, chew, or open caps

• That product may increase risk for developing high-grade prostate cancer

• To report signs/symptoms of urinary obstruction or decreased urinary flow after starting therapy; to monitor for obstructive uropathy

• **Pregnancy/breastfeeding:** do not use in pregnancy/breastfeeding; not indicated for women

---

RARELY USED

duvelisib
(Doo′-veh- lih′-sib)
Copiktra
Func. class.: Antineoplastic

USES: Relapsed/refractory CLL, SLL, follicular lymphoma in those who have received at least 2 prior therapies

CONTRAINDICATIONS: Hypersensitvity

Black Box Warning: Colitis, diarrhea, infection, pneumonitis

DOSAGE AND ROUTES
• **Adult: PO** 25 mg bid

RARELY USED

ecallantide
(ee-kal'an-tide)
Kalbitor
Func. class.: Hematological agents
Chem. class.: Kallikrein inhibitor

USES: Acute attacks of hereditary angioedema (≥12 yr)

CONTRAINDICATIONS: Hypersensitivity to the drug or its components

Black Box Warning: Anaphylaxis has occurred after administrations (usually within first hour after dosing); drug should be administered only by health care provider with medical support available to treat anaphylaxis and hereditary angioedema; monitor patient closely

DOSAGE AND ROUTES
• **Adult/adolescent ≥12 yr: SUBCUT** 30 mg given as three 10-mg injections; give additional 30-mg dose within 24 hours if attack persists

econazole
(ee-koe'na-zole)
Ecoza, Ecostatin ✦
Func. class.: Topical antifungal
Chem. class.: Imidazole derivative

ACTION: Antifungal activity results from inhibiting cell-wall permeability

USES: Tinea corporis, cruris, pedis, versicolor; cutaneous candidiasis

CONTRAINDICATIONS: Hypersensitivity
Precautions: Pregnancy

DOSAGE AND ROUTES
Tinea corporis, cruris, pedis, versicolor
• **Adult/child: TOP** rub into affected areas daily × 2 wk, or × 4 wk (pedis)
Cutaneous candidiasis
• **Adult/child:** rub into affected areas bid × 2 wk

Available forms: Topical cream/foam 1%
Administer:
Topical route
• Do not use products near the eyes, nose, or mouth
• Wash hands before and after use; wash affected area and gently pat dry
• **Foam:** shake canister for 5 seconds before use
• **Cream:** apply to the cleansed affected area; massage gently into affected areas

SIDE EFFECTS
INTEG: Burning, rash, pruritus, erythema

PHARMACOKINETICS
Unknown

NURSING CONSIDERATIONS
Assess:
• **Allergic reaction:** assess for hypersensitivity; product might need to be discontinued
• **Infection:** assess for itching, peeling
Evaluate:
• Decreased itching, peeling
Teach patient/family:
Topical route
• That product is for external use only; do not use skin products near the eyes, nose, or mouth
• To wash hands before and after use; to wash affected area and gently pat dry
• **Cream:** to apply a thin film to the cleansed affected area; massage gently into affected areas

econazole topical
See Appendix B

RARELY USED

edaravone
(e-dar'-a-vone)
Radicava
Func. class.: CNS agents

USES: Amyotrophic lateral sclerosis

DOSAGE AND ROUTES
• **Adult: IV:** 60 mg/day × 14 days then a 14-day drug-free period for an initial

treatment cycle. For subsequent cycles, give × 10 days out of 14-day periods followed by 14-day drug-free periods

---

RARELY USED

edetate calcium disodium (Rx)
(ee′de-tate)

Calcium Disodium Versenate
Func. class.: Heavy-metal antagonist (antidote)

USES: Lead poisoning, acute lead encephalopathy

CONTRAINDICATIONS: Hypersensitivity, anuria, poisoning of other metals, severe renal disease, hepatitis

Black Box Warning: Child <3 yr, increased ICP, encephalopathy

DOSAGE AND ROUTES
Lead mobilization test (lead toxicity 25-45 mcg/dL)
• **Adult/adolescent: IV INFUSION** 500 mg/m² over 1 hr or **IM**
• **Child: IV INFUSION** 500 mg/m² over 1 hr or **IM** as single dose or 2 divided doses
Acute lead encephalopathy (blood levels >70 mcg/dL)
• **Adult/adolescent/child/infant: IM/ IV** 1500 mg/m² as **IV INFUSION** over 12-24 hr in combination with dimercaprol **IM,** give 1st dose ≥4 hr after initial dimercaprol, when urine flow established

---

efavirenz (Rx)
(ef-ah-veer′enz)

Sustiva
Func. class.: Antiretroviral
Chem. class.: Nonnucleoside reverse transcriptase inhibitor (NNRTI)

ACTION: Binds directly to reverse transcriptase and blocks RNA, DNA polymerase, thus causing a disruption of the enzyme's site

USES: HIV-1 in combination with at least 2 other antivirals
Unlabeled uses: HIV prophylaxis

CONTRAINDICATIONS: Pregnancy, hypersensitivity, moderate/severe hepatic disease
Precautions: Breastfeeding, children <3 yr, renal/hepatic disease, myelosuppression, depression, seizures

DOSAGE AND ROUTES
• **Adult and child >40 kg: PO** 600 mg/day at bedtime
• **Child ≥3 mo, 32.5-39.9 kg: PO** 400 mg/day at bedtime
• **Child ≥3 mo, 25-32.4 kg: PO** 350 mg/day at bedtime
• **Child ≥3 mo, 20-24.9 kg: PO** 300 mg/day at bedtime
• **Child ≥3 mo, 15-19.9 kg: PO** 250 mg/day at bedtime
• **Child ≥3 mo, 7.5-14.9 kg: PO** 200 mg/day at bedtime
• **Child ≥3 mo, 5-<7.5 kg: PO** 150 mg/day at bedtime
• **Child ≥3 mo, 3.5-≤5 kg: PO** 100 mg/day at bedtime
Available forms: Caps 50-, 200- mg; 600-mg tabs
Administer:
• Give on empty stomach; give at bedtime to decrease CNS side effects
• Caps may be opened, added to grape jelly to disguise peppery taste, or sprinkled on food, may be mixed in formula, do not cut/break tabs

SIDE EFFECTS
CNS: Fatigue, impaired cognition, insomnia, abnormal dreams, depression,

---

headache, dizziness, anxiety, drowsiness, odd feeling, suicidal thoughts/behaviors

GI: *Diarrhea,* abdominal pain, *nausea,* vomiting, hepatotoxicity

GU: Hematuria, kidney stones

INTEG: Rash, Stevens-Johnson syndrome, toxic epidermal necrolysis, exfoliative dermatitis

SYST: Immune reconstitution syndrome

MISC: Fat accumulation/redistribution

ENDO: Hyperlipidemia

CV: QT prolongation

PHARMACOKINETICS

Peak 3-5 hr, duration up to 24 hr, well absorbed, metabolized by liver; half-life 40-76 hr; >99% protein binding, excreted in urine, feces; concentrations higher in females and 🐾 in those of African, Asian, and Hispanic descent

INTERACTIONS

• Avoid use with boceprevir, delavirdine, rilpivirine; dosage change may be needed if given with telaprevir

• Do not give together with benzodiazepines, ergots, midazolam, triazolam, pimozide

Increase: CNS depression—alcohol, antidepressants, antihistamines, opioids

Increase: levels of both products—ritonavir, estrogens, anticonvulsants

Increase: levels of warfarin, statins (except pravastatin, fluvastatin)

Decrease: levels of indinavir, amprenavir, lopinavir, oral contraceptives, ketoconazole, itraconazole, posaconazole, voriconazole, saquinavir, cyclosporine, tacrolimus, sirolimus, bupropion, sertraline

Decrease: metabolism of CYP2B6 inhibitors, CYP2C19 substrates, CYP3A4 substrates

Decrease: efavirenz metabolism—CYP3A4 inhibitors (conivaptan, ambrisentan, SORAfenib)

Decrease: efavirenz effect—CYP3A4 inducers (carBAMazepine, rifamycins)

Drug/Herb

Decrease: efavirenz level—St. John's wort; do not use together

Drug/Food

Increase: absorption—high-fat foods

Drug/Lab Test

Increase: ALT

False positive: cannabinoids

NURSING CONSIDERATIONS

Assess:

• **HIV:** monitor CBC with differential, plasma HIV RNA, absolute CD4+/CD8+ cell counts/%, serum β2 microglobulin, serum ICD+24 antigen levels, cholesterol, hepatic enzymes, blood glucose, pregnancy test, bilirubin, urinalysis

Assess for suicidal thoughts/behaviors, poor concentration, dizziness, inability to sleep, usually resolves after 4 wk, give at bedtime

• Bowel pattern before, during treatment; if severe abdominal pain with bleeding occurs, product should be discontinued; monitor hydration

• **Serious skin reactions:** Stevens-Johnson syndrome, toxic epidermal necrolysis, usually occurs during first 2 wk, mild rash may resolve within 30 days; severe skin reactions including blistering, fever, product should be discontinued immediately and corticosteroids started

• **Signs of toxicity:** severe nausea/vomiting, maculopapular rash

• **Hepatotoxicity:** LFTs in those with liver disease, hold if LFTs are moderately elevated; if severe or if LFTs increase after product is restarted, discontinue permanently, do not breastfeed

• **Pregnancy/breastfeeding:** rule out pregnancy before starting treatment; use contraception, oral/nonoral contraceptives are decreased, use barrier methods also. Avoid use in first trimester (particular caution in first 8 wk of pregnancy) and in females of childbearing potential; consider another product. Register pregnant women with Antiretroviral Pregnancy Registry at 800-258-4263.

Evaluate:

• Therapeutic response: increased CD4 cell counts; decreased viral load; slowing progression of HIV

Teach patient/family:

• To take as prescribed; if dose is missed, to take as soon as remembered; not to double dose; to take with water, juice; to take on empty stomach at bedtime; to take at same time of day; not to break tabs; to use with other antiretrovirals

• To make sure health care provider knows all medications, supplements, OTC products taken

• To notify health care provider if severe rash occurs; that adverse reactions (rash, dizziness, abnormal dreams, insomnia) lessen after 1 mo, not to stop taking

• **Pregnancy/breastfeeding:** Identify if pregnancy is planned or suspected or if breastfeeding; not to breastfeed or become pregnant if taking this product; to use nonhormonal contraception because serious birth defects have occurred, to use barrier method for ≥12 wk after last dose

• To avoid hazardous activities if dizziness, drowsiness occur

• That product does not cure disease but controls symptoms; that HIV can be transmitted to others even while taking this product; to continue with safe-sex practices, that opportunistic infections can occur

• To report all adverse reactions, insomnia, poor concentration, but usually are less in 2-4 wk

• That CNS side effects of feeling "stoned" or "drunk" usually abate in several months

---

RARELY USED

efavirenz/lamivudine/tenofovir

(ef-ah-veer′enz lam-i-voo′ deen ten-oh-foh′veer)

Symfi, Symfi Lo

Func. class.: Antiretroviral

USES: Human immunodeficiency virus (HIV) infection

CONTRAINDICATIONS: Hypersensitivity

Black Box Warning: Hepatitis B exacerbation

DOSAGE AND ROUTES

• **Adult/adolescent/child ≥35 kg: PO** (Symfi Lo) 1 tablet (efavirenz 400 mg; lamivudine 300 mg; tenofovir 300 mg) on an empty stomach daily at bedtime

• **Adult/adolescent/child ≥40 kg: PO** (Symfi) 1 tablet (efavirenz 600 mg; lamivudine 300 mg; tenofovir 300 mg) on an empty stomach daily at bedtime

---

efinaconazole topical

See Appendix B

RARELY USED

elagolix

(el′ a-goe′ lix)

Orilissa

Func. class.: Gonadotropin-releasing hormone (GnRH) receptor antagonist

---

USES: Moderate to severe pain associated with endometriosis, including endometriosis-related dyspareunia

CONTRAINDICATIONS: Hypersensitivity, osteoporosis, pregnancy

DOSAGE AND ROUTES

• **Adult female: PO** Initiate at 150 mg daily; max duration 24 mo

---

eletriptan (Rx)

(el-ee-trip′tan)

Relpax

Func. class.: Antimigraine agent, abortive

Chem. class.: 5-HT$_1$-1B/1D receptor agonist, triptan

ACTION: Binds selectively to the vascular $5-HT_1$-receptor subtype; causes vasoconstriction in cranial arteries

USES: Acute treatment of migraine with/without aura

CONTRAINDICATIONS: Hypersensitivity, coronary artery vasospasm, peripheral vascular disease, hemiplegic/basilar migraine, uncontrolled hypertension; ischemic bowel, heart disease; severe renal/hepatic disease, acute MI, stroke, angina, postmenopausal women, men >40 yr; risk factors of CAD, MI, or other cardiac disease; hypercholesterolemia, obesity, diabetes
Precautions: Pregnancy, breastfeeding, children, geriatric patients, impaired renal/hepatic function

DOSAGE AND ROUTES
• **Adult: PO** 20 or 40 mg, may increase if needed, max 40 mg (single dose); may repeat in 2 hr if headache improves but returns, max 80 mg/24 hr
Available forms: Tabs 20, 40 mg
Administer:
• Swallow tabs whole; do not break, crush, or chew; use with 8 oz of water, without regard to food
• At beginning of headache; if headache returns, repeat dose after 2 hr if 1st dose is ineffective; treat no more than 3 headaches per 30 days

SIDE EFFECTS
CNS: *Dizziness,* headache, anxiety, paresthesia, asthenia, somnolence, flushing, fatigue, hot/cold sensation, chills, vertigo, hypertonia, seizures, serotonin syndrome
CV: Chest pain, palpitations, hypertension, MI, sinus tachycardia, stroke, ventricular fibrillation/tachycardia, atrial fibrillation, AV block, bradycardia, chest pressure syndrome, coronary vasospasm
GI: Nausea, dry mouth, vomiting
MS: *Weakness,* back pain
RESP: Chest tightness, pressure

PHARMACOKINETICS
Onset of pain relief ½ hr, peak 1½-2 hr, half-life 4 hr, metabolized in the liver, 70% excreted in urine and feces

INTERACTIONS
Increase: eletriptan effect—CYP3A4 inhibitors (clarithromycin, erythromycin, itraconazole, ketoconazole, nelfinavir, ritonavir), propranolol, ergots; avoid use within 72 hr of these products
Increase: serotonin syndrome—SSRIs, SNRIs, serotonin-receptor agonists, linezolid, MAOIs
Increase: vasospastic reactions—ergots, ergot similar products; avoid use within 24 hr of these products

NURSING CONSIDERATIONS
Assess:
• **Migraine:** pain location, character, intensity, nausea, vomiting, aura; quiet, calm environment with decreased stimulation from noise, bright light, excessive talking
• B/P; signs, symptoms of coronary vasospasms, geriatric patients may be at higher risk
• Tingling, hot sensation, burning, feeling of pressure, numbness, flushing
• Stress level, activity, recreation, coping mechanisms
• Neurologic status: LOC, blurring vision, nausea, vomiting, tingling in extremities preceding headache
• Ingestion of tyramine foods (pickled products, beer, wine, aged cheese), food additives, preservatives, colorings, artificial sweeteners, chocolate, caffeine, which may precipitate these types of headaches
• Patients with CAD risk factors; 1st dose should be administered in prescriber's office or medical facility
• Determine whether CYP3A4 inhibitors or other ergot-type products are being given
Evaluate:
• Therapeutic response: decrease in frequency, severity of migraine
Teach patient/family:
• To avoid driving or hazardous activity if dizziness occurs
• To report chest pain, neck or jaw pain
• To take whole with full glass of water
• To take when migraine is starting; a second dose may be used if headache returns
• To use contraception while taking product; to inform prescriber if pregnant or intending to become pregnant

- To provide dark, quiet environment
- That product does not prevent or reduce number of migraine attacks
- To use product only short term

RARELY USED

eltrombopag
(ell-trom-bow′pag)
Promacta
Func. class.: Hematopoietic

USES: Thrombocytopenia in chronic immune thrombocytopenic purpura when unresponsive to other treatment, chronic hepatitis C–associated thrombocytopenia

CONTRAINDICATIONS: Hypersensitivity

Black Box Warning: Hepatotoxicity

DOSAGE AND ROUTES
• **Adult: PO** 50 mg/day, adjust dosage to maintain platelets at $\geq 50 \times 10^9$, max 75 mg/day; 25 mg/day chronic hepatitis C; ✹ East Asian descent reduce dose to 25 mg daily

RARELY USED

eluxadoline
(el-ux-ad′oh-leen)
Viberzi ✦
Func. class.: GI agent

USES: Irritable bowel syndrome with diarrhea

CONTRAINDICATIONS: Hypersensitivity, alcoholism, GI/biliary obstruction, constipation, pancreatitis

DOSAGE AND ROUTES
• **Adult: PO** 100 mg bid with food. Decrease to 75 mg bid with food in those who are receiving an OATP1B1 inhibitor; do not use in those without a gallbladder

RARELY USED

elvitegravir/cobicistat/emtricitabine/tenofovir disoproxil
(el-vye-teg′gra-veer/koe-bik′-i-stat/em-tra-sye′ tah-ben/ten-oh-foh′veer)
Stribild ✦
Func. class.: Antiretrovirals

USES: HIV in treatment-naive patients

CONTRAINDICATIONS: Hypersensitivity, CCr <50 mL/min, severe hepatic disease

DOSAGE AND ROUTES
• **Adult: PO** 1 Tab daily

Renal dose
• **Adult: PO** do not use in CCr <50 mL/min

emedastine ophthalmic
See Appendix B

empagliflozin
(em-pa-gli-floe′zin)
Jardiance
Func. class.: Antidiabetic
Chem. class.: Sodium-glucose cotransporter 2 (SGLT2) inhibitors

ACTION: An inhibitor of sodium-glucose cotransporter 2 (SGLT2), the transporter responsible for reabsorbing the majority of glucose filtered by the tubular lumen in the kidney

USES: Type 2 diabetes mellitus with diet and exercise

CONTRAINDICATIONS: Hypersensitivity, dialysis, renal failure
Precautions: Adrenal insufficiency, breastfeeding, children, dehydration, diabetic ketoacidosis, fever, geriatric patients, hypercholesterolemia, hypercortisolism,

---

Side effects: *italics* = common; red = life-threatening

hyperglycemia, hyperthyroidism, hypoglycemia, hypotension, hypothyroidism, hypovolemia, malnutrition, pituitary insufficiency, pregnancy, renal impairment, type 1 diabetes mellitus, vaginitis

DOSAGE AND ROUTES

• **Adult: PO** 10 mg daily, may increase to 25 mg daily

Available forms: Tabs 10, 25 mg

Administer:

• Give every day without regard to food in the AM

SIDE EFFECTS

MS: Arthralgia

ENDO: Hypercholesterolemia, hyperlipidemia, hypoglycemia (in combination)

CV: Hypotension, orthostatic hypotension, volume depletion

GU: Increased urinary frequency, nocturia, polyuria, cystitis, dehydration, diuresis

GI: Nausea

CNS: Syncope

MISC: Infection, ketoacidosis

PHARMACOKINETICS

Protein binding 82.6%, terminal elimination half-life 12.4 hr, peak 1.5 hr

INTERACTIONS

Increase: hypoglycemic effect—angiotensin II receptor antagonists, angiotensin-converting enzyme (ACE) inhibitors, loop diuretics, thiazide diuretics, fluoxetine, olanzapine, β-blockers, other antidiabetics, octreotide, fibric acid derivatives, MAOIs type A

Increase/Decrease: hypoglycemic effect—clonidine, androgens, bortezomib, lithium, alcohol, sulfonamides

Decrease: hypoglycemic effect—phenothiazines, typical antipsychotics, baclofen, carbonic anhydrase inhibitors, estrogens, progestins, oral contraceptives, dextrothyroxine, glucagon, corticosteroids, fenfluramine, dexfenfluramine, phenytoin, fosphenytoin, ethotoin, salicylates, cyclosporine, tacrolimus, tobacco

Drug/Herb/Supplements

Increase: hypoglycemia—chromium, horse chestnut

Increase/Decrease: hypoglycemia—niacin

Decrease: hypoglycemia—green tea

Drug/Lab Test

Increase: HCT, creatinine

Decrease: GFR

NURSING CONSIDERATIONS

Assess:

• **Diabetes:** monitor blood glucose, glycosylated hemoglobin A1c (HbA1c), serum cholesterol profile, serum creatinine/BUN, assess for polydipsia, other products taken by patient; assess for hypoglycemia, headache, drowsiness, hunger, weakness, sweating; have sugar source available

• **Ketoacidosis:** if patient has volume depletion, dehydration, discontinue, give insulin, glucose source

• **Renal studies:** monitor serum creatinine eGFR baseline and periodically avoid in those with eGFR <45 mL/min/1.73 m^2

• **UTI:** treat with anti-infective

• **Pregnancy/breastfeeding:** use if benefits outweigh risk to fetus; no well-controlled studies; do not breastfeed

Evaluate:

• Therapeutic response: decreasing blood glucose, A1c

Teach patient/family:

• How to check blood glucose; to continue with diet and exercise changes; to avoid smoking, alcohol

• To avoid other products unless approved by prescriber

• To take in the AM, without regard to food; that if dose is missed, to take when remembered, do not double dose; to read "medication guide" provided; that product controls symptoms but does not cure diabetes

• To follow medical regimen including diet, exercise, and weight loss

• To teach how to take blood glucose, urine ketones readings and how often

• **Hypoglycemia:** to report rapid heartbeat, dizziness, weakness; that lab testing will be needed, including blood glucose monitoring, and that a dosage change may be needed; to carry a sugar source at all times; review signs and symptoms of hypoglycemia and hyperglycemia and what to do about each

- Hypotension: to report vision changes, dizziness, fatigue; B/P should be checked regularly
- **Ketoacidosis:** to report nausea, vomiting, abdominal pain, confusion, sleepiness
- **Infections:** (usually urinary tract infections) to report burning, cloudy, foul-smelling urine, fever, back pain; antibiotics will be needed; and to report symptoms of mycotic infections, including foul-smelling vaginal discharge or penile discharge and redness
- **Pregnancy/breastfeeding:** to report if pregnancy is planned or suspected; not to breastfeed

---

⚠ HIGH ALERT

empagliflozin/ metformin (Rx)

(em′pa-gli-floe′ zin/met-for′min)

Synjardy, Synjardy XR

Func. class.: Antidiabetic

Chem. class.: Biguanide; sodium-glucose cotransporter 2 (SGLT2) inhibitor

---

ACTION: Combination products containing empagliflozin and metformin improve glycemic control in type 2 diabetes mellitus

Empagliflozin: An inhibitor of sodium-glucose cotransporter 2 (SGLT2), the transporter responsible for reabsorbing the glucose filtered by the tubular lumen in the kidney. By inhibiting SGLT2, reabsorbs filtered glucose and lowers the renal threshold for glucose (RTG), increases urinary glucose excretion

Metformin: Decreases hepatic gluconeogenesis production, decreases intestinal absorption of glucose, and improves insulin sensitivity by increasing peripheral glucose uptake and utilization

USES: Type 2 diabetes mellitus

CONTRAINDICATIONS: Hypersensitivity, diabetic ketoacidosis, dialysis, metabolic acidosis, radiographic contrast administration, renal failure

Black Box Warning: Lactic acidosis

Precautions: Pregnancy, geriatric patients, severe renal/hepatic/GI disease, pancreatitis, vit D deficiency, acidemia, acute heart failure, acute myocardial infarction, alcoholism, balanitis, breastfeeding, burns, cardiac disease, children, dehydration, diarrhea, ethanol intoxication, fever, gastroparesis, hypercholesterolemia, hypercortisolism, hyperglycemia, hyperthyroidism, hypoglycemia, hypotension, hypovolemia, hypoxemia, infection, malnutrition, pernicious anemia, pituitary insufficiency, polycystic ovary syndrome, sepsis, surgery, trauma, type 1 diabetes mellitus, vaginitis, vomiting

DOSAGE AND ROUTES
- **Adult: PO** bid with meals; individualize based on efficacy and tolerability. In geriatric patients, use lowest effective dose. Max in normal renal function is empagliflozin 25 mg/day and metformin 2000 mg/day; correct volume depletion before initiation of treatment
- **Patients currently treated with empagliflozin:** Start with metformin 500 mg with a similar total daily dose of empagliflozin; increase gradually to reduce the GI side effects
- **Patients currently treated with metformin:** Start with empagliflozin 5 mg/dose with a similar total daily dose of metformin. Patients taking an evening dose of metformin XR should check with their provider about when to take their last dose before starting empagliflozin/metformin
- **Patients already treated with both empagliflozin and metformin:** May switch to this combination product using the same doses of each component per day, then dividing the daily doses to bid dosing with meals

Renal dose:
- **Adult: PO** eGFR ≥45 mL/min/1.73 m², no change; eGFR <45 mL/min/1.73 m², do not use

Available forms: Tabs 5 mg/500 mg, 5 mg/1000 mg, 12.5 mg/500 mg, 12.5 mg/1000 mg; ext rel tabs 5 mg/1000 mg, 10 mg/1000 mg, 12.5 mg/1000 mg, 25 mg/1000 mg

Administer:
- Give bid with meals (usually at morning and evening meals) to reduce GI adverse reactions

---

Side effects: *italics* = common; red = life-threatening

Ext rel: swallow whole; take q AM with a meal

SIDE EFFECTS

ENDO: Hypoglycemia, diabetic ketoacidosis
CV: Orthostatic hypotension
GI: Nausea, vomiting, diarrhea, dyspepsia, anorexia, abdominal pain, flatulence, pyrosis (heartburn), polydipsia, metallic taste
GU: Polyuria, vaginitis, phimosis, nocturia, urinary frequency
META: Metabolic acidosis, vitamin B_{12} deficiency, hypercholesterolemia, hyperlipidemia
SYST: Lactic acidosis, infection
MS: Myalgia, arthralgia

PHARMACOKINETICS

Empagliflozin: 86% protein binding, terminal half-life 12.4 hr
Metformin: no protein binding, half-life 6.2 hr

INTERACTIONS

• Do not use with gatifloxacin
Increase: hypoglycemia
Increase: hyperglycemia—phenothiazines, corticosteroids, anabolic steroids, calcium channel blockers
Decrease: action of digoxin
Decrease: efficacy—niacin, thiazide diuretics, triamterene, estrogens, progestins, oral contraceptives

NURSING CONSIDERATIONS
Assess:

> **Black Box Warning: Lactic acidosis:** assess for nausea, vomiting, weakness, rapid breathing; notify prescriber immediately

• Fractures: assess for risk of fractures before use; do not use in those at risk for fractures; avoid SGLT 2 inhibitors in these patients
• CBC, serum cholesterol profile, serum electrolytes periodically
• Fasting blood glucose, A1c levels, postprandial glucose during treatment to determine diabetes control
• Renal studies: urinalysis, creatinine
• Hypo/hyperglycemic reaction that can occur soon after meals; for severe hypoglycemia, give IV $D_{50}W$, then IV dextrose solution

• Nausea, vomiting, diarrhea, ability to tolerate product; may cause dehydration
• **Pregnancy/breastfeeding:** use of insulin is preferred in pregnancy; do not breastfeed
Evaluate:
• Therapeutic response: decrease in polyuria, polydipsia, polyphagia, clear sensorium, improving A1c
Teach patient/family:
• About the symptoms of hypo/hyperglycemia, what to do about each; to have glucagon emergency kit available; to carry a glucose source (candy, sugar cube) to treat hypoglycemia
• That product must be continued daily; about consequences of discontinuing product abruptly
• That diabetes is a lifelong illness; product will not cure disease; to carry emergency ID with prescriber and medication information
• To continue weight control, dietary restrictions, exercise, hygiene
• That regular blood glucose monitoring and A1c testing are needed
• To notify prescriber if pregnant or intending to become pregnant
• **Infection** (usually urinary tract infection): to report burning, cloudy or foul-smelling urine, feces, fever, back pain; antibiotics will be needed; to report mycotic infection: symptoms including foul-smelling vaginal discharge or penile discharge and redness
• **Ketoacidosis:** to report nausea, vomiting, abdominal pain, confusion, sleepiness

---

emtricitabine (Rx)

(em-tri-sit'uh-bean)
Emtriva
Func. class.: Antiretroviral
Chem. class.: Nucleoside reverse transcriptase inhibitor (NRTI)

ACTION: A synthetic nucleoside analog of cytosine; inhibits replication of HIV virus by competing with the natural substrate and then becoming incorporated into cellular DNA by viral reverse transcriptase, thereby terminating cellular DNA chain

USES: HIV-1 infection with other antiretroviral

Unlabeled uses: HBV (hepatitis B virus) infection with HIV, HIV prophylaxis

CONTRAINDICATIONS: Hypersensitivity

Precautions: Pregnancy, breastfeeding, children, geriatric patients, renal disease, lactic acidosis

Black Box Warning: Hepatic insufficiency, chronic hepatitis B virus (HBV)

DOSAGE AND ROUTES
• **Adult:** PO Caps 200 mg/day; oral sol 240 mg (24 mL)/day
• **Adolescent/child >33 kg:** PO Caps 200 mg/day; **child 3 mo-17 yr:** oral sol 6 mg/kg/day, max 240 mg (24 mL)
• **Infants <3 mo:** PO oral sol 3 mg/kg daily, do not use caps
Renal dose
• **Adult: PO** Caps CCr 30-49 mL/min, 200 mg q48hr; oral sol 120 mg q24hr; caps CCr 15-29 mL/min, 200 mg q72hr; oral sol 80 mg q24hr; caps CCr <15 mL/min, 200 mg q96hr; oral sol 60 mg q24hr

Available forms: Cap 200 mg; oral sol 10 mg/mL
Administer:
• Give without regard to meals
• Oral cap and solution not interchangeable
• Store caps at 25° C (77° F); oral sol refrigerated, use within 3 mo

SIDE EFFECTS
CNS: *Headache,* abnormal dreams, *depression,* dizziness, *insomnia,* neuropathy, paresthesia, *asthenia,* weakness
GI: *Nausea, vomiting, diarrhea, anorexia, abdominal pain, dyspepsia,* hepatomegaly with steatosis (may be fatal)
INTEG: *Rash,* skin discolorization
MS: Arthralgia, myalgia
RESP: *Cough*
SYST: Change in body fat distribution, lactic acidosis, immune reconstitution syndrome

PHARMACOKINETICS
Rapidly, extensively absorbed; peak 1-2 hr; protein binding <4%; excreted unchanged in urine (86%), feces (14%); half-life 10 hr

INTERACTIONS
Decrease: emtricitabine level—interferons
• Complex interactions—ribavirin, cautious use
Drug/Lab Test
Increase: AST/ALT, glucose, amylase, bilirubin, CK, lipase
Decrease: neutrophils

NURSING CONSIDERATIONS

E

Assess:
• **HIV:** monitor for infections and improvement in symptoms of HIV
• Renal/hepatic function tests: AST, ALT, bilirubin, amylase, lipase, triglycerides periodically during treatment
• Lactic acidosis, severe hepatomegaly with steatosis: if lab reports confirm these conditions, discontinue treatment; may be fatal; more common in females or those who are overweight; monitor lactic acid levels, LFTs

Black Box Warning: Hepatotoxicity: do not use in those with risk factors such as alcoholism; discontinue if hepatotoxicity occurs

• Hepatitis B and HIV coinfection (unlabeled); perform HBV screening in any patient who has HIV to ensure appropriate treatment; avoid single-drug treatments in HBV
• **Pregnancy/breastfeeding:** use if clearly needed; register pregnant women in the Antiretroviral Pregnancy Registry at 1-800-258-4263; to reduce the risk of postnatal transmission, HIV-infected mothers are advised to avoid breastfeeding
Evaluate:
• Therapeutic response: decreased signs, symptoms of HIV; decreased viral load, increased CD4 counts
Teach patient/family:
• That GI complaints resolve after 3-4 wk of treatment
• That product must be taken at same time of day to maintain blood level; that solution and cap are not interchangeable; that if dose is missed, to take as soon as remembered; not to double doses; not to share with others

---

Side effects: *italics* = common; red = life-threatening

• That product will control symptoms but is not a cure for HIV; patient still infectious, may pass HIV virus on to others; that other products may be necessary to prevent other infections; to practice safe sex and use a condom; not to share needles or donate blood

• That changes in body fat distribution may occur

• **Lactic acidosis:** to notify prescriber immediately if fatigue, muscle aches/pains, abdominal pain, difficulty breathing, nausea, vomiting, change in heart rhythm occur

Black Box Warning: **Hepatotoxicity**: to notify prescriber of dark urine, yellowing of skin/eyes, clay-colored stools, anorexia, nausea, vomiting

• To report planned or suspected pregnancy; not to breastfeed while taking product

---

emtricitabine/rilpivirine/tenofovir disoproxil fumarate

(em-tri-sit' uh-bean/ril-pi-vir' een/ten-oh-foh'veer)

Complera

Func. class.: Antiretroviral
Chem. class.: Nucleoside reverse transcriptase inhibitor (NRTI)

ACTION:

• **Emtricitabine:** inhibits viral reverse transcriptase and is active both on HIV-1 and HBV

• **Tenofovir:** inhibits viral reverse transcriptase and acts as a DNA chain terminator

• **Rilpivirine:** inhibits HIV-1 reverse transcriptase; it does not compete for binding, nor does it require phosphorylation to be active

USES: HIV in treatment-naive patients

with HIV RNA ≤100,000 copies/mL at initiation and certain virologically stable (HIV RNA <50 copies/mL) treatment-experienced patients

CONTRAINDICATIONS: Hyper-

sensitivity, hepatotoxicity, lactic acidosis

Black Box Warning: Hepatitis B exacerbation

Precautions: Alcoholism, autoimmune disease, bone fractures, breastfeeding, children, depression, females, Graves' disease, Guillain-Barré syndrome, hepatic disease, hepatitis, hepatitis B and HIV coinfection, hepatitis C and HIV coinfection, hepatomegaly, HIV resistance, hypercholesterolemia, hyperlipidemia, hypertriglyceridemia, hypophosphatemia, immune reconstitution syndrome, obesity, osteomalacia, osteoporosis, pregnancy, QT prolongation, renal failure, renal impairment, serious rash, suicidal ideation, torsades de pointes

DOSAGE AND ROUTES

• **Adult/adolescent/child >12 yr and weighing ≥35 kg: PO** 1 tablet (200 mg emtricitabine; 25 mg rilpivirine; 300 mg tenofovir) qday. Coadministration with rifabutin, the rilpivirine dose needs to be increased to 50 mg/day; give an additional 25 mg/day of rilpivirine with a meal

HIV prophylaxis after occupational exposure to HIV (unlabeled)

• **Adult: PO** 1 tablet (200 mg emtricitabine; 25 mg rilpivirine; 300 mg tenofovir disoproxil fumarate) qday × 28 days

Renal dose

• **Adult: PO** CCr <50 mL/min: not recommended

Available forms: Tablet 200-25-300 mg
Administer:

• Give with a meal

• Antiretroviral drug resistance testing (preferably genotypic testing) before use in treatment-naive patients and before changing therapy for treatment failure

• For pregnant women, therapy should begin immediately after HIV diagnosis

• Before initiating therapy, consider the following: virologic failures occurred more frequently in those with baseline HIV RNA concentrations >100,000 copies; CD4 counts <200 cells/mm^3

• Avoid use of tenofovir-containing regimens in those with renal disease and osteoporosis

SIDE EFFECTS

CNS: *Headache*, abnormal dreams, *depression*, dizziness, *insomnia*, neuropathy, paresthesia, suicide, fatigue, drowsiness

GI: *Nausea, vomiting, anorexia, diarrhea, abdominal pain, dyspepsia*, hepatomegaly with stenosis (may be fatal), pancreatitis

INTEG: *Rash*, skin discoloration

MS: Arthralgia, myalgia, rhabdomyolysis

GU: Glomerulonephritis membranous/mesangioproliferative

SYST: Change in body fat distribution, lactic acidosis

PHARMACOKINETICS

• *Emtricitabine:* protein binding <4%, metabolized via oxidation half-life 10 hr, excreted renally (86%) and via feces (14%); peak 1-2 hr

• *Tenofovir:* protein binding <0.7%, undergoes phosphorylation, eliminated by a combination of glomerular filtration and active renal tubular secretion, 70%-80% excreted unchanged in urine half-life 17 hr, bioavailability is increased with a high-fat meal

• *Rilpivirine:* protein binding 99.7% to albumin, metabolism via oxidation by CYP3A system, half-life 50 hr, excretion 85% feces, 6.1% urine, peak 4-5 hr

INTERACTIONS

• Do not use with efavirenz, lamiVUDine; treatment duplication

Increase: rilpivirine level—CYP3A4 inhibitors (delavirdine, efavirenz, darunavir, tipranavir, atazanavir, fosamprenavir, indinavir, nelfinavir, aldesleukin IL-2, amiodarone, aprepitant, basiliximab, boceprevir, bromocriptine, chloramphenicol, clarithromycin, conivaptan, danazol, dalfopristin, dasatinib, diltiazem, dronedarone, erythromycin, ethinyl estradiol, fluconazole, fluoxetine, fluvoxamine, fosaprepitant, imatinib, isoniazid, itraconazole, ketoconazole, lantreotide, lapatinib, miconazole, nefazodone, nicardipine, octreotide, posaconazole, quinine, ranolazine, rifaximin, tamoxifen, telaprevir, telithromycin, troleandomycin, verapamil, voriconazole, zafirlukast)

Decrease: emtricitabine level—interferons

Increase: QT prolongation—class IA/III antidysrhythmics, some phenothiazines, beta agonists, local anesthetics, tricyclics, haloperidol, chloroquine, droperidol, pentamidine; CYP3A4 inhibitors (amiodarone, clarithromycin, erythromycin, telithromycin, troleandomycin), arsenic trioxide; CYP3A4 substrates (methadone, pimozide, QUEtiapine, quiNIDine, risperiDONE, ziprasidone)

Increase: rilpivirine adverse reactions, fungal infections—fluconazole, voriconazole

Decrease: rilpivirine effect, treatment failure—CYP3A4 inducers (rifAMPin, rifapentine, rifabutin, primadone, phenytoin, PHENobarbital, nevirapine, nafcillin, modafinil, griseofulvin, etravirine, efavirenz, barbiturates, bexarotene, bosentan, carBAMazepine, enzalutamide, dexamethasone), proton pump inhibitors

Drug/Lab Test

Increase: AST/ALT, glucose, amylase, bilirubin, lipase, CK

Decrease: neutrophils

NURSING CONSIDERATIONS

Assess:

• **HIV infection:** assess symptoms of HIV, including opportunistic infections before and during treatment, some may be life-threatening; monitor plasma CD4+, CD8 cell counts, serum beta-2 microglobulin, serum ICD+24 antigen levels, treatment failures occur more often in those with baseline HIV-1 RNA concentrations >100,000 copies/mL than in those <100,000 copies/mL; monitor blood glucose, CBC with differential, serum cholesterol, lipid panel

• **Hepatotoxicity/lactic acidosis:** monitor hepatitis B serology, LFTs, plasma hepatitis C RNA, lactic acidosis levels. If lab reports confirm these conditions, discontinue product. More common in females or those who are overweight. Avoid use in alcoholism

---

Side effects: *italics* = common; red = life-threatening

• **Pregnancy/breastfeeding:** obtain pregnancy testing before use

• To report suspected or planned pregnancy, not to breastfeed

Black Box Warning: Hepatitis B exacerbation: those with coexisting HBV and HIV infections who discontinue emtricitabine or tenofovir may experience severe acute hepatitis B exacerbation, with some cases resulting in hepatic decompensation and hepatic failure. Therefore patients coinfected with HBV and HIV who discontinue this product should have transaminase concentrations monitored q6wk for the first 3 mo and q3-6mo thereafter. Resumption of anti–hepatitis B treatment may be required. For patients who refuse a fully suppressive ARV regimen but still require treatment for HBV, consider 48 wk of peginterferon alfa; do not administer HIV-active medications in the absence of a fully suppressive ARV regimen

• Monitor serum bilirubin (total and direct), serum creatinine, urinalysis, LFTs, amylase, lipase, periodically

Evaluate:
• Improvement in CD4, HIV RNA counts, decreasing signs and symptoms of HIV

TEACH PATIENT/FAMILY:
• That hepatitis and HIV coinfected patients should avoid consuming alcohol; offer vaccinations against hepatitis A and hepatitis B as appropriate
• That GI complaints resolve after 2-3 wk of treatment
• To take at the same time of day to maintain blood level; not to crush, break, or chew
• That product controls the symptoms of HIV but does not cure; patient is still able to infect others, that other products may be necessary to prevent other infections
• **Lactic acidosis:** to notify prescriber if fatigue, muscle aches/pains, abdominal pain, difficulty breathing, nausea, vomiting, change in heart rhythm occurs
• **Hepatotoxicity:** to notify prescriber of dark urine, yellowing skin or eyes, clay-colored stools, anorexia, nausea, vomiting
• **Suicide:** to report severe depression, suicidal ideation to prescriber immediately

---

emtricitabine/tenofovir alafenamide fumarate
(em-tri-sit′ uh-bean/ten-oh-foh′veer)

Descovy

Func. class.: Antiretroviral
Chem. class.: Nucleoside reverse transcriptase inhibitor (NRTI)

ACTION:
• **Emtricitabine:** inhibits viral reverse transcriptase and is active both on HIV-1 and HBV
• **Tenofovir:** inhibits viral reverse transcriptase and acts as a DNA chain terminator

USES: Human immunodeficiency virus (HIV) infection used in combination with other antiretrovirals

CONTRAINDICATIONS: Hypersensitivity, CCr <30 mL/min

Precautions:

Black Box Warning: Hepatitis B exacerbation

Alcoholism, autoimmune disease, bone fractures, breastfeeding, children, depression, females, Graves' disease, Guillain-Barré syndrome, hepatic disease, hepatitis, hepatitis B and HIV coinfection, hepatitis C and HIV coinfection, hepatomegaly, HIV resistance, hypercholesterolemia, hyperlipidemia, hypertriglyceridemia, hypophosphatemia, immune reconstitution syndrome, obesity, osteomalacia, osteoporosis, pregnancy, QT prolongation, renal failure, renal impairment, serious rash, suicidal ideation, torsades de pointes, hepatotoxicity, lactic acidosis

DOSAGE AND ROUTES
• **Adult/adolescent/child ≥12 yr and weighing ≥35 kg: PO** 1 tablet (200 mg emtricitabine; 25 mg tenofovir) qday
Available forms: Tabs 200-25 mg

Administer:

• Antiretroviral drug resistance testing (preferably genotypic testing) is recommended before use in treatment-naive patients and before changing therapy for treatment failure

• For adults, use in all patients to reduce the risk of disease progression and to prevent the transmission of HIV, including perinatal transmission and transmission to sexual partners. Conditions increasing the urgency for therapy include pregnancy, AIDS-defining conditions (including HIV-associated dementia), acute or early HIV infection, acute opportunistic infections, HIV-associated nephropathy, hepatitis B (HBV) or hepatitis C (HCV) coinfection, lower CD4 counts (<200 cells/mm³), rapidly declining CD4 counts (>100 cells/mm³ decrease per year), or higher viral loads (>100,000 copies/mL)

• For pregnant women, therapy should begin immediately after HIV diagnosis, as early maternal viral suppression is associated with lower risk of perinatal effects

• Avoid use of tenofovir-containing regimens in those with renal disease and osteoporosis

SIDE EFFECTS

CNS: Weakness

GI: *Nausea*, hepatomegaly with stenosis (may be fatal), hepatic failure/decompensation, hepatitis

MS: Myalgia, bone pain, osteopenia, osteoporosis

GU: Breast enlargement, renal failure

SYST: Change in body fat distribution, lactic acidosis, Fanconi syndrome

META: Hypercholesterolemia, hypertriglyceridemia, hypophosphatemia

PHARMACOKINETICS

• **Emtricitabine:** protein binding <4%, metabolized via oxidation, half-life 10 hr, excreted renally (86%) and via feces (14%); peak 1-2 hr

• **Tenofovir:** protein binding <0.7%, undergoes phosphorylation to its active metabolite, eliminated by glomerular filtration and active renal tubular secretion, 70%-80% excreted unchanged in urine by 72 hr; half-life 17 hr, bioavailability is increased with a high-fat meal

INTERACTIONS

• Do not use with efavirenz, lamiVUDine; treatment duplication

Decrease: emtricitabine level—interferons

Increase: QT prolongation—class IA/III antidysrhythmics, some phenothiazines, beta agonists, local anesthetics, tricyclics, haloperidol, chloroquine, droperidol, pentamidine; CYP3A4 inhibitors (amiodarone, clarithromycin, erythromycin, telithromycin, troleandomycin), arsenic trioxide; CYP3A4 substrates (methadone, pimozide, quetiapine, quinidine, risperidone, ziprasidone)

NURSING CONSIDERATIONS

Assess:

• **HIV infection:** assess symptoms of HIV, including opportunistic infections before and during treatment, some may be life-threatening; monitor plasma CD4+, CD8 cell counts, serum beta-2 microglobulin; treatment failures occur more often in those with baseline HIV-1 RNA concentrations >100,000 copies/mL than in those <100,000 copies/mL; monitor blood glucose, CBC with differential, serum cholesterol, lipid panel

• **Hepatotoxicity/lactic acidosis:** monitor hepatitis B serology, LFTs, plasma hepatitis C RNA, lactic acidosis levels. If lab reports confirm these conditions, discontinue product. More common in females or those who are overweight. Avoid use in alcoholism

Black Box Warning: **Hepatitis B exacerbation:** those with coexisting HBV and HIV infections who discontinue emtricitabine or tenofovir may experience severe acute hepatitis B exacerbation with hepatic decompensation/failure. Those coinfected with HBV and HIV who discontinue this product should have transaminase concentrations monitored q6wk × the first 3 mo and q3-6mo thereafter. Resumption of anti–hepatitis B treatment may be required. For patients who refuse a fully suppressive antiretroviral regimen but still

---

require treatment for HBV, consider 48 wk of peginterferon alfa; do not administer HIV-active medications in the absence of a fully suppressive ARV regimen

• Monitor serum bilirubin (total and direct), serum creatinine, urinalysis, LFTs, amylase, lipase, periodically
• **Pregnancy/breastfeeding:** obtain pregnancy testing before use

Evaluate:
• Improvement in CD4, HIV RNC counts, decreasing signs and symptoms of HIV

Teach patient/family:
• That hepatitis and HIV coinfected patients should avoid consuming alcohol; offer vaccinations against hepatitis A and hepatitis B as appropriate.
• That GI complaints resolve after 2-3 wk of treatment
• To take at the same time of day to maintain blood level; not to crush, break, or chew
• That product controls the symptoms of HIV but does not cure; that patient is still able to infect others, that other products may be necessary to prevent other infections
• **Lactic acidosis:** to notify prescriber if fatigue, muscle aches/pains, abdominal pain, difficulty breathing, nausea, vomiting, change in heart rhythm occurs
• **Hepatotoxicity:** to notify prescriber of dark urine, yellowing skin or eyes, clay-colored stools, anorexia, nausea, vomiting
• To report suspected or planned pregnancy, not to breastfeed

---

RARELY USED

enalapril/enalaprilat (Rx)

(e-nal′a-pril)/(e-nal′a-pril-at)

Epaned, Vasotec, Vasotec IV ♦
Func. class.: Antihypertensive
Chem. class.: Angiotensin-converting enzyme (ACE) inhibitor

Do not confuse:
enalapril/ramipril/Anafranil/Eldepryl

ACTION: Selectively suppresses renin-angiotensin-aldosterone system; inhibits ACE; prevents conversion of angiotensin I to angiotensin II, dilation of arterial, venous vessels

USES: Hypertension, HF, left ventricular dysfunction

Unlabeled uses: Diabetic nephropathy, hypertensive emergency/urgency, post-MI, proteinuria, renal crisis in scleroderma

CONTRAINDICATIONS: Hypersensitivity, history of angioedema

Black Box Warning: Pregnancy

Precautions: Breastfeeding, renal disease, hyperkalemia, hepatic failure, dehydration, bilateral renal artery/aortic stenosis

DOSAGE AND ROUTES
Hypertension
• **Adult:** PO 2.5-5 mg/day, may increase or decrease to desired response, range 10-40 mg/day in 1-2 divided doses; IV 0.625-1.25 mg q6hr over 5 min
• **Child:** PO 0.08 mg/kg/day in 1-2 divided doses, max 0.58 mg/kg/day
• **Child:** IV 5-10 mcg/kg/dose q8-24hr

Heart failure
• **Adult:** PO 2.5-20 mg/day in 2 divided doses, max 40 mg/day in divided doses

Left ventricular cardiac dysfunction, asymptomatic
• **Adult:** PO 2.5 mg bid, titrate to max 10 mg bid, as tolerated; diuretic dose may require adjustment; monitor for ≥2 hr for hypotension

Renal disease
• **Adult:** PO 2.5 mg/day (CCr <30 mL/min), increase gradually; IV CCr >30 mL/min, 1.25 mg q6hr; CCr <30 mL/min, 0.625 mg as one-time dose, increase as per B/P
• **Child >1 mo:** PO/IV CCr <30 mL/min contraindicated

Hypertensive emergency/urgency (unlabeled)
• **Adult:** IV 1.25-5 mg q6hr

Available forms: *Enalapril:* tabs 2.5, 5, 10, 20 mg; oral solution 1 mg/mL; *enalaprilat:* inj 1.25 mg/mL

Administer:
PO route
• Tab may be crushed, given without regard to meals
Oral solution: May be used in those unable to swallow tabs
IV route
• Prepare in sterile environment using aseptic technique
• Dilute each dose with ≤50 mL compatible sol
• For 25 mcg/mL dilution often used for neonatal or pediatric patients, combine 1 mL enalaprilat 1.25 mg/mL and 49 mL compatible sol for IV
IV, Direct/Intermittent IV INFUSION route
• Undiluted over ≥5 min, use diluent provided or 50 mL D$_5$W, 0.9% NaCl, 0.9% NaCl in D$_5$W or LR, Isolyte E; give through Y-tube of free-flowing infusion of 0.9% NaCl, D$_5$W, LR, Isolyte E

Y-site compatibilities: Acyclovir, alemtuzumab, alfentanil, allopurinol, amifostine, amikacin, aminophylline, amphotericin B liposome, anidulafungin, ascorbic acid, atracurium, atropine, azaTHIOprine, aztreonam, benztropine, bivalirudin, bretylium, bumetanide, buprenorphine, butorphanol, calcium chloride/gluconate, CARBOplatin, ceFAZolin, cefonicid, cefotaxime, cefoTEtan, cefOXitin, cefTAZidime, ceftizoxime, cefTRIAXone, cefuroxime, chloramphenicol, cimetidine, cisatracurium, cladribine, clindamycin, cyanocobalamin, cyclophosphamide, cycloSPORINE, cytarabine, DACTINomycin, DAPTOmycin, dexamethasone, dexmedetomidine, dextran 40, digoxin, diltiazem, diphenhydrAMINE, DOBUTamine, DOCEtaxel, DOPamine, doripenem, doxacurium, DOXOrubicin, DOXOrubicin liposome, doxycycline, ePHEDrine, EPINEPHrine, epirubicin, epoetin, ertapenem, erythromycin, esmolol, etoposide, etoposide phosphate, famotidine, fenoldopam, fentaNYL, filgrastim, fluconazole, fludarabine, fluorouracil, folic acid, furosemide, ganciclovir, gemcitabine, gentamicin, granisetron, heparin, hydrocortisone, HYDROmorphone, ifosfamide, imipenem-cilastatin, indomethacin, insulin, isoproterenol, ketorolac, labetalol, levofloxacin, lidocaine, linezolid, LORazepam, magnesium sulfate, mannitol, mechlorethamine, melphalan, meperidine, meropenem, metaraminol, methicillin, methotrexate, methoxamine, methyldopate, methylPREDNISolone, metoclopramide, metoprolol, metroNIDAZOLE, mezlocillin, miconazole, midazolam, milrinone, minocycline, mitoXANtrone, morphine, moxalactam, multiple vitamin injection, nafcillin, nalbuphine, naloxone, netilmicin, niCARdipine, nitroglycerin, nitroprusside, norepinephrine, octreotide, ondansetron, oxacillin, oxaliplatin, oxytocin, PACLitaxel, palonosetron, papaverine, PEMEtrexed, penicillin G potassium, pentamidine, pentazocine, PENTobarbital, PHENobarbital, phentolamine, phenylephrine, phytonadione, piperacillin-tazobactam, potassium chloride/phosphate, procainamide, prochlorperazine, promethazine, propofol, propranolol, protamine, pyridoxime, quinupristin-dalfopristin, ranitidine, remifentanil, ritodrine, riTUXimab, rocuronium, sodium acetate, sodium bicarbonate, succinylcholine, SUFentanil, tacrolimus, teniposide, tetracycline, theophylline, thiamine, thiotepa, ticarcillin/clavulanate, tigecycline, tirofiban, tobramycin, tolazoline, trastuzumab, trimetaphan, urokinase, vancomycin, vasopressin, vecuronium, verapamil, vinCRIStine, vinorelbine, voriconazole, zoledronic acid

SIDE EFFECTS
CNS: *Insomnia, dizziness,* paresthesias, headache, fatigue, anxiety
CV: *Hypotension,* chest pain, tachycardia, dysrhythmias, syncope, angina, MI, orthostatic hypotension
EENT: *Tinnitus;* visual changes; sore throat; double vision; dry, burning eyes
GI: Nausea, vomiting, colitis, cramps, diarrhea, constipation, flatulence, dry mouth, loss of taste, hepatotoxicity
GU: Proteinuria, renal failure, increased frequency of polyuria or oliguria

---

Side effects: *italics* = common; red = life-threatening

HEMA: Agranulocytosis, neutropenia
INTEG: Rash, purpura, alopecia, hyperhidrosis, photosensitivity
META: Hyperkalemia
RESP: Dyspnea, dry cough, crackles
SYST: Toxic epidermal necrolysis, Stevens-Johnson syndrome, angioedema

PHARMACOKINETICS
• **Enalapril: PO:** Onset 1 hr, peak 4-6 hr, duration ≥24 hr
• **Enalaprilat: IV:** Onset 5-15 min, peak up to 4 hr, duration 4-6 hr, half-life 35 hr, metabolized by liver to active metabolite, excreted in urine

INTERACTIONS
Increase: hypersensitivity—allopurinol
Increase: hypotension—diuretics, other antihypertensives, phenothiazines, nitrates, acute alcohol ingestion, general anesthesia
Increase: potassium levels—salt substitutes, potassium-sparing diuretics, potassium supplements, cycloSPORINE, NSAIDs
Increase: levels of lithium, digoxin
Decrease: effects of enalapril—antacids, rifampin

Drug/Lab Test
Increase: ALT, AST, bilirubin, alk phos, glucose, uric acid, BUN, creatine
False positive: ANA titer

NURSING CONSIDERATIONS
Assess:
• **Bone marrow depression (rare):** neutrophils, decreased platelets; WBC with differential baseline, q3mo; if neutrophils <1000/mm³, discontinue treatment (recommended with collagen-vascular disease)
• **Hypertension:** B/P, peak/trough level, orthostatic hypotension, syncope when used with diuretic, pulse; note rate, rhythm, quality
• Baselines of renal, hepatic studies before therapy begins and 1 wk into therapy; electrolytes: potassium, sodium, chloride during 1st 2 wk of therapy; those with impaired renal function should be monitored for hyperkalemia
• Symptoms of heart failure: edema, dyspnea, wet crackles, weight gain, jugular venous distention, difficulty breathing

• **Serious skin disorders, angioedema:** black patients are more likely to develop angioedema; also, product is less effective; if skin rash occurs, stop product, notify prescriber

Black Box Warning: **Pregnancy:** identify whether pregnancy is planned or suspected or if breastfeeding

Evaluate:
• Therapeutic response: decreased B/P
Teach patient/family:
• Not to use OTC (cough, cold, or allergy) products unless directed by prescriber; to avoid potassium, salt substitutes
• To avoid sunlight or wear sunscreen for photosensitivity
• To comply with dosage schedule even if feeling better
• To notify prescriber of mouth sores, sore throat, fever, swelling of hands or feet, irregular heartbeat, chest pain, signs of angioedema, trouble breathing
• That excessive perspiration, dehydration, vomiting, diarrhea may lead to fall in blood pressure; to consult prescriber if these occur, maintain adequate hydration
• That product may cause dizziness, fainting; that light-headedness may occur during 1st few days of therapy, avoid activities requiring coordination
• That product may cause skin rash, impaired perspiration, or angioedema; to discontinue if angioedema occurs
• Not to discontinue product abruptly
• To rise slowly to sitting or standing position to minimize orthostatic hypotension
• **Hypertension:** continue with regimen to decrease B/P, exercise, cessation of smoking, decreasing stress, diet modification

Black Box Warning: **Pregnancy:** to notify prescriber if pregnancy is planned or suspected; to use contraception during treatment; not to breastfeed

TREATMENT OF OVERDOSE:
Lavage, IV atropine for bradycardia, IV theophylline for bronchospasm, digoxin, O₂, diuretic for cardiac failure

⚠ HIGH ALERT

RARELY USED

enasidenib
(en'-a-sid'-a-nib)
IDHIFA
Func. class.: Antineoplastic

USES: Relapsed or refractory acute myeloid leukemia (AML) with IDH2 mutation

DOSAGE AND ROUTES
• **Adult: PO:** 100 mg/day until disease progression. Treat those without disease progression for a minimum of 6 mo to allow time for clinical response

⚠ HIGH ALERT

RARELY USED

encorafenib
(en'-kor-a'-feh-nib)
Braftovi
Func. class.: Antineoplastic

USES: Treatment of unresectable or metastatic melanoma in patients with BRAF V600E or V600K mutations, in combination with binimetinib

CONTRAINDICATIONS: Hypersensitivity

DOSAGE AND ROUTES
• **Adult: PO** 450 mg daily with binimetinib **PO** 45 mg bid until disease progression

enfuvirtide (Rx)
(en-fyoo'vir-tide)
Fuzeon
Func. class.: Antiretroviral
Chem. class.: Fusion inhibitor

ACTION: Inhibitor of the fusion of HIV-1 with CD4+ cells

USES: Treatment of HIV-1 infection in combination with other antiretrovirals in those who are treatment experienced only
Unlabeled uses: HIV prophylaxis after occupational exposure

CONTRAINDICATIONS: Breastfeeding, hypersensitivity
Precautions: Pregnancy, children <6 yr, liver disease, myelosuppression, infections

DOSAGE AND ROUTES
• **Adult: SUBCUT** 90 mg (1 mL) bid
• **Child 6-16 yr and <42.6 kg: SUBCUT** 2 mg/kg bid, max 90 mg bid; **11-15.5 kg** 27 mg/0.3 mL bid; **15.6-20 kg** 36 mg/0.4 mL bid; **20.1-24.5 kg** 45 mg/0.5 mL bid; **24.6-29 kg** 54 mg/0.6 mL bid; **29.1-33.5 kg** 63 mg/0.7 mL bid; **33.6-38 kg** 72 mg/0.8 mL bid; **38.1-42.5 kg** 81 mg/0.9 mL bid
HIV prophylaxis (unlabeled)
• **Adult: SUBCUT** 90 mg bid added to PEP regimen
Available forms: Powder for inj, lyophilized 108 mg (90 mg/mL when reconstituted)
Administer:
SUBCUT route
• **Reconstitute** vial with 1.1 mL sterile water for inj; tap and roll to mix; allow to stand until completely dissolved, may take up to 45 min; after dissolved, immediately **inject** or refrigerate up to 24 hr
• Do not mix with other medications
• **SUBCUT:** Give bid, rotate sites; preferred sites: upper arm, anterior thigh, abdomen
• **Storage:** Use reconstituted product within 24 hr, refrigerated, let product come to room temperature before injecting

SIDE EFFECTS
CNS: Anxiety, peripheral neuropathy, taste disturbance, Guillain-Barré syndrome, insomnia, depression, fatigue, peripheral neuropathy
GI: Nausea, abdominal pain, anorexia, constipation, pancreatitis, dry mouth, weight loss

---

Side effects: *italics* = common; red = life-threatening

GU: Glomerulonephritis, renal failure
HEMA: Thrombocytopenia, neutropenia
INTEG: *Inj site reactions, skin papilloma*
MISC: Influenza, cough, conjunctivitis, lymphadenopathy, myalgia, hyperglycemia, bacterial pneumonia, rhinitis, fatigue, hypersensitivity

PHARMACOKINETICS

Peak 8 hr, terminal half-life 3.8 hr, well absorbed, undergoes catabolism, 92% protein binding

INTERACTIONS

Drug/Lab
Increase: LFTs, lipase, CK, triglycerides
Decrease: Hgb
Drug/Drug
Increase: effect of either product—protease inhibitor

NURSING CONSIDERATIONS

Assess:
• **Signs of infection, inj site reactions:** use analgesics; bacterial pneumonia may occur if blood counts are low or viral load is high or low CD4 counts, IV drug user, lung disease, smoker
• **Peripheral neuropathy:** may occur and last for several months, where nerves are close to the skin
• **Glomerulonephritis/renal failure:** BUN, creatinine, renal failure may occur
• Bowel pattern before, during treatment; if severe abdominal pain or constipation occurs, notify prescriber; monitor hydration
• **Hypersensitivity:** Skin eruptions, rash, urticaria, itching; assess allergies before treatment, reaction to each medication; may occur quickly or later after continued use
• **Immune reconstitution syndrome:** with combination theory
• **HIV:** CBC, blood chemistry, plasma HIV RNA, absolute CD4+/CD8+ cell counts/%, serum β_2 microglobulin, serum ICD+24 antigen levels, cholesterol
• **Pregnancy/breastfeeding:** identify if pregnancy is planned or suspected, if breastfeeding; if pregnant, register with the Antiretroviral Pregnancy Registry, 800-258-4263

Evaluate:
• Therapeutic response: increased CD4 cell counts; decreased viral load; slowing progression of HIV-1 infection
Teach patient/family:
• That pneumonia may occur; to contact prescriber if cough, fever occur
• That hypersensitive reactions may occur; rash, pruritus; to stop product, contact prescriber
• That product is not a cure for HIV-1 infection but controls symptoms; HIV-1 can still be transmitted to others; that product is to be used in combination only with other antiretrovirals
• How to prepare and give using subcut inj, watch for site reactions, rotate sites; if more information is needed, call 877-438-9366
• To notify prescriber if pregnancy is suspected; not to breastfeed

---

⚠ HIGH ALERT

enoxaparin (Rx)

(ee-nox′a-par-in)
Lovenox
Func. class.: Anticoagulant, antithrombotic
Chem. class.: Low-molecular-weight heparin (LMWH)

Do not confuse:
enoxaparin/enoxacin
Lovenox/Lotronex

ACTION: Binds to antithrombin III inactivating factors Xa/IIa, thereby resulting in a higher ratio of anti–factor Xa to IIa

USES: Prevention of DVT (inpatient or outpatient), PE (inpatient) in hip and knee replacement, abdominal surgery at risk for thrombosis; unstable angina, acute MI, coronary artery thrombosis
Unlabeled uses: Antiphospholipid antibody syndrome, arterial thromboembolism prophylaxis, cerebral thromboembolism, percutaneous coronary intervention

CONTRAINDICATIONS: Hypersensitivity to this product, heparin, pork; active major bleeding, hemophilia, leukemia with bleeding, thrombocytopenic purpura, heparin-induced thrombocytopenia

Precautions: Pregnancy, breastfeeding, children, geriatric patients, low-weight men (<57 kg), women (<45 kg), severe renal/hepatic disease, severe hypertension, subacute bacterial endocarditis, acute nephritis, recent burn, spinal surgery, indwelling catheters, hypersensitivity to benzyl alcohol

Black Box Warning: Lumbar puncture, aneurysm, coagulopathy, epidural anesthesia, spinal anesthesia

DOSAGE AND ROUTES
DVT prevention before hip or knee surgery
• **Adult:** SUBCUT 30 mg bid given 12-24 hr postop for 7-10 days
DVT prevention before hip replacement
• **Adult:** SUBCUT 40 mg/day started 9-12 hr preop or 30 mg q12hr started 12-24 hr postop
DVT prophylaxis before abdominal surgery
• **Adult:** SUBCUT 40 mg/day starting 24 hr before surgery × 7-12 days
Treatment of DVT or PE
• **Adult:** SUBCUT 1 mg/kg q12hr (without PE, outpatient); 1 mg/kg q12hr or 1.5 mg/kg/day (with or without PE, inpatient); warfarin should be started within 72 hr, continued ≥5 days until INR is 2-3 (at least 3 days)
Prevention of ischemic complications in unstable angina or non–Q-wave MI/non-ST
• **Adult:** SUBCUT/IV 1 mg/kg q12hr until stable with aspirin 100-325 mg/day
Acute MI with S-T segment elevation
• **Adult/geriatric <75 yr:** IV/SUBCUT 30 mg IV BOL plus 1 mg/kg SUBCUT, then 1 mg/kg SUBCUT q12hr, max 100 mg for first 2 doses only

• **Geriatric ≥75 yr:** SUBCUT 0.75 mg/kg q12hr, max 75 mg for first 2 doses only
Renal dose
• **Adult:** SUBCUT CCr <30 mL/min: 30 mg daily **(thrombosis prophylaxis in abdominal surgery, hip or knee replacement surgery, during acute illness);** 1 mg/kg daily **(concurrently with aspirin to treat unstable angina or non-Q-wave MI);** 1 mg/kg daily **(STEMI in those ≥75 yr),** 30 mg IV bolus plus 1 mg/kg SC, then 1 mg/kg daily **(STEMI in those <75 yr),** or 1 mg/kg daily **(concurrently with warfarin for inpatient or outpatient treatment of acute deep vein thrombosis with or without pulmonary embolism)**

Available forms: Prefilled syringes 30 mg/0.3 mL, 40 mg/0.4 mL; graduated prefilled syringes 60 mg/0.6 mL, 80 mg/0.8 mL, 100 mg/1 mL, 120 mg/0.8 mL, 150 mg/mL; multidose vials 100 mg/mL (3 mL)

Administer:
• Only after screening patient for bleeding disorders
• Do not mix with other products or infusion fluids
• Only this product when ordered; not interchangeable with heparin or other LMWHs
• At same time each day to maintain steady blood levels
• Avoid all IM inj that may cause bleeding
• Prepare in a sterile environment using aseptic technique
SUBCUT route
• Do not give IM; begin 1 hr before surgery; do not aspirate; rotate sites; do not expel bubble from syringe before administration
• To recumbent patient, give SUBCUT; rotate inj sites (left/right anterolateral, left/right posterolateral abdominal wall)
• Insert whole length of needle into skin fold held with thumb and forefinger
• If withdrawing from multidose vial, use TB syringe for proper measurement
• Prefilled syringes (30, 40 mg) not graduated; do not use for partial doses
• Do not administer if particulate is present; do not use products with benzyl alcohol in pregnant women

---

Side effects: *italics* = common; red = life-threatening

Direct IV route
- Use multidose vial for IV administration; use TB syringe, other graduated syringe to measure dose; give IV BOL through IV line, flush before and after
- Dilution may be stored for up to 4 wk in glass vial at room temperature, up to 2 wk in TB syringes with rubber stoppers at room temperature or refrigerated

SIDE EFFECTS
CNS: Fever, confusion, dizziness, headache
GI: Nausea, vomiting, constipation
HEMA: Hemorrhage from any site, hypochromic anemia, thrombocytopenia, bleeding
INTEG: Ecchymosis, inj site hematoma, alopecia, pruritus, rash
META: Hyperkalemia in renal failure
MS: Osteoporosis
SYST: Edema, peripheral edema, angioedema, anaphylaxis

PHARMACOKINETICS
SUBCUT: 90% absorbed, maximum antithrombin activity (3-5 hr), duration 12 hr half-life $4^1/_2$ hr, excreted in urine

INTERACTIONS
Increase: enoxaparin action—anticoagulants, salicylates, NSAIDs, antiplatelets, thrombolytics, RU-486, SSRIs; monitor INR/PT
Drug/Lab Test
Increase: AST, ALT
Decrease: platelet count
Drug/Herb
Increase: bleeding risk—feverfew, garlic, ginger, ginkgo, green tea, horse chestnut

NURSING CONSIDERATIONS
Assess:
- Monitor anti-factor Xa activity in chronic therapy (renal disease)
- Blood studies (Hct/Hgb, CBC, coagulation studies, platelets [for HIT], occult blood in stools), anti–factor Xa (should be checked 4 hr after inj); thrombocytopenia may occur; PT, PTT is not needed in those with adequate coagulation; discontinue use and notify prescriber if platelets <100,000/mm^3
- Renal studies: BUN/creatinine baseline and periodically

- **Bleeding:** gums, petechiae, ecchymosis, black tarry stools, hematuria; notify prescriber
- **Anaphylaxis, angioedema:** monitor for rash, swelling of face, lips, tongue, dyspnea; stop product, initiate emergency procedures
- **Neurologic status:** those with epidural catheters are at greater chance for impairments
- Injection-site reactions: inflammation, redness, hematomas

Black Box Warning: Neurologic symptoms in patients who have received spinal anesthesia, may develop spinal hematoma; those who have had trauma, spinal surgery are at greater risk

- **Beers:** reduce dose in older adults; increased bleeding risk, or if CCr <30 mL/min
- **Pregnancy/breastfeeding:** do not use in multidose vials, benzyl alcohol is present; do not breastfeed
Evaluate:
- Therapeutic response: prevention of DVT/PE
Teach patient/family:
- **Spinal anesthesia:** to report numbness, weakness in lower extremities
- To use soft-bristle toothbrush to avoid bleeding gums; to use electric razor
- To report any signs of bleeding: gums, under skin, urine, stools; do not rub injection site, easy bruising
- To report dizziness, rash, breathing changes
- To avoid OTC products containing aspirin, NSAIDs unless approved by prescriber; not to start any Rx, OTC, supplements, or herbal products unless approved by prescriber

---

RARELY USED

entacapone (Rx)
(en'ta-kah-pone)
Comtan
Func. class.: Antiparkinson agent
Chem. class.: COMT inhibitor

🔬 Genetic warning

USES: Parkinson's disease for those experiencing end-of-dose, decreased effect as adjunct to levodopa/carbidopa

CONTRAINDICATIONS: Hypersensitivity

DOSAGE AND ROUTES

• **Adult:** PO 200 mg given with carbidopa/levodopa, max 1600 mg/day; may allow for 25% dosage reduction in levodopa therapy

---

entecavir (Rx)

(en-te′ka-veer)

Baraclude

Func. class.: Antiviral

Chem. class.: Nucleoside analog

ACTION: Inhibits hepatitis B virus DNA polymerase by competing with natural substrates and by causing DNA termination after its incorporation into viral DNA; causes viral DNA death

USES: Chronic hepatitis B (HBV)

CONTRAINDICATIONS: Hypersensitivity

Precautions: Pregnancy, breastfeeding, children, geriatric patients, severe renal disease, liver transplant

Black Box Warning: Hepatic disease, hepatitis, HIV, lactic acidosis

DOSAGE AND ROUTES
Chronic hepatitis B (nucleoside treatment naive)

• **Adult and adolescent ≥16 yr:** PO Tab 0.5 mg/day

• **Adult:** PO (solution) 0.5 mg q day; **Child/adolescent ≥2 yr >30 kg:** 0.5 mg (10 mL) q day; **Child ≥2 yr, 27 to 30 kg:** 0.45 mg (9 mL) q day; **Child ≥2 yr, 24 to 26 kg:** 0.4 mg (8 mL) q day; **Child ≥2 yr, 21 to 23 kg:** 0.35 mg (7 mL) q day; **Child ≥2 yr, 18 to 20 kg:** 0.3 mg (6 mL) q day; **Child ≥2 yr, 15 to 17 kg:** 0.25 mg (5 mL) q day; **Child**

≥2 yr, 12 to 14 kg: 0.2 mg (4 mL) q day; **Child ≥2 yr,** 0.15 mg (3 mL) q day
Chronic hepatitis B with compensated liver disease

• **Adult/adolescent ≥16 yr:** PO Tab 1 mg/day

• **Adult:** PO (solution) 1 mg/day; **Child/adolescent ≥2 yr, >30 kg:** 1 mg (20 mL) q day; **Child ≥2 yr, 27 to 30 kg:** 0.9 mg (18 mL) q day; **Child ≥2 yr, 24 to 26 kg:** 0.8 mg (16 mL) q day; **Child ≥2 yr, 21 to 23 kg:** 0.7 mg (14 mL); **Child ≥2 yr, 18 to 20 kg:** 0.6 mg (12 mL) q day; **Child ≥2 yr, 15 to 17 kg:** 0.5 mg (10 mL) q day; **Child ≥2 yr, 12 to 14 kg:** 0.4 mg (8 mL) q day; **Child ≥2 yr, 10 to 11 kg:** 0.3 mg (6 mL) q day
Renal dose

• **Adult/child >16 yr:** PO CCr ≥50 mL/min, 0.5 mg/day; CCr 30-49 mL/min, 0.25 mg/day, 0.5 mg/day or 1 mg q48hr for lamiVUDine-refractory patient; CCr 10-29 mL/min, 0.15/day or 1 mg q72hr for lamiVUDine-refractory patient; CCr <10 mL/min, 0.05 mg/day, 0.1 mg/day or 1 mg q7day for lamiVUDine-refractory patient

• **Child 2-<16 yr:** PO (dosage based on weight) **10-11 kg:** 0.15 mg once daily (0.3 mg once daily if history of lamiVUDine resistance) **>11-14 kg:** 0.2 mg once daily (0.4 mg once daily if history of lamiVUDine resistance) **>14-17 kg:** 0.25 mg once daily (0.5 mg once daily if history of lamiVUDine resistance) **>17-20 kg:** 0.3 mg once daily (0.6 mg once daily if history of lamiVUDine resistance) **>20-23 kg:** 0.35 mg once daily (0.7 mg once daily if history of lamiVUDine resistance) **>23-26 kg:** 0.4 mg once daily (0.8 mg once daily if history of lamiVUDine resistance) **>26-30 kg:** 0.45 mg once daily (0.9 mg once daily if history of lamiVUDine resistance) **>30 kg:** 0.5 mg once daily (1 mg once daily if history of lamiVUDine resistance)

Available forms: Tabs, film coated 0.5, 1 mg; oral sol 0.05 mg/mL
Administer:

• After hemodialysis

• By mouth on empty stomach 2 hr before or after food

• Store at room temperature
• **Oral solution:** use calibrated oral dosing spoon provided; may be used interchangeably with tabs, do not dilute

SIDE EFFECTS
CNS: *Headache,* fatigue, dizziness, insomnia
ENDO: Hyperglycemia
GI: *Dyspepsia,* nausea, vomiting, diarrhea, elevated liver function enzymes
INTEG: Alopecia, rash
SYST: Lactic acidosis, severe hepatomegaly with steatosis

PHARMACOKINETICS
Peak 0.5-1.5 hr, steady state 6-10 days, 100% bioavailability, extensively distributed to tissues, protein binding 13%, terminal half-life 128-149 hr duration up to 24 hr, excreted unchanged (62%-73%) via kidneys

INTERACTIONS
Drug/Food
Decrease: absorption—high-fat meal
Drug/Lab Test
Increase: ALT, AST, total bilirubin, amylase, lipase, creatinine, blood glucose, urine glucose
Decrease: platelets, albumin

NURSING CONSIDERATIONS
Assess:
• **For nephrotoxicity:** increasing CCr, BUN

Black Box Warning: **For HIV** before beginning treatment because HIV resistance may occur in chronic hepatitis B patients; monitor HIV RNA; don't use in those with HIV and HBV unless receiving antiretroviral treatment for both

Black Box Warning: **For lactic acidosis and severe hepatomegaly with stenosis;** increased serum lactate, increased hepatic enzymes; discontinue if present, discontinue if signs occur; may be fatal

• Geriatric patients more carefully; may develop renal, cardiac symptoms more rapidly

Black Box Warning: **For exacerbations of hepatitis** (jaundice, pruritus, fatigue), anorexia after discontinuing treatment, and for several months monitor LFTs

• **Pregnancy/breastfeeding:** use if clearly needed; register pregnant women at the Antiretroviral Pregnancy Registry at 1-800-258-4263; to reduce risk of postnatal transmission, HIV-infected mothers are advised to avoid breastfeeding
Evaluate:
• Therapeutic response: decreased symptoms of chronic hepatitis B, improving LFTs
Teach patient/family:
• Not to take with food; to take 2 hr before or after meals
• To take exactly as prescribed, to read the "Patient Information," to take missed dose when remembered unless close to time of next dose; that compliance with dosage schedule is required; not to share product
• Not to stop medication without approval of prescriber
• That optimal duration of treatment is unknown
• To avoid use with other medications, supplements unless approved by prescriber
• To notify prescriber of decreased urinary output, blood in urine

Black Box Warning: **Symptoms of lactic acidosis:** muscle pain, severe tiredness, weakness, trouble breathing, stomach pain with nausea/vomiting, coldness in arms/legs, fast/irregular heartbeat, dizziness

Black Box Warning: **Symptoms of hepatotoxicity**: eyes/skin turning yellow, dark urine, light-colored bowel movements, no appetite for days, nausea, stomach pain; may be worsened after discontinuing treatment

• That product does not cure but lowers amount of HBV in body
• That product does not stop spread of HBV to others by sex, sharing needles, or being exposed to blood

• Not to breastfeed; to notify prescriber if pregnancy is planned or suspected

• Not to operate machinery until effect is known, dizziness may occur

• That regular follow-up and lab tests will be needed

RARELY USED

enzalutamide
(en-zal-u′ta-mide)

Xtandi

Func. class.: Antineoplastic hormone
Chem. class.: Nonsteroidal antiandrogen

USES: Metastatic, castration-resistant prostate cancer in those who have received DOCEtaxel

CONTRAINDICATIONS: Pregnancy, women, hypersensitivity

DOSAGE AND ROUTES
• **Adult:** PO 160 mg (4 × 40-mg caps) daily. If a patient experiences a grade 3 or higher toxicity or an intolerable adverse effect, withhold dosing for 1 wk or until symptoms improve to grade 2 or less, then resume at the same or a reduced dosage (120 or 80 mg), if warranted

• The concomitant use of strong CYP2C8 give 80 mg once daily; CYP3A4 inducers 240 mg daily

---

epinastine (ophthalmic)
(ep-ih-nas′teen)

Elestat

Func. class.: Antihistamine (ophthalmic)
Chem. class.: Histamine 1 receptor antagonist/mast cell stabilizer

ACTION: A topically active, direct H₁-receptor antagonist and mast cell stabilizer; by reducing these inflammatory mediators, it relieves the ocular pruritus associated with allergic conjunctivitis

USES: Prevention of ocular pruritus associated with signs and symptoms of allergic conjunctivitis

CONTRAINDICATIONS: Hypersensitivity
Precautions: Pregnancy, breastfeeding, children, contact lenses

DOSAGE AND ROUTES
• **Adult/child ≥3 yr: OPHTH** Instill 1 drop in each eye bid
Available forms: Ophthalmic sol 0.5%
Administer:
Ophthalmic route
• For topical ophthalmic use only

• The preservative benzalkonium chloride may be absorbed by soft contact lenses; wait ≥10 min after instilling the ophthalmic solution before inserting contact lenses; contact lenses should not be worn if eye is red

• Do not share ophthalmic drops with others

• Keep bottle tightly closed when not in use

• Treatment should be continued throughout the period of exposure (i.e., until the pollen season is over or until exposure to the offending allergen is terminated), even when symptoms are absent

SIDE EFFECTS
EENT: *Ocular irritation*, folliculosis, hyperemia, ocular pruritus
MISC: *Infection (including cold symptoms and upper respiratory infections)*, headache, rhinitis, sinusitis, increased cough, pharyngitis

PHARMACOKINETICS
Onset 3-5 min, peak 2 hr, duration 8 hr

NURSING CONSIDERATIONS
Assess:
• Eyes: for itching, redness, use of soft or hard contact lenses
Evaluate:
• Therapeutic response: absence of redness, itching in the eyes

---

Side effects: *italics* = common; red = life-threatening

Teach patient/family:
Ophthalmic route

• Product is for topical ophthalmic use only
• Wash hands before and after use; tilt the head back slightly and pull the lower eyelid down with the index finger; squeeze the prescribed number of drops into the conjunctival sac and gently close eyes for 1-2 min; do not blink
• Do not touch the tip of the dropper to the eye, fingertips, or other surface
• Wait ≥10 min after instilling the ophthalmic solution before inserting contact lenses; contact lenses should not be worn if eye is red
• Keep bottle tightly closed when not in use
• Do not share ophthalmic drops with others
• Remove contact lenses before use because the preservative benzalkonium chloride may be absorbed by soft contact lenses; product should not be used to treat contact lens–related irritation

---

⚠ HIGH ALERT

EPINEPHrine (Rx)
(ep-i-nef'rin)
Adrenaclick, Adrenalin, Allerjet ✤,
Auvi-Q, Anapen ✤, Anapen Jr. ✤,
EpiPen, EpiPen Jr.
Func. class.: Bronchodilator nonselective adrenergic agonist, vasopressor
Chem. class.: Catecholamine

Do not confuse:
EPINEPHrine/ePHEDrine

ACTION: β_1- and β_2-agonist causing increased levels of cAMP, thereby producing bronchodilation, cardiac, and CNS stimulation; high doses cause vasoconstriction via α-receptors; low doses can cause vasodilation via β_2-vascular receptors

USES: Acute asthmatic attacks, hemostasis, bronchospasm, anaphylaxis, allergic reactions, cardiac arrest, adjunct in anesthesia, shock

Unlabeled uses: Bradycardia, chloroquine overdose

CONTRAINDICATIONS: Hypersensitivity to sympathomimetics, sulfites, closed-angle glaucoma, nonanaphylactic shock during general anesthesia
Precautions: Pregnancy, breastfeeding, cardiac disorders, hyperthyroidism, diabetes mellitus, prostatic hypertrophy, hypertension, organic brain syndrome, local anesthesia of certain areas, labor, cardiac dilation, coronary insufficiency, cerebral arteriosclerosis, organic heart disease

DOSAGE AND ROUTES
Anaphylaxis/severe asthma exacerbation
• **Adult: IM/SUBCUT** 0.3-0.5 mg, may repeat q10-15min (anaphylaxis) or q20min-4 hr (asthma)
Severe anaphylaxis
• **Adult: IV** 0.1-0.25 mg q5-15min, then 1-4 mcg/min continuous infusion if needed
• **Child: IV** ≤0.1 mcg/kg/min, then 0.1 mcg/kg/min continuous infusion if needed
Severe allergic reactions type I
• **Adult/child ≥30 kg: IM** 0.3 mg (EpiPen/EpiPen 2-Pak)
• **Child <30 kg: IM** 0.15 mg (EpiPen Jr/ EpiPen Jr 2-Pak)
CPR (ACLS)
• **Adult: IV** 1 mg q3-5min
Bradycardia (ACLS)
• **Adult: IV** 2-10 mcg/min
Bradycardia/pulseless arrest (PALS)
• **Child: IV** 0.01 mg/kg may repeat q3-5min, may increase to 0.1-0.2 mg/kg if needed
Available forms: Nasal spray (sol) 1 mg/mL; **sol for inj** 1 mg/mL (1:1000); 0.1 mg/mL (1:10,000); inh vapor (sol) 0.22 mg/actuation; pressurized inh (sol) 0.22 mg/actuation; sol for inj 0.15 mg/0.15 mL autoinjector, 0.3 mg/0.3 mL autoinjector, 0.15 mg/0.3 mL
Administer:
• Increased dose of insulin for diabetic patients if glucose is elevated
• Check for correct concentrations, route, dosage before administering

---

• Give subcut, IM, intraosseously, IV; suspensions are for subcut use only; do not give IV

• Visually inspect parenteral products for particulate matter and discoloration before use; do not use sols that are pinkish to brownish or that contain a precipitate

• Avoid extravasation during parenteral administration; if extravasation occurs, infiltrate the affected area with phentolamine diluted in NS

• Death has occurred from drug errors; make sure the right concentration is used

• Store reconstituted sol refrigerated ≤24 hr

Inhalation route

• Place in nebulizer (10 drops of a 1% base sol)

• Dilute racepinephrine 2.25% sol

IM route

• Give in the deltoid or anterior thigh (vastus lateralis); do not administer into the gluteal muscle, may give through clothing in emergency

SUBCUT route

• Inject, taking care not to inject intradermally; massage injection site well after use to enhance absorption and to decrease local vasoconstriction; injection can cause tissue irritation

Intraosseous INFUSION route (unlabeled)

• During CPR, the same EPINEPHrine dosage may be given via the intraosseous route when IV access is not available

Intracardiac route

• Intracardiac route should be reserved for extreme emergencies; intracardiac injection should only be performed by properly trained medical personnel

Endotracheal route

• Per the ACLS or PALS guidelines, the EPINEPHrine parenteral product is administered via endotracheal (ET) route; ET administration should only be used if access to IV or intraosseous routes is not possible

• **Adult:** Dilute dose in 5-10 mL of NS or sterile distilled water; administer via ET tube; endotracheal absorption of EPINEPHrine may be improved by diluting with water instead of NS

• **Child:** After dose administration, flush the ET tube with a minimum of 5 mL NS

Direct IV INJ route

• 1:10,000 solution can be given directly without diluting: dilute 1:1000 (1 mg/0.9 mL) 0.9% NaCL (1:1000 solution)

• Inject EPINEPHrine directly into a vein over 5-10 min for adults or 1-3 min for children; may be given IV push in cardiac arrest

• In neonates, may administer via the umbilical vein

During adult cardiopulmonary resuscitation (CPR):

• Resuscitation drugs may be given IV by bolus injection into a peripheral vein, followed by an injection of 20 mL IV fluid; elevate the extremity for 10-20 sec to facilitate drug delivery to the central circulation

Continuous IV INFUSION route

• Dilute 1 mg EPINEPHrine in 250 or 500 mL of a compatible IV infusion sol to provide a concentration of 4 or 2 mcg/mL, respectively; give into a large vein, if possible; more-concentrated sols (16-32 mcg/mL) may be used in fluid-restricted patients when administered through a central line

Y-site compatibilities: Alfentanil, amikacin, amiodarone, amphotericin B liposome, anidulafungin, ascorbic acid, atracurium, atropine, aztreonam, benztropine, bivalirudin, bleomycin, bumetanide, buprenorphine, butorphanol, calcium chloride/gluconate, CARBOplatin, caspofungin, ceFAZolin, cefotaxime, cefoTEtan, cefOXitin, cefTAZidime, ceftizoxime, cefTRIAXone, cefuroxime, chloramphenicol, chlorproMAZINE, cimetidine, cisatracurium, CISplatin, clindamycin, cyanocobalamin, cyclophosphamide, cycloSPORINE, cytarabine, DACTINomycin, DAPTOmycin, dexamethasone, dexmedetomidine, digoxin, diltiazem, diphenhydrAMINE, DOBUTamine, DOCEtaxel, DOPamine, DOXOrubicin, doxycycline, enalaprilat, epirubicin, epoetin alfa, ertapenem, erythromycin, esmolol, etoposide, etoposide phosphate, famotidine, fenoldopam, fentaNYL, fluconazole,

Side effects: *italics* = common; red = life-threatening

fludarabine, folic acid, furosemide, gemcitabine, gentamicin, glycopyrrolate, granisetron, heparin, hydrocortisone, HYDROmorphone, ifosfamide, imipenem-cilastatin, isoproterenol, ketorolac, labetalol, levofloxacin, lidocaine, linezolid, LORazepam, magnesium sulfate, mannitol, mechlorethamine, meperidine, metaraminol, methicillin, methotrexate, methoxamine, methyldopa, methylPREDNISolone, metoclopramide, metoprolol, metroNIDAZOLE, midazolam, milrinone, minocycline, mitoXANtrone, morphine, multiple vitamins, nafcillin, nalbuphine, naloxone, niCARdipine, nitroglycerin, nitroprusside, norepinephrine, octreotide, ondansetron, oxacillin, oxaliplatin, oxytocin, PACLitaxel, palonosetron, pancuronium, pantoprazole, PEMEtrexed, penicillin G potassium, pentamidine, pentazocine, phentolamine, phenylephrine, phytonadione, piperacillin/tazobactam, potassium chloride, procainamide, prochlorperazine, promethazine, propofol, propranolol, protamine, pyridoxime, quinupristin/dalfopristin, ranitidine, remifentanil, ritodrine, rocuronium, sodium acetate, streptomycin, succinylcholine, SUFentanil, tacrolimus, teniposide, theophylline, thiamine, thiotepa, ticarcillin/clavulanate, tigecycline, tirofiban, tobramycin, tolazoline, trimethaphan, urokinase, vancomycin, vasopressin, vecuronium, verapamil, vinCRIStine, vinorelbine, vitamin B complex with C, voriconazole, warfarin, zoledronic acid

SIDE EFFECTS

CNS: *Tremors, anxiety,* insomnia, headache, *dizziness,* confusion, hallucinations, weakness, drowsiness
CV: *Palpitations, tachycardia,* hypertension, dysrhythmias, increased T wave
GI: *Anorexia, nausea, vomiting*
MISC: Sweating, dry eyes
RESP: *Dyspnea,* paradoxical bronchospasm (inhalation)
META: Hypoglycemia

PHARMACOKINETICS

Crosses placenta, metabolized in liver
IM: 6-10 min, duration 1-4 hr

SUBCUT: Onset 5-10 min, duration 20 min-4 hr
IV: Onset immediate, peak 20 min, duration 1-4 hr
INH: Onset 1-5 min, duration 1-3 hr

INTERACTIONS

• Do not use with MAOIs or tricyclics; hypertensive crisis may occur
• **Toxicity:** other sympathomimetics
Decrease: hypertensive effects—β-adrenergic blockers, stop β-blocker 3 days before starting product
Increase: hypotension—α-blockers
Increase: cardiac effects—antihistamines, thyroid replacement hormones
Increase: dysrhythmias—cardiac glycosides

Drug/Herb

• Increased stimulation: coffee, tea, guarana, yerba maté

NURSING CONSIDERATIONS

Assess:

• **Asthma:** auscultate lungs, pulse, B/P, respirations, sputum (color, character); monitor pulmonary function studies before and during treatment
• **Vasopressor:** ECG during administration continuously; if B/P increases, decrease dose; B/P, pulse q5min after parenteral route; CVP, ISVR, PCWP during infusion if possible; inadvertent high arterial B/P can result in angina, aortic rupture, cerebral hemorrhage
• Inj site: tissue sloughing; administer phentolamine with NS
• **Sulfite sensitivity;** may be life-threatening
• Cardiac status, I&O; blood glucose in diabetes
• **Allergic reactions, bronchospasms** (swelling of face/lips/eyelids, rash, difficulty breathing): withhold dose, notify prescriber

Evaluate:

• Therapeutic response: increased B/P with stabilization or ease of breathing, relief of bronchospasm

Teach patient/family:

• About the reason for product administration

- **Inhalation:** to rinse mouth after use to prevent dryness after inhalation, not to spray near eyes, teach correct use
- To take exactly as prescribed. If on scheduled regimen, take missed dose as soon as remembered. Space remaining doses evenly. Do not double doses. To contact prescriber immediately if shortness of breath is not relieved or diaphoresis, dizziness, or chest pain occurs
- To consult prescriber before taking any OTC, Rx medications, supplements or herbals
- To use bronchodilator before using other products
- To maintain adequate fluid intake (2000-3000 mL/day) to help liquefy secretions
- To notify prescriber if pregnancy is planned or suspected or if breastfeeding
- **Autoinjector:** how to use for anaphylaxis; remove cap, place injector end tip on thigh at 90-degree angle, hold 10 sec, remove
- **Pregnancy/breastfeeding:** Identify if pregnancy is planned or suspected or if breastfeeding

TREATMENT OF OVERDOSE: Administer α-blocker and β-blocker

EPINEPHrine nasal agent
See Appendix B

⚠ HIGH ALERT

epirubicin (Rx)
(ep-ih-roo′bi-sin)
Ellence, Pharmorubicin PFS ✦
Func. class.: Antineoplastic, antibiotic
Chem. class.: Anthracycline

Do not confuse:
epirubicin/eribulin/DOXOrubicin/ DAUNOrubicin/IDArubicin

ACTION: Inhibits DNA synthesis primarily; replication is decreased by binding to DNA, which causes strand splitting; maximum cytotoxic effects at S and for G_2 phases; a vesicant

USES: Adjuvant therapy for breast cancer with axillary node involvement after resection
Unlabeled uses: Used in combination for treatment of advanced forms of cancer: bladder, gastric, head and neck, hepatocellular, lung, ovarian, multiple myeloma, soft-tissue sarcoma

CONTRAINDICATIONS: Pregnancy, breastfeeding; hypersensitivity to product, anthracyclines, anthracenediones; baseline neutrophil count <1500 cells/mm³, severe myocardial insufficiency, recent MI, heart failure, cardiomyopathy

> **Black Box Warning:** Severe hepatic disease, IM/SUBCUT use

Precautions: Children, geriatric patients, cardiac/renal/hepatic disease, accidental exposure, angina, dental disease, herpes, hyperkalemia, hyperphosphatemia, hypertension, hyperuricemia, hypocalcemia, infection, infertility, tumor lysis syndrome, ventricular dysfunction, previous anthracycline use

> **Black Box Warning:** Bone marrow depression (severe), heart failure, extravasation, secondary malignancy, requires an experienced clinician

DOSAGE AND ROUTES
- **Adult: IV** 100 mg/m² on day 1 with fluorouracil and cyclophosphamide (FEC regimen) every 21 days × 6 cycles or 60 mg/m² on days 1 and 8 with oral cyclophosphamide and fluorouracil every 28 days × 6 cycles
Dosage adjustments based on hematologic and nonhematologic toxicities
- **Nadir platelet counts <50,000/ mm³, absolute neutrophil counts (ANC) <250/mm³, neutropenic fever,**

---

or grades 3/4 nonhematologic toxicities: Day 1 dose in subsequent cycles should be reduced by 25% of the previous dose

• For patients receiving divided-dose epirubicin (i.e., days 1 and 8): Day 8 dose should be reduced by 25% of the day 1 dose if the platelet counts are 75,000-100,000/mm^3 and the ANC is 1000-1499/mm^3; if day 8 platelet counts are <75,000/mm^3, ANC <1000/mm^3, or Grade 3/4 nonhematologic toxicity has occurred, omit the day 8 dose

Hepatic dose

• Adult: IV Bilirubin 1.2-3 mg/dL or AST 2-4 × normal upper limit, 50% of starting dose; bilirubin >3-5 mg/dL or AST >4 × normal upper limit, 25% of starting dose

Available forms: Solution for inj 2 mg/mL (250 mg/25 mL, 200 mg/100 mL)

Administer:

• Antiemetic 30-60 min before product to prevent vomiting

Black Box Warning: To be used by a clinician experienced in giving cytotoxic products

---

Black Box Warning: Do not use IM/SUBCUT because of severe tissue necrosis, give IV only, a vesicant; if extravasation occurs, stop and complete via another vein, preferably in another limb; avoid infusion into veins over joints or in extremities with compromised venous or lymphatic drainage

---

• Rapid injection can cause facial flushing or erythema along the vein; avoid administration time of <3 min

• Product should be given to those with neutrophils ≥1500/mm^3, platelet count ≥100,000/mm^3, and nonhematologic toxicities recovered to ≤grade 1

• When refrigerated, the preservative-free, ready-to-use solution can form a gelled product and will return to solution after 2-4 hr at room temperature

• Visually inspect for particulate matter and discoloration before use

IV route

• Double-check dose and product; fatalities have occurred with wrong dose or product

• Give antiinfectives before use of this product

• Use cytotoxic handling procedures; pregnant women must not handle product

• Reconstitute 50 mg and 200 mg powder for injection vials with 25 mL and 100 mL, respectively, of sterile water for injection (2 mg/mL); shake vigorously for up to 4 min; reconstituted sols are stable for 24 hr when stored refrigerated and protected from light or at room temperature in normal light

• Solution can be further diluted with sterile water for injection

IV INJ route

• Give doses of 100-120 mg/m^2 into tubing of a freely flowing 0.9% sodium chloride (NS) or D$_5$W IV infusion over 15-20 min; the infusion time may be decreased, proportionally, in those who require lower doses; infusion times <3 min are not recommended

• Direct injection into the vein is not recommended because of the risk of extravasation; avoid use with any solution of alkaline pH because hydrolysis will occur

IV INFUSION route

• Dilute dose in 0.9% sodium chloride (NS) or D$_5$W, infuse over 30-60 min, avoid use with any solution of alkaline pH because hydrolysis will occur

Y-site compatibilities: Alemtuzumab, alfentanil, amifostine, amikacin, aminocaproic acid, anidulafungin, argatroban, atracurium, aztreonam, bivalirudin, bleomycin, bumetanide, buprenorphine, butorphanol, calcium chloride/gluconate, CARBOplatin, caspofungin, ceFAZolin, cefotaxime, ceftizoxime, chlorproMAZINE, cimetidine, ciprofloxacin, cisatracurium, CISplatin, clindamycin, cyclophosphamide, cycloSPORINE, DAPTOmycin, dexrazoxane, digoxin, diltiazem, diphenhydrAMINE, DOBUTamine, DOCEtaxel, dolasetron, DOPamine, doxacurium, doxycycline, droperidol, enalaprilat, ePHEDrine, EPINEPHrine, ertapenem, erythromycin, etoposide, famotidine, fenoldopam, fentaNYL, fluconazole, gatifloxacin, gemcitabine, gentamicin, granisetron, haloperidol, hydrocortisone, HYDROmorphone, hydrOXYzine, ifosfamide, imipenem-cilastatin, inamrinone, insulin (regular), isoproterenol, labetalol, levofloxacin, levorphanol, lidocaine, linezolid, LORazepam, mannitol, meperidine, mesna, methotrexate, metoclopramide, metoprolol, metroNIDAZOLE, midazolam, milrinone, minocycline, mitoMYcin, mivacurium, morphine, moxifloxacin, nalbuphine, naloxone, nesiritide, niCARdipine, nitroglycerin, nitroprusside, norepinephrine, octreotide, ofloxacin, ondansetron, oxaliplatin, PACLitaxel, palonosetron, pamidronate, pancuronium, pentamidine, pentazocine, phenylephrine, potassium chloride, procainamide, prochlorperazine, promethazine, propranolol, quinupristin-dalfopristin, ranitidine, remifentanil, rocuronium, sodium acetate, succinylcholine, SUFentanil, tacrolimus, teniposide, theophylline, thiotepa, tigecycline, tirofiban, tobramycin, trimethobenzamide, vancomycin, vasopressin, vecuronium, verapamil, vinBLAStine, vinCRIStine, vinorelbine, voriconazole, zidovudine, zoledronic acid

SIDE EFFECTS

CV: Increased B/P, sinus tachycardia, PVCs, chest pain, bradycardia, extrasystoles, cardiomyopathy
GI: *Nausea, vomiting, anorexia, mucositis, diarrhea*
GU: *Amenorrhea, hot flashes, hyperuricemia, red urine*
HEMA: Thrombocytopenia, leukopenia, anemia, neutropenia, secondary AML
INTEG: *Rash*, necrosis, *pain at inj site, reversible alopecia*
MISC: *Infection, febrile neutropenia, lethargy, fever, conjunctivitis,* tumor lysis syndrome

PHARMACOKINETICS

Triphasic pattern of elimination; half-life 3 min, 1 hr, 30 hr; metabolized by liver,

extensively; crosses placenta; widely distributed to RBCs, excreted in urine, bile, breast milk

INTERACTIONS

• Give epiRUBicin before PACLitaxel if both are given
Increase: toxicity—other antineoplastics or radiation, cimetidine
Increase: ventricular dysfunction, HF—trastuzumab
Increase: heart failure—calcium channel blockers
Decrease: antibody response—live virus vaccine

NURSING CONSIDERATIONS
Assess:

Black Box Warning: **Bone marrow depression (severe):** CBC, differential, platelet count weekly; withhold product if baseline neutrophil ≤1500/mm³; leukocyte nadir occurs 10-14 days after administration, recovery by day 21; notify prescriber of results; assess for bleeding: hematuria, guaiac, bruising, or petechiae, or mucosa, orifices

• **Infection:** treat before receiving this product if regimens >120 mg/m², prophylactic antibiotics should be given (trimethoprim-sulfamethoxazole or a quinolone)
• Blood, urine uric acid levels; swelling, joint pain primarily in extremities; patient should be well hydrated to prevent urate deposits
• **Renal disease:** BUN, serum uric acid, urine CCr, electrolytes before, during therapy; I&O ratio; report fall in urine output to <30 mL/hr; dosage adjustment needed if serum creatinine >5 mg/dL
• Increase fluid intake to 2-3 L/day to prevent urate, calculi formation

Black Box Warning: **Hepatic studies** before, during therapy: bilirubin, AST, ALT, alk phos as needed or monthly

Black Box Warning: **Heart failure:** B/P, pulse, character, rhythm, rate, ABGs, ECG, LVEF, MUGA scan, or ECHO; watch for ST-T wave changes, low QRS and T, possible dysrhythmias (sinus tachycardia, heart block, PVCs); identify cumulative amount of anthracycline received (lifetime); reactions that follow may be delayed; assess for dyspnea, tachycardia, peripheral edema, rales/crackles, ascites

• Effects of alopecia on body image; discuss feelings about body changes

Black Box Warning: **Extravasation (vesicant):** local irritation, pain, burning, necrosis at inj site; discontinue and start at another site.

• **Stomatitis:** oral mucosa for ulceration, burning, bleeding; may lead to inability to eat and swallow
• **GI symptoms:** frequency of stools, cramping
• **Pregnancy/breastfeeding:** Women of reproductive potential should avoid becoming pregnant during therapy and should be advised to utilize effective contraceptive methods. If a woman becomes pregnant during therapy, she should be advised of the potential risks to the fetus. There is potential for male-mediated teratogenicity. Men with sexual partners of reproductive potential should use effective contraceptive methods during and after therapy. Men or women who receive this product may have a risk of infertility. Women treated may develop irreversible amenorrhea or premature menopause; discontinue breastfeeding or discontinue product

Evaluate:
• Therapeutic response: decreased tumor size, spread of malignancy

Teach patient/family:
• That hair may be lost during treatment; that wig or hairpiece may make patient feel better; that new hair may be different in color, texture; new hair growth occurs in ≤3 mo after treatment
• To avoid crowds, persons with infections when granulocyte count is low
• To avoid vaccinations because reactions may occur; to avoid cimetidine during therapy
• That urine may appear red for 2 days

• To avoid OTC medications, supplements unless approved by prescriber

Black Box Warning: That irreversible myocardial damage, leukopenia, menopause may occur

• To report rapid heartbeat, trouble breathing, fever, nausea, vomiting, oral sores
• To report pain at site immediately
• **Pregnancy/breastfeeding:** that contraceptive measures are recommended during therapy and for 4 mo thereafter for men and women; not to breastfeed

---

eplerenone (Rx)
(ep-ler-ee'known)
Inspra
Func. class.: Antihypertensive
Chem. class.: Selective aldosterone receptor antagonist

Do not confuse:
Inspra/Spiriva

ACTION: Binds to mineralocorticoid receptor and blocks the binding of aldosterone, a component of the renin-angiotensin-aldosterone system (RAAS)

USES: Hypertension, alone or in combination with thiazide diuretics, HF, post-MI

CONTRAINDICATIONS: Hypersensitivity; increased serum creatinine >2 mg/dL (male), >1.8 mg/dL (female); potassium >5.5 mEq/L, type 2 diabetes with microalbuminuria, hepatic disease, CCr <30 mL/min; CCr <50 mL/min in hypertension
Precautions: Pregnancy, breastfeeding, children, geriatric patients, impaired renal/hepatic function, hyperkalemia

DOSAGE AND ROUTES
Hypertension
• **Adult:** PO 50 mg/day initially, may increase to 50 mg bid after 4 wk, max 100 mg/day; 25 mg/day max if patient is taking CYP3A4 inhibitors

HF or post-MI
• **Adult:** PO 25 mg/day initially, may increase to 50 mg/day max after 4 wk
Dosage adjustments for those receiving moderate CYP3A4 inhibitors
• Potassium level 5 mEq/L, increase from 25 mg every other day to 25 mg q day, or increase dose from 25 mg q day to 50 mg q day; potassium level 5.1 to 5.4 mEq/L no adjustment; potassium level 5.5 to 5.9 mEq/L, decrease dose from 50 mg to 25 mg, or decrease dose from 25 mg q day to 25 mg every other day; if dose was 25 mg every other day, withhold dose; if potassium is >6 mEq/L, withhold; may restart drug at 25 mg every other day when potassium level is <5.5 mEq/L
Available forms: Tabs 25, 50 mg
Administer:
• Without regard to food
• Do not use salt substitutes containing potassium
• Store in tight container at ≤86° F (30° C)

SIDE EFFECTS
CNS: Headache, *dizziness, fatigue*
CV: Angina, MI
GI: Increased GGT, *diarrhea,* abdominal pain, increased ALT
GU: Gynecomastia, mastodynia (males), abnormal vaginal bleeding
META: *Hyperkalemia,* hyponatremia, hypercholesteremia, hypertriglyceridemia, increased uric acid
RESP: *Cough*

PHARMACOKINETICS
Peak $1^1/_2$ hr; serum protein binding 50%; half-life 4-6 hr; metabolized in liver by CYP3A4; excreted in urine <5%, feces

INTERACTIONS
Increase: hyperkalemia—ACE inhibitors, angiotensin II antagonists, NSAIDs, potassium supplements, potassium-sparing diuretics; do not use together
Increase: serum levels of lithium; monitor lithium level
Increase: eplerenone levels—erythromycin, fluconazole, verapamil; reduce dose of eplerenone

Increase: levels of eplerenone—CYP3A4 inhibitors (ketoconazole, itraconazole, saquinavir, clarithromycin, imatinib, nelfinavir, nefazodone, ritonavir, troleandomycin); do not use concurrently or reduce dose of eplerenone
Decrease: antihypertensive effect—NSAIDs
Drug/Herb
Decrease: antihypertensive effect—ephedra, St. John's wort
Drug/Food
• Grapefruit, grapefruit juice—increase product level by 25%
• Do not use salt substitutes containing potassium
Drug/Lab Test
Increase: BUN, creatinine, potassium, cholesterol, lipids, uric acid
Decrease: sodium

NURSING CONSIDERATIONS
Assess:
• **Hypertension:** B/P at peak/trough level of product, orthostatic hypotension, syncope when used with diuretic; monitor lithium level in those also taking lithium; those on CYP3A4 inhibitor should monitor potassium at baseline, within first wk, at 1 mo, and more often in diabetes, renal disease
• **Renal studies:** protein, BUN, creatinine; LFTs, uric acid may be increased; contraindicated in CCr <30 mL/min
• Potassium levels; hyperkalemia may occur
• **Pregnancy/breastfeeding:** use in pregnancy only if clearly needed; may be excreted in breast milk; do not breastfeed
Evaluate:
• Therapeutic response: decreased B/P
Teach patient/family:
• Not to discontinue product abruptly
• Not to use OTC products (cough, cold, allergy) unless directed by prescriber; not to use salt substitutes containing potassium without consulting prescriber
• To comply with dosage schedule, even if feeling better
• That product may cause dizziness, fainting, light-headedness; may occur during first few days of therapy
• How to take B/P; and about normal readings for age group

Side effects: *italics* = common; red = life-threatening

> ### ⚠ HIGH ALERT

epoetin alfa (Rx)
(ee-poe′e-tin)
Epogen, Eprex ✦, Procrit
Func. class.: Antianemic
Chem. class.: Amino acid polypeptide

ACTION: Erythropoietin is a factor controlling the rate of red cell production; product is developed by recombinant DNA technology

USES: Anemia caused by reduced endogenous erythropoietin production, primarily end-stage renal disease; to correct hemostatic defect in uremia; anemia due to AZT treatment in patients with HIV or those receiving chemotherapy; reduction of allogenic blood transfusion in surgery patients
Unlabeled uses: Anemia in premature preterm infants, anemia due to ribavirin and interferon-alfa therapy in hepatitis C

CONTRAINDICATIONS: Hypersensitivity to mammalian-cell–derived products, human albumin; uncontrolled hypertension
Precautions: Pregnancy, breastfeeding, children <1 mo, seizure disorder; multidose preserved formulation contains benzyl alcohol and should not be used in premature infants; porphyria, CV disease, hemodialysis, latex allergy, hypertension, history of CABG

Black Box Warning: Hgb >11 g/dL, surgery, neoplastic disease

DOSAGE AND ROUTES
Anemia due to chronic kidney disease:
• **Adult/adolescent ≥ 17 yr SUBCUT/IV:** initially 50-100 units/kg 3× per wk; use lowest amount to prevent need for transfusion; max Hgb 11 g/dl (dialysis) or Hgb 10 g/dl (not on dialysis); if Hgb increases by > 1 g/dl in 2 wk period,

reduce dose by 25%; if Hgb increases by 1 g/dl in 4 wk period, increase dose by 25%, do not increase dose more than q 4 wk.
• **Adolescent < 17 yr/ child >1 mo: SUBCUT/IV:** 50 units/kg 3× per wk initially use lowest amount to prevent need for transfusion; max Hgb 11 g/dl (dialysis) or Hgb 10 g/dl (not on dialysis); if Hgb increases by > 1 g/dl in 2 wk period, reduce dose by 25%; if Hgb increases by 1 g/dl in 4 wk period, increase dose by 25%, do not increase dose more than q 4 wk.
Zidovudine-induced anemia:
• **Adult: SUBCUT/IV** initially 100 units/kg 3 × per wk; × 8 wk, if needed may increase by 50-100 units/kg q 4-8 wk, max 300 units/kg 3 × per wk.
• **Child 8 mo-17 yr: SUBCUT/IV** 50-400 units/kg 2-3 × per wk.
Anemia due to chemotherapy:
• **Adult: SUBCUT** 150 units/kg 3 × per wk or 40,000 units wk, only when Hgb < 12 g/dl and only when chemotherapy course is completed; use dose to maintain Hgb (max 12 g/dl) so blood transfusion is not needed; do not start if Hgb is ≥10g/dl.
• **Adolescent/child ≥ 5 yr: SUBCUT** 600 units/kg per wk (max Hgb 12 g/dl)); if Hgb increases by > 1 g/dl in 2 wk period, reduce dose by 25%; if Hgb increases by 1 g/dl in 4 wk period, increase dose to 900 units/kg (max 60,000 units/kg), do not increase dose more than q 4 wk; do not start if Hgb ≥ 10g/dl.
• **Noncardiac, nonvascular surgery:**
Adult: SUBCUT 300units/kg/day X10 days before surgery, on day of surgery and for 4 days after surgery (15 days total) or 600 units/kg q wk 21, 14, 7 days before surgery and one dose the day of surgery.
Available forms: Inj 2000, 3000, 4000, 10,000, 20,000, 40,000 units/mL
Administer:
• Use 1 single-use vial/dose, once syringe has entered single-dose vial, sterility cannot be guaranteed, do not administer with other product, multidose vials can be stored in refrigerator up to 21 days once opened, do not use if discolored or particulates are present

SUBCUT route
• Before injecting, preservative-free, single-dose formulation may be admixed using 0.9% NaCl with benzyl alcohol 0.9% at a 1:1 ratio to reduce inj-site discomfort, store solution in refrigerator, protect from light

Direct IV route
• Additional heparin to lower chance of clots
• By direct inj or bolus into IV tubing or venous line at end of dialysis, do not shake vial, can use undiluted or diluted in 0.9% NaCl (1000-40,000 U/mL), give over ≥1 min
• Decrease dose by 25% if Hgb increases by 1 g/dL in 2 wk; increase dose if Hgb does not increase by 5-6 pts after 8 wk of therapy; suggested target Hgb range 30%-36%

Solution compatibilities: Do not dilute or administer with other sol

SIDE EFFECTS

CNS: Seizures, coldness, sweating, headache, fatigue, dizziness
CV: *Hypertension,* hypertensive encephalopathy, HF, edema, DVT, MI, stroke
INTEG: Pruritus, rash, inj site reaction
MISC: Iron deficiency
MS: Bone pain, arthralgia, myalgia
RESP: Cough

PHARMACOKINETICS

IV: Metabolized in body, extent of metabolism unknown, onset of increased reticulocyte count 2-6 wk, peak immediate
Subcut: Peak 5-24 hr

INTERACTIONS

• Need for increased heparin during hemodialysis

NURSING CONSIDERATIONS
Assess:
• Renal studies: urinalysis, protein, blood, BUN, creatinine; I&O, electrolytes, report drop in output <50 mL/hr

Black Box Warning: **Blood studies:** ferritin, transferrin, serum iron monthly; transferrin sat ≥20%, ferritin ≥100 ng/mL; Hct 2×/wk until stabilized in target range (30%-36%) then at regular intervals; those with endogenous erythropoietin levels of <500 units/L respond to product; monitor Hct 2×/wk with chronic renal failure; patients treated with zidovudine or patients with cancer should be monitored weekly, then periodically after stabilization; death may occur with Hgb >12 g/dL; monitor for blood clots

• B/P; check for rising B/P as Hct rises, antihypertensives may be needed; hypertension may occur rapidly, leading to hypertensive encephalopathy, use of antihypertensive may be needed
• CNS symptoms: coldness, sweating, pain in long bones; for seizures if Hct is increased within 2 wk by 4 points
• Hypersensitivity reactions: skin rashes, urticaria (rare), antibody development does not occur
• Pure cell aplasia (PRCA) in absence of other causes; evaluate by testing sera for recombinant erythropoetin antibodies; any loss of response to epoetin should be evaluated
• Dialysis patients: thrill, bruit of shunts; monitor for circulation impairment
• **Seizures:** place patient on seizure precautions if increase of 1 g/dL Hct in any 2-wk period, increased B/P; more common in chronic renal failure during the first 90 days of treatment
• **Pregnancy/breastfeeding:** product should be used during pregnancy only when benefits outweigh fetal risk. Multidose vials are contraindicated due to the use of benzyl alcohol as a preservative; it is not known whether epoetin alfa is distributed into breast milk

Evaluate:
• Therapeutic response: increase in reticulocyte count in 2-6 wk, Hgb/Hct; increased appetite, enhanced sense of well-being

Teach patient/family:
• How to take B/P, have patient read the "Medication Guide"; a form must be signed before each cycle
• To avoid driving or hazardous activities during beginning of treatment

---

Side effects: *italics* = common; red = life-threatening

• To take iron supplements, vit B_{12}, folic acid as directed

• To report immediately chest pain, pain in calves, confusion, inability to speak, numbness in face, arm, leg

• **Chronic renal failure (anemia):** product does not cure condition, to maintain prescribed diet, medications, dialysis follow-up appointments

• **Pregnancy/breastfeeding:** to report if pregnancy is planned or suspected or if breastfeeding

• The reason for treatment, expected results, to notify health care professional of use

---

eprosartan (Rx)

(ep-roe-sar′tan)

Teveten

Func. class.: Antihypertensive

Chem. class.: Angiotensin II–receptor antagonist (Subtype AT_1)

ACTION: Blocks the vasoconstrictive and aldosterone-secreting effects of angiotensin II; selectively blocks the binding of angiotensin II to the AT_1 receptor found in tissues

USES: Hypertension, alone or with other antihypertensives

CONTRAINDICATIONS: Hypersensitivity

Black Box Warning: Pregnancy

Precautions: Breastfeeding, children, geriatric patients, hypersensitivity to ACE inhibitors; renal/hepatic disease, angioedema, hyperkalemia

DOSAGE AND ROUTES

• **Adult: PO** 600 mg/day; dose may be divided, given bid, with total daily doses from 400-800 mg, max 800 mg/day

Renal dose

• **Adult: PO** CCr ≤30 mL/min, max 600 mg/day

Available forms: Tabs 600 mg

Administer:

• Without regard to meals

• Correct volume depletion if needed before starting treatment

SIDE EFFECTS

CNS: *Dizziness,* depression, *fatigue,* headache

CV: Chest pain, hypotension, palpitations

EENT: Sinusitis

GI: *Diarrhea, dyspepsia, abdominal pain*

GU: UTI

HEMA: Neutropenia

INTEG: Pruritus, angioedema

META: Hypertriglyceridemia

MS: *Myalgia,* arthralgia, rhabdomyolysis

RESP: *Cough, upper respiratory infection,* rhinitis, pharyngitis, viral infection

SYST: Anaphylaxis

PHARMACOKINETICS

Peak 1-2 hr, food delays absorption; protein binding 98%; moderate renal impairment increases product levels by 30%, hepatic impairment increases levels by 40%; excreted in urine and feces; half-life 5-9 hr, crosses placenta

INTERACTIONS

Increase: hyperglycemia—antidiabetics

Increase: antihypertensive effect—other antihypertensives

Increase: hyperkalemia—ACE inhibitors, angiotensin II receptor antagonists, potassium-sparing diuretics, potassium supplements

Increase: lithium toxicity—lithium

Decrease: antihypertensive effect—NSAIDs, salicylates

Drug/Herb

Decrease: antihypertensive effect—ephedra

Increase: antihypertensive effect—hawthorn

Drug/Lab Test

Increase: ALT, AST, alk phos, potassium

Decrease: Hgb

NURSING CONSIDERATIONS

Assess:

• B/P with position changes, pulse baseline and periodically; note rate, rhythm, quality

• Hypersensitivity reactions, including anaphylaxis, angioedema

• Myalgia, arthralgia; may cause rhabdomyolysis
• Baselines of renal, hepatic studies before therapy begins

Black Box Warning: Pregnancy: identify if pregnancy is planned or suspected, or if breastfeeding

Evaluate:
• Therapeutic response: decreased B/P
Teach patient/family:
• To comply with dosage schedule, even if feeling better, to take missed doses as soon as remembered if within 1 hr of next dose, do not double, use at same time of day, not to discontinue without discussing with prescriber
• To comply with treatment regimen, to avoid salt substitutes with potassium, other potassium products
• **Angioedema/hypersensitivity:** To notify health care professional immediately of swelling of face, trouble breathing, itching, rash
• To notify prescriber of fever; chest pain; swelling of hands, feet, face, lip, or tongue
• That excessive perspiration, dehydration, diarrhea may lead to fall in B/P; consult prescriber if these occur, maintain adequate hydration
• That product may cause dizziness; to avoid hazardous activities until effect is known; to rise slowly from sitting
• To take B/P; report significant changes

Black Box Warning: Not to take this product if pregnant or breastfeeding, or if have had an allergic reaction to product

• That therapeutic effect may take 2-3 wk

⚠ HIGH ALERT

eptifibatide (Rx)
(ep-tih-fib′ah-tide)
Integrilin
Func. class.: Antiplatelet agent
Chem. class.: Glycoprotein IIb/IIIa inhibitor

ACTION: Platelet glycoprotein antagonist; this agent reversibly prevents fibrinogen, von Willebrand's factor from binding to the glycoprotein IIb/IIIa receptor, thus inhibiting platelet aggregation

USES: Acute coronary syndrome including those undergoing percutaneous coronary intervention (PCI)

CONTRAINDICATIONS: Hypersensitivity, active internal bleeding; recent history of bleeding, stroke within 30 days or any hemorrhagic stroke; major surgery with severe trauma, severe hypertension, current or planned use of another parenteral GP IIb/IIIa inhibitor, dependence on renal dialysis, coagulopathy, AV malformation, aneurysm
Precautions: Pregnancy, breastfeeding, children, geriatric patients, bleeding, impaired renal function

DOSAGE AND ROUTES
Acute coronary syndrome
• **Adult:** IV BOL 180 mcg/kg as soon as diagnosed, max 22.6 mg, then **IV CONT** 2 mcg/kg/min; in CABG discontinue ≥2-4 hr before procedure
PCI in patients without acute coronary syndrome
• **Adult:** IV BOL 180 mcg/kg given immediately before PCI, then 2 mcg/kg/min × 18 hr **CONT IV INFUSION** and a second 180-mcg/kg bolus by 10 min after 1st bolus; continue infusion for up to 18-24 hr, minimum 12 hr
Renal dose
• **Adult:** IV maintenance CCr <50 mL/min, 1 mcg/kg/min, max rate 7.5 mg/hr; CCr <10 mL/min, contraindicated
Available forms: Sol for inj 2 mg/mL (10 mL), 0.75 mg/mL (100 mL)
Administer:
• Aspirin may be given with this product; check for bleeding
• D/C heparin before removing femoral artery sheath, after PCI
• Do not give discolored solutions, those with particulates; discard unused amount, protect from light
• Discontinue product before CABG

Direct IV route
• After withdrawing bolus dose from 20 mg/10 mL (2 mg/mL) vial, give IV push over 1-2 min

Continuous IV INFUSION route
• Follow bolus dose with continuous infusion using pump; give product undiluted directly from 100-mL vial, spike 100-mL vial with vented infusion set, use caution when centering spike on circle of stopper top, refrigerate vials, or may store vials ≤2 mo at room temperature

Y-site compatibilities: Alfentanil, alteplase, amikacin, aminophylline, amphotericin B lipid complex, amphotericin B liposome, ampicillin, ampicillin-sulbactam, anidulafungin, argatroban, atenolol, atracurium, atropine, azithromycin, aztreonam, bivalirudin, bumetanide, buprenorphine, butorphanol, calcium chloride/gluconate, ceFAZolin, cefepime, cefotaxime, cefoTEtan, cefOXitin, cefTAZidime, ceftizoxime, cefTRIAXone, cefuroxime, cimetidine, ciprofloxacin, cisatracurium, clindamycin, cycloSPORINE, DAPTOmycin, dexamethasone, D₅/NaCl 0.9%, diazepam, diltiazem, diphenhydrAMINE, DOBUTamine, dolasetron, DOPamine, doxycycline, droperidol, enalaprilat, ePHEDrine, EPINEPHrine, ertapenem, erythromycin, esmolol, famotidine, fentaNYL, fluconazole, fosphenytoin, ganciclovir, gatifloxacin, gentamicin, granisetron, haloperidol, heparin, hydrocortisone, HYDROmorphone, hydrOXYzine, imipenem-cilastatin, inamrinone, isoproterenol, ketorolac, labetalol, leucovorin, levofloxacin, levorphanol, lidocaine, linezolid, LORazepam, magnesium sulfate, mannitol, meperidine, meropenem, methylPREDNISolone, metoclopramide, metoprolol, metroNIDAZOLE, micafungin, midazolam, milrinone, minocycline, mivacurium, morphine, nalbuphine, naloxone, niCARdipine, nitroglycerin, nitroprusside, NS, octreotide, ofloxacin, ondansetron, oxytocin, palonosetron, pancuronium, PEMEtrexed, PENTobarbital, PHENobarbital, phenylephrine, piperacillin, piperacillin-tazobactam, potassium chloride/phosphates, procainamide, prochlorperazine, promethazine, propranolol, ranitidine, remifentanil, rocuronium, sodium bicarbonate/phosphates, succinylcholine, SUFentanil, sulfamethoxazole-trimethoprim, teniposide, theophylline, ticarcillin, ticarcillin-clavulanate, tigecycline, tirofiban, tobramycin, trimethobenzamide, vancomycin, vecuronium, verapamil, zidovudine, zoledronic acid

SIDE EFFECTS
CV: Stroke, hypotension
GU: Hematuria
HEMA: Thrombocytopenia, platelet dysfunction
SYST: Major/minor bleeding from any site, anaphylaxis

PHARMACOKINETICS
Onset within 1 hr, protein binding 25%, half-life 1.5-2 hr, steady state 4-6 hr, metabolism limited, excretion via kidneys

INTERACTIONS
• Do not give with glycoprotein inhibitors IIb, IIIa

Increase: bleeding—aspirin, heparin, NSAIDs, anticoagulants, ticlopidine, clopidogrel, dipyridamole, thrombolytics, valproate, abciximab, SSRIs, SNRIs
Drug/Herb
Increase: bleeding risk—feverfew, garlic, ginger, ginkgo, ginseng

NURSING CONSIDERATIONS
Assess:
• **Renal disease:** reduce dose if CCr >50; contraindicated in dialysis
• **Thrombocytopenia:** platelets, Hgb, Hct, creatinine, APTT baseline within 6 hr of loading dose, daily therafter, patients undergoing PCI should have ACT monitored; maintain APTT 50-70 sec unless PCI to be performed; during PCI, ACT should be 200-300 sec; if platelets drop <100,000/mm³, obtain additional platelet counts; if thrombocytopenia is confirmed, dis-

continue product; draw Hct, Hgb, serum creatinine

• **Bleeding:** gums, bruising, ecchymosis, petechiae; from GI, GU tract, cardiac cath sites, IM inj sites

• **Pregnancy/breastfeeding:** use in pregnancy only if clearly needed; it is not known if product is excreted in breast milk; consider risks and benefits

Teach patient/family:

• About reason for medication and expected results

• To report bruising, bleeding, chest pain immediately

• Not to use other Rx, OTC products or supplements without prescriber approval

---

eravacycline
(er′ a-va-sye′ kleen)
Xerava
Func. class.: Antiinfective—tetracycline
Chem. class.: Synthetic fluorocycline

ACTION: Disrupts bacterial protein synthesis by binding to the 30S ribosomal subunit and preventing the incorporation of amino acid residues into elongating peptide chains

USES: Complicated intraabdominal infections caused by *Bacteroides caccae, Bacteroides fragilis, Bacteroides ovatus, Bacteroides thetaiotaomicron, Bacteroides uniformis, Bacteroides vulgatus, Citrobacter freundii, Citrobacter koseri, Clostridium perfringens, Enterobacter aerogenes, Enterobacter cloacae, Enterococcus faecalis, Enterococcus faecium, Escherichia coli, Klebsiella oxytoca, Klebsiella pneumoniae, Parabacteroides distasonis, Staphylococcus aureus* (MRSA), *Staphylococcus aureus* (MSSA), *Streptococcus anginosus, Streptococcus salivarius*

CONTRAINDICATIONS: Hypersensitivity to this product or tetracyclines

Precautions: Breastfeeding, children, colitis, diarrhea, geriatric patients, GI/hepatic disease, increased intracranial pressure, inflammatory bowel disease/ulcerative colitis, papilledema, pregnancy, pseudomembranous colitis, UV exposure

DOSAGE AND ROUTES

• **Adult:** IV 1 mg/kg q12hr × 4-14 days

Available forms: Powder for inj 50 mg

Administer:

Intermittent IV INFUSION route

• Visually inspect for particulate matter and discoloration before use; reconstituted solution is clear, pale yellow to orange

• **Reconstitution:** Reconstitute each vial with 5 mL of sterile water for injection to a concentration of 10 mg/mL; swirl gently until powder has dissolved; avoid shaking or rapid movement. Do not give reconstituted solution by direct injection

• **Dilution:** Withdraw the full or partial reconstituted content from each vial and add it into a 0.9% Sodium Chloride Injection infusion bag to a concentration of 0.3 mg/mL (within a range of 0.2-0.6 mg/mL). Do not shake

• **Storage:** Diluted solution must be infused within 6 hr if stored at room temperature (max 25° C or 77° F) or within 24 hr if stored refrigerated at 2-8° C (36-46° F). Do not freeze

Intermittent IV infusion

• Infuse through a dedicated IV line or by Y-site. If the same IV line is used for sequential infusion of several drugs, flush the line before and after infusion with 0.9% Sodium Chloride Injection. Give over 60 min; assess IV site frequently

SIDE EFFECTS

CV: Hypotension
EENT: Tooth discoloration
GI: Nausea, vomiting, diarrhea, *pancreatitis, Clostridium difficile*
HEMA: Thrombosis
INTEG: Rash
RESP: Pleural effusion
SYST: Anaphylaxis, wound dehiscence

Side effects: *italics* = common; red = life-threatening

PHARMACOKINETICS

Metabolized primarily by CYP3A4- and FMO-mediated oxidation, excretion 47% feces, 34% urine, half-life 20 hr

INTERACTIONS

Increase: anticoagulation—anticoagulants; anticoagulant may need dosage reduction

Increase: eravacycline effect—strong CYP3A inducers (clarithromycin, telithromycin, nefazodone, itraconazole, ketoconazole, atazanavir, darunavir, indinavir, lopinavir, nelfinavir, ritonavir, saquinavir, tipranavir)

Decrease: eravacycline effect—strong CYP3A inducers (carbamazepine, rifampin)

NURSING CONSIDERATIONS
Assess:

• **Infection:** fever, condition of wound, pain, vital signs, urine, stools; monitor WBC for increased levels indicating continued infection; obtain C&S before starting treatment, may start product before receiving results

• **Bowel function:** diarrhea with mucus, blood; may indicate CDAD (*Clostridium difficile*–associated disease); report to health care provider immediately; may occur several weeks after last dose

• **Wound dehiscence:** fever, inflammation, bleeding, pain, wound opening; report any of these signs immediately

• **Anaphylaxis:** rash, dyspnea, swelling of lips/tongue; discontinue product; if severe, epinephrine is usually given; if allergic reaction is mild, discontinuing product and giving diphenhydramine may be sufficient

• **Tooth discoloration:** may occur if used in 2nd or 3rd trimester of pregnancy or in children <8 yr

Teach patient/family:

• To inform health care provider of all OTC, Rx, herbal and supplemental products taken; not to change medication without prescriber's approval

• **Pregnancy/breastfeeding:** to inform health care provider if pregnancy is planned or suspected, or if breastfeeding; that this product may cause permanent tooth discoloration and reversible inhibition of bone growth when used in the 2nd and 3rd trimesters of pregnancy; not to breast-feed during and for 4 days after last dose

• **Allergic reactions:** to identify allergies; that allergic reactions, including serious ones, could occur and that serious reactions require immediate treatment. Ask patient about any previous allergies

• **Diarrhea:** to report watery and bloody stools (with or without stomach cramps and fever), which may be a serious intestinal infection, even 2 or more mo after last dose

• That this product is used only to treat bacterial infections; to take all of the medication even if feeling better; not to skip doses or fail to complete the full course of therapy

---

erenumab
(e-ren′ ue-mab)
Aimovig
Func. class.: CNS analgesic; antimigraine agent
Chem. class.: IgG2 monoclonal antibody

ACTION: A human immunoglobulin G2 (IgG2) monoclonal antibody that binds to the calcitonin gene-related peptide (CGRP) receptor. CGRP is involved in migraine pathophysiology. Centrally, CGRP modulates pain in the brain stem; CGRP concentrations are elevated in acute migraine attacks and may be chronically elevated in those with chronic migraines

USES: For the preventive treatment of migraine in adults

CONTRAINDICATIONS: Hypersensitivity
Precautions: Breastfeeding, latex hypersensitivity, pregnancy

DOSAGE AND ROUTES

• **Adult:** SUBCUT 70 mg once monthly, may use 140 mg once monthly if needed
Available forms: SureClick 70 mg/mL autoinjector sol for injection; sol for

injection single-use 70 mg/mL prefilled syringe

Administer:

Injectable administration

• Visually inspect for particulate matter and discoloration before use; do not use if solution is cloudy or discolored or contains flakes or particles; product should be a clear to opalescent, colorless to light yellow solution

Subcutaneous route

• Product is intended for patient self-administration. Provide proper training to patients and/or caregivers

• Before use allow to sit at room temperature for at least 30 min, protected from direct sunlight. Do not warm using a heat source such as hot water or microwave

• Do not shake

• Clean injection site on the abdomen, thigh, or upper arm with an alcohol wipe; allow skin to dry

• Do not leave cap off the autoinjector or prefilled syringe for more than 5 min; product will dry out

• Do not inject into areas where skin is tender, bruised, red, or hard. Avoid injecting directly into raised, thick, red, or scaly skin patch or lesion, or into areas with scars or stretch marks

• If using the same body area for the 2 separate injections needed for the 140-mg dose, ensure that the second injection is not at same location used for the first injection

• Discard the autoinjector or prefilled syringe in sharps disposal container. Do not discard in household trash

• **Storage:** After removing the product from the refrigerator, it can be stored at room temperature between 68° and 77° F (20° to 25° C) for up to 7 days. Do not return to the refrigerator after it reaches room temperature

Single-dose, prefilled SureClick autoinjector

• Pull white cap straight off autoinjector

• Stretch or pinch skin to create a firm injection site

• Firmly push the autoinjector down onto the skin

• When ready to inject, press the purple start button; a click will be heard. The injection could take about 15 seconds. When injection is complete, a click may be heard or felt, and the window will turn yellow

• Remove autoinjector from skin

Single-dose prefilled syringe

• Always hold syringe by the barrel

• Pull gray needle cap straight out and away from body

• Pinch injection site skin firmly between thumb and fingers

• Hold the pinch, and insert the syringe into skin at a 45- to 90-degree angle

• Using slow, constant pressure, push the plunger rod all the way down with thumb until the prefilled syringe stops moving

• When finished, release thumb, and gently lift syringe off skin

SIDE EFFECTS

MISC: Antibody formation, injection site reaction, erythema

PHARMACOKINETICS

Subcut route: Peak 6 days, bioavailability 82%, half-life 28 days

INTERACTIONS

None known

NURSING CONSIDERATIONS

Assess

• **Migraines:** time of day, aggravating and ameliorating effects, auras or halos, sensitivity to light, noise, diet

• **Pregnancy/breastfeeding:** data are lacking. No adverse effects on offspring were observed when animals were given the product throughout pregnancy. Consider the developmental and health benefits of breastfeeding along with the mother's clinical need for the product and any potentially adverse effects on the breastfed infant

Evaluate:

• Therapeutic response: decrease in severity and number of migraines

Teach patient/family

• To read the FDA-approved patient labeling (Patient Information and Instructions for Use)

• Proper subcut administration technique, including aseptic technique, and how to use the single-dose prefilled autoinjector or single-dose prefilled autoinjector syringe

• To read and follow the Instructions for Use with each use of Aimovig

• That if the 140-mg once-monthly dosage is prescribed, to administer it as two separate subcut injections of 70 mg each

• **Latex sensitivity:** that the needle shield within the white cap of the Aimovig prefilled autoinjector and the gray needle cap of the Aimovig prefilled syringe contain dry natural rubber (a derivative of latex), which may cause allergic reactions in individuals sensitive to latex

---

⚠ HIGH ALERT

eribulin
(er′i-bu′lin)
Halaven
Func. class.: Antineoplastics—nontaxane
Chem. class.: Microtubule inhibitor

Do not confuse:
eribulin/epirubicin/erlotinib

ACTION: Potent antimitotic agent, different from taxanes, vinca alkaloids, epothilones; blocks cell progression during G2-M phase; inhibits the growth phase of microtubules and sequesters tubules, leading to the disruption of mitotic spindles and apoptotic cell death

USES: Metastatic breast cancer in patients who have received at least 2 chemotherapy regimens

CONTRAINDICATIONS: Hypersensitivity, pregnancy
Precautions: Breastfeeding, neonates, infants, children, bradycardia, electrolyte imbalances, heart failure, hypokalemia, hypomagnesemia, infertility, neutropenia, peripheral neuropathy, QT prolongation, hepatic/renal disease

DOSAGE AND ROUTES
• **Adult:** IV 1.4 mg/m^2 over 2-5 min on days 1 and 8, repeat q21days
• **Recommendations for dose delay:** for ANC <1000/mm^3, platelets <75,000/mm^3, or grade 3 or 4 nonhematologic toxicities: do not administer; the day 8 dose may be delayed a maximum of 1 wk; for the day 8 dose, if toxicities do not resolve to ≤ Grade 2 by day 15: omit the dose; for the day 8 dose, if toxicities resolve or improve to ≤ Grade 2 by day 15: administer eriBULin at reduced dose (see below), initiate the next cycle no sooner than 2 wk later
• **Dose adjustments for hematologic toxicity:** ANC <500/mm^3 for >7 days or ANC <1000/mm^3 with fever or infection: permanently reduce dose to 1.1 mg/m^2; platelets <25,000/mm^3 or <50,000/mm^3 requiring transfusion: permanently reduce dose to 1.1 mg/m^2; if day 8 of previous cycle omitted or delayed: permanently reduce dose to 1.1 mg/m^2; while receiving 1.1 mg/m^2, if recurrence of hematologic event occurs, or if day 8 of previous cycle omitted or delayed: permanently reduce dose to 0.7 mg/m^2; while receiving 0.7 mg/m^2, if recurrence of hematologic event occurs, or if day 8 of previous cycle omitted or delayed: discontinue
• **Dose adjustments of eribulin for nonhematologic toxicity during treatment:** any Grade 3 or 4 nonhematologic toxicity: permanently reduce dose to 1.1 mg/m^2; if day 8 of previous cycle omitted or delayed: permanently reduce dose to 1.1 mg/m^2; while receiving 1.1 mg/m^2, if recurrence of Grade 3 or 4 nonhematologic toxicity occurs, or if day 8 of previous cycle omitted or delayed: permanently reduce dose to 0.7 mg/m^2; while receiving 0.7 mg/m^2, if recurrence of Grade 3 or 4 nonhematologic toxicity occurs, or if day 8 of previous cycle omitted or delayed: discontinue
Available forms: Sol for inj 1 mg/2 mL
Administer:
IV direct, intermittent route
• Visually inspect for particulate matter, discoloration as solution and container permit; withdraw required amount (0.5 mg/mL) from single-use vial, give

---

undiluted over 2-5 min or diluted in 100 mL 0.9% NaCl and give as intermittent infusion; do not give through line with dextrose or any other product

• Store at room temperature for 4 hr or 24 hr refrigerated

SIDE EFFECTS

CNS: Depression, dizziness, *fatigue,* fever, headache, insomnia, *peripheral neuropathy*

CV: QT prolongation, peripheral edema

GI: Abdominal pain, anorexia, constipation, diarrhea, dyspepsia, nausea, vomiting, weight loss

HEMA: Anemia, neutropenia, thrombocytopenia

INTEG: *Alopecia,* rash, stomatitis, infusion-related reactions

META: Hypokalemia

MS: Arthralgia, myalgia, bone/back pain

RESP: Cough, dyspnea

SYST: Infection

PHARMACOKINETICS

Protein binding 49%-65%; inhibits CYP3A4; excreted in feces 82%; urine 9%; elimination half-life 40 hr; increased levels in hepatic/renal disease

INTERACTIONS

Increase: QT prolongation—arsenic trioxide, bepridil, chloroquine, certain phenothiazines (chlorproMAZINE, mesoridazine, thioridazine), clarithromycin, class IA antiarrhythmics (disopyramide, procainamide, quiNIDine), class III antiarrhythmics (amiodarone, bretylium, dofetilide, ibutilide, sotalol), dextromethorphan; quiNIDine, dronedarone, droperidol, erythromycin, halofantrine, haloperidol, levomethadyl, methadone, pentamidine, pimozide, posaconazole, probucol, propafenone, saquinavir, sparfloxacin, troleandomycin, and ziprasidone; also to a lesser degree abarelix, alfuzosin, amoxapine, apomorphine, artemether; lumefantrine, asenapine, β-agonists, ofloxacin, cloZAPine, cyclobenzaprine, dasatinib, dolasetron, flecainide, gatifloxacin, gemifloxacin, halogenated anesthetics, iloperidone, lapatinib, levoFLOXacin, local anesthetics, lopinavir; ritonavir, magnesium sulfate; potassium sulfate; sodium sulfate, maprotiline, mefloquine, moxifloxacin, nilotinib, norfloxacin, octreotide, ciprofloxacin, OLANZapine, ondansetron, paliperidone, palonosetron, some phenothiazines (fluPHENAZine, perphenazine, prochlorperazine, trifluoperazine), QUEtiapine, ranolazine, risperiDONE, sertindole, SUNItinib, tacrolimus, telavancin, telithromycin, tetrabenazine, tricyclic antidepressants, venlafaxine, vardenafil, vorinostat

Increase: adverse reactions—live virus vaccines; do not use together

NURSING CONSIDERATIONS

Assess:

• **Peripheral neuropathy:** pain, numbness in extremities

• **Infection:** increased temperature, sore throat, flulike symptoms

• **Electrolyte imbalances:** correct before administration; monitor during therapy

• **QT prolongation:** assess for drug interactions that may occur; monitor ECG, heart rate

• **Bone marrow depression:** CBC, differential, serum creatinine, BUN, electrolytes, LFTs at baseline, periodically; increased AST/ALT >3 × ULN or total bilirubin >1.5 × ULN involves greater chance of Grade 4 or febrile neutropenia

• **Pregnancy/breastfeeding:** may cause fetal harm; do not use in pregnancy or breastfeeding

Teach patient/family:

• **Infection:** to notify prescriber of increased temperature, sore throat, fatigue, flulike symptoms

• **QT prolongation:** to report extra heartbeats

Peripheral neuropathy:

• To report tingling, pain in extremities

• About reason for product and expected results

• To avoid other medications, supplements unless approved by provider; serious drug interactions may occur

• About hair loss, use of wig or hairpiece

• To notify prescriber if pregnancy is planned or suspected; to use contraception during treatment; to avoid breastfeeding

---

⚠ HIGH ALERT

erlotinib (Rx)
(er-loe′tye-nib)

Tarceva

Func. class.: Antineoplastic—miscellaneous

Chem. class.: Epidermal growth factor receptor inhibitor

ACTION: Not fully understood; inhibits intracellular phosphorylation of cell-surface receptors associated with epidermal growth factor receptors

USES: Non–small-cell lung cancer (NSCLC) including EGFR ex on 19 deletions or ex on 21 substitution mutations, pancreatic cancer

CONTRAINDICATIONS: Pregnancy, breastfeeding

Precautions: Children, geriatric patients, ocular/pulmonary/renal/hepatic disorders, diverticulitis

DOSAGE AND ROUTES
Non–small-cell lung cancer (NSCLC), maintenance, after failure of at least one chemotherapy regimen
• **Adult: PO** 150 mg/day
Pancreatic cancer
• **Adult: PO** 100 mg/day in combination with gemcitabine 1000 mg/m^2 cycle 1, days 1, 8, 15, 22, 29, 36, 43 of 8-wk cycle; cycle 2 and subsequent cycles, days 1, 8, 15 of 4-wk cycle, used with gemcitabine
CYP3A4 inducers concurrently (rifampin, phenytoin)
• Increase dose by 50 mg q2wk (max 450 mg/day)
CYP3A4 inhibitors (atazanavir, clarithromycin, indinavir, itraconazole, ketoconazole, telithromycin, ritonavir, saquinavir, troleandomycin, nelfinavir) or CYP3A4 and CYP1A2 inhibitors concurrently (ciprofloxacin)
• Decrease dose by 50 mg as needed
Head or neck cancer (unlabeled)
• **Adult: PO** 150 mg daily
Available forms: Tabs 25, 100, 150 mg
Administer:
• 1 hr before or 2 hr after food; at same time of day

SIDE EFFECTS
CNS: CVA, anxiety, depression, headache, rigors, insomnia
CV: MI/ischemia
EENT: Ocular changes, *conjunctivitis, eye pain,* hypertrichosis
GI: *Nausea, diarrhea, vomiting, anorexia, mouth ulceration,* hepatic failure, GI perforation
GU: Renal impairment/failure
HEMA: Deep vein thrombosis, bleeding
INTEG: *Rash,* Stevens-Johnson–like skin reaction, toxic epidermal necrolysis
MISC: *Fatigue, infection*
RESP: Interstitial lung disease, *cough, dyspnea*
SYST: Hepatorenal syndrome

PHARMACOKINETICS
Slowly absorbed (60%); peak 3-7 hr; duration up to 24 hr; excreted in feces (86%), urine (<4%); metabolized by CYP3A4; half-life 36 hr; protein binding 93%; inhibits tyrosine kinase, which is a factor in epidermal growth factor receptor (EGFR)

INTERACTIONS
Increase: GI bleeding, may be fatal—warfarin, NSAIDs
Increase: erlotinib concentrations—CYP3A4 inhibitors (ketoconazole, itraconazole, erythromycin, clarithromycin, telithromycin)
Increase: plasma concentrations of warfarin, metoprolol
Increase: myopathy—HMG-CoA reductase inhibitors
Decrease: erlotinib levels—CYP3A4 inducers (phenytoin, rifampin,

---

carBAMazepine, PHENobarbital), proton pump inhibitors

Drug/Herb

Decrease: erlotinib levels—St. John's wort

Drug/Smoking

Decrease: erlotinib level; dose may need to be increased

Drug/Food

Increase: effect of erlotinib—grapefruit juice

Drug/Lab Test

Increase: INR, PT, AST, ALT, bilirubin

NURSING CONSIDERATIONS

Assess:

• **Serious skin toxicities:** toxic epidermal necrolysis, Stevens-Johnson syndrome; check for rash, blistering; discontinue treatment, may need corticosteroids, antiinfectives

• **MI/ischemia, CVA** in patients with pancreatic cancer

• **Pulmonary changes:** lung sounds, cough, dyspnea; interstitial lung disease may occur, may be fatal; discontinue therapy if confirmed

• **Ocular changes:** eye irritation, corneal erosion/ulcer, aberrant eyelash growth, discontinue if ulcers are present in the cornea, hold for Keratitis (Grade 3 or 4)

• **GI symptoms:** frequency of stools; if diarrhea is poorly tolerated, therapy may be discontinued for ≤14 days, monitor for dehydration, fluid status during period of vomiting and diarrhea, may use antidiarrheal

• **Blood studies:** INR, LFTs, PT; elevated INR and hemorrhage are increased when used with warfarin

• **Hepatic failure:** interrupt dosing if severe changes to liver function occur (total bilirubin >3× ULN and/or transaminases >5× ULN when normal pretreatment LFTs)

• **GI perforation/bleeding:** some cases have been fatal, usually occurs in those using NSAIDs, taxanes or in those with diverticulitis or peptic ulcer disease; discontinue if these occur

• **Pregnancy/breastfeeding:** do not use in pregnancy or for 1 mo after last dose; do not breastfeed during or for 2 wk after final dose

Evaluate:

• Therapeutic response: decrease in NSCLC cells, pancreatic cancer cells

Teach patient/family:

• **To report adverse reactions immediately:** SOB, severe abdominal pain, persistent diarrhea or vomiting, ocular changes, skin eruptions (face, upper chest/back)

• About reason for treatment, expected results; to take on empty stomach 1 hr before or 2 hr after meals

• To use sunscreen, protective clothing to prevent sunburn

• To avoid use with other products, herbs, supplements unless approved by provider, not to use with grapefruit or grapefruit juice

• To avoid smoking; decreases effect of this product

• **Pregnancy/breastfeeding:** To use reliable contraception during treatment; to avoid breastfeeding

---

ertapenem (Rx)

(er-tah-pen'em)

INVanz

Func. class.: Antiinfective—miscellaneous

Chem. class.: Carbapenem

Do not confuse:

INVanz/AVINza

ACTION: Interferes with cell-wall replication of susceptible organisms; bactericidal

USES: *Bacteroides distasonis, Bacteroides fragilis, Bacteroides ovatus, Bacteroides thetaiotaomicron, Bacteroides uniformis, Bacteroides vulgatus, Citrobacter freundii, Citrobacter koseri, Clostridium clostridioforme, Clostridium perfringens, Enterobacter aerogenes, Enterobacter cloacae, Escherichia coli, Eubacterium lentum, Fusobacterium sp., Haemophilus influenzae* (beta-lactamase negative), *Haemophilus influenzae* (beta-lactamase

---

Side effects: *italics* = common; red = life-threatening

positive), *Haemophilus parainfluenzae*, *Klebsiella oxytoca*, *Klebsiella pneumoniae*, *Moraxella catarrhalis*, *Morganella morganii*, *Peptostreptococcus* sp., *Porphyromonas asaccharolytica*, *Prevotella bivia*, *Proteus mirabilis*, *Proteus vulgaris*, *Providencia rettgeri*, *Providencia stuartii*, *Serratia marcescens*, *Staphylococcus aureus* (MSSA), *Staphylococcus epidermidis*, *Streptococcus agalactiae* (group B streptococci), *Streptococcus pneumoniae*, *Streptococcus pyogenes* (group A beta-hemolytic streptococci); bacteremia, community-acquired pneumonia, diabetic foot ulcer, endometritis, gyn/intraabdominal skin/skin structure/urinary tract infections, surgical infection prophylaxis

CONTRAINDICATIONS: Hypersensitivity to this product, its components, amide-type local anesthetics (IM only); anaphylactic reactions to β-lactams, other carbapenems
Precautions: Pregnancy, breastfeeding, children, geriatric patients, GI/renal/hepatic disease, seizures

DOSAGE AND ROUTES
• **Adult/child ≥13 yr: IM/IV** 1 g/day × 14 days (IV), 7 days (IM)
• **Child 3 mo-12 yr: IM/IV** 15 mg/kg q12hr (max 1 g/day) × up to 14 days (IV) or 7 days (IM)
Renal dose
• **Adult: IM/IV** CCr ≤30 mL/min 500 mg daily

Available form: Powder, lyophilized, 1 g/vial
Administer:
IM route
• Reconstitute 1-g vial of ertapenem with 3.2 mL of 1% lidocaine HCl injection (without EPINEPHrine) (280 mg/mL), agitate; the IM reconstituted formulation is not for IV use
• IM may be used as an alternative to IV administration in the treatment of infections where IM therapy is appropriate; only give via IM injection × 7 days

• **For a 1-g dose:** immediately withdraw the contents of the vial and inject deeply into a large muscle, aspirate before injection to avoid injection into a blood vessel
• **For a dose <1 g (for pediatric patients 3 mo-12 yr):** immediately withdraw a volume equal to 15 mg/kg (max 1 g/day) and inject deeply into a large muscle, aspirate before injection to avoid injecting into a blood vessel; use the reconstituted IM sol within 1 hr after preparation
IV route
• Visually inspect for particulate matter and discoloration before use, may be colorless to pale yellow; do not mix with other products; dextrose sols are not compatible
• **1-g vial:** For each gram reconstitute with 10 mL of either NS injection, sterile water for injection, or bacteriostatic water for injection to 100 mg/mL, shake
• **1 g dose:** Immediately transfer contents of the reconstituted vial to 50 mL of NS injection; for a dose <1 g (pediatric patients 3 mo-12 yr): from the reconstituted vial, immediately withdraw a volume equal to 15 mg/kg of body weight (max 1 g/day) and dilute in NS injection to a concentration of 20 mg/mL or less
Intermittent IV INFUSION route
• Complete the infusion within 6 hr of reconstitution, infuse over 30 min; do not co-infuse with other medications
• The reconstituted IV sol may be stored at room temperature if used within 6 hr, or store under refrigeration for 24 hr and use within 4 hours after removal from refrigeration; do not freeze

Y-site compatibilities: Acyclovir, alfentanil, amifostine, amikacin, aminocaproic acid, aminophylline, amphotericin B lipid complex, amphotericin B liposome, argatroban, arsenic trioxide, atenolol, atracurium, azithromycin, aztreonam, bivalirudin, bleomycin, bumetanide, buprenorphine, busulfan, butorphanol, calcium chloride/gluconate, CARBOplatin, carmustine, chloramphenicol, cimetidine, ciprofloxacin, cisatracurium, CISplatin, cyclophosphamide, cycloSPORINE, cytarabine, dacarbazine, DACTINomycin, DAPTOmycin, dexamethasone, dexmedetomidine, dexra-zoxane, digoxin, diltiazem, diphenhydr-AMINE, DOCEtaxel, dolasetron, DOPamine, doxacurium, doxycycline, enalaprilat, ePHEDrine, EPINEPHrine, eptifibatide, erythromycin, esmolol, etoposide, etoposide phosphate, famotidine, fenoldopam, fluconazole, fludarabine, fluorouracil, foscarnet, fosphenytoin, furosemide, ganciclovir, gatifloxacin, gemcitabine, gemtuzumab, gentamicin, glycopyrrolate, granisetron, haloperidol, heparin, hydrocortisone, HYDROmorphone, ifosfamide, inamrinone, insulin (regular), irinotecan, isoproterenol, ketorolac, labetalol, lepirudin, leucovorin, levofloxacin, lidocaine, linezolid, LORazepam, magnesium sulfate, mannitol, mechlorethamine, melphalan, meperidine, mesna, metaraminol, methotrexate, methyldopate, methylPREDNISolone, metoclopramide, metroNIDAZOLE, milrinone, mitoMYcin, mivacurium, morphine, moxifloxacin, nalbuphine, naloxone, nesiritide, nitroglycerin, nitroprusside, norepinephrine, octreotide, oxaliplatin, oxytocin, PACLitaxel, pamidronate, pancuronium, pantoprazole, PEMEtrexed, PENTobarbital, PHENobarbital, phentolamine, phenylephrine, polymyxin B, potassium acetate/chloride/phosphates, procainamide, propranolol, ranitidine, remifentanil, rocuronium, sodium acetate/bicarbonate/phosphates, streptozocin, succinylcholine, SUFentanil, sulfamethoxazole-trimethoprim, tacrolimus, telavancin, teniposide, theophylline, thiotepa, tigecycline, tirofiban, tobramycin, trimethobenzamide, vancomycin, vasopressin, vecuronium, vinBLAStine, vinCRIStine, vinorelbine, voriconazole, zidovudine, zoledronic acid

SIDE EFFECTS

CNS: Insomnia, seizures, dizziness, *headache*, agitation, confusion, somnolence, disorientation, edema, hypotension
CV: Tachycardia, seizures
GI: *Diarrhea, nausea, vomiting,* CDAD, abdominal pain
GU: *Vaginitis,* dysuria
INTEG: *Rash,* pain at inj site, *phlebitis/thrombophlebitis,* erythema at inj site, dermatitis
RESP: Dyspnea, cough, pharyngitis, crackles, respiratory distress
SYST: Anaphylaxis, angioedema

PHARMACOKINETICS

IV: Onset immediate; peak dose dependent; **IM:** Peak 2.3 hr half-life 4 hr; metabolized by liver; excreted in urine, feces, breast milk

INTERACTIONS

Increase: ertapenem levels—probenecid; do not coadminister
Decrease: effect of valproic acid; monitor valproic acid level, seizure control
Drug/Lab Test
Increase: hepatic enzymes, albumin, alkaline phosphatase, bilirubin, creatinine, PT
Decrease: Hct, WBC

NURSING CONSIDERATIONS
Assess:
• Renal disease: lower dose may be required
• **CNS symptoms:** for confusion, seizures; may increase seizure risk
• **CDAD:** bowel pattern, abdominal pain, mucus or blood in stools daily; if severe diarrhea occurs, product should be discontinued
• For infection: temperature, sputum, characteristics of wound, monitor WBC before, during, after treatment
• **Allergic reactions, anaphylaxis;** rash, urticaria, pruritus; may occur a few days after therapy begins; sensitivity to carbapenem antibiotics, other β-lactam antibiotics, penicillins; have emergency equipment, epinephrine close by
• **Overgrowth of infection:** perineal itching, fever, malaise, redness, pain, swelling, drainage, rash, diarrhea, change in cough or sputum
• **Pregnancy/breastfeeding:** use only when clearly needed; use caution in breastfeeding
Evaluate:
• Therapeutic response: negative C&S; absence of signs, symptoms of infection
Teach patient/family:
• **CDAD:** To report severe diarrhea, CNS side effects

Side effects: *italics* = common; red = life-threatening

• **To report overgrowth of infection:** black, furry tongue; vaginal itching; foul-smelling stools

• **Pregnancy/breastfeeding:** Identify if pregnancy is planned or suspected or if breastfeeding to avoid breastfeeding; product is excreted in breast milk

TREATMENT OF OVERDOSE: EPINEPHrine, antihistamines; resuscitate if needed (anaphylaxis)

RARELY USED

ertugliflozin
(er-too-gli-floe'-zin)

Steglatro
Func. class.: Antidiabetic

USES: For the treatment of type 2 diabetes mellitus

DOSAGE AND ROUTES
For type 2 diabetes mellitus in combination with diet and exercise

• **Adult: PO** 5 mg/day in the morning, with or without food; max 15 mg/day

---

erythromycin (ophthalmic)
(e-rith'roe-mye'sin)
Func. class.: Ophthalmic antiinfective
Chem. class.: Macrolide

ACTION: Inhibits protein synthesis, thereby decreasing bacterial replication

USES: Conjunctivitis, eye infections, prevention of ophthalmic neonatorum

CONTRAINDICATIONS: Hypersensitivity to this product or macrolides
Precautions: Pregnancy, breastfeeding

DOSAGE AND ROUTES
Bacterial conjunctivitis

• **Adult/adolescent/child: TOP** apply 1 cm of ointment directly to the eye up to 6 times a day × 7-10 days depending on severity of infection

Prevention of ophthalmic neonatorum

• **Neonate: TOP** apply 1-cm ribbon of ointment to lower conjunctival sac of each eye once after birth
Administer:
Ophthalmic route

• Apply ribbon of ointment directly to the eye; for ophthalmic use only
Available forms: ointment/ophthalmic 0.5%

SIDE EFFECTS
EENT: Hypersensitivity, irritation, redness

PHARMACOKINETICS
Unknown

NURSING CONSIDERATIONS
Assess:
• **Allergic reaction:** assess for hypersensitivity; discontinue product
Evaluate:
• Decreased ophthalmic infection
Teach patient/family:
Ophthalmic route:
• Apply ribbon of ointment directly to the eye; for ophthalmic use only

---

erythromycin base (Rx)
(eh-rith-roh-my'sin)
Eryc ✦, Ery-Tab, Erybid ✦, PCE
erythromycin ethylsuccinate (Rx)
E.E.S., Erythro-Es ✦, Ery Ped
erythromycin lactobionate (Rx)
Erythrocin
erythromycin stearate (Rx)
Erythrocin Stearate, Erythro-S ✦
erythromycin (topical)
AKne-Mycin, Erygel
Func. class.: Antiinfective
Chem. class.: Macrolide

Do not confuse:
erythromycin/azithromycin

ACTION: Binds to 50S ribosomal subunits of susceptible bacteria and suppresses protein synthesis

USES: Mild to moderate respiratory tract, skin, soft-tissue infections caused by *Bordetella pertussis, Borrelia burgdorferi, Chlamydia trachomatis; Corynebacterium diphtheriae, Haemophilus influenzae* (when used with sulfonamides); *Legionella pneumophila,* Legionnaire's disease, *Listeria monocytogenes; Mycoplasma pneumoniae, Streptococcus pneumoniae,* syphilis: *Treponema pallidum; Staphylococcus* sp.

Unlabeled uses: Bartonellosis, burn wound infection, chancroid, cholera, diabetic gastroparesis, endocarditis prophylaxis, gastroenteritis, granuloma inguinale, Lyme disease, tetanus

CONTRAINDICATIONS: Hypersensitivity, preexisting hepatic disease (estolate)

Precautions: Pregnancy, breastfeeding, geriatric patients, hepatic disease, GI disease, QT prolongation, seizure disorder, myasthenia gravis

DOSAGE AND ROUTES
Acne
• **Adult/child >12 yr:** topical applied bid 2%

Most infections
• **Adults PO (base, Stearate):** 250 mg q6hr or 333 mg q8hr or 500 mg q12hr; (ethylsuccinate) 400 mg q6hr or 800 mg q12hr; IV 250 mg-500 mg q6hr
• **Child >1 mo: PO** (base, ethylsuccinate) 30-50 mg/kg/day divided q6-8hr, max 2 g/day (base), max 3.2 g/day (ethylsuccinate); 30-50 mg/kg/day divided q6hr, max 2 g/day (Stearate); IV 15-50 mg/kg/day divided q6hr, max 4 g/day
• **Neonates: PO** (ethylsuccinate) 20-50 mg/kg/day divided q6-8hr

Available forms: *Base:* enteric-coated tabs 250, 333, 500 mg; film-coated tabs 250, 500 mg; enteric-coated caps 250, 333 mg; *stearate:* film-coated tabs 250 mg; *ethylsuccinate:* granules for oral susp 200, 400 mg/5 mL; powder for inj 500 mg, 1 g (lactobionate), 1 g (as gluceptate)

Administer:
• Do not break, crush, or chew time rel cap or tab; chew only chewable tabs; enteric-coated tablets may be given with food
• Do not give by IM or IV push
• Oral product with full glass of water; do not give with fruit juice
• Give 1 hr before or 2 hr after meals
• Store at room temperature; store susp in refrigerator
• Adequate intake of fluids (2 L) during diarrhea episodes

IV route
• After **reconstituting** 500 mg or less/10 mL sterile water without preservatives, dilute further in 100-250 mL of 0.9% NaCl, LR, Normosol-R; may be **further diluted** to 1 mg/mL and **given** as cont infusion; run 1 g or less/100 mL over ¹/₂-1 hr; cont infusion over 6 hr, may require buffers to neutralize pH if dilution is <250 mL, use infusion pump

Lactobionate
Y-site compatibilities: Acyclovir, alfentanil, amikacin, aminocaproic acid, aminophylline, amiodarone, anidulafungin, argatroban, atenolol, atosiban, atracurium, atropine, azaTHIOprine, benztropine, bivalirudin, bleomycin, bumetanide, buprenorphine, butorphanol, calcium chloride/gluconate, CARBOplatin, caspofungin, cefotaxime, cefTRIAXone, cefuroxime, chlorproMAZINE, cimetidine, CISplatin, cyanocobalamin, cyclophosphamide, cycloSPORINE, cytarabine, DACTINomycin, DAPTOmycin, dexmedetomidine, digoxin, diltiazem, diphenhydrAMINE, DOBUTamine, DOCEtaxel, DOPamine, doxacurium, doxapram, DOXOrubicin, enalaprilat, ePHEDrine, EPINEPHrine, epirubicin, epoetin alfa, eptifibatide, ertapenem, esmolol, etoposide, famotidine, fenoldopam, fentaNYL, fluconazole, fludarabine, fluorouracil, folic acid, foscarnet, gatifloxacin, gemcitabine, gentamicin, glycopyrrolate, granisetron, hydrocortisone,

E

HYDROmorphone, hydrOXYzine, IDArubicin, ifosfamide, imipenem-cilastatin, insulin (regular), irinotecan, isoproterenol, labetalol, levofloxacin, lidocaine, LORazepam, LR, mannitol, mechlorethamine, meperidine, methicillin, methotrexate, methoxamine, methyldopate, methylPREDNISolone, metoclopramide, metroNIDAZOLE, miconazole, midazolam, milrinone, mitoXANtrone, morphine, multiple vitamins injection, mycophenolate, nafcillin, nalbuphine, naloxone, nesiritide, netilmicin, niCARdipine, nitroglycerin, norepinephrine, octreotide, ondansetron, oxacillin, oxaliplatin, oxytocin, PACLitaxel, palonosetron, pamidronate, pancuronium, papaverine, pentamidine, pentazocine, perphenazine, phenylephrine, phytonadione, piperacillin, piperacillin-tazobactam, polymyxin B, procainamide, prochlorperazine, promethazine, propranolol, protamine, pyridoxine, quiNIDine, ranitidine, Ringer's, ritodrine, sodium acetate/bicarbonate, succinylcholine, SUFentanil, tacrolimus, temocillin, teniposide, theophylline, thiamine, thiotepa, tigecycline, tirofiban, TNA, tobramycin, tolazoline, TPN, trimetaphan, urokinase, vancomycin, vasopressin, vecuronium, verapamil, vinCRIStine, vinorelbine, vitamin B complex/C, voriconazole, zidovudine, zoledronic acid

SIDE EFFECTS

CNS: Seizures

CV: Dysrhythmias, QT prolongation

GI: *Nausea, vomiting, diarrhea,* hepatotoxicity, abdominal pain, stomatitis, heartburn, anorexia, CDAD, esophagitis

GU: *Vaginitis, moniliasis*

INTEG: Rash, urticaria, pruritus, thrombophlebitis, inj-site reactions (IV site)

SYST: Anaphylaxis

PHARMACOKINETICS

Peak 1-4 hr (base); $^1/_2$-$2^1/_2$ hr (ethylsuccinate); half-life 1-2 hr, neonates 2 hr; metabolized in liver; excreted in bile, feces; protein binding 75%-90%; inhibitor of CYP3A4 and P-glycoprotein

INTERACTIONS

• Serious dysrhythmias—diltiaZEM, itraconazole, ketoconazole, nefazodone, pimozide, protease inhibitors, verapamil; do not use together

Increase: QT prolongation—products that increase QT prolongation

Increase: action, toxicity of alfentanil, ALPRAZolam, bromocriptine, busPIRone, carBAMazepine, cilostazol, clindamycin, cloZAPine, cycloSPORINE, diazePAM, digoxin, disopyramide, ergots, felodipine, HMG-CoA reductase inhibitors, ibrutinib methylPREDNISolone, midazolam, quiNIDine, rifabutin, sildenafil, tacrolimus, tadalafil, theophylline, triazolam, vardenafil, vinBLAStine, warfarin

Decrease: erythromycin effect—rifabutin, rifampin, rifapentine

Drug/Lab Test

Increase: AST/ALT

Decrease: folate assay

False increase: 17-OHCS/17-KS

Drug/Food

Decrease: erythromycin metabolism—grapefruit juice; avoid using together

NURSING CONSIDERATIONS

Assess:

• **Infection:** temperature, characteristics of wounds, urine, stools, sputum, WBCs at baseline and periodically

• I&O ratio; report hematuria, oliguria in renal disease

• Hepatic studies: AST, ALT if patient is receiving long-term therapy

• Hearing at baseline and after treatment

• Renal studies: urinalysis, protein, blood

• C&S before product therapy; product may be given as soon as culture is taken; C&S may be repeated after treatment

• **CDAD:** diarrhea with blood, mucus; abdominal pain, fever; product should be discontinued immediately, notify prescriber

• **Anaphylaxis:** generalized hives, itching, flushing, swelling of lips, tongue, throat, wheezing; have emergency equipment nearby

• **QT prolongation:** may occur (IV >15 mg/min); those with electrolyte imbalances, congenital QT prolongation, elderly at greater risk; correct electrolyte imbalances before treatment, ECG

• **Pregnancy/breastfeeding:** use only if clearly needed; use other form of erythromycin, avoid estolate salt; use caution in breastfeeding, product appears in breast milk

Evaluate:

• Therapeutic response: decreased symptoms of infection

Teach patient/family:

• To notify nurse of diarrhea stools, dark urine, pale stools, jaundice of eyes or skin, severe abdominal pain

• To take at evenly spaced intervals; to complete dosage regimen; to take without food

• To avoid use with other products unless approved by prescriber

TREATMENT OF HYPERSENSITIVITY: Withdraw product; maintain airway; administer EPINEPHrine, aminophylline, O_2, IV corticosteroids

---

erythromycin (topical)
(e-rith-roe-mye′sin)
Akne-mycin, Ery-sol ✦
Func. class.: Topical antiinfective, anti-acne
Chem. class.: Macrolide

ACTION: Antibacterial activity results from inhibition of protein synthesis; bacteriostatic

USES: Treatment of acne vulgaris

CONTRAINDICATIONS: Hypersensitivity, children

DOSAGE AND ROUTES
Acne vulgaris

• **Adult/adolescent:** TOP Apply to affected areas bid, AM, PM

Available forms: Topical gel, ointment, pledget, solution 2%

Administer:
Topical route

• For external use only; do not use skin products near the eyes, nose, or mouth

• Wash hands before and after use. Wash affected area and gently pat dry before using

• **Gel/ointment/pledget/solution:** Apply to the cleansed affected area. Massage gently into affected areas

• Each pledget should be used once and discarded

SIDE EFFECTS

INTEG: Burning, rash, pruritus, peeling, irritation

NURSING CONSIDERATIONS
Assess:

• **Allergic reaction:** assess for hypersensitivity; may need to discontinue product

• **Infection:** assess for number of lesions, severity in acne

Evaluate:

• Decreased lesions in acne

Teach patient/family:
Topical route:

• That product is for external use only; do not use skin products near the eyes, nose, or mouth

• To wash hands before and after use; wash affected area and gently pat dry before using

• **Gel/pledget/solution/ointment/lotion:**

• To apply to the cleansed affected area; to massage gently into affected areas

• That each pledget should be used once and discarded

---

escitalopram (Rx)
(es-sit-tal′oh-pram)
Cipralex ✦, Lexapro
Func. class.: Antidepressant, SSRI (selective serotonin reuptake inhibitor)

Do not confuse:
Lexapro/Loxitane

ACTION: Inhibits CNS neuron uptake of serotonin but not of norepinephrine

USES: General anxiety disorder; major depressive disorder in adults/adolescents

Unlabeled uses: Panic disorder, social phobia, hot flashes related to menopause

CONTRAINDICATIONS: Hypersensitivity to this product, citalopram, MAOIs

Precautions: Pregnancy, breastfeeding, geriatric patients, renal/hepatic disease, history of seizures, abrupt discontinuation, bleeding, anticoagulants

Black Box Warning: Children/adolescents ≤12 yr, suicidal ideation

DOSAGE AND ROUTES
• **Adult/adolescent: PO** 10 mg/day; after 1 wk, dose may be increased to 20 mg/day PM
Hepatic dose/geriatric
• **Adult/child ≤ 12 yr:** PO 10 mg/day
Hot flashes related to menopause (unlabeled)
• **Adult:** PO 10-20 mg/day × 8 wk
Available forms: Tabs 5, 10, 20 mg; oral sol 5 mg (as base)/5 mL (contains sorbitol)
Administer:
• With food or milk for GI symptoms, give with full glass of water once a day in the AM
• Crushed if patient is unable to swallow medication whole; scored tabs can be cut
• Dosage at bedtime if oversedation occurs during the day
• Gum, hard candy, frequent sips of water for dry mouth
• **Oral sol:** measure with calibrated device
• Store at room temperature; do not freeze

SIDE EFFECTS
CNS: *Insomnia,* suicidal ideation, *drowsiness, anxiety, tremor, dizziness, fatigue, sedation, abnormal dreams,* neuroleptic malignant–like syndrome

CV: Postural hypotension
GI: *Nausea, diarrhea, dry mouth, anorexia, constipation, taste changes,* hepatitis
GU: *Decreased libido,* impotence, ejaculation disorder
INTEG: *Sweating, rash, pruritus*
SYST: Serotonin syndrome, Stevens-Johnson syndrome

PHARMACOKINETICS
PO: Metabolized in liver; excreted in urine; 56% protein binding; metabolized by CYP2C19, CYP 3A4, half-life 27-32 hr; half-life increased by 50% in geriatric patients

INTERACTIONS
• Paradoxical worsening of OCD: busPIRone
Increase: serotonin syndrome—tryptophan, amphetamines, busPIRone, lithium, amantadine, bromocriptine, SSRIs, SNRIs, serotonin-receptor agonists, traMADol, trazodone, tricyclic antidepressants, linezolid, methylene blue
• Do not use pimozide, MAOIs with or 14 days before escitalopram
Increase: CNS depression—alcohol, antidepressants, opioids, sedatives
Increase: side effects of escitalopram—highly protein-bound products
Increase: levels or toxicity of carBAMazepine, lithium, warfarin, phenytoin, antipsychotics, antidysrhythmics
Increase: levels of tricyclics, phenothiazines, haloperidol, diazepam
Increase: bleeding risk—NSAIDs, salicylates, anticoagulants, SSRIs, platelet inhibitors
Drug/Herb
• **SAMe, St. John's wort:** do not use together; serotonin syndrome may occur
Increase: CNS effect—kava, valerian
Drug/Food
• Grapefruit juice—increased escitalopram effect
Drug/Lab Test
Increase: serum bilirubin, blood glucose, alk phos
Decrease: VMA, 5-HIAA, sodium
False increase: urinary catecholamines

NURSING CONSIDERATIONS
Assess:

Black Box Warning: Mental status: mood, sensorium, affect, **suicidal tendencies,** increase in psychiatric symptoms, depression, panic; not approved for use in children <12 yr, provide a limited amount of product, continuing follow-ups should be weekly × 4 wk, q3wk × next 4 wk

• Appetite with bulimia nervosa, weight daily; increase nutritious foods in diet, watch for bingeing and vomiting
• **Allergic reactions:** itching, rash, urticaria; product should be discontinued, may need to give antihistamine
• B/P (lying/standing), pulse q4hr; if systolic B/P drops 20 mm Hg, hold product, notify prescriber
• **Serotonin syndrome:** nausea, vomiting, sedation, dizziness, sweating, facial flushing, mental changes, shivering, increased B/P; discontinue product, notify prescriber
• Weight weekly; appetite may decrease with product
• Alcohol consumption; if alcohol is consumed, hold dose until AM
• **Sexual dysfunction:** ejaculation dysfunction, erectile dysfunction, decreased libido, orgasm dysfunction, priapism
• Assistance with ambulation during therapy, since drowsiness, dizziness occur; safety measures primarily for geriatric patients
• **Pregnancy/breastfeeding:** use only if benefit outweighs risk to fetus; if used during pregnancy, taper in 3rd trimester; use cautiously in breastfeeding, excreted in breast milk

Evaluate:
• Therapeutic response: decreased depression

Teach patient/family:
• That therapeutic effect may take 1-4 wk, may have increased anxiety for first 5-7 days, do not abruptly discontinue
• **Serotonin syndrome:** to report immediately nausea, vomiting, sedation, dizziness, sweating, facial flushing, mental changes, shivering
• To use caution when driving, performing other activities requiring alertness because drowsiness, dizziness, blurred vision may occur
• To avoid alcohol, other CNS depressants; to avoid all OTC, herbals, supplement products unless approved by prescriber, to take without regard to meals
• To change positions slowly; orthostatic hypotension may occur

Black Box Warning: That clinical worsening of depression and suicide risk may occur, especially in adolescents and young adults, increased depression, thoughts of dying

• To use MedGuide provided
• To notify prescriber if pregnant or planning to become pregnant or if breastfeeding, discuss sexual dysfunction

---

⚠ HIGH ALERT

eslicarbazepine
(es′lye-kar-bay′ze-peen)
Aptiom
Func. class.: Anticonvulsant
Chem. class.: Carboxamide derivative

ACTION: Exact mechanism unknown; a voltage-gated sodium-channel blocker inhibits repetitive neuronal firing

USES: Partial seizures, adjunctive treatment

CONTRAINDICATIONS: Hypersensitivity to this product or OXcarbazepine
Precautions: Breastfeeding, abrupt discontinuation, depression, driving/operating machinery, ethanol intoxication, hepatic disease, renal disease, hyponatremia, suicidal ideation, pregnancy

DOSAGE AND ROUTES
• **Adult: PO** 400 mg daily; after 1 wk, increase to 800 mg daily, max 1600 mg daily
Renal dose
• **Adult: PO** CCr <50 mL/min 200 mg daily; after 2 wk, increase to 400 mg daily, max 800 mg daily

---

Available forms: Tab 200, 400, 600, 800 mg
Administer:
- May be taken without regard to food
- May be crushed or whole
- Store at room temperature

SIDE EFFECTS

CNS: Drowsiness, dizziness, amnesia, depression, insomnia, lethargy, memory impairment, confusion, fatigue, headache, speech disturbance, suicidal thoughts/behaviors, tremors
CV: Hypertension, peripheral edema
EENT: Blurred vision, nystagmus, diplopia
GI: Nausea, constipation, diarrhea, hypercholesterolemia/hypertriglyceridemia, vomiting, hepatotoxicity
GU: Cystitis
INTEG: Rash, Stevens-Johnson syndrome, toxic epidermal necrolysis, anaphylaxis, angioedema
META: Hyponatremia
RESP: Cough

PHARMACOKINETICS

Peak 1-4 hr; metabolized by liver; moderate CYP2C19 inhibitor; weak/moderate CYP3A4 inducer; steady state 4-5 days; excreted in urine, feces; half-life 13-20 hr; protein binding <40%

INTERACTIONS

Decrease: effects of bedaquiline, boceprevir, bosutinib, cabozantinib, cobicistat, elvitegravir, emtricitabine, crizotinib, cycloSPORINE, dronedarone, erlotinib, fosamprenavir, galantamine, gefitinib, HYDROcodone, maraviroc, oxyCODONE, paliperidone, perampanel, pimozide, praziquantel, QUEtiapine, ranolazine, rilpivirine
Decrease: eslicarbazepine effect— CYP1A2, CYP2C19 substrates
Decrease: effect of CYP3A inducers

NURSING CONSIDERATIONS
Assess:
- **Hyponatremia:** nausea, vomiting, increased seizures, headache, weakness, confusion, irritability

- **Seizures:** character, location, duration, intensity, frequency, presence of aura
- **Hepatic studies:** ALT, AST, bilirubin; sodium

Black Box Warning: Mental status: mood, sensorium, affect, behavioral changes, suicidal thoughts/behaviors; if mental status changes, notify prescriber

- Eye problems: need for ophthalmic examinations before, during, after treatment (slit lamp, funduscopy, tonometry)
- **Allergic reaction:** purpura, red, raised rash; if these occur, product should be discontinued
- **Beers:** avoid in older adults unless safer alternative is unavailable; may cause ataxia, impaired psychomotor function
- **Pregnancy/breastfeeding:** use in pregnancy only if benefits outweigh risks to fetus. Patient should enroll in North American Antiepileptic Drug (NAAED) Pregnancy Registry (1-888-233-2334; www.aedpregnancyregistry.org). Product is present in breast milk; consider benefits of breastfeeding, risk of potential infant drug exposure, and risk of an untreated or inadequately treated condition
Evaluate:
- Therapeutic response: decreased seizure activity; document on patient's chart
Teach patient/family:
- To carry emergency ID stating patient's name, products taken, condition, prescriber's name, and phone number
- To avoid driving, other activities that require alertness, usually for the first 3 days of treatment
- Not to discontinue medication quickly after long-term use
- **Pregnancy:** to notify prescriber if pregnancy is planned or suspected; to use additional contraceptives if using hormonal contraceptives; to avoid breastfeeding
- Not to abruptly discontinue drug
- To report signs of decreased renal function, dizziness, increased cholesterol, ocular toxicity, suicide risk, skin rashes

---

• To take with or without food; that tablet can be crushed
• To report increased seizures, headache, nausea, vomiting, weakness, confusion, irritability (hyponatremia)

⚠ HIGH ALERT

esmolol (Rx)

(ez'moe-lole)

Brevibloc

Func. class.: β-Adrenergic blocker (antidysrhythmic II)

Do not confuse:
Brevibloc/Brevital

ACTION: Competitively blocks stimulation of β_1-adrenergic receptors in the myocardium; produces negative chronotropic, inotropic activity (decreases rate of SA node discharge, increases recovery time), slows conduction of AV node, decreases heart rate, decreases O_2 consumption in myocardium; also decreases renin-aldosterone-angiotensin system at high doses; inhibits β_2-receptors in bronchial system at higher doses

USES: Supraventricular tachycardia, noncompensatory sinus tachycardia, intraoperative and postoperative tachycardia and hypertension, atrial fibrillation/flutter

CONTRAINDICATIONS: 2nd- or 3rd-degree heart block; cardiogenic shock, HF, cardiac failure, hypersensitivity, severe bradycardia

Precautions: Pregnancy, breastfeeding, geriatric patients, hypotension, peripheral vascular disease, diabetes, hypoglycemia, thyrotoxicosis, renal disease, atrial fibrillation, bronchospasms, hyperthyroidism, myasthenia gravis, asthma, COPD, CV disease, pheochromocytoma, abrupt discontinuation

DOSAGE AND ROUTES
Atrial fibrillation/flutter
• **Adult:** IV loading dose 500 mcg/kg/min over 1 min; maintenance 50 mcg/kg/min for 4 min; if no response after 5 min, give 2nd loading dose, then increase infusion to 100 mcg/kg/min for 4 min; if no response, repeat loading dose, then increase maintenance infusion by 50 mcg/kg/min (max of 200 mcg/kg/min); titrate to patient response
• **Child:** IV total loading dose of 600 mcg/kg over 2 min, maintenance **IV INFUSION** 200 mcg/kg/min, titrate upward by 50-100 mcg/kg/min q5-10min until B/P, heart rate reduced by >10%

Perioperative hypertension/tachycardia
• **Adult:** IV immediate control 80 mg (bolus) over 30 seconds, then 150 mcg/kg/min, adjust to response, max 300 mcg/kg/min

Available forms: Inj 10 mg/mL, 10 mg/mL in 250-mLbag, 20 mg/mL in 100-mL bag

Administer:
• Do not discontinue product suddenly
• Store protected from light, moisture, in cool environment

IV route
• Check that correct concentration is being given

IV direct route
• 10 mg/mL inj sol needs no dilution, may be used as an IV loading dose using a handheld syringe

Continuous IV INFUSION route
• Ready-to-use bags of premixed isotonic sol of 10 mg/mL and 20 mg/mL available in 100-, 250-mL bags; use controlled infusion device, central line preferred; rate is based on patient's weight

Y-site compatibilities: Amikacin, aminophylline, amiodarone, atracurium, butorphanol, calcium chloride, ceFAZolin, cefTAZidime, ceftizoxime, chloramphenicol, cimetidine, cisatracurium, clindamycin, diltiazem, DOPamine, enalaprilat, erythromycin, famotidine, fentaNYL, gentamicin, insulin (regular), labetalol, magnesium sulfate, methyldopate, metroNIDAZOLE, midazolam, morphine, nitroglycerin, nitroprusside, norepinephrine, pancuronium, penicillin G

Side effects: *italics* = common; red = life-threatening

potassium, piperacillin, polymyxin B, potassium chloride, potassium phosphate, propofol, ranitidine, remifentanil, streptomycin, tacrolimus, tobramycin, trimethoprim-sulfamethoxazole, vancomycin, vecuronium, voriconazole, zoledronic acid

SIDE EFFECTS

CNS: Confusion, drowsiness, weakness, dizziness, fatigue, headache
CV: Hypotension, peripheral ischemia
GI: *Nausea*, vomiting, anorexia
INTEG: *Inflammation at site*, sweating

PHARMACOKINETICS

Onset very rapid, duration short, half-life 9 min, metabolized by hydrolysis of ester linkage, excreted via kidneys

INTERACTIONS

• Avoid use with MAOIs, Sotalol
Increase: effect of antidiabetics
Increase: possible fatal B/P increase—clonidine
Increase: potentiate suppressive effects of diltiazem, verapamil
Increase: antihypertensive effect—general anesthetics
Increase: digoxin levels—digoxin
Increase: α-adrenergic stimulation—ePHEDRine, EPINEPHrine, amphetamine, norepinephrine, phenylephrine, pseudoePHEDRine
Decrease: action of thyroid hormones
Decrease: action of esmolol—thyroid hormone, salicylates
Drug/Herb
Increase: β-blocking effect—hawthorn
Decrease: antihypertensive effect—ephedra
Drug/Lab Test
Interference: glucose/insulin tolerance test

NURSING CONSIDERATIONS
Assess:

• **Heart failure:** I&O ratio, weight daily, jugular venous distention, weight gain, crackles, edema
• **Dysrhythmias:** B/P, pulse; note rate, rhythm, quality; rapid changes can cause

shock; if systolic <100 or diastolic <60, notify prescriber before giving product; ECG continuously during infusion, hypotension common, if severe, slow or stop infusion
• **Infusion site:** monitor infusion site during infusion; do not use butterfly if irritation occurs; stop and start at another site
• **Bronchospasm:** breath sounds, respiratory pattern
• **Pregnancy/breastfeeding:** use only if benefit outweighs risk to fetus; use in the last trimester or labor or obstetric delivery has resulted in fetal bradycardia; not known if excreted in breast milk
Evaluate:
• Therapeutic response: lower B/P immediately, lower heart rate
Teach patient/family:
• Not to drive or perform other hazardous activities if drowsiness occurs
• To change positions slowly to prevent orthostatic hypotension
• About reason for use; expected results
• To notify prescriber if chest pain, SOB, wheezing, hypotension, bradycardia, pain, swelling at IV site occurs
• **Pregnancy/breastfeeding:** Identify if pregnancy is planned or suspected

TREATMENT OF OVERDOSE:
Discontinue product; IV glucagon if needed

---

esomeprazole (Rx)
(es′oh-mep′rah-zohl)
NexIUM, NexIUM 24hr
Func. class.: Antiulcer
Chem. class.: Proton pump inhibitor, benzimidazole

Do not confuse:
NexIUM/NexAVAR

ACTION: Suppresses gastric secretions by inhibiting hydrogen/potassium ATPase enzyme system in gastric parietal cell; characterized as gastric acid pump inhibitor because it blocks the final step of acid production

---

USES: Gastroesophageal reflux disease (GERD), adult/child/infant; severe erosive esophagitis, adult/child; treatment of active duodenal ulcers in combination with antiinfectives for *Helicobacter pylori* infection; long-term use for hypersecretory conditions

CONTRAINDICATIONS: Hypersensitivity to proton pump inhibitors (PPIs)
Precautions: Pregnancy, breastfeeding, children, geriatric patients, hypomagnesemia, osteoporosis

DOSAGE AND ROUTES
Active duodenal ulcers associated with *H. pylori*
• **Adult: PO** 40 mg/day × 10-14 days in combination with clarithromycin 500 mg bid × 10 days and amoxicillin 1000 mg bid × 10 days
GERD/erosive esophagitis
• **Adult: PO** 20 or 40 mg/day × 4-8 wk; no adjustment needed in renal/liver failure, geriatric patients; **IV** 20 or 40 mg/day up to 10 days
• **Adolescent and child 12-17 yr: PO** 20 or 40 mg/day 1 hr before meals for ≤8 wk
• **Child 1-11 yr and ≥20 kg: PO** 10 mg/day 1 hr before meals for ≤8 wk
• **Infant ≥1 mo: IV** 0.5 mg/kg over 10-30 min
• **Infant 1-11 mo (>7.5-12 kg): PO** 10 mg daily × up to 6 wk
• **Infant 1-11 mo (>5-7.5 kg): PO** 5 mg daily × up to 6 wk
• **Infant 1-11 mo (3-5 kg): PO** 2.5 mg daily × up to 6 wk
Gastric ulcer prophylaxis, NSAID-associated gastropathy
• **Adult: PO** 20-40 mg/day up to 6 mo
Zollinger-Ellison syndrome
• **Adult: PO** 40 mg bid, up to 240 mg/day
Hepatic dose
• **Adult: PO/IV** max 20 mg/day (severe hepatic disease)

Available forms: Del rel caps 20, 40 mg; powder for IV inj 20, 40 mg/vial; del rel powder for oral susp 2.5, 5, 10, 20, 40 mg

Administer:
PO route
• Swallow caps whole; do not crush or chew; cap may be opened and sprinkled over Tbsp of applesauce
• Same time daily, 1 hr before meal
• **Oral susp (del rel):** empty contents of packet into container with 1 Tbsp of water, let stand 2-3 min to thicken, restir, give within 30 min of mixing; any residual product should be flushed with more water, taken immediately
• **NG tube (del rel oral susp):** add 50 mL water to contents of packet in syringe, shake, leave 2-3 min to thicken, shake, inject through NG tube within 30 min, make sure granules are dissolved
IV, direct route
• Reconstitute each vial with 5 mL 0.9% NaCl, D_5W, LR; give over 3 min
Intermittent IV INFUSION route
• Dilute reconstituted sol to 50 mL, give over 30 min, do not admix, flush line with D_5W, 0.9% NaCl, LR after infusion
Continuous IV route
• Use 2 (40-mg vials) with 5 mL of 0.9% NaCL for 80-mg loading dose, further dilute in 100 mL 0.9% NaCl give over 30 min, then infusion at 8 mg/hr

Y-site compatibility: Ceftaroline, Fentanyl, furosemide, regular insulin, nitroglycerin

SIDE EFFECTS
CNS: *Headache, dizziness*
GI: *Diarrhea, flatulence,* abdominal pain, constipation, dry mouth, hepatic failure, hepatitis, microscopic colitis, *Clostridium difficile*–associated diarrhea (CDAD)
INTEG: *Rash,* dry skin
GU: Nephritis
MISC: Fractures, SLE, vitamin B_{12} deficiency
SYST: Stevens-Johnson syndrome, toxic epidermal necrolysis, exfoliative dermatitis

PHARMACOKINETICS
Well absorbed 90%; protein binding 97%; extensively metabolized in liver (CYP2C19); terminal half-life 1-1.5 hr; eliminated in urine as metabolites and in

---

Side effects: *italics* = common; red = life-threatening

feces; in geriatric patients, elimination rate decreased, bioavailability increased

INTERACTIONS

Increase: effect, toxicity of diazePAM, digoxin, penicillins, saquinavir, cilostazol, cloZAPine, those drugs metabolized by CYP2C19

Increase: effect of methotrexate, tacrolimus, warfarin

Decrease: effect—atazanavir, nelfinavir, dapsone, iron, itraconazole, ketoconazole, indinavir, calcium carbonate, vit B$_{12}$, clopidogrel, iron salts, mycophenolate

Drug/Lab Test

Interference: sodium, Hgb, WBC, platelets, magnesium

False-positive CgA

NURSING CONSIDERATIONS

Assess:

• **GI system:** bowel sounds, abdomen for pain, swelling, anorexia, bloody stools; CDAD may occur

• **Hepatic failure, hepatitis:** AST, ALT, alk phos at baseline and periodically during treatment

• **Serious skin disorders:** Stevens-Johnson syndrome, toxic epidermal necrolysis, exfoliative dermatitis

• **Pregnancy/breastfeeding:** use only if benefits clearly outweigh risks to fetus; do not breastfeed

Evaluate:

• Therapeutic response: absence of epigastric pain, swelling, fullness, decreased GERD

Teach patient/family:

• To report severe diarrhea, abdominal pain, black tarry stools, rash; product may have to be discontinued

• That hypoglycemia may occur if diabetic

• To avoid hazardous activities; dizziness may occur

• To notify provider if pregnancy is planned or suspected or if breastfeeding

• To avoid alcohol, salicylates, NSAIDs; may cause GI irritation

• To take ≥1 hr before meal; not to crush, chew del rel product; if missed, to take as soon as remembered if not almost

time for next dose; to take full course prescribed; to read "Patient Information"

• That if cap is unable to be swallowed whole, contents may be mixed with a Tbsp of applesauce

• To notify provider of all OTC, Rx, or herbal products taken

• **Hypomagnesemia:** to notify prescriber of dizziness, fast heartbeat, tremors, weakness, spasm, cramps

---

estradiol (Rx)

(es-tra-dye′ole)

Estrace

estradiol cypionate (Rx)

Depo-Estradiol

estradiol gel (Rx)

Divigel, Elestrin, Estrogel

estradiol spray (Rx)

Evamist

estradiol topical emulsion (Rx)

Estrasorb

estradiol transdermal system (Rx)

Alora, Climara, Minivelle, Vivelle-Dot

estradiol vaginal ring (Rx)

Estring, Femring

estradiol vaginal tablet (Rx)

Vagifem

estradiol valerate (Rx)

Delestrogen

Func. class.: Estrogen, progestins

Do not confuse:

Alora/Aldora

ACTION: Needed for adequate functioning of female reproductive system; affects release of pituitary gonadotropins; inhibits ovulation; adequate calcium use in bone

USES: Vasomotor symptoms (menopause), inoperable breast cancer (selected cases), prostatic cancer, atrophic vaginitis, kraurosis vulvae, hypogonadism, primary ovarian failure, prevention of osteoporosis, castration

CONTRAINDICATIONS: Pregnancy, breastfeeding, reproductive cancer, genital bleeding (abnormal, undiagnosed), protein S or C deficiency, antithrombin deficiency, angioedema, MI, stroke

Black Box Warning: Breast/endometrial cancer, thromboembolic disorders, MI, stroke

Precautions: Hypertension, asthma, blood dyscrasias, gallbladder/bone/renal/hepatic disease, HF, diabetes mellitus, depression, migraine headache, seizure disorders, family history of cancer of breast or reproductive tract, smoking, uterine fibroids, vaginal irritation/infection, history of angioedema, cardiac disease

Black Box Warning: dementia, accidental exposure pets/children (topical)

DOSAGE AND ROUTES
Hormone replacement/menopause symptoms
• **Adult:** TRANSDERMAL 1 patch delivering 0.025, 0.0375, 0.05, 0.075, or 0.1 mg/day 2×/wk (Alora, Estraderm, Vivelle-Dot); 1 patch delivering 0.025, 0.0375, 0.05, 0.06, 0.075, or 0.1 mg/day replace q7days (Climara); **GEL** apply entire unit-dose packet to 5 × 7-inch area of upper thigh/day, alternate thighs; **SPRAY** (Evamist) 1 spray to inner surface of forearm/day in AM
Menopause/hypogonadism/castration/ovarian failure
• **Adult:** PO 0.5-2 mg/day, 3 wk on, 1 wk off or continuously; **IM** (cypionate) 1-5 mg q3-4wk; (valerate) 10-20 mg q4wk
• **Adult:** TOP (Estraderm) 0.05 mg/24 hr applied 2×/wk; (Climara) 0.05 mg/hr

applied 1×/wk in cyclic regimen; women with hysterectomy may use continuously
Postmenopausal osteoporosis, prophylaxis
• **Adult female:** PO 0.5 mg/day × 23 days of a 28-day cycle; **TRANSDERMAL** (Alora, Minivelle, Vivelle-Dot) 0.025 mg/day applied to skin 2×/wk; adjust as needed based on clinical response, bone mineral density; **TRANSDERMAL** (Climara) 0.025 mg/day applied to skin qwk
Prostatic cancer (inoperable)
• **Adult:** IM (valerate) 30 mg q1-2wk; PO (oral estradiol) 1-2 mg bid-tid
Breast cancer (palliative treatment)
• **Adult:** PO 10 mg tid × 3 mo or longer
Atrophic vaginitis/kraurosis vulvae
• **Adult:** VAG CREAM 2-4 g/day × 1-2 wk, then 1 g 1-3×/wk cycled; **VAG TAB** 1/day × 2 wk, maintenance 1 tab 2×/wk; **VAG RING** inserted, left in place continuously for 3 mo
Vasomotor symptoms
• **Adult:** TOP after cleaning and drying skin on left thigh, calf, rub in contents of pouch using both hands until completely absorbed; wash hands
Available forms: *Estradiol:* tabs 0.5, 1, 2 mg; *valerate:* inj 10, 20, 40 mg/mL; *transdermal:* 0.014, 0.025, 0.0375, 0.05, 0.075, 0.1 mg/24 hr release rate; *vag cream:* 100 mcg/g; *vag tab:* 10 mcg; *vag ring:* 2 mg/90 days; *topical emulsion:* 2.5 mg; *gel* (Divigel) 0.06%, 0.1%; *spray* (Evamist) 1.53 mg/actuation
Administer:
• Titrated dose; use lowest effective dose
• IM inj deeply in large muscle mass
PO route
• With food or milk to decrease GI symptoms
Transdermal route
• May contain aluminum or other metals in backing of patch, can overheat in MRI scan and burn patients
• Apply to trunk of body 2×/wk; press firmly, hold in place for 10 sec to ensure good contact; do not apply to breasts
• On intermittent cycle schedule: 3 wk on, then 1 wk off; if patch falls off, reapply

E

Side effects: *italics* = common; red = life-threatening

Topical route

• Use Evamist daily; spray to inner upper arm; may increase to 2-3×/day based on response; allow to dry for 2 min, avoid secondary exposure to children, pets, caregivers

Vaginal route

• Use a new applicator daily, provided

SIDE EFFECTS

CNS: Dizziness, headache, migraines, depression, seizures

CV: Hypertension, thrombophlebitis, edema, thromboembolism, stroke, pulmonary embolism, MI, chest pain

EENT: Contact lens intolerance, increased myopia, astigmatism, throat swelling, eyelid edema

GI: *Nausea*, vomiting, diarrhea, anorexia, pancreatitis, cramps, constipation, increased appetite, increased weight, cholestatic jaundice, hepatic adenoma

GU: Amenorrhea, cervical erosion, breakthrough bleeding, dysmenorrhea, vaginal candidiasis, breast changes, *gynecomastia, testicular atrophy, impotence,* increased risk of breast cancer, endometrial cancer, changes in libido; toxic shock, vaginal wall ulceration/erosion (vag ring)

INTEG: Rash, urticaria, acne, hirsutism, alopecia, oily skin, seborrhea, purpura, erythema, pruritus, melasma; site irritation (transdermal)

META: Folic acid deficiency, hypercalcemia, hyperglycemia

PHARMACOKINETICS

PO/INJ/TRANSDERMAL: Degraded in liver, excreted in urine, crosses placenta, excreted in breast milk

INTERACTIONS

Increase: action of corticosteroids, tricyclics

Increase: toxicity—cycloSPORINE, dantrolene

Decrease: action of anticoagulants, oral hypoglycemics, tamoxifen

Decrease: estradiol action—anticonvulsants, barbiturates, phenylbutazone, rifampin, calcium

Drug/Herb

• Altered estrogen effect: black cohosh, DHEA

Decrease: estrogen effect—saw palmetto, St. John's wort

Drug/Food

Increase: estrogen level—grapefruit juice

Drug/Lab Test

Increase: BSP retention test, PBI, T_4, serum sodium, platelet aggregation, thyroxine-binding globulin (TBG), prothrombin; factors VII, VIII, IX, X; triglycerides

Decrease: serum folate, serum triglyceride, T_3 resin uptake test, glucose tolerance test, antithrombin III, pregnanediol, metyrapone test

False positive: LE prep, ANA

NURSING CONSIDERATIONS
Assess:

> **Black Box Warning:** For previous breast/endometrial cancer, thromboembolic disorders, MI, stroke, dementia; use adequate screening for these conditions, estrogen increases the risk

• Blood glucose of diabetic patient; hyperglycemia may occur

• Weight daily; notify prescriber of weekly weight gain >5 lb; if increase, diuretic may be ordered

• B/P q4hr; watch for increase caused by water and sodium retention

• I&O ratio; decreasing urinary output, increasing edema, report changes

• Hepatic studies, including AST, ALT, bilirubin, alk phos at baseline, periodically; periodic folic acid level

• Hypertension, cardiac symptoms, jaundice, hypercalcemia

• Mental status: affect, mood, behavioral changes, aggression

• Female patient for intact uterus; if so, progesterone should be added to estrogen therapy to decrease risk of endometrial cancer

• **Beers:** avoid oral and topical patch in older adults; evidence of carcinogenic potential (breast, endometrial)

• **Pregnancy/breastfeeding:** do not use in pregnancy; estrogens decrease milk production; use only if needed

Evaluate:

• Therapeutic response: reversal of menopause symptoms; decrease in tumor size in prostatic, breast cancer

Teach patient/family:

• To weigh weekly; to report gain >5 lb

• To report breast lumps, vaginal bleeding, edema, jaundice, dark urine, clay-colored stools, dyspnea, headache, blurred vision, abdominal pain, numbness or stiffness in legs, chest pain; tenderness, redness, and swelling in extremities; males to report impotence, gynecomastia; to report dermal rash with transdermal patch

• To avoid grapefruit or grapefruit juice (PO)

• That smoking increases CV conditions; encourage to stop

• To notify prescriber if pregnancy is planned or suspected; not to become pregnant when using estrogen

• To report changes in blood glucose if diabetic

⚠ HIGH ALERT

estrogens, conjugated (Rx)

Cenestin, Premarin, C.E.S. ✦

estrogens, conjugated synthetic B (Rx)

Enjuvia

Func. class.: Estrogen, hormone

Do not confuse:
Premarin/Provera
Enjuvia/Januvia

ACTION: Needed for adequate functioning of female reproductive system; affects release of pituitary gonadotropins, inhibits ovulation; adequate calcium use in bone

USES: Vasomotor symptoms (menopause), inoperable breast cancer, prostatic cancer, abnormal uterine bleeding, hypogonadism, primary ovarian failure, prevention of osteoporosis, castration, atrophic vaginitis

Unlabeled uses: Hyperparathyroidism, infertility

CONTRAINDICATIONS: Pregnancy, breastfeeding, thromboembolic disorders, reproductive cancer, genital bleeding (abnormal, undiagnosed), hypersensitivity, MI, stroke, thrombophlebitis

> Black Box Warning: Endometrial, breast cancer, thromboembolic diseases

Precautions: Hypertension, asthma, blood dyscrasias, HF, diabetes mellitus, depression, migraine headache, seizure disorders, gallbladder/bone/hepatic/renal disease, family history of cancer of breast or reproductive tract, smoking, hypothyroidism, obesity, SLE

> Black Box Warning: Dementia

DOSAGE AND ROUTES
Estrogens conjugated
Vasomotor symptoms (menopause)
• **Adult: PO** 0.3-1.25 mg/day 3 wk on, 1 wk off
Prevention of osteoporosis
• **Adult: PO** 0.3 mg/day or in cycle
Atrophic vaginitis
• **Adult: VAG CREAM** 0.5 g/day × 21 days, off 7 days, repeat
Prostatic cancer
• **Adult: PO** 1.25-2.5 mg tid
Advanced inoperable breast cancer
• **Adult: PO** 10 mg tid × ≥3 mo
Abnormal uterine bleeding
• **Adult: IV/IM** 25 mg q6-12hr
Castration/primary ovarian failure
• **Adult: PO** 1.25 mg/day 3 wk on, 1 wk off
Hypogonadism
• **Adult: PO** 0.3 or 0.625 mg daily (3 wk on, 1 wk off), adjust to response

Estrogens conjugated synthetic B
Vasomotor symptoms (menopause)
• **Adult: PO** 0.625 mg/day initially; may increase based on response
Dyspareunia (moderate to severe); menopausal-cyclic regimen:
• **Adult: INTRAVAGINALLY** 0.5 g daily × 21 days, then off 7 days; continuous regimen **INTRAVAGINALLY** 0.5 g bid

Available forms: Tabs 0.3, 0.45, 0.625, 0.9, 1.25, 2.5 mg; inj 25 mg/vial; vag cream 0.625 mg/g; *synthetic B:* tabs 0.625, 1.25 mg
Administer:
Titrated dose; use lowest effective dose
PO route
• Give with or immediately after food to reduce nausea
IM route
• Reconstitute after withdrawing 5 mL of air from container, inject sterile diluent on vial side, rotate to dissolve; give inj deep in large muscle mass, aspirate before inj
Vaginal route
• Use applicator provided, wash after use
Direct IV route
• IV, after reconstituting as for IM, inject into distal port of running IV line of D_5W, 0.9% NaCl at ≤5 mg/min

Y-site compatibilities: Heparin, hydrocortisone, potassium chloride, vit B/C

SIDE EFFECTS
CNS: Dizziness, headache, migraine, depression, seizures, mood disturbances
CV: Hypertension, thrombophlebitis, edema, thromboembolism, stroke, pulmonary embolism, MI, chest pain
EENT: Contact lens intolerance, increased myopia, astigmatism
GI: *Nausea*, vomiting, diarrhea, anorexia, pancreatitis, cramps, constipation, increased appetite, cholestatic jaundice, hepatic adenoma, weight gain/loss
GU: Amenorrhea, cervical erosion, breakthrough bleeding, dysmenorrhea, vaginal candidiasis, breast changes, gynecomastia, testicular atrophy, impotence, increased risk of breast cancer, endometrial cancer, libido changes
INTEG: Rash, urticaria, acne, hirsutism, alopecia, oily skin, seborrhea, purpura, melasma
META: Folic acid deficiency, hypercalcemia, hyperglycemia

PHARMACOKINETICS
PO/IM/IV: Degraded in liver, excreted in urine, crosses placenta, excreted in breast milk

INTERACTIONS
Increase: toxicity—cycloSPORINE, dantrolene
Increase: action of corticosteroids
Decrease: action of estrogens—anticonvulsants, barbiturates, phenylbutazone, rifampin, bosentan
Decrease: action of anticoagulants, oral hypoglycemics, tamoxifen, thyroid, tricyclics
Drug/Food
Increase: estrogen level—grapefruit juice
Drug/Lab Test
Increase: T_4, serum sodium, platelet aggregation, thyroxine-binding globulin (TBG), prothrombin; factors VII, VIII, IX, X; triglycerides
Decrease: serum folate, serum triglyceride, T_3 resin uptake test, glucose tolerance test, antithrombin III, metyrapone test
False positive: LE prep, antinuclear antibodies

NURSING CONSIDERATIONS
Assess:

Black Box Warning: **Breast, endometrial cancer:** estrogens should not be used in known, suspected, or history of these disorders

Black Box Warning: **Stroke, thromboembolic disease of MI:** should not be used in these conditions or known protein C deficiency, protein S deficiency, or antithrombin deficiency

---

• Blood glucose if diabetic patient; hyperglycemia may occur
• Weight daily; notify prescriber of weekly weight gain >5 lb; if increase, diuretic may be ordered; check for edema; B/P baseline and periodically
• Hepatic studies: AST, ALT, bilirubin, alk phos
• Hypertension, cardiac symptoms, jaundice, hypercalcemia
• Mental status: affect, mood, behavioral changes, aggression
• Female patient for intact uterus; if so, progesterone should be added to estrogen therapy to decrease risk of endometrial cancer; abnormal uterine bleeding, breast exam; Pap smear
• **Use lowest dose/shortest time period:** estrogen therapy should be limited to the shortest duration of therapy and lowest effective dose; individualize risks and benefits with each patient
• **Beers:** avoid oral and topical patch in older adults; evidence of carcinogenic potential (breast, endometrial)
• **Pregnancy/breastfeeding:** do not use in pregnancy; estrogens decrease milk production; use only if clearly needed

Evaluate:
• Therapeutic response: absence of breast engorgement, reversal of menopause symptoms, decrease in tumor size with prostatic cancer

Teach patient/family:
• To avoid breastfeeding; product is excreted in breast milk
• To weigh weekly; to report gain >5 lb

Black Box Warning: To report breast lumps, vaginal bleeding, edema, jaundice, dark urine, clay-colored stools, dyspnea, headache, blurred vision, abdominal pain; leg pain and redness, numbness or stiffness; chest pain; males to report impotence or gynecomastia

• To avoid sunlight or wear sunscreen; burns may occur
• To notify prescriber if pregnancy is suspected

• That vasomotor symptoms improve in 2 wk, max relief in 8 wk

---

⚠ HIGH ALERT

eszopiclone (Rx)
(es-zop′i-klone)
Lunesta
Func. class.: Sedative/hypnotic, nonbenzodiazepine
Chem. class.: Cyclopyrrolone

Controlled Substance Schedule IV

Do not confuse:
Lunesta/Neulasta

ACTION: Interacts with GABA receptors

USES: Insomnia

CONTRAINDICATIONS:
Hypersensitivity

Precautions: Pregnancy, breastfeeding, children, geriatric patients, severe hepatic disease, abrupt discontinuation, COPD, depression, labor, sleep apnea, substance abuse, suicidal ideation, ethanol intoxication

DOSAGE AND ROUTES
• **Adult: PO** 1 mg immediately before bed, may increase to 2-3 mg if needed, max 3 mg nightly

Hepatic dose/CYP3A4 inhibitors
• **Adult: PO** 1 mg immediately before bed with severe hepatic disease, max 2 mg/day

Available forms: Tabs 1, 2, 3 mg

Administer:
• Do not break, crush, or chew tab
• Immediately before bedtime; avoid use with food; for short-term use only

SIDE EFFECTS
CNS: Worsening depression, hallucinations, headache, *daytime drowsiness*, suicidal thoughts/actions, migraine, restlessness, anxiety, sleep driving, sleepwalking
CV: Peripheral edema, chest pain
GI: Dry mouth, bitter taste (dysgeusia)

Side effects: *italics* = common; red = life-threatening

GU: Gynecomastia, dysmenorrhea
INTEG: Rash, angioedema

PHARMACOKINETICS

Onset rapid; peak 1 hr; duration 6 hr; extensively metabolized in the liver by CYP3A4, CYP2E1; excreted via kidneys; half-life 6 hr, geriatric patients 9 hr, protein binding 52%-59%

INTERACTIONS

Increase: CNS depression—CNS depressants

Increase: toxicity due to decreased eszopiclone elimination—CYP3A4 inhibitors (clarithromycin, itraconazole, ketoconazole, nefazodone, nelfinavir, ritonavir, troleandomycin, SSRIs)

Decrease: eszopiclone effect—CYP3A4 inducers (dexamethasone, barbiturates, carbamazepine, oxcarbazepine, phenytoin, fosphenytoin, ethotoin)

Drug/Food
Decrease: product action—food

Drug/Herb
Decrease: eszopiclone effect—St. John's wort

NURSING CONSIDERATIONS
Assess:

• **Sleep pattern:** ability to go to sleep, stay asleep, early morning awakenings, conservative methods used

• For abuse of this product, other products

• **Anaphylaxis, angioedema:** monitor during first dose

• **CNS depression/suicidal thoughts, behaviors:** assess for these symptoms

• Alternative methods to improve sleep: reading, quiet environment, warm bath, milk

• Assistance with ambulation; night light, call bell within reach

• **Beers:** avoid in older adults with delirium or at high risk for delirium

• **Pregnancy/breastfeeding:** identify whether pregnancy is planned or suspected; avoid breastfeeding

Evaluate:

• Therapeutic response: ability to fall asleep and stay asleep throughout the night

Teach patient/family:

• That daytime drowsiness may occur; not to engage in hazardous activities until effect is known; that memory problems may occur

• That all other medications and supplements should be avoided unless approved by prescriber; to avoid alcohol

• To notify prescriber if pregnancy is suspected or planned

• To avoid use after a high-fat meal

• To swallow tab whole

• To notify prescriber of facial swelling, rash, complex sleep disorders (sleep driving, sleep eating), change in thinking or behavior

• That tolerance and dependence may occur after extended use

• To take immediately before going to bed

• To be aware of CNS depression and suicidal thoughts/behaviors, report at once

---

etanercept (Rx)
(eh-tan′er-sept)

Enbrel, Enbrel SureClick
Func. class.: Antirheumatic agent (disease modifying) (DMARDs)
Chem. class.: Anti-TNF agent

Do not confuse:
Enbrel/Levbid

ACTION: Binds tumor necrosis factor (TNF), which is involved in immune and inflammatory reactions

USES: Acute, chronic rheumatoid arthritis that has not responded to other disease-modifying agents, polyarticular course of juvenile rheumatoid arthritis (JRA), ankylosing spondylitis, plaque psoriasis, psoriatic arthritis
Unlabeled uses: Crohn's disease; plaque psoriasis (child ≥4 yr)

CONTRAINDICATIONS: Sepsis

Precautions: Pregnancy, breastfeeding, children <4 yr, geriatric patients, malignancies, HF, seizures, multiple sclerosis, latex hypersensitivity

> Black Box Warning: Infection, lymphoma, neoplastic disease, TB

DOSAGE AND ROUTES
Rheumatoid/psoriatic arthritis, ankylosing spondylitis
• **Adult:** SUBCUT 50 mg/wk or 25 mg 2×/wk, 3-4 days apart; may be used with methotrexate for psoriatic arthritis
• **Child 2-17 yr:** SUBCUT 0.8 mg/kg/wk, max 50 mg/wk
Plaque psoriasis
• **Adult:** SUBCUT 50 mg 2×/wk × 3 mo, then 50 mg q wk maintenance
• **Adolescent/child 4-17 yr (unlabeled):** SUBCUT 0.8 mg/kg/wk, max 50 mg/wk
Juvenile rheumatoid arthritis (JRA)
• **Adolescent/child 2-17 yr:** SUBCUT 0.8 mg/kg/wk, max 50 mg/wk
Available forms: Powder for inj 25 mg; inj 50 mg/mL; autoinjector, single use
Administer:
• May be administered by the patient or a caregiver. Assess the patient's or caregiver's ability to inject subcut and observe the first injection
• Administration of one 50-mg/mL prefilled syringe or autoinjector provides a dose equivalent to two 25-mg prefilled syringes or two 25-mg vials of lyophilized powder
• The needle caps on the prefilled syringe and on the SureClick autoinjector contain dry natural rubber (latex) and should not be handled by persons sensitive to this product
Route-Specific Use
Injectable Use
• Inspect for particulate matter and discoloration before use, solution should be clear and colorless, although small white particles may be noted in the autoinjector or prefilled syringe

Subcut Use
• Injection sites include front of the thigh, abdomen except the 2 in around the navel, or outer area of the upper arm; rotate injection sites; do not administer where skin is tender, bruised, red, or hard; do not inject directly into any raised, thick, red, or scaly skin patches or lesions related to psoriasis
Reconstitution and administration of the vial:
• Do not mix or transfer the contents of one vial into another vial; do not filter reconstituted product during preparation or administration; do not add other medications to solutions containing etanercept; ONLY use the supplied diluent
• A vial adapter is supplied when reconstituting the powder; the adapter should not be used if multiple doses are to be withdrawn; to reconstitute using the vial adapter, slide the plunger into the flange end of the syringe; attach the plunger to the gray rubber stopper by turning the plunger clockwise until a slight resistance is felt; remove the twist-off cap from the prefilled diluent syringe by turning counterclockwise; once the twist-off cap is removed, twist the vial adapter onto the syringe clockwise until a slight resistance is felt; place the vial adapter over the top of the vial, being careful not to bump or touch the plunger, the plastic spike inside the vial adapter should puncture the gray stopper; push the plunger down until all the liquid is in the vial, gently swirl; after the diluent is added, some foaming may occur; do not shake; dissolution takes less than 10 min; the solution should be clear and colorless. Each reconstituted vial contains 25 mg/mL of etanercept; turn the vial upside down and slowly pull the plunger down to the unit markings on the side of the syringe that correspond with the needed dose; gently tap the syringe to make any air bubbles rise to the top of the syringe, and slowly push the plunger up to remove them; remove the syringe from the vial adapter by turning the syringe counterclockwise and attach the 27-gauge needle

• If the vial will be used for multiple doses, use a 25-gauge needle for reconstituting and withdrawing; insert the 25-gauge needle or the vial adapter straight into the center of the gray stopper; a "pop" will be felt; inject the diluent very slowly; after the diluent is added, some foaming may occur; do not shake; swirl contents gently, dissolution takes less than 10 minutes; the solution should be clear and colorless; write the mixing date on the supplied sticker and attach to the vial (25 mg/mL of etanercept); withdraw the dose into the syringe; remove air bubbles; remove the 25-gauge needle from the syringe; attach a 27-gauge needle

• Hold the barrel of the syringe with one hand and pull the needle cover straight off; hold the syringe in one hand like a pencil and use the other hand to gently pinch a fold of skin at the cleaned injection site; insert the needle at a 45-degree angle to the skin; let go of the skin and hold the syringe near its base to stabilize it; push the plunger to inject all of the solution at a slow, steady rate; withdraw the needle at the same angle as insertion; do NOT rub the site

• Use as soon as possible after reconstitution; place reconstituted vials for multiple doses in the refrigerator at 36°-46° F (2°-8° C) within 4 hr of reconstitution; may be stored up to 14 days; DO NOT FREEZE

Use of the SureClick autoinjector:

• Allow to reach room temperature, do not shake; immediately before use, remove the needle shield by pulling it straight off

• Stretch the skin under and around the prefilled autoinjector, place the open end against the injection site at a 90-degree angle; without pushing the purple button on top, push the autoinjector firmly against the skin to unlock; press the purple button on top once and release the button; listen for the first click; wait for the second click or wait 15 seconds, and remove the autoinjector from injection site; do NOT rub the site

• Look at the inspection window; if it is not purple, call 1-888-436-2735; do not try to reuse the autoinjector

Use of the prefilled syringe:

• **Single-use:** allow to reach room temperature, do not shake; remove the needle shield; check to see if the amount of liquid in the prefilled syringe falls between the two purple fill level indicator lines on the syringe; if bubbles are seen, gently tap the syringe; turn the syringe so that the purple horizontal lines on the barrel are directly facing you; do not use if the syringe does not have the right amount of liquid

• Hold the barrel of the prefilled syringe with one hand and pull the needle cover straight off; holding the syringe with the needle pointing up, check the syringe for air bubbles; if there are bubbles, gently tap until the air bubbles rise to the top of the syringe; slowly push the plunger up to force the air bubbles out of the syringe

• Insert the needle at a 45-degree angle to the pinched skin; push the plunger to inject all of the solution at a slow, steady rate; withdraw the needle at the same angle as insertion; do NOT rub the site

SIDE EFFECTS

CNS: *Headache,* asthenia, dizziness, seizures

CV: Heart failure

GI: Abdominal pain, dyspepsia, vomiting, hepatitis, diarrhea

HEMA: Pancytopenia, anemia, thrombocytopenia, leukopenia, neutropenia

INTEG: Rash, *inj-site reaction*, keratoderma blenorrhagicum

RESP: *Pharyngitis, cough, URI, non-URI,* sinusitis, *rhinitis*

SYST: Serious infections, sepsis, death, malignancies, Stevens-Johnson syndrome, reactivation of hepatitis B virus, lupus-like syndrome

PHARMACOKINETICS

Elimination half-life 102 hr, 60% absorbed (SUBCUT)

INTERACTIONS

Increase: neutropenia—sulfaSALAzine
• Do not give concurrently with live virus vaccines; immunizations should be brought up to date before treatment
• Avoid use with anakinra, cyclophosphamide, rilonacept

Drug/Lab Test
Increase: LFTs

NURSING CONSIDERATIONS
Assess:
• **RA:** pain, stiffness, ROM, swelling of joints before, during, after treatment

Black Box Warning: **Secondary malignancy:** assess for lymphoma and other neoplastic diseases in children and adolescents; avoid use in those with a history of malignancy

• For inj-site pain, swelling; usually occurs after 2 inj (4-5 days)

Black Box Warning: **Infection:** patients using immunosuppressives, corticosteroids, methotrexate at greater risk; assess for fever, discontinue in those who develop a serious infection; do not use in active infection; obtain TB testing prior to use; TB must be treated prior to use

• **Hypersensitivity:** to this product, latex needle cap, benzyl alcohol; usual reactions to product last 3-5 days
• **Pregnancy/breastfeeding:** use only if clearly needed; use cautiously in breastfeeding; enroll in pregnancy surveillance program, Amgen, 1-800-772-6436
Evaluate:
• Therapeutic response: decreased inflammation, pain in joints
Teach patient/family:
• That product must be continued for prescribed time to be effective
• To use caution when driving; dizziness may occur
• Not to receive live vaccinations during treatment
• About self-administration if appropriate: inj should be made in thigh, abdo-

men, upper arm; rotate sites at least 1 inch from previous site, check for inj reactions that last 3-5 days
• To notify prescriber of possible infection (upper respiratory, other)

RARELY USED

etelcalcetide
(e-tel-kal'-se-tide)
Parsabiv
Func. class.: Parathyroid analogs

USES: For the treatment of secondary hyperparathyroidism in adults with chronic kidney disease on hemodialysis

DOSAGE AND ROUTES
Secondary hyperparathyroidism in patients with chronic kidney disease on hemodialysis
• **Adult: IV** 5 mg 3×/wk at the end of hemodialysis treatment, max 15 mg 3×/wk
For patients switching from cinacalcet to etelcalcetide
• **Adult: IV:** 5 mg 3×/wk at the end of hemodialysis treatment after discontinuing etelcalcetide for at least 7 days

ethambutol (Rx)
(e-tham′byoo-tole)
Etibi ♣, Myambutol
Func. class.: Antitubercular
Chem. class.: Diisopropylethylene diamide derivative

Do not confuse:
ethambutol/Ethmozine

ACTION: Inhibits RNA synthesis, decreases tubercle bacilli replication

USES: Pulmonary TB as an adjunct, other mycobacterial infections

CONTRAINDICATIONS: Children <13 yr, hypersensitivity, optic neuritis

Precautions: Pregnancy, breastfeeding, renal disease, diabetic retinopathy, cataracts, ocular defects, hepatic and hematopoietic disorders

DOSAGE AND ROUTES
• **Adult/child >13 yr: PO** 15-25 mg/kg/day as single dose (treatment naive) or 25 mg/kg daily (treatment experienced)
Renal disease
• **Adult: PO** CCr 10-50 mL/min, dose q24-36hr; CCr <10 mL/min, dose q48hr
Retreatment
• **Adult: PO** 25 mg/kg/day as single dose × 2 mo with at least 1 other product, then decrease to 15 mg/kg/day as single dose, max 2.5 g/day
• **Child: PO** 15 mg/kg/day
Available forms: Tabs 100, 400 mg
Administer:
• With meals to decrease GI symptoms
• Antiemetic if vomiting occurs
• After C&S completed; monthly to detect resistance
• 4 hr between this product and antacids

SIDE EFFECTS
CNS: *Headache, confusion,* fever, malaise, dizziness, *disorientation,* hallucinations, peripheral neuropathy
EENT: Blurred vision, optic neuritis, photophobia, decreased visual acuity
GI: *Abdominal distress, anorexia, nausea, vomiting*
INTEG: Dermatitis, pruritus, toxic epidermal necrolysis, erythema multiforme
META: *Elevated uric acid, acute gout,* impaired hepatic function
MISC: Thrombocytopenia, joint pain, anaphylaxis

PHARMACOKINETICS
Peak 2-4 hr, half-life 3 hr, metabolized in liver, excreted in urine (unchanged product/inactive metabolites, unchanged product in feces)

INTERACTIONS
• Delayed absorption of ethambutol: aluminum salts, separate by 4 hr
• Neurotoxicity: other neurotoxics

NURSING CONSIDERATIONS
Assess:
• Hepatic studies weekly × 2 wk, then q2mo: ALT, AST, bilirubin; decreased appetite, jaundice, dark urine, fatigue
• Signs of anemia: Hct, Hgb, fatigue
• Mental status often: affect, mood, behavioral changes; psychosis may occur
• C&S, including sputum, before treatment
• Visual status: decreased acuity, altered color perception
• **Serious skin reactions:** toxic epidermal necrolysis
• **Pregnancy/breastfeeding:** use only if benefit outweighs risk to fetus; product appears in breast milk
Evaluate:
• Therapeutic response: decreased symptoms of TB, decrease in acid-fast bacteria
Teach patient/family:
• To avoid alcohol products
• That compliance with dosage schedule, duration is necessary
• That scheduled appointments must be kept or relapse may occur
• To report to prescriber any visual changes; rash; hot, swollen, painful joints; numbness, tingling of extremities

---

etodolac
(ee-toe′doe-lak)
Ultradol ✦, Lodine
Func. class.: Nonsteroidal antiinflammatory/nonopioid analgesic

---

ACTION: Inhibits COX-1, COX-2; analgesic, antiinflammatory

USES: Mild to moderate pain, osteoarthritis, rheumatoid arthritis, arthralgia, myalgia, juvenile rheumatoid arthritis

CONTRAINDICATIONS: Hypersensitivity; patients in whom aspirin, iodides, or NSAIDs have produced

---

asthma; urticaria; coronary artery bypass graft surgery (CABG)

Precautions: Edema, renal/hepatic disease, children, GI ulcers, geriatric patients, bronchospasm, nasal polyps, alcoholism, bone marrow suppression, MI, hemophilia, neutropenia, ulcerative colitis, pregnancy, breastfeeding

> Black Box Warning: GI bleeding, perforation, MI, stroke

DOSAGE AND ROUTES

Osteoarthritis

• **Adult:** PO 300 mg bid-tid, or 400-500 mg bid initially, then adjust dosage to 600-1200 mg/day in divided doses; max 1200 mg/day; ext rel 400-1000 mg daily

Rheumatoid arthritis

• **Adult:** PO 300 mg bid-tid or 400-500 mg bid (regular release); maintenance **PO** 400-1000 mg/day (extended release) or 600-1000 mg/day divided 2-4 times, max 1200 mg/day (regular release)

Analgesia

• **Adult:** PO 200-400 mg q6-8hr up to 1000 mg daily; max 1200 mg/day; patients <60 kg, max 20 mg/kg; ext rel 400-1000 mg daily

Available forms: Caps 200, 300 mg; tabs 400, 500 mg; ext rel 400, 500, 600 mg

Administer:

Without regard to food

• Store at room temperature

SIDE EFFECTS

CNS: Dizziness, headache, drowsiness, fatigue, tremors, confusion, insomnia, anxiety, depression, light-headedness, vertigo

CV: Tachycardia, peripheral edema, fluid retention, palpitations, dysrhythmias, HF

EENT: Tinnitus, hearing loss, blurred vision, photophobia

GI: Nausea, anorexia, vomiting, diarrhea, jaundice, cholestatic hepatitis, constipation, flatulence, cramps, dry mouth, peptic ulcer, dyspepsia, GI bleeding

GU: Nephrotoxicity: dysuria, hematuria, oliguria, azotemia, cystitis, urinary tract infection

HEMA: Blood dyscrasias

INTEG: Erythema, urticaria, purpura, rash, pruritus, sweating, Stevens-Johnson syndrome

SYST: Angioedema, anaphylaxis

PHARMACOKINETICS

Peak $1\frac{1}{2}$-2 hr, serum protein binding >99%, half-life 7 hr; metabolized by liver (metabolites excreted in urine)

INTERACTIONS

Increase: toxicity—cycloSPORINE, digoxin, lithium, methotrexate, phenytoin, cidofovir, aminoglycosides

> Black Box Warning: **Increase:** GI toxicity—aspirin, NSAIDs

Decrease: effect of etodolac—antacids

Decrease: effect of—beta blockers, diuretics

Drug/Lab Test

Increase: BUN, creatinine

Decrease: Hgb/Hct, WBC

NURSING CONSIDERATIONS

Assess:

• **Pain:** location, frequency, characteristics; relief after medication

• Blood, renal, liver tests: BUN, creatinine, AST, ALT, Hgb, platelets before treatment, periodically thereafter

> Black Box Warning: **For GI bleeding:** black stools, hematemesis

• **Pregnancy/breastfeeding:** avoid use unless benefit outweighs risks; avoid in 3rd trimester due to constriction of fetal ductus arteriosus; do not breastfeed

Evaluate:

• Therapeutic response: decreased pain, stiffness, swelling in joints, ability to move more easily

Teach patient/family:

• To report blurred vision or ringing, roaring in the ears; might indicate toxicity

---

Side effects: *italics* = common; red = life-threatening

• Not to break, crush, or chew ext rel tabs

• To report change in urine pattern, weight increase, edema, pain increase in joints, fever, blood in urine; indicates nephrotoxicity

• That therapeutic effects can take up to 1 mo

Black Box Warning: To avoid aspirin, NSAIDs, acetaminophen, alcoholic beverages while taking this medication

⚠ HIGH ALERT

etoposide (Rx)
(e-toe-poe'side)
Toposar, VePesid ✦

etoposide phosphate (Rx)
Etopophos

Func. class.: Antineoplastic—miscellaneous

Chem. class.: Semisynthetic podophyllotoxin

ACTION: Inhibits cells from entering mitosis, depresses DNA/RNA synthesis, cell-cycle–specific S and G_2; binds to a complex of DNA and topoisomerase II, leading to DNA strand breaks

USES: Testicular cancer, small-cell lung cancer

Unlabeled uses: Leukemias (ALL, AML), desmoid tumor, gastric/ovarian cancer, bone marrow ablation, Hodgkin's/non-Hodgkin's lymphoma, malignant glioma, neuroblastoma, stem cell transplant preparation, trophoblastic disease

CONTRAINDICATIONS: Pregnancy, breastfeeding, hypersensitivity

Precautions: Children, renal/hepatic disease, gout, neutropenia, thrombocytopenia, infection, bleeding

Black Box Warning: Bone marrow depression, bleeding, infection; requires an experienced clinician

DOSAGE AND ROUTES
Testicular cancer
• **Adult: IV** 100 mg/m²/day on days 1, 2 in combination with bleomycin and Cisplatin (BEP) or 100 mg/m²/day on days 1, 3, 5, repeat q3-4wk

Small-cell lung carcinoma first-line treatment with ClSplatin
• **Adult: IV** 50 mg/m²/day over 5 min-3.5 hr 5 days of a 21-day cycle

Renal dose
• **Adult: IV** CCr 45-60 mL/min, reduce dose by 15%; CCr 30-44 mL/min, reduce dose by 20%; CCr <30 mL/min, reduce dose by 25%

Hepatic dose
• **Adult: IV/PO** total bilirubin 1.5-2.9 mg/dL: reduce dose by 50%; total bilirubin 3-5 mg/dL: reduce dose by 75%; total bilirubin >5 mg/dL: hold

Available forms: Inj 20 mg/mL; 100 mg powder for injection, caps 50 mg

Administer:
• Antiemetic 30-60 min before product and prn to prevent vomiting

Urate nephropathy
• Allopurinol, aggressive alkalinization to maintain uric acid levels

• Antispasmodic, EPINEPHrine, corticosteroids, antihistamines for reactions

PO route
• Give without regard to food
• Increase fluid intake to 2-3 L/day to prevent urate deposits, calculi formation
• Refrigerate oral product; do not freeze

IV route
• Do not use acrylic or ABS plastic devices; may crack, leak

Intermittent IV INFUSION route (etoposide)
• Use cytotoxic handling procedures, use Luer-Lok fittings to prevent leakage
• After **diluting** 5-mL vial with 100 mg/250 mL or more D₅W or NaCl to 0.2-0.4 mg/mL, **infuse** over 30-60 min

Y-site compatibilities: Acyclovir, alfentanil, allopurinol, amifostine, amikacin, aminocaproic acid, aminophylline, amiodarone, amphotericin B colloidal, amphotericin B lipid complex, amphotericin B liposome, ampicillin,

ampicillin-sulbactam, anidulafungin, atenolol, atracurium, aztreonam, bivalirudin, bleomycin, bumetanide, buprenorphine, butorphanol, calcium chloride/gluconate, CARBOplatin, caspofungin, ceFAZolin, cefotaxime, cefoTEtan, cefOXitin, cefTAZidime, ceftizoxime, cefTRIAXone, cefuroxime, chloramphenicol, chlorproMAZINE, cimetidine, ciprofloxacin, cisatracurium, CISplatin, cladribine, clindamycin, codeine, cyclophosphamide, cycloSPORINE, cytarabine, DACTINomycin, DAPTOmycin, DAUNOrubicin, dexamethasone, dexmedetomidine, dexrazoxane, digoxin, diltiazem, diphenhydrAMINE, DOBUTamine, DOCEtaxel, DOPamine, doxacurium, DOXOrubicin, DOXOrubicin liposomal, doxycycline, droperidol, enalaprilat, ePHEDrine, EPINEPHrine, epirubicin, ertapenem, erythromycin, esmolol, famotidine, fenoldopam, fentaNYL, floxuridine, fluconazole, fludarabine, fluorouracil, foscarnet, fosphenytoin, furosemide, ganciclovir, gatifloxacin, gemcitabine, gentamicin, glycopyrrolate, granisetron, haloperidol, heparin, hydrALAZINE, hydrocortisone, HYDROmorphone, hydrOXYzine, ifosfamide, imipenem-cilastatin, inamrinone, insulin (regular), irinotecan, isoproterenol, ketorolac, labetalol, lansoprazole, leucovorin, levofloxacin, levorphanol, lidocaine, linezolid, LORazepam, magnesium sulfate, mannitol, mechlorethamine, melphalan, meperidine, meropenem, mesna, methohexital, methotrexate, methyldopate, methylPREDNISolone, metoclopramide, metoprolol, metroNIDAZOLE, micafungin, midazolam, milrinone, minocycline, mitoXANtrone, mivacurium, morphine, nafcillin, nalbuphine, naloxone, nesiritide, nitroglycerin, nitroprusside, norepinephrine, NS, octreotide, ofloxacin, ondansetron, oxaliplatin, PACLitaxel, palonosetron, pamidronate, pancuronium, PEMEtrexed, pentamidine, pentazocine, PENTobarbital, PHENobarbital, phenylephrine, piperacillin, piperacillin-tazobactam, polymyxin B, potassium chloride/phosphates, procainamide, prochlorperazine, promethazine, propranolol, quinupristindalfopristin, ranitidine, remifentanil, rocuronium, sargramostim, sodium acetate/bicarbonate/phosphates, succinylcholine, SUFentanil, sulfamethoxazole-trimethoprim, tacrolimus, teniposide, theophylline, thiotepa, ticarcillin, ticarcillin-clavulanate, tigecycline, tirofiban, tobramycin, topotecan, trimethobenzamide, vancomycin, vasopressin, vecuronium, verapamil, vinBLAStine, vinCRIStine, vinorelbine, voriconazole, zidovudine, zoledronic acid

Intermittent IV INFUSION route (etoposide phosphate)

• **Reconstitute** each vial with 5 or 10 mL of D$_5$W, 0.9% NaCl for concentrations of 20 mg/mL or 10 mg/mL, respectively; may give diluted or undiluted to concentrations of as little as 0.1 mg/mL, **give over 5-210 min**

Y-site compatibilities: Acyclovir, alfentanil, amifostine, amikacin, aminocaproic acid, aminophylline, amiodarone, ampicillin, ampicillin-sulbactam, anidulafungin, atenolol, atracurium, aztreonam, bivalirudin, bleomycin, bumetanide, buprenorphine, butorphanol, calcium acetate/chloride/gluconate, CARBOplatin, carmustine, caspofungin, ceFAZolin, cefonicid, cefoperazone, cefotaxime, cefoTEtan, cefOXitin, cefTAZidime, ceftizoxime, cefTRIAXone, cefuroxime, chloramphenicol, cimetidine, ciprofloxacin, cisatracurium, CISplatin, clindamycin, codeine, cyclophosphamide, cycloSPORINE, cytarabine, dacarbazine, DACTINomycin, DAPTOmycin, DAUNOrubicin, dexamethasone, digoxin, diltiazem, diphenhydrAMINE, DOBUTamine, DOCEtaxel, DOPamine, doripenem, doxacurium, DOXOrubicin, HCL/liposome, doxycycline, enalaprilat, ePHEDrine, EPINEPHrine, epirubicin, ertapenem, erythromycin, esmolol, famotidine, fenoldopam, fentaNYL, floxuridine, fluconazole, fludarabine, fluorouracil, foscarnet, fosphenytoin, furosemide, ganciclovir, gatifloxacin, gemcitabine, gentamicin, glycopyrrolate, granisetron, haloperidol, heparin, hydrALAZINE, hydrocortisone, HYDROmorphone, hydrOXYzine, IDArubicin, ifosfamide, inamrinone, insulin (regular), irinotecan, isoproterenol, ketorolac, labetalol, leucovorin, levofloxacin, levorphanol, lidocaine, linezolid, LORazepam, magnesium sulfate, mannitol, mechlorethamine, meperidine, meropenem, mesna, metaraminol, methotrexate, methyldopate, metoclopramide, metoprolol, metroNIDAZOLE, midazolam, milrinone, minocycline, mitoXANTrone, mivacurium, morphine, nafcillin, nalbuphine, naloxone, nesiritide, netilmicin, nitroglycerin, nitroprusside, norepinephrine, octreotide, ofloxacin, ondansetron, oxaliplatin, PACLitaxel, palonosetron, pamidronate, pancuronium, PEMEtrexed, pentamidine, pentazocine, PENTobarbital, PHENobarbital, phenylephrine, piperacillin, piperacillin-tazobactam, plicamycin, polymyxin B, potassium chloride/phosphates, procainamide, promethazine, propranolol, quiNIDine, quinupristin-dalfopristin, ranitidine, remifentanil, riTUXimab, rocuronium, sodium acetate/bicarbonate/phosphates, streptozocin, succinylcholine, SUFentanil, sulfamethoxazole-trimethoprim, tacrolimus, teniposide, theophylline, thiopental, thiotepa, ticarcillin, ticarcillin-clavulanate, tigecycline, tirofiban, tobramycin, tolazoline, trastuzumab, trimethobenzamide, vancomycin, vasopressin, vecuronium, verapamil, vinBLAStine, vinCRIStine, vinorelbine, voriconazole, zidovudine, zoledronic acid

SIDE EFFECTS

CNS: Headache, *fever,* peripheral neuropathy, paresthesias, confusion, chills, fever
CV: *Hypotension,* MI, dysrhythmias
GI: *Nausea, vomiting, anorexia,* hepatotoxicity, dyspepsia, diarrhea, constipation
GU: Nephrotoxicity
HEMA: Thrombocytopenia, leukopenia, myelosuppression, anemia
INTEG: *Rash, alopecia,* phlebitis at IV site, Stevens-Johnson syndrome
RESP: Bronchospasm
SYST: Anaphylaxis, secondary malignancy

PHARMACOKINETICS

Half-life ½-2 hr (initial), terminal 5¼ hr, metabolized in liver, excreted in urine, feces, crosses placental barrier, protein binding 95%

INTERACTIONS

Increase: bone marrow depression—other antineoplastics, radiation, immunosuppressives
Increase: adverse reactions—live virus vaccines, toxoids
Increase: effect of etoposide, toxicity—voriconazole, conivaptan, cycloSPORINE, imatinib, nilotinib, etravirine, telithromycin
Increase: risk of bleeding—anticoagulants, NSAIDs, platelet inhibitors, thrombolytics, salicylate
Decrease: etoposide effect—sargramostim, filgrastim, separate by ≥24 hr
Drug/Food
• Decreased oral etoposide—grapefruit juice
Drug/Lab Test
Decrease: platelets, RBC, WBC, neutrophils, Hgb, calcium, phosphate
Increase: uric acid, potassium

NURSING CONSIDERATIONS
Assess:

Black Box Warning: Bone marrow depression: CBC, differential, platelet count weekly; withhold product if WBC is <500/mm³ or platelet count is <50,000/mm³; notify prescriber, treatment should be delayed

• **Nephrotoxicity:** BUN; serum uric acid; urine CCr; electrolytes before, during therapy; I&O ratio; report fall in urine output to <30 mL/hr; check B/P bid, report any significant decrease

Black Box Warning: Infection: monitor temperature, fever may indicate beginning infection; treat active infection before treatment

• **Hepatotoxicity:** hepatic studies before, during therapy (bilirubin, AST, ALT, LDH) as

---

needed or monthly; monitor jaundice of skin and sclera, dark urine, clay-colored stools, itchy skin, abdominal pain, fever, diarrhea

Black Box Warning: Bleeding: hematuria, guaiac stools, bruising or petechiae, mucosa or orifices q8hr

• Effects of alopecia on body image; discuss feelings about body changes
• B/P q15min during infusion; if systolic reading <90 mm Hg, discontinue infusion, notify prescriber
• Buccal cavity q8hr for dryness, sores or ulceration, white patches, oral pain, bleeding, dysphagia
• **Injection-site reaction:** monitor site closely for infiltration
• Local irritation, pain, burning, discoloration at inj site
• **Symptoms indicating severe allergic reaction:** rash, pruritus, urticaria, purpuric skin lesions, itching, flushing, restlessness, coughing, difficulty breathing
• **Frequency of stools, characteristics:** cramping, acidosis
• **Signs of dehydration:** rapid respirations, poor skin turgor, decreased urine output, dry skin, restlessness, weakness
• **Geriatric patients:** increased alopecia, GI effects, infection, nephrotoxicity, myelosuppression

Black Box Warning: An experienced clinician knowledgeable in the use of cytotoxic products

• **Pregnancy/breastfeeding:** do not use in pregnancy, breastfeeding unless benefits to mother outweigh risk to fetus
Evaluate:
• Therapeutic response: decreased tumor size, spread of malignancy
Teach patient/family:
• To report any changes in breathing or coughing
• That hair may be lost during treatment; that a wig or hairpiece may make patient feel better; that new hair may be different in color, texture
• That metallic taste may occur
• **Infection:** to report symptoms of infection (fever, sore throat); to avoid crowds, persons with known infections
• To avoid immunizations
• **Pregnancy/breastfeeding:** to notify prescriber if pregnancy is planned or suspected; to use reliable contraception during and for several mo after therapy; to avoid breastfeeding
• To take as prescribed (PO), not to double dose
• To report signs of infection (flulike symptoms, fever, fatigue, sore throat)
• To check B/P, hypotension occurs

etravirine (Rx)

(e-tra'veer-een)

Intelence

Func. class.: Antiretroviral
Chem. class.: Nonnucleoside reverse transcriptase inhibitor (NNRTI)

ACTION: Binds directly to reverse transcriptase, thus blocking the RNA- and DNA-dependent DNA polymerase action and causing a disruption of the enzyme's catalytic site

USES: In combination with other antiretroviral agents for HIV infection in treatment-experienced patients with evidence of HIV replication despite ongoing antiretroviral therapy

CONTRAINDICATIONS: Breastfeeding, hypersensitivity
Precautions: Pregnancy, children, geriatric patients, impaired hepatic function, antimicrobial resistance, hepatitis, hypercholesterolemia, hypertriglycerides, immune reconstitution syndrome

DOSAGE AND ROUTES
• **Adult/child/adolescent ≥6 yr, ≥30 kg:** PO 200 mg bid

- **Child/adolescent ≥6 yr, 25 to 29 kg:** PO 150 mg bid
- **Child/adolescent ≥6 yr, 20 to 24 kg:** PO 125 mg bid
- **Child/adolescent ≥6 yr, 16 to 19 kg:** PO 100 mg bid

Available forms: Tabs 25, 100, 200 mg
Administer:
In combination with other antiretrovirals with food or after a meal

- Tabs may be dispersed in ≥5 mL of water; once dispersed, stir well, give immediately, rinse glass, have patient drink to ensure all medication taken
- Store in cool environment; protect from light

SIDE EFFECTS

CNS: *Headache, insomnia,* amnesia, anxiety, confusion, fatigue, nightmares, peripheral neuropathy, seizures, stroke, tremor
CV: Atrial fibrillation, hypertension, MI
EENT: Blurred vision
GI: *Nausea, vomiting, diarrhea, anorexia,* abdominal pain, increased AST/ALT, constipation, flatulence, gastritis, GERD, hematemesis, hepatitis, hepatomegaly, pancreatitis
GU: Renal failure
HEMA: Hemolytic anemia, neutropenia, thrombocytopenia, anemia
INTEG: *Rash,* erythema multiforme, angioedema, Stevens-Johnson syndrome
MS: Rhabdomyolysis
OTHER: Diabetes mellitus, gynecomastia, hyperamylasemia, hypercholesterolemia, hyperglycemia, hyperlipidemia
RESP: Dyspnea, bronchospasm
SYST: DRESS

PHARMACOKINETICS

99.9% plasma protein binding; metabolized by CYP3A4, 2C9, 2C19; half-life 21-61 hr; excreted in feces

INTERACTIONS

- Do not use concurrently with atazanavir, carBAMazepine, delavirdine, fosamprenavir, fosphenytoin, phenytoin, PHENobarbital, rifapentine, rifAMPin, tipranavir, rilpivirine
- Altered effect of cycloSPORINE, tacrolimus, sirolimus

Increase: myopathy, rhabdomyolysis—HMG-CoA reductase inhibitors
Increase: etravirine levels—CYP3A4 inhibitors (fluconazole, itraconazole, ketoconazole, lopinavir, posaconazole, ritonavir, voriconazole)
Increase: withdrawal symptoms—methadone
Increase: levels of diazepam, rifampin, voriconazole, warfarin
Decrease: levels of CYP3A4 inducers (amiodarone, atazanavir, clarithromycin, flecainide, fosamprenavir, lidocaine, mexiletine, propafenone, quiNIDine, sildenafil, tadalafil, vardenafil)
Decrease: etravirine levels—darunavir, dexamethasone, disopyramide, efavirenz, nevirapine, ritonavir, saquinavir, tipranavir

Drug/Herb
Decrease: etravirine—St. John's wort

NURSING CONSIDERATIONS
Assess:

- **Symptoms of HIV, possible infections:** increased temperature
- **HIV:** monitor viral load, CD4 counts, plasma HIV RNA during treatment; watch for decreasing granulocytes, Hgb; if low, therapy may have to be discontinued and restarted after hematologic recovery; blood transfusions may be required; cholesterol/lipid profile
- **Fatal hypersensitivity reactions:** fever, rash, nausea, vomiting, fatigue, cough, dyspnea, diarrhea, abdominal discomfort; treatment should be discontinued and not restarted; incidence of rash may be worse in women
- **Blood dyscrasias (anemia, granulocytopenia):** bruising, fatigue, bleeding, poor healing
- **Renal failure:** BUN, serum uric acid, CCr before, during therapy; may be elevated throughout treatment
- **Hepatitis/pancreatitis:** hepatic studies before and during therapy: bilirubin,

AST, ALT, amylase, alk phos, creatine phosphokinase, creatinine, monthly

• **Pregnancy/breastfeeding:** use only if benefits outweigh risk; enroll pregnant patients in the Antretroviral Pregnancy Registry, 1-800-258-4263; do not breastfeed

Evaluate:

• Therapeutic response: increased CD4 count, decreased viral load

Teach patient/family:

• That product is not a cure but will control symptoms; that patient is still infective, may pass AIDS virus to others

• To notify prescriber of sore throat, swollen lymph nodes, malaise, fever; other infections may occur; to stop product and notify prescriber immediately if skin rash, fever, cough, SOB, GI symptoms occur; to advise all health care providers that allergic reaction has occurred with etravirine

• That follow-up visits must be continued, since serious toxicity may occur; blood counts must be performed

• To use contraception during treatment; that patient is still able to transmit disease

• About information on medication guide and warning card; discuss points on guide

• That other products may be necessary to prevent other infections

• To take medication after a meal

⚠ HIGH ALERT

everolimus (Rx)

(e-ve-ro′li-mus)

Afinitor, Afinitor Disperz, Zortress

Func. class.: Antineoplastic—miscellaneous

Chem. class.: Kinase inhibitor

Do not confuse:

everolimus/sirolimus/tacrolimus/temsirolimus

ACTION: Proliferation signal inhibitor that inhibits mammalian target of rapamycin (mTOR); this pathway is dysregulated in cancer

USES: Renal cell cancer in those with failed treatment with SORAfenib or SUNItinib kidney transplant rejection prophylaxis with cycloSPORINE, subependymal giant cell astrocytoma, progressive pancreatic neuroendocrine tumor (PNET) with unresectable locally advanced/metastatic disease, breast cancer hormone receptor positive/HER-2 negative, renal angiomyolipoma, tuberous sclerosis complex, liver transplant rejection prophylaxis

CONTRAINDICATIONS: Breastfeeding; hypersensitivity to this product, Rapamune, Torisel, pregnancy

Precautions: Children, renal/hepatic disease, diabetes mellitus, hyperlipidemia, pleural effusion

Black Box Warning: Immunosuppression, infection, renal artery thrombosis, renal impairment, renal vein thrombosis, neoplastic disease, heart transplant

DOSAGE AND ROUTES

Prophylaxis (Zortress)

• **Adult: PO** 0.75 mg q12hr with cycloSPORINE in combination with basiliximab, corticosteroids, reduced doses of cycloSPORINE

Liver transplant rejection prophylaxis

• **Adult: PO** 1 mg bid starting at least 30 days after transplant in combination with reduced-dose tacrolimus and corticosteroids

Advanced renal cancer (Afinitor)

• **Adult: PO** 10 mg daily as long as clinically beneficial; with strong 3A4 inducers 10 mg daily, then may increase by 5-mg increments to 20 mg daily

Progressive neuroendocrine tumor (PNET) (Afinitor only)

• **Adult: PO** 10 mg daily, reduce dose to 5 mg daily if intolerable adverse reactions occur

Subependymal giant-cell astrocytoma (SEGA) (Afinitor only)

• **Adult/adolescent/child:** 4.5 mg/m² daily, then titrate to a target trough of 5-15 ng/mL

Hepatic dose

• **Adult:** PO (Child-Pugh A) Afinitor: 7.5 mg/day; (Child-Pugh B) Afinitor: 5 mg/day, Zortress: 0.75 mg/day divided q12hr; (Child-Pugh C) Afinitor: 2.5 mg/day

Available forms: Tabs 0.25, 0.5, 0.75 mg (Zortress); 2.5, 5, 7.5, 10 mg (Afinitor); tablets for oral suspension 2, 3, 5 mg (Afinitor Disperg)

Administer:

Follow procedure for proper handling of antineoplastics

• Swallow tabs whole with a full glass of water; do not chew, crush, or break

• **Afinitor:** take at same time of day; if unable to swallow, consistently with or without food, disperse in 30 mL of water

• **Zortress:** must take consistently with/ without food, give at same time of day q12hr with cycloSPORINE

• Store protected from light at room temperature

Afinitor adjustments for toxicity

Noninfectious pneumonitis

• **Grade 1:** asymptomatic with radiographic findings only: no dosage change

• **Grade 2:** symptomatic but no interference with activities of daily living (ADL): consider withholding therapy, resume Afinitor at a lower dosage when symptoms improve to ≤ grade 1; discontinue Afinitor if symptoms do not improve within 4 wk

• **Grade 3:** symptomatic and interfering with ADL and oxygen therapy indicated: hold therapy; consider resuming Afinitor at a lower dosage when symptoms improve to ≤ grade 1; consider discontinuing Afinitor if grade 3 toxicity recurs

• **Grade 4:** life-threatening and ventilator support indicated: discontinue therapy

Stomatitis

• **Grade 1:** minimum symptoms and normal diet: no dosage adjustment required

• **Grade 2:** symptomatic but can eat and swallow modified diet: hold therapy until symptoms improve to ≤ grade 1 and resume Afinitor at the same dosage; if grade 2 toxicity recurs, hold therapy and resume Afinitor at a lower dosage when symptoms improve to ≤ grade 1

• **Grade 3:** symptomatic and unable to adequately eat or hydrate orally: hold therapy; resume Afinitor at a lower dosage when symptoms improve to ≤ grade 1

• **Grade 4:** symptomatic and life-threatening: discontinue therapy

Other nonhematologic toxicity (excluding metabolic events)

• **Grade 1:** No dosage adjustment required if toxicity is tolerable

• **Grade 2:** No dosage adjustment required if toxicity is tolerable; if toxicity is intolerable, hold therapy until symptoms improve to ≤ grade 1 and resume Afinitor at the same dosage; if grade 2 toxicity recurs, hold therapy and resume Afinitor at a lower dosage when symptoms improve to ≤ grade 1

• **Grade 3:** Hold therapy; consider resuming Afinitor at a lower dosage when symptoms improve to ≤ grade 1; if grade 3 toxicity recurs, consider discontinuing therapy

• **Grade 4:** Discontinue Afinitor therapy

Metabolic events (hyperglycemia, dyslipidemia)

• **Grade 1 or 2:** No dose adjustment required

• **Grade 3:** Temporarily withhold therapy; resume Afinitor at a lower dosage

• **Grade 4:** Discontinue Afinitor therapy

• **Afinitor Disperz (oral suspension):** wear gloves when preparing, use 10-mL syringe and place dose in syringe, do not crush, break, using 5-mL water and 4-mL air draw into syringe with dose, wait a few minutes until in suspension after use, use same amount of water and air, swirl, give contents

SIDE EFFECTS

CNS: *Headache, insomnia, paresthesia,* chills, fever, seizure, personality changes, insomnia, dizziness, weakness, fatigue

CV: *Hypertension, peripheral edema*

EENT: Blurred vision, photophobia, eyelid edema, epistaxis, sinusitis, cataracts, conjunctivitis

GI: Nausea, vomiting, diarrhea, constipation, stomatitis, anorexia, abdominal pain, dysgeusia, hepatic artery thrombosis

GU: Renal failure, UTI, infertility

HEMA: Anemia, leukopenia, thrombocytopenia, hemolytic uremic syndrome, thrombotic microangiopathy, thrombotic thrombocytopenia, purpura

INTEG: *Rash, acne*, leukocytoclastic vasculitis

META: Hyperglycemia, increased creatinine, *hyperlipidemia*, hypophosphatemia, weight loss, hypertriglyceridemia

RESP: Pleural effusion

SYST: Angioedema, anaphylaxis, lymphoma

PHARMACOKINETICS

Rapidly, well absorbed; peak 1-2 hr; protein binding 74%; extensively metabolized by CYP3A4 enzyme system, P-gp; half-life 30 hr; reduced by high-fat meal; excreted in feces (80%), urine (5%)

INTERACTIONS

Black Box Warning: **Increase:** nephrotoxicity—immunosuppressants

Increase: everolimus effect—CYP3A4 inhibitors (strong, moderate), antifungals, calcium channel blockers, cimetidine, danazol, erythromycin, cycloSPORINE, HIV-protease inhibitors

Decrease: everolimus effect—CYP3A4 inducers, carBAMazepine, PHENobarbital, phenytoin, rifamycin, rifapentine

Decrease: effect of live vaccines

Drug/Herb

• St. John's wort: may decrease effect of everolimus

Drug/Food

• Alters bioavailability; use consistently with/without food; do not use with grapefruit juice

Drug/Lab Test

Increase: bilirubin, calcium, cholesterol, glucose, potassium, lipids, phosphate, triglycerides, uric acid

Decrease: calcium, glucose, potassium, magnesium, phosphate

NURSING CONSIDERATIONS

Assess:

• Lipid profile: cholesterol, triglycerides, lipid-lowering agent may be needed; blood glucose

Black Box Warning: **Immunosuppression:** CBC with differential during treatment monthly; if leukocytes <3000/mm³ or platelets <100,000/mm³, product should be discontinued or reduced; decreased hemoglobin level may indicate bone marrow suppression

• Hepatic/renal studies: AST, ALT, amylase, bilirubin, creatinine, phosphate, and for hepatotoxicity: dark urine, jaundice, itching, light-colored stools; product should be discontinued

• **Pneumonitis:** continuing cough, dyspnea, pleural effusion baseline and during treatment, use corticosteroids if needed, if severe, reduce dose or discontinue

Black Box Warning: **Infection:** bacterial fungal infections can occur and are more common with combination immunosuppression therapy; assess for fever, cough, dyspnea, fatigue

Black Box Warning: May result in graft loss within 30 days after transplantation

• Obtain everolimus blood levels in kidney transplant, hepatic disease, CYP3A4 inducers, inhibitors

• **Pregnancy/breastfeeding:** avoid in pregnancy; use adequate contraception during and for 12 wk after final dose; report exposure to the National Transplant Pregnancy Registry, 1-877-955-6877; do not breastfeed

Evaluate:

• Therapeutic response: decreased spread of tumor; prevention of transplant rejection

---

Teach patient/family:

Black Box Warning: To report fever, rash, severe diarrhea, chills, sore throat, fatigue; serious infections may occur; to report clay-colored stools, cramping (hepatotoxicity)

Black Box Warning: To avoid crowds, persons with known infections to reduce risk for infection

• Not to use with grapefruit juice
• To avoid individuals recently vaccinated with live vaccines; children may require accelerated vaccine schedule before treatment
• That frequent lab tests are required
• That product may decrease male, female fertility
• That drinking alcohol is not recommended
• To take consistently with or without food
• To report vision changes, weight gain, edema, shortness of breath, impaired wound healing
• **Pregnancy:** to notify prescriber if pregnancy is planned or suspected; to use contraception before, during, and 12 wk after product discontinued; to avoid breastfeeding

---

evolocumab (Rx)

(e′-voe-lok′-ue-mab)

Repatha

Func. class.: Antilipemic
Chem. class.: Proprotein convertase subtilisin/kexin type 9 (PCSK9) inhibitor

---

ACTION: Binds to low-density lipoproteins, a human monoclonal antibody (IgG1)

USES: Heterozygous, familial hypercholesterolemia, atherosclerotic disease

CONTRAINDICATIONS: Hypersensitivity

Precautions: Pregnancy, breastfeeding, latex sensitivity

DOSAGE AND ROUTES
Primary hyperlipidemia with established clinical atherosclerosis:
• **Adult:** SUBCUT 140 mg q2wk or 420 mg monthly
Homozygous familial hypercholesterolemia:
• **Adult/adolescent:** SUBCUT 420 mg monthly
Disorder of CV system, secondary prophylaxis and primary hypercholesterolemia, alone or in combination with other lipid-lowering therapies
• **Adult:** SUBCUT 140 mg q2wk or 420 mg monthly
Available forms: Autoinjector 140 mg/mL, solutions for injection 120 mg/mL, 140 mg/mL
Administer:
• Visually inspect for particulate matter and discoloration; solution is clear, colorless to pale yellow
SUBCUT route
Prefilled Syringe or SureClick Autoinjector
• If stored in the refrigerator, warm to room temperature for ≥30 min before use. Do not shake
• Give into areas of the abdomen (except for a 2-inch area around the umbilicus), thigh, or upper arm that are not tender, bruised, red, or indurated
• To use the 420-mg dose, give 3 injections consecutively within 30 min
• Rotate the site with each injection
• Do not administer with other injectable drugs at the same injection site
Prefilled Syringe Administration
• Do not pick up or pull the prefilled syringe by the plunger rod or gray needle cap. Hold the syringe by the barrel
• Pull the gray needle cap off. It is normal to see a drop of solution at the end of the needle. Do not remove any air bubbles in the syringe
• Pinch the skin injection site to create a firm surface approximately 2 inches

wide. Hold the pinch, and insert the needle into the skin using a 45- to 90-degree angle
• Push the plunger rod all the way down until the syringe is empty
• When done, release the plunger and gently lift the syringe off skin

SureClick Autoinjector Administration
• Do not remove the orange cap until you are ready to inject
• Pull the orange cap off
• Stretch (thigh) or pinch (stomach or upper arm) the skin injection site to create a firm surface approximately 2 inches wide. Hold the stretch or pinch, and place the autoinjector on the skin at 90 degrees
• Firmly push down onto the skin when ready to inject; press the gray button. A click should be heard. Keep pushing on the skin and then lift the thumb. The injection could take about 15 sec. The window on the autoinjector will turn from clear to yellow when the injection is complete. A second click may be heard
• Remove the needle, which will be automatically covered

SIDE EFFECTS

CV: Hypertension
MS: *Myalgia, back pain, muscle spasms*
INTEG: Pruritus, injection-site reaction, erythema, rash

PHARMACOKINETICS

Absorption 40%, distribution extensive, metabolism liver (CYP3A4), excretion urine, feces; Onset 4 hr, peak 3-7 days; half-life 2-3 days

INTERACTIONS

None known
Drug/Lab Test
Increase: LFTs
Decrease: cholesterol

NURSING CONSIDERATIONS

Assess:
• **Hypercholesterolemia:** diet history: fat content, lipid levels (triglycerides, LDL, HDL, cholesterol); LFTs at baseline, periodically during treatment

• **Pregnancy/breastfeeding:** no well-controlled studies; use only if benefits outweigh fetal risk; cautious use in breastfeeding, excretion is unknown

Evaluate:
• Therapeutic response: decreased cholesterol, LDL; increased HDL

Teach patient/family:
• That compliance is needed
• That risk factors should be decreased: high-fat diet, smoking, alcohol consumption, absence of exercise
• To notify prescriber if pregnancy suspected, planned, or if breastfeeding
• To report confusion, injection-site reactions

RARELY USED

exemestane (Rx)

(ex-em′eh-stane)
Aromasin
Func. class.: Antineoplastic
Chem. class.: Aromatase inhibitor

USES: Advanced breast carcinoma not responsive to other therapy (postmenopausal), estrogen receptor–positive early breast cancer that has received tamoxifen

CONTRAINDICATIONS: Pregnancy, breastfeeding, premenopausal women, hypersensitivity

DOSAGE AND ROUTES
• **Adult:** PO 25 mg/day after meals; may need 50 mg/day if taken with a potent CYP3A4 inducer

---

⚠ HIGH ALERT

exenatide (Rx)

(ex-en′a-tide)
Bydureon, Byetta
Func. class.: Antidiabetic
Chem. class.: Incretin mimetic

ACTION: Binds and activates known human GLP-1 receptor, mimics natural physiology for self-regulating glycemic control

USES: Type 2 diabetes mellitus given in combination with metFORMIN, a sulfonylurea, thiazolidinedione, insulin glargine

CONTRAINDICATIONS: Hypersensitivity

Black Box Warning: Medullary thyroid carcinoma, multiple endocrine neoplasia syndrome type 2 (MEN-2), thyroid cancer

Precautions: Pregnancy, geriatric patients, severe renal/hepatic/GI disease, pancreatitis, vit D deficiency

DOSAGE AND ROUTES
• **Adult: SUBCUT** 5 mcg bid 1 hr before morning and evening meal; may increase to 10 mcg bid after 1 mo; ext rel **SUBCUT** (Bydureon) 2 mg q7days
Renal dose
• **Adult:** PO CCr 30-50 mL/min, use caution when increasing dose
Available forms: Inj 5, 10 mcg pen; ext rel powder for susp for inj 2 mg
Administer:
Store in refrigerator for unopened pen; may store at room temperature after opening for up to 30 days
SUBCUT route (regular release—Byetta)
• May be used as monotherapy or combined with other products
• SUBCUT only, do not give IV/IM
• Pen needles must be purchased separately, compatible; prime before use; inject into thigh, abdomen, upper arm; rotate sites
• Product 1 hr before meals, approximately 6 hr apart; if patient is NPO, may need to hold dose to prevent hypoglycemia
• If added to insulin glargine, insulin, or detemir, a dosage reduction in these products may be required
SUBCUT route (ext rel—Bydureon)
• Give every 7 days (weekly); the dose can be given at any time of day without regard to meals

• Available as a single-dose tray containing a vial of 2 mg, a prefilled syringe delivering 0.65 mL diluent, a vial connector, and two custom needles (23GX 5/16′) specific to this delivery system (one is a spare needle); do not substitute needles or any other components
• Inject immediately after the white to off-white powder is suspended in the diluent and transferred to the syringe
• Inject subcut into the thigh, abdomen, or upper arm, rotate sites to prevent lipodystrophy

SIDE EFFECTS
CNS: *Headache, dizziness,* feeling jittery, restlessness, weakness
ENDO: Hypoglycemia, thyroid hyperplasia
GI: Nausea, vomiting, diarrhea, dyspepsia, anorexia, gastroesophageal reflux, weight loss, pancreatitis
SYST: Angioedema, anaphylaxis
INTEG: Serious inj-site reactions (cellulitis, abscess, skin necrosis)

PHARMACOKINETICS
Absorption well, immediate release: Peak 2.1 hr, elimination by glomerular filtration, half-life 2.4 hr
Ext rel: Peak 2 wk

INTERACTIONS
• May decrease effect of acetaminophen
• Do not use with erythromycin, metoclopramide
Increase: hypoglycemia—ACE inhibitors, disopyramide, sulfonylureas, androgens, fibric acid derivatives, alcohol
Increase: hyperglycemia—phenothiazines, corticosteroids, anabolic steroids
Decrease: action of digoxin, lovastatin, acetaminophen (elixir)
Decrease: efficacy—niacin, dextrothyroxine, thiazide diuretics, triamterene, estrogens, progestins, oral contraceptives, MAOIs

NURSING CONSIDERATIONS
Assess:
• Fasting blood glucose, A1c levels, postprandial glucose during treatment to determine diabetes control

• **Pancreatitis:** severe abdominal pain with or without vomiting, product should be discontinued

Black Box Warning: Increased risk of thyroid tumors (medullary C-cell tumors)

• **Anaphylaxis, angioedema:** product should be discontinued immediately
• Renal studies: urinalysis, creatinine
• Hypo/hyperglycemic reaction that can occur soon after meals; for severe hypoglycemia, give IV $D_{50}W$, then IV dextrose solution
• Nausea, vomiting, diarrhea, ability to tolerate product, may cause dehydration
• **Pregnancy/breastfeeding:** use only if benefits clearly outweigh risks; if pregnant, enroll in the Exenatide Pregnancy Registry, 1-800-633-9081; do not breastfeed
Evaluate:
• Therapeutic response: decrease in polyuria, polydipsia, polyphagia, clear sensorium, improving A1c, weight; absence of dizziness, stable gait
Teach patient/family:
• About the symptoms of hypo/hyperglycemia, what to do about each; to have glucagon emergency kit available; to carry a glucose source (candy, sugar cube) to treat hypoglycemia
• That product must be continued on a daily or weekly basis (ext rel); about consequences of discontinuing product abruptly
• That diabetes is a lifelong illness; that product will not cure disease; to carry emergency ID with prescriber and medication information
• To continue weight control, dietary restrictions, exercise, hygiene
• That regular blood glucose monitoring and A1c testing are needed
• To notify prescriber if pregnant or intending to become pregnant
• About the importance of reading "Information for the Patient" and "Pen User Manual"; about self-injection
• **Pancreatitis:** if severe abdominal pain with or without vomiting occurs, seek medical attention immediately
• To review injection procedure; to store product in refrigerator, room temperature

after first use; discard 30 days after first use; do not freeze; to protect from light (Byetta)

ezetimibe (Rx)
(ehz-eh-tim′bee)
Ezetrol ♦, Zetia
Func. class.: Antilipemic; cholesterol absorption inhibitor

ACTION: Inhibits absorption of cholesterol by the small intestine, causes reduced hepatic cholesterol stores

USES: Hypercholesterolemia, homozygous familial hypercholesterolemia (HoFH), homozygous sitosterolemia

CONTRAINDICATIONS: Hypersensitivity, severe hepatic disease
Precautions: Pregnancy, breastfeeding, children, hepatic disease

DOSAGE AND ROUTES
• **Adult/adolescent/child >10 yr: PO** 10 mg/day
Available forms: Tabs 10 mg
Administer:
Without regard to meals

SIDE EFFECTS
CNS: Fatigue, dizziness, headache
GI: Diarrhea, abdominal pain
MISC: Chest pain
MS: *Myalgias, arthralgias,* back pain, myopathy, rhabdomyolysis
RESP: Pharyngitis, sinusitis, cough, *URI*
EENT: Sinusitis, nasopharyngitis
SYST: Angioedema

PHARMACOKINETICS
Absorption variable, metabolized in small intestine, liver; excreted in feces 78%, urine 11%; peak 4-12 hr; half-life 22 hr

INTERACTIONS
Increase: action of ezetimibe—fibric acid derivatives, cycloSPORINE
Decrease: action of ezetimibe—antacids, bile acid sequestrants
Drug/Lab Test
Increase: LFTs

Side effects: *italics* = common; red = life-threatening

NURSING CONSIDERATIONS
Assess:
• **Hypercholestrolemia:** diet history: fat content, lipid levels (triglycerides, LDL, HDL, cholesterol); LFTs at baseline, periodically during treatment
• **Myopathy/rhabdomyolysis:** increased CPK, myalgia, muscle cramps, musculoskeletal pain, lethargy, fatigue, fever; more common when combined with statins
• **Pregnancy/breastfeeding:** do not use in pregnancy, breastfeeding
Evaluate:
• Therapeutic response: decreased cholesterol, LDL; increased HDL
Teach patient/family:
• That compliance is needed
• That risk factors should be decreased: high-fat diet, smoking, alcohol consumption, absence of exercise
• To notify prescriber if pregnancy suspected, planned, or if breastfeeding
• To notify prescriber if unexplained weakness, muscle pain present
• To notify prescriber of dietary/herbal supplements

---

ezogabine
(e-zog′a-been)
Potiga
Func. class.: Anticonvulsant
Controlled Substance Schedule V

ACTION: The exact mechanism of anticonvulsant effects is not fully known; however, studies indicate that the drug enhances transmembrane potassium currents, which may stabilize the resting membrane potential and reduce brain excitability; may also augment GABA-mediated currents

USES: Partial seizures

CONTRAINDICATIONS:
Hypersensitivity
Precautions: Suicidal ideation/behavior, prostatic hypertrophy, dementia, psychotic disorders, QT prolongation, congestive heart failure, ventricular hypertrophy, hypokalemia, hypomagnesemia, abrupt discontinuation, renal impairment, hepatic disease, geriatric patients, pregnancy, breastfeeding, neonates, infants, children, adolescents

---

Black Box Warning: Visual impairment

DOSAGE AND ROUTES
• **Adult ≤65 yr: PO** initially, 100 mg tid, increase by ≤50 mg tid per day at weekly intervals depending on response, up to a maintenance dose of 200-400 mg tid depending on response; max is 400 mg tid (1200 mg/day)
• **Geriatric patient >65 yr: PO** initially, 50 mg tid, increase by ≤50 mg tid per day at weekly intervals depending on response; max 250 mg tid (750 mg/day)
Available forms: Film-coated tabs 50, 200, 300, 400 mg
Administer:
Tab should be swallowed whole without regard to meals
• Give in 3 equally divided doses

SIDE EFFECTS
CNS: Dizziness, drowsiness, memory impairment, tremor, vertigo, abnormal coordination, disturbance in attention, gait disturbance, aphasia, dysarthria, balance disorder, paresthesias, amnesia, dysphagia, myoclonia, hypokinesia, confusion, anxiety, hallucinations, suicidal thoughts/behaviors, fatigue, asthenia, malaise, euphoria
EENT: Diplopia, blurred vision, retinal pigment change
GI: Nausea, constipation, dyspepsia, xerostomia, constipation, weight gain, appetite stimulation
GU: Urinary retention, hydronephrosis, dysuria, urinary hesitation, hematuria, chromaturia
HEMA: Thrombocytopenia, leukopenia, neutropenia
INTEG: Rash, alopecia, blue skin discoloration
MISC: Influenza, dyspnea, QT prolongation
MS: Muscle spasms, weakness

PHARMACOKINETICS

80% protein bound; extensively distributed in the body; extensively metabolized by glucuronidation and acetylation; inactive N-glucuronides are the primary metabolites; elimination half-lives of ezogabine and its N-acetyl metabolite are 7 hr and 11 hr, respectively; 36% excreted renally as ezogabine, 18% as NAMR, 24% as the N-glucuronides of ezogabine and NAMR, 14% fecal excretion; rapidly absorbed, peak 0.5-2 hr, bioavailability 60%; high-fat food increases peak concentrations; increased in hepatic/renal disease, geriatric patients, young adult females

INTERACTIONS

Increase: QT prolongation—arsenic trioxide, chloroquine, chlorproMAZINE, mesoridazine, thioridazine, clarithromycin, Class IA antiarrhythmics (disopyramide, procainamide, quiNIDine), Class III antiarrhythmics (amiodarone, dofetilide, ibutilide, sotalol), dextromethorphan, dronedarone, droperidol, erythromycin, grepafloxacin, halofantrine, levomethadyl, methadone, pentamidine, pimozide, posaconazole, probucol, propafenone, quiNIDine, saquinavir, sparfloxacin, terfenadine, troleandomycin, ziprasidone

Decrease: effect of phenytoin

Decrease: effect of ezogabine—carBAMazepine

Increase: effect of digoxin

Increase: urinary retention—antimuscarinics, amantadine, H$_1$ blockers

Increase: CNS depression—anxiolytics, sedatives, hypnotics, buprenorphine, butorphanol, dronabinol, mirtazapine, nabilone, nalbuphine, opiate agonists, pentazocine, pregabalin, skeletal muscle relaxants, traMADol, traZODone, ethanol

Drug/Lab Test

Increase: LFTs

NURSING CONSIDERATIONS

Assess:

• **Seizures:** assess for type, duration, location, activity, presence of aura

• **QT prolongation:** monitor in those with known QT prolongation, congestive heart failure, ventricular hypertrophy, hypokalemia, hypomagnesemia, and in patients receiving medications known to cause QT prolongation; QT prolongation can occur within 3 hr of dose

• **Abrupt withdrawal:** withdraw gradually to minimize increased seizure frequency

• **Suicidal thoughts/behaviors:** assess for any unusual changes in moods or behaviors, including emotional lability or emerging or worsening depression and suicidal ideation

> Black Box Warning: **Vision changes:** obtain a baseline eye exam, then periodic eye exams; discontinue if ophthalmic changes occur unless no other treatment is available

• **Beers:** avoid in older adults unless safer alternatives are unavailable; may cause ataxia, impaired psychomotor function

Teach patient/family:

• To avoid driving or operating machinery or performing other tasks that require mental alertness until reaction is known

• To avoid concurrent use of alcohol

• To avoid abruptly discontinuing this product

• **Suicidal thoughts/behaviors:** advise patient to notify prescriber immediately of suicidal thoughts/behaviors

• That skin may turn blue; it is unknown if it is reversible

> Black Box Warning: To report vision change immediately

RARELY USED

factor Xa
Andexxa
Func. class.: Antidote

USES: For rivaroxaban reversal and apixaban reversal in patients with life-threatening or uncontrolled bleeding

CONTRAINDICATIONS: None

DOSAGE AND ROUTES
Dose based on specific factor Xa inhibitor, dose of factor Xa inhibitor, and time since the patient's last dose of factor Xa inhibitor

• **Adult:** IV For rivaroxaban ≤10 mg or apixaban ≤5 mg within 8 hr or unknown timing of last dose or for any dose of rivaroxaban or apixaban at 8 hr or more since timing of last dose, 400 mg **IV BOL** at 30 mg/min then 4 mg/min **CONT IV INFUSION** for up to 120 min

• **Adult:** IV For rivaroxaban >10 mg, apixaban >5 mg, or unknown dose of either drug within 8 hr of timing of last dose, 800 mg **IV BOL** at 30 mg/min followed by 8 mg/min **CONT IV INFUSION** for up to 120 min. Resume anticoagulant therapy as soon as medically appropriate after factor Xa treatment

---

famciclovir (Rx)
(fam-cy′clo-veer)
Famvir ✦
Func. class.: Antiviral
Chem. class.: Guanosine nucleoside

ACTION: Inhibits DNA polymerase and viral DNA synthesis by conversion of this guanosine nucleoside to penciclovir

USES: Treatment of acute herpes zoster (shingles), genital herpes; recurrent mucocutaneous herpes simplex virus (HSV) in patients with HIV; initial episodes of herpes genitalis; herpes labialis in the immunocompromised, herpes labialis prophylaxis

Unlabeled uses: Bell's palsy, postherpetic neuralgia prophylaxis

CONTRAINDICATIONS: Hypersensitivity to this product, penciclovir, acyclovir, ganciclovir, valacyclovir, valganciclovir
Precautions: Pregnancy, breastfeeding, renal disease, lactose intolerance

DOSAGE AND ROUTES
Herpes zoster
• **Adult:** PO 500 mg q8hr for 7 days
Renal dose
• **Adult:** PO CCr 40-59 mL/min, 500 mg q12hr; CCr 20-39 mL/min, 500 mg q24hr; CCr <20 mL/min, 250 mg q24hr
Suppression of recurrent herpes simplex
• **Adult:** PO 250 mg q12hr up to 1 yr
Renal dose
• **Adult:** PO CCr 20-39 mL/min, 125 mg q12hr × 5 days; CCr <20 mL/min, 125 mg q24hr × 5 days
Renal impairment: recurrent herpes labialis
• **Adult:** PO CCr ≥60 mL/min, usual dose; CCr 40-59 mL/min, 750 mg as a single dose; CCr 20-39 mL/min, 500 mg as single dose; CCr <20 mL/min, 250 mg as a single dose; hemodialysis, 250 mg as a single dose following dialysis
Renal impairment: recurrent orolabial or genital herpes in HIV-infected patients
• **Adult:** PO CCr ≥40 mL/min, usual dose; CCr 20-39 mL/min, 500 mg q24hr; CCr <20 mL/min, 250 mg q24hr; hemodialysis, 250 mg following each dialysis
Recurrent genital herpes simplex
• **Adult:** PO 1000 mg bid on a single day
Renal dose
• **Adult:** PO CCr 40-59 mL/min, 500 mg q12hr × 1 day; CCr 20-39 mL/min, 500 mg as a single dose; CCr <20 mL/min, 250 mg as a single dose
Bell's palsy (unlabeled)
• **Adult:** PO 750 mg tid × 7 days with predniSONE
Varicella zoster virus (shingles); chickenpox (unlabeled)
• **Adult:** PO 500 mg q8hr × 7 days, preferably within 48 hr of onset

---

Herpes zoster in HIV (unlabeled)
• **Adult/adolescent:** PO 500 mg tid × 7-10 days
Available forms: Tabs 125, 250, 500 mg
Administer:
• Without regard to meals
• As soon as diagnosed; for herpes zoster within 72 hr

SIDE EFFECTS
CNS: *Headache, fatigue, dizziness,* paresthesia, somnolence, fever, seizures
GI: Nausea, vomiting, diarrhea, constipation, abdominal pain, anorexia
GU: Decreased sperm count
INTEG: *Pruritus,* vasculitis
MS: Back pain, arthralgia
RESP: Pharyngitis, sinusitis
SYST: Anaphylaxis

PHARMACOKINETICS
Bioavailability 77%, 20% protein binding, 73% excreted via kidneys, half-life 2-3 hr, peak 1 hr, duration 12 hr

INTERACTIONS
Increase: effect of famciclovir—probenecid
Decrease: effect of zoster, varicella virus vaccine

NURSING CONSIDERATIONS
Assess:
• **Herpes zoster:** severity of the breakout; burning, itching, pain, which are early symptoms of herpes infection; assess daily during therapy
• **Acute renal failure:** usually in high dose or in those >65 yr; urine CCr; BUN before and during treatment if decreased renal function; dose may have to be lowered; hepatic studies: LFTs
• Bowel pattern before, during treatment; diarrhea may occur
• Postherpetic neuralgia during and after treatment
• **Pregnancy/breastfeeding:** use only if benefits outweigh fetal risk; pregnant patients should enroll in the Famvir pregnancy reporting system, 1-888-669-6682; excretion unknown
Evaluate:
• Therapeutic response: decreased size, spread of lesions

Teach patient/family:
• How to recognize beginning infection (pain, itching, tingling), use product within 48 hr of rash
• How to prevent spread of infection; that this medication does not prevent spread to others; that condoms should be used; that until crusting of lesions has taken place, not to be around those who have not had the chicken pox vaccine or those who are immunocompromised
• About the reason for medication, expected results; that product must be taken for whole course of treatment; if lactose intolerant, to notify prescriber before use
• That women with genital herpes should have yearly Pap smears; that cervical cancer is more likely
• To avoid driving or other hazardous activities until results are known; dizziness may occur

---

famotidine (otc, Rx)
(fa-moe'ti-deen)
Acid Control ✦, Pepcid, Pepcid AC, Peptic Guard Ulcidine ✦
Func. class.: H$_2$-histamine receptor antagonist

ACTION: Competitively inhibits histamine at histamine H$_2$-receptor site, thus decreasing gastric secretion while pepsin remains at a stable level

USES: Short-term treatment of duodenal ulcer, maintenance therapy for duodenal ulcer, Zollinger-Ellison syndrome, multiple endocrine adenomas, gastric ulcers; gastroesophageal reflux disease, heartburn
Unlabeled uses: GI disorders in those taking NSAIDs; urticaria; prevention of stress ulcers, aspiration pneumonitis

CONTRAINDICATIONS: Hypersensitivity
Precautions: Pregnancy, breastfeeding, children <12 yr, geriatric patients, severe renal/hepatic disease

---

Side effects: *italics* = common; red = life-threatening

DOSAGE AND ROUTES
Short-term treatment of benign gastric ulcer
• **Adult:** PO 40 mg/day at bedtime × 4-8 wk, then 20 mg/day at bedtime if needed (maintenance); IV 20 mg q12hr if unable to take PO
• **Child 1-16 yr:** PO/IV 0.25 mg/kg/dose q12hr, max 40 mg/day

Short-term treatment of duodenal ulcer
• **Adult:** PO 40 mg at bedtime or 20 mg bid; maintenance 20 mg q day at bedtime

Pathologic hypersecretory conditions
• **Adult:** PO 20 mg q6hr; may give up to 160 mg q6hr if needed; IV 20 mg q6hr if unable to take PO

GERD
• **Adult:** PO 20 mg bid ≤2 wk; 40 mg bid ≤2 wk (ulcerative esophagitis)
• **Child 1-16 yr:** PO 0.5 mg/kg bid, max 40 mg bid
• **Child 3 mo-<1 yr:** PO 0.5 mg/kg/dose bid ≤8 wk
• **Child <3 mo:** PO 0.5 mg/kg/dose q day ≤8 wk

Heartburn relief/prevention (OTC)
• **Adult:** PO 10 mg with water for relief or take 15 min-1 hr before eating for prevention

Available forms: Tabs 10, 20, 40 mg; powder for oral susp 40 mg/5 mL; inj 0.4 mg/mL premixed in normal saline, 10 mg/mL, 20 mg/50 mL

Administer:
• Store in cool environment (oral); IV sol stable for 48 hr at room temperature; do not use discolored sol; discard unused oral sol after 1 mo

PO route
• After shaking oral suspension

Direct IV route
• After diluting 2 mL of product (10 mg/mL) in 0.9% NaCl to total volume of 5-10 mL; inject over 2 min to prevent hypotension

Intermittent IV INFUSION route
• After diluting 20 mg (2 mL) of product in 100 mL of LR, 0.9% NaCl, D$_5$W, D$_{10}$W; run over 15-30 min

Continuous IV INFUSION route
• **Adults:** Dilute 40 mg of product in 250 mL D5W, NS; infuse over 24 hr, run at 11 mL/hr, use infusion device

Y-site compatibilities: Acyclovir, alfentanil, allopurinol, amifostine, amikacin, aminocaproic acid, aminophylline, amiodarone, amphotericin B lipid complex, amphotericin B liposome, amsacrine, anakinra, anidulafungin, ascorbic acid injection, atenolol, atracurium, atropine, aztreonam, benztropine, bivalirudin, bleomycin, bumetanide, buprenorphine, butorphanol, calcium chloride/gluconate, CARBOplatin, caspofungin, cefonicid, cefotaxime, cefTAZidime, cefuroxime, chlorproMAZINE, cimetidine, cisatracurium, CISplatin, cladribine, clindamycin, codeine, cyanocobalamin, cyclophosphamide, cycloSPORINE, cytarabine, DACTINomycin, DAPTOmycin, dexamethasone, dexmedetomidine, digoxin, diltiazem, diphenhydrAMINE, DOBUTamine, DOCEtaxel, DOPamine, doripenem, doxacurium, DOXOrubicin, DOXOrubicin liposomal, doxycycline, droperidol, enalaprilat, ePHEDrine, EPINEPHrine, epirubicin, epoetin alfa, eptifibatide, ertapenem, erythromycin, esmolol, etoposide, fenoldopam, fentaNYL, filgrastim, fluconazole, fludarabine, fluorouracil, folic acid, gatifloxacin, gemcitabine, gentamicin, glycopyrrolate, granisetron, heparin, hydrocortisone, HYDROmorphone, hydrOXYzine, IDArubicin, ifosfamide, imipenem-cilastatin, irinotecan, isoproterenol, ketorolac, labetalol, levofloxacin, lidocaine, linezolid, LORazepam, LR, magnesium sulfate, mechlorethamine, melphalan, meperidine, metaraminol, methicillin, methotrexate, methoxamine, methyldopa, methylPREDNISolone, metoclopramide, metoprolol, metroNIDAZOLE, miconazole, midazolam, milrinone, mitoXANtrone, morphine, moxalactam, multiple vitamins injection, mycophenolate, nafcillin, nalbuphine, naloxone, nesiritide, netilmicin, niCARdipine, nitroglycerin, nitroprusside, norepinephrine, 0.9% NaCl, octreotide, ondansetron, oxacillin, oxaliplatin, oxytocin, PACLitaxel, palonosetron, pamidronate, pancuronium, papaverine, PEMEtrexed, penicillin G potassium/sodium, pentamidine, pentazocine, PENTobarbital, perphenazine, PHENobarbital, phenylephrine, phytonadione, polymyxin B, potassium chloride/phosphates, procainamide, prochlorperazine, promethazine, propofol, propranolol, protamine, pyridoxine, quiNIDine, ranitidine, remifentanil, Ringer's, ritodrine, riTUXimab, sargramostim, sodium acetate/bicarbonate, succinylcholine, SUFentanil, tacrolimus, teniposide, theophylline, thiamine, thiotepa, ticarcillin, ticarcillin-clavulanate, tigecycline, tirofiban, TNA, tobramycin, tolazoline, TPN, trastuzumab, trimetaphan, urokinase, vancomycin, vasopressin, vecuronium, verapamil, vinCRIStine, vinorelbine, voriconazole, zoledronic acid

SIDE EFFECTS

CNS: *Headache, dizziness,* paresthesia, depression, anxiety, somnolence, insomnia, fever, seizures in renal disease
CV: Dysrhythmias, QT prolongation (impaired renal functioning)
EENT: Taste change, tinnitus, orbital edema
GI: *Constipation,* nausea, vomiting, anorexia, cramps, abnormal hepatic enzymes, diarrhea
INTEG: Rash, toxic epidermal necrolysis, Stevens-Johnson syndrome
MS: Myalgia, arthralgia
RESP: Pneumonia

PHARMACOKINETICS

Protein binding 15%-20%, metabolized in liver 30% (active metabolites), 70% excreted by kidneys, half-life $2^1/_2$-$3^1/_2$ hr
PO: Onset 60 min, duration 12 hr, peak 1-3 hr, absorption 50%
IV: Onset 60 min, peak 1-4 hr, duration 8-12 hr

INTERACTIONS

Decrease: absorption—ketoconazole, itraconazole, cefpodoxime, cefditoren
Decrease: famotidine absorption—antacids
Decrease: effect of—atazanavir, delavirdine

NURSING CONSIDERATIONS

Assess:

• **Ulcers:** epigastric pain, adominal pain, frank or occult blood in emesis, stools
• Renal function: patients with decreased renal function are at risk for prolonged QT
• Intragastric pH, serum creatinine/BUN baseline and periodically
• For bleeding, hematuria, hematuresis, occult blood in stools; abdominal pain
• Increase in bulk and fluids in diet to prevent constipation
• **Beers:** avoid in older adults with delirium or at high risk for delirium; may induce or worsen the condition; assess for confusion
• **Pregnancy/breastfeeding:** cautious use in pregnancy, breastfeeding; excreted in breast milk

Evaluate:

• Therapeutic response: decreased abdominal pain, healing of duodenal ulcers, decreased gastroesophageal reflux

Teach patient/family:

• That product must be continued for prescribed time in prescribed method to be effective; not to double dose; do not take for extended periods of time, risk of B_{12} malabsorption
• About possibility of decreased libido; that this is reversible after discontinuing therapy
• To avoid irritating foods, alcohol, aspirin, NSAIDs, extreme-temperature foods that may irritate GI system
• That smoking should be avoided because it diminishes effectiveness of product
• To avoid tasks requiring alertness because dizziness, drowsiness may occur

---

febuxostat (Rx)
(feb-ux´oh-stat)
Uloric
Func. class.: Antigout drug, antihyperuricemic
Chem. class.: Xanthene oxidase inhibitor

Side effects: *italics* = common; red = life-threatening

ACTION: Inhibits the enzyme xanthine oxidase, thereby reducing uric acid synthesis; more selective for xanthine oxidase than allopurinol

USES: Chronic gout, hyperuricemia

CONTRAINDICATIONS: Hypersensitivity

Precautions: Pregnancy, breastfeeding, children, renal/hepatic/cardiac/neoplastic disease, stroke, MI, organ transplant, Lesch-Nyhan syndrome

DOSAGE AND ROUTES
• **Adult:** PO 40 mg daily, may increase to 80 mg daily if uric acid levels are >6 mg/dL after 2 wk of therapy
Available forms: Tabs 40, 80 mg
Administer:
PO route
• Without regard to meals or antacids; may crush and add to foods or fluids

SIDE EFFECTS
CNS: Dizziness
GI: *Nausea*
INTEG: Rash
MISC: Arthralgia, gout flare

PHARMACOKINETICS
Peak 1-1.5 hr, duration up to 24 hr; metabolized extensively in the liver, excreted in feces, urine; half-life 5-8 hr; protein binding 99.2%; max lowering of uric acid 2 wk

INTERACTIONS
Increase: toxicity—azaTHIOprine, didanosine, mercaptopurine; do not use together
Increase: xanthine nephropathy, calculi—rasburicase, antineoplastics
Increase: effect of theophylline; use cautiously
Drug/Lab
Increase: LFTs, alkaline phosphatase, serum cholesterol, triglycerides, amylase, BUN, creatinine, aPTT, PT, CPK, creatine
Decrease: Hct/Hgb, RBC, platelets, lymphocytes, neutrophils, TSH, blood glucose

NURSING CONSIDERATIONS
Assess:
• **Hyperuricemia:** uric acid levels q2wk; uric acid levels should be ≤6 mg/dL, flares may occur during first 6 wk of treatment
• Hepatic studies before use, then 2, 4 mo and then periodically; assess for fatigue, anorexia, right upper abdominal discomfort, dark urine, jaundice
• **Renal disease:**
• I&O ratio; increase fluids to 2 L/day to prevent stone formation and toxicity
• For rash, hypersensitivity reactions; discontinue
Evaluate:
• Therapeutic response: decreased pain in joints, decreased stone formation in kidneys, decreased uric acid levels
Teach patient/family:
• That tabs may be crushed
• To take as prescribed; if dose is missed, to take as soon as remembered; not to double dose
• To increase fluid intake to 2 L/day unless contraindicated
• To avoid alcohol, caffeine because they will increase uric acid levels
• To report cardiovascular events to prescriber immediately (chest pain, dyspnea, slurred speech, weakness)
• **Gout:** that flares may occur during first 6 wk of treatment; continue and notify prescriber; NSAIDs or colchicine may be added to reduce the risk of flares

---

felodipine (Rx)
(fe-loe´-di-peen)
Plenedil ✦
Func. class.: Antihypertensive, calcium channel blocker, antianginal
Chem. class.: Dihydropyridine

ACTION: Inhibits calcium ion influx across cell membrane, resulting in the inhibition of the excitation and contraction of vascular smooth muscle

USES: Essential hypertension alone or with other antihypertensives

---

Unlabeled uses: Hypertension in adolescents and children, angina pectoris; Prinzmetal's angina (vasospastic)

CONTRAINDICATIONS: Hypersensitivity to this product or dihydropyridines, sick sinus syndrome, 2nd- or 3rd-degree heart block, hypotension <90 mm Hg systolic

Precautions: Pregnancy, breastfeeding, children, geriatric patients, HF, hepatic injury, renal disease, coronary artery disease

DOSAGE AND ROUTES

• **Adult:** PO 5 mg/day initially; usual range 2.5-10 mg/day; max 10 mg/day; do not adjust dosage at intervals of <2 wk

• **Geriatric:** PO 2.5 mg/day, max 10 mg/day

Hepatic disease

• **Adult:** PO 2.5-5 mg, max 10 mg/day

Hypertension in adolescent/child (unlabeled)

• **Adolescent/child:** PO 2.5 mg initially, titrate upward, max 10 mg/day

Available forms: Ext rel tabs 2.5, 5, 10 mg

Administer:

PO route

• Swallow whole; do not break, crush, or chew ext rel products

• Once daily with light meal; avoid grapefruit juice

SIDE EFFECTS

CNS: *Headache,* fatigue, drowsiness, dizziness, anxiety, depression, nervousness, insomnia, light-headedness, paresthesia, tinnitus, psychosis, somnolence, flushing

CV: Dysrhythmia, *edema,* HF, hypotension, palpitations, MI, pulmonary edema, tachycardia, syncope, AV block, angina

GI: Nausea, vomiting, diarrhea, gastric upset, constipation, dry mouth

GU: Nocturia, polyuria, sexual dysfunction, decreased libido

HEMA: Anemia

INTEG: Rash, pruritus, peripheral edema

MISC: Flushing, sexual difficulties, cough, nasal congestion, SOB, wheezing, epistaxis, respiratory infection, chest pain, angioedema, gingival hyperplasia, Stevens-Johnson syndrome

PHARMACOKINETICS

Onset 1 hr, peak 2.5-5 hr, highly protein bound >99%, metabolized in liver, 0.5% excreted unchanged in urine, elimination half-life 11-16 hr

INTERACTIONS

Increase: bradycardia, HF—β-blockers, digoxin, phenytoin, disopyramide

Increase: toxicity, hypotension—nitrates, alcohol, quiNIDine, zileuton, miconazole, diltiazem, delavirdine, quinupristin-dalfopristin, conivaptan, cycloSPORINE, cimetidine, clarithromycin, antiretroviral protease inhibitors, other antihypertensives, MAOIs, ketoconazole, erythromycin, itraconazole, propranolol

Decrease: antihypertensive effects—NSAIDs, carBAMazepine, barbiturates, phenytoin

Drug/Herb

Increase: antihypertensive effect—ginseng, ginkgo, hawthorn

Decrease: antihypertensive effect—ephedra, St. John's wort

Drug/Food

Increase: felodipine level—grapefruit juice

NURSING CONSIDERATIONS

Assess:

• **HF:** Fluid volume status, I&O, weight daily; weight gain, crackles, dyspnea, edema, jugular venous distention, adequacy of pulses, moist mucous membranes; bilateral lung sounds, peripheral pitting edema; dehydration symptoms of decreasing output, thirst, hypotension, dry mouth, and mucous membranes should be reported

• Monitor ALT, AST, bilirubin often if elevated

• Cardiac status: B/P, pulse, respiration; ECG periodically during prolonged treatment

• **Angina pain:** location, duration, intensity; ameliorating, aggravating factors

• **Hypertension:** check for compliance, number of refills

• **Pregnancy/breastfeeding:** no well-controlled studies; use only if benefits outweigh fetal risk, may cause fetal harm;

Side effects: *italics* = common; red = life-threatening

discontinue breastfeeding or product, excretion unknown

Evaluate:
• Therapeutic response: B/P, WNL, decreased anginal attacks, increased activity tolerance

Teach patient/family:
• To avoid hazardous activities until stabilized on product, dizziness no longer a problem
• To avoid OTC products, alcohol unless directed by prescriber; to limit caffeine consumption
• About the importance of complying with all areas of medical regimen: diet, exercise, stress reduction, product therapy
• That tablets may appear in stools but are insignificant
• To report dyspnea, palpitations, irregular heartbeat, swelling of extremities, nausea, vomiting, severe dizziness, severe headache
• To change positions slowly to prevent orthostatic hypotension
• To obtain correct pulse; to contact prescriber if pulse <50 bpm
• To use good oral hygiene to prevent gingival hyperplasia
• Not to stop abruptly
• To avoid grapefruit juice

TREATMENT OF OVERDOSE:
Atropine for AV block, vasopressor for hypotension

---

fenofibrate (Rx)
(fen-oh-fee′brate)

Antara, Fenoglide, Fenomax ✦, Lipidil EZ ✦, Lipidil Micro ✦, Lipidil Supra ✦, Lipofen, Lofibra, TriCor, Triglide
Func. class.: Antilipemic
Chem. class.: Fibric acid derivative

Do not confuse:
TriCor/Tracleer

ACTION: Increases lipolysis and elimination of triglyceride-rich particles from plasma by activating lipoprotein lipase, resulting in changes in triglyceride size and composition of LDL, leading to rapid breakdown of LDL; mobilizes triglycerides from tissue; increases excretion of neutral sterols

USES: Hypercholesterolemia; types IV, V hyperlipidemia that do not respond to other treatment and that increase risk for pancreatitis; Fredrickson type IV, V hypertriglyceridemia

CONTRAINDICATIONS: Hypersensitivity, severe renal/hepatic disease, primary biliary cirrhosis, preexisting gallbladder disease, breastfeeding
Precautions: Pregnancy, geriatric patients, peptic ulcer, pancreatitis, renal/hepatic disease, diabetes mellitus

DOSAGE AND ROUTES
Hypertriglyceridemia
• **Adult: PO** (Antara) 30-90 mg/day; (Fenoglide) 40-120 mg/day; (Lofibra) 67-200 mg/day; (Tricor) 48-145 mg/day; (Triglide) 50-160 mg/day; (Lipofen) 50 mg/day
Primary hypercholesterolemia/mixed hyperlipidemia
• **Adult: PO** (Antara) 90 mg/day; (Fenoglide) 120 mg/day; (Lofibra) 200 mg/day; (Tricor) 145 mg/day; (Triglide) 160 mg/day
Renal dose (geriatric)
• **Adult: PO** (Tricor) CCr 30-80 mL/min, 48 mg/day; CCr <30 mL/min, contraindicated; Adult: PO CCr 30-80 mL/min, 50 mg/day (Triglide, Lipofen), 30 mg/day (Antara), 67 mg/day (Lofibra caps), 54 mg/day (Lofibra tabs); CCr <30 mL/min, contraindicated (Antara, Lipofen, Lofibra, Triglide)
Available forms: Cap: *Antara* 30, 90 mg; *Lipofen* 50, 150 mg; Tab: *Triglide* 50, 160 mg; *Lofibra* 54, 160 mg; *TriCor* 48, 145 mg; *Fenoglide* 40, 120 mg; choline: del rel caps 45, 135 mg; acid: tabs 35, 105 mg
Administer:
• Product with meals (Lipofen, Lofibra); Triglide, Antara without regard to food; may increase q4-8wk; discontinue if there is not adequate response after 2 mo
• Caps must be swallowed whole
• Brands are not interchangeable
• Protect Lipofen, Triglide from light, moisture

SIDE EFFECTS

CNS: *Fatigue, dizziness,* headache, paresthesia

CV: Hypertension

GI: *Nausea, vomiting, dyspepsia,* flatulence, pancreatitis, cholelithiasis, diarrhea, constipation

GU: *Polyuria*

INTEG: *Rash, pruritus*

MS: *Myalgias, arthralgias,* myopathy, rhabdomyolysis

RESP: Bronchitis, cough

PHARMACOKINETICS

Peak 2 wk, protein binding 99%, converted to fenofibric acid, metabolized in liver to fenofibric acid, excreted in urine (60%), feces (25%), half-life 20 hr

INTERACTIONS

Increase: myopathy, rhabdomyolysis—colchicine

• Avoid use with HMG-CoA reductase inhibitors; rhabdomyolysis may occur

Increase: anticoagulant effects—oral anticoagulants

Decrease: absorption of fenofibrate—bile acid sequestrants; give 1 hr prior to or ≥4 hr after bile acid sequestrant

Drug/Food

Increase: absorption

Drug/Lab Test

Increase: ALT, AST, BUN, CK, creatinine

Decrease: WBC, uric acid, Hgb, paradoxical effect in HDL

NURSING CONSIDERATIONS

Assess:

• **Hypercholesterolemia/hyperlipidemia diet history:** obtain fat content; lipid levels (triglycerides, LDL, HDL, cholesterol); may cause a paradoxical decrease in HDL; LFTs at baseline, periodically during treatment, if >3 × ULN, discontinue; CPK if muscle pain occurs; CBC, Hct, Hgb, PT with anticoagulant therapy; serum bilirubin (total and direct)

• **Pancreatitis, cholelithiasis, renal failure, rhabdomyolysis** (when combined with HMG Co-A reductase inhibitors), myositis; product should be discontinued; assess often for muscle pain, weakness, fever

• **Pregnancy/breastfeeding:** identify whether pregnancy is planned or suspected; do not breastfeed

Evaluate:

• Therapeutic response: decreased triglycerides, cholesterol levels

Teach patient/family:

• That compliance is needed; not to consume chipped or broken tabs (Triglide)

• That risk factors should be decreased: high-fat diet, smoking, alcohol consumption, absence of exercise

• To notify prescriber if pregnancy is suspected or planned; not to breastfeed

• To notify prescriber of muscle pain, weakness, fever, fatigue, epigastric pain

• To report signs/symptoms of DVT (swollen, warm extremity) or PE (shortness of breath, chest pain) to provider immediately

---

⚠ HIGH ALERT

fentaNYL (Rx) REMS
(fen′ta-nill)

RAN-Fentanyl ✦, Sublimaze ✦

fentaNYL transdermal (Rx)

Duragesic, Ionsys ✦

fentaNYL nasal spray (Rx)

Lazanda

fentaNYL SL spray (Rx)

Subsys

fentaNYL SL (Rx)

Abstral

fentaNYL buccal (Rx)

Fentora

fentaNYL lozenge (Rx)

Actiq

Func. class.: Opioid analgesic

Chem. class.: Synthetic phenylpiperidine

Controlled Substance Schedule II

Do not confuse:
fentaNYL/sufentanil

ACTION: Inhibits ascending pain pathways in CNS, increases pain threshold, alters pain perception by binding to opiate receptors

USES: Controls moderate to severe pain; preoperatively, postoperatively; adjunct to general anesthetic, adjunct to regional anesthesia; **fentaNYL:** anesthesia as premedication, conscious sedation; **Actiq:** breakthrough cancer pain

CONTRAINDICATIONS: Hypersensitivity to opiates; myasthenia gravis

Black Box Warning: Headache, migraine (Actiq, ABSTRAL, Fentora, Lazanda); emergency room use (ABSTRAL, Lazanda); outpatient surgeries (Duragesic TD); opioid-naive patients, respiratory depression

Precautions: Pregnancy, breastfeeding, geriatric patients, increased intracranial pressure, seizure disorders, severe respiratory disorders, cardiac dysrhythmias

Black Box Warning: Accidental exposure, ambient temperature increase, fever, skin abrasion (TD patch), substance abuse, surgery, requires an experienced clinician

DOSAGE AND ROUTES
FentaNYL
Anesthetic (adjunct to regional anesthesia)
• **Adult:** IV 50-100 mcg/kg over 1-2 min
Anesthesia supplement to general anesthesia
• **Adult/child >12 yr:** IM/IV (low dose) 1-2 mcg/kg; **IV** (moderate dose) 2-20 mcg/kg; **IM/IV** (high dose) 20-50 mcg/kg, then 25 mcg to y₂ initial loading dose as needed
Induction and maintenance
• **Child 2-12 yr:** IV 2-3 mcg/kg
Preoperatively
• **Adult/child >12 yr:** IM/IV 50-100 mcg q30-60min before surgery
Postoperatively
• **Adult/child >12 yr:** IM/IV 50-100 mcg q1-2hr prn

Moderate/severe pain
• **Adult:** IV/IM 50-100 mcg q1-2hr; **nasal; 100 mcg spray in one nostril, titrate stepwise**

Actiq
• **Adult: TRANSMUCOSAL** 200 mcg; redose if needed 15 min after completion of 1st dose; do not give more than 2 doses during titration period, max 4 doses/day

Fentora
• **Adult: BUCCAL/SL** 100 mcg placed above rear molar between upper cheek and gum; a second 100 mcg dose, if needed, may be started 30 min after 1st dose

Abstral
• **Adult: SL** 100 mcg; another dose may be taken 30 min after 1st, max 2 doses per episode of breakthrough pain; ≥2 hr must elapse before treating again; titrate stepwise over consecutive episodes

FentaNYL transdermal
• **Adult: Duragesic:** 12.5 mcg/hr; may increase until pain relief occurs; apply patch to flat surface on upper torso and wear for 72 hr; apply new patch on different site; may use 12.5 mcg/hr if <60 mg/day morphine equivalent; **Ionsys:** use only after patient has been titrated to acceptable level of analgesia using opioid analgesia; one dose activation = 40 mcg TD over 10 min, max 6 (40 mcg doses/hr)

FentaNYL nasal spray
• **Adult:** 100 mcg (1 spray in 1 nostril), may retreat after ≥2 hr, titrate upward until adequate analgesia; treat a max of 4 episodes daily

FentaNYL SL spray
• **Adult:** 100 mcg sprayed under tongue, titrate stepwise carefully
Available forms: Inj 0.05 mg/mL; lozenges 100, 200, 300, 400, 600, 800, 1200, 1600 mcg; lozenges on a stick 200, 400, 600, 800, 1200, 1600 mcg; buccal tab 100, 200, 400, 600, 800 mcg; SL tab (ABSTRAL) 100, 200, 300, 400, 600, 800 mcg; transdermal: patch 12, 25, 50, 75, 100 mcg/hr; SL spray 100, 200, 400, 600, 800, 1200, 1600 mcg/spray; nasal spray 100, 400 mcg/actuation

Administer:

• By inj (IM, IV); give slowly to prevent rigidity

• Overdose has been fatal when confusing products/dose; recheck both before using

• Must have emergency equipment available, opioid antagonists, O₂; to be used only by those appropriately trained; IV products to be used in OR, ER, ICU

Transmucosal route

• Remove foil just before administration; instruct patient to place product between cheek and lower gum, moving it back and forth and sucking, not chewing (Actiq); place above rear molar (Fentora); place film on the inside of the cheek; all products not used or only partially used should be flushed down the toilet; this product may be used SL

Transdermal route
Duragesic:

• q72hr for continuous pain relief; dosage adjusted after at least 2 applications; apply to clean, dry skin and press firmly

• Give short-acting analgesics until patch takes effect (8-24 hr); when reducing dosage or switching to alternative IV treatment, withdraw gradually; serum levels drop gradually, give ¹/₂ the equianalgesic dose of new analgesic 12-18 hr after removal as ordered

SL spray
Ionsys:

• Open blister package with scissors immediately before use; spray contents of unit under tongue; dispose of each used unit after use by placing it into one of the disposable bags provided; seal bag, discard into a trash container out of reach of children

IV route

• IV undiluted by anesthesiologist or diluted with 5 mL or more sterile water or 0.9% NaCl given through Y-tube or 3-way stopcock at 0.1 mg or less/1-2 min. Muscular rigidity may occur with rapid IV administration

Y-site compatibilities: Abciximab, acyclovir, alfentanil, alemtuzumab alprostadil, amikacin, aminocaproic acid, aminophylline, amiodarone, amphotericin B cholesteryl, amphotericin B lipid complex, amphotericin B liposome, anidulafungin, argatroban, ascorbic acid injection, atenolol, atracurium, atropine, azaTHIOprine, aztreonam, benztropine, bivalirudin, bleomycin, bumetanide, buprenorphine, butorphanol, calcium chloride/gluconate, CARBOplatin, caspofungin, ceFAZolin, cefmetazole, cefonicid, cefotaxime, cefoTEtan, cefOXitin, cefTAZidime, ceftizoxime, ceftobiprole, cefTRIAXone, cefuroxime, cephalothin, chloramphenicol, chlorproMAZINE, cimetidine, cisatracurium, CISplatin, clindamycin, cloNIDine, cyanocobalamin, cyclophosphamide, cycloSPORINE, cytarabine, DACTINomycin, DAPTOmycin, dexamethasone, dexmedetomidine, digoxin, diltiazem, diphenhydrAMINE, DOBUTamine, DOCEtaxel, DOPamine, doripenem, doxacurium, doxapram, DOXOrubicin, doxycycline, enalaprilat, ePHEDrine, EPINEPHrine, epirubicin, epoetin alfa, eptifibatide, erythromycin, esmolol, etomidate, etoposide, famotidine, fenoldopam, fluconazole, fludarabine, fluorouracil, folic acid, furosemide, ganciclovir, gatifloxacin, gemcitabine, gentamicin, glycopyrrolate, granisetron, heparin, hydrocortisone, HYDROmorphone, hydrOXYzine, IDArubicin, ifosfamide, imipenem-cilastatin, inamrinone, insulin (regular), irinotecan, isoproterenol, ketorolac, labetalol, lansoprazole, levofloxacin, lidocaine, linezolid, LORazepam, LR, magnesium sulfate, mannitol, mechlorethamine, meperidine, metaraminol, methicillin, methotrexate, methotrimeprazine, methoxamine, methyldopate, methylPREDNISolone, metoclopramide, metoprolol, metroNIDAZOLE, mezlocillin, miconazole, midazolam, milrinone, minocycline, mitoXANtrone, mivacurium, morphine, moxalactam, multiple vitamins injection, mycophenolate, nafcillin, nalbuphine, naloxone, nesiritide, netilmicin, niCARdipine, nitroglycerin, nitroprusside, norepinephrine, octreotide, ondansetron, oxacillin, oxaliplatin, oxytocin, PACLitaxel, palonosetron, pamidronate, pancuronium, papaverine, PEMEtrexed, penicillin G potassium/sodium, pentamidine, pentazocine, PENTobarbital, PHENobarbital, phenylephrine, phytonadione, piperacillin, piperacillin-tazobactam, polymyxin B,

F

Side effects: *italics* = common; red = life-threatening

potassium chloride, procainamide, prochlorperazine, promethazine, propofol, propranolol, protamine, pyridoxine, quiNIDine, quinupristin-dalfopristin, ranitidine, remifentanil, Ringer's, ritodrine, riTUXimab, rocuronium, sargramostim, scopolamine, sodium acetate/bicarbonate, succinylcholine, SUFentanil, tacrolimus, teniposide, theophylline, thiamine, thiopental, thiotepa, ticarcillin, ticarcillin-clavulanate, tigecycline, tirofiban, TNA, tobramycin, tolazoline, TPN, trastuzumab, trimetaphan, urokinase, vancomycin, vasopressin, vecuronium, verapamil, vinCRIStine, vinorelbine, vitamin B complex/C, voriconazole, zoledronic acid

SIDE EFFECTS

CNS: Dizziness, delirium, euphoria, sedation, confusion, weakness, dizziness, seizures

CV: Bradycardia, arrest, hypo/hypertension, DVT, PE

EENT: Blurred vision, miosis

GI: Nausea, vomiting, constipation

GU: Urinary retention

INTEG: Rash, diaphoresis

MS: Muscle rigidity

RESP: Respiratory depression, arrest, laryngospasm

PHARMACOKINETICS

Metabolized by liver, excreted by kidneys, crosses placenta, excreted in breast milk; half-life: IV, 2-4 hr; transdermal, 13-22 hr; transmucosal, 7 hr; buccal, 4-12 hr; 80% bound to plasma proteins

IM: Onset 7-15 min, peak 30 min, duration 1-2 hr

IV: Onset 1 min, peak 3-5 min, duration $^1/_2$-1 hr

Intranasal: Onset 15-20 min, peak 25-30 min

Transdermal: Onset 12-24 hr, peak 1-3 days

Transmucosal: Onset 5-15 min, peak 30 min

INTERACTIONS

Black Box Warning: **Increase:** fentaNYL effect, fetal respiratory depression: CYP3A4 inhibitors (cycloSPORINE, ketoconazole, itraconazole, cimetidine, conivaptan, fluconazole, nefazodone, ranolazine), zafirlukast, zileuton

Increase: fatal reactions—MAOIs

Increase: hypotension—droperidol

Increase: CV depression—diazepam

Increase: fentaNYL effect with other CNS depressants—alcohol, opioids, sedative/hypnotics, antipsychotics, skeletal muscle relaxants, protease inhibitors

Decrease: fentaNYL effect—CYP3A4 inducers (carBAMazepine, phenytoin, PHENobarbital, rifampin)

Drug/Herb

Increase: action of fentaNYL—St. John's wort

Decrease: effect of fentaNYL—echinacea

Drug/Lab Test

Increase: amylase, lipase

NURSING CONSIDERATIONS

Assess:

• VS after parenteral route; note muscle rigidity, drug history, hepatic/renal function tests

• CNS changes: dizziness, drowsiness, hallucinations, euphoria, LOC, pupil reaction

• Allergic reactions: rash, urticaria

Black Box Warning: **Respiratory dysfunction:** respiratory depression, character, rate, rhythm; notify prescriber if respirations are <10/min

Black Box Warning: **Headache/migraine:** ABSTRAL, Actiq, Fentora, Lazanda not to be used for this condition; ABSTRAL, Lazanda not to be used in ER; Duragesic TD not to be used for outpatient surgery patients

Black Box Warning: **Apnea, respiratory arrest in opioid-naive patients:** do not use ABSTRAL, Actiq, Duragesic, Fentora, Lazanda; opioid-tolerant patients are those using ≥60 mg/day oral morphine, ≥30 mg/day oxyCODONE PO, 8 mg/day HYDROmorphone, 25 mcg TD fentaNYL/hr

Black Box Warning: **Pregnancy/breastfeeding:** no well-controlled studies; use only if benefits outweigh fetal risk; if used for prolonged periods, neonatal withdrawal syndrome may occur; discontinue breastfeeding or product, excreted in breast milk

• **Beers:** avoid in older adults unless safer alternative is unavailable; may cause ataxia, impaired psychomotor function

Evaluate:

• Therapeutic response: induction of anesthesia, relief of breakthrough cancer pain, general pain relief

Teach patient/family:

• About CNS changes: physical dependence; not to use with alcohol, other CNS depressants

Black Box Warning: **Accidental exposure:** discuss the danger of children or pets ingesting or coming in contact with product

Transdermal route

Black Box Warning: **Ambient temperature:** that excessive heat may increase absorption; do not use with heating pads, electric blankets, heat/tanning lamps, saunas, hot tubs, heated waterbeds, when sunbathing, never cut patch in half

• That excessive perspiration may alter adhesiveness

• To dispose of patch by placing sticky sides together and flushing down toilet

• That patient may need to clip hair before applying to ensure adhesion

• May add first aid tape around the edges if there is a problem with adhesion, always remove old patch before applying new patch

---

RARELY USED

ferric carboxymaltose
(fer′ik car-box-ee-mal′tose)
Injectafer

USES: Iron-deficiency anemia in those intolerant of other iron supplements or those who have had poor results with other supplements

CONTRAINDICATIONS: Hypersensitivity, iron overload

DOSAGE AND ROUTES

• **Adults ≥50 kg: IV** Give 2 doses of 750 mg/dose separated by ≥7 days, max 1500 mg of iron per course; may repeat if iron-deficiency anemia recurs

• **Adults <50 kg: IV** Give 2 doses of 15 mg/kg/dose separated by ≥7 days, max 1500 mg of iron per course; may repeat if iron-deficiency anemia recurs

---

ferrous fumarate (Rx)
Femiron, Feostat, Ferrate, Ferretts, Ferrocite Hemocyte, Palafer ♣
ferrous gluconate (Rx)
Fergon
ferrous sulfate (Rx)
Feosol, Fer-Gen-Sol, Fer-In-Sol, FeroSul, Slow Fe ♣
ferrous sulfate, dried (Rx)
Feosol, Feratab, Slow Fe, slow-release Iron
carbonyl iron (otc)
(kar′bo-nil)
ICAR Pediatric, Iron Chews
iron polysaccharide (otc)
iFerex, Niferex, Nu-Iron
Func. class.: Hematinic
Chem. class.: Iron preparation

ACTION: Replaces iron stores needed for red blood cell development as well as energy and O_2 transport and use; fumarate contains 33% elemental iron; gluconate, 12%; sulfate, 20%; iron, 30%; ferrous sulfate exsiccated

USES: Iron-deficiency anemia, prophylaxis for iron deficiency in pregnancy, nutritional supplementation

CONTRAINDICATIONS: Sideroblastic anemia, thalassemia, hemosiderosis/hemochromatosis

---

Side effects: *italics* = common; red = life-threatening

Precautions: Pregnancy, anemia (long term), ulcerative colitis/regional enteritis, peptic ulcer disease, hemolytic anemia, cirrhosis, sulfite sensitivity

> **Black Box Warning:** Accidental exposure

DOSAGE AND ROUTES
Fumarate
• **Adult:** PO 200-325 mg tid
• **Child:** PO 3 mg/kg/day (elemental iron) tid-qid
• **Infant:** PO 10-25 mg/day (elemental iron) in 3-4 divided doses, max 15 mg/day
Gluconate
• **Adult:** PO 50-100 mg elemental iron tid
• **Child:** PO 3 mg/kg/day in divided doses
Sulfate
• **Adult:** PO 0.75-1.5 g/day in divided doses tid
• **Child 6-12 yr:** PO 3 mg/kg/day in divided doses
Pregnancy
• **Adult:** PO 300-600 mg/day in divided doses
Iron polysaccharide
• **Adult:** PO 100-200 mg tid
• **Child:** PO 4-6 mg/kg/day in 3 divided doses (severe iron deficiency)
Available forms: Fumarate: tabs 90, 150, 200, 300, 324, 325 mg; chewable tabs 100 mg; ext rel tabs 18 mg; **gluconate:** tabs 225, 240, 324, 325 mg; **sulfate:** tabs 195, 300, 325 mg; elixir 220 mg/5 mL; **dried:** tabs 200 mg; ext rel tabs 160 mg; ext rel caps 160 mg; **iron polysaccharide:** tabs 50 mg; caps 150 mg; sol 100 mg/5 mL
Administer:
PO route
• Swallow tabs whole; do not break, crush, or chew unless labeled as chewable
• Between meals for best absorption; may give with juice; do not give with antacids or milk, delay at least 1 hr; if GI symptoms occur, give after meals even if absorption is decreased; eggs, milk products, chocolate, caffeine interfere with absorption
• Store in tight, light-resistant container

• **Liquid** through plastic straw to avoid discoloration of tooth enamel; dilute thoroughly
• At least 1 hr before bedtime; corrosion may occur in stomach; ferrous gluconate is less irritating to GI tract than ferrous sulfate
• For <6 mo for anemia

SIDE EFFECTS
GI: *Nausea, constipation, epigastric pain, black and red tarry stools,* vomiting, diarrhea
INTEG: Temporarily discolored tooth enamel and eyes

PHARMACOKINETICS
PO: Excreted in feces, urine, skin, breast milk; enters bloodstream; bound to transferrin; crosses placenta

INTERACTIONS
Increase: action of iron preparation—ascorbic acid, chloramphenicol
Decrease: absorption of penicillamine, levodopa, methyldopa, fluoroquinolones, L-thyroxine, tetracycline
Decrease: absorption of iron preparations—antacids, H_2-antagonists, proton pump inhibitors, cholestyramine, vit E
Drug/Food
Decrease: absorption—dairy products, caffeine, eggs
Drug/Lab Test
False positive: occult blood

NURSING CONSIDERATIONS
Assess:
• Blood studies: Hct, Hgb, reticulocytes, bilirubin before treatment, at least monthly; iron studies (iron, TIBC, ferritin); avoid use with blood transfusions, iron overload may occur
• **Toxicity:** nausea, vomiting, diarrhea (green then tarry stools), hematemesis, pallor, cyanosis, shock, coma
• Elimination: if constipation occurs, increase water, bulk, activity
• **Nutrition:** amount of iron in diet (meat, dark green leafy vegetables, dried beans, dried fruits, eggs)
• Cause of iron loss or anemia, including salicylates, sulfonamides, antimalarials, quiNIDine

• **Pregnancy/breastfeeding:** no well-controlled studies; use only if benefits outweigh fetal risk; excreted in breast milk

Evaluate:

• Therapeutic response: improvement in Hct, Hgb, reticulocytes; decreased fatigue, weakness

Teach patient/family:

• That iron will turn stools black or dark green, stain teeth

• **Accidental exposure:** to keep out of reach of children, pets; iron poisoning may occur if increased beyond recommended level

• Not to substitute 1 iron salt for another; that elemental iron content differs (e.g., 300 mg ferrous fumarate contains about 100 mg elemental iron; 300 mg ferrous gluconate contains only about 30 mg elemental iron)

• To avoid reclining position for 15-30 min after taking product to avoid esophageal corrosion

• To follow a diet high in iron; to avoid taking iron, dairy products, calcium supplements, and vit C together because they compete for absorption

TREATMENT OF OVERDOSE: Induce vomiting; give eggs, milk until lavage can be done

---

fesoterodine (Rx)

(fess'oh-ter-oh-deen)

Toviaz

Func. class.: Overactive bladder product

Chem. class.: Muscarinic receptor antagonist

ACTION: Relaxes smooth muscles in urinary tract by inhibiting acetylcholine at postganglionic sites

USES: Overactive bladder (urinary frequency, urgency), urinary incontinence

CONTRAINDICATIONS: GI obstruction, ileus, pyloric stenosis, urinary retention, gastric retention, hypersensitivity, closed-angle glaucoma

Precautions: Pregnancy, breastfeeding, children, renal/hepatic disease, urinary tract obstruction, ambient temperature increase, autonomic neuropathy, constipation, contact lenses, hazardous activity, GERD, gastroparesis, myasthenia gravis, prostatic hypertrophy, toxic megacolon, ulcerative colitis, possible cross-sensitivity with tolterodine

DOSAGE AND ROUTES

• **Adult and geriatric:** PO EXT REL 4 mg/day, may increase to 8 mg/day, max 4 mg/day in those taking potent CYP3A4 inhibitors

Renal dose

• **Adult:** PO EXT REL CCr <30 mL/min, max 4 mg/day

Available forms: EXT REL TABS 4, 8 mg

Administer:

• Do not break, crush, or chew ext rel product

• Give without regard to meals

• Store at room temperature; protect from moisture

SIDE EFFECTS

CNS: Insomnia, headache, dizziness

CV: Chest pain, angina, QT prolongation, peripheral edema

EENT: Xerophthalmia

GI: *Nausea, vomiting,* abdominal pain, constipation, dry mouth

GU: Dysuria, urinary retention, UTI

INTEG: Rash, angioedema

MISC: Peripheral edema, insomnia

MS: Back pain

RESP: Cough, URI

SYST: Infection

PHARMACOKINETICS

Peak 5 hr, duration up to 24 hr, rapidly absorbed, protein binding 50%, excreted in urine/feces, half-life 7 hr ✖ metabolized by the liver (CYP2D6, CYP3A4 converted to active metabolite)

INTERACTIONS

Increase: action of fesoterodine—CYP3A4 inhibitors (antiretroviral protease inhibitors, macrolide antiinfectives, azole antifungals), avoid use with doses >4 mg

---

Side effects: *italics* = common; red = life-threatening

Increase: anticholinergic effect—antimuscarinics, anticholinergics
Drug/Herb
Decrease: fesoterodine—caffeine, green tea, guarana
Drug/Lab
Increase: ALT

NURSING CONSIDERATIONS
Assess:
• **Urinary patterns:** distention, nocturia, frequency, urgency, incontinence
• **Allergic reactions:** angioedema; swelling of face, tongue, throat may occur anytime during treatment; have emergency equipment nearby
• **Pregnancy/breastfeeding:** no well-controlled studies; use only if benefits outweigh fetal risk
Evaluate:
• Therapeutic response: absence of urinary frequency, urgency, incontinence
Teach patient/family:
• To avoid increased temperature
• Not to drive or operate machinery until response is known
• To avoid alcohol; drowsiness may occur
• To report immediately allergic reactions including rash, swelling of mouth, face, lips, trouble breathing
• Not to drink liquids before bedtime
• About the importance of bladder maintenance
• Not to use new medications, herbs without prescriber approval

---

fexofenadine (Rx, OTC)
(fex-oh-fi′na-deen)
Allegra, Children's Allegra Allergy, Children's Allegra Hives, Mucinex Allergy
Func. class.: Antihistamine—2nd generation
Chem. class.: Piperidine, peripherally selective

Do not confuse:
Allegra/Viagra

ACTION: Acts on blood vessels, GI, respiratory system by competing with histamine for H$_1$-receptor site; decreases allergic response by blocking pharmacologic effects of histamine, less sedating

USES: Rhinitis, allergy symptoms, chronic idiopathic urticaria

CONTRAINDICATIONS: Breastfeeding, newborn or premature infants, hypersensitivity
Precautions: Pregnancy, children, geriatric patients, respiratory disease, closed-angle glaucoma, prostatic hypertrophy, bladder neck obstruction, asthma, renal failure

DOSAGE AND ROUTES
• **Adult and child >12 yr: PO** 60 mg bid or 180 mg/day
• **Child 2-11 yr: PO** 30 mg bid
• **Child 6-11 yr:** Child 6 mo-2 yr: PO 15 mg bid
Renal dose
• **Adult and child ≥12 yr: PO** CCr <80 mL/min, 60 mg/day initial
• **Child 2-11 yr: PO** CCr <80 mL/min, 30 mg daily
Available forms: Tabs 30, 60, 180 mg; oral susp 6 mg/mL, orally disintegrating tab 30 mg
Administer:
• Without regard to meals; caps/tabs should not be given with or right before grapefruit, orange, or apple juice
Store in tight, light-resistant container
• **Orally disintegrating tab:** allow to dissolve, swallow; do not remove from blister pack until time of administration
• **Oral susp:** shake well; use calibrated measuring device

SIDE EFFECTS
CNS: Headache, stimulation, drowsiness, sedation, fatigue, confusion, blurred vision, tinnitus, restlessness, tremors, paradoxical excitation in children or geriatric patients

---

PHARMACOKINETICS
Well absorbed; onset 1 hr; peak 2-3 hr; duration 12-24 hr; 80% excreted in urine; feces 11% half-life 14.5 hr, increased in renal disease

INTERACTIONS
Increase: fexofenadine effect—erythromycin, ketoconazole
Decrease: effect—magnesium-aluminum–containing antacids
Drug/Food
Decrease: absorption of product—apple, orange, grapefruit juice
Drug/Lab Test
False negative: skin allergy tests

NURSING CONSIDERATIONS
Assess:
• **Allergy:** itchy, runny, watery eyes; congested nose; before and during treatment
• Bronchial secretions, lung sounds; increase fluids to 2000 mL/day unless contraindicated to decrease thickness of secretions
• **Pregnancy/breastfeeding:** no well-controlled studies; use only if benefits outweigh fetal risk
Evaluate:
• Therapeutic response: absence of running or congested nose or rashes
Teach patient/family:
• About all aspects of product use; to notify prescriber if confusion, sedation, hypotension occur
• To avoid driving, other hazardous activity if drowsiness occurs
• To avoid alcohol, other CNS depressants
• To take with water; avoid fruit juices as they may decrease effectiveness

TREATMENT OF OVERDOSE:
Lavage, diazepam, vasopressors, IV phenytoin

---

fidaxomicin
(fye-dax′oh-mye′sin)
Dificid
Func. class.: Antiinfective-macrolide

ACTION: Bactericidal against *Clostridium difficile;* is a fermentation product obtained from *Dactylosporangium aurantiacum;* inhibits RNA synthesis by inhibiting transcription of bacterial RNA polymerases; may act at the early stages of transcription

USES: Pseudomembranous colitis, *Clostridium difficile*–associated diarrhea

CONTRAINDICATIONS: Hypersensitivity
Precautions: Pregnancy, breastfeeding, children

DOSAGE AND ROUTES
• **Adult: PO** 200 mg bid × 10 days
Available forms: Tab 200 mg
Administer:
• Without regard to food
• Store at room temperature

SIDE EFFECTS
GI: Nausea, vomiting, abdominal pain, GI bleeding, intestinal obstruction
HEMA: Anemia, neutropenia
INTEG: Rash, pruritus
META: Metabolic acidosis, hyperglycemia

PHARMACOKINETICS
Half-life 12 hr, onset <1 hr, peak 1-5 hr, excreted in feces 92%, minimal absorption, substrate of PGP efflux transporter

INTERACTIONS
Drug/Lab Test
Increase: glucose, LFTs, alk phos
Decrease: sodium bicarbonate, platelets

NURSING CONSIDERATIONS
Assess:
• **Pseudomembranous colitis:** for diarrhea, abdominal pain, fever, fatigue, anorexia, anemia, elevated WBC and low serum albumin; product may be used in place of vancomycin (PO); monitor CBC with differential and stool culture (*Clostridium difficile*), not to be used for systemic infection; obtain C&S before use; monitor glucose (diabetic patients); monitor fluid, electrolyte depletion
• **Hypersensitivity:** rash, pruritus; angioedema (rare)

Side effects: *italics* = common; red = life-threatening

• **Pregnancy/breastfeeding:** no well-controlled studies; use only if clearly needed; cautious use in breastfeeding, excretion unknown

Evaluate:

• Positive therapeutic response: resolution of *Clostridium difficile*, decreased diarrhea

Teach patient/family:

• To report GI bleeding, severe abdominal pain

• To notify if pregnancy is planned or suspected or if breastfeeding

• To take as directed; must take all of medication

• May take without regard to food

⚠ HIGH ALERT

filgrastim (Rx)

(fill-grass'stim)

Granix, Grastofil ✦,
Grastofil ✦, Neupogen, Zarxio

Func. class.: Biologic modifier
Chem. class.: Granulocyte colony-stimulating factor

Do not confuse:
Neupogen/Neumea

ACTION: Stimulates proliferation and differentiation of neutrophils

USES: To decrease infection in patients receiving antineoplastics that are myelosuppressive; to increase WBC in patients with product-induced neutropenia; bone marrow transplantation, acute radiation exposure

Unlabeled uses: Neutropenia with HIV infection, aplastic anemia, ganciclovir-induced neutropenia, zidovudine-induced neutropenia

CONTRAINDICATIONS: Hypersensitivity to proteins of *Escherichia coli*

Precautions: Pregnancy, breastfeeding, children, myeloid malignancies, radiation therapy, sepsis, sickle cell disease, chemotherapy, respiratory disease

DOSAGE AND ROUTES

After myelosuppressive chemotherapy

• **Adult and child: IV/SUBCUT** 5 mcg/kg/day in a single dose × up to 14 days; may increase by 5 mcg/kg with each cycle

After myelosuppressive doses of radiation

• **Adult and child >7 mo: SUBCUT** 10 mcg/kg/day, start as soon as possible after receiving ≥2 Gy

After bone marrow transplantation

• **Adult: IV/SUBCUT** 10 mcg/kg/day as **INFUSION (IV)** over 4 hr or 24 hr; begin 24 hr after chemotherapy and 24 hr after bone marrow transplantation

Peripheral blood progenitor cell collection/therapy

• **Adult:** 10 mcg/kg/day as bolus or **CONT INFUSION** × ≥4 days before leukapheresis, continue to last leukapheresis; may alter dose if WBC >100,000 cells/mm^3

Severe neutropenia (chronic), idiopathic/cyclical

• **Adult: SUBCUT** 5 mcg/kg daily

Neonatal neutropenia

• **Neonate: IV/SUBCUT** 5-10 mcg/kg/day × 3-5 days

Available forms: Inj 300 mcg/mL, 480 mcg/1.6 mL, 480 mcg/0.8 mL

Administer:

• Given by subcut inj, short IV infusion, or continuous SC or IV infusion

• Avoid use within 24 hr before or after chemotherapy

• Do not shake commercial single-dose vials before withdrawing the dose; if the vial is shaken and froth or bubbles form, allow the vial to stand undisturbed for a few minutes until the froth or bubbles dissipate

• Before injection, filgrastim may be allowed to reach room temperature for a maximum of 24 hr; any vial or syringe exposed to room temperature for more than 24 hr should be discarded

• Visually inspect for particulate matter and discoloration before use

• Store in refrigerator; do not freeze; may store at room temperature up to 24 hr

SUBCUT route
• **Subcut inj:** no dilution is necessary; inject by rapid subcut inj, taking care not to inject intradermally; inject into abdomen, upper outer buttock, upper outer arms, rotate sites
• **Subcut continuous infusion:** infuse subcut at a rate not to exceed 2 mL/hr

IV route
• May be diluted with 5% dextrose; do not dilute with NS; product can precipitate
• May be diluted to concentrations 5-15 mcg/mL; should be protected from adsorption to plastic by the addition of albumin to a final albumin concentration of 2 mg/mL; do not dilute filgrastim to a concentration <5 mcg/mL
• **IV infusion:** infuse IV over 15-30 min or as a continuous infusion over 24 hr

Y-site compatibilities: Acyclovir, allopurinol, amikacin, aminophylline, ampicillin, ampicillin/sulbactam, aztreonam, bleomycin, bumetanide, buprenorphine, butorphanol, calcium gluconate, CARBOplatin, carmustine, ceFAZolin, cefoTEtan, cefTAZidime, chlorproMAZINE, cimetidine, CISplatin, cyclophosphamide, cytarabine, dacarbazine, DAUNOrubicin, dexamethasone, diphenhydrAMINE, DOXOrubicin, doxycycline, droperidol, enalaprilat, famotidine, floxuridine, fluconazole, fludarabine, gallium, ganciclovir, granisetron, haloperidol, hydrocortisone, HYDROmorphone, hydrOXYzine, IDArubicin, ifosfamide, leucovorin, LORazepam, mechlorethamine, melphalan, meperidine, mesna, methotrexate, metoclopramide, miconazole, minocycline, mitoXANtrone, morphine, nalbuphine, netilmicin, ondansetron, plicamycin, potassium chloride, promethazine, ranitidine, sodium bicarbonate, streptozocin, ticarcillin, ticarcillin/clavulanate, tobramycin, trimethoprim-sulfamethoxazole, vancomycin, vinBLAStine, vinCRIStine, vinorelbine, zidovudine

SIDE EFFECTS
CNS: Fever, headache
GI: *Nausea*, vomiting, diarrhea, mucositis, anorexia, splenic rupture

HEMA: Thrombocytopenia, excessive leukocytosis
INTEG: Alopecia, exacerbation of skin conditions, urticaria, cutaneous vasculitis, allergic reactions
MS: Osteoporosis, skeletal pain
OTHER: Chest pain, hypotension
RESP: Acute respiratory distress syndrome, wheezing, alveolar hemorrhage

PHARMACOKINETICS
SUBCUT: Onset 5-60 min, peak 2-8 hr, duration up to 1 wk
IV: Onset 5-60 min, peak 24 hr, duration up to 1 wk

INTERACTIONS
Increase: adverse reactions—do not use this product concomitantly with antineoplastics, lithium
Drug/Lab Test
Increase: uric acid, LDH, alk phos, WBC

NURSING CONSIDERATIONS
Assess:
• Blood studies: CBC, platelet count before treatment and twice weekly; neutrophil counts drop by 50% if filgrastim is discontinued the next day
• B/P, respirations, pulse before and during therapy
• Bone pain; give mild analgesics
• **Respiratory distress syndrome:** fever, dyspnea; withhold product if these occur
• **Allergic reactions:** rash, wheezing, facial edema, dyspnea; may occur within 30 min of use; give antihistamines, bronchodilators, and EPINEPHrine if needed
• **Splenic rupture:** severe left upper abdominal pain
• **Pregnancy/breastfeeding:** may cause fetal harm; if used in pregnancy, enroll in Amgen's Surveillance Program, 1-800-772-6436
Evaluate:
• Therapeutic response: absence of infection
Teach patient/family:
• About the technique for self-administration: dose, side effects, disposal of containers and needles; provide instruction sheet
• That bone pain is common

Side effects: *italics* = common; red = life-threatening

finasteride (Rx)

(fin-ass′te-ride)

Propecia, Proscar

Func. class.: Hormone, androgen inhibitor, hair stimulant

Chem. class.: 5-α-Reductase inhibitor

Do not confuse:

finasteride/furosemide

Proscar/ProSom/PROzac

ACTION: Inhibits 5-α-reductase and reduction in DHT; DHT induces androgenic effects by binding to androgen receptors in the cell nuclei of the prostate gland, liver, skin; prevents development of BHP

USES: Symptomatic benign prostatic hyperplasia (Proscar); male-pattern baldness (Propecia)

Unlabeled uses: Hirsutism, prostate cancer prophylaxis

CONTRAINDICATIONS: Pregnancy, breastfeeding, children, women who are pregnant or who may become pregnant should not handle tabs, hypersensitivity

Precautions: Large residual urinary volume, severely diminished urinary flow, hepatic function abnormalities

DOSAGE AND ROUTES

BPH

• **Adult: PO** 5 mg/day × 6-12 mo (Proscar)

Male-pattern baldness

• **Adult: PO** 1 mg/day for 3 mo or more for results (Propecia)

Hirsutism (unlabeled)

• **Adult (nonpregnant): PO** 5 mg/day alone or in combination with oral contraceptives

Available forms: Tabs (Propecia) 1 mg, (Proscar) 5 mg

Administer:

• Without regard to meals

• For a minimum of 6 mo; not all patients will respond

• Store <86° F (30° C); protect from light; keep container tightly closed

SIDE EFFECTS

GU: Impotence, decreased libido, decreased volume of ejaculate, sexual dysfunction, gynecomastia

INTEG: Rash

MISC: Breast tenderness, secondary malignancy

PHARMACOKINETICS

Bioavailability 63%; readily absorbed from GI tract; protein binding 90%; metabolized in the liver; excreted in urine (metabolites) 39%, feces (57%); crosses blood-brain barrier; peak 1-2 hr; duration 24 hr

INTERACTIONS

Drug/Lab Test

Decrease: PSA levels

NURSING CONSIDERATIONS

Assess:

• **BPH:** urinary patterns, residual urinary volume, severely diminished urinary flow

• PSA levels and exclusion of prostate/urinary cancer before initiating therapy and periodically thereafter; PSA levels may be altered by this product

• Hepatic studies before treatment; extensively metabolized in liver

• **Pregnancy/breastfeeding:** not to be used in females; do not use in pregnancy/breastfeeding

Evaluate:

• Therapeutic response: increased urinary flow; decreased postvoiding dribbling, frequency, nocturia; hair growth within 3-6 mo; regression of prostate size

Teach patient/family:

• That pregnant women or women who may become pregnant should not touch crushed tabs or come into contact with the semen of a patient taking this product; that product may adversely affect developing male fetus

• That volume of ejaculate may be decreased during treatment; that impotence and decreased libido may also occur and may continue after discontinuing treatment

• That Propecia results may not occur for 3 mo

• That Proscar results may not occur for 6-12 mo

fingolimod (Rx)

(fin-gol'i-mod) (fin-go'li-mod)

Gilenya

Func. class.: Immunosuppressant
Chem. class.: Sphingosine 1-phosphate receptor modulator

ACTION: Binds with high affinity to sphingosine 1-phosphate receptors; blocks lymphocyte egress to lymph nodes, thereby reducing the number of peripheral blood lymphocytes; may reduce lymphocyte migration into the CNS

USES: To reduce frequency of exacerbation, to delay physical disability of relapsing forms of MS

CONTRAINDICATIONS: Hypersensitivity

Precautions: Pregnancy, breastfeeding, neonates/infants/children, AIDS, asthma, AV block, bradycardia, cardiac disease, COPD, diabetes mellitus, dysrhythmias, heart failure, hepatic disease, HIV, hypertension, immunosuppression, leukemia, lymphoma, QT prolongation, respiratory insufficiency, sick sinus syndrome, syncope, uveitis

DOSAGE AND ROUTES

• **Adult: PO** 0.5 mg/day

Hepatic dose

• **Adult:** PO Child-Pugh C, total score >10: closely monitor, fingolimod exposure is doubled

Available forms: Caps 0.5 mg

Administer:

PO route

Watch patient for 6 hr after initial dose or if product not given for >2 wk for development of bradycardia

• Give without regard to food

• Store at room temperature, protect from moisture

SIDE EFFECTS

CNS: Asthenia, depression, fatigue, headache, dizziness, progressive multifocal leukoencephalopathy, migraine, paresthesias, stroke

CV: AV block, bradycardia, chest pain, hypertension, palpitations, QT prolongation

EENT: Blurred vision, vision impairment, ocular pain, macular edema

GI: Abdominal pain, anorexia, diarrhea, jaundice, vomiting, weight loss, hepatotoxicity

HEMA: Leukopenia, lymphopenia, neutropenia

INTEG: Alopecia, pruritus

MS: Back pain

RESP: Dyspnea, cough

SYST: Infection, influenza, secondary malignancy

PHARMACOKINETICS

Protein binding (99.7%), distributed to RBCs (86%), steady state 1-2 mo, metabolized by CYP4F2 and CYP2D6 to a lesser extent, terminal half-life 6-9 days, excreted in urine (81% inactive metabolites), peak 12-16 hr

INTERACTIONS

Increase: risk of heart block, serious bradycardia—β-blockers, calcium channel blockers, digoxin; avoid if possible

Increase: immunosuppression—antineoplastics, immunosuppressants, immune-modulating therapies

Increase: fingolimod effect—ketoconazole

Increase: infection risk—live vaccines

Decrease: effect of—inactive vaccines, toxoids

Increase: risk of torsades de pointes—Class Ia/III antidysrhythmics

NURSING CONSIDERATIONS

Assess:

• **Multiple sclerosis:** improving paresthesia, muscle weakness, clonus, muscle spasms, difficulty with moving, difficulty with coordination of balance, speech, swallowing, vision problems, fatigue; prevention of increasing disability

• **Laboratory monitoring:** obtain before initial dose: CBC, LFTs, serum bilirubin, ophthalmologic exam, antibodies to VZV; if there is no history of chickenpox or no vaccination, may give VZV vaccination to antibody-negative patient before giving product, postpone for 1 mo after vaccination; obtain ECG for evidence of bradycardia, AV block

Side effects: *italics* = common; red = life-threatening

• **Progressive multifocal leukoencephalopathy (PML):** confusion, apathy, dizziness, unstable gait; may be fatal, discontinue product, contact prescriber

• **Bradycardia:** monitor for ≥6 hr after beginning dose, ECG before and after 1st dose, if heart rate <45 bpm or new heart block (2nd degree) occurs, do not use until resolved

• Monitor for QT prolongation

• **Pregnancy/breastfeeding:** use only if benefits outweigh fetal risk, may cause fetal harm; contraception should be used during and for 2 mo after final dose; enroll in Gilenya Pregnancy Registry (1-877-598-7237) if pregnant; discontinue breastfeeding or product, excretion unknown

Evaluate:

• Therapeutic response: improved symptoms of multiple sclerosis and prevention of increasing disability

Teach patient/family:

• About use of product and expected results; provide med guide to patient

• That continuing follow-up exams and laboratory tests will be required on a regular basis

• To use contraception during and for 2 mo after conclusion of treatment

• **Liver dysfunction:** to report jaundice, nausea, vomiting, anorexia, abdominal pain, fatigue, dark urine

• **Cardiac changes:** to report chest pain, palpitations

⚠ HIGH ALERT

flecainide (Rx)

(flek-ay′nide)

Tambocor ✦

Func. class.: Antidysrhythmic (Class IC)

Do not confuse:

Tambocor/Pamelor

ACTION: Decreases conduction in all parts of the heart, with greatest effect on the His-Purkinje system, which stabilizes cardiac membrane

USES: Life-threatening ventricular dysrhythmias, sustained ventricular tachycardia, supraventricular tachydysrhythmias, paroxysmal atrial fibrillation/flutter associated with disabling symptoms

Unlabeled uses: Atrial fibrillation, single dose

CONTRAINDICATIONS: Hypersensitivity, AV bundle branch block, cardiogenic shock

Precautions: Pregnancy, breastfeeding, children, geriatric patients, renal/hepatic disease, HF, respiratory depression, myasthenia gravis, electrolyte abnormalities, atrial fibrillation, sick sinus syndrome, torsades de pointes, MI, bundle branch block, QT prolongation

> **Black Box Warning:** Cardiac arrhythmias, atrial fibrillation, MI

DOSAGE AND ROUTES

PSVT/PAT

• **Adult:** PO 50 mg q12hr; may increase q4days by 50 mg q12hr to desired response, max 300 mg/day

Life-threatening ventricular dysrhythmias

• **Adult:** PO 100 mg q12hr; may increase by 50 mg q12hr q4days, max 400 mg/day

Renal dose

• **Adult:** PO CCr <35 mL/min, 100 mg daily or 50 mg bid initially

Available forms: Tabs 50, 100, 150 mg

Administer:

PO route

• Reduced dosage as soon as dysrhythmia is controlled

• May give with meals for GI upset

• May adjust dose q4days

• Therapeutic trough serum concentrations for adults range from 200 to 1000 ng/mL (average, 500 ng/mL); toxicity is more common with trough serum concentrations >1000 ng/mL; usual therapeutic range in children is 200-500 ng/mL; in some cases, up to 800 ng/mL is required

• Adjust dosage at intervals of ≥4 days (approximate plateau effects); however, longer intervals are needed in patients with renal or hepatic impairment

• Frequent serum drug concentration monitoring is required for patients with severe renal (CrCl <35 mL/min) or hepatic disease and may also be helpful in patients with HF or in patients with moderate renal disease

• Monitoring of flecainide serum concentrations is strongly recommended in patients receiving amiodarone therapy

SIDE EFFECTS

CNS: *Headache, dizziness,* involuntary movement, confusion, psychosis, restlessness, irritability, paresthesias, ataxia, flushing, somnolence, depression, anxiety, malaise, fatigue, asthenia, tremors

CV: *Hypotension, bradycardia,* angina, PVCs, heart block, cardiovascular collapse, arrest, dysrhythmias, HF, fatal ventricular tachycardia, palpitations, QT prolongation, torsades de pointes

EENT: Tinnitus, *blurred vision,* hearing loss, corneal deposits, dry eyes

GI: Nausea, vomiting, anorexia, constipation, abdominal pain, flatulence, change in taste, diarrhea

GU: Impotence, decreased libido, polyuria, urinary retention

HEMA: Leukopenia, thrombocytopenia

INTEG: Rash, urticaria, edema, swelling

RESP: Dyspnea, respiratory depression

PHARMACOKINETICS

Peak 3 hr, half-life 12-27 hr, metabolized by liver, excreted unchanged by kidneys (10%), excreted in breast milk

INTERACTIONS

Increase: QT prolongation—class IA/III antidysrhythmics, some phenothiazines, β-agonists, local anesthetics, tricyclics, haloperidol, chloroquine, droperidol, pentamidine; CYP3A4 inhibitors (amiodarone, clarithromycin, erythromycin, telithromycin, troleandomycin); arsenic trioxide, levomethadyl; CYP3A4 substrates (methadone, pimozide, QUEtiapine, quiNIDine, risperiDONE, ziprasidone)

Increase: of both products—propranolol

Increase: CV depressant action—β-blockers, disopyramide, verapamil

Increase: flecainide level—amiodarone, cimetidine, ritonavir

Increase: digoxin level—digoxin

Increase or decrease: effect—urinary, alkalinizing agents, acidifying agents

Drug/Herb

• Do not use with hawthorn

Drug/Lab Test

Increase: CPK

NURSING CONSIDERATIONS

Assess:

> **Black Box Warning: HF, cardiogenic shock, LVEF <30%:** should not be used in these conditions

> **Black Box Warning: Atrial fibrillation:** avoid use; risk of ventricular dysrhythmias; use only in life-threatening dysrhythmias

> **Black Box Warning: Cardiac dysrhythmias:** discontinue in those with prolonged QRS >180 ms or prolonged PR >300 ms, monitor for QT prolongation, monitor ECG before and during treatment

• **Electrolyte imbalances:** hypo/hyperkalemia before administration; correct electrolytes before use

• CNS effects: dizziness, confusion, psychosis, paresthesias, seizures; product should be discontinued

• Monitor renal studies: BUN, creatinine

• **Flecainide level:** monitor level in those with HF or renal failure; peak, trough

• **Pregnancy/breastfeeding:** no well-controlled studies; use only if benefits outweigh fetal risk; discontinue breastfeeding or product, excreted in breast milk

Evaluate:

• Therapeutic response: decreased dysrhythmias

Teach patient/family:

• To change position slowly from lying or sitting to standing to minimize orthostatic hypotension

---

Side effects: *italics* = common; red = life-threatening

• To take as prescribed; not to skip or double dose, to take missed dose as soon as remembered within 6 hr of next dose
• To avoid hazardous activities that require alertness until response is known
• To carry emergency ID with disorder, medications taken
• To notify all health care providers of treatment, that follow-up will be needed
• To report new or worsening cardiac symptoms (chest pain, trouble breathing, sweating)

TREATMENT OF OVERDOSE: O_2, artificial ventilation, ECG, DOPamine for circulatory depression, diazepam or thiopental for seizures, treat ventricular dysrhythmias

---

fluconazole (Rx)
(floo-kon′a-zole)
Canesoral ✤, Diflucan One,
Diflucan Monicure ✤
Func. class.: Antifungal, systemic; azole

Do not confuse:
Diflucan/Diprivan

ACTION: Inhibits ergosterol biosynthesis, causes direct damage to fungal membrane phospholipids

USES: Oropharyngeal candidiasis, chronic mucocutaneous candidiasis; systemic, vaginal, urinary candidiasis; cryptococcal meningitis; prevention of candidiasis in bone marrow transplant in those who receive chemotherapy and/or radiation therapy; cystitis, fungal prophylaxis, peritonitis, pneumonia, pyelonephritis
Unlabeled uses: Prophylaxis, systemic candidiasis in very-low-birthweight premature infants, blastomycosis, chemotherapy-induced neutropenia, coccidioidomycosis cryptococcosis prophylaxis, endocarditis, endophthalmitis, histoplasmosis, infectious arthritis, myocarditis, osteomyelitis, pericarditis

CONTRAINDICATIONS: Hypersensitivity to this product or azoles, pregnancy

Precautions: Breastfeeding, renal/hepatic disease, torsades de pointes

DOSAGE AND ROUTES
Vulvovaginal candidiasis
• **Adult: PO** 150 mg as a single dose; **prevention of recurrence (unlabeled)** 150 mg/day × 3 days, then weekly × 6 mo
Serious fungal infections
• **Adult: PO/IV** 50-400 mg initially, then 200-800 mg/day for 4 wk
• **Child: PO/IV** 6-12 mg/kg/day
• **Neonates <14 days, 30-36 wk gestation: PO/IV** same as child except q48hr
Oropharyngeal candidiasis
• **Adult: PO/IV** 200 mg initially, then 100 mg/day for ≥2 wk
• **Child >14 days: PO/IV** 6 mg/kg initially, then 3 mg/kg/day for ≥2 wk
• **Neonate <14 days, 30-36 wk gestation: PO/IV** 6 mg/kg/dose once, then 3 mg/kg/dose once daily
Esophageal candidiasis
• **Adult: PO/IV** 200 mg on 1st day, then 100 mg daily × ≥3 wk and for ≥2 wk after resolution of symptoms
• **Child >14 days: PO/IV** 6 mg/kg on 1st day, then 3 mg/kg × ≥3 wk and for ≥2 wk after resolution of symptoms
• **Neonate: PO/IV** 6 mg/kg q 24-48hr
Cryptococcal meningitis
• **Adult: PO/IV** 400 mg on 1st day, then 200 mg/day × 10-12 wk after CSF culture negative, suppressive therapy 200 mg/day
• **Child/infant/neonate ≥14 days: PO/IV** 12 mg/kg on 1st day, then 6-12 mg/kg daily × 10-12 wk after CSF culture negative, max 600 mg/day, suppressive therapy 6 mg/kg/day
• **Neonate 0-14 days: PO/IV** 12 mg/kg on 1st day, then 6-12 mg/kg q72hr × 10-12 wk after CSF culture negative
Prevention of candidiasis in bone marrow transplant
• **Adult: PO/IV** 400 mg/day, those anticipated to have neutrophils <500/mm³, start several days before anticipated onset of neutropenia and continue for 7 days after rise of neutrophils >1000/mm³

- **Child >14 days: PO/IV** 10-12 mg/kg/day, max 600 mg/day

Renal disease

- **Adult: PO/IV** CCr ≤50 mL/min, after loading dose, give 50% of usual dose; hemodialysis give 100% of usual dose after dialysis treatment, give dose as per CCr on non-dialysis days

Available forms: Tabs 50, 100, 150, 200 mg; inj 2 mg/mL; powder for oral susp 10 mg/mL, 40 mg/mL

Administer:

PO route

- Shake oral susp before each use, use within 2 wk

Intermittent IV INFUSION route

- After diluting according to package directions, run at ≤200 mg/hr; do not use plastic containers in connections; check for bag leaks
- Use infusion pump; check for extravasation and necrosis q2hr
- Do not use if cloudy or precipitated
- Do not admix; do not refrigerate
- Store protected from moisture and light; diluted sol stable 24 hr; do not freeze

Y-site compatibilities: Acyclovir, aldesleukin, alfentanil, allopurinol, amifostine, amikacin, aminocaproic acid, aminophylline, amiodarone, anidulafungin, ascorbic acid injection, atenolol, atracurium, atropine, azaTHIOprine, aztreonam, benztropine, bivalirudin, bleomycin, bumetanide, buprenorphine, butorphanol, calcium chloride, CARBOplatin, caspofungin, ceFAZolin, cefepime, cefmetazole, cefonicid, cefoTEtan, cefOXitin, cefpirome, cefTAZidime, ceftizoxime, ceftobiprole, cephalothin, cephapirin, chlorproMAZINE, cimetidine, cisatracurium, CISplatin, codeine, cyanocobalamin, cyclophosphamide, cycloSPORINE, cytarabine, DACTINomycin, DAPTOmycin, dexamethasone, diltiazem, dimenhyDRINATE, diphenhydrAMINE, DOBUTamine, DOCEtaxel, DOPamine, doripenem, doxacurium, DOXOrubicin, DOXOrubicin liposomal, doxycycline, droperidol, drotrecogin alfa, enalaprilat, ePHEDrine, EPINEPHrine, epirubicin, epoetin alfa, eptifibatide, ertapenem, erythromycin, esmolol, etoposide, famotidine, fenoldopam, fentaNYL, filgrastim, fludarabine, fluorouracil, folic acid, foscarnet, gallium, ganciclovir, gatifloxacin, gemcitabine, gentamicin, glycopyrrolate, granisetron, heparin, hydrocortisone, HYDROmorphone, IDArubicin, ifosfamide, IV immune globulin, inamrinone, indomethacin, insulin (regular), irinotecan, isoproterenol, ketorolac, labetalol, lansoprazole, leucovorin, levofloxacin, lidocaine, linezolid, LORazepam, LR, magnesium sulfate, mannitol, mechlorethamine, melphalan, meperidine, meropenem, metaraminol, methicillin, methotrexate, methoxamine, methyldopate, methylPREDNISolone, metoclopramide, metoprolol, metroNIDAZOLE, mezlocillin, miconazole, midazolam, milrinone, minocycline, mitoXANtrone, morphine, moxalactam, multiple vitamins injection, mycophenolate, nafcillin, nalbuphine, naloxone, nesiritide, nitroglycerin, nitroprusside, norepinephrine, octreotide, ondansetron, oxacillin, oxaliplatin, oxytocin, PACLitaxel, palonosetron, pamidronate, pancuronium, papaverine, PEMEtrexed, penicillin G potassium/sodium, pentazocine, PENTobarbital, PHENobarbital, phenylephrine, phenytoin, phytonadione, piperacillin-tazobactam, polymyxin B, potassium chloride, procainamide, prochlorperazine, promethazine, propofol, propranolol, protamine, pyridoxine, quiNIDine, quinupristin-dalfopristin, ranitidine, remifentanil, Ringer's, ritodrine, riTUXimab, rocuronium, sargramostim, sodium acetate/bicarbonate, succinylcholine, SUFentanil, tacrolimus, temocillin, teniposide, theophylline, thiotepa, ticarcillin-clavulanate, tigecycline, tirofiban, TNA, tobramycin, tolazoline, TPN, trastuzumab, trimetaphan, urokinase, vancomycin, vasopressin, vecuronium, verapamil, vinCRIStine, vinorelbine, voriconazole, zidovudine, zoledronic acid

SIDE EFFECTS

CNS: *Headache,* seizures

CV: QT prolongation, torsades de pointes

GI: *Nausea, vomiting,* diarrhea, cramping, flatus, increased AST, ALT, hepatotoxicity, abdominal pain, cholestasis

HEMA: Agranulocytosis, eosinophilia, leukopenia, neutropenia, thrombocytopenia

INTEG: Stevens-Johnson syndrome, angioedema, anaphylaxis, exfoliative dermatitis, toxic epidermal necrolysis

PHARMACOKINETICS

Peak 1-2 hr, bioavailability (PO) >90%, widely distributed (peritoneum, CSF), excreted in breast milk, excreted unchanged in urine 80%, metabolized by CYP3A enzyme system at dose >200 mg/day, half-life 30 hr (adult); child 19-25 hr (PO); premature neonates (46-74 hr)

INTERACTIONS

Increase: hypoglycemia—oral sulfonylureas (glipiZIDE)

Increase: anticoagulation—warfarin

Increase: plasma concentrations—cycloSPORINE, phenytoin, theophylline, rifabutin, tacrolimus, sirolimus, zidovudine, zolpidem

Increase: myopathy, rhabdomyolysis risk—HMG-CoA reductase inhibitors: lovastatin, simvastatin

Increase: effect of zidovudine, methadone, SUFentanil, alfentanil, buprenorphine, saquinavir, fentaNYL, ergots

Decrease: effect of calcium channel blockers

Decrease: fluconazole effect—proton pump inhibitors

Drug/Lab Test

Increase: alk phos, LFTs

Decrease: WBC, platelets

NURSING CONSIDERATIONS

Assess:

• **Infection:** clearing of CSF and other culture during treatment, obtain C&S baseline and throughout treatment, product may be started as soon as culture is taken

• **QT prolongation:** avoid with other products that cause QT prolongation

• **Hepatotoxicity:** monitor for increasing AST, ALT, baseline and periodically alk phos, bilirubin; for renal status: BUN, creatinine

• **Skin symptoms:** color, lesions, inj-site reactions; if lesions progress, stop product; monitor rash, usually appears after 2nd wk of treatment and disappears in 2 wk if continuing product

• **Pregnancy/breastfeeding:** birth defects may occur if used in 1st trimester; do not use in pregnancy, breastfeeding

Evaluate:

• Therapeutic response: decreasing oral candidiasis, fever, malaise, rash; negative C&S for infection organism

Teach patient/family:

• That long-term therapy may be needed to clear infection, not to add new medications, herbs without prescriber approval

• That medication may be taken with food to reduce GI effects

• To notify prescriber of nausea, vomiting, diarrhea, jaundice, anorexia, clay-colored stools, dark urine, skin rash, abdominal pain, fever, bruising, bleeding

---

⚠ HIGH ALERT

fludarabine (Rx)

(floo-dar'a-been)

Func. class.: Antineoplastic, antimetabolite

USES: Chronic lymphocytic leukemia

CONTRAINDICATIONS: Pregnancy, breastfeeding, hypersensitivity

Black Box Warning: Hemolytic anemia, bone marrow suppression, coma, seizures, visual disturbances

DOSAGE AND ROUTES

• **Adult: IV** 25 mg/m² over 30 min × 5 days, may repeat q28days; reconstitute with 2 mL of sterile water for inj; dissolution should occur in <15 sec, adjust dose based on toxicity; **PO** 40 mg/m² × 5 days q28days

---

RARELY USED

fludrocortisone (Rx)
(floo-droe-kor´ti-sone)
Florinef ✤
Func. class.: Corticosteroid, synthetic
Chem. class.: Mineralocorticoid

USES: Adrenal insufficiency, salt-losing adrenogenital syndrome, Addison's disease
Unlabeled uses: Idiopathic orthostatic hypotension

CONTRAINDICATIONS: Children <2 yr, hypersensitivity

DOSAGE AND ROUTES
Adrenocortical insufficiency
• **Adult: PO** 100-200 mcg/day
• **Child: PO** 50-100 mcg/day
Idiopathic hypotension (unlabeled)
• **Adult: PO** 50-200 mcg/day
Available forms: Tabs 100 mcg (0.1 mg)

flumazenil (Rx)
(flu-maz´e-nill)
Anexate ✤, Romazicon
Func. class.: Antidote: benzodiazepine receptor antagonist
Chem. class.: Imidazobenzodiazepine derivative

Do not confuse:
flumazenil/influenza virus vaccine

ACTION: Antagonizes actions of benzodiazepines on CNS, competitively inhibits activity at benzodiazepine recognition site on GABA/benzodiazepine receptor complex

USES: Reversal of sedative effects of benzodiazepines

CONTRAINDICATIONS: Hypersensitivity to this product or benzodiazepines, serious cyclic antidepressant overdose, patients given benzodiazepine for control of life-threatening conditions
Precautions: Pregnancy, breastfeeding, children, geriatric patients, status epilepticus, head injury, labor/delivery, renal/hepatic disease, hypoventilation, panic disorder, drug and alcohol dependency, ambulatory patients, benzodiazepine dependence

Black Box Warning: Seizures

DOSAGE AND ROUTES
Reversal of conscious sedation or general anesthesia
• **Adult: IV** 0.2 mg given over 15 sec; wait 45 sec, then give 0.2 mg if consciousness does not occur; may be repeated at 60-sec intervals prn (max 3 mg/hr) or 1 mg/5 min
• **Child: IV** 10 mcg (0.01 mg)/kg; cumulative dose of 1 mg or less
Management of suspected benzodiazepine overdose
• **Adult: IV** 0.2 mg given over 30 sec; wait 30 sec, then give 0.3 mg over 30 sec if consciousness does not occur; further doses of 0.5 mg can be given over 30 sec at intervals of 1 min up to cumulative dose of 3 mg
• **Child: IV** 10 mcg (0.01 mg/kg), cumulative dose of <1 mg
Available forms: Inj 0.1 mg/mL
Administer:
• Check airway and IV access before administration
• Use large vein
Direct IV route
• Give undiluted or diluted with 0.9% NaCl, D_5W, LR; give over 15-30 sec into running IV, check for extravasation
• Stable for 24 hr if drawn into a syringe or mixed with other solutions

SIDE EFFECTS
CNS: Dizziness, *agitation*, emotional lability, confusion, seizures, somnolence, panic attacks
CV: Hypertension, *palpitations*, cutaneous vasodilation, dysrhythmias, bradycardia, tachycardia, chest pain

---

Side effects: *italics* = common; red = life-threatening

EENT: Abnormal vision, blurred vision, tinnitus
GI: Nausea, vomiting, hiccups
SYST: Headache, inj site pain, increased sweating, fatigue, rigors

PHARMACOKINETICS

Half-life 41-79 min (adult), 20-75 min (child), metabolized in liver, onset 1-2 min 50% protein binding (albumin)

INTERACTIONS

• Toxicity: mixed product overdosage
• Antagonize action of benzodiazepines, zaleplon, zolpidem

NURSING CONSIDERATIONS
Assess:

• Cardiac and respiratory status using continuous monitoring

Black Box Warning: **Seizures:** protect patient from injury; most likely among those who are withdrawing from benzodiazepines; flumazenil can precipitate benzodiazepine withdrawal and onset of seizures; seizures are increased in head trauma

• GI symptoms: nausea, vomiting; place patient in side-lying position to prevent aspiration
• **Allergic reactions:** flushing, rash, urticaria, pruritus

Black Box Warning: **Seizures/benzodiazepine dependence:** do not use in those who have used these products for status epilepticus; use in intensive care setting cautiously, there may be unrecognized benzodiazepine dependence

• **Pregnancy/breastfeeding:** no well-controlled studies; use only if benefits outweigh fetal risk; discontinue breastfeeding or product
Teach patient/family:
• Not to use with alcohol or other medications for at least 24 hr
• That sedation may occur after treatment
• To avoid hazardous activities, driving until effects are known
• That amnesia may continue

---

flunisolide nasal agent
See Appendix B

---

fluocinolone topical
See Appendix B

---

fluorometholone ophthalmic
See Appendix B

⚠ HIGH ALERT

fluorouracil (Rx)
(flure-oh-yoor'a-sil)
Adrucil, Carac, Efudex, Fluoroplex, Tolak
Func. class.: Antineoplastic, antimetabolite
Chem. class.: Pyrimidine analog

Do not confuse:
Carac/Kuric

ACTION: Inhibits DNA, RNA synthesis; interferes with cell replication by competitively inhibiting thymidylate production, specific for S phase of cell cycle

USES: Systemic: cancer of breast, colon, rectum, stomach, pancreas; **topical:** multiple actinic keratoses, superficial basal cell carcinomas

CONTRAINDICATIONS: Pregnancy, breastfeeding, hypersensitivity, poor nutritional status, serious infections, dihydropyrimidine dehydrogenase deficiency, bone marrow suppression
Precautions: Children, renal/hepatic disease, angina, stomatitis, diarrhea, sunlight exposure, vaccination, occlusive dressing, GI bleeding

Black Box Warning: Requires an experienced clinician and a specialized care setting

---

DOSAGE AND ROUTES

Doses vary widely, based on actual body weight unless obese, then based on lean body weight

Colon, rectal, breast, stomach, pancreatic cancer

• **Adult: IV** 12 mg/kg/day × 4 days (max 800 mg), then 6 mg/kg on days 6, 8, 10, 12 if no toxicity, then 10-15 mg/kg as a single weekly maintenance dose (max 1 g/wk); **Poor-risk patients:** 6 mg/kg/day × 3 days, then 3 mg/kg on days 5, 7, 9 if not toxicity (max 400 mg/day)

Actinic/solar keratoses

• **Adult: TOP (Carac)** 1% cream/sol bid or 2%-5% sol for hands

Superficial basal cell carcinoma

• **Adult: TOP (Efudex)** 5% sol or cream 2×/day × 3-12 wk

Available forms: Inj 50 mg/mL; cream 0.5%, 1%, 4%, 5%; sol 2%, 5%

Administer:

• Antiemetic 30-60 min before product to prevent vomiting, for several days thereafter

Topical route

• The 1% strength is used on face; higher strengths are used on other parts of the body

• Wear gloves when applying; may use with a loose dressing; use plastic or wooden applicator, do not use occlusive dressings, may use gauze dressing

IV route

• Prepared in biologic cabinet using gloves, gown, mask; use cytotoxic handling procedures

• Double-check all dosage amounts, type of product to be used; fatalities have occurred

IV direct

• Undiluted; may inject through Y-tube or 3-way stopcock; give over 1-3 min; may be diluted in NS, D_5W and given as an **intermittent infusion;** use infusion in plastic containers; given over 2-8 hr; do not refrigerate/freeze; protect from light, discard unused portion, stable for 24 hr at room temperature, do not use discolored, cloudy solution; solution is pale yellow; for crystals, dissolve by warming slowly and shaking, let cool to body temperature before use

Y-site compatibilities: Acyclovir, alatrofloxacin, alfentanil, allopurinol, amifostine, amikacin, amphotericin B lipid complex, amphotericin B liposome, ampicillin, ampicillin-sulbactam, anidulafungin, argatroban, atenolol, atracurium, azithromycin, aztreonam, bivalirudin, bleomycin, bumetanide, butorphanol, calcium gluconate, CARBOplatin, ceFAZolin, cefepime, cefotaxime, cefoTEtan, cefOXitin, cefTAZidime, ceftizoxime, cefTRIAxone, cefuroxime, cimetidine, cisatracurium, CISplatin, clindamycin, codeine, cyclophosphamide, cycloSPORINE, DAPTOmycin, dexamethasone, digoxin, DOCEtaxel, DOPamine, doripenem, DOXOrubicin liposomal, enalaprilat, ePHEDrine, ertapenem, erythromycin, esmolol, etoposide phosphate, famotidine, fenoldopam, fentaNYL, fluconazole, fludarabine, foscarnet, fosphenytoin, furosemide, ganciclovir, gatifloxacin, gemcitabine, gentamicin, granisetron, heparin, hydrocortisone, HYDROmorphone, ifosfamide, imipenem-cilastatin, inamrinone, isoproterenol, ketorolac, labetalol, leucovorin, levorphanol, lidocaine, linezolid, magnesium sulfate, mannitol, melphalan, meperidine, meropenem, mesna, methohexital, methotrexate, methylPREDNISolone, metoprolol, metroNIDAZOLE, milrinone, mitoMYcin, mitoXANtrone, morphine sulfate, nalbuphine, naloxone, nesiritide, nitroglycerin, nitroprusside, octreotide, ofloxacin, PACLitaxel, palonosetron, pamidronate, pancuronium, pantoprazole, PEMEtrexed, PENTobarbital, PHENobarbital, phenylephrine, piperacillin, piperacillin-tazobactam, potassium chloride/phosphates, procainamide, propofol, propranolol, ranitidine, remifentanil, riTUXimab, sargramostim, sodium acetate/bicarbonate/phosphates, succinylcholine, SUFentanil, sulfamethoxazole-trimethoprim, teniposide, theophylline, thiopental, thiotepa, ticarcillin, ticarcillin-clavulanate, tigecycline, tirofiban, tobramycin, trastuzumab, vasopressin, vecuronium, vinBLAStine, vinCRIStine, vitamin B complex/C, voriconazole, zidovudine, zoledronic acid

SIDE EFFECTS
Systemic use
CNS: malaise, acute cerebellar dysfunction
EENT: Light intolerance, lacrimation
GI: *Anorexia, stomatitis,* diarrhea, nausea, vomiting, hemorrhage, enteritis, glossitis
HEMA: Thrombocytopenia, leukopenia, myelosuppression, anemia, agranulocytosis
INTEG: *Rash,* fever, photosensitivity, anaphylaxis, alopecia, hand-foot syndrome

PHARMACOKINETICS
Half-life 16 min (IV): metabolized in liver; excreted in lungs (60%-80%) urine; IV onset 1-9 days, peak 9-21 days (nadir), duration 30 days; top: onset 2-3 days, peak 2-6 wk, duration 1-2 mo; crosses blood-brain barrier (up to 15%)

INTERACTIONS
Increase: bleeding—anticoagulants, NSAIDs, platelet inhibitors, thrombolytics
Increase: toxicity—metroNIDAZOLE, irinotecan
Increase: toxicity, bone marrow depression—radiation or other antineoplastics, leucovorin
Decrease: antibody response—live virus vaccines
Decrease: effect of phenytoin
Drug/Lab Test
Increase: AST, ALT, LDH, serum bilirubin, Hct, Hgb, WBC, platelets, 5-HIAA
Decrease: albumin

NURSING CONSIDERATIONS
Assess:
• **Bone marrow suppression:** monitor daily during IV treatment: CBC, differential, platelet count daily (IV); withhold product if WBC is <3500/mm³ or platelet count is <100,000/mm³; notify prescriber of results; product should be discontinued; nadir of leukopenia within 2 wk, recovery 1 mo, if pretreatment of WBC <2000/mm³ or platelets <100,000/mm³, delay until recovery of counts above this level; nadir usually 9-14 days, recovery 30 days

Black Box Warning: Use only with an experienced clinician in a specialized care setting, for cancer chemotherapy

• **Palmar-plantar erythrodysesthesia:** hand/foot tingling changing to pain, redness
• **Infiltration:** monitor frequently for pain, redness, inflammation at site; if present, stop infusion and start at new site, may use ice at site
• Renal studies: BUN, serum uric acid, urine CCr; electrolytes before, during therapy
• Hepatic studies before, during therapy: bilirubin, alk phos, AST, ALT, LDH before, during therapy
• **Bleeding:** hematuria, guaiac, bruising, petechiae, mucosa or orifices; avoid IM injections, rectal temperatures
• Inflammation of mucosa, breaks in skin; buccal cavity q8hr for dryness, sores or ulceration, white patches, oral pain, bleeding, dysphagia
• **Infection:** fever, chills, cough, sore throat; those with current infections should be treated before receiving 5-FU, the dose reduced or discontinued if infection occurs
• **Toxicity:** hemorrhage, severe vomiting, severe diarrhea, stomatitis, WBC <3500/mm³, platelets <100,000/mm³, notify prescriber
• **Acute cerebellar dysfunction:** dizziness, weakness
• **Pregnancy:** identify pregnancy before starting therapy; do not use in pregnancy or breastfeeding; drug may cause fetal harm

Evaluate:
• Therapeutic response: decreased tumor size, spread of malignancy

Teach patient/family:
• To avoid crowds, persons with known infection
• To avoid foods with citric acid, hot temperature, or rough texture if stomatitis is present; to drink adequate fluids
• To report stomatitis: any bleeding, white spots, ulcerations in mouth; that patient should examine mouth daily,

report symptoms; viscous lidocaine may be used; rinsing of mouth tid-qid with water, club soda; brushing of teeth bid-tid with soft brush or cotton-tipped applicator for stomatitis; use unwaxed dental floss, give ice chips for mucositis
• **To report signs of infection:** fever, sore throat, flulike symptoms
• To report signs of **anemia:** fatigue, headache, faintness, shortness of breath, irritability
• To report **bleeding:** to avoid razors, commercial mouthwash, IM inj if counts are low
• Not to use aspirin products or NSAIDs
• To use contraception during therapy (men and women); to avoid breastfeeding (topical use)
• Not to receive vaccinations during therapy
• To use sunscreen or stay out of the sun to prevent photosensitivity
• About hair loss; to explore use of wigs or other products until hair regrowth occurs
• **Topical:** to apply only to affected areas, being careful around mouth, nose, eyes; to avoid occlusive dressings; to wash hands after application

---

FLUoxetine (Rx)

(floo-ox′eh-teen)

PROzac, PROzac Weekly, Sarafem, Selfemura

Func. class.: Antidepressant, SSRI (selective serotonin reuptake inhibitor)

Do not confuse:
PROzac/PriLOSEC/Prograf/Provera
Sarafem/Serophene
fluoxetine/duloxetine/loxitane/paroxetine

ACTION: Inhibits CNS neuron uptake of serotonin but not of norepinephrine

USES: Major depressive disorder, obsessive-compulsive disorder (OCD), bulimia nervosa, premenstrual dysphoric disorder (PMDD), panic disorder

Unlabeled uses: Anorexia nervosa, obesity, posttraumatic stress disorder, fibromyalgia, social phobia, ADHD, diabetic neuropathy, Raynaud's disease

CONTRAINDICATIONS: Hypersensitivity, MAOI therapy

Precautions: Pregnancy, breastfeeding, geriatric patients, diabetes mellitus, narrow-angle glaucoma, cardiac malformations in infants (exposed to FLUoxetine in utero), osteoporosis, QT prolongation

Black Box Warning: Children, suicidal ideation

DOSAGE AND ROUTES
Depression/obsessive-compulsive disorder
• **Adult: PO** 20 mg/day in AM; after 4 wk, if no clinical improvement is noted, dose may be increased to 20 mg bid in AM, PM, max 80 mg/day; **Del Rel PO** 90 mg/wk
• **Geriatric: PO** 10 mg/day, increase as needed
• **Child 7-17 yr: PO** 10 mg/day, max 20 mg/day
Premenstrual dysphoric disorder (Sarafem)
• **Adult: PO** 20 mg/day, may be taken daily 14 days before menses
Alcoholism (unlabeled)
• **Adult: PO** 20-80 mg/day, give in divided doses if >40 mg/day
Anorexia nervosa (unlabeled)
• **Adult: PO** 10 mg daily, max 60 mg/day
• **Adult: PO** 20 mg/day, max 80 mg/day
Obesity (unlabeled)
• **Adult: PO** 60 mg/day after titration
Posttraumatic stress disorder (unlabeled)
• **Adult: PO** 10-80 mg/day
Available forms: Caps 10, 20, 40 mg; tabs 10, 20, 60 mg; oral sol 20 mg/5 mL; del rel caps (PROzac Weekly) 90 mg
Administer:
• Without regard to meals

• Crushed if patient is unable to swallow medication whole (tab only)
• Immediate-release product should be given in the AM unless sedation occurs
• Gum, hard candy, frequent sips of water for dry mouth
• Sarafem is used only for premenstrual dysphoric disorder
• Store at room temperature; do not freeze
• **PROzac weekly** on the same day each wk, swallow whole; do not crush, cut, chew
• **Oral sol:** use oral syringe or calibrated measuring device

SIDE EFFECTS

CNS: *Headache, nervousness, insomnia, drowsiness, anxiety, tremor, dizziness, fatigue, sedation, poor concentration, abnormal dreams, agitation,* seizures, apathy, euphoria, hallucinations, delusions, psychosis, suicidal ideation, neuroleptic malignant syndrome–like reactions
CV: *Hot flashes, palpitations,* angina pectoris, hypertension, tachycardia, 1st-degree AV block, bradycardia, MI, thrombophlebitis, generalized edema, torsades de pointes
EENT: Visual changes, ear/eye pain, photophobia, tinnitus, increased intraocular pressure
GI: *Nausea, diarrhea, dry mouth, anorexia, dyspepsia, constipation,* taste changes, flatulence, decreased appetite
GU: *Dysmenorrhea, decreased libido, urinary frequency, UTI,* amenorrhea, cystitis, impotence, urine retention
HEMA: Hemorrhage
INTEG: *Sweating, rash, pruritus,* acne, alopecia, urticaria, angioedema, exfoliative dermatitis, Stevens-Johnson syndrome, toxic epidermal necrolysis
META: Hyponatremia
MS: *Pain,* arthritis, twitching
RESP: *Pharyngitis, cough, dyspnea, bronchitis,* asthma, hyperventilation, pneumonia
SYST: *Asthenia,* serotonin syndrome, flulike symptoms, neonatal abstinence syndrome

PHARMACOKINETICS

PO: Peak 6-8 hr, metabolized in liver to norfluoxetine active metabolite by CYP2D6 isoenzyme, ᴾᵒ some patients may be poor metabolizers; excreted in urine, half-life 2-3 days, half-life 4-16 days, protein binding 94%

INTERACTIONS

Increase: serotonin syndrome—SSRIs, SNRIs, serotonin-receptor agonists, selegiline, busPIRone, tryptophan, phenothiazines, haloperidol, loxapine, thiothixene, tricyclics
Increase: QT prolongation—pimozide, thioridiazine, antidysrhythmics class III
Increase: bleeding risk—platelet inhibitors, thrombolytics, NSAIDs, salicylates, anticoagulants
• Do not use MAOIs, linezolid, methylene blue with or 14 days before FLUoxetine
Increase: levels or toxicity of carBAMazepine, lithium, digoxin, warfarin, phenytoin, diazepam, vinBLAStine, donepezil, antidiabetics, dorifenacin, paricalcitrol, budesonide, bosentan, thioridazine
Increase: CNS depression—alcohol, antidepressants, opioids, sedatives
Decrease: FLUoxetine effect—cyproheptadine
Drug/Herb
• Do not use together; increased risk of serotonin syndrome: St. John's wort, SAM-e
Increase: CNS effect—hops, kava, lavender, valerian

NURSING CONSIDERATIONS
Assess:

Black Box Warning: Mental status: mood, sensorium, affect, suicidal tendencies (child/young adult), increase in psychiatric symptoms, depression, panic; monitor for seizures, seizure potential increased, Sarafem is not approved for children

• **Serotonin syndrome:** symptoms can occur anytime after first dose; nausea/vomiting, sedation, dizziness, diaphoresis, mental changes, elevated B/P; if these occur, product should be stopped, notify prescriber

- **QT prolongation:** may be more severe in those with history of QT prolongation; if thioridazine is being used, discontinue for 5 wk prior to using this product
- **Neuroleptic malignant syndrome:** fever, seizures, diaphoresis, dyspnea, hyper/hypotension; report immediately
- **Bulimia nervosa:** appetite, weight daily, increase nutritious foods in diet, watch for bingeing and vomiting
- Allergic reactions/serious skin reactions: angioedema, exfoliative dermatitis, Stevens-Johnson syndrome, toxic epidermal necrolysis, itching, rash, urticaria; product should be discontinued, may need to give antihistamine
- B/P (lying/standing), pulse; if systolic B/P drops 20 mm Hg, hold product, notify prescriber; ECG for flattening of T wave, bundle branch, AV block, dysrhythmias in cardiac patients
- **Blood studies:** CBC, leukocytes, differential, cardiac enzymes if patient is receiving long-term therapy; check platelets; bleeding can occur, thyroid function, growth rate (children), weight
- **Hepatic studies:** AST, ALT, bilirubin, creatinine, weight weekly; appetite may decrease with product
- Safety measures, primarily for geriatric patients
- **Beers:** avoid use in older adults unless safer alternative is unavailable; may cause ataxia, impaired psychomotor function
- **Pregnancy/breastfeeding:** no well-controlled studies; use only if benefits outweigh fetal risk; not recommended in breastfeeding

Evaluate:
- Therapeutic response: decreased depression, symptoms of OCD, absence of suicidal thoughts decreased symptoms of PMDD

Teach patient/family:
- That therapeutic effect may take 1-4 wk, not to discontinue abruptly, that follow-up will be required
- To use caution when driving, performing other activities requiring alertness because of drowsiness, dizziness, blurred vision

- To avoid alcohol, other CNS depressants
- To notify prescriber if pregnant, planning to become pregnant, or breastfeeding
- To change positions slowly because orthostatic hypotension may occur
- To avoid all OTC products unless approved by prescriber
- To notify prescriber if allergic reactions occur (rash, trouble breathing, itching)

Black Box Warning: That suicidal thoughts/behaviors may occur in young adults, children, usually during early treatment, to report immediately

- That decreased libido, erectile dysfunction may occur
- To notify prescriber of worsening symptoms, or if insomnia, anxiety, or depression continues
- **Serotonin syndrome:** to report fever, sweating, diarrhea, poor coordination, nausea/vomiting, sedation, flushing, mental changes

fluPHENAZine decanoate (Rx)
(floo-fen´a-zeen)
Modecate Concentrate ✦
fluPHENAZine hydrochloride (Rx)
Func. class.: Antipsychotic
Chem. class.: Phenothiazine, piperazine

ACTION: Depresses cerebral cortex, hypothalamus, limbic system, which control activity and aggression; blocks neurotransmission produced by DOPamine at synapse; exhibits strong α-adrenergic and anticholinergic blocking action; mechanism for antipsychotic effects is unclear

USES: Schizophrenia
Unlabeled use: Agitation

CONTRAINDICATIONS: Hypersensitivity, blood dyscrasias, coma, bone marrow depression

Precautions: Pregnancy, breastfeeding, children <12 yr, geriatric patients, seizure disorders, hypertension, cardiac/hepatic disease, abrupt discontinuation, accidental exposure, agranulocytosis, ambient temperature increase, angina, hypersensitivity to benzyl alcohol/parabens/sesame oil/tartrazine dye, QT prolongation, suicidal ideation, renal failure, Parkinson's disease, hypocalcemia, head trauma, prostatic hypertrophy, pulmonary disease, infection, ileus, chemotherapy, breast cancer

Black Box Warning: Increased mortality in elderly patients with dementia-related psychosis

DOSAGE AND ROUTES
Decanoate
• **Adult and child >12 yr: IM/SUBCUT** 12.5-25 mg q1-3wk, may increase slowly, max 100 mg/dose

HCl
• **Adult: PO** 2.5-10 mg in divided doses q6-8hr, max 40 mg/day; **IM** initially 1.25 mg, then 2.5-10 mg in divided doses q6-8hr
Available forms: *Decanoate:* inj 25, 100 ✦ mg/mL; *HCl:* tabs 1, 2.5, 5, 10 mg; inj 2.5 mg/mL; elixir 2.5 mg/5 mL; oral solution 5 mg/mL
Administer:
PO route
• Give with food, milk, or a full glass of water to minimize gastric irritation
• **Oral concentrate:** Give using a calibrated measuring device; dilute just before use with 120-240 mL of water, saline, milk, 7-Up, carbonated orange beverage, or apricot, orange, pineapple, prune, tomato, or V-8 juice; do not mix with beverages containing caffeine (coffee, cola), tannics (tea), or pectinates (apple juice) or with other liquid medications; avoid spilling the solution on the skin and clothing
• **Oral elixir:** Give using a calibrated measuring device; avoid spilling the solution on the skin and clothing

Injectable routes
• Visually inspect for particulate matter and discoloration before use, slight yellow to amber color does not alter potency, markedly discolored solutions should be discarded, protect from light
IM route (fluPHENAZine HCl only)
• No dilution necessary; if irritation occurs, subsequent IM doses may be diluted with NS for injection or 2% procaine
• Inject slowly and deeply into the upper outer quadrant of the gluteal muscle using a dry syringe and needle, aspirate before injection
• Keep patient in a recumbent position ≥30 min following injection to minimize hypotensive effects
• Rotate the site of injection to avoid irritation or sterile abscess formation with repeat use
IM injection (fluPHENAZine decanoate)
• Use a dry syringe and needle of at least 21-G, do not dilute
• Inject slowly and deeply into the upper outer quadrant of the gluteal muscle, aspirate
• Keep patient in a recumbent position for at least 30 min following the initial injection to minimize hypotensive effects; rotate the site of injection to avoid irritation or sterile abscess formation with repeat administration
Subcut injection route (fluPHENAZine decanoate)
• Use a dry syringe and a needle of at least 21-G, do not dilute
• Inject subcut, taking care not to inject intradermally
• Keep patient in a recumbent position for at least 30 min following the initial injection to minimize hypotensive effects; rotate the injection sites

SIDE EFFECTS
CNS: *EPS: pseudoparkinsonism, akathisia, dystonia, tardive dyskinesia, drowsiness, headache,* seizures, neuroleptic malignant syndrome
CV: *Orthostatic hypotension,* hypertension, cardiac arrest, ECG changes, tachycardia

EENT: Blurred vision, glaucoma, dry eyes, nasal congestion

GI: *Dry mouth, nausea, vomiting, anorexia, constipation,* diarrhea, jaundice, weight gain, paralytic ileus, hepatitis, cholecystic jaundice

GU: Urinary retention, urinary frequency, enuresis, impotence, amenorrhea, gynecomastia

HEMA: Anemia, leukopenia, leukocytosis, agranulocytosis, aplastic anemia, thrombocytopenia

INTEG: *Rash,* photosensitivity, dermatitis, hyperpigmentation (long-term use)

RESP: Laryngospasm, dyspnea, respiratory depression

PHARMACOKINETICS

Metabolized by liver, excreted in urine (metabolites), crosses placenta, enters breast milk, protein binding >90%, not dialyzable

PO/IM (HCl): Onset 1 hr, peak 90-120 min, duration 6-8 hr, half-life 15 hr

IM/SUBCUT (decanoate): Onset 1-3 days; peak 1-2 days, duration over 4 wk, single-dose half-life 7-10 days, multiple dose 14.3 days

INTERACTIONS

Increase: QT prolongation, torsades de pointes (at higher doses)—amiodarone, arsenic trioxide, astemizole, dasatinib, disopyramide, dofetilide, droperidol, erythromycin, flecainide, gatifloxacin, ibutilide, levomethadyl, ondansetron, paliperidone, palonosetron, some antidepressants, vorinostat, ziprasidone, haloperidol, phenothiazines, ARIPiprazole, lurasidone

Increase: sedation—other CNS depressants, alcohol, barbiturate anesthetics, haloperidol, metyrosine, risperiDONE

Increase: toxicity—EPINEPHrine

Increase: anticholinergic effects—anticholinergics

Decrease: effects of levodopa, lithium

Decrease: fluPHENAZine effects—smoking, barbiturates

Drug/Lab Test

Increase: LFTs, cardiac enzymes, cholesterol, blood glucose, prolactin, bilirubin, cholinesterase

Decrease: hormones (blood and urine)

False positive: pregnancy tests, PKU urinary steroids, 17-OHCS

NURSING CONSIDERATIONS
Assess:

• **QT prolongation, torsades de pointes:** ECG for changes

• Bilirubin, CBC, LFTs monthly; ophthalmic exams periodically

• Urinalysis recommended before and during prolonged therapy

• Affect, orientation, LOC, reflexes, gait, coordination, sleep pattern disturbances

• B/P standing and lying; pulse and respirations q4hr during initial treatment; establish baseline before starting treatment; report drops of 30 mm Hg

• Dizziness, faintness, palpitations, tachycardia on rising

• **EPS** including akathisia (inability to sit still, no pattern to movements), tardive dyskinesia (bizarre movements of jaw, mouth, tongue, extremities), pseudoparkinsonism (rigidity, tremors, pill rolling, shuffling gait)

• **Anticholinergic effects:** constipation, urinary retention daily; if these occur, increase bulk, water in diet

• Supervised ambulation until stabilized on medication; do not involve patient in strenuous exercise; fainting possible; patient should not stand still for long periods

Black Box Warning: **Beers:** avoid in older adults except for schizophrenia, bipolar disorder, or short-term use as an antiemetic during chemotherapy; increased risk of stroke, cognitive decline, mortality

• **Pregnancy/breastfeeding:** no well-controlled studies; use only if benefits outweigh fetal risk; may cause EPS in infant if used during 3rd trimester; excreted in breast milk

Evaluate:

• Therapeutic response: decrease in emotional excitement, hallucinations, delusions, paranoia, reorganization of patterns of thought, speech

---

Side effects: *italics* = common; red = life-threatening

Teach patient/family:

• That orthostatic hypotension occurs often; to rise from sitting or lying position gradually; to avoid hazardous activities until stabilized on medication

• To avoid hot tubs, hot showers, tub baths because hypotension may occur; that in hot weather, heat stroke may occur; to take extra precautions to stay cool

• To avoid abrupt withdrawal of this product or EPS may result; that product should be withdrawn slowly

• To avoid OTC preparations (cough, hay fever, cold) unless approved by prescriber; that serious product interactions may occur; to avoid use with alcohol, CNS depressants; that increased drowsiness may occur

• To use a sunscreen to prevent burns

• About the importance of compliance with product regimen, follow-up, lab, ophthalmic exams

• About EPS; about the need for meticulous oral hygiene because oral candidiasis may occur

• To report sore throat, malaise, fever, bleeding, mouth sores; if these occur, CBC should be drawn, product discontinued

• That urine may turn pink to reddish brown

TREATMENT OF OVERDOSE: Lavage; if orally ingested, provide an airway; *do not induce vomiting*

---

flurandrenolide topical
See Appendix B

---

flurbiprofen ophthalmic
See Appendix B

RARELY USED

flutamide (Rx)
(floo′ta-mide)
Euflex ✦
Func. class.: Antineoplastic, hormone
Chem. class.: Antiandrogen

USES: Metastatic prostatic carcinoma, stages (B_2, C, D_2) in combination with

LHRH agonistic analogs (leuprolide), B_2-C in combination with goserelin and radiation

CONTRAINDICATIONS: Pregnancy, hypersensitivity

Black Box Warning: Severe hepatic disease

DOSAGE AND ROUTES
• **Adult:** PO 250 mg q8hr for a daily dosage of 750 mg

---

fluticasone (Rx)
(floo-tic′a-sone)
ArmonAir RespiClick, Arnuity Ellipta, Avamys ✦, Flixonase ✦, Flonase, Flovent Diskus, Flovent HFA, Flutivate ✦, Veramyst (nasal spray)

Do not confuse:
Flonase/Flovent
ACTION: Decreases inflammation by inhibiting mast cells, macrophages, and leukotrienes; antiinflammatory and vasoconstrictor properties

USES: Prevention of chronic asthma during maintenance treatment in those requiring oral corticosteroids; nasal symptoms of seasonal/perennial, allergic/nonallergic rhinitis
Unlabeled uses: COPD

CONTRAINDICATIONS: Hypersensitivity to this product or milk protein, primary treatment in status asthmaticus, acute bronchospasm
Precautions: Pregnancy, breastfeeding, active infections, glaucoma, diabetes, immunocompromised patients, Cushing syndrome

DOSAGE AND ROUTES
Prevention of chronic asthma

Flovent HFA
• **Adult/child ≥12 yr:** INH 88-440 mcg bid (in those previously taking bronchodilators alone); INH 88-220 mcg bid,

---

max 440 mcg bid (in those previously taking inhaled corticosteroids); **INH** 440 mcg bid, max 880 mcg bid (in those previously taking oral corticosteroids)

• **Child 4-11 yr: INH** 88 mcg bid

Flovent Diskus

• **Adult/child ≥12 yr: INH** 100 mcg bid, max 500 mcg bid (in those previously taking bronchodilators alone); **INH** 100-250 mcg bid, max 500 mcg bid (in those previously taking inhaled corticosteroids); **INH** 500-1000 mcg bid, max 1000 mcg bid (in those previously taking oral corticosteroids)

• **Child 4-11 yr: INH** Initially 50 mcg bid, max 100 mcg bid (in those previously taking bronchodilators alone or inhaled corticosteroids)

Arnuity Ellipta

• **Adult/child ≥12 yr: INH** 100 mcg via oral inhalation daily initially; may increase to 200 mcg/day after 2 wk; max 200 mcg/day

Seasonal, perennial allergic, nonallergic rhinitis

Flonase

• **Adult: NASAL** 2 sprays initially in each nostril daily or 1 spray bid; when controlled, lower to 1 spray in each nostril daily

• **Adolescent/child >4 yr: NASAL** 1 spray in each nostril daily, may increase to 2 sprays in each nostril daily; when controlled, lower to 1 spray in each nostril daily

Veramyst

• **Adult/child ≥12 yr: NASAL** 2 sprays in each nostril daily

• **Child 2-11 yr: NASAL** 1 spray in each nostril daily

Available forms: Oral inhalation aerosol 44, 110, 220 mcg; oral inhalation powder 50, 100, 250 mcg; nasal spray (Veramyst) 27.5 mcg/actuation, (propionate) 50 mcg/actuation, 27.5 mcg/spray (furoate); inhalation powder 100, 200 mcg/actuation (Arnuity Ellipta)

Administer:

• Give at 1-min intervals; if a bronchodilator aerosol spray is used, use bronchodilator first, wait 5-15 min, then use fluticasone

• Decrease dose to lowest effective dose after desired effect; decrease dose at 2-4 wk intervals

Inhalation route (aerosol)

• Shake well, prime before 1st use, release 4 sprays into air away from face, prime using 1 spray if not used for ≥7 days; when the counter reads 000, discard; clean mouthpiece daily in warm water, dry; do not share inhaler with others

• Child <4 yr requires a face mask with spacer/VHC device for delivery; allow 3-5 INH per actuation; do not use spacer with Flovent Diskus

Inhalation route: Powder for oral inhalation (Flovent Diskus)

• Fill in the "Pouch opened" and "Use by" dates in the blank lines on the label; the "Use by" date for Flovent Diskus 50 mcg is 6 wk from the date the pouch is opened; the "Use by" date for Diskus 100 mcg and 250 mcg is 2 mo from the date the pouch is opened

• Open the diskus

• Slide the lever away from the patient as far as it will go until it clicks; the number on the dose counter will count down from 1; the diskus is now ready to use

• Before inhaling the dose, have patient breathe out, hold the diskus level and away from mouth, do not breathe out into the mouthpiece

• Instruct the patient to put the mouthpiece to the lips and breathe in through the mouth quickly and deeply through the diskus; remove the diskus from the mouth, hold breath for about 10 sec, and breathe out slowly

• After taking a dose, close the diskus by sliding the thumb grip back as far as it will go; the diskus will click shut; the lever automatically returns to its original position

F

• The counter displays how many doses are left; the counter number counts down each time the patient uses the diskus; after 55 doses (23 doses from the sample pack), numbers 5 to 0 are red to warn that there are only a few doses left

• After use, patient should rinse mouth with water and spit out the water, not swallow it

• To avoid the spread of infection, do not use the inhaler for more than one person

Intranasal

• Prime before first use

• Shake bottle gently before each use

• Rinse tip after use, dry with tissue

• Blow nose before use

SIDE EFFECTS

CNS: Fatigue, fever, headache, nervousness, dizziness, migraines

EENT: *Pharyngitis*, sinusitis, rhinitis, laryngitis, hoarseness, dry eyes, cataracts, nasal discharge, epistaxis, blurred vision

GI: Diarrhea, abdominal pain, nausea, vomiting, *oral candidiasis*

INTEG: Urticaria, dermatitis

META: Hyperglycemia, growth retardation in children, cushingoid features

MISC: Influenza, eosinophilic conditions, angioedema, Churg-Strauss syndrome, anaphylaxis, adrenal insufficiency (high doses), bone mineral density reduction

MS: Osteoporosis, muscle soreness, joint pain, arthralgia

RESP: *Upper respiratory infection*, dyspnea, cough, bronchitis, bronchospasm

PHARMACOKINETICS

Absorption 30% aerosol, 13.5% powder; protein binding 91%; metabolized in liver after absorption in lung; half-life 7.8 hr; <5% excreted in urine and feces

Oral INH: Onset 24 hr, peak several days, duration 1-2 wk

Intranasal: Onset 12 hr, peak several days

INTERACTIONS

Increase: fluticasone levels—CYP3A4 inhibitors (ketoconazole, itraconazole), darunavir, nelfinavir, ritonavir, amprenavir, fosamprenavir, atazanavir, delavirdine, saquinavir

Increase: cardiac toxicity—isoproterenol (asthma patients)

NURSING CONSIDERATIONS

Assess:

• **Respiratory status:** lung sounds, pulmonary function tests during, for several mo after change from systemic to inhalation corticosteroids

• Withdrawal symptoms from oral corticosteroids: depression, pain in joints, fatigue

• **Adrenal insufficiency:** nausea, weakness, fatigue, hypotension, hypoglycemia, anorexia; may occur when changing from systemic to inhalation corticosteroids; may be life-threatening; adrenal function tests periodically: hypothalamic–pituitary–adrenal axis suppression in long-term treatment

• Growth rate in children; blood glucose, serum potassium for all patients

• **Beers:** avoid use in older adults with delirium or at high risk of delirium; may worsen the condition

• **Pregnancy/breastfeeding:** use only if benefits outweigh fetal risk; use caution in breastfeeding, excretion unknown

Evaluate:

• Therapeutic response: decreased severity of asthma, COPD, allergies

Teach patient/family:

• To use bronchodilator 1st, before using inhalation, if taking both

• Not to use for acute asthmatic attack; acute asthma may require oral corticosteroids

• To avoid smoking, smoke-filled rooms, those with URIs, those not immunized against chickenpox or measles

• To rinse mouth after inhaled product to decrease risk of oral candidiasis

• To report immediately cushingoid symptoms: no appetite, nausea, weakness, fatigue, decreased B/P

• How to use, and when it may be empty

• To use medical ID identifying corticosteroid use

fluticasone (topical)

(floo-tic′a-sone)

Cutivate

Func. class.: Corticosteroid, topical

Do not confuse:

fluticasone/mometasone/fludrocortisone

ACTION: Crosses cell membrane to attach to receptors to decrease inflammation, itching; inhibits multiple inflammatory cytokines

USES: Inflammation/itching of corticosteroid-responsive dermatoses on the skin

CONTRAINDICATIONS: Hypersensitivity to this product or milk protein, status asthmaticus, monotherapy in primary infections, Cushing syndrome, rosacea, perioral dermatitis, diabetes mellitus
Precautions: Pregnancy, children, breastfeeding, skin infections, skin atrophy

DOSAGE AND ROUTES

• **Adult:** Apply to affected areas bid (cream/ointment) or daily (lotion) × 4 wk

Available forms: Lotion, cream 0.05%, ointment 0.005%
Administer:
Topical route
• Do not use with occlusive dressings

• **Cream/ointment/lotion:** Apply sparingly in a thin film and rub gently into the cleansed affected area; wash hands, use gloves; avoid use on face, groin, underarms
• Reassess treatment after 2 uses

SIDE EFFECTS
INTEG: Burning, *pruritus, dermatitis,* hypertrichosis, hives, rash, xerosis, irritation, hyperpigmentation, miliaria
META: Hyperglycemia, glycosuria
MISC: HPA axis suppression, Cushing syndrome

PHARMACOKINETICS
Absorption 5% but variable; half-life 7 hr

INTERACTIONS
Drug/Lab
Increase: Blood glucose

NURSING CONSIDERATIONS
Assess:
• Skin reactions: burning, pruritus, dermatitis
Evaluate:
• Decreasing itching, inflammation on the skin
Teach patient/family:
Topical route:
• Not to use with occlusive dressings

• **Cream/ointment/lotion:** to apply sparingly in a thin film and rub gently into the cleansed affected area; avoid use on face, groin, underarms; wash hands; use gloves
• To reassess treatment after each use

fluticasone/salmeterol

(floo-tic′a-sone) (sal-mee′ter-ol)

Advair Diskus, Advair HFA, AirDuo RespiClick

Func. class.: Corticosteroid, long-acting/β_2-adrenergic agonist

ACTION: Decreased inflammation in inhibiting mast cells, macrophages and leukotrienes; antiinflammatory and vasoconstrictor properties relax bronchial smooth muscles

USES: Maintenance of asthma (long term), COPD

CONTRAINDICATIONS: Hypersensitivity, acute asthma/COPD episodes, severe hypersensitivity to milk proteins
Precautions: Pregnancy, breastfeeding, active infections, diabetes mellitus, glaucoma, immunosuppression, hyperthyroidism, Cushing syndrome, hypertension, QT prolongation, pheochromocytoma, seizures, MAOIs, other long-acting β_2 agonists, inhaled corticosteroid

Black Box Warning: Asthma-related deaths

DOSAGE AND ROUTES
Asthma maintenance
• **Adult/adolescent ≥12 yr: INH** 1 inhalation of Advair Diskus q12hr, or 2 inhalations of Advair HFA q12hr
• **Child 4-11 yr: INH** 1 inhalation of fluticasone 100 mcg/salmeterol 50 mcg (Advair Diskus) q12hr, must be 12 hr apart
COPD
• **Adult: INH** 1 inhalation of Advair 250/50 Diskus q12hr, must be 12 hr apart

Available forms: Inhalation 100/50, 250/50, 500/50 mcg fluticasone/salmeterol; aerosol spray 45/21, 115/21, 230/21 mcg fluticasone/salmeterol
Administer:
Oral inhalation route
Powder for oral inhalation (Diskus):
• Most children <4 years of age do not generate sufficient inspiratory flow to activate dry powder inhalers
• Give with the Diskus device: to open and prepare mouthpiece, slide device lever to activate the first dose, do not advance the lever >1 time; holding the Diskus mouthpiece level to, but away from, the mouth, exhale; then put the mouthpiece to the lips and breathe in the dose deeply and slowly; remove the Diskus from the mouth, hold breath for at least 10 sec, and then exhale slowly; close the Diskus, which also resets the dose lever for the next scheduled dose
• Mouth should be rinsed, spit out water
• Discard device after 1 mo or when counter reads 0 (whichever comes first)
HFA aerosol:
• Shake canister; prime the inhaler before first use with 4 test sprays away from face or with 2 test sprays (away from the face) if it has not been used for more than 4 wk, or after dropping; use spacer if unable to coordinate inhalation/activation
• Rinse mouth with water after use, spit out water; clean inhaler mouthpiece at least every day; discard inhaler after 120 sprays or when the counter reads 000

Powder for inhalation (e.g., AirDuo RespiClick)
• Do not use a spacer or volume holding chamber
• Before using for the first time, check the dose counter window to ensure that the inhaler is full and the number "60" is in the window. The dose counter will count down each time the mouthpiece cap is opened and closed. The dose counter displays only even numbers
• Hold the inhaler upright while opening the cap fully. When the cap is opened, the dose will be activated for delivery. Make sure a "click" sound is heard
• The patient should breathe out through the mouth and push as much air from the lungs as he or she can. Be careful that the patient does not breathe out into the inhaler mouthpiece. Put the mouthpiece in the mouth and have patient close lips around it. The patient should breathe in deeply through the mouth, until the lungs feel completely full of air. Ensure that the vent above the mouthpiece is not blocked; hold breath for 10 seconds or as long as the patient can
• Remove inhaler; check dose counter on the back of the inhaler to make sure the dose was received
• Close cap over the mouthpiece after each use of the inhaler; make sure the cap closes firmly into place
• To inhale another dose, close cap and then repeat inhaler steps
• Following use, instruct patient to rinse mouth with water without swallowing
• The inhaler contains a powder and must be kept clean and dry at all times. Do not wash or put any part of the inhaler in water. If the mouthpiece needs cleaning, gently wipe it with a dry cloth or tissue
• When there are "20" doses left, the numbers on the dose counter will change to red; refill the prescription
• When the dose counter reaches "0," the background will change to solid red
• Throw away the inhaler 30 days after removing it from the foil pouch for the first time, when the dose counter displays "0," or after the expiration date on the package, whichever comes first

SIDE EFFECTS

CNS: Fever, headache, nervousness, dizziness, migraines, insomnia, tremors, agitation, anxiety, depression, hyperactivity, irritability

EENT: Pharyngitis, sinusitis, rhinitis, laryngitis, hoarseness, dry eyes, cataracts, nasal discharge, epistaxis, hypersalivation, eye edema, dysphonia, conjunctivitis

GI: Diarrhea, abdominal pain, nausea, vomiting, oral candidiasis

GU: UTI

INTEG: Urticaria, dermatitis

META: Hyperglycemia, growth retardation in children, cushingoid features

MISC: Influenza, eosinophilic conditions, angioedema, Churg-Strauss syndrome, anaphylaxis, adrenal insufficiency (high doses), reduced bone mineral density, HPA axis suppression

MS: Osteoporosis, muscle soreness, joint pain, decreased growth velocity

RESP: Upper respiratory infection, dyspnea, cough, bronchitis, bronchospasm

PHARMACOKINETICS

Fluticasone: half-life 8 hr, peak 1-2 hr; salmeterol: half-life 5.5 hr, peak 5 min

INTERACTIONS

Increase: CNS stimulation—theophylline

Increase: fluticasone levels—CYP3A4 inhibitors (ketoconazole, itraconazole), darunavir, nelfinavir, ritonavir, amprenavir, fosamprenavir, atazanavir, delavirdine, saquinavir, MAOIs, linezolid

Increase: tendinitis, tendon rupture—quinolones

Increase: hypokalemia—loop diuretics, thiazides, theophylline

Drug/Lab Test

Increase: LFTs

Decrease: Potassium

NURSING CONSIDERATIONS

Assess:

• **Respiratory status:** vital capacity, forced expiratory volume, ABGs, lung sounds, heart rate/rhythm

• Withdrawal symptoms from oral corticosteroids: depression, pain in joints, fatigue

• **Adrenal insufficiency:** nausea, weakness, fatigue, hypotension, hypoglycemia, anorexia; can occur when changing from systemic to inhalation corticosteroids; may be life threatening; adrenal function tests periodically: hypothalamic–pituitary–adrenal axis suppression in long-term treatment

• Growth rate in children; blood glucose, serum potassium for all patients

Black Box Warning: Asthma-related deaths: if wheezing worsens and cannot be relieved during an acute attack, provide emergency response

• **Pregnancy/breastfeeding:** use only if benefits outweigh fetal risk; use caution in breastfeeding, excretion unknown

Evaluate:

• Therapeutic response: decreased severity of asthma

Teach patient/family:

• To use bronchodilator first, before using inhalation, if taking both; may use spacer or valved chamber

• Not to use for acute asthmatic attack; acute asthma might require oral corticosteroids; may use short-acting B₂ agonists for rescue

• To avoid smoking, smoke-filled rooms, those with URIs, those not immunized against chickenpox or measles

Black Box Warning: Asthma-related deaths: seek medical attention immediately if wheezing worsens and cannot be relieved during an acute attack

• To rinse mouth after inhaled product to reduce the risk of oral candidiasis; not to swallow

fluvastatin (Rx)

(flu′vah-stay-tin)

Lescol, Lescol XL

Func. class.: Antilipemic

Chem. class.: HMG-CoA reductase inhibitor

Do not confuse:

fluvastatin/FLUoxetine

Side effects: *italics* = common; red = life-threatening

ACTION: Inhibits HMG-CoA reductase enzyme, which reduces cholesterol synthesis

USES: As an adjunct for primary hypercholesterolemia (types Ia, Ib), coronary atherosclerosis in CAD; to reduce the risk for secondary prevention of coronary events in patients with CAD; as an adjunct to diet to reduce LDL, total cholesterol, apo B levels in heterozygous familial hypercholesterolemia (LDL-C ≥190 mg/dL or LDL-C ≥160 mg/dL) with history of premature CV disease

CONTRAINDICATIONS: Pregnancy, breastfeeding, hypersensitivity, active hepatic disease
Precautions: Previous hepatic disease, alcoholism, severe acute infections, trauma, hypotension, uncontrolled seizure disorders, severe metabolic disorders, electrolyte imbalance, myopathy, rhabdomyolysis

DOSAGE AND ROUTES
• **Adult: PO** 20 mg/day in PM initially, max 80/day mg; or 60 mg/day (ext rel) dosage adjustments may be made at ≥4-wk intervals or ext rel 80 mg at bedtime
Heterozygous familial hypercholesterolemia
• **Adolescent ≥1 yr postmenarche (10-16 yr): PO** 20 mg daily at bedtime, may increase q6wk, max 40 mg bid (cap) or 80 mg (ext rel)
Renal dose
• **Adult: PO** CCr <30 L/min max 20 mg/day unless titrated
• **Child/adolescent 10-17 yr: PO** 10-40 mg/day (familial heterozygous hypercholesterolemia)
Available forms: Caps 20, 40 mg; ext rel tab 80 mg
Administer:
• Do not break, crush, or chew ext rel tabs, use at any time of day (tab), in the evening (cap)
• Bile acid sequestrant should be given at least 2 hr before fluvastatin
• Give without regard to food
• Store at room temperature, protected from light

SIDE EFFECTS
CNS: Headache, dizziness, insomnia, confusion
EENT: Lens opacities
GI: *Abdominal pain, cramps, nausea, constipation, diarrhea, dyspepsia, flatus,* hepatic dysfunction, pancreatitis
HEMA: Thrombocytopenia, hemolytic anemia, leukopenia
INTEG: Rash, pruritus
MISC: Fatigue, influenza, photosensitivity
MS: Myalgia, myositis, rhabdomyolysis, *arthritis, arthralgia*

PHARMACOKINETICS
Peak response 3-4 wk, metabolized in liver, >98% protein bound, excreted primarily in feces, enters breast milk, half-life 1.9 hr, steady state 4-5 wk

INTERACTIONS
Increase: effects of warfarin, digoxin, phenytoin; monitor closely
Increase: myopathy—cycloSPORINE, niacin, colchicine, protease inhibitors, fibric acid derivatives, erythromycin
Increase: effects of fluvastatin—alcohol, cimetidine, ranitidine, omeprazole, phenytoin, rifampin
Increase: adverse reactions—fluconazole, itraconazole, ketoconazole
Decrease: fluvastatin effect—cholestyramine, colestipol; separate by ≥4 hr
Drug/Herb
Increase: adverse reactions—red yeast rice
Drug/Lab Test
Increase: LFTs, CK
Decrease: platelets, WBC

NURSING CONSIDERATIONS
Assess:
• **Hypercholesterolemia:** diet history: fats, protein carbohydrate; nutritional analysis should see dietitian before treatment; fasting lipid profile (cholesterol, LDL, HDL, TG) before and q4-6wk, then q3-6mo when stable
• **Hepatotoxicity/pancreatitis:** monitor hepatic studies before, q12wk after dosage change, then q6mo; AST, ALT, LFTs may be increased

---

• Renal studies in patients with compromised renal system: BUN, I&O ratio, creatinine

• Myopathy, rhabdomyolysis: muscle pain, tenderness; obtain baseline CPK if elevated; if these occur, product should be discontinued

• **Pregnancy/breastfeeding:** do not use in pregnancy/breastfeeding

Evaluate:

• Therapeutic response: decrease in sLDL, VLDL, total cholesterol; increased HDL, decreased triglycerides, slowing of CAD

Teach patient/family:

• That blood work will be necessary during treatment; to take product as prescribed; that effect may take ≥4 wk

• To report severe GI symptoms, headache, muscle pain, weakness, tenderness

• That previously prescribed regimen will continue: low-cholesterol diet, exercise program, smoking cessation

• To report suspected pregnancy; not to use during pregnancy, breastfeeding

• To take without regard to meals; to take immediate-release product in the evening; separate by ≥4 hr from bile-acid product, not to cut, break, chew capsule

---

fluvoxaMINE (Rx)

(flu-vox′a-meen)

Luvox ✖, Riva-Fluvox ✖

Func. class.: Antidepressant SSRI (selective serotonin reuptake inhibitor)

Do not confuse:

Luvox/Lasix

FluvoxaMINE/FluPHENAZine/ Flavoxate

ACTION: Inhibits CNS neuron uptake of serotonin but not of norepinephrine

USES: Obsessive-compulsive disorder, social phobia

CONTRAINDICATIONS: Hypersensitivity, MAOIs

Precautions: Pregnancy, breastfeeding, geriatric patients, hepatic/cardiac disease, abrupt discontinuation, dehydration, ECT, hyponatremia, hypovolemia, bipolar disorder, seizure disorder

---

Black Box Warning: Children <8 yr, suicidal ideation

DOSAGE AND ROUTES

Obsessive-compulsive disorder (OCD)

• **Adult: PO** 50 mg at bedtime, increase by 50 mg/day at 4-7 day intervals, max 300 mg/day; doses over 100 mg should be divided; **EXT REL** 100 mg at bedtime, may titrate upward by 50 mg/wk, max 300 mg/day

• **Child 12-17 yr: PO** 25 mg at bedtime, increase by 25 mg/day q4-7days, max 300 mg/day; doses over 50 mg should be divided

• **Child 8-11 yr: PO** 25 mg/day at bedtime, may increase q4-7days, max 200 mg/day, divide doses if >50 mg

Social anxiety disorder

• **Adult: PO EXT REL CAP** (Luvox CR) 100 mg at bedtime initially, titrate as needed by 50 mg/wk to 100-300 mg/day; **PO** 50 mg at bedtime, titrate as needed by 50 mg q4-7days to 50-300 mg/day

• **Child/adolescent 12-17 yr: PO** 25 mg at bedtime, titrate by 25-50 mg q4-7days, max 300 mg/day; if total daily dose >50 mg, divide equally

Hepatic dose/geriatric

• **Adult: PO** 25 mg at bedtime, may titrate upward slowly

Available forms: Tabs 25, 50, 100 mg; ext rel cap 100, 150 mg

Administer:

• With food, milk for GI symptoms

• When discontinuing, taper by 50%, after 3 days taper by another 50% for 3 days, then discontinue

• Store at room temperature; do not freeze

• **Immediate release:** give at bedtime; doses >100 mg/day (or >50 mg/day in those aged 8-17 yr) in 2 divided doses; if doses are not equal, give larger dose at bedtime

---

Side effects: *italics* = common; red = life-threatening

• **Ext rel:** give at bedtime; do not break, crush, chew ext rel product

SIDE EFFECTS

CNS: *Headache, drowsiness, dizziness, seizures,* sleep disorders, insomnia, suicidal ideation (children/adolescents), neuroleptic malignant syndrome–like reactions, *weakness,* neuroleptic malignant syndrome, tremors

CV: Palpitation, chest pain, syncope, nervousness, agitation

GI: *Nausea, anorexia, constipation,* hepatotoxicity, *vomiting, diarrhea,* dry mouth, altered taste

GU: *Decreased libido,* anorgasmia, urinary frequency, priapism

INTEG: *Rash, sweating*

MS: Myalgia

SYST: Neonatal abstinence syndrome

PHARMACOKINETICS

Crosses blood-brain barrier, 77% protein binding, metabolism by the liver, terminal half-life 15.6 hr, peak 2-8 hr

INTERACTIONS

Increase: CNS depression—alcohol, barbiturates, benzodiazepines

Increase: effect of—ramelteon, thioridazine; do not use together

Increase: QT prolongation, death—pimozide; do not use together

Increase: fluvoxaMINE, toxicity levels—tricyclics, cloZAPine, alosetron, tiZANidine, thioridazine; do not use together

Increase: metabolism, decrease effects—smoking

Increase: serotonin syndrome, neuroleptic malignant syndrome: SSRIs, SNRIs, serotonin-receptor agonists, atypical antipsychotics, traMADol, MAOIs, methylene blue, linezolid

Increase: bleeding risk—anticoagulants, NSAIDs, salicylates, thrombolytics

Decrease: metabolism, increase action of propranolol, diazepam, lithium, theophylline, carBAMazepine, warfarin

Drug/Herb

Increase: CNS effect—kava, valerian

Increase: serotonin syndrome—tryptophan, St. John's wort; do not use together

NURSING CONSIDERATIONS
Assess:

Black Box Warning: **Suicidal thoughts/ behaviors:** risk increases in children, young adults; this group needs to be monitored more closely, weekly × 4 wk, then every other wk × 4 wk, then at 12 wk; only small amounts should be given on each refill

• **Pregnancy, breastfeeding:** neonatal abstinence syndrome can occur; do not breastfeed

• **Neuroleptic malignant syndrome:** high fever, confusion, rigid muscles, diaphoresis, tachypenia; notify prescriber immediately

• Hepatic studies: AST, ALT, bilirubin

• Mental status: mood, sensorium, affect, suicidal tendencies; increase in psychiatric symptoms: depression, panic, obsessive-compulsive symptoms

• Constipation; most likely in geriatric patients

• Growth rate (children), bone density (postmenopausal females), glucose (diabetes)

• **Serotonin syndrome:** agitation, hypothermia, hallucinations, tachycardia, nausea, vomiting, diarrhea, instability, changes in B/P

• **For toxicity:** nausea, vomiting, diarrhea, syncope, increased pulse, seizures

• **Beers:** avoid in older adults unless safer alternatives are unavailable; may cause ataxia, impaired motor function

Evaluate:

• Therapeutic response: decrease in OCD, social phobia symptoms

Teach patient/family:

• That therapeutic effects may take 2-3 wk; not to discontinue abruptly

• To use caution when driving, performing other activities requiring alertness because drowsiness, dizziness may occur

• Not to use other CNS depressants, alcohol, barbiturates, benzodiazepines, St. John's wort, kava

• **Pregnancy/breastfeeding:** to avoid use in pregnancy; not to breastfeed

• To notify prescriber if pregnancy is suspected, planned

- To notify prescriber of allergic reaction
- To increase bulk in diet if constipation occurs, especially in geriatric patients

Black Box Warning: That suicidal thoughts/behaviors may occur; that family health care providers should look closely for suicidal tendencies, especially during early therapy or in young adults, children

- **Serotonin syndrome:** to report immediately nausea, vomiting, diarrhea, agitation, instability, hallucinations
- To stop taking MAOIs at least 14 days before starting product

TREATMENT OF OVERDOSE: Gastric lavage

---

folic acid (vit B$_9$) (OTC)
(foe′lik a′sid)
Folvite ✦
Func. class.: Vit B complex group, water-soluble vitamin

ACTION: Needed for erythropoiesis; increases RBC, WBC, platelet formation with megaloblastic anemias

USES: Megaloblastic or macrocytic anemia caused by folic acid deficiency; hepatic disease, alcoholism, hemolysis, intestinal obstruction, pregnancy to reduce risk for neural tube defects
Unlabeled uses: Methotrexate toxicity prophylaxis, in those receiving methotrexate for RA

CONTRAINDICATIONS: Hypersensitivity
Precautions: Pregnancy, anemias other than megaloblastic/macrocytic anemia, vit B$_{12}$ deficiency anemia, uncorrected pernicious anemia

DOSAGE AND ROUTES
RDA
- **Adult and child ≥14 yr: PO** 400 mcg
- **Adult (pregnant/lactating): PO** 600 mcg/day
- **Child 9-13 yr: PO** 300 mcg
- **Child 4-8 yr: PO** 200 mcg
- **Child 1-3 yr: PO** 150 mcg
- **Infant 6 mo-1 yr: PO** 80 mcg
- **Neonate/infant <6 mo: PO** 65 mcg

Megaloblastic/macrocytic anemia due to folic acid or nutritional deficiency
- **Pregnant/lactating: PO** 800-1000 mcg

Therapeutic dose
- **Adult and child: PO/IM/SUBCUT/IV** up to 1 mg/day

Maintenance dose
- **Adult and child >4 yr: PO/IM/SUBCUT/IV** 0.4 mg/day
- **Pregnant and lactating: PO/IM/SUBCUT/IV** 0.8-1 mg/day
- **Child <4 yr: PO/IM/SUBCUT/IV** up to 0.3 mg/day
- **Infant: PO/IM/SUBCUT/IV** up to 0.1 mg/day

Prevention of neural tube defects during pregnancy
- **Adult: PO** 0.6 mg/day

Prevention of megaloblastic anemia during pregnancy
- **Adult: PO/IM/SUBCUT** up to 1 mg/day during pregnancy

Tropical sprue
- **Adult: PO** 3-15 mg/day

Methotrexate toxicity
- **Adult: PO/IM/SUBCUT** 1 mg daily or 5 mg weekly

Available forms: Tabs 0.1, 0.4, 0.8, 1, 5 mg; inj 5, 10 mg/mL
Administer:
SUBCUT route
- Do not inject intradermally
IM route
- Inject deeply in large muscle mass, aspirate
Direct IV route
- Direct undiluted ≤5 mg/1 min or more
Continuous IV INFUSION route
- May be added to most IV sol or TPN

Y-site compatibilities: Alfentanil, aminophylline, ascorbic acid injection, atracurium, atropine, azaTHIOprine, aztreonam, benztropine, bumetanide, calcium gluconate, ceFAZolin, cefonicid, cefotaxime, cefoTEtan, cefOXitin, cefTAZidime, ceftizoxime,

---

cefTRIAXone, cefuroxime, chloramphenicol, cimetidine, clindamycin, cyanocobalamin, cycloSPORINE, dexamethasone, digoxin, diphenhydrAMINE, DOPamine, enalaprilat, ePHEDrine, EPINEPHrine, epoetin alfa, erythromycin, esmolol, famotidine, fentaNYL, fluconazole, furosemide, ganciclovir, glycopyrrolate, heparin, hydrocortisone, hydrOXYzine, imipenem-cilastatin, indomethacin, insulin (regular), ketorolac, labetalol, lidocaine, LR, magnesium sulfate, mannitol, meperidine, methicillin, methylPREDNISolone, metoclopramide, metoprolol, mezlocillin, midazolam, moxalactam, multiple vitamins injection, naloxone, nitroglycerin, nitroprusside, ondansetron, oxacillin, oxytocin, penicillin G potassium/sodium, PENTobarbital, PHENobarbital, phenylephrine, phytonadione, piperacillin, potassium chloride, procainamide, propranolol, ranitidine, Ringer's, ritodrine, sodium bicarbonate, succinylcholine, SUFentanil, theophylline, ticarcillin, ticarcillin-clavulanate, TPN, trimetaphan, urokinase, vancomycin, vasopressin

SIDE EFFECTS

CNS: Confusion, depression, excitability, irritability
GI: Anorexia, nausea, bitter taste
INTEG: Pruritus, rash, erythema
RESP: Bronchospasm
SYST: Anaphylaxis (rare)

PHARMACOKINETICS

PO: Peak $1/2$-1 hr, bound to plasma proteins, excreted in breast milk, metabolized by liver, excreted in urine (small amounts)

INTERACTIONS

Increase: need for folic acid—estrogen, hydantoins, carBAMazepine, glucocorticoids
Decrease: folate levels—methotrexate, sulfonamides, sulfaSALAzine, trimethoprim
Decrease: phenytoin levels, fosphenytoin, may increase seizures

NURSING CONSIDERATIONS
Assess:
• **Megaloblastic anemia:** fatigue, dyspnea, weakness
• Hgb, Hct, reticulocyte count

• Nutritional status: bran, yeast, dried beans, nuts, fruits, fresh vegetables, asparagus
• Products currently taken: estrogen, carBAMazepine, methotrexate, trimethoprim, hydantoins; these products may cause increased folic acid use by the body and contribute to a deficiency if taking other neurotoxic products
• **Pregnancy/breastfeeding:** may be used in pregnancy/breastfeeding
Evaluate:
• Therapeutic response: increased weight, oriented, well-being; absence of fatigue; increase in reticulocyte count within 5 days of beginning treatment, absence of fetal neural tube defect
Teach patient/family:
• To take product exactly as prescribed; that periodic lab work is required
• To alter nutrition to include foods high in folic acid: organ meats, vegetables, fruit
• That urine will turn bright yellow
• To notify prescriber of allergic reaction
• To avoid breastfeeding

> ### ⚠ HIGH ALERT
>
> ## fondaparinux (Rx)
> (fon-dah-pair'ih-nux)
> Arixtra
> *Func. class.:* Anticoagulant, antithrombotic
> *Chem. class.:* Synthetic, selective factor Xa inhibitor

Do not confuse:
Arixtra/Anti-Xa

ACTION: Inhibits factor Xa; neutralization of factor Xa interrupts blood coagulation and thrombin formation

USES: Prevention/treatment of deep venous thrombosis, PE in hip and knee replacement, hip fracture or abdominal surgery
Unlabeled uses: Acute symptomatic superficial vein thrombosis in the legs (>= cm length)

CONTRAINDICATIONS: Hypersensitivity to this product; hemophilia, leukemia with bleeding, peptic ulcer disease, hemorrhagic stroke, surgery, thrombocytopenic purpura, weight <50 kg, severe renal disease (CCr <30 mL/min), active major bleeding, bacterial endocarditis

Precautions: Pregnancy, breastfeeding, children, geriatric patients, alcoholism, hepatic disease (severe), blood dyscrasias, heparin-induced thrombocytopenia, uncontrolled severe hypertension, acute nephritis, mild to moderate renal disease

> **Black Box Warning:** Spinal/epidural anesthesia, lumbar puncture

DOSAGE AND ROUTES
Deep venous thrombosis/PE
• **Adult <50 kg: SUBCUT** 5 mg/day × ≥5 days until INR 2-3; give warfarin within 72 hr of fondaparinux
• **Adult 50-100 kg: SUBCUT** 7.5 mg/day × ≥5 days until INR 2-3; give warfarin within 72 hr of fondaparinux
• **Adult >100 kg: SUBCUT** 10 mg/day × ≥5 days until INR 2-3; give warfarin within 72 hr of fondaparinux

Prevention of deep venous thrombosis
• **Adult: SUBCUT** 2.5 mg/day given 6 hr after surgery; (hemostasis established) continue for 5-9 days; for hip surgery, up to 32 days; for abdominal surgery, up to 24 days

Acute symptomatic superficial leg vein thrombosis (unlabeled)
• **Adult: SUBCUT** 2.5 mg daily × 45 days

Renal disease
• **Adult: SUBCUT** CCr 30-50 mL/min, use cautiously; CCr <30 mL/min, do not use

Available forms: Inj 2.5 mg/0.5 mL, 5 mg/0.4 mL, 7.5 mg/0.6 mL, 10 mg/0.8 mL prefilled syringes

Administer:
• Alone; do not mix with other products or solutions; cannot be used interchangeably (unit to unit) with other anticoagulants

• Only after screening patient for bleeding disorders

SUBCUT route
• SUBCUT only; do not give IM; do not give <6 hr after surgery
• Check for discolored sol or sol with particulate; if present, do not give
• Administer 6-8 hr after surgery; administer to recumbent patient, rotate inj sites (left/right anterolateral, left/right posterolateral abdominal wall)
• Wipe surface of inj site with alcohol swab, twist plunger cap and remove, remove rigid needle guard by pulling straight off needle; do not aspirate, do not expel air bubble from surface
• Insert whole length of needle into skinfold held with thumb and forefinger
• When product is injected, a soft click may be felt or heard
• Give at same time each day to maintain steady blood levels; observe inj site
• Avoid all IM inj that may cause bleeding
• Store at 77° F (25° C); do not freeze

SIDE EFFECTS
CNS: Confusion, headache, dizziness, *insomnia*
HEMA: *Anemia,* hematoma, thrombocytopenia, major bleeding (intracranial, cerebral, retroperitoneal hemorrhage), postoperative hemorrhage, heparin-induced thrombocytopenia
INTEG: Increased wound drainage, bullous eruption, local reaction—*rash*, pruritus, inj-site bleeding
META: Hypokalemia

PHARMACOKINETICS
Rapidly, completely absorbed; peak 3 hr, duration up to 24 hr; distributed primarily in blood; does not bind to plasma proteins except 94% to ATIII; eliminated unchanged in urine within 72 hr with normal renal function; half-life 17-21 hr

INTERACTIONS
Increase: bleeding risk—salicylates, NSAIDs, abciximab, eptifibatide, tirofiban,

---

Side effects: *italics* = common; red = life-threatening

clopidogrel, dipyridamole, quiNIDine, valproic acid, some cephalosporins
Drug/Herb
Increase: bleeding risk—feverfew, garlic, ginger, ginkgo, ginseng, green tea, horse chestnut, kava

NURSING CONSIDERATIONS
Assess:

Black Box Warning: Monitor patients who have received epidural/spinal anesthesia or lumbar puncture for neurologic impairment, including spinal hematoma; may lead to permanent disability or paralysis

• Blood studies (CBC, anti-Xa, Hgb/Hct, prothrombin time, platelets, occult blood in stools); thrombocytopenia may occur; if platelets <100,000/mm^3, treatment should be discontinued; renal studies: BUN, creatinine; contraindicated in CCr <30 mL/min; use caution in CCr 30-50 mL/min
• For bleeding: gums, petechiae, ecchymosis, black tarry stools, hematuria; decreased Hct, notify prescriber
• For risk of hemorrhage if coadministering with other products that may cause bleeding
• For hypersensitivity: rash, fever, chills; notify prescriber
• **Beers:** Avoid in older adults; increased risk of bleeding, lower creatinine clearance
• **Pregnancy/breastfeeding:** use only if benefits outweigh fetal risk; cautious use in breastfeeding, excretion unknown
Evaluate:
• Therapeutic response: prevention of DVT
Teach patient/family:
• To use soft-bristle toothbrush to avoid bleeding gums; to use electric razor
• To report any signs of bleeding: gums, under skin, urine, stools
• To avoid OTC products containing aspirin, NSAIDs

---

formoterol (Rx)
(for-moh´ter-ahl)
Foradil Aerolizer ✦, Oxeze ✦, Perforomist
Func. class.: Bronchodilator
Chem. class.: β-Adrenergic agonist

Do not confuse:
Foradil/Toradol

ACTION: Has β_1 and β_2 action; relaxes bronchial smooth muscle and dilates the trachea and main bronchi by increasing levels of cAMP, which relaxes smooth muscles; causes increased contractility and heart rate by acting on β-receptors in heart

USES: Maintenance, treatment of asthma, COPD; prevention of exercise-induced bronchospasm

CONTRAINDICATIONS: Hypersensitivity to sympathomimetics, monotherapy for asthma, COPD, status asthmaticus
Precautions: Pregnancy, geriatric patients, cardiac disorders, hyperthyroidism, diabetes mellitus, prostatic hypertrophy, hypertension, ✒ African descent, aneurysm

Black Box Warning: Asthma-related death

DOSAGE AND ROUTES
20 mcg/2 mL bid by jet nebulizer
Available form: INH powder in cap 12 mcg (Foradol Aerolizer); nebulizer sol for INH 20 mcg/2 mL (Perforomist); powder for oral inhalation (Oxeze Turbuhaler) 6 mcg/inh, 12 mcg/inh ✦
Administer:
Inhalation route
• Place cap in Aerolizer inhaler; cap is punctured; do not wash Aerolizer inhaler

---

• Pull off cover, twist mouthpiece to open, push buttons in; make sure the 4 pins are visible; remove cap from blister pack, place cap in chamber; twist to close, press (a click will be heard), release; patient should exhale, place inhaler in mouth, inhale rapidly

• Store at room temperature; protect from heat, moisture

SIDE EFFECTS

CNS: *Tremors, anxiety,* insomnia, headache, dizziness, stimulation

CV: Palpitations, tachycardia, hypertension, chest pain

GI: Nausea, vomiting, xerostomia

RESP: Bronchial irritation, dryness of oropharynx, bronchospasms (overuse), infection, inflammatory reaction (child)

PHARMACOKINETICS

Bronchodilation: Onset 15 min; peak 1-3 hr; duration 12 hr; metabolized in liver, lungs, GI tract; half-life 10 hr

INTERACTIONS

Increase: serious dysrhythmias—MAOIs, tricyclics

Increase: hypokalemia—loop/thiazide diuretics

Increase: effects of both products—other sympathomimetics, thyroid hormones

Increase: QT prolongation—class IA/III antiarrhythmics, phenothiazines, pimozide, haloperidol, risperiDONE, sertindole, ziprasidone, amoxapine, arsenic trioxide, chloroquine, clarithromycin, dasatinib, dolasetron, droperidol, erythromycin, halofantrine, halogenated anesthetics, levomethadyl, maprotiline, methadone, some quinolones, ondansetron, paliperidone, palonosetron, pentamidine, probucol, ranolazine, SUNItinib, tricyclics, vorinostat

Decrease: action when used with β-blockers

NURSING CONSIDERATIONS
Assess:

• Respiratory function: B/P, pulse, lung sounds; note sputum color, character; respiratory function tests before, during treatment; be alert for bronchospasm, which may occur with this patient

• **Cardiac status:** hypertension, palpitations, tachycardia; if CV reactions occur, product may need to be discontinued

• For paresthesias, coldness of extremities; peripheral blood flow may decrease

• **Pregnancy/breastfeeding:** use only if benefits outweigh fetal risk; use caution in breastfeeding, excretion unknown

Evaluate:

• Therapeutic response: ease of breathing

Teach patient/family:

F

Black Box Warning: Asthma-related death, severe asthma exacerbations; if wheezing worsens and cannot be relieved during an acute asthma attack, immediate medical attention should be sought

• About correct use of inhaler/nebulizer (review package insert with patient); to avoid getting aerosol in eyes

• About all aspects of product; to avoid smoking, smoke-filled rooms, persons with respiratory infections; not to swallow caps

TREATMENT OF OVERDOSE:
Administration of β-blocker

RARELY USED

fosamprenavir (Rx)
(fos-am-pren′a-veer)
Lexiva, Telzir ♣
Func. class.: Antiretroviral
Chem. class.: Protease inhibitor

USES: HIV-1 infection in combination with antiretrovirals

CONTRAINDICATIONS: Hypersensitivity to protease inhibitors

DOSAGE AND ROUTES
Therapy-naive patients

• **Adult: PO** 1400 mg bid without ritonavir or fosamprenavir 1400 mg/day with ritonavir 200 mg/day or fosamprenavir 700 mg bid and ritonavir 100 mg bid

---

Side effects: *italics* = common; red = life-threatening

• **Child >2 yr/adolescent, ≥20 kg: PO** 18 mg/kg (max: 700 mg) bid plus ritonavir 3 mg/kg (max: 100 mg) bid; 15 kg to <20 kg: 23 mg/kg bid plus ritonavir 3 mg/kg bid; 11 kg to <15 kg: 30 mg/kg/dose bid plus ritonavir 3 mg/kg/dose bid; <11 kg: 45 mg/kg/dose bid plus ritonavir 7 mg/kg/dose bid

Protease-experienced patients (PI)

• **Adult: PO** 700 mg bid and ritonavir 100 mg bid

• **Child/adolescent ≥20 kg: PO** 18 mg/kg bid with ritonavir 3 mg/kg bid

• **Child/adolescent 15 kg to <20 kg: PO** 23 mg/kg bid with ritonavir 3 mg/kg bid

• **Child/adolescent 11 kg to <15 kg: PO** 30 mg/kg bid with ritonavir 3 mg/kg bid

• **Child/adolescent <11 kg: PO** 45 mg/kg bid with ritonavir 7 mg bid

• **Infant ≥6 mo, 15 kg to <20 kg: PO** susp 23 mg/kg bid with ritonavir 3 mg/kg bid

• **Infant ≥6 mo, 11 kg to <15 kg: PO** susp 30 mg/kg bid with ritonavir 3 mg/kg bid

• **Infant ≥6 mo, <11 kg: PO** susp 45 mg/kg bid with ritonavir 7 mg/kg bid

Combination with efavirenz

• **Adult: PO** add another 100 mg/day of ritonavir for a total of 300 mg/day when all 3 products given

Hepatic dose

• **Adult: PO** (Child-Pugh 5-6) 700 mg bid without ritonavir (treatment-naive patients) or 700 mg bid with ritonavir 100 mg daily (treatment-naive or experienced patients); (Child-Pugh 7-9) 700 mg bid without ritonavir (treatment-naive patients) or 450 mg bid with ritonavir 100 mg daily (treatment-naive or experienced patients); (Child-Pugh 10-15) 350 mg bid without ritonavir (treatment-naive patients) or 300 mg bid with ritonavir 100 mg daily

---

foscarnet (Rx)

(foss-kar′net)

Foscavir

Func. class.: Antiviral

Chem. class.: Inorganic pyrophosphate organic analog

ACTION: Antiviral activity is produced by selective inhibition at the pyrophosphate binding site on virus-specific DNA polymerases and reverse transcriptases at concentrations that do not affect cellular DNA polymerases

USES: Treatment of CMV retinitis in patients with AIDS, treatment of acyclovir-resistant HSV infections; used with ganciclovir for relapsing patients

CONTRAINDICATIONS: Hypersensitivity, CCr <0.4 mL/min/kg

Precautions: Pregnancy, breastfeeding, children, geriatric patients, seizure disorders, severe anemia

> **Black Box Warning:** Nephrotoxicity, electrolyte/mineral imbalances, seizures

DOSAGE AND ROUTES

Acyclovir-resistant HSV infections

• **Adult/adolescent (unlabeled): IV** 40 mg/kg every 8-12 hr × 2-3 wk or until lesions are healed, max 120 mg/kg/day

Cytomegalovirus (CMV) retinitis (AIDS)

• **Adult/adolescent: IV** 90 mg/kg every 12 hr or 60 mg/kg every 8 hr × 3 wk (or until symptomatic improvement); maintenance IV infusion 90-120 mg/kg over 2 hr daily, max 180 mg/kg/day (initial); 120 mg/kg/day (maintenance)

Available forms: Inj 6000 mg/250 mL, 12,000 mg/500 mL (24 mg/mL)

Administer:

• Increased fluids before and during product administration to induce diuresis, minimize renal toxicity

Intermittent IV INFUSION route

• Using infusion device at no more than 1 mg/kg/min; do not give by rapid or bolus IV; give by CVL or peripheral vein; standard 24 mg/mL sol may be used without dilution if using by CVL; dilute the 24 mg/mL sol to 12 mg/mL with D_5W or NS if using peripheral vein

• Manufacturer recommends product not be given with other medications in syringe or admixed

---

SIDE EFFECTS

CNS: *Fever*, dizziness, *headache*, seizures, *fatigue*, neuropathy, asthenia, encephalopathy, malaise, meningitis, *paresthesia*, depression, *confusion, anxiety*
CV: ECG abnormalities, 1st-degree AV block, nonspecific ST-T segment changes, cerebrovascular disorder, cardiomyopathy, cardiac arrest, atrial fibrillation, HF, sinus tachycardia
GI: *Nausea, vomiting, diarrhea, anorexia,* abdominal pain, pancreatitis
GU: Acute renal failure, decreased CCr, increased serum creatinine, azotemia, diabetes insipidus, renal tubular disorders
HEMA: *Anemia,* granulocytopenia, leukopenia, thrombocytopenia, thrombosis, neutropenia, lymphadenopathy
INTEG: *Rash*, sweating, pruritus, skin discoloration
RESP: *Coughing, dyspnea,* pneumonia, pulmonary infiltration, pneumothorax, hemoptysis
SYST: *Hypokalemia, hypocalcemia, hypomagnesemia;* hypophosphatemia

PHARMACOKINETICS

14%-17% protein bound, half-life 3 hr in normal renal function, 79%-92% excreted via kidneys, onset rapid, peak infusions end, duration up to 24 hr

INTERACTIONS

Black Box Warning: **Increase:** nephrotoxicity—acyclovir, cidofovir, CISplatin, gold compounds, tacrolimus, tenofovir, vancomycin, aminoglycosides, amphotericin B, NSAIDs, lithium, cycloSPORINE, pentamidine

Increase: hypocalcemia—pentamidine, calcium products (decreases ionized calcium)

NURSING CONSIDERATIONS
Assess:
HSV: characteristics of lesions baseline and daily during treatment

Black Box Warning: **Renal tubular disorders:** I&O ratio, urine pH, serum creatinine at baseline, 3×/wk during initial therapy then 2×/wk thereafter; CCr at baseline, throughout treatment; if CCr <0.4 mL/min/kg, discontinue; provide adequate hydration before and during infusion to prevent toxicity

• Blood counts q2wk; watch for decreasing granulocytes, Hgb; if low, therapy may have to be discontinued and restarted after hematologic recovery; blood transfusions may be required
• Lesions in HSV

Black Box Warning: **Seizures:** may be caused by alterations in minerals and electrolytes, monitor for seizures; monitor electrolytes and minerals (calcium, phosphate, magnesium, potassium); watch closely for tetany during 1st administration

• Electrolytes and minerals (calcium, phosphate, magnesium, potassium); watch closely for tetany during 1st administration
• GI symptoms: nausea, vomiting, diarrhea; severe symptoms may necessitate discontinuing product
• Blood dyscrasias (anemia, granulocytopenia): bruising, fatigue, bleeding, poor healing
• **Allergic reactions:** flushing, rash, urticaria, pruritus
CMV retinitis
• Culture (blood, urine, throat) should be performed before treatment; a negative culture does not rule out CMV. Ophthalmic exam should confirm diagnosis, another exam at conclusion of induction and q4wk during treatment. Monitor closely during therapy for tingling, numbness, paresthesias; if these occur, stop infusion, obtain lab sample for electrolytes
• **Pregnancy/breastfeeding:** use only if benefits outweigh fetal risk; do not breastfeed
Evaluate:
• Therapeutic response: improvement in CMV retinitis, healing of HSV lesions
Teach patient/family:
• To call prescriber if sore throat, swollen lymph nodes, malaise, fever occur, since other infections may occur
• To report perioral tingling, numbness in extremities, and paresthesias

---

Side effects: *italics* = common; red = life-threatening

• That serious product interactions may occur if OTC products are ingested; check first with prescriber

• That product is not a cure but will control symptoms

---

fosinopril (Rx)

(foss'in-oh-pril)

Func. class.: Antihypertensive
Chem. class.: Angiotensin-converting enzyme (ACE) inhibitor

ACTION: Selectively suppresses renin-angiotensin-aldosterone system; inhibits ACE; prevents conversion of angiotensin I to angiotensin II; results in dilation of arterial, venous vessels

USES: Hypertension, alone or in combination with thiazide diuretics, systolic HF

Unlabeled uses: Proteinuria in nondiabetic nephropathy

CONTRAINDICATIONS: Breastfeeding, children, hypersensitivity to ACE inhibitors, history of ACE-inhibitor–induced angioedema

Black Box Warning: Pregnancy

Precautions: Geriatric patients, impaired hepatic function, hypovolemia, blood dyscrasias, HF, COPD, asthma, angioedema, hyperkalemia, renal artery stenosis, renal disease, aortic stenosis, autoimmune disorders, collagen vascular disease, febrile illness, black patients

DOSAGE AND ROUTES
HF
• **Adult:** PO 10 mg/day, then up to 40 mg/day increased over several wk; use lower dose for those diuresed before fosinopril, max 80 mg/day
Hypertension
• **Adult:** PO 10 mg/day initially, then 20-40 mg/day divided bid or daily, max 80 mg/day
• **Child >50 kg:** PO 5-10 mg daily, initially, max 40 mg/day

Available forms: Tabs 10, 20, 40 mg
Administer:
• May be taken without regard to meals
• Store in tight container at ≤86° F (30° C)

SIDE EFFECTS
CNS: *Headache, dizziness,* fatigue, syncope, stroke, insomnia, weakness
CV: MI, chest pain, angina, palpitations, flushing, *hypotension,* orthostatic hypotension, tachycardia
GI: *Nausea,* constipation, *vomiting,* diarrhea, hepatotoxicity, pancreatitis, red, dry mouth, abdominal pain
GU: Sexual dysfunction, urinary frequency, renal changes
HEMA: Decreased Hct, Hgb; eosinophilia, leukopenia, neutropenia, agranulocytosis
META: *Hyperkalemia*
INTEG: Rash, urticaria, photosensitivity, pruritus
RESP: *Cough,* bronchospasm
MS: Myalgia, arthralgia
SYST: Anaphylaxis, angioedema

PHARMACOKINETICS
Peak 3 hr, protein binding 99%, half-life 11.5-14 hr, metabolized by liver (metabolites excreted in urine, feces, 50%)

INTERACTIONS
Increase: hyperkalemia risk—potassium-sparing diuretics, potassium supplements
Increase: hypotension—diuretics, other antihypertensives, ganglionic blockers, adrenergic blockers, nitrates, acute alcohol ingestion
Increase: toxicity—vasodilators, hydrALAZINE, prazosin, potassium-sparing diuretics, sympathomimetics, digoxin, lithium, NSAIDs
Decrease: absorption—antacids
Decrease: antihypertensive effect—salicylates
Drug/Herb
Increase: antihypertensive effect—hawthorn
Decrease: antihypertensive effect—ephedra
Drug/Lab Test
Increase: AST, ALT, alk phos, glucose, bilirubin, uric acid, BUN, potassium

---

False positive: urine acetone
Positive: ANA titer

NURSING CONSIDERATIONS
Assess:
• **Hypertension:** B/P, orthostatic hypotension, syncope
• **Collagen vascular disease:** neutrophils, decreased platelets; obtain WBC with differential baseline and monthly × 6 mo, then q2-3mo × 1 yr; if neutrophils <1000/mm³, discontinue

Renal studies: protein, BUN, creatinine; increased levels may indicate nephrotic syndrome
• Baselines of renal, hepatic studies before therapy begins
• Potassium levels
• **HF:** edema in feet, legs daily; weigh daily
• **Allergic reactions:** rash, fever, pruritus, urticaria; product should be discontinued if antihistamines fail to help
• Supine position for severe hypotension

Black Box Warning: **Pregnancy:** identify pregnancy before starting therapy; do not use in pregnancy, breastfeeding

Evaluate:
• Therapeutic response: decrease in B/P, decreased signs, symptoms in HF, prevention of early death due to MI, stroke
Teach patient/family:
• Not to discontinue product abruptly; to take at same time of day
• Not to use OTC products (cough, cold, allergy) unless directed by prescriber; not to use salt substitutes containing potassium without consulting prescriber
• About the importance of complying with dosage schedule, even if feeling better
• To rise slowly to sitting or standing position to minimize orthostatic hypotension
• To notify prescriber of mouth sores, sore throat, fever, swelling of hands or feet, irregular heartbeat, chest pain, nonproductive cough

• To report excessive perspiration, dehydration, vomiting, diarrhea; may lead to fall in B/P
• That product may cause dizziness, fainting, light-headedness during first few days of therapy
• That product may cause skin rash or impaired perspiration
• How to take B/P; normal readings for age group

Black Box Warning: To notify prescriber if pregnancy is planned or suspected; to use contraception during treatment

TREATMENT OF OVERDOSE:
0.9% NaCl IV infusion, hemodialysis

fosphenytoin (Rx)
(foss-fen′i-toy-in)
Cerebyx
Func. class.: Anticonvulsant
Chem. class.: Hydantoin, phosphate phenytoin ester

ACTION: Inhibits spread of seizure activity in motor cortex by altering ion transport; increases AV conduction, prodrug of phenytoin

USES: Generalized tonic-clonic seizures, status epilepticus, partial seizures

CONTRAINDICATIONS: Pregnancy, hypersensitivity, bradycardia, SA and AV block, Stokes-Adams syndrome
Precautions: Breastfeeding, allergies, renal/hepatic disease, myocardial insufficiency, hypoalbuminemia, hypothyroidism, ✦ Asian patients positive for HLA-B 1502, abrupt discontinuation, agranulocytosis, alcoholism, carBAMazepine/barbiturate hypersensitivity, bone marrow suppression, CAD, geriatric patients, hemolytic anemia, hyponatremia, methemoglobinemia, myasthenia gravis, psychosis, suicidal ideation

Black Box Warning: Dysrhythmias, hypotension (rapid IV infusion)

Side effects: *italics* = common; red = life-threatening

DOSAGE AND ROUTES

All doses in PE (phenytoin sodium equivalent)

Status epilepticus
• **Adult/child:** IV 15-20 mg PE/kg

Nonemergency/maintenance dosing
• **Adult/adolescent >16 yr:** IM/IV 10-20 mg PE/kg; 4-6 mg PE/kg/day (maintenance)

Available forms: Inj 50-mg/mL vials

Administer:

Injectable routes
• Give IM/IV; the dosage, concentration, and infusion rate of fosphenytoin should always be expressed, prescribed, and dispensed in phenytoin sodium equivalents (PE); exercise extreme caution when preparing and administering fosphenytoin; the concentration and dosage should be carefully confirmed; fatal overdoses have occurred in children when the per mL concentration of the product (50 mg PE/mL) was misinterpreted as the total amount of drug in the vial
• Visually inspect for particulate matter and discoloration before use

IV INFUSION route
• Before infusion, dilute in 5% dextrose or 0.9% saline solution to a concentration ranging from 1.5 to 25 mg PE/mL

Black Box Warning: Because of the risk of hypotension, do not exceed recommended infusion rates; continuous monitoring of ECG, B/P, and respiratory function is recommended, especially throughout the period in which phenytoin concentrations peak (about 10-20 min after the end of the infusion)

• Loading doses should always be followed by maintenance doses of oral or parenteral phenytoin or parenteral fosphenytoin

Black Box Warning: **Adult:** IV Infuse at a max rate of 150 mg PE/min; **Elderly or debilitated adults:** IV Infuse at a max 3 mg PE/kg/min or 150 mg PE/min, whichever is less; **Child:** IV Infuse at a rate of 0.5-3 mg PE/kg/min or max 150 mg PE/min, whichever is less; **Infant/neonate:** IV Infuse at a rate max 0.5-3 mg PE/kg/min

Y-site compatibilities: Aminocaproic acid, amphotericin B lipid complex, amphotericin B liposome, anidulafungin, atenolol, bivalirudin, bleomycin, CARBOplatin, CISplatin, cyclophosphamide, cytarabine, DACTINomycin, DAPTOmycin, dexmedetomidine, diltiazem, DOCEtaxel, doxacurium, eptifibatide, ertapenem, etoposide, fludarabine, fluorouracil, gatifloxacin, gemcitabine, gemtuzumab, granisetron, ifosfamide, levofloxacin, linezolid, LORazepam, mechlorethamine, meperidine, methotrexate, metroNIDAZOLE, nesiritide, octreotide, oxaliplatin, oxytocin, PACLitaxel, palonosetron, pamidronate, pantoprazole, PEMEtrexed, PHENobarbital, piperacillin-tazobactam, rocuronium, sodium acetate, tacrolimus, teniposide, thiotepa, tigecycline, tirofiban, vinCRIStine, vinorelbine, voriconazole, zoledronic acid

SIDE EFFECTS

CNS: *Drowsiness,* dizziness, insomnia, paresthesias, depression, suicidal tendencies, aggression, headache, confusion, paresthesia, emotional lability, syncope, cerebral edema

CV: Hypo/hypertension, HF, shock, dysrhythmias

EENT: Nystagmus, diplopia, blurred vision

GI: Nausea, vomiting, diarrhea, constipation, anorexia, weight loss, hepatitis, jaundice, gingival hyperplasia

HEMA: Agranulocytosis, leukopenia, aplastic anemia, thrombocytopenia, megaloblastic anemia

INTEG: Rash, lupus erythematosus, Stevens-Johnson syndrome, hirsutism, hypersensitivity, pruritus

RESP: Bronchospasm, cough

SYST: Hyperglycemia, hypokalemia, ✿❀ SJS/TEN ✿❀ in Asian patients positive for HLA-B 1502; drug reaction with eosinophilia and systemic symptoms (DRESS), purple glove syndrome, anaphylaxis

PHARMACOKINETICS

Metabolized by liver, excreted by kidneys (minimal), protein binding 95%-99%, rapidly converted to phenytoin, distributed to CSF, tissue, crosses placenta;

half-life 15 min; IM: onset unknown, peak 30 min, duration 24 hr, IV onset 15-45 min, peak 15-60 min, duration 24 hr

INTERACTIONS

Increase: fosphenytoin level—cimetidine, amiodarone, chloramphenicol, estrogens, H₂ antagonists, phenothiazines, salicylates, sulfonamides, tricyclics, CYP1A2 inhibitors

Decrease: fosphenytoin effects—alcohol (chronic use), antihistamines, antacids, traMADol, antineoplastics, rifampin, folic acid, carBAMazepine, theophylline, CYP1A2 inducers

Decrease: virologic response, resistance—delavirdine; do not use concurrently

Drug/Herb
Increase: anticonvulsant effect—ginkgo
Decrease: anticonvulsant effect—ginseng, valerian

Drug/Lab Test
Increase: glucose, alk phos
Decrease: dexamethasone, metyrapone test serum, PBI, urinary steroids, potassium

NURSING CONSIDERATIONS
Assess:

Black Box Warning: **Rapid IV infusion:** risk of hypotension and dysrhythmias with rapid infusion rates

• Seizure activity, including type, location, duration, character; provide seizure precautions
• Drug level: target level 10-20 mcg/mL, toxic level 30-50 mcg/mL, wait >2 hr after dose before testing, 4 hr after IM dose; phenytoin blood levels are used for this product
• Blood studies: CBC, platelets q2wk until stabilized, then monthly × 12 mo, then q3mo; serum calcium, albumin, phosphorus, potassium
• **Mental status:** mood, sensorium, affect, memory (long, short), suicidal thoughts/behaviors
• **Serious skin reactions:** usually occurring within 28 days of treatment; if a rash develops, patient should be evaluated for DRESS

• **Pregnancy, breastfeeding:** do not use in pregnancy; birth defects have occurred; avoid breastfeeding
• Renal studies: urinalysis, BUN, urine creatinine
• Hepatic studies: ALT, AST, bilirubin, creatinine
• Allergic reaction: red, raised rash; product should be discontinued
• **Toxicity/bone marrow depression:** nausea, vomiting, ataxia, diplopia, cardiovascular collapse, slurred speech, confusion
• Respiratory depression: rate, depth, character of respirations
• Blood dyscrasias: fever, sore throat, bruising, rash, jaundice
• Continuous monitoring of ECG, B/P, respiratory function
• **Rash:** discontinue as soon as rash develops; serious adverse reactions such as Stevens-Johnson syndrome can occur

Evaluate:
• Therapeutic response: decrease in severity of seizures

Teach patient/family:
• About the reason for, expected outcomes of treatment
• Not to use machinery or engage in hazardous activity, since drowsiness, dizziness may occur
• To carry emergency ID denoting product use, name of prescriber
• To notify prescriber of rash, bleeding, bruising, slurred speech, jaundice of skin or eyes, joint pain, nausea, vomiting, severe headaches, depression, suicidal thoughts
• To keep all medical appointments, including those for lab work, physical assessment
• To notify prescriber if pregnancy is planned or suspected; not to use in pregnancy; to avoid breastfeeding
• To use contraception while using this product

fostamatinib
(fos'-tuh-ma'-tih-nib)
Tavalisse
Func. class.: Antihemorrhagics

Side effects: *italics* = common; red = life-threatening

USES: Thrombocytopenia in chronic idiopathic thrombocytopenic purpura (ITP) in patients who have had an insufficient response to previous treatment

CONTRAINDICATIONS: Hypersensitivity

DOSAGE AND ROUTES
• **Adult: PO** 100 mg bid. If platelet count has not increased to at least $50 \times 10^9/L$ after 1 mo, increase to 150 mg bid

---

fremanezumab
(free-ma-nez′ ue-mab)

Ajovy

Func. class.: Antimigraine agent
Chem. class.: Calcitonin gene-related peptide (CGRP) antagonist

---

ACTION: Binds to the calcitonin gene-related peptide (CGRP) receptor and antagonizes CGRP receptor function

USES: Migraine prophylaxis

CONTRAINDICATIONS: Hypersensitivity

Precautions: Breastfeeding, pregnancy

DOSAGE AND ROUTES
• **Adult: SUBCUT** 225 mg monthly or 675 mg q3mo

Available forms: 225 mg/1.5 mL prefilled syringe sol for injection

Administer:
SUBCUT route
• When switching between monthly and quarterly dosage options, give the first dose of the new regimen on the next scheduled date of administration
• Visually inspect for particulates, discoloration before use; do not use if solution is cloudy, discolored, or contains particles; product is clear to opalescent, colorless to slightly yellow
• Provide proper training to patients and/or caregivers on how to prepare and give product
• Allow to sit at room temperature ≥30 min, protect from direct sunlight, do not shake

• Clean injection site on the abdomen, thigh, or upper arm with an alcohol wipe, and allow skin to dry
• Do not inject into areas where skin is tender, bruised, red, or hard. Avoid injecting directly into raised, thick, red, or scaly skin patch or lesion, or into areas with scars or stretch marks
• If using the same body area for the 3 separate injections needed for the 675-mg dose, do not use the same location used for the previous injection
• Do not coadminister with other injectable drugs at the same injection site
• If a dose is missed, give the next dose as soon as possible
• **Storage:** After removing from refrigerator, may be stored at room temperature up to 77° F (25° C) for ≤24 hr; discard if not used within 24 hr after removal from refrigerator

Single-dose prefilled syringe
• Pinch injection site skin firmly between thumb and fingers
• Hold, insert syringe at a 45- to 90-degree angle for administration

SIDE EFFECTS
INTEG: Injection site reaction, rash, urticaria, pruritus, erythema
MISC: Antibody formation

PHARMACOKINETICS
Half-life 31 days, peak 5-7 days

INTERACTIONS
None known.

NURSING CONSIDERATIONS
Assess:
• **Migraine:** pain, location, intensity, duration, photophobia in the past; assess response to preventing migraine after use of this product
• Injection site reaction, rash, urticaria, pruritus, erythema; may indicate allergic reactions
• **Pregnancy/breastfeeding:** identify if pregnancy is planned or suspected, or if breastfeeding; no adequate studies are available

---

Evaluate:
• Therapeutic response: prevention of migraine

Teach patient/family:
• How to self-administer product
• Not to double, skip doses; when switching between monthly and quarterly dosage options, to give the first dose of the new regimen on the next scheduled date of administration
• To report injection site reaction, rash, itching; may indicate allergic reaction

---

frovatriptan (Rx)

(froh-vah-trip´tan)

Frova

Func. class.: Antimigraine agent
Chem. class.: 5-HT₁-Receptor agonist

ACTION: Binds selectively to the vascular 5-HT$_{1B}$, 5-HT$_{1D}$ receptor subtypes; exerts antimigraine effect; binds to benzodiazepine receptor sites, causes vasoconstriction in cranium

USES: Acute treatment of migraine with/without aura

CONTRAINDICATIONS: Hypersensitivity, angina pectoris, history of MI, documented silent ischemia, Prinzmetal's angina, ischemic heart disease; concurrent ergotamine-containing preparations; uncontrolled hypertension; basilar or hemiplegic migraine; ischemic bowel disease; peripheral vascular disease, severe hepatic disease, prophylactic migraine treatment

Precautions: Pregnancy, breastfeeding, children, geriatric patients, postmenopausal women, men >40 yr, risk factors for CAD, hypercholesterolemia, obesity, diabetes, impaired hepatic function, seizure disorder

DOSAGE AND ROUTES
• **Adult: PO** 2.5 mg; a 2nd dose may be taken after ≥2 hr; max 3 tabs (7.5 mg/day)

Available form: Tabs 2.5 mg

Administer:
• Swallow tabs whole; do not break, crush, or chew
• With fluids
• 2 days/wk or less; rebound headache may occur

SIDE EFFECTS
CNS: *Hot/cold sensation,* paresthesia, *dizziness,* headache, fatigue, insomnia, anxiety, somnolence, seizures
CV: *Flushing,* chest pain, palpitation, coronary artery vasospasm, MI, myocardial ischemia, ventricular tachycardia, ventricular fibrillation
GI: Dry mouth, dyspepsia, abdominal pain, diarrhea, vomiting, nausea
MS: Skeletal pain

PHARMACOKINETICS
Onset of pain relief 2-3 hr, terminal half-life 25-29 hr, protein binding 15%, metabolized in liver by CYP1A2

INTERACTIONS
Increase: frovatriptan levels—CYP1A2 inhibitors (cimetidine, ciprofloxacin, erythromycin), estrogen, propranolol, hormonal contraceptives
Increase: toxicity—SSRIs, other serotonin agonists (dextromethorphan, MAOIs, antidepressants)

NURSING CONSIDERATIONS
Assess:
• **Migraine symptoms:** aura, unable to view light; ingestion of tyramine-containing foods (pickled products, beer, wine, aged cheese), food additives, preservatives, colorings, artificial sweeteners, chocolate, caffeine, which may precipitate these types of headaches
• Serious cardiac reactions: may occur within a few hours of taking a 5-HT1 agent; dysrhythmias, ventricular tachycardia, ventricular fibrillation leading to death
• B/P; signs, symptoms of coronary vasospasms
• For stress level, activity, recreation, coping mechanisms
• Quiet, calm environment with decreased stimulation from noise, bright light, excessive talking

---

Side effects: *italics* = common; red = life-threatening

• **Serotonin syndrome:** agitation, confusion, diaphoresis, increased B/P, nausea, vomiting, diarrhea; product should be discontinued

• **Pregnancy/breastfeeding:** use only if benefit outweighs fetal risk; do not breastfeed, excretion unknown

Evaluate:

• Therapeutic response: decrease in frequency, severity of migraine

Teach patient/family:

• To report any side effects to prescriber
• To inform prescriber if pregnant or planning to become pregnant
• To consult prescriber if breastfeeding
• **Serious cardiac reactions:** to report immediately pain, chest tightness
• **Serotonin syndrome:** to report agitation, confusion, sweating, nausea, vomiting, diarrhea
• **Short-term use only:** That abortive migraine agents used >10 days/mo may lead to a worsening of headaches, medication overuse

---

⚠ HIGH ALERT

RARELY USED

fulvestrant (Rx)

(full-vess′trant)

Faslodex

Func. class.: Antineoplastic

Chem. class.: Estrogen-receptor antagonist

USES: Advanced breast carcinoma in estrogen receptor–positive patients (usually postmenopausal)

Unlabeled uses: Loading dose for metastatic breast cancer

CONTRAINDICATIONS: Pregnancy, breastfeeding, children, hypersensitivity

DOSAGE AND ROUTES

• **Adult:** IM 500 mg as two 5-mL injections on days 1, 15, 29, and monthly thereafter

---

furosemide (Rx)

(fur-oh′se-mide)

Lasix, Lasix special ✙

Func. class.: Loop diuretic

Chem. class.: Sulfonamide derivative

Do not confuse:

furosemide/torsemide

Lasix/Luvox/Lomotil/Lanoxin/Losec

ACTION: Inhibits reabsorption of sodium and chloride at proximal and distal tubule and in the loop of Henle

USES: Pulmonary edema; edema with HF, hepatic disease, nephrotic syndrome, ascites, hypertension

CONTRAINDICATIONS: Anuria

Precautions: Pregnancy, breastfeeding, diabetes mellitus, dehydration, severe renal disease, cirrhosis, ascites, hypersensitivity to sulfonamides/thiazides, infants, hypovolemia, electrolyte depletion, hypersensitivity

DOSAGE AND ROUTES

Acute pulmonary edema

• **Adult:** IV 40 mg slowly over 2 min, then 80 mg in 60-90 min if needed, max 200 mg/dose

Edema

• **Adult:** PO 20-80 mg/day in AM; may give another dose after 6 hr up to 600 mg/day; **IM/IV** 20-40 mg; increase by 20 mg q2hr until desired response

• **Child:** PO/IM/IV 1-2 mg/kg; may increase by 1-2 mg/kg q6-8hr up to 6 mg/kg

Hypertension

• **Adult:** PO 40 mg bid, adjust based on response

Available forms: Tabs 20, 40, 80 mg; oral sol 8 mg/mL, 10 mg/mL; inj 10 mg/mL

Administer:

• In AM to avoid interference with sleep if using product as diuretic

• Potassium replacement if potassium <3 mg/dL

PO route

• PO with food if nausea occurs; absorption may be decreased slightly; tabs may be crushed

---

✙ Canada only

⚛ Genetic warning

IV route
• Undiluted; may be given through Y-tube or 3-way stopcock; give ≤20 mg/min

Intermittent IV INFUSION route
• May be added to NS or D₅W; if large doses required and given as IV infusion, max 4 mg/min; use infusion pump

Y-site compatibilities: Acyclovir, alfentanil, allopurinol, alprostadil, amifostine, amikacin, aminocaproic acid, aminophylline, amphotericin B cholesteryl/lipid complex/liposome, anidulafungin, argatroban, ascorbic acid, atenolol, atropine, azaTHIOprine, aztreonam, bivalirudin, bleomycin, bumetanide, calcium chloride/gluconate, CARBOplatin, cefamandole, ceFAZolin, cefepime, cefonicid, cefotaxime, cefoTEtan, cefOXitin, cefTAZidime, ceftizoxime, ceftobiprole, cefTRIAXone, cefuroxime, chloramphenicol, CISplatin, cladribine, clindamycin, cyanocobalamin, cyclophosphamide, cycloSPORINE, cytarabine, DACTINomycin, DAPTOmycin, dexamethasone, dexmedetomidine, digoxin, DOCEtaxel, doripenem, doxacurium, DOXOrubicin liposome, enalaprilat, ePHEDrine, EPINEPHrine, etoposide, fentaNYL, fludarabine, fluorouracil, folic acid, foscarnet, gallium nitrate, ganciclovir, granisetron, heparin, hydrocortisone, HYDROmorphone, ifosfamide, imipenemcilastatin, indomethacin, insulin (regular), isosorbide, kanamycin, leucovorin, lidocaine, linezolid, LORazepam, LR, mannitol, mechlorethamine, melphalan, meropenem, methicillin, methotrexate, methylPREDNISolone, metoprolol, metroNIDAZOLE, mezlocillin, micafungin, miconazole, mitoMYcin, moxalactam, multiple vitamin injection, nafcillin, naloxone, nitroprusside, octreotide, oxacillin, oxaliplatin, oxytocin, PACLitaxel, palonosetron, pamidronate, pantoprazole, PEMEtrexed, penicillin G, PENTobarbital, PHENobarbital, phytonadione, piperacillin, piperacillin-tazobactam, potassium chloride, procainamide, propofol, propranolol, ranitidine, remifentanil, Ringer's, ritodrine, sargramostim, sodium acetate/bicarbonate, succinylcholine, SUFentanil, temocillin, teniposide, theophylline, thiopental, thiotepa, ticarcillin, ticarcillin-clavulanate, tigecycline, tirofiban, TNA, tobramycin, urokinase, vit B/C, voriconazole, zoledronic acid

SIDE EFFECTS
CNS: Headache, fatigue, weakness, vertigo, paresthesias
CV: Orthostatic hypotension, chest pain, ECG changes, circulatory collapse
EENT: Loss of hearing, ear pain, tinnitus, blurred vision
ELECT: *Hypokalemia, hypochloremic alkalosis, hypomagnesemia, hyperuricemia, hypocalcemia, hyponatremia,* metabolic alkalosis
ENDO: *Hyperglycemia*
GI: *Nausea,* diarrhea, dry mouth, vomiting, anorexia, cramps, oral, gastric irritations, pancreatitis
GU: *Polyuria,* renal failure, glycosuria, bladder spasms
HEMA: Thrombocytopenia, agranulocytosis, leukopenia, neutropenia, anemia
INTEG: *Rash, pruritus,* purpura, sweating, photosensitivity, urticaria
MS: Cramps, stiffness
SYST: Toxic epidermal necrolysis, erythema multiforme, Stevens-Johnson syndrome

PHARMACOKINETICS
PO: Onset 1 hr, peak 1-2 hr, duration 6-8 hr, absorbed 70%
IV: Onset 5 min; peak ½ hr; duration 2 hr (metabolized by the liver 30%); excreted in urine, some as unchanged product, and feces; crosses placenta, enters breast milk; excreted in breast milk; half-life ½-1 hr, protein binding 90%-99%

INTERACTIONS
Increase: toxicity—lithium, nondepolarizing skeletal muscle relaxants, digoxin, salicylates, aminoglycosides, CISplatin
Increase: hypotensive action of antihypertensives, nitrates
Increase: ototoxicity—aminoglycosides, CISplatin, vancomycin
Increase: effects of anticoagulants, salicylates

Side effects: *italics* = common; red = life-threatening

Decrease: furosemide effect—probenecid

Drug/Lab Test
Interference: GTT
Increase: LDL

NURSING CONSIDERATIONS
Assess:
• **HF:** weight, I&O daily to determine fluid loss; effect of product may be decreased if used daily
• **Hypertension:** B/P lying, standing; postural hypotension may occur; assess for fall risk in older adults, and implement fall prevention strategies
• Metabolic alkalosis: drowsiness, restlessness
• **Hypokalemia:** postural hypotension, malaise, fatigue, tachycardia, leg cramps, weakness; assess those who are also taking digoxin for digoxin toxicity due to hypokalemia
• Rashes, temperature elevation daily
• Confusion, especially in geriatric patients; take safety precautions if needed
• **Hearing,** including tinnitus and hearing loss, when giving high doses for extended periods or rapid infusion
• Rate, depth, rhythm of respiration, effect of exertion, lung sounds
• Electrolytes (potassium, sodium, chloride); include BUN, blood glucose, CBC, serum creatinine, blood pH, ABGs, uric acid
• Glucose in urine if patient diabetic
• Allergies to sulfonamides, thiazides
• **Serious rash:** monitor for skin rash often; Stevens-Johnson syndrome, toxic epidermal necrolysis, erythema multiforme may occur and are life threatening
• **Beers:** use with caution in older adults; may exacerbate or cause syndrome of inappropriate antidiuretic hormone secretion or hyponatremia; monitor sodium level closely when changing doses
• **Pregnancy/breastfeeding:** use only if benefit outweighs fetal risks; do not breastfeed, excretion unknown

Evaluate:
• Therapeutic response: improvement in edema of feet, legs, sacral area (HF); increased urine output, decreased B/P; decreased calcium levels (hypercalcemia)

Teach patient/family:
• To discuss the need for a high-potassium diet or potassium replacement with prescriber
• To rise slowly from lying or sitting position because orthostatic hypotension may occur; teach fall prevention strategies
• To recognize adverse reactions that may occur: muscle cramps, weakness, nausea, dizziness; teach diabetic patients to monitor blood glucose carefully; blood glucose levels can be elevated
• About the entire treatment regimen, including exercise, diet, stress relief for hypertension
• To contact prescriber if rash, cramps, nausea, dizziness, numbness, weakness occur
• To take with food or milk for GI symptoms
• To use sunscreen or protective clothing to prevent photosensitivity
• To take early in the day to prevent sleeplessness
• To avoid OTC medications unless directed by prescriber

TREATMENT OF OVERDOSE:
Lavage if taken orally; monitor electrolytes; administer dextrose in saline; monitor hydration, CV, renal status

gabapentin (Rx)

(gab′a-pen-tin)

Gralise, Horizant, Neurontin

Func. class.: Anticonvulsant

Chem. class.: GABA analogue

Do not confuse:

Neurontin/Noroxin/Motrin

ACTION: Mechanism unknown; may increase seizure threshold; structurally similar to GABA but does not bind to GABAa or GABAb; gabapentin binding sites in neocortex, hippocampus

USES: Adjunct treatment of partial seizures, with/without generalization in patients >12 yr; adjunct for partial seizures in children 3-12 yr, postherpetic neuralgia, primary restless legs syndrome in adults

Unlabeled uses: Neuropathic pain, bipolar disorder, migraine prophylaxis, fibromyalgia anxiety

CONTRAINDICATIONS: Hypersensitivity to this product

Precautions: Pregnancy, breastfeeding, children <3 yr, geriatric patients, renal disease, hemodialysis, suicidal thoughts, depression

DOSAGE AND ROUTES

Adjunctive use in partial seizures with or without secondary generalized tonic-clonic seizures (Neurontin only)

• **Adult/child >12 yr: PO** 300 mg tid; may titrate to 1800 mg/day in 3 divided doses

• **Child 3-12 yr: PO** 10-15 mg/kg/day in 3 divided doses, initially titrate dose upward over approximately 3 days; if >5 yr old, use 25-35 mg/kg/day; if 3-4 yr old, 40 mg/kg/day divided in 3 doses

Postherpetic neuralgia (PHN)

• **Adult: PO** (Neurontin) 300 mg on day 1, 600 mg daily divided bid on day 2, 900 mg/day on day 3 divided tid, may titrate to 1800-3600 mg divided tid if needed; **EXT REL** (Gralise only) 300 mg on day 1, 600 mg on day 2, 900 mg on days 3-6, 1200 mg on days 7-10, 1500 mg on days 11-14, 1800 mg on day 15 and thereafter; (Horizant only) 600 mg in AM × 3 days, day 4 give 600 mg bid

Moderate to severe restless legs syndrome (RLS) (Horizant only)

• **Adult: PO EXT REL** 600 mg daily with food at about 5 PM; if dose missed, take next day at 5 PM

Fibromyalgia (unlabeled)

• **Adult: PO** 300 mg at bedtime × 1 wk, then gradually increase (target dose 2400 mg), 300 mg bid × 1 wk, 300 mg bid and 600 mg at bedtime × 2 wk, then 600 mg bid × 2 wk with 1200 mg at bedtime; to discontinue, taper by 300 mg/day

Diabetic neuropathy pain (unlabeled)

• **Adult: PO** 900 mg-3.6 g/day in divided doses tid

Renal dose

• **Adult/child >12 yr: PO IMM REL** CCr ≥60 mL/min: no change; CCr >30-59 mL/min: total dose range 400-1400 mg/day given divided bid; CCr >15-29 mL/min: total dose range 200-700 mg/day PO given in a single daily dose; CCr = 15 mL/min: total dose range 100-300 mg/day given in one daily dose as 100, 125, 150, 200, or 300 mg; CCr <15 mL/min: reduce daily dose in proportion to CCr (CCr = 7.5 mL/min should receive half the dose that patients with CCr = 15 mL/min receive)

• **Adult: PO EXT REL tablets (Gralise tablets only):** CCr ≥60 mL/min: no change; CCr 30-59 mL/min: 600-1800 mg/day as tolerated; CCr <30 mL/min: do not use; **ext-rel tablets (Horizant tablets only)** CCr ≥60 mL/min: no change; before discontinuing, reduce the dose to 600 mg daily × 1 wk; CCr 30-59 mL/min: for RLS, start at 300 mg/day, increase to 600 mg/day as needed, for PHN, start at 300 mg in the AM × 3 days, then increase to 300 mg bid, increase to 600 mg bid as needed; for dose tapering before discontinuation, reduce the maintenance dose to daily in the AM × 1 wk before discontinuing; CCr 15-29 mL/min: for RLS, 300 mg/day; for PHN, 300 mg PO on days 1 and 3, then 300 mg daily in the AM, increase dose to 300 mg bid as needed, for dose tapering, if dose is 300 mg bid, reduce dose to 300 mg daily in AM × 1 wk before discontinuation; if the dose is 300 mg daily, no taper is required; CCr <15 mL/min: for RLS and PHN, 300 mg every other day; for PHN, dose can be increased to 300 mg daily in AM; no dose taper is required before discontinuing

Uremic pruritus in hemodialysis (unlabeled)
• **Adult: PO** 300 mg 3×/wk or 400 mg 2×/wk, at end of hemodialysis × 4 wk

Brachioradial pruritus (unlabeled)
• **Adult: PO** 300-1800 mg/day

ALS (unlabeled)
• **Adult: PO** 1000 mg/day in divided doses × 6 mo

Pendular/congenital nystagmus (unlabeled)
• **Adult: PO** 900 mg/day in divided doses initially, up to 2400 mg/day in divided doses

Spasticity in MS (unlabeled)
• **Adult: PO** 600-1200 mg/day in divided doses

Available forms: Caps 100, 300, 400 mg; tabs 600, 800 mg; Horizant: ext rel tab 300, 600 mg; oral sol 250 mg/5 mL; ext rel tab (Gralise): 300, 600 mg

Administer:
• Do not crush or chew caps, ext rel tabs; caps may be opened and contents put in applesauce or dissolved in juice; scored tabs may be cut in half
• 2 hr apart when giving antacids
• Give without regard to meals (immediate release)
• Gradually withdraw over 7 days; abrupt withdrawal may precipitate seizures
• Beginning dose at bedtime to minimize daytime drowsiness
• **Oral sol:** measure with calibrated device, refrigerate
• **Ext rel:** give with food at about 5 PM; bioavailability increased with food; swallow whole; do not interchange Gralise with Horizant
• Store at room temperature away from heat and light

SIDE EFFECTS
CNS: Dizziness, fatigue, somnolence, ataxia, amnesia, abnormal thinking, *depression;* children 3-12 yr old, emotional lability, aggression, thought disorder, hyperkinesia, hostility
CV: Vasodilation, peripheral edema
EENT: Dry mouth, blurred vision, *diplopia,* nystagmus, otitis media (child 3-12 yr)
GI: Constipation/diarrhea, weight gain, increased appetite, nausea, vomiting; diarrhea (Gralise)
GU: Impotence, *UTI*
HEMA: Leukopenia
INTEG: Pruritus, abrasion, acne vulgaris
MS: Myalgia, back pain, gout
RESP: Cough, upper respiratory infection (child 3-12 yr)
SYST: Drug reaction with eosinophilia and systemic symptoms (DRESS); dehydration (child 3-12 yr)

PHARMACOKINETICS
Protein binding <3% not metabolized; excreted in urine (unchanged); elimination half-life 5-7 hr; immediate release peak 2 hr, ext rel peak 8 hr (Gralise); 5-7 hr (Horizant)

INTERACTIONS
Increase: CNS depression—alcohol, sedatives, antihistamines, all other CNS depressants; monitor for CNS depression
Decrease: gabapentin levels—antacids, sevelamer, cimetidine; separate by 2 hr
Increase: effect of—HYDROcodone; dosage reduction may be needed

Drug/Herb
Increased: CNS depression—chamomile, kava, valerian

Drug/Lab Test
False positive: urinary protein using Ames N-multistix SG

NURSING CONSIDERATIONS
Assess:
• **Seizures:** aura, location, duration, frequency, activity at onset
• **Neuropathic Pain:** location, duration, characteristics if using for chronic pain, migraine

• **RLS:** restless leg syndrome characteristics baseline and periodically
• **Migraine:** characteristics baseline and periodically
• Mental status: mood, sensorium, affect, behavioral changes, **suicidal thoughts/behaviors;** if mental status changes, notify prescriber
• WBC, gabapentin level (therapeutic 5.9-21 mcg/mL, toxic >85 mcg/mL), serum creatinine/BUN, weight
• Drug reaction with eosinophilia and systemic symptoms
• **Seizure precautions:** padded side rails; move objects that may harm patient (Gralise)
• Increased fluids, bulk in diet for constipation
• **Beers:** avoid in older adults unless safer alternative is unavailable; ataxia, impaired psychomotor function may occur
• **Pregnancy/breastfeeding:** use only if benefits outweigh fetal risk

Evaluate:
• Therapeutic response: decreased seizure activity; decrease in chronic pain

Teach patient/family:
• To carry emergency ID stating patient's name, products taken, condition, prescriber's name and phone number
• To avoid driving, other activities that require alertness because dizziness, drowsiness may occur
• **Seizures:** not to discontinue medication quickly after long-term use; to taper over ≥1 wk because withdrawal-precipitated seizures may occur; not to double doses if dose is missed; to take if 2 hr or more before next dose
• To report changes in vision, diplopia, eye irritation to provider
• To notify providers of use before surgery
• To take as prescribed; not to interchange formulations; that ext rel product should not be crushed or chewed, if tablet is to be broken in half, use within 28 days or discard
• To report suicidal thoughts or feelings, increased depression, panic attacks, hostility, confusion to provider

• Not to use within 2 hr of antacid, may take regular release without regard to meals; ext rel should be taken with food; to take as directed, doses interval should not be ≥12 hr
• To keep oral solution refrigerated
• To notify prescriber if pregnancy is planned or suspected; to avoid breastfeeding

---

galantamine (Rx)
(gah-lan′tah-meen)
Razadyne, Razadyne ER, Reminyl ✦
Func. class.: Anti-Alzheimer agent
Chem. class.: Centrally acting cholinesterase inhibitor

Do not confuse:
Razadyne/Rozerem

ACTION: Enhances cholinergic functioning by increasing acetylcholine in cerebral cortex

USES: Mild to moderate dementia of Alzheimer's disease, dementia with Lewy bodies
Unlabeled uses: Vascular dementia, Pick's disease

CONTRAINDICATIONS: Hypersensitivity to this product, GI bleeding, jaundice, renal failure, children
Precautions: Pregnancy, geriatric patients, respiratory/renal/hepatic/cardiac disease, seizure disorder, peptic ulcer, asthma, bradycardia, heart block, surgery, urinary tract obstruction, breastfeeding

DOSAGE AND ROUTES
• **Adult: PO** 4 mg bid with morning and evening meals; after 4 wk or more, may increase to 8 mg bid; may increase to 12 mg bid after another 4 wk, usual dose 16-24 mg/day in 2 divided doses; **EXT REL** 8 mg/day in AM; may increase to 16 mg/day after 4 wk and 24 mg/day after another 4 wk
Hepatic dose
• **Adult: PO** Child-Pugh 7-9, max 16 mg/day; Child-Pugh 10-15, avoid use

---

Side effects: *italics* = common; red = life-threatening

Renal dose
- **Adult: PO** CCr 10-70 mL/min, max 16 mg/day; CCr <9 mL/min, avoid use

Available forms: Tabs 4, 8, 12 mg; ext rel caps 8, 16, 24 mg; oral sol 4 mg/mL

Administer:

PO route
- With meals; take with morning and evening meal (immediate rel); morning (ext rel)
- Dose increase after minimum of 4 wk at prior dose; if dose is interrupted for ≥3 days, restart at lower dose, titrate to current dose
- Ext rel in AM with food; do not crush, open, or chew
- **Oral sol:** use pipette provided, put in liquid and have patient consume

SIDE EFFECTS

CNS: *Tremors, insomnia,* depression, dizziness, headache, somnolence, fatigue
CV: Bradycardia, chest pain, AV block
GI: *Nausea, vomiting, anorexia, abdominal distress, flatulence,* diarrhea
GU: Urinary incontinence, bladder outflow obstruction, hematuria
HEMA: Anemia
INTEG: Stevens-Johnson syndrome, acute generalized exanthematous pustulosis

PHARMACOKINETICS

Rapidly and completely absorbed; metabolized by CYP2D6, 3A4; excreted via kidneys; clearance is lower in geriatric patients, hepatic disease; clearance is 20% lower in females; half-life 7 hr; 18% protein binding, peak 1 hr (regular release), 4.5-5 hr (extended release), duration (12 hr regular release); (24 hr ext rel)

INTERACTIONS

Increase: synergistic effect—cholinomimetics, other cholinesterase inhibitors; avoid concurrent use before anesthesia
Increase: galantamine effect—CYP3A4, CYP2D6 inhibitors (antiretroviral protease inhibitors, ketoconazole, conivaptan, delaviridine, diltiazem, efavirenz, fluconazole, fluvoxaMINE, imatinib, itraconazole, clarithromycin, troleandomycin, nefazodone, niCARdipine, verapamil,

zafirlukast); monitor for increased effect
Increase: neuromuscular blocking action succinylcholine like neuroblockers
Decrease: galantamine effect—CYP3A4, CYP2D6 inducers (bosentan, carBAMazepine, nevirapine, OXcarbazepine, phenytoin, fosphenytoin/rifabutin, rifampin, rifapentine, troglitazone), anticholinergics; monitor for decreased effect

Drug/Herb
Decrease: galantamine effect—St. John's wort

NURSING CONSIDERATIONS

Assess:
- **Alzheimer's disease:** mental status: affect, mood, behavioral changes, depression, attention, confusion; neurologic status: long- and short-term memory, cognitive functioning, baseline and periodically
- Hepatic/renal studies: AST, ALT, alk phos, LDH, bilirubin, CBC; BUN, creatinine
- For severe GI effects: nausea, vomiting, anorexia, weight loss; GU effects: urinary retention, bladder obstruction
- B/P, heart rate, respiration during initial treatment: bradycardia/AV block may occur
- Fluid status: ensure adequate hydration
- Assistance with ambulation
- **Pregnancy/breastfeeding:** use only if benefits outweigh fetal risk; cautious use in breastfeeding, excretion unknown

Evaluate:
- Therapeutic response: decreased confusion, increased language, ability to perform ADLs

Teach patient/family:
- To notify all prescribers of use
- About correct procedure for giving oral sol using instruction sheet provided
- To notify prescriber of severe GI effects; hypo/hypertension, slow heart rate
- That product is not a cure but relieves symptoms
- That results may take several wk or months to occur
- To take with food to minimize side effects
- To notify prescriber immediately and stop taking product if rash occurs

• **About CNS effects:** to avoid driving, other activities that require alertness until effects are known because drowsiness, dizziness may occur
• That follow-up exams will be needed
• To notify prescriber of use before surgery

---

galcanezumab

(gal-kuh-nezz'-you-mab)

Emgality

Func. class.: Antimigraine agent

Chem. class.: Calcitonin gene-related peptide (CGRP) antagonist

---

ACTION: Binds to the calcitonin gene-related peptide (CGRP) receptor and antagonizes CGRP receptor function

USES: Migraine prophylaxis

CONTRAINDICATIONS: Hypersensitivity

Precautions: Breastfeeding, pregnancy

DOSAGE AND ROUTES

• **Adult: SUBCUT** 240 mg once as a loading dose, then 120 mg monthly

Available forms: Prefilled pen or prefilled syringe 120 mg/mL sol for inj

Administer:

SUBCUT route

• Visually inspect for particulates, discoloration before use; do not use if solution is cloudy, discolored, or contains particles; product is clear to opalescent, colorless to slightly yellow
• Provide proper training to patients and/or caregivers on how to prepare and give product
• Allow to sit at room temperature ≥30 min, protect from direct sunlight, do not shake
• Clean injection site on the abdomen, thigh, or upper arm with an alcohol wipe, and allow skin to dry
• Do not inject into areas where skin is tender, bruised, red, or hard. Avoid injecting directly into raised, thick, red, or scaly skin patch or lesion, or into areas with scars or stretch marks
• If using the same body area for the 2 separate injections needed for the 240-mg dose, ensure that the second injection is not at the same location used for the first injection
• Do not coadminister with other injectable drugs at the same injection site
• If a dose is missed, give the next dose as soon as possible
• **Storage:** After removing from refrigerator, may be stored at room temperature up to 77° F (25° C) for ≤24 hr; discard if not used within 24 hr after removal from refrigerator

Single-dose prefilled syringe

• Pinch injection site skin firmly between thumb and fingers
• Hold, insert the syringe at 45- to 90-degree angle for administration

SIDE EFFECTS

INTEG: Injection site reaction, rash, urticaria, pruritus, erythema

MISC: Antibody formation, dyspnea

PHARMACOKINETICS

Half-life 27 days, peak 5 days

NURSING CONSIDERATIONS

Assess:

• **Migraine:** pain, location, intensity, duration, photophobia in the past; assess the response to preventing migraine after use of this product
• **Injection site reaction:** rash, urticaria, pruritus, erythema; may indicate allergic reactions
• **Pregnancy/breastfeeding:** identify if pregnancy is planned or suspected, or if breastfeeding; no adequate studies are available

Evaluate:

• Therapeutic response: prevention of migraine

Teach patient/family:

• How to self-administer product
• Not to double, skip doses
• To report injection site reaction, rash, itching; may indicate allergic reaction

---

ganciclovir (Rx)

(gan-sye′kloe-vir)

Cytovene, Vitrasert, Zirgan

Func. class.: Antiviral

Chem. class.: Synthetic nucleoside analog

Do not confuse:
Cytovene/Cytosar

ACTION: Inhibits replication of herpesviruses; competitively inhibits human CMV DNA polymerase and is incorporated, resulting in termination of DNA elongation

USES: Cytomegalovirus (CMV) retinitis in immunocompromised persons, including those with AIDS, after indirect ophthalmoscopy confirms diagnosis; prophylaxis for CMV in transplantation; ophthalmic: acute herpes keratitis

Unlabeled uses: CMV pneumonia in organ transplant patients; CMV gastroenteritis, esophagitis, colitis; CMV pneumonitis, congenital CMV disease; Epstein-Barr virus; herpes simplex types 1, 2; varicella-zoster, hepatitis B

CONTRAINDICATIONS: Hypersensitivity to acyclovir, ganciclovir

Black Box Warning: Absolute neutrophil count <500/mm³, platelet count <25,000/mm³ (intravitreal)

Precautions: breastfeeding, children <6 mo, geriatric patients, preexisting cytopenias, renal function impairment, radiation therapy, hypersensitivity to famciclovir, penciclovir, valacyclovir, valganciclovir

Black Box Warning: Secondary malignancy, bone marrow suppression, anemia, infertility, neutropenia, pregnancy, male-mediated teratogenicity

DOSAGE AND ROUTES
Prevention of CMV
• **Adult/adolescent:** IV 5 mg/kg/dose over 1 hr q12hr × 1-2 wk, then 5 mg/kg/ day 7 day/wk, or 6 mg/kg/day × 5 days/ wk; **PO** 1000 mg tid starting 10 days posttransplant × 14 wk

Induction treatment
• **Adult:** IV 5 mg/kg/dose given over 1 hr, q12hr × 2-3 wk

Maintenance treatment
• **Adult:** IV INFUSION 5 mg/kg/dose given over 1 hr, daily × 7 days/wk or 6 mg/kg/day × 5 days/wk; **PO** 1000 mg tid with food or 500 mg q3hr while awake for 6 doses; **INTRAVITREAL** 4.5 mg implant

Acute herpes keratitis
• **Adult/adolescent/child ≥2 yr: OPHTH** 1 drop in affected eye 5 times daily

Renal dose
• **Adult:** IV CCr 50-69 mL/min, reduce to 2.5 mg/kg q12hr (induction), 2.5 mg/kg q24hr (maintenance); **PO** 1500 mg/day or 500 mg tid; IV CCr 25-49 mL/min, reduce to 2.5 mg/ kg (induction); 1.25 mg/kg q24hr (maintenance); **PO** 1000 mg/day or 500 mg bid; IV CCr 10-24 mL/min, reduce to 1.25 mg/kg q24hr (induction); 0.625 mg/kg q24hr (maintenance); **PO** 500 mg/day; IV CCr <10 mL/min, reduce to 1.25 mg/kg 3×/wk after hemodialysis (induction); 0.625 mg/kg 3×/ wk after hemodialysis (maintenance); **PO** 500 mg 3×/wk after hemodialysis

Available forms: Powder for inj 500 mg/ vial; caps 250, 500 mg; implant, intravitreal 4.5 mg; ophth gel 0.15% (Zirgan)

Administer:
PO route
• With food and a full glass of water
• Do not open, crush capsules

IV route
• Mixed in biologic cabinet using gown, gloves, mask; use cytotoxic handling procedures; do not use if particulate matter is present

Intermittent IV INFUSION route
• IV after reconstituting 500 mg/10 mL sterile water for inj (50 mg/mL); shake; further dilute in 50-250 mL D₅W, 0.9% NaCl, LR, Ringer's and run over 1 hr; use infusion pump, use in-line filter, flush line well before and after product
• Do not give by bolus IV, IM, SUBCUT inj
• Use reconstituted sol within 24 hr; do not refrigerate or freeze

Y-site compatibilities: Allopurinol, amphotericin B cholesteryl, CISplatin, cyclophosphamide, DOXOrubicin liposome, enalaprilat, etoposide, filgrastim, fluconazole, gatifloxacin, granisetron, linezolid, melphalan, methotrexate, PACLitaxel, propofol, remifentanil, tacrolimus, teniposide, thiotepa

SIDE EFFECTS

CNS: *Fever,* chills, coma, *confusion,* abnormal thoughts, dizziness, bizarre dreams, *headache,* psychosis, tremors, somnolence, *paresthesia,* *weakness,* seizures, peripheral neuropathy
CV: Dysrhythmia, hypo/hypertension
EENT: Retinal detachment in CMV retinitis, ocular hypertension, ocular pain, conjunctival scarring, cataracts
GI: *Abnormal LFTs, nausea, vomiting, anorexia, diarrhea, abdominal pain,* hemorrhage, perforation, pancreatitis
GU: Hematuria, *increased creatinine,* BUN, infertility, decreased sperm count
HEMA: Granulocytopenia, thrombocytopenia, irreversible neutropenia, anemia, eosinophilia, pancytopenia
INTEG: *Rash,* alopecia, *pruritus,* urticaria, pain at site, phlebitis
RESP: Dyspnea, pneumonia

PHARMACOKINETICS

Half-life 3-4½ hr; excreted by kidneys (unchanged); crosses blood-brain barrier, CSF, increased bioavailability with fatty foods, minimal protein binding, onset rapid, peak infusions end, duration up to 24 hr

INTERACTIONS

Increase: severe granulocytopenia—zidovudine, antineoplastics, radiation; do not give together
Increase: ganciclovir toxicity—adriamycin, amphotericin B, cycloSPORINE, dapsone, DOXOrubicin, flucytosine, pentamidine, probenecid, trimethoprim-sulfamethoxazole combinations, vinBLAStine, vinCRIStine, other nucleoside analogs, mycophenolate, tenofovir, tacrolimus, aminoglycosides, NSAIDs
Increase: seizures—imipenem/cilastatin

Increase: didanosine effect—didanosine
Drug/Lab Test
Increase: LFTs, creatinine
Decrease: Hgb, WBC, platelets, neutrophils, granulocytes

NURSING CONSIDERATIONS
Assess:

Black Box Warning: **Secondary malignancy:** avoid direct contact with powder in caps/solution; if skin contact occurs, wash thoroughly with soap and water; do not get in the eyes

• **CMV retinitis:** Culture of blood, urine, and throat may be taken, CMV is not confirmed by this method; ophthalmic exam confirms diagnosis, these exams should be done baseline weekly (induction), q2wk (maintenance)
• **Infection:** Increased temperature, sore throat, chills, fever; report to prescriber

Black Box Warning: **Leukopenia/neutropenia/thrombocytopenia:** CBC, WBCs, platelets q2days during 2×/day dosing and then q1wk for leukopenia with daily WBC count in patients with prior leukopenia with other nucleoside analogs or for whom leukopenia counts are <1000 cells/mm³ at start of treatment

• Serum creatinine or CCr ≥q2wk, BUN; LFTs; ophthalmic exam
• For seizures, dysrhythmias
• **Infection:** Assess for flulike symptoms/fever, sore throat, coughing
• **Bleeding:** Assess for bleeding, thrombocytopenia, check gums, urine, emesis, avoid rectal temperature, vein punctures
• **Pregnancy/breastfeeding:** Not to be used in pregnancy, confirm by pregnancy test
Evaluate:
• Therapeutic response: decreased symptoms or prevention of CMV retinitis in transplant patients (if needed)
Teach patient/family:
• Not to wear contact lenses while using gel

• That product does not cure condition; that regular blood tests, ophthalmologic exams are necessary

• That major toxicities may necessitate discontinuing product

Black Box Warning: Pregnancy: to use contraception during treatment (males/females) and that infertility may occur; males should use barrier contraception for 90 days after treatment; may cause reversible infertility at lower doses, irreversible infertility at higher doses; not to breastfeed (IV)

• To take PO with food; do not open or crush caps

• **To report infection:** fever, chills, sore throat; blood dyscrasias: bruising, bleeding, petechiae; to avoid crowds, persons with respiratory infections

• To report itching, redness or eye pain (ophthalmic treatment)

---

ganciclovir ophthalmic
See Appendix B

---

gatifloxacin
(ga-ti-floks′a-sin)
Zymaxid
Func. class.: Ophthalmic antiinfective
Chem. class.: Fluoroquinolone

Do not confuse:
gatifloxacin/levofloxacin/moxifloxacin

ACTION: Inhibits DNA gyrase, thereby decreasing bacterial replication

USES: Bacterial conjunctivitis

CONTRAINDICATIONS: Hypersensitivity to this product or fluoroquinolones, infants <1 yr
Precautions: Pregnancy, breastfeeding

DOSAGE AND ROUTES
Bacterial conjunctivitis
• **Adult/adolescent/child ≥1 yr: OPHTH SOL** (0.5% ophthalmic solution) 1 drop

in affected eye(s) q2hr while awake (up to 8 times a day) for 1 day, then 1 drop 2-4 times a day while awake on days 2 through 7

Available forms: Ophthalmic solution 0.5%
Administer:
Ophthalmic route
• Commercially available ophthalmic solutions are not for injection subconjunctivally or into the anterior chamber of the eye
• Apply topically to the eye, taking care to avoid contamination; do not touch the tip of the dropper to the eye, fingertips, or other surface
• Apply pressure to lacrimal sac for 1 min after instillation
• Avoid wearing contact lenses during treatment

SIDE EFFECTS
EENT: Hypersensitivity, irritation, redness, tearing, keratitis, blepharitis, taste changes, ocular discharge/hemorrhage/irritation/pain
CNS: Headache
GI: Taste change

PHARMACOKINETICS
Unknown

NURSING CONSIDERATIONS
Assess:
• **Allergic reaction:** hypersensitivity, discontinue product
• **Pregnancy/breastfeeding:** use cautiously in pregnancy, breastfeeding
Evaluate:
• Decreased ophthalmic infection
Teach patient/family:
Ophthalmic route
• To apply topically to the eye, taking care to avoid contamination; for ophthalmic use only; not to share, to wash hands before use
• Not to touch the tip of the dropper to the eye, fingertips, or other surface
• To apply pressure to lacrimal sac for 1 min after instillation
• To avoid wearing contact lenses during treatment

⚠ HIGH ALERT

gemcitabine (Rx)
(jem-sit′a-been)

Gemzar

Func. class.: Antineoplastic—miscellaneous

Chem. class.: Pyrimidine analog

Do not confuse:
Gemzar/Zinecard

ACTION: Exhibits antitumor activity by killing cells undergoing DNA synthesis (S phase) and blocking G1/S-phase boundary

USES: Adenocarcinoma of the pancreas (nonresectable stage II, III, or metastatic stage IV); in combination with CISplatin for inoperable, advanced, or metastatic non–small-cell lung cancer; advanced breast cancer in combination with PACLitaxel; with CARBOplatin for ovarian cancer

Unlabeled uses: Bladder cancer, mesothelioma, adjuvant treatment of pancreatic cancer, ovarian cancer single agent, biliary tract cancer, advanced T-cell lymphoma

CONTRAINDICATIONS: Pregnancy, breastfeeding, hypersensitivity

Precautions: Children, geriatric patients, myelosuppression, radiation therapy, renal/hepatic disease, accidental exposure, alcoholism, dental disease, infection

DOSAGE AND ROUTES
Non–small-cell lung cancer
• **Adult: IV** (4-wk schedule) 1000 mg/m² given over 30 min on days 1, 8, 15, of each 28-day cycle; give CISplatin **IV** 100 mg/m² on day 1 after gemcitabine; 3-wk schedule: 1250 mg/m² given over 30 min on days 1, 8 of each 21-day cycle; give CISplatin **IV** 100 mg/m² after the infusion of gemcitabine on day 1

Advanced breast cancer
• **Adult: IV** 1250 mg/m² over 30 min on days 1 and 8 of 21-day cycle; give with PACLitaxel 175 mg/m² over 3 hr before gemcitabine on day 1

Recurrent ovarian cancer (single agent) (unlabeled)
• **Adult: IV** 1 g/m², days 1, 8, 15 of 28-day cycle

Pancreatic cancer (adjuvant therapy) unlabeled
• **Adults: IV** 1000 mg/m² on days 1, 8, 15 q28days in combination × 6 wk, beginning within 12 wk of resection

Available forms: Lyophilized powder for inj 20 mg/mL (10-, 50-mL vials); solution for inj 1 g/26.3 mL, 2 g/52.26 mL, 200 mg/2.56 mL

Administer:
Intermittent IV route
• Prepare in biologic cabinet using gown, mask, gloves; use cytotoxic handling procedures
• After reconstituting with 0.9% NaCl 5 mL/200-mg vial of product or 25 mL/1-g vial of product (38 mg/mL), shake; may be further diluted with 0.9% NaCl to concentrations as low as 0.1 mg/mL; discard unused portions, give over 30 min, do not admix
• Diluted solution stable at room temperature for 24 hr; do not refrigerate
• Infusion longer than 60 min increases toxicity; infusion-related reactions include hypotension, severe flulike symptoms, myelosuppression, asthenia
• **Bone marrow depression:** CBC, differential, platelet count before each dose; single agent: absolute granulocyte count >1000/mm³ and platelets >100,000/mm³, give complete dose; absolute granulocyte count 500-999/mm³, platelets 50,000-99,999/mm³, give 75%; absolute granulocyte count <500/mm³ or platelets <50,000/mm³, do not give; combination with PACLitaxel for breast cancer: absolute granulocyte count >1200/mm³ and platelets >75,000/mm³, give complete dose; absolute granulocyte count 1000-1199/mm³ or platelets 50,000-75,000/mm³, give 75%; absolute granulocyte count 700-999/mm³ or platelets ≥50,000/mm³, give 50%; absolute granulocyte count <700/mm³ or platelets <50,000/mm³, do not give; combination with CARBOplatin for ovarian cancer: absolute granulocyte count >1500/mm³ and platelet count

G

Side effects: *italics* = common; red = life-threatening

>100,000/mm^3, give complete dose; absolute granulocyte count 1000-1499/mm^3 or platelets 75,000-99,000/mm^3, give 75%; absolute granulocyte count <1000/mm^3 or platelets <75,000/mm^3, do not give

Y-site compatibilities: Alemtuzumab, alfentanil, allopurinol, amifostine, amikacin, aminophylline, ampicillin, anidulafungin, argatroban, aztreonam, bivalirudin, bleomycin, bumetanide, butorphanol, calcium gluconate, caspofungin, cefOXitin, cefTAZidime, ceftizoxime, cefTRIAXone, chlorproMAZINE, cimetidine, ciprofloxacin, CISplatin, clindamycin, cyclophosphamide, cytarabine, DACTINomycin, DAUNOrubicin, diphenhydrAMINE, DOBUTamine, DOCEtaxel, DOPamine, DOXOrubicin, droperidol, enalaprilat, etoposide, famotidine, floxuridine, fluconazole, fludarabine, fluorouracil, gentamicin, granisetron, haloperidol, heparin, hydrocortisone, HYDROmorphone, IDArubicin, ifosfamide, leucovorin, linezolid, LORazepam, mannitol, meperidine, mesna, metoclopramide, metroNIDAZOLE, minocycline, mitoXANtrone, morphine, nalbuphine, ondansetron, PACLitaxel, promethazine, ranitidine, streptozocin, teniposide, thiotepa, ticarcillin, tigecycline, tobramycin, topotecan, trimethoprim/sulfamethoxazole, vancomycin, vinBLAStine, vinCRIStine, vinorelbine, voriconazole, zidovudine, zoledronic acid

SIDE EFFECTS

CNS: Posterior reversible encephalopathy syndrome (PRES)

CV: Dysrthymias, hypertension

ENDO: Hyperglycemia

GI: Diarrhea, *nausea, vomiting,* anorexia, constipation, stomatitis, diarrhea, hepatotoxicity

GU: *Proteinuria,* hematuria

HEMA: Leukopenia, anemia, neutropenia, thrombocytopenia

INTEG: Irritation at site, *rash, alopecia*

META: Hypocalcemia, hypokalemia, hypomagnesemia

RESP: Dyspnea, bronchospasm, pneumonitis

OTHER: *Fever,* hemorrhage, infection, flulike symptoms, paresthesia, *peripheral edema,* myalgia, capillary leak syndrome

PHARMACOKINETICS

Half-life 2.5-18 hr; crosses placenta; excretion: renal, 92%-98%

INTERACTIONS

Increase: bleeding risk—NSAIDs, alcohol, salicylates, anticoagulants

Increase: myelosuppression, diarrhea—other antineoplastics, radiation

Decrease: antibody response—live virus vaccines

Drug/Lab Test

Increase: BUN, AST, ALT, alk phos, bilirubin, creatinine

Decrease: Hgb, WBC, neutrophils, platelets

NURSING CONSIDERATIONS

Assess:

• Assess for bruising, bleeding, petechiae

• Renal, hepatic studies before and during treatment; may increase AST, ALT, alk phos, bilirubin, BUN, creatinine, calcium, potassium, glucose, magnesium, urine protein

• Buccal cavity for dryness, sores, ulceration, white patches, oral pain, bleeding, dysphagia

• GI symptoms: frequency of stools, cramping, dark or bloody stools

• Signs of dehydration: rapid respirations, poor skin turgor, decreased urine output, dry skin, restlessness, weakness

• Increased fluid intake to 2-3 L/day to prevent dehydration unless contraindicated

• Rinsing of mouth tid-qid with water, club soda; brushing of teeth bid-tid with soft brush or cotton-tipped applicator for stomatitis; use unwaxed dental floss if stomatitis occurs

• Antiemetic agents

• **Capillary leak syndrome:** hemoconcentration, decreased albumin, B/P; discontinue if these occur

• **Hemolytic uremic syndrome (HUS):** may occur more frequently when given with bleomycin; assess renal function before use and periodically; anemia with microangiopathic hemolysis, elevated bilirubin or LDH, reticulocytosis, severe thrombocytopenia, or increases in BUN/creatinine are indications of HUS; permanently discontinue product if evidence of pulmonary toxicity, may occur ≤2 wk after last dose

• Radiation therapy risks: avoid radiation therapy 7 days before and 7 days after treatment; there is increased risk of life-threatening mucositis and toxicity at any time

Evaluate:

• Therapeutic response: decrease in tumor size; decrease in spread of cancer; symptom relief

Teach patient/family:

• To avoid foods with citric acid, hot temperature, or rough texture if stomatitis is present; to drink adequate fluids; to avoid use with NSAIDs, alcohol, salicylates

• To report stomatitis and any bleeding, white spots, ulcerations in mouth; to examine mouth daily, report symptoms

• To report signs of anemia: fatigue, headache, faintness, SOB, irritability; hematuria, dysuria

• Pregnancy/breastfeeding: to use contraception during therapy and for 4 mo after; do not breastfeed

• Not to receive vaccinations during treatment

• About possible hair loss and what can be done

• To report swelling of feet/legs

• To report bruising, bleeding: gums, blood in urine, stool, emesis

• To avoid crowds, persons with known upper respiratory infections

• To avoid use of hard-bristle toothbrush, electric razor

• Infection: to report sore throat, fever, flulike symptoms immediately

• That continuing follow-up exams and lab work will be needed

---

gemfibrozil (Rx)

(jem-fi'broe-zil)

Lopid

Func. class.: Antilipemic

Chem. class.: Fibric acid derivative

Do not confuse:

Lopid/Levbid/Slo-bid

ACTION: Inhibits biosynthesis of VLDL, decreases triglycerides, production in the liver increases HDL

USES: For use as an adjunct to diet for the treatment of hyperlipoproteinemia and for hypertriglyceridemia including Type IV (elevated triglycerides, VLDL) and Type V (elevated triglycerides, chylomicrons, VLDL) in patients who have significant risk of coronary artery disease or pancreatitis and who have not responded to diet

CONTRAINDICATIONS: Severe renal/hepatic disease, preexisting gallbladder disease, primary biliary cirrhosis, hypersensitivity, use with dasabuvir, repaglinide, or simvastatin

Precautions: Pregnancy, breastfeeding, renal disease, cholelithiasis, children

DOSAGE AND ROUTES

• **Adult: PO** 600 mg bid 30 min before AM, PM meal

Hepatic/renal dose

• Avoid use

Available forms: Tabs 600 mg; caps 300 mg ✿

Administer:

PO route

• 30 min before AM, PM meals

• Discontinue product if response does not occur within 3 mo

SIDE EFFECTS

CNS: Fatigue, vertigo, headache, paresthesia, dizziness

GI: *Dyspepsia, diarrhea, abdominal pain,* nausea, vomiting

HEMA: Leukopenia, anemia, eosinophilia, thrombocytopenia

INTEG: Rash, urticaria, pruritus

MS: Myopathy, rhabdomyolysis

PHARMACOKINETICS

Peak 1-2 hr; plasma protein binding >95%; half-life $1\frac{1}{2}$ hr; 70% excreted in urine mostly unchanged; metabolized in liver (minimal)

INTERACTIONS

• Do not use with dasabuvir, repaglinide, simvastatin

Side effects: *italics* = common; red = life-threatening

Increase: hypoglycemic effect—sulfonyl-ureas, repaglinide, metformin, glyburide, pioglitazone, other antidiabetic agents

Increase: anticoagulant effect—warfarin; monitor coagulation tests

Increase: nephrotoxicity—cyclosporine; monitor renal function

Increase: levels of CYP2C8, CYP2C9, CYP2C19; monitor for toxicities

Increase: risk of myositis, myalgia, rhabdomyolysis—HMG-CoA reductase inhibitors; avoid concurrent use

Decrease: effect of gemfibrozil—bile acid sequestrants, separate by >2 hr

Drug/Lab Test

Increase: LFTs, CK, bilirubin, alkaline phosphatase

Decrease: Hgb, Hct, WBC, potassium, eosinophils, platelets

NURSING CONSIDERATIONS
Assess:

• **Hyperlipidemia:** diet history; fats, triglycerides, cholesterol; if lipids increase, product should be discontinued; LDL, VLDL baseline and periodically

• **Myopathy, rhabdomyolysis:** for muscle pain, tenderness; obtain baseline CPK; if elevated or if these occur, product should be discontinued; at greater risk if combined with HMG-CoA reductase inhibitors

• Renal, hepatic studies, CBC, blood glucose if patient is receiving long-term therapy; if LFTs increase, therapy should be discontinued; monitor hematologic and hepatic functions

• Bowel pattern daily; watch for increasing diarrhea (common)

• **Pregnancy/breastfeeding:** use only if benefits outweigh fetal risk; do not breastfeed, excretion unknown

Evaluate:

• Therapeutic response: decreased cholesterol, triglyceride levels; HDL, cholesterol ratios improved

Teach patient/family:

• That compliance is needed for positive results; not to double or skip dose, to take missed dose as soon as remembered unless almost time for next dose

• To minimize risk factors: high-fat diet, smoking, alcohol consumption, absence of exercise

• To notify prescriber of diarrhea, nausea, vomiting, chills, fever, sore throat, muscle cramps, abdominal cramps, severe flatulence, tendon pain

• To avoid driving, hazardous activities if dizziness, blurred vision occur

---

gemifloxacin (Rx)
(gem-ah-flox′a-sin)
Factive
Func. class.: Antiinfective
Chem. class.: Fluoroquinolone

ACTION: Inhibits DNA gyrase, which is an enzyme involved in replication, transcription, and repair of bacterial DNA

USES: Acute bacterial exacerbation of chronic bronchitis caused by *Streptococcus pneumoniae, Haemophilus influenzae, Haemophilus parainfluenzae, Moraxella catarrhalis;* community-acquired pneumonia caused by *Streptococcus pneumoniae* including multiproduct-resistant strains, *H. influenzae, M. catarrhalis, Mycoplasma pneumoniae, Chlamydia pneumoniae, Klebsiella pneumoniae*

CONTRAINDICATIONS: Hypersensitivity to quinolones

Precautions: Pregnancy, breastfeeding, children, geriatric patients, hypokalemia, hypomagnesemia, renal disease, seizure disorders, excessive exposure to sunlight, psychosis, increased intracranial pressure, history of QT interval prolongation, dysrhythmias, myasthenia gravis, torsades de pointes

Black Box Warning: Tendon pain/rupture, tendinitis, myasthenia gravis, neurotoxicity

DOSAGE AND ROUTES
Adult: PO 320 mg/day × 3-5 days depending on type of infection, up to 7 days for pneumonia

---

ᴬᴰ𝕏 Genetic warning

Renal dose
• **Adult:** PO CCr ≤40 mL/min, 160 mg q24hr

Available forms: Tabs 320 mg
Administer:
• 2 hr before or 3 hr after aluminum/magnesium antacids, iron, zinc products, multivitamins, buffered products
• Without regard to food
• Provide adequate hydration

SIDE EFFECTS

CNS: *Dizziness, headache,* somnolence, depression, insomnia, nervousness, confusion, agitation, seizures, pseudotumor cerebri
CV: QT prolongation, vasodilation
EENT: Visual disturbances, retinal detachment
GI: Diarrhea, *nausea,* vomiting, anorexia, flatulence, heartburn, dry mouth; increased AST, ALT; constipation, abdominal pain, pseudomembranous colitis
INTEG: Rash, pruritus, urticaria, *photosensitivity*
MS: Tendinitis, tendon rupture
SYST: Anaphylaxis, Stevens-Johnson syndrome, toxic epidermal necrolysis, exfoliative dermatitis

PHARMACOKINETICS

Rapidly absorbed; bioavailability 71%; peak ½-2 hr; half-life 4-12 hr; excreted in urine as active product, metabolites

INTERACTIONS

Increase: CNS stimulation—NSAIDs
Increase: toxicity of gemifloxacin—probenecid

Black Box Warning: **Increase:** tendon rupture—corticosteroids

• **Increase:** QT prolongation—class IA, III antidysrhythmics, tricyclics, amoxapine, maprotiline, phenothiazines, haloperidol, pimozide, risperiDONE, sertindole, ziprasidone, β-blockers, chloroquine, cloZAPine, dasatinib, dolasetron, droperidol, dronedarone, flecainide, halogenated/local anesthetics, local anesthetics, lapatinib, methadone, erythromycin, telithromycin, troleandomycin, octreotide, ondansetron, palonosetron, pentamidine, propafenone, ranolazine, SUNitinib, tacrolimus, vardenafil, vorinostat
Decrease: absorption antacids containing aluminum, magnesium, sucralfate, zinc, iron; give 2 hr before or 3 hr after meals

NURSING CONSIDERATIONS
Assess:
• Renal, hepatic studies: BUN, creatinine, AST, ALT; I&O ratio, electrolytes
• CNS symptoms: insomnia, vertigo, headache, agitation, confusion
• **Allergic reactions and anaphylaxis:** rash, flushing, urticaria, pruritus, chills, fever, joint pain; may occur a few days after therapy begins; EPINEPHrine and resuscitation equipment should be available for anaphylactic reaction
• **Pseudomembranous colitis:** bowel pattern daily; if severe diarrhea, fever, abdominal pain occur, product should be discontinued
• **QT prolongation:** avoid use of quinolones in patients with known QT prolongation; females and those with ongoing proarrhythmic conditions (TdP) are at a greater risk; monitor ECG and/or Holter monitoring if product is used
Overgrowth of infection:
• perineal itching, fever, malaise, redness, pain, swelling, drainage, rash, diarrhea, change in cough, sputum

Black Box Warning: **Tendon rupture:** tendon pain, inflammation; if present, discontinue use; more common when used with corticosteroids; discontinue immediately if tendon pain, inflammation occur

• **Toxic psychosis/pseudotumor cerebri:** headache, blurred vision, neck/shoulder pain, nausea, vomiting, dizziness, tinnitus; discontinue immediately; may occur within hours to weeks after starting product
Pregnancy/breastfeeding: Use only if benefits outweigh fetal/infant risk
Evaluate:
• Therapeutic response: negative C&S, absence of signs, symptoms of infection
Teach patient/family:
• To take with/without food

Side effects: *italics* = common; red = life-threatening

• That fluids must be increased to 2 L/day to avoid crystallization in kidneys

• That if dizziness or light-headedness occurs, to perform activities with assistance

• To complete full course of product therapy

• To contact prescriber if adverse reactions occur

• To avoid iron- or mineral-containing supplements or aluminum/magnesium antacids, buffered products within 2 hr before and 3 hr after dosing, 2 hr before sucralfate

• That photosensitivity may occur and sunscreen should be used

• To use frequent rinsing of mouth, sugarless candy, or gum for dry mouth

• To avoid other medication unless approved by prescriber

Tendon pain:

• To immediately report pain, inflammation in tendons, weakness, tingling in extremities

Allergic reactions:

• To report rash, and stop product if it occurs

---

gentamicin (Rx)

jen-ta-mye′sin

Cidomycin ✦

Func. class.: Antiinfective
Chem. class.: Aminoglycoside

Do not confuse:

gentamicin/kanamycin

ACTION: Interferes with protein synthesis in bacterial cell by binding to 30S ribosomal subunit, thus causing misreading of genetic code; inaccurate peptide sequence forms in protein chain, thereby causing bacterial death

USES: Severe systemic infections of CNS, respiratory, GI, urinary tract, bone, skin, soft tissues caused by susceptible strains of *Pseudomonas aeruginosa, Proteus, Klebsiella, Serratia, Escherichia coli, Enterobacter, Citrobacter, Staphylococcus, Shigella, Salmonella, Acinetobacter, Bacillus anthracis*

Unlabeled uses: Bartonellosis, bronchiectasis, cystic fibrosis, endocarditis prophylaxis, febrile neutropenia, gonorrhea, granuloma inguinale, PID, plaque, surgical infection prophylaxis, tuboovarian abscess, tularemia

CONTRAINDICATIONS: Hypersensitivity to this product, other aminoglycosides

Black Box Warning: Pregnancy

Precautions: Breastfeeding, neonates, geriatric patients, pseudomembranous colitis

Black Box Warning: Myasthenia gravis, Parkinson's disease, infant botulism, tinnitus, nephrotoxicity, neurotoxicity, ototoxicity

DOSAGE AND ROUTES

Severe systemic infections

• **Adult: IV INFUSION** 3-5 mg/kg/day in divided doses q8hr; **IV** (pulse dosing, once-daily dosing) (unlabeled) 5-7 mg/kg; **IM** 3-5 mg/kg/day in divided doses q8hr

• **Child: IM/IV** 2-2.5 mg/kg q8hr; **IV** (pulse dosing, once-daily dosing) (unlabeled) 5 mg/kg

• **Neonate and infant: IM/IV** 2.5 mg/kg q8-12hr

• **Neonate <1 wk: IV** 2.5 mg/kg q12hr

Renal dose: regular dosing

• **Adult: IM/IV** CCr 70-100 mL/min, reduce dose by multiplying maintenance dose by 0.85, give q8-12hr; CCr 50-69 mL/min, reduce as above, give q12hr; CCr 25-49 mL/min, reduce as above, give q24hr; CCr <25 mL/min, reduce as above, give based on serum concentrations, give doses after dialysis

Renal dose: extended interval (unlabeled)

• **Adult: IV** CCr 40-59 mL/min 5-7 mg/kg q36hr; CCr 20-39 mL/min 5-7 mg/kg q48hr; CCr <20 mL/min 5-7 mg/kg once, then base on serial levels

Available forms: Inj 10, 40 mg/mL; premixed inj 40, 60, 70, 80, 90, 100, 120/100 mL NS

Administer:

• Obtain C&S before starting treatment, treatment may be started before results are received

IM route

• IM inj in large muscle mass; rotate inj sites

• Product in evenly spaced doses to maintain blood level

Intermittent IV INFUSION route

• After diluting in 50-200 mL NS, D₅W; decrease vol of diluent in child; maintain 0.1% sol run over $^1/_2$-1 hr (adults) or up to 2 hr (children); flush IV line with NS, D₅W after administration

Y-site compatibilities: Alatrofloxacin, aldesleukin, alemtuzumab, alfentanil, alprostadil, amifostine, amikacin, aminocaproic acid, aminophylline, amiodarone, amsacrine, anidulafungin, argatroban, arsenic trioxide, ascorbic acid injection, asparaginase, atenolol, atracurium, atropine, aztreonam, benztropine, bivalirudin, bleomycin, bumetanide, buprenorphine, butorphanol, calcium chloride/gluconate, carboplatin, carmustine, caspofungin, cefamandole, ceFAZolin, cefepime, cefotaxime, cefOXitin, cefpirome, ceftaroline, cefTAZidime, ceftizoxime, ceftRIAXone, cefuroxime, chlorothiazide, chlorpheniramine, chlorproMAZINE, cimetidine, ciprofloxacin, cisatracurium, CISplatin, clarithromycin, clindamycin, cloxacillin, codeine, colistimethate, cyanocobalamin, cyclophosphamide, cycloSPORINE, cytarabine, DACTINomycin, DAPTOmycin, DAUNOrubicin citrate liposome, DAUNOrubicin hydrochloride, dexmedetomidine, dexrazoxane, digoxin, diltiazem, dimenhyDRINATE, diphenhydrAMINE, DOBUTamine, DOCEtaxel, dolasetron, DOPamine, doripenem, doxacurium, doxapram, DOXOrubicin hydrochloride, doxorubicin hydrochloride liposomal, doxycycline, edetate calcium disodium, edetate disodium, enalaprilat, ePHEDrine, EPINEPHrine, epirubicin, epoetin alfa, eptifibatide, ergonovine, ertapenem, erythromycin lactobionate, esmolol, etoposide, etoposide phosphate, famotidine, fenoldopam, fentaNYL, fluconazole, fludarabine, fluorouracil, foscarnet, gallamine, gallium, gatifloxacin, gemcitabine, glycopyrrolate, granisetron, HYDROmorphone, hydrOXYzine, ifosfamide, imipenem-cilastatin, irinotecan, isoproterenol, ketamine, ketorolac, labetalol, lactated Ringer's injection, lansoprazole, lepirudin, leucovorin, levofloxacin, lidocaine, lincomycin, linezolid, LORazepam, magnesium sulfate, mannitol, mechlorethamine, melphalan, meperidine, mephentermine sulfate, meropenem, mesna, metaraminol, methyldopate, methylPREDNISolone sodium succinate, metoclopramide, metoprolol, metroNIDAZOLE, midazolam, milrinone, minocycline, mitoXANtrone, mivacurium, morphine, multiple vitamins injection, mycophenolate mofetil, nafcillin, nalbuphine, nalorphine, naloxone, netilmicin, niCARdipine, nitroglycerin, nitroprusside, norepinephrine, octreotide, ondansetron, oritavancin, oxaliplatin, oxytocin, PACLitaxel (solvent/surfactant), palonosetron, pamidronate, pancuronium, papaverine, penicillin G potassium/ sodium, pentazocine, perphenazine, PHENobarbital, phentolamine, phenylephrine, phytonadione, piperacillin, polymyxin B, posaconazole, potassium acetate/chloride, procainamide, prochlorperazine, promazine, promethazine, propranolol, protamine, pyridoxine, quiNIDine gluconate, ranitidine, remifentanil, Ringer's injection, riTUXimab, rocuronium, sargramostim, sodium acetate/bicarbonate/citrate, streptomycin, succinylcholine, SUFentanil, tacrolimus, telavancin, temocillin, teniposide, theophylline, thiamine, thiotepa, ticarcillin, ticarcillin-clavulanate, tigecycline, tirofiban, TNA (3-in-1), tobramycin, tolazoline, topotecan, TPN (2-in-1), trastuzumab, trimetaphan, tubocurarine, urokinase, vancomycin, vasopressin, vecuronium, verapamil, vinBLAStine, vinCRIStine, vinorelbine, vitamin B complex with C, voriconazole, zidovudine, zoledronic acid

G

SIDE EFFECTS

CNS: Confusion, depression, numbness, tremors, seizures, muscle twitching, neurotoxicity, dizziness, vertigo, encephalopathy, fever, headache, lethargy

CV: Hypo/hypertension, palpitations, edema

EENT: Ototoxicity, *deafness,* visual disturbances, tinnitus

GI: *Nausea, vomiting, anorexia;* increased ALT, AST, bilirubin; hepatomegaly, hepatic necrosis, splenomegaly

GU: Oliguria, hematuria, renal damage, azotemia, renal failure, nephrotoxicity, proteinuria

HEMA: Agranulocytosis, thrombocytopenia, leukopenia, eosinophilia, anemia

INTEG: *Rash,* burning, urticaria, dermatitis, alopecia, photosensitivity, anaphylaxis

MS: Twitching, myasthenia gravis–like symptoms

RESP: Apnea

PHARMACOKINETICS

Not metabolized, excreted unchanged in urine, crosses placental barrier

IM: Onset rapid, peak 30-60 min

IV: Onset immediate; peak 30-90 min; plasma half-life 1-2 hr, infants 6-7 hr; duration 6-8 hr

INTERACTIONS

• Do not use at the same time as or physically mix with penicillins

Black Box Warning: **Increase:** ototoxicity, neurotoxicity, nephrotoxicity—other aminoglycosides, amphotericin B, polymyxin, vancomycin, ethacrynic acid, furosemide, mannitol, methoxyflurane, CISplatin, cephalosporins, penicillins, cidofovir, acyclovir, foscarnet, cycloSPORINE, tacrolimus, ganciclovir, zoledronic acid, pamidronate

Increase: effects—nondepolarizing neuromuscular blockers, digoxin, entecavir

Drug/Lab Test

Increase: LDH, AST, ALT, bilirubin, BUN, creatinine, eosinophils

Decrease: Hgb, WBC, platelets, granulocytes

NURSING CONSIDERATIONS

Assess:

Black Box Warning: **Neurotoxicity: (myasthenia gravis, Parkinson's disease, infant botulism):** paresthesias, tetany, positive Chvostek's/Trousseau's signs, confusion (adults), tetany, muscle weakness (infants); correct electrolyte imbalance

• Weight before treatment; calculation of dosage is usually based on ideal body weight but may be calculated on actual body weight

Black Box Warning: **Nephrotoxicity:** I&O ratio, urinalysis daily for proteinuria, cells, casts; report sudden change in urine output; urine pH if product is used for UTI; urine should be kept alkaline; urine for CCr testing, BUN, serum creatinine; lower dosage should be given with renal impairment (CCr <80 mL/min); toxicity is increased in patients with decreased renal function if high doses are given

• VS during infusion; watch for hypotension, change in pulse

• IV site for thrombophlebitis, including pain, redness, swelling q30min, change site if needed; discontinue, apply warm compresses to site

• Serum peak drawn at 30-60 min after IV infusion or 60 min after IM inj and trough level drawn just before next dose; blood level should be 2-4 times bacteriostatic level; peak (5-10 mcg/mL), trough (0.5-2 mcg/mL), depending on type of infection (based on traditional dosing)

Black Box Warning: **Ototoxicity:** eighth cranial nerve dysfunction by audiometric testing; also ringing, roaring in ears, vertigo; assess hearing before, during, after treatment

• Dehydration: high specific gravity, decrease in skin turgor, dry mucous membranes, dark urine

• **Overgrowth of infection:** fever, malaise, redness, pain, swelling, perineal itching, diarrhea, stomatitis, change in cough or sputum

• C&S before starting treatment to identify infecting organism

• **Vestibular dysfunction:** nausea, vomiting, dizziness, headache; product should be discontinued if severe

• Inj sites for redness, swelling, abscesses; use warm compresses at site

• Adequate fluids of 2-3 L/day unless contraindicated to prevent irritation of tubules

Black Box Warning: **Pregnancy/ breastfeeding:** identify whether pregnancy is planned or suspected; do not use in pregnancy or breastfeeding

Evaluate:

• Therapeutic response: absence of fever, draining wounds, negative C&S after treatment

Teach patient/family:

• To report headache, dizziness, symptoms of overgrowth of infection, renal impairment

Black Box Warning: **Ototoxicity:** to report loss of hearing; ringing, roaring in ears; feeling of fullness in head

• To drink adequate fluids

• To avoid hazardous activities until reaction is known

gentamicin (ophthalmic)

(jen-ta-mye′sin)

Gentak, GenTeal

Func. class.: Ophthalmic antiinfective

Chem. class.: Aminoglycoside

Do not confuse:

gentamicin/clindamycin/tobramycin/ erythromycin/vancomycin

ACTION: Inhibits protein synthesis by binding of 30s ribosomal subunits, thereby decreasing bacterial replication

USES: External ocular infections

CONTRAINDICATIONS: Hypersensitivity to this product or aminoglycosides

Precautions: Pregnancy, breastfeeding, corneal healing, local redness/irritation

DOSAGE AND ROUTES
Ophthalmic (solution)

• **Adult/adolescent/child ≥1 mo: SOL** 1-2 drops in affected eye(s) every 4 hr while awake × 2 days, then every 4 hr; severe infections ≤2 drops every 1 hr

• **Ointment:** apply a small amount (½ in) to lower conjunctival sac bid or tid

Available forms: Ophthalmic ointment, ophthalmic solution 0.3%

Administer:

Ophthalmic route

• Commercially available ophthalmic solutions are not for injection subconjunctivally or into the anterior chamber of the eye

• Apply topically to the eye, taking care to avoid contamination

• Do not touch the tip of the dropper to the eye, fingertips, or other surface; wash hands before use

• Apply pressure to lacrimal sac for 1 min after instillation

• To apply the ointment, pull down gently on lower eyelid and apply a thin film of the ointment

SIDE EFFECTS

EENT: Burning, hypersensitivity, stinging, blurred vision, hyperemia, corneal ulcers

PHARMACOKINETICS

Unknown

NURSING CONSIDERATIONS
Assess:

• **Allergic reaction:** hypersensitivity, discontinue product

Evaluate:

• Therapeutic response: decreased ophthalmic infection

Teach patient/family:

Ophthalmic route

• To apply topically to the eye, taking care to avoid contamination; for ophthalmic use only

G

• Not to touch the tip of the dropper to the eye, fingertips, or other surface; to wash hands before use
• To apply pressure to lacrimal sac for 1 min after instillation
• To apply the ointment by pulling down gently on lower eyelid and applying a thin film of the ointment

---

gentamicin (topical)

(jen-ta-mye′sin)
Func. class.: Topical antiinfective
Chem. class.: Aminoglycoside

Do not confuse:
gentamicin/clindamycin

ACTION: Antibacterial activity results from inhibition of protein synthesis; bactericidal

USES: Superficial infections

CONTRAINDICATIONS: Hypersensitivity to this product or other aminoglycosides
Precautions: Infections, local sensitivity

DOSAGE AND ROUTES
• **Adult/child >1 yr:** apply to affected areas tid-qid
Available forms: Topical cream, ointment 0.1%
Administer:
• For external use only; do not use skin products near the eyes, nose, or mouth
• Wash hands before and after use; wash affected area and gently pat dry
• **Cream/ointment:** Apply to the cleansed affected area, massage gently into affected areas

SIDE EFFECTS
INTEG: Rash, irritation, erythema, pruritus

PHARMACOKINETICS
Unknown

NURSING CONSIDERATIONS
Assess:
• **Allergic reaction:** hypersensitivity; product may need to be discontinued

• **Infection:** skin infection
Evaluate:
• Therapeutic response: decreased skin infection
Teach patient/family:
• To use for external use only; do not use skin products near the eyes, nose, or mouth
• To wash hands before and after use; wash affected area and gently pat dry
• **Cream/ointment:** to apply to the cleansed affected area and massage gently into affected areas

---

RARELY USED

gilteritinib

(gil′ teh-rih′ tih-nib)
Xospata
Func. class.: Antineoplastic

USES: Acute myeloid leukemia-relapsed or the treatment of relapsed or refractory FLT3 mutation–positive AML

CONTRAINDICATIONS: Hypersensitivity

DOSAGE AND ROUTES
• **Adult: PO** 120 mg daily; continue for at least 6 cycles in patients who do not have unacceptable toxicity

---

⚠ HIGH ALERT

glatiramer (Rx)

(glah-tear′a-meer)
Copaxone, Glatopa
Func. class.: Multiple sclerosis agent

ACTION: Unknown; may modify the immune responses responsible for multiple sclerosis (MS) by serving as a decoy to locally generated autoantibodies

USES: Reduction of the frequency of relapses in patients with relapsing or remitting MS after first clinical episode with MRI results consistent with MS

CONTRAINDICATIONS: Hypersensitivity to this product or mannitol, IV use

Precautions: Pregnancy, breastfeeding, children <18 yr, immune disorders, renal disease, infection, vaccinations, geriatric patients

DOSAGE AND ROUTES

• 20 mg/mL and 40 mg/mL are not interchangeable

• **Adult: SUBCUT** 20 mg/day (20 mg/mL solution), on the same day 3×/wk or 40 mg (40 mg/mL solution) 3×/wk, give ≥48 hr apart

Available forms: Inj premixed 20 mg/mL in single-use syringe; sol for inj 40 mg/mL

Administer:

SUBCUT route

• Refrigerate, allow to warm for 20 min; visually inspect for particulate or cloudiness; if present, discard; prefilled syringe contents are for single use; administer SUBCUT into hip, thigh, arm; discard unused portion; if refrigeration is unavailable, may store ≤1 mo at room temperature

• Use SUBCUT route only; do not give IM or IV, do not expel air bubble in prefilled syringe

• Give 40-mg dose on same 3 days of the week, must be 48 hr apart

SIDE EFFECTS

CNS: *Anxiety, hypertonia, tremor, vertigo,* speech disorder, *agitation,* confusion, flushing

CV: *Migraine, palpitations, syncope, tachycardia, vasodilation,* chest pain, hypertension

EENT: *Ear pain, blurred vision*

GI: *Nausea, vomiting, diarrhea, anorexia, gastroenteritis*

GU: *Urinary urgency, dysmenorrhea, vaginal moniliasis,* vaginal hemorrhage

HEMA: *Ecchymosis, lymphadenopathy*

INTEG: *Pruritus, rash, sweating, urticaria, erythema,* inj-site reaction

META: *Edema, weight gain*

MS: *Arthralgia, back pain, neck pain,* increased muscle tone

RESP: *Bronchitis, dyspnea, laryngismus, rhinitis,* laryngospasm

PHARMACOKINETICS

May be hydrolyzed locally, may reach regional lymph nodes

INTERACTIONS

Increase: serious infection—denosumab, natalizumab, roflumilast; avoid using together

Increase: hematologic toxicity—leflunomide

• Avoid use with live virus vaccines

Increase: neutropenia effect—trastuzumab

Drug/Herb

Decrease: glatiramer effect—echinacea

NURSING CONSIDERATIONS

Assess:

• CNS symptoms: anxiety, confusion, vertigo

• GI status: diarrhea, vomiting, abdominal pain, gastroenteritis

• Cardiac status: tachycardia, palpitations, vasodilation, chest pain

• **Postinjection reactions:** chest pain, dyspnea, flushing, palpitations, usually dissipate on their own, may occur quickly or several months after use; usually at least one episode of chest pain occurs 1 mo after start of therapy

• **Pregnancy/breastfeeding:** use only if clearly needed; no well-controlled studies; cautious use in breastfeeding

Evaluate:

• Therapeutic response: decreased symptoms of MS

Teach patient/family:

• With written, detailed instructions about product; provide initial and return demonstrations on inj procedure; give information about use and disposal of product, inj-site reaction (hives, rash, irritation, severe pain, flushing, chest pain)

• To notify prescribers of allergic reactions including itching, trouble breathing, chest pain, dizziness, sweating

• That irregular menses, dysmenorrhea, metrorrhagia, breast pain may occur; to use contraception during treatment

G

Side effects: *italics* = common; red = life-threatening

- To notify prescriber if pregnancy is suspected or if nursing
- Not to change dosing or stop taking product without advice of prescriber
- About **immediate postinjection reaction:** flushing, chest pain, palpitations, anxiety, dyspnea, laryngeal constriction, urticaria; does not usually require treatment, may occur months after beginning treatment
- To take as directed; not to stop product or change schedule; teach on self-injection technique
- That the 20 mg/mL and 40 mg/mL are not interchangeable

⚠ HIGH ALERT

glimepiride (Rx)
(glye-me′pi-ride)
Amaryl
glipiZIDE (Rx)
(glip-i′zide)
Glucotrol, Glucotrol XL
Func. class.: Antidiabetic
Chem. class.: Sulfonylurea (2nd generation)

Do not confuse:
glipiZIDE/Glucotrol/glyBURIDE

ACTION: Causes functioning β cells in pancreas to release insulin, leading to drop in blood glucose levels; may improve insulin binding to insulin receptors or increase the number of insulin receptors with prolonged administration; may also reduce basal hepatic glucose secretion; not effective if patient lacks functioning β cells

USES: Type 2 diabetes mellitus

CONTRAINDICATIONS: Hypersensitivity to sulfonylureas/sulfonamides, type 1 diabetes, diabetic ketoacidosis
Precautions: Pregnancy, geriatric patients, cardiac disease, severe renal/hepatic disease, G6PD deficiency

DOSAGE AND ROUTES
Glimepiride
- **Adult:** PO 1-2 mg/day with breakfast, then increase by ≤2 mg/day q1-2wk, max 8 mg/day
- **Geriatric:** PO 1 mg/day; may increase if needed
Renal/hepatic dose
- **Adult:** PO 1 mg/day with breakfast; may titrate upward as needed

GlipiZIDE
- **Adult:** PO 5 mg initially before breakfast, then increase by 2.5-5 mg after several days to desired response; max 40 mg/day in divided doses; **PO** (XL) 5 mg/day with breakfast, may increase to 10 mg/day, max 20 mg/day
- **Geriatric:** PO 2.5 mg/day; may increase if needed
Hepatic disease
- **Adult:** PO 2.5 mg initially, then increase to desired response; max 40 mg/day in divided doses or 15 mg/dose

Available forms: *Glimepiride:* tabs 1, 2, 4 mg; *glipiZIDE:* tabs, scored 5, 10 mg; ext rel tabs (XL) 2.5, 5, 10 mg
Administer:
- Do not break, crush, or chew ext rel tabs; may crush tabs and mix with fluids if unable to swallow whole
- **GlipiZIDE:** give product 30 min before meals (regular release); with breakfast (ext rel); **Glimepiride:** with breakfast; if patient is NPO, may need to hold dose to prevent hypoglycemia
- Gradual conversion from other oral hypoglycemics to these products is not needed; insulin ≥20 units/day, convert using 25% reduction in insulin dose every day or every other day
- Store in tight, light-resistant container at room temperature

SIDE EFFECTS
CNS: *Headache, weakness, dizziness, drowsiness,* tinnitus, fatigue, vertigo
ENDO: Hypoglycemia
GI: Hepatotoxicity, cholestatic jaundice, nausea, vomiting, diarrhea, heartburn, weight gain

---

HEMA: Leukopenia, thrombocytopenia, agranulocytosis, aplastic anemia; increased AST, ALT, alk phos; pancytopenia, hemolytic anemia

INTEG: Rash, allergic reactions, pruritus, urticaria, eczema, photosensitivity, erythema, allergic vasculitis

SYST: Serious hypersensitivity

PHARMACOKINETICS

PO: Completely absorbed by GI route; **glipiZIDE:** onset $1-1\frac{1}{2}$ hr, peak 2-3 hr, duration 12-24 hr, half-life 2-4 hr; **glimepiride:** peak 2-3 hr, half-life 5 hr; metabolized in liver, excreted in urine, 90%-95% plasma-protein bound

INTERACTIONS

• May mask symptoms of hypoglycemia: β-blockers

Increase: action of digoxin, glycosides, cyclosporine

Increase: hypoglycemic effects—insulin, MAOIs, cimetidine, chloramphenicol, guanethidine, methyldopa, NSAIDs, salicylates, probenecid, androgens, anticoagulants, clofibrate, fenfluramine, fluconazole, gemfibrozil, histamine H_2 antagonists, magnesium salts, phenylbutazone, sulfinpyrazone, sulfonamides, tricyclics, urinary acidifiers, clarithromycin, fibric acid derivatives, voriconazole; monitor blood glucose

Decrease: hypoglycemic effect—thiazide diuretics, rifampin, isoniazid, cholestyramine, diazoxide, hydantoins, urinary alkalinizers, charcoal, corticosteroids, colesevelam; monitor blood glucose

Drug/Herb

Increase: antidiabetic effect—garlic, horse chestnut

Decrease: hypoglycemic effect—green tea

Drug/Lab Test

Increase: AST, ALT, LDH, BUN, creatinine

Decrease: platelets, WBC, sodium

NURSING CONSIDERATIONS

Assess:

• **Hypo/hyperglycemic reaction** that can occur soon after meals; for severe hypoglycemia, give IV $D_{50}W$, then IV dextrose solution

• Blood glucose, A1c levels during treatment to determine diabetes control

• **Blood dyscrasias:** CBC at baseline and throughout treatment; report decreased blood count

• For allergy to sulfonamides, potential for cross-reactivity

• For renal, hepatic dysfunction: use dose reductions, or avoidance of use may be required; increased risk of hypoglycemia in hepatic failure

• **Pregnancy/breastfeeding:** identify whether pregnancy is planned or suspected; breastfed infant may be hypoglycemic; use only if benefits outweigh fetal risk

Evaluate:

• Therapeutic response: decrease in polyuria, polydipsia, polyphagia; clear sensorium; absence of dizziness; stable gait; improved serum glucose, A1c

Teach patient/family:

• Not to drink alcohol; about disulfiram reaction (nausea, headache, cramps, flushing, hypoglycemia)

• To report bleeding, bruising, weight gain, edema, SOB, weakness, sore throat, swelling in ankles, rash

• To check for symptoms of cholestatic jaundice: dark urine, pruritus, yellow sclera; prescriber should be notified

• About symptoms of hypo/hyperglycemia, what to do about each; to have glucagon emergency kit available; to carry sugar packets

• That product must be continued on daily basis; about consequences of discontinuing product abruptly; to take product in morning to prevent hypoglycemic reactions at night

• To use sunscreen or stay out of the sun, wear protective clothing (photosensitivity)

• To avoid OTC medications unless ordered by prescriber

• That diabetes is a lifelong illness; product will not cure disease

• That all food in diet plan must be eaten to prevent hypoglycemia; to continue weight control, dietary restrictions, exercise, hygiene

• To carry emergency ID with prescriber and medication information

• To test using blood glucose meter while taking this product

• That ext rel tab may appear in stool

Side effects: *italics* = common; red = life-threatening

• To notify prescribers of use prior to surgery
• Not to drive or engage in hazardous tasks until response is known, dizziness may occur
• That continuing follow-up exams and lab work will be needed

TREATMENT OF OVERDOSE:
Use one of the following: Glucose 25 g IV via dextrose 50% sol, 50 mL, 1 mg glucagon, oral carbohydrate depending on severity

glucagon
(gloo′ka-gon)
GlucaGen
Func. class.: Antihypoglycemic

ACTION: Increases in blood glucose, relaxation of smooth muscle of the GI tract, and a positive inotropic and chronotropic effect on the heart; increases in blood glucose are secondary to stimulation of glycogenolysis

USES: Hypoglycemia, used to temporarily inhibit movement of GI tract as a diagnostic test
Unlabeled uses: Beta blocker, calcium channel toxicity

CONTRAINDICATIONS: Hypersensitivity, pheochromocytoma, insulinoma
Precautions: Pregnancy, breastfeeding, cardiac disease, adrenal insufficiency

DOSAGE AND ROUTES
Hypoglycemia in those with diabetes mellitus
• Adult/adolescent/child ≥55 lb (25 kg): **IM/IV/SUBCUT** (GlucaGen) 1 mg (1 IU)
• Child <55 lb (25 kg) or <6-8 yr: **IM/IV/SUBCUT** (Glucagon) 0.5 mg (0.5 IU)
• Adult/adolescent/child ≥44 lb (20 kg): **IM/IV/SUBCUT** (Glucagon) 1 mg (1 IU)
• Child <44 lb (20 kg): **IM/IV/SUBCUT** (Glucagon) 0.5 mg (0.5 IU) or 0.02-0.03 mg/kg (IU/kg)

Severe hypoglycemia
• **Neonate: IM/IV/SUBCUT** 0.2 mg/kg/dose, max 1 mg/dose; **CONT INFUSION** (unlabeled): 0.5-1 mg/day
Available forms: Powder for injection 1-mg vial
Administer:
• Visually inspect for particulate matter and discoloration before use
Reconstitution: Reconstitute with 1 mL of sterile water for injection or with diluent supplied by the manufacturer; the reconstituted injection should be clear and of water-like consistency (1 mg/mL); discard any unused portion
IM route
• Inject into a large muscle mass; aspirate before injection to avoid injection into a blood vessel
SUBCUT route
• Inject, taking care not to inject intradermally
IV route
• Inject directly into a vein at a rate ≤1 mg/min; may be given through line running D_5W or given at the same time as a bolus of dextrose

SIDE EFFECTS
CNS: Dizziness, headache
CV: Hypotension
GI: Nausea, vomiting
SYST: Hypersensitivity

PHARMACOKINETICS
IV: Onset immediate, peak 30 min, duration 1-1½ hr
IM/SUBCUT: Onset 5-10 min, peak 13-20 min, duration 12-30 min, half-life 8-18 min

INTERACTIONS
Increase: bleeding risk—anticoagulants
Decrease: effect of insulin, oral antidiabetics
Increase: B/P and heart rate—β-blockers

NURSING CONSIDERATIONS
Assess:
• **Hypoglycemia:** monitor glucose levels before and after product use; use other products to control hypoglycemia if patient is conscious

• **Pregnancy/breastfeeding:** use only if clearly needed

Evaluate:

• Decreased hypoglycemia

Teach patient/family:

• How to use this product, symptoms of hypoglycemia, instruct patient in use of oral glucose when hypoglycemia occurs, use this product only when patient is unable to swallow

• Not to use outdated product

• Have all patients carry a sugar source at all times

> ⚠ **HIGH ALERT**

glyBURIDE (Rx)

(glye′byoor-ide)

DiaBeta ✹, Euglucon ✹, Glynase PresTab

Func. class.: Antidiabetic

Chem. class.: Sulfonylurea (2nd generation)

Do not confuse:

glyBURIDE/Glucotrol/glipiZIDE

DiaBeta/Zebeta

ACTION: Causes functioning β cells in pancreas to release insulin, thereby leading to a drop in blood glucose levels; may improve insulin binding to insulin receptors and increase number of insulin receptors with prolonged administration; may also reduce basal hepatic glucose secretion; not effective if patient lacks functioning β cells

USES: Type 2 diabetes mellitus

Unlabeled use: Gestational diabetes not controlled by diet

CONTRAINDICATIONS: Hypersensitivity to sulfonylureas, type 1 diabetes, diabetic ketoacidosis, renal failure

Precautions: Pregnancy, geriatric patients, cardiac/thyroid disease, severe renal/hepatic disease, severe hypoglycemic reactions, sulfonamide/sulfonylurea hypersensitivity, G6PD deficiency

DOSAGE AND ROUTES

DiaBeta (nonmicronized)

To replace insulin

• **Adult:** PO if insulin was <40 U/day, switch directly; if insulin <20 U/day, give 2.5-5 mg (or 1.5-3 mg micronized); if insulin 20-40 U/day, give 5 mg (or 3 mg micronized); if insulin >40 U/day, give 5 mg (3 mg micronized) initially with 50% insulin dose, gradually taper insulin, and increase glyburide

• **Adult:** PO 1.25-5 mg initially, then increase to desired response at weekly intervals up to 20 mg/day; may be given as a single or divided dose

• **Geriatric:** PO 1.25 mg initially, then increase to desired response; max 20 mg/day, maintenance 1.25-20 mg/day

Glynase PresTab (micronized)

• **Adult:** PO 1.5-3 mg/day initially, may increase by 1.5 mg/wk, max 12 mg/day

• **Geriatric:** PO 0.75-3 mg/day, may increase by 1.5 mg/wk

Renal dose

• **Adult:** PO CCr ≤50 mL/min, use conservative dose

Gestational diabetes (unlabeled)

• **Adult (pregnant female):** PO 2.5 mg/day titrated up to 20 mg/day (conventional glyBURIDE)

Available forms: Tabs (DiaBeta) 1.25, 2.5, 5 mg (nonmicronized); (Glynase PresTab) 1.5, 3, 6 mg (micronized)

Administer:

• With breakfast as single or divided dose; hold dose if patient NPO to avoid hypoglycemia; take at same time each day

• Gradual conversion from other oral hypoglycemics to product is not needed

• Micronized glyBURIDE/nonmicronized glyBURIDE are not equivalent

• Store in tight container in cool environment

SIDE EFFECTS

CNS: *Headache, weakness,* paresthesia

ENDO: Hypoglycemia

GI: Nausea, hepatotoxicity, cholestatic jaundice, vomiting, diarrhea, weight gain

G

HEMA: Leukopenia, thrombocytopenia, agranulocytosis, aplastic anemia (rare)
INTEG: Rash, pruritus, photosensitivity, erythema
MISC: Angioedema, serious hypersensitivity

PHARMACOKINETICS
PO: Completely absorbed by GI route; onset 2 hr; peak 2-4 hr; duration 24 hr; half-life 10 hr; metabolized in liver; excreted in urine, feces (metabolites); crosses placenta; 99% plasma-protein bound

INTERACTIONS
Increase: masking symptoms of hypoglycemia—β-blockers; monitor blood glucose
Increase: level—digoxin
Increase: hypoglycemic effects—insulin, MAOIs, oral anticoagulants, chloramphenicol, guanethidine, methyldopa, NSAIDs, salicylates, probenecid, androgens, fenfluramine, fluconazole, gemfibrozil, histamine H_2 antagonists, magnesium salts, phenylbutazone, sulfinpyrazone, sulfonamides, tricyclics, urinary acidifiers, β-blockers, clarithromycin, voriconazole; monitor blood glucose
Increase: LFTs—bosentan; avoid concurrent use
Increase: triglyceride levels—colesevelam
Increase: action of—cycloSPORINE
Decrease: both products' effects—diazoxide
Decrease: glyBURIDE action—thiazide diuretics, rifampin, isoniazid, cholestyramine, hydantoins, urinary alkalinizers, charcoal, corticosteroids, phenothiazines; oral contraceptives, estrogens, thyroid; monitor blood glucose
Drug/Herb
Increase: antidiabetic effect—garlic, horse chestnut
Decrease: hypoglycemic effect—green tea
Drug/Lab Test
Increase: AST, ALT, LDH, BUN, creatinine, alkaline phosphatase
Decrease: Hgb, sodium, glucose, platelets, WBC

NURSING CONSIDERATIONS
Assess:
• Hypo/hyperglycemic reaction that can occur soon after meals; for severe hypoglycemia, give IV $D_{50}W$, then IV dextrose sol
• Blood glucose, A1c levels during treatment
• For allergy to sulfonamides, potential for cross-reactivity
• For renal, hepatic dysfunction: use dose reductions, or avoidance of use may be required; increased risk of hypoglycemia in hepatic failure
• **Blood dyscrasias:** CBC at baseline, throughout treatment; report decreased blood counts
• **Beers:** avoid in older adults; risk of severe prolonged hypoglycemia
• **Pregnancy/breastfeeding:** identify if pregnancy is planned or suspected; breastfed infant may be hypoglycemic; insulin should be used in pregnancy
Evaluate:
• Therapeutic response: decrease in polyuria, polydipsia, polyphagia; clear sensorium; absence of dizziness; stable gait; improved serum glucose, A1c
Teach patient/family:
• To check for symptoms of cholestatic jaundice: dark urine, pruritus, jaundiced sclera; if these occur, notify prescriber
• To use a blood glucose meter for testing while taking this product
• About the symptoms of hypo/hyperglycemia, what to do about each
• That product must be continued on a daily basis; about consequences of discontinuing product abruptly; that in times of stress, infection, surgery, trauma, a higher dose may be needed, also may require administration of insulin during these times
• To take product with breakfast or first meal of the day to prevent hypoglycemic reactions at night if taking once a day; if taking twice a day, not to take after last meal of the day
• To avoid OTC medications unless ordered by prescriber
• To report bleeding, bruising, weight gain, edema, shortness of breath, weakness, sore throat

• That diabetes is a lifelong illness; that product will not cure disease

• That all food included in diet plan must be eaten to prevent hypoglycemia; to have glucagon emergency kit, sugar packets always available

• To use sunscreen or stay out of the sun, wear protective clothing (photosensitivity)

• To carry an emergency ID with prescriber and medication information

• To notify prescribers of use prior to surgery

• To not drive or operate machinery until response is known, dizziness may occur

• That continuing follow-up exams and lab work will be needed

TREATMENT OF OVERDOSE:

Use one of the following: Glucose 25 g IV via dextrose 50% sol, 1 mg glucagon, oral carbohydrate depending on severity

---

golimumab (Rx)

(goal-lim'yu-mab)

Simponi, Simponi Aria

Func. class.: Antirheumatic agent (disease modifying), immunomodulator

Chem. class.: Monoclonal antibody, DMARD, tumor necrosis factor (TNF-α) modifier

---

ACTION: Monoclonal antibody specific for human tumor necrosis factor (TNF); elevated levels of TNF are found in patients with rheumatoid arthritis

USES: Rheumatoid arthritis (RA), ankylosing spondylitis, psoriatic arthritis, ulcerative colitis

CONTRAINDICATIONS: Hypersensitivity, active infections

Precautions: Pregnancy, breastfeeding, children, geriatric patients, CNS demyelinating disease, Guillain-Barré syndrome, HF, hepatitis B carriers, blood dyscrasias, surgery, MS, neurologic disease, diabetes, immunosuppression

Black Box Warning: Neoplastic disease, TB; fungal, bacterial, viral infections

DOSAGE AND ROUTES
Rheumatoid arthritis

• **Adult:** **SUBCUT** 50 mg monthly; for RA, give with methotrexate; **IV (Simponi Aria only)** 2 mg/kg over 30 min, repeat 4 wk later, then q8wk give with methotrexate

Ankylosing spondylitis/psoriasis

• **Adult:** **SUBCUT** 50 mg q mo; **IV (Simponi Aria only)** 2 mg/kg over 30 min, repeat q4wk, then q8wk therafter

Ulcerative colitis:

• **Adult:** **SUBCUT** 200 mg for 1 dose, then 100 mg in 2 wk, maintenance 100 mg q4wk starting at wk 6

Available forms: Inj 50 mg/0.5 mL, 100 mg/mL prefilled syringe, SmartJect Auto Injector; inj 50 mg/4 mL single-use vial

Administer:
SUBCUT route

• Refrigerate, do not freeze; allow to warm to room temperature before using

• Visually inspect sol for particulate or discoloration; sol should be clear to slightly opalescent and colorless to slightly yellow; there may be tiny white particles; do not shake; rotate injection sites

• **SmartJect Auto Injector:** allow to reach room temperature for 30 min before use; and inject within 5 min of removing cap; do not put cap back on; place open end against the inj site at a 90-degree angle without pushing button; push the injector firmly against the skin; press the button once and release; listen for the first click; wait for the second click or 15 sec, then remove injector; do not rub site

• **Prefilled syringe:** allow to warm to room temperature for 30 min; remove needle cover by pulling straight off; do not twist or recap; inject within 5 min of needle cover removal; hold syringe in one hand like a pencil and use other hand to pinch the skin; inject needle at a 45-degree angle; push plunger down as far as it will go; keep pressure on plunger head and remove needle from skin; remove pressure from plunger head; needle guard will cover needle; do not rub site

G

Side effects: *italics* = common; red = life-threatening

IV route
(Simponi Aria)
• Calculate number of vials needed; do not shake; dilute total volume of product in NS to yield 100 mL for infusion; slowly add product, mix gently
• Infuse over 30 min, use infusion set with in-line, sterile, nonpyrogenic, low–protein-binding filter (≤0.22 mm pore size)

SIDE EFFECTS
CNS: Dizziness, paresthesia, CNS demyelinating disorder, weakness, Guillian-Barre syndrome, MS
CV: Hypertension, HF
GI: Hepatitis
HEMA: Agranulocytosis, aplastic anemia, leukopenia, polycythemia, thrombocytopenia, pancytopenia
INTEG: Psoriasis
MISC: Increased cancer risk; antibody development to this drug; risk for infection (TB, invasive fungal infections, other opportunistic infections), may be fatal; inj-site reactions, anaphylaxis

PHARMACOKINETICS
Half-life 2 wk, IV peak 2-7 days, SUBCUT peak 2-5 days

INTERACTIONS
• Do not give concurrently with live vaccines or within 3 mo; immunizations should be brought up to date before treatment
• Dosage change may be needed: warfarin, cycloSPORINE, theophylline
Increase: infection—abatacept, etanercept, rilonacept, riTUXimab, adalimumab, anakinra, immunosuppressants, inFLIXimab; avoid concurrent use
Drug/Lab Test
Increase: LFTs
Decrease: platelets, WBC, neutrophils

NURSING CONSIDERATIONS
Assess:
• **Pain,** stiffness, ROM, swelling of joints during treatment
• Inj-site pain, swelling; usually occur after 2 inj (4-5 days)

Black Box Warning: TB: obtain TB skin test before starting treatment; treat latent TB before starting therapy; continue to monitor for TB even if TB test is negative

• **Blood dyscrasias:** CBC, differential before and periodically during treatment

Black Box Warning: Infection: fever, flulike symptoms, dyspnea, change in urination, redness/swelling around any wounds; stop treatment if present; some serious infections including sepsis may occur, may be fatal; patients with active infections should not be started on this product; obtain a chest x-ray, fungal serology, TB testing before starting treatment

• **HBV infection:** test for HBV before starting treatment; HBV can be fatal in HBV carriers; monitor LFTs; hepatitis B serology, may reactivate HBV
• **HF:** B/P, pulse, edema, SOB, may occur or worsen with treatment
• **Psoriasis:** may occur or worsen

Black Box Warning: Neoplastic disease: may occur in those <18 yr; avoid use in those with known malignancies; monitor for secondary malignancies during treatment

• **Anaphylaxis:** rash, dyspnea, wheezing, emergency equipment should be nearby, if present, discontinue product immediately
• **Pregnancy/breastfeeding:** use only if benefits outweigh fetal risk; do not breastfeed, excretion unknown
Evaluate:
• Therapeutic response: decreased inflammation, pain in joints, decreased joint destruction
Teach patient/family:
• About self-administration if appropriate: inj should be made in thigh, abdomen, upper arm; rotate sites at least 1 inch from old site; do not inject in areas that are bruised, red, hard
• That, if medication not taken when due, to inject next dose as soon as remembered and then the following dose as scheduled

• Not to receive any live virus vaccines during treatment

Black Box Warning: To report signs, symptoms of infection, allergic reaction, or lupuslike syndrome

• To notify prescriber if pregnancy is planned or suspected; not to breastfeed

goserelin (Rx)

(goe'se-rel-lin)

Zoladex

Func. class.: Gonadotropin-releasing hormone, antineoplastic (hormone)

Chem. class.: Synthetic decapeptide analog of LHRH

ACTION: Inhibitor of pituitary gonadotropin secretion; initially increases LH and FSH, with increases in testosterone, reduction in sex steroid levels

USES: Advanced and locally confined prostate cancer stage B2-C (10.8 mg), endometriosis, advanced breast cancer, endometrial thinning (3.6 mg)

CONTRAINDICATIONS: Hypersensitivity; pregnancy, breastfeeding, children, nondiagnosed vaginal bleeding; hypersensitivity to LHRH, LHRH-agonist analogs; 10.8 mg dose contraindicated in women

Precautions: Spinal cord decompression, renal disease, bone mineral density loss, hyperglycemia, diabetes mellitus, CV disease

DOSAGE AND ROUTES
Breast cancer
• **Adult: SUBCUT** 3.6 mg q28days or 10.8 mg q12wk
Endometrial thinning
• **Adult: SUBCUT** 3.6 mg 1-2 depot inj, (usually 1 depot, surgery performed at 4 wk; if 2 depots, surgery performed 2-4 wk after 2nd depot)

Available forms: Depot inj 3.6, 10.8 mg

Administer:
Depot
• SUBCUT using implant, inserted by qualified person into upper subcutaneous tissue in abdominal wall q28days or q12wk (10.8 mg); do not attempt to remove air bubbles from syringe; assess for injection site reaction

SIDE EFFECTS
CNS: *Headaches,* spinal cord compression, fatigue, weakness, *anxiety, depression, dizziness, insomnia, lethargy,* hot flashes, emotional lability

CV: Dysrhythmia, cerebrovascular accident, hypertension, chest pain, HF, MI, sudden cardiac death, stroke (men), *peripheral edema,* seizures, prolonged QT

ENDO: Gynecomastia, breast tenderness, breast enlargement, *hot flashes;* hyperglycemia, diabetes (men)

GI: *Nausea,* vomiting, constipation, diarrhea, ulcer

GU: *Spotting, breakthrough bleeding, decreased libido,* renal insufficiency, urinary obstruction, urinary tract infection, *impotence*

INTEG: Rash, pain at injection site, diaphoresis

MS: Bone pain, arthralgia, decreased bone density

PHARMACOKINETICS
Peak 12-15 days, half-life $4^1/_2$ hr, 30% protein bound, metabolism liver, excretion kidney

INTERACTIONS
Drug/Lab Test
Increase: alk phos, estradiol, FSH, LH, testosterone levels, triglycerides

Decrease: testosterone levels, progesterone

NURSING CONSIDERATIONS
Assess:
• **Reproductive studies:** pelvic ultrasound, pelvic exam, PSA, serum estradiol/testosterone, pregnancy test before therapy

• **Endometriosis:** pain, excessive menstrual period, bleeding between periods baseline and periodically

---

Side effects: *italics* = common; red = life-threatening

• I&O ratios; palpate bladder for distention in urinary obstruction

• **Cancer metastases:** for relief of bone pain (back pain), change in motor function

• Blood studies: lipid profile, acid phosphatase; calcium; hypercalcemia may occur

• **Pregnancy/breastfeeding:** do not use in pregnancy, breastfeeding

Evaluate:

• Therapeutic response: more normal levels of PSA, acid phosphatase, alk phos; testosterone level of <25 ng/dL; thinning of endometrial lining, decreased endometriosis symptoms, decreased symptoms in breast cancer

Teach patient/family:

• To continue with appointments monthly

• That hyperglycemia may occur in diabetic patients

• That gynecomastia and postmenopausal symptoms may occur but will decrease when treatment is discontinued

• That bone pain may increase then decrease, may use analgesics

• To notify prescriber of difficulty urinating, hot flashes

• **Pregnancy/breastfeeding:** Not to breastfeed; to use effective nonhormonal contraception; to notify prescriber if menstrual period continues

• To notify prescriber if chest pain, weakness, difficulty breathing occur, may indicate MI or stroke

• Reason for product, expected results; to use q3mo, to notify health care professional characteristics of periods (endometriosis)

---

granisetron (Rx)

(grane-iss′e-tron)

Kytril ♣, Sancuso, Sustol

Func. class.: Antiemetic

Chem. class.: 5-HT$_3$ receptor antagonist

ACTION: Prevents nausea, vomiting by blocking serotonin peripherally, centrally, and in the small intestine

USES: Prevention of nausea, vomiting associated with cancer chemotherapy, including high-dose CISplatin, radiation

Unlabeled uses: Acute nausea, vomiting after surgery

CONTRAINDICATIONS: Hypersensitivity to this product, benzyl alcohol

Precautions: Pregnancy, breastfeeding, children, geriatric patients, ondansetron/palonosetron/dolasetron hypersensitivity, cardiac dysrhythmias, cardiac/hepatic/GI disease, electrolyte imbalances

DOSAGE AND ROUTES

Nausea, vomiting in chemotherapy

• **Adult/child ≥2 yr:** IV 10 mcg/kg over 5 min, 30 min before the start of cancer chemotherapy; **TD** apply 1 patch (3.1 mg/24 hr) to upper outer arm 24-48 hr before chemotherapy, patch may be worn up to 7 days

• **Adult:** PO 1 mg bid, give 1st dose 1 hr before chemotherapy and next dose 12 hr after 1st or 2 mg as a single dose anytime within 1 hr before chemotherapy

Nausea, vomiting in radiation therapy

• **Adult:** PO 2 mg/day 1 hr before radiation

Available forms: Inj 0.1 mg/mL; tab 1 mg; oral sol 2 mg/10 mL; patch TD 3.1 mg/24 hr

Administer:

Chemotherapy/radiation: given on day of chemotherapy or radiation

PO route

• Give dose 1 hr before chemotherapy/radiation and another 12 hr after 1st dose

Transdermal

• Apply to clean, dry skin on upper arm q24-48 hr before chemotherapy or radiation

• Do not cut in pieces

• Apply immediately after opening pouch

Direct IV route

• May give undiluted over 30 sec via Y-site

Intermittent IV INFUSION route

• Dilute in 0.9% NaCl for inj or D$_5$W (20-50 mL); give over 5-15 min 30 min before chemotherapy

• Store at room temperature for 24 hr after dilution; do not freeze vials

• Do not admix

Solution compatibilities: D$_5$W, 0.9% NaCl

Y-site compatibilities: Acetaminophen, alemtuzumab, alfentanil, allopurinol, amifostine, amikacin, aminophylline, amphotericin B cholesteryl, ampicillin, ampicillin/sulbactam, amsacrine, aztreonam, bleomycin, bumetanide, buprenorphine, butorphanol, calcium gluconate, CARBOplatin, carmustine, ceFAZolin, cefepime, cefonicid, cefotaxime, cefoTEtan, cefOXitin, cefTAZidime, ceftizoxime, cefTRIAXone, cefuroxime, chlorproMAZINE, cimetidine, ciprofloxacin, CISplatin, cladribine, clindamycin, cyclophosphamide, cytarabine, dacarbazine, DACTINomycin, DAUNOrubicin, dexamethasone, diphenhydrAMINE, DOBUTamine, DOPamine, DOXOrubicin, DOXOrubicin liposome, doxycycline, droperidol, enalaprilat, etoposide, famotidine, filgrastim, fluconazole, fluorouracil, floxuridine, fludarabine, furosemide, gallium, ganciclovir, gentamicin, haloperidol, heparin, hydrocortisone, HYDROmorphone, hydrOXYzine, IDArubicin, ifosfamide, imipenem-cilastatin, leucovorin, LORazepam, magnesium sulfate, melphalan, meperidine, mesna, methotrexate, methylPREDNISolone, metoclopramide, metroNIDAZOLE, mezlocillin, miconazole, minocycline, mitoMYcin, mitoXANtrone, morphine, nalbuphine, netilmicin, ofloxacin, PACLitaxel, piperacillin, piperacillin/tazobactam, plicamycin, potassium chloride, prochlorperazine, promethazine, propofol, ranitidine, sargramostim, sodium bicarbonate, streptozocin, teniposide, thiotepa, ticarcillin, ticarcillin/clavulanate, tobramycin, trimethoprim-sulfamethoxazole, vancomycin, vinBLAStine, vinCRIStine, vinorelbine, voriconazole, zidovudine, zoledronic acid

Transdermal route

• Apply to dry, clean intact skin of upper outer arm 24-48 hr before chemotherapy, firmly press on skin, keep on during chemotherapy; can bathe, avoid swimming, whirlpool; remove ≥24 hr after chemotherapy completion; do not cut patch

SIDE EFFECTS

CNS: *Headache, asthenia,* anxiety, dizziness, stimulation, insomnia, drowsiness
CV: Hypertension, QT prolongation

GI: Diarrhea, *constipation,* increased AST, ALT, *nausea*
MISC: Rash, serotonin syndrome

PHARMACOKINETICS

Metabolized in liver to an active metabolite, half-life 10-12 hr, protein binding 65%, distributed to erythrocytes excreted by the kidney
PO: Peak 60 min, duration 24 hr, IV: Peak 30 min, duration up to 24 hr
TD: Peak 24 hr

INTERACTIONS

Increase: QT prolongation—amoxapine, arsenic, β-blockers, chloroquine, class IA, III antidysrhythmics, cloZAPine, dasatinib, dolasetron, dronedarone, droperidol, erythromycin, flecainide, fluconazole, halogenated/local anesthetics, haloperidol, lapatinib, maprotiline, methadone, octreotide, ondansetron, palonosetron, pentamidine, phenothiazines, pimozide, posaconazole, propafenone, ranolazine, risperiDONE, sertindole, SUNItinib, tacrolimus, telithromycin, tricyclics, troleandomycin, vardenafil, voriconazole, vorinostat, ziprasidone

NURSING CONSIDERATIONS
Assess:
• For absence of nausea, vomiting during chemotherapy
• **Hypersensitivity reaction:** rash, bronchospasm
• **Extrapyramidal symptoms:** grimacing, shuffling gait, tremors, involuntary movements, rare
• **QT prolongation:** monitor ECG in those with heart disease or renal disease or in the elderly
• **Serotonin syndrome:** hallucinations, seizures, diaphoresis, dizziness, flushing, hyperthermia, nausea, vomiting, diarrhea
• **Pregnancy/breastfeeding:** use only if benefits outweigh fetal risk
Evaluate:
• Therapeutic response: absence of nausea, vomiting during cancer chemotherapy
Teach patient/family:
• To report diarrhea, constipation, rash, changes in respirations

Side effects: *italics* = common; red = life-threatening

• That headache requiring an analgesic is common

• To take second dose of PO 12 hr after first dose

• That allergic reactions can occur up to 7 days after use (ext rel), or later (subcut)

• **Serotonin syndrome:** to report mental changes, including agitation, hallucinations, dizziness, sweating, flushing, tremors, seizures; discontinue immediately and notify prescriber

guaiFENesin (OTC, Rx)

(gwye-fen′e-sin)

Alfen, Altarussin, Balminil ♦, Benylin Chest Congestion Extra Strength ♦, Benylin E ♦, Bidex, Bronchophan, Calmylin Expectorant ♦, Cough Syrup Expectorant ♦, Diabetic Tussin, Expectorant ♦, Expectorant Syrup ♦, Guiatuss, Jack & Jill ♦, Miltuss EX, Mucinex, Naldecon Senior EX, Organidin NR, Robitussin Guaifenesin, Scot-Tussin Expectorant, Siltussin DAS, Siltussin SA, Vicks Chest Congestion Relief ♦, Vicks DayQuil Mucus Control ♦, Bidex

Func. class.: Expectorant

Do not confuse:

guaiFENesin/guanfacine
Mucinex/Mucomyst

ACTION: Increases the volume and reduces the viscosity of secretions in the trachea and bronchi to facilitate secretion removal

USES: Productive and nonproductive cough

CONTRAINDICATIONS: Hypersensitivity; chronic, persistent cough
Precautions: Pregnancy, breastfeeding, HF, asthma, emphysema, fever

DOSAGE AND ROUTES

• **Adult and adolescent: PO** 200-400 mg q4hr; **EXT REL** 600-1200 mg q12hr, max 2.4 g/day

• **Child 6-11 yr: PO** 100-200 mg q4hr; **EXT REL** 600 mg q12hr, max 1.2 g/day

• **Child 2-5 yr: PO** 50-100 mg q4hr; max 600 mg/day; ext rel 300 mg q12hr, max 600 mg/day

Available forms: Tabs 100, 200, 400 mg; oral sol 100 mg/5 mL; ext rel tabs 600, 1200 mg; syrup 100 mg/5 mL; oral granules 50, 100 mg/packet, caps 200 mg; liquid 100, 200 mg/5 mL

Administer:

Do not break, crush, chew ext rel tabs

• Store at room temperature

SIDE EFFECTS

CNS: Drowsiness, headache, dizziness
GI: Nausea, anorexia, vomiting, diarrhea

PHARMACOKINETICS

Half-life 1 hr, excreted in urine (metabolites)

NURSING CONSIDERATIONS
Assess:

• **Cough:** type, frequency, character, including sputum; fluids should be increased to 2 L/day

• Increased fluids, room humidification to liquefy secretions

• **Pregnancy/breastfeeding:** use only if benefits outweigh fetal risk
Evaluate:

• Therapeutic response: productive cough, thinner secretions
Teach patient/family:

• To avoid driving, other hazardous activities if drowsiness occurs (rare)

• To avoid smoking, smoke-filled room, perfumes, dust, environmental pollutants, cleansers

• To consult health provider if cough lasts >7 days

• To avoid if breastfeeding

• To avoid use in a child <2 yr

• To use as prescribed, not to double or skip doses

• Not to drive or operate machinery until response is known, drowsiness, dizziness may occur

• To notify health care professional of change in heartbeat or if feeling faint
TD: Not to use near heat such as heating pad or expose to sunlight, tanning, not to cut patch, or use in MRI

---

guselkumab (Rx)

(gus-elk′-ue-mab)

Tremfya

Func. class.: Antirheumatic agent (disease modifying), immunomodulator, anti-TNF

Chem. class.: Recombinant human IgG1 monoclonal antibody, DMARD

ACTION: A form of human IgG1 monoclonal antibody selectively binds to the p19 subunit of interleukin 23 (IL-23) cytokine, inhibiting its interaction with the IL-23 receptor. A naturally occurring cytokine, IL-23 is involved in normal inflammatory and immune responses. By inhibiting the interaction of IL-23 with its receptor, blocks the release of proinflammatory cytokines and chemokines

USES: For the treatment of moderate to severe plaque psoriasis in those who are candidates for phototherapy or systemic therapy

CONTRAINDICATIONS: Hypersensitivity
Precautions: Pregnancy, breastfeeding, children, geriatric patients, infection, vaccination

DOSAGE AND ROUTES
• **Adult: SUBCUT** 100 mg at week 0, week 4, and every 8 wk thereafter
Available forms: Prefilled syringe 100 mg/mL
Administer:
SUBCUT route
• Remove prefilled syringe from refrigerator; allow to reach room temperature (about 30 min) without removing needle cap
• Do not shake prefilled syringe

• Visually inspect for particulate matter and discoloration; solution should be colorless to slightly yellow and may contain a few small translucent particles. Do not use if discolored, cloudy, or if foreign particulate matter is present
• Only an individual trained in subcutaneous drug delivery should administer the injection. A patient who is properly trained in injection technique may self-inject using the prefilled syringe or vial if the prescriber deems the action appropriate. However, the first injection needs to be under the supervision of a qualified health care professional.
• Use front part of the middle thigh, the gluteal or abdominal region, and the outer area of the upper arm. Rotate injection sites. Do not use where skin is tender, bruised, red, hard, thick, scaly, or affected by psoriasis.
• Gently pinch the cleaned area of skin, and insert the needle at about a 45-degree angle subcutaneously, using a quick, dart-like motion. Push the plunger slowly and evenly to deliver the dose, remove the needle, and release the pinched skin. Do not rub injection site; slight bleeding may occur
• Each single-use prefilled syringe contains 100 mg/mL of product. Inject the entire 1 mL contents of the syringe. No preservatives are present; discard any unused portion
• Protect from light, do not freeze

SIDE EFFECTS
CNS: Headache
EENT: Sinusitis
GI: Diarrhea
MS: Arthralgia
INTEG: Erythema, pruritus, skin discoloration
HEMA: Bleeding
MISC: Infection, injection site reactions, antibody formation, pharyngitis, edema, TB

PHARMACOKINETICS
• Half-life 15-18 days

INTERACTIONS
• Avoid use with CYP2D6 substrates

Side effects: *italics* = common; red = life-threatening

• Do not give concurrently with live virus vaccines; immunizations should be brought up-to-date before treatment

Drug/Lab Test

• **Increase:** ALT, AST

NURSING CONSIDERATIONS
Assess:

• For injection site pain, swelling, redness; use cold compress to relieve pain/swelling

• **Infection:** fever, flulike symptoms, dyspnea, change in urination, redness/swelling around any wounds; stop treatment if present; serious infections including sepsis may occur, may be fatal; patients with active infections should not be started on this product

• **TB:** obtain TB test before starting product; do not use in active TB; for latent TB, give antituberculosis therapy before use of this product; monitor closely for signs and symptoms of active tuberculosis infection during and after treatment

• **Pregnancy/breastfeeding:** use only if benefits outweigh fetal risk; cautious use in breastfeeding, excretion unknown

Evaluate:

• Therapeutic response: decrease in lesions

Teach patient/family:

• About self-administration if appropriate: injection should be made in thigh, abdomen, upper arm; rotate sites at least 1 inch from old site; do not inject in areas that are bruised, red, hard

• That if medication is not taken when due, inject next dose as soon as remembered and inject next dose as scheduled

• Not to take any live virus vaccines during treatment

• To report signs of infection (fever, sweats, or chills; muscle aches; weight loss; cough; warm, red, or painful skin or sores on the body different from psoriasis; diarrhea or stomach pain; shortness of breath; blood in phlegm (mucus); burning in urination or urinating more often than normal), allergic reactions (itching, rash)

• To tell provider of all prescription, OTC medications, herbals, and supplements currently taken

halcinonide topical
See Appendix B

haloperidol (Rx)
(hal-oh-pehr'ih-dol)
Haldol Decanoate, Haldol
Func. class.: Antipsychotic, neuroleptic
Chem. class.: Butyrophenone

Do not confuse:
haloperidol/Halotestin

ACTION: Cortex, hypothalamus, limbic system, which control activity and aggression; blocks neurotransmission produced by DOPamine at synapse; exhibits strong α-adrenergic, anticholinergic blocking action; mechanism for antipsychotic effects unclear

USES: Psychotic disorders, control of tics, vocal utterances in Gilles de la Tourette's syndrome, short-term treatment of hyperactive children showing excessive motor activity, prolonged parenteral therapy in chronic schizophrenia, organic mental syndrome with psychotic features, hiccups (short-term), emergency sedation of severely agitated or delirious patients, ADHD

CONTRAINDICATIONS: Hypersensitivity, coma, Parkinson's disease
Precautions: Pregnancy, breastfeeding, geriatric patients, seizure disorders, hypertension, pulmonary/cardiac/hepatic disease, QT prolongation, torsades de pointes, prostatic hypertrophy, hyperthyroidism, thyrotoxicosis, children, blood dyscrasias, brain damage, bone marrow depression, alcohol and barbiturate withdrawal states, angina, epilepsy, urinary retention, closed-angle glaucoma, CNS depression

Black Box Warning: Increased mortality in elderly patients with dementia-related psychosis

DOSAGE AND ROUTES
Acute psychosis
• **Adult/child >12 yr: IM/IV** 2-10 mg, may repeat q1hr, convert to **PO** as soon as possible, **PO** should be 150% of total parenteral dose required
• **Child 6-12 yr: IM/IV** (unlabeled) 1-3 mg q4-8hr, max 0.15 mg/kg/day, switch to **PO** as soon as possible
Tourette's syndrome
• **Child 3-12 yr and 15-40 kg: PO** Initially, 0.5 mg/day divided and given bid or tid; may increase daily dose by 0.5 mg once q5-7days until desired response; maintenance, usual dose range of **PO** 0.05 to 0.075 mg/kg/day; upon stabilization, maintenance dose should be gradually reduced to lowest effective dose
Nonpsychotic Behavior
• **Child 3-12 yr and 15-40 kg: PO** Initially, 0.5 mg/day divided and given bid or tid; may increase daily dose by 0.5 mg once q5-7days until desired response; usual dose range of 0.05-0.075 mg/kg/day
Chronic psychosis
• **Child 3-12 yr and 15-40 kg: PO** Initially, 0.5 mg/day divided and given bid or tid; may increase daily dose by 0.5 mg once q5-7days until desired response; maintenance, usual dose range **PO** of 0.05 to 0.15 mg/kg/day; upon stabilization, dose should be gradually reduced to lowest effective dose
Available forms: Tabs 0.5, 1, 2, 5, 10, 20 mg; **lactate:** oral sol 2 mg/mL; inj 5 mg/mL, **decanoate:** 50 mg/mL, 100 mg/mL
Administer:
• Reduced dose to geriatric patients
• Antiparkinsonian agent if EPS occurs
• Avoid use with CNS depressants
PO route
• Store in tight, light-resistant container
• **Oral liquid:** use calibrated device; do not mix in coffee or tea
• PO with food or milk
• Avoid skin contact with oral suspension or solution—may cause contact dermatitis

H

IM route

• IM inj into large muscle mass, use 21-G, 2-in needle; give no more than 3 mL/inj site; patient should remain recumbent for 30 min

IV route (lactate) (unlabeled)

• Give undiluted for psychotic episode at 5 mg/min

• Only use lactate for IV

• Closely monitor ECG for QT prolongation

• Switch to oral as soon as possible if needed, give first PO dose within 12-24 hr of last parenteral dose

Y-site compatibilities: Alcohol 10%, dextrose 5%, alemtuzumab, amifostine, aminocaproic acid, amiodarone, amphotericin B liposome (ambisome), amsacrine, anidulafungin, argatroban, arsenic trioxide, asparaginase, atenolol, azithromycin, bleomycin, cangrelor, CARBOplatin, carmustine, caspofungin, ceftaroline, cisatracurium, CISplatin, cladribine, cloNIDine, codeine phosphate, cyclophosphamide, cytarabine, DACTINomycin, DAPTOmycin, DAUNOrubicin liposome, DAUNOrubicin, dexmedetomidine, dexrazoxane, diltiazem, DOCEtaxel, dolasetron, doxacurium, DOXOrubicin, doxorubicin liposomal, epirubicin, eptifibatide, ertapenem, etoposide, etoposide phosphate, fenoldopam, filgrastim, fludarabine, gatifloxacin, gemcitabine, granisetron, HYDROmorphone, IDArubicin, ifosfamide, irinotecan, ketamine, lepirudin, leucovorin, levofloxacin, linezolid, LORazepam, mechlorethamine, melphalan, mesna, methadone, metroNIDAZOLE, milrinone, mitoXANtrone, mivacurium, morphine, moxifloxacin, mycophenolate mofetil, nesiritide, niCARdipine, octreotide, oritavancin, oxaliplatin, PACLitaxel (solvent/surfactant), palonosetron, pamidronate, pancuronium, PEMEtrexed, potassium acetate, propofol, quinupristin-dalfopristin, remifentanil, riTUXimab, rocuronium, sodium acetate, tacrolimus, teniposide, thiotepa, tigecycline, tirofiban, topotecan, TPN (2-in-1), vecuronium, vinBLAStine, vinCRIStine, vinorelbine, voriconazole, zoledronic acid

SIDE EFFECTS

CNS: *EPS: pseudoparkinsonism, akathisia, dystonia, tardive dyskinesia; drowsiness, headache,* seizures, neuroleptic malignant syndrome, confusion

CV: *Orthostatic hypotension,* ECG changes, tachycardia, QT prolongation, torsades de pointes

EENT: Blurred vision, glaucoma, dry eyes

GI: *Dry mouth, nausea, vomiting, anorexia, constipation,* weight gain, ileus, hepatitis

HEMA: Agranulocytosis, anemia, neutropenia, leukopenia

GU: Urinary retention, urinary frequency, impotence

INTEG: *Rash,* photosensitivity, dermatitis

RESP: Respiratory depression

SYST: Risk for death (dementia)

PHARMACOKINETICS

Metabolized by liver; excreted in urine, bile; crosses placenta; enters breast milk; protein binding 92%; half-life 12-36 hr (metabolites)

PO: Onset erratic, peak 2-6 hr, half-life 24 hr

IM: Onset 15-30 min, peak 15-20 min, half-life 21 hr

IM (Decanoate): Peak 4-11 days, half-life 3 wk

INTERACTIONS

Increase: serotonin syndrome, neuroleptic malignant syndrome—SSRIs, SNRIs

Increase: QT prolongation—class IA, III antidysrhythmics, tricyclics, amoxapine, maprotiline, phenothiazines, pimozide, risperiDONE, sertindole, ziprasidone, β-blockers, chloroquine, cloZAPine, dasatinib, dolasetron, droperidol, dronedarone, flecainide, halogenated/local anesthetics, lapatinib, methadone, erythromycin, telithromycin, troleandomycin, octreotide, ondansetron, palonosetron, pentamidine, propafenone, ranolazine, SUNItinib, tacrolimus, vardenafil, vorinostat, usually with IV use

Increase: oversedation—other CNS depressants, alcohol, barbiturate anesthetics

Increase: toxicity—EPINEPHrine, lithium

Increase: effects of both drugs—β-adrenergic blockers, alcohol
Increase: anticholinergic effects—anticholinergics
Decrease: effects—lithium, levodopa
Decrease: haloperidol effects—PHENobarbital, carBAMazepine

Drug/Herb
Increase: CNS depression—chamomile, kava

Drug/Lab Test
Increase: LFTs

NURSING CONSIDERATIONS
Assess:
• **Mental status:** mood, behavior, orientation, presence of delusions, hallucinations; baseline, periodically
• Prolactin, CBC, urinalysis, ophthalmic exam before and during prolonged therapy

Black Box Warning: Dementia, affect, orientation, LOC, reflexes, gait, coordination, sleep pattern disturbances, risk for death in dementia-related psychosis

• B/P standing, lying; take pulse, respirations during initial treatment; establish baseline before starting treatment; report drops of 20 mm Hg
• Dizziness, faintness, palpitations, tachycardia on rising
• **Extrapyramidal symptoms,** including akathisia (inability to sit still, no pattern to movements), tardive dyskinesia (bizarre movements of jaw, mouth, tongue, extremities), pseudoparkinsonism (rigidity, tremors, pill rolling, shuffling gait)
• **Dehydration:** I&O, daily weight, lethargy, decreased thirst, low intake
• **Neuroleptic malignant syndrome/serotonin syndrome:** hyperthermia, muscle rigidity, altered mental status, increased CPK, seizures, hypo/hypertension, tachycardia; notify prescriber immediately
• Constipation, urinary retention daily; if these occur, increase bulk, water in diet
• **Abrupt discontinuation:** do not withdraw abruptly, taper

• **QT prolongation:** more common with IV use at high doses; monitor ECG in those with CV disease
• **Indication for use:** evaluate necessity if used as a chemical restraint; reevaluate patient often for adverse effects; ensure proper documentation
• Supervised ambulation until patient stabilized on medication; do not involve patient in strenuous exercise program, fainting is possible; patient should not stand still for long periods
• Sips of water, sugarless candy, gum for dry mouth
• **Beers:** avoid use in older adults except for schizophrenia, bipolar disorder; increased risk of stroke and cognitive decline, mortality
• **Pregnancy/breastfeeding:** no well-controlled studies; use in 3rd trimester results in infant extrapyramidal symptoms; avoid breastfeeding

Evaluate:
• Therapeutic response: decrease in emotional excitement, hallucinations, delusions, paranoia; reorganization of patterns of thought, speech; improvement in specific behaviors

Teach patient/family:
• That orthostatic hypotension occurs often; to rise from sitting or lying position gradually; to remain lying down after IM inj for at least 30 min
• To avoid hazardous activities until stabilized on medication and effects are known
• To avoid abrupt withdrawal of this product because EPS may result; to withdraw slowly
• To avoid OTC preparations (cough, hay fever, cold) unless approved by prescriber; serious product interactions may occur; to avoid use with alcohol, as increased drowsiness may occur
• About EPS and the necessity of meticulous oral hygiene because oral candidiasis may occur
• To report impaired vision, jaundice, tremors, muscle twitching
• To use sunscreen, protective clothing to minimize photosensitivity, avoid overheating

---

Side effects: *italics* = common; red = life-threatening

• To take as prescribed; not to use OTC, herbal products unless directed by prescriber

• To use good oral hygiene, frequent sips of water, sugarless gum, candy for dry mouth

TREATMENT OF OVERDOSE: Lavage if recently ingested orally; provide an airway; do not induce vomiting; provide supportive care

---

⚠ HIGH ALERT

heparin (Rx)

(hep′a-rin)

Hepalean ✦, Hep-Lock, Hep-Lock U/P

Func. class.: Anticoagulant, antithrombotic

Do not confuse:
heparin/Hespan

ACTION: Prevents conversion of fibrinogen to fibrin and prothrombin to thrombin by enhancing inhibitory effects of antithrombin III

USES: Prevention treatment of deep venous thrombosis, PE, MI, open heart surgery, disseminated intravascular clotting syndrome, atrial fibrillation with embolization, as an anticoagulant in transfusion and dialysis procedures, to maintain patency of indwelling venipuncture devices; diagnosis, treatment of DIC

CONTRAINDICATIONS: Bleeding, hypersensitivity to this product, corn, porcine protein (pork product)
Precautions: Pregnancy, children, geriatric patients, alcoholism, hyperlipidemia, diabetes, renal disease, heparin-induced thrombocytopenia (HIT), hemophilia, leukemia with bleeding, peptic ulcer disease, severe thrombocytopenic purpura, severe renal/hepatic disease, blood dyscrasias, severe hypertension, subacute bacterial endocarditis, acute nephritis; benzyl alcohol products in neonates/infants/pregnancy/lactation

DOSAGE AND ROUTES
Anticoagulation

• **Adult: IV BOLUS (intermittent)** 10,000 units, then 5000-10,000 q4-6hr **CONTINUOUS IV INFUSION** 5000 units, then 20,000-40,000 units give over 24 hr; **SUBCUT** 5000 units, then 10,000-20,000 units, then 8000-10,000 q8hr

• **Child >1 yr: IV bolus (intermittent)** 50-100 units/kg q4hr; **continuous IV infusion** 75 units/kg then 20 units/kg/hr, adjust to aPTT by 65-85 sc.

• **Neonates, infants <1 yr: Continuous IV infusion** 75 units/kg, then 28 units/kg/hr, adjust to aPTT 65-85 sec
Thromboembolism prevention

• **Adult: SUBCUT** 5000 units q8-12hr
CV surgery

• **Adult: IV** ≥150 units/kg (300 units) for procedure <60 min, 400 units/kg for procedure ≥ 60 min
Line flush

• **Adult/child: IV** 10-100 units/mL (10 units: infants) to fill heparin lock
TPN

• **Adult/child IV** 0.5-1 units/mL
Available forms: Sol for inj 10, 100, 1000, 2000, 5000, 7500, 10,000, 20,000 units/mL; premixed 1000 units/500 mL, 2000 units/1000 mL, 12,500 units/250 mL, 25,000 units/250 mL, 25,000 units/500 mL; lock flush preparations 10 units/mL
Administer:

• Cannot be used interchangeably (unit for unit) with LMWHs or heparinoids

• At same time each day to maintain steady blood levels; always check dose with another nurse before use or a change in dose

• Store at room temperature
Heparin lock route

• Do not mistake heparin sodium inj 10,000 units/mL and Hep-Lock U/P 10 units/mL; they have similar blue labeling; deaths in pediatric patients have occurred when heparin sodium inj vials were confused with heparin flush vials

---

- Inject to prevent clots in heparin lock; inject dilute heparin solution (10-100 units/0.5-1 mL after each injection or q8hr flush lock before and after each use with sterile water or 0.9% NaCl

SUBCUT route

- Give deeply with 25-G ³/₈-¹/₂-in needle; do not massage area or aspirate when giving SUBCUT inj; give in abdomen between pelvic bones, inject at 45- or 90-degree angle, rotate sites; do not pull back on plunger; apply gentle pressure for 1 min
- Do not give IM
- Avoid all IM inj that may cause bleeding, hematoma

Direct IV route

- Give loading dose undiluted, over ≥1 min; use before continuous infusion

Continuous IV INFUSION route

- Obtain baseline coagulation tests before use
- Use infusion pump; make sure pressure dressings are used after drawing blood
- Draw coagulation studies 30 min before next dose; never draw from tubing or from infused vein; use other arm
- Dilute 25,000 units/250-500 mL 0.9% NaCl or D₅W; 50-100 units/mL solutions are premixed and ready for use
- When product is added to infusion sol for cont IV, invert container at least 6 times to ensure adequate mixing

Y-site compatibilities: Acetaminophen, acetylcysteine, acyclovir, alcohol 10%, dextrose 5%, alemtuzumab, alfentanil, allopurinol, amifostine, aminocaproic acid, aminophylline, amphotericin B lipid complex, amphotericin B liposome, anidulafungin, argatroban, arsenic trioxide, ascorbic acid injection, asparaginase, atenolol, atropine, azaTHIOprine, azithromycin, aztreonam, benztropine, betamethasone, bivalirudin, bleomycin, bretylium, bumetanide, buprenorphine, butorphanol, caffeine, calcium chloride/gluconate, cangrelor, CARBOplatin, carmustine, cefamandole, ceFAZolin, cefotaxime, cefoTEtan, cefotiam, cefOXitin, ceftaroline, cefTAZidime,

ceftizoxime, ceftobiprole, cefTRIAXone, cefuroxime, chloramphenicol succinate, chlordiazePOXIDE, chlorothiazide, chlorpheniramine, cimetidine, CISplatin, cladribine, clindamycin, cloxacillin, codeine, colistimethate, cyanocobalamin, cyclophosphamide, cycloSPORINE, cytarabine, DACTINomycin, DAPTOmycin, DAUNOrubicin citrate liposome, dexamethasone, dexmedetomidine, dexrazoxane, digoxin, DOCEtaxel, DOPamine, doripenem, doxacurium, doxapram, DOXOrubicin liposomal, edetate calcium disodium, edrophonium, enalaprilat, ePHEDrine sulfate, EPINEPHrine, epoetin alfa, eptifibatide, ergonovine, ertapenem, esmolol, estrogens conjugated, ethacrynate, etoposide, etoposide phosphate, famotidine, fenoldopam, fentaNYL, flecainide, fluconazole, fludarabine, fluorouracil, folic acid (as sodium salt), foscarnet, gallamine, gallium, ganciclovir, gemcitabine, gemtuzumab, glycopyrrolate, granisetron, hydrocortisone, HYDROmorphone, ibuprofen lysine, ifosfamide, imipenem-cilastatin, indomethacin, irinotecan, isoproterenol, ketorolac, lactated Ringer's injection, lansoprazole, leucovorin, lidocaine, lincomycin, linezolid, LORazepam, magnesium sulfate, mannitol, mechlorethamine, melphalan, mephentermine, meropenem, mesna, metaraminol, methadone, methohexital, methotrexate, methoxamine, methyldopate, methylergonovine, metoclopramide, metoprolol, metroNIDAZOLE, micafungin, midazolam, milrinone, minocycline, mitoMYcin, mivacurium, morphine, moxifloxacin, multiple vitamins injection, nafcillin, nalbuphine, nalorphine, naloxone, neostigmine, nitroglycerin, nitroprusside, norepinephrine, octreotide, ondansetron, oxacillin, oxaliplatin, oxytocin, PACLitaxel (solvent/surfactant), palonosetron, pamidronate, pancuronium, PEMEtrexed, penicillin G potassium, sodium, PENTobarbital, PHENobarbital, phentolamine, phenylephrine, phytonadione, piperacillin sodium, piperacillin-tazobactam, potassium acetate/chloride, procainamide, prochlorperazine, promazine, propofol, propranolol, pyridostigmine, pyridoxine, raNITIdine, remifentanil,

Ringer's injection, riTUXimab, rocuronium, sargramostim, scopolamine, sodium acetate, bicarbonate/fusidate, succinylcholine, SUFentanil, tacrolimus, theophylline, thiamine, thiopental, thiotepa, ticarcillin, ticarcillin-clavulanate, tigecycline, tirofiban, tolazoline, topotecan, TPN (2-in-1), tranexamic acid, trastuzumab, trimetaphan, trimethobenzamide, tubocurarine, urokinase, vasopressin, vecuronium, verapamil, vinBLAStine, vinCRIStine, voriconazole, warfarin, zidovudine, zoledronic acid

SIDE EFFECTS

CNS: *Fever,* chills, headache
GU: Hematuria
HEMA: Hemorrhage, *thrombocytopenia,* anemia, heparin-induced thrombocytopenia (HIT)
INTEG: *Rash,* dermatitis, urticaria, pruritus, alopecia, hematoma, cutaneous necrosis (SUBCUT), inj-site reactions
META: Hyperkalemia, hypoaldosteronism, rebound hyperlipidemia, vitamin D deficiency
GI: Elevated LFTs
MS: Osteoporosis (child)
SYST: Anaphylaxis

PHARMACOKINETICS

Half-life 1-2 hr (dose dependent); excreted in urine; 95% bound to plasma proteins; does not cross placenta or alter breast milk; removed from the system via the lymph and spleen; partially metabolized in kidney, liver; excreted in urine (<50% unchanged)
SUBCUT: Onset 20-60 min, duration 8-12 hr, well absorbed >35,000 international units/24 hr
IV: Peak 5 min, duration 2-6 hr

INTERACTIONS

Increase: heparin action—oral anticoagulants, salicylates, dextran, NSAIDs, platelet inhibitors, cephalosporins, penicillins, ticlopidine, dipyridamole, antineoplastics, clopidogrel, SSRIs, SNRIs, quinidine, valproic acid
Decrease: heparin action—digoxin, tetracyclines, antihistamines, cardiac glycosides, nicotine, nitroglycerin

Drug/Herb
Increase: bleeding risk—arnica, anise, chamomile, clove, dong quai, garlic, ginger, ginkgo, feverfew, green tea, horse chestnut
Drug/Lab Test
Increase: ALT, AST, INR, PT, PTT, potassium
Decrease: platelets

NURSING CONSIDERATIONS

Assess:
• **Bleeding, hemorrhage:** gums, petechiae, ecchymosis, black tarry stools, hematuria, epistaxis, decrease in Hct, B/P; HIT may occur after product discontinuation; check periodically for sign of decreasing clots
• Blood studies (Hct, occult blood in stools) q3mo
• **Thrombosis:** monitor for increased thrombosis daily, in affected areas
• Partial prothrombin time, which should be 1.5-2.5× control; for continuous IV infusion, check aPTT baseline 6 hr after initiation and 6 hr after any dose change; use aPTT for dosing adjustments; after therapeutic aPTT has been measured 2×, check aPTT daily
• **Heparin-induced thrombocytopenia (HIT):** platelet count q2-3days; thrombocytopenia may occur on 4th day of treatment and resolves even during continued treatment; HIT may occur on the 5th-10th day of treatment, with platelets to 5000 mm³; this may lead to HITT (venous/arterial thrombosis) even after discontinued therapy
• **Hypersensitivity:** rash, chills, fever, itching; report to prescriber
Evaluate:
• Therapeutic response: prevention of DVT and pulmonary emboli; adequate anticoagulation based on aPTT, PTT 1.5-2.5× control
Teach patient/family:
• To avoid OTC preparations that may cause serious product interactions unless directed by prescriber; to notify all health care providers of heparin use
• That product may be held during active bleeding (menstruation), depending on condition
• About subcut injection technique if self-administered; to rotate sites, not to inject into irritated or broken skin

- To use soft-bristle toothbrush to avoid bleeding gums; to avoid contact sports; to use an electric razor; to avoid IM inj
- To carry emergency ID identifying product taken
- **Bleeding:** to report to prescriber any signs of bleeding: gums, under skin, urine, stools
- To report to prescriber any signs of hypersensitivity: rash, chills, fever, itching

TREATMENT OF OVERDOSE:
Withdraw product; administer 1 mg protamine/100 units heparin

---

RARELY USED

hepatitis B immune globulin (HBIG) (Rx)
HepaGam B, Hyper HEP B S/D, Nabi-HB
Func. class.: Immune globulin

USES: Prevention of hepatitis B virus in exposed patients, including passive immunity in neonates born to HBsAg-positive mother, prevention of hepatitis B recurrence after liver transplant in HBsAg-positive patients

CONTRAINDICATIONS: Hypersensitivity to immune globulins, coagulation disorders

DOSAGE AND ROUTES
Hepatitis B exposure in high-risk patients
- **Adult/child:** IM 0.06 mL/kg (usual 3-5 mL) within 7 days of exposure; repeat 28 days after exposure if patient wishes to not receive hepatitis B vaccine

Neonates born to hepatitis B surface-antigen–positive persons
- **Neonate:** IM 0.5 mL within 12 hr of birth

Prevention of hepatitis B infection recurrence after liver transplant
- **Adult:** IV (HepaGam B only) 20,000 international units concurrent with grafting transplanted liver, then 20,000 international units/day on days 1-7, then 20,000 international units q2wk starting on day 14, then 20,000 international units/mo starting with mo 4

---

homatropine ophthalmic
See Appendix B

---

hydrALAZINE (Rx)
(hye-dral′a-zeen)
Apresoline ✦
Func. class.: Antihypertensive, direct-acting peripheral vasodilator
Chem. class.: Phthalazine

Do not confuse:
hydrALAZINE/hydrOXYzine

ACTION: Vasodilates arteriolar smooth muscle by direct relaxation; reduction in blood pressure with reflex increases in heart rate, stroke volume, cardiac output

USES: Essential hypertension; hypertensive emergency/urgency
Unlabeled uses: HF, preeclampsia

CONTRAINDICATIONS: Hypersensitivity to hydrALAZINEs, mitral valvular rheumatic heart disease, CAD
Precautions: Pregnancy, breastfeeding, geriatric patients, CVA, advanced renal disease, hepatic disease, SLE, dissecting aortic aneurysm

DOSAGE AND ROUTES
Hypertension
- **Adult:** PO 10 mg qid 2-4 days, then 25 mg for rest of 1st wk, then 50 mg qid, max 300 mg/day
- **Child:** PO 0.75-1 mg/kg/day in 2-4 divided doses, max 25 mg/dose, increase over 3-4 wk to max 7.5 mg/kg/day or 200 mg, whichever is less

---

Side effects: *italics* = common; red = life-threatening

Hypertensive crisis
- **Adult: IV BOL** 10-20 mg q4-6hr, administer **PO** as soon as possible; **IM** 10-50 mg q4-6hr
- **Child: IM/IV BOL** 0.1-0.2 mg/kg/dose q4hr as needed

HF
- **Adult: PO** 10-25 mg tid, max 100 mg tid

Eclampsia
- **Adult: IM/IV** 5 mg q15-20min

Available forms: Inj 20 mg/mL; tabs 10, 25, 50, 100 mg

Administer:

PO route
- Give with meals (PO) to enhance absorption

IM route
- Do not admix, switch to PO as soon as possible, use only in those that cannot use PO
- No dilution needed, inject deeply in large muscle, aspirate

Direct IV route
- IV undiluted; give through Y-tube or 3-way stopcock, give each 10 mg over ≥1 min
- To recumbent patient, keep recumbent for 1 hr after administration

Y-site compatibilities: Alemtuzumab, anidulafungin, argatroban, atenolol, bivalirudin, bleomycin, DACTINomycin, DAPTOmycin, dexrazoxone, diltiazem, DOCEtaxel, etoposide, fludarabine, gatifloxacin, gemcitabine, granisetron, HYDROmorphone, IDArubicin, irinotecan, leucovorin, linezolid, mechlorethamine, metroNIDAZOLE, milrinone, mitoXANtrone, octreotide, oxaliplatin, PACLitaxel, palonosetron, pancuronium, potassium chloride, tacrolimus, teniposide, thiotepa, tirofiban, vecuronium, vinorelbine, vitamin B/C, voriconazole

SIDE EFFECTS
CNS: *Headache, dizziness,* drowsiness, peripheral neuritis
CV: *Palpitations, tachycardia, angina,* orthostatic hypotension
GI: *Nausea, vomiting, anorexia, diarrhea*
INTEG: Rash, pruritus
MISC: *Lupuslike symptoms*

PHARMACOKINETICS
Half-life 3-7 hr, metabolized by liver, 12%-14% excreted in urine, protein binding 89%; ▶☞ half of Mexicans, blacks, South Indians, and Caucasians are at risk for toxicity
PO: Onset 20-30 min, peak 1-2 hr, duration 2-4 hr
IM: Onset 10-30 min, peak 1 hr, duration 2-6 hr
IV: Onset 5-30 min, peak 10-80 min, duration up to 12 hr

INTERACTIONS
Increase: severe hypotension—MAOIs
Increase: tachycardia, angina—sympathomimetics (EPINEPHrine, norepinephrine)
Increase: hypotension—other antihypertensives, alcohol, thiazide diuretics
Increase: effects of β-blockers (metoprolol, propranolol)
Decrease: hydrALAZINE effects—NSAIDs, estrogens

Drug/Lab Test
Decrease: Hgb, WBC, RBC, platelets, neutrophils
Positive: ANA titer

Drug/Food
Increase: drug absorption; have patient take with food

NURSING CONSIDERATIONS
Assess:
- **Cardiac status:** B/P q15min × 2 hr, then q1hr × 2 hr, then q4hr after IV dose; pulse, jugular venous distention q4hr, after IV administration
- Electrolytes, blood studies: potassium, sodium, chloride, carbon dioxide, CBC, serum glucose, LE prep, ANA titer before, during treatment; assess for fever, joint pain, rash, sore throat (lupuslike symptoms); notify prescriber
- Number of refills to determine compliance
- Weight daily, I&O, edema in feet, legs daily, skin turgor, dryness of mucous membranes for hydration status

- For renal disease: dosage and administration are altered in reduced CCr, dialysis
- Crackles, dyspnea, orthopnea
- IV site for extravasation, rate
- Mental status: affect, mood, behavior, anxiety; check for personality changes
- **Beers:** use with caution in older adults; may exacerbate syncope in those with a history of syncope
- **Pregnancy/breastfeeding:** use only if benefits outweigh fetal risk; 3rd-trimester toxicity has occurred; use caution in breastfeeding

Evaluate:
- Therapeutic response: decreased B/P

Teach patient/family:
- To take with food to increase bioavailability (PO)
- To avoid OTC, herbals, supplements unless directed by prescriber
- To notify prescriber if chest pain, severe fatigue, fever, muscle or joint pain, rash, sore throat; tingling, pain in hands, feet, pyridoxine can be used
- To rise slowly to prevent orthostatic hypotension
- That follow-up will be needed; to comply with other requirements, such as exercise, weight loss, avoidance of smoking
- To notify providers of product use prior to surgery
- To avoid driving or other hazardous activities until response is known; drowsiness, dizziness may occur
- To weigh 2× per wk and check lower extremities for swelling
- To take as prescribed, not to skip or double doses, to take at the same time of the day, if dose is missed, take when remembered, do not discontinue abruptly
- To notify prescriber if pregnancy is suspected or planned or if breastfeeding

TREATMENT OF OVERDOSE:
Administer vasopressors, volume expanders for shock; if PO, lavage if recently ingested, digitalization

hydrochlorothiazide (Rx)
(hye-droe-klor-oh-thye′a-zide)
Apo-Hydro ♣, Neo-Codema ♣, Urozide ♣, Microzide, Oretic
Func. class.: Thiazide diuretic, antihypertensive
Chem. class.: Sulfonamide derivative

ACTION: Acts on distal tubule and ascending limb of loop of Henle by increasing excretion of water, sodium, chloride, potassium

USES: Edema, hypertension, diuresis, HF; idiopathic lower extremity edema therapy
Unlabeled uses: Diabetes insipidus, hypercalciuria, nephrolithiasis, premenstrual syndrome, renal calculus

CONTRAINDICATIONS: Hypersensitivity to thiazides or sulfonamides, preeclampsia, anuria, renal decompensation
Precautions: Pregnancy, breastfeeding, hypokalemia, renal/hepatic disease, gout, COPD, LE, diabetes mellitus, hyperlipidemia, CCr <30 mL/min, hypomagnesemia

DOSAGE AND ROUTES
Hypertension:
- **Adult/adolescent: PO** 12.5-25 mg/day, may increase to 50 mg/day in 1-2 divided doses, max 100 mg/day
- **Child 2-12 yr: PO** 1-3 mg/kg/day in divided doses, max 100 mg daily
- **Child <2 yr: PO** up to 1-3 mg/kg/day in divided doses, max 50 mg daily
- **Geriatric: PO** 12.5 mg/day

Renal dose:
- **Adult: PO** CCr <30 mL/min, do not use; not effective

Available forms: Tabs 12.5, 25, 50, 100 ♣ mg; caps 12.5 mg
Administer:
PO route
- In AM to avoid interference with sleep if using product as a diuretic; tab may be crushed, mixed with food

• Potassium replacement if potassium <3 mg/dL, replace magnesium if needed
• With food; if nausea occurs, absorption may be decreased slightly

SIDE EFFECTS

CNS: Drowsiness, paresthesia, depression, headache, *dizziness, fatigue, weakness,* fever

CV: Irregular pulse, *orthostatic hypotension,* palpitations, volume depletion, allergic myocarditis

EENT: Blurred vision

ELECT: *Hypokalemia,* hypercalcemia, hyponatremia, hypochloremia, hypomagnesemia

GI: *Nausea, vomiting, anorexia,* constipation, diarrhea, cramps, pancreatitis, GI irritation, hepatitis, jaundice

GU: *Urinary frequency,* polyuria, uremia, glucosuria, hyperuricemia, renal failure, erectile dysfunction

HEMA: Aplastic anemia, hemolytic anemia, leukopenia, agranulocytosis, thrombocytopenia, neutropenia

INTEG: *Rash,* urticaria, purpura, photosensitivity, alopecia, erythema multiforme

META: *Hyperglycemia, hyperuricemia,* increased creatinine, BUN

SYST: Stevens-Johnson syndrome

PHARMACOKINETICS

PO: Onset 2 hr, peak 4 hr, duration 6-12 hr, half-life 6-15 hr, excreted unchanged by kidneys, crosses placenta, enters breast milk

INTERACTIONS

Increase: hyperglycemia, hyperuricemia, hypotension—diazoxide

Increase: hypokalemia—corticosteroids, amphotericin B, piperacillin, ticarcillin

Increase: toxicity—lithium, non-depolarizing skeletal muscle relaxants, cardiac glycosides

Decrease: thiazide effect—NSAIDs

Increase: effects—loop diuretics

Decrease: effects—antidiabetics

Decrease: thiazides absorption—cholestyramine, colestipol

Drug/Food

Increase: severe hypokalemia—licorice

Drug/Lab Test

Increase: parathyroid test, uric acid, calcium, glucose, cholesterol, triglycerides

Decrease: potassium, sodium, Hgb, WBC, platelets

NURSING CONSIDERATIONS

Assess:

• B/P, pulse; weight, I&O, electrolytes baseline and periodically to determine fluid loss; effect of product may be decreased if used daily

• **Hypersensitivity to sulfonamides:** if skin rash occurs, discontinue product; fatal Stevens-Johnson syndrome may occur

• **Hypertension:** B/P lying, standing; postural hypotension may occur

• Blood studies: BUN, blood glucose, CBC, serum creatinine, uric acid

• **Signs of metabolic alkalosis:** drowsiness, restlessness

• **Signs of hypokalemia:** postural hypotension, malaise, fatigue, tachycardia, leg cramps, weakness, dehydration; monitor potassium

• Confusion, especially in geriatric patients; take safety precautions if needed

• **Beers:** use with caution in older adults; may exacerbate or cause syndrome of inappropriate antidiuretic hormone secretion or hyponatremia

• **Pregnancy, breastfeeding:** may affect fetus, crosses placental barrier, do not breastfeed

Evaluate:

• Therapeutic response: improvement in edema of feet, legs, sacral area daily; decreased B/P

Teach patient/family:

• To rise slowly from lying or sitting position to prevent postural hypotension

• To notify prescriber of muscle weakness, cramps, nausea, dizziness; hypokalemia is common; rash

• That product may be taken with food or milk

• To use sunscreen for photosensitivity

• That blood glucose may be increased in diabetics

- To take early in day at same time of day to avoid nocturia
- To avoid alcohol, OTC meds unless approved by prescriber
- To monitor weight and notify prescriber of changes
- To discuss dietary potassium requirements
- That follow-ups and routine lab tests will be required
- How to take B/P, to continue with other medical regimens (weight loss, exercise)

TREATMENT OF OVERDOSE: Lavage if recently ingested orally; monitor electrolytes; administer dextrose in saline; monitor hydration, CV, renal status; provide supportive care

---

⚠ HIGH ALERT

HYDROcodone (Rx)
(hye-droe-koe'done)
Hycodan ✦, Robidone ✦, Hysingla ER, Zohydro ER
HYDROcodone/acetaminophen (Rx)
Anexsia, Norco
HYDROcodone/ibuprofen (Rx)
Ibudone, Reprexain, Vicoprofen, Xylon
Func. class.: Antitussive opioid analgesic/nonopioid analgesic
Controlled Substance Schedule II

Do not confuse:
HYDROcodone/hydrocortisone/oxycodone
Hycodan/Vicodin
Reprexain/Zyprexa

ACTION: Acts directly on cough center in medulla to suppress cough; binds to opiate receptors in CNS to reduce pain

USES: Moderate to severe pain

CONTRAINDICATIONS: Abrupt discontinuation; hypersensitivity to this product, benzyl; GI obstruction; status asthmaticus

Black Box Warning: Respiratory depression

Precautions: Pregnancy, breastfeeding, neonates, addictive personality, increased intracranial pressure, MI (acute), severe heart disease, renal/hepatic disease, bowel impaction, urinary retention, viral infection, ulcerative colitis, seizures, sulfite hypersensitivity, psychosis, hypertension, hyperthyroidism

Black Box Warning: Accidental exposure; neonatal opioid withdrawal syndrome; potential for overdose or poisoning, substance abuse, ethanol ingestion

DOSAGE AND ROUTES
Analgesic
- **Adult:** PO 2.5-10 mg q3-6hr as needed; if using with acetaminophen max 4 g/day, total of 5 tablets with ibuprofen combination tablets; **ext rel (Zohydro ER)** 10 mg q12hr, may increase by 10 mg q12hr q3-7days as needed; **ext rel (Hysingla)** 20 mg daily, may increase by 10-20 mg q3-5day
- **Child 1-3 yr:** PO 0.1-0.2 mg/kg q3-4hr
Antitussive
- **Adult:** PO 5 mg q4-6hr as needed
- **Child:** PO 0.6 mg/kg/day divided q6-8hr, max <2 yr, 1.25 mg/dose; 2-12 yr, 5 mg/dose; >12 yr, 10 mg/dose
Renal dose
- **Adult:** PO CCr <45 mL/min- Hysingla decrease dose by 50% initially
Hepatic dose
- **Adult:** PO Hysingla decrease by 50% initially
Available forms: *Hydrocodone:* **Extended release (Zohydro ER)** 10, 15, 20, 30, 40, 50 mg; **(Hysingla ER)** 20, 30, 40, 60, 80, 100, 120 mg; Syrup: 1 mg/mL *Hydrocodone/acetaminophen:* **Tablet** 15 mg hydrocodone/325 acetaminophen; 10mg hydrocodone/325

Side effects: *italics* = common; red = life-threatening

acetaminophen **elixir/oral solution** 7.5 mg hydrocodone/325 acetaminophen/15 mL, 10 mg hydrocodone/325 acetaminophen/15 mL;

Hydrocodone/ibuprofen: Tabs 2.5 mg hydrocodone/200 mg ibuprofen, 5 mg hydrocodone/200 mg ibuprofen, 10 mg hydrocodone/200 mg ibuprofen, 7.5 mg hydrocodone/200 mg ibuprofen (Vicoprofen), 10 mg hydrocodone/200 mg ibuprofen

Administer:
• Check product carefully before using; fatalities have occurred using wrong dose, wrong product
• Do not break, crush, or chew tabs; only scored tabs can be broken
• With antiemetic after meals if nausea or vomiting occurs

Black Box Warning: Do not exceed 4 g acetaminophen with combination product

• Give with food or milk to prevent gastric upset
• Store in light-resistant area at room temperature

Extended-release route
• May need short- or rapid-acting opioid for breakthrough pain
• Swallow caps whole, do not crush or chew

SIDE EFFECTS

CNS: *Drowsiness*, dizziness, light-headedness, confusion, headache, sedation, euphoria, dysphoria, weakness, hallucinations, mood changes, dependence, seizures
CV: Tachycardia, bradycardia, QT prolongation (Hysingla)
EENT: Blurred vision, miosis, diplopia
GI: *Nausea, vomiting, anorexia, constipation*, esophageal obstruction, choking
GU: Urinary retention
INTEG: Rash, sweating
RESP: Respiratory depression

PHARMACOKINETICS

Onset 10-20 min, duration 4-6 hr, half-life $3^1/_2$-$4^1/_2$ hr, metabolized in liver, excreted in urine, crosses placenta

INTERACTIONS

Increase: CNS depression—alcohol, opioids, sedative/hypnotics, phenothiazines, skeletal muscle relaxants, general anesthetics, tricyclics
Black box warning: increase hydrocodone effect—CYP3A4 inhibitors
Increase: severe reactions—MAOIs, separate by ≥ 14 day
Decrease: hydrocodone effect—CYP3A4 inducers

Drug/Herb
Increase: CNS depression—lavender, valerian, chamomile, Kava
Drug/Lab Test
Increase: amylase, lipase

NURSING CONSIDERATIONS

Assess:
• **Pain:** intensity, type, location, other characteristics before, 1 hr after giving product; titrate upward by 25% until pain reduced by half; need for pain medication, physical dependence; opioid is more effective before pain is severe
• **CNS changes:** dizziness, drowsiness, hallucinations, euphoria, LOC, pupil reaction

Black Box Warning: **Respiratory depression:** do not use in those with respiratory depression; monitor for decreased respiratory rate, reduced urge to breathe, sighing breathing pattern; carbon dioxide retention from respiratory depression may worsen sedation; an opioid antagonist may be needed

Black Box Warning: **Accidental exposure:** may cause fatal overdose; do not use with ethanol; check all medications for alcohol content

• **Opioid addiction:** identify opioid addiction or use before starting product; if product has been used by snorting, fatal reactions have occurred
• B/P, pulse, respirations before, periodically; if respirations <10/min, dose may need to be reduced, oversedation may occur

• Bowel status: constipation; provide fluids, fiber in diet; may need stimulant laxatives if opioid use exceeds 3 days

Black Box Warning: Neonatal opioid withdrawal syndrome: monitor neonate for withdrawal (irritability, hyperactivity, abnormal sleep patterns, high-pitched crying, tremor, vomiting, diarrhea)

• **Allergic reactions:** rash, urticaria; stop product
• Cough and respiratory dysfunction: respiratory depression, character, rate, rhythm
• **Beers:** avoid in older adults unless safer alternative is unavailable; may cause ataxia, impaired psychomotor function

Black Box Warning: Pregnancy/breast-feeding: use only if benefits outweigh fetal risk; neonatal withdrawal syndrome may occur if used for prolonged periods in pregnancy; do not use in breastfeeding, excretion in breast milk

Evaluate:
• Therapeutic response: decrease in pain or cough
Teach patient/family:
• To report any symptoms of CNS changes, allergic reactions
• That physical dependency may result when used for extended periods
• That withdrawal symptoms may occur: nausea, vomiting, cramps, fever, faintness, anorexia
• To avoid driving, other hazardous activities because drowsiness occurs
• To avoid other CNS depressants; they will enhance sedating properties of this product
• To change positions slowly to reduce orthostatic hypotension
• To take as directed, not to double doses or exceed doses, not to discontinue abruptly, taper, there is a high abuse potential
• To notify provider if pain is not adequately controlled
• For dry mouth, use sugarless gum, frequent sips of water, use food, good oral hygiene
• To notify prescriber of relief of pain

Black Box Warning: Not to exceed 4000 mg in combination product with acetaminophen; check all other products that may contain acetaminophen

Black Box Warning: Ethanol ingestion: that a patient's use with ethanol can lead to serious overdose or death; not to use with other medications containing ethanol unless directed by prescriber

Black Box Warning: Neonatal opioid withdrawal syndrome: that this syndrome can be fatal; that it results from prolonged maternal use of long-acting opioids

• To notify prescriber if pregnancy is planned or suspected

TREATMENT OF OVERDOSE: Naloxone HCl (Narcan) 0.2-0.8 mg IV, O_2, IV fluids, vasopressors

---

hydrocortisone (Rx)
(hy-dro-kor′tih-sone)
Cortef, Cortenema
hydrocortisone acetate (Rx)
Anucort, Anusol, Hemril, Proctocort, Rectasol, Rectasol HC
hydrocortisone sodium succinate (Rx)
A-HydroCort, Solu
Func. class.: Corticosteroid
Chem. class.: Short-acting gluco-corticoid

Do not confuse:
hydrocortisone/HYDROcodone

ACTION: Decreases inflammation by suppression of migration of polymorphonuclear leukocytes, fibroblasts, reversal of increased capillary permeability, and lysosomal stabilization

USES: Severe inflammation, adrenal insufficiency, ulcerative colitis, collagen disorders, asthma, COPD, SLE, Stevens-Johnson syndrome, ulcerative colitis, TB
Unlabeled uses: Carpal tunnel syndrome, Churg-Strauss syndrome, endophthalmitis, mixed connective-tissue disease, multiple myeloma, polyarteritis nodosa, polychondritis, pulmonary edema, temporal arteritis, Wegener's granulomatosis, septic shock

CONTRAINDICATIONS: Fungal infection, hypersensitivity
Precautions: Pregnancy, breastfeeding, children <2 yr, diabetes mellitus, glaucoma, osteoporosis, seizure disorders, ulcerative colitis, HF, myasthenia gravis, renal disease, esophagitis, peptic ulcer, metastatic carcinoma, psychosis, idiopathic thrombocytopenia (IM), acute glomerulonephritis, amebiasis, nonasthmatic bronchial disease, AIDS, TB, recent MI (associated with left ventricular rupture), Cushing syndrome, hepatic disease, hypothyroidism, coagulopathy, thromboembolism

DOSAGE AND ROUTES
Most disorders
• **Adult:** PO 20-240 mg daily in divided doses; **IM/IV** 100-500 mg (succinate), may repeat q2-6hr
• **Child:** PO 2-8 mg/kg/day (60-240 mg/m²/day as a single or divided dose; **IM/IV** 0.666-4 mg/kg (20-120 mg/m²) q12-24hr
Adrenocortical insufficiency
• **Child:** PO 0.56 mg/kg/day (15-20 mg/m²/ day) as a single dose or divided dose; **IM/IV** 0.186-0.28 mg/kg/day (10-12 mg/m²/ day) in 3 divided doses
Shock prevention
• **Adult:** IM/IV (succinate) 50 mg/kg repeated after 4 hr; repeat q24hr as needed
Colitis
• **Adult:** PO 20-240 mg (base)/day in 2-4 divided doses; **ENEMA** 100 mg nightly for 21 days; **FOAM** 1 applicatorful 1-2×/day × 2-3 wk

• **Child:** PO 2-8 mg (base)/kg/day or 60-240 mg (base)/m²/day in 3-4 divided doses
Available forms: Hydrocortisone: **enema:** 100 mg/60 mL; tabs 5, 10, 20 mg; **Acetate:** rectal suppository: 25, 30 mg; **Cypionate:** tabs 5, 10, 20 mg; **Succinate:** injection 100-, 250-, 500-, 1000-mg vial
Administer:
Daily dose in AM for better results
• In one dose in AM to prevent adrenal suppression; avoid SUBCUT administration, may damage tissue
• Do not use acetate or susp for IV; salts are not interchangeable
PO route
• With food or milk for GI symptoms
IM route
• IM inj deep in large muscle mass; rotate sites; avoid deltoid; use 21-G needle
IV route
• **Succinate:** IV in mix-o-vial or reconstitute ≤250 mg/2 mL bacteriostatic water for inj; mix gently; give direct IV over ≥1 min; may be further diluted in 100, 250, 500, or 1000 mL of D₅W, D₅ 0.9%, NaCl 0.9% given over ordered rate

Sodium succinate
Y-site compatibilities: Acyclovir, acetaminophen, alemtuzumab, alfentanil, allopurinol, amifostine, amphotericin B cholesteryl, ampicillin, amrinone, amsacrine, atracurium, atropine, aztreonam, betamethasone, calcium gluconate, cefepime, cefmetazole, cephalothin, chlordiazePOXIDE, chlorproMAZINE, cisatracurium, cladribine, cyanocobalamin, cytarabine, dexamethasone, digoxin, diphenhydrAMINE, DOPamine, DOXOrubicin liposome, droperidol, edrophonium, enalaprilat, EPINEPHrine, esmolol, estrogens conjugated, ethacrynate, famotidine, fentaNYL, fentaNYL/droperidol, filgrastim, fludarabine, fluorouracil, foscarnet, furosemide, gallium, granisetron, heparin, hydrALAZINE, insulin (regular), isoproterenol, kanamycin, lidocaine, LORazepam, magnesium sulfate, melphalan, menadiol, meperidine, methicillin, methoxamine, methylergonovine,

minocycline, morphine, neostigmine, norepinephrine, ondansetron, oxacillin, oxytocin, PACLitaxel, pancuronium, penicillin G potassium, pentazocine, phytonadione, piperacillin/tazobactam, prednisoLONE, procainamide, prochlorperazine, propofol, propranolol, pyridostigmine, remifentanil, scopolamine, sodium bicarbonate, succinylcholine, tacrolimus, teniposide, theophylline, thiotepa, trimethaphan, trimethobenzamide, vecuronium, vinorelbine, zoledronic acid

SIDE EFFECTS

CNS: *Depression, flushing, sweating,* psychosis, headache, mood changes, pseudotumor cerebri, euphoria, insomnia, seizures
CV: *Hypertension,* edema
EENT: Increased intraocular pressure, blurred vision, cataracts, glaucoma
GI: *Diarrhea, nausea,* abdominal distention, GI hemorrhage, pancreatitis, vomiting
HEMA: Thrombophlebitis, thromboembolism
INTEG: Acne, poor wound healing, ecchymosis, petechiae
MISC: Adrenal insufficiency (after stress/ withdrawal), pheochromocytoma
MS: Fractures, osteoporosis, weakness

PHARMACOKINETICS

Metabolized by liver, excreted in urine (17-OHCS, 17-KS), crosses placenta
PO: Peak 1-2 hr, duration 1-1½ days
IM/IV: Onset 20 min, peak 4-8 hr, duration 1-1½ days
IV: Peak 1-2 hr
RECT: Onset 3-5 hr

INTERACTIONS

Increase: GI bleeding risk—salicylates, NSAIDs, acetaminophen
Increase: side effects—alcohol, amphotericin B, digoxin, cycloSPORINE, diuretics
Increase: neurologic reactions—live virus vaccines/toxoids
Decrease/Increase: anticoagulation—oral anticoagulants

Decrease: hydrocortisone action—bosentan, cholestyramine, colestipol, barbiturates, rifampin, phenytoin, theophylline, carBAMazepine
Decrease: anticoagulant effects, anticonvulsants, antidiabetics, calcium supplements, toxoids, vaccines
Drug/Herb
Decrease: hydrocortisone levels—ephedra
Drug/Lab Test
Increase: cholesterol, sodium, blood glucose, uric acid, calcium, glucose
Decrease: calcium, potassium, T$_4$, T$_3$, thyroid ^{131}I uptake test, urine 17-OHCS, 17-KS
False negative: skin allergy tests

NURSING CONSIDERATIONS

Assess:
• Potassium, blood glucose, urine glucose while patient receiving long-term therapy; hypokalemia and hyperglycemia; potassium depletion: paresthesias, fatigue, nausea, vomiting, depression, polyuria, dysrhythmias, weakness
• B/P, pulse; notify prescriber of chest pain
• I&O ratio; be alert for decreasing urinary output, increasing edema; weight daily, notify prescriber of weekly gain >5 lb
• **Adrenal insufficiency (cushingoid symptoms):** nausea, anorexia, SOB, moon face, fatigue, dizziness, weakness, joint pain before and during treatment; plasma cortisol levels during long-term therapy (normal level: 138-635 nmol/L SI units when drawn at 8 AM)
• **Infection:** increased temperature, WBC even after withdrawal of medication; product masks infection
• Mental status: affect, mood, behavioral changes, aggression
• **GI effects:** nausea, vomiting, anorexia or appetite stimulation, diarrhea, constipation, abdominal pain, hiccups, gastritis, pancreatitis, GI bleeding/perforation with long-term treatment

H

• **Epidural use:** vision changes, seizures, stroke, paralysis, brain edema, and death may occur (rare)

• **Beers:** avoid in older adults with delirium or at high risk for delirium

• **Pregnancy/breastfeeding:** use only if benefits outweigh fetal risk, avoid use in 1st trimester, usually compatible with breastfeeding

Evaluate:

Therapeutic response: decreased inflammation, GI symptoms

Teach patient/family:

• That emergency ID as corticosteroid user should be carried

• To immediately report abdominal pain, black tarry stools because GI bleeding/perforation can occur; if received by epidural route, to report immediately a change in vision, severe headache, seizures, weakness (emergency response needed)

• To notify prescriber if therapeutic response decreases; that dosage adjustment may be needed; about signs of infection

• Not to discontinue abruptly because adrenal crisis can result; that product should be tapered

• That supplemental calcium/vit D may be needed if patient is receiving long-term therapy

• That product can mask infection and cause hypo/hyperglycemia (diabetic)

• To avoid OTC, herbals, supplements: salicylates, alcohol in cough products, cold preparations unless directed by prescriber

• About cushingoid symptoms of adrenal insufficiency: nausea, anorexia, fatigue, dizziness, dyspnea, weakness, joint pain, moon face

• To avoid live-virus vaccines if using steroids long term

---

hydrocortisone nasal
See Appendix B

---

hydrocortisone (topical)
(hye-droe-kor'ti-sone)
Ala-Cort, Ala-Scalp, Anusol HC, Cetacort, Cortizone-5, Cortizone-10, Cortizone-10 Dermolate, Procort, Texacort
hydrocortisone cypionate
Cortef
hydrocortisone butyrate
Locoid, Locoid Lipocream
hydrocortisone probutate
Pandel
hydrocortisone valerate
Func. class.: Corticosteroid, topical

ACTION: Crosses cell membrane to attach to receptors to decrease inflammation, itching, inhibits multiple inflammatory cytokines

USES: Inflammation/itching in corticosteroid-responsive dermatoses on the skin, rectal area

CONTRAINDICATIONS: Hypersensitivity
Precautions: Pregnancy, breastfeeding, children

DOSAGE AND ROUTES
Corticosteroid-responsive dermatoses, inflammation, pruritus
• **Adult/child:** TOP apply to affected area 1 to 4 times per day
Inflammation from proctitis
• **Adult:** RECTAL 1 applicator full of foam once or twice a day × 2-3 wk, then every other day as needed; suppository: 1 bid × 2 wk
Available forms:
Hydrocortisone: cream 0.5%, 1%, 2.5%; gel 1%, 2%; lotion 0.25%, 1%, 2%,

---

2.5%; ointment 0.5%, 1%, 2.5%; rectal cream 1%; rectal ointment 1%; spray 1%; solution 1%, 2.5%; **Hydrocortisone acetate:** cream 0.5%, 1%, 2%, 2.5%; lotion 0.5%; ointment 0.5%, 1%; rectal foam 90 mg/application; suppositories 25 mg, 30 mg; **Hydrocortisone butyrate:** cream 0.1%; ointment 0.1%; lotion; **Hydrocortisone probutate:** cream 0.1%; **Hydrocortisone valerate:** cream 0.2%, ointment 0.2%

Administer:

Topical route

• May be used with dressings

Cream/ointment/lotion

• Apply sparingly in a thin film and rub gently

SIDE EFFECTS

CNS: Seizures, *increased intracranial pressure,* headache

CV: Hypertension

EENT: Cataracts, glaucoma

INTEG: Burning, folliculitis, pruritus, dermatitis, maceration

MISC: Hyperglycemia, glycosuria, HPA suppression

PHARMACOKINETICS

Unknown, minimally absorbed

NURSING CONSIDERATIONS

Assess:

• Skin reactions: burning, pruritus, folliculitis, dermatitis

Evaluate:

• Decreasing itching, inflammation on the skin, rectal area

Teach patient/family:

Topical route

• That product may be used with dressings

Cream/ointment/lotion

• To apply sparingly in a thin film and rub gently into the affected area

Gel

• To apply sparingly in a thin film and rub gently

Rectal

• To remove wrapper and insert suppository

⚠ HIGH ALERT

HYDROmorphone (Rx)

REMS

(hye-droe-mor′fone)

Dilaudid, Dilaudid HP, Exalgo, Hydromorph Contin ✦, Jurnista ✦

Func. class.: Opiate analgesic

Chem. class.: Semisynthetic phenanthrene

Controlled Substance Schedule II

Do not confuse:

HYDROmorphone/meperidine/morphine

Dilaudid/Demerol

ACTION: Inhibits ascending pain pathways in CNS, increases pain threshold, alters pain perception

USES: Moderate to severe pain

Unlabeled uses: Arthralgia, bone, dental pain, headache, migraine, myalgia

CONTRAINDICATIONS: Hypersensitivity to this product/sulfite, COPD, cor pulmonale, emphysema, GI obstruction, ileus, increased intracranial pressure, obstetric delivery, status asthmaticus

Black Box Warning: Respiratory depression, opioid-naive patients

Precautions: Pregnancy, breastfeeding, children <18 yr, addictive personality, renal/hepatic disease, abrupt discontinuation, adrenal insufficiency, angina, asthma, biliary tract disease, bladder obstruction, hypothyroidism, hypovolemia, hypoxemia, IBD, IV use, lactase/paraben deficiency, labor, latex hypersensitivity, myxedema, seizure disorders, sleep apnea

Black Box Warning: Substance abuse, accidental exposure, potential for overdose/poisoning, neonatal opioid withdrawal syndrome

---

DOSAGE AND ROUTES

Analgesic

- **Adult: PO** (oral solution) 2.5-10 mg q3-6hr or (tabs) 2-4 mg q4-6hr; **EXT REL** (Exalgo): convert to **EXT REL** by giving total daily dose of immediate release/day, in 1 daily dose, if needed titrate **EXT REL** q3-4days until adequate pain relief; use 25%-50% increase for each titration step, if more than 2 doses of rescue medication needed in 24 hr consider titration; **IV** 0.2-1 mg q2-3hr given over 2-3 min; **IM/SUBCUT** 1-2 mg q4-6hr prn, may be increased (opioid-naive patients may require lower dose); **RECT** 3 mg q6-8hr prn
- **Geriatric: PO** 1-2 mg q4-6hr
- **Child >50 kg (unlabeled): PO** 2-4 mg q3-4hr in opioid-naive patients, titrate; **IV** 0.2-1 mg q2-4hr or 0.3 mg/kg infusion (opioid-naive will require lower dose)
- **Infant >6 mo/child <50 kg (unlabeled): PO** 0.04-0.08 mg/kg q3-4hr in opioid-naive patients, titrate; **IV** 0.015-0.02 mg/kg q2-4hr or 0.006 mg/kg/hr infusion (opioid-naive)

Renal dose

- **Adult: PO (moderate impairment)** ext rel decrease dose by 50%, **Severe impairment** decrease dose by 75%

Hepatic disease

- **Adult: Child-Pugh B, or C (oral liquid, immediate rel tab, supp)** give reduced dose based on response, impairment **(parenteral)**, give 25%-50% of dose **(moderate impairment)**

Available forms: Powder for inj 250 mg; inj 1, 2, 4, 10 mg/mL; tabs 2, 4, 8 mg; supp 3 mg; oral sol 5 mg/5 mL; ext rel tab 8, 12, 16, 32 mg

Administer:

PO route

- Give with food or milk for GI irritation
- **Ext rel (Exalgo):** discontinue all other ext rel opioids, give q24hr; do not crush, break, chew
- When pain is beginning to return; determine interval by response
- Store in light-resistant area at room temperature

Black Box Warning: Do not use ext rel products in opioid-naive patients or with other ext rel opioids; do not use with other ext rel hydromorphone products; may be fatal

Extended release

- **Converting from oral opioids:** conversion ratios are approximate; initiate ext rel tabs at 50% of calculated total daily equivalent dose of ext rel, give q24hr; max increase q3-4days, consider titration increases of 25%-50% with each step
- **Converting from transdermal patch (fentaNYL):** initiate ext rel tabs 18 hr after removal of patch; for each 25 mcg/hr dose of transdermal fentaNYL dose is 12 mg q24hr, start dose at 50% of calculated HYDROmorphone ext rel dose q24hr; titrate no more often than q3-4days, consider dose increases of 25%-50% with each step; if more than 2 rescue doses are required in 24 hr, consider titration

SUBCUT route

- Use short 30-G needle; make sure not to inject ID
- Rotate inj sites

IM route

- Rotate sites

IV route

- **Direct,** diluted with 5 mL sterile water or NS; give through Y-connector or 3-way stopcock; give ≤2 mg over 3-5 min
- **IV INFUSION:** Dilute each 0.1-1 mg/mL NS (0.1-1 mg/mL), deliver by opioid syringe infuser; may be diluted in D_5W, D_5/NaCl, 0.45% NaCl, NS for larger amounts, delivery through infusion pump

Y-site compatibilities: Acyclovir, allopurinol, amifostine, amikacin, amsacrine, aztreonam, cefamandole, cefepime, cefoperazone, cefotaxime, cefOXitin, cefTAZidime, ceftizoxime, cefuroxime, chloramphenicol, cisatracurium, CISplatin, cladribine, clindamycin, cyclophosphamide, cytarabine, diltiazem, DOBUTamine, DOPamine, DOXOrubicin, DOXOrubicin liposome, doxycycline, EPINEPHrine, erythromycin lactobionate, famotidine, fentaNYL, filgrastim, fludarabine, foscarnet, furosemide, gentamicin, granisetron, heparin, kanamycin, labetalol, LORazepam, magnesium sulfate, melphalan, methotrexate, metroNIDAZOLE, midazolam, milrinone, morphine, nafcillin, niCARdipine, nitroglycerin, norepinephrine, ondansetron, oxacillin, PACLitaxel, penicillin G potassium, piperacillin, piperacillin/tazobactam, propofol, ranitidine, remifentanil, teniposide, thiotepa, ticarcillin, tobramycin, trimethoprim-sulfamethoxazole, vancomycin, vecuronium, vinorelbine

SIDE EFFECTS

CNS: *Drowsiness, dizziness, confusion, headache, sedation, euphoria, mood changes,* seizures
CV: Palpitations, bradycardia, change in B/P, hypotension, tachycardia, peripheral vasodilation
EENT: Tinnitus, blurred vision, miosis, diplopia
GI: *Nausea, vomiting, anorexia, constipation, cramps,* dry mouth, paralytic ileus
GU: Increased urinary output, dysuria, urinary retention
INTEG: *Rash,* urticaria, bruising, flushing, diaphoresis, pruritus
RESP: Respiratory depression, dyspnea
MISC: Physical/psychological dependence

PHARMACOKINETICS

IM: Onset 15-30 min, peak $^1/_2$-1 hr, duration 4-5 hr, metabolized by liver, excreted by kidneys, crosses placenta, excreted in breast milk, half-life 2-3 hr

INTERACTIONS

Increase: effects—other CNS depressants (alcohol, opiates, sedative/hypnotics, antipsychotics, skeletal muscle relaxants)
Increase: CNS, respiratory depression—MAOIs, separate by ≥ 14 days
Decrease: HYDROmorphone effects—opiate antagonists
Drug/Herb
Increase: action—chamomile, hops, kava, lavender, St. John's wort, valerian

Drug/Lab Test
Increase: amylase

NURSING CONSIDERATIONS
Assess:
• **Pain:** control, sedation by scoring on 0-10 scale, around-the-clock dosing is best for pain control

Black Box Warning: **Respiratory dysfunction:** respiratory depression, character, rate, rhythm; notify prescriber if respirations <10/min

Black Box Warning: **Substance abuse/opioid addiction:** assess for previous or current substance abuse; risk for abuse will be increased in these patients; assess for misuse of medication

• I&O ratio; check for decreasing output; may indicate urinary retention
• CNS changes: dizziness, drowsiness, hallucinations, euphoria, LOC, pupil reaction
• Bowel function, constipation
• Allergic reactions: rash, urticaria
• Need for pain medication, physical dependence
• Assistance with ambulation
• Safety measures: side rails, night-light, call bell within easy reach
• **Beers:** avoid in older adults unless safer alternative is unavailable; may cause ataxia, impaired psychomotor function
• **Pregnancy/breastfeeding:** use only if benefits outweigh fetal risk; neonatal withdrawal syndrome may occur if used in pregnancy for prolonged periods; do not breastfeed
Evaluate:
• Therapeutic response: decrease in pain
Teach patient/family:
• To report any symptoms of CNS changes, allergic reactions
• That product is contained in a hard tablet shell that may be seen in a bowel movement, which is normal
• Not to stop taking the product without discussing with provider

H

Side effects: *italics* = common; red = life-threatening

• To avoid driving, other hazardous activities because drowsiness occurs; to take with food if nausea occurs

• To notify provider if pain is not controlled adequately
• To use sugarless gum, frequent sips of water for dry mouth, use good oral hygiene

TREATMENT OF OVERDOSE:
Naloxone (Narcan) 0.2-0.8 mg IV (non-tolerant patients), O_2, IV fluids, vasopressors

---

hydroxychloroquine (Rx)
(hye-drox-ee-klor'oh-kwin)
Plaquenil
Func. class.: Antimalarial, antirheumatic (DMARDs)
Chem. class.: 4-Aminoquinoline derivative

ACTION: Impairs complement-dependent antigen–antibody reactions

USES: Malaria caused by susceptible strains of *Plasmodium vivax, P. malariae, P. ovale, P. falciparum* (some strains); SLE, rheumatoid arthritis
Unlabeled uses: Lupus nephritis, SLE in children, polymorphous light eruption

CONTRAINDICATIONS: Hypersensitivity to this product or chloroquine; retinal field changes
Precautions: Pregnancy, breastfeeding, blood dyscrasias, severe GI disease, neurologic disease, alcoholism, hepatic disease, G6PD deficiency, psoriasis, eczema, children, ocular disease

DOSAGE AND ROUTES
Malaria
• **Adult: PO Suppression or prevention:** 400 mg/wk, begin 2 wk before travel to endemic area, continue 4 wk after returning; **treatment:** 800 mg, then 400 mg after 6-8 hr, then 400 mg/day on 2nd and 3rd day, total dose 2 g
• **Child: PO Suppression or prevention:** 6.4 mg/kg (5 mg/kg base) weekly, begin 1-2 wk before travel to endemic area, continue 4 wk after returning; **treatment:** 10 mg/kg, 6.4 mg/kg (5 mg/kg base) at 6, 18, 24 hr after 1st dose
Lupus erythematosus
• **Adult: PO** 200-400 mg (310 mg base) daily or divided twice daily; length depends on patient response; maintenance: 200-400 mg/day
• **Child (unlabeled): PO** 5 mg/kg/day, max 400 mg/day; long-term therapy is contraindicated
Rheumatoid arthritis
• **Adult: PO** 400-600 mg daily or divided twice daily for 4-12 wk, then 200-400 mg/day after good response
Available forms: Tabs 200 mg
Administer:
PO route
• To be prescribed only by an experienced clinician
• Tabs may be crushed and mixed with food, fluids
• With food or milk; at same time each day to maintain product level
• For malaria, prophylaxis should be started 2 wk before exposure, continued for 4-6 wk after leaving exposure area
• Store in tight, light-resistant container at room temperature; keep inj in cool environment

SIDE EFFECTS
CNS: Headache, fatigue, irritability, seizures, bad dreams, dizziness, confusion, psychosis, anxiety, suicidal ideation
CV: HF, Torsades de pointes, QT prolongation, asystole with syncope

EENT: *Blurred vision, corneal changes,* tinnitus, vertigo, nystagmus, corneal deposits

GI: *Nausea, vomiting, anorexia,* diarrhea, cramps

HEMA: Thrombocytopenia, agranulocytosis, leukopenia, aplastic anemia

INTEG: Pruritus, exfoliative dermatitis, alopecia, Stevens-Johnson syndrome, photosensitivity, DRESS, rash, pruritus

PHARMACOKINETICS
Peak 3 hr; half-life 32-50 days; metabolized in liver; excreted in urine, feces, breast milk; crosses placenta, protein binding 45%

INTERACTIONS
Increase: digoxin, methotrexate levels
Increase: antibody titer—rabies vaccine
Decrease: hydroxychloroquine action—magnesium or aluminum compounds
Decrease: effect of—live virus vaccines, botulinum toxoids

NURSING CONSIDERATIONS
Assess:
• **SLE, malaria symptoms:** before treatment and daily
• **Rheumatoid arthritis:** pain, swelling, ROM, temperature of joints; for decreased reflexes: knee, ankle
• Ophthalmic exam at baseline for retinal toxicity then annually after 5 yr of use, or annually in those with increased risk factors
• Hepatic studies weekly: AST, ALT, bilirubin if patient receiving long-term treatment
• **Bone marrow suppression:** blood studies: CBC, platelets; WBC, RBC, platelets may be decreased; if severe, product should be discontinued; assess for malaise, fever, bruising, bleeding (rare)
• **ECG** during therapy: watch for depression of T waves, widening of QRS complex
• **Allergic reactions:** pruritus, rash, urticaria
• **Ototoxicity** (tinnitus, vertigo, change in hearing); audiometric testing should be done before, after treatment

• **Toxicity:** blurring vision, difficulty focusing, headache, dizziness, knee, ankle reflexes; product should be discontinued immediately
• **Pregnancy/breastfeeding:** increased rate of birth defects in the literature; CDC recommends this product for pregnant women with malaria or may be used in those with lupus; cautious use in breastfeeding

Evaluate:
• Therapeutic response: decreased symptoms of malaria, SLE, rheumatoid arthritis

Teach patient/family:
• To use sunglasses in bright sunlight to decrease photophobia; to wear protective clothing (photosensitivity)
• That urine may turn rust or brown; that skin may become blue-black
• To report hearing, visual problems, fever, fatigue, bruising, bleeding, which may indicate blood dyscrasias
RA: To report to provider if there is no change in condition, may need several months for results

Malaria prevention
• Discuss how to prevent mosquitoes in the environment
• Not to use with alcohol

TREATMENT OF OVERDOSE:
Induce vomiting; gastric lavage; administer barbiturate (ultrashort acting), vasopressor, ammonium chloride; tracheostomy may be necessary

---

⚠ HIGH ALERT

hydroxyurea (Rx)
(hye-drox'ee-yoo-ree-ah)
Droxia, Hydrea
Func. class.: Antineoplastic, antimetabolite
Chem. class.: Synthetic urea analog

Do not confuse:
hydroxyurea/hydrOXYzine
Hydrea/Lyrica

ACTION: Acts by inhibiting DNA synthesis without interfering with RNA or protein synthesis; incorporates thymidine into DNA, thereby causing direct damage to DNA strands; specific for S phase of cell cycle

USES: Melanoma, chronic myelogenous leukemia, recurrent or metastatic ovarian cancer, squamous cell carcinoma of the head and neck, sickle cell anemia
Unlabeled uses: Psoriasis, acute myelogenous leukemia (AML), astrocytoma, HIV, lung cancer, malignant glioma, polycythemia vera, thrombocytosis

CONTRAINDICATIONS: Pregnancy, breastfeeding, hypersensitivity, leukopenia (<2500/mm³), thrombocytopenia (<100,000/mm³), anemia (severe)
Precautions: Renal disease (severe), anemia, bone marrow suppression, dental disease, geriatric patients, HIV, hyperkalemia, hyperphosphatemia, hyperuricemia, hypocalcemia, infection, infertility, IM injection, tumor lysis syndrome, vaccinations

> **Black Box Warning:** Secondary malignancy, bone marrow suppression

DOSAGE AND ROUTES
Ovarian cancer, malignant melanoma
• **Adult: PO** 80 mg/kg as a single dose q3days or 20-30 mg/kg as a single dose daily
Ovarian cancer in combination with radiation
• **Adult: PO** 80 mg/kg as a single dose q3days
Chronic myelogenous leukemia (CML)/acute myelogenous leukemia (unlabeled)
• **Adult: PO** WBC >100,000/mm³, 50-75 mg/kg/day; WBC <100,000/mm³, 10-30 mg/kg/day; adjust for WBCs
• **Child: PO** 10-20 mg/kg/day, adjust to hematologic response
Sickle cell anemia
• **Adult: PO** 15 mg/kg/day, may increase by 5 mg/kg/day q12wk, max 35 mg/kg/day

Renal disease
• **Adult: PO** CCr <59 mL/min use 50% of dose
Available forms: Caps 200, 300, 400, 500 mg
Administer:
• Gloves should be worn when handling bottles or caps, including by caregivers; wash hands immediately and thoroughly
• Do not crush or chew caps; caps can be opened and contents mixed with water
• Antiemetic 30-60 min before product and prn

SIDE EFFECTS
CNS: Headache, confusion, hallucinations, dizziness, seizures
CV: Angina, ischemia
GI: Nausea, vomiting, anorexia, diarrhea, stomatitis, constipation, hepatotoxicity, pancreatitis
GU: Increased BUN, uric acid, creatinine, temporary renal function impairment
HEMA: Leukopenia, anemia, thrombocytopenia, megaloblastic erythropoiesis
INTEG: *Rash,* urticaria, pruritus, dry skin, facial erythema
META: Hyperphosphatemia, hyperuricemia, hypocalcemia
MISC: Fever, chills, malaise, secondary cancers, tumor lysis syndrome
RESP: Pulmonary fibrosis, diffuse pulmonary infiltrates

PHARMACOKINETICS
Readily absorbed when taken orally; peak level in 1-4 hr; degraded in liver; excreted in urine; almost totally eliminated within 24 hr; readily crosses blood-brain barrier; eliminated as CO_2; terminal half-life 3.5-4.5 hr

INTERACTIONS
Increase: pancreatitis/hepatotoxicity—didanosine, stavudine
Increase: toxicity—radiation or other antineoplastics
Increase: bleeding risk—NSAIDs, anticoagulants, thrombolytics, salicylates, platelet inhibitors

---

Increase: uric acid levels—probenecid, sulfinpyrazone

• Do not use with live virus vaccines

• Do not use hematopoietic progenitor cells (sargramostim, filgrastim) 24 hr before or after antineoplastic

Drug/Lab Test

Increase: BUN, creatinine, LFTs, uric acid

False increase: urea, uric acid, lactic acid

Decrease: Hgb, WBC, platelets, phosphate, calcium

NURSING CONSIDERATIONS
Assess:

Black Box Warning: **Bone marrow suppression:** determine the hemoglobin concentrations, total leukocyte count, and platelet count at least once a week during entire course; if the WBC is ≤2500/mm³ or platelets are ≤100,000/mm³, interrupt Hydrea until the values rise significantly toward normal concentrations; if severe anemia occurs, manage it without interrupting Hydrea receipt; for Droxia, monitor blood counts q2wk and interrupt drug receipt if neutrophils are <2000/mm³, platelets are <80,000/mm³, hemoglobin is <4.5 g/dL, or reticulocytes are <80,000/mm³ when the hemoglobin concentration is <9 g/dL; after recovery, Droxia may be resumed at lower dosage; Droxia therapy requires an experienced clinician knowledgeable in the use of this medication for the treatment of sickle cell anemia

• Renal studies: BUN, serum uric acid, urine CCr, electrolytes before, during therapy

• **Tumor lysis syndrome;** hyperkalemia, hyperphosphatemia, hyperuricemia, hypocalcemia; uric acid nephropathy, acute renal failure, metabolic acidosis can also occur; aggressive alkalinization of urine, allopurinol may help prevent this

• I&O ratio; report fall in urine output to <30 mL/hr

• Monitor temperature; fever may indicate beginning infection

• Hepatic studies before, during therapy: bilirubin, alk phos, AST, ALT, LDH; prn or monthly; pancreatitis may also occur

• **Cutaneous vasculitic toxicity and gangrene:** more common in those who are receiving interferon

• **Bleeding:** hematuria, guaiac, bruising or petechiae, mucosa or orifices q8hr

• Buccal cavity for dryness, sores or ulceration, white patches, oral pain, bleeding, dysphagia

• **Pulmonary reactions:** assess for pulmonary fibrosis, fever, dyspnea, diffuse pulmonary infiltrates

• **Symptoms indicating severe allergic reaction:** rash, urticaria, itching, flushing

• **Neurotoxicity:** headaches, hallucinations, seizures, dizziness

• Rinsing of mouth tid-qid with water, club soda; brushing of teeth bid-tid with soft brush or cotton-tipped applicators for stomatitis; use unwaxed dental floss

Black Box Warning: Secondary malignancy: leukemia may occur after extended use

• **Pregnancy/breastfeeding:** do not use in pregnancy/breastfeeding

Evaluate:

• Therapeutic response: decreased tumor size, spread of malignancy

Teach patient/family:

• To report signs of infection: elevated temperature, sore throat, flulike symptoms

• To report signs of anemia: fatigue, headache, faintness, SOB, irritability

• To report bleeding; to avoid use of razors, commercial mouthwash

• To avoid use of aspirin products, ibuprofen (thrombocytopenia)

• To avoid foods with citric acid, hot or rough texture if stomatitis is present

• To report stomatitis: any bleeding, white spots, ulcerations in the mouth; to examine mouth daily, report symptoms

• To inform provider if planning to receive vaccinations

H

- To wear gloves, wash hands before and after handling capsules
- To notify prescriber if pregnancy is planned or suspected
- To notify prescriber of fever, chills, sore throat, nausea, vomiting, anorexia, diarrhea, bleeding, bruising; may indicate blood dyscrasias; mental status changes, pancreatitis, hepatotoxicity

hydrOXYzine (Rx)

(hye-drox'i-zeen)

Atarax ✤, Vistaril

Func. class.: Antianxiety/antihistamine/sedative/hypnotic, antiemetic

Chem. class.: Piperazine derivative

Do not confuse:

hydrOXYzine/hydrALAZINE

Vistaril/Versed

ACTION: Depresses subcortical levels of CNS, including limbic system, reticular formation; competes with H_1-receptor sites

USES: Anxiety preoperatively, prevention of nausea, vomiting postoperatively; to potentiate opioid analgesics; sedation; pruritus

CONTRAINDICATIONS: Pregnancy 1st trimester, breastfeeding; hypersensitivity to this product or cetirizine; acute asthma

Precautions: Pregnancy (2nd/3rd trimester), geriatric patients, debilitated patients, renal/hepatic disease, closed-angle glaucoma, COPD, prostatic hypertrophy, asthma

DOSAGE AND ROUTES

Anxiety

- **Adult:** PO 50-100 mg qid, max 400 mg/day; IM 50-100 mg q4-6hr
- **Child ≥6 yr:** PO 50-100 mg/day in divided doses, max 100 mg/day or 2 mg/kg/day
- **Child <6 yr:** PO 50 mg/day in divided doses, max 50 mg/day or 2 mg/kg/day

Alcohol withdrawal

- **Adult:** IM 50-100 mg q4-6hr

Preoperatively/postoperatively (nausea/vomiting)

- **Adult:** IM 25-100 mg q4-6hr
- **Child:** IM 1.1 mg/kg as a single dose

Pruritus

- **Adult:** PO 25 mg tid-qid; IM 50-100 mg, then q4-6hr prn, switch to PO as soon as feasible
- **Child ≥6 yr:** PO 50-100 mg/day in divided doses; IM 0.5-1 mg/kg/dose q4-6hr prn, use PO when possible
- **Child <6 yr:** PO 50 mg/day in divided doses

Renal dose

- **Adult:** PO CCr <50 mL/min, give 50% of dose

Available forms: Tabs 10, 25, 50 mg; caps 25, 50, 100 mg; oral sol 10 mg/5 mL; inj 25, 50 mg/mL; oral susp 25 mg/5 mL

Administer:

PO route

- Without regard to meals
- Crushed if patient is unable to swallow medication whole
- Shake oral susp before giving

IM route

- Does not need to be diluted; give by Z-track inj in large muscle to decrease pain, chance of necrosis; never give IV/SUBCUT (HCl)

SIDE EFFECTS

CNS: *Dizziness, drowsiness,* confusion, headache, tremors, fatigue, depression, seizures

CV: Hypotension

GI: Dry mouth, increased appetite, nausea, diarrhea, weight gain

PHARMACOKINETICS

PO: Onset 15-60 min, duration 4-6 hr, half-life 3 hr, metabolized by liver, excreted by kidneys

INTERACTIONS

Increase: CNS depressant effect—barbiturates, opioids, analgesics, alcohol, sedative/hypnotics, other CNS depressants

Increase: anticholinergic effects—phenothiazines, quiNIDine, disopyramide, antihistamines, antidepressants, atropine, haloperidol, MAOIs

Drug/Lab Test

False negative: skin allergy testing

False increase: 17-hydroxycorticosteroids

NURSING CONSIDERATIONS

Assess:

• Anticholinergic effects: dry mouth, dizziness, confusion, hypotension, increased sedation; monitor B/P

• Assistance with ambulation during beginning therapy, since drowsiness, dizziness occurs

• **Beers:** avoid use in older adults; anticholinergic effects, toxicity may occur

• **Pregnancy/breastfeeding:** do not use in pregnancy/breastfeeding

Evaluate:

• Therapeutic response: decreased anxiety

Teach patient/family:

• To avoid OTC preparations (cold, cough, hay fever) unless approved by prescriber

• To avoid driving, activities that require alertness

• To avoid alcohol, psychotropic medications

• Not to discontinue medication quickly after long-term use

• To rise slowly because fainting may occur

• To report urinary retention, constipation, or other serious anticholinergic symptoms to provider, discontinue use

TREATMENT OF OVERDOSE:

Lavage if orally ingested; VS, supportive care; IV norepinephrine for hypotension

ibalizumab

(eye-ba-liz' ue-mab)

Trogarzo

Func. class.: HIV antiviral

Chem. class.: HIV-1 entry inhibitor/
fusion inhibitor

ACTION: An IV recombinant humanized monoclonal antibody; works by blocking HIV-1 from infecting CD4 T cells by binding to CD4 and interfering with the steps required for the entry of HIV-1 virus into host cells, preventing the viral transmission

USES: Human immunodeficiency virus type 1 (HIV-1) infection in heavily treatment-experienced adults with multidrug-resistant HIV-1 infection failing their current antiretroviral regimen

CONTRAINDICATIONS: Hypersensitivity

Precautions: Autoimmune disease, breastfeeding, Graves' disease, Guillain-Barré disease, immune reconstitution syndrome, pregnancy, progressive multifocal leukoencephalopathy, immune reconstitution syndrome

DOSAGE AND ROUTES

• **Adult:** IV 2000 mg once, then 800 mg q2wk as part of combination therapy in heavily treatment-experienced adults with multidrug-resistant HIV-1 infection failing their current antiretroviral regimen

Available forms: Sol for infusion 200 mg/1.33 mL

Administer:

IV route

• Visually inspect for particulate matter and discoloration before use

Dilution

• Select the appropriate number of vials necessary for either the loading dose (10 vials) or maintenance dose (4 vials)

• Withdraw 1.33 mL from each vial and transfer into a 250-mL IV bag of 0.9% sodium chloride for injection. Do not use other diluents

• Once diluted, solution should be given immediately

• **Storage:** If not administered immediately, diluted solution may be stored at room temperature (20°-25° C or 68°-77° F) for up to 4 hr or refrigerated (2°-8° C or 36°-46° F) for up to 24 hr. If refrigerated, allow the diluted solution to stand at room temperature for at least 30 min, but no more than 4 hr before use

Intermittent IV infusion route:

• Do not administer as an IV push or bolus

• Administer in the cephalic vein of the patient's arm or an appropriate vein located elsewhere

• Infuse the loading dose (2000 mg) over no less than 30 min

• If there are no infusion-associated adverse reactions, the maintenance doses (800 mg) can be decreased to no less than 15 min

• Flush with 30 mL of 0.9% sodium chloride for injection after the completion

• Observe for 1 hr after completion for at least the first infusion. If there are no infusion-associated adverse reactions, subsequent observation time can be reduced to 15 min

Missed doses

• If a maintenance dose (800 mg) is missed by 3 days or longer beyond the scheduled dosing day, a loading dose (2000 mg) should be given as early as possible

• Resume maintenance dosing (800 mg) q14days thereafter

SIDE EFFECTS

CNS: Dizziness

ENDO: Increased serum glucose and uric acid

GI: Nausea, diarrhea

INTEG: Rash

MISC: Thrombocytopenia, dizziness, rash, hyperglycemia, neutropenia

PHARMACOKINETICS

Half-life 64 hr

INTERACTIONS

None known

NURSING CONSIDERATIONS
Assess:
• **HIV:** monitor CD4+ T-cell count, plasma HIV RNA baseline and periodically

• **Immune reconstitution inflammatory syndrome:** has been reported when used in combination with other antiretrovirals. Monitor during beginning treatment when used with combination antiretrovirals; an inflammatory response to opportunistic infections may occur

• Blood studies: blood glucose, CBC with differential, LFTs, pregnancy testing, serum bilirubin (total and direct), serum creatinine/BUN baseline and periodically

• **Pregnancy/breastfeeding:** no adequate human data available regarding use in pregnancy. Monoclonal antibodies are transported across placenta as pregnancy progresses and may be transmitted from mother to fetus. Report cases of antenatal antiretroviral drug exposure to the Antiretroviral Pregnancy Registry, 1-800-258-4263 or http://www.apregistry.com/. Avoid breastfeeding

Evaluate:
• Therapeutic response: increased CD4+ counts, plasma HIV-1 RNA levels, decreased viral load, slowing progression of HIV-1 infection

Teach patient/family:
• That lab work will be necessary at the start of treatment and periodically thereafter

• **Pregnancy/breastfeeding:** to notify health care provider if pregnancy is planned or suspected; that pregnancy test will be required before starting treatment; to enroll in Antiretroviral Pregnancy Registry, which monitors fetal outcomes of pregnant women exposed to this product; not to breastfeed, HIV-1 can be passed to the baby in breast milk

• To report nausea, diarrhea if severe

• To read the patient information provided

• **Immune reconstitution syndrome:** that immune reconstitution syndrome has been reported in a patient receiving this product; to inform health care provider immediately of any symptoms of infection

• **Administration:** that product is given q2wk as recommended by the health care provider; not to change the dosing schedule of this product or any antiretroviral medication without consulting the health care provider

• To notify health care provider immediately if patient stops taking this product or any other drug in his or her antiretroviral regimen

• That product is not a cure for HIV-1 but controls symptoms and that disease still can be passed to others; to use in combination with other antiretrovirals

---

ibandronate (Rx)
(eye-ban′dro-nate)
Boniva
Func. class.: Bone-resorption inhibitor, electrolyte modifier
Chem. class.: Bisphosphonate

ACTION: Inhibits bone resorption, apparently without inhibiting bone formation and mineralization; absorbs calcium phosphate crystals in bone and may directly block dissolution of hydroxyapatite crystals of bone; more potent than other products

USES: Postmenopausal osteoporosis and prophylaxis
Unlabeled uses: Hypercalcemia of malignancy, osteolytic metastases, Paget's disease, osteoporosis (treatment/prevention) in those taking anastrozole

CONTRAINDICATIONS: Achalasia, esophageal stricture, hypocalcemia, intraarterial administration, renal failure, hypersensitivity to bisphosphonates, inability to stand or sit upright
Precautions: Pregnancy, breastfeeding, children, geriatric patients, anemia, chemotherapy, coagulopathy, dental disease, diabetes mellitus, dysphagia, GI/renal disease, GERD, hypertension, infection, multiple myeloma, phosphate hypersensitivity, vit D deficiency

---

Side effects: *italics* = common; red = life-threatening

DOSAGE AND ROUTES
Postmenopausal osteoporosis/ prophylaxis
• **Adult: PO** 150 mg/mo; **IV BOL** 3 mg q3mo
Paget's disease (unlabeled)
• **Adult: IV** 2 mg as a single dose
Bone metastases due to breast cancer (unlabeled)
• **Adult: IV** 6 mg over ≥15 min q3-4wk
Hypercalcemia of malignancy
• **Adult: IV INFUSION** 2 mg infused over 2 hr in moderate hypercalcemia, 4 mg in severe hypercalcemia (>3 mmol/L). The use of 6 mg should be reserved for serum calcium levels >3.5 mmol/L
Renal dose
• **Adult: PO** CCr <30 mL/min, avoid use
Available forms: Tabs 150 mg; sol for inj 1 mg/mL
Administer:
PO route
• Give early AM with a glass of water; if monthly, give on same day of each month
• Patient to remain upright for ≥1 hr after taking
• Do not suck/chew; throat ulcers may occur
• Store at room temperature
Direct IV route
• Use single-dose prefilled syringe; discard unused portion; give over 15-30 sec; give q3mo; do not use if discolored or contains particulates
• Do not admix
• Store at room temperature

SIDE EFFECTS
CNS: Fever, insomnia, dizziness, headache
CV: Hypertension, atrial fibrillation
EENT: Ocular pain/inflammation, uveitis, esophageal ulceration
GI: Constipation, nausea, vomiting, diarrhea, dyspepsia, esophageal/GI cancer
INTEG: Rash, inj-site reaction
META: *Hypomagnesemia, hypophosphatemia, hypocalcemia,* hypercholesterolemia
MS: Bone pain, myalgia, osteonecrosis of the jaw

SYST: Stevens-Johnson syndrome, erythema multiforme, dermatitis bullous

PHARMACOKINETICS
Half-life tabs 1.5-6 days, IV 4.5-25.5 hr; 91%-99% protein binding; taken up mainly by bones, primarily in areas of high bone turnover; eliminated primarily by kidneys (60%); **PO:** peak ½-2 hr; **IV:** peak 3 hr

INTERACTIONS
Increase: GI irritation—NSAIDs, salicylates
Decrease: ibandronate effect—calcium/ vit D/iron/aluminum/magnesium salts; separate by 1 hr
Drug/Food
• Do not take with food, calcium products; give product on empty stomach
Drug/Lab Test
Decrease: Alk phos, magnesium, calcium, phosphate

NURSING CONSIDERATIONS
Assess:
• **Osteoporosis:** before and during treatment; DEXA scan for bone mineral density; correct electrolyte imbalances (calcium, magnesium, phosphate) before starting therapy
• **Anaphylaxis (IV):** swelling of face, lips, mouth, rash, sweating, wheezing, trouble breathing; discontinue immediately, provide supportive treatment
• **Dental health:** before dental extraction, may require drug holiday for up to 2 mo; osteonecrosis of the jaw may occur
• Blood studies: electrolytes, creatinine/ BUN, calcium, vit D, alkaline phosphatase; correct deficiencies before treatment
• **For bone pain**; use analgesics; may begin within 24 hr or even years after treatment; pain usually subsides after treatment is discontinued
• **Esophageal irritation/ulceration:** heartburn, painful swallowing; avoid use in those with swallowing difficulties
Evaluate:
• Therapeutic response: increased bone mineral density
Teach patient/family:
• **To report hypercalcemic relapse:** nausea, vomiting, bone pain, thirst, unusual

muscle twitching, muscle spasms, severe diarrhea, constipation
• To continue with dietary recommendations, including calcium, vit D
• To obtain an analgesic from provider for bone pain, which may occur rapidly or within months
• That if nausea, vomiting occur, small, frequent meals may help
• To report vision symptoms: blurred vision, edema, inflammation
• To exercise regularly, stop smoking, decrease alcohol intake
• To notify health care professional of osteonecrosis of the jaw, after dental procedures, pain, draining, swell, to notify dentist before dental procedures
• To take PO first thing in AM at least 60 min before other medications, food, beverages; to take monthly dose on same day; that if IV dose is missed, to reschedule as soon as able and to reschedule subsequent doses on new time schedule; not to receive IV dose more than once in 3 mo
• To sit upright for ≥60 min after PO to prevent irritation; to swallow tab whole, not to chew or suck
• To report whether pregnancy is planned or suspected or if planning to breastfeed

---

⚠ HIGH ALERT

ibrutinib
(eye-broo′ti-nib)
Imbruvica
Func. class.: Antineoplastic-biologic response modifier
Chem. class.: Signal transduction inhibitor (STIs)—kinase inhibitor

---

ACTION: Irreversible inhibitor of Bruton's tyrosine kinases in B cells responsible for tumor growth

USES: Recurrent mantle cell lymphoma in patients who have received at least 1 prior treatment, Waldenström macroglobulinemia, chronic lymphocytic leukemia (CLL)

CONTRAINDICATIONS: Pregnancy, breastfeeding, hypersensitivity
Precautions: Children, geriatric patients, active infections, anticoagulant therapy (3 × 140-mg caps once daily until disease progression), bleeding, hepatic/renal disease, neutropenia, surgery

DOSAGE AND ROUTES
CLL, small lymphocytic lymphoma, Waldenström macroglobulinemia
• **Adult: PO** 420 mg/day
Mantle cell lymphoma in patients who have not received at least 1 prior treatment
• **Adult: PO** 560 mg (4 × 140-mg caps) daily

Dosage adjustment for ≥grade 3 nonhematologic toxicities, ≥grade 3 neutropenia with infection or fever, or grade 4 hematologic toxicities: Interrupt therapy; resume upon recovery to grade 1 or baseline as indicated below:
• **First occurrence:** Resume dosing at original dose (daily dose = 560 mg/day)
• **Second occurrence:** Reduce dose by 1 capsule (daily dose = 420 mg/day)
• **Third occurrence:** Reduce dose by 2 capsules (daily dose = 280 mg/day)
• **Fourth occurrence:** Discontinue
Available forms: Caps 140 mg
Administer:
• At same time of day with water; if dose is missed, take as soon as possible on same day, do not double
• Do not open, break, chew cap
• Use safe handling procedures
• Store at room temperature, avoid moisture

SIDE EFFECTS
CNS: Fatigue, fever
CV: Hypertension, atrial fibrillation, peripheral edema
EENT: Sinusitis
GI: Nausea, vomiting, dyspepsia, anorexia, abdominal pain, constipation, stomatitis, diarrhea, GI bleeding
GU: Increased serum creatinine, UTI, renal failure

Side effects: *italics* = common; red = life-threatening

HEMA: Neutropenia, thrombocytopenia, anemia, bleeding, epistaxis, transient lymphocytosis
INTEG: Rash, skin infections
MS: Pain, arthralgia, muscle cramps
RESP: Cough, dyspnea
SYST: Secondary malignancy, infection

PHARMACOKINETICS
Protein binding 97.3%; metabolized by CYP3A4/CYP2D6; primarily excreted in feces, small amount in urine; peak 1-2 hr, terminal half-life 4-8 hr

INTERACTIONS
Increase: ibrutinib effect—avoid use with moderate or strong CYP3A4 inhibitors (clarithromycin, indinavir, itraconazole, ketoconazole, nelfinavir, posaconazole, ritonavir, saquinavir, voriconazole)
Decrease: ibrutinib effect—avoid use with moderate or strong CYP3A4 inducers (carBAMazepine, phenytoin, rifAMPin)
Drug/Herb
Decrease: SUNItinib concentration—St. John's wort
Drug/Food Test
Increase: plasma concentrations—grapefruit juice; avoid use
Drug/Lab Test
Increase: lymphocytes, uric acid, creatinine

NURSING CONSIDERATIONS
Assess:
• **Bleeding:** bruising; grade 3 or higher bleeding events may occur, may be fatal; CBC
• **Hypersensitivity:** trouble breathing, fever, itching, wheezing, swelling of face, lips, tongue; stop product immediately, provide supportive treatment
• **Renal failure:** monitor for renal infection (BUN, creatinine), maintain hydration, monitor for hyperuricemia
• **Infection:** fever, sore throat, malaise; infections may be fatal
• **Cardiac changes/hypertension:** monitor B/P and for cardiac changes
• **Secondary malignancies:** monitor for new malignancies
• Hepatic/renal function; signs and symptoms of infections

• **Surgery:** may interrupt treatment a few days before surgery
• **Pregnancy/breastfeeding:** identify whether pregnancy is planned or suspected or if breastfeeding
Evaluate:
• Therapeutic response: decrease in progression of disease
Teach patient/family:
• About reason for treatment, expected result
• That many adverse reactions may occur: high B/P, bleeding, mouth swelling, shortness of breath
• To avoid persons with known upper respiratory infections; that immunosuppression is common
• To avoid grapefruit juice or medications, herbs; there are many interactions
• To report if pregnancy is planned or suspected, or if breastfeeding
• To report bleeding, severe infections, renal toxicity (maintain hydration), development of second malignancies, diarrhea (contact physician if it persists)
• To take with water at same time each day; do not open, break, or chew
• To report immediately trouble breathing, fever, itching, wheezing, swelling of face, lips, tongue; stop product

---

ibuprofen (OTC, Rx)
(eye-byoo-proe′fen)
Advil, Advil Infant, Advil Junior, Advil Migraine, Children's Advil, Children's Europrofen ✦, Children's Motrin, Ibuprohm, Ibutab, Midol, Motrin ✦, Motrin IB, Motrin Infant, Motrin Junior✦
ibuprofen lysine (Injection) (Rx)
Caldolor, NeoProfen
Func. class.: NSAID
Chem. class.: Propionic acid derivative

Do not confuse:
Motrin/neurontin

ACTION: Inhibits COX-1, COX-2 by blocking arachidonate; analgesic, antiinflammatory, antipyretic

USES: Rheumatoid arthritis, osteoarthritis, primary dysmenorrhea, dental pain, musculoskeletal disorders, fever, migraine, patent ductus arteriosus

Unlabeled uses: Ankylosing spondylitis, bone pain, cystic fibrosis, gouty arthritis, psoriatic arthritis

CONTRAINDICATIONS: Pregnancy 3rd trimester; hypersensitivity to this product, NSAIDs, salicylates; asthma; severe renal/hepatic disease; perioperative pain in CABG

Precautions: Pregnancy 1st and 2nd trimesters, breastfeeding, children, geriatric patients, bleeding disorders, GI disorders, cardiac disorders, hypersensitivity to other antiinflammatory agents, HF, CCr <25 mL/min

Black Box Warning: GI bleeding, MI, stroke

DOSAGE AND ROUTES
Self-treatment of minor aches/pains
• **Adult/adolescent:** PO (OTC product) 200 mg q4-6hr, may increase to 400 mg q4-6hr if needed, max 1200 mg/day
• **Child 11 yr (72-95 lb):** PO 300 mg q6-8hr
• **Child 9-10 yr (60-71 lb):** PO 250 mg q6-8hr
• **Child 6-8 yr (48-59 lb):** PO 200 mg q6-8hr
• **Child 4-5 yr (36-47 lb):** PO 150 mg q6-8hr
• **Child 2-3 yr (24-35 lb):** PO 100 mg q6-8hr
• **Child 12-23 mo (18-23 lb):** PO 75 mg q6-8hr
• **Child 6-11 mo (12-17 lb):** PO 50 mg q6-8hr

Analgesic
• **Adult:** PO 200-400 mg q4-6hr, max 3.2 g/day; OTC use max 1200 mg/day
• **Child:** PO 4-10 mg/kg/dose q6-8hr

Moderate to severe pain (hospitalized patients) (Caldolor)
• **Adult:** IV 400-800 mg q6hr as an adjunct to opiate-agonist therapy

Dysmenorrhea
• **Adult:** PO 400 mg q4-6hr, max 1200 mg/day

Antipyretic
• **Child 6 mo-12 yr:** PO 5 mg/kg (temperature <102.5° F or 39.2° C), 10 mg/kg (temperature >102.5° F), may repeat q6-8hr, max 40 mg/kg/day

Antiinflammatory
• **Adult:** PO 400-800 mg tid-qid, max 3.2 g/day
• **Child:** PO 30-40 mg/kg/day in 3-4 divided doses, max 50 mg/kg/day

Juvenile arthritis
• **Child:** PO 30-40 mg/kg/day (oral suspension) in 3-4 divided doses

Patent ductus arteriosus (PDA) (NeoProfen)
• **Premature neonate ≤32 wk gestation who weighs 500-1500 g:** IV 10 mg/kg initially, then, if needed, 2 doses of 5 mg/kg at 24-hr intervals; if oliguria occurs, hold dose

Cystic fibrosis (unlabeled)
• **Child 6 mo-12 yr:** PO 20-30 mg/kg/day divided bid

Available forms: Caps 200 mg; Tabs 100, 200, 300 ✽, 400, 600, 800 mg; cap, liq gels 200 mg; oral susp 40 mg/mL, 100 mg/5 mL; liq 100 mg/5 mL; chew tabs 100 mg; oral drops 50 mg/1.25 mL; inj 10 mg/mL (NeoProfen)

Administer:
PO route
• With food, milk, or antacid to decrease GI symptoms; if nausea and vomiting occur or persist, notify prescriber
• Shake susp well before use
• Do not use in pregnancy after 30 wk gestation
• Store at room temperature

IV route
• Patient must be well hydrated before administration
• Dilute to ≤4 mg/mL with 0.9% NaCl, LR, D₅W; infuse over ≥30 min; do not give IM

Side effects: *italics* = common; red = life-threatening

- Discard unused portion
- Visually inspect for particulate
- **Ibuprofen lysine:** dilute with dextrose or saline to appropriate volume (10 mg/mL of ibuprofen is recommended); give within 30 min of preparation; give via IV port nearest insertion site; give over 15 min
- Check for extravasation; do not give in same line with TPN; interrupt TPN for 15 min before and after product administration

SIDE EFFECTS

CNS: *Headache,* dizziness, drowsiness, fatigue, tremors, confusion, insomnia, anxiety, depression

CV: Tachycardia, peripheral edema, palpitations, dysrhythmias, CV thrombotic events, MI, stroke, HF

EENT: Tinnitus, hearing loss, blurred vision

GI: Nausea, *anorexia,* vomiting, diarrhea, jaundice, hepatitis, constipation, flatulence, cramps, dry mouth, peptic ulcer, GI bleeding, ulceration, necrotizing enterocolitis, GI perforation

GU: Nephrotoxicity, dysuria, hematuria, oliguria, azotemia

HEMA: Blood dyscrasias, increased bleeding time

INTEG: Purpura, rash, pruritus, sweating, urticaria, necrotizing fasciitis, photosensitivity, photophobia, toxic epidermal necrolysis, exfoliative dermatitis

META: Hyperkalemia, hyperuricemia, hypoglycemia, hyponatremia

SYST: Anaphylaxis, Stevens-Johnson syndrome

PHARMACOKINETICS

PO: Onset $1/2$ hr, peak 1-2 hr, duration 4-6 hr; IV: duration 4-6 hr, half-life 1.8-2 hr (adult), 1-2 hr (child) metabolized in liver (inactive metabolites), excreted in urine (inactive metabolites), 90%-99% protein binding, does not enter breast milk, well absorbed

INTERACTIONS

Increase: bleeding risk—valproic acid, thrombolytics, antiplatelets, anticoagulants, salicylates, SSRIs

Increase: blood dyscrasia risk—antineoplastics, radiation

Increase: toxicity—lithium, oral anticoagulants, cycloSPORINE, methotrexate

Increase: GI reactions—aspirin, corticosteroids, NSAIDs, alcohol, tobacco

Increase: hypoglycemia—oral antidiabetics

Decrease: effect of antihypertensives, thiazides, furosemide

Decrease: ibuprofen action—aspirin

Drug/Herb

Increase: bleeding risk—feverfew, garlic, ginger, ginkgo, ginseng *(Panax),* horse chestnut, red clover

Drug/Lab Test

Increase: BUN, creatinine, LFTs, potassium

Decrease: Hgb/Hct, blood glucose, WBC, platelets

NURSING CONSIDERATIONS

Assess:

Black Box Warning: **GI bleeding/ perforation:** chronic use can cause gastritis with or without bleeding; for those with a prior history of peptic ulcer disease or GI bleeding, initiate treatment at lower dose; geriatric patients are at greater risk and those who consume >3 alcoholic drinks/day

- Renal, hepatic, blood studies: BUN, creatinine, AST, ALT, Hgb, stool guaiac, before treatment, periodically thereafter; monitor electrolytes as needed; make sure patient is well hydrated
- **Perioperative pain in CABG:** MI and stroke can result for 10-14 days; can be fatal; those taking NSAIDs are at greater risk of MI and stroke even in first few weeks of therapy
- **Cardiac status:** edema (peripheral), tachycardia, palpitations; monitor B/P, pulse for character, quality, rhythm, especially in patients with cardiac disease, geriatric patients
- **Pain:** note type, duration, location, intensity with ROM 1 hr after administration
- **PDA closure:** monitor for bleeding, oliguria, infection; in preterm neonates

use only doses needed for ductus arteriosus closure, hold dose if renal output <0.6 mL/kg/hr on 2nd/3rd dose

• **Dysmenorrhea:** give at onset of menses
• Audiometric, ophthalmic exam before, during, after long-term treatment; for eye, ear problems: blurred vision, tinnitus; may indicate toxicity
• **Infection:** may mask symptoms; fever: temperature before and 1 hr after administration
• For history of peptic ulcer disorder, asthma, aspirin use, hypersensitivity; check closely for hypersensitivity reactions
• **Serious skin disorders:** for skin rash or swelling of lips, face, tongue; if present, discontinue immediately, provide supportive care
• **Beers:** avoid chronic use in older adults unless other alternatives are ineffective; increased risk of GI bleeding
• **Pregnancy:** identify if pregnancy is planned or suspected, or if breastfeeding; do not use after 30 wk gestation; use only if benefits outweigh fetal risk before 30 wk gestation; do not breastfeed

Evaluate:
• Therapeutic response: decreased pain, stiffness in joints; decreased swelling in joints; ability to move more easily; reduction in fever or menstrual cramping

Teach patient/family:
• To use sunscreen, sunglasses, and protective clothing to prevent photosensitivity, photophobia
• To report blurred vision, ringing, roaring in ears (may indicate toxicity); that eye and hearing tests should be done during long-term therapy
• To avoid driving, other hazardous activities if dizziness or drowsiness occurs
• **Nephrotoxicity:** to report change in urinary pattern, increased weight, edema, increased pain in joints, fever, blood in urine
• To avoid alcohol, NSAIDs, salicylates; bleeding may occur
• To report use of this product to all health care providers
• **Pregnancy:** to notify prescriber if pregnancy is planned or suspected; avoid after 30 wk

• To avoid driving or other hazardous activities until effect is known

> **Black Box Warning: MI/stroke:** to report signs/symptoms of MI/stroke immediately; discontinue product, seek emergency medical treatment

• To take with full glass of water; to sit upright for 30 min after use; to take with food to lessen GI effects

TREATMENT OF OVERDOSE: Lavage if recently ingested, induce diuresis

---

⚠ HIGH ALERT

ibutilide (Rx)
(eye-byoo′tih-lide)
Corvert
Func. class.: Antidysrhythmic (class III)
Chem. class.: Methane sulfonamide

ACTION: Prolongs duration of action potential and effective refractory period

USES: For rapid conversion of atrial fibrillation/flutter, including within 1 wk of coronary artery bypass or valve surgery

CONTRAINDICATIONS: Hypersensitivity
Precautions: Pregnancy, breastfeeding, children <18 yr, geriatric patients, sinus node dysfunction, 2nd- or 3rd-degree AV block, electrolyte imbalances, bradycardia, renal/hepatic disease, HF

> **Black Box Warning:** QT prolongation, torsades de pointes, ventricular arrhythmias, ventricular tachycardia, cardiac dysrhythmias, atrial fibrillation

DOSAGE AND ROUTES
Atrial fibrillation/flutter
• **Adult ≥60 kg: IV INFUSION** 1 vial (1 mg) given over 10 min, may repeat same dose after 10 min
• **Adult <60 kg: IV INFUSION** 0.01 mg/kg given over 10 min, may repeat same dose after 10 min

---

Available forms: Inj 1 mg/10 mL
Administer:

• Ice compress after stopping infusion for extravasation; tubing should be removed and attempt to aspirate product; elevate affected areas

IV route

• Undiluted or diluted in 50 mL 0.9% NaCl, or D₅W (0.017 mg/mL); give over 10 min

• Solution is stable for 48 hr refrigerated or 24 hr at room temperature

• Do not admix with other sol, products

• Reduce dosage slowly with ECG monitoring

• Stop infusion as soon as arrhythmia is controlled

• Do not use if discolored or particulate is present

SIDE EFFECTS

CNS: *Headache*

CV: *Hypotension, bradycardia,* sinus arrest, HF, dysrhythmias, torsades de pointes, hypertension, extrasystoles, ventricular tachycardia, bundle branch block, AV block, palpitations, supraventricular extrasystoles, syncope, prolonged QT interval

GI: Nausea

PHARMACOKINETICS

Elimination half-life 6 hr, metabolized by liver, excreted by kidneys

INTERACTIONS

Increase: prodysrhythmia—phenothiazines, tricyclics, tetracyclics, antidepressants, H₁-receptor antagonists, antihistamines
Increase: masking of cardiotoxicity—digoxin

• Do not use within 5 hr of ibutilide: class Ia antidysrhythmics (disopyramide, quiNIDine, procainamide), class III agents (amiodarone, sotalol); QT prolongation may occur

NURSING CONSIDERATIONS
Assess:

Black Box Warning: ECG continuously for ≥4 hr to determine product effectiveness; measure PR, QRS, QT intervals, check for PVCs, other dysrhythmias; discontinue if atrial fibrillation/flutter ceases; continue until QT interval corrected for heart rate (QTc) returned to baseline; if atrial fibrillation lasts more than 2 days, anticoagulation must be adequate >2 wk before use

• I&O ratio; electrolytes: potassium, sodium, chlorine

• Hepatic studies: AST, ALT, bilirubin, alk phos

• Dehydration or hypovolemia

• Rebound hypertension after 1-2 hr

• Cardiac rate, respiration: rate, rhythm, character, chest pain

• **Pregnancy/breastfeeding:** use only if benefits outweigh fetal risk; avoid breastfeeding, excretion unknown

Evaluate:

• Therapeutic response: decrease in atrial fibrillation/flutter

Teach patient/family:

• To report side effects immediately

• About reason for medication

RARELY USED

icosapent
(eye-koe′sa-pent)

Vascepa
Func. class.: Antilipidemic
Chem. class.: Omega-3 fatty acid ethylester

USES: As adjunct to diet in adults with severe hypertriglyceridemia (≥500 mg/dL)

CONTRAINDICATIONS: Hypersensitivity to icosapent ethyl

DOSAGE AND ROUTES
• **Adult: PO** 2 g bid
Available forms: Soft gel cap 1 g
Administer:
• Give with food, swallow whole
• Store at room temperature

A HIGH ALERT

IDArubicin (Rx)

(eye-dah-roob'ih-sin)

Idamycin PFS

Func. class.: Antineoplastic, antibiotic

Chem. class.: Anthracycline glycoside

Do not confuse:

IDArubicin/DOXOrubicin/
DAUNOrubicin/epiRUBicin
Idamycin/Adriamycin

ACTION: Non–cell-cycle specific; topoisomerase II inhibitor; vesicant; intercalating between DNA base pairs, causing shape change, low free radicals

USES: Used in combination with other antineoplastics for acute myelocytic leukemia in adults

Unlabeled uses: Breast cancer, liquid tumors, non-Hodgkin's lymphoma, ALL, CML, NHL

CONTRAINDICATIONS: Pregnancy, breastfeeding, hypersensitivity

Black Box Warning: Myelosuppression, bilirubin >5 mg/dL

Precautions: Children, gout, bone marrow depression, preexisting CV disease

Black Box Warning: Renal/hepatic disease, heart failure

DOSAGE AND ROUTES

• **Adult: IV** 8-12 mg/m²/day × 3 days in combination with cytarabine (induction)
• **Adolescent/child (unlabeled): IV** 10-12 mg/m²/day × 3 days

Black Box Warning: **Renal/hepatic dose: Adult: IV** CCr >2.5 mg/dL, reduce dose; bilirubin 2.5-5 mg/dL, reduce dose by 50%; bilirubin >5 mg/dL, do not use

Available forms: Inj 1 mg/mL

Administer:

• Ice compress after stopping infusion for extravasation
• Store at room temperature for 3 days after reconstituting or 7 days refrigerated

Intermittent IV INFUSION route

• Do not give IM/SUBCUT
• Use cytotoxic handling procedures after preparing in biologic cabinet wearing gown, gloves, mask
• Antiemetic 30-60 min before product and 6-10 hr after treatment to prevent vomiting
• After reconstituting 5-mg vial with 5 mL 0.9% NaCl (1 mg/1 mL), give over 10-15 min through Y-tube or 3-way stopcock of infusion of D₅W or NS; discard unused portion; use caution when needle inserted into vial (negative pressure)

• Use a free-flowing IV; do not give IM/SUBCUT
• A vesicant, monitor for necrosis

Y-site compatibilities: Amifostine, amikacin, aztreonam, cimetidine, cladribine, cyclophosphamide, cytarabine, diphenhydrAMINE, droperidol, erythromycin, filgrastim, granisetron, imipenem/CISplatin, magnesium sulfate, mannitol, melphalan, metoclopramide, potassium chloride, raNITIdine, sargramostim, thiotepa, vinorelbine

SIDE EFFECTS

CNS: Fever, chills, *headache,* seizures
CV: Dysrhythmias, HF, pericarditis, myocarditis, peripheral edema, angina, MI, myocardial toxicity
GI: *Nausea, vomiting, abdominal pain, mucositis, diarrhea,* hepatotoxicity
GU: Nephrotoxicity, red urine
HEMA: Thrombocytopenia, leukopenia, anemia
INTEG: Rash, extravasation, dermatitis, *reversible alopecia,* urticaria; thrombophlebitis and tissue necrosis at inj site; radiation recall
SYST: Infection, tumor lysis syndrome

PHARMACOKINETICS

Half-life 22 hr; metabolized by liver; crosses placenta; excreted in bile, urine

---

Side effects: *italics* = common; red = life-threatening

(primarily as metabolites); 97% protein binding

INTERACTIONS

Increase: bleeding risk—anticoagulants, salicylates, NSAIDs, thrombolytics; avoid concurrent use

Decrease: IDArubicin effect—corticosteroids

Increase: HF, ventricular dysfunction—trastuzumab

Increase: ECG changes (QT prolongation, changes in QRS voltage)—class IA/III antidysrhythmias, some phenothiazines, and other products that increase QT prolongation

Increase: cardiotoxicity—cyclophosphamide

Increase: toxicity—other antineoplastics or radiation

Decrease: antibody response—live virus vaccines

Drug/Lab Test

Decrease: calcium, platelets, neutrophils

Increase: uric acid, phosphate, potassium

NURSING CONSIDERATIONS
Assess:

Black Box Warning: CBC, differential, platelet count weekly; notify prescriber of results, severe myelosuppression can occur

• Renal studies: BUN, serum uric acid, urine CCr, electrolytes before, during therapy

• Tumor lysis syndrome: hyperkalemia, hyperphosphatemia, hyperuricemia, hypocalcemia

• I&O ratio; report fall in urine output to <30 mL/hr

• Monitor temperature; fever may indicate beginning infection

Black Box Warning: Hepatic studies before, during therapy: bilirubin, AST, ALT, alk phos prn or monthly; check for jaundice of skin and sclera, dark urine, clay-colored stools, itchy skin, abdominal pain, fever, diarrhea, do not use if bilirubin >5 mg/dL

Black Box Warning: **Cardiac toxicity:** HF, dysrhythmias, cardiomyopathy; cardiac studies before and periodically during treatment: ECG, chest x-ray, MUGA; ECG: watch for ST-T wave changes, low QRS and T, possible dysrhythmias (sinus tachycardia, heart block, PVCs)

• **Bleeding:** hematuria, guaiac stools, bruising or petechiae, mucosa or orifices

• Effects of alopecia on body image; discuss feelings about body changes

• Inflammation of mucosa, breaks in skin

• Buccal cavity for dryness, sores, ulceration, white patches, oral pain, bleeding, dysphagia

Black Box Warning: Local irritation, pain, burning at inj site; extravasation (vesicant)

• GI symptoms: frequency of stools, cramping

• Increase fluid intake to 2-3 L/day to prevent urate and calculi formation

• **Pregnancy/breastfeeding:** do not use in pregnancy/breastfeeding

Evaluate:

• Therapeutic response: decreased liquid tumor, spread of malignancy

Teach patient/family:

• To report signs of HF, cardiac toxicity, beginning infection

• That severe nausea/vomiting may occur; that antiemetics are usually given

• That hair may be lost during treatment; that wig or hairpiece may make patient feel better; that new hair may be different in color, texture

• To avoid foods with citric acid, hot temperature, or rough texture

• To avoid crowds, persons with upper respiratory illness

• To report any bleeding, white spots, ulcerations in mouth; to examine mouth daily

• That urine may be red-orange for 48 hr; that all body fluids will change color

• To report if pregnancy is planned or suspected

• To use contraception during treatment and for ≥4 mo after treatment

idelalisib
(eye-del′a-lis′ib)
Zydelig
Func. class.: Antineoplastic-biologic response modifier
Chem. class.: Signal transduction inhibitor (STI)

ACTION: Selective, small-molecule inhibitor of one kinase (expressed in both normal and malignant B-cells). Induces apoptosis and inhibited proliferation, inhibits several cell signaling pathways

USES: Treatment of relapsed chronic lymphocytic leukemia (CLL), in combination with riTUXimab, in those for whom riTUXimab alone should not be used; non-Hodgkin's lymphoma (NHL), relapsed follicular B-cell non-Hodgkin's lymphoma in those who have received at least 2 prior systemic therapies

CONTRAINDICATIONS: Infusion-related reaction, serious rash, pregnancy
Precautions: Serious allergic reactions, grade 3 or 4 neutropenia, breastfeeding, hyperglycemia/hypoglycemia

> **Black Box Warning:** Serious hepatotoxicity, grade 3 or higher diarrhea or colitis, fatal/serious pneumonitis

DOSAGE AND ROUTES
Small lymphocytic lymphoma (SLL) in those who have received at least 2 prior systemic therapies
• **Adult:** PO 150 mg bid until disease progression or unacceptable toxicity
Relapsed chronic lymphocytic leukemia (CLL) in combination with rituximab
• **Adult:** PO 150 mg bid with rituximab 375 mg/m² **IV**, then 500 mg/m² **IV** q2wk for 4 doses, then q4wk for 3 doses, for a total of 8 infusions

Hepatic dose
• **AST/ALT >3-5 × ULN:** No change; monitor AST/ALT at least every week until ≤1 × ULN
• **AST/ALT >5-20 × ULN:** Hold doses, monitor AST/ALT at least every week, when AST/ALT are ≤1 × ULN, resume at 100 mg bid
• **AST/ALT >20 × ULN:** Permanently discontinue
• **Bilirubin >1.5-3 × ULN:** No change; monitor bilirubin at least every week until ≤1 × ULN
• **Bilirubin >3-10 × ULN:** Hold treatment; monitor bilirubin at least every week; when bilirubin is ≤1 × ULN, resume treatment at 100 mg bid
• **Bilirubin >10 × ULN:** Permanently discontinue

Available forms: Tabs 100, 150 mg
Administer:
• Take without regard to food; do not crush or dissolve tabs
• Do not take 2 doses at the same time; if a dose is missed by <6 hr, take the dose, take next dose at usual time
Therapeutic drug monitoring: dosage adjustments due to treatment-related toxicity
• **Moderate diarrhea (4-6 stools/day over baseline):** Continue current dosing; monitor at least every week until diarrhea is resolved
• **Severe diarrhea (≥7 stools/day over baseline) or diarrhea requiring hospitalization:** Hold treatment, and monitor at least every week for resolution. When diarrhea has resolved, resume with 100 mg bid
• **Life-threatening diarrhea:** Permanently discontinue treatment
• **Neutropenia: ANC 1000-1499 cells/mm³:** no change; **ANC 500-999 cells/mm³:** continue current dosing; monitor ANC at least every week; **ANC <500 cells/mm³:** hold treatment and monitor ANC at least every week, when ANC ≥500 cells/mm³, resume treatment at 100 mg bid
• **Thrombocytopenia: Platelet count 50,000-75,000 cells/mm³:** no change; **platelet count 25,000-49,000 cells/mm³:** continue dose; monitor platelet

I

Side effects: *italics* = common; red = life-threatening

count at least every week; **platelet count <25,000 cells/mm³:** hold treatment, monitor platelet count at least every week, when platelet count ≥25,000 cells/mm³, resume treatment at 100 mg bid

• **Symptomatic pneumonitis (any severity):** Discontinue treatment

• **Other severe or life-threatening toxicities:** Hold until toxicity is resolved; if resuming treatment, reduce the dose to 100 mg bid; permanently discontinue treatment for any recurrence of severe or life-threatening toxicity after rechallenge

SIDE EFFECTS

CNS: Insomnia, fatigue, fever, headache
RESP: Pneumonitis, dyspnea, cough
ENDO: Hypoglycemia, hyperglycemia, hyponatremia
INTEG: Rash
EENT: Sinusitis
GI: Nausea, vomiting, hepatic failure, GI perforation, stomatitis, colitis, diarrhea, anorexia, abdominal pain
HEMA: Thrombocytopenia, neutropenia, anemia
SYST: Serious/fatal rashes

PHARMACOKINETICS

84% protein binding, half-life 8.2 hr, peak 1.5 hr

INTERACTIONS

Avoid use with CYP3A4 inhibitors, inducers, substrates
Drug/Lab Test
Increase: LFTs

NURSING CONSIDERATIONS
Assess:

Black Box Warning: **Hepatic failure:** increased LFTs generally occurred within the first 12 wk of treatment and were reversible with dose interruption. Monitor LFTs q2wk × 3 mo of treatment, then q4wk for 3 mo, and q1-3 mo thereafter; monitor weekly if AST or ALT are >3 times the upper limit of normal (ULN) or bilirubin >1.5 × ULN. Hepatotoxicity may require treatment interruption, dose reduction, or discontinuation of therapy

Black Box Warning: **Severe diarrhea/GI perforation:** generally responds poorly to antimotility agents. The occurrence of ≥7 stools/day over baseline or hospitalization due to diarrhea may result in interruption of therapy, dose reduction, or permanent discontinuation. Assess for new or worsening abdominal pain, chills, fever, or nausea/vomiting. If intestinal perforation occurs, permanently discontinue treatment

Black Box Warning: **Infections/pneumonitis:** monitor for cough, dyspnea, hypoxia, and bilateral interstitial infiltrates, or a decline in oxygen saturation by >5%. If pneumonitis is suspected, hold therapy. Permanently discontinue treatment for pneumonitis and consider treatment with corticosteroids

• **Pregnancy/breastfeeding:** do not use in pregnancy/breastfeeding
Evaluate:
• Therapeutic response: Decreased disease progression
Teach patient/family:
• **Pregnancy/breastfeeding:** to report planned or suspected pregnancy; to use effective contraception during treatment and for at least 1 mo after the last dose; to avoid breastfeeding
• To report new or worsening side effects
• To take tabs whole, not to crush or chew; to take with food for GI upset

---

⚠ HIGH ALERT

ifosfamide (Rx)
(i-foss′fa-mide)
Ifex
Func. class.: Antineoplastic alkylating agent
Chem. class.: Nitrogen mustard

Do not confuse:
ifosfamide/cyclophosphamide

ACTION: Alkylates DNA, inhibits enzymes that allow synthesis of amino acids in proteins; also responsible for cross-linking DNA strands; activity is not cell-cycle–stage specific

USES: Germ cell testicular cancer in combination

CONTRAINDICATIONS: Pregnancy, hypersensitivity

Black Box Warning: Bone marrow suppression

Precautions: Breastfeeding, children, renal/hepatic disease, accidental exposure, dehydration, dental disease, infection, IM injection, ocular exposure, varicella

Black Box Warning: Coma, hemorrhagic cystitis

DOSAGE AND ROUTES
Germ cell testicular cancer
• **Adult:** IV 1.2-2 g/m^2/day × 5 days, repeat course q3wk, given with mesna, in combination with 1-2 other antineoplastic agents
Sarcoma of soft tissue (orphan drug designation) (unlabeled)
• **Adult:** IV INFUSION MAID regimen: DOXOrubicin 60 mg/m^2 and dacarbazine 1000 mg/m^2, mixed or administered separately via **CONT IV INFUSION** over 4 days, ifosfamide 6000 mg/m^2 and mesna 10,000 mg/m^2 mixed or infused separately over 3 days (ifosfamide) and 4 days (mesna); repeat q21days if tolerated; OR MAID regimen: DOXOrubicin 60 mg/m^2 and dacarbazine 900 mg/m^2, mixed and administered through central venous access via **CONT IV INFUSION** over 3 days, ifosfamide 7500 mg/m^2 and mesna 10,000 mg/m^2 mixed or infused separately through a peripheral line via a **CONT IV INFUSION** over 3 days (ifosfamide) and 4 days (mesna); repeat q21days if tolerated
Renal dose
• **Adult:** IV CCr 31-60 mL/min, give 75% of dose; CCr 10-30 mL/min, give 50% of dose; CCr <10 mL/min, do not give

Available forms: Inj 1-, 3-g vials
Administer:
• Antiemetic 30-60 min before product to prevent vomiting
• Visually inspect parenteral products for particulate matter and discoloration before use
• Store powder at room temperature
Intermittant/continuous IV infusion route
• Give as an intermittent infusion or continuous infusion
• Well hydrate with ≥2 L/day of oral or IV fluids to prevent bladder toxicity
• Must be given in combination with mesna to prevent hemorrhagic cystitis
• Close hematologic monitoring is recommended; WBC count, platelet count, and hemoglobin should be obtained before each use and periodically thereafter
• A urinalysis should be performed before each dose to monitor for hematuria
Reconstitution and further dilution:
• Reconstitute 1 or 3 g with 20 or 60 mL, respectively, of sterile water for injection or bacteriostatic water for injection containing parabens or benzyl alcohol to give IV solutions containing 50 mg/mL
• Solutions may be diluted further to achieve concentrations of 0.6-20 mg/mL in the following solutions: D$_5$W, NS, LR, or sterile water for injection
• Infuse slowly over at least 30 min
• Diluted and reconstituted solutions must be refrigerated and used within 24 hr

Y-site compatibilities: Acyclovir, alatrofloxacin, alemtuzumab, alfentanil, allopurinol, amifostine, amikacin, aminocaproic acid, aminophylline, amiodarone amphotericin B cholesteryl (amphotec), amphotericin B conventional colloidal, amphotericin B lipid complex (abelcet), amphotericin B liposome (ambisome), ampicillin, ampicillin-sulbactam, anidulafungin, argatroban, arsenic trioxide, atenolol, atracurium, azithromycin, aztreonam, bivalirudin, bleomycin, bumetanide, buprenorphine, butorphanol, calcium chloride/gluconate, CARBOplatin, caspofungin, ceFAZolin, cefoperazone, cefotaxime, cefOTEtan, cefOXitin, cefTAZidime, cefTAZidime (L-arginine), ceftizoxime, cefTRIAXone, cefuroxime, chlorproMA-ZINE, cimetidine, ciprofloxacin, cisatracurium, CISplatin, clindamycin, codeine, cycloSPORINE, cytarabine, DACTINomycin, DAPTOmycin, DAUNOrubicin liposome, dexamethasone phosphate, dexmedetomidine, dexrazoxane, digoxin, diltiaZEM, diphenhydrAMINE, DOBUTamine, DOCEtaxel, dolasetron, DOPamine, doripenem, doxacurium, DOXOrubicin, DOXOrubicin liposomal, doxycycline, droperidol, enalaprilat, ePHEDrine, EPINEPHrine, epiRUBicin, ertapenem, erythromycin, esmolol, etoposide, etoposide phosphate, famotidine, fenoldopam, fentaNYL, filgrastim, fluconazole, fludarabine, fluorouracil, foscarnet, fosphenytoin, furosemide, gallium nitrate, ganciclovir, gatifloxacin, gemcitabine, gemtuzumab, gentamicin, granisetron, haloperidol, heparin, hydrocortisone phosphate/succinate, HYDROmorphone, hydrOXYzine, IDArubicin, imipenem-cilastatin, inamrinone, insulin (regular), isoproterenol, ketorolac, labetalol, lansoprazole, lepirudin, leucovorin, levoFLOXacin, levorphanol, lidocaine, linezolid, LORazepam, magnesium sulfate, mannitol, melphalan, meperidine, meropenem, mesna, methohexital, methylPREDNISolone, metoclopramide, metoprolol, metroNIDAZOLE, midazolam, milrinone, minocycline, mitoMYcin, mitoXANTRONE, mivacurium, morphine, moxifloxacin, nalbuphine, naloxone, nesiritide, niCARdipine, nitroglycerin, nitroprusside, norepinephrine, octreotide, ofloxacin, ondansetron, oxaliplatin, PACLitaxel (solvent/surfactant), palonosetron, pamidronate, pancuronium, PEMEtrexed, pentamidine, PENTobarbital, PHENobarbital, phenylephrine, piperacillin, piperacillin-tazobactam, potassium acetate/chloride, procainamide, prochlorperazine, promethazine, propofol, propranolol, quinupristin-dalfopristin, raNITIdine, rapacuronium, remifentanil, riTUXimab, rocuronium, sargramostim, sodium acetate/bicarbonate/phosphates, succinylcholine, SUFentanil, sulfamethoxazole-trimethoprim, tacrolimus, teniposide, theophylline, thiopental, thiotepa, ticarcillin, ticarcillin-clavulanate, tigecycline, tirofiban, TNA (3-in-1), tobramycin, topotecan, TPN (2-in-1), trastuzumab, vancomycin, vasopressin, vecuronium, verapamil, vinBLAStine, vinCRIStine, vinorelbine, voriconazole, zidovudine, zoledronic acid

SIDE EFFECTS

CNS: Facial paresthesia, fever, malaise, somnolence, confusion, depression, hallucinations, dizziness, disorientation, seizures, coma, cranial nerve dysfunction, encephalopathy

GI: Nausea, vomiting, anorexia, hepatotoxicity, stomatitis, dyslipidemia, hyperglycemia, constipation, diarrhea

GU: Hematuria, nephrotoxicity, hemorrhagic cystitis, dysuria, urinary frequency

HEMA: Thrombocytopenia, leukopenia, anemia, retrograde ejaculation

INTEG: Dermatitis, alopecia, pain at inj site, hyperpigmentation

META: Metabolic acidosis

PHARMACOKINETICS

Metabolized by liver; saturation occurs at high doses; excreted in urine, breast milk; half-life 15 hr, depends on dose; onset unknown, peak 1-2 wk, duration 3 wk

INTERACTIONS

Increase: myelosuppression—other antineoplastics, radiation

Increase: toxicity—CYP3A4, a weak P-gp inhibitor, inducers, barbiturates, carbamazepine, phenytoin, rifampin, allopurinol

Increase: bleeding risk—NSAIDs, anticoagulants, salicylates, thrombolytics

Decrease: antibody response—live virus vaccines

Decrease: effect of ifosfamide—CYP3A4 inhibitors

Drug/Food

Increase: levels avoid with grapefruit juice

NURSING CONSIDERATIONS

Assess:

• Hepatic studies before, during therapy (bilirubin, AST, ALT, LDH) monthly or as needed; jaundice of skin and sclera, dark urine, clay-colored stools, itchy skin, abdominal pain, fever, diarrhea

Black Box Warning: **Bone marrow suppression:** CBC, differential, platelet count weekly; withhold product if WBC <2000/mm^3 or platelet count <50,000/mm^3; notify prescriber; severe myelosuppression may occur, nadir of leukopenia, thrombocytopenia 7-14 days, recovery 21 days

• Monitor temperature, flu like symptoms (may indicate beginning infection)
• B/P, pulse, respirations, baseline and periodically during treatment
• Blood dyscrasias (anemia, granulocytopenia); bruising, fatigue, bleeding, poor healing
• Allergic reactions: dermatitis, exfoliative dermatitis, pruritus, urticaria

Black Box Warning: **Hemorrhagic cystitis:** I&O ratio; monitor for hematuria; hemorrhagic cystitis can occur; increase fluids to 3 L/day; urinalysis before each dose, not to give at night, give with mesna to prevent this condition

Black Box Warning: **Neurotoxicity:** hallucinations, confusion, disorientation, coma; product should be discontinued, usually resolves in 3-4 days

• Bleeding: hematuria, guaiac, bruising or petechiae, mucosa or orifices; avoid IM injections
• Pregnancy/breastfeeding: do not use in pregnancy/breastfeeding
Evaluate:
• Therapeutic response: decrease in size and spread of tumor
Teach patient/family:
• To notify prescriber of sore throat, swollen lymph nodes, malaise, fever; other infections may occur, to discuss encephalopathy, neurotoxicity
• Not to have live virus vaccinations during or for 3 mo-1 yr after treatment
• That hair may be lost during treatment; that wig or hairpiece may make the patient feel better; that new hair may be different in color, texture

• To report signs of anemia: fatigue, headache, faintness, SOB, irritability
• To report bleeding; to avoid use of razors, commercial mouthwash; To avoid use of aspirin products, NSAIDs, ibuprofen because hemorrhage can occur
• To avoid crowds, persons with infections
• To report confusion, hallucinations, extreme drowsiness, numbness, tingling; to avoid alcohol use for ≥4 mo after treatment
• To avoid driving, hazardous activities until reaction is known
• To use excessive fluids and urinate often to prevent hemorrhagic cystitis; to report pink or red urine
• To notify prescriber if pregnancy is planned or suspected; to use contraceptive measures during therapy; not to breastfeed

iloperidone (Rx)
(ill-o-pehr′ih-dohn)
Fanapt
Func. class.: 2nd-generation atypical antipsychotic
Chem. class.: Benzisoxazole derivative

Do not confuse:
Fanapt/Xanax

ACTION: Unknown; may be mediated through both DOPamine type 2 (D2) and serotonin type 2 (5-HT2) antagonism, high receptor binding affinity for norepinephrine (alpha 1)

USES: Schizophrenia

CONTRAINDICATIONS: Breastfeeding, hypersensitivity
Precautions: Pregnancy, children, geriatric patients, renal/hepatic disease, breast cancer, Parkinson's disease, dementia with Lewy bodies, seizure disorder, QT prolongation, bundle branch block, acute MI, ambient temperature increase, AV block, stroke, substance abuse, suicidal ideation, tardive dyskinesia, torsades de pointes, blood dyscrasias, dysphagia

Side effects: *italics* = common; red = life-threatening

DOSAGE AND ROUTES
• **Adult:** PO 1 mg bid, may increase to target dose of 6-12 mg bid with daily dose adjustment of max 2 mg bid, titrate slowly; max 24 mg/day in 2 divided doses; reduce dose by 50% 🧬 in patient who is a poor metabolizer of CYP2D6 or when used with strong CYP2D6/CYP3A4 inhibitors

Available forms: Tabs 1, 2, 4, 6, 8, 10, 12 mg; titration pack

Administer:
• Use without regard to meals
• Reduced dose in geriatric patients
• Anticholinergic agent for EPS
• Avoid use with CNS depressants
• Store in tight, light-resistant container

SIDE EFFECTS
CNS: *EPS, pseudoparkinsonism, akathisia, dystonia, tardive dyskinesia; drowsiness,* seizures, neuroleptic malignant syndrome, dizziness, delirium, depression, paranoia, fatigue, hostility, lethargy, restlessness, vertigo, tremor

CV: Orthostatic hypotension, heart failure, AV block, QT prolongation, tachycardia

EENT: Blurred vision, cataracts, nystagmus, tinnitus, nasal congestion

GI: *Nausea,* vomiting, *anorexia, constipation,* jaundice, weight gain/loss, abdominal pain, stomatitis, xerostomia, dry mouth

GU: Urinary retention/incontinence, priapism

HEMA: Agranulocytosis, leukopenia, neutropenia

MISC: 🧬, Decreased bone density hyperglycemia, dyslipidemia

SYST: Anaphylaxis, angioedema

PHARMACOKINETICS
PO: Extensively metabolized by liver to major active metabolite by 🧬 CYP2D6, CYP3A4; protein binding 95%; peak 2-4 hr; excreted in urine and feces; 🧬 terminal half-life 18 hr in extensive metabolizers; 33 hr in poor metabolizers

INTERACTIONS
Increase: sedation—other CNS depressants, alcohol

Increase: iloperidone effect, decreased clearance—CYP2D6 (fluoxetine, paroxetine), CYP3A4 inhibitors (delavirdine, indinavir, isoniazid, itraconazole, dalfopristin, ritonavir, tipranavir); reduce dose

Increase: QT prolongation—class IA/III antidysrhythmics, some phenothiazines, β-agonists, local anesthetics, tricyclics, haloperidol, methadone, chloroquine, clarithromycin, droperidol, erythromycin, pentamidine

Decrease: iloperidone action—CYP2D6, CYP3A4 inducers (carBAMazepine, barbiturates, phenytoins, rifAMPin)

Drug/Lab Test
Increase: prolactin levels, cholesterol, glucose, lipids, triglycerides

Decrease: potassium

NURSING CONSIDERATIONS
Assess:
• AIMS assessment, lipid panel, blood glucose, CBC, glycosylated hemoglobin A1c, LFTs, neurologic function, pregnancy test, serum creatinine, electrolytes, prolactin, thyroid function studies, weight
• Affect, orientation, LOC, reflexes, gait, coordination, sleep-pattern disturbances
• B/P standing and lying, pulse, respirations q4hr during initial treatment; establish baseline before starting treatment; report drops of 30 mm Hg; watch for ECG changes; QT prolongation may occur; dizziness, faintness, palpitations, tachycardia on rising
• **Extrapyramidal symptoms,** including akathisia, tardive dyskinesia (bizarre movements of the jaw, mouth, tongue, extremities), pseudoparkinsonism (rigidity, tremors, pill rolling, shuffling gait)
• Check to see the patient swallows the medication

- **Neuroleptic malignant syndrome:** hyperthermia, increased CPK, altered mental status, muscle rigidity, seizures, diaphoresis; discontinue immediately, notify prescriber
- Constipation, urinary retention daily; if these occur, increase bulk and water in diet
- Weight gain, BMI, waist circumference, hyperglycemia, metabolic changes in diabetes
- Supervised ambulation until patient is stabilized on medication; do not involve patient in strenuous exercise program because fainting is possible; patient should not stand still for long periods
- Sips of water, candy, gum for dry mouth
- **Beers:** avoid in older adults except for schizophrenia, bipolar disorder, or short-term use as an antiemetic during chemotherapy; increased risk of stroke
- **Pregnancy/breastfeeding:** use only if benefits outweigh fetal risk; infant exposed to product during 3rd trimester may exhibit EPS; do not breastfeed, excretion unknown

Evaluate:
- Therapeutic response: decrease in emotional excitement, hallucinations, delusions, paranoia; reorganization of patterns of thought, speech

Teach patient/family:
- That orthostatic hypotension may occur; to rise from sitting or lying position gradually
- To avoid hot tubs, hot showers, tub baths because hypotension may occur; that heat stroke may occur in hot weather; to take extra precautions to stay cool
- To avoid abrupt withdrawal of product because extrapyramidal symptoms may result; that product should be withdrawn slowly; to review symptoms of neuroleptic malignant syndrome
- To avoid OTC preparations (cough, hay fever, cold), herbals, supplements unless discussed by prescriber because serious product interactions may occur; to avoid use of alcohol because increased drowsiness may occur
- To use gum, lozenges for dry mouth

- To avoid hazardous activities if drowsy or dizziness occurs
- To comply with product regimen, to take as prescribed, not to skip or double doses, if medication is missed for >3 days start as initial dose
- To report impaired vision, tremors, muscle twitching
- That follow-up exams will be needed
- To use contraception; to inform prescriber if pregnancy is planned or suspected; if pregnant, should enroll in the Atypical Antipsychotic National Pregnancy Registry: 866-961-2388

TREATMENT OF OVERDOSE:
Lavage if orally ingested; provide airway; *do not induce vomiting*

---

iloprost
[eye'-loe-prost]
Ventavis
Func. class.: Pulmonary vasodilator
Chem. class.: Prostacyclin analog

ACTION: Produces vasodilation and antiproliferative effects; mechanism for vasodilation is unclear. Hemodynamic effects following relaxation of vascular smooth muscle and vasodilation include decreased pulmonary vascular resistance, increased cardiac index, increased oxygen delivery. Also decreases platelet aggregation

USES: NYHA Class III or IV symptoms

CONTRAINDICATIONS: Hypersensitivity
Precautions: Asthma, breastfeeding, children, COPD, driving, geriatrics, hepatic disease, hypotension, pregnancy, pulmonary edema

DOSAGE AND ROUTES
- **Adult:** INH 2.5 mcg using adaptive aerosol delivery (AAD) or Prodose (AAD); may increase to 5 mcg 6-9 ×/day as needed separated by ≥2 hr, max 5 mcg 9 ×/day
- **Geriatric:** INH start at low end of dose

Available forms: INH solution 10, 20 mcg/mL

Administer:

- Use only delivery devices provided
- Do not take orally; avoid ocular exposure, contact with skin
- If signs of pulmonary edema occur in those with pulmonary hypertension, treatment should be stopped immediately; this may be a sign of pulmonary venous hypertension

SIDE EFFECTS

CNS: Headache, insomnia, syncope

CV: Hypotension, chest pain, vasodilation, palpitations, heart failure, supraventricular tachycardia, edema

GI: Nausea, vomiting, mouth/tongue discomfort

GU: Renal failure

RESP: Cough, dyspnea, pneumonia, flu-like symptoms

PHARMACOKINETICS

Half-life 30 min, peak 5 min, duration 30-60 min

INTERACTIONS

Increase: bleeding risk—anticoagulants, platelet inhibitors; assess for bleeding

Increase: hypotension—antihypertensives, vasodilators; monitor B/P

Drug/Lab Test:

Increase: alkaline phosphatase

NURSING CONSIDERATIONS

Assess:

- **Pulmonary arterial hypertension (PAH):** may cause dizziness, lightheadedness, fainting because it lowers the blood pressure; these are also common symptoms of pulmonary arterial hypertension (PAH); patients should use caution when driving or operating machinery until effect is known
- **Syncope:** because of risk of syncope, vital signs should be monitored while initiating product; in those with low systemic blood pressure, avoid further hypotension; do not use in those with systolic blood pressure <85 mm Hg; if syncope occurs during physical exertion, dose may need to be adjusted

- **Renal failure:** monitor closely in patients with renal impairment; effect may be extended
- **Bronchospasm:** may occur especially in susceptible patients with hyperreactive airways; avoid use in COPD, severe asthma, acute respiratory infection
- **Pregnancy/breastfeeding:** use during pregnancy only if benefits to mother clearly outweigh potential risk to fetus; not known whether product crosses placenta

Teach patient/family:

- To take as prescribed; not to double doses; to take 2 hr before physical exertion; not to save leftover product; to always keep enough product and backup inhalation device; not to mix with other medications; not to miss doses or stop abruptly, risk of rebound hypertension
- To keep away from skin and eyes
- To avoid driving or other hazardous activities until reaction is known; dizziness, syncope may occur; to rise slowly to minimize orthostatic hypotension
- To monitor B/P; do not take if systolic B/P <85 mm Hg

⚠ HIGH ALERT

imatinib (Rx)

(im-ah-tin′ib)

Gleevec

Func. class.: Antineoplastic—miscellaneous

Chem. class.: Protein-tyrosine kinase inhibitor

ACTION: Inhibits ✲ Bcr-Abl tyrosine kinase created in patients with chronic myeloid leukemia (CML), also inhibits tyrosine kinases

USES: Treatment of ✲ CML; Philadelphia chromosome–positive (Ph+) patients in blast-cell crisis or patients in chronic failure; gastrointestinal stromal tumors (GIST) positive for c-Kit; chronic eosinophilic leukemia, Ph+ acute lymphocytic leukemia, dermatofibrosarcoma protuberans, myelodysplastic syndrome, systemic mastocytosis

CONTRAINDICATIONS: Pregnancy, hypersensitivity

Precautions: Breastfeeding, children, geriatric patients, cardiac/renal/hepatic/dental disease, GI bleeding, bone marrow suppression, infection, thrombocytopenia, neutropenia, immunosuppression

DOSAGE AND ROUTES
For the treatment of Ph+ CML chronic phase as initial therapy
• **Adult:** PO 400 mg/day, continue as long as beneficial; may increase to 600 mg/day in the absence of severe adverse reactions and severe non–leukemia-related neutropenia or thrombocytopenia
• **Adolescent/child >2 yr:** PO 340 mg/m^2/day, max 600 mg/day; the daily dose may be given as a single dose or split into 2 doses given once in the morning and once in the evening

Ph+ acute lymphocytic leukemia (ALL)
• **Adult:** PO 600 mg every day, continue as long as beneficial

GIST
• **Adult:** PO 400-600 mg every day, may increase to 400 mg bid

Adjuvant treatment of *Kit* (CD117)-positive GIST after complete gross resection
• **Adult:** PO 400 mg/day

Hypereosinophilic syndrome (HES) and/or chronic eosinophilic leukemia (CEL)
• **Adult:** PO 400 mg/day in those who are FIPL1L-PDGFR α-fusion kinase negative or unknown; for HES/CEL patients with demonstrated FIP1L1-PDGFR α-fusion kinase, 100 mg/day, may increase to 400 mg

Myelodysplastic syndrome (MDS)/myeloproliferative disease (MPD)
• **Adult:** PO 400 mg/day

Aggressive systemic mastocytosis (ASM) without D816V c-Kit mutation or with c-Kit mutation status unknown
• **Adult:** PO 400 mg/day

Renal dose
• **Adult:** PO CCr 40-59 mL/min, max 600 mg/day; CCr 20-39 mL/min, decrease initial dose by 50%, max 400 mg/day; CCr <20 mL/min, use with caution, 100 mg/day

Hepatic dose
• **Adult:** PO Total bilirubin 1.5-3 × ULN and any AST, decrease initial dose to 400 mg/day; total bilirubin >3 × ULN and any AST, decrease initial dose to 300 mg/day

Available forms: Tabs 100, 400 mg
Administer:
• With meal and large glass of water to decrease GI symptoms; doses of 800 mg should be given as 400 mg bid
• Tab may be dispersed in a glass of water or apple juice, use 50 mL of liquid for 100-mg tab, 200-mL liquid for 400-mg tab
• Use low-molecular-weight heparin for anticoagulant if needed
• Continue as long as beneficial
• Store at 77° F (25° C)

SIDE EFFECTS
CNS: Headache, dizziness, insomnia, subdural hematoma
CV: Hemorrhage, heart failure, cardiac, cardiac toxicity
EENT: Blurred vision
GI: *Nausea,* hepatotoxicity, vomiting, dyspepsia, *anorexia, abdominal pain,* GI perforation, diarrhea
HEMA: Neutropenia, thrombocytopenia, bleeding
INTEG: *Rash, pruritus,* alopecia, photosensitivity, drug rash with eosinophilia and systemic symptoms (DRESS)
META: Fluid retention, hypokalemia, edema
MISC: Fatigue, epistaxis, pyrexia, night sweats, increased weight, flulike symptoms, hypothyroidism, tumor lysis syndrome
MS: Cramps, pain, arthralgia, myalgia
RESP: Cough, dyspnea, nasopharyngitis, pneumonia

PHARMACOKINETICS
Well absorbed (98%); protein binding 95%; metabolized by CYP3A4; excreted in feces, small amount in urine; peak 2-4 hr; duration 24 hr (imatinib), 40 hr (metabolite); half-life 18-40 hr

---

Side effects: *italics* = common; red = life-threatening

INTERACTIONS

Increase: imatinib concentrations—CYP3A4 inhibitors (ketoconazole, itraconazole, erythromycin, clarithromycin)

Increase: plasma concentrations of simvastatin, calcium channel blockers, ergots

Increase: plasma concentration of warfarin; avoid use with warfarin; use low-molecular-weight anticoagulants instead

Decrease: imatinib concentrations—CYP3A4 inducers (dexamethasone, phenytoin, carBAMazepine, rifAMPin, PHENobarbital)

Drug/Herb

Decrease: imatinib concentration—St. John's wort

Drug/Food

Increase: effect of grapefruit juice, avoid use

Drug/Lab Test

Increase: bilirubin, amylase, LFTs

Decrease: albumin, calcium, potassium, sodium, phosphate, platelets, neutrophils, leukocytes, lymphocytes

NURSING CONSIDERATIONS

Assess:

• **Bone marrow suppression:** ANC, platelets; during chronic phase, if ANC <1 × 10^9/L and/or platelets <50 × 10^9/L, stop until ANC >1.5 × 10^9/L and platelets >75 × 10^9/L; during accelerated phase/blast crisis, if ANC <0.5 × 10^9/L and/or platelets <10 × 10^9/L, determine whether cytopenia related to biopsy/aspirate; if not, reduce dose by 200 mg; if cytopenia continues, reduce dose by another 100 mg; if cytopenia continues for 4 wk, stop product until ANC ≥1 × 10^9/L

• **Renal toxicity:** if bilirubin >3 × UNL, withhold imatinib until bilirubin levels return to <1.5 × UNL

• **DRESS:** swelling of face, fever, rash, later hepatitis, myocarditis may occur, discontinue if present

• **Hepatotoxicity:** monitor LFTs before and during treatment monthly; if liver transaminases >5 × UNL, withhold imatinib until transaminase levels return to <2.5 × UNL

• Monitor CBC at least weekly for first mo, biweekly next mo and periodically thereafter; may cause neutropenia (2-3 wk) and thrombocytopenia (3-4 wk) and anemia; may need dosage decrease or discontinuation

• Signs of fluid retention, edema: weigh, monitor lung sounds, assess for edema; some fluid retention is dose dependent

• **Pregnancy/breastfeeding:** do not use in pregnancy, breastfeeding

Evaluate:

• Therapeutic response: decrease in leukemic cells or size of tumor

Teach patient/family:

• To report adverse reactions immediately: shortness of breath, swelling of extremities, bleeding

• About reason for treatment, expected results

• That effect on male infertility is unknown

• Not to stop or change dose

• To avoid hazardous activities until response is known, dizziness may occur

• To take with food and water; for those unable to swallow tabs, to mix in liquid (30 mL for 100 mg) or 200 mL for 400 mg); after dissolved, stir and consume; avoid grapefruit juice

• To avoid OTC products unless approved by prescriber

• To notify prescriber if pregnancy is planned or suspected; not to breastfeed; to use effective contraception

---

imipenem/cilastatin (Rx)

(i-me-pen′em sye-la-stat′in)

Primaxin IM, Primaxin IV

Func. class.: Antiinfective—miscellaneous

Chem. class.: Carbapenem

ACTION: Interferes with cell-wall replication of susceptible organisms; osmotically unstable cell-wall swells, bursts from osmotic pressure; addition of cilastatin prevents renal inactivation that occurs with high urinary concentrations of imipenem

USES: Serious infections caused by gram-positive *Streptococcus pneumoniae,* group A β-hemolytic streptococci, *Staphylococcus aureus,* enterococcus; gram-negative *Klebsiella, Proteus, Escherichia coli, Acinetobacter, Serratia, Pseudomonas aeruginosa, Salmonella, Shigella, Haemophilus influenzae, Listeria* sp.

CONTRAINDICATIONS: Hypersensitivity to this product, amide local anesthetics, or carbapenems; AV block, shock (IM)

Precautions: Pregnancy, breastfeeding, children, geriatric patients, seizure disorders, renal disease, head trauma; hypersensitivity to cephalosporins, penicillins; pseudomembranous colitis, ulcerative colitis, diabetes mellitus

DOSAGE AND ROUTES
Doses based on imipenem content

Most infections
• **Adult ≥70 kg:** IV 250 mg every 6 hr (mild infections); 500 mg every 6-8 hr (moderate infections); 500 mg every 6 hr (severe life-threatening infections)
• **Adult 60 kg:** IV 250 mg IV every 8 hr (mild infections); 250 mg every 6 hr (moderate or severe life-threatening infections)
• **Adult 50 kg:** IV 125 mg every 6 hr (mild infections); 250 mg every 6 hr (moderate or severe life-threatening infections)
• **Adult 40 kg:** IV 125 mg every 6 hr (mild infections); 250 mg every 6-8 hr (moderate infections); 250 mg every 6 hr (severe life-threatening infections)
• **Adult 30 kg:** IV 125 mg every 8 hr (mild infections); 125 mg every 6 hr or 250 mg every 8 hr (moderate infections); 250 mg every 8 hr (severe life-threatening infections)
• **Adolescent/child/infant ≥3 mo:** IV 15-25 mg/kg every 6 hr
• **Infant 1-3 mo and ≥1500 g:** IV 25 mg/kg every 6 hr
• **Neonate 1-4 wk and ≥1500 g:** IV 25 mg/kg every 8 hr
• **Neonate <7 days and ≥1500 g:** IV 25 mg/kg every 12 hr

Renal dose
• **Adult: CCr 60-89 mL/min:** adjust to 400 mg every 6 hr for starting dose of 500 mg every 6 hr, to 500 mg every 6 hr for starting dose of 1 g every 8 hr, to 750 mg every 8 hr for starting dose of 1 g every 6 hr
CCr 30-59 mL/min: adjust to 300 mg every 6 hr for starting dose of 500 mg every 6 hr, to 500 mg every 8 hr for starting dose of 1 g every 8 hr, to 500 mg every 6 hr for starting dose of 1 g every 6 hr
CCr 15-29 mL/min: adjust to 200 mg every 6 hr for starting dose of 500 mg every 6 hr, to 500 mg every 12 hr for starting dose of 1 g every 6 or 8 hr
CCr <15 mL/min: Do not use unless unless hemodialysis is instituted within 48 hr

Available forms: Powder for sol inj 250, 500 mg; powder for inj susp 500, 750 mg

Administer:
• After C&S is taken, may start treatment before results are received

IM route
• Reconstitute 500 mg/2 mL lidocaine without EPINEPHrine; shake
• Inject deeply in large muscle, aspirate, **product for IM is not for IV use**

Intermittent IV infusion route
• After reconstitution of 250 or 500 mg with 10 mL of diluent and shake, add to ≥100 mL of same infusion sol
• 250-500 mg over 20-30 min; ≥750 mg over 40-60 min; give through Y-tube or 3-way stopcock; do not give by IV bolus or if cloudy, do not admix with other antibiotics separate by ≥1 hr (aminoglycosides)

Y-site compatibilities: Acyclovir, alfentanil, amifostine, amikacin, aminocaproic acid, anidulafungin, argatroban, ascorbic acid, atenolol, atracurium, atropine, benztropine, bivalirudin, bleomycin, bumetanide, buprenorphine, butorphanol, CARBOplatin, carmustine, caspofungin, ceFAZolin, cefotaxime, cefoTEtan, cefOXitin, cefTAZidime, cefuroxime, chloramphenicol, cimetidine, cisatracurium, CISplatin, clindamycin, codeine, cyanocobalamin, cyclophosphamide, cycloSPORINE, cytarabine, DACTINomycin, dexamethasone, dexrazoxane, digoxin, diltiaZEM, diphenhydrAMINE, DOCEtaxel, dolasetron, DOPamine, doxacurium, DOXOrubicin, DOXOrubicin liposomal, doxycycline, enalaprilat, famotidine, fludarabine, foscarnet, granisetron, IDArubicin, insulin (regular), melphalan, methotrexate, ondansetron, propofol, remifentanil, tacrolimus, teniposide, thiotepa, vinorelbine, zidovudine

SIDE EFFECTS

CNS: Fever, somnolence, seizures, confusion, dizziness, weakness, myoclonus, drowsiness
CV: Hypotension, palpitations, tachycardia
GI: *Diarrhea, nausea, vomiting,* CDAD, hepatitis, glossitis, gastroenteritis, abdominal pain, jaundice
HEMA: Eosinophilia
INTEG: Rash, urticaria, pruritus, pain at inj site, phlebitis, erythema at inj site, erythema multiforme
MISC: Hearing loss, tinnitus
SYST: Anaphylaxis, Stevens-Johnson syndrome, toxic epidermal necrolysis, angioedema

PHARMACOKINETICS

IV: Onset immediate, peak 20 min-1 hr; duration 6-8 hr
IM: Peak 1-2 hr, duration 12 hr, half-life 1 hr, 70%-80% excreted unchanged in urine

INTERACTIONS

Increase: imipenem plasma levels—probenecid
Increase: antagonistic effect—β-lactam antibiotics
Increase: seizure risk—ganciclovir, theophylline, aminophylline, cycloSPORINE
Decrease: effect of valproic acid
Decrease: effect aminoglycosides if admixed
Drug/Lab Test
Increase: AST, ALT, LDH, BUN, alk phos, bilirubin, creatinine, potassium, chloride
Decrease: sodium
False positive: direct Coombs' test

NURSING CONSIDERATIONS
Assess:
• Renal studies: creatinine/BUN, electrolytes
• **Seizures:** product decreases seizure threshold and may decrease effectiveness of seizure medications; monitor closely
• **Infection:** increased temperature, WBC, characteristics of wounds, sputum, urine or stool culture
• Sensitivity to penicillin, other β-lactams—may have sensitivity to this product
• Renal disease: lower dose may be required
• **CDAD:** Bowel pattern daily; if severe diarrhea occurs, product should be discontinued; may indicate pseudomembranous colitis
• **Allergic reactions, anaphylaxis:** rash, urticaria, pruritus, wheezing, laryngeal edema; may occur a few days after therapy begins; have EPINEPHrine, antihistamine, emergency equipment available
• **Overgrowth of infection:** perineal itching, fever, malaise, redness, pain, swelling, drainage, rash, diarrhea, change in cough, sputum
• **Pregnancy/breastfeeding:** use only if benefit outweighs fetal risk; use caution in breastfeeding, excretion unknown
Evaluate:
• Therapeutic response: negative C&S; absence of signs and symptoms of infection
Teach patient/family:
• To report severe diarrhea; may indicate CDAD

TREATMENT OF ANAPHYLAXIS: EPINEPHrine, antihistamines; resuscitate if needed

---

imipramine (Rx)

(im-ip´ra-meen)

Impril ✦, Tofranil, Tofranil PM
Func. class.: Antidepressant, tricyclic
Chem. class.: Dibenzazepine, tertiary amine

Do not confuse:
imipramine/desipramine

ACTION: Blocks reuptake of norepinephrine, serotonin into nerve endings, thereby increasing action of norepinephrine, serotonin in nerve cells

USES: Depression, enuresis in children
Unlabeled uses: Chronic pain, migraine headaches, cluster headaches as adjunct, incontinence, ADHD, neuralgia, bulimia, neuropathic pain, social phobia

CONTRAINDICATIONS: Pregnancy, hypersensitivity to this product or carBAMazepine; acute MI
Precautions: Breastfeeding, geriatric patients, suicidal patients, severe depression, increased intraocular pressure, closed-angle glaucoma, urinary retention, cardiac/hepatic disease, hyperthyroidism, electroshock therapy, elective surgery, seizure disorders, prostatic hypertrophy, MI, AV block, bundle branch block, ileus, QT prolongation, hypersensitivity to tricyclics

> **Black Box Warning:** Children other than for enuresis; suicidal ideation

DOSAGE AND ROUTES
Depression
• **Adult:** PO 75-100 mg/day in divided doses, may increase by 25-50 mg to 200 mg/day (outpatients), 300 mg/day (inpatients); may give daily dose at bedtime
• **Geriatric:** PO 25 mg at bedtime, may increase to 100 mg/day in divided doses
• **Child ≥6 yr (unlabeled):** PO 1.5 mg/kg/day in divided doses, max 2.5 mg/kg/day
Enuresis
• **Child 6-12 yr:** PO 25 mg at bedtime, max 50 mg
Social phobia/panic disorder (unlabeled)
• **Adult:** PO 10 mg at bedtime, titrate q2-4days to 100-200 mg/day
Overactive bladder (OAB) (unlabeled)
• **Adult:** PO 10-50 mg daily, may titrate to 150 mg/day
Available forms: Tabs 10, 25, 50, 75 ❦ mg; caps 75, 100, 125, 150 mg

Administer:
PO route
• Not to break, crush, or chew caps
• With food or milk for GI symptoms
• Dosage at bedtime if oversedation occurs during day; may take entire dose at bedtime; geriatric patients may not tolerate once-daily dosing
• Sugarless gum, hard candy, or frequent sips of water for dry mouth
• Do not discontinue abruptly, taper 50% × 3 days, another 50% × 3 days, then stop
• Give increased doses at bedtime to prevent sleepiness
• Store in tight container at room temperature; do not freeze

SIDE EFFECTS
CNS: *Dizziness, drowsiness,* confusion, seizures, headache, anxiety, insomnia, suicidal ideation, paresthesia
CV: *Orthostatic hypotension, ECG changes, tachycardia,* dysrhythmias
EENT: Blurred vision, mydriasis
ENDO: Hyperglycemia, hypo/hyperthyroidism
GI: *Diarrhea, dry mouth,* nausea, vomiting, paralytic ileus, increased appetite, taste change
GU: *Retention,* decreased libido
HEMA: Agranulocytosis, thrombocytopenia, eosinophilia, leukopenia
INTEG: Rash, urticaria, pruritus, photosensitivity

PHARMACOKINETICS
Metabolized to desipramine in liver by CYP2D6; excreted in urine, breast milk, feces; crosses placenta; half-life 8-16 hr, protein binding 90-95%

INTERACTIONS
• **Hyperpyretic crisis, seizures, hypertensive episode:** MAOIs, cloNIDine
• **Increase:** serotonin syndrome, neuroleptic malignant syndrome—SSRIs, SNRIs, serotonin-receptor agonists, bupropion, cyclobenzapine, trazodone, tramadil, tricyclics; avoid concurrent use, linezolid, methylene blue IV

Increase: QT interval—class IA/III antidysrhythmics, tricyclics, gatifloxacin, levoFLOXacin, moxifloxacin, ziprasidone

Increase: effects of direct-acting sympathomimetics (EPINEPHrine), alcohol, barbiturates, benzodiazepines, CNS depressants

Decrease: effects of guanethidine, cloNIDine, indirect-acting sympathomimetics (ePHEDrine)

Drug/Herb

Increase: serotonin syndrome—SAM-e, St. John's wort

Increase: sedation—chamomile, kava, valerian

Drug/Lab Test

Increase: serum bilirubin, alk phos, blood glucose, LFTs

Mental status: mood, sensorium, affect, **suicidal tendencies** especially in children, young adults; increase in psychiatric symptoms: depression, panic, monitor weekly × 1 mo, then 3 wk give limited amount of product

NURSING CONSIDERATIONS
Assess:

Black Box Warning: **Depression:** mood, behavior, sleep, lability; mental status, suicidal tendencies especially in children, young adults; increase in psychiatric symptoms, panic, monitor q wk × 1 mon, then q 3 wk, give limited amount of medication

• **Enuresis:** bedwetting frequency, stressors
• B/P (lying, standing), pulse q4hr; if systolic B/P drops 20 mm Hg, hold product, notify prescriber; take vital signs q4hr in patients with CV disease
• Blood studies: CBC, leukocytes, differential, cardiac enzymes, serum imipramine levels (125-250 ng/mL) if patient is receiving long-term therapy
• Hepatic studies: AST, ALT, bilirubin
• Weight weekly; appetite may increase with product
• **QT prolongation:** ECG for flattening of T wave, bundle branch block, AV block, dysrhythmias in cardiac patients
• EPS primarily in geriatric patients: rigidity, dystonia, akathisia
• Urinary retention, constipation; constipation is more likely to occur in children, geriatric patients; increase fluids, bulk in diet

• **Withdrawal symptoms:** headache, nausea, vomiting, muscle pain, weakness, diarrhea, insomnia, restlessness; not usual unless product is discontinued abruptly
• **Serotonin syndrome, hypertensive episodes:** identify drug interactions before use of product
• Alcohol consumption; if alcohol is consumed, hold dose until morning
• Assistance with ambulation during beginning therapy because drowsiness, dizziness, orthostatic hypotension may occur
• Safety measures, primarily for geriatric patients
• **Beers:** avoid in older adults; highly anticholinergic, high risk of delirium

Evaluate:
• Therapeutic response: decreased depression, enuresis, neurogenic pain

Teach patient/family:
• That therapeutic effects may take 2-3 wk
• That product is dispensed in small amounts because of suicide potential, especially at beginning of therapy
• To use caution when driving, performing other activities requiring alertness because of drowsiness, dizziness, blurred vision
• To report urinary retention immediately
• To avoid alcohol, other CNS depressants during treatment
• Not to discontinue medication abruptly after long-term use; may cause nausea, headache, malaise
• To wear sunscreen or large hat because photosensitivity occurs
• To rise slowly, orthostatic hypotension may occur

Black Box Warning: To report suicidal thoughts, behaviors immediately; more common in children, young adults

• **Pregnancy/breastfeeding:** Identify if pregnancy is planned or suspected or if breastfeeding

TREATMENT OF OVERDOSE:
ECG monitoring; lavage if recently ingested; sodium bicarbonate (cardiac effects); administer anticonvulsant, antidysrrhthmics

immune globulin IM (IMIG/IGIM) (Rx)

Bay Gam 15%, Flebogamma 5%, Flebogamma DIF 5%, Gammagard, GamaSTAN S/D, Gamunex 10%, Privigen 10%, Vivaglobin 10%

immune globulin IV (IGIV, IVIG) (Rx)

Bay Gam 15%, Carimune NF, Flebogamma 5%, Flebogamma 10% DIF, Gammagard S/D, Gammagard Liquid 10%, Gammaked, Gammaplex, Gammar-P IV, Gamunex, Iveegam EN, Octagam, Polygam S/D, Privigen, Vivaglobin

immune globulin SC (SCIG/IGSC)

Bay Gam 15%, Flebogamma 5%, Flebogamma DIF 5%, Gammagard 10%, Gammaked, Gammaplex, Gamunex 10%, Privigen 10%, Vivaglobin, Hizentra
Func. class.: Immune serum
Chem. class.: IgG

USES: Immunodeficiency syndrome; B-cell chronic lymphocytic leukemia; Kawasaki syndrome; bone marrow transplantation; pediatric HIV infection; agammaglobulinemia; hepatitis A, B exposure; measles exposure; measles vaccine complications; purpura; rubella exposure; chickenpox exposure; chronic inflammatory demyelinating polyneuropathy, multifocal motor neuropathy

CONTRAINDICATIONS: Hypersensitivity, coagulopathy, hemophilia, IgA deficiency, thrombocytopenia

DOSAGE AND ROUTES
Immune globulin IM (IMIG, IGIM)
Hepatitis A prophylaxis
• **Adult/geriatric/adolescent/child/infant (unlabeled):** IM 0.02 mL/kg for those who have not received hepatitis A vaccine and have been exposed during the prior 2 wk
Measles prophylaxis (exposed during prior 6 days)
• **Adult:** IM 0.25 mL/kg (immunocompetent)
• **Child (unlabeled):** IM 0.5 mL/kg as a single dose, max 15 mL (immunocompromised)
Varicella prophylaxis
• **Adult:** IM 0.6-1.2 mL/kg as soon as possible and if varicella-zoster immune globulin is not available
Rubella prophylaxis in exposed/ susceptible individual who will not consider a therapeutic abortion
• **Adult pregnant women:** IM 0.55 mL/kg
Immunoglobulin deficiency
• **Adult:** IM 1.32 mL/kg, then 0.66 mL/kg (≥100 mg/kg) q3-4wk

Immune globulin IV (IVIG, IGIV)
Primary immunodeficiency
Gammagard S/D
• **Adult/adolescent/child:** IV 300-600 mg/kg q3-4wk
Polygam S/D
• **Adult/adolescent/child:** IV 100 mg/kg/mo; initially 200-400 mg/kg may be used
Gammar-P IV
• **Adult:** IV 200-400 mg/kg q3-4wk
• **Adolescent/child:** IV 200 mg/kg q3-4wk
Gamunex
• **Adult/adolescent/child:** IV INFUSION 300-600 mg/kg (3-6 mL/kg) q3-4wk, initial infusion rate 1 mg/kg/min (max 8 mg/kg/min)
Iveegam EN
• **Adult/adolescent/child:** IV 200 mg/kg monthly, max 800 mg/kg/mo
Carimune NF
• **Adult/adolescent/child:** IV 200 mg/kg/mo
Gammagard Liquid/Flebogamma 5%
• **Adult/adolescent/child:** IV 300-600 mg/kg q3-4wk

Privigen
• Adult/adolescent/child ≥3 yr: **IV** 200-800 mg q3wk

Idiopathic thrombocytopenic purpura (ITP)

Carimune NF
• Adult/child: **IV** 400 mg/kg daily × 2-5 days; with acute ITP of childhood, only 2 of 5 days are needed if initial platelets are 30,000-50,000 microliters after 2 doses

Gammagard S/D/Polygam S/D
• Adult/adolescent/child: **IV** 1000 mg/kg as a single dose; may give on alternate days for up to 3 doses

Gamunex
• Adult/adolescent/child: **IV INFUSION** total dose of 2000 mg/kg on 2 consecutive days; initial rate is 1 mg/kg/min (max 8 mg/kg/min); if after 1st dose adequate platelets are observed after 24 hr, may withhold 2nd dose

Privigen
• Adult/adolescent ≥15 yr: **IV** 1 g/kg/day × 2 days

Kawasaki disease

Iveegam EN
• Child: **IV** 400 mg/kg daily × 4 consecutive days or a single dose of 2000 mg/kg over 10 hr, given with aspirin 100 mg/kg/day through 14th day of illness, then 3-5 mg/kg each day thereafter for 5 wk

Gammagard S/D/Polygam S/D
• Infant/child: **IV** 1000 mg/kg as a single dose or 400 mg/kg/day × 4 days beginning within 7 days of fever onset, with aspirin 80-100 mg/kg/day × 4 divided doses

Immune globulin SC (SCIG/IGSC)
• Adult/child >2 yr: **SUBCUT INFUSION** 100-200 mg/kg weekly, **Vivaglobin** brand of SCIG 160 mg IgG/mL, **SUBCUT** inj 15 mL/inj site, given at max of 20 mL/hr

Hizentra
• Adult/child: multiply the previous IVIG dose by 1.37, then divide into wk dose based on previous wk treatment

---

indacaterol
(in-da-kat′er-ol)
Arcapta Neohaler, Onbrez
Breezhal ER ✦
Func. class.: β-2 agonist, long-acting respiratory

ACTION: An agonist at β-2 receptors. Receptors are present in large numbers. Stimulation of β-2 receptors in the lung causes relaxation of bronchial smooth muscle, which produces bronchodilation and an increase in bronchial airflow. These effects may be mediated, in part, by increased activity of adenyl cyclase, an intracellular enzyme responsible for the formation of cyclic-3′,5′-adenosine monophosphate (cAMP); has >24-fold agonist activity at β-2 receptors (primarily in the lung) compared to β-1 receptors (primarily in the heart)

USES: Bronchitis, chronic obstructive pulmonary disease (COPD), emphysema

CONTRAINDICATIONS: Acute bronchospasm, acute asthma attack, status asthmaticus, acute respiratory insufficiency, monotherapy of asthma, hypersensitivity
Precautions: Ischemic cardiac disease (coronary artery disease), hypertension, cardiac arrhythmias, tachycardia, QT prolongation, congenital long QT syndrome, torsades de pointes history, hyperthyroidism (thyrotoxicosis, thyroid disease), pheochromocytoma, unusual responsiveness to other sympathomimetic amines, seizure disorder, diabetes mellitus, hypokalemia, milk protein hypersensitivity, severe hepatic disease; not indicated for neonates, infants, children, or adolescents under the age of 18 yr, pregnancy, breastfeeding

Black Box Warning: Asthma-related deaths

DOSAGE AND ROUTES
• **Adult:** INH 75 mcg (contents of 1 capsule) inhaled once daily; max 1 dose in 24 hours

Available forms: Powder in capsules for inhalation 75 mcg

Administer:

Inhalation route

• For oral inhalation use only; DO NOT swallow the capsules; always use the Neohaler Inhaler; DO NOT use with a spacer

• Use dry hands to remove a capsule from the blister pack immediately before use and place into the capsule chamber of the Neohaler Inhaler; click closed; then, holding the inhaler upright, depress buttons fully once to pierce capsule, a click will be heard; have patient breathe out fully away from inhaler, place inhaler in the mouth with buttons positioned to the left and right, close lips around mouthpiece, then breathe deeply; after inhalation, patient should hold the breath as long as comfortable while removing inhaler from the mouth; check the chamber to see if any powder remains in the capsule; repeat inhalation steps until no powder remains; most patients empty the capsule in 1 or 2 inhalations; after administration, open chamber and discard empty capsule

SIDE EFFECTS
CNS: Headache, dizziness

CV: *Tachycardia, palpitations,* peripheral edema

ENDO: Hyperglycemia

GI: *Nausea,* dry mouth

MS: Muscle cramps/spasm, musculoskeletal pain

RESP: Paradoxical bronchospasm, cough, dyspnea, upper respiratory tract infection

INTEG: Rash, pruritus

PHARMACOKINETICS:
Protein binding 94%-96%, metabolized by CYP3A4, CYP1A1, CYP2D6, UGT1A1; half-life of 45.5-126 hours; excreted renally (2%-6%), fecally (>90%); onset 5 min, peak 15 min

INTERACTIONS:
Increase: QT prolongation—class IA/III antiarrhythmics, flecainide, propafenone, some antipsychotics (phenothiazines, pimozide, haloperidol risperiDONE, sertindole, ziprasidone), amoxapine, arsenic trioxide, astemizole, bepridil, cisapride, citalopram, chloroquine, clarithromycin, dasatinib, dolasetron, dronedarone, droperidol, erythromycin, halofantrine, halogenated anesthetics, levomethadyl, maprotiline, methadone, some quinolones (ofloxacin, gatifloxacin, gemifloxacin, grepafloxacin, levoFLOXacin, moxifloxacin, sparfloxacin), ondansetron, paliperidone, palonosetron, pentamidine, probucol, propafenone, ranolazine, SUNItinib, terfenadine, thioridazine, tricyclic antidepressants, troleandomycin, vorinostat, tetrabenazine

Increase: cardiovascular reactions—MAOIs

NURSING CONSIDERATIONS
Assess

> **Black Box Warning:** Asthma-related death; not to be used in asthma

• **COPD, emphysema, bronchospasm:** monitor pulmonary function tests, respiratory status (dyspnea, rate, breath sounds before and during treatment

• **QT prolongation:** monitor ECG, ejection fraction for QT prolongation

• **Paradoxical bronchospasm:** if paradoxical bronchospasm occurs, discontinue product immediately, use a short-acting β-agonist for rescue therapy, as appropriate

• **Pregnancy/breastfeeding:** use only if benefit outweighs fetal risk; use caution in breastfeeding, excretion unknown

Teach patient/family

• To report dyspnea, wheezing, bronchospasm

• Not to use with other products unless approved by prescriber; there are many interactions; it is always prescribed with a short-acting beta-2 inhaler or steroidal inhaler

> **Black Box Warning:** Do not use for asthma

Side effects: *italics* = common; red = life-threatening

- How to use Neohaler; not to stop treatment unless approved by prescriber
- The symptoms of allergic reactions
- To inform other providers of use

---

indapamide
(in-dap'a-mide)

Lozide ✦

Func. class.: Diuretic—thiazide-like, antihypertensive
Chem. class.: Indoline

ACTION: Acts on proximal section of distal renal tubule by inhibiting reabsorption of sodium; may act by direct vasodilation caused by blocking of calcium channels

USES: Edema of HF, hypertension

CONTRAINDICATIONS: Hypersensitivity to this product or sulfonamides; anuria, hepatic coma
Precautions: Breastfeeding, hypokalemia, dehydration, ascites, hepatic disease, severe renal disease, CCr <30 mL/min (not effective), diabetes mellitus, gout, pregnancy, cardiac dysrhythmias

DOSAGE AND ROUTES
Edema
- **Adult: PO** 2.5 mg/day in AM; may be increased to 5 mg/day if needed after 1 wk
Antihypertensive
- **Adult: PO** 1.25 mg/day in AM; may increase to 2.5 mg/day after 4 wk; if not effective after 4 wk, may increase to max dose of 5 mg/day
Available forms: Tabs 1.25, 2.5 mg
Administer:
- In AM to avoid interference with sleep
- With food if nausea occurs; absorption may be decreased slightly

SIDE EFFECTS
CNS: *Headache, dizziness, fatigue,* weakness, nervousness, agitation, extremity numbness, depression
CV: Orthostatic hypotension, volume depletion, palpitations, dysrhythmias, PVCs, vasculitis

EENT: Blurred vision, nasal congestion, increased intraocular pressure
ELECT: *Hypochloremic alkalosis, hypomagnesemia, hyperuricemia, hypercalcemia, hyponatremia, hypokalemia,* hyperglycemia
GI: *Nausea,* diarrhea, dry mouth, vomiting, anorexia, cramps, constipation, abdominal pain, hypercholesterolemia
GU: *Polyuria,* nocturia, urinary frequency, impotence
HEMA: Agranulocytosis, anemia
INTEG: *Rash, pruritus,* Stevens-Johnson syndrome
MS: *Cramps*

PHARMACOKINETICS
Well absorbed (PO); widely distributed; metabolized by liver; excreted by kidney (small amounts); onset 1-2 hr; peak 2 hr; duration up to 36 hr; excreted in urine, feces; half-life 14-18 hr

INTERACTIONS
Increase: hyperglycemia—diazoxide
Increase: toxicity of muscle relaxants, steroids, lithium, digoxin
Increase: hypokalemia—corticosteroids, amphotericin B, loop diuretics, thiazide diuretics
Decrease: effects—antidiabetics, antigout agents, anticoagulants
Decrease: absorption—cholestyramine, colestipol
Decrease: hypotensive effect—indomethacin, NSAIDs
Drug/Food
Increase: severe hypokalemia—licorice
Drug/Herb
Increase: antihypertensive effect—hawthorn
Drug/Lab Test
Increase: calcium, parathyroid test, glucose, uric acid

NURSING CONSIDERATIONS
Assess:
- Weight, I&O daily to determine fluid loss; effect of product may be decreased if used daily
- Rate, depth, rhythm of respirations, effect of exertion

- B/P lying, standing; postural hypotension may occur
- Electrolytes: potassium, magnesium, sodium, chloride: include BUN, CBC, serum creatinine, blood pH, ABGs, uric acid, Ca, glucose
- Signs of metabolic alkalosis, hypokalemia
- Rashes, fever daily; allergy to sulfa products
- Confusion, especially in geriatric patients; take safety precautions if needed
- Hydration: skin turgor, thirst, dry mucous membranes
- **Beers:** use with caution in older adults; may cause or exacerbate syndrome of inappropriate antidiuretic hormone secretion
- **Pregnancy/breastfeeding:** use only if benefit outweighs fetal risk; do not breastfeed, excretion unknown

Evaluate:
- Therapeutic response: improvement in edema of feet, legs, sacral area daily; decreased B/P

Teach patient/family:
- To consume diet high in potassium; to rise slowly from lying or sitting position
- To recognize adverse reactions: muscle cramps, weakness, nausea, dizziness
- To take with food, milk for GI symptoms; to take early in day to prevent nocturia; to avoid alcohol
- To notify prescriber if urinary output decreases; to monitor daily weight
- Not to stop product abruptly

TREATMENT OF OVERDOSE:
Lavage if taken orally; monitor electrolytes, administer IV fluids; monitor hydration, CV, renal status

---

⚠ HIGH ALERT

indinavir (Rx)
(en-den′a-veer)
Crixivan
Func. class.: Antiretroviral
Chem. class.: Protease inhibitor

Do not confuse:
indinavir/Denavir

ACTION: Inhibits human immunodeficiency virus (HIV-1) protease; this prevents the maturation of the virus

USES: HIV-1 in combination with other antiretrovirals
Unlabeled uses: Prevention of HIV-1 after exposure

CONTRAINDICATIONS: Hypersensitivity, breastfeeding
Precautions: Pregnancy, children, renal/hepatic disease, history of renal stones, diabetes, hypercholesterolemia, hemophilia, autoimmune disease, immune reconstitution syndrome

DOSAGE AND ROUTES
- **Adult: PO** 800 mg q8hr; 600 mg q8hr with delavirdine 400 mg tid; 600 mg q8hr with itraconazole 200 mg bid or ketoconazole
Mild to moderate hepatic impairment
- **Adult: PO** 600 mg q8hr
Available forms: Caps 200, 400 mg
Administer:
- Do not break, crush, or chew caps
- With water, 1 hr before or 2 hr after meals; may be given with other liquids or small meal; do not give with high-fat, high-protein meals
- Dosage adjustment will need to be considered when given with other antiretrovirals
- Increase water to 1.5 L/day minimum to prevent nephrolithiasis

SIDE EFFECTS
CNS: *Headache, insomnia,* dizziness, somnolence
GI: *Diarrhea, abdominal pain, nausea, vomiting,* anorexia, dry mouth
GU: Nephrolithiasis
INTEG: Rash
MS: Pain
OTHER: Asthenia, insulin-resistant hyperglycemia, hyperlipidemia, ketoacidosis, lipodystrophy

PHARMACOKINETICS
Terminal half-life 2 hr; 60% protein binding; metabolized in liver; excreted

---

Side effects: *italics* = common; red = life-threatening

<20% unchanged in urine, 83% in feces

INTERACTIONS

• **Life-threatening dysrhythmias:** ergots, midazolam, rifAMPin, triazolam, amiodarone, pimozide, alfuzosin

Increase: myopathy—statins (atorvastatin, lovastatin, simvastatin)

Increase: indinavir levels—CYP3A4 inhibitors (arepitant, protease inhibitors, azole antifungals, nefazodone, verapamil); phosphodiesterase-5 inhibitors (sildenafil, tadalafil, vardenafil)

Increase: levels of both products—clarithromycin, zidovudine

Increase: levels of isoniazid, oral contraceptives

Decrease: indinavir levels—CYP3A4 inducers (barbiturates, carBAMazepine, nonnucleoside reverse transcriptase inhibitors, phenytoins, rifamycins, modafinil)

Decrease: effect of both products—anticonvulsants

Decrease: effect—CYP3A4 substrates (calcium channel blockers, immunosuppressants, benzodiazepines, azole antifungals, macrolides, SSRIs, statins)

Drug/Herb

Decrease: indinavir levels—St. John's wort; avoid concurrent use

Drug/Food

Decrease: indinavir absorption—grapefruit juice; high-fat, high-protein foods

Drug/Lab Test

Increase: AST, ALT, amylase, total bilirubin

NURSING CONSIDERATIONS

Assess:

• Complaints of lower back, flank pain; indicates kidney stones

• Signs of infection, anemia, presence of other sexually transmitted diseases

• Blood/hepatic studies: ALT, AST; total bilirubin, amylase, blood glucose, serum cholesterol/lipid profile, may be elevated

• Plasma HIV RNA, viral load, CD4 during treatment

• Bowel pattern before, during treatment; if severe abdominal pain with bleeding occurs, product should be discontinued; monitor hydration

• Skin eruptions; rash, urticaria, itching

• Allergies before treatment, reaction of each medication; place allergies on chart

• **Pregnancy/breastfeeding:** use only if benefit outweighs fetal risk; do not breastfeed, excretion unknown

Evaluate:

• Therapeutic response: decreasing viral load, symptoms of HIV

Teach patient/family:

• To take as prescribed; if dose is missed, to take as soon as remembered up to 1 hr before next dose; not to double dose

• That product must be taken in equal intervals around the clock to maintain blood levels for duration of therapy

• That hyperglycemia may occur; to watch for increased thirst, weight loss, hunger, and dry, itchy skin; to notify prescriber

• To increase fluids to at least 1.5 L/day to prevent kidney stones; if stone formation occurs, that treatment may need to be interrupted

• That product does not cure HIV, only controls symptoms; not to donate blood

• That fat redistribution may occur

---

indomethacin (Rx)

(in-doe-meth'a-sin)

Indocin, Tivorbex

Func. class.: Nonsteroidal antiinflammatory product (NSAID), antirheumatic

Chem. class.: Acetic acid derivative

Do not confuse:

Indocin/Endocet/minocin/Vicodin

ACTION: Inhibits prostaglandin synthesis by decreasing enzyme needed for biosynthesis; analgesic, antiinflammatory, antipyretic

USES: RA, ankylosing spondylitis, osteoarthritis, bursitis, tendinitis, acute gouty arthritis; closure of patent ductus arteriosus in premature infants (IV)

Unlabeled uses: Bone pain, headache, heterotopic ossification, juvenile rheumatoid arthritis, pericarditis

CONTRAINDICATIONS: Pregnancy 3rd trimester, aortic coarctation, bleeding, salicylate/NSAID hypersensitivity, GI bleeding

Black Box Warning: Perioperative pain in CABG

Precautions: Pregnancy 1st trimester, breastfeeding, children, bleeding disorders, GI disorders, cardiac disorders, depression, renal/hepatic disease, asthma, diabetes, acute bronchospasm, ulcerative colitis, seizures, Parkinson's disease, neonates

Black Box Warning: Stroke, GI bleeding, MI, those taking NSAIDs are at greater risk of MI and stroke, even in first few weeks of therapy

DOSAGE AND ROUTES
Arthritis/antiinflammatory
• **Adult: PO** 25-50 mg bid-tid; max 200 mg/day; **EXT REL** 75 mg/day, may increase to 75 mg bid
Acute gouty arthritis
• **Adult: PO** 50 mg tid; use only for acute attack, then reduce dose
Mild to moderate pain (Tivorbex)
• **Adult: PO** 20 mg tid or 40 mg bid/tid
• **Child >2 yr: PO** 1-2 mg/kg/day in 2-4 divided doses, max 4 mg/kg/day or 150-200 mg/day
Patent ductus arteriosus
• **Neonate >7 days: IV** Initially, 0.2 mg/kg, then, if necessary, 2 more doses of 0.25 mg/kg at 12-hr intervals if urine output is >1 mL/kg/hr after prior dose or at 24-hr intervals if urine output is <1 mL/kg/hr; hold in cases of oliguria (<0.6 mL/kg/hr) or anuria
• **Neonate 2-7 days: IV** Initially, 0.2 mg/kg, then, if necessary, 2 more doses of 0.2 mg/kg at 12-hr intervals if urine output is >1 mL/kg/hr after prior dose or at 24-hr intervals if urine output is <1 mL/kg/hr; hold in cases of oliguria (<0.6 mL/kg/hr) or anuria

• **Neonate <2 days: IV** Initially, 0.2 mg/kg, then, if necessary, 1 or 2 doses of 0.1 mg/kg at 12-hr intervals if urine output is >1 mL/kg/hr after prior dose or at 24-hr intervals if urine output is <1 mL/kg/hr; hold in cases of oliguria (<0.6 mL/kg/hr) or anuria
• **Neonate: PO** Doses of 0.3 mg/kg q day × 2 days have been used
Available forms: Caps 25, 50 mg; ext rel caps 75 mg; caps (Tivorbex 20, 40 mg); powder for inj 1-mg vial; supp 50 mg; oral susp 5 mg/mL
Administer:
PO route
• Do not break, crush, or chew sus rel cap or reg caps
• With food to decrease GI symptoms and prevent ulcerations
• Shake susp; do not mix with other liquids
• Store at room temperature
IV route
• After reconstituting 1 mg with 1 or 2 mL NS or sterile water for inj without preservative; to give 1 or 0.5 mL/mL, respectively; do not dilute further
• Infuse over 20-30 min; avoid extravasation
• Do not inject/infuse via umbilical catheter to avoid dramatic shift in cerebral blood flow

SIDE EFFECTS
CNS: Dizziness, drowsiness, fatigue, confusion, insomnia, anxiety, depression, *headache*
CV: Peripheral edema, hypertension, CV thrombotic events, MI, stroke
EENT: Tinnitus, hearing loss, blurred vision
GI: *Nausea*, anorexia, *vomiting*, diarrhea, jaundice, cholestatic hepatitis, *constipation*, flatulence, cramps, peptic ulcer, ulceration, perforation, GI bleeding
GU: Nephrotoxicity: dysuria, hematuria, oliguria, azotemia (IV)
HEMA: Blood dyscrasias, prolonged bleeding
INTEG: Purpura, rash, pruritus, sweating, phlebitis at IV site

Side effects: *italics* = common; red = life-threatening

PHARMACOKINETICS

PO: Onset 30 min; peak 2 hr; duration 4-6 hr; metabolized in liver, kidneys; excreted in urine 60%, feces 33%; crosses placenta; excreted in breast milk; 99% protein binding; half-life 1 hr 1st pass, 2.6-11.2 hr 2nd pass

INTERACTIONS

Increase: hyperkalemia—potassium-sparing diuretics

Increase: toxicity—lithium, methotrexate, cycloSPORINE, probenecid, cidofovir

Increase: effect of—digoxin, phenytoin, aminoglycosides

Increase: bleeding risk—anticoagulants, abciximab, clopidogrel, eptifibatide, plicamycin, ticlopidine, tirofiban, thrombolytics, aspirin, SSRIs, SNRIs

Decrease: effect of—antihypertensives, diuretics

Drug/Herb

Increased: bleeding risk—chamomile, clove, dong quai, garlic, ginger, ginkgo

NURSING CONSIDERATIONS

Assess:

• **Arthritis symptoms:** ROM, pain, swelling before and 2 hr after treatment

> **Black Box Warning:** Cardiac disease, CV, thrombotic events (MI, stroke) before administration, not to be used in perioperative pain in CABG surgery

• Patent ductus arteriosus: respiratory rate, character, heart sounds

• Renal, hepatic, blood studies: BUN, creatinine, AST, ALT, Hgb before treatment, periodically thereafter; if renal function has decreased, do not give subsequent doses

• Eye/ear problems: blurred vision, tinnitus; may indicate toxicity; audiometric, ophthalmic exam before, during, after treatment if patient receiving long-term therapy

• Confusion, mood changes, hallucinations, especially among geriatric patients

• Asthma, nasal polyps, aspirin sensitivity, may develop hypersensitivity to indomethacin

> **Black Box Warning:** GI bleeding/perforation: chronic use can lead to GI bleeding, use cautiously in those with a history of active GI disease

> **Black Box Warning:** MI, stroke: may be greater with longer-term use and in those with CV risk factors

• **Beers:** avoid use in older adults; more likely to cause CNS effects

• **Pregnancy/breastfeeding:** do not use after 30 wk gestation; use only if benefits outweigh fetal risk <30 wk gestation; do not breastfeed, excreted in breast milk

Evaluate:

• Therapeutic response: decreased pain, stiffness, swelling in joints; ability to move more easily, PDA closure

Teach patient/family:

• To report blurred vision, ringing, roaring in ears; may indicate toxicity

• To avoid driving, other hazardous activities if dizziness, drowsiness occurs

• To report change in urine pattern, increased weight, edema, increased pain in joints, fever, blood in urine; may indicate nephrotoxicity

• To take with food for GI upset, to use as prescribed, not to skip or double doses, to take with 8 oz of water

• **Hepatotoxicity:** diarrhea, dark urine, clay-colored stools, yellowing of skin

• To report signs of GI bleeding: dark stools, hematemesis

• To report mood changes: anxiety, depression

• To use sunscreen, protective clothing, hat to prevent burns

• That therapeutic antiinflammatory effects may take up to 1 mo

• To avoid alcohol, NSAIDs, salicylates because bleeding may occur, discuss all OTC, Rx, herbals, supplements with health care professional

• To report use to all health care providers

> **Black Box Warning:** MI/stroke: to immediately report and seek medical attention for signs/symptoms of MI/stroke; discontinue product

---

inFLIXimab (Rx)

(in-fliks′ih-mab)

Inflectra ✦, Remicade, Remsima ✦, Renflexis

Func. class.: Biologic response modifiers

Chem. class.: Tumor necrosis factor modifiers

Do not confuse:
Remicade/Renacidin/
inFLIXimab/riTUXimab

ACTION: Monoclonal antibody that neutralizes the activity of tumor necrosis factor-alpha (TNF-α) found in Crohn's disease; decreased infiltration of inflammatory cells

USES: Crohn's disease, fistulizing (moderate to severe); RA, given with methotrexate; plaque psoriasis, ankylosing spondylitis, ulcerative colitis, psoriasis
Unlabeled uses: Psoriatic arthritis, Behçet's syndrome, uveitis, juvenile arthritis

CONTRAINDICATIONS: Hypersensitivity to murines, moderate to severe HF (NYHA class III/IV)
Precautions: Pregnancy, breastfeeding, children, geriatric patients, COPD, hepatotoxicity, hematologic abnormalities, hepatitis B, Guillain-Barré syndrome, seizures, multiple sclerosis

> **Black Box Warning:** Infection, neoplastic disease, TB

DOSAGE AND ROUTES
Rheumatoid arthritis
• **Adult:** IV induction: 3 mg/kg over at least 2 hr given at week 0, 2, and 6; maintenance: 3 mg/kg IV q8wk. May increase dose up to 10 mg/kg IV OR give 3 mg/kg IV q4wk in patients with an incomplete response

Crohn's disease/ankylosing spondylitis/psoriasis/ulcerative colitis
• **Adult:** IV induction: 5 mg/kg over at least 2 hr given at week 0, 2 and 6; maintenance for Crohn's—5 mg/kg q8wk, may increase to 10 mg/kg; maintenance for ankylosing spondylitis—5 mg/kg q6wk; maintenance for psoriasis/ulcerative colitis—5 mg/kg q8wk

Available forms: Powder for inj 100 mg
Administer:
Intermittent IV INFUSION route
• Pretreat with diphenhydrAMINE, acetaminophen, predniSONE if a reaction is infusion related
• Give immediately after reconstitution; reconstitute each vial with 10 mL sterile water for inj; further dilute total dose/250 mL of 0.9% NaCl inj to a total concentration of 0.4-4 mg/mL; use 21-G or smaller needle for reconstitution; direct sterile water at glass wall of vial; gently swirl; do not shake; may foam; allow to stand for 5 min, give within 3 hr
• Give over ≥2 hr, use polyethylene-lined infusion with in-line, sterile, low–protein-binding filter
• Do not admix
• Refrigerated storage; do not freeze

SIDE EFFECTS
CNS: *Headache, dizziness, depression, vertigo, fatigue, anxiety, fever,* seizures, *chills, flulike symptoms,* demyelinating disease
CV: Chest pain, hypo/hypertension, tachycardia, HF, acute coronary syndrome
GI: *Nausea, vomiting, abdominal pain, stomatitis, constipation, dyspepsia, flatulence*
GU: Dysuria, urinary frequency
HEMA: Anemia, leukopenia, thrombocytopenia, pancytopenia
INTEG: *Rash, dermatitis, urticaria,* dry skin, sweating, flushing, hematoma, pruritus, keratoderma blenorrhagicum
MS: Myalgia, back pain, arthralgia
RESP: URI, pharyngitis, bronchitis, cough, dyspnea, sinusitis
SYST: Anaphylaxis, fatal infections, sepsis, malignancies, immunogenicity, Stevens-Johnson syndrome, toxic epidermal necrolysis, sarcoidosis

PHARMACOKINETICS
Distributed to vascular compartment, half-life 9.5 days

Side effects: *italics* = common; red = life-threatening

INTERACTIONS

Increase: infections, neutropenia—TNF blockers (abatacept, anakinra, golimumab, rilonacept); avoid concurrent use
• Do not administer live vaccines concurrently

NURSING CONSIDERATIONS
Assess:

• **RA:** pain, joints involved, ROM, aggravating ameliorating factors baseline and periodically
• **Plaque psoriasis:** lesions, body areas affected baseline and periodically
• **Ulcerative colitis/Crohn's disease:** Pain, cramping, diarrhea, change in life style baseline and periodically
• **GI symptoms:** nausea, vomiting, abdominal pain
• Periodic blood counts (CBC with differential), ANA titer, LFTs, baseline and periodically, may cause blood dyscrusia, discontinue if present
• CV status: B/P, pulse, chest pain
• **Allergic reaction, anaphylaxis:** rash, dermatitis, urticaria, dyspnea, hypotension, fever, chills; discontinue if severe, administer EPINEPHrine, corticosteroids, antihistamines; assess for allergies to murine proteins before starting therapy

Black Box Warning: Fatal infections: discontinue if infection occurs, do not administer to patients with active infection; identify TB before beginning treatment; a TB test should be obtained; if present, TB should be treated before patient receives product; exercise caution when switching from 1 DMARD to another

Black Box Warning: For neoplastic disease in those <18 yr, including hepatosplenic T-cell lymphoma; usually occurs in those with inflammatory bowel disease

• **Pregnancy/breastfeeding:** does not cross placenta during 1st trimester, but does 2nd/3rd trimester; discontinue 8-10 wk before birth; do not breastfeed. Not to breastfeed while taking this product

Evaluate:
• Therapeutic response: absence of fever, mucus in stools

Teach patient/family:
• That infusion reaction should be reported immediately
• To notify prescriber immediately if infection occurs
• To notify prescriber of GI symptoms, hypersensitivity reactions, heart symptoms
• Not to operate machinery or drive if dizziness, vertigo occur
• To avoid live virus vaccinations; bring up-to-date before use
• **Malignancy:** check skin for changes, growths, or color changes
• **Pregnancy/breastfeeding:** identify if pregnancy is planned or suspected

---

inotuzumab ozogamicin
(ih-noh-too'-zoo-mab oh'-zoh-ga-MIH-sin)
Besponsa
Func. class.: Antineoplastic monoclonal antibodies

ACTION: A CD22-directed antibody-drug conjugate; CD22 is expressed on pre–B cells and mature B cells. It consists of a cytotoxic agent; it induces double-strand DNA breaks, resulting in cell-cycle arrest and apoptotic cell death

USES: For the treatment of adults with relapsed or refractory B-cell precursor acute lymphoblastic leukemia

CONTRAINDICATIONS: Pregnancy, hypersensitivity

Black Box Warning: Hepatic disease, hepatotoxicity, mortality, sinusoidal obstructive disease, veno-occlusive disease

Precautions: Alcoholism, bleeding, breastfeeding, contraception requirements, diabetes mellitus, electrolyte imbalances, females, geriatric patients, infertility, male-mediated teratogenicity, neutropenia, bone marrow suppression, infection, reproductive risk, thrombocytopenia, thyroid disease, QT prolongation

DOSAGE AND ROUTES
Relapsed or refractory B-cell precursor ALL
• **Adult:** IV 0.8 mg/m² day 1 and 0.5 mg/m² days 8 and 15 (cycle 1). Length of cycle 1 is 21 days, may increase to 28 days

Management of treatment-related toxicity
• Do not interrupt doses within a treatment cycle (day 8 or day 15 dose) for neutropenia or thrombocytopenia. Dosing interruptions within a cycle are recommended for nonhematologic toxicity. If a dose reduction is necessary, do not re-escalate the dose

Hematologic toxicity
• **Absolute neutrophil count (ANC) of ≥1 × 10⁹ cells/L before starting therapy:** if the ANC decreases, hold next cycle of therapy until recovery of the ANC to 1 × 10⁹ cells/L or greater. Discontinue therapy if low ANC lasts >28 days and is suspected to be due to inotuzumab ozogamicin

• **Platelet count of ≥50 × 10⁹ cells/L before starting therapy:** if platelet count decreases, hold next cycle of therapy until the platelet count recovers to 50 × 10⁹ cells/L or greater. Discontinue therapy if low platelet count lasts >28 days and is suspected to be due to inotuzumab ozogamicin

• **ANC was <1 × 10⁹ cells/L and/or platelet count was <50 × 10⁹ cells/L before starting therapy:** if the ANC or platelet count decreases, hold the next cycle until at least 1 of the following occurs: the ANC and platelet counts recover to baseline or better for the prior cycle; the ANC recovers to 1 × 10⁹ cells/L or greater and the platelet count recovers to 50 × 10⁹ cells/L or greater; the patient has stable or improved disease (based on most recent bone marrow assessment) and the ANC and platelet count decrease is considered to be due to the underlying disease and not product-related toxicity

Infusion-related reactions
• **Mild to moderate reactions:** hold infusion and start medical management. Consider discontinuing or give steroids and antihistamines depending on the severity
• **Severe or life-threatening reactions:** stop infusion, permanently discontinue

Nonhematologic toxicity:
Evaluate for toxicity before each dose. For grade ≥2 toxicity, hold until toxicity recovers to grade ≤1 (or pretreatment grade level). Dose modifications depend on duration of dosing interruption as follows:
• **Less than 7 days (within a cycle):** hold the next dose; maintain a minimum of 6 days between doses
• **7 days or greater:** omit the next dose within the cycle
• **14 days or greater:** after recovery, decrease the total dose by 25% for the subsequent cycle. If further dose modification is required, reduce the number of doses to 2 per cycle for subsequent cycles. If a 25% decrease in the total dose followed by a decrease to 2 doses per cycle is not tolerated, permanently discontinue therapy
• **Greater than 28 days:** consider permanent discontinuation

Hepatic dose
• **Baseline hepatic impairment:** no change
• **Treatment-related hepatotoxicity:** evaluate for toxicity before each dose. Dosing interruptions within a cycle are recommended for hepatic impairment. If a dose reduction is necessary, do not re-escalate the dose.
• **Total bilirubin level of ≤1.5× the upper limit of normal (ULN) and AST/ALT level of ≤2.5× ULN:** no dose adjustment is necessary
• **Total bilirubin level >1.5× ULN and AST/ALT level >2.5× ULN:** hold therapy until total bilirubin level is ≤1.5× ULN and the AST/ALT level is ≤2.5× ULN unless hyperbilirubinemia is due to Gilbert's

Side effects: *italics* = common; red = life-threatening

syndrome or hemolysis. Dose modifications depend on duration of dosing interruption as follows:

• **Less than 7 days (within a cycle):** hold the next dose; maintain a minimum of 6 days between doses

• **14 days or greater:** after recovery, decrease total dose by 25% for the subsequent cycle. If further dose modification is required, reduce number of doses to 2 per cycle for subsequent cycles. If a 25% decrease in the total dose followed by a decrease to 2 doses per cycle is not tolerated, permanently discontinue

• **Greater than 28 days:** permanently discontinue

• **Hepatic veno-occlusive disease (VOD)/sinusoidal obstruction syndrome (SOS) or other severe liver toxicity:** permanently discontinue

Available forms: Powder for injection 0.9 mg

Administer:

IV route

• Visually inspect for particulate matter and discoloration before use

• Follow cytotoxic handling procedures

• Available as a single-dose, preservative-free, 0.9-mg lyophilized powder vial

• Premedication with a corticosteroid, an antipyretic agent (acetaminophen), and an antihistamine before each dose is recommended; observe patients during and for at least 1 hr after the end of the infusion for symptoms of infusion-related reactions

Reconstitution

• After calculating the number of vials needed, add 4 mL of Sterile Water for Injection to each vial for a final vial concentration of 0.25 mg/mL (0.9 mg/3.6 mL); gently swirl the vial to dissolve powder; do not shake

• The reconstitution solution should be clear to opalescent, colorless to slightly yellow, and free of visible foreign matter

• **Storage of reconstituted vials:** if not further diluted immediately, vials may be stored in the refrigerator (at 2-8° C or 36-46° F) for up to 4 hr after reconstitution; protect from light, do not freeze

Dilution:

• Add required dose/volume from the reconstituted vials to an infusion container made of polyvinyl chloride (PVC) (or non–DEHP-containing), polyolefin (polypropylene and/or polyethylene), or ethylene vinyl acetate (EVA); discard any unused portion

• Add 0.9% sodium chloride injection to the infusion container for a final total volume of 50 mL; gently invert to mix, do not shake

• **Storage of admixture:** if not infused immediately, the diluted solution may be stored at room temperature (20-25° C or 68-77° F) for up to 4 hr or refrigerated (2-8° C or 36-46° F) for up to 3 hr; protect from light and do not freeze

Intravenous (IV) Infusion:

• Allow refrigerated admixtures to warm to room temperature for 1 hr before use

• Give admixture (protected from light) as an IV infusion over 1 hr through an infusion line made of PVC, polyolefin (polypropylene and/or polyethylene), or polybutadiene

• Complete infusion within 8 hr of reconstitution

• The diluted solution does not need to be filtered; if it is filtered, use polyethersulfone (PES)-, polyvinylidene fluoride (PVDF)-, or hydrophilic polysulfone (HPS)-based filters

• Do not use filters made of nylon or mixed cellulose ester (MCE)

• Do not mix with or administer as an infusion with other drugs

SIDE EFFECTS

CNS: Fatigue, fever, headache, migraine, chills

GI: Nausea, vomiting, diarrhea, stomatitis, constipation, anorexia, abdominal pain, hepatotoxicity

HEMA: Anemia, thrombocytopenia, bleeding, hematoma, hematuria, ecchymosis, veno-occlusive disease

MISC: Infection, *asthenia*, QT prolongation, tumor lysis syndrome, sinusoidal obstruction syndrome

PHARMACOKINETICS
Protein binding 97%

INTERACTIONS
Increase: QT prolongation—other products that increase QT prolongation
Drug/Lab Test
Increase: LFTs

NURSING CONSIDERATIONS
Assess:
• **Serious infection:** some may be fatal. Monitor patients for signs and symptoms of infection; use prophylactic anti-infectives as appropriate
• **Severe myelosuppression/bone marrow suppression:** thrombocytopenia, neutropenia; obtain a CBC before each dose; therapy interruption or permanent discontinuation may be necessary in patients who develop severe myelosuppression
• **Pregnancy/breastfeeding:** product can cause fetal harm; females of reproductive potential should avoid becoming pregnant during treatment and for 8 mo after final dose; obtain pregnancy test before starting product; do not breastfeed during treatment and for at least 2 mo after last dose; men with female partners of reproductive potential should avoid fathering a child and use effective contraception during and for at least 5 mo after therapy
• **QT prolongation:** obtain an electrocardiogram (ECG) and monitor serum electrolytes before the start of treatment and periodically during therapy as needed. Use with caution in patients with a history of QT prolongation or who have an electrolyte imbalance. Avoid concomitant use with other drugs known to prolong the QT interval; if co-administration is unavoidable, monitor ECGs and serum electrolytes after starting the other QT-prolonging drug. Females, geriatric patients or patients with diabetes mellitus, thyroid disease, malnutrition, alcoholism, hepatic dysfunction, or who have received high cumulative dose anthracycline therapy may also be at increased risk for QT prolongation

Black Box Warning: Severe or life-threatening hepatotoxicity including veno-occlusive disease (VOD)/sinusoidal obstruction syndrome (SOS): monitor liver function tests (LFTs), total bilirubin, alkaline phosphatase levels before and following each dosage change; therapy interruption, dose reduction, or permanent discontinuation may be necessary in those who develop LFT abnormalities. Closely monitor for VOD/SOS (hepatomegaly, rapid weight gain, and ascites). Permanently discontinue in those who develop VOD/SOS; in those who undergo a hematopoietic stem-cell transplant (HSCT), monitor LFTs frequently during the first month post-HSCT; then, continue to monitor LFTs but less often. Time from HSCT to onset of VOD/SOS was 15 days (range, 3 to 57 days). The risk of VOD/SOS may be greater in patients who receive an HSCT or a conditioning regimen that contains 2 alkylating agents before HSCT and in patients who have an increased total bilirubin level before an HSCT; other risk factors include hepatic disease (e.g., cirrhosis, nodular regenerative hyperplasia, active hepatitis), a prior HSCT, increased age, later salvage lines, and a greater number of treatment cycles

Black Box Warning: Mortality: those who underwent a hematopoietic stem-cell transplant (HSCT) may have a higher 100-day post-HSCT nonrelapse mortality; monitor closely for post-HSCT toxicity. The most common causes of post-HSCT death were veno-occlusive disease/sinusoidal obstruction syndrome and infectious complications

Evaluate:
• Therapeutic response: improving blood counts

Teach patient/familiy:

• To report adverse reactions immediately: bleeding; report diarrhea, hepatic, hematologic symptoms/toxicity, flulike symptoms

• About reason for treatment, expected results

• That monitoring for infusion reactions will be needed for at least 1 hr after infusion has ended

• **Pregnancy/breastfeeding:** to notify provider if pregnancy is planned or suspected; to use effective contraception during treatment and for 8 mo after discontinuing treatment; not to breastfeed during treatment or for 2 mo after final dose; that men with female partners of reproductive potential should avoid fathering a child and use effective contraception during and for at least 5 mo after therapy

---

⚠ **HIGH ALERT**

insulin, inhaled

(in′su-lin)

Afrezza

Func. class.: Antidiabetic—insulin

ACTION: Endogenous insulin regulates carbohydrate, fat, and protein metabolism by the storage of and inhibiting the breakdown of glucose, fat, and amino acids. Insulin decreases glucose concentrations by the uptake of glucose in muscle and adipose tissue, and by inhibiting hepatic glucose production. Insulin also regulates fat metabolism by the storage of fat and inhibiting the mobilization of fat for energy in adipose tissues (lipolysis and free fatty acid oxidation)

USES: Diabetes mellitus types 1 and 2

CONTRAINDICATIONS: Hypersensitivity, lung cancer, hypoglycemia, smoking

Precautions: Hepatic disease, renal impairment, renal failure, diabetic ketoacidosis (DKA), hypokalemia, pregnancy, breastfeeding, child <18 yr

Black Box Warning: Asthma, COPD, pulmonary disease

Black Box Warning: Acute bronchospasm

DOSAGE AND ROUTES

• **Adult: INH:** (type 1) the average initial dose is 0.5-0.6 unit/kg/day, usually ≥3 administrations/day; (type 2) the average initial dose is 0.2-0.6 unit/kg/day. When used in combination with oral hypoglycemic agents, may only need a single dose of a longer-acting insulin at a dosage of 10 units or 0.2 unit/kg/day

Available forms: Inhalation 4 units powder in 4-, 8-, 12-unit cartridges

Administer:

• Give by inhalation only; use at beginning of a meal (blue cartridge = 4 units of regular insulin, green cartridge = 8 units of regular insulin), multiple cartridges may be needed, for single-use only, inhaler should be discarded after 15 days; store unopened cartridge packages in refrigerator; if not refrigerated, use within 10 days

• Sealed (unopened) blister cards and strips must be used within 10 days. Cartridges left over in an opened strip must be used within 3 days. Remove a blister card from the foil package. Tear along a perforation to remove one strip. Press the clear side of the strip to push the cartridge out. To load the cartridge, hold the inhaler level in one hand with the white mouthpiece on the top and purple base on the bottom; open the inhaler by lifting the white mouthpiece to a vertical position. Before placing the cartridge in the inhaler, both the cartridge and the inhaler should be at room temperature for 10 minutes. Hold the cartridge with the cup facing down and line up the cartridge with the opening in the inhaler. The pointed end of the cartridge should line up with the pointed end in the inhaler. The cartridge can be placed into the inhaler; ensure that the cartridge lies flat in the inhaler. Once the cartridge is loaded, keep level

• Remove the purple mouthpiece cover. Hold the inhaler away from the mouth and fully exhale. While keeping the head level, place the mouthpiece in the mouth and tilt the inhaler down toward the chin. Close lips around the mouthpiece to form a seal. Inhale deeply through the inhaler. Have the patient hold his or her breath for as long as comfortable and at the same time remove the inhaler from the mouth. Exhale and continue to breathe normally

SIDE EFFECTS

CNS: Headache, fatigue
GI: Nausea, diarrhea
MISC: Urinary tract infection, weight gain, hypokalemia, peripheral edema
RESP: Cough, throat irritation/pain, productive cough, decreased pulmonary function tests, bronchitis, acute bronchospasm
ENDO: Hypoglycemia

INTERACTIONS

Increase: inhaled insulin effect—bronchodilators, other inhaled products, agonists, salicylates, alcohol, fenfluramine, MAOIs
Increase: heart failure, ischemic events—pioglitazone, troglitazone
Increase: hypoglycemia—β-blockers, ACE inhibitors, angiotensin II receptor antagonists, disopyramide, guanethidine, octreotide
Increase or decrease: hypoglycemic effects—cloNIDine, metoclopramide, tegaserod, testosterone derivatives, or anabolic steroids
Increase: hyperglycemia—niacin (nicotinic acid), bumetanide, furosemide, torsemide
Decrease: hypoglycemic effects—dextrothyroxine, triamterene, thiazide diuretics; thyroid hormones, estrogens, progestins, or oral contraceptives; danazol, corticosteroids, EPINEPHrine

NURSING CONSIDERATIONS

Assess:
• Fasting blood glucose, A1c may be drawn to identify treatment effectiveness
• Urine ketones during illness, insulin requirements may increase during times of stress, trauma, illness, surgery
• Hypoglycemic reaction can occur during peak times (sweating, weakness, dizziness, chills, confusion, headache, nausea, rapid, weak pulse)

• Hyperglycemia: acetone breath, polyuria, fatigue, polydipsia, flushed dry skin, lethargy
• **Smoking status:** not recommended in current smokers or those with recent cessation
• **Beers:** avoid in older adults; higher risk of hypoglycemia without improvement in hyperglycemia management
Evaluate:
• Therapeutic response: decrease in blood glucose levels
Teach patient/family:
• That blurred vision occurs, not to operate machinery until effect is known, do not change corrective lenses for at least 1 month
• To keep all insulin equipment available at all times
• That product does not cure, but controls symptoms
• To carry ID as diabetic
• About the symptoms of hypoglycemia, hyperglycemia, ketoacidosis
• About dosage and how to use product, that the rest of the plan must be followed; do not change the dose without prescriber approval; cartridges should be at room temperature for 10 min, do not invert inhaler, do not leave used cartridge in the inhaler

---

⚠ HIGH ALERT

INSULINS

Rapid Acting

insulin aspart (Rx)
NovoLOG, NovoLOG Flexpen, NovoLOG Pen Fill, NovoMix 30 ✦, Novo Rapid ✦

insulin glulisine (Rx)
Apidra, Apidra SoloStar
Insulin Inhaled Afrezza

insulin lispro (Rx)
HumaLOG

Short Acting

insulin, regular (otc)
HumuLIN R, NovoLIN R, ReliOn R

---

insulin, regular concentrated (Rx)

Humulin R, Novolin ge Toronto ✦, Novolin R, HumuLIN R U-500

Intermediate Acting

insulin, isophane suspension (NPH) (otc)

HumuLIN N, NovoLIN ge NPH ✦, NovoLIN N, NovoLIN N Prefilled, ReliOn N

Long Acting

insulin detemir (Rx)
Levemir

insulin degludec (Rx)
Tresiba

insulin glargine (Rx)
Basaglar, Lantus, Toujeo SoloStar

Mixtures

Insulin degludec, Insulin aspart,
Ryzodeg 70/50

insulin, isophane suspension and regular insulin (Rx)
HumuLIN 70/30, NovoLIN 70/30

NPH Regular Insulin Mixture
Humalin 7/30, Novolin 7/30

insulin lispro mixture (Rx)
HumaLOG Mix 75/25, HumaLOG Mix 50/50

insulin aspart mixture (Rx)
NovoLOG 70/30, NovoLOG Mix Flexpen Prefilled Syringe 70/30

Func. class.: Antidiabetic, pancreatic hormone

Chem. class.: Modified structures of endogenous human insulin

Do not confuse
Novolog/Humalog

ACTION: Decreases blood glucose; by transport of glucose into cells and the conversion of glucose to glycogen, indirectly increases blood pyruvate and lactate, decreases phosphate and potassium; insulin may be human (processed by recombinant DNA technologies)

USES: Type 1 diabetes mellitus, type 2 diabetes mellitus, gestational diabetes; insulin lispro may be used in combination with sulfonylureas in children >3 yr

CONTRAINDICATIONS: Hypersensitivity to protamine; creosol (aspart)
Precautions: Pregnancy

DOSAGE AND ROUTES
Insulin glulisine
• **Adult/adolescent/child ≥4 yr:** SUBCUT dosage individualized, give within 15 min before or 20 min after starting a meal
• **Adult:** IV dilute to 1 unit/mL in infusion systems with 0.9% NaCl, use PVC Viaflex infusion bags and PVC tubing, use dedicated line

Insulin aspart
• **Adult/adolescent/child ≥6 yr:** INTERMITTENT SUBCUT Total daily dose is given as 2-4 inj/day just before beginning of meal; in general, 50%-70% of total daily insulin may be given as insulin aspart, remainder should be intermediate- or long-acting insulin; **CONTINUOUS SUBCUT** used with external insulin pump via cont SUBCUT insulin infusion (CSII), insulin dose should be based on insulin dose from previous regimen

Insulin lispro
• **Adult/adolescent/child ≥3 yr:** SUBCUT 15 min before meals; **CONT SUBCUT INFUSION (external insulin pump):** total daily dose should be based on insulin dose from previous regimen, 50% of total dose can be given as meal-related boluses, remainder as basal infusion

Human regular
• **Adult:** SUBCUT $^1/_2$-1 hr before meals

Insulin, isophane suspension
- **Adult: SUBCUT** dosage individualized by blood, urine glucose; usual dose 7-26 units; may increase by 2-10 units/day if needed

Insulin degludec
- **Adult: SUBCUT** dosage individualized

Insulin detemir
- **Adult/adolescent/child ≥2 yr: SUBCUT** 1-2×/day; if 1×, give with evening meal

Insulin glargine
- **Adult and child ≥6 yr: SUBCUT** 10 units/day, range 2-100 units/day, but may go much higher

Regular insulin (ketoacidosis)
- **Adult: IV** 5-10 units, then 5-10 units/hr until desired response, then switch to **SUBCUT** dose; **IV/INFUSION** 2-12 units (50 units/500 mL of normal saline)
- **Child: IV** 0.1 units/kg

Replacement
- **Adult/child: SUBCUT** 0.5-1 units/kg/day qid given 30 min before meals
- **Adolescent: SUBCUT** 0.8-1.2 units/kg/day; this dosage is used during rapid growth

Available forms: *NPH* Inj 100 units/mL; *regular* inj 100 units/mL, cartridges 100 units/mL; *insulin analog* inj 100 units/mL; *isophane insulin* inj 100 units/mL, cartridges 100 units/mL; **insulin lispro** 100 units/mL, 1.5-mL cartridges, HumaLOG Pen sol for inj 100 units/mL, Humalog KwikPen 200 U/mL prefilled pen solution for injection; *insulin glulisine* inj 100 units/mL; *insulin glargine* inj 100, 300 units/mL; *insulin degludec* solution for inj 100 units/mL (u-100), 200 units/mL (u-200); *insulin detemir* inj 100 units/mL in 10 vials, 3-mL cartridges; *insulin aspart* inj 100 units/mL (Flexpen, Pen Fill)

Administer:
- Store at room temperature for <1 mo (some insulins); keep away from heat and sunlight; refrigerate all other supply; NPH, premixed insulins are cloudy; regular, rapid-acting analogs, long-acting analogs are clear; do not freeze—IV route, regular only

SUBCUT route
- After warming to room temperature by rotating in palms; use only insulin syringes with markings or syringe matching units/mL; rotate inj sites within one area: abdomen, upper back, thighs, upper arm, buttocks; keep record of sites
- Increased dosages if tolerance occurs
- Premixed insulins, NPH are cloudy suspensions
- Regular human insulin, rapid-acting analogs, long-acting analogs are clear; do not use if cloudy, thick, or discolored

CONT SUBCUT route (insulin infusion CSII)
- Do not mix with other insulins when using a pump
- Insulin lispro 3-mL cartridges to be used in Disetronic H-TRON plus V100 pump using Disetronic rapid infusion sets; infusion set and cartridge adapter should be changed q3days; replace 3-mL cartridge q6days

IV route (insulin glulisine only)
- Dilute to 1 international unit/mL in infusion systems with 0.9% NaCl using PVC viaflex infusion bags and PVC tubing; use dedicated line; do not admix

IV route (regular only)
When regular insulin is administered IV, monitor glucose, potassium often to prevent fatal hypoglycemia, hypokalemia
- IV direct, undiluted via vein, Y-site, 3-way stopcock; give at ≤50 units/min
- By cont infusion after diluting with IV sol and run at prescribed rate; use IV infusion pump for correct dosing; give reduced dose at serum glucose level of 250 mg/100 mL

Y-site compatibilities: Amiodarone, ampicillin, ampicillin/sulbactam, aztreonam, ceFAZolin, cefoTEtan, DOBUTamine, esmolol, famotidine, gentamicin, heparin, heparin/hydrocortisone, imipenem/cilastatin, indomethacin, magnesium sulfate, meperidine, meropenem, midazolam, morphine, nitroglycerin, oxytocin, PENTobarbital, potassium chloride, propofol, ritodrine, sodium bicarbonate, sodium nitroprusside, tacrolimus, terbutaline, ticarcillin, ticarcillin/clavulanate, tobramycin, vancomycin, vit B/C

SIDE EFFECTS
EENT: Blurred vision, dry mouth
INTEG: Flushing, rash, urticaria, warmth, lipodystrophy, lipohypertrophy, swelling, redness
META: *Hypoglycemia,* rebound hyperglycemia (Somogyi effect 12-72 hr or longer)
MISC: Peripheral edema
SYST: Anaphylaxis

PHARMACOKINETICS
Rapid acting
Insulin glulisine: Onset 15-30 min, peak $^1/_2$-1$^1/_2$ hr, duration 3-4 hr
Insulin aspart: Onset 10-20 min, peak 1-3 hr, duration 3-5 hr
Insulin lispro: Onset 15-30 min, peak $^1/_2$-1$^1/_2$ hr, duration 3-5 hr
Short acting
Insulin regular: Onset 30 min, peak 2.5-5 hr, duration up to 7 hr
Intermediate acting
Insulin, isophane suspension (NPH): Onset 1.5-4 hr, peak 4-12 hr, duration ≤24 hr
Insulin degludec: Peak 12 hr, duration 42 hr after 8 doses
Long acting
Insulin detemir: Onset 0.8-2 hr, peak unknown, duration ≤24 hr (concentration dependent)
Insulin glargine: Onset 1.5 hr, no peak identified, duration ≥24 hr
Mixtures
Insulin, isophane suspension and regular insulin (70/30): Onset 10-20 min, peak 2.4 hr, duration ≤24 hr
Insophane insulin suspension (NPH) and insulin mixtures (50/50): Onset $^1/_2$-1 hr, peak dual, duration 10-16 hr

INTERACTIONS
Increase: hypoglycemia—salicylate, alcohol, β-blockers, anabolic steroids, phenylbutazone, sulfinpyrazone, guanethidine, oral hypoglycemics, MAOIs, tetracycline

Decrease: hypoglycemia—thiazides, thyroid hormones, oral contraceptives, corticosteroids, estrogens, DOBUTamine, EPINEPHrine
Drug/Lab Test
Increase: VMA
Decrease: potassium, calcium
Interference: LFTs, thyroid function studies

NURSING CONSIDERATIONS
Assess:
• Fasting blood glucose; A1c may be drawn to identify treatment effectiveness q3mo
• Urine ketones during illness; insulin requirements may increase during stress, illness, surgery
• Hypoglycemic reaction that can occur during peak time (sweating, weakness, dizziness, chills, confusion, headache, nausea, rapid weak pulse, fatigue, tachycardia, memory lapses, slurred speech, staggering gait, anxiety, tremors, hunger)
• **Hyperglycemia:** acetone breath; polyuria; fatigue; polydipsia; flushed, dry skin; lethargy
• **Beers:** avoid use of short- or rapid-acting insulin in older adults; sliding-scale insulin poses a higher risk of hypoglycemia without improvement in hyperglycemia management

Evaluate:
• Therapeutic response: decrease in polyuria, polydipsia, polyphagia; clear sensorium; absence of dizziness; stable gait, blood glucose HBA1c within normal limits

Teach patient/family:
• That blurred vision occurs; not to change corrective lenses until vision is stabilized after 1-2 mo
• To keep insulin, equipment available at all times; to carry a glucagon kit, candy, or oral glucose preparation to treat hypoglycemia
• That product does not cure diabetes but controls symptoms
• To carry emergency ID as diabetic
• To recognize hypoglycemia reaction: headache, tremors, fatigue, weakness, tachycardia

• To recognize hyperglycemia reaction: frequent urination, thirst, fatigue, hunger

• About the dosage, route, mixing instructions, diet restrictions (if any), disease process

• About the symptoms of ketoacidosis: nausea; thirst; polyuria; dry mouth; decreased B/P; dry, flushed skin; acetone breath; drowsiness; Kussmaul respirations

• That a plan is necessary for diet, exercise; that all food on diet should be eaten; that exercise routine should not vary

• About blood glucose testing; how to determine glucose level

• To avoid OTC products unless directed by prescriber

---

interferon beta-1a (Rx)

(in-ter-feer′on)

Avonex, Rebif

interferon beta-1b (Rx)

Betaseron, Extavia

Func. class.: Multiple sclerosis agent, immune modifier

Chem. class.: Interferon, *Escherichia coli* derivative

ACTION: Antiviral, immunoregulatory; action not clearly understood; biologic response-modifying properties mediated through specific receptors on cells, inducing expression of interferon-induced gene products

USES: Ambulatory patients with relapsing or remitting MS

CONTRAINDICATIONS: Hypersensitivity to natural or recombinant interferon-β or human albumin, hamster protein, rotavirus vaccine

Precautions: Pregnancy, breastfeeding, children <18 yr, chronic progressive MS, depression, mental disorders, seizure disorder, latex allergy, autoimmune disorders, bone marrow suppression, hepatotoxicity, cardiac disease, alcoholism, chickenpox, herpes zoster

DOSAGE AND ROUTES
Interferon beta-1a
Multiple sclerosis

• **Adult: IM** (Avonex) 30 mcg/wk

• **Adult: SUBCUT** (Rebif) 22 or 44 mcg 3×/wk with each dose 48 hr apart, titrate to full dose over 4-wk period

Interferon beta-1b
Multiple sclerosis

• **Adult: SUBCUT** 0.0625 mg every other day for wk 1 and 2, then 0.125 mg every other day for wk 3 and 4, then 0.1875 mg every other day for wk 5 and 6, then 0.25 mg every other day thereafter; higher doses should not be used

Available forms: *beta-1a:* (Avonex) 30 mcg (6.6 million international units/vial) (autoinjector pen); (Rebif) 22 mcg, 44 mcg/0.5 mL; *beta-1b:* powder for inj 0.3 mg kit

Administer

Interferon beta-1a

• Visually inspect parenteral products for particulate matter and discoloration before use

• Store in refrigerator; do not freeze

IM route

• Premedicate with acetaminophen or ibuprofen and give at bedtime to lessen flulike symptoms

• Interferon-β1a (Avonex) 30 mcg = 6 million IU

• If a dose is missed, give it as soon as possible; continue regular schedule but do not give 2 injections within 2 days; all products are single-use only; do not re-use needles, syringes, prefilled syringes, or autoinjectors

• Rotate injection sites to minimize injection-site reactions

• Do not inject into an area where skin is irritated, reddened, bruised, infected, or scarred

• Check site after 2 hr for redness, edema, or tenderness

• The manufacturer of Avonex offers free training on IM use for patients and health care partners; contact Above MS for more information (800-456-2255)

Side effects: *italics* = common; red = life-threatening

Reconstitution and administration of Avonex lyophilized powder for IM route

- Use aseptic technique for preparation of solution
- Sites include the thigh or upper arm
- Slowly add 1.1 mL sterile water for injection, preservative-free (supplied by manufacturer) to the vial; rapid addition of the diluent can cause foaming
- Gently swirl; do not shake; final concentration should be 30 mcg/mL (6 million IU/mL)
- The solution should be clear to slightly yellow without particles; discard if the reconstituted product contains particulate or is discolored
- Withdraw 1 mL of reconstituted solution into a syringe; attach the sterile needle and inject IM
- A 25-G 1-inch needle for IM may be substituted for the 23-G $1^1/_4$-inch needle provided
- **Storage:** Use within 6 hr of reconstitution; store reconstituted solution in refrigerator; *do not freeze;* discard any unused solution; both drug and diluent vials are single-use only

Administration of Avonex prefilled syringe

- The first injection should be performed under the supervision of an appropriately qualified person
- If self-injecting, rotate injection site between thighs
- Wash hands before handling the Dose Pack
- Remove prefilled syringe from the refrigerator to warm to room temperature (usually 30 min before use); do not use external heat sources such as hot water to warm the syringe
- Attach the needle by pressing it onto the syringe and turning it clockwise until it locks in place; be careful not to push the plunger while attaching the needle
- Use the alcohol wipe to clean the skin at the injection site you choose; then, pull the protective cover straight off the needle; do not twist the cover off
- Inject intramuscularly at a 90-degree angle into the thigh or upper arm as directed by the provider
- Dispose of used needles and syringes in a puncture-resistant container and discard appropriately
- Refer to the Patient Medication Guide for detailed instructions for preparing and giving a dose
- **Storage:** Store refrigerated; if refrigeration is unavailable, may store at 77° F or less for up to 7 days; after removing from refrigerator, do not store product above 25° C

Administration of Avonex prefilled auto-injector

- The first injection should be performed under the supervision of provider
- Remove one Administration Dose Pack from the refrigerator to warm to room temperature (about 30 min before use); do not use external heat sources such as hot water to warm the syringe Dose Pack
- Wash hands before handling Dose Pack contents
- Grasp the cap and bend it at a 90-degree angle until it snaps off; pull off the sterile foil from the needle cover
- Hold the Avonex Pen with the glass syringe tip pointing up; press the needle onto the glass syringe tip; gently turn the needle clockwise until firmly attached; do not remove plastic cover from the needle
- Hold Pen with one hand and, using other hand, hold on to the injector shield (grooved area) tightly and quickly pull up on the injector shield until the injector shield covers the needle all the way; the plastic needle cover will pop off after the injector shield has been fully extended
- When the injector shield is extended the right way, there will be a small blue rectangular area next to the oval medication display window; check the display window and make sure the Avonex is clear and colorless
- Do not use the injection if the liquid is colored, cloudy, or has lumps or particles; air bubbles will not affect the dose
- Avonex Pen should be injected into the upper outer thigh
- Hold Pen at 90-degree angle to the injection site; firmly push the body of the pen down against the thigh to release the

safety lock; safety lock is released when blue rectangle area above the oval medication display window is gone, push down on blue activation button with thumb and count to 10, you will hear a click if the injection is given the right way

• The circular display window on the Pen is yellow if the full dose is received

• Dispose of used needles and syringes in a puncture-resistant container and discard appropriately

• Refer to the Patient Medication Guide for detailed instructions for preparing and giving a dose

• **Storage:** Store at 36°-46° F (2°-8° C); if refrigeration is unavailable, may store at 77° F or less for up to 7 days; after removing from refrigerator, do not store product above 25° C; do not expose to high temperatures; do not freeze; protect from light

Subcutaneous administration

• Give at the same time (preferably late in the afternoon or evening) on the same days of the week at least 48 hours apart

• Do not give on two consecutive days; if a dose is missed, administer the dose as soon as possible, then skip the following day; return to the regular schedule the following week

• Premedication with acetaminophen or ibuprofen can lessen the severity of flu-like symptoms

• Interferon-β1a (Rebif) 44 mcg is equivalent to 12 million IU

• Rotate injection sites

• A Starter Pack containing a lower dose of Rebif syringes is available for the initial titration period

Injection (Rebif)

• Interferon-β1a (Rebif) is available in a prefilled syringe with a 29-G needle

• Inject subcut into the outer surface of the upper arm, abdomen, thigh, or buttock, do not inject the area near the navel or waistline; take care not to inject intradermally

• Discard any unused solution; prefilled syringes do not contain preservatives and are single-use only

Interferon beta-1b
SUBCUT route

• The manufacturers of Betaseron and of Extavia offer materials to assist with training on subcut use, call 1-800-788-1467 (Betaseron), 1-888-669-6682 (Extavia)

• Premedication with acetaminophen or ibuprofen and use of product at bedtime can lessen the severity of flulike symptoms

• Visually inspect parenteral products for particulate matter and discoloration before use; do not use if particulate matter is present

Reconstitution

• Add 1.2 mL of 0.54% sodium chloride injection (supplied by the manufacturer) to the vial by using the vial adapter to attach the prefilled syringe that contains the diluent

• If not used immediately, store in the refrigerator for up to 3 hr; do not freeze; discard any unused portion after 3 hr

Injection

• Withdraw the desired amount of the reconstituted solution into the syringe

• Choose an injection site on the upper back arm, abdomen, buttock, or front thigh; do not inject within 2 inches of the navel or in a site where the skin is red, bruised, infected, broken, painful, uneven, or scabbed; rotate injection sites

• Inject subcut; take care not to inject intradermally

SIDE EFFECTS

CNS: *Headache, fever, pain, chills, mental changes, depression,* hypertonia, suicide attempts, seizures

CV: *Migraine, palpitations, hypertension,* tachycardia, peripheral vascular disorders

EENT: *Conjunctivitis,* blurred vision

GI: *Diarrhea, constipation, vomiting, abdominal pain*

GU: *Dysmenorrhea, irregular menses, metrorrhagia,* cystitis, breast pain

HEMA: Decreased lymphocytes, ANC, WBC, *lymphadenopathy,* anemia

INTEG: *Sweating, inj-site reaction*

MS: *Myalgia,* myasthenia
RESP: *Sinusitis,* dyspnea

PHARMACOKINETICS

β-1a: Onset ≤12 hr, peak 16 hr, duration 4 days, half-life 8.6 hr
β-1b: Onset rapid, peak 2-8 hr, duration unknown, half-life 8 min-4.3 hr

INTERACTIONS

Increase: hepatic damage—antiretrovirals (NNRTIs, NRTIs, protease inhibitors)
Increase: myelosuppression—antineoplastics
Decrease: clearance of zidovudine
Drug/Herb
• Change in immunomodulation: astragalus, echinacea, melatonin
Drug/Lab Test
Interference: vaccines, toxoids; avoid concurrent use
Increase: LFTs

NURSING CONSIDERATIONS
Assess:
• Blood, hepatic studies: CBC, differential, platelet counts, BUN, creatinine, ALT, urinalysis; if absolute neutrophil count <750/mm^3 or if AST/ALT is 10× normal, discontinue product
• CNS symptoms: headache, fatigue, depression
• GI status: diarrhea or constipation, vomiting, abdominal pain
• Cardiac status: increased B/P, tachycardia
• Mental status: depression, depersonalization, suicidal thoughts, insomnia
• Lupus-like symptoms
• Multiple sclerosis symptoms
Evaluate:
• Therapeutic response: decreased symptoms of multiple sclerosis
Teach patient/family:
• With written, detailed information about product
• That blurred vision, hearing loss, sweating may occur
• That female patients may experience irregular menses, dysmenorrhea or metrorrhagia, breast pain

• To use sunscreen to prevent photosensitivity
• About injection technique, care of equipment
• To notify prescriber of increased temperature, chills, muscle soreness, fatigue, depression, symptoms of hepatotoxicity
• To notify prescriber if pregnancy is suspected

RARELY USED

interferon gamma-1b (Rx)
(in-ter-feer´on)
Actimmune
Func. class.: Biologic response modifier
Chem. class.: Lymphokine, interleukin type

USES: Serious infections associated with chronic granulomatous disease, osteopetrosis

CONTRAINDICATIONS: Hypersensitivity to interferon-γ, *Escherichia coli*–derived products
Precautions: Pregnancy, breastfeeding, children <1 yr, cardiac disease, seizure disorders, CNS disorders, myelosuppression

DOSAGE AND ROUTES
• **Adult:** SUBCUT 50 mcg/m^2 (1.5 million units/m^2) for patients with surface area >0.5 m^2; 1.5 mcg/kg/dose for patients with surface area <0.5 m^2; give Monday, Wednesday, Friday for 3×/wk dosing

---

⚠ HIGH ALERT

ipilimumab
(ip-i-lim´ue-mab)
Yervoy
Func. class.: Antineoplastic; biologic response modifier

ACTION: A recombinant, human monoclonal antibody that binds to the cytotoxic T-lymphocyte–associated antigen 4 (CTLA-4); action is indirect, possibly through T-cell–mediated antitumor immune responses

USES: Treatment of unresectable or metastatic malignant melanoma

CONTRAINDICATIONS:
Hypersensitivity

Precautions: Pregnancy, breastfeeding, Crohn's disease, hepatitis, immunosuppression, inflammatory bowel disease, iritis, ocular disease, organ transplant, pancreatitis, renal disease, rheumatoid arthritis, sarcoidosis, systemic lupus erythematosus, thyroid disease, ulcerative colitis, uveitis

Black Box Warning: Adrenal insufficiency, diarrhea, Guillain-Barré syndrome, hepatic disease, myasthenia gravis, hypo/hyperthyroidism, hypopituitarism, peripheral neuropathy, serious rash, hypophysitis

DOSAGE AND ROUTES
Unresectable metastatic melanoma
• **Adult/geriatric: IV** 3 mg/kg over 90 min q3wk × 4 doses
Adjuvant treatment of cutaneous melanoma
• **Adult/Child ≥12 yr: IV** 10 mg/kg over 90 min q3wk × 4 doses, followed by 10 mg/kg q12wk until disease recurrence or unacceptable toxicity, for up to 3 yr
Available forms: Sol for inj 50 mg/10 mL, 200 mg/40 mL
Administer:
Intermittent IV INFUSION route
• Visually inspect parenteral products for particulate matter and discoloration before using; sol may have a pale yellow color and have translucent to white, amorphous particles; discard the vial if sol is cloudy, if there is pronounced discoloration, or if particulate matter is present
• Allow to stand at room temperature for 5 min before infusion preparation; withdraw the required volume and transfer into an IV bag; discard partially used vials or empty vials; dilute with 0.9%

sodium chloride injection or 5% dextrose injection to a final concentration (1-2 mg/mL); mix diluted sol by gentle inversion; do not admix
• Give infusion over 90 min through an IV line with a low-protein binding in-line filter, do not give with other products; after each infusion, flush the line with 0.9% sodium chloride injection or 0.5% dextrose injection
• Store once diluted for no more than 24 hr refrigerated or at room temperature

SIDE EFFECTS
CNS: Severe and fatal immune-mediated neuropathies, fatigue, headache, fever
EENT: Uveitis, iritis, episcleritis
ENDO: Severe and fatal immune-mediated endocrinopathies
GI: Severe and fatal immune-mediated enterocolitis, hepatitis, pancreatitis, abdominal pain, nausea, diarrhea, appetite decreased, vomiting, constipation, colitis
INTEG: Severe and fatal immune-mediated dermatitis, pruritus, rash, urticaria
MISC: Cough, dyspnea, anemia, eosinophilia, nephritis
SYST: Antibody formation, Stevens-Johnson syndrome, toxic epidermal necrolysis

PHARMACOKINETICS: Steady-state by 3rd dose; terminal half-life 15.4 days

NURSING CONSIDERATIONS
Assess:
• **Serious skin disorders: Stevens-Johnson syndrome, toxic epidermal necrolysis:** permanently discontinue in these or rash complicated by full-thickness dermal ulceration or necrotic, bullous, or hemorrhagic manifestations like bullous rash; give systemic corticosteroids at a dose of 1-2 mg/kg/day of predniSONE or equivalent; when dermatitis is controlled, taper corticosteroids over a period of at least 1 mo, withhold in patients with moderate to severe reactions; for mild to moderate dermatitis (localized rash

and pruritus), give topical or systemic corticosteroids

Black Box Warning: Immune-mediated reactions: before starting treatment, assess for enterocolitis, hepatitis, dermatitis, neuropathy, endocrinopathy; take LFTs, ACTH, and thyroid function tests; permanently discontinue if these conditions occur

• **Hepatotoxicity:** LFTs baseline and before each dose to rule out infectious or malignant causes; increase the frequency of liver function test monitoring until resolution; permanently discontinue in patients with grade 3-5 toxicity; give systemic corticosteroids at a dose of 1-2 mg/kg/day of predniSONE or equivalent

• **Neuropathy:** monitor for motor or sensory neuropathy (unilateral or bilateral weakness, sensory alterations, or paresthesias) before each dose; permanently discontinue if severe neuropathy (interfering with daily activities), such as Guillain-Barré–like syndromes, occurs

• **Endocrinopathy:** monitor thyroid function tests at baseline and before each dose; monitor hypophysitis, adrenal insufficiency, adrenal crisis, hypo/hyperthyroidism (fatigue, headache, mental status changes, abdominal pain, unusual bowel habits, hypotension, or nonspecific symptoms that may resemble other causes)

• **Vision changes:** uveitis, iritis, episcleritis; corticosteroids may be used

Black Box Warning: Pregnancy/breastfeeding: do not use in pregnancy, breastfeeding

Evaluate:
• Decreasing spread or recurrence of malignant melanoma
Teach patient/family:
• To immediately report allergic reactions, skin rash, severe abdominal pain, yellowing of skin or eyes, tingling of extremities, change in bowel habits

• About the reason for treatment and expected results; to read medication guide provided
• **Pregnancy/breastfeeding:** to notify prescriber if pregnancy is planned or suspected or if breastfeeding; to use contraception during and for 3 mo after final dose

ipratropium (Rx)
(i-pra-troe′pee-um)
Atrovent ✦, Atrovent HFA, Atrovent Nasal Spray
Func. class.: Anticholinergic, bronchodilator
Chem. class.: Synthetic quaternary ammonium compound

ACTION: Inhibits interaction of acetylcholine at receptor sites on the bronchial smooth muscle, thereby resulting in decreased cGMP and bronchodilation

USES: Bronchospasm, COPD; rhinorrhea (nasal spray)

CONTRAINDICATIONS: Hypersensitivity to this product, atropine, bromide, soybean or peanut products
Precautions: Breastfeeding, children <12 yr, angioedema, heart failure, surgery, acute bronchospasm, bladder obstruction, closed-angle glaucoma, prostatic hypertrophy, urinary retention, pregnancy

DOSAGE AND ROUTES
Bronchospasm in chronic bronchitis/emphysema
• **Adult:** INH 2 sprays (17 mcg/spray) 3-4×/day, max 12 **INH**/24 hr; **SOL** 500 mcg (1 unit dose) given 3-4×/day by nebulizer; nasal spray: 2 sprays (42 mcg/spray) 3-4×/day
• **Child 5-11 yr:** INH 4-8 inhalations q20min as needed for ≤3 hr (asthma, unlabeled); **NEB** 250-500 mcg q20min as needed for ≤3 hr (asthma, unlabeled)
Rhinorrhea perennial rhinitis
• **Adult/child ≥6 yr:** INTRANASAL 2 sprays (43 mcg)/nostril bid or tid

- **Child 5-12 yr: INTRANASAL** 2 sprays (0.03%) in each nostril 3×/day

Available forms: Aerosol 17 mcg/actuation; nasal spray 0.03%, 0.06%; sol for inh 0.0125% ❦, 0.02%

Administer:
- Store at room temperature

Nebulizer route
- Use sol in nebulizer with a mouthpiece rather than a face mask

Intranasal route
- Priming pump initially requires 7 actuations of pump; priming again is not necessary if used regularly, tilt head backward after dose

SIDE EFFECTS

CNS: *Anxiety, dizziness, headache,* nervousness
CV: Palpitation
EENT: Dry mouth, blurred vision, nasal congestion
GI: *Nausea, vomiting, cramps*
INTEG: Rash
RESP: *Cough, worsening of symptoms,* bronchospasms

PHARMACOKINETICS
Half-life 2 hr, does not cross blood-brain barrier

INTERACTIONS
Increase: toxicity—other bronchodilators (INH)
Increase: anticholinergic action—phenothiazines, antihistamines, disopyramide
Drug/Herb
Increase: anticholinergic effect—belladonna
Increase: bronchodilator effect—green tea (large amts), guarana

NURSING CONSIDERATIONS
Assess:
- **Palpitations:** if severe, product may have to be changed
- Tolerance over long-term therapy; dose may have to be increased or changed
- **Atropine sensitivity:** patient may also be sensitive to this product

- **Respiratory status:** rate, rhythm, auscultate breath sounds before and after administration, vital capacity, FEV, ABGs/VBGs, heart rate, rhythm
- Hard candy, frequent drinks, sugarless gum to relieve dry mouth
- **Pregnancy/breastfeeding:** use only if benefit outweighs fetal risk; use caution in breastfeeding, excretion unknown

Evaluate:
- Therapeutic response: ability to breathe adequately

Teach patient/family:
- That compliance is necessary with number of inhalations/24 hr or overdose may occur; about spacer device for geriatric patients; that max therapeutic effects may take 2-3 mo
- How to use equipment properly and take medication as directed; to take missed doses as soon as remembered unless almost time for the next dose; to space remaining doses evenly during the day; not to double doses
- That rinsing mouth after use of the inhaler, good oral hygiene, and sugarless gum or candy may minimize dry mouth; to notify health care professional if stomatitis occurs or if dry mouth persists for more than 2 wk
- **Inhalation:** not to exceed 12 doses within 24 hr; to notify heath care professional if symptoms do not improve within 30 min after administration of medication or if condition worsens
- About the need for pulmonary function tests baseline and periodically during therapy to determine effectiveness
- To avoid spraying in eyes; may cause irritation
- To inform prescriber if cough, nervousness, headache, dizziness, nausea occurs
- **Nasal spray:** instruct patient in proper use of nasal spray. Clear nasal passages before use. Do not inhale during administration. Prime pump initially with 7 actuations. If used regularly, no further priming is needed. If not used in 24 hr, prime with 2 actuations. If not used for >7 days, prime with 7 actuations

---

• To contact prescriber if symptoms do not improve within 1-2 wk or if condition worsens

---

irbesartan (Rx)

(er-be-sartan)

Avapro

Func. class.: Antihypertensive
Chem. class.: Angiotensin II receptor blocker (Type AT$_1$)

Do not confuse:
Avapro/Anaprox

ACTION: Blocks the vasoconstrictor and aldosterone-secreting effects of angiotensin II; selectively blocks the binding of angiotensin II to the AT$_1$ receptor found in tissues

USES: Hypertension, alone or in combination; nephropathy in type 2 diabetic patients; proteinuria
Unlabeled uses: Heart failure

CONTRAINDICATIONS:
Hypersensitivity

Black Box Warning: Pregnancy

Precautions: Pregnancy 1st trimester, breastfeeding, children <6 yr, geriatric patients, hypersensitivity to ACE inhibitors; hepatic/renal disease; renal artery stenosis, ✹ African descent, angioedema

DOSAGES AND ROUTES
Hypertension
• **Adult: PO** 150 mg/day; may be increased to 300 mg/day, volume-depleted patients: start with 75 mg/day
Nephropathy in type 2 diabetic patients
• **Adult: PO** maintenance dose 300 mg/day, start 75 mg/day
Available forms: Tabs 75, 150, 300 mg
Administer:
• Without regard to meals
• May be used with other antihypertensives, diuretic

• Volume depletion should be corrected before use

SIDE EFFECTS
CNS: *Dizziness,* anxiety, *headache, fatigue,* syncope
CV: Hypotension
GI: *Diarrhea, dyspepsia,* hepatitis, cholestasis
HEMA: Thrombocytopenia
MISC: Edema, chest pain, rash, tachycardia, UTI, angioedema, hyperkalemia
RESP: *Cough, upper respiratory tract infection,* sinus disorder, pharyngitis, rhinitis

PHARMACOKINETICS
Peak 1.5-2 hr, extensively metabolized by CYP2C9, half-life 11-15 hr, highly bound to plasma proteins, excreted in urine and feces, protein binding 90%

INTERACTIONS
Increase: hyperkalemia—potassium-sparing diuretics, potassium salt substitutes, ACE inhibitors
Increase: irbesartan level—CYP2C9 inhibitors (amiodarone, delavirdine, fluconazole, FLUoxetine, fluvastatin, fluvoxaMINE, imatinib, sulfonamides, sulfinpyrazone, voriconazole, zafirlukast)
Decrease: antihypertensive effect—NSAIDs
Drug/Herb
Increase: antihypertensive effect—black cohosh, garlic, goldenseal, hawthorn, kelp
Increase or decrease: antihypertensive effect—astragalus, cola tree
Decrease: antihypertensive effect—guarana, khat, licorice, yohimbe

NURSING CONSIDERATIONS
Assess:
• **Hypotension:** for severe hypotension, place in supine position and give IV infusion of NS, drug may be continued after B/P is restored
• B/P, pulse q4hr; note rate, rhythm, quality
• Baselines of renal/hepatic studies before therapy begins; periodically monitor LFTs, total/direct bilirubin

---

• Skin turgor, dryness of mucous membranes for hydration status; edema in feet, legs daily

Evaluate:

• Therapeutic response: decreased B/P

Teach patient/family:

• To comply with dosage schedule, even if feeling better; that max therapeutic effects may take 2-3 mo, to take without regard to food

• That product may cause dizziness, fainting, light-headedness

• To rise slowly to sitting or standing position to minimize orthostatic hypotension

• Not to stop product abruptly

Black Box Warning: To notify prescriber if pregnancy is suspected; discontinue if pregnant

---

⚠ **HIGH ALERT**

irinotecan (Rx)

(ear-een-oh-tee′kan)

Camptosar

Func. class.: Antineoplastic

Chem. class.: Camptothecin analog

ACTION: Cytotoxic by producing damage to single-strand DNA during DNA synthesis; binds to topoisomerase I

USES: Metastatic carcinoma of the colon or rectum or 1st-line treatment in combination with 5-FU and leucovorin for metastatic colon or rectal carcinomas

Unlabeled uses: Cervical, gastric, lung, ovarian, pancreatic cancer, malignant glioma, rhabdomyosarcoma

CONTRAINDICATIONS: Pregnancy, hypersensitivity

Precautions: Breastfeeding, children, geriatric patients, irradiation, hepatic disease

Black Box Warning: Myelosuppression, diarrhea

DOSAGE AND ROUTES

Colorectal cancer in combination with 5-fluorouracil (5-FU):

Intravenous dosage (with bolus 5-FU/leucovorin)

• **Adult:** IV 125 mg/m^2 over 90 min followed by leucovorin 20 mg/m^2 IV bolus and then 5-FU 500 mg/m^2 IV bolus on days 1, 8, 15, and 22; the next course begins on day 43 or when toxicity has recovered to NCI grade 1 or less

IV dosage (with infusional 5-FU/leucovorin)

• **Adult:** IV 180 mg/m^2 over 90 min followed by leucovorin 200 mg/m^2 IV over 2 hr, then 5-FU bolus and continuous infusion 400 mg/m^2 IV bolus, then 600 mg/m^2 IV infusion over 22 hr on days 1, 15, and leucovorin and 5-FU are given on days 1, 2, 15, 16, 29, and 30; the next course begins on day 43 or when toxicity has recovered to NCI grade 1 or less

Available forms: Inj 20 mg/mL

Administer:

• Use cytotoxic handling precautions

IV route

• Premedicate with antiemetic dexamethasone plus another antiemetic agent, such as a 5-HT$_3$ blocker, given at least 30 min before use

• Before beginning a course of therapy, the granulocyte count should be ≥1500, the platelet count should be ≥100,000, and treatment-related diarrhea should be fully resolved

Dilution

• Dilute appropriate dose in D$_5$W (preferred) or NS injection to a final concentration of 0.12-2.8 mg/mL

• Store up to 24 hr at room temperature and room lighting; however, because of possible microbial contamination during preparation, an admixture prepared with D$_5$W or NS should be used within 6 hr, solutions prepared with D$_5$W, refrigerated, protected from light must be used within 48 hr; avoid refrigeration if prepared with NS

Intravenous infusion

• Infuse over 90 min

Side effects: *italics* = common; red = life-threatening

Y-site compatibilities: Alemtuzumab, alfentanil, amifostine, amikacin, aminocaproic acid, aminophylline, amiodarone, ampicillin, ampicillin-sulbactam, anidulafungin, argatroban, atenolol, atracurium, azithromycin, aztreonam, bivalirudin, bleomycin, bretylium, bumetanide, buprenorphine, butorphanol, calcium chloride/gluconate, capreomycin, CARBOplatin, caspofungin, ceFAZolin, cefotetan, cefOXitin, cefTAZidime, cefTAZidime (L-arginine), ceftizoxime, cefuroxime, cimetidine, ciprofloxacin, cisatracurium, CISplatin, clindamycin, cyclophosphamide, cycloSPORINE, cytarabine, dacarbazine, DAPTOmycin, DAUNOrubicin liposome, DAUNOrubicin, dexamethasone, dexrazoxane, digoxin, diltiaZEM, diphenhydrAMINE, DOBUTamine, DOCEtaxel, dolasetron, DOPamine, doxacurium, DOXOrubicin, DOXOrubicin liposomal, doxycycline, enalaprilat, ePHEDrine, EPINEPHrine, ertapenem, erythromycin, esmolol, etoposide, etoposide phosphate, famotidine, fenoldopam, fentaNYL, fluconazole, foscarnet, gallium, garenoxacin, gatifloxacin, gemtuzumab, gentamicin, granisetron, haloperidol, heparin, hydrALAZINE, hydrocortisone, HYDROmorphone, hydrOXYzine, IDArubicin, imipenem-cilastatin, inamrinone, insulin, regular, isoproterenol, ketorolac, labetalol, lepirudin, leucovorin, levoFLOXacin, LEVOleucovorin, levorphanol, lidocaine, linezolid, LORazepam, magnesium sulfate, mannitol, meperidine, meropenem, mesna, metaraminol, methadone, methyldopate, metoclopramide, metoprolol, metroNIDAZOLE, midazolam, milrinone, minocycline, mitoXANTRONE, mivacurium, morphine, moxifloxacin, nalbuphine, naloxone, nesiritide, niCARdipine, nitroglycerin, norepinephrine, octreotide, ondansetron, oxaliplatin, PACLitaxel (solvent/surfactant), palonosetron, pancuronium, pantoprazole, pentamidine, pentazocine, PHENobarbital, phentolamine, phenylephrine, polymyxin B, potassium acetate, chloride/phosphates, procainamide, prochlorperazine, promethazine, propranolol, quiNIDine, quinupristin-dalfopristin, raNITIdine, remifentanil, riTUXimab, rocuronium, sodium acetate, bicarbonate/phosphates, succinylcholine, SUFentanil, sulfamethoxazole-trimethoprim, tacrolimus, teniposide, theophylline, thiotepa, ticarcillin, ticarcillin-clavulanate, tigecycline, tirofiban, tobramycin, tolazoline, trimethobenzamide, vancomycin, vasopressin, vecuronium, verapamil, vinBLAStine, vinorelbine, voriconazole, zidovudine, zoledronic acid

SIDE EFFECTS

CNS: Fever, headache, chills, dizziness
CV: Vasodilation, edema, thromboembolism
GI: Severe diarrhea, *nausea, vomiting*, anorexia, constipation, cramps, flatus, stomatitis, dyspepsia, hepatotoxicity
HEMA: Leukopenia, anemia, neutropenia
INTEG: Irritation at site, rash, sweating, alopecia
MISC: Edema, asthenia, weight loss, back pain
RESP: Dyspnea, increased cough, rhinitis

PHARMACOKINETICS

Rapidly and completely absorbed, excreted in urine and bile as metabolites, half-life 6-12 hr, bound to plasma proteins 30%-68%, increased risk for toxicity in patients homozygous for UGT1A1 28

INTERACTIONS

Increase: toxicity—fluorouracil
Increase: bleeding risk—NSAIDs, anticoagulants
Increase: irinotecan levels—some CYP3A4 inhibitors (ketoconazole)
Increase: myelosuppression, diarrhea—other antineoplastics, radiation
Increase: lymphocytopenia, hyperglycemia—dexamethasone
Increase: akathisia—prochlorperazine
Increase: dehydration—diuretics
Decrease: irinotecan levels—CYP3A4 inducers (phenytoin, carBAMazepine, PHENobarbital)
Drug/Herb
Decrease: product level—St. John's wort; avoid concurrent use

Drug/Lab Test

Increase: alk phos, LFTs, bilirubin
Decrease: platelets, WBC, neutrophils, Hgb/HcT

NURSING CONSIDERATIONS
Assess:

• CNS symptoms: fever, headache, chills, dizziness

Black Box Warning: **Myelosuppression:** CBC, differential, platelet count weekly; use colony-stimulating factor if WBC <2000/mm^3 or platelet count <100,000/mm^3, Hgb ≤9 g/dL, neutrophil ≤1000/mm^3; notify prescriber of results; product should be discontinued

• Buccal cavity for dryness, sores or ulceration, white patches, oral pain, bleeding, dysphagia

Black Box Warning: **GI symptoms:** frequency of stools; cramping; severe, life-threatening diarrhea may occur with fluid and electrolyte imbalances, treat diarrhea within 24 hr of use with 0.25-1 mg atropine IV; treat diarrhea >24 hr of use with loperamide, diarrhea >24 hr (late diarrhea) can be fatal

• **Signs of dehydration:** rapid respirations, poor skin turgor, decreased urine output, dry skin, restlessness, weakness
• **Bone marrow depression:** bruising, bleeding, blood in stools, urine, sputum, emesis
• Increased fluid intake to 2-3 L/day to prevent dehydration unless contraindicated
Evaluate:
• Therapeutic response: decrease in tumor size, spread of cancer
Teach patient/family:
• To avoid foods with citric acid, hot temperature, or rough texture if stomatitis is present; to drink adequate fluids
• To report stomatitis; any bleeding, white spots, ulcerations in mouth; to examine mouth daily, report symptoms
• To report signs of anemia: fatigue, headache, faintness, SOB, irritability, infection, rash

• To use contraception during therapy
• To avoid salicylates, NSAIDs, alcohol because bleeding may occur; to avoid all products unless approved by prescriber
• About alopecia; that when hair grows back, it may be different in texture, thickness
• To avoid vaccinations while taking this product

Black Box Warning: To report diarrhea that occurs 24 hr after administration; severe dehydration can occur rapidly, may be fatal

• To report immediately injection site pain, irritation
• To report vomiting, dizziness
• That regular lab exams will be needed
• To report if pregnancy is planned or suspected; to use contraception during therapy

---

iron dextran (Rx)

DexFerrum, Dexiren ✦, Infufer ✦, INFeD
Func. class.: Hematinic
Chem. class.: Ferric hydroxide complex with dextran

ACTION: Iron is carried by transferrin to the bone marrow, where it is incorporated into hemoglobin

USES: Iron-deficiency anemia

CONTRAINDICATIONS:

Black Box Warning: Hypersensitivity

Precautions: Pregnancy, breastfeeding, neonates, infants <4 mo, children, acute renal disease, asthma, rheumatoid arthritis (IV), ankylosing spondylitis, lupus, hypotension, all anemias excluding iron-deficiency anemia, hepatic/cardiac/renal disease

---

Side effects: *italics* = common; red = life-threatening

DOSAGE AND ROUTES

• **Adult/child: IM** 0.5 mL as a test dose by Z-track, then no more than the following total dose including test dose per day:

• **Adult/adolescent/child (>15 kg):** Total iron dextran dose in mL = [0.0442 × (Desired Hb − observed Hb) × LBW] + (0.26 × LBW), max of undiluted is 100 mg (2 mL)/day

• **Child (10-15 kg):** Total iron dextran dose in mL = [0.0442 × (Desired Hb − observed Hb) × LBW] + (0.26 × ABW), max of undiluted iron dextran is 100 mg (2 mL)/day

• **Child/Infant >4 mo (5-9.9 kg):** Total iron dextran dose in mL = [0.0442 × (Desired Hb − observed Hb) × LBW] + (0.26 × ABW)

• **Infants >4 mo (<5 kg):** Total iron dextran dose in mL = [0.0442 × (Desired Hb − observed Hb) × LBW] + (0.26 × ABW)

Administer:

• D/C oral iron before parenteral; give only after test dose of 25 mg by preferred route; wait at least 1 hr before giving remaining portion

• Store at room temperature in cool environment

• Recumbent position 30 min after IV inj to prevent orthostatic hypotension

IM route

• IM deeply in large muscle mass; use Z-track method, 19- to 20-G 2- to 3-in needle; ensure needle long enough to place product deep in muscle; change needles after withdrawing product and before injecting to prevent skin, tissue staining

• Only with EPINEPHrine available in case of anaphylactic reaction during dose

IV route

• IV after flushing with 10 mL 0.9% NaCl; give undiluted; may be diluted in 50-250 mL NS for infusion; give ≤1 mL (50 mg) over ≥1 min; flush line after use with 10 mL 0.9% NaCl; patient should remain recumbent for $^1/_2$-1 hr

• IV inj requires single-dose vial without preservative; verify on label that IV use approved

SIDE EFFECTS

CNS: Headache, paresthesia, dizziness, shivering, weakness, seizures

CV: Chest pain, shock, hypotension, tachycardia

GI: *Nausea*, vomiting, metallic taste, abdominal pain

HEMA: Leukocytosis

INTEG: Rash, pruritus, urticaria, fever, sweating, chills, brown skin discoloration, pain at inj site, necrosis, sterile abscesses, phlebitis

OTHER: Anaphylaxis

RESP: Dyspnea

PHARMACOKINETICS

IM: Excreted in feces, urine, bile, breast milk; crosses placenta; most absorbed through lymphatics; can be gradually absorbed over weeks/months from fixed locations

INTERACTIONS

Increase: toxicity—oral iron; do not use
Decrease: reticulocyte response—chloramphenicol

Drug/Lab Test

False increase: serum bilirubin
False decrease: serum calcium
False positive: ^{99m}Tc diphosphate bone scan, iron test (large doses >2 mL)

NURSING CONSIDERATIONS

Assess:

• Observe for 1 hr after first dose to monitor for anaphylactic reactions

• Blood studies: Hct, Hgb, reticulocytes, transferrin, plasma iron concentrations, ferritin, total iron binding, bilirubin before treatment, at least monthly

Black Box Warning: Allergy: anaphylaxis, rash, pruritus, fever, chills, wheezing; notify prescriber immediately, keep emergency equipment available

• Cardiac status: anginal pain, hypotension, tachycardia

• Nutrition: amount of iron in diet (meat, dark green leafy vegetables, dried beans, dried fruits, eggs)

• Cause of iron loss or anemia, including use of salicylates, sulfonamides

- **Toxicity:** nausea, vomiting, diarrhea, fever, abdominal pain (early symptoms), cyanotic-looking lips, nailbeds, seizures, CV collapse (late symptoms)
- **Pregnancy/breastfeeding:** use only if benefit outweighs fetal risk; use caution in breastfeeding, trace amounts appear in breast milk

Evaluate:
- Therapeutic response: increased serum iron level, increased Hgb, Hct

Teach patient/family:
- That iron poisoning may occur if increased beyond recommended level; not to take oral iron preparation or vitamins containing iron
- That delayed reaction may occur 1-2 days after administration and last 3-4 days (IV), 3-7 days (IM); to report fever, chills, malaise, muscle, joint aches, nausea, vomiting, backache
- To avoid breastfeeding
- That stools may become dark

TREATMENT OF OVERDOSE:
Discontinue product, treat allergic reaction, give diphenhydrAMINE or EPINEPHrine as needed, give iron-chelating product for acute poisoning

---

iron sucrose (Rx)

Venofer
Func. class.: Hematinic
Chem. class.: Ferric hydroxide complex with dextran

ACTION: Iron is carried by transferrin to the bone marrow, where it is incorporated into hemoglobin

USES: Iron-deficiency anemia, hyperphosphatemia in chronic kidney disease on dialysis

Unlabeled uses: Dystrophic epidermolysis bullosa (DEB)

CONTRAINDICATIONS: Hypersensitivity, all anemias excluding iron-deficiency anemia, iron overload
Precautions: Pregnancy, breastfeeding, children, geriatric patients, abdominal pain,

anaphylactic shock, arthralgia, chest pain, cough, diarrhea, dizziness, dyspnea, edema, increased LFTs, fever, headache, heart failure, hypo/hypertension, infection, MS pain, nausea/vomiting, seizures, weakness

DOSAGE AND ROUTES
- **Adult:** IV 5 mL (100 mg of elemental iron) given during dialysis; most will need 1000 mg of elemental iron over 10 sequential dialysis sessions
- **Child ≥2 yr/adolescents:** IV 0.5 mg/kg by slow IV inj over 5 min (undiluted) or diluted in 25 mL of 0.9% NaCl, give over 5-60 min, max 100 mg every 2 wk × 12 wk

Hyperphosphatemia in chronic kidney disease
- **Adult:** PO 500 mg tid

Available forms: Inj 20 mg/mL; chew tab 500 mg
Administer:
- Only with EPINEPHrine, SOLU-Medrol available in case of anaphylactic reaction during dose

IV route
- Do not use if particulate is present or if discolored
- Give directly in dialysis line by slow inj or infusion; give by slow inj at 1 mL/min (5 min/vial); for infusion, dilute each vial exclusively in ≤100 mL 0.9% NaCl, give at 100 mg of iron/15 min; discard unused portions
- Do not use with IV products
- Store at room temperature in cool environment; do not freeze

SIDE EFFECTS
CNS: Headache, dizziness
CV: Chest pain, hypo/hypertension, hypervolemia, heart failure
GI: *Nausea, vomiting, abdominal pain*
INTEG: Rash, pruritus, urticaria, fever, sweating, chills
OTHER: Anaphylaxis, hyperglycemia
RESP: Dyspnea, pneumonia, cough

PHARMACOKINETICS
Excreted in urine, half-life 6 hr

INTERACTIONS
Increase: toxicity—oral iron, dimercaprol; do not use

Side effects: *italics* = common; red = life-threatening

Decrease: iron sucrose effect—chloramphenicol

Drug/Lab Test

Increase: glucose

NURSING CONSIDERATIONS

Assess:

• Blood studies: Hct, Hgb, reticulocytes, transferrin, plasma iron concentrations, ferritin, total iron binding; bilirubin before treatment, at least monthly

• **Allergy, anaphylaxis:** rash, pruritus, fever, chills, wheezing; notify prescriber immediately, keep emergency equipment available

• Cardiac status: hypo/hypertension, hypervolemia

• **Toxicity:** nausea, vomiting, diarrhea, fever, abdominal pain (early symptoms), cyanotic-looking lips, nailbeds, seizures, CV collapse (late symptoms)

• **Pregnancy/breastfeeding:** use only if clearly needed; cautious use in breastfeeding

Evaluate:

• Therapeutic response: increased serum iron levels, Hct, Hgb

Teach patient/family:

• To report itching, rash, chest pain, headache, vertigo, nausea, vomiting, abdominal pain, joint/muscle pain, numbness, tingling

• That iron poisoning may occur if dosage is increased beyond recommended level; not to take oral iron preparation

TREATMENT OF OVERDOSE:

Discontinue product, treat allergic reaction, give diphenhydrAMINE or EPINEPHrine as needed, give iron-chelating product for acute poisoning

---

isavuconazonium (Rx)

(eye-sa-vue-koe-na-zoe′nee-um)

Cresemba

Func. class.: Antifungal, systemic

Chem. class.: Azole

ACTION: Exerts antifungal activity by inhibiting the synthesis of ergosterol, an essential component of the fungal cell membrane. The depletion of ergosterol within the fungal cell membrane results in increased cellular permeability, causing leakage of cellular content

USES: *Aspergillus flavus, Aspergillus fumigatus, Aspergillus niger, Rhizopus oryzae, Mucormycetes* species; do NOT use for infections of *Candida, Blastomyces, Histoplasma*

CONTRAINDICATIONS: Hypersensitivity, short QT syndrome

Precautions: Azole hypersensitivity, pregnancy, breastfeeding, infusion-related reactions, hepatic disease

DOSAGE AND ROUTES

• **Adult: PO** loading dose of 2 caps (372 mg) q8hr × 6 doses. Then, 2 caps (372 mg) daily. Start maintenance dosing 12-24 hr after the last loading dose; treatment may last 6-12 wk up to 6 mo. **IV** loading dose of 372 mg q8hr × 6 doses, then 372 mg/day, beginning 12-24 hr after the last loading dose; use a 0.2- to 1.2-micron in-line filter and administer over a minimum of 1 hr; an additional loading dose is not needed when switching to PO

Administer:

PO route

• Swallow whole; do not chew, crush, dissolve, open the capsules; may be used without regard to food

IV route

• Visually inspect for particulate matter and discoloration; diluted solution may contain translucent to white particulates that will be removed by the in-line filter

Reconstitution

• Reconstitute the dry powder with 5 mL sterile water for injection, gently shake until dissolved

• Storage: the reconstituted solution may be stored below 77° F (25° C) for a maximum of 1 hr before further dilution

Dilution

• Remove 5 mL of the reconstituted solution and add it to 250 mL of either 0.9% NaCl or D₅W (1.5 mg/mL)

• Gently mix the solution or roll the bag. DO NOT shake. Do not place in a pneumatic transport system

- Apply an in-line filter (0.2-1.2 microns), adhere an in-line filter reminder sticker to the infusion bag
- Give within ≤6 hr of dilution
- Storage: may be stored immediately after dilution at 36° to 46° F (2° to 8° C); administration MUST be completed within 24 hr of the time of dilution. Do NOT freeze
- Product only after C&S confirms organism, product needed to treat condition; make sure product is used in life-threatening infections
- Flush IV lines with 0.9% sodium chloride or 5% dextrose in water before and after administration of the infusion
- Must be administered through a 0.2- to 1.2-micron filter; give over ≥1 hr. Do not give by bolus
- Do not admix

Available forms: Caps 186 mg; powder for injection 382 mg

SIDE EFFECTS

CNS: *Headache*, paresthesias, peripheral neuropathy, *hallucinations*, depression, insomnia, dizziness, fever, vertigo, tremor, confusion

CV: Tachypnea, supraventricular tachycardia, atrial fibrillation/flutter

EENT: Tinnitus

GI: Nausea, vomiting, anorexia, diarrhea, cramps, hepatitis, stomatitis

GU: *Hypokalemia*, renal failure

HEMA: Anemia, eosinophilia, hypomagnesemia, thrombocytopenia, leukopenia

INTEG: *Burning, irritation*, pain, necrosis at inj site with extravasation, *rash*

MISC: Cough

PHARMACOKINETICS

Metabolized by CYP3A4, CYP3A5, UGT, P-gp, OCT2 enzymes; eliminated in urine/feces; peak 2 hr (PO), Chinese patients (levels 40% lower), protein binding >99%

INTERACTIONS

Increase: effects of benzodiazepines, calcium channel blockers, cycloSPORINE, ergots, HMG-CoA reductase inhibitors, pimozide, quiNIDine, predniSOLONE, sirolimus, sulfonylureas, tacrolimus, vinca alkaloids, warfarin, rifabutin, proton pump inhibitors, NNRTIs, protease inhibitors, phenytoin

Increase: isavuconazonium effect— CYP3A4 substrates

Decrease: isavuconazonium effect— CYP3A4 inhibitors

Decrease: bupropion effect—dose may need to be increased

Drug/Herb

- Do not use with St. John's wort

Drug/Lab Test

Increase: AST/ALT, alk phos, creatinine, bilirubin

Decrease: Hgb/Hct, platelets, WBC

NURSING CONSIDERATIONS

Assess:

- **Short QT syndrome:** do not use in this condition
- VS q15-30min during first infusion; note changes in pulse, B/P
- Blood studies: CBC, potassium, sodium, calcium, magnesium, q2wk; obtain culture and sensitivity before starting first dose; may start treatment before results are received
- **Hepatotoxicity:** increases in AST, ALT, alk phos, bilirubin, baseline and periodically
- **Allergic reaction:** dermatitis, rash; product should be discontinued, antihistamines (mild reaction) or epinephrine (severe reaction) administered
- **Hypokalemia:** anorexia, drowsiness, weakness, decreased reflexes, dizziness, increased urinary output, increased thirst, paresthesias
- **Ototoxicity:** tinnitus (ringing, roaring in ears), vertigo
- **Infusion-related reactions:** dizziness, chills, fever, hypotension, dyspnea; discontinue if these occur
- **Pregnancy/breastfeeding:** test for pregnancy before starting treatment; do not use in or breastfeed

Evaluate:

- Therapeutic response: resolution of fungal infection, negative C&S

Teach patient/family:

- That long-term therapy may be needed to clear infection (2 wk-3 mo, depending on type of infection); not to discontinue unless approved by prescriber

• To notify prescriber of bleeding, bruising, soft-tissue swelling, dark urine, persistent nausea or diarrhea, headache, rash, yellow skin/eyes

• That women of childbearing age should use effective contraceptive; not to breastfeed

• To notify provider of all OTC, Rx, herbal products or supplements taken and to avoid new products unless approved by prescriber

• That lab exams will be required

---

isoniazid (Rx)

(eye-soe-nye′a-zid)

Isotamine ✦

Func. class.: Antitubercular
Chem. class.: Isonicotinic acid hydrazide

ACTION: Bactericidal interference with lipid, nucleic acid biosynthesis

USES: Treatment, prevention of TB

CONTRAINDICATIONS:
Hypersensitivity

Black Box Warning: Acute hepatic disease

Precautions: Pregnancy, renal disease, diabetic retinopathy, cataracts, ocular defects, IV drug users, >35 yr, postpartum, HIV, neuropathy

Black Box Warning: Alcoholism, females (African descent/Hispanic patients)

DOSAGE AND ROUTES

• **Adult/adolescent: PO/IM** 5 mg/kg/day up to 300 mg/day or 15 mg/kg 2-3×/wk, max 900 mg 2-3×/wk

• **Child/infant with HIV: PO/IM** 10-15 mg/kg/day, max 300 mg/day

Available forms: Tabs 100, 300 mg; inj 100 mg/mL; oral sol 10 mg/mL

Administer:

PO route

• PO with meals to decrease GI symptoms; better to take on empty stomach 1 hr before or 2 hr after meals

IM route

• IM deep in large muscle mass; massage; rotate injection site; warm inj to room temperature to dissolve crystals

SIDE EFFECTS

CNS: *Peripheral neuropathy, dizziness,* memory impairment, seizures, psychosis
EENT: Blurred vision, optic neuritis
GI: *Nausea, vomiting,* fatal hepatitis
HEMA: Agranulocytosis, hemolytic, aplastic anemia, thrombocytopenia, eosinophilia, methemoglobinemia, red
DRESS, Stevens-Johnson syndrome, toxic epidermal necrolysis, rash, fever

PHARMACOKINETICS

Metabolized in liver, 50% of patients may metabolize slowly, increasing toxicity; excreted in urine (metabolites), crosses placenta, excreted in breast milk; half life 1-4 hr (slow acetylators), 0.5-1.5 hr (fast acetylators)
PO: Peak 1-2 hr
IM: Peak 45-60 min

INTERACTIONS

Increase: toxicity—tyramine foods, alcohol, cycloSERINE, ethionamide, rifAMPin, carBAMazepine, phenytoin, benzodiazepines, meperidine
Increase: serotonin syndrome—SSRIs, SNRIs
Decrease: absorption—aluminum antacids
Decrease: effectiveness of BCG vaccine—ketoconazole

Drug/Food

• Do not give with high-tyramine foods, alcohol

Drug/Lab Test

Increase: LFTs, bilirubin, glucose
Decrease: platelets, granulocytes

NURSING CONSIDERATIONS
Assess:

Black Box Warning: **Hepatic studies weekly:** baseline in all patients, those >35 yr and all women should be monitored periodically; ALT, AST, bilirubin; increased test results may indicate hepatitis; hepatic status: decreased appetite, jaundice, dark urine, fatigue; ᴼ▣◎ᵪ those with fast acetylation may metabolize product more than 5 times faster (black, Asian patients are at greater risk than some Caucasian patients); fatal hepatitis is a greater risk in black or Hispanic patients after giving birth

• **DRESS:** fever, flulike symptoms, rash, lymphadenopathy, facial swelling, may involve other organ systems
• **Stevens-Johnson syndrome, toxic epidermal necrolysis:** rash, fever, fatigue, blistering, discontinue immediately if these occur
• Mental status often: affect, mood, behavioral changes; psychosis may occur
• Paresthesia in hands, feet
• ᴼ▣◎ᵪ **Susceptibility testing:** ᴼ▣◎ᵪ obtain susceptibility tests before treatment and periodically; half of Mexicans, blacks, Caucasians, and Native Americans may be slow acetylators; Asians, Eskimos may be fast acetylators
• **Pregnancy/breastfeeding:** use during pregnancy even 1st trimester for active TB, use only if benefits outweigh fetal risk for other indications; compatible with breastfeeding
Evaluate:
• Therapeutic response: decreased symptoms of TB
Teach patient/family:
• That compliance with dosage schedule, duration is necessary; not to skip or double dose
• That scheduled appointments must be kept or relapse may occur
• To avoid alcohol while taking product; may increase risk for hepatic injury
• If diabetic, to use blood glucose monitor to obtain correct result

• To report weakness, fatigue, loss of appetite, nausea, vomiting, jaundice of skin or eyes, tingling/numbness of hands/feet

Black Box Warning: **Fatal hepatitis:** to notify prescriber immediately of yellow skin/eyes, dark urine, loss of appetite

isosorbide dinitrate (Rx)
(eye-soe-sor'bide)
Dilatrate-SR, Isochron, IsoDitrate, Isordil
isosorbide mononitrate (Rx)
Imdur ✦, Monoket
Func. class.: Antianginal, vasodilator
Chem. class.: Nitrate

Do not confuse:
Imdur/Imuran/Inderal/K-Dur

ACTION: Relaxation of vascular smooth muscle, which leads to decreased preload, afterload, which is responsible for decreasing left ventricular end-diastolic pressure, systemic vascular resistance, and reducing cardiac oxygen demand

USES: Treatment, prevention of chronic stable angina pectoris
Unlabeled uses: Heart failure (dinitrate)

CONTRAINDICATIONS: Hypersensitivity to this product or nitrates; severe anemia, closed-angle glaucoma
Precautions: Pregnancy, breastfeeding, children, orthostatic hypotension, MI, HF, severe renal/hepatic disease, increased intracranial pressure, cerebral hemorrhage, acute MI, geriatric patients, GI disease, syncope

DOSAGE AND ROUTES
Dinitrate
• **Adult:** PO 5-20 mg bid-tid initially, maintenance 10-40 mg bid-tid; **SL,** buccal 2.5-5 mg, may repeat q5-10min × 3 doses; **EXT REL** 40-80 mg q8-12hr, max 160 mg/day

---

Mononitrate

• **Adult: PO** (Monoket) 10-20 mg bid, 7 hr apart; (Imdur) initiate at 30-60 mg/day as a single dose, increase q3days as needed, may increase to 120 mg/day, max 240 mg/day

Available forms: *Dinitrate:* sus rel caps (SR) 40 mg, ext rel tabs 40 mg; tabs 5, 10, 20, 30, 40 mg; SL tabs 2.5, 5 mg; *mononitrate:* tabs (Monoket) 10, 20 mg; ext rel (Imdur) 30, 60, 120 mg

Administer:

• Do not break, crush, or chew sus rel caps
• After checking expiration date
• PO with 8 oz water on empty stomach
• **SUS REL cap/tab:** allow dosing interval >18 hr

SIDE EFFECTS

CNS: *Vascular headache, flushing, dizziness,* weakness

CV: *Orthostatic hypotension,* tachycardia, collapse, syncope

GI: Nausea, vomiting

INTEG: Pallor, sweating, rash

MISC: Twitching, hemolytic anemia, methemoglobinemia, tolerance, xerostomia

PHARMACOKINETICS

Dinitrate

Metabolized by liver, excreted in urine as metabolites (80%-100%)

PO: Onset 15-30 min, duration 4-6 hr, half-life 5-6 hr

SUS REL: Onset ≤4 hr, duration 6-8 hr

Mononitrate

SUS REL: Onset 30-60 min, peak 1-4 hr, duration 6-8 hr, half-life 5 hr

INTERACTIONS

• Fatal hypotension: avanafil, sildenafil, tadalafil, vardenafil; do not use together

Increase: hypotension—β-blockers, diuretics, antihypertensives, alcohol, calcium channel blockers, phenothiazines

Increase: heart rate, B/P—sympathomimetics

Increase: myocardial ischemia—rosiglitazone; avoid concurrent use

NURSING CONSIDERATIONS

Assess:

• **Anginal pain:** duration, time started, activity being performed, character

• **Methemoglobinemia (rare):** cyanosis of lips, nausea/vomiting, coma, shock; usually caused by high dose of product but may occur with normal dosing

• B/P, pulse, respirations during beginning therapy and periodically thereafter

• Tolerance if taken over long period; to prevent, allow intervals of 12-14 hr/day without product

• Headache, light-headedness, decreased B/P; may indicate a need for decreased dosage, treat headache with OTC analgesics

• **Beers:** use with caution in older adults; may exacerbate episodes of syncope

• **Pregnancy/breastfeeding:** use only if benefit outweighs fetal risk; cautious use in breastfeeding, excretion unknown

Evaluate:

• Therapeutic response: decrease or prevention of anginal pain

Teach patient/family:

• To leave tabs in original container
• To avoid alcohol, OTC products unless approved by prescriber
• That product may cause headache; that taking with meals may reduce or eliminate headache; to take no later than 7 PM (last dose)
• To avoid hazardous activities if dizziness occurs
• About the importance of complying with complete medical regimen
• To make position changes slowly to prevent orthostatic hypotension
• Not to use with avanafil, sildenafil, tadalafil, vardenafil with nitrates; may cause serious drop in B/P
• Not to discontinue abruptly, may cause heart attack
• To use at beginning of angina symptoms, may repeat every 15 min; if no relief, seek medical attention immediately

---

RARELY USED

ISOtretinoin (Rx)

(eye-soe-tret'i-noyn)

Absorica, Amnesteem, Claravis, Myorisan, Sotret, Zenatane

Func. class.: Antiacne agent, retinoid

USES: Severe recalcitrant nodulocystic acne

CONTRAINDICATIONS: Hypersensitivity to this product, parabens, retinoids, inflamed skin, blood donation

Black Box Warning: Pregnancy

DOSAGE AND ROUTES
• **Adult:** PO 0.5-2 mg/kg/day in 2 divided doses × 15-20 wk; if relapse occurs, repeat after 2 mo off product

---

itraconazole (Rx)
(it-ra-con′a-zol)
Onmel, Sporanox
Func. class.: Antifungal, systemic
Chem. class.: Triazole derivative

ACTION: Alters cell membranes; inhibits several fungal enzymes

USES: Histoplasmosis, blastomycosis (pulmonary and extrapulmonary), aspergillosis, onychomycosis of toenail/fingernail
Unlabeled uses: Dermatomycosis, histoplasmosis, chromoblastomycosis, coccidioidomycosis, pityriasis versicolor, seborpsoriasis, vaginal candidiasis, cryptococcus, subcutaneous mycoses, dimorphic infections, fungal keratitis, zygomycosis, superficial mycoses (dermatophytosis), chronic mucocutaneous candidiasis

CONTRAINDICATIONS: Hypersensitivity, fungal meningitis; onychomycosis or dermatomycosis with cardiac dysfunction, in pregnant women

Black Box Warning: Heart failure, ventricular dysfunction, coadministration with other products

Precautions: Pregnancy, breastfeeding, children, cardiac/renal/hepatic disease, achlorhydria or hypochlorhydria (product-induced), dialysis, hearing loss, cystic fibrosis neuropathy

DOSAGE AND ROUTES
• **Adult:** PO 200 mg/day with food; may increase to 200 mg bid if needed; life-threatening infections may require a loading dose of 200 mg tid × 3 days
Available forms: Caps 100 mg; oral sol 10 mg/mL; tab 200 mg
Administer:
• In the presence of acid products only; do not use alkaline products, antacids within 2 hr of product; may give coffee, tea, acidic fruit juices
PO route
• Swallow caps whole; do not break, crush, or chew caps
• Give caps after full meal to ensure absorption
• Oral sol: patient should swish in mouth vigorously, use on empty stomach
• Oral sol and caps are not interchangeable on mg/mg basis
• Store in tight container at room temperature, do not freeze

SIDE EFFECTS
CNS: *Headache, dizziness,* insomnia, somnolence, depression
CV: Hypertension, HF
GI: *Nausea, vomiting, anorexia, diarrhea,* cramps, *abdominal pain,* flatulence, GI bleeding, hepatotoxicity
GU: Gynecomastia, impotence, decreased libido
INTEG: *Pruritus,* fever, *rash,* toxic epidermal necrolysis, Stevens-Johnson syndrome
MISC: *Edema, fatigue,* malaise, hypokalemia, tinnitus, rhabdomyolysis
RESP: Rhinitis, sinusitis, upper respiratory infection, pulmonary edema

PHARMACOKINETICS
PO: Peak 3-4 hr; half-life 21 hr, IV 35.4 hr; metabolized in liver; excreted in bile, feces, urine 40%; requires acid pH for absorption; distributed poorly to CSF; 99.8% protein bound; inhibits CYP3A4

INTERACTIONS
• Life-threatening CV reactions—pimozide, quiNIDine, dofetilide, levomethadyl, dronedarone

---

Side effects: *italics* = common; red = life-threatening

Increase: tinnitus, hearing loss—quiNIDine

Increase: hepatotoxicity—other hepatotoxic products

Increase: edema—calcium channel blockers

Increase: severe hypoglycemia—oral hypoglycemics

Increase: sedation—ALPRAZolam, clorazepate, diazePAM, estazolam, flurazepam, triazolam, oral midazolam

Increase: levels, toxicity—busPIRone, busulfan, clarithromycin, cycloSPORINE, diazePAM, digoxin, felodipine, fentaNYL, atorvastatin, carBAMazepine, disopyramide, indinavir, isradipine, niCARdipine, NiFEdipine, niMODipine, phenytoin, quiNIDine, QUEtiapine, ritonavir, saquinavir, tacrolimus, warfarin

Decrease: itraconazole action—antacids, H₂-receptor antagonists, rifamycins, didanosine, carBAMazepine, isoniazid, proton pump inhibitors

Drug/Food
• Food increases absorption
• Grapefruit juice decreases itraconazole level

Drug/Lab Test
Increase: LFTs, alk phos, bilirubin, triglyceride, GGT

NURSING CONSIDERATIONS
Assess:
• **HF:** if present, discontinue product
• Type of infection; may begin treatment before obtaining results
• **Infection:** temperature, WBC, sputum at baseline and periodically
• I&O ratio, potassium levels
• Hepatic studies (ALT, AST, bilirubin) if patient receiving long-term therapy
• Allergic reaction: rash, photosensitivity, urticaria, dermatitis
• **Hepatotoxicity:** nausea, vomiting, jaundice, clay-colored stools, fatigue
• **Pregnancy/breastfeeding:** do not use in onychomycosis; use for other conditions only if benefits outweigh fetal risk; do not use in breastfeeding

Evaluate:
• Therapeutic response: decreased fever, malaise, rash, negative C&S for infecting organism

Teach patient/family:
• That long-term therapy may be needed to clear infection (1 wk-6 mo, depending on infection)
• To avoid hazardous activities if dizziness occurs
• To take 2 hr before administration of other products that increase gastric pH (antacids, H₂-blockers, omeprazole, sucralfate, anticholinergics); to avoid grapefruit juice; to notify health care provider of all medications taken; to take after a full meal (caps) or on empty stomach (oral sol)
• About the importance of compliance with product regimen; to use alternative methods of contraception
• To notify prescriber of GI symptoms; signs of hepatic dysfunction (fatigue, jaundice, nausea, anorexia, vomiting, dark urine, pale stools); heart failure (trouble breathing, unusual weight gain, fatigue, swelling); hearing changes

---

RARELY USED

ivacaftor
(eye′va-kaf′tor)
Kalydeco
Func. class.: Respiratory agent

USES: Cystic fibrosis in those with G551D, G1244E, G1349D, G178R, G5515S, S1255P, S549N, S549R mutation in the CFTR gene

DOSAGE AND ROUTES
• **Adult/adolescent/child ≥6 yr: PO** 150 mg q12hr with fat-containing food
• **Child 2-5 yr, ≥14 kg: PO** 75 mg q12hr with fat-containing food
• **Child 2-5 yr, <14 kg: PO** 50 mg q12hr with fat-containing food

---

peripheral neuropathy, ventricular dysfunction

DOSAGE AND ROUTES
• **Adult: IV INFUSION** 40 mg/m² over 3 hr q3wk
Dosage reduction in those taking a strong CYP3A4 inhibitor
• **Adult: IV INFUSION** 20 mg/m² over 3 hr q3wk
Hepatic dose
• **Adult:** IV 20 mg/m² q3wk, max 30 mg/m²
Available forms: Powder for inj 15, 45 mg
Administer:
• Premedicate with histamine antagonists 1 hr before use, prevents hypersensitivity
• Antiemetic 30-60 min before product and prn
IV route
> • Let kit stand at room temperature for 30 min; to reconstitute, withdraw supplied diluent (8 mL for 15-mg vials, 23.5 mL for 45-mg vials); slowly inject sol into vial; gently swirl and invert to mix, final concentration 2 mg/mL; further dilute in LR in DEHP-free bags, final concentration should be between 0.2 and 0.6 mg/mL; after added, mix by manual rotation
> • Diluted sol stable for 6 hr at room temperature; infusion must be completed within 6 hr
> • Use in-line filter, 0.2-1.2 micron
> • Give over 3 hr

SIDE EFFECTS
CNS: *Peripheral neuropathy,* impaired cognition, chills, fatigue, fever, flushing, headache, insomnia, *asthenia*
CV: Bradycardia, *hypotension,* abnormal ECG, angina, atrial flutter, cardiomyopathy, chest pain, edema, MI, vasculitis
GI: *Nausea, vomiting, diarrhea,* abdominal pain, anorexia, colitis, constipation, gastritis, jaundice, GERD, hepatic failure, trismus
GU: Renal failure
HEMA: Neutropenia, thrombocytopenia, anemia, infections, coagulopathy
INTEG: *Alopecia,* rash, hot flashes

---

ivosidenib
(I'-voh-sih'-deh-nib)
Tibsovo
Func. class.: Antineoplastic

USES: Relapsed or refractory AML with an isocitrate dehydrogenase-1 (IDH1) mutation

CONTRAINDICATIONS: Hypersensitivity, pregnancy

Black Box Warning: Differentiation syndrome

DOSAGE AND ROUTES
• **Adult: PO** 500 mg daily until disease progression or unacceptable toxicity

⚠ HIGH ALERT

ixabepilone (Rx)
(ix-ab-ep′i-lone)
Ixempra
Func. class.: Antineoplastic—miscellaneous
Chem. class.: Epothilone, B analogue

ACTION: Microtubule stabilizing agent; microtubules are needed for cell division

USES: Breast cancer

CONTRAINDICATIONS: Pregnancy, breastfeeding, hypersensitivity to products with polyoxyethylated castor oil, neutropenia of <1500/mm³, thrombocytopenia

Black Box Warning: Hepatic disease

Precautions: Children, geriatric patients, alcoholism, bone marrow suppression, cardiac dysrhythmias, cardiac/renal disease, diabetes mellitus,

---

Side effects: *italics* = common; red = life-threatening

META: Hypokalemia, metabolic acidosis
MS: *Arthralgia, myalgia*
RESP: Bronchospasm, cough, dyspnea
SYST: *Hypersensitivity reactions,* anaphylaxis, dehydration, radiation recall reaction

PHARMACOKINETICS

Metabolized in liver by CYP3A4; excreted in feces (65%) and urine (21%); terminal half-life 52 hr

INTERACTIONS

Increase: ixabepilone level—CYP3A4 inhibitors (amiodarone, amprenavir, aprepitant, atazanavir, chloramphenicol, clarithromycin, conivaptan, cycloSPORINE, danazol, darunavir, dalfopristin, delavirdine, diltiaZEM, erythromycin, estradiol, fluconazole, fluvoxaMINE, fosamprenavir, imatinib, indinavir, isoniazid, itraconazole, ketoconazole, lopinavir, miconazole, nefazodone, nelfinavir, propoxyphene, ritonavir, RU-486, saquinavir, tamoxifen, telithromycin, troleandomycin, verapamil, voriconazole, zafirlukast)

Decrease: ixabepilone levels—CYP3A4 inducers (aminoglutethimide, barbiturates, bexarotene, bosentan, carBAMazepine, dexamethasone, efavirenz, griseofulvin, modafinil, nafcillin, nevirapine, OXcarbazepine, phenytoin, rifamycin, topiramate)

Drug/Herb
• Avoid use with St. John's wort
Drug/Food
• Avoid use with grapefruit products

NURSING CONSIDERATIONS
Assess:
• CBC, differential, platelet count before treatment and weekly; withhold product if WBC is <1500/mm³ or platelet count is <100,000/mm³, notify prescriber
• Monitor temperature q4hr (may indicate beginning infection)

Black Box Warning: **Hepatic disease:** liver function tests before, during therapy (bilirubin, AST, ALT, LDH) prn or monthly; check for jaundiced skin and sclera, dark urine, clay-colored stools, itchy skin, abdominal pain, fever, diarrhea; contraindicated in combination with capecitabine if AST or ALT is >2.5 × ULN or bilirubin >1 × ULN due to risk of toxicity and neutropenia-related death

• VS during 1st hr of infusion; check IV site for signs of infiltration
• **Hypersensitivity reactions, anaphylaxis** including hypotension, dyspnea, angioedema, generalized urticaria; discontinue infusion immediately; keep emergency equipment available
• Effects of alopecia on body image; discuss feelings about body changes
• **Pregnancy/breastfeeding:** do not use in pregnancy or breastfeeding
Evaluate:
• Therapeutic response: decreased tumor size, spread of malignancy
Teach patient/family:
• To report signs of infection: fever, sore throat, flulike symptoms
• To report signs of anemia: fatigue, headache, faintness, SOB
• To report any complaints or side effects to nurse or prescriber
• That hair may be lost during treatment; that a wig or hairpiece may make patient feel better; that new hair may be different in color, texture
• That pain in muscles and joints 2-5 days after infusion is common
• To use nonhormonal type of contraception
• To avoid receiving vaccinations while receiving product

ixekizumab
(ix' e- kiz' ue- mab)
Taltz ✦
Func. class.: Immunosuppressive

ACTION: A human IgG4 monoclonal antibody that selectively binds to the interleukin 17A (IL-17A) cytokine, inhibiting its interaction with the IL-17 receptor. Treatment inhibits the release of proinflammatory cytokines and chemokines

USES: The treatment of moderate to severe plaque psoriasis in adults who are candidates for systemic therapy or phototherapy

CONTRAINDICATIONS: Risk of serious hypersensitivity reactions or anaphylaxis

Precautions: Breastfeeding, children, Crohn's disease, immunosuppression, infection, inflammatory bowel disease, pregnancy, tuberculosis, ulcerative colitis, vaccination

DOSAGE AND ROUTES

• **Adult:** SUBCUT 160 mg at week 0 (administered as two 80-mg injections) followed by 80 mg at weeks 2, 4, 6, 8, 10, and 12, then 80 mg q4wk

• **Available forms:** Solution for injection 80 mg/mL, autoinjector 80 mg/mL

Administer:

Subcut route

• Administer by subcutaneous injection only

• Visually inspect for particulate matter and discoloration before administration whenever solution and container permit. The solution should be free of visible particles, clear, and colorless to slightly yellow

• Available as a prefilled syringe and as an autoinjector; each device contains 80 mg

• Patients may use the prefilled syringe or autoinjector after proper training

• Use upper arms, thighs, and any quadrant of the abdomen for injection sites.

• Do not use where skin is tender, bruised, erythematous, indurated, or affected by psoriasis; rotate sites with each dose.

• Does not contain preservatives; discard any unused product remaining in the prefilled syringe or autoinjector. Discard the single-dose autoinjector or syringe after use in a proper puncture-resistant container

• **Missed doses:** If a dose is missed, give as soon as possible. Then, resume dosing at the regular scheduled time

• **Preparation for use of the prefilled syringe or autoinjector:** Remove prefilled syringe or autoinjector from refrigerator and allow to warm 30 minutes at room temperature; inspect syringe or autoinjector for particulate matter and discoloration before administration

• **Storage of unopened prefilled syringes and autoinjectors:** Protect from light; store refrigerated at 2-8° C (36-46° F) until time of use. Do not freeze and do not use the injection if it has been frozen. Do not shake

SIDE EFFECTS

SYST: antibody formation, infection, angioedema

INTEG: injection site reaction, urticaria

HEMA: neutropenia

PHARMACOKINETICS

Half-life is 13 days; bioavailability 60% to 81%, injection in the thigh achieved higher bioavailability; peak 4 days

INTERACTIONS

• Do not use concurrently with vaccines; immunizations should be brought up-to-date before treatment

• Avoid use with immunosuppressives

NURSING CONSIDERATIONS

Assess:

• **TB:** TB testing should be done before use

• For injection-site reactions, redness, swelling, pain

• Bring immunizations up-to-date before use

• **Infection:** monitor for fever, sore throat, cough; do not use in active infections

• **Pregnancy/breastfeeding:** avoid in pregnancy and breastfeeding

Evaluate: Therapeutic response: decreased psoriasis

Teach Patient/Family:

• That product must be continued for prescribed time to be effective, to use as prescribed

• Not to receive vaccinations during treatment

• **Infection:** to notify prescriber of possible infections, respiratory or other, or of allergic reactions

• Injection techniques and disposal of equipment, not to reuse needles, syringes

---

Side effects: *italics* = common; red = life-threatening

RARELY USED

ketoconazole (Rx)
(kee-toe-koe′na-zole)
Func. class.: Antifungal
Chem. class.: Imidazole derivative

USES: Chronic mucocandidiasis, oral thrush, candiduria, coccidioidomycosis, histoplasmosis, chromomycosis, paracoccidioidomycosis, blastomycosis; tinea cruris, tinea corporis, tinea versicolor, *Pityrosporum ovale* in patients who are intolerant to other antifungal therapies or for whom other antifungal therapies have failed

CONTRAINDICATIONS: Breastfeeding, hypersensitivity, fungal meningitis

Black Box Warning: Coadministration with other products (ergot derivatives, cisapride, or triazolam) may cause fatal cardiac arrhythmias due to inhibition of CYP3A4 enzyme system

Black Box Warning: Hepatic disease

DOSAGE AND ROUTES
• **Adult: PO** 200-400 mg/day for 1-2 wk (candidiasis), 6 mo (other infections)
• **Child ≥2 yr: PO** 3.3-6.6 mg/kg/day as a single daily dose
Prostate cancer (unlabeled)
• **Adult: PO** 400 mg tid

ketoconazole (topical)
(kee-toe-koe′na-zole)
Extina, Ketoderm ♣, Ketozole, Nizoral, Nizoral A-D, Xolegel, Ketodan, Kuric
Func. class.: Topical antifungal
Chem. class.: Imidazole derivative

ACTION: Antifungal activity results from altering cell membrane permeability

USES: Seborrheic dermatitis (immunocompromised), tinea corporis, tinea cruris, tinea pedis, tinea versicolor, dandruff

CONTRAINDICATIONS: Hypersensitivity, sulfite allergy
Precautions: Pregnancy, breastfeeding, children

DOSAGE AND ROUTES
Seborrheic dermatitis
• **Adult/child ≥12 yr: TOP FOAM** apply to affected areas bid × 4 wk; **GEL** apply to affected areas daily × 2 wk
Tinea corporis, tinea cruris, tinea pedis, tinea versicolor
• **Adult: TOP** cover areas daily × 2 wk
Dandruff
• **Adult: SHAMPOO** wet hair, lather, massage for 1 min, rinse, repeat 2×/wk spaced by 3 days, for up to 8 wk, then as needed
Available forms: Topical gel, foam, cream 2%; shampoo 1%, 2%
Administer:
Topical route
• For external use only; do not use skin products near the eyes, nose, or mouth, wash hands before and after use
• **Cream/lotion:** Apply to the cleansed affected area, massage gently into affected areas, do not use on skin that is broken or irritated

SIDE EFFECTS
INTEG: Irritation, stinging, pustules, pruritus

NURSING CONSIDERATIONS
Assess allergic reaction:
• Assess for hypersensitivity; product may need to be discontinued
• Assess for sulfite allergy; may be life-threatening
Evaluate:
• Therapeutic response: decreased itching, scaling
Teach patient/family:
Topical route
• These products are not for intravaginal therapy and are for external use only; do not use skin products near the eyes, nose, or mouth; wash hands before and

after use; do not wash affected area for ≥3 hr after application

• **Cream/ointment/lotion:** apply a thin film to the cleansed affected area, massage gently

• **Foam formulations:** do not dispense foam directly onto hands or face; the warmth of the skin will cause the foam to melt; dispense desired amount directly into the cap or onto a cool surface; make sure enough foam is dispensed to cover the affected area(s); if the can feels warm or the foam seems runny, run the can under cold water; to apply, pick up small amounts of the foam with the fingertips and gently massage into the affected areas until the foam disappears

• To continue for prescribed time, tinea corporis/cruris ≥2 wk

---

ketoprofen (OTC, Rx)

(ke-toe-proe′fen)

Func. class.: Nonsteroidal antiinflammatory product (NSAID), antirheumatic

Chem. class.: Propionic acid derivative

ACTION: May inhibit prostaglandin synthesis; analgesic, antiinflammatory, antipyretic

USES: Mild to moderate pain, osteoarthritis, rheumatoid arthritis, dysmenorrhea; OTC relief of minor aches, pains

Unlabeled uses: Ankylosing spondylitis, bone pain, gouty arthritis

CONTRAINDICATIONS: Pregnancy 2nd/3rd trimester, hypersensitivity to this product, NSAIDs, salicylates, perioperative pain with CABG

Precautions: Pregnancy, breastfeeding, children, geriatric patients, bleeding, GI/cardiac disorders, hypersensitivity to other antiinflammatory agents; asthma, severe renal/hepatic disease, ulcer disease

Black Box Warning: GI bleeding, MI, stroke

DOSAGE AND ROUTES

Analgesic

• **Adult: PO** 25-50 mg q6-8hr, max 300 mg/day

Rheumatoid arthritis, osteoarthritis

• **Adult: PO** 50 mg qid or 75 mg tid, max 300 mg/day or **EXT REL** 200 mg/day

Dysmenorrhea

• **Adult: PO** 25-50 mg q6-8hr (immediate release) up to max 300 mg/day

Renal/hepatic dose

• **Adult: PO** GFR <25 mL/min/1.73m², albumin <3.5 g/dL, decreased hepatic function, or ESRD, max 100 mg/day

Available forms: Caps 25, 50, 75 mg; ext rel cap 100, 150, 200 mg

Administer:

• Do not break, crush, or chew ext rel caps

• Store at room temperature

• Give with a full glass of water 2 hr after meals

• Give with antacids, milk, or food for GI upset

SIDE EFFECTS

CNS: Dizziness, drowsiness, headache

CV: Peripheral edema, hypertension, CV thrombotic events, MI, stroke

GI: *Nausea, anorexia, vomiting, diarrhea,* jaundice, hepatitis, constipation, flatulence, cramps, dry mouth, peptic ulcer, GI bleeding, *dyspepsia*

GU: Nephrotoxicity, cystitis

HEMA: Blood dyscrasias

INTEG: Purpura, rash, pruritus, photosensitivity

SYST: Anaphylaxis, exfoliative dermatitis, Stevens-Johnson syndrome, toxic epidermal necrolysis

PHARMACOKINETICS

PO: Onset 1-2 hr, peak 1-2 hr; ext rel: onset 2-3 hr, peak 7 hr; half-life 2-4 hr; 3-7 hr ext rel; metabolized in liver, urine (metabolites); 99% protein binding

INTERACTIONS

Increase: toxicity—cycloSPORINE, lithium, methotrexate, phenytoin, alcohol, cidofovir

K

Increase: bleeding risk—anticoagulants, clopidogrel, eptifibatide, thrombolytics, ticlopidine, tirofiban, SSRIs

Increase: ketoprofen levels—aspirin, probenecid

Increase: adverse GI reactions—aspirin, corticosteroids, NSAIDs, alcohol

Increase: hematologic toxicity—antineoplastics

Decrease: effect of diuretics, antihypertensives

Drug/Herb

Increase: bleeding risk— dong quai, feverfew, garlic, ginger, ginkgo, horse chestnut

Drug/Lab Test

Increase: BUN, alk phos, AST, ALT, LDH, creatinine, bleeding time

NURSING CONSIDERATIONS

Assess:

• **Pain:** type, location, intensity, ROM before and 1-2 hr after treatment

• **Fever:** temperature baseline and periodically

• Renal, hepatic, blood studies: BUN, creatinine, AST, ALT, Hgb before treatment and q6mo

• **Aspirin sensitivity, asthma;** these patients may be more likely to develop hypersensitivity to NSAIDs

Black Box Warning: **GI bleeding:** blood in sputum, emesis, stools; assess for occult or frank blood

Black Box Warning: **CV thrombotic events:** MI, stroke; this product or other NSAIDs may increase the risk

• **Beers:** avoid chronic use in older adults unless other alternatives are unavailable; increased risk of GI bleeding, peptic ulcer disease

Evaluate:

• Therapeutic response: decreased pain, stiffness, swelling in joints; ability to move more easily; decreased fever

Teach patient/family:

• To avoid driving, other hazardous activities if dizziness, drowsiness occurs, especially in geriatric patients

• **Nephrotoxicity:** to report immediately change in urine pattern, increased weight, edema, increased pain in joints, fever, blood in urine; rash, itching, blurred vision, ringing in ears, flulike symptoms; blood in urine, vomit, or stools (bleeding)

• **Hepatotoxicity:** dark urine, clay-colored stools, jaundice of skin or eyes, itching, abdominal pain, fever, diarrhea, report to prescriber

• That therapeutic effects may take up to 1 mo; to take with 8 oz water; to sit upright for $1/2$ hr after administration to prevent GI irritation; not to crush, chew ext rel products

• To avoid aspirin, alcohol, corticosteroids, acetaminophen, other medications, supplements unless approved by prescriber

• To wear sunscreen, protective clothing to prevent photosensitivity

• To report product use to all health care providers

• **Pregnancy/breastfeeding:** to report planned or suspected pregnancy; to avoid breastfeeding

ketorolac (ophthalmic) (Rx)

(kee'toe-role-ak)

Acular, Acular LS, Acuvail

Func. class.: Antiinflammatory (ophthalmic)

Chem. class.: Nonsteroidal antiinflammatory drug (NSAID)

ACTION: Inhibits miosis by inhibiting the biosynthesis of ocular prostaglandins; prostaglandins play a role in the miotic response produced during ocular surgery by constricting the iris sphincter independently of cholinergic mechanisms

USES: Pain and inflammation after cataract surgery, refractive surgery, seasonal allergic conjunctivitis

CONTRAINDICATIONS: Hypersensitivity to this product, NSAIDs, salicylates

Precautions: Bleeding disorders, complicated ocular surgery, corneal denervation, diabetes mellitus, rheumatoid arthritis, dry eye syndrome, pregnancy, breastfeeding, children, contact lenses

DOSAGE AND ROUTES
Seasonal allergic conjunctivitis (Acular)
• **Adult/child ≥2 yr: OPHTH** Instill 1 drop into affected eye qid
Inflammation after cataract extraction (Acular)
• **Adult: OPHTH** 1 drop in affected eye qid beginning 24 hr after surgery × 2 wk
Corneal refracture surgery, pain, burning (Acular LS)
• **Adult: OPHTH** 1 drop in affected eye qid × ≤4 days
Incision refraction surgery, pain, photophobia (Acular PF)
• **Adult: OPHTH** 1 drop qid in affected eye × 3 days
Cataract surgery, pain, inflammation (Acuvail)
• **Adult: OPHTH** 1 drop bid in affected eye, starting 1 day before surgery, on the day of surgery, × 2 wk after surgery
Available forms: Ophthalmic solution Acular (0.5%), Acular LS (0.4%), Acuvail (0.45%)
Administer:
• Apply topically to the eye, separate by ≥5 min when using with other ophthalmics
• Remove contact lenses before instillation of solution
• Instruct patient on proper instillation of eye solution
• Do not touch the tip of the dropper to the eye, fingertips, or other surface
• Do not share bottle with other patients

SIDE EFFECTS
CNS: Headache
EENT: Abnormal sensation in eye, conjunctival hyperemia, ocular irritation, ocular pain, ocular pruritus, conjunctival hyperemia, iritis, keratitis, blurred vision, transient burning/stinging

NURSING CONSIDERATIONS
Assess:
• Eyes: for pain, inflammation, burning, redness after cataract surgery, visual acuity
Evaluate:
• Therapeutic response: decreased pain and inflammation after cataract surgery, refractive surgery, seasonal allergic conjunctivitis
Teach patient/family:
• To apply topically to the eye
• To remove contact lenses before instillation of solution, wait 10 min before reinserting
• Proper instillation of eye solution
• Not to touch the tip of the dropper to the eye, fingertips, or other surface
• Not to share bottle with other patients

K

---

ketorolac (systemic, nasal) (Rx)
(kee-toe′role-ak)
Toradol ✦, Sprix
Func. class.: Nonsteroidal antiinflammatory/nonopioid analgesic
Chem. class.: Acetic acid

Do not confuse:
Toradol/TraMADol

ACTION: Reversibly inhibits cyclooxygenase-1 and -2 (COX-1 and COX-2) enzymes; analgesic, antiinflammatory, antipyretic effects

USES: Mild to moderate pain (short term)

CONTRAINDICATIONS: Pregnancy 3rd trimester, hypersensitivity to this product, salicylates, asthma, hepatic disease, peptic ulcer disease, CV bleeding, C-section, intracranial bleeding, perioperative pain in CABG

Black Box Warning: Severe renal disease, L&D, before major surgery, epidural/intrathecal administration, GI bleeding/perforation, hypovolemia, NSAID hypersensitivity, peptic ulcer disease, CABG, hematologic disease, intracranial bleeding

---

Side effects: *italics* = common; red = life-threatening

Precautions: Pregnancy/breastfeeding, GI/cardiac disorders, hypersensitivity to other antiinflammatory agents, CCr <25 mL/min

Black Box Warning: Bleeding, MI, stroke; limit duration of use; geriatric patients, children, infants/neonates, serious hypersensitivity reactions or anaphylaxis

DOSAGE AND ROUTES
Intranasal dosage:
• **Adults ≥50 kg with normal renal function:** 1 spray (15.75 mg/spray) in each nostril (total dose of 31.5 mg) q6-8hr; max 4 doses, max 5 days; IV 30 mg; IM 60 mg
• **Adults <50 kg or who have renal impairment, and geriatric patients:**
• 1 spray (15.75 mg/spray) in one nostril q6-8hr max 4 doses, max 5 days; IV 15 mg; IM 30 mg
• **Child ≥2 yr/adolescents ≤16 yr:** IM 1 mg/kg, max 30 mg, or IV 0.5 mg/kg to a max of 15 mg
Renal dose
• Do not use in advanced renal disease
Available forms: Inj 15, 30 mg/mL (prefilled syringes), 60 mg/2 mL; tab 10 mg; nasal spray 15.75 mg/spray
Administer:
• Not to exceed 5 days
• Store at room temperature, protect from light
IM route
• IM inj deeply and slowly in large muscle mass
Nasal route
• Prime pump before using for the first time, point away from person/pets, pump activator 5 times, no need to reprime
• For single-use only, discard 24 hr after opening if not used
• Do not share with others
• Have patient blow nose, sit upright to spray
IV route
• Give undiluted over ≥15 sec

Solution compatibility: D$_5$W, 0.9% NaCl, LR, D$_5$, Plasma-Lyte A

Y-site compatibilities: Cisatracurium, remifentanil, SUFentanil

SIDE EFFECTS
CNS: Dizziness, *drowsiness,* tremors, seizures, headache
CV: Hypertension, pallor, edema, CV thrombotic events, MI, stroke
EENT: Tinnitus, hearing loss, blurred vision
GI: Nausea, anorexia, vomiting, diarrhea, constipation, flatulence, cramps, dry mouth, peptic ulcer, GI bleeding, perforation, taste change, hepatic failure
GU: Nephrotoxicity: dysuria, hematuria, oliguria
HEMA: Blood dyscrasias, prolonged bleeding
INTEG: Purpura, rash, pruritus, sweating, angioedema, Stevens-Johnson syndrome, toxic epidermal necrolysis

PHARMACOKINETICS
Half-life 6 hr, enters breast milk, metabolized by liver, excreted by kidneys
PO: Onset 30-60 min, duration 4-6 hr
IM: Onset 30 min, duration 4-6 hr

INTERACTIONS
Increase: toxicity—methotrexate, lithium, cycloSPORINE, pentoxifylline, probenecid, cidofovir
Increase: bleeding risk—anticoagulants, clopidogrel, eptifibatide, salicylates, ticlopidine, tirofiban, thrombolytics, SSRIs, SNRIs
Increase: renal impairment—ACE inhibitors
Increase: ketorolac levels—aspirin, other NSAIDs; contraindicated
Increase: GI effects—corticosteroids, alcohol, aspirin, NSAIDs
Decrease: effects—antihypertensives, diuretics
Drug/Lab Test
Increase: AST, ALT, LDH, bleeding time

NURSING CONSIDERATIONS
Assess:
• **Aspirin sensitivity, asthma:** patients may be more likely to develop hypersensitivity to NSAIDs; monitor for hypersensitivity

• **Pain:** type, location, intensity, ROM before and 1 hr after treatment

Black Box Warning: **Renal, hepatic, blood studies:** BUN, creatinine, AST, ALT, Hgb before treatment, periodically thereafter; check for dehydration

Black Box Warning: **Bleeding:** check for bruising, bleeding, occult blood in urine, stool guaiac

Black Box Warning: Do not use epidurally, intrathecally; alcohol is present in the solution

• Eye/ear problems: blurred vision, tinnitus (may indicate toxicity)
• **Hepatic dysfunction:** jaundice, yellow sclera and skin, clay-colored stools

Black Box Warning: **CV thrombotic events:** MI, stroke; do not use in perioperative pain in CABG

• Audiometric, ophthalmic exam before, during, after treatment

Black Box Warning: **Beers:** avoid in older adults; increased risk of GI bleeding, peptic ulcer disease; those >65 and 50 kg, adjust dose to CCr, risk is increased; max 60 mg/day

Evaluate:
• Therapeutic response: decreased pain, stiffness, swelling in joints, ability to move more easily

Teach patient/family:

Black Box Warning: To report blurred vision, ringing/roaring in ears (may indicate toxicity)

• To avoid driving, other hazardous activities if dizziness or drowsiness occurs

Black Box Warning: To report change in urine pattern, weight increase, edema; pain increase in joints, fever, blood in urine **(indicates nephrotoxicity)**; bruising, black tarry stools **(indicates bleeding)**; pruritus, jaundice, nausea, right upper quadrant pain, abdominal pain **(hepatotoxicity)**; to notify prescriber immediately

• To avoid alcohol, salicylates, other NSAIDs
• To report product use to all health care providers, not to use with other products unless approved by prescriber; use for ≤5 days
• **Nasal:** to discard within 24 hr of opening; may cause irritation, may drink water after dose

Black Box Warning: **Pregnancy/breastfeeding:** to notify prescriber if pregnancy is planned or suspected; not to breastfeed; contraindicated during labor and delivery

ketotifen (ophthalmic) (Rx)
(kee-toe-tye′fen)
Alaway, Zaditor, ZyrTEC Itchy Eye, Claritin Eye
Func. class.: Antihistamine (ophthalmic)
Chem. class.: Histamine 1 receptor antagonist/mast cell stabilizer

ACTION: A topically active, direct H_1-receptor antagonist and mast cell stabilizer; by reducing these inflammatory mediators, relieves the ocular pruritus associated with allergic conjunctivitis

USES: For the temporary relief of ocular pruritus due to ragweed, pollen, grass, animal hair, animal dander

CONTRAINDICATIONS: Hypersensitivity

Side effects: *italics* = common; red = life-threatening

Precautions: Pregnancy, breastfeeding, children, contact lenses

DOSAGE AND ROUTES
• **Adult/child ≥3 yr: OPHTH** instill 1 drop in affected eye(s) every 8-12 hr
Available forms: Ophthalmic solution 0.025%
Administer:
Ophthalmic route
• For topical ophthalmic use only
• Wash hands before and after use; squeeze the prescribed number of drops into the conjunctival sac
• Do not touch the tip of the dropper to the eye, fingertips, or other surface
• Wait ≥10 min after instilling the ophthalmic solution before inserting contact lenses; contact lenses should not be worn if eye is red

SIDE EFFECTS
CNS: Headache
EENT: Conjunctival hyperemia, rhinitis, allergic reactions, ocular irritation consisting of burning or stinging, conjunctivitis, eyelid disorder, flu syndrome, keratitis, lacrimation disorder, mydriasis, ocular discharge, ocular pain, pharyngitis, photophobia, pruritus, rash, xerophthalmia (dry eyes)

NURSING CONSIDERATIONS
Assess:
• Eyes: for itching, redness, tearing, use of soft or hard contact lens
Evaluate:
• Absence of redness, itching in the eyes
Teach patient/family:
Ophthalmic route
• That product is for topical ophthalmic use only
• To wash hands before and after use; tilt the head back slightly and pull the lower eyelid down with the index finger; squeeze the prescribed number of drops into the conjunctival sac and gently close eyes for 1-2 min; not to blink
• Not to touch the tip of the dropper to the eye, fingertips, or other surface
• To wait ≥10 min after instilling the ophthalmic solution before inserting contact lenses; contact lenses should not be worn if eye is red
• Not to share ophthalmic drops with others
• To remove contact lenses before use; the preservative benzalkonium chloride may be absorbed by soft contact lenses

labetalol (Rx)
(la-bet'a-lole)

Trandate ✦

Func. class.: Antihypertensive, antianginal

Chem. class.: α-1/β-Blocker

Do not confuse:
labetalol/Lamictal

ACTION: Produces decreases in B/P without reflex tachycardia or significant reduction in heart rate through mixture of α-blocking, β-blocking effects; elevated plasma renins are reduced

USES: Mild to moderate hypertension; treatment of severe hypertension (IV)
Unlabeled uses: Hypotension induction

CONTRAINDICATIONS: Hypersensitivity to β-blockers, cardiogenic shock, heart block (2nd or 3rd degree), sinus bradycardia, HF, bronchial asthma
Precautions: Pregnancy, breastfeeding, geriatric patients, major surgery, diabetes mellitus, thyroid/renal/hepatic disease, COPD, well-compensated heart failure, nonallergic bronchospasm, peripheral vascular disease

Black Box Warning: Abrupt discontinuation

DOSAGE AND ROUTES
Hypertension
• **Adult: PO Outpatient** 100 mg bid; may be given with diuretic; may increase to 200 mg bid after 2 days; may continue to increase q1-3days; max 2400 mg/day in divided doses; **Inpatient** 200 mg then 200-400 mg in 6-12 hr, depends on response; may increase by 200 mg bid at 1-day intervals
• **Child/adolescent (unlabeled): PO** 1-3 mg/kg/day, titrate to max 10-12 mg/kg/day based on B/P, max 12 mg/kg/day, max 1200 mg/day; **IV** 0.2-1 mg/kg over 2 min; **IV INFUSION** 0.25-3 mg/kg/hr, max 3 mg/kg/hr

Hypertensive crisis
• **Adult: IV Intermittent** 20 mg over 2 min; may repeat 20-80 mg over 2 min q10min, max 300 mg; **IV Cont INFUSION** after loading dose give 1-2 mg/min until desired response or max 300 mg
Available forms: Tabs 100, 200, 300 mg; inj 5 mg/mL, 20-, 40-mL vials
Administer:
PO route
• PO before meals, or with meals; tab may be crushed or swallowed whole; give with meals to increase absorption
• Take pulse before use; if <50 bpm, hold dose, notify prescriber
• Take apical pulse before use; if <50 bpm, withhold; notify prescriber
• When discontinuing IV and starting PO, begin PO when B/P rises; start at 200 mg, then 200-400 mg in 6-12 hr; adjust as needed
• Do not discontinue before surgery
• Store in dry area at room temperature; do not freeze
Direct IV route
• Give undiluted (5 mg/mL) over 2 min
Continuous IV INFUSION route
• Give at a rate of 2 mg/min after diluting in LR, D₅W, D₅ in 0.2%, 0.9%, 0.33% NaCl, Ringer's inj; infusion is titrated to patient response; 200 mg of product/160 mL sol = 1 mg/mL; 300 mg of product/240 mL sol = 1 mg/mL; 200 mg of product/250 mL sol = 2 mg/3 mL; use infusion pump
• Keep patient recumbent during and for 3 hr after administration; monitor VS q5-15min

Y-site compatibilities: Alemtuzumab, alfentanil, amikacin, aminocaproic acid, aminophylline, amiodarone, anidulafungin, argatroban, arsenic trioxide, ascorbic acid injection, atracurium, atropine, azithromycin, aztreonam, benztropine, bivalirudin, bleomycin, bretylium, bumetanide, buprenorphine, butorphanol, calcium chloride/gluconate, CARBOplatin, carmustine, caspofungin, ceFAZolin, cefotaxime, cefoTEtan, cefOXitin, ceftaroline, cefTAZidime, ceftizoxime, chlorproMAZINE, cimetidine, CISplatin, cloNIDine, cyanocobalamin, cyclophosphamide, cycloSPORINE, cytarabine, DACTINomycin, DAPTOmycin, DAUNOrubicin liposome, dexmedetomidine, dexrazoxane, digoxin, diltiazem, diphenhydrAMINE, DOBUTamine, DOCEtaxel, dolasetron, DOPamine, doripenem, doxacurium, DOXOrubicin, DOXOrubicin liposomal, doxycycline, enalaprilat, ePHEDrine, EPINEPHrine, epirubicin, epoetin alfa, eptifibatide, ertapenem, erythromycin lactobionate, esmolol, etoposide, etoposide phosphate, fenildopam, fenoldopam, fentaNYL, fluconazole, fludarabine, fluorouracil, folic acid, gallium, ganciclovir, gatifloxacin, gemcitabine, gentamicin, glycopyrrolate, granisetron, HYDROmorphone, hydroxyzine, IDArubicin, ifosfamide, imipenem-cilastatin, inamrinone, irinotecan, isoproterenol, lactated Ringer's injection, lepirudin, leucovorin, levofloxacin, lidocaine, linezolid injection, LORazepam, magnesium sulfate, mannitol, mechlorethamine, meperidine, metaraminol, methyldopate, methylPREDNISolone, metoclopramide, metoprolol, metroNIDAZOLE, midazolam, milrinone, minocycline, mitoXANtrone, morphine, moxifloxacin, multiple vitamins injection, mycophenolate, nalbuphine, naloxone, netilmicin, niCARdipine, nitroglycerin, nitroprusside, norepinephrine, octreotide, ondansetron, oxacillin, oxaliplatin, oxytocin, palonosetron, pamidronate, pancuronium, papaverine, PEMEtrexed, pentamidine, pentazocine, PENTobarbital, PHENobarbital, phentolamine, phenylephrine, phytonadione, polymyxin B, potassium acetate/chloride/phosphates, procainamide, prochlorperazine, promethazine, propofol, propranolol, protamine, pyridoxine, quiNIDine, quinupristin-dalfopristin, ranitidine, Ringer's injection, rocuronium, sodium acetate/bicarbonate, succinylcholine, SUFentanil, tacrolimus, telavancin, teniposide, theophylline, thiamine, thiotepa, ticarcillin-clavulanate, tigecycline, tirofiban, tobramycin, tolazoline, urokinase, vancomycin, vasopressin, vecuronium, verapamil, vinBLAStine, vinCRIStine, vinorelbine, voriconazole, zoledronic acid

SIDE EFFECTS

CNS: *Dizziness,* mental changes, drowsiness, *fatigue,* headache, depression, anxiety, nightmares, paresthesias, lethargy

CV: *Orthostatic hypotension, bradycardia,* HF, chest pain, ventricular dysrhythmias

EENT: Visual changes; double vision; dry, burning eyes, floppy iris syndrome; nasal congestion

ENDO: Hyperkalemia

GI: *Nausea, vomiting, diarrhea,* dyspepsia, taste distortion, hepatotoxicity

GU: Impotence, dysuria, ejaculatory failure

INTEG: Rash, urticaria, pruritus, fever

RESP: Bronchospasm, dyspnea, wheezing

PHARMACOKINETICS

Half-life 2.5-8 hr, metabolized by liver (metabolites inactive), excreted in urine, crosses placenta, excreted in breast milk, protein binding 50%

PO: Onset 30 min, peak 1-4 hr, duration 8-24 hr

IV: Onset 2-5 min, peak 5-15 min, duration 2-4 hr

INTERACTIONS

• Do not use within 2 wk of MAOIs

Increase: myocardial depression—hydantoins, general anesthetics, verapamil, class I antidysrhythmics

Increase: tremor—tricyclic antidepressants

Increase: hypotension—diuretics, other antihypertensives, cimetidine, nitroglycerin, alcohol, nitrates

Decrease: effects of—sympathomimetics, lidocaine, theophylline, β-blockers, bronchodilators, xanthines

Decrease: antihypertensive effect—NSAIDs, salicylates

Increase or decrease: effects of—antidiabetics; monitor blood glucose

Drug/Herb

Increase: antihypertensive effect—hawthorn

Decrease: antihypertensive effect—ephedra (ma huang)
Drug/Lab Test
Increase: ANA titer, blood glucose, alk phos, LDH, AST, ALT, uric acid
False increase: urinary catecholamines

NURSING CONSIDERATIONS
Assess:
• **Hypertension:** monitor B/P before starting treatment, periodically thereafter; note pulse, rate, rhythm, quality; apical/radial pulse before administration; notify prescriber of any significant changes, watch for orthostatic hypotension
• **HF:** I&O, weight daily; fluid overload: weight gain, jugular venous distention, edema, crackles in lungs; report weight gain >5 lb

Black Box Warning: **Abrupt discontinuation:** product should be tapered to prevent adverse reactions

• Baselines of renal/hepatic studies before therapy begins
• **Pregnancy/breastfeeding:** use only if benefits outweigh fetal risk; use caution in breastfeeding
Evaluate:
• Therapeutic response: decreased B/P after 1-2 wk
Teach patient/family:

Black Box Warning: Not to discontinue product abruptly; to taper over 2 wk; may cause precipitate angina

• Not to use OTC products containing α-adrenergic stimulants (nasal decongestants, OTC cold preparations) unless directed by prescriber
• To report bradycardia, dizziness, confusion, depression, fever, difficulty breathing, cold extremities, confusion, rash, sore throat
• To take pulse at home; advise when to notify prescriber
• May mask symptoms of hypoglycemia; monitor blood glucose closely in diabetes
• To avoid alcohol, smoking, increased sodium intake

• **Hypertension:** To comply with weight control, dietary adjustments, modified exercise program
• To carry emergency ID to identify product, allergies
• To avoid hazardous activities if dizziness is present
• To avoid hot baths, showers
• **To report symptoms of HF:** difficulty breathing, especially on exertion or when lying down; night cough; swelling of extremities
• To advise providers of use before surgery
• To avoid driving or other hazardous activities until response is known; dizziness, drowsiness, may occur

TREATMENT OF OVERDOSE:
Lavage, IV glucagon or atropine for bradycardia, IV theophylline for bronchospasm; digoxin, O_2, diuretic for cardiac failure; hemodialysis useful for removal/hypotension; administer vasopressor

---

lacosamide (Rx)
(la-koe′sa-mide)
Vimpat
Func. class.: Anticonvulsant
Chem. class.: Functionalized amino acid

Controlled Substance Schedule V

ACTION: May act through action at sodium channels; exact action is unknown

USES: Partial-onset seizures

CONTRAINDICATIONS: Hypersensitivity
Precautions: Pregnancy, breastfeeding, children <17 yr, geriatric patients, allergies, cardiac/renal/hepatic disease, acute MI, atrial fibrillation/flutter, AV block, bradycardia, CHD, dehydration, depression, dialysis, hazardous activity, electrolyte imbalance, heart failure, labor, PR prolongation, sick sinus syndrome, substance abuse, suicidal ideation, syncope, torsades de pointes

Side effects: *italics* = common; red = life-threatening

DOSAGE AND ROUTES

Adjunct therapy

• **Adult and adolescent ≥17 yr: PO** 50 mg bid, may increase weekly by 100 mg bid to 200-400 mg/day; **IV** 50 mg bid, infuse over 30-60 min, may be increased by 100 mg/day weekly up to 200-400 mg/day maintenance

Monotherapy

• **Adult: PO** 100 mg bid; may increase q wk by 100 mg/day in 2 divided doses, increase to 300-400 mg/day in 2 divided doses

Renal/hepatic dose

• **Adult: PO/IV** max 300 mg/day for mild to moderate hepatic disease or CCr ≤30 mL/min; do not use in severe hepatic disease; reduce dose in renal/hepatic disease in those who are taking strong CYP3A4, CYP2C9 inhibitors

Available forms: Film-coated tabs 50, 100, 150, 200 mg; solution for injection IV 20-mL single-use vials (200 mg/20 mL); oral sol 10 mg/mL

Administer:

• Store PO products/IV vials at room temperature; sol is stable for 24 hr when mixed with compatible diluents in glass or PVC bags at room temperature

PO route

• **Tablet:** give without regard to meals
• **Oral sol:** measure with calibrated measuring device

IV route

• May give undiluted or mixed in 0.9% NaCl, D$_5$W, or LR
• Infuse over 30-60 min
• Do not use if discolored or if particulates are present; discard unused portions

SIDE EFFECTS

CNS: Dizziness, syncope, tremor, drowsiness, fever, paresthesias, depression, fatigue, headache, suicidal ideation

CV: Atrial fibrillation/flutter, bradycardia, orthostatic hypotension, palpitations

EENT: Diplopia, blurred vision, tinnitus

GI: Nausea, constipation, vomiting, hepatitis, diarrhea, dyspepsia

HEMA: Anemia, neutropenia, agranulocytosis

INTEG: Rash, erythema, inj-site reaction, pruritus

SYST: Drug reaction with eosinophilia, systemic symptoms (DRESS), Stevens-Johnson syndrome, toxic epidermal necrolysis

PHARMACOKINETICS

Metabolized by liver; excreted by kidneys, 40%; protein binding <15%
PO: Peak 1-4 hr
IV: Peak 30-60 min; half-life 13 hr

INTERACTIONS

• **Increase:** PR prolongation—β-blockers, calcium channel blockers, atazanavir, dronedarone, digoxin, lopinavir, ritonavir
• **Increase:** lacosamide effect—CYP2C19 inhibitors (fluconazole, isoniazid, miconazole)

Drug/Lab Test
Increase: LFTs

NURSING CONSIDERATIONS

Assess:

• **Seizures:** duration, type, intensity, precipitating factors
• Renal function: albumin concentration
• CV status: orthostatic hypotension, PR prolongation; monitor cardiac status throughout treatment; ECG prior to therapy (IV), AV block may occur
• **Mental status:** mood, sensorium, affect, memory (long, short term), depression, suicidal ideation, psychologic dependence
• **Serious skin reactions:** discontinue product at first sign of rash
• **Pregnancy/breastfeeding:** Pregnant patient should enroll in North American Antiepileptic Drugs Pregnancy Registry, 1-888-233-2334; use only if benefits outweigh fetal risk; do not breastfeed, excretion unknown
• **Beers:** avoid in older adults unless safer alternatives are unavailable; may cause ataxia, impaired psychomotor function

Evaluate:

• Therapeutic response: increased seizure control

Teach patient/family:

• Not to discontinue product abruptly; to taper over 1 wk because seizures may occur
• To report blurred vision, nausea, dizziness, syncope; to avoid hazardous activities until stabilized on product

- To carry emergency ID stating product use
- To notify prescriber of suicidal thoughts/behaviors, syncope, cardiac changes
- To report rash, fever, fatigue, yellowing of skin, eyes, dark urine; may be hypersensitivity reaction
- To notify prescriber immediately if pregnancy is planned or suspected; to enroll in pregnancy registry at 888-233-2334, www.aedpregnancyregistry.org
- That interactions with other medications may occur; to report all OTC, Rx medications, herbals and supplements taken; not to use with alcohol
- To consult MedGuide for proper use, risks and review with patient

---

lactulose (Rx)

(lak´tyoo-lose)

Cholac, Constilac, Constulose, Enulose, Generlac, Kristalose

Func. class.: Laxative; ammonia detoxicant (hyperosmotic)

Chem. class.: Lactose synthetic derivative

Do not confuse:

lactulose/lactose

ACTION: Prevents absorption of ammonia in colon by acidifying stool; increases water, softens stool

USES: Chronic constipation, portal-systemic encephalopathy (PSE) in patients with hepatic disease

CONTRAINDICATIONS: Hypersensitivity, low-galactose diet

Precautions: Pregnancy, breastfeeding, geriatric patients, debilitated patients, diabetes mellitus

DOSAGE AND ROUTES

Constipation

- **Adult:** PO 15-30 mL/day (10-20 g), may increase to 60 mL/day prn
- **Child:** PO 7.5 mL/day after breakfast

Hepatic encephalopathy

- **Adult:** PO 30-45 mL (20-30 g) tid or qid until stools soft; **RETENTION ENEMA** 300 mL (200 g) diluted
- **Child:** PO (unlabeled) 40-90 mL/day in 3-4 divided doses
- **Infant:** PO (unlabeled) 2.5-10 mL/day in divided doses

Available forms: Oral sol 10 g/15 mL; packets 10, 20 g; rectal sol 10 g/15 mL

Administer:

PO route

- With 8 oz fruit juice, water, milk to increase palatability of oral form; for rapid effect, give on empty stomach
- Increased fluids to 2 L/day; do not give with other laxatives; if diarrhea occurs, reduce dosage
- **Kristalose:** dissolve contents of packet/4 oz water

Rectal route

- **Retention enema (no commercial product)** by diluting 300 mL lactulose/700 mL of water; administer by rectal balloon catheter; retain for >30 min; if retained for <30 min, repeat

SIDE EFFECTS

GI: *Nausea, vomiting, anorexia, abdominal cramps,* diarrhea, flatulence, distention, belching

META: Hypernatremia, hypokalemia; hyperglycemia (diabetes)

PHARMACOKINETICS

Metabolized in colon, excretion kidneys, unchanged, onset 1-2 days, peak unknown, duration unknown

INTERACTIONS

- Do not use with other laxatives (hepatic encephalopathy)

Decrease: lactulose effects—other oral antiinfectives, antacids

Drug/Herb

Increase: laxative action—flax, senna

Drug/Lab Test

Increase: blood glucose (diabetic patients)

Decrease: blood ammonia

L

NURSING CONSIDERATIONS
Assess:

- **Stool:** amount, color, consistency, frequency, abdominal pain/distention, bowel sounds prior to use and after use
- **Cause of constipation;** determine whether fluids, bulk, or exercise is missing from lifestyle; use of constipating products
- **Hepatic encephalopathy:** blood ammonia level (15-45 mcg/dL or 35-65 umol/L is normal range); may decrease ammonia level by 25%-50%; clearing of confusion, lethargy, restlessness, irritability if portal-systemic encephalopathy; monitor sodium in higher doses
- Blood, urine electrolytes if product used often; may cause diarrhea, hypokalemia, hyponatremia
- I&O ratio to identify fluid loss, replace any loss
- Cramping, rectal bleeding, nausea, vomiting; if these symptoms occur, product should be discontinued

Evaluate:

- Therapeutic response: decreased constipation, decreased blood ammonia level, clearing of mental state

Teach patient/family:

- Not to use as a laxative long term, to use as prescribed
- To dilute with water or fruit juice to counteract sweet taste
- To store in cool environment; not to freeze
- To take on an empty stomach for rapid action
- To report diarrhea, number, amount, consistency of stools; may indicate overdose

---

lamiVUDine 3TC (Rx)

(lam-i-voo′deen)

Epivir, Epivir HBV, Heptovir ♣

Func. class.: Antiretroviral

Chem. class.: Nucleoside reverse transcriptase inhibitor (NRTI)

Do not confuse:
lamiVUDine/lamoTRIgine

ACTION: Inhibits replication of HIV virus by incorporating into cellular DNA by viral reverse transcriptase, thereby terminating cellular DNA chain

USES: HIV-1–related infection in combination with at least 2 other antiretrovirals; chronic hepatitis B (Epivir HBV)
Unlabeled uses: Prophylaxis of HIV: postexposure with indinavir and zidovudine

CONTRAINDICATIONS: Hypersensitivity
Precautions: Pregnancy, breastfeeding, children, geriatric patients, granulocyte count <1000/mm^3 or Hgb <9.5 g/dL, renal disease, pancreatitis, peripheral neuropathy

> **Black Box Warning:** Severe hepatic dysfunction, lactic acidosis

DOSAGE AND ROUTES
HIV

- **Adult/adolescent >16 yr and ≥50 kg: PO** 150 mg bid or 300 mg/day; **<50 kg,** 2 mg/kg bid
- **Child 3 mo-16 yr: PO** 4 mg/kg bid, max 150 mg bid

Chronic hepatitis B with evidence of HBV replication and active liver inflammation

- **Adult: PO** 100 mg/day
- **Child/adolescent 2-17 yr: PO** 3 mg/kg/day, max 100 mg

Renal dose

- **Adult: PO** CCr 30-49 mL/min: Epivir 150 mg/day; Epivir HBV 100 mg 1st dose, then 50 mg/day; CCr 15-29 mL/min: Epivir 150 mg 1st dose, then 100 mg/day; Epivir HBV 100 mg 1st dose, then 25 mg/day; CCr 5-14 mL/min: Epivir 150 mg 1st dose, then 50 mg/day; Epivir HBV 35 mg 1st dose, then 15 mg/day; CCr <5 mL/min: Epivir 50 mg 1st dose, then 25 mg/day; Epivir HBV 35 mg 1st dose, then 10 mg/day

Available forms: **(Epivir)** oral sol 10 mg/mL; tabs 150, 300 mg; **(Epivir HBV)** oral sol 5 mg/mL; tabs 100 mg

Administer:

- PO daily or bid, without regard to meals

• Epivir and Epivir HBV are not interchangeable

• Use with other antiretrovirals only; do not use triple antiretroviral with abacavir or didanosine; resistance may occur

• Store in cool environment; protect from light

SIDE EFFECTS

CNS: *Fever, headache, malaise, dizziness, insomnia, depression, fatigue, chills,* seizures, peripheral neuropathy, paresthesias

EENT: Taste change, hearing loss, photophobia

GI: *Nausea, vomiting, diarrhea,* anorexia, cramps, dyspepsia, hepatomegaly with steatosis; pancreatitis (more common in children)

HEMA: Neutropenia, anemia, thrombocytopenia

INTEG: *Rash*

MS: *Myalgia, arthralgia, pain*

RESP: *Cough*

SYST: Lactic acidosis, anaphylaxis, Stevens-Johnson syndrome, immune reconstitution syndrome

PHARMACOKINETICS

Rapidly absorbed, distributed to extravascular space, excreted unchanged in urine, protein binding <36%, half-life 5-7 hr, child 2 hr, peak 3.2 hr

INTERACTIONS

Decrease: both products—zalcitabine; avoid concurrent use

Increase: pancreatitis—other products that cause pancreatitis

Increase: lamotrigine level—sulfamethoxazole-trimethoprim

• Do not use with emtricitabine, duplication

Decrease: lamiVUDine effect—interferons

Drug/Lab Test

Increase: ALT, bilirubin

Decrease: Hgb, neutrophil, platelet count

NURSING CONSIDERATIONS

Assess:

• **HIV:** Test for HIV before starting treatment, blood counts q2wk; watch for neutropenia, thrombocytopenia, Hgb, CD4, viral load; if low, therapy may have to be discontinued and restarted after hematologic recovery; blood transfusions may be required; assess for lessening of symptoms; if HBV is present, a higher dose of Epivir HBV is needed

Black Box Warning: Hepatitis B: fatigue, anorexia, pruritus, jaundice during and for several months after discontinuation; AST, ALT, bilirubin; amylase, lipase, triglycerides periodically during treatment

• **Children for pancreatitis:** abdominal pain, nausea, vomiting, neuropathy; discontinuing may be required; monitor amylase, lipase; use cautiously in children

Black Box Warning: Lactic acidosis, severe hepatomegaly with steatosis: obtain baseline LFTs; if elevated, discontinue treatment; discontinue even if LFTs are normal if lactic acidosis, severe hepatomegaly develops; may be fatal, especially in women

• **Pregnancy/breastfeeding:** Epivir is a drug that is used in pregnancy to treat HIV; enroll patient in the Antiretroviral Pregnancy Registry at 800-258-4263; do not breastfeed

Evaluate:

• Therapeutic response: decreasing symptoms of HIV, CD4, viral load

Teach patient/family:

• That GI complaints, insomnia resolve after 3-4 wk of treatment

• That product is not a cure for HIV but will control symptoms; that compliance is necessary; to take as directed; to complete full course of treatment even if feeling better

• To notify prescriber of sore throat, swollen lymph nodes, malaise, fever, peripheral neuropathy; other infections may occur

• To report pancreatitis, immune reconstitution syndrome immediately

• That patient is still infective, may pass HIV virus on to others

• That follow-up visits must be continued since serious toxicity may occur; that blood counts must be done

---

Side effects: *italics* = common; red = life-threatening

• That other products may be necessary to prevent other infections

• That product may cause fainting or dizziness

• **Pregnancy/breastfeeding:** to enroll in the Antiretroviral Pregnancy Registry at 800-258-4263; not to breastfeed

---

RARELY USED

lamivudine/tenofovir disoproxil

(lam-i-voo'deen ten-oh-foh'veer)

Cimduo

Func. class.: Antiretroviral

USES: In combination with other antiretrovirals for human immunodeficiency virus (HIV) infection

CONTRAINDICATIONS: Hypersensitivity

> Black Box Warning: Hepatitis B exacerbation

DOSAGE AND ROUTES

• **Adult/adolescent/child ≥35 kg: PO** 1 tablet (lamivudine 300 mg; tenofovir 300 mg) daily

---

lamoTRIgine (Rx)

(la-moe'tri-geen)

LaMICtal, LaMICtal CD, LaMICtal ODT, LaMICtal XR

Func. class.: Anticonvulsant— miscellaneous

Chem. class.: Phenyltriazine

Do not confuse:

lamoTRIgine/lamiVUDine LaMICtal/Lomotil/LamISIL

ACTION: Inhibits voltage-sensitive sodium channels, thus decreasing seizures

USES: Adjunct for the treatment of partial, tonic-clonic seizures; children with Lennox-Gastaut syndrome, bipolar disorder

Unlabeled uses: Absence seizures

CONTRAINDICATIONS: Hypersensitivity, mania

Precautions: Pregnancy (cleft lip/palate during 1st trimester), breastfeeding, geriatric patients, cardiac/renal/hepatic disease, severe depression, suicidal thoughts, blood dyscrasias, children <16 yr, risk of hemophagocytic lymphohistiocytosis (HLH)

> Black Box Warning: Serious rash

DOSAGE AND ROUTES

Seizures: monotherapy

• **Adult/adolescent ≥16 yr: PO** 50 mg/day while receiving 1 enzyme-inducing AED (carBAMazepine, PHENobarbital, phenytoin, primidone but not valproic acid) wk 1-2, then increase to 100 mg divided bid wk 3-4; maintenance 300-500 mg/day; **EXT REL** 50 mg/day × 1-2 wk, then 100 mg/day wk 3-4, then 200 mg/day wk 5, then 300 mg/day wk 6, then 400 mg/day wk 7; after wk 7, range is 400-600 mg/day

• **Adolescent <16 yr/child: PO** 0.3 mg/kg/day wk 1-2, then 0.6 mg/kg/day wk 3-4; depends on use of AED; usual dose 4.5-7.5 mg/kg/day, max 300 mg/day

Monotherapy for patients taking valproate

• **Adult/adolescent ≥16 yr receiving lamoTRIgine and valproate without enzyme-inducing drug: PO** (immediate release) stabilize on valproate, target dose of 200 mg/day lamoTRIgine; if patient is not taking lamoTRIgine 200 mg/day, increase dose by 25-50 mg/day q1-2wk to reach 200 mg/day; while maintaining lamoTRIgine 200 mg/day, decrease valproate to 500 mg/day by ≤500 mg/day/wk, maintain valproate at 500 mg/day × 1 wk, then increase lamoTRIgine to 300 mg/day while decreasing valproate 250 mg/day × 1 wk, then discontinue valproate and increase lamoTRIgine by 100 mg/day/wk to maintenance of 500 mg/day

Seizures: multiple therapy with valproate

• **Adult/adolescent ≥16 yr:** **PO** 25 mg every other day, then 25 mg/day wk 3-4, increase by 25-50 mg q1-2wk, maintenance 100-500 mg/day

• **Adolescent <16 yr/child:** **PO** 0.1-0.2 mg/kg/day initially, then increase q2wk as needed to 1-5 mg/kg/day or 200 mg/day

Hepatic dose

• **Adult: PO** moderate hepatic impairment or severe without ascites: reduce by 25%; severe hepatic impairment with ascites: reduce by 50%

Absence seizures (unlabeled)

• **Adult/child 3-13 yr: PO** 0.5 mg/kg/day in 2 divided doses × 2 wk, then 1 mg/kg/day in 2 divided doses × 2 wk, adjusted q5days

Available forms: Tabs 25, 100, 150, 200 mg; **PO** ext rel 25-50-100, 50-100-200 mg titration kit; PO 25-100 mg starter kit; **ext rel** 25, 50, 100, 250, 300 mg; **chew dispersible tabs** 5, 25 mg; **oral disintegrating tab** 25, 50, 100, 200 mg; **oral disintegrating tab** 25-50, 50-100 mg, 25-50-100 mg titration kit

Administer:

• Correct starter kit; severe side effects have occurred from incorrect starter kit

• Extended-release product is not to be used for conversion to monotherapy for ≥2 antiepileptic products

• **Orange starter kit:** for those **NOT** taking carBAMazepine, phenytoin, PHENobarbital, primidone, rifampin, valproate

• **Green starter kit:** for those taking carBAMazepine, phenytoin, PHENobarbital, primidone, rifampin but **NOT** valproate

• **Blue starter kit:** for those taking valproate

• Discontinue all products gradually over ≥2 wk; abrupt discontinuation can increase seizures

• All forms may be given without regard to meals

• **Chewable dispersible tab:** may be swallowed whole, chewed, mixed in water or fruit juice; to mix, add to small amount of liquid in glass or spoon; tabs will dissolve in 1 min, then mix in more liquid and swirl and swallow immediately; do not cut tabs in half

• **Orally disintegrating tabs:** place on tongue, move around in mouth; when disintegrated, swallow; examine blister pack before use, do not use if blisters are torn or missing

• **Extended-release tabs:** swallow whole, do not cut, break, chew; without regard to food

SIDE EFFECTS

CNS: *Dizziness,* ataxia, *headache,* fever, insomnia, tremor, depression, anxiety, suicidal ideation, seizures, poor concentration
EENT: Nystagmus, diplopia, blurred vision
GI: Nausea, vomiting, anorexia, abdominal pain, hepatotoxicity
GU: *Dysmenorrhea*
HEMA: Anemia, DIC, leukopenia, thrombocytopenia
INTEG: Rash (potentially life-threatening), alopecia, photosensitivity
CV: Chest pain, palpitations
MS: Neck pain, myalgias
SYST: Stevens-Johnson syndrome, angioedema, toxic epidermal necrolysis, DRESS

PHARMACOKINETICS

Half-life varies depending on dose; half-life 24 hr, 15 hr with enzyme inducers; rapidly, completely absorbed; metabolized by glucuronic acid conjunction; protein binding 55%; peak 1.4-2.3 hr, XR 4-10 hr; crosses placenta; excreted in breast milk

INTERACTIONS

Decrease: metabolic clearance of lamoTRIgine—valproic acid, CYP3A4 inhibitors
Decrease: lamoTRIgine concentration—carBAMazepine, acetaminophen, phenytoin, primidone, PHENobarbital, OXcarbazepine
Drug/Herb
Increase: anticonvulsant effect—ginkgo
Decrease: anticonvulsant effect—ginseng
Drug/Lab
False positive: PCP (rapid drug screen)

NURSING CONSIDERATIONS
Assess:
• **Seizure:** duration, type, intensity, halo before seizure baseline and periodically

Black Box Warning: Rash (Stevens-Johnson syndrome, toxic epidermal necrolysis) in pediatric patients: product should be discontinued at first sign of rash; more common in those taking multiple products for seizures; rash usually occurs during 2-8 wk of therapy

• **Bipolar disorder:** suicidal thoughts/behaviors
• **DRESS:** monitor for fever, rash, lymphadenopathy; may occur with hepatitis, nephritis, myocarditis; discontinue immediately, may involve multiple organ systems
• **Risk of hemophagocytic lymphohistiocytosis (HLH):** monitor for persistent fevers, rash, enlarged liver/spleen/lymph nodes, anemia, low platelets
Evaluate:
• Therapeutic response: decrease in severity of seizures or of bipolar symptoms
Teach patient/family:
• To take PO doses divided, with or after meals to decrease adverse effects; not to discontinue product abruptly because seizures may occur
• To avoid hazardous activities until stabilized on product
• To carry emergency ID; to notify prescriber of skin rash, increased seizure activity; to use sunscreen, protective clothing if photosensitivity occurs

Black Box Warning: Rash: to notify prescriber immediately if rash, fever, or swollen lymph nodes occur

• To notify prescriber immediately of suicidal thoughts/behaviors, new or worsening depression, anxiety, aggression
• **Pregnancy/breastfeeding:** to notify prescriber if pregnancy is planned or suspected; to use a nonhormonal contraceptive; to enroll with the North American Antiepileptic Drug Pregnancy Registry at 888-233-2334 (www.aedpregnancyregistry.org); that product decreases folate; to avoid breastfeeding

---

lansoprazole (Rx, OTC)
(lan-so-prey'zole)
Prevacid, Prevacid 24 hr, Prevacid SoluTab
Func. class.: Antiulcer, proton pump inhibitor
Chem. class.: Benzimidazole

Do not confuse:
Prevacid/Pravachol/Prinivil

ACTION: Suppresses gastric secretion by inhibiting hydrogen/potassium ATPase enzyme system in gastric parietal cell; characterized as gastric acid pump inhibitor because it blocks the final step of acid production

USES: Gastroesophageal reflux disease (GERD), severe erosive esophagitis, poorly responsive systemic GERD, pathologic hypersecretory conditions (Zollinger-Ellison syndrome, systemic mastocytosis, multiple endocrine adenomas); possibly effective for treatment of duodenal, gastric ulcers, maintenance of healed duodenal ulcers
Unlabeled uses: GERD (infants/neonates)

CONTRAINDICATIONS: Hypersensitivity
Precautions: Pregnancy, breastfeeding, children, hypomagnesemia, osteoporosis

DOSAGE AND ROUTES
Frequent heartburn
• **Adult:** PO (OTC) 15 mg daily up to 14 days
Duodenal ulcer
• **Adult:** PO 15 mg/day before eating for 4 wk, then 15 mg/day to maintain healing of ulcers; associated with *Helicobacter pylori:* 30 mg lansoprazole bid, 1 g amoxicillin bid; clarithromycin 500 mg bid × 10-14 day or lansoprazole tid with 1 g amoxicillin tid × 14 days
Pathologic hypersecretory conditions
• **Adult:** PO 60 mg/day, may give up to 90 mg bid, administer doses of >120 mg/day in divided doses

---

NSAID-related ulcer (continuing use)
• **Adult: PO** 30 mg daily × 8 wk
GERD/esophagitis
• **Adult/adolescent: PO** 15-30 mg/day × 8 wk
• **Child 1-11 yr (>30 kg): PO** 30 mg/day ≤12 wk
• **Child 1-11 yr (≤30 kg): PO** 15 mg/day ≤12 wk
• **Infant (unlabeled): PO** 1-1.74 mg/kg/day; limited data available
• **Neonate (unlabeled): PO** 0.5-1 mg/kg/day
Stress gastric prophylaxis
• **Adult: NG** Use 30 mg del rel caps or 30 mg disintegrating tab
Available forms: Del rel caps 15, 30 mg; orally disintegrating tabs 15, 30 mg
Administer:
PO route
• Swallow caps whole 30 min before eating; do not crush or chew caps; caps may be opened and contents sprinkled on food
Delayed-release capsules
• Swallow intact, do not chew or crush, may be opened and contents sprinkled on 1 Tbsp applesauce or other soft food, swallow immediately; or contents may be mixed into a small volume of juice, mixed and swallowed, rinse with 2 or more oz volume of liquid and have patient take
NG route
• **Oral cap:** open cap and pour ¼ of granules into NG feeding syringe with plunger removed, slowly add water and depress plunger, repeat until all granules used; flush tube with 15 mL water
• Place on tongue, allow to dissolve, use without regard to water
• **Oral syringe:** dissolve 15 mg/4 mL or 30 mg/10 mL water, use extra water in syringe to remove all of the product
NG tube
• **Oral disintegrating tab:** mix 30 mg tab in 10 mL water, give via NG tube, flush tube with 10 mL sterile water, clamp for 60 min

SIDE EFFECTS
CNS: *Headache,* dizziness
GI: Diarrhea, abdominal pain, nausea, *constipation,* flatulence, acid regurgitation, anorexia, irritable colon, CDAD

GU: Hematuria, glycosuria, impotence, kidney calculus, breast enlargement

PHARMACOKINETICS
Absorption after granules leave stomach 80%; half-life $1^1/_2$-2 hr; protein binding 97%; extensively metabolized in liver; excreted in urine, feces; clearance decreased in geriatric patients, renal/hepatic impairment, onset 1-3 hr, peak 1.7 hr duration 24 hr

INTERACTIONS
Increase: bleeding risk—warfarin
Decrease: lansoprazole absorption—sucralfate
Decrease: absorption of ketoconazole, itraconazole, iron salts, calcium carbonate, atazanavir, ampicillin
Increase: hypomagnesemia—loop/thiazide diuretics
Decrease: lansoprazole effect—antimuscarinics, H_2-blockers
• Avoid use with dasatinib, delavirdine
Drug/Herb
• Avoid use with red yeast rice, St. John's wort
Drug/Food
• Food decreases rate of absorption; use before food

NURSING CONSIDERATIONS
Assess:
• **CDAD:** bowel sounds, abdomen for pain, swelling; anorexia, blood in stool; may occur even after completion of therapy
• **Hepatic studies:** AST, ALT, alk phos during treatment
• INR and prothrombin time when taking warfarin
• **Magnesium:** low magnesium may occur, palpitations, muscle spasm, tremors
• **Beers:** avoid scheduled use for >8 wk unless for high-risk patients (oral corticosteroids/chronic NSAIDs use)
• **Pregnancy/breastfeeding:** use only if clearly needed; do not breastfeed
Evaluate:
• Therapeutic response: absence of epigastric pain, swelling, fullness

L

Teach patient/family:
• To report severe diarrhea, cramping, blood in stools, fever; product may have to be discontinued
• That hypoglycemia may occur if diabetic; to monitor blood glucose
• To avoid hazardous activities; that dizziness may occur
• To avoid alcohol, salicylates, ibuprofen; may cause GI irritation
• That if using OTC for heartburn, it may take 1-4 days to see full benefit
• Teach patient the reason for use and how to take, to take 30-60 min before eating
• Symptoms of low magnesium levels
• **Pregnancy:** to notify provider if pregnancy is planned or suspected or if breastfeeding

---

RARELY USED

lanthanum (Rx)
(lan′-tha-num)
Fosrenol
Func. class.: Phosphate binder

USES: End-stage renal disease

CONTRAINDICATIONS: Hypophosphatemia, hypersensitivity

DOSAGE AND ROUTES
• **Adult:** PO 750-1500 mg/day in divided doses with meals; titrate dose q2-3wk until an acceptable phosphate level is reached; tabs should be chewed completely before swallowing; intact tabs should not be swallowed; maintenance dose 1500-3000 mg/day divided with meals; max 3750 mg/day

---

RARELY USED

lapatinib (Rx)
(la-pa′tin-ib)
Tykerb
Func. class.: Antineoplastic—miscellaneous
Chem. class.: Biologic response modifier, signal transduction inhibitor (STIs)

USES: Advanced metastatic breast cancer patients with tumor that overexpresses HER2 protein and who have received previous chemotherapy

CONTRAINDICATIONS: Pregnancy, breastfeeding, hypersensitivity

DOSAGE AND ROUTES
Advanced/metastatic breast cancer with HER2 overexpression who have received previous therapy
• **Adult:** PO 1250 mg (5 tabs)/day 1 hr before or after food on days 1-21 plus capecitabine 2000 mg/m^2/day in 2 divided doses on days 1-14 in a repeating 21-day cycle; continue until therapeutic response or toxicity occurs
Metastatic breast cancer with HER2 overexpression for whom hormonal therapy is indicated
• **Adult:** PO 1500 mg (6 tabs) 1 hr before food with letrozole 2.5 mg/day
Hepatic dose
• **Adult:** PO (Child-Pugh C) 750 mg/day (with capecitabine); 1000 mg/day (with letrozole)

---

larotrectinib
(layr′oh-trek′tih-nib)
Vitrakvi
Func. class.: Antineoplastic—TRK inhibitor

USES: Metastatic or surgically unresectable neurotrophic receptor tyrosine kinase (NTRK) gene fusion–positive solid tumors with no known acquired resistance mutation, in patients with no satisfactory alternative treatments or in patients who have progressed following treatment

CONTRAINDICATIONS: Hypersensitivity, pregnancy

DOSAGE AND ROUTES
• **Adult/adolescent/child/infant:** PO For BSA ≥1 m^2, 100 mg bid; for BSA <1 m^2, 100 mg/m^2 bid; continue therapy until disease progression

---

latanoprost (ophthalmic)
(lah-tan′oh-prost)

Xalatan

Func. class.: Antiglaucoma agent
Chem. class.: Prostaglandin agonist

Do not confuse:
latanoprost/bimatoprost

ACTION: Increases aqueous humor outflow

USES: Increased intraocular pressure in those who have open-angle glaucoma/ocular hypertension and who do not respond to other IOP-lowering products

CONTRAINDICATIONS: Hypersensitivity to this product, benzalkonium chloride
Precautions: Eye infections, angle-closure glaucoma, renal/hepatic function impairment, children, contact lenses

DOSAGE AND ROUTES
• **Adult: OPHTH** Instill 1 drop in each affected eye (conjunctival sac) every night
Available forms: Ophthalmic solution 0.005%
Administer:
Ophthalmic route
• Wash hands before and after use; contact lenses should be removed before using the product, reinsert 15 min after use; contains benzalkonium chloride, which may be absorbed by soft contact lenses
• Tilt the head back slightly and pull the lower eyelid down with the index finger to form a pouch; squeeze the prescribed number of drops into the pouch and gently close the eyes for 1-2 min; do not blink; to avoid contamination, do not touch the tip of the dropper to the eye, fingertips, or other surface
• The solution may be used concomitantly with other topical ophthalmic drug products to lower IOP; if more than one topical ophthalmic drug is being used, the drugs should be administered at least 5 min apart
• Store unopened bottle refrigerated; once opened, it may be stored at room temperature, protected from light, for up to 6 wk

SIDE EFFECTS
EENT: *Conjunctival hyperemia, iris color change, ocular pruritus,* xerophthalmia, visual disturbance, ocular irritation/burning, foreign body sensation, ocular pain, blepharitis, cataracts, and superficial punctate keratitis
INTEG: Rash, allergic reactions
MISC: Flulike symptoms
CV: Angina

PHARMACOKINETICS
Ophthalmic: Onset 3-4 hr, peak 8-12 hr; half-life 3 hr

NURSING CONSIDERATIONS
Assess:
• **Intraocular pressure:** in those with ongoing increased IOP
Evaluate:
• Therapeutic response: decreasing IOP
Teach patient/family:
Ophthalmic route
• To wash hands before and after use; that contact lenses should be removed, reinsert 15 min after use; contains benzalkonium chloride, which may be absorbed by soft contact lenses
• Tilt the head back slightly and pull lower eyelid down to form a pouch; squeeze drops into the pouch and close the eyes for 1-2 min; not to blink; to avoid contamination, do not touch the tip of the dropper to the eye, fingertips, or other surface
• May be used concomitantly with other topical ophthalmic products to lower IOP; if more than one is used, the drugs should be administered at least 5 min apart, do not exceed dose
• To store unopened bottle refrigerated; once opened, it may be stored at room temperature, protected from light, for up to 6 wk

L

> ### ⚠ HIGH ALERT
>
> ## ledipasvir/sofosbuvir
> (le-dip′as-vir/soe-fos′bue-veer)
> Harvoni
> *Func. class.:* Antiviral, antihepatitis agent
> *Chem. class.:* NS5A inhibitor

ACTION: A combination product with an HCV NS5A inhibitor (ledipasvir) and a nucleotide analog HCV NS5B polymerase inhibitor (sofosbuvir)

USES: Chronic hepatitis C virus (HCV) genotype 1 infection in patients with compensated liver disease

CONTRAINDICATIONS: Hypersensitivity

Precautions: Decompensated hepatic disease, decompensated cirrhosis, severe renal impairment (eGFR <30 mL/min/1.73 m^2), end-stage renal failure requiring dialysis, pregnancy, breastfeeding

Black Box Warning: Hepatitis B exacerbation

DOSAGE AND ROUTES

For the treatment of chronic hepatitis C virus (HCV) genotype 1 infection:
• **Adult (treatment-naïve) without cirrhosis: PO** 1 tablet (90 mg ledipasvir; 400 mg sofosbuvir) daily with or without food; the recommended duration of treatment is 12 wk; however, 8-wk treatment can be considered for patients with a baseline HCV RNA <6 million IU/mL. Recommendation includes patients coinfected with HIV

Genotype 1
• **Adult (treatment-naïve) with compensated (Child-Pugh A) cirrhosis: PO** 1 tablet (90 mg ledipasvir; 400 mg sofosbuvir) daily with or without food; the recommended duration of treatment is 12 wk (recommendation includes patients coinfected with HIV)
• **Adult (treatment-experienced) without cirrhosis: PO** 1 tablet (90 mg ledipasvir; 400 mg sofosbuvir) daily with or without food; the recommended duration of treatment is 12 wk (recommendation includes patients coinfected with HIV)
• **Adult (treatment-experienced) with compensated (Child-Pugh A) cirrhosis: PO** 1 tablet (90 mg ledipasvir; 400 mg sofosbuvir) daily with or without food; for 24 wk
• **Adult (treatment-naïve and experienced) with decompensated (Child-Pugh B or C) cirrhosis: PO** 1 tablet (90 mg ledipasvir; 400 mg sofosbuvir) **PO** daily with ribavirin (600 mg **PO** daily) for 12 wk. Ribavirin must be administered with food
• **Adult (treatment-naïve and experienced) transplantation and is without cirrhosis or has compensated (Child-Pugh A) cirrhosis: PO** 1 tablet (90 mg ledipasvir; 400 mg sofosbuvir) daily with ribavirin for 12 wk. Ribavirin must be administered with food
• **Child/adolescent 12-17 yr (treatment-naïve) without cirrhosis or with compensated (Child-Pugh A) cirrhosis: PO** 1 tablet (90 mg ledipasvir; 400 mg sofosbuvir) daily with or without food. × 12 wk
• **Child/adolescent 12-17 yr (treatment-experienced) without cirrhosis: PO** 1 tablet (90 mg ledipasvir; 400 mg sofosbuvir) daily with or without food. × 12 wk
• **Child/adolescent 12-17 yr (treatment-experienced) with compensated (Child-Pugh A) cirrhosis: PO** 1 tablet (90 mg ledipasvir; 400 mg sofosbuvir) daily with or without food. × 24 wk

For the treatment of chronic hepatitis C virus (HCV) genotype 4, 5, 6 infection
• **Adult (treatment-naïve or experienced) without cirrhosis or who have compensated (Child-Pugh A) cirrhosis: PO** 1 tablet (90 mg ledipasvir; 400 mg sofosbuvir) daily with or without food. × 12 wk

• **Adult (treatment-naïve or experienced) who has undergone liver transplantation and is without cirrhosis or has compensated (Child-Pugh A) cirrhosis: PO** 1 tablet (90 mg ledipasvir; 400 mg sofosbuvir) daily with ribavirin for 12 wk. Ribavirin must be administered with food in 2 divided doses

• **Child/adolescent 12-17 yr (treatment-naïve or experienced) without cirrhosis or who has compensated (Child-Pugh A) cirrhosis: PO** 1 tablet (90 mg ledipasvir; 400 mg sofosbuvir) daily with or without food. × 12 wk

Available forms: Tab 90 mg ledipasir/400 mg sofosbuvir

Administer:

• Without regard to food

SIDE EFFECTS

CNS: *Fatigue, headache,* insomnia
GI: Nausea, vomiting, diarrhea

PHARMACOKINETICS

Ledipasvir: >99.8% protein binding, elimination biliary excretion, half-life 47 hr, peak 4-5 hr

Sofosbuvir: 61%-65% protein binding, elimination by the kidneys, 80% recovered in the urine, peak 0.8-1 hr, half-life 0.4 hr, metabolite 27 hr

INTERACTIONS

Increase: digoxin level—digoxin
Decrease: ledipasvir level—antacids; separate by ≥4 hr
Decrease: ledipasvir/sofosbuvir level—anticonvulsants, antimycobacterials (rifabutin, rifapentine), P-glycoprotein inducers; avoid using together
Decrease: ledipasvir level—H_2 receptor antagonists (famotidine), separate by ≥12 hr, max dose of H_2 receptor antagonist should not exceed famotidine 40 mg bid equivalent

Drug/Lab Test:
Increase: bilirubin, lipase, CK

NURSING CONSIDERATIONS
Assess:

• **Hepatitis C:** monitor hepatitis C RNA, serum bilirubin, creatinine

• **Pregnancy/breastfeeding:** use only if benefits outweigh fetal risk; cautious use in breastfeeding, excretion unknown

Black Box Warning: **Hepatitis B:** test prior to initiating therapy; risk of fulminant hepatitis and death

Evaluate:

• Therapeutic response: hepatitis C RNA reduction
• CHC is decreased

Teach patient/family:

• To report effects to the prescriber
• To notify all providers of product use
• To take at the same time each day, to use for full course even if feeling better, to take missed doses when remembered on the same day; not to double doses
• That the product will not decrease transmission of infection in others
• If antacids (magnesium, aluminum) are needed, take 4 hr before or after this product

---

leflunomide (Rx)

(leh-floo'noh-mide)
Arava
Func. class.: Antirheumatic (DMARDs)
Chem. class.: Immune modulator, pyrimidine synthesis inhibitor

ACTION: Inhibits an enzyme involved in pyrimidine synthesis; has antiproliferative, antiinflammatory effect

USES: RA: to reduce disease process and symptoms
Unlabeled uses: Juvenile RA

CONTRAINDICATIONS: Breastfeeding, hypersensitivity

Black Box Warning: Pregnancy

Precautions: Children, renal disorders, vaccinations, infection, alcoholism, immunosuppression, jaundice, lactase deficiency, hepatic disease

---

DOSAGE AND ROUTES
Rheumatoid arthritis
• **Adult:** PO Loading dose 100 mg/day × 3 days, maintenance 20 mg/day; may be decreased to 10 mg/day if not well tolerated

Juvenile rheumatoid arthritis (unlabeled)
• **Adolescent/child >40 kg: PO** 20 mg/day
• **Adolescent/child 20-40 kg: PO** 15 mg/day
• **Adolescent/child 10-19.9 kg: PO** 10 mg/day

Available forms: Tabs 10, 20 mg
Administer:
• With food for GI upset, give same time each day, loading dose is recommended
• **Drug elimination:** give cholestyramine 8 g tid × 11 days; check levels

SIDE EFFECTS
CNS: *Headache,* dizziness, insomnia, depression, paresthesia, anxiety, migraine, neuralgia
CV: Palpitations, hypertension, chest pain, angina pectoris, peripheral edema
EENT: Pharyngitis, oral candidiasis, stomatitis, dry mouth, blurred vision
GI: *Nausea, anorexia, vomiting, constipation, flatulence, diarrhea, elevated LFTs,* hepatotoxicity, weight loss
HEMA: Anemia, ecchymosis, hyperlipidemia
INTEG: Rash, pruritus, alopecia, acne, hematoma, herpes infections
RESP: Pharyngitis, rhinitis, bronchitis, cough, respiratory infection, pneumonia, sinusitis, interstitial lung disease
SYST: Opportunistic/fatal infections, Stevens-Johnson syndrome, toxic epidermal necrolysis, DRESS

PHARMACOKINETICS
Metabolized in liver to active metabolite, half-life of metabolite 2 wk, excreted in urine, protein binding, 99%, crosses placenta, onset 99 min, peak up to 6 min of RA effect

INTERACTIONS
Increase: NSAID effect—NSAIDs
Increase: hepatotoxicity—hepatotoxic agents, methotrexate
Increase: leflunomide levels—rifampin
Increase: bleeding risk—warfarin
Decrease: antibody response—live virus vaccines
Decrease: leflunomide effect—cholestyramine, use for overdose

NURSING CONSIDERATIONS
Assess:
• **Arthritic symptoms:** ROM, mobility, swelling of joints at baseline and during treatment
• Screen for latent TB before starting treatment; if TB is present, pretreat before using product
• **Interstitial lung disease:** increased or worsening cough, SOB, fever; product may need to be discontinued and drug elimination procedure initiated (rare)

• CBC with differential monthly × 6 mo, then q6-8 wk thereafter; pregnancy test; serum electrolytes
• **Infections:** fatal infections can occur
• B/P, weight; edema can occur
• **Stevens-Johnson syndrome, toxic epidermal necrolysis:** monitor for rash during treatment; if rash with fever, fatigue, joint aches, blisters is present, discontinue immediately, initiate drug elimination procedure

Evaluate:
• Therapeutic response: decreased inflammation, pain in joints

Teach patient/family:
• That continuing monitoring will be needed
• That product must be continued for prescribed time to be effective, that up to a month may be required for improvement, that other treatment may continue corticosteroids, NSAIDs
• To take with food, milk, or antacids to avoid GI upset; to take at same time of day
• To use caution when driving because drowsiness, dizziness may occur
• To take with a full glass of water to enhance absorption, may continue with correct prescribed treatment with other antiinflammatories
• To discuss with health care professional all Rx, OTC, herbals, supplements used
• That hair may be lost; review alternatives
• To avoid live virus vaccinations during treatment
• To notify prescriber of weight loss
• Overdose treatment: give cholestyramine 8 g tid × 11 days

Black Box Warning: Pregnancy/breast-feeding: not to become pregnant while taking this product; not to breastfeed while taking this product; men should also discontinue product and begin leflunomide removal protocol if pregnancy is planned

⚠ HIGH ALERT
RARELY USED

lenvatinib
(len-va′-ti-nib)
Lenvima ✦
Func. class.: Antineoplastic

USES: Locally recurrent or metastatic, progressive, radioactive iodine-refractory differentiated thyroid cancer (DTC)

CONTRAINDICATIONS: Hypersensitivity

DOSAGE AND ROUTES
Thyroid cancer
• **Adult: PO** 24 mg (two 10-mg capsules and one 4-mg capsule) daily
Advanced renal cell carcinoma after 1 prior treatment, used with everolimus
• **Adult: PO** 18 mg/day with everolimus 5 mg/day

RARELY USED

letermovir
(le-term-oh-vir)
Prevymis
Func. class.: Antiviral

USES: For the prevention of cytomegalovirus following allogenic hematopoietic stem cell transplant

DOSAGE AND ROUTES
Cytomegalovirus (CMV) disease prophylaxis
• **Adult: PO/IV** 480 mg/day started between day 0 and day 28 after transplantation (before or after engraftment) and continued through day 100 after transplantation
Cytomegalovirus (CMV) disease prophylaxis in patients with concurrent cycloSPORINE
• **Adult: PO/IV** 240 mg/day started between day 0 and day 28 after transplantation (before or after engraftment) and continued through day 100 after transplantation. If cyclosporine is initiated after starting letermovir, reduce letermovir to 240 mg with the next dose. If cyclosporine is discontinued after starting letermovir, increase the dose of letermovir to 480 mg. If cyclosporine dosing is interrupted due to high cyclosporine concentrations, no dosage adjustment of letermovir is needed

⚠ HIGH ALERT

letrozole (Rx)
(let´tro-zohl)
Femara
Func. class.: Antineoplastic, non-steroidal aromatase inhibitor

Do not confuse:
Femara/Femhrt

ACTION: Binds to the heme group of aromatase; inhibits conversion of androgens to estrogens to reduce plasma estrogen levels

USES: Early, advanced, or metastatic breast cancer in postmenopausal women who are hormone receptor positive
Unlabeled uses: Infertility, idiopathic short stature, constitutional delayed puberty

CONTRAINDICATIONS: Pregnancy, premenopausal females, hypersensitivity
Precautions: Respiratory/hepatic disease, osteoporosis

DOSAGE AND ROUTES
• **Adult: PO** 2.5 mg/day
Infertility (unlabeled)
• **Adult: PO** 2.5, 5, 7.5 mg/day × 5 days, usually days 3-7 of menstrual cycle
Idiopathic short stature, constitutional delayed puberty (unlabeled)
• **Adolescent and child ≥9 (male): PO** 2.5 mg/day; use with testosterone for delayed puberty
Available forms: Tabs 2.5 mg
Administer:
• Without regard to meals; with small glass of water
• May administer bisphosphonates to increase bone density

SIDE EFFECTS
CNS: *Headache, lethargy,* somnolence, dizziness, depression, anxiety
CV: Angina, MI, CVA, thromboembolic events, hypertension, peripheral edema
GI: *Nausea, vomiting, anorexia,* constipation, heartburn, diarrhea
GU: Endometrial cancer, vaginal bleeding, endometrial proliferation disorders
INTEG: *Rash, pruritus,* alopecia, sweating
MISC: Hot flashes, night sweats, second malignancies, anaphylaxis, angioedema, infections
MS: Arthralgia, arthritis, bone fracture, myalgia, osteoporosis
RESP: Dyspnea, cough

PHARMACOKINETICS
Metabolized in liver, excreted in urine, peak 2 days, terminal half-life 48 hr, steady state 2-6 wk

INTERACTIONS
Decrease: letrozole effect—estrogens, oral contraceptives

NURSING CONSIDERATIONS
Assess:
• **Pain:** Assess pain baseline and periodically
• Hepatic studies before, during therapy (bilirubin, AST, ALT, LDH) as needed or monthly
Evaluate:
• Therapeutic response: decrease in size of tumor
Teach patient/family:
• To report allergic reactions (rash; hives; difficulty breathing; tightness in chest; swelling of mouth, face, lips, tongue)
• To report vaginal bleeding, diarrhea, chest/bone pain
• To use adequate contraception in perimenopausal, recently postmenopausal women
• To avoid driving or other hazardous activities until response is known, dizziness may occur

RARELY USED

leucovorin (Rx)
(loo-koe-vor´in)
Func. class.: Vitamin, folic acid/methotrexate antagonist antidote
Chem. class.: Tetrahydrofolic acid derivative

USES: Megaloblastic or macrocytic anemia caused by folic acid deficiency, overdose of folic acid antagonist, methotrexate/pyrimethamine/trimetrexate/trimethoprim toxicity, pneumocystosis, toxoplasmosis

CONTRAINDICATIONS: Hypersensitivity to this product or folic acid, benzyl alcohol; anemias other than megaloblastic not associated with vit B_{12} deficiency

DOSAGE AND ROUTES
Methotrexate toxicity/leucovorin rescue
• **Adult/child: PO/IM/IV normal elimination** given 6 hr after dose of methotrexate (10 mg/m^2) until methotrexate $<5 \times 10^{-8}$ m, CCr >50% above prior level, or methotrexate level 5×10^{-8} m at 24 hr or $>9 \times 10^{-8}$ m at 48 hr; give leucovorin 100 mg/m^2 q3hr until level drops to $<10^{-8}$ m
Megaloblastic anemia caused by enzyme deficiency
• **Adult/child: PO/IV/IM** up to 6 mg/day
Pyrimethamine/trimethoprim toxicity prevention
• **Adult/child: PO/IV** 5-15 mg/day
Advanced colorectal cancer
• **Adult: IV** 200 mg/m^2, then 5-FU 370 mg/m^2 or leucovorin 20 mg/m^2, then 5-FU 425 mg/m^2; give daily × 5 days q4-5wk

---

⚠ HIGH ALERT

leuprolide (Rx)
(loo-proe′lide)
Eligard, Lupron Depot, Lupron Depot-Ped, Lupron ✦
Func. class.: Antineoplastic hormone
Chem. class.: Gonadotropin-releasing hormone

ACTION: Causes initial increase in circulating levels of LH, FSH; continuous administration results in decreased LH, FSH; in men, testosterone is reduced to castrate levels; in premenopausal women, estrogen is reduced to menopausal levels

USES: Metastatic prostate cancer (inj implant), management of endometriosis, central precocious puberty, uterine leiomyomata (fibroids)
Unlabeled uses: Breast cancer, recurrent priapism, benign prostatic hyperplasia

CONTRAINDICATIONS: Pregnancy, breastfeeding, hypersensitivity to GnRH or analogs, thromboembolic disorders, undiagnosed vaginal bleeding; Eligard should not be used in women, children
Precautions: Edema, hepatic disease, CVA, MI, seizures, hypertension, diabetes mellitus, HF, depression, osteoporosis, spinal cord compression, urinary tract obstruction

DOSAGE AND ROUTES
Advanced prostate cancer
• **Adult: SUBCUT** 1 mg/day; **IM** 7.5 mg/depot dose monthly; **IM** 22.5 mg depot q3mo; or **IM** 30 mg depot q4mo; or **IM** 45 mg depot q6mo; **SUBCUT** (Eligard) 7.5 q mo; **SUBCUT** 22.5 mg (Eligard) q 3 mo; **SUBCUT** 45 mg (Eligard) q mo
Endometriosis
• **Adult: IM** 3.75 mg depot monthly for 6 mo or 11.25 mg q3mo for 6 mo or 30 mg q4mo
Anemia related to uterine fibroids
• **Adult: IM** 3.75 mg depot q mo × 3 mo or 11.25 mg depot as a single dose
Central precocious puberty
• **Child: SUBCUT** 50 mcg/kg/day; may increase by 10 mcg/kg/day as needed
• **Child >37.5 kg: IM** Lepron Depot-Ped 15 mg q4wk
• **Child 25-37.5 kg: IM** Lepron Depot-Ped 11.25 mg q4wk
• **Child ≤25 kg: IM** Lepron Depot-Ped 7.5 mg q4wk
Benign prostatic hyperplasia (BPH) (unlabeled)
• **Adult: SUBCUT** (sol for inj) 1 mg/day, **IM**(injection susp) 3.75 mg q28day × 24 wk

Available forms: Lupron Depot inj: 3.75, 7.5, 11.25, 15, 22.5, 30, 45 mg;

Solution for Subcut Inj: 5 mg/mL (2.8-mL multidose vials)

• Never give IV

Administer:

• Store in tight container at room temperature

• **SUBCUT:** No dilution needed if patient self-administering; make sure patient is using syringes provided by manufacturer

• **SUBCUT Eligard** bring to room temperature, once mixed, give within 30 min, prepare the 2 syringes for mixing, join the 2 syringes together by pushing in and twisting until secure; mix the product by pushing the contents of both syringes back and forth between syringes until uniform; should be light tan to tan, hold syringes vertically with syringe B on the bottom, draw entire mixed product into syringe B (short, wide syringe) by depressing the syringe A plunger and slightly withdrawing syringe B plunger, uncouple syringe A, while pushing down on syringe A plunger, small air bubbles will remain, hold syringe B upright, remove pink cap, attach needle cartridge to the end of syringe B, remove needle cover, give by subcut

IM route

• **Monthly:** reconstitute single-use vial with 1 mL of diluent; if multiple vials used, withdraw 0.5 mL, inject into each vial (1 mL); withdraw all, inject at 90-degree angle (3.75 mg)

• **3-mo:** reconstitute microspheres using 1.5 mL of diluent, inject into vial; shake, withdraw, inject

SIDE EFFECTS

CNS: Memory impairment, depression, seizures

CV: MI, PE, dysrhythmias, peripheral edema

GI: Nausea, vomiting, anorexia, diarrhea, GI bleeding

GU: Edema, hot flashes, impotence, decreased libido, amenorrhea, vaginal dryness, gynecomastia, profuse vaginal bleeding

INTEG: Alopecia

MS: Bone pain

RESP: Dyspnea, pulmonary fibrosis, interstitial lung disease

PHARMACOKINETICS

IM/SUBCUT: Peak 1-2 mo, duration 1-3 mo; absorbed rapidly (SUBCUT), slowly (IM depot); half-life 3 hr

INTERACTIONS

Increase: antineoplastic action—flutamide, megestrol

Increase: seizure risk—SSRIs

Drug/Herb

• Do not use with black cohosh or chaste tree fruit; may interfere with treatment

NURSING CONSIDERATIONS

Assess:

• **Prostate cancer:** increased bone pain for first 4 wk of treatment; those with metastases in spinal column may exhibit severe back pain

• **Symptoms of endometriosis** (lower abdominal pain)/fibroids (pelvic pain, excessive vaginal bleeding, bloating) before, during, after treatment

• **Central precocious puberty (CPP)** diagnosis should have been confirmed by secondary S_4 characteristics in children <9 yr, estradiol/testosterone levels, GnRH test, tomography of head, adrenal steroids, chorionic gonadotropin, wrist x-ray, height, weight

• Hepatic studies (bilirubin, AST, ALT, LDH) before, during therapy monthly, as needed; PSA, calcium, testosterone with prostate cancer; bone mineral density; blood glucose, HbA1c

• Pituitary gonadotropic and gonadal function during therapy and 4-8 wk after therapy is discontinued

• **QT prolongation (depot):** ECG in CV patients using depot route

• **Tumor flare:** worsening of signs and symptoms; normal during beginning therapy

• Fatigue, increased pulse, pallor, lethargy; edema in feet, joints; stomach pain

• **Severe allergic reaction:** rash, pruritus, urticaria, purpuric skin lesions, itching, flushing

Evaluate:

• Therapeutic response: decreased tumor size and spread of malignancy; decrease in lesions, pain with endometriosis, fibroids, correction of CPP; increased follicle maturation

Teach patient/family:

• To notify prescriber if menstruation continues; menstruation should stop

• That bone pain will disappear after 1 wk

• To report any complaints, side effects to nurse, prescriber; that hot flashes may occur; to record weight, report gain of >2 lb/day

• How to prepare, give; to rotate sites for SUBCUT/IM inj; to use only syringes provided by manufacturer; to store depot at room temperature, to refrigerate unopened vials, to protect all from heat

• To keep accurate records of dose

• That tumor flare may occur: increase in size of tumor, increased bone pain, will subside rapidly; may take analgesics for pain, usually in prostate cancer or central precocious puberty

• That ongoing treatment is needed in central precocious puberty

• That voiding problems may increase during beginning of therapy but will decrease in several weeks

• Pregnancy: to notify prescriber if pregnancy is planned or suspected; not to breastfeed; to use nonhormonal form of contraception (women of childbearing age)

---

levalbuterol (Rx)

(lev-al-byoo′ter-ole)

Xopenex, Xopenex HFA

Func. class.: Bronchodilator, adrenergic β₂-agonist

ACTION: Causes bronchodilation by action on β_2 (pulmonary) receptors by increasing levels of cAMP, which relaxes smooth muscle; produces bronchodilation, CNS, cardiac stimulation as well as increased diuresis and gastric acid secretion

USES: Treatment or prevention of bronchospasm (reversible obstructive airway disease), asthma

CONTRAINDICATIONS: Hypersensitivity to sympathomimetics, this product, albuterol

Precautions: Pregnancy, breastfeeding, hyperthyroidism, diabetes mellitus, hypertension, prostatic hypertrophy, angle-closure glaucoma, seizures, renal disease, QT prolongation, tachydysrhythmias, severe cardiac disease, hypokalemia, children

DOSAGE AND ROUTES
Bronchospasm in reversible obstructive airway disease

• **Adult/child ≥12 yr: INH** 0.63 mg tid q6-8hr by nebulization, may increase 1.25 mg q8hr

• **Adult/adolescent/child >4 yr:** (HFA, metered dose) 90 mcg (2**INH**) q4-6hr

• **Child 6-11 yr: INH** 0.31 mg tid by nebulization, max 0.63 mg tid

Available forms: Sol, inh pediatric 0.31 mg/3 mL; 0.63 mg/3 mL; 1.25 mg/3 mL; 1.25 mg/0.5 mL; 45 mcg per actuation (HFA)

Administer:

• Every 6-8hr; wait ≥1 min between inhalation of aerosols

Inhalation route

• Keep unopened until ready for use; after opening, use within 2 wk; protect from light, heat

• Shake well before use; use a spacer device; prime with 4 test sprays in new canister or when not used for >3 days

Nebulizer route

• Dilute concentrated (1.25 mg/0.5 mL) with normal sterile saline before use

SIDE EFFECTS

CNS: *Tremors, anxiety,* insomnia, *headache,* dizziness

CV: Tachycardia

EENT: Dry nose, irritation of nose and throat, rhinitis

GI: Diarrhea, dyspepsia

INTEG: Rash

META: *Hypokalemia, hyperglycemia*

MS: Muscle cramps

RESP: Cough, dyspnea, bronchospasm

MISC: Flu-like symptoms

PHARMACOKINETICS

Metabolized in the liver and tissues; crosses placenta, breast milk, blood-brain barrier; half-life 3.3-4 hr

---

Side effects: *italics* = common; red = life-threatening

INH sol: Onset 10-17 min, peak $1^1/_2$ hr, duration 5-6 hr; **INH aerosol:** onset 4.5-10.2 min, peak 76-78 min, duration ≤6 hr

INTERACTIONS

Increase: hypokalemia—loop/thiazide diuretics

Increase: action of aerosol bronchodilators

Increase: levalbuterol action—tricyclics, MAOIs, other adrenergics; avoid use within 2 wk of MAOIs

Decrease: levalbuterol action—other β-blockers; severe bronchospasm may occur

Decrease: digoxin effect—digoxin

Drug/Herb

Increase: stimulation—black/green tea, coffee, cola nut, guarana, yerba maté

NURSING CONSIDERATIONS
Assess:

• **Respiratory function:** vital capacity, pulse oximetry, forced expiratory volume, ABGs, lung sounds, heart rate and rhythm (baseline); character of sputum: color, consistency, amount

• Cardiac status: palpitations, increase/decrease in B/P, dysrhythmias

• **For evidence of allergic reactions, paradoxic bronchospasm, anaphylaxis, angioedema;** if these occur, hold dose, notify prescriber at once; bronchospasm may occur with new canister or vial

• **Pregnancy/breastfeeding:** avoid use in pregnancy, do not breastfeed, reaction is unknown

Evaluate:

• Therapeutic response: absence of dyspnea, wheezing after 1 hr; improved airway exchange, ABGs/VBGs

Teach patient/family:

• Not to use OTC medications because excess stimulation may occur

• To avoid getting aerosol in eyes because blurring may result

• To avoid smoking, smoke-filled rooms, persons with respiratory infections

• That paradoxic bronchospasm may occur; to stop product immediately, contact prescriber

• To limit caffeine products such as chocolate, coffee, tea, colas, and herbs such as cola nut, guarana, yerba maté

• **Inhaler:** to shake well before using and to breathe normally while using and mist goes into reservoir; to spray 4 times before first use or if not used for 3 days; to wash at least weekly

• To use this product first if using other inhalers; to wait 5 min or more between products; to rinse mouth with water after each dose to prevent dry mouth

• **Diabetes:** that diabetes may be exacerbated; that medications for diabetes may need to be adjusted

TREATMENT OF OVERDOSE: Administer a $β_1$-adrenergic blocker

---

levETIRAcetam (Rx)
(lev-eh-teer-ass′eh-tam)
Keppra, Keppra XR, Spritam
Func. class.: Anticonvulsant
Chem. class.: Pyrrolidine derivative

Do not confuse:
Keppra/Kaletra
levETIRAcetam/lamotrigine/levocarnitine/levofloxacin

ACTION: Unknown; may inhibit nerve impulses by limiting influx of sodium ions across cell membrane in motor cortex

USES: Adjunctive therapy for partial-onset seizures, primary generalized tonic-clonic seizures, myoclonic seizures in juvenile patients

CONTRAINDICATIONS: Hypersensitivity, breastfeeding

Precautions: Pregnancy, children, geriatric patients, renal/cardiac disease, psychosis

DOSAGE AND ROUTES
Adjunctive treatment of partial-onset seizures

• **Adult/adolescent ≥16 yr:** IV 500 mg bid, may be titrated by 1000 mg/day q2wk, max 3000 mg/day in divided doses; **EXT REL** 1000 mg/day, may increase q2wk, max 3000 mg/day

• **Adolescent <16 yr/child: 1 mo to <6 mo** (immediate-release tablet, injection or oral solution): Initially, 7 mg/kg **IV/PO** bid; increase by 14 mg/kg/day in 2 divided doses q2wk to target dose of 42 mg/kg/day in 2 divided doses. For **PO**, use oral sol with weight of ≤20 kg

6 mo to <4 yr (immediate-release tablet, injection, or oral sol): Initially, 10 mg/kg **IV/PO** bid; increase by 20 mg/kg/day in 2 divided doses q2wk to target dose of 50 mg/kg/day in 2 divided doses as tolerated. For oral administration, use oral sol with weight of ≤20 kg

4 yr to <16 yr and 20-40 kg (immediate-release tablet): Initially, 250 mg **PO** bid; titration, increase by 500 mg/day in 2 divided doses q2wk to max 1500 mg/day in 2 divided doses

4 yr to <16 yr and >40 kg (immediate-release tablet): Initially, 500 mg **PO** bid; increase by 1000 mg/day q2wk in 2 divided doses to max 3000 mg/day in 2 divided doses

4 yr to <16 yr (oral sol): Initially, 10 mg/kg orally bid; increase by 20 mg/kg/day in 2 divided doses q2wk to target dose of 60 mg/kg/day in 2 divided doses as tolerated

Myoclonic seizures/tonic-clonic seizures/partial seizures

• **Adult/adolescent ≥16 yr: PO/IV** 500 mg bid, may increase by 1000 mg/day q2wk, max 3000 mg/day in 2 divided doses

Adjunctive treatment of partial onset seizures in those with epilepsy (Spritam)

• **Adult/child ≥4 yr and >40 kg: PO** 500 mg bid, may increase q2wk by 500 mg bid, max 1500 mg bid

Renal dose

• **Adult: PO** CCr 50-80 mL/min, 500-1000 mg q12hr or **EXT REL** 1000-2000 mg q24hr, max 2000 mg/day; CCr 30-49 mL/min, 250-750 mg q12hr or **EXT REL** 500-1500 mg q24hr, max 1500 mg/day; CCr <30 mL/min, 250-500 mg q12hr or **EXT REL** 500-1000 mg q24hr, max 1000 mg/day

Available forms: Tabs 250, 500, 750, 1000 mg; oral sol 100 mg/mL; sol for inj 100 mg/mL; ext rel tab 500, 750 mg;

premixed solution 1000 mg/100 mL 0.75% NaCl, 1500 mg/100 mL, 500 mg/100 mL 0.82% NaCl; tabs for oral suspension (Spirtam) 250, 500, 750, 1000 mg

Administer:

PO route

• Extended-release product should not be used in dialysis patients

• Swallow tab whole; do not break, crush, or chew

• With food, milk to decrease GI symptoms (rare) if needed

• Store at room temperature (PO)

Child:

• <20 kg should be given oral solution; use calibrated device

Tabs for oral suspension (Spirtam)

• Give only whole tabs

• Peel foil from blister; do not push through foil

• Place on tongue and swallow with a sip of liquid; do not swallow whole

• Tab can be added to a tablespoon of liquid in a cup; swirl gently, consume

Intermittent IV INFUSION route

• Single-use vials: dilute in 100 mL of 0.9% NaCl, D₅W, LR; give over 15 min, discard unused vial contents, do not use product with particulates or discoloration

• **Child:** max concentration of product 15 mg/mL (diluted solution); infuse over 15 min

• Diluted preparation stable for 24 hr at room temperature in polyvinyl bags

• Store vials at room temperature

Additive compatibilities: diazepam, LORazepam, valproate

SIDE EFFECTS

CNS: Dizziness, somnolence, asthenia, psychosis, suicidal ideation, nonpsychotic behavioral symptoms, headache, ataxia

EENT: Diplopia, conjunctivitis

GI: Nausea, vomiting, anorexia, diarrhea, constipation, hepatitis

HEMA: Infection, leukopenia

INTEG: Pruritus, rash

MISC: Infection, abdominal pain, pharyngitis

Side effects: *italics* = common; red = life-threatening

SYST: Stevens-Johnson syndrome, toxic epidermal necrolysis; dehydration (child <4 yr)

PHARMACOKINETICS
Rapidly absorbed; not protein bound; excreted via kidneys 66% unchanged; half-life 6-8 hr, longer in geriatric patients or with renal disease

INTERACTIONS
Increase: sedation—TCAs, antihistamines, benzodiazepines, other CNS depressants, alcohol
• Possible increased carBAMazepine toxicity: carBAMazepine
Decrease: levETIRAcetam absorption—sevelamer; separate by 1 hr before, 3 hr after sevelamer
Drug/Lab Test
Decrease: Hct/Hgb, WBC, RBC

NURSING CONSIDERATIONS
Assess:
• **Seizures:** type, location, duration, character, intensity, precipitating factors; provide seizure precautions
• Renal studies: urinalysis, BUN, urine creatinine q3mo
• Blood studies: CBC, LFTs
• **Mental status:** mood, sensorium, affect, behavioral changes, **suicidal thoughts/behaviors;** if mental status changes, notify prescriber
• Assistance with ambulation during early part of treatment; dizziness occurs
• **Beers:** avoid in older adults unless safer alternative is unavailable; may cause ataxia, impaired psychomotor function
• **Pregnancy:** if used during pregnancy, patient should enroll in the Antiepileptic Drug Pregnancy Registry at 888-233-2334; do not breastfeed
Evaluate:
• Therapeutic response: decreased seizure activity; document on patient's chart
Teach patient/family:
• To take with or without food
• Not to crush, break, chew tablets
• To carry emergency ID stating patient's name, products taken, condition, prescriber's name, phone number

• How to use oral sol; if trouble swallowing, measure oral sol in medicine cup or dropper, do not use teaspoon
• To avoid driving, other activities that require alertness until response is known; drowsiness occurs during first month
• Not to discontinue medication quickly after long-term use because withdrawal seizure may occur
• To immediately report suicidal thoughts or behaviors, mood changes, hostility, thoughts of death, dying
• **Pregnancy/breastfeeding:** to notify prescriber if pregnant, intending to become pregnant; not to breastfeed, excreted in breast milk

---

levobetaxolol ophthalmic
See Appendix B

---

levobunolol (ophthalmic)
(lee′voe-byoo′no-lahl)
Betagan
Func. class.: Antiglaucoma
Chem. class.: β-Blocker

ACTION: Can decrease aqueous humor and increase outflows

USES: Treatment of chronic open-angle glaucoma and ocular hypertension

CONTRAINDICATIONS: Hypersensitivity, AV block, heart failure, bradycardia, sick sinus syndrome, asthma
Precautions: Abrupt discontinuation, children, pregnancy, breastfeeding, COPD, depression, diabetes mellitus, myasthenia gravis, hyperthyroidism, pulmonary disease, sulfite sensitivity, angle-closure glaucoma

DOSAGE AND ROUTES
• **Adult:** Instill 1-2 drops in the affected eyes once a day (0.5% solution), bid (0.25% solution)

Available forms: Ophthalmic solution 0.25%, 0.5%

Administer:

• For ophthalmic use only

• To prevent contamination, do not touch the tip of the dropper to the eye, fingertips, or other surface

• Wash hands before and after use; tilt head back slightly and pull the lower eyelid down with the index finger to form a pouch; squeeze the prescribed number of drops into the pouch; close eyes to spread drops; to avoid excessive systemic absorption, apply finger pressure on the lacrimal sac for 1-2 min after use

• If more than one topical ophthalmic drug product is being used, the drugs should be administered at least 5 min apart

• To avoid contamination or the spread of infection, do not use dropper for more than one person

• Decreased intraocular pressure can take several weeks; monitor IOP after a month

SIDE EFFECTS

CNS: Insomnia, headache, dizziness
CV: Palpitations
EENT: Eye stinging/burning, tearing, photophobia
PULM: Bronchospasm

PHARMACOKINETICS

Onset 60 min, peak 2-6 hr, duration 24 hr

INTERACTIONS

Increase: β-blocking effect—oral β-blockers

Increase: intraocular pressure reduction—topical miotics, dipivefrin, EPINEPHrine, carbonic anhydrase inhibitors; this may be beneficial

Increase: depression of AV nodal conduction, bradycardia, or hypotension—adenosine, cardiac glycosides, disopyramide, other antiarrhythmics, class 1C antiarrhythmic drugs (flecainide, propafenone, moricizine, encainide, quiNIDine, or drugs that significantly depress AV nodal conduction

Increase: AV block nodal conduction, induce AV block—high doses of procainamide

Increase: Antihypertensive effect—other antihypertensives

NURSING CONSIDERATIONS

Assess:

• **Systemic absorption:** when used in the eye, systemic absorption is common with the same adverse reactions and interactions

• **Glaucoma:** monitor intraocular pressure

Evaluate:

• Therapeutic response: decreasing intraocular pressure

Teach patient/family:

• That product is for ophthalmic use only

• Not to touch the tip of the dropper to the eye, fingertips, or other surface to prevent contamination

• To wash hands before and after use; tilt the head back slightly and pull the lower eyelid down with the index finger to form a pouch; squeeze the prescribed number of drops into the pouch; close eyes to spread drops; to avoid excessive systemic absorption by applying finger pressure on the lacrimal sac for 1-2 min following use

• That if more than one topical ophthalmic drug product is being used, the drugs should be administered at least 5 min apart

• To avoid contamination or the spread of infection by not using dropper for more than one person

---

levocabastine ophthalmic
See Appendix B

---

levocetirizine (Rx)
(lee-voh-she-teer'ah-zeen)
Xyzal
Func. class.: Antihistamine, low sedating
Chem. class.: H₁ histamine blocker

ACTION: Acts on blood vessels, GI, respiratory system by competing with histamine for H_1-receptor site; decreases allergic response by blocking pharmacologic effects of histamine; minimal anticholinergic action

USES: Perennial or seasonal rhinitis, allergy symptoms, chronic idiopathic urticaria

CONTRAINDICATIONS: Breastfeeding; children 6-11 yr with renal disease; end-stage renal disease; dialysis; hypersensitivity to this product, cetirizine, hydrOXYzine
Precautions: Pregnancy, driving, renal disease

DOSAGE AND ROUTES
• **Adult and child ≥12 yr: PO** 2.5-5 mg/day in the evening
• **Child 6-11 yr: PO** (oral solution) 2.5 mg/day in the evening
• **Child 2-5 yr: PO** (oral solution) 1.25 mg/day in the evening
• **Geriatric: PO** 2.5-5 mg/day in the evening
Renal dose
• **Adult: PO** CCr 50-80 mL/min, 2.5 mg/day; CCr 30-49 mL/min, 2.5 mg every other day; CCr 10-29 mL/min, 2.5 mg 2×/wk; CCr <10 mL/min, do not use
Available forms: Tabs 5 mg; oral sol 2.5 mg/5 mL
Administer:
• Without regard to meals in the evening; tabs scored, may be broken in half
• Store in tight, light-resistant container

SIDE EFFECTS
CNS: *Drowsiness, fatigue,* asthenia, dizziness
GI: Dry mouth, increased LFTs, hepatitis
MISC: Urinary retention

PHARMACOKINETICS
Rapid absorption; peak 0.9 hr; protein binding 91%-92%; half-life 8 hr; excreted in urine 85.4%, feces 12.9%

INTERACTIONS
Increase: CNS depression—alcohol, other CNS depressants

Increase: anticholinergic/sedative effect—MAOIs, phenothiazines, tricyclics
Decrease: clearance of levocetirizine—ritonavir
Drug/Lab Test
False negative: skin allergy tests

NURSING CONSIDERATIONS
Assess:
• **Allergy symptoms:** pruritus, urticaria, watering eyes at baseline, during treatment
• **Respiratory status:** rate, rhythm, increase in bronchial secretions, wheezing, chest tightness
• Liver function tests, serum creatinine, BUN
• **Pregnancy/breastfeeding:** use only if clearly needed; do not breastfeed, excreted in breast milk
Evaluate:
• Therapeutic response: absence of running or congested nose or rashes
Teach patient/family:
• About all aspects of product use; to notify prescriber if confusion, sedation, hypotension occur, not to exceed recommended dose
• To avoid driving, other hazardous activities if drowsiness occurs
• To avoid alcohol, other CNS depressants
• Do not breastfeed

---

levodopa-carbidopa (Rx)
(lee-voe-doe′pa)-(kar-bi-doe′pa)
Duopa ✦, Duodopa ✦, Sinemet, Sinemet CR, Rytary, Duopa
Func. class.: Antiparkinson agent
Chem. class.: Catecholamine

ACTION: Decarboxylation of levodopa in periphery is inhibited by carbidopa; more levodopa is made available for transport to the brain and for conversion to DOPamine in the brain

USES: Parkinson's disease, parkinsonism resulting from carbon monoxide, chronic manganese intoxication, cerebral arteriosclerosis, motor fluctuations in those with advanced Parkinson's disease

Unlabeled uses: Restless legs syndrome

CONTRAINDICATIONS: Hypersensitivity, malignant melanoma, history of malignant melanoma or undiagnosed skin lesions resembling melanoma

Precautions: Pregnancy, breastfeeding, diabetes, closed-angle glaucoma, respiratory/cardiac/renal/hepatic disease, MI with dysrhythmias, seizures, peptic ulcer, depression

DOSAGE AND ROUTES

Idiopathic Parkinson's disease, post-encephalitic parkinsonism, and symptomatic parkinsonism

• **Adult: PO (immediate-release tablets)** 1 carbidopa 25 mg/levodopa 100 mg tablet tid, may increase by 1 tablet qday or every other day, max 8 tablets/day. **Maintenance:** At least 70-100 mg of carbidopa per day should be used

Converting patients from levodopa to carbidopa-levodopa

25% of the previous dose of levodopa; usual dosage is 1 carbidopa 50 mg/levodopa 200 mg ext-rel tablet bid

For the treatment of restless legs syndrome (RLS) (unlabeled)

• **Adult: PO** A bedtime dose starting at 25 mg/100 mg levodopa

Available forms: Tabs 10 mg carbidopa/100 mg levodopa, 25 mg carbidopa/100 mg levodopa, 25 mg carbidopa/250 mg levodopa; ext rel tab 25 mg carbidopa/100 mg levodopa, 50 mg carbidopa/200 mg levodopa (Sinemet CR); oral disintegrating tab 10 mg carbidopa/100 mg levodopa, 25 mg carbidopa/100 mg levodopa, 25 mg carbidopa/250 mg levodopa; ext rel caps (Rytary) 23.75 mg/95 mg, 36.25 mg/145 mg, 48.75 mg/195 mg, 61.25 mg/245 mg; enteral suspension (Duopa) 20 mg/mL levodopa/4.63 mg/mL carbidopa

Administer:

• Pyridoxine (B_6) not effective for reversing Sinemet or Sinemet CR

PO route

• Do not crush or chew **ext rel tabs;** they may be broken in half; adjust dosage to response

• **Oral disintegrating tab** by gently removing from bottle, placing on tongue and swallowing with saliva; after tab dissolves, liquid is not necessary

• With meals if GI symptoms occur; limit protein taken with product

• Only after nonselective MAOIs have been discontinued for 2 wk; if patient has been previously treated with levodopa, discontinue for at least 12 hr before change to carbidopa-levodopa

Enteral route

• Fully thaw in refrigerator; remove 1 cassette from refrigerator 20 min before use, give through NG tube or a percutaneous endoscopic gastrostomy jejunostomy tube connected to the CADD-Legacy pump; disconnect after use and flush with water; cassettes are single-use only, label in order to be used based on date

SIDE EFFECTS

CNS: *Involuntary choreiform movements, hand tremors, fatigue, headache, anxiety, twitching, numbness, weakness, confusion, agitation, insomnia, nightmares,* psychosis, hallucination, hypomania, severe depression, dizziness, impulsive behaviors, neuroleptic malignant syndrome, suicidal ideation

CV: *Orthostatic hypotension,* tachycardia, hypertension, palpitation, MI

EENT: Blurred vision, diplopia, dilated pupils

GI: *Nausea, vomiting, anorexia, abdominal distress, dry mouth, flatulence, dysphagia,* bitter taste, diarrhea, constipation, GI bleeding

HEMA: Hemolytic anemia, leukopenia, agranulocytosis, thrombocytopenia

INTEG: Rash, sweating, alopecia

MISC: Urinary retention, incontinence, weight change, dark urine, increased libido, hypersensitivity, dark sweat

---

PHARMACOKINETICS

PO: Onset 30 min, peak 1-3 hr, excreted in urine (metabolites)
EXT REL: Onset 4-6 hr
Enteral: Peak 2.5 hr

INTERACTIONS

Increase: hypertensive crisis—nonselective MAOIs
Increase: risk for sedation—CNS depressants
Increase: hypotension—antihypertensives
Increase: CV reactions—dobutamine, dopamine, epinephrine, isoproterenol, norepinephrine, TCAs
Increase: effects of levodopa—antacids, metoclopramide
Decrease: effects of levodopa—anticholinergics, hydantoins, papaverine, pyridoxine, benzodiazepines, antipsychotics
Drug/Lab Test
Increase: BUN, AST, ALT, bilirubin, alk phos, LDH, serum glucose
Decrease: BUN, creatinine, uric acid
False positive: urine ketones (dipstick), Coombs' test
False negative: urine glucose
False increase: urine protein
Drug/Food
Decrease: absorption of levodopa—protein

NURSING CONSIDERATIONS
Assess:
• **Parkinson's symptoms:** tremors, pill rolling, drooling, akinesia, rigidity, shuffling gait before, during treatment
• B/P, respiration; orthostatic B/P
• Mental status: affect, mood, behavioral changes, depression, complete suicide assessment
• **Toxicity:** muscle twitching, blepharospasm
• Renal, hepatic, hematopoietic tests; also for diabetes, acromegaly if on long-term therapy
• **Pregnancy/breastfeeding:** use only if benefits outweigh fetal risk; product is excreted in breast milk
Evaluate:
• Therapeutic response: decrease in akathisia/bradykinesis, tremor, rigidity, improved mood

Teach patient/family:
• To change positions slowly to prevent orthostatic hypotension, especially during beginning of treatment
• To report side effects: twitching, eye spasms because these indicate overdose
• To use product as prescribed; not to double doses; if discontinued abruptly, parkinsonian crisis, neuroleptic malignant syndrome (NMS) may occur; to gradually taper
• To use ODT immediately after removing from container, to dissolve on tongue, swallow with saliva
• That urine, sweat may darken
• To use physical activities to maintain mobility, lessen spasms
• To use with meals to decrease GI upset; do not use high-protein meals
• That improvement may not occur for 2-4 mo; about "on-off phenomenon"
• Not to chew or crush extended-release product
• To immediately report nausea, vomiting, abdominal pain, ongoing constipation if using enteral product

---

levofloxacin (Rx)
(lee-voh-floks′a-sin)
Levaquin
Func. class.: Antiinfective
Chem. class.: Fluoroquinolone

Do not confuse:
levofloxacin/levetiracetam

ACTION: Interferes with conversion of intermediate DNA fragments into high-molecular-weight DNA in bacteria; DNA gyrase inhibitor; inhibits topoisomerase IV

USES: Acute sinusitis, acute chronic bronchitis, community-acquired pneumonia, uncomplicated skin infections, UTI, cellulitis, prostatitis, inhalational anthrax (postexposure); acute pyelonephritis caused by *Streptococcus pneumoniae, Streptococcus pyogenes, Haemophilus influenzae, Haemophilus parainfluenzae, Moraxella catarrhalis, Escherichia coli, Serratia marcescens, Klebsiella pneumoniae, Chlamydia* *pneumoniae, Legionella pneumophila, Mycoplasma pneumoniae, Enterococcus faecalis, Staphylococcus epidermidis, Staphylococcus pyogenes, Staphylococcus aureus, Bacillus anthracis;* inhalation anthrax in children

Unlabeled uses: Adnexitis, Bartholin abscess, bartholinitis, cervicitis, epididymitis, gastroenteritis, *H. pylori* eradication, mastitis, MAC, nongonococcal urethritis, obstetric infections, PID, plague, SARS, shigellosis, TB, typhoid fever, disseminated; otitis media, otitis externa, tonsillitis, pharyngitis, sialadenitis

CONTRAINDICATIONS: Hypersensitivity to quinolones

Precautions: Pregnancy, breastfeeding, children, photosensitivity, acute MI, atrial fibrillation, colitis, dehydration, diabetes, QT prolongation, myasthenia gravis, renal disease, seizure disorder, syphilis

Black Box Warning: Tendon pain/rupture, tendinitis, myasthenia gravis, neurotoxicity

DOSAGE AND ROUTES
Most infections
• **Adult: PO/IV** 250-750 mg q24hr
Inhalational anthrax postexposure
• **Adult: PO/IV** 500 mg daily × 60 days
• **Child >50 kg: PO/IV** 500 mg daily × 60 days
• **Child <50 kg, ≥6 mo: PO/IV** 8 mg/kg q12hr × 60 days, max 250 mg/dose
Plague
• **Adult: PO/IV** 500 mg q24hr × 10-14 days
• **Child >50 kg: PO/IV** 500 mg daily × 10-14 days
• **Child <50 kg ≥6 mo: PO/IV** 8 mg/kg q12hr × 10-14 days, max 250 mg/dose
Renal disease
• **Adult: PO/IV** CCr 20-49 mL/min for 750 mg doses, give 750 mg q48hr; for 500 mg doses, give 500 mg once, then 250 mg q24hr; for 250 mg doses, no adjustment; CCr 10-19 mL/min for 750 mg dose, give 750 mg once, then 500 mg q48hr; for 500 mg dose, give 500 mg once, then 250 mg q48hr; for 250 mg dose, give 250 mg

q48hr, except when treating complicated UTI, then no dose adjustment

Available forms: Single-use vials 500, 750 mg; premixed flexible containers 250 mg/50 mL D₅W, 500 mg/100 mL D₅W, 750 mg/150 mL D₅W; tabs 250, 500, 750 mg; oral sol 25 mg/mL; ophthalmic solution 0.5%

Administer:
• Obtain C&S before treatment and periodically to determine resistance to product, treatment can start before results are obtained
• PO 2 hr before or after antacids, iron, calcium, zinc, sucralfate; give fluids
• **Oral solution:** Give 1 hr before or 2 hr after food

Intermittent IV INFUSION route
• Discard any unused sol in single-dose vial
• Visually inspect for particulate matter/discoloration before use

IV (single-use vial)
• **500 mg/20-mL vials:** To prepare a dose of 500 mg, withdraw 20 mL from a 20-mL vial and dilute with a compatible IV solution (D₅W, NS) to a total volume of 50 mL; to prepare a 500 mg dosage, withdraw all 20 mL from the vial and dilute with a compatible intravenous solution to a total volume of 100 mL
• **750 mg/30-mL vials:** To prepare a dose of 750 mg, withdraw 30 mL from a 30-mL vial and dilute with a compatible intravenous solution (D₅W, NS) to a total volume of 150 mL
• The concentration of the diluted solution should be 5 mg/mL before administration; solutions contain no preservatives; any unused portions must be discarded
• **Storage:** The diluted solution may be stored for up to 72 hr at room temperature or 14 days refrigerated; solutions may be frozen for up to 6 mo

Premixed IV solution
• No dilution is necessary

Intermittent IV injection
• Infuse doses of ≤500 mg IV over 60 min and doses of 750 mg IV over 90 min; shorter infusions or bolus inj should be avoided because of the risk of hypotension

Side effects: *italics* = common; red = life-threatening

Y-site compatibilities: Alemtuzumab, alfentanil, amifostine, amikacin, aminocaproic acid, aminophylline, ampicillin, ampicillin-sulbactam, anidulafungin, argatroban, atenolol, atracurium, aztreonam, bivalirudin, bleomycin, bumetanide, buprenorphine, busulfan, butorphanol, caffeine citrate, calcium gluconate, CARBOplatin, carmustine, caspofungin, cefepime, cefoTEtan, ceftaroline, cefTAZidime, ceftizoxime, cefTRIAXone, cefuroxime, chlorproMAZINE, cimetidine, cisatracurium, CISplatin, clindamycin, codeine, cyclophosphamide, cycloSPORINE, cytarabine, dacarbazine, DACTINomycin, DAPTOmycin, DAUNOrubicin liposomal, dexamethasone, dexrazoxane, digoxin, diltiazem, diphenhydrAMINE, DOBUTamine, DOCEtaxel, dolasetron, DOPamine, doripenem, doxacurium, doxycycline, droperidol, enalaprilat, ePHEDrine, EPINEPHrine, epirubicin, ertapenem, erythromycin, esmolol, etoposide, etoposide phosphate, famotidine, fenoldopam, fentaNYL, filgrastim, floxuridine, fluconazole, fludarabine, foscarnet, fosphenytoin, gallium, gemcitabine, gemtuzumab, gentamicin, granisetron, haloperidol, hydrocortisone, HYDROmorphone, IDArubicin, ifosfamide, imipenem-cilastatin, irinotecan, isoproterenol, labetalol, lepirudin, leucovorin, levorphanol, lidocaine, linezolid, mannitol, mechlorethamine, meperidine, mesna, methylPREDNISolone, metoclopramide, metroNIDAZOLE, midazolam, milrinone, minocycline, mitoMYcin, mitoXANtrone, mivacurium, morphine, mycophenolate mofetil, nalbuphine, naloxone, nesiritide, netilmicin, niCARdipine, octreotide, ondansetron, oxacillin, oxaliplatin, oxytocin, PACLitaxel, palonosetron, pamidronate, pancuronium, PEMEtrexed, penicillin G sodium, pentamidine, phenylephrine, plicamycin, potassium acetate/chloride, promethazine, propranolol, quinupristin-dalfopristin, ranitidine, remifentanil, rocuronium, sargramostim, sodium bicarbonate, succinylcholine, SUFentanil, sulfamethoxazole-trimethoprim, tacrolimus, teniposide, theophylline, thiotepa, ticarcillin, ticarcillin-clavulanate, tigecycline, tirofiban, tobramycin, topotecan, trimethobenzamide, vancomycin, vasopressin, vecuronium, verapamil, vinBLASTine, vinCRIStine, vinorelbine, voriconazole, zidovudine, zoledronic acid

Solution compatibilities: 0.9% NaCl, D_5W, D_5/0.9% NaCl, D_5LR, D_5/0.45% NaCl, sodium lactate, plasma-lyte 56/D_5W

Ophthalmic
• Do not share with others
• Do not touch tip to eye

SIDE EFFECTS

CNS: *Headache,* dizziness, *insomnia,* anxiety, seizures, *encephalopathy,* paresthesia, pseudotumor cerebri

CV: Chest pain, palpitations, vasodilation, QT prolongation, hypotension (rapid infusion)

EENT: Dry mouth, visual impairment, tinnitus

GI: *Nausea,* flatulence, *vomiting,* diarrhea, abdominal pain, CDAD, hepatotoxicity, esophagitis, pancreatitis

GU: Vaginitis, crystalluria

HEMA: Eosinophilia, hemolytic anemia, lymphopenia

INTEG: Rash, pruritus, *photosensitivity,* epidermal necrolysis, injection-site reaction, edema

MISC: Hypoglycemia, hypersensitivity, tendinitis, tendon rupture, rhabdomyolysis

RESP: Pneumonitis

SYST: Anaphylaxis, multisystem organ failure, Stevens-Johnson syndrome, angioedema, toxic epidermal necrolysis

PHARMACOKINETICS

Excreted in urine unchanged, half-life 6-8 hr, peak 1-2 hr

INTERACTIONS

Black Box Warning: **Increase:** tendon rupture—corticosteroids; assess for tendon pain

• Do not use with magnesium in same IV line

Increase: QT prolongation—products causing a QT prolongation; avoid concurrent use

Increase: levofloxacin levels—probenecid

Increase: CNS stimulation, seizures—NSAIDs, foscarnet, cycloSPORINE

Increase: bleeding risk—warfarin; monitor INR/PT

Decrease: levofloxacin absorption—antacids containing aluminum, magnesium; sucralfate, zinc, iron, calcium; give 2 hr before or after products

Decrease: clearance of theophylline; toxicity may result; monitor theophylline level

Drug/Herb

Increase: photosensitivity—St. John's wort

Drug/Lab Test

Increase: PT, INR

Decrease: glucose, lymphocytes

NURSING CONSIDERATIONS
Assess:
• Previous sensitivity reaction to quinolones

• **Signs, symptoms of infection:** characteristics of sputum, WBC >10,000/mm³, fever; obtain baseline information before, during treatment

• C&S before beginning product therapy to identify if correct treatment initiated

• **Allergic reactions, anaphylaxis:** rash, urticaria, pruritus, chills, fever, joint pain; may occur a few days after therapy begins; EPINEPHrine and resuscitation equipment should be available for anaphylactic reaction

• **CDAD:** bowel pattern daily; if severe diarrhea, fever occur, product should be discontinued

• **Overgrowth of infection:** perineal itching, fever, malaise, redness, pain, swelling, drainage, rash, diarrhea, change in cough, sputum

• Renal function (BUN/creatinine)

• **Peripheral neuropathy:** tingling, pain, numbness, burning in extremities, can be permanent

Black Box Warning: **Tendon rupture:** discontinue product at first sign of tendon pain or inflammation, usually the Achilles tendon is affected; can occur up to few months after treatment and may require surgical repair; risk is increased in elderly patients, transplant patients, or with use of steroids

Black Box Warning: **Myasthenia gravis:** do not use this product with this disease; may lead to life-threatening weakness of the respiratory muscles

Black Box Warning: **Neurotoxicity:** may occur within hours to weeks after starting use; may be irreversible; avoid use in those who have experienced peripheral neuropathy (numbness, tingling, burning in extremities); report to prescriber immediately

• Increased fluid intake to 2 L/day to prevent crystalluria

• **Pregnancy/breastfeeding:** avoid use in pregnancy; do not use in breastfeeding

Evaluate:
• Therapeutic response: absence of signs, symptoms of infection (WBC <10,000/mm³, temperature WNL)

Teach patient/family:
• **Superinfection:** To contact prescriber if vaginal itching; loose, foul-smelling stools; furry tongue occur (may indicate superinfection); to report itching, rash, pruritus, urticaria, change in heartbeat

• **CDAD:** To notify prescriber of diarrhea with blood or purulent discharge in stool

• To take product 2 hr before or after antacids, iron, calcium, zinc products

• To complete full course of therapy, not to skip or double doses

• To avoid driving or other hazardous activities until response is known, dizziness may occur

• To use frequent rinsing of mouth, sugarless candy, or gum for dry mouth

• To avoid other medication unless approved by prescriber

• To prevent sun exposure or to use sunscreen to prevent photosensitivity

• To monitor glucose (diabetes); to notify prescriber of changes

• Not to use contact lenses if using ophthalmic product

Black Box Warning: To notify prescriber of tendon pain, inflammation; to avoid corticosteroids with this product

• **Pregnancy/breastfeeding:** identify if pregnancy is planned or suspected or if breastfeeding

Side effects: *italics* = common; red = life-threatening

levofloxacin ophthalmic
See Appendix B

levomilnacipran
[lee'voe-mil-na'si-pran]
Fetzima
milnacipran
(mil-na'si-pran)
Savella
Func. class.: Antidepressant
Chem. class.: Serotonin-norepinephrine reuptake inhibitor (SNRI)

Do not confuse:
Fetzima/Farxiga

ACTION: May potentiate serotonergic, adrenergic activity in the CNS; is a potent inhibitor of adrenal serotonin and norepinephrine reuptake

USES: Major depressive disorder in adults

CONTRAINDICATIONS: Hypersensitivity, MAOI therapy
Precautions: Pregnancy, breastfeeding, geriatric patients, mania, hypertension, renal/cardiac disease, seizures, increased intraocular pressure, anorexia, bleeding, dehydration, diabetes, hypotension, hypovolemia, orthostatic hypotension, abrupt product withdrawal, alcohol intoxication, alcoholism, closed-angle glaucoma

Black Box Warning: Children, suicidal ideation

DOSAGE AND ROUTES
Major depressive disorder (levomilnacipran)
• **Adult:** PO 20 mg/day × 2 days, then 40 mg/day; may increase in increments of 40 mg at intervals of at least 2 days, max 120 mg/day; max 80 mg/day (strong CYP3A4 inhibitors therapy)

Major depressive disorder (milnacipran)
• **Adult:** PO 12.5-25 mg bid, may titrate to 100 mg bid, max 200 mg/day
Fibromyalgia (levomilnacipran)
• **Adult:** PO 12.5 mg daily, increase to 12.5 mg bid on days 2 and 3, then 25 mg bid on days 4 to 7; increase to 50 mg bid after day 7; may increase to 100 mg bid as needed
Fibromyalgia (milnacipran)
• **Adult/adolescent ≥17 yr:** PO 12.5 mg once on day 1, then 12.5 mg bid on days 2-3, then 25 mg bid on days 4-7, and 50 mg bid thereafter
Renal dose (levomilnacipran)
• **Adult:** PO CCr 15-29 mL/min, max 40 mg/day; CCr 30-59 mL/min, max 80 mg/day; CCr <15 mL/min, do not use
Renal dose (milnacipran)
• **Adult:** PO CCr 5-29 mL/min, reduce maintenance dose by 50% (25-50 mg bid)
Available forms: Ext rel caps 20, 40, 80, 120 mg (levomilnacipran); tabs 12.5, 25, 50, 100 mg (milnacipran)
Administer:
• Swallow cap whole; do not break, crush, or chew; do not sprinkle on food or mix with liquid
• Without regard to food
• Give at the same time each day

SIDE EFFECTS
CNS: Dizziness, agitation, hallucinations, seizures, drowsiness, mania, migraine, paresthesias, suicidal ideation, syncope
CV: Hypertension, palpitations, dysrhythmia, sinus tachycardia
EENT: Teeth grinding, blurred vision
GI: Constipation, diarrhea, nausea, vomiting, anorexia, dry mouth, abdominal pain
GU: Urinary retention
SYST: Serotonin syndrome, Stevens-Johnson syndrome

PHARMACOKINETICS
Peak 6-8 hr metabolized (CYP2D6) in the liver; excretion 58% (urine), 22% protein binding, half-life 12 hr (levomilnacipran) 6-10 hr (milnacipran)

INTERACTIONS

• Do not use with linezolid or methylene blue IV, or within 14 days of MAOIs

• **Increase:** levomilnacipran effect—CYP34A inhibitors

Increase: serotonin syndrome—SSRIs, serotonin receptor agonists, SNRIs, lithium

Increase: bleeding risk—anticoagulants, antiplatelets, salicylates, NSAIDs

Increase: risk of neuroleptic malignant syndrome—antipsychotics, DOPamine antagonists; avoid concurrent use

Increase: bleeding risk—alfalfa, feverfew, dong quai, fish oil, ginseng, garlic, ginkgo biloba

Drug/Herb

• **Serotonin syndrome:** St. John's wort

Increase: CNS depression—kava, valerian

NURSING CONSIDERATIONS

Assess:

• **Neuroleptic malignant syndrome:** hyperthermia, rigidity, rapid fluctuations of vital signs, mental status changes; MAOIs: coadministration contraindicated within 14 days of MAOI

Black Box Warning: **Depression:** mood, sensorium, affect, suicidal tendencies, increase in psychiatric symptoms; panic; monitor children weekly face to face during first 4 wk, or dosage change, then every other week for the next 4 wk, then at 12 wk

• B/P lying, standing; pulse; if systolic B/P drops 20 mm Hg, hold product, notify prescriber; take VS more often in patients with CV disease

• **Hepatic studies:** AST, ALT, bilirubin baseline and periodically

• **Withdrawal symptoms:** headache, nausea, vomiting, muscle pain, weakness; not common unless product is discontinued abruptly

Black Box Warning: **Serotonin syndrome:** nausea, vomiting, dizziness, facial flush, shivering, sweating

• **Beers:** use with caution in older adults; may exacerbate or cause SIADH; monitor for hyponatremia

• **Pregnancy/breastfeeding:** use only if benefits outweigh fetal risk; SSRIs should not be used; do not use in 3rd trimester; do not breastfeed

Evaluate:

• Therapeutic response: decreased depression

Teach patient/family:

• About signs and symptoms of bleeding (GI bleeding, nosebleed, ecchymosis, bruising)

• To use with caution when driving and performing other activities requiring alertness because of drowsiness and blurred vision

• To avoid ingestion of alcohol, MAOIs, other CNS depressants; not to use within 14 days of MAOIs; to notify all providers of use of this product

• Not to discontinue medication quickly after long-term use; may cause headache, malaise; taper

• That product may be used with or without food

• To swallow caps whole; do not break, crush, chew

Black Box Warning: That clinical worsening and suicidal risk may occur, usually worse in first few months of treatment; to notify prescriber immediately if suicidal thoughts/behaviors, aggression, hostility, agitation, panic attacks occur

• That improvement may occur in 4-8 wk or up to 12 wk (geriatric patients)

• To report trouble with urination

• **Serotonin syndrome:** to report immediately nausea, vomiting, dizziness, facial flush, shivering, sweating

• **Pregnancy/breastfeeding:** to notify prescriber if pregnancy is planned or suspected or if breastfeeding

L

levothyroxine (T₄) (Rx)

(lee-voe-thye-rox′een)

Eltroxin ✤, Levo-T, Levoxyl, Synthroid, Tirosint, Unithroid, Euthyrox ✤, Levo-T ✤

Func. class.: Thyroid hormone
Chem. class.: Levoisomer of thyroxine

Do not confuse:

Synthroid/Symmetrel
levothyroxine/lamatrigine/Lanoxin/
liothyronine

ACTION: Increases metabolic rate; controls protein synthesis; increases cardiac output, renal blood flow, O_2 consumption, body temperature, blood volume, growth, development at cellular level via action on thyroid hormone receptors

USES: Hypothyroidism, myxedema coma, thyroid hormone replacement, thyrotoxicosis, congenital hypothyroidism, some types of thyroid cancer, pituitary TSH suppression

CONTRAINDICATIONS: Adrenal insufficiency, recent MI, thyrotoxicosis, hypersensitivity to beef, alcohol intolerance (inj only)

Black Box Warning: Obesity treatment

Precautions: Pregnancy, breastfeeding, geriatric patients, angina pectoris, hypertension, ischemia, cardiac disease, diabetes

DOSAGE AND ROUTES—NTI
Hypothyroidism

• **Adult ≤50 yr:** PO 1.6 mcg/kg/day, 6-8 wk, average dose 100-200 mcg/day; **IM/IV** 50-100 mcg/day as single dose or 50% of usual oral dosage
• **Adult >50 yr without heart disease or <50 yr with heart disease:** PO 25-50 mcg/day, titrate q6-8wk
• **Adult >50 yr with heart disease:** PO 12.5-25 mcg/day, titrate by 12.5-25 mcg q6-8wk
• **Child (puberty complete):** PO 1.7 mcg/kg/day

• **Child >12 yr (incomplete puberty):** PO 2-3 mcg/kg/day as single dose in AM
• **Child 6-12 yr:** PO 4-5 mcg/kg/day as single dose in AM
• **Child 1-5 yr:** PO 5-6 mcg/kg/day as single dose in AM
• **Child 6-12 mo:** PO 6-8 mcg/kg/day as single dose in AM
• **Child 3-6 mo:** PO 8-10 mcg/kg/day as single dose in AM
• **Infant/neonate to age 3 mo:** PO 10-15 mcg/kg/day; use in lower dose in those at risk for cardiac failure; may increase q4-6wk if needed

Myxedema coma

• **Adult:** IV 300-500 mcg initially, may increase by 100-300 mcg after 24 hr; give oral medication as soon as possible

Subclinical hypothyroidism

• **Adult:** PO 1 mcg/kg/day

Available forms: Powder for inj 100, 200, 500 mcg/vial; tabs 25, 50, 88, 100, 112, 125, 137, 150, 175, 200, 300 mcg; cap (liquid filled) 13, 25, 50, 75, 88, 100, 112, 125, 137, 150 mcg

Administer:

• Store in tight, light-resistant container; sol should be discarded if not used immediately
• Withdrawal of medication 4 wk before RAIU test

PO route

• In AM if possible as single dose to decrease sleeplessness; at same time each day to maintain product level; take on empty stomach
• Only for hormone imbalances; not to be used for obesity, male infertility, menstrual conditions, lethargy
• Use 8 oz of water with on empty stomach
• Lowest dose that relieves symptoms; lower dose to geriatric patients and for those with cardiac diseases
• Crush and mix with water, nonsoy formula (decreased absorption), or breast milk for infants, children; give by spoon or dropper; may crush and sprinkle over applesauce or other food
• Separate antacids, iron, calcium products by 4 hr

Direct IV route
• IV after reconstituting with 5 mL normal saline injection (500 mcg/5 mL, 200 mcg/2 mL); shake; give through Y-tube or 3-way stopcock; give ≤100 mcg/1 min; do not add to IV infusion
• Considered to be incompatible in syringe with all other products

SIDE EFFECTS

CNS: *Anxiety, insomnia, tremors,* headache, thyroid storm, excitability
CV: *Tachycardia, palpitations, angina, dysrhythmias,* hypertension, cardiac arrest
GI: Nausea, diarrhea, increased or decreased appetite, cramps
MISC: Menstrual irregularities, weight loss, sweating, heat intolerance, fever, alopecia, decreased bone mineral density

PHARMACOKINETICS

Half-life euthyroid 6-7 days, hypothyroid 9-10 days, hyperthyroid 3-4 days, distributed throughout body tissues, protein binding 99%
PO: Onset 24 hr
IV: Onset 6-8 hr

INTERACTIONS

Increase: levothyroxine need—SSRIs, antiepileptics (carbamazepine, oxcarbazepine, phenobarbital, primidone, phenytoin), antimicrobials (rifampin, efavirenz, rifabutin, rifapentine); monitor levels of levothyroxine
Increase or Decrease: glucose levels—insulin, antidiabetics; monitor blood glucose, adjust levels
Increase: cardiac insufficiency risk—EPINEPHrine products
Increase: effects of both products—tricyclics, tetracyclics
Increase: effects of anticoagulants, sympathomimetics, tricyclics; monitor PT, INR if using with anticoagulants
Decrease: levothyroxine absorption—bile acid sequestrants, orlistat, ferrous sulfate
Decrease: levothyroxine effect—estrogens, antacids, sucralfate, aluminum, magnesium, calcium, iron, rifampin, rifabutin

Drug/Herb
Decrease: thyroid hormone effect—soy, horseradish
Drug/Lab Test
Increase: blood glucose
Decrease: thyroid function tests

Drug/Food
Decrease: product absorption—fiber, walnuts; avoid concurrent use or adjust dose

NURSING CONSIDERATIONS
Assess:
• B/P, pulse periodically during treatment
• Weight daily in same clothing, using same scale, at same time of day
• Height, growth rate of child
• Patient may require decreased anticoagulant; check for bleeding, bruising
• Cardiac status: angina, palpitation, chest pain, change in VS
• **CAD:** monitor for coronary insufficiency; also watch for cardiac changes in those receiving high, rapid dosing
• **Bone density:** test bone density baseline and periodically; bone loss may occur with long-term therapy
• **Pregnancy/breastfeeding:** may be used in pregnancy and breastfeeding
Hypothyroidism:
• T_3, T_4, FTIs, which are decreased; radioimmunoassay of TSH, which is increased; radio uptake, which is increased if patient is receiving too low a dose of medication
• Increased nervousness, excitability, irritability, which may indicate too high a dose of medication, usually after 1-3 wk of treatment
Evaluate:
• Therapeutic response: absence of depression; increased weight loss, diuresis, pulse, appetite; absence of constipation, peripheral edema, cold intolerance; pale, cool, dry skin; brittle nails, alopecia, coarse hair, menorrhagia, night blindness, paresthesias, syncope, stupor, coma, rosy cheeks
Teach patient/family:
• That hair loss will occur in child, is temporary; that hypothyroid child will

show almost immediate behavior/personality change

• To report excitability, irritability, anxiety, which indicate overdose

• Not to switch brands unless approved by prescriber; to protect from light, moisture

Black Box Warning: That product is not to be taken to reduce weight

• To avoid OTC preparations with iodine; to read labels; to separate antacids, iron, calcium products by 4 hr

• To take in AM on empty stomach, at least 30 min before food

• To avoid iodine-rich food, iodized salt, soybeans, tofu, turnips, high-iodine seafood, some bread products

• That product is not a cure but controls symptoms; that treatment is lifelong, full effect may take up to 6 wk

• That all products are not interchangeable

• **Pregnancy/breastfeeding:** to continue using during pregnancy, breastfeeding

• **Anticoagulants:** to have anticoagulant level monitored, dose adjusted as needed

---

⚠ HIGH ALERT

lidocaine (parenteral) (Rx)

(lye'doe-kane)

LidoPen Auto-Injector, Xylocaine, Xylocard ✦

Func. class.: Antidysrhythmic (Class Ib)
Chem. class.: Aminoacyl amide

ACTION: Increases electrical stimulation threshold of ventricle, His-Purkinje system, which stabilizes cardiac membrane, decreases automaticity

USES: Ventricular tachycardia, ventricular dysrhythmias during cardiac surgery, digoxin toxicity, cardiac catheterization
Unlabeled uses: Attenuation of intracranial pressure increased during intubation/endotracheal tube suctioning

CONTRAINDICATIONS: Hypersensitivity to amides, severe heart block, supraventricular dysrhythmias, Adams-Stokes syndrome, Wolff-Parkinson-White syndrome
Precautions: Pregnancy, breastfeeding, children, geriatric patients, renal/hepatic disease, HF, respiratory depression, malignant hyperthermia, myasthenia gravis, weight <50 kg

DOSAGE AND ROUTES
Ventricular arrhythmias caused by MI, cardiac manipulation/ glycosides
• **Adult:** IV BOL 50-100 mg (1-1.5 mg/ kg) 25-50 mg/min, repeat q5min until arrhythmias are controlled, max 300 mg in 1 hr; begin **IV INFUSION; IV INFUSION** 1-4 mg/min (20-50 mcg/kg/min)
• **Child:** IV/INTRAOSSEUS BOL 1 mg/ kg; start infusion at 30 mcg/kg/min
Renal/hepatic dose with heart failure
• **Adult <50 kg:** IV reduce dose
Available forms: IV INFUSION 0.2% (2 mg/mL), 0.4% (4 mg/mL), 0.8% (8 mg/mL); IV 4% (40 mg/mL), 10% (100 mg/mL), 20% (200 mg/mL); IV dir 1% (10 mg/mL), 2% (20 mg/mL); Inj (to IV admix) 20% (200 mg/mL)
Administer:
• IM inj in deltoid; aspirate to avoid intravascular administration; check IV site daily for infiltration or extravasation; do not use in shock, usually used if ECG monitoring cannot be done
IV route
• Bolus undiluted (1%, 2% only), give ≤50 mg/1 min or dilute 1 g/250-500 mL D₅W; titrate to patient response; use infusion pump; pediatric infusion 120 mg lidocaine/100 mL D₅W; 1-2.5 mL/kg/hr = 20-50 mcg/kg/min; use only 1%, 2% sol for IV bol
• Use a cardiac monitor
• Additive syringes/single-use vials are for infusions and must be diluted

Y-site compatibilities: Acetaminophen, alemtuzumab, alfentanil, alteplase, amikacin, aminocaproic acid, aminophylline, amiodarone, amphotericin B lipid/

liposome, anidulafungin, argatroban, ascorbic acid injection, atenolol, atropine, atracurium, azithromycin, aztreonam, benztropine, bivalirudin, bleomycin, bumetanide, buprenorphine, butorphanol, calcium chloride/gluconate, CARBOplatin, carmustine, ceFAZolin, cefotaxime, cefoTEtan, cefOXitin, ceftaroline, cefTAZidime, ceftizoxime, cefTRIAXone, cefuroxime, chloramphenicol, chlorproMAZINE, cimetidine, ciprofloxacin, cisatracurium, CISplatin, clarithromycin, clindamycin, cyanocobalamin, cyclophosphamide, cycloSPORINE, cytarabine, DACTINomycin, DAPTOmycin, DAUNOrubicin, dexamethasone, dexmedetomidine, dexrazoxane, digoxin, diltiazem, diphenhydrAMINE, DOBUTamine, DOCEtaxel, dolasetron, DOPamine, doxacurium, DOXOrubicin, DOXOrubicin liposomal, doxycycline, enalaprilat, EPINEPHrine, epirubicin, epoetin alfa, eptifibatide, ertapenem, erythromycin, esmolol, etomidate, etoposide, etoposide phosphate, famotidine, fenoldopam, fentaNYL, fluconazole, fludarabine, fluorouracil, folic acid, furosemide, gentamicin, granisetron, haloperidol, heparin, hydrocortisone, imipenem/cilastatin, inamrinone, insulin, isoproterenol, ketorolac, labetalol, levofloxacin, linezolid, LORazepam, magnesium sulfate, meperidine, methylPREDNISolone sodium succinate, metoclopramide, metoprolol, metroNIDAZOLE, micafungin, midazolam, morphine, nafcillin, niCARdipine, nitroglycerin, nitroprusside, norepinephrine, ondansetron, palonosetron, penicillin G potassium, phenylephrine, phytonadione, piperacillin/tazobactam, potassium chloride, procainamide, prochlorperazine, promethazine, propofol, propranolol, protamine, quinupristin/dalfopristin, ranitidine, remifentanil, sodium bicarbonate, streptokinase, tacrolimus, theophylline, ticarcillin/clavulanate, tigecycline, tirofiban, tobramycin, vancomycin, vasopressin, verapamil, vitamin B complex with C, voriconazole, warfarin

SIDE EFFECTS

CNS: *Headache, dizziness,* involuntary movement, confusion, tremor, drowsiness, euphoria, seizures, shivering

CV: *Hypotension, bradycardia,* heart block, CV collapse, arrest
EENT: Tinnitus, blurred vision
GI: Nausea, vomiting, anorexia
HEMA: Methemoglobinemia
INTEG: Rash, urticaria, edema, swelling, petechiae, pruritus
MISC: Febrile response, phlebitis at inj site
RESP: Dyspnea, respiratory depression

PHARMACOKINETICS

Half-life 8 min, 1-2 hr (terminal); metabolized in liver; excreted in urine; crosses placenta
IM: Onset 5-15 min, duration $1^1/_2$ hr
IV: Onset 2 min, duration 20 min

INTERACTIONS

Increase: cardiac depression, toxicity—amiodarone, phenytoin, procainamide, propranolol, quiNIDine
Increase: hypotensive effects—MAOIs, antihypertensives
Increase: neuromuscular blockade—neuromuscular blockers, tubocurarine; monitor for adverse effects
Increase: lidocaine effects, toxicity—cimetidine, β-blockers, protease inhibitors, ritonavir
Increase: hypotension—ergots; avoid concurrent use
Decrease: lidocaine effects—barbiturates, ciprofloxacin, voriconazole
Decrease: effect of—cycloSPORINE

NURSING CONSIDERATIONS
Assess:

• ECG continuously to determine increased PR or QRS segments; if these develop, discontinue or reduce rate; watch for increased ventricular ectopic beats, may have to rebolus; B/P
• **Drug levels:** therapeutic level, 1.5-5 mcg/mL
• I&O ratio, electrolytes (potassium, sodium, chlorine)
• **Toxicity:** monitor for seizures, confusion, tremors; if these occur, discontinue immediately; notify prescriber; keep emergency equipment nearby
• **Malignant hyperthermia:** tachypnea, tachycardia, changes in B/P, increased temperature

Side effects: *italics* = common; red = life-threatening

• **Respiratory status:** rate, rhythm, lung fields for crackles, watch for respiratory depression; lung fields, bilateral crackles may occur with HF; increased respiration, pulse; product should be discontinued

• **CNS effects:** dizziness, confusion, psychosis, paresthesias, convulsions; product should be discontinued

• **Pregnancy/breastfeeding:** use only if clearly needed; use caution in breastfeeding, excreted in breast milk

Evaluate:

• Therapeutic response: decreased dysrhythmias

Teach patient/family:

• About the use of automatic lidocaine injection device if ordered for personal use

• To report signs of toxicity immediately

TREATMENT OF OVERDOSE: O_2, artificial ventilation, ECG; administer DOPamine for circulatory depression, diazepam or thiopental for seizures; decrease product if needed

---

lidocaine ophthalmic
See Appendix B

---

lidocaine topical
See Appendix B

⚠ **HIGH ALERT**

linagliptin
(lin′a-glip′tin)
Tradjenta, Trajenta ✦
Func. class.: Antidiabetic
Chem. class.: Didipeptidyl peptidase-4 inhibitor

ACTION: Slows the inactivation of incretin hormones; concentrations of the active, intact hormones are increased, thereby increasing and prolonging the action of these hormones; incretin hormones are released by the intestine throughout the day, and levels are increased in response to a meal

USES: Type 2 diabetes mellitus with diet and exercise

CONTRAINDICATIONS: Hypersensitivity to linagliptin, type 1 diabetes mellitus, diabetic ketoacidosis (DKA)
Precautions: Pregnancy, breastfeeding, adolescents or children <18 yr, debilitated physical condition, malnutrition, uncontrolled adrenal insufficiency, pituitary insufficiency, hypo/hyperthyroidism, diarrhea, gastroparesis, GI obstruction, ileus, female hormonal changes, high fever, severe psychological stress, uncontrolled hypercortisolism

DOSAGE AND ROUTES
• **Adult: PO** 5 mg daily; when used with a sulfonylurea or insulin, a lower dose of the sulfonylurea may be necessary to minimize the risk of hypoglycemia
Available forms: Tab 5 mg
Administer:
• Once daily; may give without regard to food
• May require an increased dose in stress, fever, surgery, trauma
• Store at room temperature

SIDE EFFECTS
CNS: Headache
EENT: Nasopharyngitis
ENDO: Hypoglycemia, hyperuricemia, hypertriglyceridemia
GI: Body weight loss, pancreatitis
INTEG: Serious hypersensitivity reactions, urticaria, angioedema, exfoliative dermatitis
MISC: Arthralgia, back pain
RESP: Bronchial hyperreactivity (with bronchospasm), nasopharyngitis, cough

PHARMACOKINETICS
Extensively distributed to tissues, protein binding is concentration-dependent, weak to moderate inhibitor of

CYP3A4, half life of >100 hr; effective half-life 12 hr, 90% excreted unchanged, 85% excreted enterohepatic system urine (5%), rapidly absorbed, peak in 1.5 hr; bioavailability 30%

INTERACTIONS

Increase: hypoglycemia—sulfonylureas, β-blockers, ACE inhibitors, angiotensin II receptor antagonists, disopyramide, guanethidine, cloNIDine, octreotide, fenfluramine, dexfenfluramine, fibric acid derivatives, monoamine oxidase inhibitors (MAOIs), FLUoxetine, salicylates

Increase: masking of the signs and symptoms of hypoglycemia—reserpine, β-blockers

Increase: need for dosing change—cisapride, metoclopramide, tegaserod, androgens, alcohol, lithium, quinolones

Decrease: hypoglycemic effect—dextrothyroxine, bumetanide, furosemide, ethacrynic acid, torsemide, estrogens, progestins, oral contraceptives, thyroid hormones, glucocorticoids, glucagon, carbonic anhydrase inhibitors, phenytoin, fosphenytoin, or ethotoin; atypical antipsychotics (ARIPiprazole, cloZAPine, OLANZapine, QUEtiapine, risperiDONE, and ziprasidone), phenothiazine, niacin (nicotinic acid), triamterene, thiazide diuretics

Decrease: effect of linagliptin—CYP3A4 inducers (topiramate, rifabutin, pioglitazone, OXcarbazepine, carBAMazepine, nevirapine, modafinil, metyrapone, etravirine, efavirenz, bosentan, barbiturates, aprepitant, fosaprepitant)

Drug/Herb

Decrease: linagliptin effect—St. John's wort

Drug/Lab Test

Increase: uric acid

Decrease: HbA1c level, fasting blood glucose

NURSING CONSIDERATIONS
Assess

• **Diabetes:** blood glucose, A1c during treatment to determine diabetes control; monitor for hypoglycemia: confusion, sweating, tachycardia, anxiety; hyperglycemia: polydipsia, polyuria, polyphagia

• CBC baseline and periodically during treatment; report decreased blood counts

• **Pancreatitis (rare):** severe abdominal pain, nausea, vomiting; may be fatal; discontinue product immediately; use supportive therapy; monitor amylase, lipase, electrolytes

• **Arthralgia:** may be severe, but temporary

• **Pregnancy/breastfeeding:** use only if clearly needed; use caution in breastfeeding, excretion is unknown

Evaluate:

• Therapeutic response: improving blood glucose level, A1c; decreasing polydipsia, polyphagia, polyuria, clear sensorium, absence of dizziness

Teach patient/family:

• About the symptoms of hypo/hyperglycemia and what to do about each; to have glucagon emergency kit available, to carry sugar packets

• That product must be continued on a daily basis, about the consequences of discontinuing product abruptly; to take only as directed

• To avoid OTC products unless approved by prescriber

• That diabetes is a lifelong illness, that product will not cure diabetes

• To carry emergency ID with prescriber, condition and medications taken

• To immediately report skin disorders, swelling, difficulty breathing, or severe abdominal pain

• **Pregnancy/breastfeeding:** to notify provider if pregnancy is planned or suspected, or if breastfeeding

---

lindane (Rx)

(lin′dane)

Hexit

Func. class.: Scabicide, pediculicide
Chem. class.: Chlorinated hydrocarbon (synthetic)

ACTION: Stimulates nervous system of arthropods, resulting in seizures, death

USES: Scabies, lice (head/pubic/body), nits in those intolerant to or who do not respond to other agents

CONTRAINDICATIONS: Hypersensitivity, patients with known seizure disorders, Norwegian (crusted) scabies

Black Box Warning: Seizure disorder

Precautions: Pregnancy, breastfeeding, infants, children <10 yr, avoid contact with eyes

Black Box Warning: Neurotoxicity

DOSAGE AND ROUTES
Lice
• **Adult/child: CREAM/LOTION** shampoo using 30 mL: work into lather, rub for 5 min, rinse, dry with towel; comb with fine-toothed comb to remove nits; most require 1 oz, max 2 oz
Scabies
• **Adult/child: TOP** apply 1% cream/lotion to skin, from neck to bottom of feet, toes; wash area with soap, water; remove visible crusts; apply to skin surfaces; remove with soap, water in 8-12 hr; repeat after 1 wk prn; most require 1 oz, max 2 oz
Available forms: Lotion, shampoo, cream (1%)
Administer:
• Caregivers should wear gloves less permeable to lindane, thoroughly clean hands after application; avoid natural latex gloves
• **Cream/ointment/lotion:** use for scabies only; skin should be clean without other products on it, wait 1 hr after bathing or showering before application, shake well, apply under fingernails after trimming; toothbrush can be used to apply; after application, wrap toothbrush in paper and throw away; use only a single application, apply as thin layer over all skin from neck down, close bottle containing leftover lotion, throw away
• Do not cover, wash off after 8-12 hr
• Use warm, not hot, water; do not leave on >12 hr

• **Shampoo:** for lice only; do not use other hair products before use; shake well; hair should be completely dry; use only enough shampoo to lightly coat hair and scalp, work into hair, do not use water; allow to remain only 4 min, rinse, lather away, towel briskly
• To scalp only; do not apply to face, lips, mouth, eyes, any mucous membrane, anus, or meatus
• Topical corticosteroids as ordered to decrease contact dermatitis; antihistamines
• Lotions of menthol or phenol to control itching
• Topical antibiotics for infection

SIDE EFFECTS
CNS: Seizures, CNS toxicity, stimulation, dizziness
INTEG: *Pruritus, rash, irritation, contact dermatitis*

PHARMACOKINETICS
Onset 3 hr, half-life 18-22 hr

INTERACTIONS
• Oils may increase absorption; if oil-based hair dressing used, shampoo, rinse, dry hair before applying lindane shampoo

NURSING CONSIDERATIONS
Assess:

Black Box Warning: **Abrasions, skin inflammation, breaks in skin:** do not use on these areas, increased risk of neurotoxicity

• **Infestation:** head, hair for lice, nits before and after treatment; if scabies present, check all skin surfaces; identify source of infection: school, family, sexual contacts
• **Isolation** until areas on skin, scalp have cleared, treatment completed
• **Removal** of nits with fine-toothed comb rinsed in vinegar after treatment; use gloves

Black Box Warning: **Seizures:** avoid use in children with uncontrolled seizure disorders

• **Pregnancy/breastfeeding:** avoid in pregnancy, breastfeeding
Evaluate:
• Therapeutic response: decreased crusts, nits, brownish trails on skin, itching papules in skin folds, decreased itching after several weeks
Teach patient/family:
• To wash all inhabitants' clothing using insecticide; that preventive treatment may be required of all persons living in same house, using lotion or shampoo to decrease spread of infection; to use rubber gloves when applying product
• That itching may continue for 4-6 wk
• That product must be reapplied if accidentally washed off or treatment will be ineffective
• Not to apply to face; if accidental contact with eyes occurs, flush with water

• To treat sexual contacts simultaneously

linezolid (Rx)

(line-zoe′lide)

Zyvox, Zyvoxam ✤
Func. class.: Broad-spectrum antiinfective
Chem. class.: Oxazolidinone

Do not confuse:
Zyvox/Vioxx/Zovirax

ACTION: Inhibits protein synthesis by interfering with translation; binds to bacterial 23S ribosomal RNA of the 50S subunit, thus preventing formation of the bacterial translation process in primarily gram-positive organisms

USES: Vancomycin-resistant *Enterococcus faecium* infections, hospital-acquired pneumonia caused by *Staphylococcus aureus* or *Streptococcus pneumoniae*, uncomplicated or complicated skin and skin-structure infections, community-acquired pneumonia, *Pasteurella multocida*, viridans streptococci, *E. faecium* infections, *S. aureus, S. pyogenes;* can be used for MSSA/MRSA/MDRSP strains

CONTRAINDICATIONS: Hypersensitivity
Precautions: Pregnancy, breastfeeding, children, thrombocytopenia, bone marrow suppression, hypertension, hyperthyroidism, pheochromocytoma, seizure disorder, ulcerative colitis, MI, PKU, renal/GI disease

DOSAGE AND ROUTES
Vancomycin-resistant *Enterococcus faecium* infections
• **Adult/adolescent/child ≥12 yr: IV/PO** 600 mg q12hr × 14-28 days; max 1200 mg/day
• **Child <12 yr/infant/term neonate: IV/PO** 10 mg/kg q8hr × 14-28 days
Pneumonia/complicated skin infections
• **Adult: IV/PO** 600 mg q12hr × 10-14 days; max 1200 mg/day
• **Child birth-11 yr: PO/IV** 10 mg/kg q8hr × 10-14 days
Uncomplicated skin infections caused by *S. aureus* (MSSA only) or *S. pyogenes*
• **Adult: PO** 400 mg q12hr × 10-14 days; max 1200 mg/day
• **Adolescent: PO** 600 mg q12hr × 10-14 days; max 1200 mg/day
• **Child 5-11 yr: PO** 10 mg/kg q12hr × 10-14 days
• **Neonate ≥7 days old/infant/child <5 yr: PO** 10 mg/kg q8hr × 10-14 days
• **Infant preterm <7 days old: PO** 10 mg/kg q12hr × 10-14 days
Available forms: Tabs 600 mg; oral susp 100 mg/5 mL; premixed infusion

L

200 mg/100 mL, 400 mg/200 mL, 600 mg/mL (2 mg/mL)

Administer:

• Obtain culture and sensitivity before starting treatment, may give before results are received

PO route

• With/without food

• Store reconstituted oral susp at room temperature; use within 3 wk

Intermittent IV INFUSION route

• Do not use if particulate is present, yellow color is normal

• Premixed sol ready to use (2 mg/mL), give over 30-120 min; do not use IV infusion bag in series connections; do not use with additives in sol; do not use with another product, administer separately, flush line before and after use

• Store at room temperature in original packaging

Y-site compatibilities: Acyclovir, alfentanil, amikacin, aminophylline, ampicillin, aztreonam, buprenorphine, butorphanol, calcium gluconate, CARBOplatin, ceFAZolin, cefoTEtan, cefOXitin, cefTAZidime, ceftizoxime, cefuroxime, cimetidine, ciprofloxacin, cisatracurium, CISplatin, clindamycin, cyclophosphamide, cycloSPORINE, cytarabine, digoxin, furosemide, ganciclovir, gemcitabine, gentamicin, heparin, HYDRO-morphone, ifosfamide, labetalol, leucovorin, levofloxacin, lidocaine, LORazepam, magnesium sulfate, mannitol, meperidine, meropenem, mesna, methotrexate, methyl-PREDNISolone, metoclopramide, metro-NIDAZOLE, midazolam, minocycline, mito-XANtrone, morphine, nalbuphine, naloxone, nitroglycerin, ofloxacin, ondansetron, PACLitaxel, PENTobarbital, PHENo-barbital, piperacillin, potassium chloride, prochlorperazine, promethazine, propran-olol, ranitidine, remifentanil, SUFentanil, theophylline, ticarcillin, tobramycin, vancomycin, vecuronium, verapamil, vinCRIStine, zidovudine

Solution compatibilities: D_5W, 0.9% NaCl, LR

SIDE EFFECTS

CNS: *Headache,* dizziness, insomnia

GI: *Nausea, diarrhea,* CDAD, increased ALT/AST, *vomiting,* taste change, tongue-color change

EENT: Optic neuropathy

HEMA: Myelosuppression

MISC: Vaginal moniliasis, fungal infection, oral moniliasis, lactic acidosis, anaphylaxis, angioedema, Stevens-Johnson syndrome, serotonin syndrome

PHARMACOKINETICS

Peak 1-2 hr, terminal half-life 4-5 hr, rapidly and extensively absorbed, protein binding 31%, metabolized by oxidation of the morpholine ring

INTERACTIONS

Do not use with MAOIs (or within 2 wk) or with products that possess MAOI-like action (furazolidone, isoniazid, INH, procarbazine); hypertensive crisis may occur

Increase: hypertensive crisis, seizures, coma—amoxapine, maprotiline, mirtaza-pine, traZODone, cyclobenzaprine, tricyclics, methyldopa

Increase: serotonin syndrome—bupropion, cyclobenzaprine, tramadol, trazodone, SSRIs, SNRIs, serotonin receptor agonists; notify prescriber immediately

Increase: effects of adrenergic agents (DOPamine, EPINEPHrine, pseudoephedrine); monitor B/P

Drug/Herb

• Avoid use with green tea, valerian, ginseng, yohimbine, kava, guarana, St. John's wort

Drug/Food

• Tyramine foods: avoid; increased pressor response

Drug/Lab Test

Increase: LFTs, alkaline phosphatase, amylase, lipase, BUN

Decrease: WBC, platelets, blood glucose

NURSING CONSIDERATIONS

Assess:

• **Infection:** VS, characteristics of sputum, wounds, stool, emesis; WBC baseline, periodically

• Vision change, optic neuritis may occur

• CBC with differential weekly, assess for myelosuppression (anemias, leukopenia, pancytopenia, thrombocytopenia)

• **Serotonin syndrome:** at least 2 wk should elapse between discontinuing linezolid and starting serotonergic agents; assess for increased heart rate, shivering, sweating, dilated pupils, tremor, high B/P, hyperthermia, headache, confusion; if these occur, stop linezolid, administer a serotonin antagonist if needed

• **Lactic acidosis:** repeated nausea/vomiting, unexplained acidosis, low bicarbonate level; notify prescriber immediately

• **Anaphylaxis/angioedema/Stevens-Johnson syndrome:** rash, pruritus, difficulty breathing, fever; have emergency equipment nearby

• CNS symptoms: headache, dizziness

• Hepatic studies: AST, ALT

• **Diabetes mellitus:** monitor those receiving insulin or oral antidiabetics for increased hypoglycemia

• **CDAD:** diarrhea, abdominal pain, fever, fatigue, anorexia, possible anemia, elevated WBC, low serum albumin; stop product, usually either vancomycin or IV metroNIDAZOLE given

• **Pregnancy/breastfeeding:** avoid use in pregnancy and breastfeeding

Evaluate:

• Therapeutic response: decreased symptoms of infection, blood cultures negative

Teach patient/family:

• If dizziness occurs, to ambulate, perform activities with assistance

• To complete full course of product therapy, use as directed, not to skip or double dose when remembered, unless close to next dose

• **Serotonin syndrome:** to notify prescriber immediately of fever, sweating, diarrhea, confusion

• To contact prescriber if adverse reaction occurs

• To inform prescriber if SSRIs or cold products, decongestants being used

• To inform prescriber of history of hypertension

• To avoid large amounts of high-tyramine foods (aged cheeses, red wine), drinks; provide list

• To report diarrhea, signs/symptoms of superinfection

• **Pregnancy/breastfeeding:** Identify if pregnancy is planned or suspected or if breastfeeding

• To notify health care professional of vision change

• To avoid large amounts of tyramine (cereal meats, pickled products, beer, wine, chocolate)

• To discuss with health care professional all Rx, OTC, herbals, supplements used

---

RARELY USED

liothyronine (T₃) (Rx)

(lye-oh-thye'roe-neen)

Cytomel, Triostat

Func. class.: Thyroid hormone

Chem. class.: Synthetic T_3

USES: Hypothyroidism, myxedema coma, thyroid hormone replacement, congenital hypothyroidism, nontoxic goiter, T_3 suppression test

CONTRAINDICATIONS: Adrenal insufficiency, MI, thyrotoxicosis, untreated hypertension

Black Box Warning: Obesity treatment

DOSAGE AND ROUTES

• **Adult:** PO 25 mcg/day, increase by 12.5-25 mcg q1-2wk until desired response, maintenance dose 25-75 mcg/day, max 100 mcg/day

• **Geriatric:** PO 5 mcg/day, increase by 5 mcg/day q1-2wk, maintenance 25-75 mcg/day

Congenital hypothyroidism

• **Child >3 yr:** PO 50-100 mcg/day

• **Child <3 yr:** PO 5 mcg/day, increase by 5 mcg q3-4days titrated to response, infant maintenance 20 mcg/day; 1-3 yr 50 mcg/day

Myxedema, severe hypothyroidism

• **Adult:** PO 25-50 mcg, then may increase by 5-10 mcg q1-2wk; maintenance dose 50-100 mcg/day

---

Myxedema coma/precoma
• **Adult:** IV 25-50 mcg initially, 5 mcg in geriatric patients, 10-20 mcg with cardiac disease; give doses q4-12hr

Nontoxic goiter
• **Adult:** **PO** 5 mcg/day, increase by 12.5-25 mcg q1-2wk; maintenance dose 75 mcg/day

Suppression test
• **Adult:** **PO** 75-100 mcg/day × 1 wk; radioactive ^{131}I given before and after 1-wk dose

---

RARELY USED

liotrix (Rx)
(lye'oh-trix)
Thyrolar, T$_3$/T$_4$
Func. class.: Thyroid hormone
Chem. class.: Levothyroxine/liothyronine (synthetic T$_4$, T$_3$)

USES: Hypothyroidism, thyroid hormone replacement

CONTRAINDICATIONS: Adrenal insufficiency, MI, thyrotoxicosis

Black Box Warning: Obesity treatment

DOSAGE AND ROUTES
• **Adult:** PO single dose of Thyrolar, $^1/_4$ or $^1/_2$ tab, adjust as needed at 2-wk intervals
• **Geriatric:** PO $^1/_4$ tab initially; adjust q6-8wk

⚠ HIGH ALERT

liraglutide (Rx)
(lir'a-gloo'tide)
Saxenda, Victoza
Func. class.: Antidiabetic agent
Chem. class.: Incretin mimetics

ACTION: Improved glycemic control and potential weight loss via activation of the glucagon-like peptide-1 (GLP-1) receptor

USES: Type 2 diabetes mellitus in combination with diet/exercise, obesity

CONTRAINDICATIONS: Hypersensitivity, medullary thyroid carcinoma (MTC), multiple endocrine neoplasia syndrome type 2 (MEN 2), thyroid cancer, pregnancy
Precautions: Breastfeeding, children, geriatric patients, alcoholism, cholelithiasis, ketoacidosis, diarrhea, fever, gastroparesis, hepatic/renal disease, hypoglycemia, infection, surgery, thyroid disease, trauma, vomiting, pancreatitis

Black Box Warning: Thyroid C-cell tumors

DOSAGES AND ROUTES
• **Adult:** SUBCUT (Victoza) 0.6 mg/day × 1 wk, then increase to 1.2 mg/day, max 1.8 mg/day; **Saxenda:** 0.6 mg/day × 1 wk, then 1.2 mg/day × 1 wk then 1.8 mg × 1 wk, then 2.4 mg/day × 1 wk, then 3 mg/day

Available forms: Solution for injection 0.6, 1.2, 1.8, 2.4, 3 mg prefilled pen (Saxenda); solution for injection 0.6, 1.2, 1.8 mg prefilled pen (Victoza)
Administer:
SUBCUT route
• Use safe handling procedures
• Give subcut only, inspect for particulate matter, discoloration; do not use if unusually viscous, cloudy, discolored, or if particles present; give daily anytime, without regard to meals; pen needles must be purchased separately, use Novo Nordisk needle; before first use, prime, see manual for directions; give in thigh, abdomen, or upper arm; lightly pinch fold of skin, insert needle at 90-degree angle (45-degree angle if thin), release skin; aspiration is not needed, give over 6 sec, rotate injection sites
• If dose is missed, resume once-daily dosing at next scheduled dose; if >3 days have elapsed since last dose, reinitiate at 0.6 mg, titrate

• Storage: do not store pen with needle attached; avoid direct heat and sunlight; discard 30 days after first use; after first use may be stored at room temperature or refrigerated; do not freeze

SIDE EFFECTS
CNS: Dizziness, headache
CV: Hypertension
ENDO: Hypoglycemia
EENT: Sinusitis
GI: Abdominal pain, anorexia, constipation, diarrhea, dyspepsia, nausea, vomiting, *pancreatitis*
INTEG: erythema, injection site reaction, urticaria
MS: Back pain
SYST: Antibody formation, infection, influenza, secondary thyroid malignancy, anaphylaxis, angioedema

INTERACTIONS
Increase: hypoglycemic reactions—angiotensin II receptor antagonists, ACE inhibitors, other antidiabetics, β-blockers, dexfenfluramine, fenfluramine, disopyramide, FLUoxetine, fibric acid derivatives, mecasermin, MAOIs, octreotide, pegvisomant, salicylates
Decrease: liraglutide effect—protease inhibitors, phenothiazines, baclofen, atypical antipsychotics, corticosteroids, cycloSPORINE, tacrolimus, carbonic anhydrase inhibitors, dextrothyroxine, diazoxide, phenytoin, fosphenytoin, ethotoin, isoniazid, INH, niacin, nicotine, estrogens, progestins, oral contraceptives, growth hormones, sympathomimetics
Increase or decrease: hypoglycemic reactions—androgens, bortezomib, quinolones, cloNIDine, alcohol, lithium, pentamidine
Increase or decrease: effects of—atorvastatin, acetaminophen, griseofulvin
Decrease: levels of digoxin
Drug/Lab Test
Increase: calcitonin, lipase
Decrease: glucose

PHARMACOKINETICS
Protein binding (98%); half-life 12-13 hr; binds to albumin, then released into circulation; peak 8-12 hr; body weight significantly affects pharmacokinetics

NURSING CONSIDERATIONS
Assess:

Black Box Warning: **Thyroid C-cell tumors;** monitor during treatment; if calcitonin is elevated or if nodules can be felt, referral is needed; do not use in those with a family history of MTC or in those with multiple endocrine neoplasia syndrome type 2

• **Diabetes:** that may occur soon after meals: hunger, sweating, weakness, dizziness, tremors, restlessness, tachycardia; serum glucose, A1c, CBC during treatment
• Hypersensitivity to this product
• **Insulin use with Victoza:** monitor for hypoglycemic reactions often
• **Stress:** those diabetic patients exposed to stress, surgery, fever, infections may require insulin administration temporarily
• **Serious skin reactions:** angioedema
• **Pancreatitis:** monitor for nausea, vomiting, severe abdominal pain; product should be discontinued; give supportive care; monitor amylase, lipase, electrolytes
Evaluate:
• Therapeutic response: stable and improved serum glucose, A1c, weight loss
Teach patient/family:
• **Hypersensitivity:** to report any allergic symptoms
• About symptoms of hypoglycemia/hyperglycemia and what to do for each; to have glucagon emergency kit available; to carry a carbohydrate source at all times
• About side effects associated with therapy, such as nausea and vomiting; that upward dose titration can be delayed or ignored, depending on tolerance
• That diabetes is a lifelong illness; that product does not cure disease and must be continued on a daily basis
• To carry emergency ID with prescriber's phone number and medications taken
• To continue with other recommendations: diet, exercise
• To test blood glucose using a blood glucose meter

• To avoid other medications, herbs, supplements unless approved by prescriber

• To report serious skin effects, abdominal pain with nausea/vomiting immediately

• To consult written instructions if self-administration is ordered; to discard pen after 30 days

• That continuing follow-up exams will be needed

• That secondary malignancy is possible; that routine monitoring may be needed; to report trouble breathing, continuous hoarseness, lump in neck region immediately

• Not to share product with others; infections such as hepatitis may occur

• **Pregnancy/breastfeeding:** that product is not to be used in pregnancy or breastfeeding, that insulin is usually used in pregnancy, to notify health care professional if pregnancy is planned or suspected or if breastfeeding

---

lisdexamfetamine (Rx)

(lis-dex′am-fet′a-meen)

Vyvanse

Func. class.: CNS stimulant

Chem. class.: Amphetamine

Controlled Substance Schedule II

ACTION: Increases release of norepinephrine, DOPamine in cerebral cortex to reticular activating system

USES: Attention-deficit/hyperactivity disorder (ADHD), binge eating disorder

CONTRAINDICATIONS: Breastfeeding, hyperthyroidism, hypertension, glaucoma, severe arteriosclerosis, hypersensitivity to sympathomimetic amines

Black Box Warning: Substance abuse

Precautions: Pregnancy, children <6 yr, Gilles de la Tourette's disorder, depression, anorexia nervosa, psychosis, seizure disorder, suicidal ideation, MI, heart failure, alcoholism, aortic stenosis, bipolar disorder, CV disease

DOSAGE AND ROUTES

ADHD

• **Adult/child 6-17 yr: PO** 30 mg/day in AM; may increase by 10-20 mg/day at weekly intervals, max 70 mg/day

Moderate to severe binge eating disorder

• **Adult: PO** 30 mg/day in AM, increase by 20 mg q wk to target of 50-70 mg/day

Renal dose

• **Adult: PO** Severe impairment (GFR 15-<30 mL/min/1.73 m^2): max 50 mg/day; ESRD (GFR <15 mL/min/1.73 m^2): max 30 mg/day

Available forms: Caps 10, 20, 30, 40, 50, 60, 70 mg

Administer:

• Give daily in AM

• Without regard to meals

• Caps: may take whole or opened and contents dissolved in water, take immediately

SIDE EFFECTS

CNS: *Hyperactivity, insomnia, restlessness, talkativeness,* dizziness, headache, dysphoria, irritability, CNS tumor, dependence, addiction, mild euphoria, somnolence, lability, psychosis, mania, hallucinations, aggression; movement disorders, psychiatric events (child)

CV: *Palpitations, tachycardia,* hypertension, decrease in heart rate, dysrhythmias, MI, cardiomyopathy

EENT: Blurred vision, mydriasis, diplopia

ENDO: Growth inhibition

GI: *Anorexia,* dry mouth, diarrhea, weight loss

GU: Impotence, change in libido

INTEG: Urticaria, angioedema, Stevens-Johnson syndrome, toxic epidermal necrolysis

MISC: Rhabdomyolysis

PHARMACOKINETICS

Metabolized by liver; urine excretion pH dependent; crosses placenta, breast milk; half-life <1 hr

INTERACTIONS

• **Hypertensive crisis:** MAOIs or within 14 days of MAOIs

Increase: serotonin syndrome, neuroleptic malignant syndrome—SSRIs, SNRIs, serotonin-receptor agonists

Increase: lisdexamfetamine effect—acetaZOLAMIDE, antacids, sodium bicarbonate, urinary alkalinizers

Increase: CNS effect—haloperidol, tricyclics, phenothiazines, modafinil, meperidine, PHENobarbital, phenytoin

Increase: CNS stimulation—melatonin

Decrease: absorption of phenytoin

Decrease: lisdexamfetamine effect—ascorbic acid, ammonium chloride, urinary acidifiers

Decrease: effect of—adrenergic blockers, antidiabetics

Drug/Herb

• **Serotonin syndrome:** St. John's wort

Increase: stimulant effect—khat, melatonin, green tea, guarana

Decrease: stimulant effect—eucalyptus

Drug/Food

Increase: amine effect—caffeine

NURSING CONSIDERATIONS

Assess:

• **ADHD:** obtain history from parents, patient, counselors, as well as testing; confirm diagnosis before use

• **Binge eating disorder:** obtain history of diet bingeing times and food

• VS, B/P; product may reverse antihypertensives; check patients with cardiac disease often

• CBC, urinalysis; in diabetes: blood glucose; insulin changes may be required because eating may decrease

• Height, growth rate in children; growth rate may be decreased; treatment should be discontinued if this is present

• Mental status: mood, sensorium, affect, stimulation, insomnia, irritability

• **Serotonin syndrome, neuroleptic malignant syndrome:** increased heart rate, shivering, sweating, dilated pupils, tremors, high B/P, hyperthermia, headache, confusion; if these occur, stop product, administer serotonin antagonist if needed; at least 2 wk should elapse between discontinuation of serotonergic agents and start of product

• **Tolerance or dependency:** increased amount of product may be used to get same effect; will develop after long-term use

• Overdose: pain, fever, dehydration, insomnia, hyperactivity

Black Box Warning: Before giving this product, identify presence of substance abuse; high potential for abuse, may be fatal

• **Psychotic manic episodes:** may occur when patients have underlying psychiatric conditions

• Gum, hard candy, frequent sips of water for dry mouth

• **Pregnancy/breastfeeding:** avoid use in pregnancy and breastfeeding

Evaluate:

• Therapeutic response: increased CNS stimulation, decreased drowsiness

Teach patient/family:

• **Seizures:** that product may decrease seizure threshold; those with a seizure disorder should notify prescriber if seizure occurs

• To report CNS changes, blurred vision; decrease in dose may be needed

• To decrease caffeine consumption (coffee, tea, cola, chocolate); may increase irritability, stimulation

• To avoid OTC preparations unless approved by prescriber

• To taper product over several weeks; depression, increased sleeping, lethargy may occur

• To avoid alcohol ingestion

• To avoid breastfeeding

• To avoid hazardous activities until stabilized on medication

• To get needed rest; patient will feel more tired at end of day

Black Box Warning: Serious CV effects may occur from increasing dose

• **Pregnancy/breastfeeding:** to avoid use in pregnancy, breastfeeding

TREATMENT OF OVERDOSE:

Administer fluids, antihypertensive for increased B/P, ammonium chloride for increased excretion, chlorproMAZINE for antagonizing CNS effects

---

lisinopril (Rx)

(lyse-in′oh-pril)

Prinivil, Zestril

Func. class.: Antihypertensive, angiotensin-converting enzyme 1 (ACE) inhibitor

Chem. class.: Enalaprilat lysine analog

Do not confuse:
lisinopril/RisperDAL/Lipitor
Prinivil/Plendil/Proventil/PriLOSEC
Zestril/Zetia/Zyprexa

ACTION: Selectively suppresses renin-angiotensin-aldosterone system; inhibits ACE, thereby preventing conversion of angiotensin I to angiotensin II

USES: Mild to moderate hypertension, adjunctive therapy of systolic HF, acute MI
Unlabeled uses: Diabetic nephropathy/retinopathy, proteinuria, post MI

CONTRAINDICATIONS: Hypersensitivity, angioedema

Black Box Warning: Pregnancy

Precautions: Breastfeeding, renal disease, hyperkalemia, renal artery stenosis, HF, aortic stenosis

DOSAGE AND ROUTES
Hypertension
• **Adult: PO** initially 10 mg, 10-40 mg/day; max 80 mg/day
• **Child ≥6 yr: PO** 0.07 mg/kg/day up to 5 mg/day; titrate q1-2wk up to 0.6 mg/kg/day or 40 mg/day
• **Geriatric: PO** 2.5-5 mg/day, increase q7days
Renal dose
• **Adult: PO** CCr <30 mL/min, reduce dose by 50%, initially 5 mg/day, max 40 mg/day; CCr <10 mL/min, 2.5 mg/day, max 40 mg/day
Heart failure
• **Adult: PO** 5 mg/day, increase if needed to max 20 mg/day or 40 mg/day (Zestril);

in hypernatremia of <130 mEqL or creatinine >3 mg/dL or CCr <30 mL/min, 2.5 mg/day initially
Acute myocardial infarction
• **Adult: PO** give 5 mg within 24 hr of onset of symptoms, then 5 mg after 24 hr, 10 mg after 48 hr, then 10 mg daily
Available forms: Tabs 2.5, 5, 10, 20, 30, 40 mg
Administer:
• Severe hypotension may occur after 1st dose of product; may be prevented by reducing or discontinuing diuretic therapy 3 days before beginning lisinopril therapy
• Without regard to food

SIDE EFFECTS
CNS: *Vertigo,* depression, stroke, insomnia, paresthesias, *headache, fatigue,* asthenia, *dizziness*
CV: Chest pain, *hypotension,* sinus tachycardia
EENT: Blurred vision, nasal congestion
GI: Nausea, vomiting, anorexia, constipation, flatulence, GI irritation, diarrhea, hepatic failure, hepatic necrosis, pancreatitis
GU: Proteinuria, renal insufficiency, sexual dysfunction, impotence
HEMA: Neutropenia, agranulocytosis
INTEG: Rash, pruritus
MISC: Muscle cramps, *hyperkalemia*
RESP: Dry cough, dyspnea
SYST: Angioedema, anaphylaxis, toxic epidermal necrolysis

PHARMACOKINETICS
Onset 1 hr, peak 6-8 hr, duration 24 hr, excreted unchanged in urine, half-life 12 hr

INTERACTIONS
Increase: hyperkalemia—potassium salt substitutes, potassium-sparing diuretics, potassium supplements, cycloSPORINE
Increase: possible toxicity—lithium
Increase: hypotensive effect—diuretics, other antihypertensives, probenecid, phenothiazines, nitrates, acute alcohol ingestion
Increase: hypersensitivity—allopurinol
Decrease: lisinopril effects—aspirin, indomethacin, NSAIDs; dose may need adjustment

---

Drug/Food

• High-potassium diet (bananas, orange juice, avocados, nuts, spinach) should be avoided; hyperkalemia may occur; monitor potassium levels

Drug/Lab Test

Interference: glucose/insulin tolerance tests, LFTs, BUN, creatinine

NURSING CONSIDERATIONS

Assess:

• **Heart failure:** edema in feet, legs daily; weight daily; dyspnea, wet crackles

• Skin turgor, dryness of mucous membranes for hydration status

• **Acute MI:** can be used in combination with salicylates, β blockers, thrombolytics

• **Hypertension:** B/P, pulse q4hr during beginning treatment and periodically; black patients should take in combination with diuretics thereafter; note rate, rhythm, quality; apical/pedal pulse before administration; notify prescriber of any significant changes

• Blood studies, platelets; WBC with differential at baseline, periodically q3mo; if neutrophils <1000/mm³, discontinue treatment (recommended with collagen-vascular disease)

• Baselines of renal, hepatic studies before therapy begins, periodically; LFTs, uric acid, glucose may be increased

• **Angioedema, anaphylaxis, toxic epidermal necrolysis:** facial swelling, dyspnea, tongue swelling (rare); have emergency equipment nearby; may be more common in black patients

• Electrolytes: potassium, sodium, chlorine

Black Box Warning: **Pregnancy/breastfeeding:** assess pregnancy, breastfeeding status before giving this product; if pregnant, do not use; do not breastfeed

Evaluate:

• Therapeutic response: decreased B/P, HF symptoms

Teach patient/family:

• Not to discontinue product abruptly; to taper

• To rise slowly to sitting or standing position to minimize orthostatic hypotension

• To avoid increasing potassium in the diet

• To report dry cough

Black Box Warning: **Pregnancy/breastfeeding:** to report if pregnancy is planned or suspected; not to breastfeed

TREATMENT OF OVERDOSE:

Lavage, IV atropine for bradycardia, IV theophylline for bronchospasm, digoxin, O₂, diuretic for cardiac failure

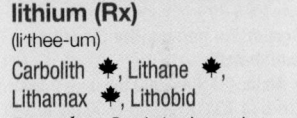

lithium (Rx)

(li′thee-um)

Carbolith ✦, Lithane ✦, Lithamax ✦, Lithobid

Func. class.: Psychotropic agent—antimanic

Chem. class.: Alkali metal ion salt

Do not confuse:

lithium/lanthanum

ACTION: May alter sodium, potassium ion transport across cell membrane in nerve, muscle cells; may balance biogenic amines of norepinephrine, serotonin in CNS areas involved in emotional responses

USES: Bipolar disorders (manic phase), prevention of bipolar manic-depressive psychosis

Unlabeled uses: Borderline personality disorder

CONTRAINDICATIONS: Pregnancy, breastfeeding, children <12 yr, hepatic disease, brain trauma, organic brain syndrome, schizophrenia, severe cardiac/renal disease, severe dehydration

Precautions: Geriatric patients, thyroid disease, seizure disorders, diabetes mellitus, systemic infection, urinary retention, QT prolongation

Black Box Warning: Lithium level >1.5 mmol/L

Side effects: *italics* = common; red = life-threatening

DOSAGE AND ROUTES—NTI

Bipolar disorder (mania)

• **Adult:** PO 600 mg tid, maintenance 300 mg tid or qid; **EXT REL** 900 mg q12hr; dose should be individualized to maintain blood levels at 1-1.5 mEq/L or 0.6-1.2 mEq/L (maintenance)

• **Geriatric:** PO 300 mg bid, increase q7days by 300 mg to desired dose

• **Child:** PO 15-20 mg/kg/day in 3-4 divided doses; increase as needed; do not exceed adult doses; maintain blood levels at 0.4-0.5 mEq/L

Renal dose

• **Adult:** PO CCr 10-50 mL/min give 50%-75% of normal dose, CCr <10 mL/min give 25%-50% of normal dose

Borderline personality disorder (unlabeled)

• **Adult:** PO 900-2400 mg in 3-4 divided doses or **EXT REL** 900-1800 mg in 2 divided doses, maintain levels 0.8-1 mEq/L

Available forms: Caps 150, 300, 600 mg; tabs 300 mg; ext rel tabs 300, 450 mg; syr 300 mg/5 mL (8 mEq/5 mL)

Administer:

• Do not break, crush, chew caps, ext rel tabs

• Reduced dose to geriatric patients

• With meals to avoid GI upset

• Adequate fluids (2-3 L/day) to prevent dehydration during initial treatment, 1-2 L/day during maintenance

SIDE EFFECTS

CNS: *Headache, drowsiness, dizziness,* tremors, twitching, ataxia, seizure, slurred speech, restlessness, confusion, stupor, memory loss, clonic movements, fatigue

CV: *Hypotension,* ECG changes, dysrhythmias, circulatory failure, edema, Brugada syndrome, QT prolongation

EENT: Tinnitus, blurred vision

ENDO: Hyponatremia, goiter, hyperglycemia, hypo/hyperthyroidism

GI: *Dry mouth, anorexia, nausea, vomiting, diarrhea,* incontinence, abdominal pain, metallic taste

GU: Polyuria, glycosuria, proteinuria, albuminuria, urinary incontinence, polydipsia

HEMA: Leukocytosis

INTEG: Drying of hair, alopecia, rash, pruritus, hyperkeratosis, acneiform lesions, folliculitis

MS: Muscle weakness

PHARMACOKINETICS

PO: Onset rapid, peak ½-3 hr, half-life 18-36 hr depending on age, crosses blood-brain barrier, 80% of filtered lithium reabsorbed by renal tubules, excreted in urine, crosses placenta, enters breast milk, well absorbed by oral method

INTERACTIONS

Increase: hypothyroid effects—antithyroid agents, calcium iodide, potassium iodide, iodinated glycerol

Increase: effects of neuromuscular blocking agents

Increase: renal clearance—sodium bicarbonate, acetaZOLAMIDE, mannitol, aminophylline

Increase: lithium level—ACE inhibitors

Increase: QT interval—antiarrhythmics, other QT prolongation products

Increase: masking of lithium toxicity—β-blockers used for lithium tremor

Increase: toxicity—indomethacin, diuretics, NSAIDs

Increase: lithium effect/toxicity—carBAMazepine, FLUoxetine, methyldopa, thiazide diuretics, probenecid; monitor drug levels

Decrease: lithium effects—calcium channel blockers

Drug/Herb

• Avoid use with kava, St. John's wort, valerian

Decrease: lithium levels—black/green tea, guarana

Drug/Food

• Significant changes in sodium intake will alter lithium excretion

Decrease: lithium levels—caffeine; adjust dose as needed

Drug/Lab Test

Increase: potassium excretion, urine glucose, blood glucose, protein, BUN

Decrease: VMA, T_3, T_4, ^{131}I

NURSING CONSIDERATIONS
Assess:
• **Mental status:** manic symptoms, mood, behavior before, during treatment

Black Box Warning: **Lithium toxicity:** diarrhea, vomiting, tremor, twitching, poor coordination, lassitude; **major toxicity,** coarse tremors, severe thirst, tinnitus, dilute urine; serum lithium levels wk initially, then q2mo (therapeutic level: 0.5-1.5 mEq/L); toxic level >1.5 mcg/L; the drug has a narrow therapeutic index (NTI), measure level before AM dose

• Weight daily; check for, report edema in legs, ankles, wrists
• Sodium intake; decreased sodium intake with decreased fluid intake may lead to lithium retention; increased sodium, fluids may decrease lithium retention
• Skin turgor at least daily
• Urine for albuminuria, glycosuria, uric acid during beginning treatment, q2mo thereafter; specific gravity, any level <1.005 may indicate diabetes insipidus and should be reported to prescriber
• Neurologic status: LOC, gait, motor reflexes, hand tremors
• ECG in those >50 yr with CV disease; cardiology consult is recommended in those with risk factor; QT prolongation may occur
• **Pregnancy/breastfeeding:** do not use in pregnancy, breastfeeding
Evaluate:
• Therapeutic response: decrease in excitement, manic phase
Teach patient/family:
• **About the symptoms of minor toxicity:** vomiting, diarrhea, poor coordination, fine motor tremors, weakness, lassitude; major toxicity: coarse tremors, severe thirst, tinnitus, diluted urine; to seek medical care immediately
• To monitor urine specific gravity, emphasize need for follow-up care to determine lithium levels; to monitor lithium levels to ensure effective levels and treatment
• Not to operate machinery until lithium levels are stable

• To use emergency ID with diagnosis, product used
• That beneficial effects may take 1-3 wk
• About products that interact with lithium (provide list); about need for adequate, stable intake of salt and fluids; not to use OTC products unless approved by prescriber
• **Pregnancy/breastfeeding:** that contraception is necessary because lithium may harm fetus; not to breastfeed

TREATMENT OF OVERDOSE:
Induce emesis or lavage, maintain airway, respiratory function; dialysis for severe intoxication

> ## ⚠ HIGH ALERT
>
> ## lixisenatide
> (lix' i-sen' a-tide)
>
> Adlyxin
> *Func. class.:* Antidiabetic
> *Chem. class.:* Incretin mimetic

L

ACTION: An incretin mimetic; a glucagon-like peptide-1 (GLP-1) receptor agonist; binds and activates the GLP-1 receptor. GLP-1 is an important, gut-derived, glucose homeostasis regulator that is released after the oral ingestion of carbohydrates or fats

USES: Treatment of type 2 diabetes mellitus in combination with diet and exercise

CONTRAINDICATIONS: Angioedema
Precautions: Alcoholism, breastfeeding, children, cholelithiasis, diabetic ketoacidosis, gastroparesis, hypoglycemia, pancreatitis, pregnancy, renal failure, renal impairment, risk of serious hypersensitivity reactions or anaphylaxis, type 1 diabetes mellitus

DOSAGE AND ROUTES
• **Adult:** SUBCUT Initially, 10 mcg/day within 1 hr before the morning meal. If a dose is missed, give within 1 hr before

the next meal. Continue 10 mcg/day × 14 days; on day 15, increase the dose to the maintenance dose of 20 mcg/day, max 20 mcg/day

Renal dose

• Adult: eGFR 30 to 89 mL/min/1.73 m^2: no dosage adjustment needed; eGFR 15 to 29 mL/min/1.73 m^2: monitor closely for adverse reactions, especially hypoglycemia, nausea, and vomiting, and for changes in renal function. Dehydration and acute renal failure and worsening of chronic renal failure may occur in these patients. eGFR less than 15 mL/min/1.73 m^2: do not use

Available forms: Solution for injection 10 mcg, 20 mcg prefilled pen starter pack, maintenance pack

Administer:

• May be used as monotherapy or with other antidiabetic medications. Dose adjustment of metformin or a thiazolidinedione is not usually required. A reduction in the dose of a sulfonylurea may be needed to reduce the risk of hypoglycemia

• Give subcut injection only. Do not give IV/IM

• Visually inspect for particulate matter and discoloration before use; do not use if unusually viscous, cloudy, discolored, or if particles are present

• Available as a prefilled pen. Each pen must be activated before the first use

• Administer daily within 1 hr before the first meal of the day, preferably the same meal each day. If a dose is missed, give within 1 hr before the next meal

• Inject subcut into the thigh, abdomen, or upper arm

• Double-check dosage before use

• Rotate sites with each injection to prevent lipodystrophy

• **Storage:** Protect pen from light and keep in its original packaging; discard pen 14 days after its first use

SIDE EFFECTS

GI: Nausea, vomiting, diarrhea, constipation, abdominal pain, dyspepsia, pancreatitis (rare)

CNS: Dizziness, headache

MISC: Antibody formation, hypoglycemia, injection site reactions, hypotension; anaphylactoid reaction, bronchospasm, renal failure, laryngeal edema

PHARMACOKINETICS

Eliminated through glomerular filtration and proteolytic degradation, terminal half-life 1-3 hr; peak 1-3.5 hr; elimination prolonged in renal disease, with mild (CCr 60 to 89 mL/min), moderate (CCr 30 to 59 mL/min), and severe renal impairment (CCr 15 to 29 mL/min) was increased by approximately 34%, 69%, and 124%, respectively; use with caution in renal disease

INTERACTIONS

Increase: effect of—sulfonylureas

Increase: hypoglycemia—antidiabetes

Decrease: effect of hormonal contraceptives, to be taken 1 hr before

NURSING CONSIDERATIONS

Assess:

• **Diabetes:** fasting blood glucose, A1c level during treatment to determine diabetic control

• **Pancreatitis:** severe abdominal pain with or without nausea and vomiting, product should be discontinued immediately

• **Renal disease:** monitor BUN, creatinine in mild renal disease; do not use in severe renal disease

• Hypoglycemia/hyperglycemia: reaction can occur soon after meals; for severe hypoglycemia, give IV D$_{50}$W, IV dextrose solution

Evaluate:

• Therapeutic response: decreasing polydipsia, polyuria, polyphagia, clear sensorium, improving A1c, weight

Teach patient/family:

• Not to share among patients. Even if the disposable needle is changed, sharing may result in transmission of hepatitis viruses, HIV, or other blood-borne pathogens

• How to prepare and use the pen; include a practice injection

---

- About the signs and symptoms of hypoglycemia/hyperglycemia and what to do about each; to have emergency glucagon kit available at all times, to carry glucose source (sugar, candy)
- That product must be taken on a continuing basis; not to discontinue without prescriber's approval
- That diabetes is a lifelong condition; that product will not cure condition; to carry emergency ID with condition, products taken, prescriber's phone number and name
- To continue weight control, dietary restrictions, exercise, hygiene
- That regular lab testing and A1c will be necessary
- **Pancreatitis:** to seek medical care immediately if severe abdominal pain occurs with or without nausea, vomiting
- **Pregnancy:** to notify prescriber if pregnant or planning to become pregnant; if taking oral contraceptives, to take at least 1 hr before this product

---

Iodoxamide ophthalmic
See Appendix B

Iofexidine
(loe FEX i deen)
Lucemyra
Func. class.: Opioid withdrawal agent
Chem. class.: Central alpha-2 agonist

ACTION: A central alpha-2 agonist that binds to adrenergic receptors, resulting in a reduction in the release of norepinephrine and a decrease in sympathetic tone

USES: For the mitigation of opioid withdrawal symptoms to facilitate abrupt opioid discontinuation in adults

CONTRAINDICATIONS: Hypersensitivity
Precautions: Abrupt discontinuation, acute MI, alcoholism, bradycardia, breastfeeding, cardiac dysrhythmias, CV disease, children, coadministration with other CNS depressants, coronary artery disease, dehydration, diabetes mellitus, dialysis, driving or operating machinery, electrolyte imbalance, ethanol ingestion, females, geriatric patients, heart failure, hepatic disease, hypertension, hypocalcemia, hypomagnesemia, hypotension, infertility, long QT syndrome, malnutrition, poor metabolizers, pregnancy, renal disease, syncope, thyroid disease

DOSAGE AND ROUTES
- **Adult: PO** Initially, 0.54 mg (3 × 0.18 mg tablets) 4× daily during peak withdrawal symptoms (first 5-7 days after last use of opioid), with dosing based on opiate withdrawal symptoms and tolerability; may use up to 14 days. Space dosing 5-6 hr apart; max 0.72 mg (4 tabs) as a single dose; max 2.88 mg (16 tabs) per day. To discontinue, gradually taper dose over 2-4 days to reduce drug withdrawal symptoms (reduce by 1 tab per dose every 1-2 days)
Available forms: Tabs 0.18 mg
Administer:
- May administer orally without regard to meals

PHARMACOKINETICS
Protein binding 55%, 30% of dose is converted to inactive metabolites during first-pass metabolism by CYP2D6, CYP1A2 and CYP2C19, excretion kidney 15-20%, half-life 17-22 hr after repeated dosing, peak 3-5 hr

INTERACTIONS
- **Increase:** QT prolongation—type IA, IC, III antidysrhythmics, antihistamines, antidepressants; monitor ECG if used concurrently
- **Increase:** CNS effects and sedation—other CNS depressants; if used concurrently, monitor for increased sedation
- **Increase:** hypotension—antihypertensives; avoid concurrent use if possible
- **Increase:** hypotension, bradycardia—CYP2D6 inhibitors

NURSING CONSIDERATIONS

Assess:

• **QT prolongation:** this product can cause QT prolongation and should be avoided in those with congenital long QT syndrome. Use with caution in those with cardiac disease, cardiac dysrhythmias, heart failure, bradycardia, MI, hypertension, coronary artery disease, hypomagnesemia, hypokalemia, hypocalcemia, or in patients receiving medications known to prolong the QT interval or cause an electrolyte imbalance. Monitor ECG in heart failure, bradyarrhythmias, liver or kidney impairment, or during concurrent use of other medications that lead to QT prolongation

• **Electrolyte imbalances** (hypokalemia, hypomagnesemia) should be corrected before use; monitor electrolytes for changes

• **Somnolence and sedation** are common and may cause impairment of cognitive and motor skills; may be increased when coadministered with other CNS depressants (benzodiazepines, ethanol, and barbiturates)

• **Abrupt discontinuation:** monitor B/P during tapering; a significant increase in B/P may occur with abrupt discontinuation. May also cause diarrhea, insomnia, anxiety, chills, hyperhidrosis, and extremity pain

• **Hepatic disease:** may reduce drug clearance. Dosage reductions are recommended based on degree of hepatic impairment

• **Renal impairment:** may reduce drug clearance. Dosage reductions may be needed based on degree of renal impairment, including renal failure (end-stage renal disease, patients on dialysis); may be used without regard to timing of dialysis

• **Geriatric patients:** caution is recommended when administering to patients over age 65. Dose adjustments may be needed

• **Fertility:** infertility has been noted in some animal studies

• **Pregnancy/breastfeeding:** safety not established. Consider the benefits of breastfeeding, the risk of potential infant drug exposure, and the risk of an untreated or inadequately treated condition

Teach patient/family

• About self-monitoring for hypotension, bradycardia, and related symptoms; that moving from a supine to upright position may increase the risk for hypotension or orthostatic effects

• To stay hydrated; to recognize symptoms of hypotension; if hypotension occurs, to sit or lie down; to carefully rise from a sitting or lying position

• To withhold doses when experiencing hypotension or bradycardia and to contact health care provider for guidance on dose adjustments

• To use caution or avoid performing activities that require mental alertness, such as driving or operating machinery, until effect of product is known

• Not to discontinue without consulting health care provider. That when discontinuing the drug, a gradual reduction in dose is recommended

• To inform health care provider of other medications being taken, including ethanol ingestion

• That patients who complete opioid discontinuation are at an increased risk of fatal overdose should they resume opioid use

---

loperamide (OTC, Rx)

(loe-per′a-mide)

Imodium ♥, Imodium A-D

Func. class.: Antidiarrheal

Chem. class.: Piperidine derivative

Do not confuse:
Imodium/Indocin
Loperamide/furosemide

ACTION: Direct action on intestinal muscles to decrease GI peristalsis; reduces volume, increases bulk; electrolytes not lost

USES: Diarrhea (cause undetermined), travelers' diarrhea, chronic diarrhea, to decrease amount of ileostomy discharge

---

Unlabeled uses: Irritable bowel syndrome, irinotecan-induced diarrhea

CONTRAINDICATIONS: Hypersensitivity, CDAD, constipation, dysentery, GI bleeding/obstruction/perforation, ileus, vomiting

Precautions: Pregnancy, breastfeeding, children <2 yr, hepatic disease, dehydration, gastroenteritis, toxic megacolon, geriatric patients, severe ulcerative colitis

DOSAGE AND ROUTES

• **Adult:** PO 4 mg, then 2 mg after each loose stool, max 16 mg/day
• **Child 9-11 yr:** PO 2 mg, then 1 mg after each loose stool, max 6 mg/24 hr
• **Child 6-8 yr:** PO 2 mg, then 0.1 mg/kg after each loose stool, max 4 mg/day
• **Child 2-5 yr:** PO 1 mg, then 0.1 mg/kg after each loose stool, max 4 mg/24 hr

Available forms: Caps 2 mg; liq 1 mg/5 mL; tabs 2 mg, chew tabs 2 mg

Administer:
• Do not break, crush, or chew caps
• For 48 hr only
• Do not mix oral sol with other sol

SIDE EFFECTS

CNS: Dizziness, drowsiness, fatigue
GI: *Nausea, dry mouth, vomiting, constipation,* abdominal pain, anorexia, toxic megacolon, bacterial enterocolitis, flatulence
INTEG: Rash
MISC: Hyperglycemia
SYST: Anaphylaxis, angioedema, toxic epidermal necrolysis

PHARMACOKINETICS

PO: Duration 24 hr, protein binding 97%, half-life 9-14 hr, metabolized in liver, excreted in feces as unchanged product, small amount in urine

INTERACTIONS

Increase: CNS depression—alcohol, antihistamines, analgesics, opioids, sedative/hypnotics
Drug/Herb
Increase: CNS depression—chamomile, hops, kava, valerian

NURSING CONSIDERATIONS

Assess:
• **Stools:** volume, color, characteristics, frequency; bowel pattern before product; rebound constipation
• Electrolytes (potassium, sodium, chlorine) if receiving long-term therapy
• Response after 48 hr; if no response, product should be discontinued
• **Pregnancy/breastfeeding:** use only if benefits outweigh fetal risk; breastfeeding is not recommended

Evaluate:
• Therapeutic response: decreased diarrhea (48 hr); decreased chronic diarrhea (10 days)

Teach patient/family:
• To avoid OTC products unless directed by prescriber
• That ileostomy patient may take product for extended time
• Not to operate machinery if drowsiness occurs
• To use hard candy, sips of water for dry mouth
• To notify health care professional if diarrhea continues over 48 hr or 10 days if distention, fever, or abdominal pain occurs

---

lopinavir/ritonavir
(low-pin′ah-ver/ri-toe′na-veer)
Kaletra
Func. class.: Antiretroviral
Chem. class.: Protease inhibitor

ACTION: Inhibits human immunodeficiency virus (HIV-1) protease and prevents maturation of the infectious virus

USES: HIV-1 in combination with or without other antiretrovirals

CONTRAINDICATIONS: Hypersensitivity to this product or polyoxyethylated castor oil (oral solution), CYP3A4 metabolized products
Precautions: Pregnancy, breastfeeding, hepatic disease, pancreatitis, diabetes,

---

hemophilia, AV block, hypercholesterolemia, immune reconstitution syndrome, neonates, cardiomyopathy, congenital long-QT prolongation, hypokalemia, elderly patients, Graves' disease, polymyositis, Guillain-Barré syndrome, children, HBV/HCV coinfection

DOSAGE AND ROUTES
HIV infection
• **Adult:** PO 400 mg lopinavir/100 mg ritonavir bid or 800 mg lopinavir/200 mg ritonavir per day
• **Pregnant adult:** PO 400 mg lopinavir/100 mg ritonavir bid, may need 600 mg lopinavir/150 mg ritonavir bid in the 2nd/3rd trimesters; once-daily dosing is not recommended
• **Adult receiving concomitant efavirenz, nelfinavir, or nevirapine: PO TABS,** 500 mg lopinavir/125 mg ritonavir bid; **CAPS/SOL,** 533 mg lopinavir/133 mg ritonavir bid
• **Adolescent/child/infant >6 mo:** 300 mg lopinavir/75 mg ritonavir/m²/dose bid. The once-daily regimen is not recommended in pediatric patients; capsules are not recommended for use in patients ≤40 kg

Available forms: Oral solution 400 mg lopinavir/100 mg ritonavir/5 mL; tablets 100 mg lopinavir/25 mg ritonavir, 200 mg lopinavir/50 mg ritonavir
Administer:
PO route
• **TAB:** take without regard to food; swallow whole; do not crush, break, chew
• **ORAL SOL:** shake well, use calibrated measuring device
• Drug resistance testing should be done before beginning therapy in antiretroviral-naive patients and before changing therapy for treatment failure

SIDE EFFECTS
CNS: Paresthesia, headache, seizures, fever, dizziness, insomnia, asthenia, intracranial bleeding, encephalopathy
CV: QT, PR interval prolongation, deep vein thrombosis
EENT: Blurred vision, otitis media, tinnitus

GI: Diarrhea, buccal mucosa ulceration, abdominal pain, nausea, taste perversion, dry mouth, vomiting, anorexia
INTEG: Rash
MISC: Asthenia, angioedema, anaphylaxis, Stevens-Johnson syndrome, increased lipids, lipodystrophy
MS: Pain, rhabdomyolysis, myalgias

PHARMACOKINETICS
Well absorbed, 98% protein binding, hepatic metabolism, peak 4 hr, terminal half-life 6 hr

INTERACTIONS
Increase: toxicity—amiodarone, avanafil, azole antifungals, benzodiazepines, buPROPion, cloZAPine, desipramine, dihydroergotamine, encainide, ergotamine, flecainide, HMG-CoA reductase inhibitors, interleukins, meperidine, midazolam, pimozide, piroxicam, propafenone, quiNIDine, ranolazine, rivaroxaban, saquinavir, triazolam, zolpidem
Increase: QT prolongation—class IA/III antidysrhythmics, some phenothiazines, β-agonists, local anesthetics, tricyclics, haloperidol, chloroquine, droperidol, pentamidine, CYP3A4 inhibitors (amiodarone, clarithromycin, erythromycin, telithromycin, troleandomycin), arsenic trioxide, levomethadyl, CYP3A4 substrates (methadone, pimozide, QUEtiapine, quiNIDine, risperiDONE, ziprasidone)
Increase: ritonavir levels—fluconazole
Increase: level of both products—clarithromycin, ddI
Increase: levels of bosentan
Decrease: ritonavir levels—rifamycins, nevirapine, barbiturates, phenytoin, budesonide, predniSONE
Decrease: levels of anticoagulants, atovaquone, divalproex, ethinyl estradiol, lamoTRIgine, phenytoin, sulfamethoxazole, theophylline, voriconazole, zidovudine
Drug/Lab Test
Increase: AST, ALT, CPK, cholesterol, GGT, triglycerides, uric acid, glucose
Decrease: Hct, Hgb, RBC, neutrophils, WBC
Drug/Herb
Decrease: ritonavir levels—St. John's wort; avoid concurrent use

- Avoid use with red yeast rice, evening primrose oil

NURSING CONSIDERATIONS
Assess:
- **HIV:** viral load, CD4 at baseline, throughout therapy; blood glucose, plasma HIV RNA, serum cholesterol/lipid profile; resistance testing before starting therapy and after treatment failure
- Signs of infection, anemia
- Hepatic studies: ALT, AST
- Bowel pattern before, during treatment; if severe abdominal pain with bleeding occurs, discontinue product; monitor hydration
- Skin eruptions; rash
- **Rhabdomyolysis:** muscle pain, increased CPK, weakness, swelling of affected muscles, tea-colored dark urine; if these occur and if confirmed by CPK, product should be discontinued
- **QT prolongation:** ECG for QT prolongation, ejection fraction; assess for chest pain, palpitations, dyspnea
- **Serious skin disorders:** Stevens-Johnson syndrome, angioedema, anaphylaxis
- **Pregnancy/breastfeeding:** all pregnant women who experience adverse reactions should have provider report the reactions to Antiretroviral Pregnancy Registry, 800-258-4263; avoid breastfeeding

Evaluate:
- Therapeutic response: improvement in HIV symptoms; improving viral load, CD4+ T cells

Teach patient/family:
- To take as prescribed; if dose is missed, to take as soon as remembered up to 1 hr before next dose; not to double dose
- That product is not a cure for HIV; that opportunistic infections can continue to be acquired
- That redistribution of body fat or accumulation of body fat may occur
- That others can continue to contract HIV from patient
- To avoid OTC, prescription medications, herbs, supplements unless approved by prescriber; not to use St. John's wort because it decreases product's effect; that taking this product with ED drugs may increase adverse reactions
- That regular follow-up exams and blood work will be required
- To report a change in heart rhythm or abnormal heartbeats

---

loratadine (OTC, Rx)
(lor-a′ti-deen)
Alavert, Claritin, Claritin Children's, Claritin RediTabs, Clear-Atadine, Dimetapp, Triaminic AllerChews
Func. class.: Antihistamine, 2nd generation
Chem. class.: Selective histamine (H$_1$)-receptor antagonist

Do not confuse:
loratadine/lovastatin/
LORazepam/losartan

ACTION: Binds to peripheral histamine receptors, thereby providing antihistamine action without sedation

USES: Seasonal rhinitis, chronic idiopathic urticaria for those ≥2 yr

CONTRAINDICATIONS: Hypersensitivity, acute asthma attacks, lower respiratory tract disease
Precautions: Pregnancy, breastfeeding, increased intraocular pressure, bronchial asthma, hepatic/renal disease

DOSAGE AND ROUTES
- **Adult and child ≥6 yr: PO** 10 mg/day
- **Child 2-5 yr: PO** 5 mg/day
- Renal/hepatic dose
- **Adult: PO** CCr <30 mL/min or hepatic disease, 10 mg every other day
- **Child 2-5 yr: PO** GFR <50 mL/min; 5 mg every other day
Available forms: Tabs 10 mg; rapid-disintegrating tabs 10 mg; orally disintegrating tabs 10 mg; syr 1 mg/mL; susp 5 mg/mL, ext rel tab 10 mg

---

Administer:
- **Rapid-disintegrating tabs** by placing on tongue, to be swallowed after disintegrated with/without water
- Use within 6 mo of opening pouch and immediately after opening blister pack
- On empty stomach daily

Ext Rel Tab
- Do not break, crush, or chew

SIDE EFFECTS

CNS: Sedation (more common with increased doses), headache, fatigue, restlessness
EENT: Dry mouth

PHARMACOKINETICS

Onset 1-3 hr, peak 8-12 hr, duration 24 hr, metabolized in liver to active metabolites, excreted in urine, active metabolite desloratadine half-life 20 hr

INTERACTIONS

Increase: CNS depressant effects—alcohol, antidepressants, other antihistamines, sedative/hypnotics, MAOIs
Increase: loratadine level—cimetidine, ketoconazole, macrolides (clarithromycin, erythromycin)

Drug/Herb
Increase: CNS depression—chamomile, kava, valerian

Drug/Lab Test
False negative: skin allergy tests (discontinue antihistamine 3 days before testing)

NURSING CONSIDERATIONS

Assess:
- **Allergy:** hives, rash, rhinitis; monitor respiratory status
- **Beers:** avoid in older men; may decrease urinary flow and cause urinary retention
- **Pregnancy/breastfeeding:** use only if clearly needed; cautious use in breastfeeding

Evaluate:
- Therapeutic response: absence of running or congested nose, other allergy symptoms

Teach patient/family:
- To avoid driving, other hazardous activities if drowsiness occurs
- To avoid use of other CNS depressants

⚠ HIGH ALERT

LORazepam (Rx)

(lor-a′ze-pam)

Ativan

Func. class.: Sedative, hypnotic; antianxiety
Chem. class.: Benzodiazepine, short acting

Controlled Substance Schedule IV

Do not confuse:
LORazepam/ALPRAZolam/clonazePAM

ACTION: Potentiates the actions of GABA, especially in the limbic system and the reticular formation

USES: Anxiety, irritability with psychiatric or organic disorders, preoperatively; insomnia; adjunct for endoscopic procedures, status epilepticus, insomnia
Unlabeled uses: Antiemetic before chemotherapy, rectal use, alcohol withdrawal, seizure prophylaxis, agitation, insomnia, sedation maintenance

CONTRAINDICATIONS: Pregnancy, breastfeeding, hypersensitivity to benzodiazepines, benzyl alcohol; closed-angle glaucoma, psychosis, history of drug abuse, COPD, sleep apnea
Precautions: Children <12 yr, geriatric patients, debilitated patients, renal/hepatic disease, addiction, suicidal ideation, abrupt discontinuation

Black Box Warning: Coadministration with other CNS depressants

---

DOSAGE AND ROUTES

Anxiety

• **Adult/adolescent ≥12 yr:** PO 2-3 mg/day in divided doses, max 10 mg/day
• **Geriatric:** PO 1-2 mg/day in divided doses or 0.5-1 mg at bedtime
• **Child <11 yr (unlabeled):** PO 0.025-0.05 mg/kg/dose (max q4hr)

Preoperatively for sedation

• **Adult:** IM 50 mcg/kg 2 hr before surgery; IV 44 mcg/kg 15-20 min before surgery, max 2 mg 15-20 min before surgery
• **Child ≥12 yr:** IV 0.05 mg/kg, max 4 mg

Status epilepticus

• **Adult:** IM/IV 4 mg, may repeat after 10-15 min
• **Neonate:** IV 0.05 mg/kg
• **Child:** IV 0.1 mg/kg up to 4 mg/dose; RECT(unlabeled) 0.05-0.1 mg × 2; wait 7 min before giving 2nd dose

Insomnia

• **Adult:** PO 2-4 mg at bedtime; only minimally effective after 2 wk continuous therapy
• **Geriatric:** PO 0.5-1 mg initially

Sedation in mechanically ventilated patients (unlabeled)

• **Adult/adolescent:** INTERMITTENT IV 0.044 mg/kg q2-4hr, prn, max 4 mg single dose
• **Adult/adolescent:** IV INFUSION 0.5-8 mg/hr, titrate, use loading dose of 2-4 mg

Alcohol withdrawal (unlabeled)

• **Adult:** PO 2 mg q6hr × 4 doses, then 1 mg q6hr for 8 doses

Available forms: Tabs 0.5, 1, 2 mg; inj 2, 4 mg/mL; oral sol 2 mg/mL

Administer:

PO route
• With food or milk for GI symptoms; crushed if patient is unable to swallow medication whole
• Sugarless gum, hard candy, frequent sips of water for dry mouth
• Give largest dose before bedtime if giving in divided doses
• **Oral solution:** use calibrated dropper; add to food/drink; consume immediately

IM route
• Deep into large muscle mass
• Use this route when IV is not feasible

Direct IV route
• Prepare immediately before use; short stability time
• IV after diluting in equal vol sterile water, 5% dextrose, or 0.9% NaCl for inj; give through Y-tube or 3-way stopcock; give at ≤2 mg/1 min; do not give rapidly
• To reduce amount of benzyl alcohol to a neonate, dilute with preservative-free sterile water injection (0.4 mg/mL) for IV use

Y-site compatibilities: Acetaminophen, acyclovir, albumin, allopurinol, amifostine, amikacin, amoxicillin, amoxicillin/clavulanate, amphotericin B cholesteryl, amsacrine, atenolol, atracurium, bivalirudin, bleomycin, bumetanide, butorphanol, calcium chloride/gluconate, CARBOplatin, ceFAZolin, cefepime, cefotaxime, cefoTEtan, cefOXitin, cefTAZidime, ceftizoxime, ceftobiprole, cefTRIAXone, cefuroxime, chloramphenicol, chlorproMAZINE, cimetidine, ciprofloxacin, cisatracurium, CISplatin, cladribine, clindamycin, cloNIDine, cyclophosphamide, cycloSPORINE, cytarabine, DACTINomycin, DAPTOmycin, dexamethasone, dexmedetomidine, diltiazem, DOBUTamine, DOCEtaxel, DOPamine, doripenem, DOXOrubicin, DOXOrubicin liposomal, droperidol, enalaprilat, ePHEDrine, EPINEPHrine, epirubicin, eptifibatide, erythromycin, esmolol, etomidate, famotidine, fenoldopam, fentaNYL, filgrastim, fluconazole, fludarabine, fosphenytoin, furosemide, ganciclovir, gatifloxacin, gemcitabine, gentamicin, glycopyrrolate, granisetron, haloperidol, heparin, hydrocortisone, HYDROmorphone, hydrOXYzine, ifosfamide, inamrinone, insulin (regular), irinotecan, isoproterenol, ketorolac, labetalol, lidocaine, linezolid, magnesium sulfate, mannitol, mechlorethamine, melphalan, meropenem, metaraminol, methadone, methotrexate, methyldopate, methylPREDNISolone, metoclopramide, metoprolol, metroNIDAZOLE, micafungin, midazolam, milrinone, minocycline, mitoXANtrone, morphine, mycophenolate, nafcillin, nalbuphine, naloxone, nesiritide, niCARdipine, nitroglycerin, nitroprusside, norepinephrine, octreotide, oxaliplatin,

---

Side effects: *italics* = common; red = life-threatening

oxytocin, PACLitaxel, palonosetron, pamidronate, pancuronium, PEMEtrexed, pentamidine, PENTobarbital, PHENobarbital, piperacillin, piperacillin-tazobactam, polymyxin B, potassium chloride, propofol, ranitidine, remifentanil, tacrolimus, teniposide, theophylline, thiotepa, ticarcillin, ticarcillin-clavulanate, tigecycline, tirofiban, tobramycin, TPN, trastuzumab, trimethobenzamide, trimethoprim-sulfamethoxazole, vancomycin, vasopressin, vecuronium, verapamil, vinCRIStine, vinorelbine, voriconazole, zidovudine

SIDE EFFECTS

CNS: *Dizziness, drowsiness,* confusion, headache, anxiety, tremors, stimulation, fatigue, depression, insomnia, hallucinations, weakness, unsteadiness
CV: *Orthostatic hypotension,* ECG changes, tachycardia, hypotension, apnea, cardiac arrest (IV, rapid)
EENT: *Blurred vision,* tinnitus, mydriasis
GI: Constipation, dry mouth, nausea, vomiting, anorexia, diarrhea
INTEG: Rash, dermatitis, itching
MISC: Acidosis

PHARMACOKINETICS

Metabolized by liver; excreted by kidneys; crosses placenta, excreted in breast milk; half-life 42 hr (neonates), 10.5 hr (older child), 12 hr (adult), 91% protein bound
PO: Onset 1 hr, peak 2 hr, duration 12-24 hr
IM: Onset 15-30 min, peak 1-1^1/$_2$ hr, duration 6-8 hr
IV: Onset 5 min, peak 1-1^1/$_2$ hr, duration 6-8 hr

INTERACTIONS

Black Box Warning: **Increase:** LORazepam effects—CNS depressants, opioids, alcohol, disulfiram

Increase: delirium, sedation—cloZAPine
Increase: LORazepam effect of probenecid, valproate reduce dose by 50%
Decrease: LORazepam effects—oral contraceptives; change dose as needed
Drug/Herb
Increase: CNS depression—chamomile, kava, valerian

Drug/Lab Test
Increase: AST, ALT

NURSING CONSIDERATIONS
Assess:
• **Anxiety:** decrease in anxiety; mental status: mood, sensorium, affect, sleeping pattern, drowsiness, dizziness, suicidal tendencies

Black Box Warning: Coadministration with other CNS depressants (especially opioids) should be avoided; if used together, use lower dose

• Renal/hepatic/blood status if receiving high-dose therapy
• **Physical dependency, withdrawal symptoms:** headache, nausea, vomiting, muscle pain, weakness, tremors, seizures, after long-term, excessive use
• **Beers:** avoid in older adults; may increase cognitive impairment, delirium
• **Pregnancy/breastfeeding:** use only if clearly needed; neonatal withdrawal syndrome may occur; do not breastfeed unless benefits outweigh risk; excreted in breast milk
Evaluate:
• Therapeutic response: decreased anxiety, restlessness, insomnia
Teach patient/family:
• That product may be taken with food
• Not to take more than prescribed amount; may be habit forming
• To avoid OTC preparations (cough, cold, hay fever) unless approved by prescriber
• To avoid driving, activities that require alertness since drowsiness may occur

Black Box Warning: To avoid alcohol, other psychotropic medications, opioids unless directed by prescriber; to notify prescriber immediately of trouble breathing, dizziness, coma, or if no response

• Not to discontinue medication abruptly after long-term use, taper
• To rise slowly because fainting may occur, especially among geriatric patients
• That drowsiness may worsen at beginning of treatment

• To report suicidal ideation

• **Pregnancy/breastfeeding:** not to use in pregnancy or breastfeeding; to use contraception while using this product

TREATMENT OF OVERDOSE:
Lavage, VS, supportive care, flumazenil

---

lorcaserin

(lor-ca-ser'in)

Belviq, Belviq XR

Func. class.: Appetite suppressant
Chem. class.: Serotonin 2C (5-HT$_{2C}$) receptor agonist

Controlled Substance Schedule IV

ACTION: Decreases food consumption and decreases hunger by selectively activating 5-HT$_{2C}$ receptors

USES: Obesity management

CONTRAINDICATIONS: Pregnancy, breastfeeding, hypersensitivity, severe renal impairment
Precautions: Children, other organic causes of obesity, anemia, AV block, bradycardia, bundle branch block, depression, dialysis, liver/kidney disease, multiple myeloma, neutropenia, suicidal ideation, Peyronie's disease, pulmonary hypertension, sick sinus syndrome

DOSAGE AND ROUTES
• **Adult: PO** 10 mg bid; do not exceed recommended dosage; discontinue after 12 wk if at least 5% weight loss has not been achieved by 12 wk; **ext rel** 20 mg daily
Available forms: Tabs, film-coated 10 mg; ext rel tabs 20 mg
Administer:
• For obesity if patient is on weight reduction program that includes dietary changes, exercise
• May give without regard to food

SIDE EFFECTS
CNS: *Insomnia, depression,* serotonin syndrome, *anxiety,* suicidal ideation, *dizziness, headache, fatigue*
CV: Bradycardia, hypertension

GI: *Diarrhea, constipation, nausea*
HEMA: Neutropenia, leukopenia, lymphopenia
INTEG: Rash
MS: Back pain

PHARMACOKINETICS
70% protein binding, half-life 11 hr

INTERACTIONS
Increase: life-threatening serotonin syndrome or NMS—SSRIs, SNRIs, serotonin-receptor agonists, sibutramine, MAOIs, linezolid, tricyclic antidepressants, buPROPion, lithium, DOPamine antagonist, traMADol
Increase: risk of hypoglycemia with sulfonylureas and insulin
Drug/Herb
Increase: serotonin syndrome—St. John's wort
Drug/Lab
Increase: prolactin
Decrease: glucose, Hct, WBC, RBC

NURSING CONSIDERATIONS
Assess:
• Weight weekly; oral hypoglycemic dosage might need to be reduced in diabetic patients
• Monitor blood glucose, CBC with differential, Hct/Hgb, serum prolactin, baseline and periodically
• **Suicidal ideation:** use caution in psychiatric disorders with emotional lability; assess for depression, suicidal thoughts/behaviors, hostility, irritability
• **Serotonin syndrome:** nausea, vomiting, diarrhea, confusion, tachycardia, hyperthermia; if these occur, stop product, notify prescriber
• **Pregnancy/breastfeeding:** do not use in pregnancy, breastfeeding
Evaluate:
• Therapeutic response: decrease in weight
Teach patient/family:
• To avoid hazardous activities until stabilized on medication
• To discuss unpleasant side effects
• To notify prescriber if pregnancy is planned or suspected; not to use in pregnancy or breastfeeding
• To use in conjunction with diet, exercise

Side effects: *italics* = common; red = life-threatening

RARELY USED

lorlatinib
(lor-la'ti-nib)
Lorbrena
Func. class.: Antineoplastic

USES: Metastatic ALK-positive non–small-cell lung cancer (NSCLC) with disease progression on either alectinib or ceritinib as the first ALK inhibitor for metastatic disease, or disease progression on crizotinib and at least one other ALK inhibitor for metastatic disease

CONTRAINDICATIONS: Hypersensitivity

DOSAGE AND ROUTES
• **Adult: PO** 100 mg daily until disease progression or unacceptable toxicity

---

losartan
(lo-zar'tan)
Cozaar
Func. class.: Antihypertensive
Chem. class.: Angiotensin II receptor (type AT$_1$) antagonist

Do not confuse:
losartan/valsartan
Cozaar/Zocor

ACTION: Blocks the vasoconstrictor and aldosterone-secreting effects of angiotensin II; selectively blocks the binding of angiotensin II to the AT$_1$ receptor found in tissues

USES: Hypertension, alone or in combination; nephropathy in type 2 diabetes; proteinuria; stroke prophylaxis for hypertensive patients with left ventricular hypertrophy
Unlabeled uses: Heart failure

CONTRAINDICATIONS: Hypersensitivity

Black Box Warning: Pregnancy

Precautions: breastfeeding, children, geriatric patients, hypersensitivity to ACE inhibitors, hepatic disease, angioedema, renal artery stenosis, ✿ African descent, hyperkalemia, hypotension

DOSAGE AND ROUTES
Hypertension
• **Adult: PO** 50 mg/day alone or 25 mg/day in combination with diuretic; maintenance 25-100 mg/day
• **Child ≥6 yr: PO** 0.7 mg/kg/day, max 50 mg/day
Hypertension with left ventricular hypertrophy
• **Adult: PO** 50 mg/day; add hydrochlorothiazide 12.5 mg/day and/or increase losartan to 100 mg/day, then increase hydrochlorothiazide to 25 mg/day
Nephropathy in type 2 diabetic patients/proteinuria
• **Adult: PO** 50 mg/day, may increase to 100 mg/day
Heart failure
• **Adult: PO** 25-50 mg/day initially, then titrate to max 50-150 mg/day maintenance
Hepatic dose/volume depletion
• **Adult: PO** 25 mg/day as starting dose
Available forms: Tabs 25, 50, 100 mg
Administer:
• Without regard to meals
• If product is compounded into suspension, store in refrigerator and shake well before use
• May use alone or in combination

SIDE EFFECTS
CNS: *Dizziness, insomnia,* anxiety, confusion, abnormal dreams, migraine, tremor, vertigo, headache, malaise, depression, fatigue
CV: Angina pectoris, 2nd-degree AV block, cerebrovascular accident, *hypotension,* MI, dysrhythmias
EENT: Blurred vision, burning eyes, conjunctivitis
GI: *Diarrhea, dyspepsia,* anorexia, constipation, dry mouth, flatulence, gastritis, vomiting

GU: Impotence, nocturia, urinary frequency, UTI, renal failure
HEMA: Anemia, thrombocytopenia
INTEG: Alopecia, dermatitis, dry skin, flushing, photosensitivity, rash, pruritus, sweating, angioedema
META: Gout, hyperkalemia, hypoglycemia
MS: Cramps, myalgia, pain, stiffness
RESP: *Cough, upper respiratory infection*, congestion, dyspnea, bronchitis
MISC: Diabetic vascular disease

PHARMACOKINETICS
Peak 1 hr, extensively metabolized, half-life 2 hr, metabolite 6-9 hr, excreted in urine/feces, protein binding 98.7%

INTERACTIONS
Increase: lithium toxicity—lithium; monitor lithium level
Increase: antihypertensive effect—garlic
Increase: hyperkalemia—potassium-sparing diuretics, potassium supplements, ACE inhibitors
Decrease: antihypertensive effect—NSAIDs

Drug/Herb
Decrease: antihypertensive effects—ma huang, black licorice

Drug/Lab Test
Increase: AST, ALT

NURSING CONSIDERATIONS
Assess:
• B/P with position changes, pulse before and periodically during treatment; note rate, rhythm, quality; ♦ black patients should use combination therapy for better control of B/P
• Baselines of renal, hepatic, electrolyte studies before therapy begins and periodically thereafter
• Skin turgor, dryness of mucous membranes for hydration status
• Angioedema: facial swelling, dyspnea, wheezing; may occur rapidly; tongue swelling (rare)
• **HF:** jugular venous distention; edema in feet/legs, weight daily
• **Blood dyscrasias:** thrombocytopenia, anemia (rare)

Black Box Warning: **Pregnancy/breastfeeding:** assess for pregnancy before starting treatment; do not use in pregnancy; do not breastfeed

Evaluate:
• Therapeutic response: decreased B/P, slowing diabetic neuropathy
Teach patient/family:
• To avoid sunlight or to wear sunscreen if in sunlight; that photosensitivity may occur
• To comply with dosage schedule, even if feeling better; not to discontinue abruptly; not to share with others
• To notify prescriber of mouth sores, fever, swelling of hands or feet, irregular heartbeat, chest pain
• That excessive perspiration, dehydration, vomiting, diarrhea may lead to fall in B/P; to consult prescriber if these occur
• That product may cause dizziness, fainting, light-headedness; to avoid hazardous activities until reaction is known
• To rise slowly to sitting or standing position to minimize orthostatic hypotension

Black Box Warning: **Pregnancy/breastfeeding:** to use contraception while taking this product; not to breastfeed

• To avoid salt substitutes, alcohol, OTC products unless approved by prescriber

loteprednol ophthalmic
See Appendix B

lovastatin (Rx)
(loh-vah-stat′in)
Altoprev
Func. class.: Antilipemic
Chem. class.: HMG-CoA reductase inhibitor

Do not confuse:
lovastatin/Lotensin

Side effects: *italics* = common; red = life-threatening

ACTION: Inhibits HMG-CoA reductase enzyme, which reduces cholesterol synthesis

USES: As an adjunct for primary hypercholesterolemia (types IIa, IIb), atherosclerosis; heterozygous familial hypercholesterolemia (adolescents)

CONTRAINDICATIONS: Pregnancy, breastfeeding, hypersensitivity, active hepatic disease

Precautions: Children, past hepatic disease, alcoholism, severe acute infections, trauma, hypotension, uncontrolled seizure disorders, severe metabolic disorders, electrolyte imbalances, visual disorder

DOSAGE AND ROUTES
To prevent/treat CAD, hyperlipidemia
• **Adult: PO** 20 mg/day with evening meal; may increase to 20-80 mg/day in single or divided doses at 4-wk intervals, max 80 mg/day; **EXT REL** 20-60 mg/day at bedtime, max 60 mg/day

Heterozygous familial hypercholesterolemia ✖️📧✖️
• **Adolescent 10-17 yr: PO** 10-40 mg with evening meal

Primary prevention of CV disease
• **Adult 40-75 yr with type 1 or 2 diabetes: PO** 40 mg immediate release q day

Secondary prevention of CV disease
• **Adult >75 yr (not candidate for high-intensity use): PO** 40 mg immediate release q day

Renal dose
• **Adult: PO** CCr <30 mg/min, max 20 mg/day unless titrated

Available forms: Tabs 10, 20, 40 mg; ext rel tab 20, 40, 60 mg

Administer:
• In evening with meal; if dose is increased, take with breakfast and evening meal (immediate release); use at bedtime (extended release)
• Altroprev is not equivalent to Mevacor
• Do not crush, chew ext rel tab
• Store in cool environment in airtight, light-resistant container

SIDE EFFECTS
CNS: *Dizziness, headache, tremor,* insomnia, paresthesia
EENT: *Blurred vision,* lens opacities
GI: Flatus, nausea, constipation, diarrhea, dyspepsia, abdominal pain, heartburn, hepatic dysfunction, vomiting, acid regurgitation, dry mouth, dysgeusia
HEMA: Thrombocytopenia, hemolytic anemia, leukopenia
INTEG: *Rash, pruritus,* photosensitivity
MS: *Muscle cramps, myalgia,* myositis, rhabdomyolysis; leg, shoulder, or localized pain

PHARMACOKINETICS
PO: Peak 2 hr; peak response 4-6 wk, ext rel peak 14 hr; metabolized in liver (metabolites); highly protein bound; excreted in urine 10%, feces 83%; crosses blood-brain barrier, placenta; excreted in breast milk; half-life 1 hr

INTERACTIONS
Increase: myalgia, myositis, rhabdomyolysis—azole antifungals, clarithromycin, clofibrate, cycloSPORINE, danazol, diltiazem, erythromycin, gemfibrozil, niacin, protease inhibitors, quinupristin-dalfopristin, telithromycin, verapamil; avoid concurrent use
Increase: bleeding—warfarin
Increase: lovastatin effects—diltiazem
Decrease: effects of lovastatin—bile acid sequestrants, exenatide, bosentan
Decrease: lovastatin metabolism, avoid combining with >40 mg/day amiodarone

Drug/Herb
Decrease: effect—pectin, St. John's wort
Increase: adverse reactions—red yeast rice

Drug/Food
• Possible toxicity: grapefruit juice
Increase: levels of lovastatin with food; must be taken with food
Decrease: absorption—oat bran

Drug/Lab Test
Increase: CK, LFTs
Interference: T_3, T_4, T_7, TSH

NURSING CONSIDERATIONS
Assess:
• **Diet:** obtain diet history including fat, cholesterol in diet
• Fasting cholesterol, LDL, HDL, triglycerides periodically during treatment
• **Pregnancy/breastfeeding:** not to be used in pregnancy, breastfeeding
• Hepatic studies at initiation, 6 wk, 12 wk after initiation or change in dose, periodically thereafter; AST, ALT, LFTs may increase
• Renal function in patients with compromised renal system: BUN, creatinine, I&O ratio
Evaluate:
• Therapeutic response: decreased triglycerides, sLDL, total cholesterol; increased HDL; slowing CAD
Teach patient/family:
• **Pregnancy/breastfeeding:** to report suspected pregnancy; not to breastfeed
• That blood work, ophthalmic exam will be necessary during treatment
• To report blurred vision, severe GI symptoms, dizziness, headache, muscle pain, weakness
• To use sunscreen or to stay out of the sun to prevent photosensitivity
• That previously prescribed regimen will continue: low-cholesterol diet, exercise program, smoking cessation
• That product should be taken with food; not to crush, chew ext rel product; to take immediate-release product in the AM, PM if used bid; to take ext rel product at bedtime
• Not to use with grapefruit juice, large amounts of alcohol
• To protect product from light and moisture

RARELY USED

loxapine (Rx)
(lox'a-peen)
Adasuve, Loxapac ✦
Func. class.: Antipsychotic, neuroleptic
Chem. class.: Dibenzoxazepine

USES: Schizophrenia, bipolar disorder
Unlabeled uses: Anxiety

CONTRAINDICATIONS: *Hypersensitivity, coma*

Black Box Warning: Acute bronchospasm, asthma, COPD, emphysema

DOSAGE AND ROUTES
• **Adult: PO** 10 mg bid-qid initially, may be rapidly increased depending on severity of condition, maintenance 60-100 mg/day; inhalation powder 10 mg as a single dose in 24 hr
• **Geriatric: PO** 5-10 mg daily-bid, increase q4-7days by 5-10 mg, max 250 mg/day

---

RARELY USED

L

lucinactant
(loo'sin-ak'tant)
Surfaxin
Func. class.: Synthetic lung surfactant

USES: Prevention of respiratory distress syndrome in premature neonates (RDS)

DOSAGE AND ROUTES
• **Premature neonate: INTRATRACHEAL** 5.8 mL/kg birth weight divided in 4 doses; give each dose with neonate in a different position; provide positive pressure ventilation when stable; dosage may be repeated 4 times in first 48 hr

---

luliconazole topical
See Appendix B

---

lurasidone (Rx)

(loo-ras'i-done)

Latuda

Func. class.: Atypical antipsychotic
Chem. class.: Dopamine-serotonin receptor antagonist derivative

Do not confuse:
Latuda/Lantus

ACTION: May modulate central DOPaminergic and serotonergic activity; high affinity for DOPamine-D2 receptors, serotonin 5-HT2A receptors; partial agonist at serotonin 5-HT1A receptor

USES: Schizophrenia, depression associated with bipolar disorder I

CONTRAINDICATIONS: Hypersensitivity

Precautions: Pregnancy, breastfeeding, geriatric patients, abrupt discontinuation, ambient temperature increase, breast cancer, cardiac disease, dehydration, diabetes, ketoacidosis, driving, operating machinery, dysphagia, heart failure, hematologic/hepatic/renal disease, hypotension, hypovolemia, MI, infertility, obesity, Parkinson's disease, seizures, strenuous exercise, stroke, substance abuse, syncope, tardive dyskinesia

Black Box Warning: Dementia: antipsychotics (e.g., lurasidone) not approved for treatment of dementia-related psychosis in geriatric patients; may increase risk of death in this population, children, suicidal ideation

DOSAGE AND ROUTES
Schizophrenia

• **Adult: PO** 40 mg/day, range 40-160 mg/day; for those receiving CYP3A4 inhibitors max 80 mg/day, do not use with strong CYP3A4 inducers/inhibitors

• **Child 13-17 yr: PO** 40 mg daily, may increase to max 80 mg daily

Bipolar Disorder I

• **Adult: PO** 20 mg daily, max 120 mg/day

Hepatic/renal dose

• **Adult: PO** CCr <50 mL/min, hepatic disease CTP A start dose 20 mg/day, max 80 mg/day; hepatic disease CTP B start dose 20 mg/day, max 40 mg/day

Available forms: Tabs 20, 40, 80, 120 mg

Administer:

• Give with meal of ≥350 calories

SIDE EFFECTS

CNS: Agitation, akathisia, anxiety, dizziness, drowsiness, fatigue, hyperthermia, insomnia, dystonic reactions, pseudoparkinsonism, restlessness, seizures, suicidal ideation, syncope, tardive dyskinesia, vertigo

CV: Angina, AV block, bradycardia, hypertension, orthostatic hypotension, sinus tachycardia, stroke

EENT: Blurred vision

ENDO: Diabetes mellitus, ketoacidosis, hyperglycemia, hyperprolactinemia

GI: Abdominal pain, diarrhea, dyspepsia, nausea, vomiting, gastritis, weight gain/loss

GU: Amenorrhea, breast enlargement, dysmenorrhea, impotence, dysuria, renal failure

HEMA: Agranulocytosis, anemia, leukopenia, neutropenia

INTEG: Pruritus, rash

MS: Back pain, dysarthria; rhabdomyolysis (rare)

SYST: Angioedema

PHARMACOKINETICS

99% protein binding; excreted 80% in feces, 9% in urine; elimination half-life 18 hr; 9%-19% absorbed; peak 1-3 hr, steady-state 7 days

INTERACTIONS

• Do not use with metoclopramide

Increase: hypertensive risk—antihypertensive

Increase: lurasidone effect—strong CYP3A4 inhibitors; do not use concurrently

Increase: serotonin syndrome, neuroleptic malignant syndrome—SSRIs, SNRIs

Increase: sedation, respiratory depression—other CNS depressants, alcohol, opioids; avoid using together

Decrease: lurasidone effect—CYP3A4 inducers (carbamazepine, rifampin); do not use concurrently

Drug/Herb

Decrease: product effect—St. John's wort; do not use together

Drug/Food

• Do not use with grapefruit, grapefruit juice

NURSING CONSIDERATIONS
Assess:

• **Schizophrenia:** hallucinations, delusions, agitation, social withdrawal; monitor orientation, behavior, mood before and periodically during therapy

• **Temperature regulation:** avoid strenuous activities, excessive heat, dehydration, concomitant anticholinergic medications; risk of hyperthermia

• **Coadministration with other CNS depressants (opioids):** if given together, assess for excessive sedation, slow breathing; avoid concurrent use

• AIMS assessment, thyroid function tests, LFTs, lipid panel, electrolytes

• **EPS:** restlessness, difficulty speaking, loss of balance, pill rolling, masklike face, shuffling gait, rigidity, tremors, muscle spasms; monitor before and periodically during therapy; report tardive dyskinesia immediately

Black Box Warning: **Dementia:** this product is not approved for geriatric patients with dementia-related psychosis

Black Box Warning: **Suicidal ideation/children:** avoid use in children; there may be increased risk of suicide in young adults (<24 yr) and children; assess for worsening depression, suicidal thoughts/behaviors; product should be dispensed in small quantities

• Weight gain, hyperglycemia, metabolic changes in diabetes

• **Beers:** avoid in older adults except for schizophrenia, bipolar disorder, or short-term use as an antiemetic for chemotherapy; increased risk of stroke, cognitive decline

• **Pregnancy/breastfeeding:** use only if clearly needed; cautious use in breastfeeding; excretion is unknown

Evaluate:

• Therapeutic response: decreasing hallucinations, delusions, agitation, social withdrawal

Teach patient/family:

• About reason for treatment, expected results; not to use grapefruit juice, alcohol

• That lab work will be needed regularly

• To avoid hazardous activities until response is known

• To avoid OTC products unless approved by prescriber; serious reactions may occur

• To report fast heartbeat, extra beats, trouble breathing, sweating, stiffness, thirst, urinating more than usual

• To report EPS symptoms, blood dyscrasias: sore throat, fever, unusual bleeding/bruising

Black Box Warning: **Suicidal ideation/children:** to be aware of and report immediately any worsening depression, suicidal thoughts/behaviors, hostility, irritability

---

lusutrombopag
(lew-soo-trom′ bow-pag)
Mulpleta
Func. class.: Antihemorrhagic

USES: Thrombocytopenia in chronic hepatic disease in patients who are scheduled to undergo a procedure

CONTRAINDICATIONS: Hypersensitivity

DOSAGE AND ROUTES

• **Adult: PO** 3 mg daily × 7 days beginning 8 to 14 days before a scheduled procedure. Schedule the procedure for 2 to 8 days after the last dose

---

mafenide topical
See Appendix B

MAGNESIUM SALTS

magnesium chloride (Rx)

(12% mg, 9.8 Eq mg/g)

Chloromag, Slo-mag

magnesium citrate (OTC)

(16.2% mg, 4.4 mEq mg/g)

Citrate of magnesia, Citroma, Citromag ✦

magnesium gluconate (OTC)

(5.4% mg, 4.4 mEq mg/g)

Magtrate, Magonate

magnesium oxide (OTC)

(60.3% mg, 49.6 mEq mg/g)

Mag-Ox 400, Uro-Mag

magnesium hydroxide (OTC)

(41.7% mg, 34.3 mEq mg/g)

Dulcolax magnesium tablets, MOM, Phillips' Milk of Magnesia

⚠ HIGH ALERT

magnesium sulfate (OTC, Rx)

(9.9% mg, 8.1 mEq mg/g)

Func. class.: Electrolyte; anticonvulsant; saline laxative, antacid

ACTION: Increases osmotic pressure, draws fluid into colon, neutralizes HCl

USES: Constipation, dyspepsia; bowel preparation before surgery or exam; anticonvulsant for preeclampsia, eclampsia (magnesium sulfate); electrolyte; cardiac glycoside–induced arrhythmias, nutritional supplement

Unlabeled uses: Magnesium sulfate: persistent pulmonary hypertension of the newborn (PPHN), cardiac arrest, CPR, digitoxin/digoxin toxicity, premature labor, seizure prophylaxis, status asthmaticus, torsades de pointes, ventricular fibrillation/tachycardia

CONTRAINDICATIONS: Hypersensitivity, abdominal pain, nausea/vomiting, obstruction, acute surgical abdomen, rectal bleeding, heart block, myocardial damage
Precautions: Pregnancy (magnesium sulfate), renal/cardiac disease

DOSAGE AND ROUTES
Laxative
• **Adult: PO** (milk of magnesia) 15-60 mL at bedtime
• **Adult/child >12 yr: PO** (magnesium sulfate) 15 g in 8 oz water; **PO** (concentrated milk of magnesia) 5-30 mL; **PO** (magnesium citrate) 5-10 oz at bedtime
• **Child 2-6 yr: PO** (milk of magnesia) 5-15 mL/day
Prevention of magnesium deficiency (mg of magnesium)
• **Adult/child ≥10 yr: PO** (male) 350-400 mg/day; (female) 280-300 mg/day; (breastfeeding) 335-350 mg/day; (pregnancy) 320 mg/day
• **Child 8-10 yr: PO** 170 mg/day
• **Child 4-7 yr: PO** 120 mg/day
Magnesium sulfate deficiency (mg of magnesium)
• **Adult: PO** 200-400 mg in divided doses tid-qid; **IM** 1 g q6hr × 4 doses; **IV** 5 g (severe)
• **Child 6-12 yr: PO** 3-6 mg/kg/day in divided doses tid-qid
Preeclampsia/eclampsia (magnesium sulfate)
• **Adult: IM/IV** 4-5 g IV infusion; with 5 g **IM** in each gluteus, then 5 g q4hr or 4 g **IV INFUSION,** then 1-3 g/hr **CONT INFUSION,** max 30-40 g/24 hr or 20 g/48 hr in severe renal disease
Persistent pulmonary hypertension of the newborn (PPHN) in mechanically ventilated neonates (unlabeled)
• **Premature infants >33 wk and term neonates: IV** (magnesium sulfate) 200 mg/kg

over 20-30 min, then **CONT IV INFUSION** 20-150 mg/kg/hr to maintain blood magnesium levels at 3.5-5.5 mmol/L

Status asthmaticus (unlabeled)

• **Adult: IV** (magnesium sulfate) 2 g
• **Child: IV INFUSION** (PALS) (magnesium sulfate) 25-50 mg/kg diluted in D_5W, given over 10-20 min, max 2 g/dose

Premature labor (unlabeled)

• **Adult: IV INFUSION** (magnesium sulfate) 4-6 g given as a loading dose over 20-30 min, then 2-4 g/hr **CONT INFUSION;** use infusion pump until contractions cease; continue infusion at lowest dose over 12-24 hr; **PO** (magnesium chloride/gluconate/oxide) 648-1200 mg/ day elemental magnesium in divided doses

Torsades de pointes/cardiac dysrhythmias with hypomagnesemia (unlabeled)

• **Adult: IV** (magnesium sulfate) use ACLS guidelines or 1-2 g in 50-100 mL D_5W given over 5-20 min in emergent cases or over 5-60 min

Available forms: Chloride: sus rel tabs 535 mg (64 mg Mg); enteric tabs 833 mg (100 mg Mg); **citrate:** oral sol 240-, 296-, 300-mL bottles (77 mEq/100 mL); **gluconate:** tabs 500 mg; liquid 54 mg/5 mL; **oxide:** tabs 400 mg; caps 140 mg; **hydroxide:** liq 400 mg/5 mL; concentration liq 800 mg/5 mL; chew tabs 300, 600 mg; **sulfate:** 500 mg/mL; premixed infusion 1 g/100 mL, 2 g/100 mL, 4 g/50 mL, 4 g/100 mL, 20 g/500 mL, 40 g/1000 mL

Administer:

PO route

• With 8 oz water
• Refrigerate magnesium citrate before giving
• Shake susp before using as antacid at least 2 hr after meals
• Tablets should be chewed thoroughly before patient swallows; give 4 oz of water afterward
• **Laxative:** give on empty stomach with full glass of liquid, do not give at bedtime

IM route (magnesium sulfate)

• Give deeply in gluteal site

IV route (magnesium sulfate)

• Only when calcium gluconate is available for magnesium toxicity

Direct IV route

• Dilute 50% sol to ≤20%, give at ≤150 mg/min

Continuous IV INFUSION route

• May dilute to 20% sol, infuse over 3 hr
• IV at less than 125 mg/kg/hr; circulatory collapse may occur; use INFUSION pump

Y-site compatibilities: Acyclovir, aldesleukin, alemtuzumab, alfentanil, amifostine, amikacin, aminocaproic acid, argatroban, arsenic trioxide, ascorbic acid injection, asparaginase, atenolol, atosiban, atracurium, atropine, azithromycin, aztreonam, benztropine, bivalirudin, bleomycin, bumetanide, buprenorphine, butorphanol, calcium gluconate, cangrelor, CARBOplatin, carmustine, caspofungin, cefotaxime, cefoTEtan, cefOXitin, cefTAZidime, ceftizoxime, cephapirin, chloramphenicol, chlorproMAZINE, cimetidine, cisatracurium, CISplatin, clindamycin, cloNIDine, codeine, cyanocobalamin, cyclophosphamide, cytarabine, DACTINomycin, DAPTOmycin, DAUNOrubicin liposome, DAUNOrubicin, dexmedetomidine, dexrazoxane, digoxin, diltiaZEM, dimenhyDRINATE, diphenhydrAMINE, DOBUTamine, DOCEtaxel, dolasetron, DOPamine, doripenem, doxacurium chloride, DOXOrubicin liposomal, doxycycline, enalaprilat, ePHEDrine, EPINEPHrine, epoetin alfa, eptifibatide, ertapenem, esmolol, etoposide, etoposide phosphate, famotidine, fenoldopam, fentaNYL, fluconazole, fludarabine, fluorouracil, folic acid (as sodium salt), foscarnet, gallium, gatifloxacin, gemcitabine, gemtuzumab, gentamicin, glycopyrrolate, granisetron, heparin, HYDROmorphone, hydrOXYzine, IDArubicin, ifosfamide, imipenem-cilastatin, insulin (regular), irinotecan, isoproterenol, kanamycin, ketamine, ketorolac, labetalol, lactated Ringer's injection, lepirudin, leucovorin, lidocaine, linezolid, LORazepam, mannitol, mechlorethamine, mesna, metaraminol, methotrexate, methyldopa, metoclopramide, metoprolol, metroNIDAZOLE, micafungin, midazolam, milrinone, minocycline, mitoMYcin, mitoXANTRONE,

M

mivacurium, morphine, moxifloxacin, multiple vitamins injection, mycophenolate mofetil, nafcillin, nalbuphine, nesiritide, netilmicin, niCARdipine, nitroglycerin, nitroprusside, norepinephrine, octreotide, ondansetron, oxaliplatin, oxytocin, PACLitaxel, palonosetron, pamidronate, pancuronium, papaverine, PEMEtrexed, penicillin G potassium/sodium, pentazocine, PENTobarbital, PHENobarbital, phentolamine, phenylephrine, piperacillin, piperacillin tazobactam, polymyxin B, potassium acetate/chloride, procainamide, prochlorperazine, promethazine, propranolol, protamine, pyridoxine, quiNIDine, quinupristin-dalfopristin, raNITIdine, remifentanil, Ringer's injection, riTUXimab, rocuronium, sargramostim, sodium acetate/bicarbonate, succinylcholine, SUFentanil, tacrolimus, telavancin, teniposide, theophylline, thiamine, thiotepa, ticarcillin, ticarcillin-clavulanate, tigecycline, tirofiban, TNA (3-in-1), tobramycin, tolazoline, topotecan, TPN (2-in-1), trastuzumab, urokinase, vancomycin, vasopressin, vecuronium, verapamil, vinBLAStine, vinCRIStine, vinorelbine, vitamin B complex with C, voriconazole, zoledronic acid

SIDE EFFECTS

CNS: Muscle weakness, flushing, sweating, confusion, sedation, depressed reflexes, flaccid paralysis, hypothermia
CV: Hypotension, heart block, circulatory collapse, vasodilation
GI: *Nausea, vomiting, anorexia, cramps,* diarrhea
HEMA: Prolonged bleeding time
META: Electrolyte, fluid imbalances
RESP: Respiratory depression/paralysis

PHARMACOKINETICS

PO: Onset 1-2 hr
IM: Onset 1 hr, duration 4 hr
IV: Duration 1/2 hr
Excreted by kidney, effective anticonvulsant serum levels 2.5-7.5 mEq/L

INTERACTIONS

Increase: effect of neuromuscular blockers

Increase: hypotension—antihypertensives, calcium channel blockers
Decrease: absorption of tetracyclines, fluoroquinolones, nitrofurantoin
Decrease: effect of digoxin

NURSING CONSIDERATIONS
Assess:
• **Laxative:** cause of constipation; lack of fluids, bulk, exercise; cramping, rectal bleeding, nausea, vomiting; product should be discontinued
• **Eclampsia:** seizure precautions, B/P, ECG (magnesium sulfate); magnesium toxicity: thirst, confusion, decrease in reflexes; I&O ratio; check for decrease in urinary output
• **Pregnancy/breastfeeding:** use only if clearly needed (chloride), contraindicated in labor, toxemia during 2 hr prior to delivery, appears in breast milk
Evaluate:
• Therapeutic response: decreased constipation, absence of seizures (eclampsia), normal serum calcium levels
Teach patient/family:
• Not to use laxatives for long-term therapy because bowel tone will be lost
• That chilling improves taste of magnesium citrate
• To shake suspension well
• Not to give at bedtime as a laxative, may interfere with sleep; that milk of magnesia is usually given at bedtime
• To give citrus fruit after administering to counteract unpleasant taste
• About reason for product, expected results

mannitol (Rx)
(man´i-tole)
Osmitrol, Resectisol
Func. class.: Diuretic, osmotic
Chem. class.: Hexahydric alcohol

ACTION: Acts by increasing osmolarity of glomerular filtrate, which inhibits reabsorption of water and electrolytes and increases urinary output

USES: Edema; promotion of systemic diuresis in cerebral edema; decrease in

intraocular/intracranial pressure; improved renal function in acute renal failure, chemical poisoning, urinary bladder irrigation, kidney transplant
Unlabeled uses: Traumatic brain injury

CONTRAINDICATIONS: Active intracranial bleeding, hypersensitivity, anuria, severe pulmonary congestion, edema, severe dehydration, progressive heart/renal failure, acute MI, aneurysm, stroke

Precautions: Pregnancy, breastfeeding, geriatric patients, dehydration, severe renal disease, HF, electrolyte imbalances

Black Box Warning: Acute bronchospasm (inhalation test kit), asthma

DOSAGE AND ROUTES
Oliguria, prevention, in acute renal failure
• **Adult:** IV after initial test dose; if urine output is 30-50 mL/hr × 2 hr, give 20-100 g over a 24-hr period of 15% or 20% sol
Oliguria, treatment
• **Adult:** IV after initial test dose; give balance of 50 g of a 20% sol over 1 hr then 5% via **CONT IV INFUSION** to maintain output at 50 mL/hr
• **Child (unlabeled):** IV 0.5-2 g/kg as 15%-20% sol, run over 30-60 min; maintenance 0.25-0.5 g/kg q4-6hr
Edema
• **Adult:** IV after test dose, use product 10%-20% at a rate of 25-75 mL/hr; give loop diuretics before mannitol
• **Child (unlabeled):** IV 0.5-2 g/kg of 15%-20% mannitol over 2-6 hr
Intraocular pressure
• **Adult:** IV 1.5-2 g/kg of 15%-20% sol over 30-60 min
ICP
• **Adult:** IV 1-2 g/kg, then 0.25-1 g/kg q4hr
Diuresis with drug intoxication
• **Adult/child >12 yr:** 5%-25% sol continuously up to 200 g IV while maintaining 100-500 mL urine output/hr
Available forms: Inj 5%, 10%, 15%, 20%, 25%; GU irrigation: 5%; inhalation capsule challenge kit

Administer:
Intermittent/continuous IV route
• Precipitate may occur with PVC
• Change IV set q24hr
• May warm solution to dissolve crystals
• In 15%-25% sol with filter; rapid infusion may worsen HF; warm in hot water, shake to dissolve, use in-line filter; do not give as direct injection; to redissolve, run bottle under hot water and shake vigorously; cool to body temperature before using
• Run at 30-50 mL/hr in oliguria; 30-60 min in ICP; increased over 30 min in intraocular pressure; 60-90 min after surgery
• Give 20 mEq NaCl/L of product solution if blood is given concurrently
• Monitor for infiltration during use
• **Test dose** with severe oliguria, 0.2 g/kg over 3-5 min; if continued oliguria, give 2nd test dose; if no response, reassess patient

Y-site compatibilities: Acetaminophen, acyclovir, aldesleukin, alemtuzumab, amifostine, amikacin, ampicillin, asparaginase, atropine, aztreonam, bivalirudin, bumetanide, calcium gluconate, caspofungin, ceFAZolin, cefotaxime, cefOXitin, cefTAZidime, ceftizoxime, chloramphenicol, cimetidine, cisatracurium, clindamycin, DAPTOmycin, dexmedetomidine, digoxin, diltiaZEM, diphenhydrAMINE, DOBUTamine, DOCEtaxel, DOPamine, DOXOrubicin liposome, doxycycline, enalaprilat, EPINEPHrine, ertapenem, esmolol, famotidine, fenoldopam, fentaNYL, fluconazole, fludarabine, gentamicin, granisetron, heparin, HYDROmorphone, hydrOXYzine, IDArubicin, imipenem/cilastatin, insulin, isoproterenol, ketorolac, labetalol, levoFLOXacin, lidocaine, linezolid, LORazepam, meperidine, metoclopramide, metoprolol, metroNIDAZOLE, micafungin, midazolam, milrinone, morphine, nafcillin, niCARdipine, nitroglycerin, nitroprusside, norepinephrine, ondansetron, oxaliplatin, PACLitaxel, palonosetron, pantoprazole, penicillin G potassium, phenylephrine, piperacillin/tazobactam, potassium

Side effects: *italics* = common; red = life-threatening

chloride, procainamide, prochlorpera-zine, promethazine, propofol, proprano-lol, protamine, quinupristin/dalfopristin, raNITIdine, remifentanil, sargramostim, sodium bicarbonate, tacrolimus, thio-tepa, ticarcillin/clavulanate, tirofiban, tobramycin, trimethoprim/sulfamethoxa-zole, vancomycin, vasopressin, verap-amil, vinCRIStine, vit B complex with C, voriconazole, zoledronic acid

SIDE EFFECTS

CNS: *Dizziness, headache,* confusion
CV: Edema, thrombophlebitis, hypo/hypertension, tachycardia, angina-like chest pains, fever, chills, HF, circulatory overload
ELECT: Fluid, electrolyte imbalances, electrolyte loss, dehydration, hypo/hyperkalemia
GI: *Nausea, vomiting,* dry mouth
GU: Marked diuresis, urinary retention, thirst
INTEG: Injection-site reaction

PHARMACOKINETICS

IV: Onset 1-3 hr for diuresis, $^{1}/_{2}$-1 hr for intraocular pressure, 15 min for cere-brospinal fluid; duration 4-8 hr for intra-ocular pressure, 3-8 hr for cerebrospinal fluid; excreted in urine; half-life 100 min

INTERACTIONS

Increase: elimination of mannitol—lith-ium; monitor lithium level
Increase: excretion of imipramine
Increase: hypokalemia—cardiac glyco-sides
Increase or Decrease: sodium, potas-sium, magnesium
Drug/Lab Test
Interference: inorganic phosphorus, eth-ylene glycol

NURSING CONSIDERATIONS
Assess:
• Monitor I&O, B/P, pulse q hr; report decreasing urine output; monitor weight, electrolytes: potassium, sodium, chloride q day; BUN, serum creatinine q day, blood pH, PAP
• Use urinary catheter in those who are comatose; I&O must be precise

• **Metabolic acidosis:** drowsiness, rest-lessness
• **Hypokalemia:** postural hypotension, malaise, fatigue, tachycardia, leg cramps, weakness, or hyperkalemia
• Rashes, temperature daily
• Confusion, especially in geriatric pa-tients; take safety precautions if needed
• Hydration including skin turgor, thirst, dry mucous membranes; provide ade-quate fluids, mouth care frequently
• Blurred vision, pain in eyes before, during treatment **(increased intraocu-lar pressure)**; neurologic checks, in-tracranial pressure during treatment **(increased intracranial pressure)**
• **Pregnancy/breastfeeding:** use only if clearly needed; cautious use in breast-feeding, unknown if excreted in breast milk

> **Black Box Warning: Bronchospasm/asthma (inhalation test kit):** test for bronchial hyperresponsiveness should not be performed in any person with asthma or baseline pulmonary function test FEV1 <1-1.5 liters or <70% of pre-dicted values

• **Beers:** use with caution in older adults; may cause or exacerbate SIADH
Evaluate:
• Therapeutic response: improvement in edema of feet, legs, sacral area daily if medication being used with HF; de-creased intraocular pressure, prevention of hypokalemia, increased excretion of toxic substances; decreased ICP
Teach patient/family:
• To rise slowly from lying or sitting po-sition
• About the reason for, method of treat-ment
• To report signs of electrolyte imbal-ance, confusion, pain at injection site, hearing loss, blurred vision

TREATMENT OF OVERDOSE:
Discontinue infusion; correct fluid, elec-trolyte imbalances; hemodialysis; moni-tor hydration, CV status, renal function

A HIGH ALERT

maraviroc (Rx)
(mah-rav′er-rock)

Selzentry
Func. class.: Antiretroviral
Chem. class.: Fusion inhibitor,
CCR5-receptor antagonist

ACTION: Interferes with entry into HIV-1 by inhibiting the fusion of the virus and the cell membrane

USES: CCR5-tropic HIV in combination with other antiretroviral agents for treating experienced patients

CONTRAINDICATIONS: Hypersensitivity, dialysis, renal impairment
Precautions: Pregnancy, 🐾 Asian patients, breastfeeding, renal/hepatic/cardiac disease, electrolyte imbalance, dehydration, immune reconstitution syndrome, infection, MI, orthostatic hypotension, children, geriatric patients, Graves' disease, Guillain-Barré syndrome, polymyositis, fever, serious rash

Black Box Warning: Hepatitis

DOSAGE AND ROUTES
Those not taking any CYP3A inducers/inhibitors
• **Adult/adolescent ≥16 yr: PO** 300 mg bid
Those taking CYP3A4 inhibitors with/without a CYP3A inducer
• **Adult/adolescent ≥16 yr: PO** 150 mg bid
Those taking CYP3A4 inducers without a strong CYP3A inhibitor
• **Adult/adolescent ≥16 yr: PO** 600 mg bid
Renal dose
• **Adult: PO** CCr ≥30 mL/min, no dose adjustment; CCr <30 mL/min, use is contraindicated
Available forms: Tabs 150, 300 mg
Administer:
• May give without regard to meals, with 8 oz water; swallow whole; do not crush, chew, break
• Store at room temperature

SIDE EFFECTS
CV: MI, cardiac ischemia, orthostatic hypotension
CNS: Dizziness, depression, viral meningitis, disturbances in consciousness, peripheral neuropathy, paresthesia, dysesthesia, fever
EENT: Gingival hyperplasia, visual changes
GI: Diarrhea, constipation, dyspepsia, pseudomembranous colitis, hepatotoxicity
INTEG: Rash, urticaria, pruritus, folliculitis
MS: Joint pain, leg pain, muscle cramps
RESP: Cough, upper respiratory tract infection, sinusitis, bronchitis, pneumonia, bronchospasm, obstruction, dyspnea
SYST: Herpes virus, lipodystrophy, malignancy

PHARMACOKINETICS
Metabolized by P450 system; CYP3A metabolism; excreted 20% urine, 76% feces; protein binding 76%; terminal half-life 14-18 hr

INTERACTIONS
Increase: maraviroc levels—CYP3A inhibitors (amiodarone, aprepitant, chloramphenicol, clarithromycin, conivaptan, cycloSPORINE, dalfopristin, danazol, diltiaZEM, erythromycin, estradiol, fluconazole, fluvoxaMINE, imatinib, isoniazid, itraconazole, ketoconazole, miconazole, nefazodone, niCARDipine, propoxyphene, RU-486, tamoxifen, telithromycin, troleandomycin, verapamil, voriconazole, zafirlukast); reduce dose
Decrease: maraviroc levels—CYP3A4 inducers (efavirenz, aminoglutethimide, barbiturates, bexarotene, bosentan, carBAMazepine, dexamethasone, griseofulvin, modafinil, nafcillin, OXcarbazepine, phenytoin, fosphenytoin, rifabutin, rifAMPin, rifapentine, topiramate, tipranavir); increase dose
Drug/Herb
• Decreased maraviroc effect: St. John's wort

M

Side effects: *italics* = common; red = life-threatening

Drug/Food

• High-fat meal decreases absorption 33%

Drug/Lab Test

Increase: AST, ALT, bilirubin, amylase, lipase, CK

Decrease: ANC

NURSING CONSIDERATIONS

Assess:

• **HIV:** CD4, T-cell count, plasma HIV RNA, CCR5-tropic HIV-1; assess for changes in symptoms, other infections during treatment

• Severe renal disease (ESRD CCr <30 mL/min): for those taking CYP3A inhibitors/inducers and with severe renal disease, drug is contraindicated

• Bowel pattern before, during treatment

• **Allergies:** skin eruptions, rash, urticaria, itching; discontinue product

• **Serious skin rash (Stevens-Johnson syndrome, toxic epidermal necrolysis, DRESS):** assess for serious rash; if symptoms develop, discontinue product immediately, provide supportive treatment

• **Pregnancy/breastfeeding:** provide during pregnancy in those who are HIV positive; avoid breastfeeding to reduce risk of HIV transmission; register pregnant patient with Antiretroviral Pregnancy Registry, 1-800-258-4263

Evaluate:

• Therapeutic response: improvement in CD4, viral load, T-cell count

Teach patient/family:

• To take as prescribed; if dose is missed, to take as soon as remembered up to 1 hr before next dose; not to double dose; that product does not cure condition, should not be shared with others

• To take every day with other antiretrovirals as directed, not to stop product without approval of prescriber

• That product does not cure infection, just controls symptoms and does not prevent infecting others

• To report sore throat, fever, fatigue (may indicate superinfection); yellow skin/eyes, abdominal pain, vomiting, dark urine, nausea (hepatitis); itching, SOB (allergic reaction)

• That product must be taken in equal intervals around the clock to maintain blood levels for duration of therapy

• To avoid all OTC products unless approved by prescriber

• To avoid driving, other hazardous activities until reaction is known; that dizziness may occur

• To make position changes slowly to prevent postural hypotension

• To notify prescriber if pregnancy is planned or suspected; not to breastfeed

---

RARELY USED

mecasermin (Rx)

(mec-a′sir-men)

Increlex

Func. class.: Biologic response modifier; insulin-like growth factor

USES: Growth failure in children with severe primary insulin-like growth factor-1 (IGF-1) deficiency (primary IGFD) or with growth hormone (GH) gene deletion who have developed neutralizing antibodies to GH

Unlabeled uses: ALS

CONTRAINDICATIONS: Hypersensitivity, benzyl alcohol, closed epiphyses, active/suspected neoplasia, IV use

DOSAGE AND ROUTES

• **Child ≥2 yr: SUBCUT** 0.04-0.08 mg/kg (40-80 mcg/kg) bid; if well tolerated for 1 wk, may increase by 0.04 mg/kg/dose, max 0.12 mg/kg bid

---

meclizine (OTC, Rx)

(mek′li-zeen)

Bonine, Dramamine Less Drowsy Formula

Func. class.: Antiemetic, antihistamine, anticholinergic

Chem. class.: H$_1$-receptor antagonist, piperazine derivative

---

ACTION: Suppresses vestibular end-organ receptors and inhibits activation of cholinergic pathways

USES: Vertigo, motion sickness

CONTRAINDICATIONS: Hypersensitivity to cyclizines

Precautions: Pregnancy, breastfeeding, children, geriatric patients, closed-angle glaucoma, prostatic hypertrophy, hepatic/renal disease, urinary retention, GI obstruction, contact lenses

DOSAGE AND ROUTES
Vertigo
• **Adult/adolescent:** PO 25-100 mg/day in divided doses
Motion sickness
• **Adult/adolescent:** PO 25-50 mg 1 hr before traveling, repeat dose q24hr prn
Available forms: Tabs 12.5, 25, 50 mg
Administer:
PO route
• May give without regard to food
• **Chew tab:** give without regard to water or may be swallowed whole with water
• Lowest possible dose for geriatric patients; anticholinergic effects

SIDE EFFECTS
CNS: *Drowsiness,* fatigue
EENT: Blurred vision
GI: Dry mouth

PHARMACOKINETICS
PO: Onset 1 hr, duration 8-24 hr, half-life 6 hr

INTERACTIONS
Increase: sedation—CYP2D6, inhibitors
Increase: anticholinergic effects—other antihistamines, atropine, antidepressants, phenothiazines
Increase: effect of alcohol, opioids, other CNS depressants
Drug/Lab Test
False negative: allergy skin testing (allergen extracts)

NURSING CONSIDERATIONS
Assess:
• **Vertigo/motion sickness:** nausea, vomiting after 1 hr; assess vertigo periodically

• **Signs of toxicity:** CNS depression, constipation; consider other causes of symptoms; may mask symptoms of other diseases, such as brain tumor, intestinal obstruction
• For urinary disease obstruction, decreased urinary output; may exacerbate symptoms; monitor urinary output
• **Hepatic impairment:** accumulation and severe effects may occur; monitor
• Observe for drowsiness, dizziness, level of consciousness
• **Pregnancy/breastfeeding:** use only if needed; occasional doses should not pose a risk in breastfeeding
• **Beers:** use caution in older adults; higher risk of anticholinergic effects
Evaluate:
• Therapeutic response: absence of dizziness, vomiting
Teach patient/family:
• That a false-negative result may occur with skin testing for allergies; that these procedures should not be scheduled for ≤4 days after discontinuing use
• To avoid hazardous activities, activities requiring alertness because dizziness may occur; to request assistance with ambulation
• To avoid alcohol, other depressants; not to breastfeed; to report severe side effects
• To use sugarless gum, frequent sips of water for dry mouth
• **Motion sickness prophylaxis:** to take ≥1 hr before event that may cause motion sickness

---

medroxyPROGESTERone (Rx)

(me-drox´ee-proe-jess´te-rone)
Depo-Provera, Depo-SubQ Provera 104, Provera
Func. class.: Antineoplastic, hormone, contraceptive
Chem. class.: Progesterone derivative

Do not confuse:
medroxyPROGESTERone/
methylPREDNISolone
Provera/Premarin/Covera

ACTION: Inhibits secretion of pituitary gonadotropins, which prevents follicular maturation and ovulation; antineoplastic action against endometrial cancer

USES: Uterine bleeding (abnormal); secondary amenorrhea; prevention of endometrial changes associated with estrogen replacement therapy (ERT); contraceptive; inoperable, recurrent, metastatic endometrial/renal cancer, endometriosis

Unlabeled uses: Hot flashes; symptoms of menopause; paraphilia (men); hot flashes (men) with prostate cancer

CONTRAINDICATIONS: Pregnancy, hypersensitivity, reproductive cancer, genital bleeding (abnormal, undiagnosed), missed abortion, stroke, cerebrovascular disease, cervical cancer, hepatic disease, uterine/vaginal cancer

Black Box Warning: Breast cancer, MI, stroke, thromboembolic disease, thrombophlebitis

Precautions: Breastfeeding, hypertension, asthma, blood dyscrasias, gallbladder disease, HF, diabetes mellitus, bone disease, depression, migraine headache, seizure disorders, renal/hepatic disease, family history of cancer of breast or reproductive tract, bone mineral density loss, ocular disorders, AIDS/HIV, alcoholism, children, hyperlipidemia, cardiac disease

Black Box Warning: Dementia, osteoporosis

DOSAGE AND ROUTES
Secondary amenorrhea
• **Adult:** PO 5-10 mg/day × 5-10 days, start during any time of menstrual cycle
Uterine bleeding
• **Adult:** PO 5-10 mg/day × 5-10 days starting on 16th or 21st day of menstrual cycle
With ERT
• **Adult:** PO 5-10 mg daily × 10-14 or more days/mo (sequential estrogen); 2.5-5 mg daily (continuous estrogen)

Contraceptive
• **Adult (women):** IM (contraceptive inj) 150 mg (Depo-Provera) q12wk; SUBCUT (depot SUBCUT; Depo-SubQ Provera 104 inj) 104 mg q3mo, give first dose during the first 5 days of menstrual period, only within the first 5 days postpartum (no breastfeeding), only at 6th postpartum wk (breastfeeding)
Endometrial/renal cancer, inoperable, reccurent metastatic
• **Adult:** IM 400 mg–1 g (using 400 mg/mL depot inj susp) weekly
Endometriosis pain
• **Adult:** SUBCUT 104 mg q12-14wk; begin on day 5 of normal menses; avoid use >2 yr; **PO** (unlabeled) 10 mg/day starting on 16th-25th day of menstrual cycle
Hot flashes/symptoms of menopause (unlabeled)
• **Adult (female):** PO 20 mg/day; **IM** 150 mg monthly
Hot flashes (men) in prostate cancer (unlabeled)
• **Adult (male):** IM Depot 150 or 400 mg
Available forms: Tabs 2.5, 5, 10 mg; inj susp, 104 mg/0.65 mL; 150, 400 mg/mL
Administer:
• Store in dark area
PO route
• Give without regard to food
IM route
• Visually inspect for particulate matter or discoloration before use
Depo-Provera contraceptive injection suspension
• IM only, *never* IV; use only 150 mg/mL vial
• Instruct patient on risks and warnings associated with hormonal contraceptives (see Patient Information)
• The possibility of pregnancy should be excluded before giving the first dose of medroxyPROGESTERone or whenever >14 wk has passed since the last dose
• Do not dilute
• Shake vigorously immediately before administration
• Inject deeply into the gluteal or deltoid muscle; aspirate before injection to avoid injection into a blood vessel

Depo-Provera sterile aqueous suspension, preserved

• IM only, *never* IV

• Instruct patient on risks and warnings associated with progestin use (see Patient Information)

• Shake vigorously immediately before use

• When multidose vials are used, take special care to prevent contamination

• Inject deeply into the gluteal or deltoid muscle; aspirate before injection

SUBCUT route

Depo-SubQ Provera 104 contraceptive injection suspension only

• For subcut only, *never* give IM or IV

• Instruct patient on risks and warnings associated with hormonal contraceptives (see Patient Information)

• Shake vigorously for at least 1 min before use

• Inject the entire contents of the pre-filled syringe subcut into the anterior thigh or abdomen, avoiding bony areas and the umbilicus; gently grasp and squeeze a large area of skin in the chosen injection area, ensuring that the skin is pulled away from the body; insert the needle at a 45-degree angle; inject until the syringe is empty; this usually requires 5-7 sec; following use, press lightly on the injection site with a clean cotton pad for a few seconds; do not rub the area

SIDE EFFECTS

CNS: Dizziness, *headache*, migraines, depression, fatigue, nervousness

CV: Thrombophlebitis, edema, thromboembolism, stroke, PE, MI

GI: *Nausea, increased weight, abdominal pain*

GU: *Amenorrhea*, cervical erosion, breakthrough bleeding, dysmenorrhea, vaginal candidiasis, breast changes, vaginitis

INTEG: Acne, hirsutism, alopecia, injection-site reaction

META: Hyperglycemia

MS: Decreased bone density

SYST: Angioedema, anaphylaxis, breast cancer

PHARMACOKINETICS

PO: Duration 3-5 days; **IM** duration 3-4 mo; excreted in urine and feces, breast milk; metabolized in liver, half-life 14.5 hr

INTERACTIONS

Decrease: medroxyPROGESTERone action—strong CYP3A4 inducers (carBAMazepine, phenytoin, rifAMPin, rifabutin, PHENobarbital); avoid concurrent use

Increase: medroxyPROGESTERone level—strong CYP3A4 inhibitors (clarithromycin, ketoconazole, itraconazole, atazanavir, indinavir, ritonavir, voriconazole), avoid using together

Increase or Decrease: medroxyPROGESTERone levels—NNRTIs, protease inhibitors; may diminish progestin level; to provide contraception use nonhormonal method

Decrease: bone mineral density—anticoagulants, corticosteroids

Decrease: contraception—carBAMazepine, phenytoin, rifAMPin, rifabutin; avoid concurrent use, or use additional nonhormonal method of contraception

Drug/Lab Test

Increase: LFTs, HDL, triglycerides, coagulation tests

Decrease: GTT

Drug/Herb

Decreased levels—St. John's wort; avoid concurrent use

NURSING CONSIDERATIONS

Assess:

• **Menstrual history:** duration of menses, bleeding, spotting, age at menarche, regularity; start on any day in those with amenorrhea, or on day 16 or 21 in dysfunctional bleeding

• Pelvic exam, Pap smear, pregnancy test before treatment, periodically

• **Severe allergic reaction, angioedema;** have EPINEPHrine and resuscitative equipment available

• Weight daily; notify prescriber of weekly weight gain >5 lb; bone mineral density

• B/P at beginning of treatment and periodically

M

• Hepatic studies: ALT, AST, bilirubin baseline and periodically during long-term therapy; triglycerides, caution if preexisting elevation, product may exacerbate levels

• Mental status: affect, mood, behavioral changes, depression

Black Box Warning: This product should not be given to those with breast cancer, MI, stroke, thromboembolic disorders; assess for these conditions before using

• **Bone mineral density loss:** those taking anticoagulants, corticosteroids with Depo-Provera or Depo-SubQ Provera are at greater risk

Black Box Warning: Use of product shown to increase dementia in women ≥65 yr old; use may increase osteoporosis in long-term treatment; those who smoke also at greater risk; adequate calcium and vit D should be taken

• Ectopic pregnancy: severe abdominal pain may indicate ectopic pregnancy if patient is pregnant

Evaluate:

• Therapeutic response: decreased abnormal uterine bleeding, absence of amenorrhea

Teach patient/family:

• To take with food if nausea occurs

• To have complete physical exam, including reproductive exam, yearly

• To avoid sunlight or to use sunscreen; photosensitivity can occur

• To report breast lumps, vaginal bleeding, edema, jaundice, dark urine, clay-colored stools, dyspnea, headache, blurred vision, abdominal pain, sudden change in speech/coordination, numbness or stiffness in legs, chest pain; males to report impotence, gynecomastia immediately

• That product doesn't protect against sexually transmitted diseases, including HIV

• That injection (subcut) must be given q3mo for contraception; missing dose may lead to pregnancy

Black Box Warning: Long-term use decreases bone density; exercise, calcium, vitamin D, supplements can help lessen osteoporosis

• Review package insert with patient; patient must understand all possible adverse reactions

• **Pregnancy/breastfeeding:** not to use in pregnancy; to report suspected pregnancy; that fertility returns 6-12 mo after discontinuing; not to breastfeed

---

⚠ HIGH ALERT

megestrol (Rx)

(me-jess′trole)

Megace, Megace ES, Megace OS ✦

Func. class.: Antineoplastic hormone

Chem. class.: Progestin

ACTION: Affects endometrium with antiluteinizing effect; thought to bring about cell death, stimulates appetite by unknown action

USES: Breast, endometrial cancer; cachexia, anorexia, weight loss with AIDS

CONTRAINDICATIONS: Pregnancy, hypersensitivity

Precautions: Diabetes, thrombosis, adrenal insufficiency

DOSAGE AND ROUTES

Endometrial/ovarian carcinoma (palliative)

• **Adult: PO** 40-320 mg/day in divided doses

Breast carcinoma (palliative)

• **Adult: PO** 40 mg qid or 160 mg/day

Available forms: Tabs 20, 40, 160 ✦ mg; oral susp 40, 125 mg/mL

Administer:

• Oral susp for AIDS patients; shake well

• Tablets for carcinoma

• Without regard to food

• Store in tight container at room temperature

SIDE EFFECTS

CNS: Mood swings, insomnia, fever, lethargy, depression
CV: Thrombophlebitis, thromboembolism, hypertension
ENDO: Adrenal insufficiency
GI: Nausea, vomiting, *diarrhea*, abdominal cramps, *weight gain*, flatus, indigestion
GU: Gynecomastia, fluid retention, vaginal bleeding, discharge, *impotence*, decreased libido, menstruation disorders
INTEG: Alopecia, *rash*, pruritus
MISC: Tumor flare leukopenia

PHARMACOKINETICS

PO: Half-life 13-105 hr; metabolized in liver; excreted in feces, urine, breast milk; food increases bioavailability of oral sol

INTERACTIONS

• **Increase:** serious arrhythmias—dofetilide; avoid using concurrently
• **Increase:** megestrol metabolism, decreasing effect—antidiabetics; may need to increase megestrol dose
• **Decrease:** effect of indinavir; may need to increase indinavir dose

Drug/Lab Test
Increase: glucose

NURSING CONSIDERATIONS
Assess:

• PSA levels in men (prostate cancer); blood glucose, LFTs, serum calcium, weight
• Effects of alopecia on body image; feelings about body changes
• Frequency of stools, characteristics: cramping, acidosis, signs of dehydration (poor skin turgor, decreased urine output, dry skin, restlessness, weakness), rapid respirations
• Anorexia, nausea, vomiting, constipation, weakness, loss of muscle tone
• **Thrombophlebitis:** unilateral increase in leg girth; edema; warm, red skin; pain in extremity; notify prescriber immediately
• **HPA axis suppression:** in chronic users, do not discontinue abruptly; wear medical ID; monitor for hypotension during stress, trauma, acute illness
• **Beers:** avoid in older adults as an appetite stimulant; minimal effect on weight; increased risk of thrombotic events

• **Pregnancy/breastfeeding:** do not use in pregnancy or breastfeeding
Evaluate:
• Therapeutic response: decreased tumor size, spread of malignancy; weight gain in AIDS patients; resolved dysfunctional uterine bleeding
Teach patient/family:
• To report vaginal bleeding
• That gynecomastia, alopecia can occur; reversible after discontinuing treatment
• To recognize signs of fluid retention, thromboemboli; to report these immediately
• To monitor blood glucose if diabetic
• That products may be taken without food
• **Pregnancy/breastfeeding:** that nonhormonal contraception should be used during and for 4 mo after treatment

---

⚠ HIGH ALERT   M

melphalan (Rx)
(mel′fa-lan)
Alkeran, Evomela
Func. class.: Antineoplastic, alkylating agent
Chem. class.: Nitrogen mustard

Do not confuse:
melphalan/Myleran/Leukeran

ACTION: Responsible for cross-linking DNA strands, thereby leading to cell death; activity is not cell-cycle–phase specific

USES: Multiple myeloma, advanced ovarian cancer

CONTRAINDICATIONS: Pregnancy, breastfeeding, hypersensitivity
Precautions: Children, radiation therapy, infections, renal disease

Black Box Warning: Bone marrow depression, secondary malignancy, radiation therapy, bleeding, infection, risk of serious hypersensitivity reaction; requires an experienced clinician

---

Side effects: *italics* = common; red = life-threatening

DOSAGE AND ROUTES
Multiple myeloma (palliative)
• **Adult: PO** 6 mg daily × 2-3 wk, stop for ≤4 wk or until WBC/platelets begin to rise, maintenance 2 mg/day or 10 mg daily × 7-10 days, then 2 mg/day when WBC >4000 cells/mm³ and platelets >100,000 cells/mm³, adjust dose daily between 1-3 mg/day based on response, or 0.15 mg/kg/day × 7 days, then a rest period of ≥14 days, maintenance ≤0.05 mg/kg/day or 0.25 mg/kg/day × 4 days, repeat 4-6 wk

Multiple myeloma conditioning treatment before stem cell transplantation (Evomela only)
• **Adult: IV INFUSION** 100 mg/m²/day over 30 min for 2 days before stem cell transplant (day 3, day 2; day 0 [transplant])

Amyloidosis (unlabeled)
• **Adult: PO** 0.22 mg/kg/day × 4 days q28days in combination with dexamethasone or 10 mg/m²/day × 4 days q28days with dexamethasone; >130% of ideal weight or renal disease (BUN ≥30 mg/dL), reduce dose by 50%
• **Adult: IV INFUSION** 16 mg/m², reduce with renal insufficiency, give over 15-20 min, give at 2-wk intervals × 4 doses, then at 4-wk intervals

Ovarian carcinoma
• **Adult: PO** 0.2 mg/kg/day × 5 days q4-5wk; repeat q4-5wk depending on blood counts

Available forms: Tabs 2 mg, powder for inj 50 mg

Administer:
• Antiemetic 30-60 min before product to prevent vomiting

PO route
• Give on empty stomach
• Protect from light; store refrigerated

Intermittent IV INF route
• Use gloves during administration; if skin exposure occurs, wash immediately with soap and water, use cytotoxic handling procedures

Evomela
Reconstitution:
• Add 8.6 mL of 0.9% sodium chloride injection to the vial for a final vial concentration of 5 mg/mL

• Negative pressure should be present in the vial; discard any vial that does not have a vacuum present during reconstitution
• Storage after reconstitution: Store at room temperature for up to 1 hr or refrigerated up to 24 hr

IV infusion:
• Dilute the appropriate dose with 0.9% sodium chloride to a final concentration not to exceed 0.45 mg/mL
• The diluted solution may be stored at room temperature for up to 4 hr (in addition to 1 hr after reconstitution)
• Administer IV over 30 min when used as conditioning treatment before an autologous stem cell transplant or IV over 15-20 min when used as palliative treatment in multiple myeloma patients
• Infuse into an injection port or by injecting slowly into a fast-running IV infusion via a central venous line to avoid extravasation

Alkeran and generic melphalan
Reconstitution:
• Using a 20-gauge or larger needle, rapidly inject 10 mL of the supplied diluent into a 50-mg vial for a final vial concentration of 5 mg/mL
• Immediately shake the vial well until the solution becomes clear and all material is dissolved
• Dilute the reconstituted vial immediately; the solution is unstable
• Do NOT refrigerate the reconstituted vial; a precipitate forms if the solution is stored at 5° C

IV infusion:
• Dilute the appropriate dose in 0.9% sodium chloride to a final concentration not to exceed 0.45 mg/mL
• Administer IV over 15-20 min; do NOT give over less than 15 min, and complete the infusion within 60 min from vial reconstitution
• The diluted solution is unstable; about 1% of the labeled dose hydrolyzes every 10 min after dilution with sodium chloride
• Infuse through a central line to avoid extravasation

Y-site compatibilities: Acyclovir, amikacin, aminophylline, ampicillin, aztreonam, bleomycin, bumetanide, buprenorphine, butorphanol, calcium gluconate, CARBOplatin, carmustine, ceFAZolin, cefepime, cefoperazone, cefotaxime, cefoTEtan, cefTAZidime, ceftizoxime, cefTRIAXone, cefuroxime, cimetidine, CISplatin, clindamycin, cyclophosphamide, cytarabine, dacarbazine, DACTINomycin, DAUNOrubicin, dexamethasone, diphenhydrAMINE, DOXOrubicin, doxycycline, droperidol, enalaprilat, etoposide, famotidine, floxuridine, fluconazole, fludarabine, fluorouracil, furosemide, gallium, ganciclovir, gentamicin, granisetron, haloperidol, heparin, hydrocortisone, hydrocortisone sodium phosphate, HYDROmorphone, hydrOXYzine, IDArubicin, ifosfamide, imipenem-cilastatin, LORazepam, mannitol, mechlorethamine, meperidine, mesna, methotrexate, methylPREDNISolone, metoclopramide, metroNIDAZOLE, miconazole, minocycline, mitoMYcin, mitoXANTRONE, morphine, nalbuphine, netilmicin, ondansetron, pentostatin, piperacillin, plicamycin, potassium chloride, prochlorperazine, promethazine, raNITIdine, sodium bicarbonate, streptozocin, teniposide, thiotepa, ticarcillin, ticarcillin/clavulanate, tobramycin, trimethoprim-sulfamethoxazole, vancomycin, vinBLAStine, vinCRIStine, vinorelbine, zidovudine

SIDE EFFECTS

GI: *Nausea, vomiting, stomatitis, diarrhea,* hepatotoxicity, *abdominal pain, anorexia, constipation*
GU: *Amenorrhea,* infertility
HEMA: Thrombocytopenia, neutropenia, leukopenia, anemia
INTEG: Pruritus, necrosis, extravasation, alopecia, rash
RESP: Dyspnea, pneumonitis, bronchospasm
SYST: Anaphylaxis, allergic reactions, secondary malignancies, edema
CNS: *Fatigue, fever,* dizziness
META: *Hypokalemia, hypophosphatemia*
ENDO: Menstrual irregularities

PHARMACOKINETICS

Metabolized in liver, excreted in urine, half-life 2 hr, protein binding ≤30%

INTERACTIONS (IV MELPHALAN)

Increase: toxicity—antineoplastics, radiation
Increase: bleeding risk—NSAIDs, anticoagulants, salicylates, thrombolytics, platelet inhibitors; avoid concurrent use
Decrease: antibody response—live virus vaccines; bring up-to-date before use or postpone 3 mo after conclusion of treatment
Increase: uric acid, HIAA
Drug/Lab Test
Decrease: Hgb, RBC, WBC, platelets
False-positive: Direct Coombs' test

NURSING CONSIDERATIONS
Assess:

Black Box Warning: **Bone marrow depression:** full nadir 2-3 wk; CBC, differential, platelet count weekly; notify prescriber, withhold product if WBC is <3000/mm^3 or platelet count is <100,000/mm^3; recovery usually occurs in 6 wk

• Renal studies: BUN, serum uric acid before, during therapy
• I&O ratio; report fall in urine output to 30 mL/hr

Black Box Warning: **Infection:** fever, cough, temperature, chills, sore throat; notify prescriber

Black Box Warning: **Secondary malignancy:** acute leukemia, myeloproliferative syndrome may occur due to chromosome damage; risk is increased when using long-term treatment

Black Box Warning: **Requires an experienced clinician:** product should be used only by clinician knowledgeable in use of chemotherapy

M

Side effects: *italics* = common; red = life-threatening

• **Hepatotoxicity:** hepatic studies before, during therapy (bilirubin, AST, ALT, LDH) as needed; jaundiced skin and sclera, dark urine, clay-colored stools, itchy skin, abdominal pain, fever, diarrhea

Black Box Warning: IV product causes more myelosuppression

Black Box Warning: Bleeding: hematuria, guaiac, bruising or petechiae, mucosa or orifices often, no rectal temperature, IM injections if possible

• Buccal cavity q8hr for dryness, sores, ulceration, white patches, oral pain, bleeding, dysphagia
• Local irritation, pain, burning, discoloration at inj site

Black Box Warning: Severe allergic reaction: rash, pruritus, urticaria, purpuric skin lesions, itching, flushing; assess allergy to chlorambucil; cross-sensitivity may occur in 2% of patients; avoid

• **Gout:** Increased uric acid, joint pain, especially in extremities, provide fluids to 2L/day, may use with anti-gout medications such as allopurinol
• Increase fluid intake to 2-3 L/day to prevent urate deposits, calculi formation
• Rinsing of mouth tid-qid with water, club soda; brushing of teeth bid-tid with soft brush or cotton-tipped applicators for stomatitis; use unwaxed dental floss

Black Box Warning: Pregnancy/breastfeeding: Do not use during pregnancy or breastfeeding

Evaluate:
• Therapeutic response: decreased tumor size, spread of malignancy
Teach patient/family:
• That usually sterility, amenorrhea occur; reversible after discontinuing treatment
• To avoid foods with citric acid, hot temperature, or rough texture

• To report any bleeding, white spots, or ulcerations in mouth to prescriber; to examine mouth daily

Black Box Warning: To report signs of infection: fever, sore throat, flulike symptoms

• To report signs of anemia: fatigue, headache, faintness, SOB, irritability, nausea/vomiting, dehydration, decreased urine output
• To avoid use of aspirin products, NSAIDs, alcohol
• **Hepatotoxicity:** to report immediately yellowing of skin or eyes, dark urine, clay-colored stools, itchy skin, abdominal pain, fever, diarrhea
• **Pregnancy/breastfeeding:** to report suspected pregnancy; to use contraception during treatment

---

memantine (Rx)

(me-man′teen)

Ebixa ✦, Namenda, Namenda XR
Func. class.: Anti-Alzheimer's agent
Chem. class.: *N*-methyl-D-aspartate receptor antagonist

ACTION: Antagonist action of CNS NMDA receptors that may contribute to the symptoms of Alzheimer's disease

USES: Moderate to severe dementia in Alzheimer's disease

CONTRAINDICATIONS: Children, hypersensitivity
Precautions: Pregnancy, breastfeeding, renal disease, GU conditions that raise urine pH, seizures, severe hepatic disease, renal failure

DOSAGE AND ROUTES
• **Adult: PO** 5 mg/day, may increase dose in 5-mg increments ≥1-wk intervals over a 3-wk period; recommended target dose is 10 mg bid at wk 4; ext rel 7 mg daily, increased by 7 mg ≥1 wk up to target dose of 28 mg daily

---

Renal dose
• **Adult: PO** CCr 5-29 mL/min, a target of 5 mg bid immediate release or 14 mg/day extended release

Conversion from immediate-release to extended-release product

When switching from the immediate-release (IR) tablets to the extended-release (ER) capsules, the following conversion is recommended: 10 mg bid of the IR tablets should be converted to 28 mg daily of the ER capsules beginning the day after the last dose of the IR tablet. Those with severe renal impairment receiving 5 mg bid of the IR tablets may be converted to the ER capsules at a dose of 14 mg daily beginning the day after the last dose of the IR tablet

Available forms: Tabs 5, 10 mg; tab (Namenda Titration Pak) 5, 10 mg; oral sol 2 mg/mL (10 mg/5 mL); cap ext rel 7, 14, 21, 28 mg

Administer:
• Can be taken without regard to meals
• Twice a day if dose >5 mg
• Dosage adjusted to response no more than q1wk
• **Ext rel caps:** do not crush, chew, divide; swallow whole or open and sprinkle on applesauce
• When switching from immediate-release product, begin the ext rel the day after the last dose of immediate-release product. Those on 10 mg bid should be switched to ext rel 28 mg daily
• **Oral sol:** using device provided; remove dosing syringe, green cap, plastic tube from plastic; attach tube to green cap; open cap by pushing down on cap, turning counterclockwise; remove unscrewed cap; remove seal from bottle, discard; insert plastic tube fully into bottle, screw green cap tightly onto bottle by turning cap clockwise; keeping bottle upright on table, remove lid; with plunger fully depressed, insert tip of syringe into cap; while holding syringe, gently pull up on plunger; remove syringe, invert syringe, slowly press plunger to level that removes large air bubbles; keep plunger in inverted position; few small air bubbles may be present

SIDE EFFECTS

CNS: *Dizziness, confusion,* headache
CV: Hypertension
GI: Vomiting, constipation, diarrhea
HEMA: Anemia
INTEG: Rash
MISC: Back pain, fatigue

PHARMACOKINETICS

Rapidly absorbed PO, 44% protein binding, very little metabolism, 57%-82% excreted unchanged in urine, half-life 60-80 hr; peak 3-7 hr (tabs), 9-12 hr (caps)

INTERACTIONS

Increase/decrease: both products: hydro-CHLOROthiazide, triamterene, cimetidine, quiNIDine, raNITIdine, nicotine; monitor for effect
Increase: effect—levodopa, some ergots
Decrease: clearance of memantine—products that make urine alkaline (sodium bicarbonate, carbonic anhydrase inhibitors); monitor for effect
• Use cautiously with amantadine, dextromethorphan, ketamine; reaction unknown

Drug/Food
Increase: product level—foods that cause urine alkalinity (fruits, vegetables, nuts, dairy)

Drug/Lab Test
Increase: alkaline phosphatase
Decrease: Hct, Hgb

NURSING CONSIDERATIONS

Assess:
• **Alzheimer's dementia:** affect, mood, behavioral changes; hallucinations, confusion, attention, orientation, memory; monitor serum creatinine
• Provide assistance with ambulation during beginning therapy; dizziness may occur
• **Adverse reactions:** patient may be unable to verbalize reactions

Evaluate:
• Therapeutic response: decrease in confusion, improved mood, maintenance of function, even with no improvement in symptoms

Teach patient/family:
• To report side effects: restlessness, psychosis, visual hallucinations, stupor, LOC; may indicate overdose

M

- To use product exactly as prescribed; to avoid alcohol, nicotine
- To use oral sol dispenser provided
- To avoid OTC, herbal products unless approved by prescriber
- That product doesn't cure Alzheimer's disease but controls symptoms
- Not to smoke or use alcohol
- Not to crush, chew ext rel caps, may be opened and sprinkled on applesauce; do not mix oral sol with other liquids
- That product may cause dizziness

⚠ HIGH ALERT

meperidine (Rx)

(me-per′i-deen)

Demerol

Func. class.: Opioid analgesic

Chem. class.: Phenylpiperidine derivative

Controlled Substance Schedule II

Do not confuse:
meperidine/HYDROmorphone/
meprobamate/morphine
Demerol/Dilaudid

ACTION: Depresses pain impulse transmission at the spinal cord level by interacting with opioid receptors

USES: Moderate to severe pain preoperatively, postoperatively, general anesthesia maintenance, sedation induction
Unlabeled uses: Obstetric/regional analgesic, acute severe headache/migraine, shaking chills induced by IV amphotericin B or postoperative shivering

CONTRAINDICATIONS: Hypersensitivity, GI obstruction, ileus

Black Box Warning: MAOI therapy, respiratory depression

Precautions: Pregnancy, breastfeeding, children, geriatric patients, addictive personality, increased intracranial pressure, renal/hepatic disease, seizure disorder, abrupt discontinuation, chronic pain, cardiac disease, adrenal insufficiency, alcoholism, angina, anticoagulant therapy, asthma, atrial flutter, biliary tract disease, bladder obstruction, cardiac dysrhythmias, COPD, CNS depression, coagulopathy, constipation, cor pulmonale, dehydration, diarrhea, driving, epidural use, geriatric patients, GI obstruction, head trauma, heart failure, hypotension, hypothyroidism, ileus, IBS, IM/intrathecal/IV use, labor, myxedema, thrombocytopenia

Black Box Warning: Coadministration with other CNS depressants, accidental exposure, neonatal opioid withdrawal syndrome, potential for overdose or poisoning, substance abuse

DOSAGE AND ROUTES
Moderate to severe pain
- **Adult: PO/SUBCUT/IM** 50-150 mg q3-4hr prn; **IV CONT INF** 15-35 mg/hr
- **Child: PO/SUBCUT/IM** 1-1.8 mg/kg q3-4hr prn, max single dose 150 mg; **IV CONT INF** 0.5-1 mg/kg loading dose then 0.3 mg/kg/hr

Labor analgesia
- **Adult: SUBCUT/IM** 50-100 mg given when contractions regularly spaced, repeat q1-3hr prn

Preoperative analgesia
- **Adult: IM/SUBCUT** 50-100 mg 30-90 min before surgery
- **Child: IM/SUBCUT** 1-2.2 mg/kg 30-90 min before surgery, max 100 mg

PCA
- **Adult: IV** 10 mg, range 1-5 mg increments, lock out interval 6-10 min

Coadministration with other CNS depressants
- **Adult: PO/IM/SUBCUT/IV** Reduce dose by 25%-50%

Renal dose
- **Adult: PO/IM/SUBCUT/IV** CCr 10-50 mL/min give 75% of dose; CCr <10 mL/min give 50% of dose

Available forms: Inj 10, 25, 50, 75, 100 mg/mL; tabs 50, 100 mg; oral sol 50 mg/5 mL
Administer:
- Doses given regularly before pain returns are more effective

---

PO route

- May give with food or milk to decrease GI irritation
- Do not use in severe respiratory insufficiency
- **Oral solution:** dilute in 4 oz water; less effective than IM
- Store in light-resistant container at room temperature

IM/SUBCUT route

- Patient should remain recumbent for 1 hr after IM/SUBCUT route
- With antiemetic for nausea, vomiting
- When pain beginning to return; determine dosage interval by patient response
- In gradually decreasing dose after long-term use; withdrawal symptoms may occur
- Inject IM into large muscle mass; IM preferred route for multiple inj

Direct IV route

- Dilute to concentration of ≤10 mg/mL with sterile water for inj or NS
- Inject slowly ≤25 mg/min over at least 5 min, rapid administration may cause respiratory depression, hypotension, circulatory collapse
- Have emergency equipment and opiate antagonist on hand

Intermittent IV INFUSION route

- Dilute to concentration of 1 mg/mL
- Infuse using infusion pump over 15-30 min, titrate

Y-site compatibilities: Abelcet, acetaminophen, amifostine, amikacin, anidulafungin, atenolol, aztreonam, bumetanide, ceFAZolin, cefotaxime, cefOXitin, cefTAZidime, ceftizoxime, cefTRIAXone, cefuroxime, cisatracurium, cladribine, clindamycin, diltiaZEM, diphenhydrAMINE, DOBUTamine, DOPamine, DOXOrubicin hydrochloride, doxycycline, droperidol, erythromycin, famotidine, filgrastim, fluconazole, fludarabine, gallium, gentamicin, granisetron, hydrocortisone, insulin (regular), kanamycin, labetalol, lidocaine, methyldopa, melphalan, metoclopramide, metoprolol, metroNIDAZOLE, ondansetron, oxytocin, PACLitaxel, penicillin G potassium, piperacillin, potassium chloride, propofol, propranolol, raNITIdine, remifentanil, sargramostim, teniposide, thiotepa, ticarcillin, ticarcillin/clavulanate, tobramycin, vancomycin, verapamil, vinorelbine

Continuous intrathecal INFUSION route

- Use controlled infusion device; implantable controlled microinfusion device used for highly concentrated infusion; monitor for several days after implantation
- Filling of infusion reservoir should be done only by those fully qualified
- To prevent pain, depletion of reservoir should be avoided

SIDE EFFECTS

CNS: *Drowsiness, dizziness, confusion, headache, sedation, euphoria,* increased intracranial pressure, seizures, serotonin syndrome

CV: Palpitations, bradycardia, hypotension, change in B/P, tachycardia (IV)

EENT: Tinnitus, blurred vision, miosis, diplopia, depressed corneal reflex

GI: Nausea, vomiting, anorexia, constipation, cramps, biliary spasm, paralytic ileus

GU: Urinary retention, dysuria

INTEG: Rash, urticaria, bruising, flushing, diaphoresis, pruritus

RESP: Respiratory depression

SYST: Anaphylaxis

PHARMACOKINETICS

Metabolized by liver (to active/inactive metabolites), excreted by kidneys; crosses placenta, excreted in breast milk; half-life 3-4 hr; toxic by-product accumulation can result from regular use or renal disease; protein binding 65%-75%

PO: Onset 15 min, peak 1.5 hr, duration 2-4 hr, absorption 50%

SUBCUT/IM: Onset 10 min, peak 30-60 min, duration 2-4 hr, well absorbed

IV: Onset immediate, peak 5-7 min, duration 2 hr

INTERACTIONS

Black Box Warning: **May cause fatal reaction:** MAOIs, procarbazine within 14 days

Increase: serotonin syndrome, neuroleptic malignant syndrome—SSRIs, SNRIs, serotonin-receptor agonists, tricyclics, 5-HT3 receptor antagonists

Side effects: *italics* = common; red = life-threatening

Increase: effects, severe respiratory depression with other CNS depressants, alcohol, opioids, sedative/hypnotics, antipsychotics, skeletal muscle relaxants

Increase: adverse reactions—protease inhibitor antiretrovirals

Increase: opioid toxicity—CYP3A4 inhibitors (fluconazole, ketoconazole, itraconazole, clarithromycin, nefazodone, verampamil), avoid using together

Decrease: meperidine effect—phenytoin, nalbuphine, pentazocine

Increase: sedation—kava, hawthorn, lavender, valerian

Drug/Herb

Increase: CNS depression, serotonin syndrome—St. John's wort, avoid using together

Drug/Lab Test

Increase: amylase, lipase

NURSING CONSIDERATIONS
Assess:
• **Pain:** location, type, character; give product before pain becomes extreme; reassess after 60 min (IM, SUBCUT, PO) and 5-10 min (IV)
• B/P, pulse, respirations baseline and during use
• Monitor BUN, serum creatinine

Black Box Warning: Opioids/benzodiazepines: use only if alternative products cannot be used; excessive sedation and death may occur; if used, monitor closely

• **Abrupt discontinuation:** withdraw slowly; if stopped abruptly, assess for withdrawal
• **Sex hormone changes:** assess for libido, changes in menstrual cycle, erectile dysfunction, infertility; if androgen deficiency is suspected, lab tests should be done
• **Adrenal insufficiency:** assess for anorexia, nausea, vomiting, decreased B/P, weakness; if suspected, confirm with cortisol, sodium, potassium levels; if present, do not abruptly discontinue meperidine, but gradually withdraw
• Renal function before initiating therapy; poor renal function can lead to accumulation of toxic metabolite and seizures

Black Box Warning: Serotonin syndrome when given with SSRIs, SNRIs, and serotonin receptor agonists: monitor for hyperthermia, hypertension, rigidity, delirium, coma; do not use within 14 days of MAOIs

• I&O ratio; check for decreasing output; may indicate urinary retention
• **Bowel function:** for constipation; increase fluids, bulk in diet; give stimulant laxatives if needed
• **CNS changes:** dizziness, drowsiness, hallucinations, euphoria, LOC, pupil reactions with chronic or high-dose use; risk of toxicity increases with >600 mg/day

Black Box Warning: P450 3A4 inhibitors: avoid concomitant use as increased plasma concentrations of meperidine may occur, resulting in serious effects, respiratory depression, or death

• Allergic reactions: rash, urticaria

Black Box Warning: Respiratory dysfunction: depression, character, rate, rhythm; notify prescriber if respirations are <12/min

• CNS stimulation with chronic or high doses
• **Children:** monitor for restlessness; changes in respirations may occur more frequently than in adults
• **Beers:** avoid in older adults, especially those with chronic disease; may cause neurotoxicity; monitor for delirium frequently

Black Box Warning: Pregnancy/breastfeeding: Avoid prolonged use during pregnancy, risk of neonatal opioid withdrawal syndrome; notify prescriber of intended or suspected pregnancy; do not breastfeed

Evaluate:
• Therapeutic response: decrease in pain
Teach patient/family:
• To report any symptoms of CNS changes, allergic reactions
• That physical dependency may result from extended use; use should be short-term only

- That drowsiness, dizziness may occur
- That withdrawal symptoms may occur: nausea, vomiting, cramps, fever, faintness, anorexia
- To make position changes slowly; orthostatic hypotension can occur
- To avoid OTC medications, alcohol, herbals unless directed by prescriber
- Not to be used long term
- That nausea may be decreased by lying down

Black Box Warning: **Serotonin syndrome:** to report symptoms immediately

TREATMENT OF OVERDOSE:
Naloxone (Narcan) 0.2-0.8 mg IV, caution in physically dependent patients, O_2, IV fluids, vasopressors

---

⚠ HIGH ALERT

mercaptopurine (6-MP) (Rx)

(mer-kap-toe-pyoor′een)

Purixan

Func. class.: Antineoplastic-antimetabolite

Chem. class.: Purine analog

ACTION: Inhibits purine metabolism at multiple sites, which inhibits DNA and RNA synthesis; specific for S phase of cell cycle

USES: Acute lymphocytic leukemia
Unlabeled uses: Ulcerative colitis, Crohn's disease

CONTRAINDICATIONS: Pregnancy, breastfeeding, patients with prior product resistance, hypersensitivity
Precautions: Renal/hepatic disease, tumor lysis syndrome, dental disease, herpes, radiation therapy, leukopenia, thrombocytopenia, anemia, requires an experienced clinician, secondary malignancy, infection, hypocalcemia, hyperuricemia, hyperphosphatemia, hyperkalemia

DOSAGE AND ROUTES
Acute lymphocytic leukemia
- **Adult/child: PO** 1.5-2.5 mg/kg/day in combination with other agents; start mercaptopurine therapy after a complete hematologic remission
Renal dose
- **Adult: PO** CCr <50 mL/min, give dose q48hr; if used with allopurinol, reduce usual dose by at least 25%

Crohn's disease/ulcerative colitis (unlabeled)
- **Adult: PO** 1.5-2 mg/kg/day
Available forms: Tabs 50 mg; oral susp 20 mg/mL
Administer:
- Store in tightly closed container in cool environment
- Give product after evening meal, before bedtime, on an empty stomach; risk of relapse is lower with evening dose
- Use cytotoxic handling procedures
- **Suspension:** Shake well, wash syringe with warm, soapy water, rinse, move plunger up and down several times, use only after dry; after opening, use within 6 wk

SIDE EFFECTS
GI: *Nausea, vomiting, anorexia, diarrhea, stomatitis,* hepatotoxicity (high doses), jaundice, gastritis, pancreatitis
GU: Hyperuricemia
HEMA: Thrombocytopenia, leukopenia, myelosuppression, anemia
INTEG: *Rash,* dry skin, urticaria, alopecia

PHARMACOKINETICS
Incompletely absorbed when taken orally, metabolized in liver, excreted in urine, peak 1-2 hr, terminal half-life 47 min (adult), 21 min (child)

INTERACTIONS
Increase: effects of mercaptopurine—allopurinol; avoid use or decrease dose by at least 25%

Increase: effects—radiation or other antineoplastics, immunosuppressants

Increase: bone marrow suppresion—azaTHIOprine, sulfamethoxazole-trimethoprim; avoid concurrent use or monitor blood counts

---

Side effects: *italics* = common; red = life-threatening

Increase: anticoagulant action—anticoagulants, NSAIDs, thrombolytics, platelet inhibitors, salicylates; monitor PT, INR
Decrease: antibodies—live virus vaccines; bring vaccinations up-to-date before use
Decrease: TPMT, rapid bone marrow suppression—balsalazide, olsalazine, mesalamine, sulfaSALAzine; use cautiously

Drug/Lab Test
Increase: alk phos, bilirubin, uric acid
Decrease: platelets, WBC, RBC

NURSING CONSIDERATIONS
Assess:
• **Bone marrow suppression:** CBC, differential, platelet count weekly during induction and monthly during maintenance; withhold product at first sign of abnormally large decrease in blood counts unless bone marrow aplasia is the goal

• **Thiopurine methyltransferase (TPMT) deficiency:** individuals are prone to rapid bone marrow suppression; dosage reduction may be required in homozygous TPMT–deficient persons

• **Tumor lysis syndrome:** monitor for increased potassium, uric acid, phosphate; decreased urine output, calcium

• Renal studies: BUN, serum uric acid, urine CCr, electrolytes before, during therapy

• I&O ratio; report fall in urine output to <30 mL/hr; increase fluids to 3 L/day unless contraindicated

• Monitor temperature; fever may indicate beginning infection; no rectal temperature

• **Pregnancy/breastfeeding:** identify whether pregnancy is planned or suspected, or if breastfeeding; do not use in pregnancy or breastfeeding, excreted in breast milk

• **Hepatotoxicity:** hepatic studies before, during therapy: bilirubin, alk phos, AST, ALT weekly during beginning therapy; hepatic encephalopathy, toxic hepatitis, ascites can be fatal; monitor for jaundice, dark urine, clay-colored stools, abdominal pain; reversible after completion of treatment

• **Bleeding:** hematuria, guaiac, bruising, petechiae, mucosa, or orifices; avoid IM inj if platelets are <100,000/mm³; blood transfusions may be needed

• **Stomatitis:** buccal cavity for dryness, sores, ulceration, white patches, oral pain, bleeding, dysphagia

• Increase fluid intake to 2-3 L/day to prevent urate deposits, calculi formation, unless contraindicated

• Rinsing of mouth tid-qid with water, club soda; brushing of teeth bid-tid with soft brush or cotton-tipped applicators for stomatitis; use unwaxed dental floss

Evaluate:
• Therapeutic response: decreased size of tumor, spread of malignancy

Teach patient/family:
• To avoid foods with citric acid, hot temperature, or rough texture for stomatitis; to report stomatitis: any bleeding, white spots, ulcerations in mouth; to examine mouth daily, report symptoms

• **Pregnancy/breastfeeding:** that contraceptive measures are recommended during therapy; not to breastfeed

• To drink 10-12 8-oz glasses of fluid/day

• To notify prescriber of fever, chills, sore throat, nausea, vomiting, anorexia, diarrhea, bleeding, bruising, all of which may indicate blood dyscrasias/infection

• To report signs of infection: fever, sore throat, flulike symptoms

• To report signs of anemia: fatigue, headache, faintness, SOB, irritability

• To report bleeding; to avoid use of razors, commercial mouthwash

• To avoid use of aspirin products, NSAIDs

• To take entire dose at one time; how to safely handle and dispose of product

---

meropenem (Rx)
(mer-oh-pen′em)
Merrem
Func. class.: Antiinfective—miscellaneous
Chem. class.: Carbapenem

ACTION: Bactericidal; interferes with cell-wall replication of susceptible organisms

USES: *Acinetobacter* sp., *Aeromonas hydrophila, Bacteroides distasonis,*

Bacteroides fragilis, Bacteroides ovatus, Bacteroides thetaiotaomicron, Bacteroides uniformis, Bacteroides ureolyticus, Bacteroides vulgatus, Campylobacter jejuni, Citrobacter diversus, Citrobacter freundii, Clostridium difficile, Clostridium perfringens, Enterobacter cloacae, Enterococcus faecalis, Escherichia coli, Eubacterium lentum, Fusobacterium sp., *Haemophilus influenzae* (beta-lactamase negative), *Haemophilus influenzae* (beta-lactamase positive), *Hafnia alvei, Klebsiella oxytoca, Klebsiella pneumoniae, Moraxella catarrhalis, Morganella morganii, Neisseria meningitidis, Pasteurella multocida, Peptostreptococcus* sp., *Porphyromonas asaccharolytica, Prevotella bivia, Prevotella intermedia, Prevotella melaninogenica, Propionibacterium acnes, Proteus mirabilis, Proteus vulgaris, Pseudomonas aeruginosa, Salmonella* sp., *Serratia marcescens, Shigella* sp., *Staphylococcus aureus* (MSSA), *Staphylococcus epidermidis, Streptococcus agalactiae* (group B streptococci), *Streptococcus pneumoniae, Streptococcus pyogenes* (group A beta-hemolytic streptococci), viridans streptococci, *Yersinia enterocolitica;* appendicitis, bacteremia, intraabdominal infections, meningitis, peritonitis, skin/skin structure infections

Unlabeled uses: Febrile, neutropenic, community-acquired pneumonia

CONTRAINDICATIONS: Hypersensitivity to this product, carbapenems, hypersensitivity to cephalosporins, penicillins

Precautions: Pregnancy, breastfeeding, geriatric patients, renal disease, seizure disorder, gram-negative infection, hypersensitivity to pneumonia

DOSAGE AND ROUTES
Intraabdominal infections (complicated appendicitis, peritonitis)
• Adult/child/adolescent >50 kg: **IV** 1 g q8hr or adult 500 mg q6hr

• Infant ≥3 mo/child/adolescent ≤50 kg: **IV** 20 mg/kg q8hr
• Term neonates/infants <3 mo (unlabeled): **IV** 30 mg/kg/dose q8hr
Extended dose (infusion over 3-4 hours) (unlabeled)
• Adult: **IV** 1 g over 3 hr, q8hr
Complicated skin and skin structure infections
• Adult/adolescents/child >50 kg: **IV** 500 mg q8hr over 15-30 min, 1 g q8hr for *Pseudomonas aeruginosa,* max 500 mg
• Infants ≥3 mo/children/adolescents ≤50 kg: **IV** 10 mg/kg q8hr over 15-30 min; 20 mg/kg q8hr for *Pseudomonas aeruginosa,* max 1 g
Bacterial meningitis
• Adult/child/adolescent >50 g: **IV** 2 g q8hr
• Infant/child/adolescent ≤50 kg: **IV** 40 mg/kg q8hr, max 2 g
Renal disease
• Adult: **IV** CCr 26-50 mL/min, give dose q12hr; CCr 10-25 mL/min, give $1/2$ dose q12hr; CCr <10 mL/min, give $1/2$ dose q24hr
Febrile neutropenia (unlabeled)
• Adult: **IV** 1 g q8hr
Community-acquired pneumonia (CAP) (unlabeled)
• Adult: **IV** 1 g q8hr with ciprofloxacin/levaquin or with aminoglycoside plus fluoroquinolone
Available forms: Powder for inj 500 mg, 1 g
Administer:
• Monitor injection site periodically for redness, inflammation, phlebitis
Direct IV route
• Reconstitute 500-mg or 1-g vials with 10, 20 mL of sterile water for inj, respectively; shake to dissolve; let stand until clear (average concentration 50 mg/mL); reconstituted sol may be stored for 3 hr at room temperature or for 13 hr refrigerated; inject up to 1 g in 5-20 mL over 3-5 min
Intermittent IV INFUSION route
• Vials may be directly reconstituted with compatible infusion fluid (NS, D_5W) to 2.5-50 mg/mL; vials with NS can be

M

stored 2 hr at room temperature or for ≤18 hr refrigerated, D₅W solutions may be stored for up to 1 hr at room temperature or ≤15 hr refrigerated; infuse over 15-30 min

Continuous IV INFUSION (unlabeled)
• **3 g/day continuous IV infusion:** Constitute a 1-g vial according to manufacturer recommendations; further dilute in 50 mL or 250 mL of NS and run over 8 hr; for continuous infusion, administer a new infusion bag q8hr
• **4 g/day continuous IV infusion:** Constitute a 1-g vial according to manufacturer recommendations; further dilute in 100 mL of NS and administer over 6 hr; for continuous infusion, administer a new infusion bag q6hr
• **3 g/day IV continuous infusion in ambulatory infusion pump with freezer packs:** Reconstitute 1-g vial according to manufacturer recommendations by adding 20 mL of NS into each vial; add 3 g (60 mL) to a 100 mL medication cassette reservoir and bring the final volume to 100 mL (final concentration, 30 mg/mL), run over 24 hr

Y-site compatibilities: Alemtuzumab, aminocaproic acid, aminophylline, anidulafungin, argatroban, atenolol, atropine, azithromycin, bivalirudin, bleomycin, CARBOplatin, carmustine, caspofungin, cimetidine, CISplatin, cyclophosphamide, cycloSPORINE, cytarabine, DACTINomycin, DAPTOmycin, dexamethasone, dexmedetomidine, dexrazoxane, digoxin, diltiaZEM, diphenhydrAMINE, DOCEtaxel, doxacurium, DOXOrubicin liposomal, enalaprilat, eptifibatide, etoposide, etoposide phosphate, fluconazole, fludarabine, fluorouracil, foscarnet, furosemide, gallium, gatifloxacin, gemcitabine, gemtuzumab, gentamicin, granisetron, heparin sodium, HYDROmorphone, ifosfamide, insulin (regular), irinotecan, lepirudin, leucovorin, linezolid injection, LORazepam, mechlorethamine, methotrexate, metoclopramide, metroNIDAZOLE, milrinone, mitoXANTRONE, morphine, nesiritide, norepinephrine, octreotide, oxaliplatin,

oxytocin, PACLitaxel, palonosetron, pamidronate, pancuronium, PEMEtrexed, PHENobarbital, potassium acetate/chloride, rocuronium, teniposide, thiotepa, tigecycline, tirofiban, TNA (3-in-1) total nutrient admixture, vancomycin, vasopressin, vecuronium, vinBLAStine, vinCRIStine, vinorelbine, voriconazole, zoledronic acid

SIDE EFFECTS
CNS: Seizures, dizziness, *headache*
CV: Hypotension, tachycardia
ENDO: Hypoglycemia
GI: Diarrhea, nausea, vomiting, CDAD; thrush (child), hepatitis, glossitis, jaundice
INTEG: *Rash*, urticaria, *pruritus*, pain at inj site, phlebitis, erythema at inj site, DRESS
RESP: Apnea, pneumonia
SYST: Anaphylaxis, Stevens-Johnson syndrome, angioedema

PHARMACOKINETICS
IV: Onset immediate, peak dose dependent, half-life 1 hr, excreted unchanged in urine (70%), duration 8 hr

INTERACTIONS
Increase: meropenem plasma levels—probenecid; avoid concurrent use
Decrease: effect of valproic acid; monitor for seizures

Drug/Lab Test
Increase: AST, ALT, LDH, BUN, alk phos, bilirubin, creatinine
Increase or decrease: INR, platelets, PT, PTT
False positive: direct Coombs' test, urine glucose

NURSING CONSIDERATIONS
Assess:
• C&S before starting treatment, may give before results are received
• Sensitivity to carbapenem antibiotics, penicillins, cephalosporins before starting this product
• **Blood studies:** LFTs, HCT, BUN, LDH, alkaline phosphatase, Coom's test baseline and periodically if on long-term therapy

• Renal disease: lower dose may be required; monitor serum creatinine/BUN before, during therapy; monitor weight, fluid balance
• **CDAD:** bowel pattern daily; if severe diarrhea, fever, abdominal pain, fatigue occurs, product should be discontinued
• **Infection:** temperature, sputum, characteristics of wound, WBC, stool, vital signs before, during, and after treatment
• **Allergic reactions, anaphylaxis:** rash, laryngeal edema, wheezing, urticaria, pruritus; may occur immediately or several days after therapy begins; identify if there has been hypersensitivity to penicillins, cephalosporins, beta-lactams; cross-sensitivity may occur; have emergency equipment nearby
• **DRESS:** Rash, fever, swelling of face, lymphadenopathy, may lead to other organ systems
• **Seizures:** may occur in those with brain lesions, seizure disorder, bacterial meningitis, or renal disease; stop product, notify prescriber if seizures occur, seizure threshold is lowered
• **Overgrowth of infection:** perineal itching, fever, malaise, redness, pain, swelling, drainage, rash, diarrhea, change in cough, sputum
• **Pregnancy/breastfeeding:** use only if clearly needed; no well-controlled studies; use cautiously in breastfeeding, excreted in breast milk
Evaluate:
• Therapeutic response: negative C&S; absence of symptoms and signs of infection
Teach patient/family:
• CDAD: to report severe diarrhea
• To avoid driving or other hazardous activities until response is known, dizziness may occur
• To discuss all OTC, Rx, herbals, supplements with prescriber
• To report sore throat, bruising, bleeding, joint pain; may indicate blood dyscrasias (rare)
• **To report overgrowth of infection:** black, furry tongue; vaginal itching; foul-smelling stools; seizures
• To avoid breastfeeding; product is excreted in breast milk

TREATMENT OF ANAPHYLAXIS: EPINEPHrine, antihistamines; resuscitate if necessary

meropenem/vaborbactam (Rx)
(mer-oh-pen'em/va-bor-bak'tam)
Vabomere
Func. class.: Antiinfective—miscellaneous
Chem. class.: Carbapenem

ACTION: Bactericidal; interferes with cell-wall replication of susceptible organisms

USES: For the treatment of complicated urinary tract infections caused by *Citrobacter freundii, Citrobacter koseri, Enterobacter aerogenes, Enterobacter cloacae, Escherichia coli, Klebsiella oxytoca, Klebsiella pneumoniae, Morganella morganii, Proteus mirabilis, Providencia sp., Pseudomonas aeruginosa, Serratia marcescens*

CONTRAINDICATIONS: Hypersensitivity to this product, carbapenems
Precautions: Pregnancy, breastfeeding, geriatric patients, renal disease, seizure disorder, gram-negative infection, pneumonia; hypersensitivity to cephalosporins, penicillins

DOSAGE AND ROUTES
Complicated urinary tract infection (UTI), including pyelonephritis
• **Adult: IV** 4 g (2 g meropenem and 2 g vaborbactam) q8hr for up to 14 days
Renal dose
• **Adult: IV** eGFR ≥50 mL/min/1.73 m²: no change; eGFR 30-49 mL/min/1.73 m²: 2 g (1 g meropenem and 1 g vaborbactam) q8hr; eGFR 15-29 mL/min/1.73 m²: 2 g (1 g meropenem and 1 g vaborbactam) q12hr; eGFR <15 mL/min/1.73 m²: 1 g (0.5 g meropenem and 0.5 g vaborbactam) q12hr

Intermittent hemodialysis
• Meropenem and vaborbactam are removed by hemodialysis; give drug after hemodialysis

Available forms: Powder for inj 2 g
Administer:
IV route
• Visually inspect for particulate matter and discoloration before use
• **Reconstitution:** Constitute the appropriate number of vials as needed for the dose
• 2 vials are used for 4-g dose (2 g meropenem and 2 g vaborbactam)
• 1 vial is used for 2-g (1 g meropenem and 1 g vaborbactam) or 1-g (0.5 g meropenem and 0.5 g vaborbactam) doses
• **Withdraw** 20 mL of 0.9% sodium chloride injection from an infusion bag, and constitute each vial
• For 4-g (2 g meropenem and 2 g vaborbactam) dose/250 to 1000 mL
• For 2-g (1 g meropenem and 1 g vaborbactam) dose/125 to 500 mL
• For 1-g (0.5 g meropenem and 0.5 g vaborbactam) dose/70 to 250 mL
• Mix gently to dissolve
• The constituted solution is concentrations of 0.05 g/mL meropenem /0.05 g/mL vaborbactam; the final volume is 21.3 mL
• Further dilute before use; do not use by direct injection
• **Dilution:** withdraw the full or partial constituted vial contents from each vial and add back into the 0.9% sodium chloride injection infusion bag
• The final concentration of meropenem and vaborbactam will be between 2 and 8 mg/mL
• **Storage:** complete infusion within 4 hr if stored at room temperature or 22 hr if refrigerated at 2-8° C (36-46° F)
Intermittent IV Infusion:
• Give over 3 hr

SIDE EFFECTS

GI: Diarrhea, nausea, vomiting, CDAD, hepatitis, glossitis, jaundice
RESP: Dyspnea, hyperventilation, cough, sputum
SYST: Anaphylaxis, Stevens-Johnson syndrome, angioedema

INTEG: Rash, urticaria, pruritus, pain at inj site, phlebitis, erythema at inj site
CNS: Seizures, dizziness, weakness, headache, insomnia, agitation, confusion, drowsiness
CV: Hypotension, tachycardia
ENDO: Hypoglycemia

PHARMACOKINETICS

Protein binding 2% for meropenem, 33% for vaborbactam; excreted by kidneys; half-life 1.22 hr meropenem, 1.68 hr vaborbactam; meropenem is a substrate of OAT1 and OAT3 transporters; use after hemodialysis

INTERACTIONS

Increase: effect of—valproic acid
Drug/Lab Tests
Increase: AST, ALT, LDH, BUN, alk phos, bilirubin, creatinine
Decrease: prothrombin time
False positive: direct Coombs test

NURSING CONSIDERATIONS

Assess:
• Obtain culture and sensitivity before first dose; product can be given while waiting for results
• **Infusion site reactions:** assess for redness, inflammation, pain and phlebitis at infusion site
• Sensitivity to carbapenem antibiotics, penicillins, cephalosporins
• Renal disease: lower dose may be required; monitor serum creatinine/BUN, sodium, before, during therapy
• **CDAD:** bowel pattern daily; if severe diarrhea, abdominal pain, fatigue occurs, product should be discontinued
• **Infection:** temperature, sputum, characteristics of wound before, during, and after treatment
• **Allergic reactions, anaphylaxis:** rash, laryngeal edema, wheezing, urticaria, pruritus; may occur immediately or several days after therapy begins; identify whether there has been hypersensitivity to penicillins, cephalosporins, beta-lactams; cross-sensitivity may occur
• **Seizures:** may occur in those with brain lesions, seizure disorder, bacte-

rial meningitis, or renal disease; stop product, notify prescriber if seizures occur

• **Overgrowth of infection:** perineal itching, fever, malaise, redness, pain, swelling, drainage, rash, diarrhea, change in cough, sputum

Evaluate:

• Therapeutic response: negative C&S; absence of symptoms and signs of infection

Teach patient/family:

• **CDAD:** to report severe diarrhea
• To report sore throat, bruising, bleeding, joint pain; may indicate blood dyscrasias (rare)
• To report overgrowth of infection: black furry tongue, vaginal itching, foul-smelling stools

---

mesalamine, 5-ASA (Rx)

me-sal′ a-meen)

Apriso, Asacol, Asocol 800 ✦, Asacol HD, Canasa, Delzicol, Lialda, Mesasal ✦, Mezavant ✦, Pentasa, Rowasa ✦, Salofalk ✦, Teva-5-ASA ✦

Func. class.: GI antiinflammatory
Chem. class.: 5-Aminosalicylic acid

Do not confuse:
Asacol/Os-Cal

ACTION: May diminish inflammation by blocking cyclooxygenase, inhibiting prostaglandin production in colon; local action only

USES: Mild to moderate active distal ulcerative colitis, proctitis

CONTRAINDICATIONS: Hypersensitivity to this product or salicylates, 5-aminosalicylates

Precautions: Pregnancy, breastfeeding, children, geriatric patients, renal disease, sulfite sensitivity, pyloric stenosis, GI obstruction

DOSAGE AND ROUTES

Treatment of ulcerative colitis

• **Adult: RECT** 60 mL (4 g) at bedtime, retained for 8 hr × 3-6 wk; **DEL REL TAB (Lialda)** 2.4-4.8 g/day × 8 wk; **DEL REL TAB (Asacol HD)** 1.6 g × 6 wk; **DEL REL TAB (Asacol)** 800 mg tid × 6 wk; **CONTROLLED REL CAP (Pentasa)** 1 g qid up to 8 wk; **RECT SUPP** 500 mg bid retained for 1-3 hr × 3-6 wk until remission, may increase tid if needed; **DEL REL CAP (Delzicol)** 800 mg tid × 6 wk

• **Child ≥5 yr and 54-90 kg: PO** Delzicol 27-44 mg/kg/day in divided doses × 6 wk, max 2.4 g/day

• **Child ≥5 yr and 33-53 kg: PO** Delzicol 37-61 mg/kg/day in 2 divided doses × 6 wk, max 2 g/day

• **Child ≥5 yr and 17-32 kg PO:** Delzicol 36-71 mg/kg/day in 2 divided doses × 6 wk, max 1.2 g/day

Maintenance of remission

• **Adult: DEL REL TAB (Asacol)** 800 mg bid or 400 mg qid; **DEL REL TAB (Apriso)** 1500 mg (4 caps) each AM; **DEL REL TAB (Lialda)** 2.4 g (2 tabs) daily with meal; **DEL REL TAB (Delzicol)** 800 mg bid

Treatment of ulcerative proctosis-moiditis/proctitis

• **Adult:** Rectal Rowasa 4 g enema (60 mL) at bedtime retained for 8 hr × 3-6 wk

Available forms: Rectal susp 4 g/60 mL (Rowasa); ext rel tab 500 mg; ext rel cap 250, 500 mg (Pentasa); 0.375 g (Apriso); del rel tab 400 mg (Asacol), 800 mg (Asacol HD); del rel tab (Lialda) 1.2 g; rectal supp 1000 mg (Canasa); del rel cap (Delzicol) 400 mg; enema suspension 4 g/60 mL (sf Rowasa)

Administer:

PO route

• Swallow tabs whole; do not break, crush, or chew tabs; give with a full glass of water
• **Lialda:** take with meal
• **Apriso caps:** take without regard to meals in AM
• **Delzicol caps:** give ≥1 hr before a meal or 2 hr after a meal

---

Rectal suspension

• Product should be given at bedtime, retained until morning (8 hr); empty bowel before insertion, shake well

Rectal suppository

• Moisten before insertion; suppository should be retained for 1-3 hr

SIDE EFFECTS

CNS: *Headache, fever, dizziness,* insomnia, asthenia, weakness, fatigue

CV: Chest pain, palpitations, pericarditis

EENT: Pharyngitis, rhinitis

GI: *Cramps, gas, nausea, diarrhea,* rectal pain, constipation, vomiting, pancreatitis

GU: Nephrotoxicity, interstitial nephritis

INTEG: *Rash, itching,* acne, Stevens-Johnson syndrome, hair loss

SYST: Anaphylaxis, acute intolerance syndrome, angioedema, DRESS

PHARMACOKINETICS

RECT: Primarily excreted in feces unchanged but some in urine as metabolite; half-life 1 hr, metabolite half-life 12 hr PO, ½-1 ½ hr rectal

INTERACTIONS

Increase: action, adverse reactions of azaTHIOprine, mercaptopurine

Decrease: mesalamine absorption—lactulose, antacids

Decrease: effect of—warfarin

Drug/Lab Test

Increase: AST, ALT, alk phos, LDH, GGTP, amylase, lipase, BUN, serum creatinine

NURSING CONSIDERATIONS

Assess:

• **Allergy to salicylates, sulfonamides, sulfites:** if allergic reactions occur, discontinue product

• Renal studies: BUN, creatinine before, periodically during treatment; renal toxicity may occur; increase fluids to maintain urine at ≥1200 mL/day to prevent crystalluria

• **Bowel disorders:** cramps, gas, nausea, diarrhea, rectal pain; if severe, product should be discontinued

• **Pregnancy/breastfeeding:** avoid in pregnancy; excreted in breast milk, avoid use

Evaluate:

• Therapeutic response: absence of pain, bleeding from GI tract, decrease in number of diarrhea stools

Teach patient/family:

• To report immediately trouble breathing, rash, hives

• To use rectal dose at bedtime, teach how to use

• That follow-up exams and blood work will be needed, including possible proctoscopy or sigmoidoscopy

• Not to drive or engage in other hazardous activities until response is known, dizziness may occur

• That usual initial course of therapy is 3-6 wk; to notify prescriber if symptoms do not improve after 2 mo of treatment; to continue to take even if feeling better; not to miss doses; if a dose is missed, to take when remembered, if almost time for next dose, skip it; do not double doses

• To shake bottle well (rectal susp)

• About method of rectal administration

• To inform prescriber of GI symptoms

• To report abdominal cramping, pain, diarrhea with blood, headache, fever, rash, chest pain, bruising, bleeding, mouth sores; product should be discontinued

---

⚠ HIGH ALERT

metFORMIN (Rx)

(met-for′min)

Fortamet, Glucophage, Glucophage XR, Glumetza, Glycon ✦, Riomet

Func. class.: Antidiabetic, oral

Chem. class.: Biguanide

Do not confuse:

metformin/metroNIDAZOLE

Glucophage/Glucovance/Glucotrol

ACTION: Inhibits hepatic glucose production and increases sensitivity of peripheral tissue to insulin

USES: Type 2 diabetes mellitus

CONTRAINDICATIONS: Diabetic ketoacidosis, metabolic acidosis, renal failure, radiographic contrast use

Precautions: Pregnancy, breastfeeding, geriatric patients, previous hypersensitivity, thyroid disease, HF, type 1 diabetes mellitus, hepatic disease, alcoholism, cardiopulmonary disease, acidemia, acute MI, cardiogenic shock, renal disease, heart failure, lactic acidosis

DOSAGE AND ROUTES
Type 2 diabetes mellitus
• **Adult: PO** 500 mg bid or 850 mg/day initially, then 500 mg weekly or 850 mg q2wk up to 2000 mg/day in divided doses with morning meal, with dosage increased every other wk, max 2550 mg/day, **EXT REL** (Glucophage XR) 500 mg daily with evening meal, may increase by 500 mg per wk, max 2000 mg/day; (Glumetza) 1000 mg daily with food, preferably with PM meal, may increase by 500 mg per wk, max 2000 mg daily; (Fortamet) 500-1000 mg daily with PM meal, may increase by 500 mg per wk, max 2500 mg daily

Renal dose
• **Adult: PO** eGFR 30-45 mL/min/1.73 m², avoid use; if eGFR >45 mL/min/1.73 m² then falls <45 mL/min/1.73 m², assess benefits/risks of treatment; discontinue if eGFR falls <30 mL/min/1.73 m²

Available forms: Tabs 500, 850, 1000 mg; ext rel tab 500, 850, 1000 mg; oral sol 500 mg/5 mL

Administer:
PO route
• Conversion from other oral hypoglycemic agents; change may be made without gradual dosage change; monitor serum glucose, urine ketones tid during conversion
• Store in tight container in cool environment
• Monitor eGFR at least annually
• Do not use in dialysis
• **Immediate rel product:** twice a day given with meals to decrease GI upset and provide the best absorption; immediate rel tabs crushed, mixed with meal, fluids for patients with difficulty swallowing

• **Ext rel product** may also be taken as single dose; titrate slowly to therapeutic response, side effect tolerance
• **Ext rel tabs:** do not chew, break, crush; may be given with evening meal
• **Oral solution:** use calibrated spoon, oral syringe or container to measure; give with meals

SIDE EFFECTS
ENDO: Lactic acidosis
GI: *Nausea, vomiting, diarrhea,* heartburn, anorexia, metallic taste

PHARMACOKINETICS
Excreted by kidneys unchanged 35%-50%, half-life 6 hr, peak 2-3 hr (immediate release); 7 hr (ext release); $2^{1}/_{2}$ hr (solution)

INTERACTIONS
• Do not give with radiologic contrast media; may cause renal failure
• Do not use with dofetilide; may cause lactic acidosis
Increase: digoxin levels—digoxin; monitor digoxin level
Increase: metFORMIN level—cimetidine, digoxin, morphine, procainamide, quiNIDine, raNITIdine, triamterene, vancomycin; monitor blood glucose
Increase: hyperglycemia—calcium channel blockers, corticosteroids, estrogens, oral contraceptives, phenothiazines, sympathomimetics, diuretics, phenytoin, β-blockers; monitor blood glucose
Drug/Herb
Increase: hyperglycemia—glucosamine
Increase: hypoglycemia—chromium, coenzyme Q10, garlic, green tea, horse chestnut
Drug/Lab Test
Decrease: vit B$_{12}$

NURSING CONSIDERATIONS
Assess:
• **Hypoglycemic reactions** (sweating, weakness, dizziness, anxiety, tremors, hunger); hyperglycemic reactions soon after meals; these occur rarely with product, may occur when product combined with sulfonylureas

---

Side effects: *italics* = common; red = life-threatening

• CBC (baseline, q3mo) during treatment; check LFTs periodically, AST, LDH, renal studies: BUN, creatinine during treatment; glucose, A1c; folic acid, vit B_{12} q1-2yr

• **Surgery:** product should be discontinued temporarily for surgical procedures when patient is NPO or if contrast medium is used; resume when patient is eating

Black Box Warning: **Lactic acidosis:** malaise, myalgia, abdominal distress; risk increases with age, poor renal function; monitor electrolytes, lactate, pyruvate, blood pH, ketones, glucose; suspect in any diabetic patient with metabolic acidosis, with ketoacidosis; immediately stop product if hypoxemia or significant renal dysfunction occurs; do not use in those >80 yr unless CCr is normal; alcohol use may increase lactic acidosis risk

• **Renal status:** obtain BUN, creatinine before use; if elevated, a dose reduction is required

• **Pregnancy/breastfeeding:** avoid use in pregnancy, do not use in breastfeeding; if an antidiabetic is needed during pregnancy, use insulin

Evaluate:

• Therapeutic response: decrease in polyuria, polydipsia, polyphagia; clear sensorium; absence of dizziness; stable gait; blood glucose, A1c at normal level

Teach patient/family:

Black Box Warning: **Lactic acidosis:** hyperventilation, fatigue, malaise, chills, myalgia, somnolence; to notify prescriber immediately, stop product; not to use in excessive alcohol intake that is chronic

• To regularly self-monitor blood glucose with blood-glucose meter

• About signs, symptoms of hypoglycemia/hyperglycemia; what to do about each (rare)

• That product must be continued on daily basis; about consequences of discontinuing product abruptly; to take as prescribed; not to double doses

• To avoid OTC medications, alcohol unless approved by prescriber

• That diabetes is a lifelong illness; that product is not a cure, only controls symptoms

• To carry emergency ID and glucagon emergency kit

• That Glucophage XR tab may appear in stool

• To report adverse reactions; if GI upset occurs, it usually decreases over time

• To take with meals; not to break, crush, chew ext rel product

• **Pregnancy:** that PCOS patients with insulin resistance may be at risk of conception; to use adequate contraception if pregnancy is not desired

---

⚠ HIGH ALERT

methadone (Rx) REMS
(meth′a-done)

Dolophine, Metadol ♣, Metadol-D ♣, Methadose

Func. class.: Opioid analgesic
Chem. class.: Synthetic diphenylheptane derivative

Controlled Substance Schedule II

Do not confuse:
methadone/methylphenidate

ACTION: Depresses pain impulse transmission at the spinal cord level by interacting with opioid receptors; produces CNS depression

USES: Severe pain, opioid withdrawal
Unlabeled uses: Neonatal abstinence syndrome

CONTRAINDICATIONS: Hypersensitivity, asthma, ileus

Black Box Warning: Respiratory depression

Precautions: Breastfeeding, children <18 yr, geriatric patients, addictive personality, increased intracranial pressure,

MI (acute), severe heart disease, respiratory depression, pulmonary/renal/hepatic disease, respiratory insufficiency, torsades de pointes, COPD, seizures

> **Black Box Warning:** QT prolongation, pain, substance abuse, potential for overdose, poisoning, accidental exposure, coadministration with other CNS depressants, IV use, pregnancy, requires an experienced clinician

DOSAGE AND ROUTES
Severe pain
• **Adult:** PO 2.5 mg q8-12hr in opioid-naive, titrate; **IV/IM/SUBCUT** 2.5-10 mg q8-12hr in opioid-naive
Opioid withdrawal
• **Adult including pregnant woman:** PO 20-30 mg initially unless low opioid tolerance expected; additional 5-10 mg q2-4hr as needed after initial dose; if symptoms continue, may give for ≤5 days
Analgesic
• **Adult/child <50 kg:** PO 0.1 mg/kg/dose q4hr × 2-3 doses, then q6-8hr prn, max 10 mg q6-8hr; **≥ 50 kg IM/IV/SUBCUT** 10 mg q 6-8 hr, max 10 mg/dose
Narcotic dependency
• **Adult/child <50 kg:** PO 0.05-0.1 mg/kg/dose q6hr, increase by 0.05 mg/kg/dose until withdrawal, if controlled after 1-2 days lengthen dosing interval to q12-24hr, taper by 0.05 mg/kg/day; **≥50 kg IM/IV SUBCUT** 15-40 mg daily, decrease dose q1-2days
Available forms: Inj 10 mg/mL; tabs 5, 10 mg; oral sol 5, 10 mg/5 mL; 10 mg/mL (concentrate); dispersible tabs 40 mg
Administer:
PO route
• When using during a methadone maintenance program, use only PO according to NATA guidelines
• PO is half as potent as parenteral
IM route
• Rotating inj sites, give deep in large muscle mass (IM)
• Protect from light

IV route
• Used as PCA
• Protect from light
SUBCUT route
• Pain and induration may occur at site

SIDE EFFECTS
CNS: *Drowsiness, dizziness, confusion, headache, sedation,* euphoria, seizures
CV: Bradycardia, change in B/P, hypotension, torsades de pointes, QT prolongation
EENT: Blurred vision, miosis, diplopia
ENDO: adrenal insufficiency
MISC: Dependence, tolerance
GI: *Nausea, vomiting, anorexia, constipation*
GU: Urinary retention
INTEG: *Rash,* flushing, diaphoresis
RESP: Respiratory depression

PHARMACOKINETICS
Metabolized by liver; excreted by kidneys; crosses placenta; excreted in breast milk; half-life 15-23 hr, extended interval with continued dosing; 90% bound to plasma proteins
PO: Onset 30-60 min, peak 1-1.5 hr, duration 6-8 hr, cumulative 22-48 hr; PO half as active as INJ
SUBCUT/IM: Onset 10-20 min, peak $1\frac{1}{2}$-2 hr, duration 4-6 hr, cumulative 22-48 hr

INTERACTIONS
• **Unpredictable reactions:** MAOIs; do not use together
• Do not use within 2 wk of selegiline
Increase: serotonin syndrome—linezolid, methylene blue, mirtazapine, tramadol, trazadone, SSRIs, SNRIs, MAOIs, tricyclics, 5-HT3 receptor antagonists
Increase: fatal reaction: benzodiazapines
Increase: effects with other CNS depressants—alcohol, opiates, sedative/hypnotics, antipsychotics, skeletal muscle relaxants
Increase: toxicity—CYP2C9 inhibitors, CYP2C19 inhibitors, CYP2D6 inhibitors, CYP3A4 inhibitors (aprepitant, antiretroviral protease inhibitors, clarithromycin, danazol, delavirdine, diltiaZEM, erythromycin,

M

fluconazole, FLUoxetine, fluvoxaMINE, imatinib, ketoconazole, mibefradil, nefazodone, telithromycin, voriconazole)

Increase: QT prolongation—class IA antiarrhythmics (disopyramide, procainamide, quiNIDine), class III antiarrhythmics (amiodarone, dofetilide, ibutilide, sotalol), astemizole, arsenic trioxide, cisapride, chloroquine, clarithromycin, levomethadyl, pentamidine, some phenothiazines, pimozide, terfenadine

Decrease: analgesia—rifAMPin, phenytoin, nalbuphine

Decrease: methadone effect—CYP2C9 inducers, CYP2C19 inducers CYP3A4 inducers (barbiturates, bosentan, carBAMazepine, efavirenz, phenytoins, nevirapine, rifabutin, rifAMPin); withdrawal symptoms may occur

Drug/Food
• Avoid use with grapefruit juice

Drug/Herb
• Avoid use with St. John's wort; withdrawal may result

Increase: CNS depression—chamomile, hops, kava, valerian

Drug/Lab Test
Increase: amylase, lipase

NURSING CONSIDERATIONS
Assess:
• **Pain:** type, location, intensity, grimacing before, $1^1/_2$-2 hr after administration; use pain scoring; monitor for cumulative reactions; use during entire 24-hr period for severe pain
• I&O ratio; check for decreasing output; may indicate urinary retention
• CNS changes: dizziness, drowsiness, hallucinations, euphoria, LOC, pupil reaction
• Allergic reactions: rash, urticaria

Black Box Warning: **Respiratory dysfunction:** respiratory depression, character, rate, rhythm; notify prescriber if respirations are <10/min; avoid use with other CNS depressants (benzodiazepines)

Black Box Warning: **QT prolongation:** may be dose related or use with other products that increase QT; titrate doses carefully, may be fatal

Black Box Warning: **Accidental exposure:** make sure product is not accessible to children, pets

Black Box Warning: **Overdose, poisoning:** advise persons involved in correct use

Black Box Warning: **Substance abuse:** may occur but has less psychological dependence than other opiate agonists

• **Opioid detoxification:** goal in detoxification is only prevention of withdrawal symptoms, not to provide analgesia or pain relief

Black Box Warning: B/P, pulse, ECG; hypotension, palpitations may occur

• Bowel changes, bulk, fluids, laxatives should be used for constipation
• **Beers:** avoid in older adults unless safer alternatives are unavailable; may cause ataxia, impaired psychomotor function
• **Pregnancy/breastfeeding:** do not use in pregnancy, neonatal opioid withdrawal syndrome may result; do not use in breastfeeding, serious sedation of the infant may occur, with respiratory depression

Evaluate:
• Therapeutic response: decrease in pain, successful opioid withdrawal

Teach patient/family:
• To report any symptoms of CNS changes, allergic reactions, extreme sedation, trouble breathing
• That physical dependency may result from extended use
• **That withdrawal symptoms may occur:** nausea, vomiting, cramps, fever, faintness, anorexia
• To maintain proper hydration; to avoid alcohol use
• To avoid use with other products without approval of prescriber; many drug interactions
• To use correctly, exactly as directed; not to increase unless directed by prescriber

- That drowsiness, dizziness may occur; not to perform hazardous tasks until effect is known; to ask for assistance when getting out of bed
- That regular ECGs will be needed
- To change positions slowly to minimize orthostatic hypotension
- To advise all providers of product taken
- **Pregnancy/breastfeeding:** not to use in pregnancy, breastfeeding

TREATMENT OF OVERDOSE: Naloxone (Narcan) 0.2-0.8 mg IV, O_2, IV fluids, vasopressors

---

methimazole (Rx)

(meth-im′a-zole)

Tapazole

Func. class.: Thyroid hormone antagonist

Chem. class.: Thioamide

Do not confuse:
methimazole/metoprolol/minoxidil

ACTION: Inhibits synthesis of thyroid hormones by decreasing iodine use in manufacture of thyroglobulin and iodothyronine; does not affect circulatory T_4, T_3

USES: Hyperthyroidism, preparation for thyroidectomy

CONTRAINDICATIONS: Pregnancy, breastfeeding, hypersensitivity
Precautions: Infection, bone marrow suppression, hepatic disease, bleeding disorders

DOSAGE AND ROUTES
Hyperthyroidism
- **Adult:** PO 15 mg/day (mild hyperthyroidism); 30-40 mg/day (moderate to severe); 60 mg/day (severe); maintenance 5-15 mg/day; may be divided
- **Child:** PO 0.4 mg/kg/day in divided doses q8hr; continue until euthyroid; maintenance dose 0.2 mg/kg/day in divided doses q8hr, max 30 mg/24 hr; may be divided

Preparation for thyroidectomy
- **Adult/child:** PO same as above; iodine may be added × 10 days before surgery
Thyrotoxic crisis
- **Adult/child:** PO 15-20 mg q4 hr × 24 hr with other products
Available forms: Tabs 5, 10 mg
Administer:
- With meals to decrease GI upset
- At same time each day to maintain product level
- Lowest dose that relieves symptoms; discontinue before RAIU

SIDE EFFECTS
CNS: *Drowsiness, headache, vertigo, fever,* paresthesias, neuritis
ENDO: *Enlarged thyroid*
GI: *Nausea, diarrhea, vomiting,* jaundice, hepatitis, loss of taste
GU: Nephritis
HEMA: Agranulocytosis, leukopenia, thrombocytopenia, hypothrombinemia, lymphadenopathy, bleeding, vasculitis
INTEG: *Rash, urticaria, pruritus, alopecia, hyperpigmentation,* lupuslike syndrome
MS: Myalgia, arthralgia, nocturnal muscle cramps

PHARMACOKINETICS
Onset rapid; peak 1-2 hr; half-life 4-6 hr; excreted in urine, breast milk; crosses placenta

INTERACTIONS
Increase: bone marrow depression—radiation, antineoplastic agents
Increase: response to digoxin; monitor digoxin level, reduce dose if needed
Decrease: effectiveness—amiodarone, potassium iodide; methIMAzole dose may need to be increased
Decrease: anticoagulant effect—warfarin; monitor PT, INR
Drug/Lab Test
Increase: PT, AST, ALT, alk phos

NURSING CONSIDERATIONS
Assess:
- **Hyperthyroidism:** palpitations, nervousness, loss of hair, insomnia, heat intolerance, weight loss, diarrhea; product adjustment may be needed

M

• **Hypothyroidism:** constipation, dry skin, weakness, fatigue, headache, intolerance to cold, weight gain; adjustment may be needed; check for edema: puffy hands, feet, periorbits; these indicate hypothyroidism

• Pulse, B/P, temperature

• Weight daily; same clothing, scale, time of day; weight increase or decrease is a sign of need to adjust product dose

• Monitor lab work: T_3, T_4, which are increased; serum TSH, which is decreased; free thyroxine index, which is increased if dosage too low; discontinue product 3-4 wk before RAIU

• **Blood dyscrasias:** CBC; monitor leukopenia, thrombocytopenia, agranulocytosis; if these occur, product should be discontinued and other treatment initiated; may occur at doses >40 mg/day

• **Hypersensitivity:** rash, enlarged cervical lymph nodes; product may have to be discontinued

• **Hypoprothrombinemia:** bleeding, petechiae, ecchymosis

• **Clinical response:** after 3 wk should include increased weight; decreased T_4, pulse

• **Bone marrow suppression:** sore throat, fever, fatigue

• **Pregnancy/breastfeeding:** may cause fetal harm; do not use in pregnancy; avoid use in breastfeeding

Evaluate:

• Therapeutic response: weight gain, decreased pulse, decreased T_4, B/P

Teach patient/family:

• Not to breastfeed

• To take pulse daily

• To report redness, swelling, sore throat, mouth lesions, fever, which indicate blood dyscrasias

• To keep graph of weight, pulse, mood

• To avoid OTC products, seafood that contain iodine, other iodine products

• Not to discontinue product abruptly because thyroid crisis may occur; stress patient response

• That response may take several months if thyroid is large

• **Symptoms and signs of overdose:** periorbital edema, cold intolerance, mental depression

• **Symptoms of inadequate dose:** tachycardia, diarrhea, fever, irritability

• To take medication as prescribed; not to skip or double dose

• To report yellowing of skin/eyes, dark urine, anorexia, right upper abdominal pain; may indicate hepatic dysfunction

---

⚠ HIGH ALERT

methotrexate (Rx)
(meth-oh-trex′ate)

Metoject ♦, Otrexup, Rasuvo, Rheumatrex, Trexall, Xatmep

Func. class.: Antineoplastic-antimetabolite (vesicant)

Chem. class.: Folic acid antagonist

Do not confuse:
methotrexate/metOLazone/ MTX Patch

ACTION: Inhibits an enzyme that reduces folic acid, which is needed for nucleic acid synthesis in all cells; specific to S phase of cell cycle; immunosuppressive

USES: Acute lymphocytic leukemia; in combination for breast, lung, head, neck carcinoma; lymphoma, sarcoma, gestational choriocarcinoma, hydatidiform mole, psoriasis, RA, mycosis fungoides, osteosarcoma

Unlabeled uses: Burkitt's lymphoma, bladder or ovarian cancer, carcinomatous meningitis, desmoid tumor, fibromatosis, asthma, active Crohn's disease, ulcerative colitis, GVHD prophylaxis, ectopic pregnancy, pregnancy termination, psoriatic arthritis, pruritus due to cholestasis or primary biliary cirrhosis, SLE, sarcoidosis

CONTRAINDICATIONS: Hypersensitivity, leukopenia (<3500/mm³), thrombocytopenia (<100,000/mm³), anemia; psoriatic patients with severe renal disease, alcoholism, AIDS, hepatic disease

---

Black Box Warning: Pregnancy, bone marrow suppression

Precautions: Breastfeeding, children, exfoliative dermatitis

Black Box Warning: Renal disease, ascites, diarrhea, infection, intrathecal administration, lymphoma, pleural effusion, pulmonary toxicity, radiation therapy, stomatitis, tumor lysis syndrome, gastroenteritis, GI bleeding/perforation, hepatotoxicity, intrauterine fetal death, nephrotoxicity, requires an experienced clinician

DOSAGE AND ROUTES
Acute lymphocytic leukemia (except Otrexup, Rasuvo)
• **Adult/child:** IM/IV 3.3 mg/m²/day × 4-6 wk or until remission, with predniSONE 60 mg/m²/day, then 30 mg/m² **PO/IM** weekly in 2 divided doses or 2.5 mg/kg **IV**× q2wk; **IT adult:** 12 mg/m²
• **Child ≥3 yr:** 12 mg; **2 yr,** 10 mg; **1 yr,** 8 mg; **<1 yr,** 6 mg

Choriocarcinoma hydatidiform mole (except Otrexup, Rasuvo)
• **Adult/child:** PO/IM 15-30 mg/day × 5 days, then off 1 wk; may repeat, max 5 courses

Meningeal leukemia (except Otrexup, Rasuvo)
• **Adult:** ≤12 mg/m² **INTRATHECALLY** q2-5days until CSF is normal, then 1 additional dose, max 15 mg
• **Child ≥3 yr:** Intrathecally 12 mg q2-5days
• **Child 2-3 yr:** 10 mg q2-5days
• **Child 1-2 yr:** 8 mg q2-5days

Osteosarcoma (except Otrexup, Rasuvo)
• **Adult/child:** IV 12 g/m² given over 4 hr, then leucovorin rescue

Mycosis fungoides (except Otrexup, Rasuvo)
• **Adult:** PO 5-50 mg weekly or 15-37.5 mg twice weekly; **IV/IM** 50 mg weekly or 15-37.5 mg twice weekly

Psoriasis
• **Adult:** PO/IM/IV 10-25 mg/wk or 2.5 mg PO q12hr × 3 doses/wk, may increase to 25 mg/wk, max 30 mg/wk

Breast cancer (except Otrexup, Rasuvo)
• **Adult:** IV 40-60 mg/m² on day 1 of every 21-28 days with other antineoplastics

Epidermal head/neck cancer (except Otrexup, Rasuvo)
• **Adult/child:** IV 40 mg/m² on days 1 and 15, q21days alone or in combination with bleomycin, CISplatin
• **Adult:** PO 25-50 mg/m² q7days
• **Child:** PO 7.5-30 mg/m² q7-14days

Rheumatoid arthritis
• **Adult:** PO 7.5 mg/wk or in divided doses of 2.5 mg q12hr × 3 doses once a wk; max 20 mg/wk

Polyarticular-course juvenile RA
• **Child:** PO/IM 10 mg/m²/wk

Burkitt's lymphoma (stages I, II, III) (except Otrexup, Rasuvo)
• **Adult/adolescent/child:** IV 200 mg/m² days 8 and 15 q21days with bleomycin, cyclophosphamide, vinCRIStine, dexamethasone

Renal dose
• **Adult:** PO/IM/IV CCr 46-60 mL/min, give 65% of standard dose; CCr 31-45 mL/min, give 50% of standard dose; CCr ≤30 mL/min, not recommended

Bladder cancer (unlabeled)
• **Adult:** IV 30 mg/m² on days 1, 15, 22 q28days in combination with vinBLAStine, DOXOrubicin, CISplatin (MVAC regimen)

Active Crohn's disease/ulcerative colitis (unlabeled)
• **Adult:** IM 25 mg/wk; **SUBCUT** 15 mg/kg/wk × 16 wk

Ectopic pregnancy (unlabeled)
• **Adult:** IM 50 mg/m² may be used in combination with miFEPRIStone

Pregnancy termination before 63rd day of pregnancy (unlabeled)
• **Adult:** IM 50 mg/m², then intravaginal miSOPROStol 5-7 days later

Psoriatic arthritis (unlabeled)
• **Adult:** PO 5-7.5 mg weekly

Available forms: Tabs 2.5, 5, 7.5, 10, 15 mg; inj 25 mg/mL (2, 4, 8, 10, 20, 40 mL single-use vials); 25 mg/mL (2-, 10-mL vials with benzyl alcohol);

M

lyophilized powder: 2.5 mg/mL, 25 mg/mL in 1000-mg preservative-free vials; oral solution 2.5 mg/mL

Single-use autoinjector: 7.5 mg/0.15 mL, 7.5 mg/0.4 mL, 10 mg/0.2 mL, 10 mg/0.4 mL, 12.5 mg/0.25 mL, 15 mg/0.3 mL, 15 mg/0.4 mL, 17.5 mg/0.35 mL, 20 mg/0.4 mL, 22.5 mg/0.46 mL, 25 mg/0.4 mL, 25 mg/0.5 mL, 27.5 mg/0.55 mL, 30 mg/0.6 mL

Administer:
Intrathecal route

> **Black Box Warning:** Use preservative-free sol, reconstitute with NS; dose should be drawn into 5- to 10-mL syringe after LP, vol of CSF should be withdrawn equal to vol of methotrexate; allow CSF to flow into syringe and mix, inject over 15-30 sec with bevel of needle upward

• Use safe handling procedures for chemotherapeutic agents

PO route
• This route is preferred for low-dose therapy
• Methotrexate absorption is dose-dependent; absorption of single doses more than 40 mg/m² is significantly less than that of lower doses
• Weekly therapy with Rheumatrex Dose Packs is not intended for doses more than 15 mg PO/wk
• **Oral liquid formulations:** Mistaken daily use of the recommended dose has led to fatal toxicity
• Measure using a calibrated oral measuring device
• **Storage:** store at room temperature (68-77° F) for up to 60 days

Injectable route
• Visually inspect parenteral products for particulate matter and discoloration before use
• The preserved solutions contain benzyl alcohol and should not be used for intrathecal, intermediate-, or high-dose therapy
• **Reconstitution of lyophilized powders:** reconstitute each vial with an appropriate sterile, preservative-free solution such as 5% dextrose injection or 0.9% sodium chloride injection. Reconstitute the 25-mg vial to a concentration no greater than 25 mg/mL. The 1-g vial should be reconstituted with 19.4 mL to a concentration of 50 mg/mL; prepare immediately before use. Discard any unused portions

Intravenous route
• **Direct IV injection:** inject as a slow push via Y-site or 3-way stopcock into a free-flowing IV infusion
• **Intermittent/continuous IV infusion:** further dilute solution in 5% dextrose injection, 5% dextrose and 0.9% sodium chloride injection, or 0.9% sodium chloride injection; before infusion, check vein patency by flushing with 5 to 10 mL of 5% dextrose injection or 0.9% sodium chloride injection; infuse at prescribed rate. Following infusion, flush IV tubing

IV infusion of intermediate- or high-dose methotrexate (500 mg/m² over <4 hr or more than 1 g/m² over >4 hr)
• Before use, the following laboratory parameters should be confirmed: WBC >1,500/mm³, neutrophil count >200/mm³, platelet count >75,000/mm³, serum bilirubin <1.2 mg/dL, normal serum creatinine, and SGPT <450 U. Creatinine clearance should be >60 mL/min. If serum creatinine has increased by 50% or more compared to a prior value, creatinine clearance should be measured and documented as more than 60 mL/min even if the serum creatinine is still within normal limits
• Give 1 L/m² of IV fluids over 6 hr before initiation of the methotrexate infusion; continue hydration at 125 mL/m²/hr during the methotrexate infusion and for 2 days after the infusion has been completed
• Alkalinize the urine using sodium bicarbonate to maintain the urine pH more than 7 during the methotrexate infusion and leucovorin therapy
• Repeat serum creatinine and methotrexate serum level determinations 24 hr after starting methotrexate and at least daily until the methotrexate level is below 5×10^{-8} mol/L (0.05 micro-M)

IM route
- Inject deeply into a large muscle
- Aspirate before injection

Subcut route
- Otrexup and Rasuvo are methotrexate formulations for subcutaneous use only
- Both Otrexup and Rasuvo are single-use auto-injectors. Otrexup is available in 5-mg increments for doses between 10 and 25 mg; Rasuvo is available in 2.5-mg increments for doses between 7.5 and 30 mg. Neither formulation should have lumps or particles floating in it
- Administer Otrexup and Rasuvo in the abdomen or thigh; do NOT administer within 2 inches of the navel, on the arms, on any other areas of the body, or on skin that is tender, bruised, red, scaly, hard, or has scars or stretch marks
- If self-injection is deemed appropriate, patients or caregivers should practice injections using a training device with guidance from a health care professional

Use of Otrexup auto-injector
- Immediately before use, twist cap to remove; flip the safety clip
- Place needle end of Otrexup against thigh or stomach (abdomen) at a 90-degree angle and firmly push until you hear a click; hold for 3 sec before removing

Use of Rasuvo auto-injector:
- Pull the yellow cap straight off. Do not twist
- Position the uncapped end of the auto-injector at a 90-degree angle to the skin. Without pressing the button, push firmly onto the skin until the stop point is felt, which will unlock the yellow injection button
- Press the yellow injection button until a click is heard. Hold Rasuvo against the skin until all medication is injected. This can take up to 5 sec
- Visually inspect the transparent control zone to ensure there is no liquid left in the syringe

Intrathecal administration
- Use preservative-free solutions. The preserved solutions contain benzyl alcohol and should NOT be used for intrathecal therapy
- Reconstitute the preservative-free powder for injection with preservative-free 0.9% sodium chloride injection. The desired dose should be drawn into a 5- to 10-mL syringe
- After lumbar puncture is complete, withdraw an amount of CSF equivalent to the volume of methotrexate injection to be administered. If puncture was traumatic, wait 2 days before attempting to administer methotrexate intrathecally
- Allow CSF (approximately 10% of estimated CSF total volume) to flow into the syringe and mix with the product
- Inject intrathecally over 15 to 30 sec with the bevel of the needle directed upward

SIDE EFFECTS
CNS: Dizziness, seizures, leukoencephalopathy, headache, confusion, encephalopathy, hemiparesis, malaise, fatigue, chills, fever; arachnoiditis (intrathecal)
EENT: Blurred vision, optic neuropathy
GI: *Nausea, vomiting, anorexia, diarrhea, ulcerative stomatitis,* hepatotoxicity, cramps, ulcer, gastritis, GI hemorrhage, abdominal pain, hematemesis, hepatic fibrosis, acute toxicity
GU: Urinary retention, renal failure, menstrual irregularities, defective spermatogenesis, hematuria, azotemia, uric acid nephropathy
HEMA: Leukopenia, thrombocytopenia, myelosuppression, anemia
INTEG: *Rash, alopecia,* dry skin, urticaria, photosensitivity, folliculitis, vasculitis, petechiae, ecchymosis, acne, alopecia, severe fatal skin reaction
RESP: Methotrexate-induced lung disease
SYST: Sudden death, *Pneumocystis jiroveci,* tumor lysis syndrome, secondary malignancy

PHARMACOKINETICS
Not metabolized; excreted in urine (unchanged); crosses placenta, blood-brain barrier; 50% plasma protein bound; terminal half-life 10-12 hr
PO: Readily absorbed
PO/IM/IV: Onset, duration unknown
IT: Onset, peak, duration unknown

M

Side effects: *italics* = common; red = life-threatening

INTERACTIONS

Do not use with proton pump inhibitors

Increase: toxicity—salicylates, sulfa products, other antineoplastics, radiation, alcohol, probenecid, NSAIDs, phenylbutazone, theophylline, penicillins

Increase: hypoprothrombinemia—oral anticoagulants

Increase: hepatitis—acitretin; avoid concurrent use

Decrease: effect of oral digoxin, vaccines, phenytoin, fosphenytoin

Decrease: antibody response—live virus vaccines

Decrease: effect of methotrexate—folic acid supplements, asparaginase

NURSING CONSIDERATIONS
Assess:
• Make sure product is taken weekly in RA, JRA

Black Box Warning: **Infection:** those with active infections should be treated for infection before product use; monitor temperature, fever may indicate beginning of infection; more common during neutropenia

• **Rheumatoid arthritis:** ROM, pain, joint swelling before, during treatment
• **Psoriasis:** skin lesions before, during treatment
• Make sure drug–drug interacting products are discontinued before therapy, and do not resume until methotrexate level is safe
• **Bone marrow suppression:** CBC, differential, platelet count weekly; avoid use until WBC is >1500/mm^3 or platelet count is >75,000/mm^3, neutrophils >200/mm^3; notify prescriber; WBC, platelet nadirs occur on day 7

Black Box Warning: **Nephrotoxicity:** avoid use in renal failure; BUN, serum uric acid, urine CCr, electrolytes before, during therapy; I&O ratio; report fall in urine output to <30 mL/hr

• Monitor vital signs during use; report changes if significant

• Monitor for stomatitis, diarrhea, abdominal cramping or pain; if severe, product may need to be discontinued
• **Anemia:** extreme fatigue, increased heart rate, dyspnea, headache, dizziness, pale skin
• **Gout:** joint warmth, pain, edema, increased uric acid level; use of allopurinol and alkalinization of urine will decrease uric acid
• **Bleeding:** bleeding time, coagulation time during treatment; bleeding: hematuria, guaiac, bruising, petechiae, hematemesis, assess in mucosa or orifices; avoid IM injections, rectal temperature when platelets are low

Black Box Warning: **Pulmonary toxicity:** may start with dry, nonproductive cough; those with ascites or pleural effusion at greater risk for toxicity; fluid should be removed before treatment; monitor plasma methotrexate levels

Black Box Warning: **Tumor lysis syndrome:** hyperkalemia, hyperphosphatemia, hyperuricemia, hypocalcemia, decreased urine output; use aggressive hydration, allopurinol to correct severe electrolyte imbalances, renal toxicity

Black Box Warning: **Hepatotoxicity:** jaundiced skin and sclera, dark urine, clay-colored stools, pruritus, abdominal pain, fever, diarrhea, hepatic studies before and during therapy: bilirubin, alk phos, AST, ALT; liver biopsy should be done before start of therapy (psoriasis)

• Monitor methotrexate levels; adjust leucovorin dose based on level
• Buccal cavity for dryness, sores, ulceration, white patches, oral pain, bleeding, dysphagia

Black Box Warning: **Serious skin reaction:** Stevens-Johnson syndrome, exfoliative dermatitis, skin necrosis, erythema multiforme may occur within days of receiving product by any route; product should be discontinued

- **Stroke-like encephalopathy:** common in high-dose therapy; assess for confusion, hemiparesis, seizures, coma; usually transient
- Increased fluid intake to 2-3 L/day to prevent urate deposits, calculi formation unless contraindicated
- Rinsing of mouth tid-qid with water, club soda; brushing of teeth bid-tid with soft brush or cotton-tipped applicators for stomatitis; use unwaxed dental floss
- **Pregnancy/breastfeeding:** do not use in pregnancy or breastfeeding

Evaluate:
- Therapeutic response: decreased tumor size, spread of malignancy; decreased joint inflammation, pain in RA

Teach patient/family:

Black Box Warning: To report any complaints, side effects to nurse or prescriber: black tarry stools, chills, fever, sore throat, bleeding, bruising, cough, shortness of breath, dark or bloody urine, seizures, rash

- That hair may be lost during treatment; that wig or hairpiece may make patient feel better; that new hair may be different in color, texture (alopecia rare)
- To avoid foods with citric acid, hot temperature, or rough texture if stomatitis is present
- To report stomatitis and any bleeding, white spots, ulcerations in mouth to prescriber; to examine mouth daily; to report symptoms to nurse; to use good oral hygiene

Black Box Warning: **Pregnancy:** that contraceptive measures are recommended during therapy and for at least 8 wk after cessation of therapy for women and men; to discontinue breastfeeding; that toxicity to infant may occur

- To drink 10-12 glasses of fluid/day
- To avoid alcohol, salicylates, live vaccines
- To avoid use of razors, commercial mouthwash; to use soft-bristle toothbrush
- To use sunblock to prevent burns

- To use good dental care to prevent overgrowth of infection in the mouth
- How to use this product with leucovorin rescue
- To continue leucovorin until told it is safe to stop
- To report CNS symptoms, vision changes
- To report fever, other symptoms of infection
- To report decreased urine output
- To avoid crowds, persons with known infections
- To advise all health care providers that methotrexate is being taken; not to use Rx, OTC medications, herbs, or supplements unless approved by prescriber
- **Subcut route:** Teach patient self-injection technique and use and disposal of equipment

---

⚠ HIGH ALERT

M

methyldopa/methyldopate (Rx)
(meth-ill-doe′pa)
Func. class.: Antihypertensive
Chem. class.: Centrally acting α-adrenergic inhibitor

Do not confuse:
methyldopa/L-dopa/levodopa

ACTION: Stimulates central inhibitory α-adrenergic receptors or acts as false transmitter, resulting in reduction of arterial pressure

USES: Hypertension, hypertensive crisis

CONTRAINDICATIONS: Active hepatic disease, hypersensitivity, MAOI therapy

Precautions: Pregnancy, geriatric patients, cardiac disease, autoimmune disease, depression, dialysis, hemolytic anemia, Parkinson's disease, pheochromocytoma, sulfite hypersensitivity

DOSAGE AND ROUTES
Hypertension/hypertensive crisis
- **Adult: PO** 250-500 mg bid or tid, then adjusted q2days as needed, 0.5-2 g/day

---

Side effects: *italics* = common; red = life-threatening

in 2-4 divided doses (maintenance), max 3 g/day; **IV** 250-500 mg in 100 mL D$_5$W q6hr, run over 30-60 min, max 1 g q6hr; switch to oral as soon as possible

• **Child:** PO 10 mg/kg/day in 2-4 divided doses, max 65 mg/kg or 3 g/day, whichever is less; **IV** 20-40 mg/kg/day in 4 divided doses, max 65 mg/kg or 3 g, whichever is less

Renal dose

• **Adult:** PO CCr 10-50 mL/min dose q8-12hr; CCr <10 mL/min dose q12-24hr

Available forms: Methyldopa: tabs 125 ✦, 250, 500 mg; **methyldopate:** inj 50 mg/mL

Administer:

PO route

• Increase in dose should be done in the evening to minimize drowsiness

• Product should not be withdrawn abruptly

Intermittent IV INFUSION route

• After diluting with 100 mL D$_5$W; infuse over $^1/_2$-1 hr

Y-site compatibilities: Alemtuzumab, alfentanil, amikacin, aminophylline, anidulafungin, ascorbic acid, atenolol, atracurium, atropine, aztreonam, benztropine, bivalirudin, bleomycin, bumetanide, buprenorphine, butorphanol, calcium chloride/gluconate, caspofungin, cefamandole, ceFAZolin, cefmetazole, cefonicid, cefotaxime, cefoTEtan, cefOXitin, cefTAZidime, ceftizoxime, cefTRIAXone, cefuroxime, cephalothin, chlorproMAZINE, cimetidine, clindamycin, cyanocobalamin, cycloSPORINE, DACTINomycin, DAPTOmycin, dexamethasone, digoxin, diltiaZEM, diphenhydrAMINE, DOCEtaxel, DOPamine, doxycycline, enalaprilat, ePHEDrine, EPINEPHrine, epoetin alfa, ertapenem, erythromycin, esmolol, etoposide, etoposide phosphate, famotidine, fenoldopam, fentaNYL, fluconazole, fludarabine, gatifloxacin, gemcitabine, gentamicin, glycopyrrolate, granisetron, heparin, hydrocortisone, HYDROmorphone, hydrOXYzine, IDArubicin, insulin (regular), irinotecan, isoproterenol, labetalol, lidocaine, linezolid, LORazepam, magnesium sulfate, mannitol, mechlorethamine, meperidine, metaraminol, methicillin, methoxamine, methylPREDNISolone, metoclopramide, metoprolol, metroNIDAZOLE, mezlocillin, miconazole, midazolam, milrinone, minocycline, mitoXANTRONE, morphine, moxalactam, multiple vitamins, mycophenolate mofetil, nafcillin, nalbuphine, naloxone, netilmicin, nitroglycerin, nitroprusside, norepinephrine, octreotide, ondansetron, oxacillin, oxaliplatin, oxytocin, PACLitaxel, palonosetron, pamidronate, pancuronium, pantoprazole, papaverine, PEMEtrexed, penicillin G potassium/sodium, pentazocine, phentolamine, phenylephrine, phytonadione, piperacillin, polymyxin B, potassium chloride, procainamide, prochlorperazine, promethazine, propranolol, protamine, pyridoxine, quiNIDine, raNITIdine, ritodrine, sodium bicarbonate, succinylcholine, SUFentanil, tacrolimus, teniposide, theophylline, thiamine, thiotepa, ticarcillin, ticarcillin-clavulanate, tigecycline, tirofiban, tobramycin, tolazoline, trimetaphan, urokinase, vancomycin, vasopressin, vecuronium, verapamil, vinorelbine, voriconazole, zoledronic acid

SIDE EFFECTS

CNS: *Drowsiness, weakness, dizziness, sedation, headache,* depression, psychosis, paresthesias, parkinsonism, Bell's palsy, nightmares, drug fever

CV: Bradycardia, myocarditis, orthostatic hypotension, angina, edema, weight gain, HF, paradoxic pressor response (IV)

EENT: Nasal congestion

ENDO: Breast enlargement, gynecomastia, amenorrhea

GI: Nausea, vomiting, diarrhea, constipation, hepatic dysfunction, sore or "black" tongue, pancreatitis, colitis, flatulence

GU: Impotence, failure to ejaculate

HEMA: Leukopenia, thrombocytopenia, hemolytic anemia, granulocytopenia, positive Coombs' test

INTEG: Rash, toxic epidermal necrolysis, lupuslike syndrome

PHARMACOKINETICS
PO: Onset 4-6 hr, duration 24-48 hr
IV: Onset 4-6 hr, duration 10-16 hr
Metabolized by liver, excreted in urine,
half-life 2 hr

INTERACTIONS
• **Lithium toxicity:** lithium
Increase: pressor effect—sympathomi-
metic amines, MAOIs; do not use concur-
rently with MAOIs
Increase: hypotension, CNS toxicity—
levodopa
Increase: hypotension—diuretics, other
antihypertensives
Increase: psychosis—haloperidol
Increase: CNS depression—alcohol,
antihistamines, antidepressants, analge-
sics, sedative/hypnotics
Increase: B/P—phenothiazines, β-
blockers, amphetamines, NSAIDs, tricy-
clics, barbiturates
Increase: hypoglycemia—TOLBUTamide
Decrease: methyldopa absorption—iron

Drug/Lab Test
Increase: creatinine, LFTs
Decrease: platelets, WBC, Hgb/HcT
Interference: urinary uric acid, serum
creatinine, AST
False increase: urinary catecholamines

NURSING CONSIDERATIONS
Assess:
• Blood studies: neutrophils, decreased
platelets, CBC
• **Hemolytic anemia:** direct Coombs'
test before, after 6, 12 mo of therapy; a
positive test may indicate hemolytic anemia; usually reverses within weeks to
months after discontinuing treatment;
monitor Hgb/Hct and RBC; do not start
therapy in those with hemolytic anemia
• Baselines of renal, hepatic studies before therapy begins
• **Drug-induced hepatitis/drug fever:**
usually subsides within 3 mo of discontinuing therapy
• **Hypertension:** B/P when beginning
treatment, periodically thereafter; report
significant changes

• **Allergic reaction:** rash, fever, pruritus,
urticaria; product should be discontinued if antihistamines fail to help
• CNS symptoms, especially in geriatric
patients; depression, change in mental
status
• **HF:** edema, dyspnea, wet crackles, B/P
• Renal symptoms: polyuria, oliguria,
urinary frequency; I&O ratio, weight; report weight gain >5 lb
• **Product tolerance:** may occur within 3
mo of starting treatment; a dosage change
and other products may be needed
• **Beers:** avoid in older adults; high risk
of CNS effects; may cause bradycardia
and orthostatic hypotension
• **Pregnancy/breastfeeding:** use cautiously
in pregnancy, breastfeeding; has been used
for pregnancy-induced hypertension
Evaluate:
• Therapeutic response: decrease in B/P
Teach patient/family:
• To avoid hazardous activities
• Not to discontinue product abruptly
because withdrawal symptoms may occur: anxiety, increased B/P, headache,
insomnia, increased pulse, tremors, nausea, sweating
• To rise slowly to sitting or standing
position to minimize orthostatic hypotension
• To notify prescriber of mouth sores,
sore throat, fever, swelling of hands or
feet, irregular heartbeat, chest pain, signs
of angioedema
• That excessive perspiration, dehydration, vomiting, diarrhea may lead to fall
in B/P; to consult prescriber
• That dizziness, fainting, light-headedness may occur during first few days of
therapy
• Not to use OTC (cough, cold, allergy)
products unless directed by prescriber;
that compliance is necessary; not to skip or
stop product unless directed by prescriber
• That product may cause skin rash

TREATMENT OF OVERDOSE:
Gastric evacuation, sympathomimetics
may be indicated; if severe, hemodialysis

M

methylergonovine (Rx)

(meth-ill-er-goe-noe´veen)

Methergine

Func. class.: Oxytocic

Chem. class.: Ergot alkaloid

ACTION: Stimulates uterine, vascular, and smooth muscle, thereby causing contractions; decreases bleeding; arterial vasoconstriction

USES: Prevention, treatment of hemorrhage postpartum or postabortion, uterine contractions

CONTRAINDICATIONS: Pregnancy (other than obstetric delivery/abortion), hypertension, preeclampsia, eclampsia, elective induction of labor, hypersensitivity to ergot preparations
Precautions: Severe renal/hepatic disease, jaundice, diabetes mellitus, seizure disorders, sepsis, CAD, last stage of labor

DOSAGE AND ROUTES

• **Adult: PO** 200 mcg tid-qid × ≤7 days; **IM/IV** 200 mcg q2-4hr × 1-5 doses
Available forms: Inj 200 mcg/mL; tabs 200 mcg

Administer:

PO route

• Do not exceed dosage limits
• Store tabs at room temperature
• Give with water
• Only during 4th stage of labor; not to be used to augment labor

IM route

• Protect from light
• IM in deep muscle mass; rotate inj sites for additional doses, aspirate

Direct IV route

• Undiluted through Y-tube or 3-way stopcock; give ≤0.2 mg/min or diluted in 5 mL 0.9% NaCl given through Y-site
• With crash cart available on unit; IV route used only in emergencies
• Refrigerated storage of ampules; protect from light; give only if solution is clear, colorless

Y-site compatibilities: Heparin, hydrocortisone sodium succinate, potassium chloride, vit B/C

SIDE EFFECTS

CNS: *Headache, dizziness,* seizures, hallucinations; stroke (IV)
CV: Hypotension, chest pain, palpitation, hypertension, dysrhythmias, CVA (IV)
EENT: Tinnitus
GI: *Nausea, vomiting*
GU: Cramping
INTEG: Sweating, rash, allergic reactions
MS: Leg cramps
RESP: Dyspnea

PHARMACOKINETICS

Metabolized in liver, excreted in urine
PO: Onset 5-15 min, duration 3 hr
IM: Onset 2-5 min, duration 3 hr
IV: Onset immediate, duration 45 min-3 hr

INTERACTIONS

Increase: vasoconstriction—DOPamine, ergots, anesthetics (regional), vasopressors, nicotine
Increase: ergot toxicity—CYP3A4 inhibitors; do not use together

NURSING CONSIDERATIONS

Assess:

• B/P, pulse, character and amount of vaginal bleeding; watch for indications of hemorrhage
• Uterine relaxation; observe for severe cramping
• **Ergot toxicity:** tinnitus, hypertension, palpitations, chest pain, nausea, vomiting, weakness; cold, numb extremities
• **Pregnancy/breastfeeding:** do not use in pregnancy except following obstetric delivery or abortion to reduce postpartum hemorrhagic risk; may breastfeed 1 wk postpartum

Evaluate:

• Therapeutic response: absence of postpartum hemorrhage

Teach patient/family:

• To report increased blood loss, severe abdominal cramps, fever, or foul-smelling lochia

---

methylnaltrexone (Rx)

(meth-il-nal-trex′one)

Relistor

Func. class.: GI agent
Chem. class.: Opioid antagonist

ACTION: Peripheral μ-opioid receptor antagonist that reduces constipation associated with opiate agonists

USES: Treatment of opioid-induced constipation in patients with advanced illness who are receiving palliative care when response to laxative therapy has been insufficient; treatment of opioid-induced constipation in chronic noncancer pain

Unlabeled uses: Pruritus; nausea, vomiting related to morphine; urinary retention from opioids

CONTRAINDICATIONS: Hypersensitivity, GI obstruction, IV route, eclampsia, elective induction of labor, hypertension, preeclampsia, pregnancy

Precautions: Pregnancy, breastfeeding, children, geriatric patients, renal disease, diarrhea, driving, operating machinery, neoplastic disease, Crohn's disease, peptic ulcer, ulcerative colitis

DOSAGE AND ROUTES

Opiate-agonist–induced constipation

• **Adult >114 kg:** SUBCUT 0.15 mg/kg every other day prn

• **Adult 62-114 kg:** SUBCUT 12 mg every other day prn, max 12 mg/24 hr

• **Adult 38-<62 kg:** SUBCUT 8 mg every other day prn, max 8 mg/24 hr

• **Adult <38 kg:** SUBCUT 0.15 mg/kg every other day prn, max 0.15 mg/kg/24 hr

Opioid-induced constipation with noncancer pain

• **Adult:** PO 450 mg daily in the AM SUBCUT 12 mg q day; discontinue laxative before starting this product

Renal dose

• **Adult:** SUBCUT CCr <60 mL/min, reduce normal adult dose by 50%; PO 150 mg/day

Available forms: Sol for inj 12 mg/0.6 mL (single-use vials), 8 mg/0.4 mL (prefilled syringes); tab 150 mg

Administer:

PO route

• Take on empty stomach at least 30 min before first meal of the day

SUBCUT route

Do not give IV; IV dosing for urinary retention investigational

• Store at 59° F-86° F (15° C-30° C); do not freeze

• Store away from light

• Inspect sol before use; should be clear, colorless to pale yellow aqueous sol; do not use if particulate matter or discoloration is present

• Withdraw needed amount of sol into sterile syringe; if immediate administration is impossible, syringe may be kept at room temperature for ≤24 hr; immediately discard any unused portion in vial; no preservatives are present

• Administer into upper arm, abdomen, or thigh ≤1×/24 hr; rotate inj sites; do not inject same spot each time; do not inject into areas where skin is tender, bruised, red, or hard; avoid areas with scars or stretch marks

• If using with retractable needle, slowly push down on plunger past resistance point until the syringe is empty and click is heard

PO route

• Give with water on empty stomach 30 min before morning meal

SIDE EFFECTS

CNS: Dizziness

GI: Nausea, vomiting, diarrhea, flatulence, abdominal pain, GI perforation

PHARMACOKINETICS

Half-life 8 hr, protein binding 11%-15.3%; renal impairment has marked

M

effect on renal excretion of methylnaltrexone; dose adjustment is required for patients with CCr <60 mL/min; renal clearance decreased and total systemic exposure increased in patients with severe renal impairment who receive single SUBCUT dose of 0.3 mg/kg
SUBCUT: Peak 30 min

NURSING CONSIDERATIONS
Assess:
• Serum creatinine, BUN, baseline and periodically
• **Opioid-induced constipation:** stool characteristics, bowel sounds during treatment
• **Pain:** monitor characteristics of pain; this product does not affect analgesics
• **Beers:** avoid in older adults unless safer alternatives are unavailable; may cause ataxia, impaired psychomotor function
• **Pregnancy/breastfeeding:** avoid use in pregnancy, withdrawal in fetus may occur; do not breastfeed
Evaluate:
• Therapeutic response: decreasing constipation
Teach patient/family:
• That, after 30 min, to remain near toilet facilities because bowel relaxation occurs; not to use more than 1 dose in 24 hr
• To notify prescriber of abdominal pain, continuous or severe diarrhea, nausea, vomiting
• **Pregnancy/breastfeeding:** to avoid use in pregnancy unless absolutely necessary; to avoid in breastfeeding
• To notify prescriber before taking all other OTC, prescription, or herbal products
• Not to drive or perform other hazardous activities until response is known; dizziness may occur
• To continue other products for constipation unless directed by prescriber not to
• **Opioid withdrawal:** to report severe diarrhea, abdominal pain, chills

---

methylphenidate (Rx)
(meth-ill-fen′i-date)
Aptensio XR, Biphentin ✦,
Concerta, Cotempla XR-ODT,
Daytrana, Jornay PM, Metadate
CD, Metadate ER, Methylin,
Methylin ER, Quillivant XR,
Ritalin, Ritalin LA, QuilliChew
Func. class.: Cerebral stimulant
Chem. class.: Piperidine derivative

**Controlled Substance
Schedule II**

Do not confuse:
methylphenidate/methadone
Metadate ER/methadone
Ritalin/ritodrine/Ritalin LA

ACTION: Increases release of norepinephrine, DOPamine in cerebral cortex to reticular activating system; exact action not known

USES: Attention deficit disorder (ADD), attention-deficit/hyperactivity disorder (ADHD); narcolepsy (except Concerta, Metadate CD, Ritalin LA)
Unlabeled uses: Management of depression

CONTRAINDICATIONS: Hypersensitivity, anxiety, history of Gilles de la Tourette's syndrome; glaucoma, hereditary fructose intolerance
Precautions: Pregnancy, breastfeeding, hypertension, depression, seizures, abrupt discontinuation, acute MI, aortic stenosis, arteriosclerosis, bipolar disorder, cardiac dysrhythmias, cardiomyopathy, chemical leukoderma, child depression, dysphagia, esophageal stricture, growth inhibition, heart failure, hepatic disease, hypertension, hyperthyroidism, ileus, mania, peripheral vascular disease, PKU, psychosis, Raynaud's disease, schizophrenia, stroke, suicidal ideation, visual disturbances

---

Black Box Warning: Substance abuse, alcoholism

DOSAGE AND ROUTES
Attention-deficit/hyperactivity disorder (ADHD) initial treatment, not currently on methylphenidate

Regular release: Ritalin, Methylin, Methylin oral sol, Methylin chew tabs
• **Adult:** PO 20-30 mg/day, range 10-60 mg/day in 2-3 divided doses, 30-45 min before meals
• **Child ≥6 yr:** PO 5 mg bid initially, increase 5-10 mg/day weekly, usual dose 0.3-2 mg/kg/day, max 60 mg/day

Extended release: Ritalin SR, Metadate ER, Methylin ER
• **Adult/adolescent/child ≥6 yr:** PO max 20-30 mg tid

Extended-release once-daily tabs: Concerta
• **Adult:** PO 18-36 mg/day initially, then adjust by 18 mg/wk, max 72 mg/day
• **Adolescent:** PO 18 mg/day initially, then adjust by 18 mg/wk, max 72 mg/day
• **Child ≥6 yr:** PO 18 mg/day initially, then adjust by 18 mg/wk, max 54 mg/day

Extended-release once-daily capsules: Ritalin LA
• **Adult/adolescent/child ≥6 yr:** PO 10-20 mg daily in AM initially, adjust by 10 mg/wk, max 60 mg/day

Extended release once-daily PM capsule:
• **Child >9 yr and adolescents:** PO 20 mg in evening; may increase q wk by 20 mg, max 100 mg/day

Transdermal: Daytrana
• **Adolescent/child ≥6 yr:** TD wk 1: 10 mg/day (9-hr patch); wk 2: 15 mg/day (9-hr patch); wk 3: 20 mg/day (9-hr patch); wk 4: 30 mg/day (9-hr patch)

Conversion to once-daily treatment from other forms for ADHD

Extended-release once-daily capsules: Ritalin LA
• **Adult/adolescent/child ≥6 yr:** PO give no more than total daily dose of other

forms, may adjust by 10 mg/wk, max 60 mg/day

Extended-release once-daily tablets: Concerta
• **Adult/adolescent/child ≥6 yr (currently on 10-15 mg/day):** PO 18 mg every AM initially, adjust by 18 mg/wk, max 72 mg/day (adult); max 72 mg/day, 2 mg/kg/day (adolescent); 54 mg/day (child)
• **Adult/adolescent/child ≥6 yr (currently receiving 20-30 mg/day):** PO 36 mg every AM, adjust by 18 mg/wk, max 72 mg/day (adult); 72 mg/day, 2 mg/kg/day (adolescent); 54 mg/day (child)
• **Adult/adolescent/child ≥6 yr (currently receiving 30-45 mg/day):** PO 54 mg every AM, adjust by 18 mg/wk, max 72 mg/day (adult); 72 mg/day, 2 mg/kg/day (adolescent); 54 mg/day (child)
• **Adult/adolescent/child ≥6 yr (currently receiving 40-60 mg/day):** PO 72 mg every AM, 72 mg/day

Extended-release once-daily suspension: Quillivant XR
• **Adolescent/child ≥6 yr:** PO give 20 mg in AM, increase in 10-20 mg increments weekly

Narcolepsy

Immediate release: Ritalin, Methylin oral sol, Methylin chew tabs
• **Adult:** PO 20-30 mg/day, range 10-60 mg/day in 2-3 divided doses
• **Child ≥6 yr:** PO 5 mg bid, may increase by 5-10 mg/wk, max 60 mg/day

Extended-release tabs: Ritalin SR, Metadate ER
• **Adult/adolescent/child ≥6 yr:** PO max 20 mg tid
• **Adult and geriatric:** PO (immediate rel tabs) 2.5 mg morning/noon, may increase by 2.5-5 mg q2-3days

Available forms: Tabs 5, 10, 20 mg; ext rel tabs 10, 20 mg; ext rel tabs (Concerta) 18, 27, 36, 54 mg; ext rel caps 10, 20, 30, 40 mg; ext rel chewable tabs (QuillChew ER) 20, 30, 40 mg; oral sol 5 mg/5 mL, 10 mg/5 mL; chew tabs (Methylin) 2.5, 5, 10 mg; transdermal

M

patch 12.5 cm^2 (10 mg), 18.75 cm^2 (15 mg), 25 cm^2 (20 mg), 37.5 cm^2 (30 mg); ext rel oral susp 300 mg/60 mL, 600 mg/120 mL, 750 mg/150 mL, 900 mg/180 mL; capsule (Journay PM) 20 mg

Administer:

PO route

• **Methylin chewable tablets:** give with at least 8 oz of fluid to avoid choking

• **Immediate-release dosage forms (Ritalin, Methylin, Metadate):** give 30-45 min before meal; twice-daily dosages may be used in AM and noon

• **Ext-rel tablets (Ritalin SR, Metadate ER):** may be given without regard to meals. Give whole; do not cut, crush, or chew. Give the last dose of the day several hours before bedtime. Ext-rel tablets may be used when the determined 8-hr dose of immediate-release methylphenidate tablets equals the 8-hr dosage of the ext-rel tablets

• **Once-daily ext-rel tablets (Concerta):** may be given without regard to meals. Give whole; do not cut, crush, or chew; portion of this tablet may appear intact in the stool

• **Once-daily ext-rel capsules (Ritalin LA, Aptensio XR):** may be given without regard to meals; establish a routine pattern with regard to meals. Give with an adequate amount of fluid. Do not cut, crush, or chew. If swallowing is difficult, capsule may be opened and the contents sprinkled on 1 tablespoon of applesauce and swallowed immediately. The capsule contents (beads) should not be crushed or chewed. Instruct patient to drink fluids (water, milk, or juice) after taking sprinkles with applesauce

• **Once-daily ext-rel chewable tablets (QuilliChew ER):** give q day in the AM with or without food. The tablet may be broken in half for 10-mg and 15-mg doses

• **Immediate-release oral solution (Methylin):** measure dose with oral syringe or calibrated measuring device. Give 30-45 min before meals in divided doses 2 to 3 times/day. Twice-daily dosages may be administered in AM and around noon. Give last dose of day before 6 PM

• **Once-daily ext-rel oral suspension (Quillivant XR):** vigorously shake before use; measure dose with calibrated oral dosing dispenser provided. Give in AM without regard to meals

• **Reconstitution of once-daily ext-rel oral suspension (Quillivant XR):** review manufacturer's instructions for the particular product and package size; before reconstitution, tap bottle several times to loosen powder. To prepare suspension, add specified amount of water to bottle, fully insert the bottle adapter into the bottle neck, replace the cap, and vigorously shake bottle for at least 10 sec. Store reconstituted suspension at 77° F; dispense in original packaging (bottle in container). Reconstituted suspension is stable for 4 mo from date of reconstitution

Topical route

• **Daytrana transdermal system:** apply patch 2 hr before effect is needed

• Do not cut or trim patch

• Apply patch immediately after opening. Do not use if pouch seal is broken. Do not touch adhesive side of patch during application to avoid absorption. Wash hands immediately if adhesive side of patch is touched. Discard patch if difficulty is encountered in separating patch from the release liner, or if tearing or other damage occurs. Discard patch if adhesive containing medication has transferred to the liner during removal of patch from the liner

• Place on a dry, clean area of the hip, and hold in place for 30 sec with palm of hand. Do not apply to oily, damaged, or irritated skin. Do not apply topical preparations to the application site immediately before patch application. Avoid waistline area where patch could be rubbed by clothing

• Application sites should be alternated from one hip to the next each day

• Adherence of patch may be affected by showering, bathing, or swimming

• Avoid exposing the application site to hair dryers, heating pads, electric blankets, heated water beds, or other direct external heat sources

• Do not apply or reapply the patch with dressings, tape, or adhesives. If the patch is not fully adhered to the skin during application or wear time, discard patch according to disposal instructions, and apply a new patch

• Total daily wear time should not exceed 9 hr, regardless of patch replacement

• Patches should be peeled off slowly. Patch removal may be aided by applying an oil-based product (petroleum jelly, mineral oil, olive oil) to the patch edges

• **For disposal,** instruct patient and/or caregiver to fold used patch so that the adhesive side of the patch adheres to itself, and then flush it down the toilet or dispose of in an appropriate lidded container

SIDE EFFECTS

CNS: *Hyperactivity, insomnia, restlessness, talkativeness,* dizziness, drowsiness, toxic psychosis, headache, akathisia, dyskinesia, masking or worsening of Tourette's syndrome, seizures, hallucinations, malignant neuroleptic syndrome, aggression; cerebral vasculitis, hemorrhage, stroke (rare)

CV: *Palpitations, tachycardia,* B/P changes, angina, dysrhythmias, sudden death

ENDO: Growth retardation

GI: Nausea, anorexia, dry mouth, weight loss, abdominal pain

HEMA: Leukopenia, anemia, thrombocytopenic purpura

INTEG: Exfoliative dermatitis, urticaria, rash, erythema multiforme, hypersensitivity reactions; patch: permanent loss of skin color, anaphylaxis, angioedema

MISC: Fever, arthralgia, scalp hair loss, rhabdomyolysis

PHARMACOKINETICS

PO: Varies with formulation, metabolized by liver, excreted by kidneys, half-life 3-4 hr

INTERACTIONS

Increase: hypertensive crisis—MAOIs or within 14 days of MAOIs, vasopressors

Increase: effects of tricyclics, SSRIs, anticonvulsants, SNRIs, CNS stimulants; monitor for adverse reactions

Decrease: effect of antihypertensives

Drug/Herb

Increase: CNS stimulation—cola nut, guarana, horsetail, yerba maté, yohimbe

Drug/Food

Increase: stimulation—caffeine

NURSING CONSIDERATIONS

Assess:

• **ADHD:** attention span, decreased hyperactivity, impulsivity, socialization

Black Box Warning: Substance abuse: there is a high potential for abuse; use caution in those with history of substance abuse

• VS, B/P; may reverse antihypertensives; check patients with cardiac disease more often for increased B/P

• CBC with differential, platelets, LFTs, urinalysis; in diabetes: blood glucose, urine glucose; insulin changes may have to be made because eating will decrease

• Height, growth rate q3mo in children; growth rate may be decreased, but normal growth will resume when product is discontinued

• Mental status: mood, sensorium, affect, stimulation, insomnia, aggressiveness; may produce euphoria, rebound depression after product wears off

• **Withdrawal symptoms:** headache, nausea, vomiting, muscle pain, weakness; usually not associated with drug holidays

• Appetite, sleep, speech patterns

• **Narcolepsy:** identify frequency, length of narcoleptic episodes

• Skin pigmentation when using TD product; may cause loss of pigmentation around site

• **Beers:** avoid use in older adults; CNS stimulant effects

• **Pregnancy/breastfeeding:** use only if benefit outweighs risk to fetus; no well-controlled studies; cautious use in breastfeeding

Evaluate:

• Therapeutic response: decreased hyperactivity (ADHD); increased ability to stay awake (narcolepsy)

Teach patient/family:
• To decrease caffeine consumption (coffee, tea, cola, chocolate); may increase irritability, stimulation; not to use guarana, yerba maté, cola nut
• To avoid OTC preparations unless approved by prescriber
• To always use dosing dispenser provided for oral suspension dose
• To taper off product over several weeks because depression, increased sleeping, lethargy will occur
• To avoid driving, hazardous activities if dizziness, blurred vision occur
• To avoid alcohol
• To get needed rest; patients will feel more tired at end of day
• That shell of Concerta tab may appear in stools
• To take regular tab at least 6 hr before sleep, 10 hr for ext rel; to use dosing syringe, not household teaspoon, to measure liquid
• **Seizures:** that those with seizure disorders may have lower seizure threshold
• **Transdermal:** to use in AM; after tray is opened, to use within 2 mo; not to store patches without protective covering; to notify prescriber if skin irritation or rash occurs; that if patch comes off, to use a new one on a different skin site; to tell child not to remove or share with others
• **Sus rel:** not to chew tabs

TREATMENT OF OVERDOSE: Administer fluids; hemodialysis or peritoneal dialysis; antihypertensive for increased B/P; administer short-acting barbiturate before lavage

---

methylPREDNISolone (Rx)

(meth-il-pred-niss'oh-lone)

A-Methapred, Depo, Medrol, Solu
Func. class.: Corticosteroid, synthetic
Chem. class.: Glucocorticoid, intermediate acting

Do not confuse:
methylPREDNISolone/predniSONE/
medroxyPROGESTERone/
methylTESTOSTERone

ACTION: Decreases inflammation by suppression of migration of polymorphonuclear leukocytes, fibroblasts; reversal of increased capillary permeability and lysosomal stabilization

USES: Severe inflammation, shock, adrenal insufficiency, collagen disorders, management of acute spinal cord injury, multiple sclerosis, acute lymphocytic leukemia, anaphylaxis, angioedema, asthma, Crohn's disease, eczema, gouty arthritis
Unlabeled uses: Multiple myeloma, bronchospasm prophylaxis, airway-obstructing hemangioma, noncardiogenic pulmonary edema, idiopathic pulmonary fibrosis, carpal tunnel syndrome, temporal arteritis, Churg-Strauss syndrome, mixed connective-tissue disease, polyarteritis nodosa, relapsing polychondritis, polymyalgia rheumatica, vasculitis, Wegener's granulomatosis, *Pneumocystis jiroveci* pneumonia in AIDS patients, acute spinal cord injury, severe acute respiratory syndrome (SARS), acute interstitial nephritis

CONTRAINDICATIONS: Hypersensitivity, intrathecal use, neonates
Precautions: Pregnancy, breastfeeding, diabetes mellitus, glaucoma, osteoporosis, seizure disorders, ulcerative colitis, HF, myasthenia gravis, renal disease, esophagitis, peptic ulcer, tartrazine, benzyl alcohol, corticosteroid hypersensitivity, viral infection, TB, traumatic brain injury, Cushing syndrome, measles, varicella, fungal infections

DOSAGE AND ROUTES
Adrenal insufficiency/inflammation
• **Adult:** PO 4-48 mg in 4 divided doses; **IM** 10-120 mg (acetate); **IM/IV** 10-40 mg (succinate); **INTRAARTICULAR** 4-80 mg (acetate)
• **Child:** IV 0.5-1.7 mg/kg in 3-4 divided doses (succinate)
Multiple sclerosis
• **Adult:** PO/IM/IV 160 mg/day × 1 wk, then 64 mg every other day × 30 days
Most uses
• **Adult:** IM/IV 40-250 mg q4-6hr; pulse therapy IV 2 mg/kg, then 0.5-1 mg/kg q6hr × up to 5 days

Acute spinal cord injury (succinate)
• **Adult/child:** IV 30 mg/kg over 15 min, then continuous infusion after 45 min, 5.4 mg/kg/hr × 23 hr

Pneumocystitis jirovecii pneumona (AIDS) (Succinate)
• **Adult:** IV 30 mg bid × 5 days, then 30 mg daily × 5 days, then 15 mg daily × 10 days

Available forms: Tabs 2, 4, 8, 16, 32 mg; inj 20, 40, 80 mg/mL acetate; inj 40, 125, 500, 1000, 2000 mg/vial succinate

Administer:
• Titrated dose; use lowest effective dose

PO route
• With food or milk to decrease GI symptoms (PO)
• Once-a-day dose should be given in AM to coincide with body's normal cortisol secretion

IM route
• IM inj deep in large muscle mass; rotate sites; avoid deltoid; use 21-G needle; after shaking suspension (parenteral); inj-site reaction may occur (induration, pain at site, atrophy)
• In one dose in AM to prevent adrenal suppression; avoid SUBCUT administration; may damage tissue

IV route
• Use only methylprednisolone sodium succinate; never use acetate product

Direct IV route
• After diluting with diluent provided; agitate slowly; give ≤500 mg/≥1 min directly over 3-15 min; doses ≥2 mg/kg or 250 mg should be given by intermittent IV infusion unless potential benefits outweigh risks

Intermittent/continuous INFUSION route
• Dilute further in D₅W, NS, D₅NS; haze may form; give over 15-60 min; large dose (≥500 mg) should be given over 30-60 min

Y-site compatibilities: Acetaminophen, acyclovir, amifostine, amphotericin B cholesteryl, amrinone, aztreonam, cefepime, CISplatin, cladribine, cyclophosphamide, cytarabine, DOPamine, DOXOrubicin, enalaprilat, famotidine, fludarabine, granisetron, heparin, melphalan, meperidine, methotrexate, metroNIDAZOLE, midazolam, morphine, piperacillin/tazobactam, remifentanil, sodium bicarbonate, tacrolimus, teniposide, theophylline, thiotepa

SIDE EFFECTS
CNS: Depression, flushing, sweating, headache, mood changes
CV: Hypertension, circulatory collapse, thrombophlebitis, embolism, tachycardia
EENT: Fungal infections, increased intraocular pressure, blurred vision, cataracts
GI: Diarrhea, nausea, abdominal distention, GI hemorrhage, increased appetite, pancreatitis
HEMA: Thrombocytopenia
INTEG: Acne, poor wound healing, ecchymosis, petechiae
MS: Fractures, osteoporosis, weakness
MISC: Hypernatremia

PHARMACOKINETICS
Half-life >3½ hr (plasma), 18-36 hr (tissue); crosses placenta, enters breast milk in small amounts; metabolized in liver; excreted by kidneys (unchanged)
PO: Peak 1-2 hr, duration 1½ days, well absorbed
IM: Peak 4-8 days, duration 1-4 wk, well absorbed
Intraarticular: Peak 1 wk

INTERACTIONS
Increase: side effects—amphotericin B, diuretics
Increase: GI bleeding—salicylates, NSAIDs; assess for GI bleeding
Increase: methylPREDNISolone action—oral contraceptives, estrogens
Increase: adrenal suppression—CYP3A4 inhibitors (aprepitant, antiretroviral protease inhibitors, clarithromycin, danazol, delavirdine, diltiaZEM, erythromycin, fluconazole, FLUoxetine, fluvoxaMINE, imatinib, ketoconazole, mibefradil, nefazodone, telithromycin, voriconazole); dose may need to be decreased
Decrease: methylPREDNISolone effect—CYP3A4 inducers (barbiturates,

M

Side effects: *italics* = common; red = life-threatening

bosentan, carBAMazepine, efavirenz, phenytoins, nevirapine, rifabutin, rifAMPin); dose may need to be increased
Decrease: effects of antidiabetics, vaccines, somatrem

Drug/Herb
• Avoid use with St. John's wort

Drug/Food
• Do not use with grapefruit/grapefruit juice; level of methylPREDNISolone will be increased

Drug/Lab Test
Increase: cholesterol, blood glucose
Decrease: calcium, potassium, T_4, T_3, thyroid ^{131}I uptake test, urine 17-OHCS, 17-KS
False negative: skin allergy tests

NURSING CONSIDERATIONS
Assess:
• **Potassium depletion:** parethesias, fatigue, nausea, vomiting, depression, polyuria, dysrhythmias, weakness
• Edema, hypertension, cardiac symptoms
• Mental status: affect, mood, behavioral changes, aggression
• Monitor potassium, blood glucose, urine glucose while receiving long-term therapy; hypokalemia and hyperglycemia
• Assess joint mobility, pain, edema if product given intraarticularly
• B/P q4hr, pulse; notify prescriber of chest pain, crackles
• I&O ratio; be alert for decreasing urinary output, increasing edema; weight daily; notify prescriber of weekly gain >5 lb
• **Adrenal insufficiency:** weight loss, nausea, vomiting, confusion, anxiety, hypotension, weakness; plasma cortisol levels during long-term therapy (normal level: 138-635 nmol/L SI units when drawn at 8 AM)
• Growth in children receiving long-term treatment
• **Infection:** increased temperature, WBC, even after withdrawal of product; product masks infection
• **Beers:** avoid in older adults with delirium or at high risk for delirium; assess for confusion, delirium frequently
• **Pregnancy/breastfeeding:** use only if benefits outweigh risk to fetus, no well-controlled studies; do not breastfeed, excreted in breast milk

Evaluate:
• Therapeutic response: ease of respirations, decreased inflammation; decreased symptoms of adrenal insufficiency

Teach patient/family:
• To increase intake of potassium, calcium, protein
• To carry emergency ID as corticosteroid user, with product used and prescriber's information
• To notify prescriber if therapeutic response decreases; that dosage adjustment may be needed
• Not to discontinue abruptly because adrenal crisis can result
• To take PO with food, milk to decrease GI symptoms
• To avoid OTC products: salicylates, alcohol in cough products, cold preparations unless directed by prescriber; to avoid vaccinations because immunosuppression occurs
• **Adrenal insufficiency:** nausea, anorexia, fatigue, dizziness, dyspnea, weakness, joint pain
• **Cushingoid symptoms:** buffalo hump, moon face, rapid weight gain, excess sweating, when to notify prescriber
• **Infection:** to avoid persons with known infections; corticosteroids can mask symptoms of infection

---

metipranolol ophthalmic
See Appendix B

---

metoclopramide (Rx)
(met-oh-kloe-pra′mide)
Metonia ✦, Metozolv ODT, Reglan
Func. class.: Cholinergic, antiemetic, GI stimulant
Chem. class.: Central dopamine receptor antagonist

Do not confuse:
metoclopramide/metOLazone
Reglan/Megace/Renagel

ACTION: Enhances response to acetylcholine of tissue in upper GI tract, which causes the contraction of gastric muscle; relaxes pyloric, duodenal segments; increases peristalsis without stimulating secretions; blocks DOPamine in chemoreceptor trigger zone of CNS

USES: Prevention of nausea, vomiting induced by chemotherapy, radiation, delayed gastric emptying, gastroesophageal reflux

Unlabeled uses: Hiccups, migraines, breastfeeding induction, lung cancer

CONTRAINDICATIONS: Hypersensitivity to this product, procaine, or procainamide; seizure disorder, pheochromocytoma, GI obstruction

Precautions: Pregnancy, breastfeeding, GI hemorrhage, Parkinson's disease, breast cancer (prolactin dependent), abrupt discontinuation, cardiac disease, children, depression, diabetes mellitus, G6PD deficiency, geriatrics, heart failure, hypertension, infertility, malignant hyperthermia, methemoglobinemia, procainamide/paraben hypersensitivity, renal impairment

Black Box Warning: Tardive dyskinesia

DOSAGE AND ROUTES
Nausea/vomiting (chemotherapy)
• **Adult: IV** 1-2 mg/kg 30 min before administration of chemotherapy, then q2hr × 2 doses, then q3hr × 3 doses
• **Child (unlabeled): IV** 1-2 mg/kg/dose
Facilitate small-bowel intubation for radiologic exams
• **Adult and child >14 yr: IV** 10 mg over 1-2 min
• **Child <6 yr: IV** 0.1 mg/kg
• **Child 6-14 yr: IV** 2.5-5 mg
Diabetic gastroparesis
• **Adult: PO** 10 mg 30 min before meals, at bedtime × 2-8 wk
• **Geriatric: PO** 5 mg 30 min before meals, at bedtime, increase to 10 mg if needed
Gastroesophageal reflux
• **Adult: PO** 10-15 mg qid 30 min before meals and at bedtime

• **Child: PO** 0.4-0.8 mg/kg/day in 4 divided doses
Renal dose
• **Adult: PO** CCr <60 mL/min, 5 mg qid, max 20 mg/day, or CCr 10-15 mL/min give 75% of normal dose; CCr <10 mL/min give 50% of normal dose
Lactation induction (unlabeled)
• **Adult: PO** 10 mg bid-tid, may increase to 20-45 mg/day in divided doses
Non–small-cell lung cancer (NSCLC) radiation sensitizer (unlabeled)
• **Adult: IV** (Sensamide IV) 2 mg/kg given 1 hr before radiation therapy 3×/wk
Hiccups (unlabeled)
• **Adult: PO/IM/IV** 10 mg q6hr
Available forms: Tabs 5, 10 mg; syr 1 mg/mL ✿, 5 mg/5 mL; solution for inj 5 mg/mL; oral sol 5 mg/5 mL; orally disintegrating tab 5, 10 mg
Administer:
PO route
• $^{1}/_{2}$-1 hr before meals and at bedtime for better absorption
• Gum, hard candy, frequent rinsing of mouth for dry oral cavity
• **Oral disintegrating:** place on tongue, allow to dissolve, swallow; remove from blister immediately before use; give ≥30 min before meals and at bedtime; do not use if tablet breaks
IM route
• Give for postoperative nausea, vomiting before end of surgery
Direct IV route
• DiphenhydrAMINE IV or benztropine IM for EPS
• Undiluted if dose ≤10 mg; give over 2 min
Intermittent IV INFUSION route
• >10 mg may be diluted in ≥50 mL D_5W, NaCl, Ringer's, LR, given over ≥15 min
• Protect from light with aluminum foil during infusion
• Discard open ampules

Y-site compatibilities: Acetaminophen, alfentanil, amifostine, amikacin, aminophylline, ascorbic acid, atracurium, atropine, azaTHIOprine, aztreonam, bivalirudin,

M

bleomycin, bumetanide, buprenorphine, butorphanol, calcium chloride/gluconate, CARBOplatin, caspofungin, ceFAZolin, cefonicid, cefoperazone, cefotaxime, cefoTEtan, cefOXitin, cefTAZidime, ceftizoxime, cefTRIAXone, cefuroxime, chloramphenicol, chlorproMAZINE, cimetidine, ciprofloxacin, cisatracurium, CISplatin, cladribine, clindamycin, cyanocobalamin, cyclophosphamide, cycloSPORINE, cytarabine, DACTINomycin, DAPTOmycin, dexamethasone, dexmedetomidine, digoxin, diltiaZEM, diphenhydrAMINE, DOBUTamine, DOCEtaxel, DOPamine, doripenem, doxapram, DOXOrubicin hydrochloride, doxycycline, droperidol, enalaprilat, ePHEDrine, EPINEPHrine, epiRUBicin, epoetin alfa, ertapenem, erythromycin, esmolol, etoposide, etoposide phosphate, famotidine, fenoldopam, fentaNYL, filgrastim, fluconazole, fludarabine, folic acid, foscarnet, gallium nitrate, gemcitabine, gentamicin, glycopyrrolate, granisetron, heparin, hydrocortisone, HYDROmorphone, IDArubicin, ifosfamide, imipenem/cilastatin, indomethacin, insulin, isoproterenol, ketorolac, labetalol, leucovorin, levoFLOXacin, lidocaine, linezolid, LORazepam, magnesium sulfate, mannitol, mechlorethamine, melphalan, meperidine, meropenem, metaraminol, methadone, methotrexate, methoxamine, methyldopa, methylPREDNISolone, metoprolol, metroNIDAZOLE, miconazole, midazolam, milrinone, minocycline, mitoMYcin, morphine, moxalactam, multiple vitamins, nafcillin, nalbuphine, naloxone, nesiritide, nitroglycerin, nitroprusside, norepinephrine, octreotide, ondansetron, oxaliplatin, oxytocin, PACLitaxel, palonosetron, pantoprazole, papaverine, PEMEtrexed, penicillin G, pentamidine, pentazocine, PENTobarbital, PHENobarbital, phentolamine, phenylephrine, phytonadione, piperacillin/tazobactam, potassium chloride, procainamide, prochlorperazine, promethazine, propranolol, protamine, pyridoxine, quinupristin/dalfopristin, raNITIdine, remifentanil, riTUXimab, rocuronium, sargramostim, sodium acetate/bicarbonate, succinylcholine, SUFentanil, tacrolimus, teniposide, theophylline, thiamine, thiotepa, ticarcillin/clavulanate, tigecycline, tirofiban, tobramycin, tolazoline, topotecan, trastuzumab, trimethaphan, urokinase, vancomycin, vasopressin, vecuronium, verapamil, vinBLAStine, vinCRIStine, vinorelbine, voriconazole, zidovudine

SIDE EFFECTS

CNS: *Sedation, fatigue, restlessness, headache, sleeplessness, dystonia,* dizziness, drowsiness, suicidal ideation, seizures, EPS, neuroleptic malignant syndrome; tardive dyskinesia (>3 mo, high doses)

CV: Hypotension, supraventricular tachycardia

GI: Dry mouth, constipation, nausea, anorexia, vomiting, diarrhea

GU: Decreased libido, prolactin secretion, amenorrhea, galactorrhea

HEMA: Neutropenia, leukopenia, agranulocytosis

INTEG: Urticaria, rash

PHARMACOKINETICS

Metabolized by liver, excreted in urine, half-life $2\frac{1}{2}$-6 hr

PO: Onset $\frac{1}{2}$-1 hr, duration 1-2 hr

IM: Onset 10-15 min, duration 1-2 hr

IV: Onset 1-3 min, duration 1-2 hr

INTERACTIONS

• Avoid use with MAOIs; may increase hypertension in those patients

Increase: sedation—alcohol, other CNS depressants; avoid concurrent use

Increase: risk for EPS—haloperidol, phenothiazines; assess for EPS

Decrease: action—anticholinergics, opiates; avoid using together or assess carefully

Drug/Lab Test

Increase: prolactin, aldosterone, thyrotropin

NURSING CONSIDERATIONS
Assess:

Black Box Warning: **EPS, tardive dyskinesia;** more likely to occur in treatment >3 mo, geriatric patients and may be irreversible; assess for involuntary movements often; avoid using phenothiazines, haloperidol

• **Neuroleptic malignant syndrome:** hyperthermia, change in B/P, pulse, tachycardia, sweating, rigidity, altered consciousness (rare)

• ECG for QT prolongation, B/P, especially in renal patients

• Mental status: depression, anxiety, irritability

• GI complaints: nausea, vomiting, anorexia, constipation; assess bowel sounds

• **Pregnancy/breastfeeding:** use only if clearly needed; no studies in pregnancy; do not breastfeed, appears in breast milk

• **Beers:** avoid in older adults unless for gastroparesis; can cause extrapyramidal effects; monitor for EPS frequently

Evaluate:

• Therapeutic response: absence of nausea, vomiting, anorexia, fullness; decreased GERD

Teach patient/family:

• To avoid driving, other hazardous activities until stabilized on product

• To avoid alcohol, other CNS depressants that will enhance sedating properties of this product

Black Box Warning: Symptoms of EPS, tardive dyskinesia; to report to prescriber

• How to use oral disintegrating product

---

metolazone (Rx)

(me-tole′a-zone)
Func. class.: Diuretic, antihypertensive
Chem. class.: Thiazide-like quinazoline derivative

Do not confuse:
metolazone/methotrexate/ metoclopramide

ACTION: Acts on distal tubule by increasing excretion of water, sodium, chloride, potassium, magnesium, bicarbonate; decreases GFR

USES: Edema, hypertension
Unlabeled uses: Heart failure, nephrotic syndrome

CONTRAINDICATIONS: Pregnancy (preeclampsia, intrauterine growth retardation), hypersensitivity to thiazides, sulfonamides; anuria, coma, hepatic encephalopathy

Precautions: Pregnancy, breastfeeding, geriatric patients, hypokalemia, renal/hepatic disease, gout, COPD, lupus erythematosus, diabetes mellitus, hypotension, history of pancreatitis; hypersensitivity to sulfonamides, thiazides; electrolyte imbalance

DOSAGE AND ROUTES
Edema in heart failure/renal disease
• **Adult:** PO 5-10 mg/day; max 20 mg/day
Hypertension
• **Adult:** PO 2.5-5 mg/day
• **Child:** PO 0.2-0.4 mg/kg/day in divided doses q12-24hr
Available forms: Tabs 2.5, 5, 10 mg
Administer:
• In AM to avoid interference with sleep if using product as diuretic
• Potassium replacement if potassium <3 mg/dL
• With food if nausea occurs; absorption may be decreased slightly

SIDE EFFECTS
CNS: Drowsiness, lethargy
CV: *Orthostatic hypotension,* palpitations, hypotension, chest pain
ELECT: *Hypokalemia,* hypercalcemia, hyponatremia, hyperuricemia, hypomagnesemia, hypophosphatemia, hypovolemia
GI: *Nausea, vomiting, anorexia,* constipation, diarrhea, cramps, pancreatitis, GI irritation, dry mouth, jaundice, hepatitis
GU: *Urinary frequency,* polyuria, uremia, glucosuria, nocturia, impotence, *hyperuricemia*
HEMA: Aplastic anemia, hemolytic anemia, leukopenia, agranulocytosis, neutropenia
INTEG: *Rash,* urticaria, purpura, photosensitivity, fever, dry skin, toxic epidermal necrolysis, Stevens-Johnson syndrome
META: *Hyperglycemia,* increased creatinine, BUN
MS: Muscle cramps

M

Side effects: *italics* = common; red = life-threatening

PHARMACOKINETICS

Protein binding 33%, peak 8 hr, duration 12-24 hr, excreted unchanged by kidneys, crosses placenta, enters breast milk, half-life 14 hr

INTERACTIONS

Increase: hyperglycemia—antidiabetics

Increase: hypokalemia—mezlocillin, piperacillin, amphotericin B, glucocorticoids, digoxin, stimulant laxatives

Increase: hypotension—alcohol (large amounts), nitrates, antihypertensives, barbiturates, opioids

Increase: toxicity—lithium

Increase: metOLazone effects—loop diuretics

Decrease: action of metOLazone, increase renal failure risk—NSAIDs, salicylates

Drug/Food

Increase: severe hypokalemia—licorice

Drug/Herb

Decrease: antihypertensive effect—ephedra (ma huang)

Increase: antihypertensive effect—hawthorn

Drug/Lab Test

Increase: calcium, cholesterol, glucose, triglycerides

Decrease: potassium, sodium, chloride, magnesium, WBC, Hb

Interference: parathyroid function tests

NURSING CONSIDERATIONS

Assess:

• Weight, I&O daily to determine fluid loss; effect of product may be decreased if used daily

• **HF:** improvement in edema of feet, legs, sacral area daily if product being used

• **Hypertension:** B/P lying, standing; postural hypotension may occur

• **Electrolytes:** potassium, magnesium, sodium, chloride; include BUN, blood glucose, CBC, serum creatinine, blood pH, ABGs, uric acid, calcium

• **Hypokalemia:** postural hypotension, malaise, fatigue, tachycardia, leg cramps, weakness

• Rashes, temperature daily

• Confusion, especially among geriatric patients; take safety precautions if needed

• **Hepatic encephalopathy:** do not use in hepatic coma or precoma; fluctuations in electrolytes can occur rapidly and precipitate hepatic coma; use caution in patients with impaired hepatic function

• **Pregnancy/breastfeeding:** use in pregnancy only if needed, no well-controlled studies; do not breastfeed, appears in breast milk

• **Beers:** use with older adults may exacerbate or cause SIADH; monitor sodium level frequently

Evaluate:

• Therapeutic response: decreased edema, B/P

Teach patient/family:

• To rise slowly from lying or sitting position

• To notify prescriber of muscle weakness, cramps, nausea, dizziness

• That product may be taken with food or milk

• To use sunscreen, protective clothing for photosensitivity

• That blood glucose may be increased in diabetics

• To take early in day to avoid nocturia, to take at same time of day, not to skip or double doses, that skipped dose should be taken when remembered if not close to next dose

• To avoid alcohol

• To avoid sodium foods; to increase potassium foods in diet

• Not to stop product abruptly

TREATMENT OF OVERDOSE:

Lavage if taken orally; monitor electrolytes; administer dextrose in saline; monitor hydration, CV, renal status

---

⚠ HIGH ALERT

metoprolol (Rx)

(meh-toe′proe-lole)

Betaloc ✦, Lopressor, Toprol-XL

Func. class.: Antihypertensive, antianginal

Chem. class.: β₁-Blocker

Do not confuse:

Lopressor/Lyrica

Toprol-XL/Topamax

ACTION: Lowers B/P by β-blocking effects; reduces elevated renin plasma levels; blocks $β_2$-adrenergic receptors in bronchial, vascular smooth muscle only at high doses; negative chronotropic effect

USES: Mild to moderate hypertension, acute MI to reduce cardiovascular mortality, angina pectoris, NYHA class II, III heart failure, cardiomyopathy

Unlabeled uses: Migraine prevention, heart rate control for atrial fibrillation/flutter without accessory pathway, essential tremor, unstable angina

CONTRAINDICATIONS: Hypersensitivity to β-blockers, cardiogenic shock, heart block (2nd, 3rd degree), sinus bradycardia, sick sinus syndrome

Precautions: Pregnancy, breastfeeding, geriatric patients, major surgery, diabetes mellitus, thyroid/renal/hepatic disease, COPD, CAD, nonallergic bronchospasm, bronchial asthma, CVA, children, depression, vasospastic angina, pheochromocytoma

Black Box Warning: Abrupt discontinuation

DOSAGE AND ROUTES
Hypertension
• **Adult: PO** 50 mg bid or 100 mg/day; may give up to 100-450 mg in divided doses; **EXT REL** 25-100 mg daily, titrate at weekly intervals; max 400 mg/day
• **Geriatric: PO** 25 mg/day initially, increase weekly as needed
• **Child and adolescent 6-16 yr: PO EXT REL** 1 mg/kg up to 50 mg daily
Myocardial infarction
• **Adult: IV BOL** (early treatment) 5 mg q2min × 3, then 50 mg **PO** 15 min after last dose and q6hr × 48 hr; (late treatment) **PO** maintenance 50-100 mg bid for 1-3 yr
Heart failure (NYHA class II/III)
• **Adult: PO EXT REL** 25 mg daily × 2 wk (class II); 12.5 mg daily (class III)
Angina
• **Adult: PO** 100 mg/day as a single dose or in 2 divided doses, increase weekly prn or 100 mg **EXT REL** daily, max 400 mg/day ext rel
Migraine prevention (unlabeled)
• **Adult: PO** 25-100 mg bid; 50-200 mg daily (XL)
Heart rate control for atrial fibrillation/flutter without accessory pathway (unlabeled)
• **Adult: IV BOL** (acute setting) 2.5-5 mg over 2 min, may repeat dose × 3; **PO** (nonacute setting) 25-100 mg bid
Essential tremor (unlabeled)
• **Adult: PO** 50 mg/day, may increase, max 300 mg/day in divided doses; **EXT REL** 100 mg/day, max 400 mg/day

Available forms: Tabs 25, 50, 100 mg; inj 1 mg/mL; ext rel tab (succinate) (XL) 25, 50, 100, 200 mg; ext rel tabs, tartrate: 100 mg

Administer:
PO route
• Take apical pulse before giving; if <50 bpm, hold and notify prescriber
• Do not break, crush, or chew ext rel tabs
• Regular release tab after meals, at bedtime; tab may be crushed or swallowed whole; take at same time each day
• Store in dry area at room temperature; do not freeze
Direct IV route
• IV, undiluted, give 1 mg/mL over 1 min × 3 doses at 2- to 5-min intervals; start **PO** 15 min after last IV dose
• Check dose with another person to prevent errors that could be fatal

Y-site compatibilities: Abciximab, acyclovir, alemtuzumab, alfentanil, alteplase, amikacin, aminophylline, amiodarone, amphotericin B liposome, anidulafungin, argatroban, ascorbic acid, atracurium, atropine, azaTHIOprine, aztreonam, benztropine, bivalirudin, bleomycin, bumetanide, buprenorphine, butorphanol, calcium chloride/gluconate, CARBOplatin, caspofungin, ceFAZolin, cefonicid, cefoperazone, cefotaxime, cefoTEtan, cefOXitin, cefTAZidime, ceftizoxime, cefTRIAXone, cefuroxime, chloramphenicol, chlorproMAZINE, cimetidine, CISplatin, clindamycin, cyanocobalamin, cyclophosphamide, cycloSPORINE, cytarabine,

M

Side effects: *italics* = common; red = life-threatening

DACTINomycin, DAPTOmycin, dexamethasone, dexmedetomidine, digoxin, diltiaZEM, diphenhydrAMINE, DOBUTamine, DOCEtaxel, DOPamine, doxacurium, DOXOrubicin, doxycycline, enalaprilat, ePHEDrine, EPINEPHrine, epiRUBicin, epoetin alfa, eptifibatide, esmolol, etoposide, etoposide phosphate, famotidine, fenoldopam, fentaNYL, fluconazole, fludarabine, fluorouracil, folic acid, furosemide, ganciclovir, gemcitabine, gentamicin, glycopyrrolate, granisetron, heparin, hydrocortisone, HYDROmorphone, IDArubicin, ifosfamide, imipenem/cilastatin, indomethacin, insulin, isoproterenol, ketorolac, labetalol, linezolid, LORazepam, magnesium sulfate, mannitol, mechlorethamine, meperidine, metaraminol, methotrexate, methoxamine, methyldopate, methylPREDNISolone, metoclopramide, metroNIDAZOLE, midazolam, milrinone, mitoXANTRONE, morphine, multivitamins, nafcillin, nalbuphine, naloxone, nitroprusside, norepinephrine, octreotide, ondansetron, oxacillin, oxaliplatin, oxytocin, PACLitaxel, palonosetron, pancuronium, papaverine, PEMEtrexed, penicillin G, pentamidine, pentazocine, PENTobarbital, PHENobarbital, phentolamine, phenylephrine, phytonadione, piperacillin/tazobactam, potassium chloride, procainamide, prochlorperazine, promethazine, propranolol, protamine, pyridoxime, quinupristin/dalfopristin, raNITIdine, rocuronium, sodium bicarbonate, succinylcholine, SUFentanil, tacrolimus, teniposide, theophylline, thiamine, thiotepa, ticarcillin/clavulanate, tigecycline, tirofiban, tobramycin, tolazoline, trimetaphan, urokinase, vancomycin, vasopressin, vecuronium, verapamil, vinCRIStine, vinorelbine, voriconazole

SIDE EFFECTS

CNS: *Insomnia, dizziness,* mental changes, hallucinations, depression, anxiety, headaches, nightmares, confusion, fatigue, weakness

CV: *Hypotension,* bradycardia, HF, *palpitations,* dysrhythmias, cardiac arrest, AV block, pulmonary/peripheral edema, chest pain

EENT: Blurred vision

GI: *Nausea, vomiting,* colitis, cramps, *diarrhea,* constipation, flatulence, dry mouth, *hiccups*

GU: Impotence, urinary frequency

HEMA: Agranulocytosis, eosinophilia, thrombocytopenia, purpura

INTEG: Rash, purpura, alopecia, dry skin, urticaria, pruritus

RESP: Bronchospasm, dyspnea, wheezing

ENDO: Hyper/hypoglycemia

PHARMACOKINETICS

Half-life 3-7 hr, metabolized in liver (metabolites) by CYP2D6 🐾 some may be poor metabolizers, excreted in urine; crosses placenta, enters breast milk

PO: Peak 2-4 hr, duration 13-19 hr

PO-ER: Peak 6-12 hr, duration 24 hr

IV: Onset immediate, peak 20 min, duration 6-8 hr

INTERACTIONS

Increase: hypoglycemic digoxin, diltiazem, bradycardia effects—verapamil, insulin, oral antidiabetics

Increase: metoprolol level—cimetidine

Increase: effects of benzodiazepines

Decrease: antihypertensive effect—salicylates, NSAIDs

Decrease: metoprolol level—barbiturates

Decrease: effects of—xanthines

Decrease: effects of each—dopamine, theophylline

Drug/Food

Increase: absorption with food

Drug/Lab Test

Increase: blood glucose, BUN, potassium, ANA titer, serum lipoprotein, triglycerides, uric acid, alk phos, LDH, AST, ALT

NURSING CONSIDERATIONS

Assess:

Black Box Warning: **Abrupt withdrawal:** may cause MI, ventricular dysrhythmias, myocardial ischemia; taper dose over 7-14 days

• **Hypertension/angina:** ECG directly when giving IV during initial treatment

• I&O, weight daily; check for heart failure (weight gain, jugular venous distention, crackles, edema, dyspnea)

• Monitor B/P during initial treatment, periodically thereafter; pulse; note rate, rhythm, quality; apical/radial pulse before administration; notify prescriber of any significant changes or pulse <50 bpm; atropine 0.25-0.5 mg IV may be given for heart rate <40 bpm

• Baselines of renal, hepatic studies before therapy begins

• **Pregnancy/breastfeeding:** use only if clearly needed, no well-controlled studies, excreted in breast milk in small quantities; American Academy of Pediatrics considers this product to be compatible with breastfeeding

Evaluate:

• Therapeutic response: decreased B/P after 1-2 wk, decreased anginal pain

Teach patient/family:

• To take immediately after meals; to take medication at bedtime to prevent effect of orthostatic hypotension

Black Box Warning: Not to discontinue product abruptly; to taper over 2 wk; may cause angina

• Not to use OTC products containing α-adrenergic stimulants (nasal decongestants, OTC cold preparations) unless directed by prescriber; to avoid alcohol, smoking, sodium intake

• To report bradycardia, dizziness, confusion, depression, fever, sore throat, SOB, decreased vision to prescriber

• To take pulse, B/P at home; when to notify prescriber

• To comply with weight control, dietary adjustments, modified exercise program

• To carry emergency ID to identify product, allergies, prescriber

• To monitor blood glucose closely if diabetic, hypo/hyperglycemia

• To avoid hazardous activities if dizziness is present

• To report symptoms of heart failure: difficult breathing, especially on exertion or when lying down; night cough; swelling of extremities

• To rise slowly to decrease orthostatic hypertension

• To report Raynaud's symptoms

• That product may increase sensitivity to cold

TREATMENT OF OVERDOSE:
Lavage, IV atropine for bradycardia, IV theophylline for bronchospasm, digoxin, O₂, diuretic for cardiac failure, hemodialysis, administer vasopressor

---

RARELY USED

metreleptin
(met′-re-lep′-tin)
Myalept
Func. class.: Hormone replacement-leptin receptor agonist

USES: Complications caused by leptin deficiency in patients with congenital or acquired generalized lipodystrophy

CONTRAINDICATIONS: Hypersensitivity

Black Box Warning: Secondary malignancy, antimetreleptin antibodies

DOSAGE AND ROUTES

• **Adult/adolescent/child >40 kg: SUB-CUT** 2.5 mg/day (0.5 mL) initially, may increase or decrease dose by 1.25-2.5 mg/day (0.25-0.5 mL) as needed, max 10 mg/day (2 mL/day). **Females:** 5 mg/day (1 mL) initially; may increase or decrease dose by 1.25-2.5 mg/day (0.25-0.5 mL) as needed, max 10 mg/day (2 mL/day)

• **Adult/adolescent/child/neonate ≤40 kg: SUBCUT** 0.06 mg/kg/day (0.012 mL/kg) initially. Increase or decrease dose by 0.02 mg/kg/day (0.004 mL/kg) as needed, max 0.13 mg/kg/day (0.026 mL/kg/day). Give daily at the same time every day

metroNIDAZOLE (Rx)

(me-troe-ni′da-zole)

Flagyl, Flagyl ER

Func. class.: Antiinfective— miscellaneous

Chem. class.: Nitroimidazole derivative

Do not confuse:
metroNIDAZOLE/metFORMIN

ACTION: Direct-acting amebicide/ trichomonacide binds and disrupts DNA structure, thereby inhibiting bacterial nucleic acid synthesis

USES: Intestinal amebiasis, amebic abscess, trichomoniasis, refractory trichomoniasis, bacterial anaerobic infections, giardiasis, septicemia, endocarditis; bone, joint, lower respiratory tract infections; rosacea

CONTRAINDICATIONS: Pregnancy 1st trimester, breastfeeding, hypersensitivity to this product

Precautions: Pregnancy, geriatric patients, *Candida* infections, heart failure, fungal infection, dental disease, bone marrow suppression, hematologic disease, GI/renal/hepatic disease, contracted visual or color fields, blood dyscrasias, CNS disorders

Black Box Warning: Secondary malignancy

DOSAGE AND ROUTES
Trichomoniasis
• **Adult: PO** 500 mg bid × 7 days or 2 g as single dose; do not repeat treatment for 4-6 wk
• **Child ≥45 kg (unlabeled): PO** 2 g once
• **Child <45 kg (unlabeled): PO** 15 mg/ kg/day in 3 divided doses × 7-10 days
• **Infant (unlabeled): PO** 15 mg/kg/day divided in 3 doses × 7 days
Amebic hepatic abscess
• **Adult: PO** 750 mg tid × 7-10 days
• **Child: PO** 35-50 mg/kg/day in 3 divided doses × 7-10 days

Intestinal amebiasis
• **Adult: PO** 750 mg tid × 7-10 days
• **Child: PO** 35-50 mg/kg/day in 3 divided doses × 7-10 days, then oral iodoquinol
Anaerobic bacterial infections
• **Adult: IV INFUSION** 15 mg/kg over 1 hr, then 7.5 mg/kg **IV** or **PO** q6hr, not to exceed 4 g/day; 1st maintenance dose should be administered 6 hr after loading dose
Bacterial vaginosis
• **Adult: PO** regular rel 500 mg bid or 250 mg tid × 7 days; ext rel 750 mg/day × 7 days

Available forms: Tabs 250, 500 mg; ext rel tab (ER) 750 mg; caps 375 mg; injection solution 5 mg/mL
Administer:
• Store in light-resistant container; do not refrigerate
PO route
• Do not break, crush, or chew ext rel product, give on empty stomach
• PO with or after meals to avoid GI symptoms, metallic taste; crush tabs if needed
IV route
Intermittent INFUSION
• **Premixed infusion bags:** prediluted, ready to use 500 mg/100 mL (5 mg/mL); infusion over 30-60 min
• **Lyophilized vials:** dilute 500 mg with 4.4 mL sterile water, 0.9% NaCl; must be diluted further with ≤8 mg/mL with 0.9% NaCl, D_5W, or LR; must neutralize with 5 mEq $NaCO_3$/500 mg; CO_2 gas will be generated and may require venting; run over 30-60 min; primary IV must be discontinued; may be given as cont infusion; do not use aluminum products; IV may require venting
• Do not use aluminum needles or other products to prepare product

Y-site compatibilities: Acyclovir, alemtuzumab, alfentanil, allopurinol, amifostine, amikacin, aminophylline, amiodarone, ampicillin, ampicillin/sulbactam, anidulafungin, atracurium, bivalirudin, bumetanide, buprenorphine, busulfan, butorphanol, calcium acetate/chloride/

gluconate, CARBOplatin, ceFAZolin, cefepime, cefoperazone, cefotaxime, cefoTEtan, cefTRIAXone, cefuroxime, chloramphenicol, chlorproMAZINE, cimetidine, ciprofloxacin, cisatracurium, CISplatin, clindamycin, codeine, cyclophosphamide, cycloSPORINE, cytarabine, DACTINomycin, dexamethasone, dexmedetomidine, dexrazoxane, digoxin, diltiaZEM, dimenhyDRINATE, diphenhydrAMINE, DOBUTamine, DOCEtaxel, DOPamine, doripenem, doxacurium, doxapram, DOXOrubicin, DOXOrubicin liposome, doxycycline, droperidol, enalaprilat, ePHEDrine, EPINEPHrine, epiRUBicin, eptifibatide, ertapenem, erythromycin, esmolol, etoposide, etoposide phosphate, famotidine, fenoldopam, fentaNYL, fluconazole, fludarabine, fluorouracil, foscarnet, fosphenytoin, furosemide, gemcitabine, gentamicin, glycopyrrolate, granisetron, haloperidol, heparin, hydrALAZINE, hydrocortisone, HYDROmorphone, IDArubicin, ifosfamide, imipenem/cilastatin, inamrinone, insulin, isoproterenol, ketorolac, labetalol, leucovorin, levoFLOXacin, lidocaine, linezolid, LORazepam, magnesium sulfate, mannitol, mechlorethamine, melphalan, meperidine, meropenem, mesna, metaraminol, methotrexate, methyldopate, methylPREDNISolone, metoclopramide, metoprolol, midazolam, milrinone, mitoXANTRONE, morphine, nafcillin, nalbuphine, naloxone, nesiritide, niCARdipine, nitroglycerin, nitroprusside, norepinephrine, octreotide, ondansetron, oxaliplatin, oxytocin, PACLitaxel, palonosetron, pancuronium, pentamidine, pentazocine, PENTobarbital, perphenazine, PHENobarbital, phentolamine, phenylephrine, piperacillin/tazobactam, potassium chloride/phosphates, prochlorperazine, promethazine, propranolol, raNITIdine, remifentanil, riTUXimab, rocuronium, sargramostim, sodium acetate/bicarbonate/phosphates, streptozocin, succinylcholine, SUFentanil, tacrolimus, teniposide, theophylline, thiopental, thiotepa, ticarcillin/clavulanate, tigecycline, tirofiban, tobramycin, trastuzumab, trimethobenzamide, trimethoprim/sulfamethoxazole, vancomycin, vasopressin, vecuronium, verapamil, vinCRIStine, vinorelbine, voriconazole, zidovudine, zoledronic acid

SIDE EFFECTS

CNS: *Headache, dizziness,* confusion, irritability, restlessness, ataxia, depression, fatigue, drowsiness, insomnia, paresthesia, peripheral neuropathy, seizures, incoordination, depression, encephalopathy, aseptic meningitis (IV)

CV: Flattening of T waves

EENT: Blurred vision, sore throat, retinal edema, dry mouth, metallic taste, furry tongue, glossitis, stomatitis, photophobia, optic neuritis

GI: *Nausea, vomiting, diarrhea,* epigastric distress, *anorexia,* constipation, *abdominal cramps,* CDAD, xerostomia, metallic taste, abdominal pain, pancreatitis

HEMA: Leukopenia, bone marrow supression, aplasia, thrombocytopenia

GU: Genital candida infection

INTEG: Rash, pruritus, urticaria, flushing, Stevens-Johnson syndrome, phlebitis at injection site, toxic epidermal necrolysis

PHARMACOKINETICS

Crosses placenta, enters breast milk, metabolized by liver 30%-60%, excreted in urine (60%-80%), half-life 6-8 hr

PO: Peak 2 hr, absorbed 80%-85%

IV: Onset immediate, peak end of infusion

INTERACTIONS

• Do not use with zalcitabine, disulfiram

Decrease: metroNIDAZOLE level—cholestyramine

Increase: disulfiram reaction—alcohol, oral ritonavir, any product with alcohol

Increase: busulfan toxicity—busulfan; avoid concurrent use

Increase: metroNIDAZOLE level, toxicity—cimetidine

Increase: lithium, CYP3A4 substrates

Increase: action of warfarin, phenytoin, lithium, fosphenytoin

Increase: leukopenia—azaTHIOprine, fluorouracil

Drug/Lab Test

Altered: AST, ALT, LDH, glucose

Decrease: WBC, neutrophils

False decrease: triglycerides

Side effects: *italics* = common; red = life-threatening

NURSING CONSIDERATIONS
Assess:

• **Infection:** WBC, wound symptoms, fever, skin or vaginal secretions; start treatment after C&S is obtained, waiting for results is not needed; for opportunistic fungal infections; superinfection: fever, monilial growth, fatigue, malaise

• Stools during entire treatment; should be clear at end of therapy; stools should be free of parasites for 1 yr before patient considered cured (amebiasis)

• Vision by ophthalmic exam during, after therapy; vision problems often occur

• **Allergic reaction:** fever, rash, itching, chills; product should be discontinued if these occur, if fever, facial swelling, blisters occur, discontinue immediately

• Renal, reproductive dysfunction: dysuria, polyuria, impotence, dyspareunia, decreased libido, I&O; weight daily

Black Box Warning: Secondary malignancy: use only when indicated; avoid unnecessary use

• **Giardiasis:** stool samples before starting to confirm diagnosis, then 3-4 week after treatment

• I&O, weight, sodium, other electrolytes, product contains sodium

• **Pregnancy/breastfeeding:** not to be used in breastfeeding or 1st trimester of pregnancy

Evaluate:

• Therapeutic response: decreased symptoms of infection

Teach patient/family:

• That urine may turn dark reddish brown; that product may cause metallic taste; that both are normal

• About proper hygiene after bowel movement; handwashing technique

• To notify physician about numbness or tingling of extremities

• To avoid hazardous activities because dizziness can occur

• About need for compliance with dosage schedule, duration of treatment; to take extended-release tabs 1 hr before or 2 hr after meals; to take PO with meals to prevent GI upset

• To discuss all OTC, Rx, herbals, supplements taken with provider

• To notify provider immediately of rash, fever, facial swelling, blisters

• To use condoms if treatment for trichomoniasis or cross-contamination may occur; to notify prescriber if pregnant or planning to become pregnant; that treatment of both partners is necessary for trichomoniasis

• To use frequent sips of water, sugarless gum, candy for dry mouth

• Not to drink alcohol or use preparations containing alcohol during use or for 48 hr after use of product; disulfiram-like reaction can occur

• To notify if pregnancy is planned or suspected, or if breastfeeding

---

metroNIDAZOLE (topical, vaginal)
(met-roe-ni′da-zole)

MetroCream, MetroGel, MetroGel Vaginal, MetroLotion, Noritate, Rosasol ✦, Rosadan, Vandazole

Func. class.: Antiprotozoal, antibacterial

Chem. class.: Nitroimidazole

ACTION: Antibacterial and antiprotozoal activity may result from interacting with DNA

USES: Acne rosacea, bacterial vaginosis

CONTRAINDICATIONS: Hypersensitivity to this product or nitroimidazoles, parabens

Precautions: Hepatic disease, blood dyscrasias; CNS conditions (vaginal), children, pregnancy

DOSAGE AND ROUTES
Acne rosacea

• **Adult: TOP** apply to affected areas bid (0.75%) or daily (1%); adjust therapy based on response

Bacterial vaginosis

• **Adult: VAG** 1 applicatorful daily × 5 days

Available forms: Topical cream 0.75%, 1%; gel 0.75%, 1%; lotion 0.75%; vaginal gel 0.75%

Administer:
Topical route
• Topical skin products are not for intravaginal therapy and are for external use only; do not use skin products near the eyes, nose, or mouth
• Wash hands before and after use; wash affected area and gently pat dry
• **Cream/gel/lotion:** Apply a thin film to the cleansed affected area; massage gently into affected areas

Intravaginal route
• Only use dosage formulations specified for intravaginal use; intravaginal dosage forms are not for topical therapy; do not ingest
• Avoid vaginal intercourse during treatment
• **Cream:** Use applicator(s) supplied by the manufacturer

SIDE EFFECTS
GU: Vaginitis, cervicitis
GI: Nausea, vomiting, cramping
INTEG: Redness, burning, dermatitis, rash, pruritus

INTERACTIONS
• MetroNIDAZOLE may increase warfarin anticoagulant effect
• Caution with drinking alcohol or using disulfiram while using metroNIDAZOLE products(vaginal gel)
• Possible lithium toxicity (vaginal gel)

NURSING CONSIDERATIONS
Assess:
• **Allergic reaction:** assess for hypersensitivity; product may need to be discontinued
• **Infection:** assess for number of lesions and severity of acne rosacea, itching in vaginosis
• **Pregnancy/breastfeeding:** not to be used in breastfeeding, systemic absorption; use in pregnancy only if clearly needed, no adequate studies

Evaluate:
• Decreased severity of acne rosacea, infection in vaginosis

Teach patient/family:
• That topical skin products are not for intravaginal therapy and are for external use only; not to use skin products near the eyes, nose, or mouth
• To wash hands before and after use; to wash affected area and gently pat dry
• **Cream/gel/lotion:** to apply a thin film to the cleansed affected area and massage gently into affected areas
• **Intravaginal route:** to use only dosage formulations specified for intravaginal use; not to ingest intravaginal dosage forms because these are not for topical therapy; to avoid vaginal intercourse during treatment
• **Cream:** to use applicator(s) supplied by the manufacturer

---

micafungin (Rx)
(my-ca-fun′gin)
Mycamine
Func. class.: Antifungal, systemic
Chem. class.: Echinocandin

M

ACTION: Inhibits an essential component of fungal cell walls; causes direct damage to fungal cell wall

USES: Treatment of esophageal candidiasis; prophylaxis for *Candida* infections in patients undergoing hematopoietic stem-cell transplantation (HSCT); susceptible *Candida* sp.: *C. albicans, C. glabrata, C. krusei, C. parapsilosis, C. tropicalis*

CONTRAINDICATIONS: Hypersensitivity to this product or other echinocandins
Precautions: Pregnancy, breastfeeding, children, geriatric patients, severe hepatic disease, renal impairment, hemolytic anemia

DOSAGE AND ROUTES
Esophageal candidiasis
• **Adult: IV INFUSION** 150 mg/day given over 1 hr × 15 days
• **Child ≥4 mo, >30 kg: IV INFUSION** 2.5 mg/kg/day, max 150 mg/day

---

Side effects: *italics* = common; red = life-threatening

• **Child ≥4 mo, ≤30 kg: IV INFUSION**
3 mg/kg/day

Candidemia/acute disseminated candidiasis, abscess/peritonitis

• **Adult: IV** 100 mg/day over 1 hr × 15 days
• **Child ≥4 mo and >30 kg: IV** 2 mg/kg/day, max 100 mg/day; **≥4 mo and ≤30 kg:** 2 mg/kg/day

Prophylaxis for *Candida* infections in hemapoietic stem-cell transplant patients

• **Adult: IV INFUSION** 50 mg/day given over 1 hr
• **Child ≥4 mo: IV INFUSION** 2 mg/kg/day, max 100 mg/day
• **Adolescent/child/infant ≥4 mo: IV INFUSION** 1 mg/kg/day, max 50 mg/day

Administer:

Available forms: Powder for inj 50 mg, in single-dose vials 50-, 100-mg vial

IV Route

Intermittent IV Infusion

• For adults: Reconstitute 50 mg vial/5 mL 0.9% NaCl or D5W (10mg/mL); or 100mg vial/ 5 mL 0.9% NaCl or D5W (20mg/mL), dissolve by swirling, do not shake; **Prophylaxis of *Candida* infections:** 50mg/100mL of 0.9%NaCl or D5W; **Esophageal candidiasis:** 150mg/100 mL of 0.9% NaCL or D5W; stable for 24 hr at room temperature, protect from light; Child: take ordered dose and divide final concentration either 10 mg/mL for the 50mL vial or 20 mg/mL for the 100ml vial, add volume withdrawn to IV bag/syringe with 0.9% NaCl or D5W, ensure concentration is between 0.5-4 mg/mL, flush line before and after use with 0.9% NaCl, give over 1 hr, > 1.5mg/mL concentrations should be given by central line, do not give rapidly as histamine reactions may occur

Y-site compatibilities: Aminophylline, bumetanide, calcium chloride/gluconate, cycloSPORINE, DOPamine, eptifibatide, esmolol, fenoldopam, furosemide, heparin, HYDROmorphone, lidocaine, LORazepam, magnesium sulfate, milrinone, nitroglycerin, nitroprusside, norepinephrine, phenylephrine, potassium chloride, potassium phosphate, tacrolimus, vasopressin

SIDE EFFECTS

GI: Abdominal pain, *nausea, anorexia, vomiting, diarrhea, hyperbilirubinemia,* hepatitis
GU: Renal failure
HEMA: Hemolytic anemia
INTEG: *Rash, pruritus, inj-site pain*
MISC: Allergic reactions

PHARMACOKINETICS

Metabolized in liver; excreted in feces, urine; terminal half-life 14-17.2 hr; protein binding 99%

INTERACTIONS

Increase: plasma concentrations—CYP3A4 substrates (aripiprazole, dofetilide, pimozide); itraconazole, sirolimus, NIFEdipine; may need dosage reduction

Drug/Lab Test

Increase: ALT/AST, alk phos, bilirubin, potassium, sodium, LDH, BUN, creatinine
Decrease: blood glucose platelets, Hgb, WBCs

NURSING CONSIDERATIONS

Assess:

• **Infection,** clearing of cultures during treatment; obtain culture at baseline and during treatment; product may be started as soon as culture is taken (esophageal candidiasis); monitor cultures during HSCT for prevention of *Candida* infections
• CBC (RBC, Hct, Hgb), differential, platelet count baseline, periodically; notify prescriber of results
• Renal studies: BUN, urine CCr, electrolytes before and during therapy
• Hepatic studies before and during treatment: bilirubin, AST, ALT, alk phos as needed
• **For hypersensitivity:** rash, pruritus, facial swelling, phlebitis
• For hemolytic anemia
• **GI symptoms:** frequency of stools, cramping; if severe diarrhea occurs, electrolytes may need to be given
• **Pregnancy/breastfeeding:** use cautiously in breastfeeding; use in pregnancy if benefit outweighs risk to fetus, no adequate studies

Evaluate:

• Therapeutic response: prevention of *Candida* infection with HSCT or de-

creased symptoms of *Candida* infection, negative culture
Teach patient/family:
• To avoid breastfeeding while taking this product
• To report bleeding, facial swelling, wheezing, difficulty breathing, itching, rash, hives, increasing warmth, flushing
• To report signs of infection: increased temperature, sore throat, flulike symptoms

---

miconazole
(mi-kon′a-zole)
Oravig
miconazole nitrate
Baza, Desenex, Fungoid, Lotrimin AF, Micaderm, Micatin, Micozole ✦, Monistat-1, Monistat-3, Monistat-7, M-Zole 3, Vagistat-3, Zeasorb-AF
Func. class.: Antifungal
Chem. class.: Imidazole

Do not confuse:
miconazole/clotrimazole/
metroNIDAZOLE

ACTION: Antifungal activity results from disruption of cell membrane permeability

USES: Treatment of topical fungal infection, vulvovaginal candidiasis; athlete's foot (tinea pedis), jock itch (tinea cruris), and ringworm (tinea corporis)

CONTRAINDICATIONS: Hypersensitivity to this product or imidazoles; pregnancy first trimester (vaginal)
Precautions: Breastfeeding, children

DOSAGE AND ROUTES
Oropharyngeal candidiasis (thrush)
• Adult/adolescent ≥16 yr: BUCCAL apply 1 tab (50 mg) to upper gum region, just above incisor daily × 14 days
Tinea corporis, cruris, pedis; cutaneous candidiasis
• Adult/child >2 yr: TOP apply bid × 2-4 wk

Tinea versicolor
• Adult/child >2 yr: TOP use bid × 2 wk, apply sparingly every day
Vulvovaginal candidiasis
• Adult/child ≥12 yr: VAG 1 applicatorful of Monistat-7 (100 mg) or 1 supp (100 mg) at bedtime × 7 days, repeat if needed, or Monistat-3 (200 mg) × 3 days or a 1200 mg supp × 1 day
Available forms: Topical cream, ointment, solution, lotion, powder, aerosol, powder 2%; aerosol spray 2%; vag cream 2, 4%; vag supp 100, 200, 1200 mg; buccal tab 50 mg
Administer:
Transmucosal use (adhesive buccal tablet)
• Apply tab in the morning after brushing teeth, use dry hands
• Place the rounded surface of the tab against the upper gum just above the incisor tooth, hold in place with slight pressure over the upper lip for 30 sec to assure adhesion
• Although the tab is rounded on one side for comfort, the flat side may also be applied to the gum
• The tab will gradually dissolve
• Administration of subsequent tab should be made to alternate sides of the mouth
• Before applying the next tab, clear away any remaining tab material
• Do not crush, chew, or swallow; food and drink can be taken normally; avoid chewing gum
• If tab does not adhere or falls off within the first 6 hr, the same tab should be repositioned immediately; if the tab still does not adhere, a new tab should be used
• If the tab falls off or is swallowed after it was in place for 6 hr or more, a new tab should not be applied until the next regularly scheduled dose
Topical route
• Topical skin products are not for intravaginal therapy and are for external use only; do not use skin products near the eyes, nose, or mouth
• Wash hands before and after use; wash affected area and gently pat dry
• **Cream/ointment/lotion/solution:** apply a thin film to the cleansed affected area; massage gently into affected areas

• **Solution formulations:** apply a thin film to the cleansed affected area; massage gently into affected areas; if using a solution-soaked pledget, patient may use more than 1 pledget per application as needed to treat affected areas, but each pledget should be used only once and then discarded

• **Intravaginal route:** only use dosage formulations specified for intravaginal use; intravaginal dosage forms are not for topical therapy; do not ingest

• **Suppository:** unwrap vaginal ovule (suppository) before insertion; use applicator(s) supplied by the manufacturer

• **Cream:** use applicator(s) supplied by the manufacturer

SIDE EFFECTS

CNS: Headache
GI: Diarrhea, nausea
GU: Pruritus, irritation, vaginal burning
INTEG: Burning, dermatitis, rash

DRUG INTERACTIONS

Increase: anticoagulant effect—(buccal) monitor PT, INR
Decrease: effect (vaginal)—progesterone
Drug/Lab
Decrease: WBC, RBC (buccal)

NURSING CONSIDERATIONS
Assess:

• **Allergic reaction:** assess for hypersensitivity; product may need to be discontinued
• **Infection:** assess for severity of infection
• **Pregnancy/breastfeeding:** use cautiously in breastfeeding; use PO form in pregnancy only if benefits outweigh risk to fetus, no adequate studies
Evaluate:
• Decreasing severity of infection
Teach patient/family:
Topical route
• That topical skin products are not for intravaginal therapy and are for external use only; not to use skin products near the eyes, nose, or mouth
• To wash hands before and after use; wash affected area and gently pat dry
• **Cream/ointment/lotion/solution:** to apply a thin film to the cleansed affected area and massage gently into affected areas

• **Solution formulations:** to shake well before use, apply a thin film to the cleansed affected area, and massage gently into affected areas
Intravaginal route
• To only use dosage formulations specified for intravaginal use; not to ingest intravaginal dosage forms; not to use tampons, douches, spermicides; not to engage in sexual activity; product may damage condoms, diaphragms, cervical caps

• **Suppository:** to unwrap vaginal ovule (suppository) before inserting; to use applicator(s) supplied by the manufacturer

• **Cream:** to use applicator(s) supplied by the manufacturer

---

⚠ HIGH ALERT

midazolam (Rx)
(mid'ay-zoe-lam)
Func. class.: Anxiolytic
Chem. class.: Benzodiazepine, short-acting

Controlled Substance Schedule IV

ACTION: Depresses subcortical levels in CNS; may act on limbic system, reticular formation; may potentiate γ-aminobutyric acid (GABA) by binding to specific benzodiazepine receptors

USES: Preoperative sedation, general anesthesia induction, sedation for diagnostic endoscopic procedures, intubation, anxiety
Unlabeled uses: Refractory status epilepticus

CONTRAINDICATIONS: Pregnancy, hypersensitivity to benzodiazepines, acute closed-angle glaucoma, epidural/intrathecal use
Precautions: Breastfeeding, children, geriatric patients, COPD, HF, chronic renal failure, chills, debilitated patients, hepatic disease, shock, coma, alcohol intoxication, status asthmaticus

---

Black Box Warning: Neonates (contains benzyl alcohol), IV administration, respiratory depression/insufficiency, specialized care setting, experienced clinician, coadministration with other CNS depressants

DOSAGE AND ROUTES
Preoperative sedation/amnesia induction
• **Adult/child ≥12 yr:** IM 0.07-0.08 mg/kg $^1/_2$-1 hr before general anesthesia
• **Child 6 yr-12 yr:** IV 0.025-0.05 mg/kg; total dose of 0.4 mg/kg may be necessary
• **Child 6 mo-5 yr:** IV 0.05-0.1 mg/kg; total dose of 0.6 mg/kg may be necessary
Induction of general anesthesia
• **Adult >55 yr:** (ASA I/II) IV 150-300 mcg/kg over 30 sec; (ASA III) IV limit dose to 250 mcg/kg (nonpremedicated) or 150 mcg/kg (premedicated)
• **Adult <55 yr:** IV 200-350 mcg/kg over 20-30 sec; if patient has not received premedication, may repeat by giving 20% of original dose; if patient has received premedication, reduce dose by 50 mcg/kg
• **Child:** no safe and effective dose established; however, doses of 50-200 mcg/kg IV have been used
Continuous infusion for mechanical ventilation (critical care)
• **Adult:** IV 0.01-0.05 mg/kg over several min; repeat at 10- to 15-min intervals until adequate sedation, then 0.02-0.10 mg/kg/hr maintenance; adjust as needed
• **Child:** IV 0.05-0.2 mg/kg over 2-3 min then 0.06-0.12 mg/kg/hr by cont infusion; adjust as needed
• **Neonate:** IV 0.03 mg/kg/hr, titrate using lowest dose
Status epilepticus (unlabeled)
• **Child and infant >2 mo:** IV 0.15 mg/kg then **CONT IV** 1 mcg/kg/min, titrate upward q5min until seizures controlled
Available forms: Inj 1, 5 mg/mL (preservative free); injection 1 mg/mL, 5 mg/mL; syr 2 mg/mL

Administer:
• Store at room temperature; protect from light
PO route (syrup)
• **Press-in-bottle adaptor (PIBA)** Remove cap of press-in bottle adapter, push adapter into neck of bottle; close with cap; remove cap, insert tip of dispenser, insert into adapter; turn upside-down, withdraw correct dose; place in mouth
IM route
• IM deep into large muscle mass
IV route
• May be given diluted or undiluted 1 mg/mL or 5 mg/mL (undiluted) or 0.03-3 mL (diluted)
• After diluting with D_5W or 0.9% NaCl, give over 2-5 min (conscious sedation) or over 30 sec (anesthesia induction)

Continuous IV infusion route
• Dilute in 0.9% NaCl or D5W to 0.5-1 mg/mL, dose is calculated on patient's weight and use

Black Box Warning: Do not use rapid injection in neonates

Y-site compatibilities: Abciximab, acetaminophen, alemtuzumab, alfentanil, amikacin, amiodarone, anidulafungin, argatroban, atracurium, atropine, aztreonam, benzotropine, calcium gluconate, ceFAZolin, cefotaxime, cefOXitine, cefTRIAXone, cimetidine, ciprofloxacin, CISplatin, clindamycin, cloNIDine, cyanocobalamin, cycloSPORINE, DACTINomycin, digoxin, diltiaZEM, diphenhydrAMINE, DOCEtaxel, DOPamine, doxycycline, enalaprilat, EPINEPHrine, erythromycin, esmolol, etomidate, etoposide, famotidine, fentaNYL, fluconazole, folic acid, gatifloxacin, gemcitabine, gentamicin, glycopyrrolate, granisetron, heparin, hetastarch, HYDROmorphone, hydrOXYzine, inamrinone, isoproterenol, labetalol, lactated Ringer's, levoFLOXacin, lidocaine, linezolid, LORazepam, magnesium, mannitol, meperidine, methadone, methyldopa, methylPREDNISolone, metoclopramide, metoprolol,

M

Side effects: *italics* = common; red = life-threatening

metroNIDAZOLE, milrinone, morphine, nalbuphine, naloxone, niCARdipine, nitroglycerin, nitroprusside, norepinephrine, ondansetron, oxacillin, oxytocin, PACLitaxel, palonosetron, pancuronium, papaverine, phytonadione, piperacillin, potassium chloride, propranolol, protamine, pyridoxine, raNITIdine, remifentanil, sodium nitroprusside, succinylcholine, SUFentanil, teniposide, theophylline, thiotepa, ticarcillin, tobramycin, vancomycin, vasopressin, vecuronium, verapamil, voriconazole, zoledronic acid

SIDE EFFECTS

CNS: Retrograde amnesia, headache, paresthesia, chills, paradoxic reactions
CV: Hypotension, PVCs
EENT: Nystagmus
GI: *Nausea, vomiting*
INTEG: Urticaria; pain, swelling, pruritus at inj site; rash
RESP: Coughing, apnea, respiratory depression

PHARMACOKINETICS

Protein binding 97%; half-life 1-5 hr, metabolized in liver; by CYP3A4 to metabolites excreted in urine; crosses placenta, blood-brain barrier
PO: Onset 10-30 min
IM: Onset 15 min, peak $^1/_2$-1 hr, duration 2-3 hr
IV: Onset 1.5-5 min, onset of anesthesia $1^1/_2$-$2^1/_2$ min, duration 2 hr

INTERACTIONS

Increase: extended half-life—CYP3A4 inhibitors (cimetidine, erythromycin, raNITIdine), adjust dose if needed
Increase: respiratory depression—other CNS depressants, alcohol, barbiturates, opiate analgesics, verapamil, ritonavir, indinavir, fluvoxaMINE, protease inhibitors
Decrease: midazolam metabolism—CYP3A4 inducers (azole antifungals, theophylline), adjust dose if needed
Drug/Herb
Increase: sedation—kava, valerian

Decrease: midazolam effect—St. John's wort
Drug/Food
Increase: (PO) midazolam effect—grapefruit juice, do not use together

NURSING CONSIDERATIONS
Assess:
• B/P, pulse, respirations during IV; emergency equipment should be nearby
• Inj site for redness, pain, swelling

> **Black Box Warning:** Should be used only in a specialized care setting by those trained in use

> **Black Box Warning: Respiratory depression/insufficiency:** apnea, respiratory depression may be increased in geriatric patients

• Assistance with ambulation until drowsy period ends
• Immediate availability of resuscitation equipment, O_2 to support airway; do not give by rapid bolus
• **Beers:** avoid in older adults with delirium or at high risk for delirium; assess frequently for confusion, delirium; degree of amnesia in geriatric patients may be increased
• **Pregnancy/breastfeeding:** do not use in pregnancy; avoid use in breastfeeding, excreted in breast milk
Evaluate:
• Therapeutic response: induction of sedation, general anesthesia
Teach patient/family:
• That amnesia occurs; that events may not be remembered; to give with instructions
• To avoid driving, other hazardous activities until effects are known
• Reason for product, expected results

TREATMENT OF OVERDOSE:
Flumazenil, O_2

midostaurin
(mye-doe-staw´-rin)
Rydapt
Func. class.: Antineoplastic

USES: Newly diagnosed FLT3 mutation–positive AML in combination with standard cytarabine and DAUNOrubicin induction and consolidation therapy and for the treatment of aggressive systemic mastocytosis, systemic mastocytosis with associated hematologic neoplasm, or mast cell leukemia

DOSAGE AND ROUTES
Newly diagnosed FLT3 mutation–positive AML
• **Adult: PO** 50 mg bid on days 8 to 21 of each cycle of induction therapy with cytarabine and DAUNOrubicin; additionally, give midostaurin 50 mg bid on days 8 to 21 of each cycle of consolidation with high-dose cytarabine therapy

Aggressive systemic mastocytosis, systemic mastocytosis
• **Adult: PO** 100 mg bid until disease progression

miglitol (Rx)
(mig´lih-tol)
Glyset
Func. class.: Oral hypoglycemic
Chem. class.: α-Glucosidase inhibitor

ACTION: Delays digestion and absorption of ingested carbohydrates, which results in a smaller rise in blood glucose after meals; does not increase insulin production

USES: Type 2 diabetes mellitus
Unlabeled uses: Type 1 diabetes mellitus

CONTRAINDICATIONS: Hypersensitivity, diabetic ketoacidosis, cirrhosis, inflammatory bowel disease, colonic ulceration, partial intestinal obstruction, chronic intestinal disease, ileus

Precautions: Pregnancy, breastfeeding, children, diarrhea, hiatal hernia, hypoglycemia, renal disease, type 1 diabetes, vomiting

DOSAGE AND ROUTES
• **Adult: PO** 25 mg tid initially, with 1st bite of meal; maintenance dose may be increased to 50 mg tid; may be increased to 100 mg tid if needed with dosage adjustment at 4- to 8-wk intervals

Available forms: Tabs 25, 50, 100 mg
Administer:
• Tid with first bite of each meal
• Store in tight container at room temperature

SIDE EFFECTS
GI: *Abdominal pain, diarrhea, flatulence,* hepatotoxicity
INTEG: Rash

PHARMACOKINETICS
Peak 2-3 hr, not metabolized, excreted in urine as unchanged product, half-life 2 hr

INTERACTIONS
Increase: hypoglycemia risk—insulin, other antidiabetics
Decrease: levels of digoxin, propranolol, raNITIdine; adjust dose as needed
Decrease: miglitol levels—digestive enzymes, intestinal adsorbents; do not use together

Drug/Food
Increase: diarrhea—carbohydrates

NURSING CONSIDERATIONS
Assess:
• **Hypo/hyperglycemia;** even though product does not cause hypoglycemia, if patient receiving sulfonylureas or insulin, hypoglycemia may be additive (rare)
• Blood glucose levels, hemoglobin, A1c, LFTs; if hypoglycemia occurs with monotherapy, treat with glucose
• Identify medical regimen prescribed—diet, exercise, lab work

M

• Monitor blood glucose testing more often in stress, trauma, surgery

• **Pregnancy/breastfeeding:** use of insulin during pregnancy is recommended, don't use this product unless clearly needed; excreted in breast milk, avoid use

Evaluate:

• Therapeutic response: decreased signs, symptoms of diabetes mellitus (polyuria, polydipsia, polyphagia; clear sensorium, absence of dizziness; stable gait); improved blood glucose, A1c

Teach patient/family:

• About the symptoms of hypo/hyperglycemia; what to do about each; that during periods of stress, infection, or surgery, insulin may be required

• To carry oral glucose or glucagon to treat low blood sugar, do not use simple sugar in fruit juices, candy, table sugar

• How to use a glucose monitor and when to monitor; how to identify low blood glucose levels

• That medication must be taken as prescribed, tid with first bite of each meal; about consequences of discontinuing medication abruptly

• To avoid OTC medications unless approved by health care provider

• That diabetes is lifelong; that product is not a cure; to continue with medical regimen of diet, exercise, lab work

• To carry ID for emergency purposes

• About GI side effects that are common during several weeks of treatment, that they improve with continued treatment

---

⚠ **HIGH ALERT**

milrinone (Rx)

(mill′rih-nohn)

Func. class.: Inotropic/vasodilator agent

Chem. class.: Bipyridine phosphodiesterase inhibitor

ACTION: Positive inotropic agent; increases contractility of cardiac muscle with vasodilator properties; reduces preload and afterload by direct relaxation on vascular smooth muscle

USES: Short-term management of advanced heart failure that has not responded to other medication

Unlabeled uses: Adolescents, children, infants

CONTRAINDICATIONS: Hypersensitivity to this product, severe aortic disease, severe pulmonic valvular disease, acute MI

Precautions: Pregnancy, breastfeeding, children, geriatric patients, renal/hepatic disease, atrial flutter/fibrillation

DOSAGE AND ROUTES

Short-term treatment of acutely decompensated heart failure

• **Adult:** IV BOL 50 mcg/kg given over 10 min (loading dose); start infusion of 0.375-0.75 mcg/kg/min, titrate based on response

• **Adolescent/child/infant (unlabeled):** IV 50 mcg/kg over 10-60 min, then 0.5-0.75 mcg/kg/min

Renal dose

• **Adult:** IV CCr 41-50 mL/min, 0.43 mcg/kg/min, titrate up; CCr 31-40 mL/min, 0.38 mcg/kg/min, titrate up; CCr 21-30 mL/min, 0.33 mcg/kg/min, titrate up; CCr 11-20 mL/min, 0.28 mcg/kg/min; CCr 6-10 mL/min, 0.23 mcg/kg/min; CCr ≤5 mL/min, 0.20 mcg/kg/min; max for all doses 0.75 mcg/kg/min

Available forms: Inj 1 mg/mL; premixed inj 200 mcg/mL in D₅W

Administer:

• Potassium supplements if ordered for potassium levels <3 mg/dL

Direct IV route

• Give IV loading dose undiluted over 10 min, use infusion device

Continuous IV route

• Dilute 20-mg vial with 80, 113, 180 mL of 0.45% NaCl, 0.9% NaCl, or D₅W to a concentration of 200, 150, 100 mcg/mL, respectively

• Titrate rate based on hemodynamic and clinical response, use infusion device

• Precipitation will form when furosemide is injected into line with milrinone

---

Y-site compatibilities: Acyclovir, alfentanil, allopurinol, amifostine, amikacin, aminocaproic acid, aminophylline, amiodarone, amphotericin B liposome, ampicillin, ampicillin-sulbactam, anidulafungin, argatroban, atenolol, atracurium, aztreonam, bivalirudin, bleomycin, bumetanide, buprenorphine, busulfan, butorphanol, calcium chloride/gluconate, CARBOplatin, caspofungin, ceFAZolin, cefepime, cefotaxime, cefoTEtan, cefOXitin, cefTAZidime, ceftizoxime, cefTRIAXone, cefuroxime, chloramphenicol, chlorproMAZINE, cimetidine, ciprofloxacin, cisatracurium, CISplatin, clindamycin, cyclophosphamide, cycloSPORINE, cytarabine, DACTINomycin, DAPTOmycin, dexamethasone, digoxin, diltiaZEM, DOBUTamine, DOCEtaxel, DOPamine, doripenem, doxacurium, DOXOrubicin, doxycycline, droperidol, enalaprilat, ePHEDrine, EPINEPHrine, epiRUBicin, eptifibatide, ertapenem, erythromycin, etoposide, famotidine, fenoldopam, fentaNYL, fluconazole, fludarabine, fluorouracil, gallium, ganciclovir, gatifloxacin, gemcitabine, gentamicin, glycopyrrolate, granisetron, haloperidol, heparin, hydrALAZINE, hydrocortisone, HYDROmorphone, IDArubicin, ifosfamide, insulin (regular), irinotecan, isoproterenol, ketorolac, labetalol, levoFLOXacin, linezolid, LORazepam, magnesium sulfate, mannitol, mechlorethamine, melphalan, meperidine, meropenem, methohexital, methotrexate, methyldopate, methylPREDNISolone, metoclopramide, metoprolol, metroNIDAZOLE, micafungin, midazolam, mitoXANTRONE, morphine, mycophenolate, nafcillin, nalbuphine, naloxone, nesiritide, niCARDipine, nitroglycerin, nitroprusside, norepinephrine, octreotide, oxacillin, oxaliplatin, oxytocin, PACLitaxel, palonosetron, pamidronate, pancuronium, PEMEtrexed, pentamidine, pentazocine, PENTobarbital, PHENobarbital, phenylephrine, piperacillin, piperacillin-tazobactam, polymyxin B, potassium chloride/phosphates, prochlorperazine, promethazine, propofol, propranolol, quiNIDine, quinupristin-dalfopristin, raNITI-dine, remifentanil, rocuronium, sodium acetate/bicarbonate/phosphates, streptozocin, succinylcholine, SUFentanil, sulfamethoxazole-trimethoprim, tacrolimus, teniposide, theophylline, thiopental, thiotepa, ticarcillin, ticarcillin-clavulanate, tigecycline, tirofiban, tobramycin, torsemide, vancomycin, vasopressin, vecuronium, verapamil, vinCRIStine, vinorelbine, voriconazole, zidovudine, zoledronic acid

SIDE EFFECTS
CNS: Headache
CV: Dysrhythmias, hypotension, chest pain, *PVCs, palpitations, angina*
HEMA: Thrombocytopenia
MISC: Inj site reactions

PHARMACOKINETICS
IV: Onset 2-5 min, peak 10 min, duration variable; terminal half-life 2.3 hr; metabolized in liver; excreted in urine as product (83%), metabolites (12%)

INTERACTIONS
None significant

NURSING CONSIDERATIONS
Assess:
• Monitor ECG continuously during IV; ventricular dysrhythmia can occur, PEWP, CVP index often during infusion; B/P, pulse q5min during infusion; if B/P drops 30 mm Hg, stop infusion, call prescriber
• Electrolytes: potassium, sodium, chloride, calcium, correct as needed; renal studies: BUN, creatinine; blood studies: platelet count
• ALT, AST, bilirubin daily
• **Digoxin toxicity:** may occur if given with this product, diuretics; potassium loss may occur; check digoxin level, electrolytes. Product may be given with digoxin in atrial flutter/fibrillation; some diuretics may be used

• I&O ratio, weight daily; diuresis should increase with continuing therapy

• **Pregnancy/breastfeeding:** use in pregnancy if benefit outweighs risk to fetus; no well-controlled studies; cautious use in breastfeeding, not known if excreted in breast milk

Evaluate:

• Therapeutic response: increased cardiac output, decreased PCWP, adequate CVP; decreased dyspnea, fatigue, edema, ECG

Teach patient/family:

• To report angina, palpitations immediately during infusion

• To report headache, which can be treated with analgesics

TREATMENT OF OVERDOSE: Discontinue product, support circulation

---

RARELY USED

miltefosine

(mil′-te-foe′-seen)

Impavido

Func. class.: Antiprotozoal/antileishmanial

USES: Treatment of visceral leishmaniasis caused by *L. donovani*, mucosal leishmaniasis caused by *L. braziliensis*, and cutaneous leishmaniasis caused by *L. braziliensis*, *L. guyanensis*, and *L. panamensis*

CONTRAINDICATIONS: Hypersensitivity, pregnancy

DOSAGE AND ROUTES

• **Adult/adolescent/child ≥12 yr and ≥45 kg: PO** 50 mg tid × 28 days

• **Adult/adolescent/child ≥12 yr and 30-44 kg: PO** 50 mg bid × 28 days; HIV guidelines suggest 100 mg daily × 4 wk in adults and adolescents regardless of weight

---

minocycline (Rx)

(min-oh-sye′kleen)

Dynacin, Minocin, Minolira, Solodyn

Func. class.: Broad-spectrum antiinfective

Chem. class.: Tetracycline

Do not confuse:

Dynacin/Dynacirc

Minocin/Minoxidil

ACTION: Inhibits protein synthesis, phosphorylation in microorganisms by binding to ribosomal subunits, reversibly binding to ribosomal subunits; bacteriostatic

USES: *Acinetobacter* sp., *Actinomyces israelii*, *Actinomyces* sp., *Bacillus anthracis*, *Bartonella bacilliformis*, *Bordetella pertussis*, *Borrelia burgdorferi*, *Borrelia recurrentis*, *Brucella* sp., *Burkholderia mallei*, *Burkholderia pseudomallei*, *Campylobacter fetus*, *Chlamydia trachomatis*, *Chlamydophila psittaci*, *Clostridium perfringens*, *Clostridium* sp., *Clostridium tetani*, *Coxiella burnetii*, *Eikenella corrodens*, *Entamoeba* sp., *Enterobacter aerogenes*, *Escherichia coli*, *Francisella tularensis*, *Fusobacterium fusiforme*, *Fusobacterium nucleatum*, *Haemophilus ducreyi*, *Haemophilus influenzae (beta-lactamase negative)*, *Haemophilus influenzae (beta-lactamase positive)*, *Klebsiella granulomatis*, *Klebsiella* sp., *Legionella pneumophila*, *Leptospira* sp., *Leptotrichia buccalis*, *Listeria monocytogenes*, *Mycobacterium marinum*, *Mycoplasma hominis*, *Mycoplasma pneumoniae*, *Neisseria gonorrhoeae*, *Neisseria meningitidis*, *Nocardia* sp., *Pasteurella multocida*, *Porphyromonas gingivalis*, *Prevotella intermedia*, *Propionibacterium acnes*, *Propionibacterium propionicum*, *Rickettsia akari*, *Rickettsia prowazekii*, *Rickettsia rickettsii*, *Rickettsia tsutsugamushi*, *Shigella* sp., *Spirillum minus*, *Staphylococcus aureus* (MRSA), *Staphylococcus aureus* (MSSA), *Streptobacillus moniliformis*, *Streptococcus* *pneumoniae, Treponema pallidum, Treponema pertenue, Ureaplasma urealyticum, Vibrio cholerae, Vibrio parahaemolyticus, Yersinia enterocolitica, Yersinia pestis*

CONTRAINDICATIONS: Pregnancy, children <8 yr, hypersensitivity to tetracyclines

Precautions: Hepatic disease, breastfeeding

DOSAGE AND ROUTES
Most infections
• **Adult:** PO/IV 200 mg, then 100 mg q12hr, max 400 mg/24 hr IV; **SUBGINGIVAL** inserted into periodontal pocket
• **Child >8 yr:** PO/IV 4 mg/kg, then 4 mg/kg/day PO in divided doses q12hr
Rickettsial infections
• **Adult:** PO/IV 200 mg, then 100 mg q12hr
• **Child ≥8 yr/adolescent:** PO/IV 4 mg/kg, then 2 mg/kg q12hr, max adult dose
Gonorrhea (allergic to penicillin)
• **Adult:** PO 200 mg, then 100 mg q12hr × ≥4 days
Syphilis (allergic to penicillin)
• **Adult:** PO 200 mg, then 100 mg q12hr × 10-15 days
Meningococcal carrier state
• **Adult:** PO 100 mg q12hr × 5 days
• **Child ≥8 yr:** PO 4 mg/kg initially (max 200 mg), then 2 mg/kg dose q12hr × 5 days, max 100 mg/dose
Uncomplicated gonococcal urethritis in men
• **Adult:** PO 100 mg q12hr × 5 days
Acne vulgaris (Solodyn only)
• **Adult/adolescent/child ≥12 yr:** PO ext rel 1 mg/kg/day × 12 wk or those weighing 126-136 kg—135 mg/day; 111-125 kg—115 mg/day; 97-110 kg—105 mg/day; 85-96 kg—90 mg/day; 72-84 kg—80 mg/day; 60-71 kg—65 mg/day; 50-59 kg—55 mg/day; 45-49 kg—45 mg/day
Acne vulgaris (all except Solodyn)
• **Adult/adolescent/child ≥12 yr:** PO ext rel 1 mg/kg/day × 12 wk or those weighing 91-136 kg—135 mg/day; 60-90 kg—90 mg/day; 45-59 kg—45 mg/day

Available forms: Caps 50, 75, 100 mg; powder for inj 100 mg; caps, pellet filled 50, 100 mg; tabs 50, 75, 100 mg; ext rel tabs 45, 55, 65, 80, 90, 105, 115, 135 mg

Administer:
• After C&S obtained before first dose; begin treatment as soon as drawn
• Store in airtight, light-resistant container at room temperature; do not expose to light
• **Fanconi's syndrome:** do not use outdated products; may cause nephrotoxicity

PO route
• With full glass of water; with food for GI symptoms
• Use pellet-filled caps/tabs 1 hr before or 2 hr after a meal
• Use extended-release tabs at same time each day, without regard to food
• Swallow caps, extended-release tabs whole; do not crush, chew
• 2 hr before or after laxative or ferrous products; 3 hr after antacid

IV route
• After reconstituting 100 mg/5 mL sterile water for inj; further dilute in 100-1000 mL of NaCl, dextrose sol; give over 1-6 hr, do not give rapidly or 250-1000 mL with Ringer's or LR, do not admix
• Change to PO dose as soon as possible to reduce thrombophlebitis risk

Y-site compatibilities: Alfentanil, amikacin, atracurium, benztropine, buprenorphine, butorphanol, calcium chloride, CARBOplatin, caspofungin, cefonicid, chlorproMAZINE, cimetidine, cisatracurium, codeine, cyclophosphamide, cycloSPORINE, cytarabine, DACTINomycin, dexmedetomidine, diltiaZEM, diphenhydrAMINE, DOBUTamine, DOCEtaxel, doxacurium, doxycycline, enalaprilat, ePHEDrine, EPINEPHrine, eptifibatide, etoposide, fenoldopam, fentaNYL, filgrastim, fludarabine, gatifloxacin, gemcitabine, gentamicin, glycopyrrolate, granisetron, heparin, hetastarch, IDARubicin, ifosfamide, inamrinone, isoproterenol, labetalol, levoFLOXacin, lidocaine, linezolid, LORazepam, magnesium sulfate, mannitol, melphalan, metaraminol, methotrexate, methyldopa, metoclopramide,

M

metoprolol, midazolam, mitoXANTRONE, nalbuphine, naloxone, perphenazine, potassium chloride, remifentanil, sargramostim, teniposide, vinorelbine, vit B/C

SIDE EFFECTS

CNS: *Dizziness*, fever, light-headedness, vertigo, seizures, increased intracranial pressure, headache

CV: Pericarditis, thrombophlebitis

EENT: Permanent discoloration of teeth, oral candidiasis, tinnitus

GI: *Nausea, vomiting, diarrhea,* anorexia, hepatotoxicity, CDAD

GU: Renal failure

HEMA: Eosinophilia, neutropenia, thrombocytopenia, hemolytic anemia, pancytopenia

RESP: Bronchospasm, cough, dyspnea

INTEG: *Rash, urticaria, photosensitivity, increased pigmentation,* exfoliative dermatitis, pruritus, blue-gray color of skin, mucous membranes

MS: Myalgia, arthritis; bone growth retardation (<8 yr)

SYST: Angioedema, Stevens-Johnson syndrome, DRESS

PHARMACOKINETICS

PO: Peak 1-4 hr, half-life 11-22 hr; excreted in urine, feces, breast milk; crosses placenta

INTERACTIONS

Increase: effect of warfarin, digoxin, insulin, oral anticoagulants, theophylline, neuromuscular blockers

Increase: chance of pseudomotor cerebri—retinoids; do not use concurrently

Decrease: effect of hormonal contraceptives, use another form of contraception

Decrease: effect of live virus vaccines, bring up to date before use

Decrease: minocycline absorption, give 2 hr before or 3 hr after iron products; laxatives (calcium, aluminum, magnesium) antidiarrhea

Decrease: effect of penicillins, avoid using together

Drug/Lab Test

False negative: urine glucose with Clinistix or Tes-Tape

Increase: BUN, FTs, eosinophils

Decrease: Hb, platlets, neutrophils

NURSING CONSIDERATIONS

Assess:

• **CDAD:** diarrhea, abdominal cramps, fever; may start up to 2 mo after treatment ends; if diarrhea occurs, evaluate

• I&O ratio

• Age and tooth development

• Blood tests: PT, CBC, AST, ALT, BUN, creatinine

• Signs of anemia: Hct, Hgb, fatigue

• **Serious allergic reactions (anaphylaxis, Stevens-Johnson syndrome, DRESS):** assess for rash, fever, fatigue, fluid-filled blisters, abnormal LFTs; product should be discontinued immediately

• Nausea, vomiting, diarrhea; administer antiemetic, antacids as ordered

• **Overgrowth of infection:** fever, malaise, redness, pain, swelling, drainage, perineal itching, diarrhea; changes in cough or sputum; black, furry tongue in long-term therapy

• Beers: Avoid in older adults, may exacerbate syncope, monitor frequently

• **Pregnancy/breastfeeding:** do not use in pregnancy, can cause fetal harm; if pregnancy occurs, stop immediately; do not breastfeed, excreted in breast milk

Evaluate:

• Therapeutic response: decreased temperature, absence of lesions, negative C&S

Teach patient/family:

• To avoid sunlight, wear protective clothing; that sunscreen does not seem to decrease photosensitivity

• That all prescribed medication must be taken to prevent superinfection; not to use outdated product because Fanconi's syndrome may occur

• To report diarrhea that can occur several months after discontinuing product

• To avoid taking antacids, iron, cimetidine; to use 2 hr before, 6 hr after this product, absorption may be decreased; to take with a full glass of water; to take with food; not to take at bedtime, esophageal irritation may occur

• That teeth discoloration, joint or muscle pain may occur

• To use backup contraception; effectiveness may be decreased

---

• Not to use during pregnancy, breastfeeding; not to use for acne if trying to conceive
• To avoid driving, other hazardous activities until reaction is known
• To swallow extended-release product whole, do not crush, chew, split; not to increase, double doses, take at same time of day

---

minoxidil (Rx, OTC)
(mi-nox′i-dill)
Rogaine (topical)
Func. class.: Antihypertensive
Chem. class.: Vasodilator, peripheral

ACTION: Directly relaxes arteriolar smooth muscle, causing vasodilation; reduces peripheral vascular resistance, decreases B/P

USES: Severe hypertension unresponsive to other therapy (use with diuretic and β-blocker); topically to treat alopecia
Unlabeled uses: Scleroderma renal crisis (SRC) to control hypertension, anal fissures

CONTRAINDICATIONS: Dissecting aortic aneurysm, hypersensitivity, pheochromocytoma
Precautions: Pregnancy, breastfeeding, children, geriatric patients, renal disease, CVD, acute MI

> Black Box Warning: CAD, HF, cardiac disease, cardiac tamponade, edema, hypotension, orthostatic hypotension, pericardial effusion

DOSAGE AND ROUTES
Severe hypertension
• **Adult:** PO 5 mg/day in 1-2 divided doses; max 100 mg/day; usual range 10-40 mg/day divided in 1-2 doses
• **Geriatric:** PO 2.5 mg/day, may be increased gradually
• **Child <12 yr:** PO (initial) 0.1-0.2 mg/kg/day; (effective range) 0.25-1 mg/kg/day; (max) 50 mg/day

Alopecia
• **Adult:** TOP 1 mL bid, rub into scalp daily, max 2 mL/day
Renal dose
• **Adult:** PO CCr 10-15 mL/min extend interval to q24hr; CCr <10 mL/min not recommended
Anal fissures (unlabeled)
• **Adult/adolescent:** TOP (0.5% minoxidil in white paraffin base) 0.5 g each compounded minoxidil and lignocaine ointment q8hr
Scleroderma renal crisis (unlabeled)
• **Adult:** PO 5 mg/day in 1-2 divided doses, increase after 3 days by 10-20 mg/day to reach desired B/P, max 100 mg/day
Available forms: Tabs 2.5, 10 mg; topical 2%, 5% sol; topical foam 5%
Administer:
• Store protected from light and heat
PO route
• Without regard to meals
• With β-blocker and/or diuretic for hypertension
Topical route
• 1 mL no matter how much balding has occurred; increasing dosage does not speed growth

SIDE EFFECTS
Systemic
CNS: Headache, fatigue
CV: *Severe rebound hypertension on withdrawal in children,* tachycardia, angina, increased T wave, HF, pulmonary edema, pericardial effusion, edema, sodium, water retention, *hypotension*
GI: Nausea, vomiting
GU: Breast tenderness
HEMA: Hct, Hgb; erythrocyte count may decrease initially, leukopenia
INTEG: Pruritus, Stevens-Johnson syndrome, rash, hirsutism, contact dermatitis

PHARMACOKINETICS
PO: Onset 30 min, peak 2-3 hr, duration 48-120 hr; half-life 4.2 hr; metabolized

in liver; metabolites excreted in urine, feces; protein binding minimal

INTERACTIONS

Increase: hypotension—antihypertensives, MAOIs

Decrease: antihypertensive effect—NSAIDs, salicylates, estrogens

Drug/Herb

Increase: antihypertensive effect—hawthorn

Drug/Lab Test

Increase: renal studies

Decrease: Hgb/Hct/RBC

NURSING CONSIDERATIONS

Assess:

• Monitor closely; usually given with β-blocker to prevent tachycardia and increased myocardial workload; usually given with diuretic to prevent serious fluid accumulation; patient should be hospitalized during beginning treatment

• Nausea, edema in feet, legs daily

• Skin turgor, dryness of mucous membranes for hydration status

• Crackles, dyspnea, orthopnea

• Electrolytes: potassium, sodium, chloride, CO_2

• Renal studies: catecholamines, BUN, creatinine

• Hepatic studies: AST, ALT, alk phos

• B/P, pulse

• Weight daily, I&O

Black Box Warning: **Cardiac disease:** may cause reflex increase in heart rate and decrease in B/P

• **Beers:** avoid use in older adults; may exacerbate syncope; monitor frequently for syncope

• **Pregnancy/breastfeeding:** use only if benefits outweigh risk to fetus; do not use in breastfeeding

Evaluate:

• Therapeutic response: decreased B/P, increased hair growth

Teach patient/family:

• That body hair will increase but is reversible after discontinuing treatment

• Not to discontinue product abruptly

• To report pitting edema, dizziness, weight gain >5 lb, SOB, bruising or bleeding, heart rate >20 beats/min over normal, severe indigestion, dizziness, light-headedness, panting, new or aggravated symptoms of angina

• To take product exactly as prescribed because serious side effects may occur

Topical:

• That for topical use, treatment must continue for the long term, or new hair will be lost

• Not to use except on scalp; use on clean, dry scalp before styling aids; wash hands after each use

TREATMENT OF OVERDOSE: Administer normal saline IV, vasopressors

---

mipomersen (Rx)

(mye'poe-mer-sen)

Kynamro

Func. class.: Antilipemics

Chem. class.: Antisense oligonucleotide

ACTION: Inhibits synthesis of the principal apolipoprotein of LDL, VLDL; binds to messenger ribonucleic acid (mRNA)

USES: Decreasing LDL, total cholesterol, apolipoprotein B, non–high-density lipoprotein cholesterol to reduce LDL, total cholesterol, apolipoprotein B, non–high-density lipoprotein cholesterol (homozygous familial hypercholesterolemia)

CONTRAINDICATIONS:

Black Box Warning: Hepatic disease

Precautions: Pregnancy, breastfeeding, dialysis, alcohol ingestion, geriatric patients, proteinuria, renal disease, low-density lipoprotein apheresis

DOSAGE AND ROUTES

Homozygous familial hypercholesterolemia

• **Adult:** SUBCUT 200 mg weekly

Renal/hepatic dose
• **Adult:** SUBCUT do not use in severe renal or hepatic disease
Available forms: Solution for injection 200 mg/mL

Black Box Warning: Enroll in Kynamro REMS program at 1-877-596-2676; only prescribers who enroll are able to use product

Administer:
• Give on the same day weekly; if a dose is missed, give ≥3 days from the next weekly dose
• Monitor ALT, AST, alkaline phosphatase, and total bilirubin before start of therapy; monitor lipid levels q3-4mo for the first year
• Monitor LDL-C level after 6 mo

Black Box Warning: Dose adjustments for elevated transaminases during treatment

Subcut route
• Visually inspect parenteral products for particulate matter and discoloration before use
• The first injection given by the patient or caregiver should be performed under the guidance and supervision of a qualified health care professional
• Remove vial or prefilled syringe from refrigerated storage; allow to reach room temperature for at least 30 min before use
• Inject into abdomen, thigh region, or outer area of upper arm. Do not inject in areas of active skin disease or injury such as sunburns, skin rashes, inflammation, skin infections, active areas of psoriasis; areas of tattooed skin and scarring should also be avoided

Black Box Warning: ALT or AST ≥3× and <5× ULN: confirm elevation with a repeat test within 1 wk; if confirmed, withhold product; obtain other tests if not already obtained (total bilirubin, alkaline phosphatase, INR) to identify the probable cause; if resuming product after transaminases resolve to <3× ULN, consider monitoring liver-related tests more frequently

Black Box Warning: ALT or AST ≥5× ULN: withhold, obtain additional liver-related tests if not already obtained (total bilirubin, alkaline phosphatase, INR), and identify the probable cause; if resuming product after transaminases resolve to <3× ULN, monitor liver-related tests more frequently

SIDE EFFECTS
CNS: Fatigue, headache, fever, chills
CV: Hypertension, palpitations, angina
GI: abdominal pain, vomiting, nausea
GU: Glomerulonephritis, proteinuria
MS: Musculoskeletal pain
SYST: Angioedema
INTEG: Injection site reaction, malignancy
MISC: Flulike symptoms

PHARMACOKINETICS
Half-life 1-2 mo, protein binding >90%

INTERACTIONS
Increase: hepatotoxicity risk—acetaminophen, methotrexate, tetracyclines, tamoxifen; monitor LFTs for increase

Drug/Lab
Increase: LFTs, urine protein

NURSING CONSIDERATIONS
Assess:

Black Box Warning: **Hepatic disease:** obtain LFTs monthly × 1 yr, then q3mo; assess for nausea, vomiting, jaundice, dark urine; product may need to be discontinued

• Determine whether the LDL-C reduction achieved is sufficient to warrant the potential risk of liver toxicity
• **Geriatric patients:** increased risk for hypertension, peripheral edema, hepatic steatosis
• **Hypercholesterolemia:** diet history: fat content, lipid levels (triglycerides, LDL, HDL, cholesterol); LFTs at baseline, periodically during treatment

M

Side effects: *italics* = common; red = life-threatening

• **Pregnancy/breastfeeding:** use effective contraception during therapy; if pregnancy occurs, stop product; no well-controlled studies; discontinue breastfeeding or product

Evaluate:

• Therapeutic response: decreasing LDL, total cholesterol, apolipoprotein B, non–high-density lipoprotein cholesterol

Teach patient/family:

• That risk factors should be decreased: high-fat diet, smoking, alcohol consumption, absence of exercise

• To notify prescriber if pregnancy is suspected, planned, or if breastfeeding

• To notify prescriber of dietary/herbal supplements

• Not to use alcohol

• To report fever, chills, fatigue, other flulike symptoms, usually 2 days after subcut injection

• How to use subcut injection; not to reuse needles, syringes

• That injection site may be red, inflamed, and usually resolves

Black Box Warning: Hepatic disease: to report yellowing of skin/eyes, nausea, vomiting, anorexia, dark urine; to report immediately

---

mirabegron

(mir′a-beg′ron)

Myrbetriq

Func. class.: Bladder antispasmodic
Chem. class.: β₃-Adrenergic receptor agonist

ACTION: Relaxes smooth muscles in urinary tract, increase bladder capacity

USES: Overactive bladder (urinary frequency, urgency), urinary incontinence

CONTRAINDICATIONS: Hypersensitivity

Precautions: Pregnancy, breastfeeding, children, kidney/liver disease, bladder obstruction, dialysis, hypertension

DOSAGE AND ROUTES
Overactive bladder

• **Adult: PO** 25 mg/day, may increase to 50 mg/day if needed

Hepatic/renal dose

• **Adult: PO** Child-Pugh B or CCr 15-29 mL/min, max 25 mg/day; Child-Pugh C or CCr <15 mL/min, not recommended

Available forms: Tabs ext rel 25, 50 mg
Administer:

• Give whole; take with liquids; do not crush, chew, or break ext rel product; use without regard to meals

SIDE EFFECTS
CNS: Fatigue, dizziness, headache
CV: Hypertension, tachycardia
EENT: Xerophthalmia, blurred vision
GI: Anorexia, abdominal pain, constipation, diarrhea
GU: Urinary retention, frequency, UTI, bladder discomfort
SYST: Stevens-Johnson syndrome

PHARMACOKINETICS
71% protein binding, excretion 25% unchanged in urine, half-life 50 hr, peak 3.5 hr

INTERACTIONS
Increase: effect of CYP2D6 substrates
Increase: effect of digoxin, warfarin, desipramine

Drug/Lab Test
Increase: LFTs, digoxin, INR, LDH

NURSING CONSIDERATIONS
Assess:

• **Urinary patterns:** distention, nocturia, frequency, urgency, incontinence

• **Angioedema:** swelling of face, lips, tongue, dyspnea; discontinue immediately, have emergency equipment nearby

• LFTs at baseline, periodically

• Monitor B/P, pulse often

• **Pregnancy/breastfeeding:** use only if benefits outweigh risks to fetus; no well-controlled studies, discontinue product, not known if excreted in breast milk

Evaluate:

• Decreasing dysuria, frequency, nocturia, incontinence

Teach patient/family:

- **Hypertension:** to report fast heartbeat; monitor B/P, P at home
- **Angioedema:** to report immediately swelling of face, lips, tongue
- To avoid hazardous activities; dizziness can occur; may take up to 8 wk for full effect
- Not to drink liquids before bedtime
- About the importance of bladder maintenance
- Not to breastfeed; to report if pregnancy is planned or suspected
- Not to crush, chew, split; to take without regard to food, not to skip, double doses, if missed take at regularly scheduled next day, provide "Patient Information Materials"
- To discuss all OTC, Rx, herbals, supplements with provider

---

mirtazapine (Rx)

(mer-ta'za-peen)
Remeron, Remeron RD ✦,
Remeron SolTab
Func. class.: Antidepressant
Chem. class.: Tetracyclic

ACTION: Blocks reuptake of norepinephrine and serotonin into nerve endings, thereby increasing action of norepinephrine and serotonin in nerve cells; antagonist of central α_2-receptors; blocks histamine receptors

USES: Depression; dysthymic disorder; bipolar disorder: depressed, agitated depression
Unlabeled uses: Panic disorder, PTSD, generalized anxiety disorder (GAD)

CONTRAINDICATIONS: Hypersensitivity to tricyclics, recovery phase of MI, agranulocytosis, jaundice, MAOIs
Precautions: Pregnancy, geriatric patients, suicidal patients, severe depression, increased intraocular pressure, closed-angle glaucoma, urinary retention, cardiac/renal/hepatic disease, hypo/hyperthyroidism, electroshock therapy, elective surgery, seizure disorder, bone marrow suppression, thrombocytopenia

Black Box Warning: Suicidal ideation, children

DOSAGE AND ROUTES
Major depressive disorder

- **Adult:** PO 15 mg/day at bedtime, maintenance to continue for 6 mo, titrate up to 45 mg/day; **ORALLY DISINTEGRATING** tabs: open blister pack, place tab on tongue, allow to disintegrate, swallow
- **Geriatric:** PO 7.5 mg at bedtime, increase by 7.5 mg q1-2wk to desired dose, max 45 mg/day

Renal dose
- **Adult:** PO CCr 11-39 mL/min, use lowest dose, titrate slowly to 30% reduction in normal drug clearance; CCr ≤10 mL/min, use lowest dose, titrate slowly to 50% reduction in normal drug clearance

Available forms: Tabs 7.5, 15, 30, 45 mg; orally disintegrating tab (SolTab) 15, 30, 45 mg
Administer:
- Increased fluids, bulk in diet for constipation, especially for geriatric patients
- Without regard to meals
- Dosage at bedtime if oversedation occurs during day; may take entire dose at bedtime; geriatric patients may not tolerate once-daily dosing
- Gum, hard candy, or frequent sips of water for dry mouth
- Store in tight container at room temperature; do not freeze
- **Orally disintegrating tab:** no water needed; allow to dissolve on tongue, do not split; contains phenylalanine

SIDE EFFECTS
CNS: *Dizziness, drowsiness,* confusion, nightmares, abnormal dreams, neuroleptic malignant syndrome, suicidal thoughts
CV: *Orthostatic hypotension, ECG changes,* tachycardia, twitching
EENT: *Blurred vision,* tinnitus, mydriasis
GI: *Dry mouth,* nausea, vomiting, increased appetite, cramps, epigastric distress, constipation, weight gain
GU: Urinary frequency

M

Side effects: *italics* = common; red = life-threatening

HEMA: Agranulocytosis, thrombocytopenia, eosinophilia, leukopenia
META: Hyponatremia, hypercholesterolemia
INTEG: Rash, urticaria, sweating, pruritus, photosensitivity
MS: Back pain, myalgia
RESP: Cough, dyspnea
SYST: Flulike symptoms, serotonin syndrome

PHARMACOKINETICS
PO: Peak 2 hr, metabolized by CYP1A2, 2D6, 3A4 in liver; excreted in urine, feces; crosses placenta; half-life 20-40 hr, protein binding 85%

INTERACTIONS
Increase: hyperpyretic crisis, seizures, hypertensive episode—MAOIs; avoid within 14 days
Increase: CNS depression—alcohol, barbiturates, benzodiazepines, other CNS depressants
Increase: serotonin syndrome—SSRIs, buspropion, SNRIs, serotonin-receptor agonists, fentanyl, triptans, tricyclics, linezolid, methylene blue; monitor for symptoms
Decrease: effects of cloNIDine, indirect-acting sympathomimetics (ePHEDrine)
Drug/Herb
• **Serotonin syndrome:** St. John's wort; monitor for symptoms
Increase: CNS depression—kava
Drug/Lab Test
Increase: cholesterol, triglycerides

NURSING CONSIDERATIONS
Assess:
• B/P (lying, standing), pulse often; if systolic B/P drops 20 mm Hg, hold product, notify prescriber; vital signs more frequently in patients with CV disease
• **Seizures:** in those with seizure disorder, may be increased, provide seizure precautions
• **Neuroleptic malignant syndrome:** fever, dyspnea, sweating, change in B/P, discontinue immediately

• Blood studies: ECG, lipid profile, blood glucose, LFTs, serum creatinine/BUN if patient is receiving long-term therapy
• Weight weekly; appetite may increase with product

Black Box Warning: Mental status: mood, sensorium, affect, suicidal tendencies (especially among adolescents, young adults), increase in psychiatric symptoms: depression, panic; product should be discontinued in those who exhibit worsening depression, emergent suicidality; EPS primarily in geriatric patients: rigidity, dystonia, akathisia

• **Serotonin syndrome:** hyperthermia, hypertension, myoclonus, rigidity, delirium, coma (if using other serotonergic products)
• Alcohol consumption; if alcohol consumed, hold dose until morning
• Assistance with ambulation during beginning therapy because drowsiness, dizziness occurs
• **Pregnancy/breastfeeding:** use only if clearly needed; excreted in breast milk, discontinue product or breastfeeding
Evaluate:
• Therapeutic response: decreased depression
Teach patient/family:
• That therapeutic effects may take 2-3 wk; to take at bedtime; that there is decreased sedation with increased doses; not to discontinue abruptly
• To use caution when driving, performing other activities requiring alertness because of drowsiness, dizziness, blurred vision
• To avoid alcohol, other CNS depressants without prescriber approval
• **Infection:** to report flulike symptoms, other signs of infection
• **Serotonin syndrome:** to report immediately symptoms that include fever, delirium, rigidity; may occur in combination with other products
• About how to take orally disintegrating tabs; dissolve on tongue, swallow
• Not to crush, break, chew ODT product

• To notify prescriber immediately if pregnancy is suspected, or if breast-feeding
• Not to use within 14 days of MAOIs
• That follow-up exams will be needed

Black Box Warning: To notify prescriber immediately of suicidal thoughts, behavior

TREATMENT OF OVERDOSE: ECG monitoring, lavage; administer anticonvulsant, IV fluids

RARELY USED

misoprostol (Rx)
(mye-soe-prost'ole)
Cytotec
Func. class.: Gastric mucosa protectant, antiulcer
Chem. class.: Prostaglandin E₁ analog

Do not confuse:
miSOPROStol/metoprolol

USES: Prevention of NSAID-induced gastric ulcers
Unlabeled uses: Pregnancy termination, postpartum hemorrhage, cervical ripening/labor induction (vaginal), active duodenal/gastric ulcer

CONTRAINDICATIONS: Hypersensitivity to this product or prostaglandins

Black Box Warning: Pregnancy, females

DOSAGE AND ROUTES
• **Adult: PO** 200 mcg qid with food for duration of NSAID therapy, with last dose given at bedtime; if 200 mcg is not tolerated, 100 mcg may be given
Active duodenal/gastric ulcer (unlabeled)
• **Adult: PO** 100-200 mcg qid with meals at bedtime × 4-8 wk

Pregnancy termination before 63rd day (unlabeled)
• **Adult: INTRAVAGINALLY** 800 mcg 5-7 days after methotrexate IM
Cervical ripening induction for term pregnancy (unlabeled)
• **Adult: INTRAVAGINALLY** 25 mcg q3-6hr

⚠ HIGH ALERT

mitoMYcin (Rx)
(mye-toe-mye'sin)
Func. class.: Antineoplastic, antibiotic

Do not confuse:
mitoMYcin/mitoXANTRONE

ACTION: Inhibits DNA synthesis, primarily; derived from *Streptomyces caespitosus;* appears to cause cross-linking of DNA; vesicant

USES: Pancreatic, stomach, colorectal, bladder cancer
Unlabeled uses: Palliative treatment of anal, bladder, head, neck, colon, breast, biliary, cervical, lung malignancies; bone marrow ablation, desmoid tumor, mesothelioma, stem cell transplant preparation

CONTRAINDICATIONS: Pregnancy, breastfeeding, hypersensitivity, as single agent, coagulation disorders, thrombocytopenia
Precautions: Accidental exposure, acute bronchospasm, anemia, children, dental disease/work, extravasation, females, infection, radiation therapy, surgery, vaccines, renal/respiratory disease

Black Box Warning: Bone marrow suppression, hemolytic uremic syndrome, leukopenia; requires an experienced clinician and specialized care setting

M

DOSAGE AND ROUTES
Disseminated adenocarcinoma of stomach/pancreas in combination
• **Adult:** IV 20 mg/m^2 q6-8wk
Available forms: Inj 5, 20, 40 mg/vial
Administer:
• **Cytotoxic:** use safe handling and disposal procedures
• **Vesicant:** check for extravasation; do not give IM/subcut, may result in extreme tissue damage
Direct IV route
• Use port or central line if possible
• Antiemetic 30-60 min before product to prevent vomiting
• IV after reconstituting 5 mg/10 mL, 20 mg/40 mL, 40 mg/80 mL (0.5 mg/mL) sterile water for inj; shake, allow to stand, protect from light, give through Y-tube or 3-way stopcock; give slow IV push or infuse over 15-30 min; color of reconstituted sol is gray
• Avoid excessive heat; store unreconstituted product at room temperature

Y-site compatibilities: Amifostine, amphotericin B lipid complex, amphotericin B liposome, anidulafungin, argatroban, atenolol, bivalirudin, bleomycin, caspofungin, CISplatin, cyclophosphamide, DACTINomycin, dolasetron, DOXOrubicin, droperidol, epiRUBicin, ertapenem, fluorouracil, furosemide, granisetron, heparin, leucovorin, melphalan, methotrexate, metoclopramide, nesiritide, octreotide, ondansetron, oxaliplatin, PACLitaxel, palonosetron, PEMEtrexed, riTUXimab, teniposide, thiotepa, tigecycline, tirofiban, trastuzumab, vinBLAStine, vinCRIStine, voriconazole, zoledronic acid

SIDE EFFECTS
CNS: Fever, headache, confusion, drowsiness, syncope, fatigue
CV: Edema
EENT: Blurred vision
GI: *Nausea, vomiting, anorexia, stomatitis*, hepatotoxicity, diarrhea
GU: Urinary retention, renal failure, infertility
HEMA: Thrombocytopenia, leukopenia, anemia
INTEG: *Rash*, alopecia, extravasation, nail discoloration
MISC: Hemolytic uremic syndrome
RESP: Fibrosis, pulmonary infiltrate

PHARMACOKINETICS
Half-life 1 hr, metabolized in liver, 10% excreted in urine (unchanged)

INTERACTIONS
Increase: toxicity—other antineoplastics, radiation
Increase: bleeding risk—NSAIDs, anticoagulants
• Avoid use with vaccines

Drug/Lab Test
Increase: BUN, creatinine
Decrease: platelets, WBCs

NURSING CONSIDERATIONS
Assess:

Black Box Warning: Bone marrow suppression: monitor CBC, differential, platelet count weekly; withhold product if WBC is <4000/mm^3, serum creatinine >1.7 mg/dL, or platelet count is <100,000/mm^3, nadir of leukopenia, thrombocytopenia is 4-8 wk, recovering within 10 wk; notify prescriber; bleeding: hematuria, guaiac, bruising, petechiae, mucosa, or orifices, avoid IM injections when platelets are low

Black Box Warning: Fatal hemolytic uremic syndrome: assess for hypertension, thrombocytopenia, microangiopathic hemolytic anemia; occurs in those receiving long-term therapy; most cases are caused by doses ≥60 mg; transfusion may worsen syndrome

• **Nephrotoxicity:** Renal studies: BUN, uric acid, urine CCr, before, during therapy; adjust dose based on renal function; I&O ratio; report fall in urine output to <30 mL/hr

• Monitor temperature; fever may indicate beginning infection

• **Hepatotoxicity:** hepatic studies before, during therapy: bilirubin, AST, ALT, alk phos as needed or monthly; check for jaundiced skin and sclera, dark urine, clay-colored stools, itchy skin, abdominal pain, fever, diarrhea

• **Pulmonary fibrosis:** bronchospasm, dyspnea, crackles, unproductive cough; chest pain, tachypnea, fatigue, increased pulse, pallor, lethargy; pulmonary function tests; chest x-ray before, during therapy; chest x-ray should be obtained q2wk during treatment

• Effects of alopecia on body image; discuss feelings about body changes

• Buccal cavity q8hr for dryness, sores, ulceration, white patches, oral pain, bleeding, dysphagia

• Local irritation, pain, burning at inj site

• GI symptoms: frequency of stools, cramping

• Adequate fluids (2-3 L/day) unless contraindicated

• Rinsing of mouth tid-qid with water; brushing of teeth with baking soda bid-tid with soft brush or cotton-tipped applicators for stomatitis; use unwaxed dental floss

• **Cardiac toxicity (rare):** HF may be treated with diuretics, cardiac glycosides; most with this condition received doxorubicin

• **Pregnancy/breastfeeding:** do not use in pregnancy or breastfeeding

Evaluate:

• Therapeutic response: decreased tumor size, spread of malignancy

Teach patient/family:

• That hair may be lost during treatment; that wig or hairpiece may make patient feel better; that new hair may be different in color, texture

• To avoid foods with citric acid, hot temperature, or rough texture

• To report any bleeding, white spots, ulcerations in mouth; to examine mouth daily

• To report sign of IV site reaction: redness, inflammation, burning, pain

• To avoid crowds, persons with infections if granulocyte count is low

• **Infection:** to report fever, flulike symptoms, sore throat

• To immediately report urine retention, absence of urine, dyspnea, bleeding, jaundice, signs of pulmonary toxicity

• **Pregnancy/breastfeeding:** to report if pregnancy is planned or suspected; not to breastfeed

---

⚠ **HIGH ALERT**

mitoXANTRONE (Rx)

(mye-toe-zan′trone)
Func. class.: Antineoplastic, antiinfective, immunomodulator
Chem. class.: Synthetic anthraquinone

Do not confuse:
mitoXANTRONE/mitoMYcin

ACTION: DNA reactive agent; cytocidal effect on both proliferating and nonproliferating cells; topoisomerase II inhibitor (vesicant)

USES: Acute myelogenous leukemia (adult), relapsed leukemia; used with steroids to treat bone pain (advanced prostate cancer), multiple sclerosis (MS)

Unlabeled uses: Liver malignancies, non-Hodgkin's lymphoma, breast cancer

CONTRAINDICATIONS: Pregnancy, hypersensitivity

Precautions: Breastfeeding, children; myelosuppression, renal/cardiac/hepatic disease; gout

Black Box Warning: Secondary malignancy, neutropenia, intrathecal adminis-

---

tration, extravasation, heart failure

DOSAGE AND ROUTES
Acute myelogenous leukemia/induction
• **Adult:** IV INFUSION 12 mg/m²/day on days 1-3 and 100 mg/m² cytarabine × 7 days as continuous 24-hr infusion may use 2nd induction
Consolidation
• **Adult:** IV 12 mg/m² given as short 5- to 15-min infusion for 2 days with cytarabine × 5 days, use 6 wk after induction, and another course after 4 wk
Advanced prostate cancer
• **Adult:** IV 12-14 mg/m² as single dose or short infusion q21days
Multiple sclerosis, relapsing
• **Adult:** IV INFUSION 12 mg/m² as 5- to 15-min infusion q3mo, cumulative lifetime dose 140 mg/m²

Available forms: Solution for inj 2 mg/mL

Administer:
• Other medications by oral route if possible; avoid IM, SUBCUT, IV routes
• Antiemetic 30-60 min before product to prevent vomiting
• **Cytotoxic:** use precautions for handling, preparing, and disposal of this product; use goggles, gloves, gown during preparation and administration; rinse accidentally exposed skin with warm water
• Undiluted solution may be stored for 7 days (room temperature), 14 days (refrigerated); do not freeze

Direct IV route
• IV after diluting with ≥50 mL NS or D₅W; discard unused portion immediately; do not mix in same infusion with heparin; give over 3-5 min into running IV of D₅W or NS; check for extravasation; do not give IM, SUBCUT, or intraarterially

Intermittent IV INFUSION route
• May be diluted further in D₅W, NS (0.02-0.5 mg/mL), run over 15-30 min

Continuous IV INFUSION route
• Give over 24 hr

Y-site compatibilities: Acyclovir, alemtuzumab, alfentanil, allopurinol, amikacin, aminocaproic acid, aminophylline, amiodarone, anidulafungin, argatroban, arsenic trioxide, atracurium, bivalirudin, bleomycin, bretylium, bumetanide, buprenorphine, butorphanol, calcium chloride, calcium gluconate, CARBOplatin, carmustine, caspofungin, cefoTEtan, ceftizoxime, chloramphenicol, chlorproMAZINE, cimetidine, ciprofloxacin, cisatracurium, CISplatin, cladribine, codeine, cyclophosphamide, cycloSPORINE, cytarabine, DACTINomycin, DAPTOmycin, DAUNOrubicin citrate liposome, dexmedetomidine, dexrazoxane, diltiaZEM, diphenhydrAMINE, DOBUTamine, DOCEtaxel, dolasetron, DOPamine, doxacurium, doxycycline, droperidol, enalaprilat, ePHEDrine, EPINEPHrine, erythromycin, esmolol, etoposide, etoposide phosphate, famotidine, fenoldopam, fentaNYL, filgrastim, fluconazole, fludarabine, fluorouracil, ganciclovir, gatifloxacin, gemcitabine, gentamicin, glycopyrrolate, granisetron, haloperidol, hydrALAZINE, hydrocortisone sodium succinate, HYDROmorphone, hydrOXYzine, ifosfamide, imipenem-cilastatin, inamrinone, insulin (regular), irinotecan, isoproterenol, ketorolac, labetalol, leucovorin, levoFLOXacin, levorphanol, lidocaine, linezolid, LORazepam, magnesium sulfate, mannitol, melphalan, meperidine, meropenem, mesna, metaraminol, methohexital, methotrexate, methyldopa, metoclopramide, metoprolol, metroNIDAZOLE, midazolam, milrinone, minocycline, mivacurium, morphine sulfate, nalbuphine, naloxone, nesiritide, niCARdipine, nitroglycerin, norepinephrine, octreotide, ondansetron, oxaliplatin, palonosetron, pamidronate, pancuronium, pentamidine, pentazocine, PENTObarbital, PHENObarbital, phentolamine, phenylephrine, polymyxin B, potassium acetate, potassium chloride, procainamide, prochlorperazine, promethazine hydrochloride, propranolol, quiNIDine gluconate, quinupristin-dalfopristin, raNITIdine, remifentanil, riTUXimab, rocuronium, sargramostim, sodium acetate, sodium bicarbonate, succinylcholine, SUFentanil, sulfamethoxazole-trimethoprim, tacrolimus, teniposide, theophylline, thiopental, thiotepa, tigecycline, tirofiban, tobramycin, tolazoline, trastuzumab, trimethobenzamide, vancomycin, vasopressin, vecuronium, verapamil, vinCRIStine, vinorelbine, zidovudine, zoledronic acid

SIDE EFFECTS

CNS: Headache, seizures, fatigue
CV: Cardiotoxicity, dysrhythmias
EENT: Conjunctivitis, blue/green sclera, blurred vision
GI: *Nausea, vomiting, diarrhea, anorexia, stomatitis,* hepatotoxicity, abdominal pain, constipation
GU: Amenorrhea, menstrual disorders, blue-green urine, renal failure
HEMA: Thrombocytopenia, leukopenia, myelosuppression, anemia, secondary leukemia
INTEG: *Rash, necrosis at inj site,* dermatitis, thrombophlebitis at inj site, alopecia
MISC: Fever, hyperuricemia, infections
RESP: Cough, dyspnea
SYST: Tumor lysis syndrome, sepsis

PHARMACOKINETICS

Protein binding 78%; excreted via renal, hepatobiliary systems; half-life 23-215 hr

INTERACTIONS

Increase: bone marrow depression toxicity—radiation, other antineoplastics
Increase: adverse reactions—live virus vaccines, trastuzumab
Increase: oral mucositis—palifermin, do not use within 24 hr of mitoxantrone
Increase: immunosuppression—tofacitinib, avoid using together
Increase: infection risk—natalizumab
Increase: bleeding risk—NSAIDs, anticoagulants
Increase: mitoXANTRONE, effects of—cyclosporine
Decrease: digoxin, hydration level—monitor levels, adjust dose
Drug/Lab Test

Increase: LFTs, uric acid, bilirubin
Decrease: HcT/Hgb, platelets, WBC, calcium, sodium, granulocytes

NURSING CONSIDERATIONS
Assess:

• **Bone marrow depression:** CBC, differential, platelet count weekly; withhold product if WBC is <1500/mm^3; leukopenia, neutropenia, thrombocytopenia are expected, leukocyte nadir 10-14 days, recovers in 2-3 wk

Black Box Warning: **Extravasation:** avoid extravasation; not traditionally considered a vesicant; serious skin necrosis requiring debridement, skin graft has occurred; if extravasation occurs, stop product, place ice packs on area

• **Hepatotoxicity:** hepatic studies before, during therapy: bilirubin, AST, ALT, alk phos prn or monthly; dose reduction needed with hepatic disease; jaundiced skin and sclera, dark urine, clay-colored stools, itchy skin, abdominal pain, fever, diarrhea
• **Renal studies:** BUN, serum uric acid, urine CCr, electrolytes before, during therapy
• Bleeding, hematuria, guaiac, bruising or petechiae, mucosa or orifices q8hr

Black Box Warning: **Cardiotoxicity:** ECG, ECHO, chest x-ray, MUGA, RAI angiography; assess ejection fraction before and during treatment; cardiotoxicity may develop during treatment or months to years after treatment; use vigilant cardiac monitoring in MS; risk is greater in cumulative dose >140 mg/m^2

Black Box Warning: **Secondary acute myelogenous leukemia (AML)** can develop after taking this product

Black Box Warning: **Multiple sclerosis:** obtain MUGA, LVEF baselines; repeat LVEF if symptoms of HF occur or if cumulative dose is >100 mg/m^2; do not administer to patients who have received lifetime dose of ≥140 mg/m^2 or if LVEF <50% or significant LVEF or if neutrophils <1500/mm^3

M

• **Pregnancy/breastfeeding:** do not use in pregnancy, breastfeeding; obtain pregnancy test for all women of childbearing age, even if birth control is used

• Rinsing of mouth tid-qid with water, club soda; brushing of teeth bid-qid with soft brush or cotton-tipped applicators for stomatitis; use unwaxed dental floss

• Provide increased fluids to 2-3 L/day unless contraindicated

Black Box Warning: Requires a specialized care setting with an experienced clinician: use only in a setting with emergency equipment, those trained in administration of cytotoxic products

Evaluate:

• Therapeutic response: decreased tumor size, spread of malignancy, prevention of relapse in MS

Teach patient/family:

• To immediately report bleeding, dyspnea, possible infections, seizure, jaundice, fever, cough, or dyspnea

• To avoid hot foods or those with citric acid, rough texture

• To report any bleeding, white spots, ulcerations in mouth; to examine mouth daily

• To avoid crowds, persons with infections

• To provide package insert and review with patient

• To report immediately yellow eyes, skin, clay-colored stools, dark urine, diarrhea

• That follow-up exams and blood work will be needed

• That sclera, urine may turn blue or green; that hair loss may occur

• To notify prescriber if pregnancy is suspected or planned; to use effective contraception

---

modafinil (Rx)

(mo-daf'i-nil)

Alertec ✦, Provigil

Func. class.: CNS stimulant

Chem. class.: Racemic compound

Controlled Substance Schedule IV

ACTION: Similar action as that of sympathomimetics; does not alter release of DOPamine, norepinephrine

USES: Narcolepsy, shift-work sleep disturbance, obstructive sleep apnea

CONTRAINDICATIONS: Hypersensitivity, ischemic heart disease, left ventricular hypertrophy, chest pain, dysrhythmias

Precautions: Pregnancy, breastfeeding, child <16 yr, geriatric patients, unstable angina, history of MI, severe hepatic disease

DOSAGE AND ROUTES

To improve wakefulness with daytime sleepiness

• **Adult/adolescent ≥16 yr: PO** 200 mg daily

Hepatic dose (severe hepatic disease)

• **Adult: PO** 100 mg daily

Available forms: Tabs 100, 200 mg

Administer:

• Give 1 hr before start of shift work or in AM for those with narcolepsy or sleep apnea

• Store at room temperature

• Give without regard to food

SIDE EFFECTS

CNS: *Headache,* anxiety, cataplexy, depression, dizziness, insomnia, amnesia, confusion, ataxia, tremors, paresthesia, dyskinesia, suicidal ideation

CV: Dysrhythmias, hypo/hypertension, chest pain, vasodilation

EENT: Change in vision, *rhinitis,* pharyngitis, epistaxis

GI: Nausea, vomiting, changes in LFTs, anorexia, diarrhea, thirst, mouth ulcers

GU: Ejaculation disorder, urinary retention, albuminuria

HEMA: Eosinophilia

INTEG: Rash, dry skin, herpes simplex, Stevens-Johnson syndrome

MISC: Infection, hyperglycemia, neck pain

RESP: *Dyspnea,* lung changes

PHARMACOKINETICS

Absorbed rapidly, 60% protein binding, metabolized by the liver (90%), half-life 15 hr, peak 2-4 hr

INTERACTIONS

Increase: altered levels of CYP3A4 inhibitors (azole antibiotics, some SSRIs); reaction difficult to predict; monitor for reaction

Increase: levels of CYP2C19 substrates (diazePAM, phenytoin, some tricyclics), adjust dose if needed

Decrease: effects of—cycloSPORINE, hormonal contraceptives, theophylline, estrogens

Delayed effect modafinil by 1 hr: methylphenidate

Altered: levels of CYP3A4 inducers (carBAMazepine, phenytoin, rifAMPin, cycloSPORINE, theophylline)

Drug/Herb

Increase: stimulation—cola nut, guarana, yerba maté, coffee, tea

Drug/Lab Test

Increase: LFTs, glucose, eosinophils

NURSING CONSIDERATIONS

Assess:

• Narcolepsy, shift work, history of sleep apnea

• **Stevens-Johnson syndrome:** rash, fever, fatigue, blisters; discontinue immediately if these occur; provide supportive therapy

• Depression, suicidal ideation

• Monitor B/P in those with hypertension

• **Pregnancy/breastfeeding:** pregnant patients should enroll in the pregnancy registry, 1-866-404-4106; use only when benefits outweigh risk to the fetus; avoid use in breastfeeding

• **Beers:** avoid in older adults; CNS stimulant effects

Evaluate:

• Ability to stay awake

Teach patient/family:

• To take only as directed; that product may be taken with/without food

• To use other form of contraception during and for ≥30 days after discontinuing medication if using hormonal birth control; to notify prescriber if pregnancy is planned or suspected or if breastfeeding

• To notify prescriber of allergic reaction, tremors, confusion, trouble breathing

• To avoid all OTC medications unless approved by prescriber; not to use alcohol

• To avoid hazardous activities until drug effect is known

RARELY USED

moexipril (Rx)

(moe-ex′ih-prill)

Univasc

Func. class.: Antihypertensive

Chem. class.: Angiotensin-converting enzyme inhibitor

USES: Hypertension, alone or in combination with thiazide diuretics

CONTRAINDICATIONS: Breastfeeding, children, hypersensitivity, heart block, bilateral renal stenosis, history of angioedema

Black Box Warning: Pregnancy

DOSAGE AND ROUTES

• **Adult: PO** 7.5 mg 1 hr before meals initially; may be increased or divided depending on B/P response; maintenance dosage 7.5-30 mg/day in 1-2 divided doses 1 hr before meals

Renal dose

• **Adult: PO** CCr <40 mL/min, 3.75 mg/day; titrate to desired dose; max 15 mg/day

---

RARELY USED

mogamulizumab
(moh-gam'-yoo-lih'-zoo-mab)
Poteligeo
Func. class.: Antineoplastic

USES: Cutaneous T-cell lymphoma (CTCL) (mycosis fungoides or Sézary syndrome) in those who have received at least 1 prior systemic therapy

CONTRAINDICATIONS: Hypersensitivity, pregnancy

DOSAGE AND ROUTES
• **Adult:** IV 1 mg/kg on days 1, 8, 15, and 22 in cycle 1, then 1 mg/kg on days 1 and 15 in subsequent cycles until disease progression; therapy cycles are repeated q28days

---

montelukast (Rx)
(mon-teh-loo'kast)
Singulair
Func. class.: Bronchodilator
Chem. class.: Leukotriene receptor antagonist, cysteinyl

Do not confuse:
Singulair/SINEquan

ACTION: Inhibits leukotriene (LTD_4) formation; leukotrienes exert their effects by increasing neutrophil, eosinophil migration; aggregation of neutrophils, monocytes; smooth muscle contraction, capillary permeability; these actions further lead to bronchoconstriction, inflammation, edema

USES: Chronic asthma in adults and children, seasonal allergic rhinitis, bronchospasm prophylaxis

CONTRAINDICATIONS: Hypersensitivity

Precautions: Pregnancy, breastfeeding, children <6 yr, acute attacks of asthma, alcohol consumption, severe hepatic disease, corticosteroid withdrawal, phenylketonuria, suicidal ideation, depression

DOSAGE AND ROUTES
Asthma, seasonal/perennial allergic rhinitis
• **Adult/child ≥15 yr:** PO 10 mg/day in PM
• **Child 6-14 yr:** PO 5-mg chew tab/day in PM
• **Child 2-5 yr:** PO (chew tab/granules) 4 mg/day
Asthma
Child 6-23 mo: PO 1 packet (4 mg) granules taken in PM
Exercise-induced bronchoconstriction prevention
• **Adult/child ≥15 yr:** PO 10 mg 2 hr before exercise; do not take another dose within 24 hr
• **Child 6 yr-<15 yr:** PO 5 mg once given 2 hr before exercise, max 1 dose/24 hr
Available forms: Tabs 10 mg; chew tabs 4, 5 mg; oral granules 4 mg/packet
Administer:
PO route
• In PM daily for all uses except exercise-induced bronchoconstriction; then take 2 hr before exercise
• Granules directly in mouth or mixed with spoonful of soft food (carrots, applesauce, ice cream, rice)
• Do not open granules packet until ready to use; mix whole dose; give within 15 min

SIDE EFFECTS
CNS: *Dizziness, fatigue, headache,* behavior changes, hallucinations, seizures, agitation, anxiety, depression, fever, drowsiness, suicidal ideation, memory impairment, hostility, somnambulism
GI: *Abdominal pain,* dyspepsia, nausea, vomiting, diarrhea, pancreatitis
HEMA: Thrombocytopenia
INTEG: Rash, pruritus, erythema
MS: Asthenia, myalgia, muscle cramps

RESP: *Influenza, cough,* nasal congestion
SYST: Churg-Strauss syndrome, Stevens-Johnson syndrome, toxic epidermal necrosis

PHARMACOKINETICS
Rapidly absorbed; peak 3-4 hr, chew tab (5 mg) 2-2.5 hr; half-life 2.7-5.5 hr, extended in hepatic disease; protein binding 99%; metabolized by liver; excreted via bile

INTERACTIONS
Increase: adverse reactions of CYP2C8 substrates
Decrease: montelukast levels—barbiturates, rifabutin, rifapentine, carBAMazepine, fosphenytoin, phenytoin, rifAMPin
Drug/Herb
Increase: stimulation—black, green tea, guarana
Drug/Lab Test
Increase: ALT, AST

NURSING CONSIDERATIONS
Assess:
• **Respiratory symptoms:** wheezing, decrease in asthma exacerbations, rhinitis, urticaria
• **Churg-Strauss syndrome (rare):** assess adult patients carefully for symptoms: eosinophilia, vasculitic rash, worsening pulmonary symptoms, cardiac complications, neuropathy
• For behavioral changes, suicidal ideation, other neuropsychiatric reactions
• **Severe hepatic disease:** use cautiously
• **Stevens-Johnson syndrome:** rash, fever, blisters, fatigue, muscle/joint aches; if these occur, discontinue, provide supportive therapy
• **Pregnancy/breastfeeding:** use in pregnancy only if clearly needed, no well-controlled studies; use cautiously in breastfeeding, unknown if excreted in breast milk
Evaluate:
• Therapeutic response: ability to breathe more easily

Teach patient/family:
• To check OTC medications, stimulation; to avoid alcohol
• To avoid hazardous activities; dizziness may occur
• If aspirin sensitivity is known, not to take NSAIDs while taking this product
• To report mood, behavioral changes to prescriber
• Not to use for acute asthma/acute exercise-induced bronchospasm; not effective
• To take even if no symptoms are present
• To continue to use inhaled β-agonists if exercise-induced asthma occurs
• **Granules:** to give directly in mouth or mixed in a spoonful of room temperature soft food (use only applesauce, carrots, rice, or ice cream); use within 15 min of opening packets; discard unused portions

M

⚠ HIGH ALERT

morphine (Rx)
(mor′feen)
Arymo ER, Doloral ✤, Duramorph PF, Infumorph, Kadian, MorphaBond ER, M-Eslon ✤, M-Eslon IR✤, Morphabond, Morphine LP Epidural ✤, MS IR ✤, MS Contin, MSIR ✤, Oramorph SR, Ratio-Morphine ✤, Simplist, Statex ✤
Func. class.: Opioid analgesic
Chem. class.: Alkaloid
Controlled Substance Schedule II

Do not confuse:
morphine/HYDROmorphone
MS Contin/OxyCONTIN

ACTION: Depresses pain impulse transmission at the spinal cord level by interacting with opioid receptors

USES: Moderate to severe pain
Unlabeled uses: Agitation, bone/dental pain, dyspnea in end-stage cancer or pulmonary disease, sedation induction, rapid-sequence intubation

CONTRAINDICATIONS: Hypersensitivity, addiction (opioid/alcohol), hemorrhage, bronchial asthma, increased intracranial pressure, paralytic ileus, hypovolemia, shock, MAOI therapy

Black Box Warning: Respiratory depression

Precautions: Pregnancy, breastfeeding, children <18 yr, geriatric patients, addictive personality, acute MI, severe heart disease, renal/hepatic disease, bowel impaction, abrupt discontinuation, seizures

Black Box Warning: Accidental exposure, epidural/intrathecal/IM/subcut administration, opioid-naïve patients, substance abuse, coadministration with other CNS depressants, ethanol ingestion, neonatal opioid withdrawal syndrome, potential for overdose or poisoning, requires a specialized care setting

Acute and chronic moderate pain or severe pain
PO Route (regular-release)
Adults: Initially, 10-30 mg q4hr as needed in opioid-naive patients. Titrate to pain relief. Only use the concentrated oral morphine solution (20 mg/mL) in opioid-tolerant patients. When converting parenteral to oral morphine, an oral dose that is 3 times the parenteral dose is generally sufficient. When converting from extended-release morphine, give the same 24-hr total as a divided regimen given at appropriate intervals. When converting from other oral or parenteral opioids, calculate the 24-hr total dose of the current opioid and consult pub-lished relative potency information for conversion.

Infants, children, and adolescents 6 mo to 17 yr (unlabeled): Initially, 0.2-0.3 mg/kg/dose q3-6 hr as needed; max initial dose of 5 mg/dose for children or the adult initial dose of 10 mg/dose for larger adolescents. Titrate to pain relief
Intermittent IV, IM, or SUBCUT
Adults: Initially, 2-10 mg/70 kg q3-4 hr as needed, titrated to pain relief. Higher doses (10 mg) are recommended for IM or SUBCUT; dosage may range from 5-20 mg IM or SUBCUT every 4 hr depending on patient requirements and response
Infants >6 mo and older, children, and adolescents: 0.05-0.2 mg/kg/dose q2-4 hr as needed; begin at the lower end of dosage range and titrate to effect (usual max dose: 4 mg for children or 8 mg for adolescents
Neonates (unlabeled) and infants<6 mo: Initially, 0.03-0.1 mg/kg/dose q3-4 hr as needed. Titrate upward as needed for adequate pain relief
Continuous IV infusion dosage (unlabeled)
Continuous infusions should only be used in acute care settings (ICU) where trained personnel are continuously monitoring the patient and emergency medications and equipment are readily available
Adults: Loading dose by slow IV infusion at a rate of 2 mg/min. Loading doses of 15-20 mg may be required; higher doses may be needed in opioid-tolerant patients. Initial infusion rates of 2-5 mg/hr have been used, with usual rates of 2-30 mg/hour used in critically ill patients. Higher infusion rates may be required in opioid-tolerant patients. Titrate dose to pain relief
Infants, children, and adolescents: A bolus of 0.05-0.2 mg/kg IV (or 5-10 mg for patients weighing more than 60 kg) followed by a continuous infusion. Initial infusion rates of 0.01-0.03 mg/kg/hr, but initial doses up to 0.06 mg/kg/hr may be appropriate for some patients. Alternatively, rates of 0.8-3 mg/hr IV may be

used for patients over 60 kg. Titrate to pain relief

Neonates: 0.01-0.02 mg/kg/hr and titrate to effect. May increase up to 0.03 mg/kg/hr if needed

Continuous subcut infusion dosage (unlabeled)

Adults: Initial infusion rates of 2-5 mg/hr may be used, with usual rates of 2-30 mg/hr used in critically ill patients

Infants, children, and adolescents: Initial rate of 0.03 mg/kg/hr. The mean infusion rate was 0.0175 mg/kg/hr over the first 24 hr after surgery in 60 patients (aged 7 mo to 20 yr) and decreased to 0.011-0.0133 mg/kg/hr over the next 48 hr. Titrate dose to pain relief

IV dosage (patient-controlled analgesia [PCA])

Adults: Starting dose should be based on the patient's recent exposure to opioids. Titrate the regimen to patient response. Larger doses may be needed in opioid-tolerant patients. For OPIOID-NAIVE patients, start with a demand dose of 1 mg (range: 0.5-2.5 mg) and lockout interval of 6 min (range: 5-10 min), with a maximal dosing rate of 10 mg/hr. For OPIOID TOLERANT patients, start with a demand dose of 2-5 mg IV and lockout interval of 6 min (range: 5-10 min), with a maximal dosing rate of 30 mg/hr

Children >7 yr and adolescents

Demand dose: 0.01-0.025 mg/kg IV (max: 1 mg/dose)

Lockout interval: 5-10 min

Doses per hour: 5

Epidural dosage (morphine sulfate injection, but NOT DepoDur)

Adults: Initially, inject 5 mg epidurally in the lumbar region and assess the patient in 1 hr; if pain relief is not adequate at that time, administer incremental doses of 1-2 mg, with sufficient time between injections to appropriately assess for efficacy. Max: 10 mg per 24 hr. For continuous epidural infusion, initiate at 2-4 mg per 24 hr, with additional doses of 1-2 mg given if pain relief is not initially achieved

Intrathecal dosage (morphine sulfate injection, but NOT DepoDur)

Adults: 0.2-1 mg in the lumbar area as a single dose or to establish dosage for continuous intrathecal infusion

Rectal dosage

Adults: 10-20 mg q4hr, as needed

PO [extended-release tablets (Arymo ER, Morphabond, MS Contin) or capsules (Kadian, Avinza)] in opioid nontolerant adult patients

Adults: 15 mg q8hr or q12hr (Arymo ER, Morphabond, or MS Contin) or 30 mg q24hr (Avinza) for use as the first opioid analgesic. Do not use Kadian capsules as a first opioid analgesic; initiate with an immediate-release formulation and then convert patients to Kadian. For opioid nontolerant patients, initiate with 15 mg q12hr (MS Contin), 15 mg q8hr or q12hr (Arymo ER or Morphabond), or 30 mg q24hr (Avinza or Kadian). With the exception of Avinza, adjust the dose every 1-2 days based upon the total daily morphine requirements (extended-release dose plus breakthrough doses). Adjust the dose of Avinza q3-4 days in increments of 30 mg or less.

PO dosage [extended-release tablets (Arymo ER, Morphabond, MS Contin) or capsules (Kadian, Avinza)] in adult patients receiving other opioid agonist therapy

Adults: Discontinue all other around-the-clock opioids. To convert from other morphine formulations, calculate the morphine 24-hr oral requirement; in general, the 24-hr oral requirement is 3 times the 24-hr parenteral requirement. Initiate dosing, using the 24-hr oral requirement (round down to the closest available tablet/capsule strength), for: Arymo ER, Morphabond, or MS Contin at one-half of the requirement every 12 hr or one-third q8hr; Avinza at the total requirement once q24hr; and Kadian at one-half q12hr or the total once q24hr. When initiating extended-release morphine, anticipate

M

and treat breakthrough pain with adequate doses of immediate-release morphine as needed. When converting from other opioids, established conversion ratios to extended-release formulations have not been defined by clinical trials. Initiate dosing for: Arymo ER, Morphabond, or MS Contin at 15 mg q8hr or q12hr; and Avinza or Kadian at 30 mg q24hr. Alternatively, initiate with one-half of the calculated morphine 24-hr oral requirement estimate, anticipating breakthrough pain and providing adequate doses of immediate-release morphine as needed.

Available forms: Immediate release tablets 15, 30 mg; extended release tablets (Arymo ER) 15, 30, 60 mg; extended release tablets (MS Contin) 15, 30, 60, 100, 200 mg; extended release tablets (Morphabond ER) 15, 30, 60, 100 mg; extended release capsules (Kadian) 10, 20, 30, 40, 50, 60, 70, 80, 100, 130, 150, 200 mg; extended release capsules 30, 45, 60, 75, 90, 120 mg; oral solution 1 mg/mL ♥, 2 mg/mL, 4 mg/mL, 5 mg/mL ♥, 20 mg/mL; rectal suppositories 5, 10, 20, 30 mg; solution for injection (IM, IV, SUBCUT) 1 mg/mL, 2 mg/mL, 4 mg/mL, 5 mg/mL, 8 mg/mL, 10 mg/mL, 15 mg/mL, 25 mg/mL, 50 mg/mL; solution for epidural, IV (no preservative) 0.5 mg/mL, 1 mg/mL; solution for IT or epidural, continuous microinfusion device no preservative 10 mg/mL, 25 mg/mL; solution for IV (PCA device) 1 mg/mL, 2 mg/mL, 3 mg/mL, 5 mg/mL

Administer:

PO route

• Give with food or milk to minimize GI effects

• Begin with immediate-release products and titrate to correct dose and convert to a sustained-release product

• **Immediate-release cap:** may swallow whole, or cap may be opened and contents sprinkled on cool food (pudding or applesauce) or added to juice; give immediately or delivered via gastric or NG tube by either adding to or following with liquid

• **Extended-release and controlled-release tabs:** swallow whole; do not crush, break, dissolve, or chew

• The use of MS Contin 100-mg or 200-mg tabs should be limited to opioid-tolerant patients requiring oral doses equivalent to ≥200 mg/day; use of the 100-mg or 200-mg tablet is only recommended for patients who have already been titrated to a stable analgesic regimen using lower strengths of MS Contin or other opioids

• **Sustained-release caps:** swallow; do not chew, crush, or dissolve; caps may be opened and contents sprinkled on applesauce (at room temperature or cooler) immediately before ingestion; do not chew, crush, or dissolve the pellets/beads inside the cap; the applesauce should be swallowed without chewing; if the pellets/beads are chewed, an immediate release of a potentially fatal morphine dose may be delivered; rinse mouth

• **Kadian caps:** may be given through a 16-F gastrostomy tube; flush with water, and sprinkle the cap contents into 10 mL of water; using a funnel and a swirling motion, pour the pellets and water into the tube; rinse the beaker with 10 mL of water, and pour the water into the funnel; repeat until no pellets remain in the beaker; *do not administer Kadian through a nasogastric tube*

• Kadian 100 mg, 130 mg, 150 mg, or 200 mg caps are given only to opioid-tolerant patients

Oral liquid

• Check dose before use because many concentrations of oral solution are available; may be diluted in fruit juice; protect from light

Injectable administration

• Visually inspect for particulate matter, discoloration before use; do not use if a precipitate is present after shaking; do not use the Duramorph solution if a precipitate is present or if the color is darker than pale yellow

SUBCUT route

• Inject, taking care not to inject intradermally

• **Continuous SC infusion:** morphine is not approved by the FDA for subcut use; dilute to an appropriate concentration in D₅W; give using a portable, controlled, subcut device; adjust rate based on patient response and tolerance; max subcut rate is 2 mL/hour/site

Intrathecal/epidural route

• Morphine sulfate injection is not interchangeable with morphine sulfate extended-release liposome injection (DepoDur); DepoDur is only for epidural administration

• Do not use Infumorph (10 mg/mL or 25 mg/mL) for single-dose neuraxial injection because lower doses can be more reliably administered with Duramorph (0.5 mg/mL or 1 mg/mL)

Rectal route

• Moisten the suppository with water before insertion; if suppository is too soft, chill in the refrigerator for 30 min or run cold water over it before removing the wrapper

IV route

• Before use, an opiate antagonist and emergency facilities should be available

• Do not use the highly concentrated morphine injections (i.e., 10-25 mg/mL) for IV, IM, or SC administration of single doses; these injection solutions are intended for use via continuous, controlled microinfusion devices

• **Direct IV route:** dilute dose with ≥5 mL of sterile water for injection or NS injection; inject 2.5-15 mg directly into a vein or into the tubing of a freely flowing IV solution over 4-5 min; do not give rapidly

• **Continuous IV infusion:** dilute in 5% dextrose; use a controlled-infusion device; adjust dosage and rate based on patient response

• **Patient-controlled analgesia (PCA):** a compatible patient-controlled infusion device must be used; dilute solutions to a concentration of 1 or 10 mg/mL for ease in calculations and programming of PCA pumps; adjust dosage and rate based on patient response; consult the patient-controlled infusion device manual for directions on rate of infusion

Y-site compatibilities: Acetaminophen, aldesleukin, allopurinol, amifostine, amikacin, aminophylline, amiodarone, amsacrine, atenolol, atracurium, aztreonam, bumetanide, calcium chloride, cefamandole, ceFAZolin, cefotaxime, cefoTEtan, cefOXitin, cefTAZidime, ceftizoxime, cefTRIAXone, cefuroxime, cephalothin, chloramphenicol, cisatracurium, cladribine, clindamycin, cyclophosphamide, cytarabine, dexamethasone, digoxin, diltiaZEM, DOBUTamine, DOPamine, doxycycline, enalaprilat, EPINEPHrine, erythromycin, esmolol, etomidate, famotidine, fentaNYL, filgrastim, fluconazole, fludarabine, foscarnet, gentamicin, granisetron, heparin, hydrocortisone, HYDROmorphone, kanamycin, labetalol, lidocaine, LORazepam, magnesium sulfate, melphalan, meropenem, methotrexate, methyldopate, methylPREDNISolone, metoclopramide, metoprolol, metroNIDAZOLE, midazolam, milrinone, nafcillin, niCARdipine, nitroglycerin, norepinephrine, ondansetron, oxacillin, oxytocin, PACLitaxel, pancuronium, penicillin G potassium, piperacillin, piperacillin/tazobactam, potassium chloride, propranolol, raNITIdine, remifentanil, sodium bicarbonate, teniposide, thiotepa, ticarcillin, ticarcillin/clavulanate, tigecycline, tobramycin, vancomycin, vecuronium, vinorelbine, vit B/C, warfarin, zidovudine, zoledronic acid

SIDE EFFECTS

CNS: Drowsiness, dizziness, confusion, headache, sedation, euphoria, insomnia, *seizures*

CV: Palpitations, *bradycardia*, change in B/P, *shock*, *cardiac arrest*, chest pain, hypo/hypertension, edema, *tachycardia*

EENT: Blurred vision, miosis, diplopia

ENDO: Gynecomastia

M

GI: Nausea, vomiting, anorexia, constipation, cramps, biliary tract pressure
GU: Urinary retention, impotence, gonadal suppression
HEMA: Thrombocytopenia
INTEG: Rash, urticaria, bruising, flushing, diaphoresis, pruritus
RESP: Respiratory depression, respiratory arrest, apnea

PHARMACOKINETICS
PO: Onset variable, peak 60 min, duration 4-5 hr
IM: Onset $1/2$ hr, peak 30-60 min, duration 4-5 hr
SUBCUT: Onset 15-20 min, peak 50-90 min, duration 4-5 hr
IV: Peak 20 min, duration 4-5 hr
RECT: Peak $1/2$-1 hr, duration 3-7 hr
Intrathecal: Onset rapid, duration ≤24 hr
Metabolized by liver, crosses placenta; excreted in urine, breast milk; half-life IM 3-4 hr; Kadian 11-13 hr

INTERACTIONS
• **Unpredictable reaction, avoid use:** MAOIs
Increase: serotonin syndrome risk—SSRIs, SNRIs, tricyclics, MAOIs, amoxapine, dolasetron, palonosetron, antimigraine agents, linezolid, lithium, methylene blue, traZODone; monitor for serotonin syndrome
Increase: effects with other CNS depressants—alcohol, opiates, sedative/hypnotics, antipsychotics, skeletal muscle relaxants, general anesthetics, benzodiazepine; avoid using together; increased respiratory depression
Decrease: morphine effect—butorphanol, nalbuphine, pentazocine; consider using another product; withdrawal symptoms may occur
Decrease: morphine action—rifAMPin
Drug/Herb
Increase: CNS depression—chamomile, hops, kava, St. John's wort, valerian
Drug/Lab Test
Increase: amylase, lipase

NURSING CONSIDERATIONS
Assess:
• **Pain:** location, intensity, type, charac-

ter; check for pain relief 20 min following IV, 1 hr following PO/IM/Subcut; titrate to relieve pain; give dose before pain becomes severe
• Bowel status; constipation common, use stimulant laxative if needed; provide increased bulk, fluids in diet
• I&O ratio; check for decreasing output; may indicate urinary retention; monitor serum sodium
• B/P, pulse, respirations (character, depth, rate)
• CNS changes: dizziness, drowsiness, hallucinations, euphoria, LOC, pupil reaction
• **Abrupt discontinuation:** gradually taper to prevent withdrawal symptoms; decrease by 50% q1-2days; avoid use of narcotic antagonists
• Allergic reactions: rash, urticaria

Black Box Warning: Accidental exposure: if Duramorph or Infumorph gets on skin, remove contaminated clothing, rinse affected area with water

Black Box Warning: Requires a specialized care setting: patient should be observed for ≥24 hr; have emergency equipment nearby

Black Box Warning: Respiratory dysfunction: depression, character, rate, rhythm; notify prescriber if respirations are <12/min; accidental overdose has occurred with high-potency oral sols

• Gradual withdrawal after long-term use

Black Box Warning: Pregnancy/breastfeeding: use only if benefits outweigh risk to fetus; longer use can result in neonatal opioid withdrawal syndrome; do not breastfeed

Evaluate:
• Therapeutic response: decrease in pain intensity
Teach patient/family:

Black Box Warning: To keep out of the reach of children, pets

Black Box Warning: To notify health care professional if pregnancy is planned or suspected

• To avoid driving, hazardous activities until response is known
• To turn, cough and deep breathe if on bed rest
• To report constipation, as other products will need to be used
• To change position slowly; orthostatic hypotension may occur
• To report any symptoms of CNS changes, allergic reactions
• That physical dependency may result from long-term use
• To avoid use of alcohol, CNS depressants
• That withdrawal symptoms may occur: nausea, vomiting, cramps, fever, faintness, anorexia
• To take exactly as directed; do not crush, break, chew, or dissolve caps or tabs

TREATMENT OF OVERDOSE: Naloxone (Narcan) 0.2-0.8 mg IV (caution with opioid-tolerant individuals), O_2, IV fluids, vasopressors

⚠ HIGH ALERT

RARELY USED

moxetumomab pasudotox
(mox-e-toom'oh-mab pa-soo'doe-tox)
Lumoxiti
Func. class.: Antineoplastic

USES: Relapsed or refractory hairy-cell leukemia in patients who have received at least 2 prior systemic therapies, including treatment with a purine nucleoside analog

CONTRAINDICATIONS: Hypersensitivity

Black Box Warning: Capillary leak syndrome, hemolytic-uremic syndrome

DOSAGE AND ROUTES
• **Adult: IV** 0.04 mg/kg (actual body weight) over 30 min on days 1, 3, and 5 repeated q28days until disease progression or a maximum of 6 cycles

moxifloxacin (Rx)
(mocks-ah-flox' a-sin)
Avelox, Avelox IV, Moxeza, Vigamox
Func. class.: Antiinfective
Chem. class.: Fluoroquinolone

ACTION: Interferes with conversion of intermediate DNA fragments into high-molecular-weight DNA in bacteria; DNA gyrase inhibitor

USES: Acute bacterial sinusitis: *Streptococcus pneumoniae, Haemophilus influenzae, Moraxella catarrhalis;* acute bacterial exacerbation of chronic bronchitis: *S. pneumoniae, H. influenzae, Haemophilus parainfluenzae, Klebsiella pneumoniae, Staphylococcus aureus, M. catarrhalis;* community-acquired pneumonia: *S. pneumoniae, H. influenzae, Mycoplasma pneumoniae, Chlamydia pneumoniae, M. catarrhalis;* uncomplicated skin/skin-structure infections: *S. aureus, Streptococcus pyogenes;* complicated intraabdominal infections including polymicrobial infections: *E. coli, Bacterioides fragilis, S. anginosus, S. constellatus, Enterococcus faecalis, Proteus mirabilis, Clostridium perfringens, Bacteroides thetaiotaomicron, Peptostreptococcus* sp; complicated skin, skin-structure infections caused by methicillin-susceptible bacteria: *S. aureus, E. coli, K. pneumoniae,*

M

Enterobacter cloacae; prophylaxis and treatment of plague caused by *Yersinia pestis,* including pneumonic and septicemic plague

Unlabeled uses: Anthrax treatment/prophylaxis, gastroenteritis, MAC, nongonococcal urethritis, shigellosis, surgical infection prophylaxis, TB

CONTRAINDICATIONS: Hypersensitivity to quinolones

Precautions: Pregnancy, breastfeeding, children, hepatic/cardiac/renal/GI disease, epilepsy, uncorrected hypokalemia, prolonged QT interval; patients receiving class IA, III antidysrhythmics; seizure disorder, pseudomembranous colitis, diabetes mellitus

Black Box Warning: Tendon pain, rupture; tendinitis, myasthenia gravis

DOSAGE AND ROUTES
Acute bacterial sinusitis
• **Adult: PO/IV** 400 mg q24hr × 10 days
Acute bacterial exacerbation of chronic bronchitis
• **Adult: PO/IV** 400 mg q24hr × 5 days
Community-acquired pneumonia
• **Adult: PO/IV** 400 mg q24hr × 7-14 days
Uncomplicated skin/skin-structure infections
• **Adult: PO/IV** 400 mg q24hr × 7 days
Complicated intraabdominal infections
• **Adult: IV** 400 mg/day × 7-21 days
Complicated skin, skin-structure infections
• **Adult: PO/IV** 400 mg/day × 7-21 days
Plague
• **Adult: PO/IV** 400 mg q24hr × 10-14 days
Bacterial conjunctivitis
• **Adult/child ≥1 yr** (Vigamox): 1 drop into affected eye(s) tid × 7 days
• **Adult/child ≥4 mo** (Moxeza): 1 drop into affected eye(s) bid × 7 days
Available forms: Tabs 400 mg; inj premix 400 mg/250 mL; opthalmic solution 0.5%

Administer:
PO route
• 4 hr before or 8 hr after antacids, zinc, iron, calcium, sucralfate, multivitamins
• Without regard to food
• Store at room temperature; do not refrigerate, do not use if particulate is present
IV route
• Do not use if particulate matter is present
• Give PO 4 hr before or 8 hr after antacids, sucrasulfate, multivitamins
• Do not give SUBCUT, IM
• Available as premixed sol; may be diluted at ratios from 1:10 to 10:1; do not refrigerate; give by direct infusion or through Y-type infusion set; do not add other medications to sol or infusion through same IV line at same time
• Flush line with compatible sol before and after use
• Do not admix

Solution compatibilities: 0.9% NaCl, D_5, D_{10}, LR, sterile water for inj
Opthalmic route
• After instilling use gentle pressure on lacrimal duct for 2 min

SIDE EFFECTS
CNS: *Headache,* dizziness, fatigue, insomnia, depression, *restlessness,* seizures, confusion, increased intracranial pressure, peripheral neuropathy, pseudotumor cerebri, fever
CV: Prolonged QT interval, dysrhythmias, torsades de pointes, tachycardia
EENT: Blurred vision, tinnitus, taste changes
GI: *Nausea, diarrhea,* increased ALT, AST, flatulence, heartburn, *vomiting,* oral candidiasis, dysphagia, pseudomembranous colitis, abdominal pain, dyspepsia, constipation, gastroenteritis, xerostomia
GU: Renal failure
INTEG: *Rash,* pruritus, urticaria, photosensitivity, flushing, fever, chills, injection-site reactions
MISC: Candidiasis vaginitis
MS: Tremor, arthralgia, tendinitis, tendon rupture, myalgia

SYST: Anaphylaxis, Stevens-Johnson syndrome, angioedema, toxic epidermal necrolysis

PHARMACOKINETICS
Excreted in urine as active product, metabolites; parent product excreted in urine (20%), feces (25%); half-life PO 12-16 hr, IV 8-15 hr, peak 1 hr (PO), 1-3 hr (IV)

INTERACTIONS
Increase: QT prolongation—drugs that increase QT interval; avoid using concurrently

Increase: moxifloxacin serum levels—probenecid

Increase: warfarin, cycloSPORINE effect

Increase: seizure risk—NSAIDs; monitor, adjust or use different product

Black Box Warning: **Increase:** tendon rupture—corticosteroids

Increase: anticoagulant level—warfarin; monitor PT/INR

Decrease: moxifloxacin absorption—magnesium antacids, aluminum hydroxide, zinc, iron, sucralfate, calcium, enteral feeding, didanosine

Drug/Lab Test
Increase: glucose, lipids, triglycerides, uric acid, LDH ALT, ionized calcium, chloride, globulin, albumin, PT, INR, WBC

Decrease: potassium, glucose, amylase, RBC, eosinophils, Hb, Hct

NURSING CONSIDERATIONS
Assess:
• CNS symptoms: headache, dizziness, fatigue, insomnia, depression, seizures
• Renal, hepatic studies: BUN, creatinine, AST, ALT, electrolytes
• I&O ratio, urine pH <5.5 is ideal
• **Allergic reactions, Stevens-Johnson syndrome, toxic epidermal necrolysis, anaphylaxis:** fever, flushing, rash, urticaria, pruritus, sore throat, fatigue, ulcers, other lesions; keep EPINEPHrine, emergency equipment nearby for anaphylaxis

Black Box Warning: Tendon pain, rupture, tendinitis; if tendon becomes inflamed, product should be discontinued; more common in Achilles tendon

• **Cardiac status:** prolonged QT or use of products that increase QT prolongation
• **CDAD:** assess for diarrhea, abdominal pain, fever, fatigue, anorexia; possible anemia, elevated WBC, low serum albumin; stop product; usually either vancomycin or IV metroNIDAZOLE given
• Increased fluids to 3 L/day to avoid crystallization in kidneys

Black Box Warning: **Myasthenia gravis:** assess for increased weakness when using this product; avoid using in this condition

Black Box Warning: **Peripheral neuropathy:** assess for pain, numbness, tingling in extremities; report

• **Pregnancy/breastfeeding:** risks to fetus are unknown; adverse events observed in some animal studies; discuss risks, benefits of treatment
Evaluate:
• Therapeutic response: decreased pain, C&S; absence of infection
Teach patient/family:

Black Box Warning: To notify prescriber of tendon pain, inflammation, or burning, tingling, weakness; stop drug

• Not to take any products containing magnesium or calcium (such as antacids), iron, or aluminum with this product or 4 hr before or 8 hr after
• That photosensitivity may occur; to avoid sunlight or use sunscreen to prevent burns
• To use frequent rinsing of mouth, sugarless candy or gum for dry mouth
• To take as prescribed; not to double or miss doses; to take without regard to meals
• To report immediately rash, diarrhea, rapid heartbeat

M

Side effects: *italics* = common; red = life-threatening

• If dizziness occurs, to ambulate, perform activities with assistance
• To complete full course of product therapy
• To contact prescriber if abnormal heart rhythm or seizures occur

moxifloxacin (ophthalmic)

(mocks-ih-floks'a-sin)

Vigamox, Moxeza

Func. class.: Ophthalmic antiinfective
Chem. class.: Fluoroquinolone

Do not confuse:

moxifloxacin/ciprofloxacin/gatifloxacin/levoFLOXacin

ACTION: Inhibits DNA gyrase, thereby decreasing bacterial replication

USES: Bacterial conjunctivitis (aerobic gram-positive/negative organisms), *Chlamydia trachomatis*

CONTRAINDICATIONS: Hypersensitivity to this product or fluoroquinolones
Precautions: Pregnancy, breastfeeding

DOSAGE AND ROUTES
Bacterial conjunctivitis
• **Adult/adolescent/child ≥1 yr: ophthalmic SOL** 1 drop in affected eye(s) bid (Moxeza) or tid (Vigamox) × 7 days
Available forms: Ophthalmic solution 0.5%
Administer:
Ophthalmic route
• Commercially available ophthalmic solutions are not for injection subconjunctivally or into the anterior chamber of the eye
• Apply topically to the eye, taking care to avoid contamination
• Do not touch the tip of the dropper to the eye, fingertips, or other surface
• Apply pressure to lacrimal sac for 1 min after instillation
• Avoid wearing contact lenses during treatment

SIDE EFFECTS
EENT: Hypersensitivity, pruritus, blurred vision, tearing

PHARMACOKINETICS
Half-life 13 hr

NURSING CONSIDERATIONS
Assess:
• **Allergic reaction:** assess for hypersensitivity; discontinue product
Evaluate:
• Decreased ophthalmic infection
Teach patient/family:
Ophthalmic route
• To apply topically to the eye, taking care to avoid contamination
• That product is for ophthalmic use only
• Not to touch the tip of the dropper to the eye, fingertips, or other surface
• To apply pressure to lacrimal sac for 1 min after installation
• To avoid wearing contact lenses during treatment

mupirocin (topical, nasal)

(myoo-pihr'oh-sin)

Bactroban, Centany

Func. class.: Topical antiinfective

ACTION: Antibacterial activity results from inhibition of protein synthesis; bacteriostatic at low concentration, bactericidal at high concentration

USES: Impetigo, skin lesions *(Staphylococcus aureus/Streptococcus pyogenes)*; nasal: methicillin-resistant *S. aureus*

CONTRAINDICATIONS: Hypersensitivity to this product
Precautions: Open wounds, burns, severe kidney disease, children, pregnancy, breastfeeding

DOSAGE AND ROUTES
Impetigo
• **Adult/child: TOP** apply to affected area tid × 1-2 wk

Skin lesions

• **Adult/child: TOP** apply to affected area tid × 10 days

Methicillin-resistant *S. aureus* in the nose

• **Adult/child ≥12 yr: NASAL** divide ointment in single use tube in half; use in each nostril bid × 5 days

Available forms: Topical cream, ointment 2%; intranasal ointment 2%

Administer:

Topical route

• Do not use skin products near the eyes, nose, or mouth

• Wash hands before and after use; wash affected area and gently pat dry

• May cover treated areas with gauze dressing

Cream/ointment

• Apply a thin film to the cleansed affected area; massage gently into affected areas, do not use near eyes, mouth

• **Nasal:** Close nostrils by squeezing and releasing and gently massaging over 1 min

SIDE EFFECTS

CNS: Headache

EENT: Burning, pharyngitis, rhinitis (nasal)

GI: Taste change, nausea

INTEG: Burning, rash, pruritus

INTERACTIONS

Decrease: Effect of other nasal products

NURSING CONSIDERATIONS

Assess:

• **Allergic reaction:** assess for hypersensitivity; product may need to be discontinued

• **Infection:** assess for number of lesions, severity in impetigo, other skin disorders

Evaluate:

• Decreased lesions in impetigo, other skin disorders

Teach patient/family:

Topical route

• Not to use skin products near the eyes, nose, or mouth

• To wash hands before and after use and to wash affected area and gently pat dry

• **Cream/ointment:** to apply a thin film to the cleansed affected area; to cover treated areas with gauze dressing if desired

• **Nasal:** to close nostrils by squeezing and releasing and gently massaging over 1 min

---

mycophenolate mofetil (Rx)

(mye-koe-phen'oh-late)

CellCept,

Mycophenolate acid

Myfortic

Func. class.: Immunosuppressant

ACTION: Inhibits inflammatory responses that are mediated by the immune system

USES: Prophylaxis for organ rejection in allogenic cardiac, hepatic, renal transplants

Unlabeled uses: Nephrotic syndrome

CONTRAINDICATIONS: Hypersensitivity to this product or mycophenolic acid

Black Box Warning: Pregnancy

Precautions: Breastfeeding, lymphomas, neutropenia, renal disease, accidental exposure, anemia

Black Box Warning: Infection, neoplastic disease; requires an experienced clinician and a specialized care setting

DOSAGE AND ROUTES

For kidney transplant rejection prophylaxis with or without antithymocyte induction

• **Adult: IV** 1 g over at least 2 hr bid in combination with corticosteroids and cycloSPORINE; initial dose should be given within 24 hr of transplantation

Oral dosage

The delayed-release tablets (mycophenolate sodium) and the capsules, oral suspension, and tablets (mycophenolate mofetil) are not interchangeable on an mg basis.

• **Adult: PO** (regular release) 1 g mycophenolate mofetil or **PO** (extended release) 720 mg mycophenolate sodium bid in combination with corticosteroids and cyclosporine

• **Child: PO** (oral suspension) 600 mg/m^2 bid, max 2 g/day. Mycophenolate mofetil capsules may be given at dose of 750 mg bid for those with a body surface area (BSA) of 1.25–1.5 m^2 or 1 g bid for those with a BSA >1.5 m^2; mycophenolate sodium delayed-release tablets 400 mg/m^2 bid, max 720 mg bid

• **Infant ≥3 mo: PO** (oral suspension) 600 mg/m^2 bid, max 2 g/day

For heart transplant rejection prophylaxis

• **Adult: IV** 1.5 g over at least 2 hr bid in combination with corticosteroids and cycloSPORINE. The first dose may be administered within 24 hr after transplantation

• **Adult: PO** (regular release) (mycophenolate mofetil) 1.5 g bid in combination with corticosteroids and cycloSPORINE. Initial oral dose should be administered as soon as possible after transplantation

For liver transplant rejection prophylaxis

• **Adult: IV** 1 g over at least 2 hr bid in combination with corticosteroids and cycloSPORINE; the first dose may be administered within 24 hr after transplantation

• **Adult: PO** (mycophenolate mofetil) 1.5 g bid in combination with corticosteroids and cycloSPORINE; give initial dose as soon as possible after transplantation

Available forms: Caps 250 mg; tabs 500 mg; inj (powder) 500 mg/20-mL vial; powder for oral susp 200 mg/mL; delayed rel tab (Myfortic) 180, 360 mg

Administer:

• May be given in combination with corticosteroids, cycloSPORINE

• **Cytotoxic:** Use safe handling procedures; avoid inhalation or direct contact with skin, mucous membranes; terato-genic in animals; wash skin if product comes in contact with skin

PO route

• Do not break, crush, or chew tabs; do not open caps

• Give at same time each day

• **Oral susp:** tap closed bottle several times to loosen powder; use 94 mL of water in graduated cylinder; add $^1/_2$ total amount of water for reconstitution and shake the closed bottle; add remaining water and shake again; remove child-resistant cap; push adapter into neck of bottle; close tightly, may give by NG tube ≥8 French catheter

• Give alone for better absorption

Intermittent IV INFUSION route

• Reconstitute each vial with 14 mL D$_5$W; shake gently; further dilute to 6 mg/mL; dilute 1 g/140 mL D$_5$W, 1.5 g/210 mL D$_5$W; give by slow IV infusion ≥2 hr; never give by bolus or rapid IV inj

• Do not give with other medications or sol, do not use if particulates are present

Y-site compatibilities: Alemtuzumab, alfentanil, amikacin, anidulafungin, argatroban, bivalirudin, caspofungin, cefepime, DAPTOmycin, DOPamine, norepinephrine, octreotide, oxytocin, tacrolimus, tigecycline, tirofiban, vancomycin, zoledronic acid

SIDE EFFECTS

CNS: *Tremor, dizziness, insomnia, headache, fever,* anxiety, pain, progressive multifocal leukoencephalopathy, asthenia, paresthesia

CV: *Hypertension, chest pain,* hypotension, edema

GI: *Diarrhea, constipation, nausea, vomiting,* stomatitis, GI bleeding, abdominal pain, anorexia, dyspepsia

GU: *UTI, hematuria,* renal tubular necrosis, polyomavirus-associated nephropathy

HEMA: Leukopenia, thrombocytopenia, anemia, pancytopenia, pure red cell aplasia, neutropenia

INTEG: *Rash*

META: *Peripheral edema, hypercholesterolemia, hypophosphatemia, edema, hyperkalemia, hypokalemia, hyperglycemia,* hypocalcemia, hypomagnesemia

MS: Arthralgia, muscle wasting, back pain, weakness
RESP: *Dyspnea, respiratory infection, increased cough, pharyngitis, bronchitis, pneumonia,* plural effusion, pulmonary fibrosis
SYST: Lymphoma, *nonmelanoma skin carcinoma,* sepsis

PHARMACOKINETICS
Rapidly and completely absorbed; metabolized to active metabolite (MPA); excreted in urine, feces; protein binding (MPA) 97%; half-life (MPA) 17.9 hr

INTERACTIONS
Increase: bone marrow suppression—azaTHIOprine; do not use concurrently
Increase: bleeding risk—anticoagulants, NSAIDs, thrombolytics, salicylates
Increase: toxicity—acyclovir, ganciclovir, valACYclovir; monitor if used together
Increase: effects of both products—phenytoin, theophylline
Increase: mycophenolate levels—probenecid, immunosuppressives, salicylates; monitor for adverse reactions
Decrease: mycophenolate levels—antacids (magnesium, aluminum), cholestyramine, cycloSPORINE, rifamycin; separate dosing times by several hr
Decrease: protein binding of phenytoin, theophylline
Decrease: effect of live attenuated vaccines, oral contraceptives
Drug/Herb
Interference with immunosuppression: astragalus, cat's claw, echinacea, melatonin
Drug/Food
Decrease: absorption if taken with food
Drug/Lab Test
Increase: serum creatinine, BUN, cholesterol, potassium, WBC

NURSING CONSIDERATIONS
Assess:
• **Progressive multifocal leukoencephalopathy:** may be fatal; ataxia,

confusion, apathy, hemiparesis, visual problems, weakness; side effects should be reported to FDA
• **Pure red cell aplasia (PRCA):** occurs when used in combination with other immunosuppressants; assess for fatigue, pulmonary tachycardia; may cause graft rejection
• Blood studies: CBC during treatment monthly, may monitor mycophenolate levels in those at high risk for organ rejection
• Hepatic studies: alk phos, AST, ALT, bilirubin
• Renal studies: BUN, CCr, electrolytes

> **Black Box Warning: Pregnancy/breastfeeding:** pregnancy test within 1 wk before initiation of treatment; confirm negative pregnancy test; if patient becomes pregnant, enroll in Mycophenolate Pregnancy Registry 1-800-617-8191; do not breastfeed during treatment and for 6 wk after final dose

> **Black Box Warning: Requires a specialized setting and experienced clinician:** should be used by those experienced in the use of immunosuppressive therapy in a facility equipped for transplants

Evaluate:
• Therapeutic response: absence of graft rejection
Teach patient/family:
• About the need for repeated lab tests and follow-up exams

> **Black Box Warning: Pregnancy/breastfeeding:** to use 2 forms of contraception before, during, and for 6 wk after therapy; not to breastfeed during and for 6 wk after final dose; that pregnancy test is required the wk before start of therapy and 8-10 days later

M

• To take at same time each day; not to crush, chew caps, or ext rel tab; swallow whole, take on empty stomach

Black Box Warning: Infection: to report fever, chills, sore throat, fatigue; serious infections may occur; avoid crowds, persons with known infections

Black Box Warning: Neoplastic disease: lymphoma and other neoplastic diseases may occur, particularly skin cancer; limit UV exposure by wearing protective clothing, sunscreen

RARELY USED

nabumetone (Rx)
(na-byoo′me-tone)

Relafen ✦

Func. class.: Nonsteroidal antiinflammatory

Chem. class.: Acetic acid derivative

USES: Osteoarthritis, rheumatoid arthritis, acute or chronic treatment

CONTRAINDICATIONS: Hypersensitivity to this product or aspirin, NSAIDs

Black Box Warning: Perioperative pain with CABG surgery

DOSAGE AND ROUTES
• **Adult: PO** 1 g as single dose or divided bid; max 2 g/day if needed
Renal dose
• **Adult: PO** CCr 31-49 mL/min, 750 mg daily, max 1500 mg/day; CCr <30 mL/min, 500 mg daily, max 1000 mg/day

⚠ HIGH ALERT

nadolol (Rx)
(nay-doe′lole)

Corgard, Syn-Nadol ✦

Func. class.: Antihypertensive, antianginal

Chem. class.: β-Adrenergic receptor blocker

Do not confuse:
Corgard/Cognex/Coreg
Nadolol/Mandol

ACTION: Long-acting, nonselective β-adrenergic receptor blocking agent, blocks β_1 in the heart and β_2 in the lungs, uterus, and circulatory system; mechanism is similar to that of propranolol

USES: Chronic stable angina pectoris, mild to moderate hypertension

Unlabeled uses: Tachydysrhythmias, anxiety, tremors, esophageal varices (rebleeding only), migraines, reduction of intraocular pressure

CONTRAINDICATIONS: Hypersensitivity to this product, cardiac failure, cardiogenic shock, 2nd-/3rd-degree heart block, bronchospastic disease, sinus bradycardia, HF, COPD, asthma
Precautions: Pregnancy, breastfeeding, diabetes mellitus, renal disease, hyperthyroidism, peripheral vascular disease, myasthenia gravis, major surgery, nonallergic bronchospasm

Black Box Warning: Abrupt discontinuation

DOSAGE AND ROUTES
Angina pectoris/hypertension
• **Adult: PO** 40 mg/day, increase by 40-80 mg q7 days; maintenance 40-240 mg/day for angina, 40-320 mg/day for hypertension
• **Geriatric: PO** 20 mg/day, may increase by 20 mg until desired dose

Renal dose
• **Adult: PO** CCr 31-50 mL/min, give q24-36hr; CCr 10-30 mL/min, give q24-48hr; CCr <10 mL/min, give q40-60hr
Esophageal varices (unlabeled)
• **Adult: PO** 40 mg q day
Available forms: Tabs 20, 40, 80, 160 ✦ mg
Administer:
• With 8 oz water; check apical pulse before use; if <50 bpm, withhold; notify prescriber
• Give without regard to food
• Tabs may be crushed and mixed with food
• Discontinue other antihypertensives gradually

Black Box Warning: Taper over 1-2 wk to discontinue product; do not stop abruptly

SIDE EFFECTS
CNS: Depression, *dizziness, fatigue,* anxiety, drowsiness, lethargy, paresthesias, headache, *weakness,* insomnia, memory loss, nightmares

Side effects: *italics* = common; red = life-threatening

CV: *Bradycardia, hypotension,* HF, palpitations, chest pain, peripheral ischemia, flushing, edema, vasodilation
EENT: Blurred vision, dry eyes, nasal congestion
ENDO: Hyperglycemia, hypoglycemia
GI: Nausea, vomiting, diarrhea, constipation, dry mouth, flatulence, pancreatitis, taste distortion
GU: *Impotence,* decreased libido
INTEG: Rash, pruritus, fever
RESP: Bronchospasm, cough, wheezing

PHARMACOKINETICS

PO: Onset variable, peak 3-4 hr, duration 10-24 hr; half-life 20-24 hr; not metabolized; excreted in urine 70% (unchanged), bile, breast milk; protein binding 30%

INTERACTIONS

Increase: orthostatic hypertension—MAOIs; monitor B/P
Increase: peripheral ischemia—ergots
Increase: bradycardia—digoxin; monitor for bradycardia
Increase: hypotension, bradycardia—cloNIDine, EPINEPHrine
Increase: lack of stability of dose—antidiabetics, insulin
Increase: hypotensive effects—other hypotensive agents, phenothiazines, general anesthetics
Decrease: β-blocking effect—thyroid hormones
Decrease: antihypertensive effect—NSAIDs

Drug/Herb

Increase: orthostatic hypertension—dong quai, garlic, ginseng, yohimbe; avoid concurrent use

Drug/Lab Test

Increase: serum potassium, serum uric acid, ALT, AST, alk phos, LDH, blood glucose, cholesterol, ANA, triglycerides

NURSING CONSIDERATIONS
Assess:

• **Hypertension:** check that prescriptions have been filled
• B/P, pulse, respirations during beginning therapy and periodically thereafter; orthostatic hypotension may occur

• **Angina:** monitor frequency of angina, alleviating factors; duration, time started, activity being performed, character
• **HF:** Weight daily; report gain of >5 lb; I&O ratio, CCr if kidney damage diagnosed; crackles, jugular venous distention, fatigue, dyspnea
• Headache, light-headedness, decreased B/P; may indicate a need for decreased dosage

> **Black Box Warning: Abrupt discontinuation:** can result in MI, myocardial ischemia, ventricular dysrhythmias, severe hypertension; withdraw slowly by tapering over 1-2 wk; if symptoms return, restart

• **Pregnancy/breastfeeding:** use only if benefits outweigh risk to fetus; discontinue product or breastfeeding, excreted in breast milk
Evaluate:
• Therapeutic response: decreased B/P, heart rate, symptoms of angina
Teach patient/family:
• That product may mask signs of hypoglycemia or alter blood glucose in patients with diabetes
• To avoid OTC products unless prescriber approves; to take as prescribed, at same time each day, do not double; to take missed dose as soon as remembered if less than 8 hr before next dose
• To avoid hazardous activities if dizziness occurs
• **Hypertension:** to comply with complete medical regimen; to report weight gain of >5 lb, swelling, unusual bruising, bleeding
• To rise slowly to prevent orthostatic hypotension
• About how and when to check B/P, pulse; to hold dose, contact prescriber if pulse ≤50 bpm, systolic B/P <90 mm Hg; to take missed dose as soon as possible if less than 8 hr before next dose

> **Black Box Warning:** Not to discontinue abruptly; may cause life-threatening cardiac changes, taper over 1-2 wk

nafcillin (Rx)

(naf-sill'in)

Func. class.: Antiinfective, broad-spectrum

Chem. class.: Penicillinase-resistant penicillin

ACTION: Bacteriocidal, interferes with cell-wall replication of susceptible organisms; cell lysis mediated by cell wall autolytic enzymes

USES: Effective for gram-positive cocci (*Staphylococcus aureus, Streptococcus viridans, Streptococcus pneumoniae*), infections caused by penicillinase-producing *Staphylococcus*

CONTRAINDICATIONS: Hypersensitivity to penicillins

Precautions: Pregnancy, breastfeeding, neonates; hypersensitivity to cephalosporins or carbapenems; GI disease, asthma, electrolyte imbalances, hepatic/renal disease, pseudomembranous colitis

DOSAGE AND ROUTES

• **Adult:** IV 500-1000 mg q4hr; **IM** 500-1000 mg q4hr, max 12 g/day

• **Child and infant >1 mo:** IV 100-200 mg/kg/day in divided doses

• **Neonate >7 days (weight >2 kg):** IV/IM 25 mg/kg q6hr

• **Neonate 0-7 days (weight >2 kg):** IV 25 mg/kg q8hr

• **Neonates 0-7 days (weight ≤2 kg):** IV 25 mg/kg q12hr

Available forms: Powder for inj 1 g/vial, 2 g/vial, 10 g/vial

Administer:

• Product after C&S has been drawn, begin therapy while waiting for results

IM route

• Reconstitute vials: add 1.7, 3.4, or 6.4 mL sterile water for inj, 0.9% NaCl, bacteriostatic water for inj with benzyl alcohol or parabens to vials with 500 mg, 1 g, 2 g of nafcillin, respectively (250 mg/mL)

• No further dilution needed; after reconstitution, inject in deep muscle mass

IV route

• Reconstitute vials: add 1.7, 3.4, or 6.4 mL sterile water for inj, 0.9% NaCl, bacteriostatic water for inj with benzyl alcohol or parabens to vials with 500 mg, 1 g, 2 g of nafcillin, respectively (250 mg/mL); pharmacy bulk pack reconstitute 10 g/93 mL sterile water inj or 0.9% NaCl (100 mg/mL)

Direct IV INJ route

• Further dilute reconstituted sol in 15-30 mL sterile water inj, 0.45% NaCl, 0.9% NaCl; inj slowly over 5-10 min into tubing of free-flowing compatible IV solution

Intermittent IV route

• Vials, further dilute reconstituted sol to 2-40 mg/mL for peripheral vein infusion ≤20 mg/mL (preferred); infuse ≥ 30-60 mins

• Extravasation management: stop infusion and disconnect, leave needle/cannula in place, gently aspirate extravasated solution, do not flush line, use hyaluronidase, remove cannula/needle, apply dry cold compresses, elevate extremity

Y-site compatibilities: Acyclovir, alfentanil, amikacin, aminophylline, amphotericin B lipid complex (Abelcet), anidulafungin, argatroban, ascorbic acid injection, atenolol, atracurium, atropine, aztreonam, benztropine, bivalirudin, bleomycin, bretylium, bumetanide, buprenorphine, butorphanol, calcium chloride/gluconate, CARBOplatin, carmustine, cefamandole, ceFAZolin, cefoperazone, cefotaxime, cefoTEtan, cefOXitin, cefTAZidime, ceftizoxime, cefTRIAXone, cefuroxime, chlorproMAZINE, cimetidine, CISplatin, clindamycin, cyanocobalamin, cyclophosphamide, cycloSPORINE, DACTINomycin, DAPTOmycin, DAUNOrubicin liposome, dexamethasone, digoxin, DOBUTamine, DOCEtaxel, DOPamine, DOXOrubicin liposomal, enalaprilat, EPHEDrine, EPINEPHrine, epoetin alfa, erythromycin, etoposide, etoposide phosphate, famotidine, fenoldopam, fentaNYL, fluconazole, fludarabine, foscarnet, furosemide, gallium, ganciclovir, gatifloxacin, gemtuzumab, gentamicin, glycopyrrolate, granisetron, heparin, hydrocortisone,

Side effects: *italics* = common; red = life-threatening

HYDROmorphone, imipenem-cilastatin, indomethacin, isoproterenol, ketorolac, lactated Ringer's, lepirudin, leucovorin, lidocaine, linezolid injection, LORazepam, magnesium sulfate, mannitol, methyldopate, methylPREDNISolone, metoclopramide, metoprolol, metroNIDAZOLE, milrinone, morphine, multiple vitamins injection, naloxone, niCARdipine, nitroglycerin, nitroprusside, norepinephrine, octreotide, ondansetron, oxacillin, oxaliplatin, oxytocin, PACLitaxel (solvent/surfactant), pamidronate, pancuronium, pantoprazole, PEMEtrexed, penicillin G potassium/sodium, PENTobarbital, perphenazine, PHENobarbital, phentolamine, phenylephrine, phytonadione, piperacillin, polymyxin B, potassium acetate/chloride, procainamide, prochlorperazine, propofol, propranolol, ranitidine, Ringer's injection, sodium bicarbonate, SUFentanil, tacrolimus, teniposide, theophylline, thiamine, thiotepa, ticarcillin, ticarcillin-clavulanate, tigecycline, tirofiban, TNA (3-in-1), tobramycin, tolazoline, TPN (2-in-1), urokinase, vasopressin, vinBLAStine, voriconazole, zidovudine, zoledronic acid

SIDE EFFECTS

CNS: Lethargy, hallucinations, anxiety, depression, twitching, seizures
GI: *Nausea, vomiting, diarrhea,* CDAD, hepatitis
GU: Oliguria, proteinuria, hematuria, vaginitis, moniliasis, glomerulonephritis, interstitial nephritis
HEMA: Neutropenia
INTEG: Tissue necrosis, extravasation at inj site, rash, pruritus, exfoliative dermatitis
SYST: Anaphylaxis, serum sickness, Stevens-Johnson syndrome

PHARMACOKINETICS

Half-life 30-90 min; metabolized by liver; excreted in bile, urine; 70%-90% protein bound; peak 30-120 min (PO); peak 30-60 min (IM)

INTERACTIONS

Increase: nafcillin concentrations—probenecid

Decrease: effect of cycloSPORINE—warfarin
Decrease: nafcillin effect—chloramphenicol, macrolides, sulfonamides, tetracyclines, aminoglycosides
Decrease: effect of live virus vaccines, do not use together
Decrease: effect of hormonal contraceptives, use additional contraceptives

Drug/Food
Decrease: absorption—food, carbonated drinks, citrus fruit juices
Decrease: Hgb/HcT, neutrophils

Drug/Lab Test
False positive: urine glucose, urine protein
Decrease: potassium

NURSING CONSIDERATIONS
Assess:
Infection: signs, symptoms of infection, including characteristics of wounds, sputum, urine, stool, WBC >10,000/mm³, earache, fever, obtain information baseline, during treatment

• I&O ratio; report hematuria, oliguria; high doses are nephrotoxic

• **CDAD:** diarrhea, abdominal pain, fever, fatigue, anorexia; possible anemia, elevated WBC, low serum albumin; stop product; usually either vancomycin or IV metroNIDAZOLE given

• **Renal studies:** urinalysis, BUN, creatinine; abnormal urinalysis may indicate nephrotoxicity

• C&S before product therapy; product may be given as soon as culture is taken

• **Allergies before initiation of treatment;** monitor for anaphylaxis, dyspnea, rash, laryngeal edema; stop product; keep emergency equipment nearby; skin eruptions after administration of penicillin to 1 wk after discontinuing product; cross-sensitivity with cephalosporins may occur

• **IV site:** for redness, swelling, pain at site; if extravasation occurs, aspirate from IV catheter after disconnecting, administer hyaluronidase as an antidote, elevate extremity

• **Pregnancy/breastfeeding:** use only if clearly needed; use caution in breastfeeding

Evaluate:

• Therapeutic response: absence of fever, draining wounds

Teach patient/family:

• To report vaginal itching; loose, foul-smelling stools; furry tongue; sore throat; fever; fatigue (may indicate superinfection); CNS reactions; CDAD (diarrhea, fever, abdominal pain, fatigue)

• To wear or carry emergency ID if allergic to penicillins

• To avoid use with other products unless approved by prescriber

• To take all medication prescribed for the length of time ordered

TREATMENT OF ANAPHYLAXIS: Withdraw product; maintain airway; administer EPINEPHrine, aminophylline, O$_2$, IV corticosteroids

---

⚠ HIGH ALERT

nalbuphine (Rx)

(nal′byoo-feen)

Nubain ✦

Func. class.: Opioid analgesic

Chem. class.: Synthetic opioid agonist, antagonist

Do not confuse:

nalbuphine/naloxone

ACTION: Depresses pain impulse transmission at the spinal cord level by interacting with opioid receptors

USES: Moderate to severe pain, supplement to anesthesia, sedation prior to surgery

CONTRAINDICATIONS: Hypersensitivity to this product or parabens, addiction (opiate)

Precautions: Pregnancy, breastfeeding, addictive personality, increased intracranial pressure, MI (acute), severe heart disease, respiratory depression, renal/hepatic disease, bowel impaction, abrupt discontinuation

Black Box Warning: Coadministration with other CNS depressants, respiratory depression

DOSAGE AND ROUTES

Analgesic

• **Adult: SUBCUT/IM/IV** 10 mg q3-6hr prn (based on 70-kg body weight), max 160 mg/day; max 20 mg/dose if opiate naïve

Balanced anesthesia adjunct

• **Adult: IV** 0.3-3 mg/kg given over 10-15 min; may give 0.25-0.5 mg/kg as needed for maintenance

Available forms: solution for Inj 10, 20 mg/mL

Administer:

• With antiemetic if nausea, vomiting occur

• When pain beginning to return; determine dosage interval by response

• Store in light-resistant area at room temperature

IM route

• IM deep in large muscle mass, rotate inj sites, protect from light

Direct IV route

• Undiluted ≤10 mg over 3-5 min into free-flowing IV line of D$_5$W, NS, or LR

SIDE EFFECTS

CNS: *Drowsiness, dizziness, confusion, headache, sedation, euphoria,* dysphoria (high doses), hallucinations, dreaming, tolerance, physical, psychologic dependency

CV: Bradycardia, change in B/P

EENT: Blurred vision, miosis, diplopia

GI: *Nausea, vomiting, anorexia, constipation, cramps,* abdominal pain, dyspepsia, xerostomia, bitter taste

GU: Urinary urgency

INTEG: *Rash,* urticaria, flushing, diaphoresis, pruritus

RESP: Respiratory depression, pulmonary edema

PHARMACOKINETICS

SUBCUT/IM/IV: Peak 30 min, onset 2-15 min, IV 2-3 min, duration 3-6 hr, metabolized by liver, excreted by kidneys, half-life 3-6 hr

---

Side effects: *italics* = common; red = life-threatening

N

INTERACTIONS

Increase: effects with other CNS depressants—alcohol, opiates, sedative/hypnotics, antipsychotics, skeletal muscle relaxants

Increase: severe reactions—MAOIs; decrease dose to 25%

Drug/Herb

Increase: CNS depression—kava, valerian, hops, chamomile

NURSING CONSIDERATIONS

Assess:

• **Pain:** type, location, intensity before and 30-60 min after administration; titrate upward with 25%-50% until 50% of pain reduced; need for pain medication by pain sedation scoring, physical dependency, can repeat if initial dose is not adequately effective, not for long-term use

• Bowel status; constipation is common; may need laxative or stool softener

• **Withdrawal reactions** in opiate-dependent individuals: PE, vascular occlusion; abscesses, ulcerations, nausea, vomiting, seizures; low potential for dependence

• **CNS changes:** dizziness, drowsiness, hallucinations, euphoria, LOC, pupil reaction

• Allergic reactions: rash, urticaria

• Monitor VS after parenteral route, note muscle rigidity, product history, liver, kidney function tests

Black Box Warning: Avoid coadministration with other CNS depressants: coadministration increases the risk for respiratory depression, low B/P, and death

Black Box Warning: Respiratory dysfunction: respiratory depression, character, rate, rhythm; notify prescriber if respirations are <10/min

• **Pregnancy/breastfeeding:** use only if clearly needed; cautious use in breastfeeding

Evaluate:

• Therapeutic response: decrease in pain without respiratory depression

Teach patient/family:

• To report any symptoms of CNS changes, allergic reactions

• That physical dependency may result from long-term use; low potential for dependency

• **That withdrawal symptoms may occur:** nausea, vomiting, cramps, fever, faintness, anorexia, profuse sweating, twitching; without treatment symptoms resolve in 5-14 days, chronic abstinence syndrome may last 2-6 mo

• To avoid CNS depressants, alcohol

• To avoid driving, operating machinery if drowsiness occurs

• To use sugarless gum or candy and good oral hygiene for dry mouth

TREATMENT OF OVERDOSE:

Naloxone (Narcan) 0.2-0.8 mg IV, O_2, IV fluids, vasopressors

---

naloxone (Rx)

(nal-oks′one)

Evzio, Narcan

Func. class.: Opioid antagonist, antidote

Chem. class.: Thebaine derivative

Do not confuse:

naloxone/naltrexone/nalbuphine
Narcan/Norcuron

ACTION: Competes with opioids at opiate receptor sites

USES: Respiratory depression induced by opioids, opiate agonist overdose

Unlabeled uses: IBS, opiate agonist dependence, opiate agonist–induced constipation, pruritus, urinary retention, coma, nausea, vomiting

CONTRAINDICATIONS: Hypersensitivity

Precautions: Pregnancy, breastfeeding, children, neonates, CV disease, opioid dependency, seizure disorder, drug dependency, hepatic disease

DOSAGE AND ROUTES
Opioid-induced respiratory depression (known for suspected opiate agonist overdose)
• **Adult: IV/SUBCUT/IM** 0.4-2 mg, repeat q2-3min if needed, max 10 mg; **IV INFUSION** loading dose 0.005 mg/kg, then 0.0025 mg/kg/hr
• **Child <5 yr or ≤20 kg: IV/INTRAOSSEOUS** 0.01 mg/kg slowly followed by 0.1 mg/kg if needed; **IV INFUSION** (PALS) 0.04-0.16 mg/kg/hr, titrate
• **Adult/adolescent/child: NASAL** 1 spray, may repeat q2-3min if needed
Postoperative opioid-induced respiratory depression
• **Adult: IV** 0.1-0.2 mg q2-3min prn
• **Child: IV** 0.005-0.01 mg/kg q2-3min prn
• **Neonates: IM/IV/SUBCUT** 0.01 mg/kg, repeat q2-3min until adequate response
Diagnosis of opiate-agonist dependence (unlabeled)
• **Adult: IM** 0.16 mg; if no withdrawal symptoms after 20-30 min, give 0.24 mg **IV**
Nausea/vomiting from continuous morphine infusion (unlabeled)
• **Adult: IV** 0.2 mg
Opioid-induced pruritus (unlabeled)
• **Child:** continuous IV infusion 2 mcg/kg/hr, may increase by 0.5 mcg/kg/hr q4hr
Available forms: Inj 0.4, 0.4 mg/0.4 mL auto injector; nasal spray 4 mg/0.1 mL
Administer:
• Only with resuscitative equipment, O_2 nearby
• Only sol prepared within 24 hr
• Store in dark area at room temperature
• Double-check dose; those taking opioids >1 wk are sensitive to this product
• Solution should be clear
Direct IV route
• Undiluted (suspected opioid overdose) or diluted with sterile water for inj; give ≤0.4 mg over 15 sec; (respiratory depression) dilute with sterile water for injection (0.1 mg/mL); <40 kg; in neonates, may give via umbilical vein

Continuous IV INFUSION route
• Dilute 2 mg/500 mL 0.9% NaCl or D_5W (4 mcg/mL); titrate to response
• Do not admix with bisulfite, sulfites
IM route with standard syringe
• Inject deeply into a large muscle mass; aspirate
IM route with autoinjector (Evzio)
• Remove red safety guard; Evzio must be used immediately or disposed of properly. Give quickly into the anterolateral aspect of the thigh, through clothing if necessary. Press firmly and hold in place 5 sec
• For neonates and infants: caregiver should pinch the middle of the outer thigh muscle before and during drug administration. Carefully observe administration site for evidence of residual needle parts and/or signs of infection
• Upon activation, the needle is automatically inserted, delivers the injection, and then retracts fully
• After initial injection, seek immediate medical attention. Keep patient under continued surveillance because the duration of action of most opioids is longer than that of naloxone. Repeat doses q2-3min as needed
• Do NOT attempt to reuse Evzio; each device contains a single dose of naloxone
Subcut with standard syringe
• Inject undiluted solution, taking care not to inject intradermally
Subcut route with autoinjector (Evzio)
• Once the red safety guard is removed, Evzio must be used immediately or disposed of properly. Do not attempt to replace the red safety guard once it is removed
• Administer as quickly as possible into the anterolateral aspect of the thigh, through clothing if necessary. Press firmly and hold in place for 5 sec
• For neonates and infants: caregiver should pinch the middle of the outer thigh muscle before and during drug administration. Carefully observe administration site for evidence of residual needle parts and/or signs of infection
• Upon activation, the needle is automatically inserted, delivers the injection, and then retracts fully

Side effects: *italics* = common; red = life-threatening

• After initial injection, seek immediate medical attention

• Do NOT attempt to reuse Evzio; each device contains a single dose of naloxone. Additional supportive and/or resuscitative measures may be helpful while awaiting emergency assistance

Nasal route

• Give as quickly as possible if a patient is unresponsive and an opioid overdose is suspected

• Place the patient in the supine position. Assure that the device nozzle is inserted into one of the patient's nostrils and provide support to the back of the neck to allow the head to tilt back. Do NOT prime or test the device before administration

• Press firmly on the device plunger

• Turn the patient on his or her side (recovery position) and seek immediate medical assistance after the first dose of naloxone

• Do NOT attempt to reuse the naloxone nasal spray device; each device contains a single dose

• Using a new nasal spray device, readminister naloxone q2-3min if the patient does not respond or responds and then relapses into respiratory depression

• Administer the nasal spray in alternate nostrils with each dose

Y-site compatibilities: Acyclovir, alfentanil, amikacin, aminocaproic acid, aminophylline, anidulafungin, ascorbic acid, atenolol, atracurium, atropine, azaTHIOprine, aztreonam, benztropine, bivalirudin, bleomycin, bumetanide, buprenorphine, butorphanol, calcium chloride/gluconate, CARBOplatin, caspofungin, cefamandole, ceFAZolin, cefmetazole, cefonicid, cefoperazone, cefotaxime, cefoTEtan, cefOXitin, cefTAZidime, ceftizoxime, cefTRIAXone, cefuroxime, cephalothin, cephapirin, chloramphenicol, chlorproMAZINE, cimetidine, CISplatin, clindamycin, cyanocobalamin, cyclophosphamide, cycloSPORINE, cytarabine, DACTINomycin, DAPTOmycin, dexamethasone, digoxin, diltiazem, diphenhydrAMINE, DOBUTamine, DOCEtaxel, DOPamine, doxacurium, DOXOrubicin, doxycycline, enalaprilat, ePHEDrine, EPINEPHrine, epirubicin, epoetin alfa, eptifibatide, ertapenem, erythromycin, esmolol, etoposide, etoposide phosphate, famotidine, fenoldopam, fentaNYL, fluconazole, fludarabine, fluorouracil, folic acid, furosemide, ganciclovir, gatifloxacin, gemcitabine, gentamicin, glycopyrrolate, granisetron, heparin, hydrocortisone, hydrOXYzine, IDArubicin, ifosfamide, imipenem-cilastatin, inamrinone, indomethacin, insulin (regular), irinotecan, isoproterenol, ketorolac, labetalol, levofloxacin, lidocaine, linezolid, LORazepam, mannitol, mechlorethamine, meperidine, metaraminol, methicillin, methotrexate, methoxamine, methyldopate, methylPREDNISolone, metoclopramide, metoprolol, metroNIDAZOLE, mezlocillin, miconazole, midazolam, milrinone, minocycline, mitoXANtrone, morphine, moxalactam, multiple vitamins, mycophenolate, nafcillin, nalbuphine, nesiritide, netilmicin, nitroglycerin, nitroprusside, norepinephrine, octreotide, ondansetron, oxacillin, oxaliplatin, oxytocin, PACLitaxel, palonosetron, pamidronate, pancuronium, papaverine, PEMEtrexed, penicillin G potassium/sodium, pentamidine, pentazocine, PENTobarbital, PHENobarbital, phentolamine, phenylephrine, phytonadione, piperacillin, piperacillin-tazobactam, polymyxin B, potassium chloride, procainamide, prochlorperazine, promethazine, propofol, propranolol, protamine, pyridoxine, quiNIDine, quinupristin-dalfopristin, ranitidine, ritodrine, rocuronium, sodium acetate/bicarbonate, succinylcholine, SUFentanil, tacrolimus, teniposide, theophylline, thiamine, ticarcillin, ticarcillin-clavulanate, tigecycline, tirofiban, tobramycin, tolazoline, trimetaphan, urokinase, vancomycin, vasopressin, vecuronium, verapamil, vinCRIStine, vinorelbine, voriconazole, zoledronic acid

SIDE EFFECTS
CV: Rapid pulse, *ventricular tachycardia, fibrillation, hypo/hypertension*
GI: Nausea, vomiting

PHARMACOKINETICS
Well absorbed IM, SUBCUT; metabolized by liver, crosses placenta; excreted in urine, breast milk; half-life 30-81 min
IM/SUBCUT: Onset 2-5 min, duration 45-60 min
IV: Onset 1 min, duration 45 min
Nasal: Peak 20 min

INTERACTIONS
Decrease: effect of opioid analgesics

NURSING CONSIDERATIONS
Assess:
• **Withdrawal:** cramping, hypertension, anxiety, vomiting; signs of withdrawal in drug-dependent individuals may occur ≤2 hr after administration; severity depends on length of time opioids were taken, naloxone dose
• **Respiratory dysfunction:** respiratory depression, character, rate, rhythm; if respirations are <10/min, administer naloxone; probably due to opioid overdose; monitor LOC, ECG, B/P
• **Pain:** duration, intensity, location before and after administration; analgesia will be decreased; may be used for respiratory depression
• **Acute opioid reversal:** patients may become very agitated and violent after use
• **Pregnancy/breastfeeding:** use only if clearly needed, cautious use in breastfeeding
Evaluate:
• Therapeutic response: reversal of respiratory depression; LOC—alert
Teach patient/family:
• When patient is lucid, about the reasons for, expected results of product; for nasal administration, teach family, caregivers correct use

---

naltrexone (Rx)
(nal-trex´one)
ReVia, Vivitrol
Func. class.: Opioid antagonist, antidote
Chem. class.: Thebaine derivative

Do not confuse:
naltrexone/naloxone

ACTION: Competes with opioids at opioid-receptor sites

USES: Blockage of opioid analgesics; used for treatment of opiate addiction, alcoholism, opiate agonist overdose
Unlabeled uses: Nicotine withdrawal, opiate-agonist withdrawal, pruritus

CONTRAINDICATIONS: Hypersensitivity, opioid dependence
Precautions: Pregnancy, breastfeeding, children, renal disease, depression, suicidal ideation, coagulopathy, respiratory depression, IV use, hepatic failure, hepatitis

DOSAGE AND ROUTES
Adjunct in opiate-agonist dependence
• **Adult:** PO 25 mg; if no withdrawal symptoms in 1 hr, then 25 mg additionally; if no withdrawal symptoms, then 50-150 mg/day or in divided doses
Adjunct in alcoholism treatment
• **Adult:** PO 50 mg/day with food × 12 wk; **IM** (Vivitrol) 380 mg q4wk
Pruritus (unlabeled)
• **Adult:** PO 50 mg/day × 7 days to 4 wk
Nicotine withdrawal (unlabeled)
• **Adult:** PO 50 mg/day
Ultrarapid opiate detoxification (unlabeled)
• **Adult:** PO 50 mg before sedation with midazolam; various titration regimens leading up to a full dose of naltrexone have been used
Available forms: Tabs 50 mg; powder for inj 380 mg

Administer:

PO route

• Give with food or after meals, antacid to prevent nausea, vomiting

• Store in tight container

IM route

• Do not give until opioid-free for 7-10 days to prevent opioid withdrawal (relapse only)

• IM deep in gluteal, alternate inj sites; use supplied needle to prevent inj-site reaction; aspirate before inj

• Only if resuscitative equipment is nearby

• Do not use IV or SUBCUT

SIDE EFFECTS

CNS: *Stimulation, drowsiness,* dizziness, confusion, seizures, headache, flushing, hallucinations, nervousness, irritability, suicidal ideation, syncope, anxiety

CV: Rapid pulse, pulmonary edema, hypertension, DVT

EENT: Tinnitus, hearing loss, blurred vision

GI: *Nausea, vomiting, diarrhea, heartburn,* hepatotoxicity, constipation, abdominal pain

GU: Delayed ejaculation, impotence

INTEG: *Rash,* urticaria, bruising, oily skin, acne, pruritus, inj-site reactions

MISC: Increased thirst, chills, fever

MS: Joint and muscle pain

RESP: Wheezing, hyperpnea, nasal congestion, rhinorrhea, sneezing, sore throat, pneumonia

PHARMACOKINETICS

Metabolized by liver, excreted by kidneys; crosses placenta, excreted in breast milk; half-life 4 hr; IM half-life 5-10 days; extensive first-pass metabolism; protein binding 21%-28%

PO: Onset 15-30 min, peak 1 hr

IM: Peak 2-3 days, duration >1 month

INTERACTIONS

Increase: lethargy—phenothiazines

Increase: hepatotoxicity—disulfiram

Increase: bleeding risk—anticoagulants

NURSING CONSIDERATIONS

Assess:

• **Hepatic status:** LFTs, jaundice, hepatitis, hepatic failure

• ABGs including PO_2, PCO_2, LFTs, VS q3-5min

• Signs of withdrawal in drug-dependent individuals; use naltrexone challenge to test opioid dependence; must be free of opioids for 7-10 days before using this product, or withdrawal symptoms can occur

• Cardiac status: tachycardia, hypertension

• **Respiratory dysfunction:** respiratory depression, character, rate, rhythm; if respirations <10/min, respiratory stimulant should be administered

• Mental status: depression, suicidal ideation

• **Beers:** avoid in older adults unless safer alternatives are unavailable; may cause ataxia, impaired psychomotor function

• **Pregnancy/breastfeeding:** use only if clearly needed; do not breastfeed

Evaluate:

• Therapeutic response: blocking opiate ingestion; successful nicotine, alcohol withdrawal

Teach patient/family:

• That patient must be drug-free to start treatment

• That using opioid while taking this product could prove fatal because high dose is needed to overcome this antagonist; not to self-dose with OTC products unless approved by prescriber

• To carry emergency ID stating product used

• That, if surgery is needed, all involved should be aware of this product

• To use caution while driving or performing other hazardous tasks until effect is known

• That suicidal thoughts/behaviors may occur; to report these immediately

• About IM injection sites; monitor for injection site reactions; about duration of effects and need for repeat injections q4wk

naphazoline (ophthalmic)

(na-faz'oh-leen)

Advanced Eye Relief, Redness Maximum Relief, Ak-Con, All Clear, Clear Eyes, Naphcon Forte ✦, VasoClear

Func. class.: Ophthalmic vasocon-strictor

Chem. class.: Sympathomimetic

ACTION: Acts on the blood vessels in the eye to produce vasoconstriction

USES: Ocular congestion, irritation, itching of the eye

CONTRAINDICATIONS: Hyper-sensitivity, acute angle-closure glaucoma, 0.1% solution in children/infants
Precautions: Hyperthyroidism, diabetes mellitus, hypertension, cardiac conditions

DOSAGE AND ROUTES
• **Adult:** OPHTH instill 1-2 drops in affected eye in the conjunctival sac every 3-4 hr, up to qid
Available forms: ophthalmic solution 0.012%, 0.1%
Administer:
• Store at room temperature; keep tightly closed

SIDE EFFECTS
CNS: Headache
EENT: Blurred vision, irritation, photophobia, dilation, stinging, elevated IOP, keratitis

PHARMACOKINETICS
Onset 10 min, duration up to 6 hr

INTERACTIONS
Increase: Systemic effects—β-blockers
• Do not use within 14 days of MAOIs

NURSING CONSIDERATIONS
Assess:
• Ocular itching, congestion, irritation: should show improvement quickly; avoid using more than 3 consecutive days; long-term use or exceeding dosage can

lead to rebound congestion; report eye pain, blurred vision
Evaluate:
• Decreasing ocular itching, congestion, irritation
Teach patient/family:
• Method for instilling drops
• To notify prescriber of eye pain, blurred vision
• That ocular itching, congestion, irritation should show improvement quickly
• To avoid using longer than 3 days; that long-term use or exceeding dosage can lead to rebound congestion
• To wait for at least 15 min before wearing contact lenses

naproxen (Rx, OTC)

Aleve, Anaprox, Anaprox DS, EC-Naprosyn, Maxidol ✦, Naprelan, Naprosyn

Func. class.: Nonsteroidal antiinflam-matory, nonopioid analgesic

Chem. class.: Propionic acid derivative

ACTION: Inhibits COX-1, COX-2 by blocking arachidonate; analgesic, antiin-flammatory, antipyretic

USES: Osteoarthritis; rheumatoid, gouty arthritis; primary dysmenorrhea; ankylosing spondylitis, bursitis, tendinitis, myalgia, dental pain, juvenile rheumatoid arthritis
Unlabeled uses: Bone pain, migraine/migraine prophylaxis, heterotropic ossification

CONTRAINDICATIONS: Pregnancy 3rd trimester; hypersensitivity to NSAIDs, salicylates; perioperative pain in CABG surgery; MI; stroke
Precautions: Pregnancy, breastfeeding, children <2 yr, geriatric patients, bleeding disorders, GI disorders, cardiac disorders, hypersensitivity to other antiinflammatory agents, CCr <30 mL/min, asthma, renal failure, hepatic disease

---

Side effects: *italics* = common; red = life-threatening

Black Box Warning: GI bleeding, thromboembolism

DOSAGE AND ROUTES

200 mg base = 220 mg naproxen sodium

Antiinflammatory/analgesic/antidysmenorrheal

• **Adult: PO** 250-500 mg bid, max 1500 mg/day; **DEL REL** 375-500 mg bid

• **Child ≥2 yr: PO** 7 mg/kg q12hr

Antigout

• **Adult: PO** 750 mg, then 250 mg q8hr

OTC use

• **Adult: PO** 220 mg q8-12hr or 440 mg, then 220 mg q12hr; max 660 mg/24 hr taken ≤10 days

• **Geriatric >65 yr: PO** max 220 mg q12hr

Available forms: Naproxen: tabs 250, 375, 500 mg; del rel tabs (EC-Naprosyn, Naprosyn-E) 250 ❖, 375, 500 mg; oral susp 125 mg/5 mL; ext rel tabs (CR) 375, 500, 750 mg; **naproxen sodium:** tabs 220, 275, 550 mg tab

Administer:

• Store at room temperature

• With food to decrease GI symptoms; take on empty stomach to facilitate absorption; give with full glass of liquid

• Do not crush, break, or chew ext rel tabs

• OTC for ≤10 days unless approved by prescriber

• Adequately hydrate in those taking angiotensin receptor blockers/angiotensin-converting enzyme inhibitors

• **Oral susp:** shake well; use measuring cup provided or other calibrated device

SIDE EFFECTS

CNS: Dizziness, drowsiness, fatigue, tremors, confusion, insomnia, anxiety, depression

CV: Tachycardia, peripheral edema, palpitations, dysrhythmias, MI, stroke

EENT: Tinnitus, hearing loss, blurred vision

GI: Nausea, anorexia, vomiting, diarrhea, jaundice, hepatitis, constipation, flatulence, cramps, peptic ulcer, bleeding

GU: Nephrotoxicity: dysuria, hematuria, oliguria, azotemia

HEMA: Blood dyscrasias

INTEG: Purpura, rash, pruritus, sweating

SYST: Anaphylaxis, Stevens-Johnson syndrome

PHARMACOKINETICS

PO: Peak 2-4 hr, half-life 12-17 hr; metabolized in liver; excreted in urine (metabolites), breast milk; 99% protein binding

INTERACTIONS

Increase: renal impairment—ACE inhibitors, angiotensin II antagonists

Increase: toxicity risk—methotrexate, lithium, antineoplastics, probenecid, radiation treatment

Black Box Warning: **Increase:** bleeding risk—oral anticoagulants, thrombolytic agents, eptifibatide, tirofiban, clopidogrel, ticlopidine, plicamycin, SSRIs, SNRIs, tricyclics

Increase: GI side effects risk—aspirin, corticosteroids, alcohol, NSAIDs

Decrease: effect of antihypertensives, loop/thiazide diuretics

Decrease: absorption of naproxen—antacids, sucralfate, cholestyramine

Drug/Herb

• Bleeding risk: feverfew, garlic, ginger, ginkgo, ginseng *(Panax)*

Drug/Lab Test

Increase: BUN, alk phos, LFTs, potassium, glucose, cholesterol

Decrease: potassium, sodium

False increase: 5-HIAA, 17KS

NURSING CONSIDERATIONS

Assess:

• **Pain:** frequency, characteristics, intensity; relief before and 1-2 hr after product

• **Arthritis:** range of motion, pain, swelling before and 1-2 hr after use

• **Fever:** before, 1 hr after use

• **Cardiac status:** CV thrombotic events, MI, stroke; may be fatal; not to be used with CABG

Black Box Warning: GI status: ulceration, bleeding, perforation; may be fatal; obtain stool guaiac

❖ Canada only   ⚕ Genetic warning

• Asthma, aspirin hypersensitivity or nasal polyps; increased risk of hypersensitivity
• **Renal, hepatic blood studies:** BUN, creatinine, AST, ALT, Hgb, LDH, blood glucose, Hct, WBC, platelets, CCr before treatment, periodically thereafter during long-term therapy
• Monitor B/P baseline and periodically
• **Beers:** avoid chronic use in older adults unless other alternatives are unavailable; increased GI bleeding risk, peptic ulcer disease
• **Pregnancy/breastfeeding:** use only if benefits outweigh fetal risk; avoid in ≥30 wk gestation; cautious use in breastfeeding

Evaluate:
• Therapeutic response: decreased pain, stiffness, swelling in joints; ability to move more easily

Teach patient/family:
• To report ringing, roaring in ears
• To avoid driving, other hazardous activities if dizziness or drowsiness occurs
• To report change in urine pattern, weight increase, edema (face, lower extremities), pain increase in joints, fever, blood in urine (indicates nephrotoxicity); black stools, flu-like symptoms, signs of MI, stroke
• That therapeutic effects may take up to 1 mo in arthritis

Black Box Warning: To avoid aspirin, alcohol, steroids, or other OTC medications without prescriber approval; increased risk of GI bleeding

• To report use to all health care providers
• To notify prescriber if pregnancy is planned or suspected; to avoid breastfeeding

---

naratriptan (Rx)

(nair'ah-trip-tan)

Amerge

Func. class.: Antimigraine agent
Chem. class.: 5-HT₁ receptor agonist

ACTION: Binds selectively to the vascular 5-HT₁ B/D receptor subtype; exerts antimigraine effect; causes vasoconstriction in cranial arteries

USES: Acute treatment of migraine with/without aura

CONTRAINDICATIONS: Hypersensitivity, angina pectoris, history of MI, documented silent ischemia, ischemic heart disease, concurrent ergotamine-containing preparations, uncontrolled hypertension, CV syndromes, hemiplegic or basilar migraines, severe renal disease (CCr <15 mL/min); severe hepatic disease (Child-Pugh grade C)
Precautions: Pregnancy, breastfeeding, children, geriatric patients, postmenopausal women, men >40 yr, CAD risk, hypercholesterolemia, obesity, diabetes, impaired renal/hepatic function, peripheral vascular disease overuse

DOSAGE AND ROUTES
• **Adult: PO** 1 or 2.5 mg with fluids; if headache returns, repeat 1× after 4 hr; max 5 mg/24 hr
Hepatic/renal dose
• **Adult: PO** CCr 15-39 mL/min or mild to moderate hepatic disease max 2.5 mg/24 hr

Available forms: Tabs 1, 2.5 mg
Administer:
With fluids as soon as symptoms appear; may take another dose after 4 hr; do not take >5 mg during any 24-hr period

SIDE EFFECTS
CNS: Dizziness, sedation, fatigue
CV: Increased B/P, palpitations, tachydysrhythmias, PR, QTc prolongation, ST/T wave changes, PVCs, atrial flutter/fibrillation, coronary vasospasm
EENT: EENT infections, photophobia
GI: *Nausea, vomiting*
MISC: Temperature change sensations; tightness, pressure sensations
MS: *Weakness, neck stiffness,* myalgia

PHARMACOKINETICS
Onset 2-3 hr; peak 2-3 hr; 28%-31% protein binding; half-life 6 hr; metabolized in liver (metabolite); excreted in urine, feces; may be excreted in breast milk

N

Side effects: *italics* = common; red = life-threatening

INTERACTIONS

Increase: serotonin syndrome, neuroleptic malignant syndrome—SSRIs (FLUoxetine, fluvoxaMINE, PARoxetine, sertraline), SNRIs, serotonin receptor agonists, sibutramine

Increase: vasospastic effects—ergot, ergot derivatives, other 5-HT$_1$ agonists

Increase: adverse reactions risk—MAOIs; do not use together

Drug/Herb

• **Serotonin syndrome:** SAM-e, St. John's wort

NURSING CONSIDERATIONS

Assess:

• **Migraine symptoms:** aura, duration, effect on lifestyle, aggravating/alleviating factors

• **Serotonin syndrome, neuroleptic malignant syndrome:** increased heart rate, shivering, sweating, dilated pupils, tremors, high B/P, hyperthermia, headache, confusion; if these occur, stop product, administer serotonin antagonist if needed; at least 2 wk should elapse between discontinuation of serotonergic agents and start of product

• **Cardiac status:** ECG, increased B/P, dysrhythmias, monitor for PR, QT prolongation, ST-T wave changes, PVCs in those with cardiac disease

• Stress level, activity, recreation, coping mechanisms

• Neurologic status: LOC, blurred vision, nausea, vomiting, tingling in extremities preceding headache

• Quiet, calm environment with decreased stimulation (noise, bright light, excessive talking)

• **Pregnancy/breastfeeding:** use only if benefits outweigh fetal risk; has been shown to increase birth defects; cautious use in breastfeeding

Evaluate:

• Therapeutic response: decrease in frequency, severity of headache

Teach patient/family:

• To report pain, tightness in chest, neck, throat, or jaw; to notify prescriber immediately if sudden, severe abdominal pain occurs

• Not to use if another 5-HT$_1$ agonist or ergot preparation has been used during past 24 hr; to avoid using >2 days/wk because rebound headache may occur

• To notify prescriber if pregnancy is planned or suspected; to avoid breastfeeding

• To discuss all OTC, Rx, herbals, supplements with health care professional

• To take as soon as headache is starting, only use to treat, not prevent, migraine

• That drowsiness, dizziness may occur, not to drive or perform other hazardous tasks until response is known

---

natalizumab (Rx)

(na-ta-liz'u-mab)

Tysabri

Func. class.: Biologic response modifier, immunoglobulins, monoclonal antibody

---

ACTION: Biologic-response-modifying properties mediated through specific receptors on cells; may be secondary to blockade of the interaction of inflammatory cells with vascular endothelial cells

USES: Ambulatory patients with relapsing/remitting MS who have not responded to other treatment; those with moderate to severe Crohn's disease

CONTRAINDICATIONS: Hypersensitivity, immunocompromised individuals (HIV, AIDS, leukemia, lymphoma, transplants), PML, murine (mouse) protein allergy

Black Box Warning: Progressive multifocal leukoencephalopathy

Precautions: Pregnancy, breastfeeding, geriatric patients, chronic progressive MS, depression, mental disorders, diabetes, TB, active infections, hepatotoxicity

DOSAGE AND ROUTES

• **Adult:** IV INFUSION 300 mg q4wk; give over 1 hr q4wk; observe during and for 1 hr after infusion

• **Adolescent and child ≥11 yr (unlabeled):** IV INFUSION pediatric Crohn's disease activity index (PCDAI) >30, 3 mg/kg q4wk

Available forms: Single-use vial, 300 mg/100 mL 0.9% NaCl

Administer:
- Acetaminophen for fever, headache
- Only after being enrolled in the TOUCH Prescribing Program

Intermittent IV INFUSION route
- Use only clear, colorless solution, without particulates
- Withdraw 15 mL from the vial using aseptic technique: inj concentration into 100 mL 0.9% NaCl; do not use other diluents; mix completely; do not shake; infuse immediately or refrigerate for ≤8 hr; warm to room temperature before using; flush with 0.9% NaCl before, after infusion; do not admix or use in same line with other agents
- Withhold product at first sign of PML
- Prescribers must be registered in the TOUCH Prescribing Program (1-800-456-2255)
- Store sol in refrigerator; do not freeze or shake; protect from light

SIDE EFFECTS

CNS: *Headache, fatigue,* rigors, syncope, tremors, *depression,* progressive multifocal leukoencephalopathy (PML), suicidal ideation, anxiety

CV: Chest discomfort, hypo/hypertension, tachycardia

GI: *Abdominal discomfort,* abnormal LFT, gastroenteritis, severe hepatic injury

GU: Amenorrhea, *UTI, irregular menses,* vaginitis, urinary frequency

INTEG: *Rash,* dermatitis, pruritus, skin melanoma, infusion-related reactions

MS: *Arthralgia,* myalgia

RESP: *Lower respiratory tract infection,* dyspnea

SYST: Anaphylaxis, angioedema

PHARMACOKINETICS
Half-life approximately 11 days

INTERACTIONS
- Do not use with vaccines

Increase: infection—immunosuppressants, antineoplastics, immunomodulators, tumor necrosis factors

NURSING CONSIDERATIONS
Assess:

Black Box Warning: Progressive multifocal leukoencephalopathy (weakness, paralysis, vision loss, impaired speech, cognitive deterioration; obtain gadolinium-enhanced MRI scan of the brain, possibly cerebrospinal fluid for JC viral DNA; signs, symptoms of PML (decreased cognition, vision; ataxia, dysphagia), incidence increases with number of doses, over 2 yr immunosuppressants and anti-JC virus antibody; consider testing for the anti-JC virus and periodically retest

- **Infection:** report serious opportunistic infections to the manufacturer; those with Crohn's disease and chronic oral corticosteroids may be at greater risk of infection
- Blood, renal, hepatic studies: CBC, differential, platelet counts, BUN, creatinine, ALT, urinalysis, antibody testing
- CNS symptoms: headache, fatigue, depression, rigors, tremors
- GI status: abdominal discomfort, gastroenteritis, severe hepatic injury, abnormal LFTs
- Mental status: depression, depersonalization, suicidal thoughts, insomnia
- **MS symptoms;** product should be used only by patients who have not responded to other treatments and for relapsing forms of MS and Crohn's disease; restricted prescribing program; discuss risks, benefits
- **Anaphylaxis:** SOB, hives; swelling, tightness in throat, chest pain; usually within 2 hr of infusion
- **Pregnancy/breastfeeding:** use only if benefits outweigh fetal risk; avoid breastfeeding

Evaluate:
- Therapeutic response: decreased symptoms of MS, Crohn's disease

Teach patient/family:
- Provide patient or family member with written, detailed information about product (med guide)
- That female patients may experience irregular menses, amenorrhea; may worsen over several days; to notify

---

Side effects: *italics* = common; red = life-threatening

prescriber if pregnancy is suspected; to avoid breastfeeding while taking this product; if pregnant, call the Tysabri Pregnancy Exposure Registry (1-800-456-2255)

• **To notify prescriber of possible infection:** sore throat, cough, increased temperature, infusion-site reactions

• That continuing follow-up will be needed at 3, 6 mo after first dose, then every 6 mo

• To inform all prescribers of product use

---

natamycin ophthalmic
See Appendix B

⚠ HIGH ALERT

nebivolol (Rx)
(ne-biv′oh-lol)
Bystolic
Func. class.: Antihypertensive
Chem. class.: β$_1$-blocker, selective

ACTION: Competitively blocks stimulation of β-adrenergic receptors within vascular smooth muscle; decreases rate of SA node discharge; increases recovery time; slows conduction of AV node, thereby resulting in decreased heart rate (negative chronotropic effect), which decreases O$_2$ consumption in myocardium due to β$_1$-receptor antagonism

USES: Hypertension alone or in combination

CONTRAINDICATIONS: Cardiogenic shock, acute heart failure, severe hepatic disease, severe bradycardia, sick sinus syndrome, AV heart block; hypersensitivity to product, β-blockers
Precautions: Pregnancy, breastfeeding, children, major surgery, peripheral vascular disease, diabetes mellitus, thyrotoxicosis disease, COPD, asthma, well-compensated heart failure, renal/hepatic

disease, abrupt discontinuation, acute bronchospasm

DOSAGE AND ROUTES
Hypertension
• **Adult: PO** 5 mg/day, may be increased to desired response q2wk; max 40 mg/day
• **Geriatric: PO** max 40 mg/day
Renal/hepatic dose
• **Adult: PO** CCr <30 mL/min, 2.5 mg/day; may increase cautiously; (Child-Pugh class B) 2.5 mg daily; use dose escalation cautiously
Available forms: Tabs 2.5, 5, 10, 20 mg
Administer:
PO route
• Without regard to meals; tab may be crushed or swallowed whole; give with food to prevent GI upset
• Taper over 1-2 wk when discontinuing, minimize physical exertion, if angina recurs, give nebivolol
• Store protected from light, moisture; place in cool environment

SIDE EFFECTS
CNS: *Insomnia, fatigue, dizziness, mental changes,* drowsiness, *headache*
CV: Bradycardia, MI, AV heart block, edema
GI: *Nausea, diarrhea,* vomiting, abdominal pain
GU: *Impotence*
HEMA: Thrombocytopenia
INTEG: Rash, pruritus, vasculitis, urticaria, psoriasis, angioedema
MISC: Renal failure, pulmonary edema, hyperuricemia, hypercholesterolemia, withdrawal symptoms
RESP: Bronchospasm, dyspnea

PHARMACOKINETICS
Peak 1.5-4 hr; half-life 12 hr; metabolized in liver by CYP2D6; 38% excreted in urine, 44% in feces, protein binding 98%

INTERACTIONS
Increase: nebivolol action—CYP2D6 inhibitors (amiodarone, buPROPion, chloroquine, chlorpheniramine, chlorproMAZINE, cinacalcet, diphenhydrAMINE, DULoxetine, FLUoxetine, haloperidol,

imatinib, PARoxetine, promethazine, propoxyphene, quiNIDine, quiNINE, ritonavir, terbinafine, thioridazine), cimetidine, calcium channel blockers (nondihydropyridine), SSRIs

Decrease: nebivolol action—CYP2D6 inducers (rifampin), sildenafil

Drug/Herb
• May increase nebivolol effect—hawthorn
• May decrease nebivolol effect—ephedra

Drug/Lab Test
Increase: serum lipoprotein levels, BUN, potassium, triglycerides, uric acid, LDH, AST, ALT, alk phos
Decrease: platelets

NURSING CONSIDERATIONS
Assess:
• **Hypertension:** B/P, pulse, ECG during beginning treatment, periodically thereafter; apical/radial pulse before administration; notify prescriber of any significant changes (pulse <50 bpm); signs of HF (dyspnea, crackles, weight gain, jugular venous distention)
• Blood glucose in patients with diabetes
• Baselines of renal, hepatic function tests before therapy begins and periodically; do not use in Child-Pugh class C
• Edema in feet, legs daily: monitor I&O, weight
• **Pregnancy/breastfeeding:** use only if benefits outweigh fetal risk; avoid breastfeeding
Evaluate:
• Therapeutic response: decreased B/P after 1-2 wk; decreased dysrhythmias
Teach patient/family:
• Not to discontinue product abruptly because severe cardiac reactions may occur; to taper over 2 wk; not to double dose; if dose is missed, to take as soon as remembered up to 4 hr before next dose
• That product may mask signs of hypoglycemia or alter blood glucose levels
• Not to use OTC products containing α-adrenergic stimulants (nasal decongestants, OTC cold preparations) unless directed by prescriber

• To report low pulse, dizziness, confusion, depression, fever
• To take pulse, B/P at home; advise patient when to notify prescriber
• To comply with weight control, dietary adjustments, modified exercise program
• To carry emergency ID to identify product, allergies
• To avoid hazardous activities if dizziness, drowsiness present
• **To report symptoms of HF:** difficulty breathing, especially on exertion or when lying down; night cough; swelling of extremities
• To continue with required lifestyle changes (exercise, diet, weight loss, stress reduction)

TREATMENT OF OVERDOSE:
Lavage, IV atropine for bradycardia, IV theophylline for bronchospasm, digoxin, O_2, diuretic for cardiac failure, IV glucose for hypoglycemia, IV diazepam (or phenytoin) for seizures, IV fluids, IV pressors

---

nelfinavir (Rx)

(nell-fin′a-ver)

Viracept
Func. class.: Antiretroviral
Chem. class.: Protease inhibitor

Do not confuse:
Viracept/Viramune

ACTION: Inhibits human immunodeficiency virus (HIV-1) protease, which prevents maturation of the infectious virus
Uses: HIV-1 in combination with other antiretrovirals

CONTRAINDICATIONS: Hypersensitivity to protease inhibitors
Precautions: Pregnancy, breastfeeding, renal/hepatic disease, hemophilia, PKU, pancreatitis, diabetes, infection, immune reconstitution syndrome

DOSAGE AND ROUTES
HIV infection
• **Adult/child >13 yr: PO** 750 mg tid or 1250 mg bid, max 2500 mg/day in combination

---

Side effects: *italics* = common; red = life-threatening

• **Child 2-12 yr: PO** 25-35 mg/kg tid or 45-55 mg/kg bid, max 2500 mg/day in combination

Prevention of HIV infection after exposure (unlabeled)

• **Adult: PO** 1250 mg bid with 2 other antiretroviral agents × 4 wk

Available forms: Tabs 250, 625 mg

Administer:

PO route

Do not mix with juice or acidic fluids

• **Tabs** may be crushed and dispersed in water or mixed with food; consume immediately

SIDE EFFECTS

CNS: Headache, asthenia, poor concentration, seizures, suicidal ideation

CV: Bleeding

ENDO: Hyperglycemia, hyperlipidemia

GI: *Diarrhea*, anorexia, dyspepsia, *nausea, flatulence*, hepatitis, pancreatitis

HEMA: Anemia, leukopenia, thrombocytopenia, Hgb abnormalities

INTEG: *Rash*, dermatitis, anaphylaxis

MISC: Hypoglycemia, redistribution/ accumulation of body fat, immune reconstitution syndrome

MS: Pain, arthralgia, myalgia, myopathy

PHARMACOKINETICS

Half-life $3^1/_2$-5 hr, excreted in feces (87%), peak 2-4 hr, 98% protein binding; metabolized by CYP3A4 enzyme system; potent inhibitor of CYP3A4

INTERACTIONS

Increase: serious dysrhythmias—amiodarone, ergots, lovastatin, midazolam, pimozide, quiNIDine, simvastatin, triazolam, salmeterol

Increase: effect of—atorvastatin, azithromycin, rifabutin, indinavir, saquinavir, cycloSPORINE, tacrolimus, sirolimus, sildenafil, alfentanil, alosetron, buprenorphine, busPIRone, bortezomib, calcium channel blockers, cilostazol, disopyramide, dofetilide, DOCEtaxel, donepezil, ethosuximide, fentaNYL, galantamine, gefitinib, levomethadyl, systemic lidocaine, PACLitaxel, sibutramine, SUFentanil, vinca alkaloids, ziprasidone,

zonisamide, traZODone, tricyclic antidepressants, sildenafil

Increase: nelfinavir levels—ketoconazole, indinavir, ritonavir; delavirdine, other HIV protease inhibitors

Decrease: nelfinavir levels—rifamycins, nevirapine, PHENobarbital, phenytoin, carBAMazepine

Decrease: effect of—didanosine, methadone, oral contraceptives, phenytoin

Drug/Herb

• **Decrease:** antiretroviral effect—St. John's wort; do not use concurrently

Drug/Food

Increase: absorption with food

Drug/Lab Test

Increase: AST, ALT, alk phos, total bilirubin, CPK, LDH, lipids, uric acid

Decrease: WBC, platelets

NURSING CONSIDERATIONS

Assess:

• Resistance testing at initiation, with failure of treatment

• Signs of infection, anemia

• Hepatic studies: ALT, AST

• Bowel pattern before, during treatment; if severe abdominal pain with bleeding occurs, product should be discontinued; monitor hydration

• **Immune reconstitution syndrome:** occurs with combination therapy, including MAC, CMV, PCP, TB, requiring treatment

• **Anaphylaxis, hypersensitivity reaction:** wheezing, flushing; swelling of lips, tongue, throat, skin eruptions, rash, urticaria, itching

• **HIV:** serum lipid profile, plasma HIV RNA, blood glucose, viral load, CD4 cell counts at baseline and throughout treatment

• **Pregnancy/breastfeeding:** enroll pregnant patients in Antiretroviral Pregnancy Registry; use only if potential benefit is greater than risk; do not breastfeed

Teach patient/family:

• To avoid taking with other medications unless directed by prescriber

• **Diarrhea** is most common side effect; may use loperamide to control

• That product does not cure but does manage symptoms; that product does not prevent transmission of HIV to others

• **Pregnancy:** to use a nonhormonal form of birth control while taking this product if using contraceptives

• If dose is missed, to take as soon as remembered up to 1 hr before next dose; not to double dose; to take with food

• To report symptoms of hyperglycemia, bleeding, abdominal pain, yellowing of skin, eyes

• **Phenylketonuria:** that powder contains phenylalanine

• To advise all providers of this product; to advise prescriber of all OTC products, prescription products, or herbal products taken

---

RARELY USED

neomycin (Rx)

(nee-oh-mye′sin)
Neo-Fradin
Func. class.: Antiinfective—aminoglycoside

USES: Severe systemic infections of CNS, respiratory, GI, urinary tract, eye, bone, skin, soft tissues; hepatic coma, preoperatively to sterilize bowel, infectious diarrhea caused by enteropathogenic *E. coli, Enterobacter* sp., *Escherichia coli, Klebsiella* sp. May be effective for *Acinetobacter* sp., *Bacillus anthracis, Citrobacter* sp., *Haemophilus influenzae* (beta-lactamase negative), *Haemophilus influenzae* (beta-lactamase positive), *Neisseria* sp., *Proteus mirabilis, Proteus vulgaris, Providencia* sp., *Salmonella* sp., *Serratia* sp., *Shigella* sp., *Staphylococcus aureus* (MSSA), *Staphylococcus epidermidis*

CONTRAINDICATIONS: Infants, children, bowel obstruction (oral use), severe renal disease, hypersensitivity, GI disease

Precautions: Dehydration, geriatric patients, respiratory insufficiency

Black Box Warning: Hearing impairment, neuromuscular disease, renal disease

---

DOSAGE AND ROUTES
Hepatic encephalopathy

• **Adult: PO** 4-12 g/day in divided doses q6hr × 5-6 days

• **Child: PO** 50-100 mg/kg/day in divided doses q6hr × 5-6 days

Preoperative intestinal antisepsis

• **Adult: PO** 1 g/hr × 4 hr, then 1 g q4hr for remaining 24 hr

---

⚠ HIGH ALERT

RARELY USED

nepafenac ophthalmic
See Appendix B

---

neratinib

(ne-ra′-ti-nib)
Nerlynx
Func. class.: Antineoplastic
Chem. class.: Protein kinase inhibitors

ACTION: It is an irreversible inhibitor of the epidermal growth factor receptor (EGFR) and the human epidermal receptor type 2 (HER2) and HER4. It is a protein kinase inhibitor

USES: For the extended adjuvant treatment of early-stage HER2-positive breast cancer after completion of adjuvant trastuzumab

CONTRAINDICATIONS: Hypersensitivity

Precautions: Breastfeeding, contraception requirements, geriatric patients, hepatic disease, hepatotoxicity, infertility, pregnancy, pregnancy testing, reproductive risk

DOSAGE AND ROUTES
For the extended adjuvant treatment of early-stage HER2-positive breast cancer after completion of adjuvant trastuzumab-based therapy

• **Adult: PO** 240 mg/day with food, × 1 yr

Side effects: *italics* = common; red = life-threatening

Hepatic dose
• **Adult: PO Child-Pugh A or B:** no change; **Child-Pugh C:** reduce starting dose to 80 mg/day; **grade 3 elevations in ALT (5-20× ULN) or bilirubin (3-10× ULN):** hold and evaluate causes; first occurrence, if LFTs resolve to grade ≤1 (ALT ≤3× ULN or bilirubin ≤1 to 1.5× ULN) in ≤3 wk, resume at the next lower dose; discontinue if hepatotoxicity does not recover to ≤1, if hepatotoxicity results in a treatment delay of >3 wk, or if grade 3 ALT or bilirubin occurs again despite 1 dose reduction

Available forms: Tabs 40 mg
Administer:
• With food at the same time every day
• Swallow tablets whole; do not chew, crush, or split
• If a dose is missed, do not replace the missed dose. Resume with the next scheduled daily dose
• Antidiarrheal prophylaxis is recommended during the first 2 cycles (56 days) of treatment, and should be initiated with the first dose of neratinib; loperamide should be taken as directed below, titrating to 1 to 2 bowel movements/day; additional antidiarrheal agents may be required to manage patients with loperamide-refractory diarrhea
• Weeks 1 to 2 (days 1 to 14): take loperamide 4 mg tid
• Weeks 3 to 8 (days 15 to 56): take loperamide 4 mg bid
• Weeks 9 to 52 (days 57 to 365): take loperamide 4 mg as needed (max 16 mg/day)

SIDE EFFECTS
GI: Diarrhea, abdominal pain, anorexia, nausea, vomiting
MS: Muscle cramps
INTEG: Rash
GU: Renal failure (rare)
MISC: Infection

PHARMACOKINETICS
Protein binding >99%; half-life after 7 days was 14.6 hr, half-life of active metabolites 21.6 hr, 13.8 hr, 10.4 hr, respectively; fecal excretion 97.1%; metabolized in the liver by CYP3A4; avoid with strong and moderate CYP3A4 inhibitors and inducers

INTERACTIONS
Decrease: neratinib effect—gastric acid–reducing agents; avoid concomitant use with proton pump inhibitors (PPI) and H₂-receptor antagonists; separate by 3 hr after antacid dosing
Increase: neratinib effect—strong or moderate CYP3A4 inhibitors; avoid concomitant use
Decrease: neratinib effect—strong or moderate CYP3A4 inducers; avoid concomitant use
Increase: CNS and CV adverse reactions—P-glycoprotein (P-gp) substrates; monitor for adverse reactions of narrow therapeutic agents that are P-gp substrates

NURSING CONSIDERATIONS
Assess
• **Hepatotoxicity:** use with caution in those with preexisting hepatic disease; a dose reduction is required for patients with severe (Child-Pugh C) hepatic disease at baseline. Monitor LFTs (total bilirubin, AST, ALT, alkaline phosphatase) baseline, q month × 3 mo and then q3mo thereafter and as needed. Monitor LFTs (including fractionated bilirubin and prothrombin time) in those experiencing grade 3 diarrhea or any signs of hepatotoxicity (fatigue, nausea, vomiting, right upper quadrant tenderness, fever, rash, eosinophilia)
• **Geriatric patients >65 yr:** monitor geriatric patients more closely for toxicities (vomiting, diarrhea, renal failure, dehydration) during treatment
• **Infection:** may occur after completion of adjuvant trastuzumab-based therapy; assess for urinary tract infection, cellulitis and erysipelas
• **Pregnancy/breastfeeding:** avoid drug in females of reproductive potential; use contraception during treatment and for at least 1 mo after the last dose; can cause fetal harm or death; discontinue breastfeeding during treatment and for 1 mo after the final dose. Presence in breast milk unknown. Obtain a pregnancy test

before starting treatment. Males with female partners of reproductive potential should avoid pregnancy and use effective contraception during treatment and ≥3 mo after last dose

Evaluate:
• Therapeutic outcome: decrease in size of cancerous tumor

Teach patient/family
• That infection may occur; to report urinary pain, hesitancy; skin redness, pain, heat; fever, shaking, chills
• **Diarrhea:** to report number of loose stools per day or change in stools to provider
• **Pregnancy/breastfeeding:** not to use in pregnancy, breastfeeding; to use contraception during treatment and for at least 1 mo after last dose; men with a partner who may become pregnant should use contraception during treatment and for at least 3 mo after last dose

---

⚠ HIGH ALERT

nesiritide (Rx)
(neh-seer'ih-tide)
Natrecor
Func. class.: Vasodilator
Chem. class.: Human B-type natriuretic peptide

ACTION: Uses DNA technology; human B-type natriuretic peptide binds to the receptor in vascular smooth muscle and endothelial cells, thereby leading to smooth muscle relaxation

USES: Acutely decompensated HF

CONTRAINDICATIONS: Hypersensitivity to this product or *Escherichia coli* protein; cardiogenic shock, B/P <90 mm Hg as primary therapy
Precautions: Pregnancy, breastfeeding; children; mitral stenosis; significant valvular stenosis, restriction, or obstructive cardiomyopathy, or any condition dependent on venous return; renal disease; constrictive pericarditis

DOSAGE AND ROUTES
• **Adult: IV BOL** 2 mcg/kg, then **CONT IV INFUSION** 0.01 mcg/kg/min
Available forms: Powder for inj, 1.5-mg single-use vial
Administer:
IV route
• Do not give through a central catheter containing other products; administer other products through separate catheter or central line heparin-coated catheter because nesiritide binds to heparin
• If hypotension develops, reduce or discontinue
• Reconstitute one 1.5-mg vial/5 mL of diluent from prefilled 250-mL plastic IV bag with diluent of choice (preservative free D_5, 0.9% NaCl, $D_5/^1/_2$ NaCl, $D_5/0.2\%$ NaCl); do not shake vial; roll gently; use only clear sol
• Withdraw all contents of reconstituted vial and add to 250-mL plastic IV bag (6 mcg/mL), invert bag several times
• Use within 24 hr of reconstituting
• Prime IV fluid with infusion of 5 mL before connecting to patient's vascular access port and before bolus dose or IV infusion
Direct IV route
• Prime tubing with 5 mL infusion sol; calculate dose based on patient's weight, $0.33 \times$ patient weight (kg) = bolus vol (mL) (6 mcg/mL); withdraw prescribed bolus dose (volume) from prepared infusion bag; give over 1 min through IV port
Intermittent IV INFUSION route
• After bolus dose, use infusion, give at 0.1 mL/kg/hr (0.01 mcg/kg/min)

Y-site compatibilities: Acyclovir, alfentanil, allopurinol, amifostine, aminocaproic acid, aminophylline, amiodarone, amphotericin B colloidal, amphotericin B lipid complex, amphotericin B liposome, anidulafungin, argatroban, atenolol, atracurium, azithromycin, aztreonam, bivalirudin, bleomycin, buprenorphine, busulfan, butorphanol, calcium acetate/chloride/gluconate, CARBOplatin, carmustine, ceFAZolin, cefotaxime, cefoTEtan, cefOXitin, cefTAZidime, ceftizoxime, cefTRIAXone, cefuroxime, chloramphenicol, cimetidine, ciprofloxacin, cisatracurium, CISplatin, clindamycin, cyclophosphamide, cycloSPORINE, cytarabine, dacarbazine, DACTINomycin, DAUNOrubicin, digoxin, diltiazem, diphenhydrAMINE, DOCEtaxel, dolasetron, doxacurium, DOXOrubicin, doxycycline, droperidol, ePHEDrine, epirubicin, ertapenem, erythromycin, esmolol, etoposide, etoposide phosphate, famotidine, fenoldopam, fentaNYL, filgrastim, fluconazole, fludarabine, fluorouracil, foscarnet, fosphenytoin, ganciclovir, gatifloxacin, gemcitabine, gemtuzumab, glycopyrrolate, granisetron, haloperidol, hydrocortisone, HYDROmorphone, hydrOXYzine, IDArubicin, ifosfamide, imipenem-cilastatin, irinotecan, ketorolac, leucovorin, levofloxacin, lidocaine, linezolid, LORazepam, magnesium sulfate, mannitol, mechlorethamine, melphalan, meropenem, mesna, metaraminol, methohexital, methotrexate, methylPREDNISolone, metoclopramide, metroNIDAZOLE, midazolam, milrinone, minocycline, mitoMYcin, mitoXANtrone, mivacurium, moxifloxacin, mycophenolate, nalbuphine, naloxone, niCARdipine, nitroglycerin, nitroprusside, octreotide, ondansetron, oxaliplatin, oxytocin, PACLitaxel, palonosetron, pamidronate, pancuronium, PEMEtrexed, pentamidine, PENTobarbital, PHENobarbital, phentolamine, phenylephrine, polymyxin B sulfate, potassium chloride/phosphates, prochlorperazine, propranolol, quiNIDine, quinupristin-dalfopristin, ranitidine, remifentanil, rocuronium, sodium acetate/bicarbonate/phosphates, streptozocin, succinylcholine, SUFentanil, tacrolimus, teniposide, theophylline, thiotepa, ticarcillin, tigecycline, tirofiban, tolazoline, topotecan, torsemide, trimethobenzamide, vancomycin, vasopressin, vecuronium, verapamil, vinBLAStine, vinCRIStine, vinorelbine, zidovudine, zoledronic acid

SIDE EFFECTS

CNS: Headache, insomnia, dizziness, anxiety, confusion, paresthesia, tremor
CV: *Hypotension,* tachycardia, dysrhythmias, bradycardia, ventricular tachycardia, ventricular extrasystoles, atrial fibrillation

GI: Vomiting, nausea
INTEG: Rash, sweating, pruritus, inj-site reaction
MISC: Abdominal pain, back pain
RESP: Increased cough, hemoptysis, apnea

PHARMACOKINETICS

Half-life 18 min

INTERACTIONS

Increase: hypotension—ACE inhibitors, antihypertensives, IV nitrates
Drug/Lab
Increase: creatinine

NURSING CONSIDERATIONS
Assess:
• **Hypotension:** monitor B/P closely and decrease dose or discontinue if hypotension occurs
• PCWP, RAP, cardiac index, MPAP, respiratory rate, CVP, B/P, pulse during treatment until stable
• Daily serum creatinine, BUN
• **Heart failure:** weight gain, dyspnea, crackles, I&O ratios, peripheral edema
• **Pregnancy/breastfeeding:** use only if benefits outweigh fetal risk; cautious use in breastfeeding, excretion unknown
Evaluate:
• Therapeutic response: improvement in HF with improved PCWP, RAP, MPAP
• **Allergic reactions to peptides:** rash, pruritus, wheezing; discontinue immediately, keep emergency equipment available
Teach patient/family:
• About purpose of medication, expected results; to report pain at IV site
• To report dizziness, blurred vision, lightheadedness, sweating, allergic reaction

---

nevirapine (Rx)
(ne-veer′a-peen)
Viramune, Viramune XR
Func. class.: Antiretroviral
Chem. class.: Nonnucleoside reverse transcriptase inhibitor (NNRTI)

Do not confuse:
nevirapine/nelfinavir
Viramune/Viracept

ACTION: Binds directly to reverse transcriptase and blocks RNA, DNA, thus causing a disruption of the enzyme's site

USES: HIV-1 in combination with other highly active antiretroviral therapy (HAART)

CONTRAINDICATIONS: Hypersensitivity

Black Box Warning: Hepatic disease

Precautions: Pregnancy, breastfeeding, children, renal disease, ⚕ Hispanic patients, hepatitis

Black Box Warning: Females, serious rash

DOSAGE AND ROUTES
Treatment of HIV infection in combination with other antiretrovirals
• **Adult/adolescent: PO** 200 mg/day × 2 wk, then 200 mg bid in combination; **EXT REL** tab (adults not currently taking immediate rel nevirapine) 200 mg/day (immediate rel tab) × 14 days with other antiretrovirals; if rash develops during lead-in periods and persists beyond 14 days, do not use ext rel tab; if no consistent rash present, then give 400 mg/day ext rel tab with other antiretrovirals; if interrupted >7 days, restart 14 day lead-in dosing; for adults switched from immediate rel tab, give 400 mg/day ext rel tab
• **Child/adolescent ≥6 yr: PO EXT REL** not currently taking immediate release 150 mg/m^2 (immediate release) daily (max 200 mg/day) × 14 days, then BSA 0.58-0.83 m^2 200 mg/day; BSA 0.84-1.16 m^2 300 mg/day
• **Child/infant/neonate ≥15 days old: PO** 150 mg/m^2/day × 14 days, then 150 mg/m^2 bid, max 400 mg/day
Perinatal transmission prophylaxis (unlabeled)
• **Females with no previous antiretroviral therapy: PO** 200 mg as a single dose at onset of labor with zidovudine 2 mg/kg over 1 hr followed by zidovudine 1 mg/kg/hr until delivery
• **Neonate ≥34 wk gestation: PO** Nevirapine 12 mg (>2 kg) or 8 mg (1.5-2 kg) × 3 doses; 1st dose 48 hr after birth, 2nd dose 48 hr after 1st dose, 3rd dose 96 hr after 2nd dose and **PO** zidovudine
Hepatic dose
• **Adult: PO** do not use with Child-Pugh grade B or C

Available forms: Tabs 200 mg; oral susp 50 mg/5 mL; ext rel 400 mg
Administer:
• Do not initiate treatment in females when CD4 counts >250 cells/mm^3 or in males when >400 cells/mm^3 unless benefits outweigh risks
• Without regard to meals
• Use in combination with at least 1 other antiretroviral
• **Oral susp** should be shaken before giving

SIDE EFFECTS
CNS: *Paresthesia, headache, fever, peripheral neuropathy*
GI: *Diarrhea*, abdominal pain, *nausea, stomatitis*, hepatotoxicity, hepatic failure
HEMA: Neutropenia, anemia, thrombocytopenia
INTEG: *Rash*, toxic epidermal necrolysis
MISC: Stevens-Johnson syndrome, anaphylaxis
MS: Pain, myalgia, rhabdomyolysis

PHARMACOKINETICS
Rapidly absorbed, peak 4 hr, 60% bound to plasma proteins, metabolized by liver; metabolized by hepatic P450 enzyme system, excreted 91% in urine, terminal half-life 25-30 hr, 50% removed by peritoneal dialysis; with hepatic disease and in ⚕ Hispanic patients, African-American patients, slower rate of clearance

INTERACTIONS
Increase: nevirapine levels—cimetidine, macrolide antiinfectives
Decrease: effects of protease inhibitors, oral contraceptives, ketoconazole, methadone, itraconazole

Side effects: *italics* = common; red = life-threatening

Decrease: nevirapine levels—rifamycins, anticonvulsants, clonazePAM, diazepam, warfarin

Drug/Herb

Decrease: action of antiretroviral—St. John's wort; do not use concurrently

Drug/Lab Test

Increase: ALT, AST, GGT, bilirubin, Hgb

Decrease: neutrophil count

NURSING CONSIDERATIONS
Assess:

• Resistance testing before therapy and when therapy fails

• Signs of infection, anemia, hepatotoxicity, immune reconstitution syndrome; hepatitis B or C, liver toxicity may occur

• **HIV:** blood studies during treatment: ALT, AST, viral load, CD4, plasma HIV RNA, renal studies; if LFTs elevated significantly, product should be withheld; glucose levels in patients with diabetes; if treatment is interrupted by >1 wk, restart at initial dose

Black Box Warning: **Hepatotoxicity:** may be fatal; usually occurs within the first 18 wk of treatment; higher risk in females

• **Rhabdomyolysis:** pain, tenderness, weakness, edema; product should be discontinued

• Bowel pattern before, during treatment; if severe abdominal pain with bleeding occurs, product should be discontinued; monitor hydration

Black Box Warning: **Stevens-Johnson syndrome, toxic epidermal necrolysis:** allergies before treatment, reaction to each medication; skin eruptions; rash, urticaria, itching; if rash is severe or systemic symptoms occur, discontinue immediately

• **Pregnancy/breastfeeding:** use only if benefits outweigh fetal risk, cautious use in breastfeeding

Evaluate:

• Therapeutic response: absence of AIDS-defining symptoms, improvement in quality of life; decreased viral load, increase in CD4 count

Teach patient/family:

Black Box Warning: To report immediately any right quadrant pain, yellowing of eyes or skin, dark urine, nausea, anorexia, muscle pain or tenderness, rash

• That product may be taken with food, antacids

• To take as prescribed; if dose is missed, to take as soon as remembered up to 1 hr before next dose; not to double dose

• That product is not a cure, does not prevent transmission; controls symptoms of HIV

• To avoid OTC agents unless approved by prescriber

• To use a nonhormonal form of contraception during treatment in those using contraceptives

---

RARELY USED

niacin (OTC, Rx)
(nye′a-sin)
Equaline Niacin, Niaspan, Ni-Odan ✦, Slo-Niacin

niacinamide (OTC, Rx)
Func. class.: Vit B₃, antihyperlipidemic
Chem. class.: Water-soluble vitamin

USES: Pellagra, hyperlipidemias (types 4, 5), peripheral vascular disease that presents a risk for pancreatitis

CONTRAINDICATIONS: Breastfeeding, hypersensitivity, peptic ulcer, hepatic disease, hemorrhage, severe hypotension

DOSAGE AND ROUTES
Niacin deficiency

• **Adult: PO** 100-500 mg/day in divided doses; **IM/SUBCUT** 50-100 mg ≥5×/ day; **IV** 25-100 mg bid or tid

• **Child: PO** ≤300 mg/day in divided doses

Adjunct in hyperlipidemia

• **Adult: PO** 250 mg after evening meal; may increase dose at 1-4 wk intervals to

1-2 g tid, max 6 g/day; **EXT REL** 500 mg at bedtime × 4 wk, then 1000 mg at bedtime for wk 5-8; do not increase by >500 mg q4wk, max 2000 mg/day

Pellagra

• **Adult:** PO 300-500 mg/day in divided doses; IM 50-100 mg 5×/day or IV 25-100 mg bid by slow **IV INFUSION**

• **Child:** PO 100-300 mg/day in divided doses; IV ≤300 mg/day by slow **IV INFUSION**

Peripheral vascular disease

• **Adult:** PO 250-800 mg/day in 3-5 divided doses

---

niCARdipine (Rx)

(nye-card′i-peen)

Cardene IV

Func. class.: Calcium channel blocker, antianginal, antihypertensive

Chem. class.: Dihydropyridine

Do not confuse:
niCARdipine/NIFEdipine
Cardene/Cardizem

ACTION: Inhibits calcium ion influx across cell membrane during cardiac depolarization; produces relaxation of coronary vascular smooth muscle, peripheral vascular smooth muscle; dilates coronary vascular arteries; increases myocardial oxygen delivery in patients with vasospastic angina

USES: Chronic stable angina pectoris, hypertension

CONTRAINDICATIONS: Sick sinus syndrome, 2nd-/3rd-degree heart block; hypersensitivity to this product or dihydropyridine; advanced aortic stenosis

Precautions: Pregnancy, breastfeeding, children, geriatric patients, HF, hypotension, hepatic injury, renal disease

DOSAGE AND ROUTES

Hypertension

• **Adult:** PO 20 mg tid initially; may increase after 3 days (range 20-40 mg tid)

may increase to 60 mg bid or **IV** 5 mg/hr; may increase by 2.5 mg/hr q15min; max 15 mg/hr

Angina

• **Adult:** PO 20 mg tid; may be adjusted q3days; may use 20-40 mg tid

Renal dose

• **Adult:** PO adjust based on response

Hepatic dose

• **Adult:** PO 20 mg bid

Available forms: Caps 20, 30 mg; inj 2.5 mg/mL, premixed 20 mg/200 mL, 40 mg/200 mL

Administer:

PO route

• Without regard to meals

• To start PO, give 1 hr prior to discontinuing IV nicardipine

• Avoid use with grapefruit, grapefruit juice

IV route

• To convert from PO to IV for adults: if PO 20 mg q8hr, start infusion at 0.5 mg/hr; if PO 30 mg q8hr, start infusion at 1.2 mg/hr; if PO 40 mg q8hr, start infusion at 2.2 mg/hr

Continuous IV INFUSION

• Dilute each 25 mg/240 mL of compatible sol (0.1 mg/mL), give slowly, titrate to patient response, change IV site q12hr

• Stable at room temperature for 24 hr

Solution compatibilities: D_5W, D_5/0.45% NaCl, D_5/0.9% NaCl

Y-site compatibilities: Alemtuzumab, amikacin, aminophylline, aztreonam, bivalirudin, butorphanol, calcium gluconate, CARBOplatin, caspofungin, ceFAZolin, ceftizoxime, chloramphenicol, cimetidine, CISplatin, clindamycin, cytarabine, DAPTOmycin, dexmedetomidine, diltiazem, DOBUTamine, DOCEtaxel, DOPamine, DOXOrubicin hydrochloride, enalaprilat, EPINEPHrine, epirubicin, erythromycin, esmolol, famotidine, fenoldopam, fentaNYL, gentamicin, hydrocortisone, HYDROmorphone, labetalol, lidocaine, linezolid, LORazepam, magnesium sulfate, mechlorethamine, methylPREDNISolone, metroNIDAZOLE, midazolam, milrinone, morphine, nafcillin, nesiritide,

---

nitroglycerin, nitroprusside, norepinephrine, octreotide, oxaliplatin, oxytocin, palonosetron, penicillin G potassium, potassium chloride/phosphate, quinupristin/dalfopristin, ranitidine, rocuronium, tacrolimus, tirofiban, tobramycin, trimethoprim/sulfamethoxazole, vancomycin, vasopressin, vecuronium, vinCRIStine, voriconazole, zoledronic acid

SIDE EFFECTS

CNS: *Headache, dizziness,* anxiety, depression, confusion, paresthesia
CV: Edema, hypotension, palpitations, tachycardia, angina
GI: Nausea, vomiting, abdominal cramps, dry mouth
INTEG: Rash, infusion-site discomfort, Stevens-Johnson syndrome
OTHER: Myalgia (IV)

PHARMACOKINETICS

Metabolized by liver, excreted in urine 60%, feces 35%, half-life 2-5 hr
PO: Onset 20 min, peak 1-2 hr, duration 8 hr
PO-SR: Onset unknown, duration 10-12 hr
IV: Onset 1 min, peak 45 min

INTERACTIONS

Increase: effects of digoxin, neuromuscular blocking agents, theophylline, other antihypertensives, nitrates, alcohol, quiNIDine
Increase: hypotension—antihypertensives, neuromuscular blockers, nitrates, protease inhibitors, fentanyl
Increase: toxicity —cycloSPORINE, prazosin, carBAMazepine, quiNIDine, propranolol, cimetidine
Decrease: antihypertensive effect—NSAIDs, rifampin

Drug/Herb
Increase: effect—ginkgo, ginseng, hawthorn
Decrease: effect—ephedra, melatonin, St. John's wort, yohimbe

Drug/Food
Increase: hypotensive effect—grapefruit, grapefruit juice
Decreased: absorption of high-fat foods

Drug/Lab Test
Decrease: potassium (IV), phosphate, platelets
Increase: LFTs

NURSING CONSIDERATIONS
Assess:
• **Anginal pain:** intensity, location, duration; alleviating, precipitating factors
• **HF:** weight gain, crackles, peripheral edema, jugular venous distention, dyspnea, I&O
• **Cardiac status:** B/P baseline and frequent intervals, pulse, respiration, ECG during long-term treatment
• Potassium, renal, hepatic studies periodically if on long-term treatment
• **Allergic reactions (Stevens-Johnson syndrome):** if rash is severe, with joint aches, mouth lesions, discontinue immediately
• **Hypertension:** decreasing B/P; assess salt in diet, smoking, exercise, weight, monitor B/P often
• **Pregnancy/breastfeeding:** use only if benefits outweigh fetal risk; cautious use in breastfeeding
Evaluate:
• **Therapeutic response:** decreased anginal pain, decreased B/P
Teach patient/family:
• How to take pulse and what to report
• To avoid hazardous activities until stabilized on product, dizziness is no longer a problem
• To limit caffeine consumption; to avoid alcohol products; to take without regard to food, avoid high-fat foods, to avoid grapefruit, grapefruit juice
• **Hypertension:** to comply in all areas of medical regimen: diet, exercise, stress reduction, product therapy
• To notify prescriber of irregular heartbeat, SOB, swelling of feet and hands, pronounced dizziness, constipation, nausea, hypotension, change in severity/pattern/incidence of angina
• To rise slowly from sitting or lying down to prevent orthostatic hypotension

TREATMENT OF OVERDOSE:
Defibrillation, β-agonists, IV calcium,

diuretics, atropine for AV block, vasopressor for hypotension

---

nicotine
(nik′o-teen)
nicotine chewing gum
Nicorette, Thrive
nicotine inhaler (OTC, Rx)
Nicotrol
nicotine lozenge (OTC)
Commit, Nicorette
nicotine nasal spray (Rx)
Nicotrol NS
nicotine transdermal (OTC, Rx)
Nicoderm CQ
Func. class.: Smoking deterrent
Chem. class.: Ganglionic cholinergic agonist

ACTION: Agonist at nicotinic receptors in peripheral, central nervous systems; acts at sympathetic ganglia, on chemoreceptors of aorta, carotid bodies; also affects adrenalin-releasing catecholamines

USES: Deter cigarette smoking

CONTRAINDICATIONS: Pregnancy (transdermal, inhaler); hypersensitivity, immediate post-MI recovery period, severe angina pectoris
Precautions: Pregnancy (gum); breastfeeding, vasospastic disease, dysrhythmias, diabetes mellitus, hyperthyroidism, pheochromocytoma, esophagitis, peptic ulcer, coronary/renal/hepatic disease; MRI (patch); soy hypersensitivity (mint lozenge)

DOSAGE AND ROUTES
Nicotine chewing gum
• **Adult:** chew 1 piece of gum (2 mg nicotine) whenever urge to smoke occurs; dose varies; usually 20 mg/day during first mo, max 24 pieces/day, max 3 mo

Nicotine inhaler
• **Adult:** INH 6 cartridges/day (24-64 mg) for up to 12 wk, then gradual reduction over 12 wk
Nicotine lozenge
• **Adult:** if cigarette is desired >30 min after awakening, start with 2-mg lozenge; if <30 min after awakening, start with 4-mg lozenge, then again q1-2hr, max 20 lozenges/day or 5 lozenges/6 hr × 6 wk, then 1 lozenge q2-4hr × 2 wk, then 1 lozenge q4-8hr × 2 wk, then discontinue
Nicotine nasal spray
• **Adult:** 1 spray in each nostril 1-2×/hr, max 5×/hr or 40×/day, max 3 mo
Nicotine transdermal/inhaler system
• **Nicoderm:** 21 mg/day × 4-8 wk; 14 mg/day × 2-4 wk; 7 mg/day × 2-4 wk
• **Nicotrol:** 15 mg/day × 12 wk; 10 mg/day × 2 wk; 5 mg/day × 2 wk
• **Nicotrol inhaler:** delivers 30% of nicotine that smoker receives from an actual cigarette
Available forms: Transdermal patch (Habitrol ✦, Nicoderm, nicotine transdermal system) delivering 7, 14, 21 mg/day; (Nicoderm) 5, 10, 15 mg/day; **nicotine inhaler** 4 mg delivered; **nasal spray** 0.5 mg nicotine/actuation; **gum** 2, 4 mg/piece; **lozenge** 2 mg, 4 mg
Administer:
• **Gum:** chew gum slowly for 30 min to promote buccal absorption of product; do not chew >45 min
• Do not expose to light; gum will turn color
• Begin product withdrawal after 3 mo of use; do not exceed 6 mo
• **Transdermal patch:** 1 × day to nonhairy, clean, dry area of skin on upper body or upper outer arm; rotate sites to prevent skin irritation; can remove before bed if patient has strange dreams
• **Nasal spray/inhaler:** puffing on mouthpiece delivers nicotine through mouth
• **Lozenge:** allow to dissolve slowly

SIDE EFFECTS
CNS: Dizziness, vertigo, insomnia, headache, confusion, seizures, numbness, tinnitus, strange dreams

---

CV: Dysrhythmias, tachycardia, palpitations, edema, flushing, hypertension
EENT: Jaw ache, irritation in buccal cavity
GI: *Nausea, vomiting, anorexia, indigestion,* diarrhea, abdominal pain, constipation, eructation, irritation
RESP: Breathing difficulty, cough, hoarseness, sneezing, wheezing, bronchial spasm

PHARMACOKINETICS
Onset 15-30 min, metabolized in liver, excreted in urine, half-life 2-3 hr, 30-120 hr (terminal)

INTERACTIONS
Increase: vasoconstriction—ergots, bromocriptine, cabergoline
Increase: effect after smoking cessation—adrenergic antagonists, β blockers
Increase: effect of—adenosine
Increase: B/P—buPROPion
Decrease: effect of—α-blockers, insulin
Decrease: nicotine clearance—cimetidine
Drug/Food
• Avoid use of gum with acidic foods (colas, coffee) and for 15 min after

NURSING CONSIDERATIONS
Assess:
• **Smoking:** number of cigarettes smoked, years used, brand; **withdrawal:** headache, cravings, restlessness, irritation, drowsiness, insomnia, sore throat, periodic increase in appetite
• **Adverse reaction:** irritation of buccal cavity, dislike of taste, jaw ache, gum should not be used if temporomandibular condition exists
• **Toxicity:** nausea, vomiting, diarrhea, headache, dizziness, dyspnea, hypertension
• **Pregnancy/breastfeeding:** whenever possible, avoid in pregnancy; cautious use in breastfeeding
Evaluate:
• Therapeutic response: decrease in urge to smoke, decreased need for gum after 3-6 mo
Teach patient/family:
• To discontinue if patient is unable to stop smoking after 4th week of therapy

• **Gum:** about all aspects of product use; give package insert to patient and explain
• That gum will not stick to dentures, dental appliances
• That gum is as toxic as cigarettes; that it is to be used only to deter smoking; to call prescriber immediately, stop use if difficulty breathing or rash occurs
• To avoid use during pregnancy
• **Transdermal patch:** that patch is as toxic as cigarettes; to be used only to deter smoking
• Not to use during pregnancy because birth defects may occur; not to breastfeed
• To keep used and unused system out of reach of children and pets
• To stop smoking immediately when beginning patch treatment
• To apply promptly after removing from protective patch because system may lose strength
• **Nasal spray:** to tilt head back; not to swallow or inhale during administration; after smoking is stopped, to use spray up to 8 wk, then discontinue over 6 wk by tapering
• **Lozenges:** to allow to dissolve; to avoid swallowing; not to chew
• **Inhalation:** to use by inhaler for 20 min by frequent puffs

---

NIFEdipine (Rx)
(nye-fed′i-peen)
Adalat CC, Adalat XL ✦, Afeditab CR, Procardia, Procardia XL, Nifedical XL
Func. class.: Calcium channel blocker, antianginal, antihypertensive
Chem. class.: Dihydropyridine

Do not confuse:
NIFEdipine/niCARdipine/niMODipine
Procardia XL/Protain XL

ACTION: Inhibits calcium ion influx across cell membrane during cardiac depolarization; relaxes coronary vascular smooth muscle; dilates coronary arteries; increases myocardial oxygen delivery in patients with vasospastic angina; dilates peripheral arteries

USES: Chronic stable angina pectoris, variant angina, hypertension
Unlabeled uses: Migraines, migraine prophylaxis; preterm labor, acute hypertension (pediatrics), diabetic nephropathy, proteinuria, hiccups

CONTRAINDICATIONS: Hypersensitivity to this product or dihydropyridine; cardiogenic shock
Precautions: Pregnancy, breastfeeding, children, hypotension, sick sinus syndrome, 2nd-/3rd-degree heart block, hypotension <90 mm Hg systolic, hepatic injury, renal disease, acute MI, aortic stenosis, GERD, heart failure

DOSAGE AND ROUTES
• **Adult: PO** Immediate release 10 mg tid, increase in 10-mg increments q7-14days, max 180 mg/24 hr or single dose of 30 mg; **SUS REL** 30-60 mg/day, may increase q7-14days, max 90 mg/day
Hypertension
• **Adult: PO EXT REL** 30-60 mg daily, titrate upward as needed, max 90 mg/day (Adalat CC), 120 mg/day (Procardia XL)
• **Child/adolescent (unlabeled): PO EXT REL** 0.25-0.5 mg/kg/day, max 3 mg/kg/day
Acute hypertensive episodes in pediatric patients (unlabeled)
• **Adolescent/child/infant: PO** 0.2-0.5 mg/kg/dose up to 10 mg (total dose)
Migraine prophylaxis (unlabeled)
• **Adult: PO** 30-180 mg/day
Preterm labor (unlabeled)
• **Pregnant female: PO** Immediate release (Procardia, Adalat) 30-mg loading dose, then 10-20 mg q4-6hr; use in monitored settings
Hiccups (unlabeled)
• **Adult:** 10-20 mg tid
Available forms: Caps 10, 20 mg; ext rel tabs (CC, XL) 30, 60, 90 mg
Administer:
• Do not break, crush, or chew ext rel tabs, do not use immediate-release caps

within 7 days of MI, coronary syndrome; do not use caps (SL) to reduce severe hypertension, may cause death
• Without regard to meals; avoid grapefruit juice
• Protect caps from direct light, keep in dry area, do not freeze

SIDE EFFECTS
CNS: *Headache,* fatigue, drowsiness, *dizziness,* anxiety, depression, weakness, insomnia, light-headedness, paresthesia, tinnitus, blurred vision, nervousness, tremor, *flushing*
CV: Dysrhythmias, edema, hypotension, palpitations, tachycardia
GI: Nausea, vomiting, diarrhea, gastric upset, constipation, increased LFTs, dry mouth, flatulence, gingival hyperplasia
GU: *Nocturia, polyuria*
HEMA: Bruising, bleeding, petechiae
INTEG: Rash, pruritus, flushing, hair loss, Stevens-Johnson syndrome, toxic epidermal necrolysis, exfoliative dermatitis
MISC: Sexual difficulties, cough, fever, chills

PHARMACOKINETICS
Metabolized by liver; excreted in urine 60%-80% (metabolites), feces 15%; protein binding 92%-98%, half-life 2-5 hr, well absorbed
PO: Onset 20 min, duration 6-8 hr
PO-ER: Duration 24 hr
PO-CC, XL: Peak 6 hr, duration 24 hr

INTERACTIONS
• Contraindicated with strong CYP3A4 inducers
Increase: level of digoxin, phenytoin, cycloSPORINE, prazosin, carBAMazepine
Increase: NIFEdipine, toxicity—cimetidine, raNITIdine
Increase: effects of β-blockers, antihypertensives
Decrease: antihypertensive effect—NSAIDs
Decrease: effects of quiNIDine
Decrease: NIFEdipine level—smoking
Drug/Herb
Increase: effect—ginkgo biloba, ginseng, hawthorn
Decrease: effect—ephedra, melatonin, St. John's wort, yohimbe

Drug/Food
Increase: NIFEdipine level—grapefruit juice
Drug/Lab Test
Increase: CPK, LDH, AST
Positive: ANA, direct Coombs' test

NURSING CONSIDERATIONS
Assess:

• **Anginal pain:** location, intensity, duration, character, alleviating, aggravating factors

• **HF:** peripheral edema, dyspnea, weight gain >5 lb, jugular venous distention, rales; monitor I&O ratios, daily weight

• Cardiac status: B/P, pulse, respiration, ECG at baseline and periodically, in those taking antihypertensives, β-blockers, monitor B/P often

• Potassium, renal, hepatic studies periodically during treatment

• For bruising, petechiae, bleeding

• **GI obstruction:** ext rel products have been associated with rare reports of obstruction in those with strictures and no known GI disease

• **Serious skin disorders:** rash that starts suddenly, fever, cutaneous lesions that may have pustules present; discontinue product if fever present or if rash is severe

• **Beers:** avoid in older adults; potential for hypotension, myocardial ischemia

• **Pregnancy/breastfeeding:** use only if benefits outweigh fetal risk; do not breastfeed
Evaluate:

• Therapeutic response: decreased anginal pain, B/P, activity tolerance
Teach patient/family:

• To avoid hazardous activities until stabilized on product, dizziness is no longer a problem

• To limit caffeine consumption; to avoid alcohol products

• To avoid OTC products unless directed by prescriber; give without regard to meals, Adelat CC should be taken on empty stomach

• That empty tab shells may appear in stools and are not significant

• **Hypertension:** to comply with all areas of medical regimen: diet, exercise, stress reduction, product therapy

• To change position slowly because orthostatic hypotension is common

• To notify prescriber of dyspnea, edema of extremities, nausea, vomiting, severe ataxia, severe rash; changes in pattern, frequency, severity of angina

• To increase fluid intake and fiber to prevent constipation

• To check for gingival hyperplasia and report promptly

• Not to discontinue abruptly; to gradually taper

• About fall risk for older adults

TREATMENT OF OVERDOSE:
Defibrillation, atropine for AV block, vasopressor for hypotension

---

⚠ HIGH ALERT

nilotinib (Rx)
(nye-loe'ti-nib)
Tasigna
Func. class.: Antineoplastic—miscellaneous
Chem. class.: Protein-tyrosine kinase inhibitor

ACTION: Inhibits BCR-ABL tyrosine kinase created in patients with chronic myeloid leukemia (CML)

USES: Chronic phase/accelerated phase Philadelphia chromosome–positive CML that is resistant or intolerant to imatinib

CONTRAINDICATIONS: Pregnancy, breastfeeding, hypersensitivity

Black Box Warning: Hypokalemia, hypomagnesemia, QT prolongation

Precautions: Children, females, geriatric patients, active infections, anemia, cardiac disease, bone marrow suppression, cholestasis, diabetes, gelatin hypersensitivity, infertility, galactose-free diet, lactase deficiency, neutropenia, pancreatitis, thrombocytopenia, hepatic disease, alcoholism, angina, ascites, tumor lysis syndrome

DOSAGE AND ROUTES

• **Adult: PO** 300 mg q12hr, continue until disease progression (chronic phase, newly diagnosed); 400 mg q12hr, continue until disease progression or unacceptable toxicity (accelerated phase)

• **Child/adolescent: PO** 230 mg/m² q12hr until disease progression or unacceptable toxicity. Round the dose to the nearest 50 mg to a max single dose of 400 mg

Adjustment after discontinuation of a strong CYP3A4 inducer

• **Adult: PO** reduce to 400 mg bid

Use with a strong CYP3A4 inhibitor

• **Adult: PO** reduce dose to 300 mg/day

QT prolongation

• QTcF >480 msec: withhold dose

Myelosuppression

• ANC 1 × 10⁹/L or platelets <50 × 10⁹/L: withhold dose

Hepatic dose

• **Adult: PO** (Child-Pugh A/B/C) newly diagnosed CML 200 mg bid, then escalation to 300 mg bid initially

Available forms: Caps 150, 200 mg

Administer:

• Do not break, crush, or chew caps; if whole capsule cannot be swallowed, disperse capsule contents in 1 tsp applesauce

• On empty stomach; separate doses by 12 hr; make-up dose should not be taken if dose is missed

• Store at 59° F-86° F (15° C-30° C)

SIDE EFFECTS

CNS: Headache, dizziness, fatigue, fever, flushing, paresthesia

CV: QT prolongation, palpitations, torsades de pointes, AV block

GI: *Nausea,* hepatotoxicity, vomiting, dyspepsia, *anorexia, abdominal pain,* constipation, pancreatitis, diarrhea, xerostomia

HEMA: Neutropenia, thrombocytopenia, anemia, pancytopenia

INTEG: *Rash,* alopecia, erythema

META: Hyperamylasemia, hyperbilirubinemia, hyperglycemia, hyperkalemia, hypocalcemia, hyponatremia, hypomagnesemia

MISC: Diaphoresis, anxiety

MS: Arthralgia, myalgia, back or bone pain, muscle cramps

RESP: Cough, dyspnea

SYST: Bleeding, tumor lysis syndrome

PHARMACOKINETICS

Protein binding 98%, metabolized by CYP3A4, plasma levels 3 hr, elimination half-life 17 hr

INTERACTIONS

• Product interactions are numerous

• Do not use with phenothiazines, pimozide, ziprasidone

Increase: QT prolongation—class IA/III antidysrhythmics, some phenothiazines, β agonists, local anesthetics, tricyclics, haloperidol, chloroquine, droperidol, pentamidine; CYP3A4 inhibitors (amiodarone, clarithromycin, erythromycin, telithromycin, troleandomycin), arsenic trioxide, levomethadyl; CYP3A4 substrates (methadone, pimozide, QUEtiapine, quiNIDine, risperiDONE, ziprasidone)

Increase: hepatotoxicity—acetaminophen

Increase: concentrations—ketoconazole, itraconazole, erythromycin, clarithromycin

Increase: plasma concentrations of simvastatin, calcium channel blockers

Increase: plasma concentration of warfarin; avoid use with warfarin, use low-molecular-weight anticoagulants instead

Decrease: concentrations—dexamethasone, phenytoin, carBAMazepine, rifampin, PHENobarbital

Drug/Herb

Decrease: concentration—St. John's wort

Drug/Food

Increase: plasma concentrations—grapefruit juice

NURSING CONSIDERATIONS

Assess:

• **Tumor lysis syndrome:** maintain hydration, correct uric acid before use with this product

Black Box Warning: QT prolongation can occur; monitor ECG, left ventricular ejection fraction (LVEF) at baseline, periodically; hypertension, assess for chest pain, palpitations, dyspnea

N

Side effects: *italics* = common; red = life-threatening

Black Box Warning: Hepatotoxicity: monitor LFTs before treatment and monthly; if liver transaminases >5 × IULN, withhold until transaminase levels return to <2.5 × IULN

• **Myelosuppression:** Monitor CBC ×2 mo, then monthly, differential, platelet count; for bleeding: epistaxis, rectal, gingival, upper GI, genital and wound bleeding; tumor-related hemorrhage may occur rapidly

• ANC and platelets: if ANC <1 × 10^9/L and/or platelets <50 × 10^9/L, stop until ANC >1.5 × 10^9/L and platelets >75 ×10^9/L

• **Electrolytes:** calcium, potassium, magnesium, sodium; lipase, phosphate; hypokalemia, hypomagnesemia should be corrected before use

• AST/ALT/bilirubin/lipase/amylase: if increased to grade 3, withhold product; resume at 400 mg daily when levels return to grade 1 or below

• **Pregnancy/breastfeeding:** do not use in pregnancy, breastfeeding

Evaluate:

• Therapeutic response: decrease in progression of disease

Teach patient/family:

• **Infection:** to report immediately cough, fever, chills

• To report bleeding gums; blood in stools, urine, emesis

• About reason for treatment, expected results

• That many adverse reactions may occur

• To avoid persons with known upper respiratory tract infections; immunosuppression is common

• To watch for signs, symptoms of low potassium or magnesium

• To notify prescriber of all OTC, prescription, and herbal products used; not to receive vaccinations without prescriber's approval

• **Pregnancy/breastfeeding:** to use contraception during treatment; not to breastfeed

A HIGH ALERT

RARELY USED

niraparib
(nye-rap′-a-rib)
Zejula
Func. class.: Antineoplastic

USES: Recurrent epithelial ovarian, fallopian tube, or primary peritoneal cancer

DOSAGE AND ROUTES
• **Adult:** PO 300 mg/day until disease progression or unacceptable toxicity. Begin therapy no later than 8 wk after last platinum-containing regimen

RARELY USED

nisoldipine (Rx)
(nye-sole′dih-peen)
Sular
Func. class.: Calcium channel blocker, antihypertensive
Chem. class.: Dihydropyridine

USES: Essential hypertension, alone or in combination with other antihypertensives, ischemic heart disease

CONTRAINDICATIONS: Hypersensitivity to this product or dihydropyridines; sick sinus syndrome; 2nd-/3rd-degree heart block; aortic stenosis

DOSAGE AND ROUTES
Hypertension
• **Adult:** PO 17 mg/day initially, may increase by 8.5 mg/wk, usual dose 17-34 mg/day, max 34 mg/day
• **Geriatric/hepatic dose:** PO 8.5 mg/day, increase based on patient response
Variant (Prinzmetal's) angina/ stable angina pectoris (unlabeled)
• **Adult:** PO 17-34 mg/day, max 34 mg/day

Hepatic dose
• **Adult:** PO 8.5 mg/day

---

nitrofurantoin (Rx)

(nye-troe-fyoor′an-toyn)

Furadantin, Macrobid, Macrodantin, Novo-Furantoin ✚

Func. class.: Urinary tract antiinfective

Chem. class.: Synthetic nitrofuran derivative

ACTION: Inhibits bacterial acetyl-CoA intereference with carbohydrate metabolism

USES: Urinary tract infections caused by *Escherichia coli, Klebsiella, Pseudomonas, Proteus vulgaris, Proteus morganii, Serratia, Citrobacter, Staphylococcus aureus, Staphylococcus epidermidis, Enterococcus, Salmonella, Shigella*

CONTRAINDICATIONS: Infants <1 mo, hypersensitivity, anuria, severe renal disease CCr <60 mL/min, at term pregnancy (38-42 wk), labor, delivery, cholestatic jaundice due to nitrofurantoin therapy

Precautions: Pregnancy, breastfeeding, geriatric patients, ⚕ G6PD deficiency, GI disease, diabetes

DOSAGE AND ROUTES
Active infections
• **Adult:** PO 50-100 mg qid after meals
• **Child:** PO 5-7 mg/kg/day in 4 divided doses
Chronic suppression
• **Adult:** PO 50-100 mg q PM
• **Child:** PO 1-2 mg/kg/day in PM or 0.5-1 mg/kg q12hr if dose not well tolerated
Available forms: Caps 25, 50, 100 mg; susp 25 mg/5 mL; macrocrystal caps (Macrodantin) 25, 50, 100 mg; Macrobid cap 100 mg (25 macrocrystals, 75 monohydrate)
Administer:
PO route
• Give with meals
• Do not break, crush, chew, or open tabs, caps, store in original container

• Two daily doses if urine output is high or if patient has diabetes
• Use calibrated device to measure liquid product; may mix water, fruit juice; rinse mouth after liquid product; staining of teeth may occur

SIDE EFFECTS
CNS: *Dizziness, headache,* drowsiness, peripheral neuropathy, chills, confusion, vertigo
CV: Bundle branch block, chest pain
GI: *Nausea, vomiting, abdominal pain, diarrhea,* cholestatic jaundice, loss of appetite, CDAD, hepatitis, pancreatitis
HEMA: Anemia, agranulocytosis, hemolytic anemia, leukopenia, thrombocytopenia
INTEG: Pruritus, rash, urticaria, angioedema, alopecia, tooth staining, exfoliative dermatitis, Stevens-Johnson syndrome
MS: Arthralgia, myalgia, numbness, peripheral neuropathy
RESP: Cough, dyspnea, pneumonitis, pulmonary fibrosis or infiltrate
SYST:
Superinfection, SLE-like syndrome

PHARMACOKINETICS
PO: Half-life 20-60 min; crosses blood-brain barrier, placenta; enters breast milk; excreted as inactive metabolites in liver, unchanged in urine; protein binding 60%-90%

INTERACTIONS
Increase: antagonistic effect—norfloxacin
Increase: levels of nitrofurantoin—probenecid
Decrease: absorption of magnesium trisilicate antacid
Drug/Lab Test
Increase: BUN, alk phos, bilirubin, creatinine, blood glucose

NURSING CONSIDERATIONS
Assess:
• **Urinary tract infection:** burning, pain on urination; fever; cloudy, foul-smelling urine; I&O ratio: C&S before treatment, after completion; serum creatinine, BUN

Side effects: *italics* = common; red = life-threatening

- Blood count during chronic therapy, LFTs, pulmonary function tests
- **CDAD:** diarrhea with mucus, abdominal pain, fever, fatigue, anorexia; may be treated with vancomycin or metroNIDAZOLE
- CNS symptoms: insomnia, vertigo, headache, drowsiness, seizures
- **Hepatotoxicity:** yellowing of skin or eyes, dark urine, clay-colored stools; monitor AST, ALT
- **Pulmonary fibrosis, pneumonitis:** dyspnea, tachypnea, persistent cough
- **Serious skin disorders:** fever, flushing, rash, urticaria, pruritus
- **Peripheral neuropathy:** paresthesias (more common in diabetes mellitus, electrolyte imbalances, vit B deficiency, debilitated patients)
- **Beers:** avoid in older adults; potential for pulmonary, hepatic toxicity, peripheral neuropathy
- **Pregnancy/breastfeeding:** do not use in gestation of 38-42 wk or in labor/delivery; cautious use in breastfeeding, excreted in breast milk

Evaluate:
- Therapeutic response: decreased dysuria, fever; negative C&S

Teach patient/family:
- To notify prescriber of continued symptoms of UTI, fever, myalgias, arthralgias, numbness or tingling of extremities
- To take with food or milk; to avoid alcohol
- To protect susp from freezing; shake well before taking
- That product may cause drowsiness; to seek aid with walking, other activities; not to drive or operate machinery while taking medication
- That patients with diabetes should monitor blood glucose levels
- That product may turn urine rust-yellow to brown
- **CDAD:** to report immediately symptoms of fever; diarrhea with mucus, pus, or blood

---

nitroglycerin (Rx)

Nitrojet ♣, Nitronal

extended release caps (Rx)

Nitro-Time, Nitrogard SR ♣

topical ointment (Rx)

Nitro-Bid, Nitrol ♣

rectal ointment

Rectiv

SL (Rx)

Nitrostat

SL Powder (Rx)

Go Nitro

translingual spray (Rx)

Nitrolingual, NitroMist, Rho-Nitro ♣

transdermal (Rx)

Minitran, Nitro-Dur, Trinipatch ♣

Func. class.: Coronary vasodilator, antianginal

Chem. class.: Nitrate

ACTION: Decreases preload and afterload, which are responsible for decreasing left ventricular end-diastolic pressure, systemic vascular resistance; dilates coronary arteries, improves blood flow through coronary vasculature, dilates arterial and venous beds systemically

USES: Chronic stable angina pectoris, prophylaxis of angina pain, HF, acute MI, controlled hypotension for surgical procedures, anal fissures

Unlabeled uses: Pulmonary hypertension, hemorrhoids, retained placenta

CONTRAINDICATIONS: Hypersensitivity to this product or nitrites; severe anemia, increased intracranial pressure, cerebral hemorrhage, closed-angle glaucoma, cardiac tamponade, cardiomyopathy, constrictive pericarditis

Precautions: Pregnancy, breastfeeding, children, postural hypotension, severe renal/hepatic disease, acute MI, abrupt discontinuation, hyperthyroidism

---

DOSAGE AND ROUTES

• **Adult: SL** Dissolve tab under tongue when pain begins; may repeat q5min until relief occurs; take ≤3 tabs/15 min; use 1 tab prophylactically 5-10 min before activities; **SUS CAP** q6-12hr on empty stomach; **TOP** 1-2 inches q8hr, increase to 4 inches q4hr as needed; **IV** 5 mcg/min, then increase by 5 mcg/min q3-5min; if no response after 20 mcg/min, increase by 10-20 mcg/min until desired response; **TRANS PATCH** apply a patch daily to a site free of hair; remove patch at bedtime to provide 10-12 hr nitrate-free interval to avoid tolerance

• **Child: IV** Initially 0.25-0.5 mcg/kg/min, titrate to patient response, usual dose 1-3 mcg/kg/min transmucosal

Anal fissures (Rectiv)

• **Adult: Rectal** Apply 1 inch of 0.4% ointment q12hr × 3 wk

Available forms: Translingual aero 0.4 mg/metered spray; sus rel tabs 2.5, 6.5, 9 mg; SL tabs 0.3, 0.4, 0.6 mg; topical oint 2%; trans syst 0.1, 0.2, 0.3, 0.4, 0.6, 0.8 mg/hr; inj sol 25 mg/250 mL, 50 mg/250 mL, 50 mg/500 mL, 100 mg/250 mL, 200 mg/500 mL; rectal ointment 0.4% (Rectiv)

Administer:

• **Topical ointment** should be measured on papers supplied; use paper to spread on nonhairy area of chest, abdomen, thigh skin; thin layer spread over 2-3 inches; do not rub

PO route

• Swallow sus rel products whole; do not break, crush, or chew

• With 8 oz water on empty stomach (oral tablet) 1 hr before or 2 hr after meals

• **SL:** should be dissolved under tongue, or between gum and cheek, not swallowed

• **Aerosol** sprayed under tongue (**nitrolingual**), not inhaled; prime before 1st-time use or if product has not been used in >6 wk; press valve head with forefinger

Transdermal route

• Apply new TD patch daily; remove after 12-14 hr to prevent tolerance

Rectal route

• Cover finger with plastic wrap, disposable glove, or finger cot; lay finger alongside 1-inch dosing line on carton; squeeze tube until equal to 1-inch dosing line; insert covered finger gently into anal canal no further than 1st finger joint and apply to sides; wash hands thoroughly; if too painful, apply directly to outside of anus

Continuous IV INFUSION route

• Diluted in D_5, D_5W, 0.9% NaCl for infusion to 200-400 mcg/mL, depending on patient's fluid status; common dilution 50 mg/250 mL, use controlled infusion device; use glass infusion bottles, non–polyvinyl-chloride infusion tubing; titrate to patient response; do not use filters

Y-site compatibilities: Acyclovir, alfentanil, amikacin, aminocaproic acid, aminophylline, amiodarone, amphotericin B cholesteryl, amphotericin B lipid complex, amphotericin B liposome, anidulafungin, argatroban, ascorbic acid, atenolol, atracurium, atropine, azaTHIOprine, aztreonam, benztropine, bivalirudin, bleomycin, bumetanide, buprenorphine, butorphanol, calcium chloride/gluconate, CARBOplatin, caspofungin, cefamandole, ceFAZolin, cefmetazole, cefonicid, cefoperazone, cefotaxime, cefoTEtan, cefOXitin, cefTAZidime, ceftizoxime, cefTRIAXone, cefuroxime, cephalothin, cephapirin, chloramphenicol, chlorproMAZINE, cimetidine, cisatracurium, CISplatin, clindamycin, cloNIDine, cyanocobalamin, cyclophosphamide, cycloSPORINE, cytarabine, DACTINomycin, dexamethasone, digoxin, diltiazem, diphenhydrAMINE, DOBUTamine, DOCEtaxel, DOPamine, doxacurium, DOXOrubicin, doxycycline, drotrecogin alfa, enalaprilat, ePHEDrine, EPINEPHrine, epirubicin, epoetin alfa, eptifibatide, ertapenem, erythromycin, esmolol, etoposide, famotidine, fenoldopam, fentaNYL, fluconazole, fludarabine, fluorouracil, folic acid, ganciclovir, gatifloxacin, gemcitabine, gemtuzumab, gentamicin, glycopyrrolate, granisetron, heparin, hydrocortisone, HYDROmorphone, hydrOXYzine, IDArubicin, ifosfamide, imipenem-cilastatin, indomethacin, insulin (regular), irinotecan, isoproterenol, ketorolac, labetalol, lidocaine, linezolid, LORazepam, magnesium sulfate, mannitol, mechlorethamine, meperidine, metaraminol, methicillin, methotrexate, methoxamine, methyldopate, methylPREDNISolone, metoclopramide, metroNIDAZOLE, mezlocillin, micafungin, miconazole, midazolam, milrinone, minocycline, mitoXANtrone, morphine, moxalactam, mycophenolate, nafcillin, nalbuphine, naloxone, nesiritide, netilmicin, niCARdipine, nitroprusside, norepinephrine, octreotide, ondansetron, oxacillin, oxaliplatin, oxytocin, PACLitaxel, palonosetron, pamidronate, pancuronium, pantoprazole, papaverine, PEMEtrexed, penicillin G potassium/ sodium, pentamidine, pentazocine, PENTobarbital, PHENobarbital, phentolamine, phenylephrine, phytonadione, piperacillin, piperacillin-tazobactam, polymyxin B, potassium chloride, procainamide, prochlorperazine, promethazine, propofol, propranolol, protamine, pyridoxine, quiNIDine, quinupristin-dalfopristin, ranitidine, remifentanil, ritodrine, rocuronium, sodium bicarbonate, succinylcholine, SUFentanil, tacrolimus, teniposide, theophylline, thiamine, thiopental, thiotepa, ticarcillin, ticarcillin-clavulanate, tigecycline, tirofiban, tobramycin, tolazoline, trimetaphan, urokinase, vancomycin, vasopressin, vecuronium, verapamil, vinCRIStine, vinorelbine, voriconazole, warfarin, zoledronic acid

SIDE EFFECTS

CNS: *Headache, flushing, dizziness*
CV: *Postural hypotension,* tachycardia, collapse, syncope, palpitations
GI: Nausea, vomiting
INTEG: Pallor, sweating, rash

PHARMACOKINETICS

Metabolized by liver, excreted in urine, half-life 1-4 min
SUS REL: Onset 20-45 min, duration 3-8 hr
SL: Onset 1-3 min, duration 30 min

TRANSDERMAL: Onset 30 min-1 hr, duration 12-24 hr
AEROSOL: Onset 2 min, duration 30-60 min
TOPICAL OINT: Onset 30-60 min, duration 2-12 hr
IV: Onset 1-2 min, duration 3-5 min

INTERACTIONS

• **Severe hypotension, CV collapse:** alcohol

Increase: effects of β-blockers, diuretics, antihypertensives, calcium channel blockers
Increase: fatal hypotension—avanafil, sildenafil, tadalafil, vardenafil; do not use together
Increase: nitrate level—aspirin
Decrease: heparin—IV nitroglycerin
Drug/Lab Test
Increase: urine catecholamine, urine VMA
False increase: cholesterol

NURSING CONSIDERATIONS

Assess:
• **Chest pain/angina:** duration, time started, activity being performed, character
• Orthostatic B/P, pulse before and after administration
• Tolerance if taken over long period
• Headache, light-headedness, decreased B/P; may indicate a need for decreased dosage
• **Pregnancy/breastfeeding:** use only if clearly needed; cautious use in breastfeeding
Evaluate:
• Therapeutic response: decrease, prevention of anginal pain
Teach patient/family:
• To place buccal tab between lip and gum above incisors or between cheek and gum
• To keep tabs in original container; to replace q6mo because effectiveness is lost; to keep away from heat, moisture, light
• That if 3 SL tabs in 15 min do not relieve pain, to seek immediate medical attention
• To avoid alcohol
• That product may cause headache; that tolerance usually develops; to use nonopioid analgesic

• That product may be taken before stressful activity: exercise, sexual activity
• That SL may sting when product comes in contact with mucous membranes
• To avoid hazardous activities if dizziness occurs
• To comply with complete medical regimen
• To make position changes slowly to prevent fainting
• Never to use erectile dysfunction products (sildenafil, tadalafil, vardenafil); may cause severe hypotension, death

---

⚠ HIGH ALERT

nitroprusside (Rx)
(nye-troe-pruss′ide)
Nitropress
Func. class.: Antihypertensive, vasodilator

ACTION: Directly relaxes arteriolar, venous smooth muscle, thereby resulting in reduction in cardiac preload and afterload

USES: Hypertensive crisis/urgency/induction; to decrease bleeding by creating hypotension during surgery; acute HF
Unlabeled uses: Postoperative hypertension, mitral regurgitation

CONTRAINDICATIONS: Hypersensitivity, hypertension (compensatory) due to aortic coarctation or AV shunting, acute HF associated with reduced peripheral vascular resistance, toxic amblyopia, hypothyroidism
Precautions: Anemia, increased intracranial pressure, pregnancy, breastfeeding, children, geriatric patients, hypovolemia, electrolyte imbalances, renal/hepatic disease, hypothyroidism

Black Box Warning: Hypotension, cyanide toxicity

DOSAGE AND ROUTES
• **Adult/child: IV INFUSION** 0.25-10 mcg/kg/min; max 10 mcg/kg/min × 10 min
Renal dose
• **Adult: IV INFUSION** CCr <60 mL/min, maintain doses <3 mcg/kg/min to reduce thiocyanate accumulation
Available forms: Inj 50 mg/2 mL
Administer:
• Antidote is sodium thiosulfate
Continuous IV INFUSION route
• Depending on B/P reading q15min
• Reconstitute 50 mg/2-3 mL of D₅W, further dilute in 250, 500, or 1000 mL of D₅W to 200, 100, 50 mcg/mL, respectively; use infusion pump only; wrap bottle with aluminum foil to protect from light; observe for color change in infusion; discard if highly discolored (blue, green, dark red); titrate to patient response, protect from light
• Do not exceed max dose as cyanide may accumulate

Y-site compatibilities: Alfentanil, alprostadil, amikacin, aminocaproic acid, aminophylline, amphotericin B lipid compex, amphotericin B liposome, anidulafungin, argatroban, atenolol, atropine, aztreonam, benztropine, bivalirudin, bleomycin, bumetanide, buprenorphine, butorphanol, calcium chloride/gluconate, CARBOplatin, cefamandole, ceFAZolin, cefmetazole, cefonicid, cefoperazone, cefotaxime, cefoTEtan, cefOXitin, cefTAZidime, ceftizoxime, cefTRIAXone, cefuroxime, cephalothin, chloramphenicol, cimetidine, CISplatin, clindamycin, cyanocobalamin, cyclophosphamide, cycloSPORINE, cytarabine, DACTINomycin, DAPTOmycin, dexamethasone, digoxin, diltiazem, DOCEtaxel, DOPamine, doxacurium, DOXOrubicin, doxycycline, enalaprilat, ePHEDrine, EPINEPHrine, epirubicin, epoetin alfa, eptifibatide, ertapenem, esmolol, etoposide, famotidine, fenoldopam, fentaNYL, fluconazole, fludarabine, fluorouracil, folic acid, furosemide, ganciclovir, gatifloxacin, gemcitabine, gemtuzumab,

N

---

gentamicin, glycopyrrolate, granisetron, heparin, hydrocortisone, HYDROmorphone, IDArubicin, ifosfamide, inamrinone, indomethacin, insulin (regular), isoproterenol, ketorolac, labetalol, lidocaine, linezolid, LORazepam, magnesium sulfate, mannitol, mechlorethamine, meperidine, metaraminol, methicillin, methoxamine, methyldopate, methylPREDNISolone, metoclopramide, metoprolol, metroNIDAZOLE, mezlocillin, micafungin, miconazole, midazolam, milrinone, minocycline, morphine, moxalactam, multiple vitamins injection, nafcillin, nalbuphine, naloxone, nesiritide, netilmicin, niCARDipine, nitroglycerin, norepinephrine, octreotide, ondansetron, oxacillin, oxaliplatin, oxytocin, PACLitaxel, palonosetron, pamidronate, pancuronium, pantoprazole, penicillin G potassium/sodium, pentamidine, PENTobarbital, PHENobarbital, phentolamine, phenylephrine, phytonadione, piperacillin, piperacillin-tazobactam, polymyxin B, potassium chloride/phosphates, procainamide, propofol, propranolol, protamine, pyridoxine, ranitidine, ritodrine, rocuronium, sodium acetate/bicarbonate, succinylcholine, SUFentanil, tacrolimus, teniposide, theophylline, thiamine, ticarcillin, ticarcillin-clavulanate, tigecycline, tirofiban, tobramycin, tolazoline, trimetaphan, urokinase, vancomycin, vasopressin, vecuronium, verapamil, vinCRIStine, zoledronic acid

SIDE EFFECTS

CNS: *Dizziness, headache,* agitation, twitching, decreased reflexes, *restlessness*
CV: *Bradycardia,* ECG changes, tachycardia, *hypotension*
GI: Nausea, vomiting, abdominal pain
INTEG: Pain, irritation at inj site, sweating
MISC: Cyanide, thiocyanate toxicity, flushing, hypothyroidism

PHARMACOKINETICS

IV: Onset 1-2 min, duration 1-10 min, half-life 2 min; metabolized in liver, excreted in urine

INTERACTIONS

Increase: severe hypotension—ganglionic blockers, volatile liquid anesthetics, halothane, enflurane, circulatory depressants
Drug/Herb
Increase: antihypertensive effect—hawthorn

NURSING CONSIDERATIONS
Assess:
• Electrolytes: potassium, sodium, chloride, CO_2, CBC, serum glucose, serum methemoglobin if pulmonary O_2 levels are decreased; use IV 1-2 mg/kg methylene blue given over several min for methemoglobinemia, ABGs
• Renal studies: catecholamines, BUN, creatinine
• Hepatic studies: AST, ALT, alk phos

Black Box Warning: Hypotension: B/P by direct means if possible; check ECG continuously; pulse, jugular venous distention; PCWP; rebound hypertension may occur after nitroprusside is discontinued, give only with emergency equipment nearby, rapid decrease in B/P may occur; check weight, I&O daily

Black Box Warning: Thiocyanate, lactate, cyanide toxicity: obtain levels daily if infusion >3 mcg/kg/min; thiocyanate toxicity occurs at plasma levels of 50-100 mcg/mL; thiocyanate toxicity includes confusion, weakness, seizures, hyperreflexia, psychosis, tinnitus, coma

• Nausea, vomiting, diarrhea
• Edema in feet, legs daily; skin turgor, dryness of mucous membranes for hydration status
• Crackles, dyspnea, orthopnea q30min
• For decrease in bicarbonate, $PaCO_2$, blood pH, acidosis
• **Pregnancy/breastfeeding:** prolonged use may result in death of the fetus (cyanide toxicity); do not breastfeed
Evaluate:
• Therapeutic response: decreased B/P, decreasing symptoms of cardiogenic shock or cardiac pump failure

Teach patient/family:
• To report headache, dizziness, loss of hearing, blurred vision, dyspnea, faintness, pain at IV site
• About the reason for giving product and expected results

RARELY USED

nivolumab
(nye-vol´ ue-mab)
Opdivo ✤
Func. class.: Antineoplastic, monoclonal antibody

USES: Treatment of BRAF V600 mutation-positive unresectable/metastatic melanoma, Hodgkin's disease, non–small-cell lung cancer (NSCLC), renal cell cancer

CONTRAINDICATIONS: Hypersensitivity

DOSAGE AND ROUTES
• **Adult:** IV INFUSION 240 mg over 30 min q2wk OR 480 mg over 30 min q4wk, until disease progression or unacceptable toxicity
Available forms: Injection 10 mg/mL

---

nizatidine (OTC, Rx)
(ni-za´ti-deen)
Axid, Axid AR
Func. class.: H$_2$-receptor antagonist
Chem. class.: Substituted thiazole

USES: Benign gastric and duodenal ulceration, prevention of duodenal ulcer recurrence, symptomatic relief of gastroesophageal reflux, heartburn prevention

CONTRAINDICATIONS: Hypersensitivity

DOSAGE AND ROUTES
Gastric and duodenal ulcer
• **Adult:** PO 300 mg at night or 150 mg bid for 4-8 wk; maintenance 150 mg at night
Prophylaxis of duodenal ulcer
• **Adult:** PO 150 mg/day at bedtime

Gastroesophageal reflux
• **Adult and child ≥12 yr:** PO 150 mg bid × ≤12 wk, max 300 mg/day
Heartburn prevention
• **Adult:** PO 75 mg before eating bid
Renal dose
• **Adult:** PO CCr 20-50 mL/min, give 150 mg every other day; CCr <20 mL/min, give 150 mg q72hr

---

⚠ HIGH ALERT

norepinephrine (Rx)
(nor-ep-i-nef´rin)
Levophed
Func. class.: Adrenergic
Chem. class.: Catecholamine

Do not confuse:
norepinephrine/EPINEPHrine

ACTION: Causes increased contractility and heart rate by acting on β-receptors in heart; also acts on α-receptors, thereby causing vasoconstriction in blood vessels; B/P is elevated, coronary blood flow improves, and cardiac output increases

USES: Acute hypotension, shock

CONTRAINDICATIONS: Hypersensitivity to this product or cyclopropane/halothane anesthesia, hypovolemia, mesenteric thrombosis
Precautions: Pregnancy, breastfeeding, geriatric patients, arterial embolism, peripheral vascular disease, hypertension, hyperthyroidism, cardiac disease, ventricular fibrillation, tachydysrhythmias, pheochromocytoma, hypotension, sulfite hypersensitivity

Black Box Warning: Extravasation

DOSAGE AND ROUTES
• **Adult:** IV INFUSION 0.5-1 mcg/min titrated to B/P; maintenance 2-4 mcg/min; max 30 mcg/min
• **Child:** IV INFUSION 0.1 mcg/kg/min titrated to B/P; max 2 mcg/kg/min

---

Side effects: *italics* = common; red = life-threatening

Available forms: Inj 1 mg/mL
Administer:
Plasma expanders for hypovolemia; correct volume depletion before starting treatment

Continuous IV INFUSION route
• Dilute with 500-1000 mL D$_5$W or D$_5$/0.9% NaCl; average dilution 4 mg/1000 mL diluent (4 mcg base/mL); give as infusion 2-3 mL/min; titrate to response; discontinue gradually
• Store reconstituted sol in refrigerator ≤24 hr, protect from light, store unopened product at room temperature, do not use discolored sol

Y-site compatibilities: Alemtuzumab, alfentanil, amikacin, amiodarone, anidulafungin, argatroban, ascorbic acid, atenolol, atracurium, atropine, aztreonam, benztropine, bivalirudin, bleomycin, bumetanide, buprenorphine, butorphanol, calcium chloride/gluconate, CARBOplatin, caspofungin, cefamandole, ceFAZolin, cefmetazole, cefonicid, cefoperazone, cefotaxime, cefoTEtan, cefOXitin, cefTAZidime, ceftizoxime, ceftobiprole, cefTRIAXone, cefuroxime, cephalothin, chloramphenicol, chlorproMAZINE, cimetidine, cisatracurium, CISplatin, clindamycin, cloNIDine, cyanocobalamin, cyclophosphamide, cycloSPORINE, cytarabine, DAPTOmycin, dexamethasone, digoxin, diltiazem, diphenhydrAMINE, DOBUTamine, DOCEtaxel, DOPamine, doripenem, doxycycline, enalaprilat, ePHEDrine, EPINEPHrine, epirubicin, epoetin alfa, ertapenem, erythromycin, esmolol, etoposide, famotidine, fenoldopam, fentaNYL, fluconazole, fludarabine, gatifloxacin, gemcitabine, gentamicin, glycopyrrolate, granisetron, heparin, hydrocortisone, HYDROmorphone, hydrOXYzine, IDArubicin, ifosfamide, imipenem-cilastatin, irinotecan, isoproterenol, ketorolac, labetalol, lidocaine, linezolid, LORazepam, magnesium sulfate, mannitol, mechlorethamine, meperidine, meropenem, metaraminol, methicillin, methotrexate, methoxamine, methyldopate, methylPREDNISolone, metoclopramide, metoprolol, metroNIDAZOLE, mezlocillin, micafungin, miconazole, midazolam, milrinone, minocycline, mitoXANtrone, morphine, moxalactam, multiple vitamins injection, mycophenolate, nafcillin, nalbuphine, naloxone, netilmicin, niCARdipine, nitroglycerin, nitroprusside, octreotide, ondansetron, oxacillin, oxaliplatin, oxytocin, PACLitaxel, palonosetron, pamidronate, pancuronium, papaverine, PEMEtrexed, penicillin G potassium/sodium, pentamidine, pentazocine, phenylephrine, phytonadione, piperacillin, piperacillin-tazobactam, polymyxin B, potassium chloride, procainamide, prochlorperazine, promethazine, propofol, propranolol, protamine, pyridoxine, quiNIDine, ranitidine, remifentanil, ritodrine, succinylcholine, SUFentanil, tacrolimus, teniposide, theophylline, thiamine, thiotepa, ticarcillin, ticarcillin-clavulanate, tigecycline, tirofiban, tobramycin, tolazoline, trimetaphan, urokinase, vancomycin, vasopressin, vecuronium, verapamil, vinCRIStine, vinorelbine, vitamin B complex with C, voriconazole, zoledronic acid

SIDE EFFECTS
CNS: *Headache,* anxiety, dizziness, insomnia, restlessness, tremor, cerebral hemorrhage
CV: *Palpitations, tachycardia, hypertension, ectopic beats, angina*
GI: *Nausea, vomiting*
GU: Decreased urine output
INTEG: Necrosis, tissue sloughing with extravasation, gangrene
RESP: Dyspnea
SYST: Anaphylaxis

PHARMACOKINETICS
IV: Onset 1-2 min; metabolized in liver; excreted in urine (inactive metabolites); crosses placenta

INTERACTIONS
• Do not use within 2 wk of MAOIs, antihistamines, ergots, methyldopa, oxytocics, tricyclics because hypertensive crisis may result
Increase: B/P—oxytocics
Increase: pressor effect—tricyclics, MAOIs

Decrease: norepinephrine action—α-blockers

NURSING CONSIDERATIONS
Assess:
• I&O ratio; notify prescriber if output <30 mL/hr
• B/P, pulse q2-3min after parenteral route, ECG during administration continuously; if B/P increases, product is decreased, CVP or PWP during infusion if possible
• Paresthesias and coldness of extremities; peripheral blood flow may decrease

Black Box Warning: **Extravasation:** inj site: tissue sloughing; change injection sites if blanching or vasoconstriction occurs

• Sulfite sensitivity, which may be life-threatening
• **Pregnancy/breastfeeding:** use only if clearly needed; cautious use in breastfeeding
Evaluate:
• Therapeutic response: increased B/P with stabilization, adequate tissue perfusion
Teach patient/family:
• About the reason for product administration; to report dyspnea, dizziness, chest pain

TREATMENT OF OVERDOSE:
Administer fluids, electrolyte replacement

---

norethindrone (Rx)
(nor-eth-in′drone)
Aygestin, Camila, Errin ♣, Jencycla, Jolivette, Micronor, Nor-QD
Func. class.: Progestogen

ACTION: Inhibits the secretion of pituitary gonadotropins, which prevents follicular maturation and ovulation; stimulates growth of mammary tissue; antineoplastic action against endometrial cancer

USES: Uterine bleeding (abnormal), amenorrhea, endometriosis, contraception

CONTRAINDICATIONS: Pregnancy, breast cancer, hypersensitivity, thromboembolic disorders, reproductive cancer, genital bleeding (abnormal, undiagnosed), liver tumors, hepatic disease
Precautions: Breastfeeding, hypertension, asthma, blood dyscrasias, HF, diabetes mellitus, depression, migraine headache, seizure disorders, bone/gallbladder/renal/hepatic disease, family history of breast or reproductive tract cancer, smoking, HIV

DOSAGE AND ROUTES
Amenorrhea, abnormal uterine bleeding (Aygestin)
• **Adult: PO** 2.5-10 mg/day on days 5-25 of menstrual cycle
Endometriosis (Aygestin)
• **Adult: PO** 5 mg/day × 2 wk, then increased by 2.5 mg/day × 2 wk up to 15 mg/day, may continue for 6-9 mo
Contraception
• **Adult: PO** 0.35 mg on 1st day of menses, then 0.35 mg/day
Available forms: Tabs (Aygestin) 5 mg; tabs 0.35 mg
Administer:
• Titrated dose; use lowest effective dose
• One dose in AM; do not interrupt between pill packs; give at roughly same time of day
• Without regard to meals
• Store in dark area

SIDE EFFECTS
CNS: *Dizziness, headache,* migraines, depression, fatigue
CV: Hypotension, thrombophlebitis, edema, thromboembolism, CVA, stroke, PE, MI
EENT: Diplopia
GI: *Nausea,* vomiting, anorexia, cramps, increased weight, cholestatic jaundice
GU: Amenorrhea, cervical erosion, breakthrough bleeding, dysmenorrhea, vaginal candidiasis, breast changes, (gynecomastia, testicular atrophy, impotence), endometriosis, spontaneous abortion, *breast tenderness*

Side effects: *italics* = common; red = life-threatening

INTEG: Rash, urticaria, acne, hirsutism, alopecia, oily skin, seborrhea, purpura, melasma
META: Hyperglycemia

PHARMACOKINETICS
Excreted in urine, feces; metabolized in liver, half-life 5-14 hr

INTERACTIONS
Decrease: progestin effect—barbiturates, carBAMazepine, fosphenytoin, phenytoin, rifampin
Drug/Herb
Decrease: contraception—St. John's wort
Drug/Food
Increase: caffeine level—caffeine
Drug/Lab Test
Increase: LDL
Decrease: GTT, HDL, alk phos

NURSING CONSIDERATIONS
Assess:
• Weight daily: notify prescriber of weekly weight gain >5 lb
• B/P at beginning of treatment and periodically
• I&O ratio; be alert for decreasing urinary output, increasing edema
• Hepatic studies: ALT, AST, bilirubin periodically during long-term therapy
• Edema, hypertension, cardiac symptoms, jaundice, thromboembolism
• Mental status: affect, mood, behavioral changes, depression
• Hypercalcemia
• Pap smear
Evaluate:
• Therapeutic response: decreased abnormal uterine bleeding, absence of amenorrhea
Teach patient/family:
• About cushingoid symptoms (fatigue, weakness, increased thirst/urination, anxiety, weight gain, facial puffiness)
• To report vaginal bleeding, amenorrhea, edema, jaundice, dark urine, clay-colored stools, dyspnea, headache, blurred vision, abdominal pain, numbness or stiffness in legs, chest pain; impotence or gynecomastia (men)
• To take at same time of day; not to interrupt between pill packs

• **Pregnancy:** to report suspected pregnancy immediately; to wait ≥3 mo after stopping product to become pregnant; to use backup contraception methods for 48 hr if treatment is not begun on the first day of menstruation
• To avoid smoking; CV reactions may occur
• That product does not protect against HIV, STDs
• That product may mask onset of menopause

---

nortriptyline (Rx)
(nor-trip′ti-leen)
Arentyl ✦, Norrentyl ✦, Pamelor
Func. class.: Antidepressant, tricyclic
Chem. class.: Dibenzocycloheptene—secondary amine

Do not confuse:
nortriptyline/amitriptyline
Pamelor/Panlor DC/Tambocol

ACTION: Blocks reuptake of norepinephrine and serotonin into nerve endings, thereby increasing action of norepinephrine and serotonin in nerve cells

USES: Major depression
Unlabeled uses: Chronic pain management, PMDD, social phobia, panic disorder, enuresis, migraine prophylaxis

CONTRAINDICATIONS: Hypersensitivity to tricyclics, carBAMazepine; recovery phase of MI
Precautions: Breastfeeding, suicidal patients, severe depression, increased intraocular pressure, closed-angle glaucoma, urinary retention, cardiac/hepatic disease, hyperthyroidism, electroshock therapy, elective surgery, pregnancy, seizure disorders, prostatic hypertrophy

Black Box Warning: Children, suicidal ideation

DOSAGE AND ROUTES
• **Adult:** PO 25 mg tid or qid; may increase to 150 mg/day; may give daily dose at bedtime

- **Adolescent: PO** 1-3 mg/kg/day in 3-4 divided doses or daily at bedtime, max 150 mg/day
- **Child 6-12 yr (unlabeled): PO** 1-3 mg/kg/day in 3-4 divided doses, max 150 mg/day
- **Geriatric: PO** 10-25 mg at bedtime, increase by 10-25 mg at weekly intervals to desired dose; usual maintenance 75 mg/day, max 150 mg/day

Available forms: Caps 10, 25, 50, 75 mg; sol 10 mg/5 mL

Administer:
- Store in tight, light-resistant container at room temperature
- Increased fluids, bulk in diet if constipation occurs
- Without regard to meals
- Dosage at bedtime to avoid oversedation during day; may take entire dose at bedtime; geriatric patients may not tolerate once-daily dosing
- Gum, hard candy, frequent sips of water for dry mouth
- **Oral solution:** with fruit juice, water, or milk to disguise taste

SIDE EFFECTS

CNS: *Dizziness, drowsiness,* confusion, headache, anxiety, tremors, stimulation, weakness, insomnia, nightmares, EPS (geriatric patients), increased psychiatric symptoms, seizures

CV: *Orthostatic hypotension,* ECG changes, *tachycardia,* hypertension, palpitations, dysrhythmias

EENT: *Blurred vision,* tinnitus, mydriasis, dry eyes

ENDO: SIADH, hyponatremia, hypothyroidism

GI: *Constipation, dry mouth,* nausea, vomiting, paralytic ileus, increased appetite, cramps, epigastric distress, jaundice, hepatitis, stomatitis, weight gain

GU: *Urinary retention,* acute renal failure, sexual dysfunction

HEMA: Agranulocytosis, thrombocytopenia, eosinophilia, leukopenia

INTEG: Rash, urticaria, sweating, pruritus, photosensitivity

SYST: Serotonin syndrome

PHARMACOKINETICS

PO: Steady-state 4-19 days; metabolized by liver; excreted by kidneys; crosses placenta; excreted in breast milk; half-life 18-28 hr, protein binding 93%-95%

INTERACTIONS

Increase: QT prolongation—class IA/III antidysrhythmics, some phenothiazines, β agonists, local anesthetics, tricyclics, haloperidol, chloroquine, droperidol, pentamidine; CYP3A4 inhibitors (amiodarone, clarithromycin, erythromycin, telithromycin, troleandomycin), arsenic trioxide, levomethadyl; CYP3A4 substrates (methadone, pimozide, QUEtiapine, quiNIDine, risperiDONE, ziprasidone)

- **Heavy smoking:** decreased product effect
- **Hyperpyretic crisis, seizures, hypertensive episode:** MAOI

Increase: effects of direct-acting sympathomimetics (EPINEPHrine), alcohol, barbiturates, benzodiazepines, CNS depressants, products increasing QT interval, other anticholinergics

Increase: serotonin syndrome, neuroleptic malignant syndrome—SSRIs, SNRIs, serotonin receptor agonists, linezolid; methylene blue (IV)

Decrease: effects of guanethidine, cloNIDine, indirect-acting sympathomimetics (ePHEDrine)

Drug/Herb
Increase: CNS effect—kava, valerian
Decrease: nortriptyline level—St. John's wort

Drug/Lab Test
Increase: serum bilirubin, blood glucose, alk phos
Decrease: VMA, 5-HIAA
False increase: urinary catecholamines

NURSING CONSIDERATIONS
Assess:

> **Black Box Warning: Suicidal thoughts/ behaviors in children/young adults:** not approved for children; monitor for suicidal ideation in depression, adolescents, young adults

N

Side effects: *italics* = common; red = life-threatening

• Monitor for glaucoma exacerbation and paralytic ileus

• B/P (lying, standing), pulse q4hr; if systolic B/P drops 20 mm Hg, hold product, notify prescriber; VS q4hr in patients with CV disease

• Blood studies: thyroid function tests, LFTs, serum nortriptyline level/target 50-150 mg/mL if patient is receiving long-term therapy

• Weight weekly; appetite may increase with product

• **PR, QT prolongation:** ECG for flattening of T wave, bundle branch block, AV block, QT prolongation, dysrhythmias in cardiac patients; assess for chest pain, palpitations, dyspnea

• EPS primarily in geriatric patients: rigidity, dystonia, akathisia, preferred tricyclic in geriatric patients

• Mental status changes: mood, sensorium, affect, suicidal tendencies, increase in psychiatric symptoms, depression, panic

• Urinary retention, constipation; constipation is more likely to occur in children

• **Withdrawal symptoms:** headache, nausea, vomiting, muscle pain, weakness; do not usually occur unless product was discontinued abruptly

• Alcohol intake; if alcohol is consumed, hold dose until AM

• **Serotonin syndrome, neuroleptic malignant syndrome:** assess for increased heart rate, shivering, sweating, dilated pupils, tremors, high B/P, hyperthermia, headache, confusion; if these occur, stop product, administer serotonin antagonist if needed (rare)

• Assistance with ambulation during beginning therapy because drowsiness/dizziness occurs; safety measures including side rails, primarily for geriatric patients

• **Beers:** avoid in older adults; highly anticholinergic, sedating, and may cause orthostatic hypotension

• **Pregnancy/breastfeeding:** use only if benefits outweigh fetal risk; cautious use in breastfeeding

Evaluate:

• Therapeutic response: decreased depression

Teach patient/family:

• That therapeutic effects may take 2-3 wk; only small quantities may be dispersed

• To use caution when driving, during other activities requiring alertness because of drowsiness, dizziness, blurred vision

• To avoid alcohol ingestion, other CNS depressants; to avoid MAOIs within 14 days

• Not to discontinue medication quickly after long-term use; may cause nausea, headache, malaise

• To wear sunscreen or large hat because photosensitivity occurs

• To immediately report urinary retention, worsening depression, suicidal thoughts/behaviors

TREATMENT OF OVERDOSE:
ECG monitoring; lavage; administer anticonvulsant

---

nusinersen (Rx)

(neu-si-ner'sen)

Spinraza

Func. class.: Miscellaneous CNS agent muscular dystrophy

Chem. class.: Antisense oligonucleotide

Do not confuse:
Nusinersen/Neurontin, Nucynta, Sprinraza/Spriva

ACTION: Increases exon 7 inclusion in SMN2 messenger ribonucleic acid (mRNA) transcripts and production of full-length SMN protein

Therapeutic outcome: Increasing muscle strength and movement

USES: Spinal muscular atrophy

CONTRAINDICATIONS: Hypersensitivity **PRECAUTIONS:** Pregnancy, breastfeeding, bleeding, nephrotoxicity, requires a specialized care setting and clinician, thrombocytopenia

DOSAGE AND ROUTES
Adult/child: Intrathecal 12 mg q14days 3 doses, then 12 mg q30days after third dose; maintenance 12 mg q4mo thereafter

Available forms: Injection 12 mg/5 mL single-use vials

Implementation

Intrathecal Route

Preparation
• Allow the vial to warm to room temperature (25° C or 77° F) prior to use; do not use external heat sources to warm
• Do not administer if visible particulates are observed or if the liquid in the vial is discolored; product should be clear and colorless; a filter is not required
• Use aseptic technique; each vial is for single use only
• Withdraw 12 mg (5 mL) from the vial into a syringe; discard unused contents
• Give within 4 hr of removal from the vial

Intrathecal administration
• Administered by, or under the direction of, healthcare professionals experienced in performing lumbar punctures
• Consider sedation as indicated by the clinical condition of the patient
• Consider ultrasound or other imaging techniques to guide intrathecal administration, particularly in younger patients
• Prior to use, remove 5 mL of cerebrospinal fluid (CSF)
• Give as an intrathecal bolus injection over 1 to 3 min using a spinal anesthesia needle. Do not administer in areas of the skin where there are signs of infection or inflammation

ADVERSE EFFECTS
CNS: *Headache, fever*
GI: *Constipation*, feeding difficulties, *vomiting*
GU: Renal toxicity
Hema: *Thrombocytopenia*, coagulation changes
Resp: URI, aspiration, atelectasis
EENT: Ear infection, teething, dysphagia
MS: Back pain, scoliosis, post-lumbar puncture syndrome
Misc: *Infection*, growth inhibition

PHARMACOKINETICS
Absorption Unknown **Distribution** Unknown **Metabolism** Unknown **Excretion** Unknown **Half-life** 133-177 days CSF, 63-87 days plasma **Onset** Unknown **Peak** 1.7-6 hr **Duration** Unknown

INTERACTIONS
Drug classifications: None known
Drug/lab test
Increase: PT, PTT Decrease: Platelets

NURSING CONSIDERATIONS
Assessment
• **Coagulation studies:** Obtain platelets and PT, aPTT baseline and before each dose; monitor for bleeding
• **Nephrotoxicity:** Quantitative spot urine protein testing is required at baseline and prior to each dose; for a urinary protein concentration more than 0.2 grams/L, consider repeat testing and further evaluation; monitor for changes in urinary patterns, blood in urine
Patient/family education
• Reason for medication and expected results
• **Pregnancy/breastfeeding:** to notify healthcare professional if pregnancy is planned or suspected or if breastfeeding
• That continuing blood and lab tests will be required
• To report bleeding or bruising
• **Renal toxicity:** change in urinary patterns, blood in urine
Evaluation
• Increasing muscle strength and movement

N

---

nystatin (Rx)
(nye-stat′in)
Mycostatin, Nadostine ✦, Nilstat
Func. class.: Antifungal
Chem. class.: Amphoteric polyene

ACTION: Interferes with fungal DNA replication; binds sterols in fungal cell membrane, which increases permeability, leaking of cell nutrients

Side effects: *italics* = common; red = life-threatening

USES: *Candida* species causing oral, intestinal infections

CONTRAINDICATIONS: Hypersensitivity
Precautions: Pregnancy

DOSAGE AND ROUTES
Oral infection
• **Adult/adolescent/child:** SUSP 400,000-600,000 units qid; use $1/2$ dose in each side of mouth; swish and swallow; use for at least 48 hr after symptoms resolved
• **Infant:** SUSP 200,000 units qid (100,000 units in each side of mouth)
• **Newborn and premature infant:** SUSP 100,000 units qid
• **Adult/child:** TROCHES 200,000-400,000 units qid × ≤2 wk
GI infection
• **Adult:** PO 500,000-1,000,000 units tid
Cutaneous candidiasis
• **Adult/child:** Top cream/ointment apply to affected area bid; **powder** apply to affected area bid-tid
Available forms: Tabs 500,000 units; oral caps 500,000, 1,000,000 units, bulk powder; suspension 100,000 mg/mL
Administer:
Store at room temperature for oral susp; tabs in tight, light-resistant containers at room temperature
PO route
• Oral susp dose by placing $1/2$ in each cheek, then swallow; do not mix with food
• Topical dose after cleansing area; mouth may be swabbed; very moist lesions best treated with topical powder

SIDE EFFECTS
GI: Nausea, vomiting, anorexia, diarrhea, cramps
INTEG: Rash, urticaria (rare)

PHARMACOKINETICS
PO: Little absorption, excreted in feces

NURSING CONSIDERATIONS
Assess:
• **Allergic reaction:** rash, urticaria, irritated oral mucous membranes; product may have to be discontinued
• Obtain culture, histologic tests to confirm organism
• Predisposing factors: antibiotic therapy, pregnancy, diabetes mellitus, sexual partner infection (vaginal infections)
• **Pregnancy/breastfeeding:** use only if clearly needed; may breastfeed
Evaluate:
• Therapeutic response: culture negative for *Candida*
Teach patient/family:
• That long-term therapy may be needed to clear infection; to complete entire course of medication
• To avoid commercial mouthwashes for mouth infection
• To shake susp before measuring each dose
• To notify prescriber of irritation; product may have to be discontinued

---

nystatin topical
See Appendix B

RARELY USED

obiltoxaximab ♣
(oh-bil-tox-ax′ i-mab)
Func. class.: Monoclonal antibody

USES: Treatment of inhalational anthrax and for inhalational anthrax prophylaxis when alternative therapies are not available or appropriate

CONTRAINDICATIONS: Hypersensitivity reactions or anaphylaxis

DOSAGE AND ROUTES
• **Adult weighing >40 kg: IV** 16 mg/kg as a single dose in combination with appropriate antibacterial agents
• **Adult weighing ≤40 kg: IV** 24 mg/kg as a single dose in combination with appropriate antibacterial agents
• **Adolescent/child weighing >40 kg: IV** 16 mg/kg as a single dose in combination with appropriate antibacterial agents
• **Adolescent/child/infant weighing >15-40 kg: IV** 24 mg/kg as a single dose in combination with appropriate antibacterial agents
• **Child/infant/neonate weighing ≤15 kg: IV** 32 mg/kg IV as a single dose in combination with appropriate antibacterial agents

⚠ HIGH ALERT

obinutuzumab
(oh′bi-nue-tooz′ue-mab)
Gazyva
Func. class.: Antineoplastic; biologic response modifier; monoclonal antibody

ACTION: A recombinant, human monoclonal antibody that binds to the gastric B-lymphocyte–associated antibody; action is indirect, possible through T-cell–mediated anti-tumor responses

USES: Chronic lymphocytic leukemia, previously untreated in combination; non-Hodgkin's lymphoma (follicular lymphoma) in relapse or refractory to rituximab-containing regimen, used in combination

CONTRAINDICATIONS: Hypersensitivity
Precautions: Pregnancy, breastfeeding, cardiac disease, children, human antichimeric antibody (HACA), human antimurine antibody (HAMA), infection, infusion-related reactions, neutropenia, pulmonary disease, thrombocytopenia, tumor lysis syndrome, vaccination

Black Box Warning: Hepatitis B exacerbation, progressive multifocal leukoencephalopathy

DOSAGE AND ROUTES
• **Adult: IV cycle 1** 100 mg over 4 hr (day 1); then 900 mg (50 mg/hr, increased by 50 mg/hr q30min, to max 400 mg/hr) (day 2); then 1000 mg (100 mg/hr, increased by 100 mg/hr q30min to max 400 mg/hr (day 8, day 15); **cycle 2-6** 1000 mg (100 mg/hr increased by 100 mg/hr q30min to max 400 mg/hr (day 1 repeat q28days)
Available forms: Sol for inj 1000 mg/40 mL
Administer:
IV intermittent INFUSION route
• Due to the risk of hypotension, consider withholding antihypertensive medications for 12 hr before, during, and for the 1st hr after use until blood pressure is stable
• Single-use vials do not contain preservatives
• Do not mix with other products
• Give antimicrobial prophylaxis to neutropenic patients throughout treatment; consider antiviral and antifungal prophylaxis as needed
• **Premedication for cycle 1, days 1 and 2:** acetaminophen 650-1000 mg, and diphenhydrAMINE 50 mg at least 30 min before infusion, dexametha-

Side effects: *italics* = common; red = life-threatening

sone 20 mg IV or methylPREDNISolone 80 mg IV at least 1 hr before infusion

• **Premedication for cycle 1, days 8 and 15, and cycles 2-6, day 1:** acetaminophen 650-1000 mg at least 30 min before infusion; those with any infusion-related reaction with the previous infusion should also receive diphenhydrAMINE 50 mg at least 30 min before the infusion; if the patient had a grade 3 infusion-related reaction with the previous dose or has a lymphocyte count >25 × 10⁹/L, additionally administer dexamethasone 20 mg IV or methylPREDNISolone 80 mg IV at least 1 hr before infusion

• Use in a facility to adequately monitor and treat infusion reactions

• Visually inspect parenteral products for particulate matter and discoloration before use

• Prepare all doses in 0.9% NaCl; do not admix; use a final concentration of 0.4-4 mg/mL; give as an IV infusion only

Reconstitution: Cycle 1, days 1 and 2:
• Withdraw 4 mL (100 mg) from the vial and dilute into 100 mL 0.9% NaCl for use on day 1; mix by gentle inversion; do not shake, use immediately

• Withdraw the remaining 36 mL (900 mg) and dilute into 250 mL 0.9% NaCl for use on day 2; mix by gentle inversion; do not shake

Cycle 1, days 8 and 15; cycles 2-6:
• Withdraw 40 mL (1000 mg) from the vial and dilute into 250 mL 0.9% NaCl; mix by gentle inversion; do not shake

• Store following reconstitution: store at 2° C-8° C (36° F-46° F) for up to 24 hr; do not freeze; allow to come to room temperature before administration; use a dedicated line, protect from light

• **Day 1 (100-mg dose):** give at initial rate of 25 mg/hr over 4 hr; do not increase the infusion rate

• **Day 2 (900-mg dose):** give at 50 mg/hr × 30 min; if no hypersensitivity or infusion-related events occur, increase the rate by 50 mg/hr q30min to a max rate of 400 mg/hr

• **Subsequent infusions (1000-mg dose):** give at rate of 100 mg/hr for 30 min; if no hypersensitivity or infusion-related events occur, increase the infusion rate by 100 mg/hr q30min, max rate of 400 mg/hr

SIDE EFFECTS
CNS: Headache, *fever*, chills, flushing
CV: Cardiac arrest, MI, sinus tachycardia, hypertension
GI: *Constipation*, decreased appetite, diarrhea, hepatitis/hepatic failure, nausea, vomiting
HEMA: Neutropenia, thrombocytopenia, lymphopenia, leukopenia, *anemia*
META: Lower potassium/*sodium*/calcium, aluminum, higher *potassium*/uric acid
RESP: Wheezing, dyspnea, *cough*
SYST: Tumor lysis syndrome, *infection*
MISC: *Arthralgia*

PHARMACOKINETICS
Terminal half-life 29 days

INTERACTIONS
Increase: adverse reactions—abciximab, belimumab, cloZAPine, pimecrolimus; avoid concurrent use
Increase: infection—denosumab, natalizumab, live virus vaccines
Increase: hypotension—antihypertensives
Increase: thrombocytopenia—chlorambucil
Increase: hematologic toxicity—leflunomide
Increase: immunosuppression—tofacitinib; avoid concurrent use

Drug/Herb
Decrease: obinutuzumab—echinacea
Drug/Lab
Increase: LFTs

NURSING CONSIDERATIONS
Assess:

Black Box Warning: **Hepatitis B**: reactivation of HBV in those who are HBsAg positive, HBsAg negative, and core antibody anti-HBc positive; may result in fulminant hepatitis, hepatic failure, or death, screen high-risk patients before use, monitor carriers for active HBV infection during and for several months after therapy completion, discontinue treatment of any other antineoplastics if infection is reactivated

Black Box Warning: **Progressive multifocal leukoencephalopathy (PML)**: notify prescriber of any new, worsening neurological signs/symptoms (ataxia, visual changes, confusion)

• **Tumor lysis syndrome:** can occur within 24 hr of 1st infusion; those with high tumor burden or lymphocyte count $>25 \times 10^9$/L are at increased risk; monitor serum creatinine, potassium, calcium, uric acid, phosphate closely
• **Severe/life-threatening infusion reactions:** $^2/_3$ have a reaction to 1st dose; consider withholding antihypertensives for 12 hr before, during, and for 1 hour after infusion
• **Bone marrow suppression:** CBC with differential before infusion and regularly, platelets
• **Infection:** signs of infection; provide neutropenia precautions
• **Pregnancy/breastfeeding:** use only if benefits outweigh fetal risk; do not breastfeed, excretion unknown

Evaluate:
• Therapeutic response: decreased disease progression
Teach patient/family:
• About the reason for treatment and expected results
• To avoid live virus vaccines, that vaccinations should be brought up-to-date before treatment

Black Box Warning: **Hepatitis B:** to report yellow skin, eyes, fatigue, dark urine; that continuing follow-up will be needed

Black Box Warning: **Progressive multifocal leukoencephalopathy (PML):** to report confusion, visual changes, dizziness, difficulty walking or talking

---

RARELY USED

ocrelizumab (Rx)
(oc″-re-liz′-ue-mab)
Ocrevus
Func. class.: Multiple sclerosis agent

O

USES: For the treatment of multiple sclerosis

CONTRAINDICATIONS: Hypersensitivity

DOSAGE AND ROUTES
For the treatment of relapsing or primary progressive forms of multiple sclerosis
• **Adult: IV INFUSION** 300 mg as a single dose, followed by a second 300 mg 2 wk later
• Subsequent infusions of 600 mg are given q6mo. The first 600-mg dose is due 6 mo after infusion 1 of the initial dose

---

octreotide (Rx)

(ok-tree′oh-tide)

SandoSTATIN, SandoSTATIN LAR Depot

Func. class.: Growth hormone, antidiarrheal

Chem. class.: Synthetic analog of somatostatin

Do not confuse:
SandoSTATIN/SandIMMUNE

ACTION: A potent growth hormone similar to somatostatin

USES: **SandoSTATIN:** acromegaly, improves symptoms of carcinoid tumors, vasoactive intestinal peptide tumors (VIPomas); **LAR Depot:** long-term maintenance of acromegaly, carcinoid tumors, VIPomas

Unlabeled uses: GI fistula, variceal bleeding, diarrheal conditions, pancreatic fistula, irritable bowel syndrome, dumping syndrome, short bowel syndrome, insulinoma, hepatorenal syndrome

CONTRAINDICATIONS: Hypersensitivity

Precautions: Pregnancy, breastfeeding, children, geriatric patients, diabetes mellitus, hypothyroidism, renal disease

DOSAGE AND ROUTES
Acromegaly
• **Adult: SUBCUT/IV** (SandoSTATIN) 50-100 mcg bid-tid, adjust q2wk based on growth hormone levels or **IM** (SandoSTATIN LAR) 20 mg q4wk × 3 mo, adjust based on growth hormone levels
VIPomas
• **Adult: SUBCUT/IV** (SandoSTATIN) 200-300 mcg/day in 2-4 doses for 2 wk, or **IM** (SandoSTATIN LAR) 20 mg q4wk × 2 mo, adjust dose
Flushing/diarrhea in carcinoid tumors
• **Adult: SUBCUT/IV** (SandoSTATIN) 100-600 mcg/day in 2-4 doses for 2 wk, titrated to patient response or **IM** (SandoSTATIN LAR) 20 mg q4wk × 2 mo, adjust dose

GI fistula
• **Adult: SUBCUT** (SandoSTATIN) 50-200 mcg q8hr
Antidiarrheal in AIDS patients (unlabeled)
• **Adult: SUBCUT** (SandoSTATIN) 50 mcg q8hr prn, increase to 500 mcg q8hr
Irritable bowel syndrome (unlabeled)
• **Adult: SUBCUT** (SandoSTATIN) 100 mcg in single dose, up to 125 mcg bid
Dumping syndrome (unlabeled)
• **Adult: SUBCUT** (SandoSTATIN) 50-150 mcg/day
Variceal bleeding (unlabeled)
• **Adult: IV bolus** 50 mcg;
Continuous IV infusion 50 mcg/hr for 2-5 days

Available forms: Inj (SandoSTATIN) 0.05, 0.1, 0.2, 0.5, 1 mg/mL; inj powder for susp (LAR depot) 10, 20, 30 mg/5 mL

Administer:
• Store in refrigerator for unopened amps, vials or at room temperature for 2 wk; protect from light; do not use discolored or cloudy sol
• Do not use if discolored or if particulates are present
IM route
• Reconstitute with diluent provided; give in gluteal region, immediately after reconstitution rotate injection sites
SUBCUT route
• Rotate inj site; use hip, thigh, abdomen
• Avoid using medication that is cold; allow to reach room temperature; do not use LAR depot, do not use if discolored or if particulates are present
IV route
• **IV direct:** give over 3 min; during an emergency carcinoid crisis, give rapid bolus, may give undiluted
• **Intermittent IV infusion:** dilute in 50-200 mL D$_5$W, 0.9% NaCl; give over 15-30 min
• Solution is stable for 24 hr

Y-site compatibilities: Acyclovir, alfentanil, allopurinol, amifostine, amikacin, aminocaproic acid, aminophylline, amiodarone, amphotericin B colloidal, amphotericin B lipid complex, amphotericin B liposome, ampicillin,

ampicillin-sulbactam, anidulafungin, argatroban, arsenic trioxide, atenolol, atracurium, azithromycin, aztreonam, bivalirudin, bleomycin, bumetanide, buprenorphine, busulfan, butorphanol, calcium chloride/gluconate, capreomycin, CARBOplatin, carmustine, caspofungin, ceFAZolin, cefepime, cefotaxime, cefoTEtan, cefOXitin, cefTAZidime, ceftizoxime, cefTRIAXone, cefuroxime, chloramphenicol, chlorproMAZINE, cimetidine, ciprofloxacin, cisatracurium, CISplatin, clindamycin, cyclophosphamide, cycloSPORINE, cytarabine, dacarbazine, DACTINomycin, DAPTOmycin, DAUNOrubicin, DAUNOrubicin liposome, dexamethasone, digoxin, diltiaZEM, diphenhydrAMINE, DOBUTamine, DOCEtaxel, dolasetron, DOPamine, DOXOrubicin, DOXOrubicin liposomal, doxycycline, droperidol, enalaprilat, ePHEDrine, EPINEPHrine, epiRUBicin, eptifibatide, ertapenem, erythromycin, esmolol, etoposide, famotidine, fenoldopam, fentaNYL, fluconazole, fludarabine, fluorouracil, foscarnet, fosphenytoin, furosemide, gallium nitrate, ganciclovir, gatifloxacin, gemcitabine, gentamicin, glycopyrrolate, granisetron, haloperidol, heparin, hydrALAZINE, hydrocortisone, HYDROmorphone, hydrOXYzine, IDArubicin, ifosfamide, imipenem-cilastatin, insulin (regular), irinotecan, isoproterenol, ketorolac, labetalol, lansoprazole, leucovorin, levoFLOXacin, lidocaine, linezolid, LORazepam, magnesium sulfate, mannitol, mechlorethamine, melphalan, meperidine, meropenem, mesna, methohexital, methotrexate, methyldopate, methylPREDNISolone, metoclopramide, metoprolol, metroNIDAZOLE, midazolam, milrinone, minocycline, mitoMYcin, mitoXANTRONE, mivacurium, morphine, moxifloxacin, mycophenolate, nafcillin, nalbuphine, naloxone, nesiritide, niCARdipine, nitroglycerin, nitroprusside, norepinephrine, ondansetron, oxaliplatin, PACLitaxel, palonosetron, pamidronate, pancuronium, PEMEtrexed, pentamidine, pentazocine, PENTobarbital, PHENobarbital, phenylephrine, piperacillin, piperacillin-tazobactam, polymyxin B, potassium acetate/chloride/phosphates, procainamide, prochlorperazine, promethazine, propranolol, quiNIDine, quinupristin-dalfopristin, raNITIdine, remifentanil, rocuronium, sodium acetate/bicarbonate/phosphates, streptozocin, succinylcholine, SUFentanil, sulfamethoxazole-trimethoprim, tacrolimus, teniposide, thiopental, thiotepa, ticarcillin, ticarcillin-clavulanate, tigecycline, tirofiban, tobramycin, topotecan, vancomycin, vasopressin, vecuronium, verapamil, vinBLAStine, vinCRIStine, vinorelbine, voriconazole, zidovudine, zoledronic acid

SIDE EFFECTS

CNS: *Headache, dizziness, fatigue, weakness,* depression, anxiety, tremors, seizure, paranoia

CV: *Sinus bradycardia, conduction abnormalities,* dysrhythmias, chest pain, SOB, thrombophlebitis, ischemia, HF, hypertension, palpitations, QT prolongation

ENDO: *Hypo/hyperglycemia, ketosis, hypothyroidism,* galactorrhea, diabetes insipidus

GI: *Diarrhea, nausea, abdominal pain, vomiting, flatulence, distention, constipation,* increased LFTs, cholelithiasis, ileus

GU: UTI

HEMA: Hematoma of inj site, bruise

INTEG: Rash, urticaria, pain; inflammation at inj site

PHARMACOKINETICS

Absorbed rapidly, completely; peak $^{1}/_{2}$ hr (subcut/IV), 2-3 wk (IM); half-life 1.7 hr, duration 12 hr, excreted unchanged in urine 32%, protein binding 65%

INTERACTIONS

Increase: QT prolongation—class IA/III antidysrhythmics, some phenothiazines, β agonists, local anesthetics, tricyclics, haloperidol, chloroquine, droperidol, pentamidine; CYP3A4 inhibitors (amiodarone, clarithromycin, erythromycin, telithromycin, troleandomycin); arsenic trioxide; CYP3A4 substrates (methadone, pimozide, QUEtiapine, quiNIDine, risperiDONE, ziprasidone)

Increase: effect of β-blockers, reduction of dose may be required

---

Decrease: effect of insulin, oral antidiabetics, monitor blood glucose
Decrease: effect of—bromocriptine
Decrease: effect of—cycloSPORINE
Drug/Food
Decrease: absorption of dietary fat, vit B_{12} levels
Drug/Lab Test
Increase: glucose
Decrease: T_4, thyroid function tests, vit B_{12}, glucose

NURSING CONSIDERATIONS
Assess:

• Growth hormone antibodies, IGF-1 at 1- to 4-hr intervals for 8-12 hr after dose **(acromegaly)**; 5-HIAA, plasma serotonin; blood glucose, serotonin levels **(carcinoid tumors)**, plasma substance P, plasma vasoactive intestinal peptide (VIP) **(VIPoma)**

• Thyroid function tests: T_3, T_4, T_7, TSH to identify hypothyroidism

• Vital signs B/P, pulse, hydration status

• Fecal fat, serum carotene, somatomedin-C q14days, glucose; plasma serotonin levels (carcinoid tumors); plasma vasoactive intestinal peptide levels (VIPoma); serum growth hormone, serum IGF-1 baseline and periodically, diabetes to monitor blood glucose

• Chronic therapy may cause B_{12} absorption issues; monitor B_{12} and replace if necessary

• **Allergic reaction:** rash, itching, fever, nausea, wheezing

• **Cardiac status:** bradycardia, conduction abnormalities, dysrhythmias; monitor ECG for QT prolongation, low voltage, axis shifts, early repolarization, R/S transition, early wave progression

• Gallbladder disease, monitor for abdominal pain, ultrasound of gallbladder baseline, periodically

• **Ileus:** assess character of stools, bowel sounds, baseline and throughout treatment

• **Pregnancy/breastfeeding:** use only if benefits outweigh fetal risk; cautious use in breastfeeding, excreted in breast milk
Evaluate:

• Therapeutic response: relief of diarrhea in patients with AIDS; improved symptoms of carcinoid or VIP tumors; decreasing symptoms of acromegaly
Teach patient/family:

• That regular assessments are required; that diabetics need to monitor blood glucose

• About SUBCUT inj if patient or other persons will be giving inj

• That product may cause dizziness, drowsiness, weakness; to avoid hazardous activities if these occur; to report abdominal pain immediately

• That pregnancy may occur in acromegaly because fertility may be restored

• That patients with diabetes need to monitor glucose regularly

---

ofloxacin (Rx)
(o-flox′a-sin)
Func. class.: Antiinfective
Chem. class.: Fluoroquinolone

ACTION: Interferes with conversion of intermediate DNA fragments into high-molecular-weight DNA in bacteria; inhibits DNA gyrase

USES: Treatment of lower respiratory tract infections (pneumonia, bronchitis), genitourinary infections (prostatitis, UTIs) caused by *Escherichia coli, Klebsiella pneumoniae, Chlamydia trachomatis,* skin and skin-structure infections; otitis media, PID
Unlabeled uses: Epididymitis, meningococcal infection, prophylaxis, plague, traveler's diarrhea, typhoid fever, TB

CONTRAINDICATIONS: Hypersensitivity to quinolones
Precautions: Pregnancy, breastfeeding, children, geriatric patients, renal disease, seizure disorders, excessive sunlight, hypokalemia, colitis, QT prolongation

Black Box Warning: Tendon pain/rupture, tendinitis, myasthenia gravis, psychiatric event, peripheral neuropathy, neurotoxicity

---

DOSAGE AND ROUTES
Lower respiratory tract infections/ skin and skin-structure infections
• **Adult: PO** 400 mg q12hr × 10 days
Prostatitis from *E. coli*
• **Adult: PO** 300 mg q12hr × 6 wk
Urinary tract infection
• **Adult: PO** 200 mg q12hr × 3-7 days depending on organism 10 days (complicated)
Pelvic inflammatory disease
• **Adult: PO** 400 mg q12hr with metronidazole × 10-14 days
Traveler's diarrhea (unlabeled)
• **Adult: PO** 400 mg as a single dose or q d X 3 days
Epididymitis (unlabeled)
• **Adult: PO** 300 mg bid × 10 days
• **Adult: PO** 400 mg bid
Renal dose
• **Adult: PO** CCr 20-50 mL/min, give q24hr; CCr <20 mL/min, give 50% of dose q24hr
Hepatic dose
• **Adult (Child-Pugh class C): PO** max 400 mg/day
Available forms: Tabs 200, 300, 400 mg
Administer:
PO route
• 2 hr before or 2 hr after antacids, calcium, iron, zinc products, without regard to food, maintain hydration
• Store at room temperature, protect from light

SIDE EFFECTS
CNS: *Dizziness, headache, fatigue, somnolence,* depression, insomnia, lethargy, malaise, seizures, vertigo
CV: QT prolongation, dysrhythmias, chest pain
EENT: Visual disturbances, pharyngitis
GI: *Diarrhea, nausea, vomiting,* anorexia, flatulence, heartburn, dry mouth, increased AST, ALT, abdominal pain, constipation, CDAD, abnormal taste, xerostomia
HEMA: Blood dyscrasias
INTEG: Rash, pruritus, photosensitivity
MS: Tendinitis, tendon rupture, rhabdomyolysis
SYST: Anaphylaxis, Stevens-Johnson syndrome, toxic epidermal necrolysis

PHARMACOKINETICS
PO: Peak 1-2 hr; half-life 4-8 hr; steady-state 2 days; excreted in urine as active product, metabolites; 90%-95% bioavailability

INTERACTIONS

Black Box Warning: **Increase:** tendon rupture/tendinitis—corticosteroids

• May alter blood glucose levels: antidiabetics
• **Possible theophylline toxicity:** theophylline
Increase: QT prolongation—class IA/III antidysrhythmics, some phenothiazines, β-agonists, local anesthetics, tricyclics, haloperidol, methadone, chloroquine, clarithromycin, droperidol, erythromycin, pentamidine
Increase: CNS stimulation, seizures—NSAIDs
Increase: anticoagulation—warfarin
Decrease: ofloxacin—sevelamer
Decrease: absorption—antacids with aluminum, magnesium, iron products, sucralfate, zinc products; separate by 2 hr
Drug/Lab Test
Increase: INR

NURSING CONSIDERATIONS
Assess:

Black Box Warning: **Tendon rupture/ tendinitis:** more common in lung, heart, kidney transplants or geriatric patients; assess for pain or inflammation; product should be discontinued; steroids may increase risk

• Blood studies: BUN, creatinine, AST, ALT, CBC, blood glucose, INR (warfarin use)
• **CNS symptoms:** insomnia, vertigo, headache, agitation, confusion

Black Box Warning: **Myasthenia gravis**: product may increase weakness; avoid use in patients with myasthenia gravis

• For overgrowth of infection in long-term treatment

Side effects: *italics* = common; red = life-threatening

• **Anaphylaxis, Stevens-Johnson syndrome, toxic epidermal necrolysis:** rash, flushing, urticaria, pruritus, peripheral neuropathy; may be fatal; may occur even after first dose; have emergency equipment nearby

Evaluate:

• Therapeutic response: culture negative, absence of symptoms of infection

Teach patient/family:

• To ambulate, perform activities using assistance if dizziness or light-headedness occurs

• To complete full course of therapy; to take with plenty of fluids

• To avoid iron- or mineral-containing supplements within 2 hr before or after dose; to take without regard to meals

• **Anaphylaxis, Stevens-Johnson syndrome, toxic epidermal necrolysis:** that allergic reactions usually occur after first dose but may occur later; to stop product; to report to prescriber rash, fever

• To avoid sun exposure; photosensitivity can occur

• To avoid use with other products unless approved by prescriber

• To notify prescriber immediately if tingling, pain in extremities occurs

---

ofloxacin ophthalmic
See Appendix B

OLANZapine (Rx) REMS
(oh-lanz´a-peen)
ZyPREXA, ZyPREXA Relprevv,
ZyPREXA Zydis, ZyPREXA
Intramuscular
Func. class.: Antipsychotic (1st generation), neuroleptic
Chem. class.: Thienobenzodiazepine

Do not confuse:
OLANZapine/osalazine
ZyPREXA/CeleXA/ZyrTEC

ACTION: May mediate antipsychotic activity by both DOPamine and serotonin type 2 (5-HT2) antagonists; may antagonize muscarinic receptors, histaminic (H_1)- and α-adrenergic receptors

USES: Schizophrenia, acute manic episodes with bipolar disorder, acute agitation

Unlabeled uses: Chemotherapy-related breakthrough nausea, vomiting, diarrhea

CONTRAINDICATIONS: Hypersensitivity

Precautions: Pregnancy, breastfeeding, geriatric patients, hypertension, cardiac/renal/hepatic disease, diabetes, agranulocytosis, abrupt discontinuation, ✖◕ Asian patients, closed-angle glaucoma, coma, leukopenia, QT prolongation, tardive dyskinesia, torsades de pointes, suicidal ideation, stroke history, TIA

> **Black Box Warning:** Increased mortality in elderly patients with dementia-related psychosis, postinjection delirium/sedation syndrome

DOSAGE AND ROUTES
Schizophrenia

• **Adult:** PO 5-10 mg/day initially, may increase dosage by 5 mg at ≥1 wk intervals, max 20 mg/day; **ORALLY DISINTEGRATING** tabs: daily, open blister pack, place tab on tongue, let disintegrate, swallow; **ext rel inj** (Zyprexa Relprevv) **IM** 150-300 mg q2wk or 405 mg q4wk

• **Geriatric/debilitated:** PO 5 mg/day, may increase cautiously at 1-wk intervals, max 20 mg/day

• **Adolescent:** PO 2.5 or 5 mg/day, target 10 mg/day, max 20 mg

• **Child 6-12 yr (unlabeled):** PO 2.5 mg daily, may increase to 5 mg/day after 4-7 days

Acute mania or mixed episodes associated with bipolar I disorder

• **Adult:** PO 10-15 mg/day, may increase dose after >24 hr by 5 mg, max 20 mg/day

• **Adolescent:** PO 2.5 or 5 mg/day, target 10 mg/day, max 20 mg/day

Acute agitation associated with schizophrenia, bipolar I mania
- **Adult: IM** (reg rel) 10 mg once
- **Geriatric: IM** (reg rel) 2.5-5 mg once

Severe behavioral disturbances in geriatric patients (unlabeled)
- **Adult: PO** 2.5-5 mg/day; **acute psychosis PO** 5-10 mg every night

Available forms: Tab 2.5, 5, 7.5, 10, 15, 20 mg; **orally disintegrating tabs** 5, 10, 15, 20 mg (ZyPREXA Zydis); **powder for inj** 210, 300, 405 mg base/vial (ZyPREXA Relprevv)

Administer:
- Decreased dose in geriatric patients

PO route
- With full glass of water, milk, food to decrease GI upset, may give without regard to food
- Store in tight, light-resistant container
- **Orally disintegrating tabs:** open blister pack; place tab on tongue until dissolved; swallow; no water needed; do not break, crush, chew

IM route (ZyPREXA intramuscular)
- Inspect for particulate, discoloration before use; if present, do not use
- Dissolve contents of vials with 2.1 mL sterile water for inj (5 mg/mL); use immediately
- Do not use IV or subcut
- Inject slowly, deep into muscle mass

IM route (ZyPREXA Relprevv)

Black Box Warning: Available only through restricted distribution program (Zyprexa Relprevv Patient Care Program, 877-772-9390) due to postinjection delirium/sedation syndrome; given at a facility with emergency services; continuous observation; monitor for 3 hr after injection

- Use gloves to prepare; irritating to skin
- Use deep IM gluteal inj only
- Use only diluent provided in kit; give q2-4wk using 19-G, 1.5-inch needle in kit; for obese patients, use 19-G, 2-inch or larger needle

SIDE EFFECTS

CNS: EPS (pseudoparkinsonism, akathisia, dystonia, tardive dyskinesia), seizures, headache, neuroleptic malignant syndrome (rare), agitation, nervousness, hostility, *dizziness,* hypertonia, *tremor,* euphoria, confusion, *drowsiness,* fatigue, abnormal gait, insomnia, fever, suicidal thoughts

CV: Hypotension, tachycardia, chest pain, heart failure, sudden death (geriatric patients, IM), orthostatic hypotension, peripheral edema

ENDO: Increased prolactin levels, hypo/hyperglycemia

GI: *Dry mouth, nausea, vomiting, appetite, dyspepsia,* anorexia, *constipation,* abdominal pain, *weight gain,* jaundice, hepatitis

GU: Urinary retention, urinary frequency, enuresis, impotence, amenorrhea, gynecomastia, breast engorgement, premenstrual syndrome

HEMA: Neutropenia, agranulocytosis, leukopenia

INTEG: Rash

MISC: Peripheral edema, accidental injury, hypertonia, hyperlipidemia

MS: *Joint pain,* twitching

RESP: *Cough, pharyngitis;* fatal pneumonia (geriatric patients, IM)

PHARMACOKINETICS

Well absorbed (60%), metabolized by liver, glucuronidation/oxidation by CYP1A2 and CYP2D6; excreted in urine (57%), feces (30%); 93% bound to plasma proteins; half-life 21-54 hr, extended in geriatric patients; clearance decreased in women, increased in smokers, peak PO 6 hr, IM 15-45 min

INTERACTIONS

Increase: sedation—other CNS depressants, alcohol, barbiturate anesthetics, antihistamines, sedatives/hypnotics, antidepressants

Increase: OLANZapine levels—CYP1A2 inhibitors (fluvoxaMINE)

Increase: hypotension—antihypertensives, alcohol, diazePAM

Increase: anticholinergic effects—anticholinergics

O

Black Box Warning: **Increase:** respiratory depression—opioids

Decrease: OLANZapine levels—CYP1A2 inducers: carBAMazepine, omeprazole, rifAMPin

Decrease: antiparkinson activity—levodopa, bromocriptine, other DOPamine agonists

Drug/Lab Test

Increase: LFTs, prolactin, CPK

Drug/Herb

Increase: toxicity—kava

Decrease: olanzapine effect—St. John's wort; avoid concurrent use

NURSING CONSIDERATIONS
Assess:

Black Box Warning: **Postinjection delirium/sedation syndrome (ZyPREXA Relprevv):** monitor continuously for ≥3 hr after injection; patient must be accompanied when leaving; assess for sedation, coma, delirium, EPS, slurred speech, altered gait, aggression, dizziness, weakness, hypertension, seizures; before leaving, confirm that patient is alert, oriented, and free of any other symptoms

• Mental status: assess orientation, affect, LOC, reflexes, coordination, sleep pattern disturbances, mood, behavior, presence of hallucinations and type before initial administration, monthly; EPS, including akathisia (inability to sit still, no pattern to movements), tardive dyskinesia (bizarre movements of jaw, mouth, tongue, extremities), pseudoparkinsonism (rigidity, tremors, pill rolling, shuffling gait), suicidal thoughts, behaviors

• **Renal status:** I&O ratio; palpate bladder if low urinary output occurs; urinary retention may be cause, especially in geriatric patients; urinalysis recommended before, during prolonged therapy

• Bilirubin, CBC, LFTs

• B/P sitting, standing, lying: take pulse, respirations during initial treatment; establish baseline before starting treatment; report drops of 30 mm Hg; obtain baseline ECG

• Dizziness, faintness, palpitations, tachycardia on rising

Black Box Warning: Geriatric patients for serious reactions: fatal pneumonia, heart failure, stroke leading to death (IM); do not use in dementia-related psychosis

• **Neuroleptic malignant syndrome:** hyperpyrexia, muscle rigidity, increased CPK, altered mental status, acute dystonia (cheek chewing, swallowing, eyes, pill rolling), stop drug immediately

• Constipation, urinary retention daily; increase bulk, water in diet

• Weight gain, hyperglycemia, metabolic changes in diabetic patients

• Supervised ambulation until patient stabilized on medication; do not involve patient in strenuous exercise program because fainting is possible; patient should not stand still for long periods

• **Hyperglycemia:** increased in diabetic patient, monitor FBS baseline and periodically

• **Metabolic syndrome:** large weight gain, increased B/P, FBS, cholesterol, and triglycerides

• **DRESS:** may be fatal; fever, hepatitis, cutaneous reactions, eosinophilia, nephritis, pneumonia, discontinue immediately

• **Beers:** avoid in older adults except for schizophrenia, bipolar disorder, or short-term use as an antiemetic during chemotherapy; increased risk of stroke

• **Pregnancy/breastfeeding:** use only if benefits outweigh fetal risk, may cause EPS in infant if used in 3rd trimester; those pregnant should enroll women in the National Pregnancy Registry for Atypical Antipsychotics, 1-866-961-2388; excreted in breast milk

Evaluate:

• Therapeutic response: decrease in emotional excitement, hallucinations, delusion, paranoia, reorganization of patterns of thought, speech

Teach patient/family:

Black Box Warning: About postinjection delirium/sedation syndrome: all symptoms

• To use good oral hygiene; frequent rinsing of mouth; sugarless gum, hard candy, ice chips for dry mouth

- To avoid hazardous activities until product response is determined
- That orthostatic hypotension occurs often; to rise from sitting or lying position gradually
- To avoid hot tubs, hot showers, tub baths because hypotension may occur
- To avoid abrupt withdrawal of this product because EPS may result; product should be withdrawn slowly
- To avoid OTC preparations (cough, hay fever, cold) unless approved by prescriber because serious product interactions may occur; to avoid use with alcohol, CNS depressants, opioids because increased drowsiness may occur
- **Suicidal thoughts, behaviors:** report immediately suicidal thoughts/behaviors
- That in hot weather, heat stroke may occur; to take extra precautions to stay cool
- To take PO without regard to food
- To notify prescriber if pregnancy is planned or suspected; not to breastfeed

TREATMENT OF OVERDOSE: Lavage if orally ingested; provide airway; do not induce vomiting or use EPINEPHrine

⚠ HIGH ALERT

RARELY USED

olaparib
(oh-lap′a-rib)
Lynparza
Func. class.: Antineoplastic-PARP

USES: Treatment of deleterious or suspected deleterious germline BRCA-mutated advanced ovarian cancer in patients who have not responded successfully to ≥3 prior courses of chemotherapy, as monotherapy

CONTRAINDICATIONS: Hypersensitivity

DOSAGE AND ROUTES
- **Adult female:** **PO** 400 mg bid, (tablets) 300 mg bid (capsules) until disease

progression or unacceptable toxicity. Avoid use of concomitant strong and moderate CYP3A4 inhibitors if possible

⚠ HIGH ALERT

RARELY USED

olaratumab
(oh-lar-at′ ue-mab)
Lartruvo ✿
Func. class.: Antineoplastic, monoclonal antibody

USES: The treatment of soft-tissue sarcoma not amenable to curative treatment with radiotherapy or surgery, in combination with DOXOrubicin

CONTRAINDICATIONS: Hypersensitivity, pregnancy

DOSAGE AND ROUTES
- **Adult:** **IV INFUSION** 15 mg/kg over 60 min on days 1 and 8 repeated q21days until disease progression or unacceptable toxicity in combination with doxorubicin 75 mg/m^2 **IV** on day 1 repeated q21days for up to 8 cycles

olmesartan (Rx)
(ol-meh-sar′tan)
Benicar, Olmetec ✿
Func. class.: Antihypertensive
Chem. class.: Angiotensin II receptor (type AT$_1$) antagonist

Do not confuse:
Benicar/Mevacor

ACTION: Blocks the vasoconstrictor and aldosterone-secreting effects of angiotensin II; selectively blocks the binding of angiotensin II to the AT$_1$ receptor found in tissues

USES: Hypertension, alone or in combination with other antihypertensives

CONTRAINDICATIONS: Hypersensitivity

Side effects: italics = common; red = life-threatening

Precautions: Breastfeeding, children, geriatric patients, hepatic disease, HF, renal artery stenosis, ✆ African descent, hyperkalemia

DOSAGE AND ROUTES

• **Adult: PO** single agent 20 mg/day initially in patients who are not volume depleted; may be increased to 40 mg/day if needed after 2 wk; **in volume depletion:** start with lower dose

• **Child ≥6 yr/adolescent ≤16 yr weighing ≥35 kg: PO** 20 mg/day; may increase to max 40 mg/day after 2 wk

• **Child ≥6 yr/adolescent ≤16 yr weighing 20-<35 kg: PO** 10 mg daily; may increase to max 20 mg/day after 2 wk

Available forms: Tabs 5, 20, 40 mg

Administer:

• Without regard to meals

• Compounded suspension may be made in the pharmacy; refrigerate up to 1 mo, shake well before use

SIDE EFFECTS

CNS: *Dizziness*, fatigue, *headache*, insomnia, syncope

CV: Chest pain, peripheral edema, tachycardia, *hypotension*

EENT: Sinusitis, rhinitis, pharyngitis

GI: *Diarrhea*, abdominal pain

META: Hyperkalemia

MS: Arthralgia, pain, rhabdomyolysis

RESP: *Upper respiratory infection*, bronchitis

SYST: Angioedema

PHARMACOKINETICS

Peak 1-2 hr; excreted in urine, (50% unchanged) feces; half-life 13 hr; protein binding 99%

INTERACTIONS

Increase: antihypertensive effects—other antihypertensives, diuretics

Increase: hyperkalemia—potassium supplements, potassium-sparing diuretics, ACE inhibitors

Increase: effect of lithium, antioxidants

Decrease: antihypertensive effect—NSAIDs, colesevelam, COX-2 inhibitors

Drug/Herb

Increase: antihypertensive effect—hawthorn, garlic

Decrease: antihypertensive effect—ephedra, black licorice

NURSING CONSIDERATIONS

Assess:

• **Volume depletion:** correct volume depletion before starting therapy

• **Hypertension:** B/P, pulse; note rate, rhythm, quality; electrolytes: sodium, potassium, chloride; baselines for renal, hepatic studies before therapy begins; may use antihypertensives to control B/P if needed

• **Hypotension:** place supine; may occur with hyponatremia or in those with volume depletion; more common in those taking a diuretic also

• **Heart failure:** monitor for edema, jugular vein distention, dyspnea; monitor weight daily

Evaluate:

• Therapeutic response: decreased B/P

Teach patient/family:

• To comply with dosage schedule, not to double or skip dose, to take missed dose when remembered if not close to next dose

• To notify prescriber of mouth sores, fever, swelling of hands or feet, irregular heartbeat, chest pain, severe chronic diarrhea, severe weight loss

• That excessive perspiration, dehydration, vomiting, diarrhea may lead to fall in B/P; to consult prescriber if these occur; to maintain adequate hydration

• That product may cause dizziness, fainting, light-headedness; to avoid hazardous activities

• To rise slowly to sitting or standing position to minimize orthostatic hypotension

---

• To notify provider immediately of swelling of the face, lips, tongue, trouble breathing
• That follow-up exams will be needed
• To avoid all OTC medications unless approved by prescriber
• That blood glucose may increase and antidiabetic product may need dosage change
• To inform all health care providers of medication use
• To use proper technique for obtaining B/P, and discuss acceptable parameters

Black Box Warning: To notify prescriber immediately if pregnant; not to use during breastfeeding

---

olopatadine nasal agent
See Appendix B

---

olopatadine ophthalmic
See Appendix B

---

olsalazine (Rx)
(ohl-sal′ah-zeen)
Dipentum
Func. class.: GI antiinflammatory
Chem. class.: Salicylate derivative

Do not confuse:
olsalazine/OLANZapine

ACTION: Bioconverted to 5-amino-salicylic acid, which decreases inflammation

USES: Maintenance of remission of ulcerative colitis in patients intolerant to sulfasalazine

CONTRAINDICATIONS: Hypersensitivity to this product or salicylates
Precautions: Pregnancy, breastfeeding, children <14 yr; impaired renal/hepatic function; severe allergy; bronchial asthma

DOSAGE AND ROUTES
• **Adult:** **PO** 500 mg bid, max 3 g/day
Available forms: Caps 250 mg
Administer:
• Total daily dose evenly spaced to minimize GI intolerance; give with food
• Store in tight, light-resistant container at room temperature

SIDE EFFECTS
CNS: Headache, hallucinations, depression, vertigo, fatigue, dizziness
GI: Nausea, vomiting, abdominal pain, diarrhea, bloating
INTEG: Rash, dermatitis, urticaria

PHARMACOKINETICS
Partially absorbed, peak $1^1/_2$ hr, half-life 30-90 min (rectal), 2-15 hr (PO), excreted in urine as 5-aminosalicylic acid and metabolites, crosses placenta

INTERACTIONS
Increase: azaTHIOprine toxicity—azaTHIOprine
Increase: myelosuppression—mercaptopurine, thioguanine
Increase: bleeding risk—low-molecular-weight heparins; discontinue before using this product
Increase: Reye's syndrome development—varicella vaccine; do not use within 6 wk of olsalazine
Increase: PT, INR—warfarin
Drug/Lab Test
Increase: AST, ALT

NURSING CONSIDERATIONS
Assess:
• **Colitis:** bowel pattern, number of stools, consistency, frequency, pain, mucus, abdominal pain before treatment and periodically
• **Allergic reaction:** rash, dermatitis, urticaria, pruritus, dyspnea, bronchospasm; allergy to salicylates, sulfonamides
• BUN, creatinine in those with renal disease; LFTs (liver disease); monitor I&O, output of 1500 mL/day is needed to prevent crystals in urine
• **Pregnancy/breastfeeding:** use only if benefits outweigh fetal risk; avoid breastfeeding, excreted in breast milk

O

Side effects: *italics* = common; red = life-threatening

Evaluate:

• Therapeutic response: absence of fever, mucus in stools, decreased diarrhea, abdominal pain

Teach patient/family:

• To report diarrhea, rash, bleeding, bruising, fever, hallucinations, or if symptoms do not improve after 2 mo of therapy

• That product may cause dizziness; to avoid hazardous activities until reaction is known

• To take even if feeling better; to take as directed; to take missed dose when remembered, but not to double

• That lab work and exams will be needed during treatment

---

omalizumab (Rx)

(oh-mah-lye-zoo′mab)

Xolair

Func. class.: Antiasthmatic

Chem. class.: Monoclonal antibody

ACTION: Recombinant DNA-derived humanized IgG murine monoclonal antibody that selectively binds to IgE to limit the release of mediators in the allergic response

USES: Moderate to severe persistent asthma, chronic idiopathic urticaria

Unlabeled uses: Seasonal allergic rhinitis, food allergy

CONTRAINDICATIONS: Hypersensitivity to hamster protein

Black Box Warning: Hypersensitivity to this product

Precautions: Pregnancy, breastfeeding, children <12 yr, acute attacks of asthma, lymphoma, nephrotic disease, bronchospasm, neoplastic disease, status asthmaticus

DOSAGE AND ROUTES

Moderate to severe asthma

• Adult/adolescent/child ≥12 yr: SUBCUT 150-300 mg × 2-4 wk; divide inj into 2 sites if dose >150 mg; dose is adjusted based on IgE levels, significant changes in body weight

Chronic idiopathic urticaria

• Adult/adolescent >12 yr: SUBCUT 150-300 mg q4wk

Available forms: Powder for inj, lyophilized 202.5 mg (150 mg/1.2 mL after reconstitution)

Administer:

SUBCUT route

• Reconstitute using 1.4 mL sterile water for inj (150 mg/1.2 mL or 125 mg/mL); gently swirl to dissolve; allow vial to stand and q5min gently swirl for 5-10 sec to dissolve; some vials may take ≥20 min; do not use if contents do not dissolve within 40 min; should be clear or slightly opalescent; use large-bore needle to withdraw medication; replace needle with small-bore needle

• Given q2-4wk; product is viscous; if >150 mg is given, divide into 2 sites; inj may take 5-10 sec to administer

SIDE EFFECTS

CV: Heart failure, cardiomyopathy, hypotension, MI, PE, thrombosis

HEMA: Serious systemic eosinophilia

INTEG: Pruritus, dermatitis, inj-site reactions, rash

MISC: Earache, dizziness, fatigue, pain, malignancies, viral infections, anaphylaxis, thrombocytopenia, headache

MS: Arthralgia, fracture, leg, arm pain

RESP: Sinusitis, upper respiratory infections, pharyngitis, pulmonary hypertension, bronchospasm

PHARMACOKINETICS

Slowly absorbed, peak 7-8 days, half-life 26 days, degradation by liver, excretion in bile

INTERACTIONS

• Use cautiously with live virus vaccines

Drug/Lab Test

Increase: IgE

NURSING CONSIDERATIONS

Assess:

• **Asthma:** respiratory rate, rhythm, depth; auscultate lung fields bilaterally; notify prescriber of abnormalities; monitor pulmonary function tests; serum IgE (may increase and continue for 1 yr)

• **Inj-site reactions:** inflammation, edema, redness, warmth at site; may occur within 60 min of inj; may decrease with repeated dosing

Black Box Warning: **Anaphylaxis, allergic reactions:** rash, urticaria, inability to breathe, edema of throat; product should be discontinued; have emergency equipment available; observe for 2 hr; reaction can occur ≤24 hr

• **Pregnancy/breastfeeding:** use only if clearly needed; pregnant patients should enroll in the EXPECT Pregnancy Registry, 1-866-496-5247; cautious use in breastfeeding, excretion unknown
Evaluate:
• Therapeutic response: ability to breathe more easily
Teach patient/family:
• That improvement will not be immediate
• Not to stop taking or decrease current asthma medications unless instructed by prescriber
• To avoid live virus vaccines while taking this product

Black Box Warning: To report signs of allergic reaction immediately, can be life-threatening

omeprazole (OTC, Rx)
(oh-mep′ray-zole)
Losec ✦, Olex ✦ PriLOSEC, PriLOSEC OTC
Func. class.: Antiulcer, proton pump inhibitor
Chem. class.: Benzimidazole

Do not confuse:
PriLOSEC/Prinivil/PROzac/predniSONE/ Pristiq
omeprazole/fomepizole

ACTION: Suppresses gastric secretion by inhibiting hydrogen/potassium ATPase enzyme system in gastric parietal cells; characterized as gastric acid pump inhibitor because it blocks the final step of acid production

USES: Gastroesophageal reflux disease (GERD), severe erosive esophagitis, poorly responsive systemic GERD, pathologic hypersecretory conditions (Zollinger-Ellison syndrome, systemic mastocytosis, multiple endocrine adenomas); treatment of active duodenal ulcers with/without antiinfectives for *Helicobacter pylori*
Unlabeled uses: NSAID-induced ulcer prophylaxis, stress gastritis prophylaxis

CONTRAINDICATIONS: Hypersensitivity to this product or benzimidazoles
Precautions: Pregnancy; breastfeeding; children; ⚫ Asian, black patients, hepatic disease

DOSAGE AND ROUTES
Active duodenal ulcers
• **Adult: PO** 20 mg/day × 4-8 wk; associated with *H. pylori* 40 mg q AM and clarithromycin 500 mg tid on days 1-14, then 20 mg/day on days 15-28
Severe erosive esophagitis/poorly responsive GERD
• **Adult: PO** (del rel cap/del rel susp) 20 mg/day × 4-8 wk
Pathologic hypersecretory conditions
• **Adult: PO** 60 mg/day; may increase to 120 mg tid; daily doses >80 mg should be divided
Gastric ulcer
• **Adult: PO** 40 mg/day 4-8 wk
• **Geriatric: PO** ≤20 mg/day
Heartburn (OTC)
• **Adult: PO** 1 del rel tab (20 mg)/day before AM meal with glass of water × 14 days
Available forms: Del rel caps 10, 20, 40 mg; del rel tabs 20 mg; granules for oral susp 2.5, 10 mg (del rel)
Administer:
• Swallow caps whole; do not crush or chew; caps may be opened and sprinkled over applesauce
• Before eating, usually in the AM, separate with other medications
• **Oral susp powder:** give on empty stomach ≥1 hr before food; if there is NG or enteral feeding tube, do not feed 3 hr before or 1 hr after giving product: contents of packet should be mixed with

O

Side effects: *italics* = common; red = life-threatening

1-2 tbsp water; add 20 mL water for NG tube; for oral, stir well, drink, add more water, and drink

SIDE EFFECTS

CNS: *Headache, dizziness, asthenia*
GI: *Diarrhea, abdominal pain, vomiting, nausea, constipation, flatulence, acid regurgitation,* abdominal swelling, anorexia, irritable colon, esophageal candidiasis, dry mouth, hepatic failure, *Clostridium difficile*–associated diarrhea (CDAD)
INTEG: *Rash,* dry skin, urticaria, pruritus, alopecia
MISC: *Back pain,* fever, fatigue, malaise
RESP: *Upper respiratory infections, cough,* epistaxis, pneumonia

PHARMACOKINETICS

Bioavailability 30%-40%; peak $^1/_2$-$3^1/_2$ hr; half-life $^1/_2$-1 hr; protein binding 95%; eliminated in urine as metabolites and in feces; in geriatric patients, elimination rate decreased, bioavailability increased; metabolized by CYP2C19 enzyme system; some Asian, black, and Caucasian patients are poor metabolizers

INTERACTIONS

Increase: bleeding—warfarin
Increase: serum levels of diazePAM, phenytoin, flurazepam, triazolam, cycloSPORINE, disulfiram, digoxin
Decrease: effect of iron salts, ketoconazole, cyanocobalamin, calcium carbonate, ampicillin, indinavir, gefitinib
Drug/Lab Test
Increase: alk phos, AST, ALT, bilirubin, gastrin

NURSING CONSIDERATIONS
Assess:

• **GI system:** bowel sounds, abdomen for pain, swelling, anorexia, blood in stools, diarrhea, emesis
• *Clostridium difficile*–associated diarrhea (CDAD): assess for fever, abdominal pain, bloody stool; may occur up to several wk after conclusion of therapy; report to the prescriber immediately
• **Electrolyte imbalances:** hyponatremia; hypomagnesemia in patients using product 3 mo-1 yr; if hypomagnesemia occurs,

use of magnesium supplements may be sufficient; if severe, discontinue product
• **Hepatic enzymes:** AST, ALT, alk phos during treatment; **blood studies:** CBC, differential during treatment, blood dyscrasias may occur; vit B$_{12}$ in long-term treatment
• **Fractures:** use over 1 yr has been associated with fractures
• **Beers:** avoid scheduled use >8 wk in patients with hypersecretory condition, esophagitis, risk of *Clostridium difficile*, and fractures
• **Pregnancy/breastfeeding:** use only if benefits outweigh fetal risk; cautious use in breastfeeding, excreted in breast milk
Evaluate:
• Therapeutic response: absence of epigastric pain, swelling, fullness, bleeding; decreased GERD, esophagitis symptoms
Teach patient/family:
• To report severe diarrhea; black, tarry stools; abdominal cramps/pain; or continuing headache; product may have to be discontinued
• That, if diabetic, hypoglycemia may occur
• To avoid hazardous activities because dizziness may occur
• To avoid alcohol, salicylates, NSAIDs; may cause GI irritation
• To take as directed, even if feeling better; to take missed dose as soon as remembered; not to double; PriLOSEC OTC takes up to 4 days for full effect
• Not to use OTC, prescription, or herbal products without prescriber's consent
• To take as directed at lowest dose possible for shortest time needed
• To report if pregnancy is planned or suspected or if breastfeeding

---

ondansetron (Rx)
(on-dan-seh′tron)
Zofran, Zofran ODT, Zuplenz, Ondissolve ✦
Func. class.: Antiemetic
Chem. class.: 5-HT$_3$ antagonist

Do not confuse:
Zofran/Zantac

ACTION: Prevents nausea, vomiting by blocking serotonin peripherally, centrally, and in the small intestine

USES: Prevention of nausea, vomiting associated with cancer chemotherapy, radiotherapy; prevention of postoperative nausea, vomiting

Unlabeled uses: Pruritus (rectal use), alcoholism, severe vomiting in pregnancy, gastroenteritis, postoperative nausea/vomiting

CONTRAINDICATIONS: Hypersensitivity; phenylketonuric hypersensitivity (oral disintegrating tab), torsades de pointes

Precautions: Pregnancy, breastfeeding, children, geriatric patients, granisetron hypersensitivity, QT prolongation, torsades de pointes

DOSAGE AND ROUTES
Prevention of nausea/vomiting (cancer chemotherapy)
• **Adult/child 4-18 yr:** IV 0.15 mg/kg infused over 15 min given 30 min before start of cancer chemotherapy, max 16 mg/dose; 0.15 mg/kg given 4 hr and 8 hr after 1st dose or 16 mg as single dose; dilute in 50 mL of D₅ or 0.9% NaCl before giving; **oral dissolving film** 24 mg dissolved on the tongue 30 min prior to single-day chemotherapy; **RECT**(unlabeled) 16 mg/day 2 hr before chemotherapy; **PO** 8 mg ½ hr before chemotherapy, repeat 4, 8 hr after 1st dose
• **Child ≥4 yr:** PO 4 mg tid, first dose ½ hr before chemotherapy
Prevention of nausea/vomiting (radiotherapy)
• **Adult:** PO 8 mg tid, may repeat q8hr
Prevention of postoperative nausea/vomiting
• **Adult:** IV/IM 4 mg undiluted over >30 sec before induction of anesthesia
• **Child 2-12 yr:** IV 0.1 mg/kg (≤40 kg); IV 4 mg (≥40 kg), give over ≥30 sec
Hepatic dose
• **Adult:** PO/IM/IV max dose 8 mg/day

Severe vomiting in pregnancy (unlabeled)
• **Adult:** PO/IV 4-8 mg bid-tid
Pruritus (unlabeled)
• **Adult:** PO 8 mg bid
Alcoholism (unlabeled)
• **Adult PO** 4 mcg/kg bid
Available forms: Inj 2 mg/mL, 32 mg/50 mL (premixed); tabs 4, 8 mg; oral sol 4 mg/5 mL; oral disintegrating tabs 4, 8 mg; oral dissolving film 4, 8 mg
Administer:
PO route
• **Regular tab:** protect from light (4 mg tab)
• **Oral disintegrating tab:** do not push through foil; gently remove; immediately place on tongue to dissolve; swallow with saliva
• **Oral dissolving film:** fold pouch along dotted line to expose tear notch; tear and remove film; place film on tongue until dissolved; swallow after dissolved; to reach desired dose, administer successive films, allowing each to dissolve before using another
• **Oral solution:** protect from light; measure in calibrated oral syringe or other calibrated device
IM route
• Visually inspect for particulate or discoloration
• May give 4 mg undiluted IM; inject deeply in large muscle mass; aspirate
Direct IV route
• Give undiluted 2 mg/mL immediately proceeding anesthesia induction
Intermittent IV infusion
• Check for discoloration or particulate; if particulate is present, shake to dissolve
• After diluting single dose in 50 mL NS or D₅W, 0.45% NaCl or NS; give over 15 min
• Do not use IV 32 mg/dose in chemotherapy nausea/vomiting due to QT prolongation, max 16 mg/dose (adult)
• Store at room temperature for 48 hr after dilution

Y-site compatibilities: Aldesleukin, amifostine, amikacin, aztreonam, bleomycin, CARBOplatin, carmustine, ceFAZolin, cefmetazole, cefotaxime, cefOXitin, cefTAZidime, ceftizoxime, cefuroxime, chlorproMAZINE, cimetidine, cisatracurium, CISplatin, cladribine, clindamycin, cyclophosphamide, cytarabine, dacarbazine, DACTINomycin, DAUNOrubicin, dexamethasone, diphenhydrAMINE, DOPamine, DOXOrubicin, DOXOrubicin liposome, doxycycline, droperidol, etoposide, famotidine, filgrastim, floxuridine, fluconazole, fludarabine, gallium, gentamicin, haloperidol, heparin, hydrocortisone, HYDROmorphone, hydrOXYzine, ifosfamide, imipenem-cilastatin, magnesium sulfate, mannitol, mechlorethamine, melphalan, meperidine, mesna, methotrexate, metoclopramide, miconazole, mitoMYcin, mitoXANTRONE, morphine, PACLitaxel, pentostatin, piperacillin/tazobactam, potassium chloride, prochlorperazine, promethazine, raNITIdine, remifentanil, streptozocin, teniposide, thiotepa, ticarcillin, ticarcillin-clavulanate, vancomycin, vinBLAStine, vinCRIStine, vinorelbine, zidovudine

SIDE EFFECTS

CNS: *Headache, dizziness, drowsiness, fatigue, EPS*

GI: *Diarrhea, constipation,* abdominal pain, dry mouth

MISC: Rash, bronchospasm (rare), *musculoskeletal pain, wound problems, shivering, fever, hypoxia, urinary retention*

PHARMACOKINETICS

IV: Mean elimination half-life 3.5-4.7 hr, plasma protein binding 70%-76%, extensively metabolized in the liver, excreted 45%-60% in urine

INTERACTIONS

Increase: unconsciousness, hypotension—apomorphine, do not use together

Increase: QT prolongation—other products that prolong QT

Decrease: ondansetron effect—rifampin, carBAMazepine, phenytoin

Drug/Lab Test

Increase: LFTs

NURSING CONSIDERATIONS

Assess:
• Absence of nausea, vomiting during chemotherapy

• Hypersensitivity reaction: rash, bronchospasm (rare)

• **EPS:** shuffling gait, tremors, grimacing, rigidity periodically

• **Pregnancy/breastfeeding:** identify whether pregnancy is planned or suspected; avoid use in pregnancy, cardiac malformations, oral clefts may occur if used in 1st trimester; cautious use in breastfeeding

• **QT prolongation:** monitor ECG in those with hypokalemia, hypomagnesemia, cardiac disease or in those receiving other products that increase QT

• **Serotonin syndrome:** occurs when other products are given that increase CNS or peripheral serotonin levels; assess for agitation, confusion, dizziness, diaphoresis, flushing, tremor, seizures, nausea, vomiting, diarrhea; product should be discontinued

Evaluate:
• Therapeutic response: absence of nausea, vomiting due to chemotherapy, surgery

Teach patient/family:
• To report diarrhea, constipation, rash, changes in respirations, discomfort at insertion site, serotonin symptoms, EPS symptoms

• That headache requiring analgesic is common

• Drink with whole glass of water (PO)

• **Oral disintegrating tabs:** remove strip from pouch, place on tongue, and allow to dissolve; drink water

---

oritavancin

(or-it'a-van'sin)
Orbactiv
Func. class.: Antiinfective agents
Chem. class.: Glycopeptides

ACTION: Inhibits bacterial cell wall biosynthesis by preventing transglycosylation (polymerization) due to binding to precursors, as well as by preventing crosslinking by binding to the peptide bridging segments of the cell wall, also disrupts the bacterial cell membrane integrity, resulting in depolarization, increased permeability, and eventual cell death

USES: *Enterococcus faecalis, Enterococcus faecium, Staphylococcus aureus* (MRSA), *Staphylococcus aureus* (MSSA), *Streptococcus agalactiae* (group B streptococci), *Streptococcus anginosus, Streptococcus constellatus, Streptococcus dysgalactiae, Streptococcus intermedius, Streptococcus pyogenes* (group A β-hemolytic streptococci); treatment of acute bacterial skin and skin structure infections due to gram-positive organisms, including cellulitis/erysipelas, major cutaneous abscesses, and wound infections

CONTRAINDICATIONS: Hypersensitivity

Precautions: Anticoagulant therapy, antimicrobial resistance, breastfeeding, colitis, diarrhea, inflammatory bowel disease, infusion reactions, pregnancy, CDAD, vancomycin hypersensitivity, viral infection

DOSAGE AND ROUTES
• **Adult: IV** 1200 mg as a single dose
Available forms: Powder for injection: 400 mg
Administer:
• Visually inspect for particulate matter and discoloration beforehand; the reconstituted solution is clear, colorless to pale yellow
• **Reconstitution:** Reconstitute each 400-mg vial with 40 mL sterile water for injection. Three vials are necessary for a single dose; gently swirl until dissolved
• **Dilution:** Withdraw and discard 120 mL from a 1000-mL intravenous bag of D₅W; transfer 40 mL solution from each of the 3 reconstituted vials to the D₅W IV bag (1.2 mg/mL)
• **Storage:** Refrigerate or store at room temperature. The combined storage time (from reconstitution to dilution) and 3-hour infusion time should not exceed 6 hr at room temperature or 12 hr if refrigerated
Intermittent IV INFUSION
• Infuse over 3 hr; do not infuse with other medications or electrolytes; do not use saline-based solution

• Avoid heparin for 5 days after use of this product; false elevated aPTT and coagulation studies will occur

SIDE EFFECTS
CNS: Dizziness, flushing, headache
CV: Sinus tachycardia, phlebitis
GI: Nausea, vomiting, diarrhea, CDAD
HEMA: Anemia, eosinophilia
MS: Myalgia, osteomyelitis
INTEG: Rash, vasculitis, pruritus, angioedema, infusion-related reaction
MISC: Wheezing, bronchospasm

PHARMACOKINETICS
85% protein binding, half-life 245 hr, excretion urine, unchanged, peak infusion's end

INTERACTIONS
Increase: toxicity—products metabolized by CYP2D6, CYP3A4
Increase: bleeding risk—warfarin; avoid concurrent use
Drug/Lab Test
Increase: LFTs, uric acid, INR, aPTT

NURSING CONSIDERATIONS
Assess:
• **Infection:** wounds, fever, sputum, urine, monitor WBC baseline and periodically report changes
• CBC and differential
• C&S before therapy; may give product before receiving results
• **Infusion-related reactions:** symptoms of red man syndrome (flushing, urticaria, pruritus); slow or stop infusion
• **Bowel function:** for diarrhea, bloody stools, cramping; assess for fever; report to health care professional, may be *Clostridium difficile*–associated diarrhea (CDAD), may start up to 8 wk after completion of treatment
• **Anticoagulant use:** may increase effects of warfarin; monitor closely, avoid use with heparin; heparin effects may be reduced and lab results altered
• **Pregnancy/breastfeeding:** use only if benefits outweigh fetal risk; cautious use in breastfeeding, excreted in breast milk
Evaluate:
• Therapeutic response: resolution of infection

O

Side effects: *italics* = common; red = life-threatening

Teach patient/family:
- Reason for product, expected result
- Used only once to resolve infection
- **Hypersensitivity reactions:** to notify prescriber of rash, facial swelling, dyspnea
- To avoid use of other prescription products, OTC products, or herbal products unless approved by prescriber
- **Bowel function:** to notify health care professional of diarrhea, bloody stools, cramping, fever; do not self-treat
- To notify prescriber if pregnancy is planned or suspected

RARELY USED

orlistat (Rx, OTC)
(or′lih-stat)
Alli, Xenical
Func. class.: Weight-control agent
Chem. class.: Lipase inhibitor

ACTION: Inhibits the absorption of dietary fats

USES: Obesity management

CONTRAINDICATIONS: Hypersensitivity, chronic malabsorption syndrome, cholestasis

DOSAGE AND ROUTES
- **Adult:** PO (Alli) 60 mg, (Xenical) 120 mg tid with each main meal containing fat, max 360 mg/day

oseltamivir (Rx)
(oss-el-tam′ih-veer)
Tamiflu
Func. class.: Antiviral
Chem. class.: Neuraminidase inhibitor

ACTION: Inhibits influenza virus neuraminidase with possible alteration of virus particle aggregation and release

USES: Prevention and treatment of influenza type A or B
Unlabeled uses: Avian flu (H5N1)

CONTRAINDICATIONS: Hypersensitivity
Precautions: Pregnancy, neonates, breastfeeding, infants, children, geriatric patients, renal/hepatic/pulmonary/cardiac disease, psychosis, viral infection

DOSAGE AND ROUTES
Treatment of influenza
- **Adult/child >40 kg:** PO 75 mg bid × 5 days, begin treatment within 2 days of onset of symptoms
- **Child 23-40 kg and ≥1 yr:** PO 60 mg bid × 5 days
- **Child 15-23 kg and ≥1 yr:** PO 45 mg bid × 5 days
- **Child ≤15 kg and ≥1 yr:** PO 30 mg bid × 5 days
- **Neonate ≥14 days/infant:** PO 3 mg/kg/dose bid × 5 days

Prevention of influenza
- **Adult/child ≥13 yr:** PO 75 mg/day × 10 days; begin treatment within 2 days of contact, max use 6 wk

Renal dose
- **Adult: PO** Treatment: CCr 10-30 mL/min, 30 mg/day × 5 days; CCr 30-60 mL/min, 30 mg bid × 5 days; Prophylaxis: CCr 10-30 mL/min, 30 mg every other day; CCr 30-60 mL/min, 30 mg daily

H1N1 influenza A virus (unlabeled)
- **Adult/adolescent/child >40 kg:** PO 75 mg bid × 5 days
- **Adolescent/child 24-40 kg:** PO 60 mg bid × 5 days
- **Child >1 yr and 15-23 kg:** PO 45 mg bid × 5 days
- **Child >1 yr and ≤15 kg:** PO 30 mg bid × 5 days

Available forms: Caps 30, 45, 75 mg; powder for oral susp 6 mg/mL
Administer:
- Within 2 days of symptoms of influenza; continue for 5 days
- At least 4 hr before bedtime to prevent insomnia
- Without regard to food; give with food for GI upset
- Take with full glass of water
- Store in tight, dry container
- **Oral susp:** 6 mg/mL concentration, take care to administer correct dose;

---

loosen powder from side of bottle, add 55 mL, shake well (6 mg/mL), remove push bottle adapter into neck of bottle, close tightly to ensure sealing, use within 17 days of preparation when refrigerated or within 10 days at room temperature, write expiration date on bottle, shake well before use, use oral syringe provided but only with markings for 30, 45, 60 mg, confirm that dosing instructions are in same units as syringe provided

SIDE EFFECTS

CNS: *Headache, dizziness,* fatigue, *insomnia,* seizures, delirium, self-injury (children)
GI: *Nausea, vomiting*
INTEG: Toxic epidermal necrolysis, Stevens-Johnson syndrome, erythema multiforme
RESP: Cough

PHARMACOKINETICS

Rapidly absorbed, protein binding 3%, converted to oseltamivir carboxylate (active form), active forms half-life 1-3 hr, metabolite 6-10 hr, excreted in urine (99%)

INTERACTIONS

• **Decrease:** effect, influenza virus vaccine, avoid prior to use (2 days before or after 14 days)

NURSING CONSIDERATIONS
Assess:
• Bowel pattern before, during treatment
• **Influenza:** fever, fatigue, sore throat, headache, muscle soreness, aches
• **Behavioral symptoms:** hallucinations, abnormal behaviors, delirium (rare)
Evaluate:
• Therapeutic response: absence of fever, malaise, cough, dyspnea in infection
Teach patient/family:
• About all aspects of product therapy
• To avoid hazardous activities if dizziness occurs
• To take as soon as symptoms appear; to take full course even if feeling better
• To take missed dose as soon as remembered if within 2 hr of next dose
• To stop immediately; to report to prescriber skin rash, delirium, psychosis, hallucinations (child)

• That this product should not be substituted for flu shot
• That this product will not treat the common cold
• To avoid other products unless approved by prescriber

⚠ HIGH ALERT

oxaliplatin (Rx)
(ox-al-i′plat-in)
Eloxatin
Func. class.: Antineoplastic
Chem. class.: 3rd-generation platinum analog, alkylating agent

---

ACTION: Forms crosslinks, thereby inhibiting DNA replication and transcription; not specific to cell cycle

USES: Metastatic carcinoma of the colon or rectum in combination with 5-FU/leucovorin
Unlabeled uses: Relapsed or refractory non-Hodgkin's lymphoma; advanced ovarian cancer; breast, head/neck, testicular, pancreatic, gastric cancer; mesothelioma

CONTRAINDICATIONS: Pregnancy, breastfeeding, radiation therapy or chemotherapy within 1 mo, thrombocytopenia, smallpox vaccination

Black Box Warning: Hypersensitivity to this product or other platinum products

Precautions: Children, geriatric patients, pneumococcus vaccination, renal disease

DOSAGE AND ROUTES
Dosage protocols may vary
• **Adult:** IV INFUSION *Day 1:* oxaliplatin 85 mg/m^2 in 250-500 mL D$_5$W and leucovorin 200 mg/m^2 in D$_5$W; give both over 2 hr at the same time in separate bags using a Y-line, followed by 5-FU 400 mg/m^2 **IV BOL** over 2-4 min, then 5-FU 600 mg/m^2 **IV INFUSION** in 500 mL D$_5$W as a 22-hr **CONT INFUSION**; *day 2:* leucovorin 200 mg/m^2 IV

INFUSION over 2 hr, then 5-FU 400 mg/m^2 **IV BOL** over 2-4 min, then 5-FU 600 mg/m^2 **IV INFUSION** in 500 mL D$_5$W as a 22-hr **CONT INFUSION**; repeat cycle q2wk

Renal dose
• **Adult:** IV CCr <30 mL/min, reduce starting dose to 65 mg/m^2

Gastric cancer (unlabeled)
• **Adult:** IV 130 mg/m^2 over 2 hr on day 1 with epirubicin in 50 mg/m^2 and capecitabine

Available forms: Powder for inj 50, 100-mg single-use vials (5 mg/mL); solution for inj 50 mg/10 mL, 100 mg/20 mL, 200 mg/40 mL

Administer:

Intermittent IV INFUSION route
• Premedicate with antiemetics including 5HT$_3$ blockers, with or without dexamethasone; prehydration not needed
• Do not reconstitute or dilute with sodium chloride or any chloride-containing sol; do not use aluminum equipment during any preparation or administration; will degrade platinum; do not refrigerate unopened powder or sol; do not freeze; protect from light
• Use cytotoxic handling procedures; prepare in biologic cabinet using gown, gloves, mask; do not allow product to come in contact with skin; use soap and water if contact occurs
• EPINEPHrine, antihistamines, corticosteroids for hypersensitivity reaction
• **Lyophilized powder:** reconstitute vial 50 mg/10 mL or 100 mg/20 mL sterile water for inj or D$_5$W; after reconstitution, sol may be stored for ≤24 hr in refrigerator; after dilution in 250-500 mL D$_5$W, may store ≤24 hr in refrigerator or 6 hr at room temperature; infuse over 2 hr
• **Aqueous solution:** dilute in 250-500 mL of D$_5$W; after dilution, may store ≤24 hr refrigerator, 6 hr at room temperature, infuse over 2 hr

Y-site compatibilities: Alfentanil, amifostine, amikacin, aminocaproic acid, amiodarone, amphotericin B colloidal, amphotericin B lipid complex, amphotericin B liposome, ampicillin, ampicillin-sulbactam, anidulafungin, atenolol, atracurium, azithromycin, aztreonam, bivalirudin, bleomycin, bumetanide, buprenorphine, butorphanol, calcium chloride/gluconate, CARBOplatin, caspofungin, ceFAZolin, cefotaxime, cefoTEtan, cefOXitin, cefTAZidime, ceftizoxime, cefTRIAXone, cefuroxime, chloramphenicol, chlorproMAZINE, cimetidine, ciprofloxacin, cisatracurium, CISplatin, clindamycin, cyclophosphamide, cycloSPORINE, cytarabine, dacarbazine, DACTINomycin, DAPTOmycin, DAUNOrubicin, dexamethasone, digoxin, diltiaZEM, diphenhydrAMINE, DOBUTamine, DOCEtaxel, dolasetron, DOPamine, doxacurium, DOXOrubicin, doxycycline, droperidol, enalaprilat, ePHEDrine, EPINEPHrine, epiRUBicin, ertapenem, erythromycin, esmolol, etoposide, famotidine, fenoldopam, fentaNYL, fluconazole, fludarabine, foscarnet, fosphenytoin, furosemide, gatifloxacin, gemcitabine, gemtuzumab, gentamicin, glycopyrrolate, granisetron, haloperidol, heparin, hydrALAZINE, hydrocortisone, HYDROmorphone, hydrOXYzine, IDArubicin, ifosfamide, imipenem-cilastatin, inamrinone, insulin (regular), irinotecan, isoproterenol, ketorolac, labetalol, leucovorin, levoFLOXacin, levorphanol, lidocaine, linezolid, LORazepam, magnesium sulfate, mannitol, meperidine, meropenem, mesna, metaraminol, methyldopate, methylPREDNISolone, metoclopramide, metoprolol, metroNIDAZOLE, midazolam, milrinone, minocycline, mitoMYcin, mitoXANTRONE, mivacurium, morphine, nafcillin, nalbuphine, naloxone, nesiritide, niCARdipine, nitroglycerin, nitroprusside, norepinephrine, octreotide, ondansetron, PACLitaxel, palonosetron, pancuronium, PEMEtrexed, pentamidine, pentazocine, phenylephrine, piperacillin, polymyxin B, potassium chloride/phosphates, procainamide, prochlorperazine, promethazine, propranolol, quiNIDine, quinupristin-dalfopristin, raNITIdine, rocuronium, sodium acetate/phosphates, succinylcholine, SUFentanil, sulfamethox-azole-trimethoprim, tacrolimus, tenipo-side, theophylline, thiotepa, ticarcillin, ticarcillin-clavulanate, tigecycline, tirofi-ban, tobramycin, tolazoline, topotecan, trimethobenzamide, vancomycin, vaso-pressin, vecuronium, verapamil, vinBLAS-tine, vinCRIStine, vinorelbine, voriconazole, zidovudine, zoledronic acid

SIDE EFFECTS

CNS: Peripheral neuropathy, fatigue, headache, dizziness, insomnia, reversible posterior leukoencephalopathy syndrome
CV: Cardiac abnormalities, thromboembolism
EENT: *Decreased visual acuity, tinnitus, hearing loss*
GI: *Severe nausea, vomiting, diarrhea, weight loss,* stomatitis, anorexia, gastro-esophageal reflux, constipation, dyspep-sia, mucositis, flatulence
GU: Hematuria, dysuria, creatinine
HEMA: Thrombocytopenia, leukopenia, pancytopenia, neutropenia, anemia, hemolytic uremic syndrome
INTEG: Rash, flushing, extravasation, redness, swelling, pain at inj site
META: Hypokalemia
RESP: Fibrosis, dyspnea, cough, rhinitis, URI, pharyngitis
SYST: Anaphylaxis, angioedema

PHARMACOKINETICS

Metabolized in liver, excreted in urine; after administration, 15% of platinum in systemic circulation, 85% either in tis-sues or being eliminated in urine; half-life 390 hr; protein binding >90%

INTERACTIONS

• **Increase:** QT prolongation: class Ia/III antidysrhythmics, monitor ECG
Increase: bleeding risk—NSAIDs, alco-hol, anticoagulants, platelet inhibitors, thrombolytics, salicylates
Increase: oxaliplatin toxicity—tannins
Increase: myelosuppression—myelo-suppressive agents, radiation
Increase: nephrotoxicity—aminoglyco-sides, loop diuretics
Decrease: antibody response—live virus vaccines

Drug/Lab Test
Increase: ALT, AST, bilirubin, creatinine
Decrease: potassium, neutrophils, WBC, platelets

NURSING CONSIDERATIONS
Assess:
• **Bone marrow depression:** CBC, differ-ential, platelet count each cycle; withhold product if WBC is <4000/mm³ or platelet count is <100,000/mm³; notify prescriber of results
• Renal/hepatic studies: BUN, creatinine, serum uric acid, urine CCr before, elec-trolytes during therapy; dose should not be given if BUN >19 mg/dL; creatinine <1.5 mg/dL; I&O ratio; report fall in urine output of <30 mL/hr; LFTs

Black Box Warning: **Anaphylaxis:** wheezing, tachycardia, facial swelling, fainting, rash, dyspnea, hives; discon-tinue product, report to prescriber; resus-citation equipment should be nearby with epinephrine, corticosteroids

• **Pulmonary fibrosis:** cough, crackles, dyspnea, pulmonary infiltrate; discontinue immediately; death may occur
• **Reversible posterior leukoencepha-lopathy syndrome:** assess for headache, seizures, diarrhea, infection, abnormal vision, change in mental functioning; dis-continue immediately
• Monitor temperature; may indicate be-ginning infection
• Hepatic studies before each cycle (bilirubin, AST, ALT, LDH) as needed or monthly
• **Bleeding:** hematuria, guaiac, bruising or petechiae, mucosa or orifices; obtain pre-scription for viscous lidocaine (Xylocaine)
• All medications PO if possible; avoid IM inj when platelets <100,000/mm³
• **Pregnancy/breastfeeding:** do not use in pregnancy, breastfeeding
Evaluate:
• Therapeutic response: decreased tu-mor size, spread of malignancy
Teach patient/family:
• **To report signs of infection:** increased temperature, sore throat, flulike symptoms

- To report signs of **anemia:** fatigue, headache, faintness, SOB, irritability
- To report **bleeding;** to avoid use of razors, commercial mouthwash
- To avoid aspirin, ibuprofen, NSAIDs, alcohol; may cause GI bleeding
- To report any changes in breathing, coughing
- To report numbness, tingling in face or extremities, poor hearing, or joint pain or swelling
- Not to receive live virus vaccines during treatment
- **Dysesthesias:** to avoid contact with cold (air, ice, liquid)
- To use contraception during treatment and for 4 mo after; that product may cause infertility

---

⚠ HIGH ALERT

oxazepam (Rx)

(ox-ay′ze-pam)

Novoxapam ♥, Oxpam ♥, Serax, Zapex ♥

Func. class.: Sedative/hypnotic; antianxiety

Chem. class.: Benzodiazepine, short acting

Controlled Substance Schedule IV

ACTION: Potentiates the actions of GABA, especially in the limbic system and the reticular formation

USES: Anxiety, alcohol withdrawal
Unlabeled uses: Insomnia

CONTRAINDICATIONS: Pregnancy, breastfeeding, children <6 yr, hypersensitivity to benzodiazepines, closed-angle glaucoma, psychosis
Precautions: Geriatric patients, debilitated patients, renal/hepatic disease, depression, suicidal ideation, dementia, sleep apnea, seizure disorder

Black Box Warning: Depressants, respiratory depression

DOSAGE AND ROUTES
Anxiety
- **Adult: PO** 10-15 mg tid-qid, max 120 mg/day
- **Geriatric: PO** 10 mg daily-bid, max 60 mg/day tid
Alcohol withdrawal
- **Adult: PO** 15-30 mg tid-qid
Severe anxiety syndrome, agitation, anxiety with depression
- **Adult/child >12 yr: PO** 15-30 mg tid
Available forms: Caps 10, 15, 30 mg
Administer:
- Without regard to food
- Taper product (0.5 mg q3days) before discontinuing

SIDE EFFECTS
CNS: *Dizziness, drowsiness,* confusion, headache, anxiety, tremors, fatigue, depression, insomnia, hallucinations, paradoxical excitement, transient amnesia
CV: *Orthostatic hypotension,* ECG changes, tachycardia, hypotension
EENT: *Blurred vision,* tinnitus, mydriasis
GI: Nausea, vomiting, anorexia, drug-induced hepatitis
HEMA: Leukopenia
INTEG: Rash, dermatitis, itching
SYST: Dependence

PHARMACOKINETICS
Peak 2-4 hr; metabolized by liver; excreted by kidneys; half-life 5-15 hr; crosses placenta, breast milk; protein binding 97%

INTERACTIONS

Black Box Warning: **Increase:** oxazepam effects, respiratory depression—CNS depressants, alcohol, disulfiram

Decrease: oxazepam effects—oral contraceptives, phenytoin, theophylline, valproic acid
Decrease: effects of levodopa
Drug/Herb
Increase: CNS depression—kava, melatonin, valerian
Drug/Lab Test
Increase: AST, ALT, serum bilirubin
Decrease: WBC

NURSING CONSIDERATIONS
Assess:
- CBC and LFTs periodically
- B/P (lying, standing), pulse; if systolic B/P drops 20 mm Hg, hold product, notify prescriber

Black Box Warning: **Respiratory depression:** not to be used in preexisting respiratory depression; use cautiously in severe pulmonary disease; monitor respirations

- Mental status: mood, sensorium, affect, sleeping pattern, drowsiness, dizziness, sedation, suicidal thoughts/behaviors
- **Physical dependency, withdrawal symptoms:** headache, nausea, vomiting, muscle pain, weakness, tremors, seizures (long-term use)
- **Beers:** avoid in older adults; delirium, cognitive impairment may occur
- **Pregnancy/breastfeeding:** assess for pregnancy before use; do not use in pregnancy; do not breastfeed

Evaluate:
- Therapeutic response: decreased anxiety, restlessness, insomnia

Teach patient/family:
- That product may be taken without regard to food
- That medication is not to be used for everyday stress or used >4 mo unless directed by prescriber; not to take more than prescribed dose because product may be habit forming
- To avoid OTC preparations (cough, cold, hay fever) unless approved by prescriber
- To avoid driving, activities that require alertness because drowsiness may occur
- To avoid alcohol, other psychotropic products unless directed by prescriber
- Not to discontinue product abruptly after long-term use
- To rise slowly because fainting may occur, especially among geriatric patients
- That drowsiness may worsen at beginning of treatment
- To notify prescriber if pregnancy is planned or suspected

OXcarbazepine (Rx)
(ox′kar-baz′uh-peen)
Trileptal, Oxtellar XR
Func. class.: Anticonvulsant
Chem. class.: CarBAMazepine analog

Do not confuse:
OXcarbazepine/carBAMazepine

ACTION: May inhibit nerve impulses by limiting influx of sodium ions across cell membrane in motor cortex

USES: Partial seizures
Unlabeled uses: Trigeminal neuralgia, atypical panic disorder, bipolar disorder

CONTRAINDICATIONS: Hypersensitivity
Precautions: Pregnancy, breastfeeding, children <4 yr, hypersensitivity to carBAMazepine, renal disease, fluid restriction, hyponatremia, abrupt discontinuation, suicidal ideation, ⚘ positive for HLA-B 1502 allele

DOSAGE AND ROUTES
Seizures, adjunctive therapy
- **Adult:** PO 300 mg bid, may be increased by 600 mg/day in divided doses bid at weekly intervals; maintenance 1200 mg/day; ext rel: 600 mg daily × 1 wk, increase weekly in 600 mg/day increments to 1200-2400 mg daily
- **Child 4-16 yr:** PO 8-10 mg/kg/day divided bid; dose determined by weight, increase by 5 mg/kg/day q3days, max doses weight dependent
- **Child 2 to <4 yr:** PO 8-10 mg/kg divided in 2 doses, max 600 mg/day

Conversion to monotherapy for partial seizures
- **Adult:** PO 300 mg bid with reduction in other anticonvulsants; increase OXcarbazepine by 600 mg/day each week over 2-4 wk; withdraw other anticonvulsants over 3-6 wk; max 2400 mg/day

Initiation of monotherapy for partial seizures
- **Adult:** PO 300 mg bid, increase by 300 mg/day q3days to 1200 mg in divided doses bid, max 2400 mg/day

---

Side effects: *italics* = common; red = life-threatening

Renal dose
• **Adult: PO** CCr <30 mL/min, 150 mg bid, increase slowly

Trigeminal neuralgia (unlabeled)
• **Adult: PO** 300 mg bid, may increase by ≤600 mg/day

Available forms: Film-coated tabs 150, 300, 600 mg; oral susp 300 mg/5 mL; ext rel tab 150, 300, 600 mg

Administer:

PO route
• Without regard to meals
• **Oral susp:** shake well, use calibrated oral syringe provided, use or discard within 7 days of opening
• **Ext rel:** do not crush, break, or chew
• Store at room temperature

SIDE EFFECTS

CNS: *Headache, dizziness, confusion, fatigue,* feeling abnormal, ataxia, abnormal gait, tremors, anxiety, agitation, worsening of seizures, suicidal thoughts/behaviors

CV: *Hypotension,* chest pain, edema, bradycardia, syncope

EENT: *Blurred vision, diplopia, nystagmus,* rhinitis, sinusitis

ENDO: Hypothyroidism, hot flashes

GI: *Nausea, constipation, diarrhea,* anorexia, vomiting, abdominal pain, gastritis

GU: Urinary frequency, hematuria, menses change

INTEG: Purpura, rash, acne

META: Hyponatremia

RESP: Flulike symptoms

SYST: Angioedema, anaphylaxis, Stevens-Johnson syndrome, toxic epidermal necrolysis, drug reaction with eosinophilia and systemic symptoms (DRESS)

PHARMACOKINETICS

PO: Onset unknown; peak 4-6 hr; metabolized by liver to active metabolite; terminal half-life 7-9 hr metabolite; inhibits P450 CYP2C19, induces CYP3A4/5, 95% renal extraction

INTERACTIONS

Increase: CNS depression—alcohol
Decrease: effects—felodipine, oral contraceptive, carBAMazepine

Decrease: OXcarbazepine levels—carBAMazepine, PHENobarbital, phenytoin, valproic acid, verapamil
Decrease: effect of substrates—CYP3A4 substrates (cycloSPORINE, itraconazole, rivaroxaban)

Drug/Herb
Increase: anticonvulsant effect—ginkgo
Decrease: anticonvulsant effect—ginseng, santonica

Drug/Lab Test
Decrease: sodium

NURSING CONSIDERATIONS

Assess:
• Description of seizures: frequency, duration, aura
• Hyponatremia: headache, nausea, confusion, usually within the first 3 mo of treatment, but may occur ≤1 yr, if this product is being used with other products that decrease sodium, monitor sodium levels
• Electrolyte: sodium; T_4; phenytoin (when given together)
• **Serious reactions:** angioedema, anaphylaxis, Stevens-Johnson syndrome
• CNS/mental status: mood, sensorium, affect, behavioral changes, confusion, suicidal thoughts/behaviors; if mental status changes, notify prescriber
• **Beers:** avoid in older adults unless safer alternatives are unavailable; ataxia, impaired psychomotor function may occur
• **Pregnancy/breastfeeding:** use only if benefits outweigh fetal risk; may cause lack of seizure control due to a metabolite of OXcarbazepine; monitor seizure control; enroll in the North American Antiepileptic Drug (NAAED) Pregnancy Registry, 888-233-2334; do not breastfeed

Evaluate:
• Therapeutic response: decreased seizure activity

Teach patient/family:
• To avoid driving, other activities that require alertness
• **Pregnancy/breastfeeding:** if pregnant, to enroll in North American Antiepileptic Drug Pregnancy Registry, 1-888-233-2334; not to breastfeed, excreted in breast milk

• Not to discontinue medication quickly after long-term use; seizures may increase

• To inform prescriber if hypersensitive to carBAMazepine; multisystem hypersensitivity may occur; to report fever, other allergic symptoms

• To avoid use of alcohol while taking product

• To use alternative contraception if using hormonal method; to report if pregnancy is planned or suspected

• To report skin rashes immediately; serious skin reactions can occur

• To report suicidal thoughts/behavior immediately

TREATMENT OF OVERDOSE:
Give 0.9% NaCl (hypotensive state), atropine (bradycardia); use benzodiazepines, barbiturates for seizures

---

oxybutynin (Rx, OTC)

(ox-i-byoo´ti-nin)

Ditropan XL, Gelnique, Oxyt ✤, Oxytrol, Oxytrol for Women Transdermal, Uromax ✤

Func. class.: Anticholinergic, urinary antispasmodic

Chem. class.: Synthetic tertiary amine

Do not confuse:
Ditropan/diazePAM/Diprivan

ACTION: Relaxes smooth muscles in urinary tract by inhibiting acetylcholine at postganglionic sites

USES: Antispasmodic for neurogenic bladder, overactive bladder in females (OTC)

CONTRAINDICATIONS: Hypersensitivity, GI obstruction, urinary retention, glaucoma, severe colitis, myasthenia gravis, unstable CV disease

Precautions: Pregnancy, breastfeeding, children <12 yr, geriatric patients, suspected glaucoma, cardiac disease, dementia

DOSAGE AND ROUTES

• **Adult: PO** 5 mg bid-tid, max 5 mg qid; **EXT REL** 5-10 mg/day, may increase by 5 mg, max 30 mg/day; **TD** apply 1 patch to abdomen, hip, buttock 2×/wk (q3-4 days); **GEL** apply contents of 1 packet to abdomen, upper arms, shoulders, thighs daily

• **Geriatric: PO** 2.5-5 mg bid-tid, increase by 2.5 mg q several days

• **Child >6 yr: PO** 5 mg bid, max 5 mg tid; **EXT REL** 5 mg/day, max 20 mg/day

• **Child 1-5 yr: PO** 0.2 mg/kg/dose bid-tid

Available forms: Syr 5 mg/5 mL; tabs 5 mg; ext rel tabs 5, 10, 15 mg; TD 3.9 mg/day; top gel 10% (Gelnique)

Administer:

PO route

• Do not crush, break, or chew ext rel tabs

• Without regard to meals

Topical route

• Wash hands; apply to clean, dry intact skin on abdomen, upper arms/shoulders, thighs; avoid navel, rotate sites

• Squeeze contents into palm of hand or directly on site, rub gently

• Do not bathe, exercise, swim for 1 hr after application

• Allow to dry before putting on clothing

• Do not be near flame, fire, or smoke until gel has dried

• Delivers 100 mg

Transdermal route

• Apply to clean, dry intact skin on abdomen, hip, buttock; use firm pressure; not affected by showering/bathing; rotate sites

• Delivers 3.9 mg/day

SIDE EFFECTS

CNS: *Anxiety, restlessness, dizziness, somnolence, insomnia, nervousness,* seizures, headache, *drowsiness,* confusion

CV: *Palpitations, sinus tachycardia,* hypertension, peripheral edema, QT prolongation

EENT: *Blurred vision, dry eyes,* increased intraocular tension, *dry mouth,* dry throat

GI: *Nausea, vomiting, anorexia,* abdominal pain, *constipation, dyspepsia,* diarrhea, taste perversion, GERD

Side effects: *italics* = common; red = life-threatening

GU: Dysuria, impotence, *urinary retention, hesitancy*

MISC: Hyperthermia, anaphylaxis, angioedema

PHARMACOKINETICS

Onset $1/_2$-1 hr, peak 3-6 hr, duration 6-10 hr; metabolized by liver, excreted in urine; terminal half-life 2-3 hr

INTERACTIONS

• Altered pharmacokinetic parameters: CYP3A4 inhibitors

Increase: CNS depression—benzodiazepines, sedatives, hypnotics, opioids

Increase: levels of atenolol, digoxin, nitrofurantoin

Increase: anticholinergic effects—antihistamines, amantidine, other anticholinergics

Increase or decrease: levels of phenothiazines

Decrease: levels of acetaminophen, haloperidol, levodopa

Decrease: effects of oxybutynin—CYP3A4 inducers

NURSING CONSIDERATIONS
Assess:

• **Urinary patterns:** distention, nocturia, frequency, urgency, incontinence, I&O ratios; cystometry to diagnose dysfunction, urinary tract infections should be treated

• **Allergic reactions:** rash, urticaria; if these occur, product should be discontinued; **angioedema:** swelling of face, tongue, throat

• **QT prolongation:** ECG for QT prolongation, ejection fraction; assess for chest pain, palpitations, dyspnea

• **CNS effects:** confusion, anxiety; anticholinergic effects in geriatric patients

• **Beers:** avoid in older adults; delirium risk is increased

• **Pregnancy/breastfeeding:** use only if benefit outweighs risks; cautious use in breastfeeding, excretion unknown

Evaluate:

• Absence of dysuria, frequency, nocturia, incontinence

Teach patient/family:

• To avoid hazardous activities because dizziness, blurred vision may occur

• To avoid OTC medications with alcohol, other CNS depressants

• To avoid hot weather, strenuous activity because product decreases perspiration

• About the correct application of each product form

• **Transdermal:** change patch 2×/wk; do not use same site within 7 days; dispose of and use container not accessible to pets/children

• To open patch immediately before using

• Do not use during MRI, remove

• **Topical gel:**

• Rotate sites

• Apply to clean, dry skin on abdomen, upper arm/shoulders/thighs

• Gel is flammable

⚠ HIGH ALERT

oxyCODONE (Rx)
(ox-i-koe′done)

Oxado, OxyCONTIN, Oxy IR ✦, RoxyBond, Supeudol ✦, Xtampza

oxyCODONE/acetaminophen (Rx)

Endocet, Nalocet, Percocet, Primlev, Roxicet

oxyCODONE/aspirin (Rx)

Endodan, Percodan

oxyCODONE/ibuprofen (Rx)

Func. class.: Opiate analgesic
Chem. class.: Semisynthetic derivative

Controlled Substance Schedule II

Do not confuse:
oxyCODONE/HYDROcodone

ACTION: Inhibits ascending pain pathways in CNS, increases pain threshold, alters pain perception

USES: Moderate to severe pain
Unlabeled uses: Postherpetic neuralgic (cont rel)

CONTRAINDICATIONS: Hypersensitivity, addiction (opiate), asthma, ileus

Black Box Warning: Respiratory depression

Precautions: Pregnancy, breastfeeding, child <18 yr, addictive personality, increased intracranial pressure, MI (acute), severe heart disease, renal/hepatic disease, bowel impaction

Black Box Warning: Opioid-naïve patients, substance abuse, accidental exposure, potential for overdose/poisoning, status asthmaticus

DOSAGE AND ROUTES
Severe Pain
• **Adult: PO** 10-30 mg q4hr (5-15 mg q4-6hr for opiate-naïve patients) Concentrated sol is extremely concentrated; do not use interchangeably; **CONT REL** 10 mg q12hr for opiate-naïve patients
• **Child >5 yr/adolescent: PO (unlabeled)** 0.2 mg/kg given 30 min preprocedural
Available forms: OxyCODONE: *cont rel tabs* (OxyCONTIN) 10, 15, 20, 30, 40, 80, 160 mg; *immediate rel tabs* 5, 7.5, 10, 15, 20, 30 mg; *immediate rel caps* 5 mg; *oral sol* 5 mg/5 mL, 20 mg/mL; **oxyCODONE with acetaminophen:** 2.5 mg/325 mg, 5 mg/325 mg, 7.5 mg/325 mg, 7.5 mg/300 mg, 10 mg/325 mg, *oral sol* 5 mg/325 mg/5 mL; *ext rel caps* 9, 13.5, 18, 27, 36 mg; **oxyCODONE with aspirin:** 4.835 mg/325 mg; **oxyCODONE with ibuprofen:** 5 mg/400 mg
Administer:
• Clarify all orders; fatalities have occurred
• Regular administration is more effective than PRN; give before pain becomes severe
• Discontinue gradually after long-term use
• Store in light-resistant area at room temperature

• OxyCODONE should be titrated from the initial recommended dosage to the dosage required to relieve pain
• There is no maximum dosage of oxyCODONE; however, careful titration is required until tolerance develops to some of the side effects (drowsiness, respiratory depression)
Oral solid formulations
Immediate-release tablets route
• May be administered with food or milk to minimize GI irritation
Extended-release caps route
• **Xtampza ER brand capsules:** take with food and the same amount of food
• Capsule contents may be sprinkled onto soft foods (applesauce, pudding, yogurt, ice cream, or jam) or into a cup and then given directly into the mouth; swallow immediately and rinse mouth
• Capsule contents may be given through an NG or gastrostomy tube. Flush tube with water. Open a capsule and pour the contents directly into the tube. Do not premix capsule contents with the liquid that will be used to flush the tube. Draw up 15 mL of water into a syringe, insert the syringe into the tube, and flush the contents through the tube. Repeat flushing twice using 10 mL of water with each flush. Extended-release 36-mg capsules are for use ONLY in opioid-tolerant patients
• Monitor patients closely for respiratory depression, particularly within the first 24-72 hr after initiation or dose escalation
Controlled-release tablets route (OxyCONTIN)
• Administer whole; do not crush, chew, or break in half; taking chewed, broken, or crushed controlled-release tablets could lead to the rapid release and absorption of a potentially toxic dose of oxyCODONE
• **OxyCONTIN brand tablets:** do not presoak, lick, or otherwise wet tablet before administering dose; administer 1 tablet at a time; allow patient to swallow each tablet separately with sufficient liquid
• **OxyCODONE controlled-release (OxyCONTIN)** 60-mg and 80-mg tablets are for use only in opioid-tolerant patients
• May be administered without food

Side effects: *italics* = common; red = life-threatening

Oral liquid formulations
Oral concentrate solution route

• Is a highly concentrated sol (20 mg oxyCODONE/mL), and care should be taken in dispensing and administering this medication; the sol may be added to 30 mL of a liquid or semisolid food; if the medication is placed in liquid or food, consume immediately; do not store diluted oxyCODONE for future use

SIDE EFFECTS

CNS: *Drowsiness, dizziness, confusion, headache, sedation, euphoria,* fatigue, abnormal dreams/thoughts, hallucinations
CV: Palpitations, bradycardia, change in B/P
EENT: Tinnitus, blurred vision, miosis, diplopia
GI: *Nausea, vomiting, anorexia, constipation, cramps,* gastritis, dyspepsia, biliary spasms
GU: Increased urinary output, dysuria, urinary retention
INTEG: *Rash,* urticaria, bruising, flushing, diaphoresis, pruritus
RESP: Respiratory depression

PHARMACOKINETICS

PO: Onset 15-30 min, peak 1 hr, duration reg rel 2-6 hr, cont rel 12 hr, metabolized by liver, excreted in urine, crosses placenta, excreted in breast milk, half-life 3-5 hr, protein binding 45%

INTERACTIONS

Increase: effects with other CNS depressants—alcohol, opioids, sedative/hypnotics, antipsychotics, skeletal muscle relaxants
Increase: oxyCODONE level—CYP3A4 inhibitors
Increase: toxicity—cimetidine, MAOIs
Drug/Herb
Increase: sedative effect—kava, St. John's wort, valerian
Drug/Lab Test
Increase: amylase, lipase

NURSING CONSIDERATIONS
Assess:

• **Pain:** intensity, location, type, characteristics; need for pain medication by pain/sedation scoring; physical dependence

• I&O ratio; check for decreasing output; may indicate urinary retention
• **CNS changes:** dizziness, drowsiness, hallucinations, euphoria, LOC, pupil reaction
• **Allergic reactions:** rash, urticaria

Black Box Warning: **Respiratory dysfunction:** respiratory depression, character, rate, rhythm; notify prescriber if respirations are <10/min; monitor B/P, pulse baseline and periodically

• **Bowel status:** constipation; stimulant laxative may be needed with fluids, fiber

Black Box Warning: **Substance abuse:** assess for substance abuse in patient/family/friends before prescribing; monitor for abuse, may crush, chew, snort, or inject ext rel product; may be fatal

Black Box Warning: **Accidental exposure:** dispose of properly away from pets, children

Black Box Warning: **Pregnancy/breastfeeding:** use only if benefits outweigh fetal risk; neonatal opioid withdrawal syndrome may occur with extended use; avoid breastfeeding, excreted in breast milk

• **Beers:** avoid in older adults; ataxia, impaired psychomotor function may occur
• Assistance with ambulation
• Safety measures: night-light, call bell within easy reach
Evaluate:
• Therapeutic response: decrease in pain without dependence
Teach patient/family:
• To report any symptoms of CNS changes, allergic reactions
• That physical dependency may result from extended use
• That withdrawal symptoms may occur after long-term use: nausea, vomiting, cramps, fever, faintness, anorexia

- To avoid CNS depressants, alcohol
- To avoid driving, operating machinery if drowsiness occurs

TREATMENT OF OVERDOSE: Naloxone (Narcan) 0.2-0.8 mg IV, O₂, IV fluids, vasopressors, caution with patients physically dependent on opioids

---

oxymetazoline nasal agent
See Appendix B

---

oxymetazoline ophthalmic
See Appendix B

⚠ HIGH ALERT

oxyMORphone (Rx)
(ox-i-mor′fone)
Opana, Numorphan ✦
Func. class.: Opiate analgesic
Chem. class.: Semisynthetic phenanthrene derivative

Controlled Substance Schedule II

Do not confuse:
oxyMORphone/oxyCODONE

ACTION: Inhibits ascending pain pathways in CNS, increases pain threshold, alters pain perception

USES: Moderate to severe pain

CONTRAINDICATIONS: Hypersensitivity, addiction (opiate), asthma, hepatic disease, ileus, intrathecal use, surgery

Black Box Warning: Respiratory depression

Precautions: Pregnancy (short-term), breastfeeding, children <18 yr, addictive personality, increased intracranial

pressure, MI (acute), severe heart disease, respiratory depression, renal/hepatic disease, bowel impaction

Black Box Warning: Alcoholism, opioid-naive patients, substance abuse

DOSAGE AND ROUTES
- **Adult:** 5-20 mg q4-6hr prn
Available forms: Tabs 5, 10 mg
Administer:
- 1 hr before or 2 hr after food (PO)
- With antiemetic for nausea, vomiting
- When pain is beginning to return; determine interval by response
- Store in light-resistant area at room temperature

SIDE EFFECTS
CNS: *Drowsiness, dizziness, confusion, headache,* hallucinations, increased intracranial pressure, *sedation,* seizures, *euphoria (geriatric patients)*
CV: Palpitations, bradycardia, change in B/P, hypotension
EENT: Tinnitus, blurred vision, miosis, diplopia
GI: *Nausea, vomiting, anorexia, constipation, cramps*
GU: Dysuria, urinary retention
INTEG: *Rash,* urticaria, bruising, flushing, diaphoresis, pruritus
RESP: Respiratory depression

PHARMACOKINETICS
Metabolized by liver, excreted in urine, crosses placenta, half life: PO: 7-9 hr, ext rel: 9-11 hr
PO: Peak 1 hr (fasting)

INTERACTIONS
- **Increase:** effects with other CNS depressants—alcohol, opiates, sedative/hypnotics, antipsychotics, skeletal muscle relaxants
- **Increase:** unpredictable effects/reactions—MAOIs

Drug/Herb
Increase: sedative effect—kava, St. John's wort, valerian
Drug/Lab Test
Increase: amylase

O

Side effects: *italics* = common; red = life-threatening

NURSING CONSIDERATIONS
Assess:
- **Pain:** location, intensity, type, other characteristics before and after need for pain medication, physical dependence, give 25%-50% until pain reduction of 50% on pain rating scale, repeat dose may be given at time of peak if previous dose does not control pain and respiratory depression has not occurred
- **I&O ratio** for decreasing output; may indicate urinary retention
- **Bowel status:** constipation; may need stimulative laxative if use ≥3 days; increased fluids, fiber for prevention
- **CNS changes:** dizziness, drowsiness, hallucinations, euphoria, LOC, pupil reaction
- **Allergic reactions:** rash, urticaria

Black Box Warning: **Respiratory dysfunction:** respiratory depression, character, rate, rhythm; notify prescriber if respirations are <10/min; dose may need to be decreased by 25%-50%; monitor B/P, pulse also

Black Box Warning: **Accidental exposure:** dispose of properly, away from children/pets

Black Box Warning: **Overdose/poisoning:** avoid alcohol ingestion, do not crush, chew, snort, or inject tabs, high abuse potential

Black Box Warning: **Opioid-naive patients:** ext rel tabs are not to be used immediately postop (12-24 hr after surgery) in these patients

- **Pregnancy/breastfeeding:** use only if benefits outweigh fetal risk; neonatal opioid withdrawal syndrome may occur with extended use; avoid breastfeeding
- **Beers:** avoid use in older adults; ataxia, impaired psychomotor function may occur

Evaluate:
- Therapeutic response: decrease in pain

Teach patient/family:
- To report any symptoms of CNS changes, allergic reactions
- That physical dependency may result from extended use
- That withdrawal symptoms may occur: nausea, vomiting, cramps, fever, faintness, anorexia
- Not to drive or operate machinery if drowsiness occurs
- Not to use other CNS depressants, alcohol
- To make position changes slowly to prevent orthostatic hypotension
- To notify health care professional if pregnancy is planned or suspected; avoid breastfeeding
- To notify prescriber of all OTC, Rx, herbs, supplements being taken; not to take new products unless approved by prescriber

TREATMENT OF OVERDOSE:
Naloxone (Narcan) 0.2-0.8 mg IV (caution with patients physically dependent on opioids), O₂, IV fluids, vasopressors

---

⚠ HIGH ALERT

oxytocin (Rx)
(ox-i-toe′sin)
Pitocin, Syntocinon ✦
Func. class.: Hormone
Chem. class.: Oxytocic, uterine-active agent

ACTION: Acts directly on myofibrils, thereby producing uterine contraction; stimulates milk ejection by the breast; vasoactive antidiuretic effect

USES: Stimulation, induction of labor; missed or incomplete abortion; postpartum bleeding

CONTRAINDICATIONS: Hypersensitivity, serum toxemia, cephalopelvic disproportion, fetal distress, hypertonic uterus, prolapsed umbilical cord, active genital herpes

Precautions: Cervical/uterine surgery, uterine sepsis, primipara >35 yr, 1st/2nd stage of labor

Black Box Warning: Elective induction of labor

DOSAGE AND ROUTES
Postpartum hemorrhage
- **Adult: IV** 10-40 units in 1000 mL non-hydrating diluent infused at 20-40 mU/min
- **Adult: IM** 3-10 units after delivery of placenta

Contraction stress test (CST)
- **Adult: IV** 0.5 mU/min, increase q20min until 3 contractions within 10 min

Stimulation of labor
- **Adult: IV** 0.5-2 mU/min, increase by 1-2 mU q15-60min until contractions occur, then decrease dose

Incomplete abortion
- **Adult: IV INFUSION** 10 units/500 mL D$_5$W or 0.9% NaCl at 10-20 mU/min, max 30 units/12 hr

Available forms: Inj 10 units/mL
Administer:
- Give by IV infusion or IM
- Before use, an IV infusion of NS should be already running for use in case of adverse reactions. Magnesium sulfate should be readily available if relaxation of the myometrium is needed
- Visually inspect parenteral product for particulate matter and discoloration before use

IV infusion route
- Administer using an infusion pump to ensure accurate dosing

Induction of labor
- Dilute 1 mL (10 units) in 1000 mL of a compatible IV infusion solution. Rotate infusion bottle for thorough mixing. The resultant infusion should contain 10 milliunits/mL

Control of postpartum uterine bleeding
- Dilute 10-40 units in a compatible IV solution or to an already infusing solution. The maximum concentration is 40 units in 1000 mL of solution

Incomplete, inevitable, or elective abortion
- Dilute 10 units in 500 mL of a compatible IV solution

IM route
- Inject into a large muscle mass; aspirate before injection to avoid injection into a blood vessel

Y-site compatibilities: Acyclovir, alfentanil, allopurinol, amikacin, aminocaproic acid, aminophylline, amphotericin B liposome (ambisome), anidulafungin, argatroban, ascorbic acid injection, atenolol, atracurium, atropine, azaTHIOprine, azithromycin, aztreonam, benztropine, bivalirudin, bumetanide, buprenorphine, butorphanol, calcium chloride/gluconate, capreomycin, caspofungin, cefamandole, ceFAZolin, cefepime, cefoperazone, cefotaxime, cefoTEtan, cefOXitin, cefTAZidime, ceftizoxime, cefTRIAXone, cefuroxime, chloramphenicol, chlorothiazide, chlorpheniramine, cimetidine, ciprofloxacin, cisatracurium, clindamycin, cloxacillin, colistimethate, cyanocobalamin, cyclophosphamide, cycloSPORINE, DAPTOmycin, dexamethasone, dexmedetomidine, digoxin, dilTIAZem, diphenhydrAMINE, DOBUTamine, dolasetron, DOPamine, doxycycline, droperidol, edetate calcium disodium, enalaprilat, ePHEDrine, EPINEPHrine, epoetin alfa, eptifibatide, ergonovine, ertapenem, erythromycin, esmolol, famotidine, fenoldopam, fentaNYL, fluconazole, folic acid (as sodium salt), foscarnet, fosphenytoin, furosemide, gallamine, ganciclovir, gatifloxacin, gentamicin, glycopyrrolate, granisetron, heparin, hydrocortisone sodium succinate, HYDROmorphone, hydrOXYzine, imipenem-cilastatin, isoproterenol, kanamycin, ketamine, ketorolac, labetalol, lactated Ringer's injection, lansoprazole, lepirudin, leucovorin, levoFLOXacin, lidocaine, lincomycin, linezolid, LORazepam, magnesium sulfate, mannitol, mechlorethamine, meperidine, mephentermine, meropenem, metaraminol, methyldopa, methylPREDNISolone, metoclopramide, metoprolol, metroNIDAZOLE, midazolam, milrinone, minocycline, morphine, moxifloxacin, multiple vitamins injection, mycophenolate mofetil, nafcillin, nalbuphine, nalorphine, naloxone, nesiritide, netilmicin, niCARdipine, nitroglycerin, nitroprusside, norepinephrine, ondansetron, oxacillin, palonosetron, pamidronate, papaverine, penicillin G potassium/sodium, pentamidine, pentazocine, PENTobarbital, PHENobarbital, phentolamine, phenylephrine, phytonadione, piperacillin sodium, piperacillin-tazobactam, polymyxin B, potassium acetate/chloride/phosphates, procainamide, prochlorperazine, promazine, promethazine, propranolol, protamine, pyridoxine, quinupristin-dalfopristin, raNITIdine, Ringer's injection, sodium acetate/bicarbonate/phosphates, streptomycin, succinylcholine, SUFentanil, tacrolimus, theophylline, thiamine hydrochloride, ticarcillin disodium, ticarcillin disodium-clavulanate potassium, tigecycline, tirofiban hydrochloride, tobramycin sulfate, tolazoline, trimetaphan, tubocurarine, urokinase, vancomycin, vasopressin, verapamil, vitamin B complex with B, voriconazole, warfarin, zidovudine, zoledronic acid.

SIDE EFFECTS

CNS: Seizures, tetanic contractions
CV: Hypo/hypertension, dysrhythmias, increased pulse, bradycardia, tachycardia, PVC
FETUS: Dysrhythmias, jaundice, hypoxia, intracranial hemorrhage
GI: Anorexia, nausea, vomiting, constipation
GU: Abruptio placentae, decreased uterine blood flow
HEMA: Increased hyperbilirubinemia
INTEG: Rash
RESP: Asphyxia
SYST: Water intoxication of mother

PHARMACOKINETICS

IM: Onset 3-7 min, duration 1 hr, half-life 12-17 min
IV: Onset 1 min, duration 30 min, half-life 12-17 min

INTERACTIONS

• **Increase:** hypertension—vasopressors
Drug/Herb
• **Increase:** hypertension—ephedra

NURSING CONSIDERATIONS
Assess:

• Assess for fetal presentation, pelvic dimensions before use
• B/P, pulse; watch for changes that may indicate hemorrhage
• Respiratory rate, rhythm, depth; notify prescriber of abnormalities
• Monitor continuously, discontinue immediately if fetal distress occurs or uterine hyperactivity occurs
• Length, intensity, duration of contraction; notify prescriber of contractions lasting >1 min or absence of contractions; turn patient on her left side; discontinue oxytocin
• **FHTs, fetal distress;** watch for acceleration, deceleration; notify prescriber if problems occur; fetal presentation, pelvic dimensions; turn patient on left side if FHT change in rate, give O_2
• **Water intoxication:** confusion, anuria, drowsiness, headache; monitor I&O

Black Box Warning: Elective induction of labor: use for induction only when medically necessary

Evaluate:
• Therapeutic response: stimulation of labor, control of postpartum bleeding
Teach patient/family:
• To report increased blood loss, abdominal cramps, fever, foul-smelling lochia, nausea, blurred vision, itching, swelling
• That contractions will be similar to menstrual cramps, gradually increasing in intensity

⚠ HIGH ALERT

PACLitaxel (Rx)

(pa-kli-tax′el)

PACLitaxel Protein Bound particle (Rx)

Abraxane

Func. class.: Antineoplastic—miscellaneous

Chem. class.: Taxane

Do not confuse:
PACLitaxel/PARoxetine/Paxil

ACTION: Inhibits reorganization of microtubule network needed for interphase and mitotic cellular functions; causes abnormal bundles of microtubules during cell cycle and multiple esters of microtubules during mitosis

USES: **PACLitaxel:** metastatic carcinoma of the ovary, breast; AIDS-related Kaposi's sarcoma (2nd-line), non–small-cell lung cancer (1st-line), adjuvant treatment for node-positive breast cancer, prostate cancer, esophageal cancer, melanoma
PACLitaxel Protein Bound Particles: metastatic breast cancer after failure or relapse, metastatic pancreatic adenocarcinoma refractory prostate cancer, bladder cancer

CONTRAINDICATIONS: Pregnancy; hypersensitivity to PACLitaxel or other products with polyoxyethylated castor oil, albumin

Black Box Warning: Neutropenia <1500/mm³

Precautions: Breastfeeding, children, females, geriatric patients, cardiovascular/hepatic/renal disease, CNS disorder, bone marrow suppression, dental disease, dental work, extravasation, herpes, infection, infertility, jaundice, ocular exposure, radiation therapy, thrombocytopenia, vaccination

Black Box Warning: Taxane hypersensitivity, bone marrow suppression, requires a specialized care setting, requires an experienced clinician

DOSAGE AND ROUTES
PACLitaxel
Ovarian carcinoma
• **Adult: IV INFUSION** 135 mg/m² given over 24 hr q3wk, then CISplatin 75 mg/m²; or (refractory or metastatic) 175 mg/m² over 3 hr q3wk; or 175 mg/m² over 3 hr
Advanced ovarian carcinoma
• **Adult: IV INFUSION** 175 mg/m² with CISplatin 75 mg/m² using a 3-hr regimen q3wk
Breast carcinoma
• **Adult: IV INFUSION** 175 mg/m² over 3 hr q3wk × 4 courses
AIDS-related Kaposi's sarcoma
• **Adult: IV INFUSION** 135 mg/m² over 3 hr q3wk or 100 mg/m² over 3 hr q2wk
First-line non–small-cell lung cancer
• **Adult: IV INFUSION** 135 mg/m²/24 hr infusion with CISplatin 75 mg/m² × 3 wk
Hepatic dose
• **Adult:** Dose reduction for 135 mg/m² 24-hr **IV INFUSION**—AST/ALT 2-10 × ULN, total bilirubin ≤1.5 mg/dL: give 100 mg/m²; AST/ALT <10 × ULN, total bilirubin 1.6-7.5 mg/dL: 50 mg/m²; AST/ALT ≥10 × ULN or total bilirubin >7.5 mg/dL: avoid use
• **Adult:** Dose reduction for 175 mg/m² 3-hr **IV INFUSION**—AST/ALT <10 × ULN, total bilirubin 1.26-2 × ULN: give 135 mg/m²; AST/ALT <10 × ULN, total bilirubin 2.01-5 × ULN: 90 mg/m²; AST/ALT ≥10 × ULN or total bilirubin >5 × ULN: avoid use

PACLitaxel protein-bound particles
Non–small-cell lung cancer, advanced or metastatic, first-line treatment, in combination with carboplatin
• **Adult: IV** 100 mg/m² over 30 min on days 1, 8, and 15 of each 21-day cycle; carboplatin dosed to an AUC 6 mg × mL/min on day 1 only of each 21-day cycle, beginning immediately after completion of paclitaxel

P

Side effects: *italics* = common; red = life-threatening

Breast cancer
• **Adult:** IV 260 mg/m^2 q3wk

Pancreatic cancer
• **Adult:** IV 125 mg/m^2 over 30-40 min on days 1, 8, 15 of each 28-day cycle

Available forms: Inj 6 mg/5mL, powder for inj, lyophilized 100 mg in single-use vials (Abraxane)

Administer:
• If CISplatin is given, use after taxane
• Confirmation that dexamethasone was given 12 hr and 6 hr before infusion begins
• Store prepared sol up to 27 hr in refrigerator

Continuous IV INFUSION route
• After premedicating with dexamethasone 20 mg PO 12 hr and 6 hr before PACLitaxel, diphenhydrAMINE 50 mg IV $^1/_2$-1 hr before PACLitaxel and cimetidine 300 mg or ranitidine 50 mg IV $^1/_2$-1 hr before PACLitaxel
• Assess for extravasation if given by regular IV, not port

PACLitaxel

Continuous IV INFUSION
• Dilute 30 mg vial/5 mL
• After diluting in 0.9% NaCl, D$_5$W, D$_5$ and 0.9% NaCl, D$_5$LR (0.3-1.2 mg/mL), chemo dispensing pin or similar devices with spikes should not be used in vials of Taxol; use in-line filter ≤0.22 micron; give as 3-hr (breast cancer, Kaposi sarcoma) or 24-hr infusion (ovarian cancer)
• Using only glass bottles, polypropylene, polyolefin bags, and administration sets; do not use PVC infusion bags or sets

Y-site compatibilities: Acyclovir, amikacin, aminophylline, ampicillin/sulbactam, bleomycin, butorphanol, calcium chloride, CARBOplatin, cefepime, cefoTEtan, cefTAZidime, cefTRIAXone, cimetidine, CISplatin, cladribine, cyclophosphamide, cytarabine, dacarbazine, dexamethasone, diphenhydrAMINE, DOXOrubicin, droperidol, etoposide, famotidine, floxuridine, fluconazole, fluorouracil, furosemide, ganciclovir, gentamicin, granisetron, haloperidol, heparin, hydrocortisone, HYDROmorphone, ifosfamide, LORazepam, magnesium sulfate, mannitol, meperidine, mesna, methotrexate, metoclopramide, morphine, nalbuphine, ondansetron, pentostatin, potassium chloride, prochlorperazine, propofol, raNITIdine, sodium bicarbonate, thiotepa, vancomycin, vinBLAStine, vinCRIStine, zidovudine

PACLitaxel Protein Bound Particles

Intermittent IV INFUSION route
• No premedication for allergic reaction is needed
• Reconstitute vial by injecting 20 mL of 0.9% NaCl; slowly inject 20 mL of 0.9% NaCl over at least 1 min to direct sol flow on wall of vial (5 mg/mL); do not inject 0.9% NaCl directly onto lyophilized cake (foaming will occur); allow vial to sit for at least 15 min to ensure proper wetting of lyophilized cake; gently swirl or invert vial slowly for ≥2 min until completely dissolved, should look milky
• Calculate dose by dosing vol/mL = total dose (mg) ÷ 5 (mg/mL)
• Use PVC IV bag, do not use filter
• Solution is stable for 8 hr refrigerated
• Give over 30 min

SIDE EFFECTS

CNS: *Peripheral neuropathy, dizziness, headache, seizures*
CV: Bradycardia, *hypotension,* abnormal ECG, supraventricular tachycardia (SVT)
GI: *Nausea, vomiting, diarrhea, mucositis, stomatitis,* pancreatitis
HEMA: Neutropenia, leukopenia, thrombocytopenia, anemia
INTEG: *Alopecia,* tissue necrosis, generalized urticaria, *flushing*
MS: *Arthralgia, myalgia*
RESP: Pulmonary embolism, dyspnea, cough
SYST: *Hypersensitivity reactions,* anaphylaxis, Stevens-Johnson syndrome, toxic epidermal necrolysis, angioedema
GU: Renal failure

PHARMACOKINETICS

89%-98% of product serum protein bound, metabolized in liver, excreted in bile and urine; terminal half-life 5.3-17.4 hr

INTERACTIONS
Increase: myelosuppression—other anti-neoplastics, radiation

Increase: DOXOrubicin levels—DOXOrubicin

Increase: toxicity—gemfibrozil

Increase: effect, toxicity—CYP3A4 inhibitors (clarithromycin, indinavir, ketoconazole, ritonavir, saquinavir)

Decrease: effect, treatment failure—CYP3A4 inducers (carBAMazepine, phenytoin, rifAMPin)

Decrease: immune response—live virus vaccines

Drug/Lab Test
Increase: AST/ALT, alk phos, triglycerides

Decrease: neutrophils, platelets, WBC, Hgb

NURSING CONSIDERATIONS
Assess:

Black Box Warning: Requires a specialized care setting such as a hospital or facility with management of complications; should be used by a clinician experienced in cytotoxic agents

Black Box Warning: **Bone marrow suppression:** CBC, differential, platelet count before treatment and weekly; withhold product if WBC is <1500/mm^3 or platelet count is <100,000/mm^3; notify prescriber

• **Cardiovascular status:** ECG continuously in CV conditions; monitor for hypotension, sinus bradycardia/tachycardia

• **Peripheral neuropathy:** paresthesias, numbness; during infusion, use ice packs on extremities to lessen continued neuropathy; may use acupuncture for some relief; use of ice on extremities when infusing

• **Arthralgia, myalgia:** may begin 2-3 days after infusion and continue for 4-5 days; may use analgesics

• **Nausea, vomiting:** premedicate with antiemetics; nausea and vomiting occur often

• **Stevens-Johnson syndrome:** rash, fever, blisters, discontinue immediately if these occur

• **PACLitaxel:** CBC and differential baseline and periodically, leukocytes <1500/mm, platelets 100,000/mm^3 hold, nadir is 11 days (leukopenia) recovery 15-21 days

• **PACLitaxel Protein Bound Particles:** CBC and differential on days 1, 8, 15, hold if neutrophils <1500/mm^3 x 1 wk, reduce all doses

• Hepatic studies before, during therapy (bilirubin, AST, ALT, LDH) prn or monthly, check for jaundiced skin and sclera, dark urine, clay-colored stool, itchy skin, abdominal pain, fever, diarrhea

• VS during 1st hr of infusion, check IV site for signs of infiltration

Black Box Warning: **Hypersensitivity reactions, anaphylaxis:** hypotension, dyspnea, angioedema, generalized urticaria; discontinue infusion immediately; keep emergency equipment available, monitor continuously during first 30-60 min, then periodically, usually occurs in first few minutes, pretreat with dexamethasone, diphenhydramine

• **Flush:** for mild to moderate flush, may continue diphenhydrAMINE for ≤48 hr

• Effects of alopecia on body image; discuss feelings about body changes

• **Pregnancy/breastfeeding:** do not use in pregnancy, breastfeeding

Evaluate:
• Therapeutic response: decreased tumor size, spread of malignancy

Teach patient/family:
• To report signs of infection: fever, sore throat, flulike symptoms

• To report signs of anemia: fatigue, headache, faintness, SOB, irritability

• To report bleeding; to avoid use of razors, commercial mouthwash; to use soft-bristle toothbrush; to use viscous xylocaine or compounded formula for stomatitis

• To avoid use of aspirin, ibuprofen

• To avoid crowds, persons with known infections

• That hair may be lost during treatment; that a wig or hairpiece may make patient feel better; that new hair may be different in color, texture

P

• That pain in muscles and joints 2-5 days after infusion is common
• To notify prescriber if pregnancy is planned or suspected; do not breastfeed
• To avoid receiving vaccinations while taking product

⚠ HIGH ALERT

palbociclib

(pal-boe-sye′klib)

Ibrance

Func. class.: Antineoplastic
Chem. class.: Signal transduction inhibitor, kinase inhibitor

---

ACTION: Inhibits progression of the cell cycle from G_1 into S phase, decreased proliferation of ER-positive breast cancer cell lines. When combined with antiestrogen therapy (letrozole), decreases retinoblastoma protein (Rb) phosphorylation, reducing E2F expression and signaling and increasing growth arrest

USES: Treatment of estrogen receptor (ER)–positive, HER2-negative advanced breast cancer in postmenopausal women, in combination with letrozole as initial endocrine-based therapy

CONTRAINDICATIONS: Hypersensitivity, pregnancy, lactation
Precautions: children, fungal/viral infection, infants, infertility, neutropenia, testicular failure, thromboembolic disease

DOSAGE AND ROUTES
Hormone receptor (HR)-positive, HER2-negative advanced or metastatic breast cancer
• **Adult females: PO** 125 mg daily with food × 21 days, followed by 7 days off
Available forms: Caps 75, 100, 125 mg
Administer:
• Give at the same time of the day with food and letrozole, capsules should be swallowed whole, do not cut, open, chew, do not use if capsule is not intact
Treatment-related hepatotoxicity:
• **Grade 1 or 2 hepatotoxicity:** No dosage change

• **Grade ≥3 hepatotoxicity (AST or ALT >5 × ULN or total bilirubin >3 × ULN) that persists despite medical treatment:** Hold until toxicity resolves to grade ≤2 (AST or ALT ≤5 × ULN or total bilirubin ≤3 × ULN), resume treatment at the next lower dose level if not considered a safety risk for the patient; discontinue if grade ≥3 toxicity occurs at a dose of 75 mg/day
Treatment-related nephrotoxicity:
• **Grade 1 or 2 nephrotoxicity:** No change
• **Grade ≥3 nephrotoxicity (CCr >3 × baseline or >4 mg/dL, or requiring hospitalization or dialysis) that persists despite medical treatment:** Hold therapy. When toxicity resolves to grade ≤2 (CCr <3 × baseline or <4 mg/dL), resume at the next lower dose level if not considered a safety risk for the patient, discontinue if grade ≥3 toxicity occurs at a dose of 75 mg/day
Other dosage adjustments
• **Strong CYP3A4 inhibitors:** Avoid concomitant use. If a strong CYP3A4 inhibitor is needed, consider reducing the dose to 75 mg daily; if the strong CYP3A4 inhibitor is discontinued, increase the dose upward to the previously tolerated/recommended dose after a washout period of 3-5 half-lives of the inhibitor
• **Strong CYP3A4 inducers:** Avoid use

SIDE EFFECTS
CNS: Weakness, fever, fatigue
EENT: Stomatitis, oral ulceration, glossitis, pharyngitis, sinusitis, epistaxis
GI: Vomiting, nausea, anorexia, diarrhea
HEMA: Thrombocytopenia, neutropenia, leukopenia, lymphopenia, anemia
MISC: Peripheral neuropathy, alopecia, infection, pulmonary embolism, thromboembolism

PHARMACOKINETICS
85% protein bound, elimination half-life was 24-34 hr, metabolized by CYP3A, peak 6-12 hr

INTERACTIONS
Avoid use with CYP3A inhibitors and inducers
Drug/Herb
• Avoid use with St. John's wort

Drug/Food
• Avoid use with grapefruit juice

NURSING CONSIDERATIONS
Assess:
• **Pulmonary embolism/thromboembolic events:** dyspnea/shortness of breath, chest pain, arm or leg swelling, sudden numbness or weakness, severe headache or confusion, or problems with vision, speech, or balance
• **Blood dyscrasias:** CBC/differential prior to and q2wk first 2 cycles, then before each cycle or if change in symptoms
• **Pregnancy:** product can cause fetal harm; identify if the patient is pregnant or if pregnancy is planned
Evaluate: Therapeutic response: decreased progression of disease
Teach patient/family:
• Identify if pregnancy is planned or suspected. Discuss the need for contraception due to possible fetal harm; avoid breastfeeding
• That laboratory testing will be needed during treatment
• Do not take with grapefruit juice
• **Pulmonary/thromboembolic events:** to seek medical attention if dyspnea/shortness of breath, chest pain, arm or leg swelling, sudden numbness or weakness, severe headache or confusion, or problems with vision, speech, or balance develop
• To take as prescribed, not to double or skip dose, review "Patient Information Sheet"
• To notify provider of infection
• To discuss all OTC, Rx, herbals, supplements taken

---

paliperidone (Rx)
(pal-ee-per'i-done)
Invega, Invega Sustenna, Invega Trinza
Func. class.: Antipsychotic, 2nd generation
Chem. class.: Benzisoxazole derivative

Do not confuse:
Invega/Iveegam
paliperidone/risperiDONE

ACTION: Mediated through both DOPamine type 2 (D_2) and serotonin type 2 (5-HT_2) antagonism

USES: Schizophrenia, schizoaffective disorder

CONTRAINDICATIONS: Breastfeeding, geriatric patients, seizure disorders, AV block, QT prolongation, torsades de pointes; hypersensitivity to this product, risperidone
Precautions: Pregnancy, children, renal/hepatic disease, obesity, Parkinson's disease, suicidal ideation, diabetes mellitus, hematological disease

Black Box Warning: Dementia-related psychosis (mortality)

DOSAGE AND ROUTES
• **Adult: PO** 6 mg/day, max 12 mg/day; **IM (Invega Sustenna)** 234 mg on day 1, then 156 mg 1 wk later; after 2nd dose, give 117 mg each mo; range 39-234 mg; **(Invega Trinza)** dose based on previous 1-mo injection dose of Invega Sustenna; if last dose of Invega Sustenna was 78 mg, give 273 mg of Invega Trinza; if last dose of Invega Sustenna was 117 mg, give 410 mg of Invega Trinza; if last dose of Invega Sustenna was 156 mg, give 546 mg of Invega Trinza; if last dose of Invega Sustenna was 234 mg, give 819 mg of Invega Trinza; give dose q3mo, adjust as needed
• **Child/adolescent ≥12 yr and ≥51 kg: PO** 3 mg daily, may increase if needed by 3 mg/day in intervals of >5 days, up to max 12 mg/day; <51 kg max 6 mg/day
Renal dose
• **Adult: PO** CCr 50-79 mL/min, 3 mg/day, max 6 mg/day; **EXT REL/IM** 156 mg on day 1, 117 mg 1 wk later, then 78 mg each mo; CCr 10-49 mL/min, 1.5 mg/day, max 3 mg/day; **IM** not recommended
Available forms: Ext rel tabs 1.5, 3, 6, 9 mg; ext rel susp for inj 39 mg/0.25 mL, 78

P

Side effects: *italics* = common; red = life-threatening

mg/0.5 mL, 117 mg/0.75 mL, 156 mg/mL, 234 mg/1.5 mL; Invega Trinza extended-release suspension 273, 410, 546, 819 mg

Administer:
• Avoid use with CNS depressants

PO route
• Do not break, crush, or chew ext rel tabs; use plenty of water
• Without regard for food
• Reduced dose for geriatric patients

IM route
• Use for IM only; do not use IV or subcut; inj kits contain prefilled syringe and 2 safety needles; for single use only; shake for 10 sec; **deltoid inj:** ≥90 kg, use 1.5-inch, 22-G needle; <90 kg, use 1-inch, 23-G needle; alternate injections between deltoid muscles; **gluteal inj:** use 1.5-inch, 22-G needle; attach needle to Luer connection in clockwise motion; pull needle sheath away using straight pull; bring syringe with attached needle upright to de-aerate, de-aerate, inject; after inj, use finger, thumb, or flat surface to activate needle protection system until click heard; use deltoid × 2 doses

SIDE EFFECTS

CNS: *EPS, pseudoparkinsonism, akathisia, dystonia, tardive dyskinesia; drowsiness, insomnia, agitation, anxiety, headache,* seizures, neuroleptic malignant syndrome, dizziness, suicidal thoughts/behaviors

CV: Orthostatic hypotension, tachycardia; heart failure, QT prolongation, dysrhythmias

EENT: Blurred vision, cough

ENDO: Hyperinsulinemia, weight gain, hyperglycemia, dyslipidemia

GI: *Nausea,* vomiting, *anorexia, constipation,* weight gain in adolescents, xerostomia

GU: Priapism, menstrual irregularities, impotence, priapism

MS: Back pain

MISC: Angioedema, anaphylaxis

HEMA: Agranulocytosis, leukopenia, neutropenia

PHARMACOKINETICS

Peak 24 hr; elimination half-life 23 hr; excreted 80% urine, 11% feces, protein binding >74%

INTERACTIONS

Increase: sedation—other CNS depressants, alcohol, sedative/hypnotics, opiates

Increase: QT prolongation—class IA, III antidysrhythmics, azole antifungals, tricyclics (high doses), some phenothiazines, β-blockers, chloroquine, pimozide, droperidol, some antipsychotics, abarelix, alfuzosin, amoxapine, apomorphine, dasatinib, dolasetron, flecainide, halogenated anesthetics

Increase: neurotoxicity—lithium

Increase: orthostatic hypotension—antihypertensives, nitrates

Increase: effect of paliperidone, dose may need to be decreased

Increase: serotonin syndrome, neuroleptic malignant syndrome—SSRIs, SNRIs

Decrease: levels of carBAMazepine, increased dose of paliperidone may be needed

Decrease: effect of paliperidone—carBAMazepine, other CYP3A4 inducers

Decrease: levodopa effect—levodopa

Drug/Lab Test
Increase: prolactin levels

NURSING CONSIDERATIONS
Assess:

> Black Box Warning: **Mental status:** mood, behavior, confusion, orientation, suicidal thoughts/behaviors; dementia, especially in geriatric patients before initial administration and periodically

• **QT prolongation:** ECG for QT prolongation, ejection fraction; chest pain, palpitations, dyspnea
• AIMS assessment, blood glucose, CBC, glycosylated hemoglobin A1c (HbA1c), LFTs, neurologic function, pregnancy testing, serum creatinine/electrolytes/lipid profile/prolactin, thyroid function tests, weight
• Swallowing of PO medication; check for hoarding, giving of medication to others
• Affect, orientation, LOC, reflexes, gait, coordination, sleep pattern disturbances
• B/P (standing, lying), pulse, respirations; q4hr during initial treatment; establish baseline before starting treatment; report drops of 30 mm Hg; watch for ECG changes

- **Hyperprolactinemia:** sexual dysfunction, decreased menstruation, breast pain
- Dizziness, faintness, palpitations, tachycardia on rising
- **EPS:** akathisia, tardive dyskinesia (bizarre movements of jaw, mouth, tongue, extremities), pseudoparkinsonism (rigidity, tremors, pill rolling, shuffling gait)
- *Serotonin syndrome, neuroleptic malignant syndrome:* monitor for hyperthermia, increased CPK, altered mental status, muscle rigidity, fever, seizures; discontinue
- Constipation, urinary retention daily; if these occur, increase bulk and water in diet; monitor for weight gain, especially among adolescents
- Supervised ambulation until patient is stabilized on medication; do not involve patient in strenuous exercise program because fainting is possible; patient should not stand still for a long time
- Increased fluids to prevent constipation
- Sips of water, candy, gum for dry mouth
- **Beers:** avoid in older adults except for schizophrenia, bipolar disorder, or short-term use as an antiemetic in chemotherapy; increase in stroke risk
- *Pregnancy/breastfeeding:* use only if benefits outweigh fetal risk; EPS may result; pregnant patients should enroll in the National Pregnancy Registry for Atypical Antipsychotics, 1-866-961-2388; do not breastfeed

Evaluate:
- Therapeutic response: decrease in emotional excitement, hallucinations, delusions, paranoia; reorganization of patterns of thought, speech

Teach patient/family:
- That orthostatic hypotension may occur; to rise gradually from sitting or lying position
- To avoid abrupt withdrawal of this product, EPS may result; that product should be withdrawn slowly
- To avoid OTC preparations (cough, hay fever, cold) unless approved by prescriber because serious product interactions may occur; to avoid alcohol because increased drowsiness may occur

- To avoid hazardous activities if drowsy or dizzy
- About compliance with product regimen; that nonabsorbable tab shell is expelled in stool
- To report impaired vision, tremors, muscle twitching
- To avoid hot tubs, hot showers, tub baths because hypotension may occur
- That heat stroke may occur in hot weather; to take extra precautions to stay cool
- To use contraception; to inform prescriber if pregnancy is planned or suspected; not to breastfeed

Black Box Warning: Suicidal thoughts/ behaviors: to notify prescriber of suicidal thoughts/behaviors, other changes in behavior; identify dementia in the elderly

TREATMENT OF OVERDOSE: Lavage if orally ingested; provide airway; *do not induce vomiting*

---

palonosetron (Rx)

(pa-lone-o′se-tron)

Aloxi
Func. class.: Antiemetic
Chem. class.: 5-HT$_3$ receptor antagonist

P

ACTION: Prevents nausea, vomiting by blocking serotonin peripherally, centrally, and in the small intestine at the 5-HT$_3$ receptor

USES: Prevention of nausea, vomiting associated with cancer chemotherapy, postoperative nausea/vomiting

CONTRAINDICATIONS: Hypersensitivity

Precautions: Pregnancy, breastfeeding, children, geriatric patients, hypokalemia, hypomagnesemia, patients taking diuretics

DOSAGE AND ROUTES
Prevention of chemotherapy-induced nausea/vomiting
• **Adult:** IV 0.25 mg as single dose over 30 sec ½ hr before chemotherapy

Child 1 mo to <17 yr: IV 20 mcg/kg, max 1.5 mg given 30 min before chemotherapy

Postoperative nausea/vomiting prophylaxis for ≤24 hr after surgery
• **Adult:** IV 0.075 mg given over 10 sec immediately before induction

Available forms: Inj 0.075 mg/1.5 mL, 0.25 mg/5 mL single use

Administer:
Direct IV route
• Give 30 min before chemotherapy or immediately before anesthesia
• Do not admix with other products, flush IV line with 0.9% NaCL before and after use
• **Chemotherapy nausea/vomiting:** give as single dose over 30 sec
• **Postoperative nausea/vomiting:** give over 10 sec immediately before anesthesia induction

Y-site compatibilities: Alemtuzumab, alfentanil, amifostine, amikacin, aminocaproic acid, aminophylline, amiodarone, amphotericin B liposome, ampicillin, ampicillin/sulbactam, atracurium, atropine, azithromycin, aztreonam, bivalirudin, bleomycin, bumetanide, buprenorphine, busulfan, butorphanol, calcium acetate/chloride/gluconate, CARBOplatin, carmustine, caspofungin, ceFAZolin, cefepime, cefotaxime, cefoTEtan, cefOXitin, cefTAZidime, ceftizoxime, cefTRIAXone, cefuroxime, chloramphenicol, chlorproMAZINE, cimetidine, ciprofloxacin, cisatracurium, CISplatin, clindamycin, cyclophosphamide, cycloSPORINE, cytarabine, dacarbazine, DACTINomycin, dantrolene, DAPTOmycin, DAUNOrubicin, dexamethasone, dexmedetomidine, dexrazoxane, digoxin, diltiaZEM, diphenhydrAMINE, DOBUTamine, DOCEtaxel, DOPamine, doxacurium, DOXOrubicin hydrochloride, droperidol, enalaprilat, ePHEDrine, EPINEPHrine, epiRUBicin, eptifibatide, erythromycin, esmolol, etoposide, etoposide phosphate, famotidine, fenoldopam, fentaNYL, fluconazole, fludarabine, fluorouracil, foscarnet, fosphenytoin, furosemide, gemcitabine, gentamicin, glycopyrrolate, haloperidol, heparin, hydrALAZINE, hydrocortisone, HYDROmorphone, IDArubicin, ifosfamide, inamrinone, insulin, irinotecan, isoproterenol, ketorolac, labetalol, leucovorin, levoFLOXacin, lidocaine, linezolid, LORazepam, magnesium sulfate, mannitol, mechlorethamine, melphalan, meperidine, meropenem, mesna, metaraminol, methotrexate, methyldopate, metoclopramide, metoprolol, metroNIDAZOLE, midazolam, milrinone, mitoMYcin, mitoXANTRONE, mivacurium, morphine, nalbuphine, naloxone, neostigmine, nesiritide, niCARdipine, nitroglycerin, nitroprusside, norepinephrine, octreotide, oxaliplatin, oxytocin, PACLitaxel, pamidronate, pancuronium, pentazocine, PHENobarbital, phentolamine, phenylephrine, piperacillin/tazobactam, potassium acetate/chloride/phosphates, procainamide, prochlorperazine, promethazine, propranolol, quinupristin/dalfopristin, raNITIdine, remifentanil, rocuronium, sodium acetate/bicarbonate/phosphates, streptozocin, succinylcholine, SUFentanil, tacrolimus, teniposide, theophylline, thiotepa, ticarcillin/clavulanate, tigecycline, tirofiban, tobramycin, topotecan, trimethobenzamide, trimethoprim/sulfamethoxazole, vancomycin, vasopressin, vecuronium, verapamil, vinBLAstine, vinCRIStine, vinorelbine, zidovudine

SIDE EFFECTS
CNS: *Headache, dizziness, drowsiness*
GI: *Diarrhea, constipation*
MISC: Serotonin syndrome

PHARMACOKINETICS
62% protein bound; metabolized by liver; unchanged product and metabolites excreted by kidney; terminal elimination half-life 40 hr

INTERACTIONS
• **Increase: QT prolongation:** class IA antidysrhythmics (disopyramide, procainamide, quiNIDine), class III antidysrhyth-

mics (amiodarone, dofetilide, ibutilide, sotalol), chloroquine, clarithromycin, droperidol, erythromycin, haloperidol, methadone, pentamidine, some phenothiazines, diuretics (except potassium sparing)

Increase: hypotension, severe—apomorphine

Increase: serotonin syndrome: buspirone, fentanyl, lithium, methylene blue, Tramadol, SSRIs, SNRIs, MAOIs, tricyclics, triptans

Drug/Lab

Increase: potassium

NURSING CONSIDERATIONS
Assess:
• For agents that cause QT prolongation, even if manufacturer has removed QT prolongation from warnings
• Absence of nausea, vomiting during chemotherapy
• **Hypersensitivity reaction:** rash, bronchospasm (rare)
• **Pregnancy/breastfeeding:** use only if clearly needed; do not breastfeed

Evaluate:
• Therapeutic response: absence of nausea, vomiting during cancer chemotherapy, postoperatively

Teach patient/family:
• To report diarrhea, constipation, rash, changes in respirations, or discomfort at insertion site
• To avoid alcohol, barbiturates
• Use other antiemetics if nausea occurs
• Reason for product, expected results

---

pamidronate (Rx)
(pam-i-drone′ate)
Aredia ✽
Func. class.: Bone-resorption inhibitor, electrolyte modifier
Chem. class.: Bisphosphonate

Do not confuse:
Aredia/Adriamycin

ACTION: Inhibits bone resorption, apparently without inhibiting bone formation and mineralization; adsorbs calcium phosphate crystals in bone and may directly block the dissolution of hydroxyapatite crystals of bone

USES: Moderate to severe Paget's disease, hypercalcemia, osteolytic bone metastases in breast cancer, patients with multiple myeloma

Unlabeled uses: Postmenopausal osteoporosis and prevention, osteoporosis prophylaxis, ankylosing spondylitis

CONTRAINDICATIONS: Pregnancy, hypersensitivity to bisphosphonates
Precautions: Children, nursing mothers, renal dysfunction, poor dentition

DOSAGE AND ROUTES
Hypercalcemia of malignancy
• **Adult:** IV INFUSION 60-90 mg as single dose for moderate hypercalcemia; 90 mg for severe hypercalcemia over 2-24 hr; dose should be diluted in 1000 mL 0.45% NaCl, 0.9% NaCl, or D₅W; wait 7 days before 2nd course

Osteolytic lesions
• **Adult:** IV 90 mg/500 mL of D₅W, 0.45% NaCl, or 0.9% NaCl given over 4 hr each mo (multiple myeloma) or over 2 hr q3-4wk (breast carcinoma)

Paget's disease
• **Adult:** IV INFUSION 30 mg/day given over 4 hr × 3 days

Corticosteroid-induced osteoporosis (unlabeled)
• **Adult:** IV 30 mg q3mo × 1 yr

Ankylosing spondylitis (unlabeled)
• **Adult:** IV INFUSION 60 mg over 4 hr; 6-hr infusion for 1st dose

Available forms: Powder for inj 30, 90 mg/vial; inj 3, 6, 9 mg/mL

Administer:
IV route
• Use saline hydration to produce 2000 mL/24 hr of urine output
• Avoid diuretics before treatment
• After reconstituting by adding 10 mL sterile water for inj to each vial (30 mg/10 mL or 90 mg/10 mL, depending on vial

P

used); add to 1000 mL of sterile 0.45%, 0.9% NaCl, D₅W, run over 2-24 hr **(hypercalcemia)**; dilute reconstituted sol in 500 mL of 0.9% NaCl, 0.45% NaCl, or D₅W, give over 4 hr **(multiple myeloma, Paget's disease)**; dilute reconstituted sol in 250 mL of 0.9% NaCl, 0.45% NaCl, or D₅W; give over 2 hr **(osteolytic bone metastases of breast cancer)**

• Do not mix with calcium-containing infusion sol such as Ringer's sol
• Monitor IV site for pain, redness
• Store infusion sol up to 24 hr at room temperature
• Reconstituted sol with sterile water may be refrigerated for ≤24 hr

Y-site compatibilities: Acyclovir, alfentanil, allopurinol, amifostine, amikacin, aminocaproic acid, aminophylline, amphotericin B lipid complex, amphotericin B liposome, ampicillin, anidulafungin, atenolol, atracurium, azithromycin, aztreonam, bivalirudin, bleomycin, bumetanide, buprenorphine, butorphanol, CARBOplatin, carmustine, ceFAZolin, cefepime, cefoperazone, cefotaxime, cefoTEtan, cefOXitin, cefTAZidime, ceftizoxime, cefTRIAXone, cefuroxime, chloramphenicol, chlorproMAZINE, cimetidine, ciprofloxacin, cisatracurium, CISplatin, clindamycin, cyclophosphamide, cycloSPORINE, cytarabine, dacarbazine, DAPTOmycin, dexamethasone, dexmedetomidine, dexrazoxane, digoxin, diltiaZEM, diphenhydrAMINE, DOBUTamine, DOCEtaxel, dolasetron, DOPamine, doxacurium, DOXOrubicin, doxycycline, droperidol, enalaprilat, ePHEDrine, EPINEPHrine, epirubicin, ertapenem, erythromycin, esmolol, etoposide, famotidine, fenoldopam, fentaNYL, fluconazole, fludarabine, fluorouracil, foscarnet, fosphenytoin, furosemide, gallium, ganciclovir, gatifloxacin, gemcitabine, gentamicin, glycopyrrolate, granisetron, haloperidol, heparin, hetastarch 6%, hydrALAZINE, hydrocortisone, HYDROmorphone, hydrOXYzine, ifosfamide, imipenem-cilastatin, inamrinone, insulin (regular), isoproterenol, ketorolac, labetalol, levoFLOXacin, levorphanol, lidocaine, linezolid, LORazepam, magnesium sulfate, mannitol, mechlorethamine, melphalan, meperidine, meropenem, mesna, metaraminol, methotrexate, methyldopate, methylPREDNISolone, metoclopramide, metoprolol, metroNIDAZOLE, midazolam, milrinone, minocycline, mitoXANTRONE, mivacurium, morphine, mycophenolate, nafcillin, nalbuphine, naloxone, nesiritide, niCARdipine, nitroglycerin, nitroprusside, norepinephrine, octreotide, ondansetron, oxytocin, PACLitaxel, palonosetron, pancuronium, PEMEtrexed, pentamidine, pentazocine, PENTobarbital, PHENobarbital, phenylephrine, piperacillin, polymyxin B, potassium chloride/phosphates, procainamide, prochlorperazine, promethazine, propranolol, quiNIDine, quinupristin-dalfopristin, raNITIdine, remifentanil, rocuronium, sodium acetate/bicarbonate/phosphates, succinylcholine, SUFentanil, sulfamethoxazole-trimethoprim, teniposide, theophylline, thiopental, thiotepa, ticarcillin, ticarcillin-clavulanate, tigecycline, tirofiban, tobramycin, tolazoline, topotecan, trimethobenzamide, vancomycin, vasopressin, vecuronium, verapamil, vinBLAStine, vinCRIStine, vinorelbine, voriconazole, zidovudine

SIDE EFFECTS

CNS: *Fever,* fatigue
CV: Hypertension, atrial fibrillation
EENT: Ocular pain, inflammation, vision impairment
GI: Abdominal pain, anorexia, constipation, nausea, vomiting, dyspepsia
GU: Renal failure
HEMA: Thrombocytopenia, anemia, leukopenia
INTEG: Redness, swelling, induration, pain on palpation at site of catheter insertion
META: *Hypokalemia, hypomagnesemia, hypophosphatemia, hypocalcemia,* hypothyroidism
MS: Severe bone pain, myalgia, osteonecrosis of the jaw

RESP: Coughing, dyspnea, upper respiratory tract infection
SYST: Angioedema, anaphylaxis

PHARMACOKINETICS
Rapidly cleared from circulation and taken up mainly by bones, primarily in areas of high bone turnover; eliminated primarily by kidneys; half-life 21-35 hr, terminal half-life in bone is 300 days

INTERACTIONS
None known
Drug/Lab Test
Increase: creatinine
Decrease: potassium, magnesium, phosphate, calcium, WBC, platelets

NURSING CONSIDERATIONS
Assess:
• **Hypocalcemia:** nausea, vomiting, constipation, thirst, dysrhythmias, hypocalcemia, paresthesia, twitching, laryngospasm, Chvostek's sign, Trousseau's sign; **hypercalcemia:** thirst, nausea, vomiting, dysrhythmias
• **Dehydration/hypovolemia:** should be corrected during treatment of hypercalcemia, before therapy, maintain adequate urine output
• Monitor WBCs, platelets, electrolytes, creatinine, BUN, Hgb/Hct before beginning treatment
• **Dental health:** optimal dental health should be obtained before treatment with this product; cover with antiinfectives for dental extractions
• Temperature may be elevated during the first 3 days after a dose; risk of fever increases as dose increases
• **Renal disease:** max 90-mg single dose, longer infusions >2 hr may increase risk for renal toxicity
• Bone pain; use analgesics
• I&O, check for fluid overload, edema, crackles, increased B/P; BUN, creatinine, electrolytes (calcium, potassium, magnesium)
• **Pregnancy/breastfeeding:** do not use in pregnancy/breastfeeding; use contraception

Evaluate:
• Therapeutic response: decreased calcium levels
Teach patient/family
• To notify prescriber if pregnancy is planned or suspected; to use contraception while taking this product
• To report hypercalcemic relapse: nausea, vomiting, bone pain, thirst; unusual muscle twitching, muscle spasms; severe diarrhea, constipation
• To continue with dietary recommendations, including calcium and vit D
• To obtain analgesic from provider for bone pain
• That small, frequent meals may help if nausea, vomiting occur
• To report ocular symptoms to prescriber: blurred vision, edema, inflammation
• To maintain good oral hygiene; to get regular dental checkups
• To report dental or jaw pain to prescriber

---

pancrelipase (Rx)
(pan-kre-li'pase)
Creon, DMH ✦, Pancrease ✦, Pancreaze, Pertzye, Ultresa, Viokase, Zenpep, Cotazym ✦
Func. class.: Digestant
Chem. class.: Pancreatic enzyme—bovine/porcine

ACTION: Pancreatic enzyme needed for the breakdown of substances released from the pancreas

USES: Exocrine pancreatic secretion insufficiency, cystic fibrosis (digestive aid), steatorrhea, pancreatic enzyme deficiency

CONTRAINDICATIONS: Allergy to pork
Precautions: Pregnancy, ileus, pancreatitis, Crohn's disease, diabetes mellitus

DOSAGE AND ROUTES
• **Adult/adolescent/child ≥4 yr (del rel caps) Creon Caps, Zenpep Caps, Pancreaze Caps: PO** 500 lipase units/kg/meal,

---

Side effects: *italics* = common; red = life-threatening

titrate based on patient response, max 2500 lipase units/kg/meal

• **Child 1-4 yr: PO** 1000 lipase units/kg/meal, titrate based on patient response, max 2500 lipase units/kg/meal

Available forms: Tabs (Viokase) 10, 20; cap, del rel 4, 8, 16 (Pancrecarb MS), 12, 18, 20 (Ultrase MT); Ultrase: cap 3000, 4200, 5000, 6000, 8000, 10,500, 12,000, 15,000, 16,000, 16,800, 24,000, 25,000 units

Administer:

• After antacid or cimetidine; decreased pH inactivates product

• Low-fat diet for GI symptoms

• Have patient sit up during administration; give with meals

• Do not crush, chew del rel products, caps

• Viokase is not interchangeable with other products

• Store in tight container at room temperature

SIDE EFFECTS

ENDO: Hypo/hyperglycemia

GI: Anorexia, nausea, vomiting, diarrhea, cramping, bloating

GU: Hyperuricuria, hyperuricemia

INTERACTIONS

Decrease: absorption—cimetidine, antacids, oral iron

Decrease: effect of acarbose, miglitol

NURSING CONSIDERATIONS

Assess:

• Appropriate height, weight development before and periodically; may be delayed

• I&O ratio; watch for increasing urinary output

• Fecal fat, nitrogen, PT during treatment

• **Diabetes mellitus:** for polyuria, polydipsia, polyphagia; monitor glucose level more frequently

• Pork sensitivity; cross-sensitivity may occur

• Adequate hydration

• **Pregnancy/breastfeeding:** use only if clearly needed; do not breastfeed

Evaluate:

• Therapeutic response: improved digestion of carbohydrates, protein, fat; absence of steatorrhea

Teach patient/family:

• To notify prescriber of allergic reactions, abdominal pain, cramping, or blood in urine

• To always take with food; not to crush, chew del rel product, caps

• To store at room temperature, away from moisture

• Not to sprinkle capsule contents onto alkaline foods

⚠ HIGH ALERT

pancuronium (Rx)

(pan-kyoo-roe′nee-um)

Func. class.: Neuromuscular blocker (nondepolarizing)

Chem. class.: Synthetic curariform

ACTION: Inhibits transmission of nerve impulses by binding with cholinergic receptor sites, antagonizing action of acetylcholine

USES: Facilitation of endotracheal intubation, skeletal muscle relaxation during mechanical ventilation, surgery, or general anesthesia

CONTRAINDICATIONS: Hypersensitivity to bromide ion

Precautions: Pregnancy, breastfeeding, children <2 yr, neuromuscular/cardiac/renal/hepatic disease, electrolyte imbalances, dehydration, previous anaphylactic reactions (other neuromuscular blockers), respiratory insufficiency

Black Box Warning: Requires an experienced clinician

DOSAGE AND ROUTES

• **Adult/child/infant >1 mo: IV** 0.04-0.1 mg/kg initially or 0.05 mg/kg after initial dose of succinylcholine; maintenance 0.01 mg/kg 60-100 min after initial dose, then 0.01 mg/kg q25-60min as needed; for obese patients, use ideal body weight

• **Neonate <1 mo: IV** test dose 0.02 mg/kg, then 0.03 mg/kg/dose initially, repeat 2× as needed at 5-10 min intervals; maintenance 0.03-0.09 mg/kg/dose q30min-4 hr as needed

Available forms: Inj 1, 2 mg/mL
Administer:
Direct IV route
• May be given undiluted over 1-2 min (1 mg/mL [10-mL vial], 2 mg/mL [2-, 5-mL vial])

Intermittent IV INFUSION route
• Add 100 mg of product to 250 mL D₅W, NS, LR (0.4 mg/mL)
• Store in refrigerator; do not store in plastic; use only fresh sol
• Reassurance if communication is difficult during recovery from neuromuscular blockade
• Frequent (q2hr) instillation of artificial tears, covering of eyes to prevent drying of cornea

Additive compatibilities: Verapamil, ciprofloxacin
Y-site compatibilities: Aminophylline, ceFAZolin, cefuroxime, cimetidine, DOBUTamine, DOPamine, EPINEPHrine, esmolol, fenoldopam, fentaNYL, fluconazole, gentamicin, heparin, hydrocortisone, isoproterenol, levoFLOXacin, LORazepam, midazolam, morphine, nitroglycerin, raNITIdine, trimethoprim-sulfamethoxazole, vancomycin

SIDE EFFECTS
CV: Bradycardia; tachycardia; increased, decreased B/P; ventricular extrasystoles, edema, hypertension
EENT: Increased secretions
INTEG: Rash, flushing, pruritus, urticaria, sweating, salivation
MS: Weakness to prolonged skeletal muscle relaxation
RESP: Prolonged apnea, bronchospasm, cyanosis, respiratory depression, dyspnea
SYST: Anaphylaxis

PHARMACOKINETICS
IV: Onset 3-5 min, dose dependent, peak 3-5 min; metabolized (small amounts), excreted in urine (unchanged), crosses placenta

INTERACTIONS
Increase: dysrhythmias—theophylline
Increase: neuromuscular blockade—aminoglycosides, clindamycin, enflurane, isoflurane, lincomycin, lithium, local anesthetics, opioid analgesics, polymyxin antiinfectives, quiNIDine, thiazides
Drug/Lab Test
Decrease: cholinesterase

NURSING CONSIDERATIONS
Assess:
• **Respiratory recovery:** decreased paralysis of face, diaphragm, leg, arm, rest of body; allow to recover fully before neurologic assessment
• Electrolyte imbalances (K, Mg); may lead to increased action of product
• VS (B/P, pulse, respirations, airway) until fully recovered; rate, depth, pattern of respirations, strength of hand grip
• I&O ratio; check for urinary retention, frequency, hesitancy
• **Allergic reactions, anaphylaxis:** rash, fever, respiratory distress, pruritus; product should be discontinued
• **Pregnancy/breastfeeding:** use only if benefits outweigh fetal risk; breast milk excretion is unknown
Evaluate:
• Therapeutic response: paralysis of jaw, eyelid, head, neck, rest of body

TREATMENT OF OVERDOSE:
Neostigmine, atropine, monitor VS; may require mechanical ventilation

> ⚠ **HIGH ALERT**
>
> **panitumumab (Rx)**
> (pan-i-tue′moo-mab)
> Vectibix
> *Func. class.:* Antineoplastic—miscellaneous
> *Chem. class.:* Multikinase inhibitor, signal transduction inhibitor

P

ACTION: Decreases growth and survival of cancer cells by competitive inhibition of EGF receptor

USES: ✖️ᴼᴇ EGFR expressing metastatic colorectal cancer; not beneficial with KRAS mutations in codon 12 or 13

CONTRAINDICATIONS: Hypersensitivity

Precautions: Pregnancy, breastfeeding, children, hepatic disease, acute bronchospasm, diarrhea, hamster protein allergy, hypomagnesemia, hypotension, pulmonary fibrosis, sepsis, ✖️ᴼᴇ KRAS mutations, soft tissue toxicities, infusion-related reactions

> **Black Box Warning:** Exfoliative dermatitis

DOSAGE AND ROUTES
• **Adult: IV INFUSION** 6 mg/kg over 60 min every 2 wk; doses >1000 mg over 90 min

Available forms: Sol for inj 20 mg/mL (100 mg/5 mL, 400 mg/20 mL)

Administer:

Intermittent IV INFUSION route
• Assess for KRAS before use
• Give in hospital or clinic setting with full resuscitation equipment
• Only as IV infusion using controlled IV infusion pump; do not give IV push or bolus; use low–protein binding 0.2- or 0.22-micron in-line filter; flush line with 0.9% NaCl before and after administration
• Give over 60 min through a peripheral line or indwelling catheter; infuse doses of >1000 mg over 90 min
• Dilute in 100 mL of 0.9% NaCl; dilute doses >1000 mg in 150 mL of 0.9% NaCl; mix by inverting; do not exceed 10 mg/mL; use within 6 hr if stored at room temperature; can be stored between 2° C and 8° C for up to 24 hr
• **Dosage adjustment for infusion/dermatologic reaction:** Grade 1 or 2: reduce infusion by 50%; Grade 3 or 4: terminate,

permanently discontinue depending on severity/resistance
• Store unopened vials in refrigerator; do not shake; protect from direct sunlight; do not freeze

SIDE EFFECTS
CNS: Fatigue
CV: Peripheral edema
EENT: Ocular irritation, ocular toxicity
GI: *Nausea, diarrhea, vomiting,* anorexia, mouth ulceration, abdominal pain, constipation
HEMA: Thrombophlebitis
INTEG: *Rash,* pruritus, exfoliative dermatitis, skin fissure, angioedema, severe/fatal infusion reactions
META: Hypocalcemia, hypomagnesemia, antibody formation
RESP: Bronchospasm, cough, dyspnea, hypoxia, pulmonary fibrosis/embolism, pneumonitis, wheezing, interstitial lung disease

PHARMACOKINETICS
Bioavailability 38%-49%; elimination half-life 7.5 days; peak 3 hr; high-fat meal decreases bioavailability; plasma protein binding 99.5%; metabolized in liver; oxidative metabolism by CYP3A4, glucuronidation by UGT1A9; 77% excreted in feces

INTERACTIONS
• Do not use in combination with other antineoplastics

NURSING CONSIDERATIONS
Assess:

> **Black Box Warning: Serious skin disorders:** fever, sore throat, fatigue, then lesions in mouth, lips; withhold product, notify prescriber

• Serum electrolytes periodically (calcium, magnesium)
• **Infection:** increased temperature
• Assess for diarrhea

Black Box Warning: Infusion reactions:
bronchospasm, fever, chills, hypotension;
may require discontinuation, have emergency equipment available

• **Ocular toxicity:** ocular irritation, hyperemia
• **Pulmonary fibrosis:** dyspnea, cough, wheezing; may require discontinuation
• **Pregnancy/breastfeeding:** do not use in pregnancy/breastfeeding
Evaluate:
• Therapeutic response: decrease in colon carcinoma progression
Teach patient/family:
• **To report adverse reactions immediately:** difficulty breathing, mouth sores, skin rash, ocular toxicity
• About reason for treatment, expected results, adverse reactions
• To use contraception while taking product, for 6 mo after treatment; not to breastfeed for ≥2 mo after stopping treatment; to enroll in Amgen Pregnancy Surveillance Program, 1-800-772-6436
• To avoid the sun, use sunscreen while taking product

⚠ HIGH ALERT

RARELY USED

panobinostat
(pan′-oh-bin′-oh-stat)
Farydak
Func. class.: Antineoplastic: biologic response modifiers

USES: Multiple myeloma in those who have received at least 2 prior therapies (including bortezomib and an immunomodulatory agent), in combination with bortezomib and dexamethasone; an orphan drug

CONTRAINDICATIONS: Hypersensitivity

DOSAGE AND ROUTES
• **Adult: PO** 20 mg every other day × 3 times per wk (on days 1, 3, 5, 8, 10, and 12) for the first 2 wk of each 21-day cycle. Continue for up to 8 cycles; may give up to another 8 cycles (max of 16 treatment cycles) in those who experience clinical benefit without unresolved severe or medically significant toxicity, give with bortezomib (cycles 1-8: 1.3 mg/m^2 on days 1, 4, 8, and 11; cycles 9-16: 1.3 mg/m^2 on days 1 and 8) and dexamethasone (cycles 1-8: 20 mg **PO** on days 1, 2, 4, 5, 8, 9, 11, and 12; cycles 9-16: 20 mg **PO** on days 1, 2, 8, and 9). Avoid concomitant use with strong CYP3A4 inducers

pantoprazole (Rx)
(pan-toe-pray′zole)
Panto IV ✦, Pantoloc ✦, Protonix, Prontonix IV, Tecta ✦
Func. class.: Proton pump inhibitor
Chem. class.: Benzimidazole

Do not confuse:
Protonix/Lotronex/protamine

ACTION: Suppresses gastric secretion by inhibiting hydrogen/potassium ATPase enzyme system in gastric parietal cell; characterized as gastric acid pump inhibitor because it blocks the final step of acid production

USES: Gastroesophageal reflux disease (GERD), severe erosive esophagitis; maintenance of long-term pathologic hypersecretory conditions, including Zollinger-Ellison syndrome
Unlabeled uses: Duodenal/gastric ulcer, NSAID ulcer prophylaxis, *Helicobacter pylori*–associated ulcer, dyspepsia

CONTRAINDICATIONS: Hypersensitivity to this product or benzimidazole
Precautions: Pregnancy, breastfeeding, children, proton pump hypersensitivity

DOSAGE AND ROUTES
GERD
• **Adult:** PO 40 mg/day × 8 wk, may repeat course

Erosive esophagitis
• **Adult:** IV 40 mg/day × 7-10 days; PO 40 mg/day × 8 wk; may repeat PO course
Child ≥5 yr and >40 kg: PO 40 mg daily for up to 8 wk; **15-39 kg:** 20 mg daily for up to 8 wk

Pathologic hypersecretory conditions
• **Adult:** PO 40 mg bid; IV 80 mg q12hr, max 240 mg/day

Duodenal ulcer/gastric ulcer/ NSAID ulcer prophylaxis (unlabeled)
• **Adult:** PO 40 mg/day

H. pylori–associated ulcers (unlabeled)
• **Adult:** PO 40 mg bid; may be used with other products
Available forms: Del rel tabs 20, 40 mg; powder for inj 40 mg/vial; del rel granules for susp 40 mg

Administer:
PO route
• Swallow del rel tabs whole; do not break, crush, or chew; take del rel tabs at same time of day
• May take with/without food
• **Suspension:** give in apple juice 30 min before a meal or sprinkled on 1 tbsp of applesauce

IV route
• Use of Protonix IV vials with spiked IV system adapters is not recommended
• Visually inspect for particulate matter and discoloration before use
• Give as an IV infusion over 15 min either through a dedicated line or a Y-site; a 2-min slow-injection regimen is also approved; do not give fast IV push
• When using a Y-site, immediately stop use if a precipitation or discoloration occurs
• **Reconstitution of vial:** use 40-mg vial/10 mL NS; do not freeze
• **Two-minute slow IV infusion injection:** dilute one or two 40-mg vials with 10 mL NS per vial to 4 mg/mL; store ≤24 hr at room temperature before use; infuse slowly over ≥2 min; do not give with other IV fluids or medications; flush line with D_5W, NS, or LR before and after each dose
• **Fifteen-minute IV infusion:** dilute each 40-mg dose with 10 mL NS; the reconstituted vial should be further admixed with 100 mL (for one vial) or 80 mL (for 2 vials) of D_5W, NS, or LR (to 0.4 mg/mL or 0.8 mg/mL, respectively); store ≤6 hr at room temperature before further dilution; the admixed solution (0.4 mg/mL or 0.8 mg/mL) may be stored at room temperature and must be used within 24 hr from the time of initial reconstitution; infuse over 15 min at 7 mL/min; do not administer with other IV fluids or medications; flush IV line with D_5W, NS, or LR before and after each dose

Y-site compatibilities: Acyclovir, allopurinol, amifostine, amikacin, aminocaproic acid, aminophylline, amoxicillin-clavulanate, amphotericin B liposome, ampicillin, ampicillin-sulbactam, anidulafungin, azithromycin, bleomycin, bumetanide, calcium gluconate, CARBOplatin, carmustine, ceFAZolin, cefOXitin, cefTAZidime, ceftizoxime, cefTRIAXone, cefuroxime, clindamycin, cyclophosphamide, cycloSPORINE, cytarabine, dextrose 3.3% in sodium chloride 0.3%, digoxin, dimenhyDRINATE, DOCEtaxel, DOPamine, doripenem, doxycycline, enalaprilat, EPINEPHrine, ertapenem, fluorouracil, foscarnet, fosphenytoin, furosemide, ganciclovir, gentamicin, granisetron, heparin, hydrocortisone HYDROmorphone, imipenem-cilastatin, inamrinone, insulin (regular), irinotecan, isoproterenol, magnesium, mannitol, mesna, methohexital, methyldopate, metoclopramide, nafcillin, nitroglycerin, nitroprusside, ofloxacin, oxytocin, PACLitaxel, pentazocine, PENTobarbital, phenylephrine, piperacillin-tazobactam, potassium chloride, procainamide, rifAMPin, sodium bicarbonate, succinylcholine, SUFentanil, sulfamethoxazole-trimethoprim, teniposide, theophylline, thiopental, ticarcillin,

ticarcillin-clavulanate, tigecycline, tirofiban, tobramycin, traMADol, vasopressin, zidovudine

SIDE EFFECTS

CNS: *Headache,* insomnia, asthenia, fatigue, malaise, insomnia, somnolence
GI: *Diarrhea, abdominal pain,* flatulence, pancreatitis, weight changes, CDAD
INTEG: *Rash*
META: Hyperglycemia, weight gain/loss, hyponatremia, hypomagnesemia, vitamin B_{12} deficiency
MS: Myalgia

PHARMACOKINETICS

Peak 2.4 hr, duration >24 hr, half-life 1.5 hr, protein binding 97%, eliminated in urine as metabolites and in feces; in geriatric patients, elimination rate decreased; some Asian patients (15%-20%) may be poor metabolizers

INTERACTIONS

Decrease: effect of each of these drugs: protease inhibitors (atazanavir, indinavir, nelfinavir)
Increase: bleeding—warfarin
Decrease: absorption of these products—sucralfate, calcium carbonate, vit B_{12}, ketoconazole, itraconazole, atazanavir, ampicillin, iron salts, separate doses
Decrease: clopidogrel effect

Drug/Herb
Decrease: effect of pantoprazole—St. John's wort

NURSING CONSIDERATIONS
Assess:
• **CDAD:** bowel sounds; abdomen for pain, swelling; anorexia; diarrhea with blood, mucus
• **Hepatic studies:** AST, ALT, alk phos during treatment
• For vit B_{12} deficiency in patients receiving long-term therapy
• **Serious skin reactions:** toxic epidermal necrolysis, Stevens-Johnson syndrome, exfoliative dermatitis: fever, sore throat, fatigue, thin ulcers; lesions in the mouth, lips

• **Electrolyte imbalances:** hyponatremia; hypomagnesemia in patients using product 3 mo to 1 year; if hypomagnesemia occurs, use of magnesium supplements may be sufficient; if severe, discontinuation of product may be required
• **Rhabdomyolysis, myalgia:** muscle pain, increased CPK; weakness, swelling of affected muscles
• **Beers:** avoid in older adults for >8 wk unless for high-risk patients; risk of *Clostridium difficile,* fractures
• **Pregnancy/breastfeeding:** use only if clearly needed; do not breastfeed
Evaluate:
• Therapeutic response: absence of epigastric pain, swelling, fullness
Teach patient/family:
• To report severe diarrhea; black, tarry stools; abdominal pain; product may have to be discontinued; do not treat diarrhea with OTC products without approval of provider (CDAD)
• That hyperglycemia may occur in diabetic patients
• To take as directed, not to skip or double dose
• To avoid alcohol, salicylates, NSAIDs; may cause GI irritation
• To continue taking even if feeling better
• To notify prescriber if pregnant or planning to become pregnant; not to breastfeed

PARoxetine (Rx)
(par-ox′e-teen)
Paxil, Paxil CR
PARoxetine mesylate
Pexeva, Brisdelle
Func. class.: Antidepressant, SSRI
Chem. class.: Phenylpiperidine derivative

Do not confuse:
PARoxetine/FLUoxetine/Piroxicam/PACLitaxel
Paxil/PACLitaxel/Taxol/doxil

ACTION: Inhibits CNS neuron uptake of serotonin but not of norepinephrine or DOPamine

Side effects: *italics* = common; red = life-threatening

USES: Major depressive disorder, obsessive-compulsive disorder, panic disorder, generalized anxiety disorder, posttraumatic stress disorder, premenstrual disorders, social anxiety disorder, hot flashes, menopause

Unlabeled uses: Premature ejaculation

CONTRAINDICATIONS: Pregnancy, hypersensitivity, MAOI use, alcohol use

Precautions: Breastfeeding, geriatric patients, seizure history; patients with history of mania, renal/hepatic disease

Black Box Warning: Children, suicidal ideation

DOSAGE AND ROUTES
Generalized anxiety disorder
• **Adult: PO** 20 mg/day in AM, range 20-50 mg/day

Posttraumatic stress disorder
• **Adult: PO** 20 mg/day, range 20-60 mg/day

Depression
• **Adult: PO** 20 mg/day in AM; after 4 wk, if no clinical improvement is noted, dose may be increased by 10 mg/day each wk to desired response, max 50 mg/day or **CONT REL** 25 mg/day, may increase by 12.5 mg/day/wk up to 62.5 mg/day
• **Geriatric: PO** 10 mg/day, increase by 10 mg to desired dose, max 40 mg/day

Obsessive-compulsive disorder
• **Adult: PO** 40 mg/day in AM, start with 20 mg/day, increase in 10-mg/day increments, max 60 mg/day

Panic disorder
• **Adult: PO** start with 10 mg/day, increase in 10-mg/day increments to 40 mg/day, max 60 mg/day or **CONT REL** 12.5 mg/day, max 75 mg/day

Premenstrual disorders
• **Adult: CONT REL** 12.5 mg/day in AM

Menopause symptoms/hot flashes
• **Adult: PO (CONT REL)** 12.5 mg/day, may increase to 25 mg/day after 1 wk

Renal dose
• **Adult: PO** CCr 30-60 mL/min, lower doses may be needed; CCr <30 mL/min, 10 mg/day initially, **REGULAR REL,** max 40 mg/day; **CONT REL** 12.5 mg/day initially, max 50 mg/day

Hepatic dose
• **Adult: PO** 10 mg/day initially, max 40 mg **(REGULAR REL)**; 12.5 mg/day initially, max 50 mg/day **(CONT REL)**

Premature ejaculation (unlabeled)
• **Adult: PO** 20 mg/day

Available forms: Tabs 10, 20, 30, 40 mg; oral susp 10 mg/5 mL; cont rel tab 12.5, 25, 37.5 mg; cap 7.5 mg

Administer:
• Do not substitute Pexeva with Paxil, Paxil CR, or generic PARoxetine
• Store at room temperature; do not freeze
• Increased fluids, bulk in diet for constipation, urinary retention
• With food, milk for GI symptoms
• Crushed if patient is unable to swallow medication whole (regular rel only)
• Gum, hard candy, frequent sips of water for dry mouth
• Avoid use with other CNS depressants
• **Oral susp:** shake, measure with oral syringe or calibrated measuring device
• **Cont rel tab:** do not cut, chew, crush; do not give concurrently with antacids

SIDE EFFECTS
CNS: *Headache,* nervousness, insomnia, *drowsiness, anxiety, tremors, dizziness,* fatigue, *sedation,* abnormal dreams, agitation, apathy, euphoria, hallucinations, delusions, psychosis, seizures

CV: Vasodilation, postural hypotension, palpitations, bleeding, chest pain

EENT: Visual changes

GI: *Nausea, diarrhea, dry mouth,* anorexia, dyspepsia, *constipation,* cramps, vomiting, taste changes, flatulence, decreased appetite, weight gain

GU: Dysmenorrhea, decreased libido, urinary frequency, UTI, amenorrhea, cystitis, impotence; decreased sperm quality, decreased fertility, *abnormal ejaculation (male)*

INTEG: *Sweating,* rash, photosensitivity

MS: Pain, arthritis, myalgia, myopathy

RESP: Infection, pharyngitis, nasal congestion, sinus headache, sinusitis, cough, dyspnea, yawning

SYST: Fever, abrupt withdrawal syndrome, Stevens-Johnson syndrome, neuroleptic malignant syndrome, suicidal thoughts/behaviors

PHARMACOKINETICS

PO: Peak 5.2 hr, ext rel peak 6-10 hr; metabolized in liver by CYP2D6 enzyme system, ◆ 7% may be poor metabolizers; unchanged products and metabolites excreted in feces and urine; half-life 21 hr (reg rel); 15-20 hr (cont rel); protein binding 95%

INTERACTIONS

Increase: serotonin syndrome—SSRIs, SNRIs, atypical psychotics, serotonin-receptor agonists, tricyclics, amphetamines, bupropion, cyclobenzaprine, linezolid, traMADol

Decrease: level of digoxin

• Do not use with MAOIs, pimozide, thioridazine; potentially fatal reactions can occur

Increase: bleeding—NSAIDs, thrombolytics, salicylates, platelet inhibitors, anticoagulants

Increase: PARoxetine plasma levels—cimetidine

Increase: agitation—L-tryptophan

Increase: side effects—highly protein-bound products

Increase: theophylline levels—theophylline

Increase: toxicity—CYP2D6 inhibitors (aprepitant, delavirdine, imatinib, nefazodone)

Decrease: PARoxetine levels—PHENobarbital and phenytoin

Drug/Herb

• SAMe

• Possible serotonin syndrome: St. John's wort, tryptophan

• **Hypertensive crisis:** ephedra

NURSING CONSIDERATIONS

Assess:

Black Box Warning: Depression/OCD/anxiety/panic attacks: mental status: mood, sensorium, affect, suicidal tendencies (especially in child/young adult), increase in psychiatric symptoms, decreasing obsessive thoughts, compulsive behaviors, restrict amount available

• **Postural hypotension:** B/P (lying/standing), pulse q4hr; if systolic B/P drops 20 mm Hg, hold product, notify prescriber; take vital signs q4hr for patients with CV disease

• Hepatic/renal studies: AST, ALT, bilirubin, creatinine

• Weight weekly; appetite may decrease with product, but weight gain may occur; constipation

• EPS, primarily in geriatric patients: rigidity, dystonia, akathisia

• **Renal status:** BUN, creatinine, urinary retention

• **Withdrawal symptoms:** headache, nausea, vomiting, muscle pain, weakness; not usual unless product discontinued abruptly, taper over 1-2 wk

• Alcohol intake; if alcohol is consumed, hold dose until morning

• **Serotonin, neuroleptic malignant syndrome:** hallucinations, coma, headache, agitation, shivering, sweating, tachycardia, diarrhea, tremors, hypertension, hyperthermia, rigidity, delirium, coma, myoclonus, agitation, nausea, vomiting

• **Pregnancy/breastfeeding:** use only if clearly needed; do not breastfeed

Evaluate:

• Therapeutic response: decreased depression

Teach patient/family:

• That therapeutic effect may take 1-4 wk

• To use caution when driving, performing other activities requiring alertness because of drowsiness, dizziness, blurred vision

• Not to discontinue medication quickly after long-term use; may cause nausea, headache, malaise (abrupt withdrawal syndrome)

Black Box Warning: That depression, suicidal thoughts/behaviors in children/adolescents or young adults may worsen, to notify prescriber immediately

P

• To avoid alcohol ingestion, OTC products unless approved by prescriber
• To report bleeding, headache, nausea, anxiety, or if depression continues
• To discuss sexual side effects: impotence, possible male infertility while taking product

TREATMENT OF OVERDOSE:
Gastric lavage, airway; for seizures, give diazepam, symptomatic treatment

---

⚠ HIGH ALERT

pazopanib
(paz-oh′pa-nib)
Votrient
Func. class.: Antineoplastic biologic response modifiers/multikinase angiogenesis inhibitor
Chem. class.: Kinase inhibitor

Do not confuse:
pazopanib/penatinib

ACTION: Targets vascular endothelial growth factor receptors; a multikinase angiogenesis inhibitor

USES: Advanced renal cell carcinoma; soft-tissue sarcoma patients who have received prior chemotherapy
Unlabeled uses: Breast, ovarian cancer

CONTRAINDICATIONS: Pregnancy, hypothyroidism, QT prolongation, MI, wound dehiscence, hypertension
Precautions: Breastfeeding, children, cardiac/renal/hepatic/dental disease, GI bleeding

Black Box Warning: Hepatic disease

DOSAGE AND ROUTES
• **Adult: PO** 800 mg/day without food (1 hr before, 2 hr after a meal), may decrease to 400 mg/day if not tolerated (renal cell cancer); or adjust in 200-mg increments based on toxicity (soft-tissue sarcoma); **use with strong CYP3A4 inhibitors** 400 mg daily
Hepatic dose
Adult: PO 200 mg daily (moderate hepatic disease)
Available forms: Tabs 200 mg
Administer:
• Give on an empty stomach (1 hr before or 2 hr after a meal); separate doses by ~24 hr
• Do not crush tablets owing to the potential for an increased rate of absorption, which can affect systemic exposure; only intact, whole tablets should be used
• If a dose is missed, it should not be taken if it is <12 hr until the next dose
• Store at 77° F (25° C)

SIDE EFFECTS
CNS: Intracranial bleeding, headache
CV: Heart failure, hypertension, hypertensive crisis, chest pain, MI, QT prolongation, torsades de pointes
GI: Nausea, hepatotoxicity, vomiting, dyspepsia, GI hemorrhage, anorexia, abdominal pain, GI perforation, pancreatitis, diarrhea; hepatotoxicity (geriatric)
HEMA: Neutropenia, thrombocytopenia, bleeding
INTEG: Rash, alopecia
MISC: Fatigue, epistaxis, pyrexia, hot sweats, increased weight, flulike symptoms, hypothyroidism, hand-foot syndrome, retinal tear/detachment

PHARMACOKINETICS
Protein binding 99%, peak 2-4 hr, duration 24 hr, half-life 31 hr

INTERACTIONS
Increase: QT prolongation—class IA/III antidysrhythmics, some phenothiazines, β-agonists, local anesthetics, tricyclics, haloperidol, chloroquine, droperidol, pentamidine; CYP3A4 inhibitors (amiodarone, clarithromycin, erythromycin, telithromycin, troleandomycin), arsenic trioxide; CYP3A4 substrates (methadone, pimozide, QUEtiapine, quiNIDine, risperiDONE, ziprasidone)

Increase: pazopanib concentrations—CYP3A4 inhibitors (ketoconazole, itraconazole, erythromycin, clarithromycin)
Increase: plasma concentrations of simvastatin, calcium-channel blockers, ergots
Increase: plasma concentration of warfarin; avoid use with warfarin; use low-molecular-weight anticoagulants instead
Decrease: PAZOPanib concentrations—CYP3A4 inducers (dexamethasone, phenytoin, carBAMazepine, rifampin, PHENobarbital)

Drug/Food
Increase: PAZOPanib effect—grapefruit juice; avoid use while taking product

Drug/Herb
Decrease: PAZOPanib concentration—St. John's wort

NURSING CONSIDERATIONS
Assess:

Black Box Warning: **Hepatic disease:** fatal hepatotoxicity can occur; obtain LFTs baseline and at least every 2 wk × 2 mo, then monthly

• **Fatal bleeding:** from GI, respiratory, GU tracts, permanently discontinue in those with severe bleeding

• **Palmar-plantar erythrodysesthesia (hand-foot syndrome):** more common in those previously treated; reddening, swelling, numbness, desquamation on palms and soles

• **GI perforation/fistula:** discontinue if this occurs, assess for pain in epigastric area, dyspepsia, flatulence, fever, chills

• **Hypertension/hypertensive crisis:** hypertension usually occurs in the first cycle; in those with preexisting hypertension, do not start treatment until B/P is controlled; monitor B/P every wk × 6 wk, then at start of each cycle or more often if needed, temporarily or permanently discontinue for severe uncontrolled hypertension

• **Pregnancy/breastfeeding:** do not use in pregnancy, breastfeeding

Evaluate:
• Therapeutic response: decrease in size, spread of tumor

Teach patient/family:

• To report adverse reactions immediately: heart attack, stroke
• About reason for treatment, expected results
• That effect on male fertility is unknown
• Not to crush or chew tabs; to take on an empty stomach 1 hr before or 2 hr after meals; to avoid grapefruit juice

• **Blood clots:** Pain in legs, chest pain, swelling in legs, arms, notify provider immediately

• **Hepatotoxicity:** To notify provider immediately of yellow skin, eyes, clay-colored stools, dark urine, monitor LFTs before and at 3, 5, 7, 9 wk, then 3 mo, 4 mo if symptoms are present

---

⚠ HIGH ALERT

pegfilgrastim (Rx)
(peg-fill-grass′stim)
Neulasta, Neulata Onpro Kit
pegfilgrastim-cbqv
Udenyca (biosimilar)
pegfilgrastim-jmdb
Fulphia (biosimilar)
Func. class.: Hematopoietic agent
Chem. class.: Granulocyte colony-stimulating factor

Do not confuse:
Neulasta/Lunesta/Neumega/Nuedexta

ACTION: Stimulates proliferation and differentiation of neutrophils

USES: To decrease infection in patients receiving antineoplastics that are myelosuppressive; to increase WBC count in patients with product-induced neutropenia

CONTRAINDICATIONS: Hypersensitivity to proteins of *Escherichia coli,* filgrastim
Precautions: Pregnancy, breastfeeding, children <45 kg, adolescents, myeloid malignancies, sickle cell disease, leukocytosis, splenic rupture, ARDS, allergic-type reactions, peripheral blood stem cell (PBSC) mobilization

P

Side effects: *italics* = common; red = life-threatening

DOSAGE AND ROUTES
• **Adult/child >45 kg: SUBCUT** 6 mg per chemotherapy cycle

Available forms: Sol for inj 6 mg/0.6 mL

Administer:
SUBCUT route
• Using single-use vials; after dose is withdrawn, do not reenter vial
• Do not use 6-mg fixed dose in infants, children, or others <45 kg
• Inspect sol for discoloration, particulates; if present, do not use
• Do not administer during the period 14 days before and 24 hr after cytotoxic chemotherapy
• Store in refrigerator; do not freeze; may store at room temperature up to 6 hr; avoid shaking, protect from light

SIDE EFFECTS
CNS: Fever, fatigue, headache, dizziness, insomnia, peripheral edema
GI: Splenic rupture
HEMA: Leukocytosis
INTEG: Alopecia
MISC: Chest pain, hyperuricemia, anaphylaxis, capillary leak syndrome
GU: Glomerulonephritis
MS: Skeletal pain
RESP: Respiratory distress syndrome

PHARMACOKINETICS
Half-life: 15-80 hr; 20-38 hr (children)

INTERACTIONS
• Do not use product concomitantly, 2 wk before, or 24 hr after administration of cytotoxic chemotherapy
Increase: release of neutrophils—lithium
Drug/Lab Test
Increase: uric acid, LDH, alk phos

NURSING CONSIDERATIONS
Assess:
• **Allergic reactions, anaphylaxis:** rash, urticaria; discontinue product, have emergency equipment nearby
• **ARDS:** dyspnea, fever, tachypnea, occasionally confusion; obtain ABGs, chest x-ray; product may need to be discontinued
• **Bone pain:** give mild analgesics

• Blood studies: CBC with differential, platelet count before treatment, 2× weekly; neutrophil counts may be increased for 2 days after therapy
• B/P, respirations, pulse before and during therapy
• **Pregnancy/breastfeeding:** use only if benefits outweigh fetal risk; pregnant women should enroll in Amgen's Pregnancy Surveillance Program, 1-800-772-6436; cautious use in breastfeeding, excretion unknown

Evaluate:
• Therapeutic response: absence of infection

Teach patient/family:
• How to perform the technique for self-administration if product to be given at home: dose, side effects, disposal of containers and needles; provide instruction sheet
• To notify prescriber immediately of allergic reaction, trouble breathing, abdominal pain

---

⚠ HIGH ALERT

peginterferon alfa-2a (Rx)
(peg-in-ter-feer'on)
Pegasys
peginterferon alfa-2b (Rx)
PegIntron, Sylatron
Func. class.: Immunomodulator

ACTION: Stimulates genes to modulate many biologic effects, including the inhibition of viral replication; inhibits ion cell proliferation, immunomodulation; stimulates effector proteins; decreases leukocyte, platelet counts

USES: Chronic hepatitis C infections in adults with compensated liver disease; chronic hepatitis B in adults who are HBe AG positive, HBe AG negative; HCV patients coinfected with HIV;

nonresponders or relapsers with chronic hepatitis C, malignant melanoma
Unlabeled uses: Adenovirus, coronavirus, encephalomyocarditis virus, herpes simplex types 1 and 2, hepatitis D, acute hepatitis C, HIV, HPV, polio virus, rhinovirus, varicella zoster, variola, vesicular stomatitis

CONTRAINDICATIONS: Neonates, infants, sepsis; hypersensitivity to interferons, benzyl alcohol, *Escherichia coli* protein
Precautions: Pregnancy, breastfeeding, children <18 yr, geriatric patients, thyroid disorders, myelosuppression, renal/hepatic disease, suicidal/homicidal ideation, preexisting ophthalmologic disorders, pancreatitis, hemodialysis

Black Box Warning: Cardiac disease, depression, autoimmune disease, infection, use with ribavirin

DOSAGE AND ROUTES
Pegasys
• **Adult:** SUBCUT 180 mcg weekly × 48 wk; if poorly tolerated, reduce dose to 135 mcg weekly; in some cases, reduction to 90 mcg may be needed
Peg-Intron
(chronic hepatitis C with compensated liver disease)
• **Adult >105 kg:** SUBCUT 1.5 mcg/kg/wk plus ribavirin 600 mg in AM and 800 mg in PM plus a HCV NS3/4A protease inhibitor; **86-105 kg:** 150 mcg/0.5 mL (0.5 mL of 150 mcg vial or Redipen) per wk plus ribavirin 1200 mg/day in 2 divided doses plus a HCV NS3/4A protease inhibitor; **81-85 kg:** 120 mcg/0.5 mL (0.5 mL of 120 mcg vial or Redipen) per wk plus ribavirin 1200 mg/day in 2 divided doses plus a HCV NS3/4A protease inhibitor; **76-80 kg:** 120 mcg/0.5 mL (0.5 mL of 120 mcg vial or Redipen) per wk plus ribavirin 400 mg in AM and 600 mg in PM plus a HCV NS3/4A protease inhibitor; **66-75 kg:** 96 mcg/0.4 mL (0.4 mL of 120 mcg vial or Redipen) per wk plus ribavirin 400 mg in AM and 600 mg in PM plus a HCV NS3/4A protease inhibitor; **61-65 kg:** 96 mcg/0.4 mL (0.4 mL of 120 mcg vial or Redipen) per wk plus ribavirin 800 mg/day in 2 divided doses plus a HCV NS3/4A protease inhibitor; **51-60 kg:** 80 mcg/0.5 mL (0.5 mL of 80 mcg vial or Redipen) per wk plus ribavirin 800 mg/day in 2 divided doses plus a HCV NS3/4A protease inhibitor; **40-50 kg:** 64 mcg/0.4 mL (0.4 mL of 80 mcg vial or Redipen) per wk plus ribavirin 800 mg/day in 2 divided doses plus a HCV NS3/4A protease inhibitor; **<40 kg:** 50 mcg/0.5 mL (0.5 mL of 50 mcg vial or Redipen) per wk plus ribavirin 800 mg/day in 2 divided doses plus a HCV NS3/4A protease inhibitor
Malignant melanoma (Sylatron only)
• **Adult:** SUBCUT 6 mcg/kg/wk × 8 wk then 3 mcg/kg/wk × ≤5 yr, premedicate with acetaminophen 500-1000 mg 30 min before first dose, prn for subsequent doses
Available forms: Pegasys: inj 135, 180 mcg/0.5 mL; **Pegintron:** 50, 80, 120, 150 mcg/0.5 mL; **Sylatron:** 200, 300, 600 mcg powder for inj
Administer:
• In evening to reduce discomfort, to allow patient to sleep through some side effects
• Continue pediatric dose in those who turn 18 yr
Interferon alfa-2a
• Use prefilled syringes; store in refrigerator
Interferon alfa-2b
SUBCUT/IM route
• Reconstitute with 1 mL of provided diluent/10-, 18-, or 50-million unit vials, swirl; sol for inj vials do not need reconstitution

SIDE EFFECTS
CNS: *Headache, insomnia, dizziness,* anxiety, hostility, lability, nervousness, depression, fatigue, poor concentration, pyrexia, suicidal ideation, homicidal ideation, relapse of drug addiction, emotional lability, mania, psychosis
CV: Ischemic CV events

ENDO: Hypothyroidism, diabetes
GI: *Abdominal pain, nausea, diarrhea, anorexia, vomiting,* dry mouth, fatal colitis, fatal pancreatitis
HEMA: Thrombocytopenia, neutropenia, anemia, lymphopenia
INTEG: *Alopecia, pruritus, rash,* dermatitis
MISC: Blurred vision, inj-site reaction, rigors
MS: *Back pain,* myalgia, arthralgia
RESP: Cough, dyspnea

PHARMACOKINETICS
Half-life 15-80 hr, large variability in other pharmacokinetics

INTERACTIONS
• Use caution when giving with theophylline, myelosuppressive agents
Increase: hepatic damage—NNRTIs, NRTIs, protein inhibitors
Drug/Lab Test
Increase: triglycerides, ALT
Decrease: Hgb, platelets, WBCs, neutrophils
Abnormal: thyroid function test

NURSING CONSIDERATIONS
Assess:
• **Neuropsychiatric symptoms:** severe depression with suicidal ideation; monitor q3wk then 8 wk, then q6mo
• B/P, blood glucose, ophthalmic exam, pulmonary function
• ALT, HCV viral load; patients who show no reduction in ALT, HCV unlikely to show benefit of treatment after 6 mo
• Platelet counts, heme concentration, ANC, serum creatinine concentration, albumin, bilirubin, TSH, T_4, AFP
• **Myelosuppression:** hold dose if neutrophil count is $<500 \times 10^6$/L or if platelets are $<50 \times 10^9$/L
• **Hypersensitivity:** discontinue immediately if hypersensitivity occurs
• **Infection:** vital signs, increased WBCs, fever; product may need to be discontinued
• **Colitis/pancreatitis:** may be fatal; diarrhea, fever, nausea, vomiting, severe abdominal pain; if these occur, product should be discontinued
• **Pregnancy/breastfeeding:** may cause birth defects if alfa-2b is used with ribavarin; do not use in pregnancy, contraception is needed; do not breastfeed
Evaluate:
• Therapeutic response: decreased chronic hepatitis C signs, symptoms; undetectable viral load
Teach patient/family:
• Provide patient or family member with written, detailed information about product
• Use 2 forms of effective contraception throughout treatment and for 6 mo after treatment (men and women) (combination therapy with ribavirin)
• To avoid driving, other hazardous activity if dizziness, confusion, fatigue, somnolence occur
• To use puncture-resistant container for disposal of needles/syringes if using at home
• To report suicidal/homicidal ideation, visual changes, bleeding/bruising, pulmonary symptoms

---

pegloticase (Rx)
(peg-loe'ti-kase)
Krystexxa
Func. class.: Antigout agent
Chem. class.: Pegylated, recombinant, mammalian urate oxidase enzyme

---

ACTION: Lowers plasma uric acid concentration by converting uric acid to allantoin, which is readily excreted by the kidneys

USES: Chronic gout in patients experiencing treatment failure

CONTRAINDICATIONS:

Black Box Warning: Hypersensitivity, ⚠️ G6PD deficiency

Precautions: Pregnancy, breastfeeding, children/infants/neonates, ✖ African-American patients, heart failure

Black Box Warning: Requires specialized setting, experienced clinician; serious hypersensitivity; methemoglobinemia

DOSAGE AND ROUTES
• **Adult: IV INFUSION** 8 mg over 2 hr q2wk
Available forms: Sol for inj 8 mg/mL
Administer:
Intermittent IV INFUSION route
• **Reconstitute:** visually inspect for particulate matter, discoloration whenever sol/container permits; use aseptic technique; withdraw 8 mg (1 mL) of product/250 mL 0.9% NaCl or 0.45% NaCl; invert several times to mix, do not shake; discard remaining product in vial
• **Premedicate:** with antihistamines and corticosteroids in all patients and acetaminophen if deemed necessary to prevent anaphylaxis, infusion site reactions
• **Infusion:** if refrigerated, allow to come to room temperature; do not warm artificially; give over 120 min; do not give IV push or bolus; use infusion by gravity feed, syringe-type pump, or infusion pump; given in a specialized setting by those who can manage anaphylaxis or inj-site reactions; monitor during and for 1 hr after infusion; if reaction occurs, slow or stop infusion, may be restarted at a slower rate; do not admix
• Store diluted product in refrigerator or at room temperature for up to 4 hr; refrigerator is preferred; protect from light; do not freeze; use within 4 hr of preparation

SIDE EFFECTS
CNS: Dizziness, fatigue, fever
CV: *Chest pain*, heart failure, hypotension
GI: *Nausea*, vomiting, diarrhea, constipation
GU: Nephrolithiasis
HEMA: Anemia
INTEG: Ecchymosis, *erythema*, *pruritus*, *urticaria*
MS: Back pain, arthralgia, muscle spasm

SYST: Antibody formation, infection, anaphylaxis, infusion-related reactions
RESP: *Dyspnea*, upper respiratory infection

PHARMACOKINETICS
Remains primarily in intravascular space after administration, elimination half-life 2 wk, mean nadir uric acid concentration 24-72 hr

INTERACTIONS
Do not use with urate-lowering agents (allopurinol, probenecid, febuxostat, sulfinpyrazone)

NURSING CONSIDERATIONS
Assess:
• **Gout:** pain in big toe, feet, knees, redness, swelling, tenderness lasting a few days to weeks; intake of alcohol, purines, if patient is overweight or taking diuretics
• Obtain uric acid levels at baseline, before administration; 2 consecutive uric acid levels of >6 mg/dL may indicate therapy failure; greater chance of anaphylaxis; infection-related reactions

Black Box Warning: Specialized care setting: use only in facility where emergency equipment is available, anaphylaxis may occur

Black Box Warning: Infusion reactions: monitor for reactions for ≥1 hr after use

Black Box Warning: Assess for G6PD deficiency, methemoglobinemia

• **Pregnancy/breastfeeding:** use only if benefits outweigh fetal risk; avoid breastfeeding, excretion unknown
Evaluate:
• Therapeutic response: decrease uric acid levels; relief of pain, swelling, redness in toes, feet, knees
Teach patient/family:
• About reason for infusion, expected results

P

• To notify prescriber during infusion of allergic reactions or redness, swelling, pain at infusion site

• That continuing follow-up exams and uric acid levels will be needed

---

> ### ⚠ HIGH ALERT
>
> ## pembrolizumab
> (pem′broe-liz′ue-mab)
> Keytruda
> *Func. class.:* Antineoplastics, biologic response modifiers
> *Chem. class.:* Monoclonal antibodies

ACTION: A human monoclonal antibody that binds to the programmed death receptor-1 (PD-1) found on T-cells and blocks the interaction of PD-1 with its ligands, PD-L1 and PD-L2, on the tumor cell

USES: Unresectable or metastatic malignant melanoma in those who have disease progression after ipilimumab or in BRAF V600 mutation–positive patients who have disease progression after ipilimumab and a BRAF inhibitor, metastatic non-small-cell lung cancer with high PD-L1 expression, lacking EGFR or ALK, recurrent head and neck squamous cell carcinoma, Hodgkin lymphoma

CONTRAINDICATIONS: Hypersensitivity, pregnancy, breastfeeding
Precautions: Immune-mediated colitis, immune-mediated hepatitis, immune-mediated hyperthyroidism/hypothyroidism; immune-mediated nephritis, acute interstitial nephritis, and renal failure; immune-mediated pneumonitis, adrenocortical insufficiency, arthritis, exfoliative dermatitis, hemolytic anemia, hypophysitis, myasthenia syndrome, myositis, optic neuritis, pancreatitis, partial seizures after inflammatory foci identified in brain

parenchyma, rhabdomyolysis, uveitis, incidence of abortion/stillbirths

DOSAGE AND ROUTES
• **Adult:** IV 200 mg over 30 min q3wk until disease progression up to 24 mo
Available forms: Powder for injection 50 mg/vial; solution for injection 25 mg/mL
Administer:
Intermittent IV INFUSION route
• Add 2.3 mL of sterile water for injection, 50-mg vial (25 mg/mL); inject sterile water along the walls of the vial and not directly on the powder
• Gently swirl and allow up to 5 min for bubbles to clear, do not shake, solution will be clear to slightly opalescent, colorless to slightly yellow
• Add the required amount of product to a bag of normal saline (0.9% sodium chloride injection) to a final diluted concentration between 1 and 10 mg/mL; mix by gentle inversion
• Discard any unused solution left in the vial
• **Storage after reconstitution and dilution:** Store at room temperature up to 4 hr or refrigerate up to 24 hr (includes reconstitution, dilution, and administration time). If refrigerated, allow the diluted solution to warm to room temperature before use, give over 30 min
• Use a sterile, nonpyrogenic, low–protein binding 0.2- to 5-micron in-line or add-on filter
• Do not use with other drugs through the same infusion line
• **Grade 2 or 3 toxicity:** Withhold and give corticosteroids; resume when the adverse event recovers to grade ≤1. Permanently discontinue if there is no recovery within 12 wk, if the corticosteroid dose cannot be reduced to ≤10 mg/day of predniSONE (or equivalent) within 12 wk, or for recurrent severe or grade 3 colitis
• **Grade 4 toxicity:** Permanently discontinue, give corticosteroids
Hepatitis:
• **Grade 2 toxicity (AST or ALT >3-5 × upper limit of normal [ULN] or total**

---

bilirubin >1.5-3 × ULN): Withhold and give corticosteroids; resume when adverse event recovers to grade 1 or less. Permanently discontinue if there is no recovery within 12 wk or if the corticosteroid dose cannot be reduced to ≤10 mg/day of predniSONE (or equivalent) within 12 wk

• **Grade 3 or 4 toxicity (AST or ALT >5 × ULN or total bilirubin >3 × ULN):** Permanently discontinue; give corticosteroids

• **Liver metastases and grade 2 elevated transaminase levels at baseline:** Permanently discontinue if AST/ALT levels increase by ≥50% over baseline and transaminase level elevations persist for at least 1 wk

SIDE EFFECTS

CNS: Seizures, *myasthenia, headache, fever, insomnia, chills, dizziness, fatigue*
ENDO: Hyponatremia, hypothyroidism/hyperthyroidism, hyperglycemia, hypocalcemia, immune-mediated hypophysis
EENT: Optic neuritis
GI: Nausea, vomiting, *abdominal pain,* pancreatitis, colitis, *diarrhea,* hepatitis, constipation
GU: Interstitial nephritis, renal failure
RESP: *Cough, dyspnea,* immune-mediated pneumonitis
INTEG: *Rash, pruritus,* skin discoloration
MS: Myalgia, immune-mediated rhabdomyolysis
SYST: Exfoliative dermatitis

INTERACTIONS
None known
Drug/Lab Test
Increase: LFTs, renal function studies

NURSING CONSIDERATIONS
Assess:

• For hyperthyroidism/hypothyroidism, renal function studies baseline, periodically during therapy, CCr, BUN; monitor for nephritis

• For pneumonitis (new or worsening cough, chest pain, shortness of breath); confirm with radiographic imaging, give

corticosteroids ≥ grade 2, withhold in grade 2, resume grade 0-1

• **Immune-mediated hepatitis:** liver function tests and hepatitis, jaundice, severe nausea/vomiting, easy bleeding or bruising; withhold and give corticosteroids if grade 2 hepatitis (AST or ALT >3-5 × ULN or total bilirubin >1.5-3 × ULN)

• **Pregnancy:** assess whether pregnancy is planned or suspected or if breastfeeding; do not use in pregnancy, breastfeeding

• **Immune-mediated hypophysis:** headache, weakness, fainting, dizziness, blurred vision; use corticosteroids if >grade 2, discontinue >grade 3

• **Hyperglycemia:** may cause diabetes mellitus 1 or diabetic ketoacidosis
Evaluate:

• Therapeutic response: decreased progression of multiple myeloma
Teach patient/family:

• To notify prescriber immediately of signs of colitis, pneumonitis, hepatitis, hypophysis

• **Hyperglycemia:** about signs and symptoms of hyperglycemia, diabetes; how to ensure tight glucose control; to report hyperglycemia immediately

• **Pregnancy:** to use highly effective contraceptive methods during and for 4 mo after treatment; to contact health care provider if pregnancy is suspected or confirmed; not to breastfeed

---

⚠ **HIGH ALERT**

PEMEtrexed (Rx)
(pem-ah-trex'ed)
Alimta
Func. class.: Antineoplastic-antimetabolite
Chem. class.: Folic acid antagonist

Do not confuse:
PEMEtrexed/PRALAtrexate

ACTION: Inhibits multiple enzymes that reduce folic acid, which is needed for cell replication

USES: Malignant pleural mesothelioma in combination with CISplatin; non–small-cell lung cancer as single agent; nonsquamous non–small-cell lung cancer (1st-line treatment)
Unlabeled uses: Bladder, breast, colorectal, gastric, head/neck, renal cancers

CONTRAINDICATIONS: Pregnancy, hypersensitivity, ANC <1500 cells/mm^3, CCr <45 mL/min, thrombocytopenia (<100,000/mm^3), anemia
Precautions: Breastfeeding, children, renal/hepatic disease

DOSAGE AND ROUTES
• **Adult:** IV INFUSION 500-600 mg/m^2 given over 10 min on day 1 of 21-day cycle with CISplatin 75 mg/m^2 infused over 2 hr beginning $^1/_2$ hr after end of PEMEtrexed infusion
Renal dose
• **Adult:** IV INFUSION CCr <45 mL/min, not recommended
Available forms: Inj, single-use vials, 100, 500 mg
Administer:
• Store at 77° F, excursions permitted at 59° F to 86° F, not light sensitive, discard unused portions
• Vit B$_{12}$ and low-dose folic acid as prophylactic measure to treat related hematologic, GI toxicity; 400-1000 mcg/day × 7 days before 1st dose and × 21 days after last dose, vit B$_{12}$ 1 mg IM 1 wk before 1st dose and q 3 cycles (9 wk) thereafter
• Premedicate with corticosteroid (dexamethasone) given PO bid day before, day of, and day after administration of PEMEtrexed

Intermittent IV INFUSION route
• Use cytotoxic handling procedures
• Reconstitute 500-mg vial/20 mL 0.9% NaCl inj (preservative free) = 25 mg/mL, swirl until dissolved, further dilute with 100 mL 0.9% NaCl inj (preservative free), give as IV infusion over 10 min
• Use only 0.9% NaCl inj (preservative free) for reconstitution, dilution
• Do not begin a new cycle unless neutrophils (ANC) are ≥1500 cells/mm^3, platelets are ≥100,000 cells/mm^3, CCr is ≥45 mL/min
• **Platelet nadir <50,000/mm^3 regardless of the ANC:** if necessary, delay until platelet count recovery, reduce PEMEtrexed and CISplatin by 50%; if grade 3/4 toxicity occurs after 2 reductions, discontinue both products
• **ANC nadir <500/mm^3 when platelet nadir is ≥50,000/mm^3:** if necessary, delay until ANC recovery, reduce PEMEtrexed and CISplatin by 75%; if grade 3/4 toxicity occurs after 2 reductions, discontinue both products
• **CTC Grade 3/4 nonhematologic toxicity including diarrhea requiring hospitalization and excluding neurotoxicity, mucositis, and grade 3 transaminase elevations:** withhold therapy until pretherapy value or condition, reduce by 75% both products; if grade 3 or 4 toxicity occurs after 2 reductions, discontinue both products
• **CTC grade 3/4 mucositis:** withhold therapy until pretherapy condition, reduce 50% of PEMEtrexed; if grade 3 or 4 mucositis occurs after 2 dosage reductions, discontinue both products
• **CTC grade 2 neurotoxicity:** withhold therapy until pretherapy value or condition, reduce dose of CISplatin by 50%
• **CTC grade 3/4 neurotoxicity:** discontinue both products

Y-site compatibilities: Acyclovir sodium, alfentanil, allopurinol, amifostine, amikacin, aminocaproic acid, aminophylline, amiodarone, amphotericin B lipid complex, amphotericin B liposome, ampicillin, ampicillin-sulbactam, atenolol, atracurium, azithromycin, aztreonam, bivalirudin, bleomycin, bumetanide, buprenorphine, butorphanol, CARBOplatin, carmustine, ceftizoxime, cefTRIAXone, cefuroxime, cimetidine, cisatracurium, CISplatin, clindamycin, cyclophosphamide, cycloSPORINE, cytarabine, DACTINomycin, DAPTOmycin, dexamethasone, digoxin, diltiaZEM, diphenhydrAMINE, DOCEtaxel, dolasetron, DOPamine, doxacurium, enalaprilat, ePHEDrine, EPINEPHrine, eptifibatide, ertapenem, esmolol, etoposide, famotidine, fenoldopam, fentaNYL, fluconazole, fludarabine, fluorouracil, foscarnet, fosphenytoin, furosemide, ganciclovir, gatifloxacin, glycopyrrolate, granisetron, haloperidol, heparin, hydrocortisone, HYDROmorphone, hydrOXYzine, ifosfamide, imipenem-cilastatin, insulin (regular), isoproterenol, ketorolac, labetalol, leucovorin, levo-FLOXacin, lidocaine, linezolid, LORazepam, magnesium, mannitol, meperidine, meropenem, mesna, methyldopate, methylPREDNISolone, metoclopramide, metoprolol, midazolam, milrinone, mito-MYcin, mivacurium, morphine, moxifloxacin, nafcillin, naloxone, nesiritide, nitroglycerin, norepinephrine, octreotide, oxaliplatin, PACLitaxel, pamidronate, pancuronium, PENTobarbital, PHENobarbital, piperacillin-tazobactam, polymyxin B, potassium chloride/phosphates, procainamide, promethazine, propranolol, raNITIdine, remifentanil, rocuronium, sodium acetate/bicarbonate/phosphates, succinylcholine, SUFentanil, sulfamethoxazole-trimethoprim, tacrolimus, theophylline, thiopental, thiotepa, ticarcillin, ticarcillin-clavulanate, tigecycline, tirofiban, trimethobenzamide, vancomycin, vecuronium, verapamil, vinBLAStine, vinCRIStine, vinorelbine, zidovudine, zoledronic acid

SIDE EFFECTS

CNS: *Fatigue, fever, mood alteration, neuropathy*

CV: Thrombosis, embolism, *chest pain,* arrhythmia exacerbation

GI: *Nausea, vomiting, anorexia, diarrhea, ulcerative stomatitis, constipation, dehydration*

GU: Renal failure, creatinine elevation

HEMA: Neutropenia, leukopenia, thrombocytopenia, myelosuppression, anemia

INTEG: *Rash, desquamation*

RESP: *Dyspnea*

SYST: Infection with/without neutropenia, radiation recall reaction, toxic epidermal necrolysis, Stevens-Johnson syndrome, anaphylaxis

PHARMACOKINETICS

Not metabolized; excreted in urine (unchanged 70%-90%); not known if excreted in breast milk; half-life 3.5 hr, 81% protein binding

INTERACTIONS

Decrease: clearance of PEMEtrexed—nephrotoxic products, avoid NSAIDs for 2-8 days before use

NURSING CONSIDERATIONS

Assess:

• Previous radiation treatments; radiation recall reactions have occurred (erythema, exfoliative dermatitis, pain, burning)

• **Bone marrow depression:** CBC, differential, platelet count; monitor for nadir, recovery on days 8, 15 of the cycle; new cycle should not begin if ANC <1500 cells/mm^3, platelets <100,000 cells/mm^3, CCr <45 mL/min

• **Nephrotoxicity:** Renal studies: BUN, serum uric acid, urine CCr, electrolytes before, during therapy; I&O ratio; report fall in urine output to <30 mL/hr

• Monitor temperature; fever may indicate beginning infection; no rectal temperature

• **Neurotoxicity:** CTC grade 2: withhold until resolution to at least pretherapy value/condition, reduce CISplatin by 50%; CTC grade 3-4: immediately discontinue

P

product and CISplatin if given in combination

• **Mucositis:** CTC 3/4: withhold until resolution to at least pretherapy value/condition, reduce dose by 50%; if grade 3/4 occurs after 2 dosage reductions, discontinue product and CISplatin

• **Bleeding:** bleeding time, coagulation time during treatment; bleeding: hematuria, guaiac, bruising or petechiae, mucosa or orifices

• Buccal cavity for dryness, sores, ulceration, white patches, oral pain, bleeding, dysphagia

• **Severe allergic reaction, toxic epidermal necrolysis:** rash, urticaria, itching, flushing

• Rinsing of mouth tid-qid with water, club soda; brushing of teeth bid-tid with soft brush or cotton-tipped applicators for stomatitis; use unwaxed dental floss

• **Pregnancy/breastfeeding:** do not use in pregnancy, breastfeeding

Evaluate:

• Therapeutic response: decreased spread of malignancy

Teach patient/family:

• To report any complaints, side effects to nurse or prescriber: black, tarry stools, chills, fever, sore throat, bleeding, bruising, cough, SOB, dark or bloody urine

• To discuss with provider all OTC, Rx, herbals, supplements taken, to avoid alcohol

• To avoid foods with citric acid, hot temperature, or rough texture if stomatitis is present

• To report stomatitis: any bleeding, white spots, ulcerations in mouth to prescriber; to examine mouth daily; to report symptoms to nurse; to use good oral hygiene

• That prophylactic folic acid and B_{12} injections may be necessary 1 wk before therapy to prevent bone marrow suppression and GI symptoms

• To avoid use of razors, commercial mouthwash

• To eat foods high in folic acid; to take supplements as prescribed

• That contraceptive measures are recommended during therapy, for ≥8 wk after cessation of therapy; to discontinue breastfeeding because toxicity to infant may occur

---

penciclovir topical
See Appendix B

PENICILLINS

penicillin G benzathine (Rx)
(pen-i-sill′in)
Bicillin L-A

penicillin G potassium (Rx)
Pfizerpen

penicillin G procaine (Rx)

Penicillin Sodium ✦,
Crystapen ✦

penicillin V (Rx)
Apo-Pen-VK ✦, Penicillin VK, Novo-Pen-VK ✦, Pen-VK ✦

Func. class.: Broad-spectrum antiinfective
Chem. class.: Natural penicillin

ACTION: Interferes with cell-wall replication of susceptible organisms; lysis is mediated by cell-wall autolytic enzymes, results in cell death

USES: Respiratory infections, scarlet fever, erysipelas, otitis media, pneumonia, skin and soft-tissue infections, gonorrhea; effective for gram-positive cocci *(Staphylococcus, Streptococcus pyogenes, S. viridans, S. faecalis, S. bovis, S. pneumoniae),*

---

gram-negative cocci (*Neisseria gonorrhoeae*), gram-positive bacilli (*Actinomyces, Bacillus anthracis, Clostridium perfringens, C. tetani, Corynebacterium diphtheriae, Listeria monocytogenes*), gram-negative bacilli (*Escherichia coli, Proteus mirabilis, Salmonella, Shigella, Enterobacter, Streptobacillus moniliformis*), spirochetes (*Treponema pallidum*)

CONTRAINDICATIONS: Hypersensitivity to penicillins, corn

Precautions: Pregnancy, breastfeeding; hypersensitivity to cephalosporins, carbapenem, sulfites; severe renal disease, GI disease, asthma

Black Box Warning: Penicillin G benzathine: IV use

DOSAGE AND ROUTES
Penicillin G benzathine
Early syphilis
• **Adult: IM** 2.4 million units in single dose
Congenital syphilis
• **Child <2 yr: IM** 50,000 units/kg in single dose, max 2.4 million units as single inj
Prophylaxis of rheumatic fever, glomerulonephritis
• **Adult: IM** 1.2 million units every month or 600,000 units q2wk
• **Child >27 kg: IM** 900,000-1.2 million units as single dose
• **Child ≤27 kg: IM** 300,000-600,000 units as single dose
Upper respiratory infections (group A streptococcal)
• **Adult: IM** 1.2 million units as single dose
• **Child >27 kg: IM** 900,000-1.2 million units as single dose
• **Child ≤27 kg: IM** 300,000-600,000 units as single dose
Available forms: Inj 600,000 units/mL
Penicillin G Potassium
Pneumococcal/streptococcal infections (serious)
• **Adult: IM/IV** 5-24 million units in divided doses q4-6hr

• **Child <12 yr: IV** 150,000-300,000 units/kg/day in 4-6 divided doses; max 24 million units/day
Most infections
• **Adult: IM/IV** 1-5 million units q4-6hr
• **Child: IM/IV** 8333-16,667 units/kg q4hr; 12,550-25,000 units/kg q6hr; up to 250,000 units/kg daily in divided doses, if more serious 300,000 units/kg daily
• **Infant >7 days: IV** 25,000 units/kgq 8hr; meningitis up to 75,000 units/kg q6hr
• **Infant <7 days: IV** 25,000 units/kg q12hr, meningitis 100,000-150,000 units/kg daily in divided doses
Renal dose
• CCr <10 mL/min, give full loading dose then $^1/_2$ of loading dose q8-10hr
Available forms: Powder for inj 1, 5, 20 million units/vial; inj 1, 2, 3 million units/50 mL
Penicillin G procaine
Moderate to severe pneumococcal infections
• **Adult: IM** 600,000-1 million units as single dose or divided bid doses/day for 10 days to 2 wk
• **Child: IM** 50,000 units/kg daily × 10-14 days (congenital syphilis)
Available forms: Inj 600,000, units/mL
Penicillin V
Most infections
• **Adult/adolescent/child >12 yr: PO** 125-500 mg q6-8hr
• **Child <12 yr: PO** 125 mg q12hr (streptococcus pneumonia in sickle cell); 12.5 mg/kg q6hr (Lyme disease) unlabeled
Rheumatic fever/chorea
• **Adult: PO** 125-250 mg bid continuously
Available forms: Tabs 250, 500 mg; powder for oral sol 125, 250 mg/5 mL
Administer:
• Store in dry, tight container; oral susp refrigerated 2 wk
Penicillin G benzathine
• No dilution needed, shake well, deep IM inj in large muscle mass; avoid intravascular inj; aspirate; do not give IV

P

Penicillin G

• Penicillin G sodium or potassium can be given IM or IV, vials containing 10 or 20 million units not for IM use

Intermittent IV INFUSION route ○

• Vials/bulk packages: dilute according to manufacturer's directions

• Frozen bags: thaw at room temperature, do not force thaw, no reconstitution needed

• Final concentration (100,000-500,000 units/mL—adults; 50,000 units/mL—neonate/infant)

• Total daily dose divided q4-6hr and given over 1-2 hr (adult), 15 min (infant/neonate)

Penicillin G potassium

Y-site compatibilities: Acyclovir, amiodarone, atropine, aztreonam, benztropine, bumetanide, buprenorphine, butorphanol, calcium chloride, calcium gluconate, ceFAZolin, cefotaxime, cefTAZidime, cefTRIAXone, cefuroxime, chloramphenicol, clindamycin, cyclophosphamide, diltiaZEM, enalaprilat, esmolol, fluconazole, foscarnet, heparin, HYDROmorphone, labetalol, magnesium sulfate, meperidine, morphine, perphenazine, potassium chloride, tacrolimus, theophylline, verapamil, vit B/C

Penicillin G procaine

• No dilution needed; give deep IM inj; avoid intravascular inj; aspirate; do not give IV

Penicillin V

• Orally on empty stomach for best absorption

• Oral susp: tap bottle to loosen, add $1/2$ total amount of water, shake, add remaining water, shake; final concentration 125 or 250 mg/mL, store in refrigerator after reconstitution, discard after 14 days

SIDE EFFECTS

CNS: Lethargy, hallucinations, anxiety, depression, twitching, coma, seizures, hyperreflexia

GI: *Nausea, vomiting, diarrhea,* increased AST, ALT, abdominal pain, glossitis, colitis, CDAD

GU: Oliguria, proteinuria, hematuria, *vaginitis, moniliasis,* glomerulonephritis, renal tubular damage

HEMA: Anemia, increased bleeding time, bone marrow depression, granulocytopenia, hemolytic anemia

META: Hypo/hyperkalemia, alkalosis, hypernatremia

MISC: Anaphylaxis, serum sickness, Stevens-Johnson syndrome, *local pain,* tenderness and fever with IM inj

PHARMACOKINETICS

Penicillin G benzathine: IM: Very slow absorption; time to peak 12-24 hr; duration 21-28 days; excreted in urine, feces, breast milk; crosses placenta

Penicillin G: IV: Peak immediate

IM: Peak $1/4$-$1/2$ hr

PO: Peak 1 hr, duration 6 hr

Excreted in urine unchanged, excreted in breast milk, crosses placenta, half-life 30-60 min

Penicillin G procaine: IM: Peak 1-4 hr, duration 15 hr, excreted in urine

Penicillin V: PO: Peak 30-60 min, half-life 30 min, excreted in urine, breast milk

INTERACTIONS

Increase: penicillin effect—aspirin, probenecid

Increase: effect of heparin, methotrexate

Decrease: effect of oral contraceptives, typhoid vaccine

Decrease: antimicrobial effect of penicillin—tetracyclines

Drug/Lab Test

False positive: urine glucose, urine protein

NURSING CONSIDERATIONS

Assess:

• **Infection:** temperature; characteristics of sputum, wounds, urine, stools before, during, after treatment; C&S before therapy; product may be given as soon as culture is taken

• I&O ratio; report hematuria, oliguria because penicillin in high doses is nephrotoxic; renal tests: urinalysis, protein, blood

• **Renal disease:** any patient with compromised renal system because product is excreted slowly with poor renal system function; toxicity may occur rapidly

• Hepatic studies: AST, ALT

• Blood studies: WBC, RBC, Hct, Hgb, bleeding time

• **CDAD:** diarrhea, mucus, pus; bowel pattern before, during treatment

• Respiratory status: rate, character, wheezing, tightness in chest

• Allergies before initiation of treatment, reaction to each medication; because of prolonged action, allergic reaction may be prolonged and severe; watch for anaphylaxis: rash, dyspnea, pruritus, laryngeal edema; skin eruptions after administration of penicillin to 1 wk after discontinuing product

• EPINEPHrine, suction, tracheostomy set, endotracheal intubation equipment

• Scratch test to assess allergy after securing order from prescriber; usually done when penicillin is only product of choice

• Adequate fluid intake (2 L) during diarrhea episodes

Evaluate:

• Therapeutic response: resolution of infection

Teach patient/family:

• To report sore throat, fever, fatigue; may indicate superinfection; CNS effects: depression, hallucinations, seizures

• To wear or carry emergency ID if allergic to penicillins

• **CDAD:** To report diarrhea with blood, pus, mucus to prevent dehydration

• To shake susp well before each dose; to store in refrigerator for up to 2 wk

• To use all medication prescribed

TREATMENT OF ANAPHY-LAXIS: Withdraw product; maintain airway; administer EPINEPHrine, aminophylline, O_2, IV corticosteroids

---

pentamidine (Rx)

(pen-tam′i-deen)

NebuPent, Pentam 300

Func. class.: Antiprotozoal

Chem. class.: Aromatic diamide derivative

ACTION: Interferes with DNA/RNA synthesis in protozoa

USES: Treatment/prevention of *Pneumocystis jiroveci* infections

Unlabeled uses: PJP (inhalation)

CONTRAINDICATIONS: Hypersensitivity

Precautions: Pregnancy, breastfeeding, children, blood dyscrasias, cardiac/renal/hepatic disease, diabetes mellitus, hypocalcemia, hypo/hypertension, anemia

DOSAGE AND ROUTES

• **Adult and child ≥4 mo: IV/IM** 4 mg/kg/day × 2-3 wk; **NEB** 300 mg via Repirgard II Jet (Nebupent); or 150 mg q2wk given q4wk for prevention

Available forms: Inj, aerosol 300 mg/vial; sol for aerosol 300 mg ✦

Administer:

• Store in refrigerator protected from light

Inhalation route

• Through nebulizer, using Respirgard II jet nebulizer; mix contents in 6 mL of sterile water; do not use low pressure (<20 psi); flow rate should be 5-7 L/min (40-50 psi) air or O_2 source over 30-45 min until chamber is empty

IM route

• 300 mg diluted in 3 mL sterile water (100 mg/mL), give deep IM by Z-track; if painful by this route, rotate inj site

Intermittent IV INFUSION route

• Check IV site frequently (vesicant properties)

• Reconstitute 300 mg/3-5 mL of sterile water for inj, D_5W, withdraw dose and further dilute in 50-250 mL D_5W, give over 1-2 hr with patient lying down; check B/P often

Y-site compatibilities: alemtuzumab, alfentanil, aminocaproic acid, anidulafungin, argatroban, atracurium, atropine, benztropine, buprenorphine, calcium gluconate, CARBOplatin, caspofungin, chlorproMAZINE, cimetidine, CISplatin, cyclophosphamide, cycloSPORINE,

P

cytarabine, DACTINomycin, diltiaZEM, gatifloxacin, zidovudine

SIDE EFFECTS

CNS: Disorientation, hallucinations
CV: Hypotension, chest pain
GI: *Nausea, anorexia;* metallic taste
HEMA: Anemia, leukopenia, thrombocytopenia
INTEG: Sterile abscess, pain at inj site, pruritus, urticaria, *rash*
MISC: Night sweats, anaphylaxis, Stevens-Johnson syndrome
RESP: Cough, SOB, bronchospasm (with aerosol), sore throat

PHARMACOKINETICS

IV: Peak 1 hr
IM: Peak 30 min
Excreted unchanged in urine (66%); half-life 9-12 hr (IM), 6 hr (IV)

INTERACTIONS

• Nephrotoxicity: aminoglycosides, amphotericin B, CISplatin, NSAIDs, vancomycin

• **Fatal dysrhythmias: erythromycin IV**
Increase: QT prolongation—class IA/III antidysrhythmics, some phenothiazines, β-agonists, local anesthetics, tricyclics, haloperidol, chloroquine, droperidol, pentamidine; CYP3A4 inhibitors (amiodarone, clarithromycin, erythromycin, telithromycin, troleandomycin, arsenic trioxide); CYP3A4 substrates (methadone, pimozide, QUEtiapine, quiNIDine, risperiDONE, ziprasidone)
Increase: myelosuppression—antineoplastics, radiation

Drug/Lab Test
Decrease: WBC, platelets, Hgb, Hct, calcium, magnesium
Increase: BUN, creatinine, potassium, LFTs, bilirubin, alkaline phosphatase

NURSING CONSIDERATIONS

Assess:
• Blood tests, blood glucose, CBC, platelets, calcium, magnesium

• I&O ratio; report hematuria, oliguria
• ECG for cardiac dysrhythmias in cardiac patients; patient should be lying down when receiving product; severe hypotension may develop; monitor B/P during administration and until B/P stable
• Hepatic studies: AST, ALT
• Renal studies: urinalysis, BUN, creatinine; nephrotoxicity may occur; any patient with compromised renal system; product is excreted slowly with poor renal system function; toxicity may occur rapidly
• Signs of infection, anemia
• Bowel pattern before, during treatment
• Sterile abscess, pain at inj site
• Respiratory status: rate, character, wheezing, dyspnea
• Dizziness, confusion, hallucination
• **Serious skin reactions, allergic reactions:** rash, fever, fatigue, muscle or joint aches, oral lesions, blisters; discontinue product immediately if these occur
• **Pancreatitis:** nausea, vomiting, severe abdominal pain; monitor lab values of lipase and amylase (elevated in pancreatitis); if these signs or symptoms occur, product may need to be discontinued
• Diabetic patients, hypoglycemia may occur, then hyperglycemia with prolonged therapy
• **Pregnancy/breastfeeding:** use only if benefits outweigh fetal risk; cautious use in breastfeeding
Evaluate:
• Therapeutic response: resolution of AIDS-related PCP
Teach patient/family:
• To report sore throat, fever, fatigue (may indicate superinfection)
• To maintain adequate fluid intake
• That IM injection is painful
• To complete entire course of medication

• **Pancreatitis:** To report to provider immediately nausea, vomiting, severe abdominal pain

• To report immediately rash, bleeding, fever, sore throat, or flulike symptoms, to avoid crowds, persons with known infections

---

⚠ HIGH ALERT

RARELY USED

pentazocine (Rx)
(pen-taz′oh-seen)
Talwin
Func. class.: Opiate analgesic, antagonist
Chem. class.: Synthetic benzomorphan

Controlled Substance Schedule IV

USES: Moderate to severe pain

CONTRAINDICATIONS: Hypersensitivity to this product or sulfites; addiction (opiate)

DOSAGE AND ROUTES
• **Adult: IV/IM/SUBCUT** 30 mg q3-4hr prn, max 360 mg/day
Labor
• **Adult: IM** 30 mg as a single dose; **IV** 20 mg q2-3hr when contractions are regular, max 2-3 times
Renal dose
• **Adult:** CCr 10-50 mL/min, reduce dose by 25%; CCr <10 mL/min, reduce dose by 50%

---

peramivir
(per-am′i-vir)
Rapivab
Func. class.: Antiviral

ACTION: Competitively binds to the active site of the influenza virus, inhibits the activity of strains of influenza A and B viruses

USES: Treatment of uncomplicated acute influenza (seasonal influenza A virus infection or seasonal influenza B virus infection)
Unlabeled uses: Treatment of H1N1 influenza A virus (swine influenza) infection in pediatric patients requiring hospitalization

CONTRAINDICATIONS: Hypersensitivity
Precautions: Breastfeeding, children, dialysis, infants, infection, pregnancy, psychosis, renal impairment

DOSAGE AND ROUTES
Influenza
• **Adult: IV** 600 mg as a single dose infused over 15-30 min, give within 48 hr of onset of influenza symptoms
Available forms: Solution for injection 200 mg/20 mL
Administer:
• For IV use only, do not give IM, visually inspect parenteral products for particulate matter and discoloration
• **Dilute** the 10 mg/mL to a max volume of 100 mL, use only 0.9% or 0.45% NaCl, 5% dextrose, or LR
• **Storage of diluted solution:** Use immediately or refrigerate up to 24 hr. Refrigerated solution should be allowed to reach room temperature before administration. Discard any unused diluted solution after 24 hr
• Give over 15-30 min, do not mix or coadminister with other IV products

SIDE EFFECTS
CNS: Delirium, psychosis, hallucinations, insomnia
GI: Constipation, diarrhea, vomiting
MISC: Rash, Stevens-Johnson syndrome

PHARMACOKINETICS
Protein binding <30%

INTERACTIONS
Avoid use with intranasal influenza vaccines, H1N1 vaccines

NURSING CONSIDERATIONS
Assess:
• Hypersensitivity reactions/Stevens-Johnson syndrome

P

Side effects: *italics* = common; red = life-threatening

• **Neuropsychiatric reactions:** delirium, psychosis, hallucinations
• **Renal disease:** reduced dosing is required
Evaluate:
• Therapeutic response: absence of developing influenza A or B
Teach patient/family:
• That product is for use only within 48 hr of symptoms

⚠ HIGH ALERT

pertuzumab
(per-too'zoo-mab)
Perjeta
Func. class.: Antineoplastic
Chem. class.: HER-2/new antagonist

ACTION: Blocks liquid-dependent action of human epidermal growth factor-2 (HER2), inhibiting signal pathways

USES: First-line treatment of ⚕ HER2-positive metastatic breast cancer with trastuzumab and DOCEtaxel

CONTRAINDICATIONS HYPERSENSITIVITY:

Black Box Warning: Pregnancy

Precautions: Breastfeeding, children, infants, neonates, cardiac arrhythmias, MI, cardiac disease, heart failure, hypertension, infusion-related reactions, ⚕ Asian patients

Black Box Warning: Heart failure, ventricular dysfunction

DOSAGE AND ROUTES
• **Adult:** IV 840 mg over 60 min, then after 3 wk 420 mg over 30-60 min every 3 wk; give with trastuzumab 8 mg/kg IV over 90 min, then after 3 wk 6 mg/kg over 30-90 min every 3 wk and DOCEtaxel 75 mg/m² IV every 3 wk; dosage may be escalated to 100 mg/m²
Available forms: Solution for inj 420 mg/14 mL (single-use vials) (30 mg/mL)

♦ Canada only

Administer:
• Visually inspect for particulate matter and discoloration
Dilution and preparation
• Withdraw the calculated dose from the vial and add to a 250 mL 0.9% sodium chloride PVC or non-PVC polyolefin infusion bag; do not dilute with dextrose 5% solution
• Dilute in normal saline only; do not mix or dilute with other drugs or dextrose solutions
• Mix the diluted solution by gentle inversion; do not shake
IV infusion
• Administer the diluted solution immediately
• Do not administer as an IV push or bolus
• Give the first dose of 840 mg over 60 min and subsequent 420-mg doses over 30-60 min
• If the diluted solution is not used immediately, store at 2°-8° C for up to 24 hr
Delayed or missed doses
• If time since previous dose is <6 wk, give 420 mg IV (do not wait for next scheduled dose)
• If time since previous dose is ≥6 wk, give 840 mg IV over 60 min, followed 3 wk later by 420 mg IV over 30-60 min repeated every 3 wk
• If DOCEtaxel is discontinued, this product and trastuzumab may continue

SIDE EFFECTS
CNS: *Headache,* fever, *peripheral neuropathy,* chills, *fatigue,* asthenia
CV: Heart failure
EENT: Lacrimation, *stomatitis*
GI: *Nausea, vomiting,* diarrhea, dysgeusia, *stomatitis, constipation, anorexia*
HEMA: *Anemia,* neutropenia
MS: *Arthralgia*
RESP: Upper respiratory infection, cough
SYST: Anaphylaxis, antibody formation
INTEG: *Alopecia*

PHARMACOKINETICS
Median half-life 18 days

⚕ Genetic warning

NURSING CONSIDERATIONS
Assess:
• **HER2 overexpression:** testing should be done to identify HER2 overexpression before using this product

• **Decreased left ventricular ejection fraction (LVEF):** can occur and is increased in those with a history of prior anthracycline use or radiotherapy to the chest; evaluate LVEF at baseline and every 3 mo; withhold therapy ×3 wk if LVEF is <40% or LVEF is 40%-45% with a 10% or greater absolute decrease from baseline; resume therapy if the LVEF is recovered to >45% or to 40%-45% with <10% absolute decrease at reassessment; if the LVEF has not improved or has declined further, consider permanently discontinuing pertuzumab and trastuzumab after a risk/benefit assessment

• **Infusion-related reactions/hypersensitivity:** assess anaphylactoid reaction, acute infusion reaction, cytokine-release syndrome 60 min after the first infusion, 30 min after other infusions; monitor for pyrexia, chills, fatigue, headache, asthenia, hypersensitivity, and vomiting; if a significant reaction occurs, slow or interrupt the infusion; permanent discontinuation may be needed in severe reactions

• **Neutropenia:** can occur, but occurs more commonly when trastuzumab is also used and in ☥ Asian patients; monitor CBC with differential baseline and periodically

• **Upper respiratory infection:** monitor for dyspnea, shortness of breath, fever

Black Box Warning: **Pregnancy:** determine whether pregnancy is planned or suspected; patients who become pregnant during therapy should report exposure to the Genentech Adverse Event line at 888-835-2555 and enroll in the MotHER Pregnancy Registry at 800-690-6720

Evaluate:
• Decreased size, spread of tumor

Teach patient/family:
• To notify prescriber immediately of **infection** (cough, fever, chills, sore throat); **bleeding** (gums, bruising, blood in urine/stools/sputum); to avoid persons with known infections

• To avoid all OTC, prescription, herbal, and supplement products unless approved by prescriber; not to use aspirin, NSAIDs, alcohol

• To notify prescriber of peripheral neuropathy

• That hair loss is common

Black Box Warning: **Pregnancy/breastfeeding:** counsel women of childbearing age on the need for contraception during and for 6 mo after therapy; advise patients who suspect pregnancy to contact their health care provider immediately; discontinue breastfeeding

phenylephrine nasal agent
See Appendix B

phenylephrine ophthalmic
See Appendix B

phenytoin (Rx)
(fen′i-toh-in)
Dilantin, Phenytek, Tremytoine
✦

Func. class.: Anticonvulsant; antidysrhythmic (IB)
Chem. class.: Hydantoin

ACTION: Inhibits spread of seizure activity in motor cortex by altering ion transport; increases AV conduction

USES: Generalized tonic-clonic seizures; status epilepticus; nonepileptic seizures

---

Side effects: *italics* = common; red = life-threatening

associated with Reye's syndrome or after head trauma; complex partial seizures

Unlabeled uses: Migraines, diabetic neuropathy, neuropathic pain, paroxysmal atrial tachycardia, ventricular tachycardia

CONTRAINDICATIONS: Pregnancy, hypersensitivity, bradycardia, SA and AV block, Stokes-Adams syndrome

Precautions: Geriatric patients, allergies, renal/hepatic disease, petit mal seizures, hypotension, myocardial insufficiency, ✋ Asian patients positive for HLA-B1502, hepatic failure, acute intermittent porphyria, psychiatric condition

Black Box Warning: IV use

DOSAGE AND ROUTES—NTI

Seizures

• **Adult:** PO 15-20 mg/kg (ext rel) in 3-4 divided doses given q2hr or 400 mg, then 300 mg q2hr × 2 doses; maintenance 4-7 mg/kg/day; IV 15-20 mg/kg, max 25-50 mg/min, then 100 mg q6-8hr

• **Child:** PO 5 mg/kg/day in 2-3 divided doses, maintenance 4-8 mg/kg/day in 2-3 divided doses, max 300 mg/day; IV 15-20 mg/kg at 1-3 mg/kg/min

Status epilepticus

• **Adult:** IV 15-20 mg/kg, max 25-50 mg/min, may give 100 mg q6-8hr thereafter

• **Child:** IV 15-20 mg/kg, max in divided doses 1-3 mg/kg/min

Ventricular dysrhythmias

• **Adult:** PO loading dose 1 g divided over 24 hr, then 500 mg/day × 2 days; IV 250 mg over 5 min until dysrhythmias subside or until 1 g is given or 100 mg q15min until dysrhythmias subside or until 1 g is given

• **Child:** PO 3-8 mg/kg or 250 mg/m²/day as single dose or 2 divided doses; IV 3-8 mg/kg over several min or 250 mg/m²/day as single dose or 2 divided doses

Renal/hepatic dose

• Do not use loading dose if CCr <10 mL/min or hepatic failure

Neuropathic pain/diabetic neuropathy (unlabeled)

• **Adult:** PO 300 mg/day in divided doses

Migraine prophylaxis (unlabeled)

• **Adult:** PO 200-400 mg/day

Available forms: Susp 25 mg/5 mL; chewable tabs 50 mg; inj 50 mg/mL; ext rel caps 100, 200, 300 mg; prompt rel caps 100 mg

Administer:

PO route

• Do not interchange chewable product with caps, not equivalent; only ext rel caps to be used for once-a-day dosing

• **Oral susp:** shake well before each dose given via G tube/NG tube; dilute susp before administration; flush tube with 20 mL water after dose; hold tube feedings 1 hr before and 1 hr after dose

• Allow 7-10 days between dosage changes

• Divided PO doses with or after meals to decrease adverse effects

• 2 hr before or after antacid, enteral feeding

Direct IV route

Black Box Warning: Give undiluted at ≤50 mg/min (adult) 1-3 mg/kg/min; 0.5-1 mg/kg/min (neonates), monitor for CV reactions

Intermittent IV INFUSION route

Black Box Warning: Dilute dose in NS to ≤6.7 mg/mL; complete infusion within 1 hr of preparation; use 0.22- or 0.55-micron in-line particulate final filter between IV catheter and tubing; flush IV line or catheter with NS before and after use; give at ≤50 mg/min (adult), 0.5-1 mg/kg/min (child, infant, neonate)

Additive compatibilities: Do not admix

SIDE EFFECTS

CNS: Dizziness, insomnia, paresthesias, depression, suicidal tendencies, aggression, headache, confusion, slurred speech, peripheral neuropathy

CV: Hypotension, ventricular fibrillation, bradycardia, cardiac arrest

EENT: Nystagmus, diplopia, blurred vision

ENDO: Diabetes insipidus

GI: Nausea, vomiting, constipation, anorexia, weight loss, hepatitis, jaundice, gingival hyperplasia, abdominal pain

GU: Nephritis, urine discoloration, sexual dysfunction

HEMA: Agranulocytosis, leukopenia, aplastic anemia, thrombocytopenia, megaloblastic anemia

INTEG: Rash, lupus erythematosus, Stevens-Johnson syndrome, hirsutism, toxic epidermal necrolysis

SYST: Hypocalcemia, purple glove syndrome (IV), DRESS, anaphylaxis, exacerbates myasthenia gravis

PHARMACOKINETICS

Metabolized by liver, excreted by kidneys, protein binding 90%-95%, half-life 7-42 hr, dose dependent

PO: Onset 2-24 hr, peak $1^{1}/_{2}$-$2^{1}/_{2}$ hr, duration 6-12 hr

PO-ER: Onset 2-24 hr, peak 4-12 hr, duration 12-36 hr

IV: Onset 1-2 hr, duration 12-24 hr

INTERACTIONS

• Do not use with delavirdine; decreased response, resistance

Increase: phenytoin effect—benzodiazepines, cimetidine, tricyclics, salicylates, valproate, cycloSERINE, diazePAM, chloramphenicol, disulfiram, alcohol, amiodarone, sulfonamides, FLUoxetine, gabapentin, H_2 antagonists, azole antifungals, estrogens, succinamides, phenothiazines, methylphenidate, felbamate, traZODone

Decrease: phenytoin effects—alcohol carBAMazepine, rifAMPin, calcium (high dose), folic acid

Drug/Food

Enteral tube feeding: may decrease absorption of oral product; do not use enteral feedings 2 hr before or 2 hr after dose

Drug/Lab Test

Increase: glucose, alk phos, GGT

Decrease: dexamethasone, metyraPONE test serum, PBI, urinary steroids

NURSING CONSIDERATIONS

Assess:

• **Phenytoin hypersensitivity syndrome** 3-12 wk after start of treatment: rash, temperature, lymphadenopathy; may cause hepatotoxicity, renal failure, rhabdomyolysis

• **Serious skin disorders:** for beginning rash that may lead to Stevens-Johnson syndrome or toxic epidermal necrolysis; phenytoin should not be used again; may occur more often among Asian patients with HLA-B 1502

• Purple glove syndrome with IV use

• **Phenytoin level:** toxic level 30-50 mcg/mL; therapeutic level 7.5-20 mcg/mL

• **Seizures:** duration, type, intensity, precipitating factors; obtain EEG periodically; monitor therapeutic level

• Blood studies: CBC, platelets q2wk until stabilized, then monthly × 12, then q3mo; discontinue product if neutrophils <1600/mm^3; renal function: albumin concentration; folic acid levels, LFTs

• **Mental status:** mood, sensorium, affect, memory (long, short), suicidal thoughts/behaviors

• Monitor EKG, B/P, respiratory function during IV loading dose; verify potency of IV access port before IV infusion

• Monitor EEG function and serum levels periodically

• **Blood dyscrasias:** fever, sore throat, bruising, rash, jaundice

• **Beers:** avoid use in older adults unless safer alternatives are unavailable; ataxia, impaired psychomotor function may occur

• **Pregnancy/breastfeeding:** pregnant women should enroll in the Antiepileptic Drug Pregnancy Registry, 1-888-233-2334; may cause fetal malformations; use other options when possible; breastfeeding is not recommended

Evaluate:

• Therapeutic response: decrease in severity of seizures, ventricular dysrhythmias

Teach patient/family:

• That, if diabetic, blood glucose should be monitored

• That urine may turn pink

• Not to discontinue product abruptly because seizures may occur

---

Side effects: *italics* = common; red = life-threatening

• **Oral hygiene:** about the proper brushing of teeth using a soft toothbrush, flossing to prevent gingival hyperplasia; about the need to see dentist frequently

• To avoid hazardous activities until stabilized on product

• To carry emergency ID stating product use

• That heavy use of alcohol may diminish effect of product; to avoid OTC medications

• Not to change brands or forms once stabilized on therapy because brands may vary

• Not to use antacids within 2 hr of product

• To notify prescriber of unusual bleeding, bruising, petechiae (bleeding), clay-colored stools, abdominal pain, dark urine, yellowing of skin or eyes (hepatotoxicity); slurred speech, headache, drowsiness

• To report suicidal thoughts/behaviors immediately

• **Pregnancy/breastfeeding:** to use nonhormonal contraception; to notify prescriber if pregnancy is planned or suspected

---

RARELY USED

phosphate/biphosphate (OTC)

Fleet Enema, Phospho-Soda
Func. class.: Laxative, saline

ACTION: Increases water absorption in the small intestine by osmotic action; laxative effect occurs by increased peristalsis and water retention

USES: Constipation, bowel or rectal preparation for surgery, exam

CONTRAINDICATIONS: Hypersensitivity, rectal fissures, abdominal pain, nausea, vomiting, appendicitis, acute surgical abdomen, ulcerated hemorrhoids, sodium-restricted diet, renal failure, hyperphosphatemia, hypocalcemia, hypokalemia, hypernatremia, Addison's disease, HF, ascites, bowel perforation, megacolon, imperforate anus

> **Black Box Warning:** GI obstruction, renal failure

Precautions: Pregnancy

> **Black Box Warning:** Colitis, geriatric hypovolemia, renal disease

DOSAGE AND ROUTES
• **Adult: PO** 20-30 mL (Phospho-Soda)
• **Child: PO** 5-15 mL (Phospho-Soda)
• **Adult/child >12 yr: RECT** 1 enema (118 mL)
• **Child 2-12 yr: RECT** $1/2$ enema (59 mL)

Available forms: Enema 7 g phosphate/19 g biphosphate/118 mL; oral sol 18 g phosphate/48 g biphosphate/100 mL

Administer:
• Alone for better absorption; do not take within 1-2 hr of other products

SIDE EFFECTS
CV: Dysrhythmias, cardiac arrest, hypotension, widening QRS complex
GI: *Nausea, cramps,* diarrhea
META: Electrolyte, fluid imbalances

PHARMACOKINETICS
Onset 30 min-3 hr, excreted in feces

NURSING CONSIDERATIONS
Assess:
• **Stools:** color, amount, consistency; bowel pattern, bowel sounds, flatulence, distention, fever, dietary patterns, exercise; cramping, rectal bleeding, nausea, vomiting; if these occur, product should be discontinued
• Blood, urine electrolytes if product used often

Evaluate:
• Therapeutic response: decrease in constipation

Teach patient/family:
• Not to use laxatives for long-term therapy because bowel tone will be lost

---

- That normal bowel movements do not always occur daily
- Not to use in presence of abdominal pain, nausea, vomiting
- To notify prescriber if constipation unrelieved or if symptoms of electrolyte imbalance occur: muscle cramps, pain, weakness, dizziness, excessive thirst
- To maintain fluid consumption

physostigmine ophthalmic
See Appendix B

phytonadione (Rx)
(fye-toe-na-dye′one)
Mephyton, Vit K
Func. class.: Vit K$_1$, fat-soluble vitamin

Do not confuse:
Mephyton/methadone

ACTION: Needed for adequate blood clotting (factors II, VII, IX, X)

USES: Vit K malabsorption, hypoprothrombinemia, prevention of hypoprothrombinemia caused by oral anticoagulants, prevention of hemorrhagic disease of the newborn

CONTRAINDICATIONS: Hypersensitivity, severe hepatic disease, last few weeks of pregnancy
Precautions: Pregnancy, neonates, hepatic disease, IV use

Black Box Warning: Risk of anaphylaxis

DOSAGE AND ROUTES
Hypoprothrombinemia caused by vit K malabsorption
- Adult: PO/IM 2.5-25 mg, may repeat or increase to 50 mg
- Child: PO 2.5-5 mg
- Infant: PO/IM 2 mg

Prevention of hemorrhagic disease of the newborn
- **Neonate:** IM 0.5-1 mg within 1 hr after birth, repeat after 2-3 wk if required
Hypoprothrombinemia caused by oral anticoagulants
- **Adult/child:** PO/SUBCUT/IM 1-10 mg, may repeat 12-48 hr after PO dose or 6-8 hr after SUBCUT/IM dose based on INR
Available forms: Tabs 5 mg; inj 10 mg/mL, 1 mg/0.5 mL
Administer:
- Store in tight, light-resistant container (PO)
IM route
- Use this route only when other routes cannot be used (deaths may occur due to allergic reactions)
Intermittent IV INFUSION route
- After diluting with ≥10 mL D$_5$NS; give max 1 mg/min
- IV only when other routes not possible (deaths have occurred)

Y-site compatibilities: Alfentanil, amikacin, aminophylline, ascorbic acid, atracurium, atropine, azaTHIOprine, aztreonam, bumetanide, buprenorphine, butorphanol, calcium chloride/gluconate, ceFAZolin, cefonicid, cefoperazone, cefotaxime, cefoTEtan, cefOXitin, cefTAZidime, ceftizoxime, cefTRIAXone, cefuroxime, chloramphenicol, chlorproMAZINE, cimetidine, clindamycin, cyanocobalamin, cycloSPORINE, dexamethasone, digoxin, diphenhydrAMINE, DOPamine, doxycycline, enalaprilat, ePHEDrine, EPINEPHrine, epoetin alfa, erythromycin, esmolol, famotidine, fentaNYL, fluconazole, folic acid, furosemide, ganciclovir, gentamicin, glycopyrrolate, heparin, hydrocortisone, imipenem/cilastatin, indomethacin, insulin, isoproterenol, ketorolac, labetalol, lidocaine, mannitol, meperidine, metaraminol, methoxamine, methyldopate, metoclopramide, metoprolol, metroNIDAZOLE, midazolam, morphine, multivitamins, nafcillin, nalbuphine, naloxone, nitroglycerin, nitroprusside, norepinephrine, ondansetron, oxacillin, oxytocin, papaverine, penicillin G potassium,

P

Side effects: *italics* = common; red = life-threatening

pentamidine, pentazocine, PENTobarbital, PHENobarbital, phentolamine, phenylephrine, potassium chloride, procainamide, prochlorperazine, propranolol, pyridoxime, raNITIdine, sodium bicarbonate, succinylcholine, SUFentanil, theophylline, thiamine, ticarcillin/clavulanate, tobramycin, tolazoline, trimetaphan, urokinase, vancomycin, vasopressin, verapamil, vit B with C

SIDE EFFECTS

CNS: Headache, brain damage (large doses)
GI: Nausea, decreased LFTs
HEMA: Hemolytic anemia, hemoglobinuria, hyperbilirubinemia
INTEG: Rash, urticaria
RESP: Bronchospasm, dyspnea, feeling of chest constriction, respiratory arrest

PHARMACOKINETICS
PO/INJ: Metabolized, crosses placenta

INTERACTIONS
Decrease: action of phytonadione—bile acid sequestrants, sucralfate, antiinfectives, salicylates, mineral oil
Decrease: action of warfarin—large dose of product

NURSING CONSIDERATIONS
Assess:
• **Increased bleeding risk:** emesis, stools, urine; pressure on all venipuncture sites; avoid all inj if possible
• PT, INR during treatment (2-sec deviation from control time, bleeding time, clotting time, INR); monitor for bleeding, pulse, and B/P
• **Pregnancy/breastfeeding:** usually not needed in pregnancy; may breastfeed
Evaluate:
• Therapeutic response: cessation of bleeding
Teach patient/family:
• Not to take other supplements, OTC products, prescription products unless directed by prescriber
• About the necessary foods for associated diet

• To avoid IM inj; to use soft toothbrush; not to floss; to use electric razor until coagulation defect corrected
• To report symptoms of bleeding
• About the importance of frequent lab tests to monitor coagulation factors
• To notify all health care providers of use of this product
• To carry emergency ID describing condition and products used

---

pilocarpine ophthalmic
See Appendix B

---

pimecrolimus topical
See Appendix B

---

pimavanserin
(pim-a-van′ ser-in)
Nuplazid ✴
Func. class.: Atypical antipsychotic

ACTION: The exact mechanism of action is unknown; may be mediated through inverse agonist and antagonist activity at serotonin 5-HT2A receptors and to a lesser extent at 5-HT2C receptors.

USES: The treatment of hallucinations and delusions associated with Parkinson's disease psychosis

CONTRAINDICATIONS: Hypersensitivity
Precautions: Alcoholism, bradycardia, breastfeeding, cardiac arrhythmias, cardiac disease, children, coronary artery disease, diabetes mellitus, females, geriatric patients, heart failure, hepatic disease, hypertension, hypocalcemia, hypokalemia, hypomagnesemia, long QT syndrome, malnutrition, myocardial infarction, pregnancy, QT prolongation, renal failure, renal impairment, stroke, thyroid disease

---

DOSAGE AND ROUTES
• **Adult: PO** 34 mg (taken as two 17-mg tablets) daily, without titration
Hepatic dose
• **Adult: PO** Not recommended
Renal dose
• **Adult: PO** CCr ≥30 mL/min, no dosage adjustment needed; CCr <30 mL/min, not recommended
Other dosage adjustments
• Patients receiving a strong CYP3A4 inhibitor: 17 mg/day
• Patients receiving a strong CYP3A4 inducer: monitor for reduced effect, increase dose if needed
Available forms:
Tab 17 mg
Administer:
• Give without regard to food

SIDE EFFECTS
CNS: Confusion, hallucinations, fatigue, stroke, dizziness
GI: Nausea, constipation
MISC: Peripheral edema, infection, QT prolongation

PHARMACOKINETICS
Protein binding 95%, hepatic metabolism occurs through CYP3A4 and CYP3A5 and to a lesser extent CYP2J2, CYP2D6 with a major active metabolite; peak 6 hr, plasma half-lives of drug and metabolite are 57 hr and 200 hr, respectively; 0.55% eliminated unchanged in the urine and 1.53% was eliminated in feces after 10 days

INTERACTIONS
Increase: effects of pimavanserin—CYP3A4 inhibitors (ketoconazole, erythromycin), CYP2D6 inhibitors (quiNIDine, FLUoxetine, PARoxetine); reduce dose of pimavanserin
Increase: sedation—other CNS depressants
Increase: QT prolongation—products that cause QT prolongation

Decrease: pimavanserin effects—famotidine, valproate, CYP3A4 inducers (carbamazepine)
Decrease: pimavanserin effect—St. John's wort

NURSING CONSIDERATIONS
Assess:

• Swallowing of medication; check for hoarding, giving product to other patients
• AIMS assessment, neurologic function, LFTs, serum electrolytes, creatinine monthly
• Constipation daily; if this occurs, increase bulk, water in diet; stool softeners, laxatives may be needed
• **QT prolongation:** avoid in those with cardiac disease or other risk factors for QT prolongation, torsades de pointes (TdP), and/or sudden death such as cardiac arrhythmias, congenital long QT syndrome, heart failure, bradycardia, myocardial infarction, hypertension, coronary artery disease, hypomagnesemia, hypokalemia, hypocalcemia, or in patients receiving medications known to prolong the QT interval. Females, elderly patients, patients with diabetes mellitus, thyroid disease, malnutrition, alcoholism, or hepatic impairment may also be at increased risk for QT prolongation
• **Renal disease:** product not recommended for patients with severe renal impairment (CCr <30 mL/min)
• **Hepatic disease:** product is extensively metabolized in the liver; use is not recommended in patients with mild, moderate, or severe hepatic impairment
• **Stroke:** avoid antipsychotics to treat delirium- or dementia-related behavioral problems unless nonpharmacologic options have failed or are not possible and the patient is a substantial threat to self or others; avoid use in those with a history of falls or fractures

P

• **Hyponatremia:** product can cause hyponatremia and SIADH and elderly patients are at increased risk of developing these conditions; sodium levels should be closely monitored when starting or changing dosages of antipsychotics in older adults

Evaluate:

• Therapeutic response: decrease in hallucinations, delusions, paranoia; reorganization of patterns of thought and speech

Teach Patient/Family:

• To avoid hazardous activities until response is known, dizziness may occur
• That compliance with dose is needed
• To avoid OTC products unless approved by prescriber

⚠ HIGH ALERT

pioglitazone (Rx)

(pie-oh-glye′ta-zone)

Actos

Func. class.: Antidiabetic, oral

Chem. class.: Thiazolidinedione

Do not confuse:
Actos/Actonel

ACTION: Specifically targets insulin resistance; an insulin sensitizer; regulates the transcription of a number of insulin-responsive genes

USES: Type 2 diabetes mellitus

CONTRAINDICATIONS: Breastfeeding, children, hypersensitivity to thiazolidinedione, diabetic ketoacidosis

Black Box Warning: NYHA Class III/IV heart failure

Precautions: Pregnancy, geriatric patients, geriatric patients with CV disease, renal/hepatic/thyroid disease, edema, polycystic ovary syndrome, bladder cancer, osteoporosis, pulmonary disease, secondary malignancy

DOSAGE AND ROUTES
Monotherapy

• **Adult: PO** 15 or 30 mg/day, may increase to 45 mg/day; with strong CYP2C8, max 15 mg/day; with NYHA class I/II heart failure, max 15 mg/day

Combination therapy

• **Adult: PO** 15 or 30 mg/day with a sulfonylurea, metFORMIN, or insulin; decrease sulfonylurea dose if hypoglycemia occurs; decrease insulin dose by 10%-25% if hypoglycemia occurs or if plasma glucose is <100 mg/dL, max 45 mg/day

Hepatic dose

• Do not use in active hepatic disease or if ALT >2.5 times ULN

Available forms: Tabs 15, 30, 45 mg

Administer:

• Once a day; without regard to meals
• Tabs crushed and mixed with food or fluids for patients with difficulty swallowing

SIDE EFFECTS

CNS: *Headache*

CV: MI, heart failure, death (geriatric patients)

ENDO: Hypo/hyperglycemia

MISC: *Sinusitis, upper respiratory tract infection, pharyngitis,* hepatotoxicity, edema, weight gain, anemia, macular edema; risk of bladder cancer (use >1 yr), peripheral/pulmonary edema

MS: Rhabdomyolysis, fractures (females), myalgia

PHARMACOKINETICS

Maximal reduction in FBS after 12 wk; half-life 3-7 hr, terminal 16-24 hr; protein binding >99%

INTERACTIONS

Decrease: effect of atorvastatin

Decrease: effect of oral contraceptives; use alternative contraceptive method

Decrease: pioglitazone effect—CYP2C8 inducers (ketoconazole, fluconazole, itraconazole, miconazole, voriconazole)

Drug/Herb

Increase: hypoglycemia—garlic, green tea, horse chestnut

Drug/Lab Test

Increase: CPK, LFTs, HDL, cholesterol

Decrease: glucose, Hct/Hgb

NURSING CONSIDERATIONS
Assess:

Black Box Warning: Heart failure: do not use in NYHA Class III/IV; excessive/rapid weight gain >5 lb, dyspnea, edema; may need to be reduced or discontinued; monitor daily weights

• **Bladder cancer:** avoid use in a history of bladder cancer; use of pioglitazone >1 yr has shown an increase in bladder cancer

• **Hypoglycemic reactions:** sweating, weakness, dizziness, anxiety, tremors, hunger; hyperglycemic reactions soon after meals (rare); may occur more often with insulin or other antidiabetics

• **Hepatic disease:** check LFTs periodically: AST, LDH; do not start treatment in active heart disease or if ALT >2.5× upper limit of normal; if treatment has already begun, follow closely with continuing ALT levels; if ALT increases to >3× upper limit of normal, recheck ALT as soon as possible; if ALT remains >3× upper limit of normal, discontinue

• FBS, glycosylated HbA1c, plasma lipids/lipoproteins, B/P, body weight during treatment

• CBC with differential before and during therapy; more necessary in those with anemia; Hct/Hgb (may be decreased in first few months of treatment)

• **Beers:** avoid use in older adults; may promote fluid retention and/or exacerbate heart failure

• **Pregnancy/breastfeeding:** use only if benefits outweigh fetal risk; usually insulin is used in pregnancy; do not breastfeed, excretion unknown

Evaluate:

• Therapeutic response: decrease in polyuria, polydipsia, polyphagia; clear sensorium; absence of dizziness; stable gait; blood glucose A1c improvement

Teach patient/family:

• To self-monitor using a blood glucose meter

• About the symptoms of hypo/hyperglycemia; what to do about each

• That product must be continued on daily basis; about the consequences of discontinuing product abruptly

• To avoid OTC medications or herbal preparations unless approved by prescriber

• That diabetes is a lifelong illness; that product is not a cure, it only controls symptoms

• **To report symptoms of hepatic dysfunction:** nausea, vomiting, abdominal pain, fatigue, anorexia, dark urine, jaundice

• To report weight gain, edema

• That lab work, eye exams will be needed periodically

• To notify prescriber if oral contraceptives are used, effect may be decreased; not to use product if breastfeeding

---

piperacillin/tazobactam (Rx)

(pip′er-ah-sill′in/ta-zoe-bak′tam)

Tazocin ✦, Zosyn

Func. class.: Antiinfective, broad spectrum

Chem. class.: Extended-spectrum penicillin, β-lactamase inhibitor

ACTION: Interferes with cell-wall replication of susceptible organisms; tazobactam is a β-lactamase inhibitor that protects piperacillin from enzymatic degradation

USES: Moderate to severe infections: piperacillin-resistant, β-lactamase–producing strains causing infections in respiratory, skin, urinary tract, bone, gonorrhea, pneumonia; effective for resistant *Staphylococcus aureus*, resistant *Escherichia coli, Bacteroides fragilis, Bacteroides ovatus, Bacteroides thetaiotaomicron, Bacteroides vulgatus, Haemophilus influenzae*

Unlabeled uses: Endocarditis

CONTRAINDICATIONS: Hypersensitivity to penicillins; neonates; carbapenem allergy

Precautions: Pregnancy, breastfeeding, renal insufficiency in neonates, hypersensitivity to cephalosporins, seizures, GI disease, electrolyte imbalances, biliary obstruction

DOSAGE AND ROUTES
Nosocomial pneumonia
• **Adult:** IV 4.5 g q6hr or 3.375 g q4hr with an aminoglycoside or antipseudomonal fluoroquinolone × 1-2 wk

Infection of skin and/or subcutaneous tissue (moderate to severe), uncomplicated or complicated; pelvic inflammatory disease (moderate to severe); puerperal endometritis (moderate to severe)
• **Adult:** IV 3.375 g q6hr × 7-10 days

Appendicitis/peritonitis
• **Adult/adolescent/child ≥40 kg (88 lb):** IV 3.375 g q6hr × 7-10 days
• **Child ≥9 mo and <40 kg:** IV 100 mg/kg (piperacillin) q8hr × 7-10 days
• **Infant 2 mo to <9 mo:** IV 80 mg/kg (piperacillin) q8hr × 7-10 days

Renal dose
• **Adult:** IV CCr 20-40 mL/min, give 3.375 g q6hr (nosocomial pneumonia); give 2.25 g q6hr (all other indications); CCr <20 mL/min, give 2.25 g q6hr (nosocomial pneumonia); give 2.25 g q8hr (all other indications)

Available forms: Powder for inj 2 g piperacillin/0.25 g tazobactam, 3 g piperacillin/0.375 g tazobactam, 4 g piperacillin/0.5 g tazobactam, 36 g piperacillin/4.5 g tazobactam

Administer:
• Separate aminoglycoside from piperacillin to avoid inactivation
• Product after C&S is complete

Intermittent IV INFUSION route
• Reconstitute each 1 g of product/5 mL 0.9% NaCl for inj or sterile water for inj, dextrose 5%; shake well; further dilute in ≥50 mL compatible IV sol, run as int infusion over ≥30 min

ADD-Vantage IV solution: Reconstitution:
• Reconstitute with 0.9% sodium chloride or D₅W in the appropriate flexible diluent container provided; for 500-mg vials, use at least a 100 mL diluent container and for 750 mg and 1-g vials, use only the 250-mL diluent container
• Remove the protective covers from the top; remove vial cap (do not access with a syringe) and vial port cover; screw the vial into the vial port; to activate the contents of the vial, squeeze the bottom of the diluent container gently; with the other hand, push the drug vial down into the container; pull the inner cap from the drug vial; mix the container contents thoroughly
• *Storage after reconstitution:* the admixture solution may be stored for up to 24 hr at room temperature; do not refrigerate or freeze after reconstitution
• Do not use in series connections with flexible containers

Premixed Galaxy IV solution:
• Thaw frozen containers at room temperature (20-25° C or 68-77° F) or under refrigeration (2-8° C or 36-46° F); do not force thaw by immersion in water baths or by microwaving; check for leaks by squeezing bag firmly
• Do not admix
• **Storage:** the thawed solution is stable for 24 hr at room temperature or for 14 days under refrigeration; do not refreeze thawed product
• Do not use plastic containers in series connections, as this could result in an embolism due to residual air being drawn from the primary container before administration of the fluid from the secondary container is complete

IV INFUSION:
• Infuse IV over at least 30 min; ambulatory intravenous infusion pumps can be used; the solution is stable for up to 12 hr at room temperature

Y-site compatibilities: Alfentanil, allopurinol, amifostine, amikacin, aminocaproic acid, aminophylline, amphotericin B lipid complex, amphotericin B liposome, anidulafungin, argatroban, atenolol, aztreonam, bivalirudin, bleomycin, bumetanide, buprenorphine, busulfan, butorphanol, calcium acetate/chloride/gluconate, CARBOplatin, carmustine, cefepime, chloramphenicol, cimetidine, clindamycin, cyclophosphamide, cycloSPORINE, cytarabine, DACTINomycin, DAPTOmycin, dexamethasone, dexrazoxane, diazePAM, digoxin, diphenhydrAMINE, DOCEtaxel, DOPamine, doxacurium, enalaprilat, ePHEDrine, EPINEPHrine, eptifibatide, erythromycin, esmolol, etoposide, fenoldopam, fentaNYL, floxuridine, fluconazole, fludarabine, fluorouracil, foscarnet, fosphenytoin, furosemide, gallium, granisetron, heparin, hydrocortisone, HYDROmorphone, ifosfamide, isoproterenol, ketorolac, lansoprazole, lepirudin, leucovorin, lidocaine, linezolid, LORazepam, magnesium sulfate, mannitol, mechlorethamine, melphalan, meperidine, mesna, metaraminol, methotrexate, methylPREDNISolone, metoclopramide, metoprolol, metroNIDAZOLE, milrinone, morphine, naloxone, nitroglycerin, nitroprusside, norepinephrine, octreotide, ondansetron, oxytocin, PACLitaxel, palonosetron, pamidronate, pancuronium, PEMEtrexed, PENTobarbital, PHENobarbital, phentolamine, phenylephrine, plicamycin, potassium chloride/phosphates, procainamide, raNITIdine, remifentanil, riTUXimab, sargramostim, sodium acetate/bicarbonate/phosphate, succinylcholine, SUFentanil, sulfamethoxazole-trimethoprim, tacrolimus, telavancin, teniposide, theophylline, thiotepa, tigecycline, tirofiban, trimethobenzamide, vasopressin, vinBLAStine, vinCRIStine, voriconazole, zidovudine, zoledronic acid

SIDE EFFECTS
CNS: Lethargy, hallucinations, anxiety, depression, twitching, insomnia, headache, fever, dizziness, seizures, vertigo

CV: Cardiac toxicity, edema
GI: *Nausea, vomiting, diarrhea;* increased AST, ALT; abdominal pain, glossitis, CDAD, constipation, pancreatitis
GU: Oliguria, proteinuria, hematuria, *vaginitis, moniliasis,* glomerulonephritis, renal failure
HEMA: Anemia, increased bleeding time, bone marrow depression, agranulocytosis, hemolytic anemia
INTEG: Rash, pruritus, exfoliative dermatitis
META: Hypokalemia, hypernatremia
SYST: Serum sickness, anaphylaxis, Stevens-Johnson syndrome

PHARMACOKINETICS
Half-life 0.7-1.2 hr; excreted in urine, bile, breast milk; crosses placenta; 33% bound to plasma proteins
IV: Peak completion of IV

INTERACTIONS
Increase: effect of neuromuscular blockers, oral anticoagulants, methotrexate
Increase: piperacillin concentrations—aspirin, probenecid
Decrease: antimicrobial effect of piperacillin—tetracyclines, aminoglycosides IV

Drug/Lab Test
Increase: eosinophilia, neutropenia, leukopenia, serum creatinine, PTT, AST, ALT, alk phos, bilirubin, BUN, electrolytes
Decrease: Hct, Hgb, electrolytes
False positive: urine glucose, urine protein, Coombs' test

NURSING CONSIDERATIONS
Assess:
• **Infection:** temperature, stools, urine, sputum, wounds
• I&O ratio; report hematuria, oliguria because penicillin in high doses is nephrotoxic; maintain hydration unless contraindicated

P

• Hepatic studies: AST, ALT before treatment and periodically thereafter

• Blood studies: WBC, RBC, Hct, Hgb, bleeding time before treatment and periodically thereafter; serum potassium

• Renal studies: urinalysis, protein, blood, BUN, creatinine before treatment and periodically thereafter

• C&S before product therapy; product may be given as soon as culture is taken

• **CDAD:** diarrhea, bloody stools, fever, abdominal cramps; may occur ≤2 mo after treatment; bowel pattern before and during treatment

• Skin eruptions after administration of penicillin to 1 wk after discontinuing product

• Respiratory status: rate, character, wheezing, tightness in chest

• **Anaphylaxis:** wheezing, laryngeal edema, rash, itching; discontinue product, have emergency equipment nearby

• Adequate intake of fluids (2 L) during diarrhea episodes

• **Pregnancy/breastfeeding:** use only if clearly needed; cautious use in breastfeeding

Evaluate:

• Therapeutic response: absence of fever, purulent drainage, redness, inflammation; culture shows decreased organisms

Teach patient/family:

• That culture may be taken after completed course of medication

• To report sore throat, fever, fatigue (superinfection); CNS effects (anxiety, depression, hallucinations, seizures); pseudomembranous colitis (fever, diarrhea with blood, pus, mucus)

• To wear or carry emergency ID if allergic to penicillins

• CDAD: to notify nurse of diarrhea with blood, pus

TREATMENT OF OVERDOSE:

Withdraw product, maintain airway, administer EPINEPHrine, aminophylline, O₂, IV corticosteroids for anaphylaxis

---

RARELY USED

pirfenidone
(pir-fen′i-done)
Esbriet
Func. class.: Respiratory agent

USES: Pulmonary fibrosis

CONTRAINDICATIONS: Hypersensitivity

DOSAGE AND ROUTES

• **Adult: PO** Titrate over 2 wk to a maintenance dose of 801 mg tid. Give 267 mg tid on days 1-7, 534 mg tid on days 8-14, and 801 mg tid from day 15 onward

---

pitavastatin (Rx)
(pit′a-va-stat′-in)
Livalo, Zypitamag
Func. class.: Antilipidemic
Chem. class.: HMG-CoA reductase inhibitor

Do not confuse:
pitavastatin/pravastatin

ACTION: Inhibits HMG-CoA reductase enzyme, which reduces cholesterol synthesis; high doses lead to plaque regression

USES: As an adjunct for primary hypercholesterolemia (types Ia, Ib), dysbetalipoproteinemia, elevated triglyceride levels, prevention of CV disease by reduction of heart risk in those with mildly elevated cholesterol
Unlabeled uses: Atherosclerosis

CONTRAINDICATIONS: Pregnancy, breastfeeding, hypersensitivity, active hepatic disease, cholestasis
Precautions: Past hepatic disease, alcoholism, severe acute infections, trauma, severe metabolic disorders, electrolyte imbalance, seizures, surgery, organ transplant, endocrine disease, females, hypotension, renal disease

---

DOSAGE AND ROUTES

• **Adult: PO** 2 mg/day, usual range 1-4, max 4 mg/day

Renal dose

• **Adult: PO** CCr 30-<60 mL/min, 1 mg daily, max 2 mg daily; CCr <30 mL/min on hemodialysis, 1 mg daily, max 2 mg daily; CCr <30 mL/min, not recommended

Atherosclerosis (unlabeled)

• **Adult: PO** 4 mg/day

Available forms: Tabs 1, 2, 4 mg

Administer:

• Total daily dose any time of day without regard to meals

• Store in cool environment in tight container protected from light

SIDE EFFECTS

CNS: Headache

GI: Constipation, diarrhea

INTEG: Rash, pruritus, alopecia

MS: Arthralgia, myalgia, rhabdomyolysis

RESP: Pharyngitis

PHARMACOKINETICS

Peak 1 hr; metabolized in liver, excreted in urine, feces; half-life 12 hr; protein binding 99%; ⚭ concentrations lower in healthy African Americans

INTERACTIONS

Increase: risk for possible rhabdomyolysis—azole antifungals, cycloSPORINE, erythromycin, niacin, gemfibrozil, clofibrate

Increase: levels of pitavastatin—erythromycin

Drug/Herb

Increase: pitavastatin—red yeast rice

Drug/Lab Test

Increase: bilirubin, alk phos, ALT, AST

Interference: thyroid function tests

NURSING CONSIDERATIONS

Assess:

• **Diet;** obtain diet history including fat, cholesterol in diet

• Cholesterol, triglyceride levels periodically during treatment; check lipid panel 6 wk after changing dose

• Hepatic studies baseline and when clinically indicated; if AST >3× normal,

reduce or discontinue; AST, ALT, LFTs may be increased

• Renal studies in patients with compromised renal system: BUN, I&O ratio, creatinine

• **Rhabdomyolysis:** muscle pain, tenderness; obtain CPK if clinically indicated; if markedly increased, product may need to be discontinued

• **Pregnancy/breastfeeding:** do not use in pregnancy, breastfeeding

Evaluate:

• Therapeutic response: decrease in cholesterol to desired level after 6 wk

Teach patient/family:

• That blood work will be necessary during treatment

• To report blurred vision, severe GI symptoms, headache, muscle pain, weakness, tenderness

• That previously prescribed regimen will continue: low-cholesterol diet, exercise program, smoking cessation

• That product may increase blood glucose level

• Not to take product if pregnant or if pregnancy is planned or suspected (notify prescriber); to avoid breastfeeding

P

---

plazomicin

(pla-zoe-mye′ sin)

Zemdri

Func. class.: Antiinfective—aminoglycoside

ACTION: Bactericidal; inhibits bacterial protein synthesis through irreversible binding to the 30S ribosomal subunit of susceptible bacteria

USES: Complicated urinary tract infection (UTI), including pyelonephritis

CONTRAINDICATIONS: Aminoglycoside hypersensitivity, pregnancy

Precautions: Breastfeeding, colitis, diarrhea, geriatrics, GI disease, hearing

---

impairment, myasthenia gravis, pseudo-membranous colitis, renal disease

Black Box Warning: Nephrotoxicity, neuromuscular blockade, ototoxicity, pregnancy

DOSAGE AND ROUTES
• **Adult: IV** 15 mg/kg q24hr for 4-7 days

SIDE EFFECTS
CNS: Headache
CV: Hypo/hypertension
GI: Nausea, vomiting, diarrhea
GU: Decreased renal function, nephrotoxicity
MISC: Ototoxicity

PHARMACOKINETICS
Plasma protein binding 20%, not metabolized, excreted by kidneys

INTERACTIONS

Black Box Warning: **Increase:** nephrotoxicity—cephalosporins, acyclovir, vancomycin, amphotericin B, cyclosporine, loop diuretics, cidofovir

Black Box Warning: **Increase:** ototoxicity—IV loop diuretics

Black Box Warning: **Increase:** neuromuscular blockade, respiratory depression—anesthetics, nondepolarizing neuromuscular blockers

NURSING CONSIDERATIONS
Assess:
• Weight before treatment; calculation of dosage is usually based on ideal body weight but may be calculated on actual body weight
• Vital signs during infusion; watch for hypotension, change in pulse
• IV site for thrombophlebitis (pain, swelling, redness); change site if needed; apply warm compress to discontinued site

Black Box Warning: **Nephrotoxicity** is greater in those with impaired renal function, the elderly, and in those receiving other nephrotoxic medications; monitor creatinine clearance in all patients before starting therapy and daily; therapeutic drug monitoring (TDM) is recommended for complicated urinary tract infection patients with CCr <90 mL/min to avoid potentially toxic levels; I&O ratio, urinalysis daily for casts, protein; report sudden drop in urinary output

Black Box Warning: **Ototoxicity:** hearing loss, tinnitus, and/or vertigo; assess hearing baseline and throughout treatment; may be irreversible and may not become evident until after completion of therapy; usually in patients with a family history of hearing loss, with renal impairment, or in those receiving higher doses and/or longer durations of therapy than recommended

Black Box Warning: **Neuromuscular blockade** in those with neuromuscular disorders (myasthenia gravis) or in those receiving neuromuscular blocking agents; respiratory paralysis may occur

• **Pregnancy/breastfeeding:** can cause fetal harm when administered to a pregnant woman; do not use in pregnancy; considered compatible with breastfeeding
• For dehydration; provide adequate hydration of 1500-2000 mL/day
Teach patient/family:

Black Box Warning: **Ototoxicity:** to report hearing loss, ringing, roaring in ears; feeling of fullness in the head

• To report headache, dizziness, symptoms of overgrowth of infection, renal impairment, symptoms of nephrotoxicity
• To report redness, swelling at infusion site
• To drink plenty of fluids each day

• **Pregnancy/breastfeeding:** to notify health care provider if pregnancy is planned or suspected, or if breastfeeding

plecanatide
(ple-kan′-a-tide)
Trulance
Func. class.: Laxative
Chem. class.: Guanylate cyclase-C agonist

ACTION: Binds to GC-C and acts locally on the luminal surface of the intestinal epithelium. Activation of GC-C results in an increase in both intracellular and extracellular concentrations of cyclic guanosine monophosphate (cGMP); this action results in increased intestinal fluid and accelerated gastrointestinal (GI) transit

USES: Chronic idiopathic constipation, IBS-C

CONTRAINDICATIONS: Hypersensitivity, GI obstruction

Black Box Warning: Child <6 yr

Precautions: Pregnancy, breastfeeding

DOSAGE AND ROUTES
• **Adult: PO** 3 mg daily
Available forms: Tabs 3 mg
Administer:
• Give without regard to food
• Swallow whole; tablets may be crushed and given with applesauce or in water, may be given orally or via NG tube

SIDE EFFECTS
CNS: Dizziness
GI: *Diarrhea,* flatulence, abdominal distention, abdominal tenderness, nausea
GU: UTI
RESP: Sinusitis, upper respiratory tract infection

PHARMACOKINETICS
Unknown

INTERACTIONS

Drug/Lab Test
Increase: AST/ALT

NURSING CONSIDERATIONS
Assess:
Bowel pattern: frequency, consistency, baseline and periodically; provide adequate hydration if diarrhea occurs
Evaluate:
• Therapeutic response: complete bowel movements
Teach patient/family:
• **Pregnancy/breastfeeding:** to notify health care professional if pregnancy is planned or suspected or if breastfeeding
• To notify all health care professionals of all OTC, Rx, herbals or supplements taken
• To take as directed, not to double or skip doses; that if dose is missed, to take next regularly scheduled dose when due

RARELY USED

pomalidomide
(pom–a-lid′oh-mide)
Pomalyst
Func. class.: Antineoplastic, biologic response modifier, hormone
Chem. class.: TNF modifier

USES: Multiple myeloma in those who have received ≥2 treatments including lenalidomide and bortezomib and disease has progressed within 60 days of completion of the treatment or in BRAF V600 mutation-positive patients who have disease progression following ipilimumab and a BRAF inhibitor

CONTRAINDICATIONS: Breastfeeding, hypersensitivity

Black Box Warning: Pregnancy, thrombocytopenia

DOSAGE AND ROUTES
• **Adult: PO** 4 mg on days 1-21
Hepatic/renal dose:
• **Adult: PO** bilirubin >2 mg/dL and AST/ALT >3 × ULN or CCr >3 mg/dL, do not use

P

Side effects: *italics* = common; red = life-threatening

posaconazole (Rx)

(poe′sa-kon′a-zole)

Noxafil, Posanol ✦

Func. class.: Antifungal—systemic
Chem. class.: Triazole derivative

ACTION: Inhibits a portion of cell-wall synthesis; alters cell membranes and inhibits several fungal enzymes

USES: Prevention of aspergillus, candida infection, oropharyngeal candidiasis in immunocompromised patients, chemotherapy-induced neutropenia, mucocutaneous candidiasis

Unlabeled uses: Aspergillosis, cellulitis, coccidioidomycosis, endocarditis, endophthalmitis, esophageal candidiasis, febrile neutropenia, fungal keratitis, fusariosis, histoplasmosis, infectious arthritis, myocarditis, osteomyelitis, pericarditis, sinusitis, tracheobronchitis

CONTRAINDICATIONS: Hypersensitivity to this product or other systemic antifungals or azoles; fungal meningitis, onychomycosis or dermatomycosis in cardiac dysfunction; use with ergots, sirolimus, CYP3A4 substrates

Precautions: Pregnancy, breastfeeding, children, cardiac/hepatic/renal disease

DOSAGE AND ROUTES

Adult/adolescent: PO 600 mg/day in 2-4 divided doses

Oropharyngeal candidiasis

Adult: PO 100 mg bid × 1 day, then 100 mg/day × 13 days

Oropharyngeal candidiasis resistant to fluconazole or itraconazole

Adult/child ≥13 yr: PO 400 mg bid

Available forms: Oral susp 200 mg/5 mL; del rel tab 100 mg; sol for inj 300 mg/16.7 mL

Administer: Delayed-release tab: do not divide, chew, crush; give with food

IV route

Intermittent IV INFUSION route

• **Dilution:** bring to room temperature; transfer 16.7 mL of posaconazole to IV solution that is sufficient for final concentration of 1-2 mg/mL; use immediately

• Store divided solution up to 24 hr refrigerated

• Use 0.22-micron PES or PVDF filter; give slowly over 90 min through central line; if central line is unavailable, may give a single dose through a peripheral line over 30 min; do not give multiple doses by this method

PO route

Oral susp: shake well; use calibrated measuring device; take only with full meal or liquid nutritional supplements such as Ensure; rinse measuring device after each use

• Store in tight container in refrigerator; do not freeze

SIDE EFFECTS

CNS: *Headache, dizziness,* insomnia, fever, rigors, weakness, anxiety

CV: Hypo/hypertension, tachycardia, anemia, QT prolongation, torsades de pointes

GI: *Nausea, vomiting, anorexia, diarrhea,* cramps, abdominal pain, flatulence, GI bleeding, hepatotoxicity

GU: Gynecomastia, impotence, decreased libido

INTEG: *Pruritus,* fever, *rash,* toxic epidermal necrolysis

MISC: *Edema, fatigue,* malaise, hypokalemia, tinnitus, rhabdomyolysis, hypokalemia

PHARMACOKINETICS

Well absorbed, enhanced by food, protein binding 98%-99%, peak 3-5 hr, half-life 35 hr, metabolized in liver, excreted in feces (77% unchanged)

INTERACTIONS

• Do not use with lovastatin, atorvastatin

• **Increase:** QT prolongation—class IA/III antidysrhythmics, some phenothiazines, β agonists, local anesthetics, tricyclics, haloperidol, chloroquine, droperidol, pentamidine; CYP3A4 inhibitors (amiodarone, clarithromycin, erythromycin, telithromycin, troleandomycin), arsenic trioxide; CYP3A4 substrates (methadone, pimozide, QUEtiapine, quiNIDine, risperiDONE, ziprasidone)

Increase: tinnitus, hearing loss—quiNIDine

Increase: hepatotoxicity—other hepatotoxic products

Increase: severe hypoglycemia—oral hypoglycemics

Increase: sedation—triazolam, oral midazolam

Increase: levels, toxicity—busPIRone, busulfan, calcium-channel blockers, clarithromycin, cycloSPORINE, diazePAM, digoxin, felodipine, HMG-CoA reductase inhibitors, indinavir, isradipine, midazolam, niCARdipine, NIFEdipine, niMODipine, phenytoin, quiNIDine, ritonavir, saquinavir, sirolimus, tacrolimus, vinca alkaloids, warfarin

Decrease: posaconazole level—cimetidine, phenytoin

Decrease: posaconazole action—antacids, H₂-receptor antagonists, rifamycin, didanosine

Drug/Food

• Food increases absorption

NURSING CONSIDERATIONS
Assess:

• **Infection:** type of, may begin treatment before obtaining results; temperature, WBC, sputum at baseline and periodically, breakthrough infections may occur when used with fosamprenavir

• I&O ratio, electrolytes; correct electrolyte imbalances before starting treatment

• For allergic reaction: rash, photosensitivity, urticaria, dermatitis

• **Rhabdomyolysis:** muscle pain, increased CPK; weakness, swelling of affected muscles; if these occur and if confirmed by CPK, product should be discontinued

• **Hepatotoxicity:** nausea, vomiting, jaundice, clay-colored stools, fatigue; hepatic studies (ALT, AST, bilirubin) if patient receiving long-term therapy

• **QT prolongation:** ECG for QT prolongation, ejection fraction; assess for chest pain, palpitations, dyspnea

• **Pregnancy/breastfeeding:** use only if benefits outweigh fetal risk, may cause malformations; use in breastfeeding is not recommended

Evaluate:

• Therapeutic response: decreased symptoms of fungal infection, negative C&S for infecting organism

Teach patient/family:

• That long-term therapy may be needed to clear infection (1 wk-6 mo, depending on infection)

• To avoid hazardous activities if dizziness occurs

• To take 2 hr before administration of other products that increase gastric pH (antacids, H₂ blockers, omeprazole, sucralfate, anticholinergics); to notify health care provider of all medications taken (many interactions)

• About the importance of compliance with product regimen; to use alternative method of contraception

• To notify prescriber of GI symptoms, signs of hepatic dysfunction (fatigue, nausea, anorexia, vomiting, dark urine, pale stools)

• To take during or within 20 min of eating

---

potassium acetate
potassium bicarbonate (OTC, Rx)
K Effervescent, Klor-Con EF, K-Vescent
potassium bicarbonate and potassium chloride (OTC, Rx)
potassium bicarbonate and potassium citrate (OTC, Rx)
potassium gluconate (OTC, Rx)

⚠ HIGH ALERT

potassium chloride (OTC, Rx)
Klor-Con, K-Tab, Micro-K Micro-K10
Func. class.: Electrolyte, mineral replacement
Chem. class.: Potassium

P

ACTION: Needed for the adequate transmission of nerve impulses and cardiac contraction, renal function, intracellular ion maintenance

USES: Prevention and treatment of hypokalemia

CONTRAINDICATIONS: Renal disease (severe), severe hemolytic disease, Addison's disease, hyperkalemia, acute dehydration, extensive tissue breakdown
Precautions: Pregnancy, cardiac disease, potassium-sparing diuretic therapy, systemic acidosis

DOSAGE AND ROUTES
Hypokalemia (prevention) (bicarbonate, chloride, gluconate)
• **Adult:** PO 20 mEq/day in 1-2 divided doses
• **Child:** PO 1-2 mEq/kg/day in 1-2 divided doses
Hypokalemia, digoxin toxicity (acetate, chloride)
• **Adult:** serum potassium concentration >2.5 mEq/L: IV max 10 mEq/1 hr with 24-hr max dose 200 mEq, initial dose of 20-40 mEq has been recommended; PO 40-100 mEq/day in 2-4 divided doses
• **Child:** IV 0.25-0.5 mEq/kg/dose at 0.25-0.5 mEq/kg/hr; PO 2-5 mEq/day in divided doses
Available forms: Tabs for sol 6.5, 25 mEq; ext rel caps 8, 10 mEq; powder for sol 3.3, 5, 6.7, 10, 13.3 mEq/5 mL; tabs 2, 4, 5, 13.4 mEq; ext rel tabs 6.7, 8, 10 mEq; elix 6.7 mEq/5 mL; oral sol 2.375 mEq/5 mL; inj for prep of IV 1.5, 2, 2.4, 3, 3.2, 4.4, 4.7 mEq/mL
Administer:
PO route
• Do not break, crush, or chew ext rel tabs, caps, or enteric products
• With or after meals; dissolve effervescent tabs, powder in 8 oz cold water or juice; do not give IM, SUBCUT
• Caps with full glass of liquid

IV route
• Through large-bore needle to decrease vein inflammation; check for extravasation; in large vein, avoid scalp vein in child (IV); never give IV bolus

Potassium acetate
Y-site compatibilities: Ciprofloxacin
Potassium chloride
• Must be diluted; concentrated potassium injections fatal
Continuous IV INFUSION route
• Concentration max 80 mcg/L for peripheral line; 120 mEq/L for central line
• Dehydrated patients should receive 1 L of potassium-free hydrating solution, then infuse 10 mEq/hr; in severe hypokalemia, rate may be 40 mEq/hr

Y-site compatibilities: Acyclovir, aldesleukin, allopurinol, amifostine, aminophylline, amiodarone, ampicillin, amrinone, atropine, aztreonam, betamethasone, calcium gluconate, cephalothin, cephapirin, chlordiazePOXIDE, chlorproMAZINE, ciprofloxacin, cladribine, cyanocobalamin, dexamethasone, digoxin, diltiaZEM, diphenhydrAMINE, DOBUTamine, DOPamine, droperidol, edrophonium, enalaprilat, EPINEPHrine, esmolol, estrogens, ethacrynate, famotidine, fentaNYL, filgrastim, fludarabine, fluorouracil, furosemide, gallium, granisetron, heparin, hydrALAZINE, IDArubicin, indomethacin, insulin (regular), isoproterenol, kanamycin, labetalol, lidocaine, LORazepam, magnesium sulfate, melphalan, meperidine, methicillin, methoxamine, methylergonovine, midazolam, minocycline, morphine, neostigmine, norepinephrine, ondansetron, oxacillin, oxytocin, PACLitaxel, penicillin G potassium, pentazocine, phytonadione, piperacillin/tazobactam, prednisoLONE, procainamide, prochlorperazine, propofol, propranolol, pyridostigmine, remifentanil, sargramostim, scopolamine, sodium bicarbonate, succinylcholine, tacrolimus, teniposide, theophylline, thiotepa, trimethaphan, trimethobenzamide, vinorelbine, warfarin, zidovudine

SIDE EFFECTS
CNS: Confusion
CV: Bradycardia, cardiac depression, dysrhythmias, arrest; peaking T waves, lowered R, depressed RST, prolonged P-R interval, widened QRS complex
GI: *Nausea, vomiting, cramps,* pain, *diarrhea,* ulceration of small bowel
GU: Oliguria
INTEG: Cold extremities, rash

PHARMACOKINETICS
PO: Excreted by kidneys and in feces; onset of action ≈30 min
IV: Immediate onset of action

INTERACTIONS
Increase: hyperkalemia—potassium phosphate IV; products containing calcium or magnesium; potassium-sparing diuretic or other potassium products; ACE inhibitors

NURSING CONSIDERATIONS
Assess:
• **Hyperkalemia:** indicates toxicity; fatigue, muscle weakness, confusion, dyspnea, palpitation; ECG for peaking T waves, lowered R, depressed RST, prolonged P-R interval, widening QRS complex, hyperkalemia; product should be reduced or discontinued, administer sodium bicarbonate (metabolic acidosis); potassium level during treatment (3.5-5 mg/dL is normal level)
• Determine hydration status, I&O ratio; watch for decreased urinary output; notify prescriber immediately
• Cardiac status: rate, rhythm, CVP, PWP, PAWP if being monitored directly
• IV site for irritation; decrease rate if irritation occurs
• **Pregnancy/breastfeeding:** use only if clearly needed; cautious use in breastfeeding
Evaluate:
• Therapeutic response: absence of fatigue, muscle weakness; decreased thirst, urinary output; cardiac changes
Teach patient/family:
• To add potassium-rich foods to diet: bananas, orange juice, avocados, whole grains, broccoli, carrots, prunes, cocoa after product is discontinued
• To avoid OTC products: antacids, salt substitutes, analgesics, vitamin preparations unless specifically directed by prescriber; to avoid licorice in large amounts because it may cause hypokalemia, sodium retention
• To report hyperkalemia symptoms (lethargy, confusion, diarrhea, nausea, vomiting, fainting, decreased output) or continued hypokalemia symptoms (fatigue, weakness, polyuria, polydipsia, cardiac changes)
• To dissolve powder or tablet completely in ≥120 mL water or juice
• About the importance of regular follow-up visits
• That potassium levels will need to be monitored periodically

potassium iodide (Rx)
SSKI, Thyro-Block ✿
Func. class.: Thyroid hormone antagonist
Chem. class.: Iodine product

ACTION: Inhibits secretion of thyroid hormone, fosters colloid accumulation in thyroid follicles, decreases vascularity of gland

USES: Preparation for thyroidectomy, thyrotoxic crisis, neonatal thyrotoxicosis, radiation protectant, thyroid storm
Unlabeled uses: Erythema multiforme, erythema nodosum leprosum (ENL), sporotrichosis, thyroid involution induction

CONTRAINDICATIONS: Pregnancy, pulmonary edema, pulmonary TB, bronchitis, hypersensitivity to iodine
Precautions: Breastfeeding, children

DOSAGE AND ROUTES
Hyperthyroidism/thyrotoxicosis
• **Adult/child: PO** (SSKI) 250 mg tid × 10-14 days preoperatively

---

Preparation for thyroidectomy
• **Adult/child: PO** 3-5 gtt strong iodine sol tid or 1-5 drops SSKI in water tid after meals for 10 days before surgery

Radiation exposure (radioactive iodine)
• **Adult: PO** 130 mg/day (distribution by government/public health officials or OTC purchase)
• **Child ≥3 yr: PO** 65 mg daily
• **Child/infant >1 mo-3 yr: PO** 32 mg/day
• **Neonate: PO** 16 mg/day

Available forms: Oral sol (Lugol's solution) iodine 5%/potassium iodide 10%; oral sol (SSKI) 1 g/mL (Thyro-Shield) 65 mg/mL; syrup (PIMA) 325 mg/5 mL; tabs 65, 130 mg

Administer:
• Products are not interchangeable
• Strong iodine solution after diluting with water or juice to improve taste
• Through straw to prevent tooth discoloration
• With meals to decrease GI upset
• At same time each day to maintain product level
• At lowest dose that relieves symptoms; discontinue before RAIU

SIDE EFFECTS

CNS: Headache, confusion, paresthesias
EENT: Metallic taste, stomatitis, salivation, periorbital edema, sore teeth and gums, cold symptoms
ENDO: Hypothyroidism, hyperthyroid adenoma
GI: *Nausea, diarrhea, vomiting,* small-bowel lesions, upper gastric pain, metallic taste
INTEG: Rash, urticaria, angioneurotic edema, acne, mucosal hemorrhage, fever
MS: Myalgia, arthralgia, weakness

PHARMACOKINETICS

PO: Onset 24-48 hr, peak 10-15 days after continuous therapy, uptake by thyroid gland or excreted in urine, crosses placenta

INTERACTIONS

Increase: hypothyroidism—lithium, other antithyroid agents

Increase: hyperkalemia—angiotensin II receptor antagonist, ACE inhibitors, potassium salts, potassium-sparing diuretics

NURSING CONSIDERATIONS

Assess:
• Pulse, B/P, temperature; serum potassium
• I&O ratio; check for edema: puffy hands, feet, periorbit; indicate hypothyroidism
• Weight daily; same clothing, scale, time of day
• T_3, T_4, which is increased; serum TSH, which is decreased; free thyroxine index, which is increased if dosage is too low; discontinue product 3-4 wk before RAIU
• **Overdose:** peripheral edema, heat intolerance, diaphoresis, palpitations, dysrhythmias, severe tachycardia, fever, delirium, CNS irritability
• **Hypersensitivity:** rash; enlarged cervical lymph nodes may indicate product should be discontinued
• **Hypoprothrombinemia:** bleeding, petechiae, ecchymosis
• Clinical response: after 3 wk should include increased weight, pulse; decreased T_4
• Fluids to 3-4 L/day unless contraindicated
• **Pregnancy/breastfeeding:** do not use in pregnancy, breastfeeding

Evaluate:
• Therapeutic response: weight gain; decreased pulse, T_4, size of thyroid gland

Teach patient/family:
• To abstain from breastfeeding after delivery
• To keep graph of weight, pulse, mood
• To avoid OTC products that contain iodine
• That seafood, other iodine products may be restricted
• Not to discontinue product abruptly; that thyroid crisis may occur as part of stress response
• That response may take several mo if thyroid is large
• To discontinue product, notify prescriber of fever, rash, metallic taste, swelling of throat; burning of mouth, throat;

sore gums, teeth; severe GI distress, enlargement of thyroid, cold symptoms

pramipexole (Rx)

(pra-mi-pex′ol)

Mirapex, Mirapex ER

Func. class.: Antiparkinson agent
Chem. class.: DOPamine-receptor agonist, non-ergot

Do not confuse:
Mirapex/Miralax

ACTION: Selective agonist for D_2 receptors (presynaptic/postsynaptic sites); binding at D_3 receptor contributes to antiparkinson effects

USES: Idiopathic Parkinson's disease, restless legs syndrome

CONTRAINDICATIONS: Hypersensitivity
Precautions: Pregnancy, cardiac/renal disease, MI with dysrhythmias, affective disorders, psychosis, preexisting dyskinesias, history of falling asleep during daily activities, rapid dose reduction

DOSAGE AND ROUTES
Parkinson's disease
• **Adult: PO** 0.125 mg tid; increase gradually by 0.125 mg/dose at 5- to 7-day intervals until total daily dose of 4.5 mg/day reached; ER 0.375 mg daily initially, then up to 0.75 mg/day; may increase by 0.75 mg/day no more than q5-7days as needed, max 4.5 mg/day
Restless legs syndrome
• **Adult: PO** 0.125 mg 2-3 hr before bedtime, increase gradually, max 0.5 mg/day
Renal dose
• **Adult: PO** CCr 35-59 mL/min, 0.125 mg bid, may increase q5-7days to 1.5 mg bid if required; CCr 15-34 mL/min, 0.125 mg/day, increase q5-7days to 1.5 mg/day
Available forms: Tabs 0.125, 0.25, 0.5, 0.75, 1, 1.5 mg; ER tab 0.375, 0.75, 1.5, 2.25, 3.0, 3.75, 4.5 mg
Administer:
• Adjust dosage to patient response, titrate slowly, taper when discontinuing

• With meals to minimize GI symptoms
• Do not crush, chew, or break ext rel product

SIDE EFFECTS
CNS: *Agitation, insomnia,* psychosis, hallucinations, depression, dizziness, headache, confusion, amnesia, dream disorder, asthenia, dyskinesia, hypersomnolence, sudden sleep onset, impulse control disorders
CV: *Orthostatic hypotension,* edema, syncope, tachycardia, increased B/P, heart rate, heart failure
EENT: Blurred vision, retinal/vision deterioration
ENDO: Antidiuretic hormone secretion (SIADH)
GI: *Nausea, anorexia,* constipation, dysphagia, dry mouth
GU: Impotence, urinary frequency
HEMA: Hemolytic anemia, leukopenia, agranulocytosis
INTEG: Pruritus

PHARMACOKINETICS
Minimally metabolized, peak 2 hr, half-life 8 hr, 8.5-12 hr in geriatric patients

INTERACTIONS
Increase: pramipexole levels—levodopa, cimetidine, raNITIdine, diltiaZEM, triamterene, verapamil, quiNIDine
Decrease: pramipexole levels—DOPamine antagonists, phenothiazines, metoclopramide, butyrophenones

NURSING CONSIDERATIONS
Assess:
• **Parkinson's disease:** involuntary movements: bradykinesia, tremors, staggering gait, muscle rigidity, drooling
• B/P, ECG, respiration during initial treatment; hypo/hypertension should be reported
• **Mental status:** affect, mood, behavioral changes, depression; complete suicide assessment, worsening of symptoms of restless legs syndrome, impulse control disorders
• **Somnolence:** may fall asleep during activities without warning; may need to discontinue medication

Side effects: *italics* = common; red = life-threatening

- Assistance with ambulation during beginning therapy
- Testing for diabetes mellitus, acromegaly if receiving long-term therapy
- **Pregnancy/breastfeeding:** use only if benefits outweigh fetal risk, may cause fetal harm; do not breastfeed

Evaluate:
- Therapeutic response: movement disorder improves

Teach patient/family:
- That therapeutic effects may take several weeks to a few months
- To change positions slowly to prevent orthostatic hypotension
- To use product exactly as prescribed; if product is discontinued abruptly, parkinsonian crisis may occur; to avoid alcohol, OTC sleeping products
- To notify prescriber if pregnancy is planned or suspected
- To notify prescriber of impulse control disorders: shopping

---

⚠ HIGH ALERT

pramlintide (Rx)
(pram'lin-tide)
SymlinPen
Func. class.: Antidiabetic
Chem. class.: Synthetic human amylin analog

ACTION: Modulates and slows stomach emptying, prevents postprandial rise in plasma glucagon, decreases appetite, leads to decreased caloric intake and weight loss

USES: As an adjunct prandial to insulin therapy for uncontrolled type 1 or type 2 diabetes

CONTRAINDICATIONS: Hypersensitivity to this product or cresol; gastroparesis

Black Box Warning: Hypoglycemia

Precautions: Pregnancy, breastfeeding, osteoporosis, thyroid disease, trauma, vomiting, renal failure, fever, diarrhea

DOSAGE AND ROUTES
Type 1 diabetes
- **Adult: SUBCUT** 15 mcg before each meal (≥30 g carbohydrate), titrate up in 15-mcg increments to target dose of 60 mcg/dose; each dose titration should occur after no nausea for 3 days

Type 2 diabetes
- **Adult: SUBCUT** 60 mcg before each meal (≥30 g CHO), titrate up to 120 mcg **SUBCUT** with each meal after no nausea for 3-7 days

Available forms: PEN 60, 120 (1000 mcg/mL solution for injection)

Administer:
- Store at room temperature for ≤30 days; keep away from heat and sunlight; refrigerate all other supply
- Premeal insulin should be decreased by 50% when starting and adjusted to therapeutic dose to prevent hypoglycemia

SUBCUT route
- Rotate injection sites, allow solution to warm to room temperature before use
- Take immediately before mealtime or if 30 g of carbohydrates will be consumed
- Do not use if a meal is skipped
- Do not use if discolored; do not give in arm; absorption is variable

SIDE EFFECTS
CNS: *Headache,* fatigue, dizziness, confusion
EENT: Blurred vision
GI: *Nausea, vomiting, anorexia,* abdominal pain
INTEG: Inj-site reactions, diaphoresis
META: Hypoglycemia
MS: Arthralgia
RESP: *Cough,* pharyngitis
SYST: *Systemic allergy*

PHARMACOKINETICS
Bioavailability 30%-40%, not extensively bound to blood cells or albumin, 40% bound in plasma, half-life 48 min, metabolized by kidneys, peak 20 min, duration 3 hr

---

INTERACTIONS
• Do not use with erythromycin, metoclopramide

Increase: effect of acetaminophen

Increase: pramlintide action—antimuscarinics, α-glucosidase inhibitors, diphenoxylate, loperamide, octreotide, opiate agonist, tricyclics

Increase: hypoglycemia—ACE inhibitors, disopyramide, anabolic steroids, androgens, fibric acid derivatives, alcohol, corticosteroids, insulin

Increase: hyperglycemia—phenothiazines

Decrease: hypoglycemia—niacin, dextrothyroxine, thiazide diuretics, triamterene, estrogens, progestins, oral contraceptives, MAOIs

NURSING CONSIDERATIONS
Assess:

Black Box Warning: Fasting blood glucose, 2 hr postprandial (80-150 mg/dL, normal fasting level; 70-130 mg/dL, normal 2 hr level); A1c may also be drawn to identify treatment effectiveness; also monitor weight, appetite

• **Hypoglycemic reaction:** sweating; weakness; dizziness; chills; confusion; headache; nausea; rapid, weak pulse; fatigue; tachycardia; memory lapses; slurred speech; staggering gait; anxiety; tremors; hunger
• **Hyperglycemia:** acetone breath; polyuria; fatigue; polydipsia; flushed, dry skin; lethargy
• **Pregnancy/breastfeeding:** use only if benefits outweigh fetal risk, usually insulin is used in pregnancy; avoid breastfeeding

Evaluate:
• Therapeutic response: decrease in polyuria, polydipsia, polyphagia; clear sensorium; absence of dizziness; stable gait; improving blood glucose, A1c

Teach patient/family:
• That product does not cure diabetes but rather controls symptoms
• To carry emergency ID as diabetic
• To recognize hypoglycemia reaction: headache, fatigue, weakness, fast pulse

• About the dosage, route, mixing instructions, diet restrictions, disease process

Black Box Warning: To carry a glucose source (candy or lump sugar, glucose tabs) to treat hypoglycemia

• About the symptoms of ketoacidosis: nausea; thirst; polyuria; dry mouth; decreased B/P; dry, flushed skin; acetone breath; drowsiness; Kussmaul respirations
• That a plan is necessary for diet, exercise; that all food on diet should be eaten; that exercise routine should not vary
• About blood glucose testing; how to determine glucose level
• To avoid OTC products, alcohol unless directed by prescriber
• Not to operate machinery or drive until effect is known
• About how to use pen

TREATMENT OF OVERDOSE:
Glucose 25 g IV or 50 mL dextrose 50% sol or 1 mg glucagon SUBCUT

pramoxine topical
See Appendix B

P

⚠ HIGH ALERT

prasugrel (Rx)
(pra′soo-grel)
Effient
Func. class.: Platelet aggregation inhibitor
Chem. class.: ADP receptor antagonist

ACTION: Inhibits ADP-induced platelet aggregation

USES: Reducing the risk of stroke, MI, vascular death, peripheral arterial disease in high-risk patients

CONTRAINDICATIONS: Hypersensitivity, stroke, TIA

Side effects: *italics* = common; red = life-threatening

Black Box Warning: Active bleeding

Precautions: Pregnancy, breastfeeding, children, geriatric patients, hepatic disease, increased bleeding risk, neutropenia, agranulocytosis, renal disease, surgery, trauma, thrombotic thrombocytopenic purpura, ✣ Asian patients, weight <60 kg, CABG, abrupt discontinuation

DOSAGE AND ROUTES
• **Adult/geriatric <75 yr and ≥60 kg: PO** 60 mg loading dose, then 10 mg daily with aspirin (75-325 mg/day)
• **Adult/geriatric <75 yr and <60 kg: PO** 60 mg loading dose, then 5 mg daily
• **Geriatric ≥75 yr:** not recommended
Available forms: Tabs 5, 10 mg
Administer:
• With food to decrease gastric symptoms
• Do not break tablets, tablet may be crushed and mixed in food, fluids
• Do not discontinue therapy abruptly

SIDE EFFECTS
CNS: Headache, dizziness
CV: Edema, atrial fibrillation, bradycardia, chest pain, hypo/hypertension
GI: Nausea, vomiting, diarrhea
HEMA: Epistaxis, leukopenia, thrombocytopenia, neutropenia, anaphylaxis, angioedema, anemia
INTEG: Rash, hypercholesterolemia
MISC: Fatigue, intracranial hemorrhage, secondary malignancy, angioedema
MS: Back pain

PHARMACOKINETICS
Rapidly absorbed; peak 30 min; metabolized by liver (CYP3A4; CYP2B6); excreted in urine, feces; half-life 7 hr

INTERACTIONS
Increase: bleeding risk—anticoagulants, aspirin, NSAIDs, abciximab, eptifibatide, tirofiban, thrombolytics, ticlopidine, SSRIs, treprostinil, rifAMPin

NURSING CONSIDERATIONS
Assess:
• **Thrombotic/thrombocytic purpura:** fever, thrombocytopenia, neurolytic anemia

• Hepatic studies: AST, ALT, bilirubin, creatinine with long-term therapy
• Blood studies: CBC, differential, Hct, Hgb, PT, cholesterol with long-term therapy

Black Box Warning: **Bleeding:** may be fatal, decreased B/P in those who have had CABG may be the first indication; bleeding should be controlled while continuing product; may use transfusion; do not use within 1 wk of CABG; may use lower doses in those <60 kg

• **Pregnancy/breastfeeding:** use only if benefits outweigh fetal risk
• **Beers:** avoid use in those age ≥75 yr; increased bleeding risk
Evaluate:
• Therapeutic response: absence of stroke, MI
Teach patient/family:
• That blood work will be necessary during treatment

Black Box Warning: To report any unusual bruising, bleeding to prescriber; that it may take longer to stop bleeding

• To take with food or just after eating to minimize GI discomfort
• To report diarrhea, skin rashes, subcutaneous bleeding, chills, fever, sore throat
• To tell all health care providers that prasugrel is being used; that product may be held before surgery

---

pravastatin (Rx)
(pra′va-sta-tin)
Pravachol, PravASA ✣
Func. class.: Antilipemic
Chem. class.: HMG-CoA reductase enzyme

Do not confuse:
Pravachol/Prevacid/propranolol

ACTION: Inhibits HMG-CoA reductase enzyme, which reduces cholesterol synthesis

---

USES: As an adjunct for primary hypercholesterolemia (types IIa, IIb, III, IV), to reduce the risk for recurrent MI, atherosclerosis, primary/secondary CV events, stroke, TIAs

CONTRAINDICATIONS: Pregnancy, breastfeeding, hypersensitivity, active hepatic disease

Precautions: Past hepatic disease, alcoholism, severe acute infections, trauma, severe metabolic disorders, electrolyte imbalances, renal disease

DOSAGE AND ROUTES

• **Adult: PO** 40 mg/day at bedtime (range 10-80 mg/day); start at 10 mg/day if patient also taking immunosuppressants

• **Adolescent 14-18 yr: PO** 40 mg/day

• **Child 8-13 yr: PO** 20 mg/day

• **Geriatric/renal/hepatic disease: PO** 10 mg/day initially

Renal dose

• **Adult: PO** 10-20 mg daily at bedtime, increase at 4-wk intervals

Available forms: Tabs 10, 20, 40, 80 mg

Administer:

• Without regard to meals, at bedtime

• Give 4 hr after bile acid sequestrants

• Store in cool environment in tight container protected from light

SIDE EFFECTS

CNS: Headache, dizziness, fatigue, confusion

CV: Chest pain

EENT: Lens opacities

GI: Nausea, constipation, diarrhea, flatus, abdominal pain, heartburn, hepatic dysfunction, pancreatitis, hepatitis

GU: Renal failure (myoglobinuria)

INTEG: Rash, pruritus

MS: Muscle cramps, myalgia, myositis, rhabdomyolysis

RESP: Common cold, rhinitis, cough

PHARMACOKINETICS

Peak $1-1^1/_2$ hr; metabolized by liver; protein binding 50%; excreted in urine 20%, feces 70%, breast milk; crosses placenta; half-life 1.25-2.25 hr

INTERACTIONS

Increase: myopathy, rhabdomyolysis risk—erythromycin, niacin, cycloSPORINE, gemfibrozil, clofibrate, clarithromycin, itraconazole, protease inhibitors

Decrease: bioavailability of pravastatin—bile acid sequestrants

Drug/Herb

Increase: adverse reactions—red yeast rice

Increase: hepatotoxicity—eucalyptus

Decrease: effect—St. John's wort

Drug/Lab Test

Increase: CK, LFTs

Altered: thyroid function tests

NURSING CONSIDERATIONS

Assess:

• Fasting lipid profile: LDL, HDL, triglycerides, cholesterol at baseline, q12wk, then q6mo when stable; obtain diet history

• Hepatic studies: baseline, then when clinically indicated; LFTs may increase

• **Rhabdomyolysis:** muscle tenderness, pain; obtain CPK if clinically indicated; therapy should be discontinued

• **Pregnancy/breastfeeding:** do not use in pregnancy, breastfeeding

Evaluate:

• Therapeutic response: decrease in LDL total cholesterol, triglycerides; increase in HDL

Teach patient/family:

• That blood work will be necessary during treatment

• To report blurred vision, severe GI symptoms, dizziness, headache, muscle pain, weakness, fever

• That regimen will continue: low-cholesterol diet, exercise program; that if taking a product like cholestyramine, to take this product at least 1 hr prior to or 4 hr after the bile acid resin

• To report suspected, planned pregnancy; not to use product during pregnancy; not to breastfeed

• **Hepatic disease:** to notify prescriber of lack of appetite, yellow sclera/skin, dark urine, abdominal pain, weakness

P

prazosin (Rx)

(pray´zoe-sin)

Minipress

Func. class.: Antihypertensive
Chem. class.: α_1-Adrenergic blocker, peripheral

Do not confuse:
prazosin/predniSONE

ACTION: Blocks α-mediated vasoconstriction of adrenergic receptors, thereby inducing peripheral vasodilation

USES: Hypertension, benign prostatic hypertrophy to decrease urine outflow obstruction

Unlabeled uses: Heart failure, hypertensive urgency, Raynaud's phenomenon, posttraumatic stress disorder (PTSD)

CONTRAINDICATIONS: Hypersensitivity

Precautions: Pregnancy, breastfeeding, children, geriatric patients, prostate cancer, ocular surgery, orthostatic hypotension

DOSAGE AND ROUTES
Hypertension
• **Adult: PO** 1 mg bid or tid increasing to 20 mg/day in divided doses, if required; usual range 6-15 mg/day, max 40 mg/day
• **Child (unlabeled): PO** 5 mcg/kg q6hr; max 400 mcg/kg/day or 15 mg/day
Benign prostatic hyperplasia
• **Adult: PO** 2 mg bid
Posttraumatic stress disorder (unlabeled)
• **Adult: PO** 1 mg at bedtime, then titrated to max 15 mg/day
Available forms: Caps 1, 2, 5 mg
Administer:
• 1st dose at bedtime to avoid fainting
• Without regard to meals
• Store at room temperature

SIDE EFFECTS
CNS: *Dizziness, headache, drowsiness,* anxiety, depression, vertigo, *weakness,* fatigue, syncope
CV: *Palpitations, orthostatic hypotension,* tachycardia, edema, rebound hypertension
EENT: Blurred vision, epistaxis, tinnitus, dry mouth, red sclera
GI: *Nausea,* vomiting, diarrhea, constipation, abdominal pain, pancreatitis
GU: Urinary frequency, incontinence, impotence, priapism; water, sodium retention

PHARMACOKINETICS
Onset 2 hr, peak 2-4 hr, duration 6-12 hr, half-life 2-4 hr; metabolized in liver, excreted via bile, feces (>90%), urine (<10%); protein binding 97%

INTERACTIONS
Increase: hypotensive effects—β-blockers, nitroglycerin, alcohol, phosphodiesterase inhibitors (vardenafil, tadalafil, sildenafil); diuretics, other antihypertensives, MAOIs
Decrease: antihypertensive effect—NSAIDs
Increase: antihypertensive effect—hawthorn
Drug/Lab Test
Increase: urinary norepinephrine, VMA, BUN, uric acid, LFTs
Positive: ANA titer

NURSING CONSIDERATIONS
Assess:
• **Hypertension/HF:** B/P (sitting, standing) during initial treatment, periodically thereafter; pulse, jugular venous distention, orthostatic hypotension usually occurs on first dose
• BUN, uric acid if patient receiving long-term therapy
• Weight daily, I&O; edema in feet, legs daily
• **Benign prostatic hypertrophy (unlabeled):** urinary patterns, frequency, stream, dribbling; flow before, during, and after therapy

---

- **Beers:** avoid use as an antihypertensive in older adults; high risk of orthostatic hypotension
- **Pregnancy/breastfeeding:** use only if benefits outweigh fetal risk; cautious use in breastfeeding, excreted in breast milk

Evaluate:
- Therapeutic response: decreased B/P

Teach patient/family:
- That fainting occasionally occurs after 1st dose; to take 1st dose at bedtime; to not drive or operate machinery for 4 hr after 1st dose; that full effect may take 4-6 wk
- To change positions slowly to prevent orthostatic hypotension
- To avoid OTC medications, alcohol unless approved by prescriber; not to crush, chew caps
- Not to discontinue abruptly

TREATMENT OF OVERDOSE: Administer volume expanders or vasopressors, discontinue product, place patient in supine position

prednisoLONE (Rx)
(pred-niss'oh-lone)
Orapred, Orapred ODT, Prelone, Pediapred
Func. class.: Corticosteroid, synthetic
Chem. class.: Glucocorticoid, immediate acting

Do not confuse:
prednisoLONE/predniSONE

ACTION: Decreases inflammation by the suppression of migration of polymorphonuclear leukocytes, fibroblasts; reversal to increase capillary permeability and lysosomal stabilization

USES: Severe inflammation, immunosuppression, neoplasms, asthma

CONTRAINDICATIONS: Hypersensitivity, fungal infections, viral infection, varicella

Precautions: Pregnancy, breastfeeding, children, diabetes mellitus, glaucoma, osteoporosis, seizure disorders, ulcerative colitis, HF, myasthenia gravis, abrupt discontinuation, children, acute MI, GI ulcers, hypertension, hepatitis, psychosis, thromboembolism, peptic ulcer disease, renal disease, Cushing syndrome

DOSAGE AND ROUTES
Most conditions
- **Adult:** PO 5-60 mg PO per day as a single dose or divided doses
- **Infant/child/adolescent:** PO 0.14-2 mg/kg or 4-60 mg/m² per day in 3-4 divided doses

Multiple sclerosis
- **Adult:** PO 200 mg/day x 7 day, then 80 mg every other day x 1 mo

Antiinflammatory
- **Adult:** PO 5-60 mg/day as a single dose or in divided doses
- **Infant/child/adolescent:** PO 0.14-2 mg/kg or 4-60 mg/m² per day in 3-4 divided doses

Acute asthma exacerbation
- **Adult/adolescent:** PO 40-60 mg per day as a single dose or in 2 divided doses for 3-10 days
- **Child 5-12 yr:** PO 1-2 mg/kg (up to 60 mg) per day in 2 divided doses for 3-10 days
- **Infant/child ≤4 yr:** PO 1-2 mg/kg (up to 30 mg) per day in 2 divided doses for 3-10 days

Available forms: Tabs 5 mg; oral disintegrating tab 10, 15, 30 mg; oral sol 5 mg/5 mL, 10 mg/5 mL, 15 mg/5 mL, 25 mg/5 mL; oral suspension 15 mg/mL

Administer:
- **Oral sol:** use calibrated measuring device
- **Orally disintegrating tabs:** place on tongue; allow to dissolve, swallow or swallow whole; do not cut, split

SIDE EFFECTS

CNS: *Depression,* headache, mood changes

CV: *Hypertension,* circulatory collapse, thrombophlebitis, embolism, tachycardia

EENT: Fungal infections, increased intraocular pressure, blurred vision

GI: *Diarrhea, nausea, abdominal distention,* GI hemorrhage, increased appetite, pancreatitis

INTEG: Acne, poor wound healing, ecchymosis, petechiae, sweating

MS: Fractures, osteoporosis, weakness, arthralgia, myopathy, tendon rupture

MISC: Hyperglycemia

PHARMACOKINETICS

PO: Peak 1-2 hr, duration 2 days

INTERACTIONS

Increase: tendon rupture—quinolones

Increase: side effects—alcohol, salicylates, indomethacin, amphotericin B, digitalis, cycloSPORINE, diuretics

Increase: prednisoLONE action—salicylates, estrogens, indomethacin, oral contraceptives, ketoconazole, macrolide antibiotics

Increase: prednisoLONE effect—CYP3A4 inhibitors

Increase: toxicity—azole antifungals, cycloSPORINE, NSAIDs

Decrease: prednisoLONE action—cholestyramine, colestipol, barbiturates, rifAMPin, ePHEDrine, phenytoin, theophylline

Decrease: effects of anticoagulants, anticonvulsants, antidiabetics, ambenonium, neostigmine, isoniazid, toxoids, vaccines, anticholinesterases, salicylates, somatrem

Decrease: prednisoLONE effect—CYP3A4 inducers

Drug/Lab Test

Increase: cholesterol, sodium, blood glucose, uric acid, calcium, urine glucose

Decrease: calcium, potassium, T_4, T_3, thyroid ^{131}I uptake test, urine 17-OHCS, 17-KS, PBI

False negative: skin allergy tests

NURSING CONSIDERATIONS

Assess:

• Potassium, blood glucose, urine glucose while patient receiving long-term therapy; hypokalemia, hyperglycemia

• Weight daily; notify prescriber if weekly gain of >5 lb

• B/P q4hr, pulse; notify prescriber if chest pain occurs

• I&O ratio; be alert for decreasing urinary output, increasing edema

• Plasma cortisol levels with long-term therapy; normal level: 138-635 nmol/L SI units when drawn at 8 AM

• **Infection:** increased temperature, WBC, even after withdrawal of medication; product masks infection

• **Potassium depletion:** paresthesias, fatigue, nausea, vomiting, depression, polyuria, dysrhythmias, weakness

• Edema, hypertension, cardiac symptoms

• Mental status: affect, mood, behavioral changes, aggression

• **Adrenal insufficiency:** nausea, vomiting, lethargy, restlessness, confusion, weight loss, hypotension before, during treatment baseline and periodically; HPA suppression may be precipitated by abrupt withdrawal

• **Beers:** avoid in older adults with delirium or at high risk of delirium

• **Pregnancy/breastfeeding:** not recommended in pregnancy; cautious use in breastfeeding

Evaluate:

• Therapeutic response: ease of respirations, decreased inflammation

Teach patient/family:

• That emergency ID as steroid user should be carried

• To notify prescriber if therapeutic response decreases; that dosage adjustment may be needed

• Not to discontinue abruptly; that adrenal crisis can result; to take product exactly as prescribed

• To avoid OTC products: salicylates, cough products with alcohol, cold preparations unless directed by prescriber

• About cushingoid symptoms: moon face, buffalo hump, rapid weight gain, excessive sweating, stretch marks
• **About the symptoms of adrenal insufficiency:** nausea, anorexia, fatigue, dizziness, dyspnea, weakness, joint pain

---

prednisoLONE ophthalmic (Rx)
See Appendix B

---

predniSONE (Rx)
(pred'ni-sone)
Rayos, Winpred ✤
Func. class.: Corticosteroid
Chem. class.: Intermediate-acting glucocorticoid

Do not confuse:
predniSONE/methylPREDNISolone/ prednisoLONE/PriLOSEC

ACTION: Decreases inflammation by increasing capillary permeability and lysosomal stabilization, minimal mineralocorticoid activity

USES: Severe inflammation, neoplasms, multiple sclerosis, collagen disorders, dermatologic disorders, pulmonary fibrosis, asthma
Unlabeled uses: Adjunct for refractory seizures, infantile spasms, acute interstitial nephritis, amyloidosis, autoimmune hepatitis, Behçet's syndrome, Bell's palsy, carpal tunnel syndrome, Churg-Strauss syndrome, dermatomyositis, Duchenne muscular dystrophy, endophthalmitis, Lennox-Gastaut syndrome, lupus nephritis, mixed connective-tissue disease, pericarditis, pneumonia, polyarteritis nodosa, polychondritis, polymyositis, rheumatic carditis, temporal arteritis, TB, Wegener's granulomatosis

CONTRAINDICATIONS: Fungal infections, hypersensitivity
Precautions: Pregnancy, diabetes mellitus, glaucoma, osteoporosis, seizure disorders, ulcerative colitis, HF, myasthenia gravis, renal disease, esophagitis, peptic ulcer, cataracts, coagulopathy, abrupt discontinuation, children, corticosteroid hypersensitivity, Cushing syndrome, diabetes mellitus, ulcerative colitis, thromboembolism, geriatric patients, acute MI

DOSAGE AND ROUTES
Most uses
• **Adult: PO** 5-60 mg/day or divided bid-qid
• **Child: PO** 0.05-2 mg/kg/day divided 1-4×/day
Nephrotic syndrome
• **Child: PO** 2 mg/kg/day in divided doses, until urine is protein-free for 3 consecutive days, then 1-1.5 mg/kg/day every other day × 4 wk
Multiple sclerosis
• **Adult: PO** 200 mg/day × 1 wk, then 80 mg every other day × 1 mo
Asthma
• **Adult/adolescent: PO** 40-80 mg/day in 1-2 divided doses until PEF is 70% of predicted or personal best
• **Child: PO** 1 mg/kg (max 60 mg)/day in 2 divided doses until PEF is 70% of predicted or personal best
Available forms: Tabs 1, 2.5, 5, 10, 20, 50 mg; oral sol 5 mg/5 mL; del rel tab 1, 2, 5 mg
Administer:
• Regular tabs may be crushed and given with foods or fluids
• For long-term use, alternate-day therapy recommended to decrease adverse reactions; give in AM to coincide with normal cortisol secretion
• Titrated dose; use lowest effective dose
• With food or milk to decrease GI symptoms
• **Oral sol:** use calibrated measuring device
• **Del rel tab:** swallow whole; do not break, crush, chew; give once a day

SIDE EFFECTS
CNS: Depression, flushing, sweating, headache, mood changes
CV: Hypertension, thrombophlebitis, embolism, tachycardia, fluid retention

---

Side effects: *italics* = common; red = life-threatening

EENT: Fungal infections, increased intra-ocular pressure, blurred vision

GI: Diarrhea, nausea, abdominal distention, GI hemorrhage, increased appetite, pancreatitis

INTEG: Acne, poor wound healing, ecchymosis, petechiae

META: Hyperglycemia

MS: Fractures, osteoporosis, weakness

MISC: Decreased immune response

PHARMACOKINETICS

PO: Well absorbed PO, peak 1-2 hr; del rel peak $6-6^1/_2$ hr; half-life $3^1/_2$-4 hr, crosses placenta, enters breast milk, metabolized by liver after conversion, excreted in urine

INTERACTIONS

Increase: tendon rupture—quinolones

Increase: side effects—alcohol, salicylates, NSAIDs, amphotericin B, digoxin, cycloSPORINE, diuretics

Increase: predniSONE action—salicylates, estrogens, NSAIDs, oral contraceptives, ketoconazole, macrolide antiinfectives

Increase: predniSONE effect—CYP3A4 inhibitors

Decrease: predniSONE effect—CYP3A4 inducers

Decrease: predniSONE action—cholestyramine, colestipol, barbiturates, rifAMPin, phenytoin, theophylline

Decrease: effects of anticoagulants, anticonvulsants, antidiabetics, neostigmine, isoniazid, toxoids, vaccines, anticholinesterases, salicylates, somatrem

Drug/Herb

Decrease: predniSONE effect—ephedra (ma huang)

Drug/Lab Test

Increase: cholesterol, sodium, blood glucose, uric acid, calcium, urine glucose

Decrease: calcium, potassium, T_4, T_3, thyroid ^{131}I uptake test, urine 17-OHCS, 17-KS, PBI

False negative: skin allergy tests

NURSING CONSIDERATIONS
Assess:

• **Adrenal insufficiency:** nausea, vomiting, anorexia, confusion, hypotension, weight loss before or during treatment; HPA suppression may be precipitated by abrupt withdrawal

• Potassium, blood glucose, urine glucose while patient receiving long-term therapy; hypokalemia and hyperglycemia; plasma cortisol with long-term therapy, normal: 138-635 nmol/L SI units drawn at 8 AM

• Weight daily; notify prescriber of weekly gain of >5 lb

• B/P, pulse; notify prescriber of chest pain; monitor for crackles, dyspnea if edema is present; hypertension, cardiac symptoms

• I&O ratio; be alert for decreasing urinary output, increasing edema, rales, crackles; notify provider if present

• **Infection:** increased temperature, WBC, even after withdrawal of medication; product masks infection

• **Potassium depletion:** paresthesias, fatigue, nausea, vomiting, depression, polyuria, dysrhythmias, weakness

• **Mental status:** affect, mood, behavioral changes, aggression

• **Pregnancy/breastfeeding:** use only if benefits outweigh fetal risk; do not breastfeed

• **Beers:** avoid in older adults with a high risk of delirium

Evaluate:

• Therapeutic response: ease of respirations, decreased inflammation

Teach patient/family:

• That emergency ID as corticosteroid user should be carried; provide information about product being taken and condition

• To notify prescriber if therapeutic response decreases; that dosage adjustment may be needed

• To avoid vaccinations

• Not to discontinue abruptly; adrenal crisis can result

• To avoid OTC products: salicylates, cough products with alcohol, cold preparations unless directed by prescriber

• **Cushingoid symptoms:** moon face, weight gain; symptoms of adrenal insufficiency: nausea, anorexia, fatigue, dizziness, dyspnea, weakness, joint pain

- That product causes immunosuppression; to report any symptoms of infection (fever, sore throat, cough)
- To notify provider before surgery
- That continuing follow-up and blood work will be needed
- That antidiabetic agents may need adjustment in diabetic patients
- **Pregnancy:** to notify prescriber if pregnancy is planned or suspected; cleft palate, stillbirth, abortion reported

pregabalin (Rx)

(pre-gab′a-lin)
Lyrica, Lyrica CR
Func. class.: Anticonvulsant
Chem. class.: γ-Aminobutyric acid (GABA) analog

Controlled Substance Schedule V

Do not confuse:
Lyrica/Lopressor

ACTION: Binds to high-voltage–gated calcium channels in CNS tissues; this may lead to anticonvulsant action similar to the inhibitory neurotransmitter GABA; anxiolytic, analgesic, and antiepileptic properties

USES: Neuropathic pain associated with spinal cord injury/diabetic peripheral neuropathy, partial-onset seizures, postherpetic neuralgia, fibromyalgia

CONTRAINDICATIONS: Hypersensitivity to this product or gabapentin, abrupt discontinuation

Precautions: Pregnancy, breastfeeding, children <12 yr, geriatric patients, renal disease, PR interval prolongation, creatine kinase elevations, HF (class III, IV), decreased platelets, substance abuse, dependence, glaucoma, myopathy, angioedema history, suicidal behavior

DOSAGE AND ROUTES
Diabetic peripheral neuropathic pain
- **Adult:** PO/ORAL SOL 50 mg tid, may increase to 300 mg/day (max) within 1 wk, adjust in patients with renal disease; **EXT REL** 165 mg/day, may increase to 330 mg/day (treatment-naive patients)

Partial-onset seizures
- **Adult:** PO/ORAL SOL 75 mg bid or 50 mg tid; may increase to 600 mg/day (max)

Postherpetic neuralgia
- **Adult:** PO/ORAL SOL 150 mg/day in 2-3 divided doses, may increase to 300 mg/day in 2-3 divided doses; if higher dose is required after 2-4 wk, may increase to 600 mg/day in 2-3 divided doses

Fibromyalgia, spinal cord injury pain
- **Adult:** PO/ORAL SOL 75 mg bid, may increase to 150 mg bid within 1 wk and 225 mg bid after 1 wk

Renal dose
- **Adult:** PO CCr 30-60 mL/min, 75-300 mg/day in 2-3 divided doses; CCr 15-30 mL/min, 25-150 mg/day in 1-2 divided doses; CCr <15 mL/min, 25-75 mg/day as a single dose

Social phobia (unlabeled)
- **Adult:** PO 150-600 mg/day in 3 divided doses

Available forms: Caps 25, 50, 75, 100, 150, 200, 225, 300 mg; oral sol 20 mg/mL; ext rel tabs 82.5, 165, 330 mg

Administer:
- Do not crush or chew caps; caps may be opened and contents put in applesauce or dissolved in juice
- Give without regard to meals
- Gradually withdraw over 7 days; abrupt withdrawal may precipitate seizures
- **Ext rel tablets:** do not split, crush, chew; to be taken after evening meal
- **Oral sol:** should be written in mg and calculated to mL

SIDE EFFECTS
CNS: *Dizziness*, drowsiness abnormal thinking, suicidal ideation
EENT: *Dry mouth*, blurred vision, sinusitis
GI: Constipation, abdominal pain, weight gain, nausea, vomiting, increased appetite
GU: Gynecomastia

P

Side effects: *italics* = common; red = life-threatening

HEMA: Thrombocytopenia
MS: Back pain, rhabdomyolysis, myopathy
OTHER: Pruritus, *peripheral edema*, angioedema

PHARMACOKINETICS
Well absorbed, peak 1.5 hr; 90% recovered in urine unchanged; negligible metabolism; not bound to plasma proteins; half-life 6 hr

INTERACTIONS
Increase: weight gain/fluid retention—pioglitazone, rosiglitazone; avoid use if possible
Increase: CNS depression—anxiolytics, sedatives, hypnotics, barbiturates, general anesthetics, opiate agonists, phenothiazines, sedating H$_1$ blockers, thiazolidinediones, tricyclics, alcohol
Increase: angioedema—ACE inhibitors
Drug/Lab Test
Increase: creatine kinase
Decrease: platelets

NURSING CONSIDERATIONS
Assess:
• **Seizures:** aura, location, duration, activity at onset, use seizure precautions
• **Pain:** location, duration, characteristics if using for diabetic neuropathy, spinal cord injury, neuralgia
• Renal studies: urinalysis, BUN, urine creatinine q3mo, creatine kinase; if markedly increased, discontinue product
• **Mental status:** mood, sensorium, affect, behavioral changes, suicidal thoughts/behaviors; if mental status changes, notify prescriber
• **Angioedema/hypersensitivity:** (rare) monitor for blisters, hives, rash, dyspnea, wheezing; angioedema; if these occur, discontinue; cross-hypersensitivity with this product and gabapentin may occur
• **Rhabdomyolysis and creatinine kinase elevations (rare):** monitor for muscle pain, tenderness, weakness accompanied by malaise or fever; product should be discontinued

• **Beers:** avoid in older adults unless safer alternative is unavailable; may cause ataxia, impaired psychomotor function
• **Pregnancy/breastfeeding:** use only if benefits outweigh fetal risk, may cause fetal toxicity; pregnant patients should enroll in the Antiepileptic Drug Pregnancy Registry, 1-888-233-2334; do not breastfeed
Evaluate:
• Therapeutic response: decreased seizure activity; decrease in neuropathic pain
Teach patient/family:
• To carry emergency ID stating patient's name, products taken, condition, prescriber's name and phone number
• To avoid driving, other activities that require alertness because dizziness, drowsiness may occur, to obtain clearance from provider if driving is acceptable
• Not to discontinue medication quickly after long-term use; to taper over ≥1 wk; that withdrawal-precipitated seizures may occur; not to double doses if dose is missed, to take if 2 hr or more before next dose
• To notify prescriber if pregnancy is planned or suspected; to avoid breastfeeding
• To report muscle pain, tenderness, weakness when accompanied by fever, malaise, suicidal thoughts/behaviors
• To avoid alcohol, live virus vaccines

TREATMENT OF OVERDOSE:
Lavage, VS, hemodialysis

---

primaquine (Rx)
(prim′a-kween)
Func. class.: Antimalarial
Chem. class.: Synthetic 8-aminoquinolone

ACTION: Unknown; thought to destroy exoerythrocytic forms by gametocidal action

USES: Malaria caused by *Plasmodium vivax;* in combination with clindamycin for *Pneumocystis jiroveci* pneumonia

CONTRAINDICATIONS: Lupus erythematosus, rheumatoid arthritis; hypersensitivity to this product or iodoquinol

Precautions: Pregnancy, breastfeeding, methemoglobin reductase deficiency, bone marrow suppression, ⚕ hemolytic anemia, ⚕ G6PD deficiency

DOSAGE AND ROUTES
• **Adult:** PO 15-30 mg (base)/day × 2 wk or 45 mg (base)/wk × 8 wk; 26.3-mg tab is 15-mg base
• **Child:** PO 0.5 mg/kg (0.3 mg/base/day) daily × 2 wk

Available forms: Tabs 26.3 mg

Administer:

PO route
• Before or after meals at same time each day to maintain product level; take with food to decrease GI upset

SIDE EFFECTS
CNS: Headache, dizziness
CV: Hypertension, dysrhythmias
EENT: *Blurred vision, difficulty focusing*
GI: *Nausea, vomiting, anorexia,* cramps
HEMA: Agranulocytosis, granulocytopenia, leukopenia, hemolytic anemia, leukocytosis, mild anemia, methemoglobinemia
INTEG: Pruritus, skin eruptions, pallor, weakness

PHARMACOKINETICS
PO: Metabolized by liver (metabolites), half-life 3.7-9.6 hr

INTERACTIONS
• Toxicity: quinacrine
Decrease: effect of carBAMazepine, PHENobarbital, phenytoins, rifamycins, nafcillin

Drug/Food
Increase: primaquine effect—food
Decrease: primaquine effect—grapefruit juice

Drug/Lab Test
Increase: WBC
Decrease: WBC, RBC, Hgb

NURSING CONSIDERATIONS
Assess:
• Hepatic studies weekly: AST, ALT, bilirubin if patient receiving long-term therapy
• Blood studies: CBC; blood dyscrasias occur
• Allergic reactions: pruritus, rash, urticaria
• Blood dyscrasias: malaise, fever, bruising, bleeding (rare)
• Renal status: dark urine, hematuria, decreased output
• **Hemolytic reaction:** chills, fever, chest pain, cyanosis; product should be discontinued immediately; ⚕ hemolytic anemia, G6PD deficiency may be severe in patients of Asian, Mediterranean descent
• **Pregnancy/breastfeeding:** do not use in pregnancy/breastfeeding; pregnancy testing should be completed in sexually active females of childbearing age; adequate contraception should be used while taking this product

Evaluate:
• Therapeutic response: decreased symptoms of malaria

Teach patient/family:
• To report visual problems, fever, fatigue, dark urine, bruising, bleeding; may indicate blood dyscrasias
• To complete full course of therapy; to take with food to decrease GI upset; if vomiting occurs within 30 min of taking dose, to repeat the dose

P

---

probenecid (Rx)
(proe-ben′e-sid)
Func. class.: Uricosuric, antigout agent
Chem. class.: Sulfonamide derivative

ACTION: Inhibits tubular reabsorption of urates, with increased excretion of uric acids

USES: Hyperuricemia in gout, gouty arthritis, adjunct to penicillin treatment

---

Side effects: *italics* = common; red = life-threatening

CONTRAINDICATIONS: Hypersensitivity, severe renal/hepatic disease, CCr <50 mg/min, history of uric acid calculus

Precautions: Pregnancy, children <2 yr, sulfonamide hypersensitivity, peptic ulcer

DOSAGE AND ROUTES
Adjunct to penicillin
• **Adult/adolescent >15 yr, >50 kg (110 lb): PO** 500 mg qid
Gout/gouty arthritis
• **Adult: PO** 250 mg bid for 1 wk, then 500 mg bid, max 2 g/day; maintenance 500 mg/day × 6 mo
Adjunct in penicillin treatment
• **Adult and adolescent >50 kg: PO** 500 mg qid
• **Child <50 kg: PO** 25 mg/kg, then 40 mg/kg in divided doses qid
Renal dose
• Avoid use if CCr <50 mL/min
Available forms: Tabs 500 mg
Administer:
• After meals or with milk if GI symptoms occur
• Increase fluid intake to 2-3 L/day to prevent urinary calculi

SIDE EFFECTS
CNS: Drowsiness, headache, flushing
CV: Bradycardia
GI: *Gastric irritation, nausea, vomiting, anorexia,* hepatic necrosis
GU: Glycosuria, thirst, frequency, nephrotic syndrome
INTEG: Rash, dermatitis, pruritus, fever
META: *Acidosis, hypokalemia, hyperchloremia,* hyperglycemia
RESP: Apnea, irregular respirations

PHARMACOKINETICS
Peak 2-4 hr, duration 8 hr, half-life 5-8 hr; metabolized by liver; excreted in urine

INTERACTIONS
Increase: effect of acyclovir, barbiturates, allopurinol, benzodiazepines, dyphylline, zidovudine, cephalosporins, penicillins, sulfonamides

Increase: toxicity—sulfa products, dapsone, clofibrate, indomethacin, rifAMPin, naproxen, methotrexate
Decrease: action of probenecid—salicylates
Drug/Lab Test
Increase: theophylline levels

NURSING CONSIDERATIONS
Assess:
• Uric acid levels (3-7 mg/dL); mobility, joint pain, swelling, maintain fluid intake at 2-3 L/day
• Respiratory rate, rhythm, depth; notify prescriber of abnormalities
• Electrolytes; CO_2 before, during treatment
• Urine pH, output, glucose during beginning treatment, poor effect in GFR <30 mL/min
• **For CNS symptoms:** confusion, twitching, hyperreflexia, stimulation, headache; may indicate overdose
• **Beers:** avoid in older adults with creatinine clearance <30 mL/min
Evaluate:
• Therapeutic response: absence of pain, stiffness in joints
Teach patient/family:
• To avoid OTC preparations (aspirin) unless directed by prescriber; to increase water intake, avoid alcohol, caffeine

---

⚠ **HIGH ALERT**

procainamide (Rx)
(proe-kane-ah'mide)
Procan SR ✦
Func. class.: Antidysrhythmic (class IA)
Chem. class.: Procaine HCl amide analog

ACTION: Depresses excitability of cardiac muscle to electrical stimulation and slows conduction velocity in atrium, bundle of His, and ventricle; increases refractory period

---

USES: Life-threatening ventricular dysrhythmias

Unlabeled uses: Atrial fibrillation/flutter, paroxysmal atrial tachycardia, PSVT, Wolff-Parkinson-White (WPW) syndrome

CONTRAINDICATIONS: Hypersensitivity, severe heart block, torsades de pointes

Black Box Warning: Lupus erythematosus

Precautions: Pregnancy, breastfeeding, children, renal/hepatic disease, HF, respiratory depression, cytopenia, dysrhythmia associated with digoxin toxicity, myasthenia gravis, digoxin toxicity

Black Box Warning: Bone marrow failure, cardiac arrhythmias

DOSAGE AND ROUTES—NTI
Ventricular tachycardia during CPR
• **Adult:** IV loading dose 20 mg/min; either ventricular tachycardia resolves or patient becomes hypotensive; QRS complex is widened by 50% of original width or total is 17 mg/kg (1.2 g for a 70-kg patient); may give up to 50 mg/min in urgent situations; maintenance: 1-4 mg/min **CONT IV INFUSION;** **IM** 50 mg/kg/day in divided doses q3-6hr
• **Child:** IV PALS 15 mg/kg over 30-60 min
Renal dose
• **Adult:** IV CCr 35-59 mL/min, give 70% maintenance dose; CCr 15-34 mL/min, give 40%-60% maintenance dose; CCr <15 mL/min, individualize dose
Available forms: Inj 100, 500 mg/mL
Administer:
IM route
• IM inj in deltoid; aspirate to avoid intravascular administration; use only when unable to use IV
Direct IV route
• Dilute each 100 mg/10 mL of 0.9% NaCl; give at max 50 mg/min
Intermittent IV INFUSION route
• Dilute 0.2-1 g/50-500 mL of D₅W (2-4 mg/mL); give over 30-60 min at max 25-50 mg/min; use infusion pump

Y-site compatibilities: Alfentanil, amikacin, aminocaproic acid, aminophylline, amiodarone, amphotericin B lipid complex, amphotericin B liposome, anidulafungin, ascorbic acid, atenolol, atracurium, atropine, aztreonam, benztropine, bivalirudin, bleomycin, bumetanide, buprenorphine, butorphanol, calcium chloride/gluconate, caspofungin, ceFAZolin, cefmetazole, cefonicid, cefoperazone, cefotaxime, cefoTEtan, cefOXitin, cefTAZidime, cefTRIAXone, cefuroxime, cephalothin, chlorproMAZINE, cimetidine, cisatracurium, CISplatin, clindamycin, cyanocobalamin, cyclophosphamide, cycloSPORINE, cytarabine, DACTINomycin, DAPTOmycin, dexamethasone, digoxin, diphenhydrAMINE, DOBUTamine, DOCEtaxel, DOPamine, doxacurium, DOXOrubicin, doxycycline, enalaprilat, ePHEDrine, EPINEPHrine, epiRUBicin, epoetin alfa, eptifibatide, ertapenem, erythromycin, esmolol, etoposide, etoposide phosphate, famotidine, fenoldopam, fentaNYL, fluconazole, fludarabine, fluorouracil, folic acid, furosemide, gatifloxacin, gemcitabine, gentamicin, glycopyrrolate, granisetron, heparin, hydrocortisone, HYDROmorphone, IDArubicin, ifosfamide, indomethacin, insulin (regular), irinotecan, isoproterenol, ketorolac, labetalol, lidocaine, linezolid, LORazepam, magnesium sulfate, mannitol, mechlorethamine, meperidine, metaraminol, methicillin, methotrexate, methoxamine, methyldopate, methylPREDNISolone, metoclopramide, metoprolol, mezlocillin, miconazole, midazolam, mitoXANTRONE, morphine, moxalactam, multivitamins, mycophenolate, nafcillin, nalbuphine, naloxone, netilmicin, nitroglycerin, nitroprusside, norepinephrine, octreotide, ondansetron, oxacillin, oxaliplatin, oxytocin, PACLitaxel, palonosetron, pamidronate, pancuronium, pantoprazole, papaverine, PEMEtrexed, penicillin G potassium/sodium, pentamidine, pentazocine, PENTobarbital, PHENobarbital, phenylephrine, phytonadione, piperacillin, piperacillin-tazobactam, polymyxin B, potassium chloride, prochlorperazine,

P

promethazine, propranolol, protamine, pyridoxine, quiNIDine, quinupristin-dalfopristin, raNITIdine, remifentanil, ritodrine, rocuronium, sodium bicarbonate, succinylcholine, SUFentanil, tacrolimus, teniposide, theophylline, thiamine, thiotepa, ticarcillin, ticarcillin-clavulanate, tigecycline, tirofiban, tobramycin, tolazoline, trimetaphan, urokinase, vancomycin, vasopressin, vecuronium, verapamil, vinCRIStine, vinorelbine, vitamin B complex/C, voriconazole, zoledronic acid

SIDE EFFECTS

CNS: *Headache, dizziness,* confusion, psychosis, restlessness, irritability, weakness, depression

CV: *Hypotension,* heart block, cardiovascular collapse, arrest, torsades de pointes

GI: Nausea, vomiting, anorexia, diarrhea, hepatomegaly, pain, bitter taste

HEMA: SLE syndrome, agranulocytosis, thrombocytopenia, neutropenia, hemolytic anemia

INTEG: Rash, urticaria, edema, swelling (rare), pruritus, flushing, angioedema

SYST: SLE

PHARMACOKINETICS

Metabolized in liver to active metabolites, excreted unchanged by kidneys (60%), protein binding 15%

IM: Peak 10-60 min, half-life 3 hr

INTERACTIONS

Increase: effects of neuromuscular blockers

Increase: procainamide effects—cimetidine, quiNIDine, trimethoprim, β-blockers, raNITIdine

Increase: toxicity—other antidysrhythmics, thioridazine, quinolones

Drug/Lab Test

Increase: ALT, AST, alk phos, LDH, bilirubin

NURSING CONSIDERATIONS

Assess:

Black Box Warning: **Cardiac dysrhythmias:** ECG continuously if using IV

to determine increased PR or QRS segments; discontinue immediately; watch for increased ventricular ectopic beats, maximum need to rebolus

• Therapeutic blood levels, 4-10 mcg/mL or NAPA levels 10-20 mcg/mL

Black Box Warning: **Bone marrow suppression:** CBC q2wk × 3 mo; leukocyte, neutrophil, platelet counts may be decreased, treatment may need to be discontinued

• I&O ratio; electrolytes (K, Na, Cl), weight weekly, report gain of >2 lb

• **Toxicity:** confusion, drowsiness, nausea, vomiting, tachydysrhythmias, oliguria

• ANA titer; during long-term treatment, watch for lupuslike symptoms

• Respiratory status: rate, rhythm, character, lung fields; bilateral crackles may occur in HF patient; watch for respiratory depression

• **CNS effects:** dizziness, confusion, psychosis, paresthesias, seizures; product should be discontinued

• **Pregnancy/breastfeeding:** use only if clearly needed; do not breastfeed

Evaluate:

• Therapeutic response: decreased dysrhythmias

Teach patient/family:

• That wax matrix may appear in stools

• Not to discontinue without provider's approval

Black Box Warning: To notify prescriber immediately if lupuslike symptoms appear (joint pain, butterfly rash, fever, chills, dyspnea)

Black Box Warning: To notify prescriber of leukopenia (sore mouth, gums, throat) or thrombocytopenia (bleeding, bruising)

• How to take pulse and when to report to prescriber

• To avoid driving, other hazardous activities until product effect is known

TREATMENT OF OVERDOSE: O_2, artificial ventilation, ECG, administer DOPamine for circulatory depression, diazePAM or thiopental for seizures, isoproterenol

⚠ HIGH ALERT

procarbazine (Rx)
(proe-kar′ba-zeen)
Matulane, Natulan ✦
Func. class.: Antineoplastic, alkylating agent
Chem. class.: Hydrazine derivative

Do not confuse:
Matulane/Materna

ACTION: Inhibits DNA, RNA, protein synthesis; has multiple sites of action; nonvesicant

USES: Lymphoma, Hodgkin's disease, cancers resistant to other therapy
Unlabeled uses: Brain, lung malignancies; other lymphomas; multiple myeloma, malignant melanoma, polycythemia vera

CONTRAINDICATIONS: Pregnancy, breastfeeding, hypersensitivity, thrombocytopenia, bone marrow depression
Precautions: Cardiac/renal/hepatic disease, radiation therapy, seizure disorder, anemia, bipolar disorder, Parkinson's disease

Black Box Warning: Requires a specialized care setting and an experienced clinician

DOSAGE AND ROUTES
• **Adult:** PO 2-4 mg/kg/day for 1st wk; maintain dosage of 4-6 mg/kg/day until platelets, WBC fall; after recovery, 1-2 mg/kg/day

• **Child:** PO 50 mg/m²/day for 7 days, then 100 mg/m² until desired response, leukopenia, or thrombocytopenia occurs; 50 mg/m²/day maintenance after bone marrow recovery
Available forms: Caps 50 mg
Administer:
• In divided doses and at bedtime to minimize nausea and vomiting
• Nonphenothiazine antiemetic 30-60 min before product and 4-10 hr after treatment to prevent vomiting

SIDE EFFECTS
CNS: Headache, dizziness, insomnia, hallucinations, confusion, coma, pain, chills, fever, sweating, paresthesias, seizures, peripheral neuropathy
EENT: Retinal hemorrhage, nystagmus, photophobia, diplopia, dry eyes
GI: *Nausea, vomiting,* anorexia, diarrhea, constipation, dry mouth, stomatitis, elevated hepatic enzymes
GU: Azoospermia, cessation of menses
HEMA: Thrombocytopenia, anemia, leukopenia, myelosuppression, bleeding tendencies, purpura, petechiae, epistaxis, hemolysis
INTEG: *Rash,* pruritus, dermatitis, alopecia, herpes, hyperpigmentation
MS: Arthralgias, myalgias
RESP: Cough, pneumonitis, hemoptysis
SYST: Secondary malignancy

PHARMACOKINETICS
Half-life 1 hr; concentrates in liver, kidney, skin; metabolized in liver, excreted in urine

INTERACTIONS
Increase: hypotension—meperidine; do not use together
Increase: neuroleptic malignant syndrome, seizures, hyperpyrexia—alcohol, MAOIs, tricyclics, sympathomimetic products, SSRIs, SNRIs
Increase: hypertension—guanethidine, levodopa, methyldopa, reserpine, caffeine
Life-threatening hypertension: sympathomimetics

P

Increase: bleeding risk—NSAIDs, anticoagulants, platelet inhibitors, thrombolytics

Increase: CNS depression—barbiturates, antihistamines, opioids, hypotensive agents, phenothiazines

Drug/Food
• **Hypertensive crisis:** tyramine foods

NURSING CONSIDERATIONS
Assess:
• **Bone marrow suppression:** CBC, differential, platelet count weekly; withhold product if WBC is <4000/mm³ or platelet count is <100,000/mm³; notify prescriber
• **Hepatic/renal disease:** can cause accumulation of drug, increased toxicity; renal studies: BUN; serum uric acid; urine CCr; electrolytes before, during therapy; I&O ratio, report fall in urine output to <30 mL/hr; hepatic studies before, during therapy: bilirubin, AST, ALT, alk phos, LDH prn or monthly
• Monitor temperature; fever may indicate beginning infection

Black Box Warning: To be used only in a specialized care setting with emergency equipment

Black Box Warning: To be given only by an experienced clinician knowledgeable in cytotoxic products

• CNS changes: confusion, paresthesias, neuropathies; product should be discontinued
• Tyramine foods in diet; hypertensive crisis can occur
• **Toxicity:** facial flushing, epistaxis, increased PT, thrombocytopenia; product should be discontinued
• **Bleeding:** hematuria, guaiac stools, bruising or petechiae, mucosa or orifices q8hr
• Effects of alopecia on body image; discuss feelings about body changes
• Jaundiced skin, sclera; dark urine, clay-colored stools, itchy skin, abdominal pain, fever, diarrhea
• Buccal cavity for dryness, sores or ulceration, white patches, oral pain, bleeding, dysphagia

• GI symptoms: frequency of stools, cramping
• **Acidosis, signs of dehydration:** rapid respirations, poor skin turgor, decreased urine output, dry skin, restlessness, weakness
• **Pregnancy/breastfeeding:** do not use in pregnancy, breastfeeding

Evaluate:
• Therapeutic response: decreasing malignancy

Teach patient/family:
• **To report any complaints, side effects to nurse or prescriber:** CNS changes, diarrhea, cough, SOB, fever, chills, sore throat, bleeding, bruising, vomiting blood; black, tarry stools
• That hair may be lost during treatment and wig or hairpiece may make patient feel better; that new hair may be different in color, texture
• To avoid sunlight or UV exposure; to wear sunscreen or protective clothing
• To avoid foods with citric acid, hot temperature, or rough texture
• To report any bleeding, white spots, ulcerations in mouth to prescriber; to examine mouth daily
• To avoid driving, activities requiring alertness because dizziness may occur
• **Pregnancy/breastfeeding:** to use effective contraception; to avoid breastfeeding; that product may cause infertility
• To avoid the ingestion of alcohol, caffeine, tyramine-containing foods; that cold, hay fever, and weight-reducing products may cause serious product interactions; to avoid smoking
• To avoid crowds, persons with infections if granulocytes are low
• To avoid vaccines

---

prochlorperazine (Rx)
(proe-klor-pair′a-zeen)
Compro, Prochlorazine ✿
Func. class.: Antiemetic, antipsychotic
Chem. class.: Phenothiazine, piperazine derivative

Do not confuse:

prochlorperazine/chlorproMAZINE

ACTION: Decreases DOPamine neurotransmission by increasing DOPamine turnover through the blockade of the D_2 somatodendritic autoreceptor in the mesolimbic system

USES: Nausea, vomiting, psychotic disorders

Unlabeled uses: Migraine

CONTRAINDICATIONS: Hypersensitivity to phenothiazines, coma; infants, neonates, children <2 yr or <20 lb; surgery

Precautions: Pregnancy, breastfeeding, geriatric patients, seizure, encephalopathy, glaucoma, hepatic disease, Parkinson's disease, BPH

Black Box Warning: Increased mortality in elderly patients with dementia-related psychosis

DOSAGE AND ROUTES
Postoperative nausea/vomiting
• **Adult:** IM 5-10 mg 1-2 hr before anesthesia; may repeat after 30 min; IV 5-10 mg 15-30 min before anesthesia; IV INFUSION 20 mg/L D₅W or NS 15-30 min before anesthesia, max 40 mg/day
Severe nausea/vomiting
• **Adult:** PO 5-10 mg tid-qid; SUS REL 15 mg/day in AM or 10 mg q12hr; RECT 25 mg/bid; IM 5-10 mg q3-4hr prn, max 40 mg/day
• **Child 18-39 kg:** PO 2.5 mg tid or 5 mg bid; IM 0.132 mg/kg q3-4hr prn, max 15 mg/day
• **Child 14-17 kg:** PO/RECT 2.5 mg bid-tid; IM 0.132 mg/kg q3-4hr prn, max 10 mg/day
• **Child 9-13 kg:** PO/RECT 2.5 mg/day-bid; IM 0.132 mg/kg q3-4hr prn, max 7.5 mg/day
Antipsychotic
• **Adult/child ≥12 yr:** PO 5-10 mg tid-qid; may increase q2-3days, max 150 mg/day; IM 10-20 mg q2-4hr up to 4 doses, then 10-20 mg q4-6hr
• **Child 2-12 yr:** PO 2.5 mg bid-tid; IM 0.132 mg/kg change to oral ASAP
Antianxiety
• **Adult/child ≥12 yr:** PO 5 mg tid-qid, max 20 mg/day
• **Child 2-12 yr:** IM 0.132 mg/kg change to oral ASAP

Available forms: Tabs 5, 10 mg; supp 10 ✿, 25 mg; sol for inj 5 mg/mL
Administer:
• Avoid other CNS depressants
IM route
• IM inj in large muscle mass; aspirate to avoid IV administration
• Keep patient recumbent for ¹/₂ hr
Direct IV route
• May give diluted or undiluted; inject directly in a vein ≤5 mg/min; do not give as bolus
Intermittent IV INFUSION route
• May dilute 20 mg/L NaCl and give as infusion 15-30 min before anesthesia induction

Continuous IV INFUSION
• May give using 20 mg/L of compatible solution

Y-site compatibilities: Amsacrine, calcium gluconate, cisatracurium, CISplatin, cladribine, cyclophosphamide, cytarabine, DOXOrubicin, DOXOrubicin liposome, fluconazole, granisetron, heparin, hydrocortisone, melphalan, methotrexate, ondansetron, PACLitaxel, potassium chloride, propofol, remifentanil, sargramostim, SUFentanil, teniposide, thiotepa, vinorelbine, vit B/C

SIDE EFFECTS
CNS: Neuroleptic malignant syndrome, *extrapyramidal reactions, tardive dyskinesia, euphoria,* depression, *drowsiness,* restlessness, tremor, dizziness, headache
CV: tachycardia, hypotension, ECG changes
EENT: Blurred vision
GI: Nausea, vomiting, anorexia, dry mouth, diarrhea, constipation, weight loss, metallic taste, cramps
HEMA: Agranulocytosis
MISC: Impotence; urine color change
RESP: Respiratory depression

Side effects: *italics* = common; red = life-threatening

PHARMACOKINETICS

Metabolized by liver; excreted in urine, breast milk; crosses placenta; 91%-99% protein binding

IM: Onset 10-20 min, duration 4-6 hr; children: 12 hr
PO: Onset 30-40 min, duration 3-4 hr
RECT: Onset 60 min, duration 3-4 hr

INTERACTIONS

Increase: anticholinergic action—anticholinergics, antiparkinson products, antidepressants
Increase: CNS depression—CNS depressants
Increase: serotonin syndrome, neuroleptic malignant syndrome—SSRIs, SNRIs
Decrease: prochlorperazine effect—barbiturates, antacids, lithium

Drug/Herb
Increase: CNS depression—chamomile, hops, kava, St. John's wort, valerian
Increase: EPS—kava

Drug/Lab Test
Increase: LFTs, cardiac enzymes, cholesterol, blood glucose, prolactin, bilirubin, PBI, ^{131}I, alk phos, leukocytes, granulocytes, platelets
Decrease: hormones (blood and urine)
False positive: pregnancy tests, urine bilirubin
False negative: urinary steroids, 17-OHCS, pregnancy tests

NURSING CONSIDERATIONS
Assess:
• **EPS:** abnormal movement, tardive dyskinesia, akathisia
• VS, B/P; check patients with cardiac disease more often
• **Neuroleptic malignant syndrome:** seizures, hypo/hypertension, fever, tachycardia, dyspnea, fatigue, muscle stiffness, loss of bladder control; notify prescriber immediately
• CBC, LFTs during course of treatment; blood dyscrasias, hepatotoxicity may occur
• Respiratory status before, during, after administration of emetic; check rate, rhythm, character; respiratory depression can occur rapidly among geriatric or debilitated patients
• **Beers:** avoid in older adults with a high risk of delirium
• **Pregnancy/breastfeeding:** use only if benefits outweigh fetal risk; EPS may result; cautious use in breastfeeding, excreted in breast milk

Evaluate:
• Therapeutic response: absence of nausea, vomiting; reduced anxiety, agitation, excitability

Teach patient/family:
• To avoid hazardous activities, activities requiring alertness because dizziness may occur
• To avoid alcohol
• Not to double or skip doses
• That urine may be pink to reddish brown
• That suppositories may contain coconut/palm oil
• To report dark urine, clay-colored stools, bleeding, bruising, rash, blurred vision
• To avoid sun; wear sunscreen, protective clothing

---

progesterone (Rx)
(proe-jess'ter-one)
Crinone, Endometrin, Prometrium, Utrogestran ♣
Func. class.: Hormone, Progestogen
Chem. class.: Progesterone derivative

ACTION: Inhibits secretion of pituitary gonadotropins, which prevents follicular maturation, ovulation; stimulates growth of mammary tissue; antineoplastic action against endometrial cancer

USES: Contraception, amenorrhea, premenstrual syndrome, abnormal uterine bleeding, endometrial hyperplasia prevention, assisted reproductive technology (ART) gel

---

Unlabeled uses: Corpus luteum insufficiency, early pregnancy failure, PMS, preterm delivery prophylaxis

CONTRAINDICATIONS: Pregnancy, ectopic pregnancy; hypersensitivity to this product, peanuts, or peanut oil; thromboembolic disorders, reproductive cancer, genital bleeding (abnormal, undiagnosed), cerebral hemorrhage, PID, STDs, thrombophlebitis

Black Box Warning: Breast cancer

Precautions: Breastfeeding, hypertension, asthma, blood dyscrasias, HF, diabetes mellitus, bone disease, depression, migraine headache, seizure disorders, gallbladder/renal/hepatic disease, family history of breast/reproductive tract cancer

Black Box Warning: Cardiac disease, dementia

DOSAGE AND ROUTES
Infertility
• **Adult: VAG** 90 mg/day (micronized gel); 100 mg 2-3 times/day starting day after oocyte retrieval and for ≤10 wk total (insert)
Amenorrhea/functional uterine bleeding
• **Adult: IM** 5-10 mg/day × 6-8 doses
Endometrial hyperplasia prevention
• **Adult: PO** 200 mg/day × 14 days
Assisted reproductive therapy
• **Adult: GEL** 90 mg (8%) vaginally daily for supplementation; 90 mg (8%) vaginally bid for replacement; if pregnancy occurs, continue × 10-12 wk
Corpus luteum insufficiency (unlabeled)
• **Adult: VAG INSERT** 90-100 mg bid-tid starting at oocyte retrieval and continuing up to 10-12 wk gestation
Available forms: Inj 50 mg/mL; vag gel 4%, 8%; caps 100, 200 mg; vag insert 100 mg; vag supp 25, 100, 200, 500 mg; compounding kit 25, 50, 100, 200, 400 mg; oil for IM injection 50 mg/mL

Administer:
PO route
• Do not break, crush, or chew caps
• Titrated dose; use lowest effective dose
• In 1 dose in AM
• With food or milk to decrease GI symptoms
• Start progesterone 14 days after estrogen dose if given concomitantly
Vaginal route
• Wait at least 6 hr after any vaginal treatment before using vaginal gel, use applicator provided
IM route
• Shake vial, inject deeply into large muscle, aspirate
• Check for particulate matter and discoloration before injecting

SIDE EFFECTS
CNS: *Dizziness, headache,* depression, *fatigue,* mood swings
CV: Hypotension, thrombophlebitis, edema, thromboembolism, stroke, pulmonary embolism, MI
EENT: Diplopia, retinal thrombosis
GI: *Nausea,* vomiting, anorexia, cramps, increased weight, cholestatic jaundice, *constipation,* abdominal pain
GU: Amenorrhea, cervical erosion, breakthrough bleeding, dysmenorrhea, nocturia, breast changes, *gynecomastia,* endometriosis, spontaneous abortion, breast pain, ectopic pregnancy
INTEG: Rash, urticaria, acne, hirsutism, alopecia, photosensitivity
META: Hyperglycemia
SYST: Angioedema, anaphylaxis

PHARMACOKINETICS
Excreted in urine, feces; metabolized in liver
IM/RECT/VAG: Duration 24 hr

INTERACTIONS
Decrease: effect—bromocriptine
Drug/Lab Test
Increase: alk phos, nitrogen (urine), pregnanediol, amino acids, factors VII, VIII, IX, X
Decrease: GTT, HDL

P

Side effects: *italics* = common; red = life-threatening

NURSING CONSIDERATIONS
Assess:
• **Abnormal uterine bleeding:** vaginal bleeding; obtain pad count, patient menstrual history, breast exam, cervical cytology
• Weight daily; notify prescriber of weekly weight gain of >5 lb
• B/P at beginning of treatment and periodically
• I&O ratio; be alert for decreasing urinary output, increasing edema
• Hepatic studies: ALT, AST, bilirubin periodically during long-term therapy
• Edema, hypertension, cardiac symptoms, jaundice, thromboembolism
• Mental status: affect, mood, behavioral changes, depression
• **Pregnancy/breastfeeding:** do not use in pregnancy, breastfeeding

Evaluate:
• Therapeutic response: decreased abnormal uterine bleeding, absence of amenorrhea

Teach patient/family:
• To report breast lumps, vaginal bleeding, edema, jaundice, dark urine, clay-colored stools, dyspnea, headache, blurred vision, abdominal pain, numbness or stiffness in legs, chest pain
• To avoid gel with other vaginal products; if to be used together, to separate by ≥6 hr; for vaginal route, on proper insertion technique
• To report suspected pregnancy
• To monitor blood glucose if diabetic
• To avoid activities requiring mental alertness until effects are realized; can cause dizziness

---

⚠ HIGH ALERT

promethazine (Rx)
(proe-meth′a-zeen)
Histanil ✦
Func. class.: Antihistamine, H₁-receptor antagonist, antiemetic
Chem. class.: Phenothiazine derivative

ACTION: Acts on blood vessels, GI, respiratory system by competing with histamine for H_1-receptor sites; decreases allergic response by blocking histamine

USES: Motion sickness, rhinitis, allergy symptoms, sedation, nausea, preoperative and postoperative sedation
Unlabeled uses: Allergic rhinitis, acute peripheral vestibular nystagmus, hyperemesis gravidarum

CONTRAINDICATIONS: Hypersensitivity, breastfeeding, agranulocytosis, bone marrow suppression, coma, jaundice, Reye's syndrome

Black Box Warning: Infants, neonates, children, intraarterial/SUBCUT administration, extravasation

Precautions: Pregnancy, cardiac/renal/hepatic disease, asthma, seizure disorder, prostatic hypertrophy, bladder obstruction, glaucoma, COPD, GI obstruction, ileus, CNS depression, diabetes, sleep apnea, urinary retention, IV use

Black Box Warning: Tissue necrosis (IV use)

DOSAGE AND ROUTES
Nausea/vomiting
• **Adult:** PO/IM/IV/RECT 12.5-25 mg; q4-6hr prn
• **Child >2 yr:** PO/IM/IV/RECT 0.25-0.5 mg/kg q4-6hr prn
Motion sickness
• **Adult:** PO 25 mg bid, give ¹/₂-1 hr before departure, then q8-12hr prn
• **Child ≥2 yr:** PO/IM/RECT 12.5-25 mg bid, give ¹/₂-1 hr before departure, then q8-12hr prn
Sedation
• **Adult:** PO/IM 25-50 mg at bedtime
• **Child ≥2 yr:** PO/IM/RECT 12.5-25 mg at bedtime
Sedation (preoperative/postoperative)
• **Adult:** PO/IM/IV 25-50 mg

- **Child >2 yr: PO/IM/IV** 0.5-1.1 mg/kg

Allergy/rhinitis (unlabeled)
- **Adult: PO** 12.5 mg qid or 25 mg at bedtime
- **Child ≥2 yr: PO** 6.25-12.5 mg tid or 25 mg at bedtime

Hyperemesis gravidarum (unlabeled)
- **Pregnant female: PO/RECT/IM/IV** 12.5-25 mg q4hr

Nystagmus (unlabeled)
- **Adult: PO** 12.5-25 mg q4-6hr for ≤48 hr

Available forms: Tabs 12.5, 25, 50 mg; supp 12.5, 25, 50 mg; inj 25, 50 mg/mL; oral solution 6.25, 10 mg/mL

Administer:
Avoid use with other CNS depressants

PO route
- With meals for GI symptoms; absorption may slightly decrease
- When used for motion sickness, 30 min-1 hr before travel

IM route
- IM inj deep in large muscle; rotate site, necrosis may occur from subcut injection, give only IM

Direct IV route

Black Box Warning: Check for extravasation: burning, pain, swelling at IV site; can cause tissue necrosis

- Do not use if precipitate is present
- Rapid administration may cause transient decrease in B/P
- After diluting each 25-50 mg/9 mL of NaCl for inj; give ≤25 mg/2 min

Y-site compatibilities: Alfentanil, amifostine, amikacin, aminocaproic acid, amsacrine, anidulafungin, ascorbic acid, atenolol, atracurium, atropine, aztreonam, benztropine, bivalirudin, bleomycin, bumetanide, buprenorphine, butorphanol, calcium chloride/gluconate, CARBOplatin, caspofungin, chlorproMAZINE, cimetidine, ciprofloxacin, cisatracurium, CISplatin, cladribine, codeine, cyanocobalamin, cyclophosphamide, cycloSPORINE, cytarabine, DACTINomycin, DAPTOmycin,

dexmedetomidine, digoxin, diltiaZEM, diphenhydrAMINE, DOBUTamine, DOCEtaxel, DOPamine, doxacurium, DOXOrubicin, doxycycline, enalaprilat, ePHEDrine, EPINEPHrine, epirubicin, epoetin, eptifibatide, erythromycin, esmolol, etoposide, famotidine, fenoldopam, fentaNYL, filgrastim, fluconazole, fludarabine, gemcitabine, gentamicin, glycopyrrolate, granisetron, HYDROmorphone, hydrOXYzine, IDArubicin, ifosfamide, insulin (regular), irinotecan, isoproterenol, labetalol, levoFLOXacin, lidocaine, linezolid, LORazepam, magnesium sulfate, mannitol, mechlorethamine, melphalan, meperidine, metaraminol, methoxamine, methyldopate, metoclopramide, metoprolol, metroNIDAZOLE, miconazole, midazolam, milrinone, mitoXANTRONE, morphine, mycophenolate, nalbuphine, naloxone, netilmicin, nitroglycerin, norepinephrine, octreotide, ondansetron, oxaliplatin, oxytocin, PACLitaxel, palonosetron, pamidronate, pancuronium, PEMEtrexed, pentamidine, pentazocine, phenylephrine, polymyxin B, procainamide, prochlorperazine, propranolol, protamine, pyridoxine, quiNIDine, quinupristin-dalfopristin, raNITIdine, remifentanil, Ringer's, ritodrine, riTUXimab, rocuronium, sargramostim, sodium acetate, succinylcholine, SUFentanil, tacrolimus, teniposide, theophylline, thiamine, thiotepa, tigecycline, tirofiban, TNA, tobramycin, tolazoline, trastuzumab, trimetaphan, vancomycin, vasopressin, vecuronium, verapamil, vinCRIStine, vinorelbine, voriconazole

SIDE EFFECTS
CNS: *Dizziness, drowsiness,* poor coordination, fatigue, anxiety, euphoria, confusion, paresthesia, neuritis, EPS, neuroleptic malignant syndrome
CV: Hypo/hypertension, palpitations, tachycardia, orthostatic hypotension
EENT: Blurred vision, dilated pupils, tinnitus, nasal stuffiness; dry nose, throat, mouth; photosensitivity

---

Side effects: *italics* = common; red = life-threatening

GI: *Constipation,* dry mouth, nausea, vomiting, anorexia, diarrhea
GU: *Urinary retention,* dysuria, frequency
INTEG: Rash, urticaria, photosensitivity, tissue necrosis (infiltration IV site)
RESP: Increased thick secretions, wheezing, chest tightness; apnea in neonates, infants, young children

PHARMACOKINETICS

Metabolized in liver; excreted by kidneys, GI tract (inactive metabolites)
PO: Onset 20 min, duration 4-12 hr
IV: Onset 3-5 min

INTERACTIONS

Increase: CNS depression—barbiturates, opioids, hypnotics, tricyclics, alcohol
Increase: promethazine effect—MAOIs
Decrease: oral anticoagulants effect—heparin

Drug/Lab Test
Increase: glucose
False negative: skin allergy test, urine pregnancy test
False positive: urine pregnancy test
Interference: blood grouping (ABO), GTT

NURSING CONSIDERATIONS
Assess:

> Black Box Warning: **Child:** not to be used in children <2 yr, fatal respiratory depression may occur; use cautiously in children >2 yr, seizures, paradoxical CNS stimulation may occur

• **Antiemetic/motion sickness:** nausea, vomiting before, after dose
• I&O ratio; be alert for urinary retention, frequency, dysuria; product should be discontinued
• **Respiratory depression/sedation:** degree of sedation, respiratory risk, CNS depressants may cause increased sedation
• **EPS:** pseudoparkinsonism, dystonia, akathisia, may be worse in geriatric patients
• **Anticholinergic effects:** dry mouth, confusion, urinary retention, more common in geriatric patients

• CBC with differential, LFTs during long-term therapy; blood dyscrasias, jaundice may occur
• Respiratory status: rate, rhythm, increase in bronchial secretions, wheezing, chest tightness
• Cardiac status: palpitations, increased pulse, hypo/hypertension, B/P in those receiving IV doses
• **Neuroleptic malignant syndrome:** fever, confusion, diaphoresis, rigid muscles, elevated CPK, encephalopathy; discontinue product, notify prescriber
• Hard candy, gum, frequent rinsing of mouth for dryness
Evaluate:
• Therapeutic response: absence of running, congested nose; rashes; absence of motion sickness, nausea; sedation
Teach patient/family:
• That product may cause photosensitivity; to avoid prolonged exposure to sunlight
• To notify prescriber of confusion, sedation, hypotension, jaundice, fever
• To avoid driving, other hazardous activity if drowsy
• To avoid concurrent use of alcohol or other CNS depressants
• That product may reduce sweating; that there is a risk of heat stroke
• How to use frequent sips of water, gum to decrease dry mouth

---

⚠ HIGH ALERT

propafenone (Rx)
(pro-paff′e-nown)
Rythmol, Rythmol SR
Func. class.: Antidysrhythmic (class IC)

ACTION: Slows conduction velocity; reduces membrane responsiveness; inhibits automaticity; increases ratio of effective refractory period to action potential duration; β-blocking activity

USES: Sustained ventricular tachycardia, atrial fibrillation (single dose), paroxysmal

---

supraventricular tachycardia (PSVT) prophylaxis, supraventricular dysrhythmias
Unlabeled uses: Wolff-Parkinson-White (WPW) syndrome

CONTRAINDICATIONS: 2nd/3rd-degree AV block, right bundle branch block, cardiogenic shock, hypersensitivity, bradycardia, uncontrolled HF, sick-sinus syndrome, marked hypotension, bronchospastic disorders, electrolyte imbalance, Brugada syndrome
Precautions: Pregnancy, breastfeeding, children, geriatric patients, HF, hypo/hyperkalemia, nonallergic bronchospasm, renal/hepatic disease, hematologic disorders, myasthenia gravis, COPD

Black Box Warning: Recent MI, cardiac arrhythmias, QT prolongation, torsades de pointes

DOSAGE AND ROUTES
PSVT
• **Adult: PO** 150 mg q8hr; allow 3-4 day interval before increasing dose, max 900 mg/day
Atrial fibrillation
• **Adult: PO** 450 or 600 mg as single dose; SR 225 mg q12hr, may increase to 325 q12hr, max 425 mg q12hr
Available forms: Tabs 150, 225, 300 mg; SR cap 225, 325, 425 mg
Administer:
• Do not break, crush, or chew tabs; swallow whole
• To hospitalized patients because heart monitoring is required
• After hypo/hyperkalemia is corrected
• With dosage adjustment q3-4days
• Without regard to meals

SIDE EFFECTS
CNS: Headache, dizziness, abnormal dreams, syncope, confusion, seizures, insomnia, tremor, anxiety, fatigue
CV: Supraventricular dysrhythmia, ventricular dysrhythmia, bradycardia, prodysrhythmia, palpitations, AV block, intraventricular conduction delay, AV dissociation, hypotension, chest pain, asystole
EENT: Blurred vision, altered taste, tinnitus
GI: *Nausea, vomiting,* constipation, dyspepsia, cholestasis, abnormal hepatic studies, dry mouth, diarrhea, anorexia
HEMA: Leukopenia, agranulocytosis, granulocytopenia, thrombocytopenia, anemia, bruising
INTEG: Rash
RESP: Dyspnea

PHARMACOKINETICS
Peak 3-8 hr, half-life 2-10 hr, poor metabolizers 10-32 hr; metabolized in liver; excreted in urine (metabolite)

INTERACTIONS
Increase: propafenone effects—CYP1A2, CYP2D6, CYP3A4 inhibitors (protease inhibitors, quiNINE, PARoxetine, saquinavir, erythromycin, azole antifungals, sertraline, tricyclics)
Increase: QT prolongation—other class IA/IC antidysrhythmics, arsenic trioxide, chloroquine, clarithromycin, droperidol, erythromycin, haloperidol, methadone, pentamidine, chlorproMAZINE, mesoridazine, thioridazine
Increase: anticoagulation—warfarin
Increase: CNS effects—local anesthetics
Increase: digoxin level—digoxin
Increase: β-blocker effect—propranolol, metoprolol
Increase: cycloSPORINE levels—cycloSPORINE
Decrease: propafenone effect—rifAMPin, cimetidine, quiNIDine
Drug/Food
Increase: propafenone effect—grapefruit juice
Drug/Herb
Decrease: propafenone effect—St. John's wort
Drug/Lab Test
Increase: CPK, Hct, Hgb
Decrease: WBC, platelets

P

NURSING CONSIDERATIONS
Assess:
• GI status: bowel pattern, number of stools

Black Box Warning: **QT/PR prolongation:** ECG or Holter monitor before and during therapy

Black Box Warning: **HF:** dyspnea, jugular venous distention, crackles, edema in extremities, I&O ratio; check for decreasing output; daily weight

• CBC, ANA titer, LFTs
• Chest x-ray, pulmonary function test during treatment
• Lung fields; bilateral crackles, dyspnea, peripheral edema, weight gain; jugular venous distention may occur in patient with HF
• **Toxicity:** fine tremors, dizziness, hypotension, drowsiness, abnormal heart rate
• **Pregnancy/breastfeeding:** use only if benefits outweigh fetal risk; do not breastfeed, excreted in breast milk
Evaluate:
• Therapeutic response: absence of ventricular dysrhythmias; decreasing recurrence of PAF, PSVT
Teach patient/family:
• To avoid hazardous activities until response is known
• To report fever, chills, sore throat, bleeding, SOB, chest pain, palpitations, blurred vision
• To take tab with food; alterations in taste sensation may occur; not to use with grapefruit juice or St. John's wort
• To carry emergency ID identifying medication and prescriber
• To avoid abrupt discontinuation of product; to take as prescribed; not to miss, double doses
• **Pregnancy/breastfeeding:** to notify prescriber if pregnancy is planned or suspected; not to breastfeed

TREATMENT OF OVERDOSE:
O_2, artificial ventilation, defibrillation ECG; administer DOPamine for circulatory depression, diazePAM or thiopental for seizures, isoproterenol

---

proparacaine ophthalmic
See Appendix B

⚠ HIGH ALERT

propofol (Rx)
(pro′poh-fole)
Diprivan
Func. class.: General anesthesia
Chem. class.: Phenol derivative

Do not confuse:
Diprivan/Diflucan/Ditropan

ACTION: Produces dose-dependent CNS depression by activation of GABA receptor, hypnotic

USES: Induction or maintenance of anesthesia as part of balanced anesthetic technique; sedation in mechanically ventilated patients

CONTRAINDICATIONS: Hypersensitivity to this product or soybean oil, egg, benzyl alcohol (some products)
Precautions: Pregnancy, breastfeeding, children, geriatric patients, respiratory depression, severe respiratory disorders, cardiac dysrhythmias, labor and delivery, renal disease, hyperlipidemia

DOSAGE AND ROUTES
Anesthesia
• **Adult <55 yr:** IV 40 mg q10sec until induction onset, maintenance 100-200 mcg/kg/min or IV BOL 20-50 mg prn, allow 3-5 min between adjustments
• **Child ≥3 yr:** IV induction 2.5-3.5 mg/kg over 20-30 sec when not premedicated or lightly premedicated
• **Child 2 mo-16 yr maintenance:** IV 125-300 mcg/kg/min, lower dose for ASA III or IV
Monitored anesthesia care (MAC) sedation
• **Adult <55 yr:** IV 100-150 mcg/kg infusion or 0.5 mg/kg by slow infusion;

maintenance 25-75 mcg/kg/min infusion or boluses of 10-20 mg
• **Geriatric debilitated, ASA III/IV:** IV initial, use slower rates; maintenance use 20% less than adult dose

ICU sedation
• **Adult:** IV 5 mcg/kg/min over 5 min; may increase by 5-10 mcg/kg/min over 5-10 min until desired response (Diprivan or generic)

Available forms: Inj 10 mg/mL in 20-mL ampule, vials, syringes

Administer:

IV route
• Shake well before use; dilution is not necessary, but if diluted, use only D₅W to ≥2 mg/mL; give over 3-5 min, titrate to needed level of sedation; use only glass containers when mixing, not stable in plastic; use aseptic technique when transferring from original container
• Only with resuscitative equipment available; only by qualified persons trained in anesthesia
• Store in light-resistant area at room temperature, use within 6 hr of opening
• If transferred from original container to another container, complete infusion within 12 hr (Diprivan), 6 hr (generic propofol)

Y-site compatibilities: Acyclovir, alfentanil, aminophylline, ampicillin, aztreonam, bumetanide, buprenorphine, butorphanol, calcium gluconate, CARBOplatin, ceFAZolin, cefoperazone, cefotaxime, cefoTEtan, cefOXitin, ceftizoxime, cefTRIAXone, cefuroxime, chlorproMAZINE, cimetidine, CISplatin, clindamycin, cyclophosphamide, cycloSPORINE, cytarabine, dexamethasone, diphenhydrAMINE, DOBUTamine, DOPamine, doxycycline, droperidol, enalaprilat, ePHEDrine, EPINEPHrine, esmolol, famotidine, fentaNYL, fluconazole, fluorouracil, furosemide, ganciclovir, glycopyrrolate, granisetron, haloperidol, heparin, hydrocortisone, HYDROmorphone, hydrOXYzine, ifosfamide, imipenem/cilastatin, inamrinone, insulin (regular), isoproterenol, ketamine, labetalol, levorphanol, lidocaine, LORazepam,

magnesium sulfate, mannitol, meperidine, mezlocillin, miconazole, morphine, nafcillin, nalbuphine, naloxone, nitroglycerin, norepinephrine, ofloxacin, PACLitaxel, PENTobarbital, PHENobarbital, piperacillin, potassium chloride, prochlorperazine, propranolol, raNITIdine, scopolamine, sodium bicarbonate, sodium nitroprusside, succinylcholine, SUFentanil, thiopental ticarcillin, ticarcillin/clavulanate, vecuronium, verapamil

Solution compatibilities: if given together via Y-site: D₅W, D₅LR, LR, D₅/0.45% NaCl, D₅/0.2% NaCl

SIDE EFFECTS

CNS: Involuntary movement, headache, fever, dizziness, shivering, abnormal dreams, euphoria, fatigue
CV: *Bradycardia, hypotension,* hypertension
GI: *Nausea, vomiting, abdominal cramping,* dry mouth
GU: Urine retention, green urine, *phlebitis, hives, burning/stinging at inj site,* rash
RESP: Apnea, *cough, hiccups*
SYST: Propofol infusion syndrome

PHARMACOKINETICS

Onset 15-30 sec, rapid distribution, half-life 1-8 min, half-life 3-12 hr; 70% excreted in urine; metabolized in liver by conjugation to inactive metabolites, 95%-99% protein binding, crosses placenta, enters breast milk, crosses blood brain barrier

INTERACTIONS

• Do not use within 10 days of MAOIs
Increase: CNS depression—alcohol, opioids, sedative/hypnotics, antipsychotics, skeletal muscle relaxants, inhalational anesthetics
Drug/Herb
Increase: propofol effect—St. John's wort

NURSING CONSIDERATIONS

Assess:
• Inj site: phlebitis, burning, stinging
• **ECG** for changes: PVC, PAC, ST segment changes; monitor VS , B/P, pulse, respirations

---

Side effects: *italics* = common; red = life-threatening

- **Neurologic excitatory symptoms:** movement, tremors, dizziness, LOC, pupil reaction
- Avoid general anesthetic use in child <3 yr; may negatively affect the brain
- Allergic reactions: hives
- **Respiratory dysfunction:** respiratory depression, character, rate, rhythm; notify prescriber if respirations are <10/min, apnea may occur ≥1 min, check airway, ventilation, determine level of sedation
- **Propofol infusion syndrome:** rhabdomyolysis, renal failure, hyperkalemia, metabolic acidosis, cardiac dysrhythmias, heart failure usually between 35 and 93 hr after infusion begun at >5 mg/kg/hr for >48 hr
- **ICU sedation:** test wake up on a daily basis to determine needed dose for sedation, do not discontinue abruptly during test
- **For lipids:** adjust enteral nutrition if receiving; monitor for signs and symptoms of pancreatitis (elevated lipids); propofol contains 1.1 Kcal/mL
- **Pregnancy/breastfeeding:** use only if clearly needed; avoid breastfeeding, excreted in breast milk

Evaluate:
- Therapeutic response: induction of anesthesia

Teach patient/family:
- That product will cause dizziness, drowsiness, sedation; to avoid hazardous activities until drug effect wears off
- That drug may cause burning sensation during administration

TREATMENT OF OVERDOSE: Discontinue product; administer vasopressor agents or anticholinergics, artificial ventilation

---

> **⚠ HIGH ALERT**
>
> **propranolol (Rx)**
> (proe-pran'oh-lole)
> Inderal LA, InnoPran XL, Hemangeol
> *Func. class.:* Antihypertensive, antianginal, antidysrhythmic (class II)
> *Chem. class.:* β-Adrenergic blocker

Do not confuse:
propranolol/Pravachol

ACTION: Nonselective β-blocker with negative inotropic, chronotropic, dromotropic properties

USES: Chronic stable angina pectoris, hypertension, supraventricular dysrhythmias, migraine prophylaxis, pheochromocytoma, cyanotic spells related to hypertrophic subaortic stenosis, essential tremor, acute MI, vascular headache prophylaxis

Unlabeled uses: Anxiety, prevention of variceal bleeding caused by portal hypertension, akathisia induced by antipsychotics, portal hypertension, sclerodermal renal crisis, unstable angina, infantile capillary hemangioma, lithium-induced tremor, attenuation of hypermetabolism in severe burns

CONTRAINDICATIONS: Hypersensitivity to this product; cardiogenic shock, AV heart block; bronchospastic disease; sinus bradycardia; bronchospasm; asthma

Precautions: Pregnancy, breastfeeding, children, diabetes mellitus, hyperthyroidism, COPD, renal/hepatic disease, myasthenia gravis, peripheral vascular disease, hypotension, cardiac failure, Raynaud's disease, sick sinus syndrome, vasospastic angina, smoking, Wolff-Parkinson-White syndrome, thyrotoxicosis

> **Black Box Warning:** Abrupt discontinuation

DOSAGE AND ROUTES
Dysrhythmias
- **Adult:** PO 10-30 mg tid-qid; **IV BOL** 1-3 mg give 1 mg/min; may repeat after 2 min, may repeat q4hr thereafter
- **Child:** PO 1 mg/kg/day in 2 divided doses; **IV** 0.01-0.1 mg/kg over 5 min

Hypertension
- **Adult:** PO 40 mg bid or 80 mg/day (ext rel) initially; usual dose 120-240 mg/day bid-tid or 120-160 mg/day (ext rel)
- **Child:** PO 0.5-1 mg/kg/day divided q6-12hr

Angina
- **Adult:** PO 10-20 mg bid-qid, increase at 3-7 day intervals up to 160-320 mg/day or **EXT REL** 80 mg daily

MI prophylaxis
- **Adult:** PO 180-240 mg/day tid-qid starting 5 days to 2 wk after MI

Pheochromocytoma
- **Adult:** PO 60 mg/day × 3 days preoperatively in divided doses or 30 mg/day in divided doses (inoperable tumor)

Migraine
- **Adult:** PO 80 mg/day (ext rel) or in divided doses; may increase to 160-240 mg/day in divided doses
- **Child >35 kg (unlabeled):** PO 20-40 mg tid
- **Child ≤35 kg (unlabeled):** PO 10-20 mg tid

Essential tremor
- **Adult:** PO 40 mg bid; usual dose 120 mg/day

Acute MI
- **Adult:** PO 180-320 mg/day in 3-4 divided doses; **IV** 0.1 mg/kg in 3 divided doses at 2-3 min intervals

Anxiety (unlabeled)
- **Adult:** PO 10-80 mg given 1 hr before anxiety-producing event

Scleroderma renal crisis (unlabeled)
- **Adult:** PO 40 mg bid, may increase q3-7days, max 160-480 mg/day

Esophageal varices (portal hypertension) (unlabeled)
- **Adult:** PO 40 mg bid, titrate to heart rate reduction of 25%

Infantile capillary hemangioma (unlabeled)
- **Infant:** PO 2-3 mg/kg/day

Available forms: Ext rel caps 60, 80, 120, 160 mg; tabs 10, 20, 40, 60, 80, 90 mg; inj 1 mg/mL; oral sol 20 mg, 40 mg/mL; oral sol (Hemangeol) 4.28 mg/mL

Administer:
PO route
- Do not break, crush, chew, or open ext rel cap
- Do not use ext rel cap for essential tremor, MI, cardiac dysrhythmias; do not use InnoPran XL in hypertropic subaortic stenosis, migraine, angina pectoris
- Ext rel caps should be taken daily; InnoPran XL should be taken at bedtime
- May mix oral sol with liquid or semisolid food; rinse container to get entire dose
- With 8 oz water with food; food enhances bioavailability
- Do not give with aluminum-containing antacid; may decrease GI absorption

Direct IV route
> IV undiluted or diluted 10 mL D$_5$W for inj; give 0.5 mg/min (adult), over 10 min (child)

Intermittent IV INFUSION route
- May be diluted in 50 mL NaCl and run over 10-15 min

Y-site compatibilities: Acyclovir, alfentanil, alteplase, amikacin, aminocaproic acid, aminophylline, anidulafungin, ascorbic acid, atracurium, atropine, azaTHIOprine, aztreonam, benztropine, bivalirudin, bleomycin, bumetanide, buprenorphine, butorphanol, calcium chloride/gluconate, CARBOplatin, carmustine, caspofungin, cefamandole, ceFAZolin, cefmetazole, cefonicid, cefoperazone, cefotaxime, cefoTEtan, cefOXitin, cefTAZidime, ceftizoxime, cefTRIAXone, cefuroxime, cephalothin, cephapirin, chloramphenicol, chlorproMAZINE, cimetidine, CISplatin, clindamycin, cyanocobalamin, cyclophosphamide, cycloSPORINE, cytarabine, DACTINomycin, DAPTOmycin, dexamethasone, digoxin, diltiaZEM, diphenhydrAMINE, DOBUTamine, DOCEtaxel, DOPamine, doxacurium, DOXOrubicin, doxycycline, enalaprilat, ePHEDrine, EPINEPHrine, epirubicin, epoetin alfa, eptifibatide, ertapenem, erythromycin, esmolol, etoposide, etoposide phosphate, famotidine, fenoldopam, fentaNYL, fluconazole, fludarabine, fluorouracil, folic acid, furosemide, ganciclovir, gatifloxacin, gemcitabine, gemtuzumab, gentamicin, glycopyrrolate, granisetron, heparin, hydrocortisone, HYDROmorphone, hydrOXYzine, IDArubicin, ifosfamide, imipenem-cilastatin, inamrinone,

P

irinotecan, isoproterenol, ketorolac, labetalol, levoFLOXacin, lidocaine, linezolid, LORazepam, magnesium, mannitol, mechlorethamine, meperidine, metaraminol, methicillin, methotrexate, methoxamine, methyldopa, methylPREDNISolone, metoclopramide, metoprolol, metroNIDAZOLE, mezlocillin, miconazole, midazolam, milrinone, minocycline, mitoXANTRONE, morphine, moxalactam, multiple vitamins, mycophenolate, nafcillin, nalbuphine, naloxone, nesiritide, netilmicin, nitroglycerin, nitroprusside, norepinephrine, octreotide, ondansetron, oxacillin, oxaliplatin, oxytocin, palonosetron, pamidronate, pancuronium, papaverine, PEMEtrexed, penicillin G potassium/sodium, pentamidine, pentazocine, PENTobarbital, PHENobarbital, phenylephrine, phytonadione, piperacillin, polymyxin B, potassium chloride, procainamide, prochlorperazine, promethazine, propofol, protamine, pyridoxine, quiNIDine, quinupristin-dalfopristin, raNITIdine, ritodrine, rocuronium, sodium acetate/bicarbonate, succinylcholine, SUFentanil, tacrolimus, teniposide, theophylline, thiamine, thiotepa, ticarcillin, ticarcillin-clavulanate, tigecycline, tirofiban, tobramycin, tolazoline, trimetaphan, urokinase, vancomycin, vasopressin, vecuronium, verapamil, vinCRIStine, vinorelbine, vitamin B complex/C, voriconazole, zoledronic acid

SIDE EFFECTS

CNS: Depression, hallucinations, *dizziness, fatigue,* lethargy, paresthesias, bizarre dreams, disorientation
CV: Bradycardia, hypotension, HF, palpitations, AV block, peripheral vascular insufficiency, vasodilation, cold extremities, pulmonary edema, dysrhythmias
EENT: Sore throat, laryngospasm, blurred vision, dry eyes
GI: Nausea, vomiting, diarrhea, colitis, constipation, cramps, dry mouth, hepatomegaly, gastric pain, acute pancreatitis

GU: Impotence, decreased libido, UTIs
HEMA: Agranulocytosis, thrombocytopenia
INTEG: Rash, pruritus, fever, Stevens-Johnson syndrome, toxic epidermal necrolysis
META: Hyperglycemia, hypoglycemia
MISC: Facial swelling, weight change, Raynaud's phenomenon
MS: Joint pain, arthralgia, muscle cramps, pain
RESP: Dyspnea, respiratory dysfunction, *bronchospasm,* cough

PHARMACOKINETICS

Metabolized by liver; crosses placenta, blood-brain barrier; excreted in breast milk; protein binding 90%; ✖ CYP2D6 enzyme system causes 7% of population to be poor metabolizers
PO: Onset 30 min, peak 1-1$^1/_2$ hr, duration 12 hr, half-life 3-8 hr
PO-ER: Peak 6 hr, duration 24 hr, half-life 8-11 hr
IV: Onset 2 min, peak 1 min, duration 2-4 hr

INTERACTIONS

Increase: toxicity—phenothiazines
Increase: propranolol level—propafenone
Increase: effect of calcium channel blockers, neuromuscular blocker
Increase: negative inotropic effects—disopyramide
Increase: β-blocking effect—cimetidine
Increase: hypotension—quiNIDine, haloperidol, prazosin
Decrease: β-blocking effects—barbiturates
Decrease: propranolol levels—smoking
Drug/Herb
• Avoid use with feverfew
Increase: antihypertensive effect—hawthorn
Decrease: antihypertensive effect—ma huang
Drug/Lab Test
Increase: serum potassium, serum uric acid, ALT, AST, alk phos, LDH
Decrease: blood glucose
Interference: glaucoma testing

NURSING CONSIDERATIONS
Assess:

Black Box Warning: **Abrupt withdrawal:** taper over 1-2 wk, do not discontinue abruptly; dysrhythmias, angina, myocardial ischemia, or MI may recur

- B/P, pulse, respirations during beginning therapy; notify prescriber if pulse <50 bpm or systolic B/P <90 mm Hg
- **ECG** continuously if using as antidysrhythmic IV, PCWP (pulmonary capillary wedge pressure), CVP (central venous pressure)
- Hepatic enzymes: AST, ALT, bilirubin; blood glucose (diabetes mellitus)
- **Angina pain:** duration, time started, activity being performed, character
- Tolerance with long-term use
- Headache, light-headedness, decreased B/P; may indicate need for decreased dosage; may aggravate symptoms of arterial insufficiency
- **Fluid overload:** weight daily; report gain of >5 lb
- I&O ratio, CCr if kidney damage is diagnosed; fatigue, weight gain, jugular distention, dyspnea, peripheral edema, crackles
- **Pregnancy/breastfeeding:** use only if benefits outweigh fetal risk, cautious use in breastfeeding

Evaluate:

- Therapeutic response: decreased B/P, dysrhythmias

Teach patient/family:

- Not to discontinue abruptly; may precipitate life-threatening dysrhythmias, exacerbation of angina, MI; to take product at same time each day, either with or without food consistently; to decrease dosage over 2 wk
- To avoid OTC products unless approved by prescriber; to avoid alcohol
- To avoid hazardous activities if dizzy
- About the importance of compliance with complete medical regimen; to monitor blood glucose, may mask symptoms of hypoglycemia
- To make position changes slowly to prevent fainting

- That sensitivity to cold may occur
- How to take pulse, B/P; to withhold product if <50 bpm or systolic B/P <90 mm Hg

---

⚠ HIGH ALERT

propylthiouracil (Rx)
(proe-pill-thye-oh-yoor′a-sill)

Propyl-Thyracil ✦

Func. class.: Thyroid hormone antagonist (antithyroid)

Chem. class.: Thioamide

Do not confuse:
propylthiouracil/purinethol

ACTION: Blocks synthesis peripherally of T_3, T_4 (triiodothyronine, thyroxine), inhibits organification of iodine

USES: Preparation for thyroidectomy, thyrotoxic crisis, hyperthyroidism, thyroid storm

CONTRAINDICATIONS: Pregnancy, breastfeeding, hypersensitivity

Precautions: Infants, bone marrow depression, fever, agranulocytosis, hepatitis, jaundice

Black Box Warning: Hepatic disease, pregnancy

DOSAGE AND ROUTES
Thyrotoxic crisis
- **Adult/child:** PO 200-400 mg q4hr for 1st 24 hr

Preparation for thyroidectomy
- **Adult:** PO 600-1200 mg/day
- **Child:** PO 10 mg/kg/day in divided doses

Hyperthyroidism
- **Adult:** PO 100 mg tid increasing to 300 mg q8hr if condition is severe; continue to euthyroid state, then 100 mg daily tid
- **Child >6 yr:** PO 50 mg/day divided q8hr, titrate based on TSH/free T_4 levels
- **Neonate (unlabeled):** PO 5-10 mg/kg/day in divided doses q8hr

P

Available forms: Tabs 50, 100 ✚ mg
Administer:
• With meals to decrease GI upset
• At same time each day to maintain product level
• At lowest dose that relieves symptoms

SIDE EFFECTS

CNS: *Drowsiness, headache, vertigo, fever,* paresthesias, neuritis
GI: *Nausea, diarrhea, vomiting,* jaundice, hepatitis, loss of taste, liver failure, death
GU: Nephritis
HEMA: Agranulocytosis, leukopenia, thrombocytopenia, hypothrombinemia, lymphadenopathy, bleeding, vasculitis, periarteritis
INTEG: *Rash, urticaria, pruritus, alopecia, hyperpigmentation,* lupuslike syndrome
MS: Myalgia, arthralgia, nocturnal muscle cramps, osteoporosis

PHARMACOKINETICS

Onset up to 3 wk, peak 6-10 wk, duration 1 wk to 1 mo, half-life 1-2 hr; excreted in urine, bile, breast milk; crosses placenta; concentration in thyroid gland

INTERACTIONS

• Bone marrow suppression: radiation, antineoplastics
• Agranulocytosis: phenothiazines
Increase: effects—potassium/sodium iodide, lithium
Decrease: anticoagulant effect—heparin, oral anticoagulants
Drug/Lab Test
Increase: PT, AST, ALT, alk phos

NURSING CONSIDERATIONS

Assess:

• **Hyperthyroidism:** weight loss, nervousness, insomnia, fever, diaphoresis, tremors; **hypothyroidism:** constipation, dry skin, weakness, headache; monitor T_3, T_4, which are increased; serum TSH, which is decreased; free thyroxine index, which is increased if dosage is too low; discontinue product 3-4 wk before RAIU
• Pulse, B/P, temperature

• I&O ratio; check for edema: puffy hands, feet, periorbits; indicates hypothyroidism
• Weight daily; same clothing, scale, time of day
• **Blood dyscrasias:** CBC with differential; leukopenia, thrombocytopenia, agranulocytosis; monitor periodically; agranulocytosis may develop in first 2 mo of treatment; discontinue treatment
• **Overdose:** peripheral edema, heat intolerance, diaphoresis, palpitations, dysrhythmias, severe tachycardia, increased temperature, delirium, CNS irritability
• **Hypersensitivity:** rash, enlarged cervical lymph nodes; product may have to be discontinued
• **Hypoprothrombinemia:** bleeding, petechiae, ecchymosis
• Clinical response: after 3 wk should include increased weight, pulse; decreased T_4
• **Bone marrow suppression:** sore throat, fever, fatigue

Black Box Warning: **Hepatotoxicity:** LFTs before, during treatment; jaundice, nausea, vomiting, abdominal pain, anorexia, diarrhea, fatigue

• Fluids to 3-4 L/day unless contraindicated

Black Box Warning: **Pregnancy/breastfeeding:** do not use in pregnancy, breastfeeding

Evaluate:
• Therapeutic response: weight gain, decreased pulse, decreased T_4, decreased B/P
Teach patient/family:
• To take pulse daily
• To report redness, swelling, sore throat, mouth lesions, which indicate blood dyscrasias; to report symptoms of hepatic dysfunction (yellow skin or eyes, clay-colored stools, dark urine)
• To keep graph of weight, pulse, mood
• To avoid OTC products that contain iodine

• That seafood, other iodine products may be restricted

• Not to discontinue product abruptly because thyroid crisis may occur; about stress response

• That response may take several months if thyroid is large

• About the symptoms/signs of overdose: periorbital edema, cold intolerance, mental depression

• About the symptoms of an inadequate dose: tachycardia, diarrhea, fever, irritability

• To take medication as prescribed; not to skip or double dose; that missed doses should be taken when remembered up to 1 hr before next dose

• To carry emergency ID listing conditions, medication

Black Box Warning: **Pregnancy:** to notify prescriber immediately if pregnancy is planned or suspected; not to breastfeed

protamine (Rx)

(proe'ta-meen)

Func. class.: Heparin antagonist
Chem. class.: Low-molecular-weight protein

Do not confuse:
protamine/Protonix

ACTION: Binds heparin, thereby making it ineffective

USES: Heparin, LMWH toxicity, hemorrhage

CONTRAINDICATIONS:

Black Box Warning: Hypersensitivity

Precautions: Pregnancy, breastfeeding, fish allergy, diabetes, previous exposure to protamine, insulins, heparin rebound or bleeding

Black Box Warning: Requires a specialized care setting

DOSAGE AND ROUTES
Heparin overdose

• **Adult/child:** IV 1 mg of protamine/100 units heparin given; administer slowly over 1-3 min; max 50 mg/10 min

Enoxaparin overdose

• **Adult:** IV 1 mg protamine/1 mg enoxaparin

Dalteparin overdose

• **Adult:** IV 1 mg protamine/100 anti-Xa unit

Available forms: Inj 10 mg/mL
Administer:

• Store at 36° F-46° F (2° C-8° C)

Direct IV route

• May give diluted or undiluted

• After reconstituting 50 mg/5 mL sterile bacteriostatic water for inj; shake, give ≤20 mg over 1-3 min, do not give rapidly

Y-site compatibilities: Alfentanil, amikacin, aminophylline, ascorbic acid, atracurium, atropine, azaTHIOprine, aztreonam, benztropine, bumetanide, buprenorphine, butorphanol, calcium chloride/gluconate, cefTAZidime, chlorproMAZINE, cimetidine, clindamycin, cyanocobalamin, cycloSPORINE, digoxin, diphenhydrAMINE, DOBUTamine, DOPamine, doxycycline, enalaprilat, ePHEDrine, EPINEPHrine, epoetin alfa, erythromycin, esmolol, famotidine, fentaNYL, fluconazole, ganciclovir, gentamicin, glycopyrrolate, hydrOXYzine, imipenem-cilastatin, inamrinone, iohexol, iopamidol, iothalamate, isoproterenol, labetalol, lidocaine, magnesium, mannitol, meperidine, metaraminol, methoxamine, methyldopate, metoclopramide, metoprolol, miconazole, midazolam, minocycline, morphine, multiple vitamins, nalbuphine, naloxone, netilmicin, nitroglycerin, nitroprusside, norepinephrine, ondansetron, oxytocin, papaverine, pentazocine, phenylephrine, polymyxin B, potassium chloride, procainamide, prochlorperazine, promethazine, propranolol, pyridoxine, quiNIDine, raNITIdine, Ringer's, ritodrine, sodium bicarbonate, succinylcholine, SUFentanil, theophylline, thiamine, tobramycin, tolazoline, trimetaphan, urokinase, vancomycin, vasopressin, verapamil

P

SIDE EFFECTS

CV: Hypotension, bradycardia, circulatory collapse, capillary leak
GI: Nausea, vomiting
HEMA: Bleeding, heparin rebound (cardiac surgery)
INTEG: *Rash,* dermatitis, urticaria
RESP: Dyspnea, pulmonary edema, severe respiratory distress, bronchospasm
SYST: Anaphylaxis, angioedema

PHARMACOKINETICS

IV: Onset 5 min, duration 2 hr, half-life unknown

NURSING CONSIDERATIONS
Assess:

• **Bleeding:** 30 min to 18 hr after dose in cardiac surgery

Black Box Warning: Hypersensitivity: urticaria, cough, wheezing, have emergency equipment nearby; allergy to fish; use with caution; men who have had vasectomies may be more prone to hypersensitivity, also high doses

• Blood studies (Hct, platelets, occult blood in stools)
• Coagulation tests (aPTT, ACT) 15 min after dose, then again after several hours
• VS, B/P, pulse after 30 min, then 3 hr after dose
• Skin rash, urticaria, dermatitis
• **Pregnancy/breastfeeding:** use only if clearly needed; cautious use in breastfeeding
Evaluate:
• Therapeutic response: reversal of heparin overdose
Teach patient/family:
• Not to take if allergic to fish
• The purpose of product, expected result
• To avoid activities in which bleeding may occur—shaving, use of hard-bristle toothbrush, injections, rectal temperature—until risk for bleeding has passed

---

pseudoephedrine (OTC, Rx)

(soo-doh-eh-fed′rin)

Eltor ♣, Nasofed, Sudafed, Sudafed 24 Hour, Sudogest
Func. class.: Adrenergic
Chem. class.: Substituted phenylethylamine

Controlled Substance Schedule V

Do not confuse:
Sudafed/sotalol

ACTION: Primary activity through α-effects on respiratory mucosal membranes reducing congestion, hyperemia, edema; minimal bronchodilation secondary to β-effects

USES: Nasal decongestant, adjunct for otitis media; with antihistamines

CONTRAINDICATIONS: Hypersensitivity to sympathomimetics, closed-angle glaucoma
Precautions: Pregnancy, breastfeeding, cardiac disorders, hyperthyroidism, diabetes mellitus, prostatic hypertrophy, hypertension, child <4 yr

DOSAGE AND ROUTES
Adult and child >12 yr: PO 60 mg q6hr; **EXT REL** 120 mg q12hr or 240 mg q24hr
Geriatric: PO 30-60 mg q6hr prn
Child 6-12 yr: PO 30 mg q6hr, max 120 mg/day
Child 4-6 yr: PO 15 mg q6hr, max 60 mg/day
Available forms: Ext rel caps 120, 240 mg; oral sol 15 mg, 30 mg/5 mL; tabs 30, 60 mg; ext rel tabs 120, 240 mg
Administer:
• Avoid taking at or near bedtime; stimulation can occur
• OTC preparations require an ID for sale; tracked, Schedule V

SIDE EFFECTS
CNS: *Tremors, anxiety,* stimulation, insomnia, headache, dizziness, hallucinations, seizures (geriatric patients)

CV: Palpitations, tachycardia, hypertension, chest pain, dysrhythmias, CV collapse
EENT: Dry nose; irritation of nose and throat
GI: *Anorexia, nausea, vomiting,* dry mouth, ischemic colitis
GU: Dysuria

PHARMACOKINETICS
PO: Onset 15-30 min; duration 4-6 hr, 8-12 hr (ext rel); metabolized in liver; excreted in feces and breast milk; half-life 7 hr (adult), 3 hr (child)

INTERACTIONS
• Do not use with MAOIs or tricyclics; hypertensive crisis may occur
Increase: effect of this product—urinary alkalizers, adrenergics, β-blockers, phenothiazines, tricyclics
Decrease: effect of this product—urinary acidifiers

NURSING CONSIDERATIONS
Assess:
• **Nasal congestion**: auscultate lung sounds; check for tenacious bronchial secretions
• B/P, pulse throughout treatment
• **Beers:** avoid in older adults; CNS stimulant effects, seizures, hallucinations, excitation
• **Pregnancy/breastfeeding:** avoid in pregnancy; cautious use in breastfeeding
Evaluate:
• Therapeutic response: decreased nasal, eustachian tube, congestion
Teach patient/family:
• About the reason for product administration
• Ext rel: do not divide, crush, chew, or dissolve
• Do not use within 14 days of MAOIs
• Not to use continuously or to take more than recommended dose because rebound congestion may occur
• To notify prescriber immediately of anxiety, slow or fast heart rate, dyspnea, seizures

• To check with prescriber before using other products because product interactions may occur
• To avoid taking near bedtime because stimulation can occur
• Not to use if stimulation, restlessness, tremors occur
• That use in children may cause excessive agitation
• To notify provider if symptoms do not improve within 7 days or if having a fever

---

psyllium (OTC, Rx)
(sill′ee-um)
Hydrocil, Leader Fiber Laxative, Metamucil, Natural Fiber, Natural Vegetable Fiber, Reguloid, Wal-Mucil, Karacil ✤, Konsyl
Func. class.: Bulk laxative
Chem. class.: Psyllium colloid

ACTION: Bulk-forming laxative

USES: Chronic constipation, ulcerative colitis
Unlabeled uses: Diarrhea, diverticulosis, irritable bowel syndrome, hypercholesterolemia

CONTRAINDICATIONS: Hypersensitivity, intestinal obstruction, abdominal pain, nausea, vomiting, fecal impaction
Precautions: Pregnancy

DOSAGE AND ROUTES
• **Adult: PO** 1-2 tsp in 8 oz water bid or tid, then 8 oz water or 1 premeasured packet in 8 oz water bid or tid, then 8 oz water
• **Child >6 yr: PO** 1 tsp in 4 oz water at bedtime
Available forms: Chew pieces 1.7, 3.4 g/piece; effervescent powder 3.4, 3.7 g/packet; powder 3.3, 3.4, 3.5, 4.94 g/tsp; wafers 3.4 g/wafer

Administer:
PO route
- Alone for better absorption, separate from other products by 1-2 hr
- In morning or evening (oral dose)
- Immediately after mixing with water or will congeal
- With 8 oz water or juice followed by another 8 oz of fluid

SIDE EFFECTS
GI: *Nausea, vomiting, anorexia, diarrhea,* cramps, intestinal or esophageal blockage

PHARMACOKINETICS
Onset 12-72 hr, excreted in feces, not absorbed in GI tract

INTERACTIONS
Decrease: absorption of cardiac glycosides, oral anticoagulants, salicylates
Drug/Herb
Increase: laxative effect—flax, senna

NURSING CONSIDERATIONS
Assess:
- Blood, urine electrolytes if used often
- I&O ratio to identify fluid loss
- **Constipation:** cause of constipation; fluids, bulk, exercise missing; bowel sounds, distention, usual bowel function; color, consistency, amount, cramping; rectal bleeding, nausea, vomiting; product should be discontinued
- **Pregnancy/breastfeeding:** generally considered safe in pregnancy, breastfeeding
Evaluate:
- Therapeutic response: decrease in constipation, decreased diarrhea with colitis
Teach patient/family:
- To maintain adequate fluid consumption
- That normal bowel movements do not always occur daily
- Not to use in presence of abdominal pain, nausea, vomiting
- To notify prescriber if constipation unrelieved or if symptoms of electrolyte imbalance occur: muscle cramps, pain, weakness, dizziness, excessive thirst

pyridostigmine (Rx)
(peer-id-oh-stig′meen)
Mestinon, Mestinon SR ✦,
Mestinon Tinespan, Regonol
Func. class.: Cholinergic; anticholinesterase
Chem. class.: Tertiary amine carbamate

ACTION: Inhibits destruction of acetylcholine, which increases concentration at sites where acetylcholine is released; this facilitates the transmission of impulses across the myoneural junction

USES: Nondepolarizing muscle relaxant antagonist, myasthenia gravis, pretreatment for nerve gas exposure (military only)

CONTRAINDICATIONS: Bradycardia; hypotension; obstruction of intestine, renal system; bromide, benzyl alcohol sensitivity; adrenal insufficiency; cholinesterase inhibitor toxicity
Precautions: Pregnancy, seizure disorders, bronchial asthma, coronary occlusion, hyperthyroidism, dysrhythmias, peptic ulcer, megacolon, poor GI motility

DOSAGE AND ROUTES
Myasthenia gravis
- **Adult: PO** 600 mg/day in 5-6 divided doses, max 1.5 g/day; **IM/IV** 2 mg; **SUS REL** 180-540 mg/day or bid at intervals of ≥6 hr
- **Child: PO** 7 mg/kg/day in 5-6 divided doses; **IM/IV** 0.05-0.15 mg/kg/dose
Nondepolarizing neuromuscular blocker antagonist
- **Adult:** 0.6-1.2 mg **IV** atropine, then 0.1-0.25 mg/kg/dose
- **Child: IV** 0.1-0.25 mg/kg/dose
Nerve gas exposure prophylaxis (military)
- **Adult: PO** 30 mg q8hr if threat of exposure to Soman gas is anticipated; start several hours before exposure and discontinue upon exposure; after product is

discontinued, give antidotes (atropine, pralidoxime)

Available forms: Tabs 60 mg; ext rel tabs 180 mg; syr 60 mg/5 mL; inj 5 mg/mL

Administer:

• Only with atropine sulfate available for cholinergic crisis

• Only after all other cholinergics have been discontinued

• Increased doses for tolerance as ordered

• Larger doses after exercise or fatigue as ordered

• Do not break, crush, or chew sus rel tabs

PO route

• On empty stomach for better absorption

Direct IV route

• Undiluted (5 mg/mL), give through Y-tube or 3-way stopcock, give ≤0.5 mg/min (myasthenia gravis); 5 mg/min (reversal of nondepolarizing neuromuscular blockers)

Y-site compatibilities: Heparin, hydrocortisone, potassium chloride, vit B/C

SIDE EFFECTS

CNS: Dizziness, headache, sweating, weakness, seizures, incoordination, paralysis, drowsiness, LOC

CV: Tachycardia, dysrhythmias, bradycardia, AV block, hypotension, ECG changes, cardiac arrest, syncope

EENT: Miosis, blurred vision, lacrimation, visual changes

GI: *Nausea, diarrhea, vomiting, cramps, increased salivary and gastric secretions, peristalsis*

GU: Urinary frequency, incontinence, urgency

INTEG: Rash, urticaria, flushing

RESP: Respiratory depression, bronchospasm, constriction, laryngospasm, respiratory arrest

SYST: Cholinergic crisis

PHARMACOKINETICS

Metabolized in liver, excreted in urine (unchanged)

PO: Onset 20-30 min, duration 3-6 hr
PO-EXT REL: Onset 30-60 min, duration 6-12 hr
IM/IV/SUBCUT: Onset 2-15 min, duration $2^1/_2$-4 hr

INTERACTIONS

Increase: action—succinylcholine

Decrease: action—gallamine, metocurine, pancuronium, tubocurarine, atropine

Decrease: pyridostigmine action—aminoglycosides, anesthetics, procainamide, quiNIDine, mecamylamine, polymyxin, magnesium, corticosteroids, antidysrhythmics, quinolones

NURSING CONSIDERATIONS

Assess:

• **Myasthenia gravis:** fatigue, ptosis, diplopia, difficulty swallowing, SOB, hand/gait before, after product; improvement should be seen after 1 hr

• VS, respiration q8hr

• I&O ratio; check for urinary retention or incontinence

• **Toxicity:** bradycardia, hypotension, bronchospasm, headache, dizziness, seizures, respiratory depression; product should be discontinued if toxicity occurs

• **Pregnancy/breastfeeding:** use only if benefits outweigh fetal risk; cautious use in breastfeeding

Evaluate:

• Therapeutic response: increased muscle strength, hand grasp, improved gait, absence of labored breathing (if severe), negative inspiratory force, and vital capacity; reversal of nondepolarizing neuromuscular blockers; prevention of nerve gas toxicity

Teach patient/family:

• **Myasthenia gravis:** that product is not a cure, only relieves symptoms

• To wear emergency ID specifying myasthenia gravis, products taken

• To avoid driving, other hazardous activities until effect is known

• To report muscle weakness (cholinergic crisis or underdosage), bradycardia

• Not to drink alcohol

• To take with food to decrease gastric side effects

P

• That doses are highly individualized, often 5-6 times per day, and will be based on response to the product

TREATMENT OF OVERDOSE:
Discontinue product, atropine 1-4 mg IV

---

pyridoxine (vit B$_6$) (Rx, OTC)
(peer-i-dox′een)
Pyri 500, Neuro-K
Func. class.: Vit B$_6$, water soluble

ACTION: Needed for fat, protein, carbohydrate metabolism; enhances glycogen release from liver and muscle tissue; needed as coenzyme for metabolic transformations of a variety of amino acids

USES: Vit B$_6$ deficiency of inborn errors of metabolism, seizures, isoniazid therapy, oral contraceptives, alcoholic polyneuritis

CONTRAINDICATIONS: Hypersensitivity
Precautions: Pregnancy, breastfeeding, children, Parkinson's disease; patients taking levodopa should avoid supplemental vitamins with >5 mg pyridoxine

DOSAGE AND ROUTES
RDA
• **Adult: PO** (male) 1.7-2 mg; (female) 1.4-1.6 mg
• **Child 9-13 yr: PO** 1 mg/day
• **Child 4-8 yr: PO** 0.6 mg/day
• **Child 1-3 yr: PO** 0.5 mg/day
• **Infant 7-12 mo: PO** 0.3 mg/day
Vit B$_6$ deficiency
• **Adult: PO** 5-25 mg/day × 3 wk
• **Child: PO** 10 mg until desired response
Pyridoxine deficiency neuritis/ seizure (not drug induced)
• **Adult: PO** *without neuritis* 2.5-10 mg/day, after corrected 2-5 mg/day; *with neuritis* 100-200 mg/day × 3wk, then 2-5 mg/day

• **Child: PO** *without neuritis* 5-25 mg/day × 3wk, then 1.5-2.5 mg/day in a multivitamin; *with neuritis:* 10-50 mg/day × 3wk, then 1-2 mg/day
• **Neonate with seizures: IM/IV** 50-100 mg as single dose
Deficiency caused by isoniazid, cycloSERINE, hydrALAZINE, penicillAMINE
• **Adult: PO** 100-300 mg/day
• **Child: PO** 10-50 mg/day
Prevention of deficiency caused by isoniazid, cycloSERINE, hydrALAZINE, penicillAMINE
• **Adult: PO** 25-100 mg/day
• **Child: PO** 1-2 mg/kg/day
Available forms: Tabs 25, 50, 100, 250, 500 mg; ext rel tabs 200, 500 mg; inj 100 mg/mL; ext rel caps 200, 500 mg; capsules 250 mg
Administer:
PO route
• Do not break, crush, or chew ext rel tabs/caps
IM route
• Rotate sites; burning or stinging at site may occur
• Z-track to minimize pain
IV route
• Undiluted or added to most IV sol; give ≤50 mg/1 min if undiluted
Syringe compatibilities: Doxapram

SIDE EFFECTS
CNS: Paresthesia, flushing, warmth, lethargy (rare with normal renal function)
INTEG: Pain at inj site

PHARMACOKINETICS
PO/INJ: Half-life 2-3 wk, metabolized in liver, excreted in urine

INTERACTIONS
Decrease: effects of levodopa
Decrease: effects of pyridoxine—oral contraceptives, isoniazid, cycloSERINE, hydrALAZINE, penicillamine, chloramphenicol, immunosuppressants

NURSING CONSIDERATIONS
Assess:
• **Pyridoxine deficiency:** seizures, irritability, cheilitis, conjunctivitis, anemia,

confusion, red tongue, weakness, fatigue before and during treatment; monitor pyridoxine levels
• Nutritional status: yeast, liver, legumes, bananas, green vegetables, whole grains
• Blood studies: Hct, Hgb
• **Malabsorption:** may require injection if abdominal resection has occurred or in malabsorption syndromes
• **Pregnancy/breastfeeding:** safe in pregnancy, breastfeeding

Evaluate:
• Therapeutic response: absence of nausea, vomiting, anorexia, skin lesions, glossitis, stomatitis, edema, seizures, restlessness, paresthesia

Teach patient/family:
• To avoid vitamin supplements unless directed by prescriber
• To increase meat, bananas, potatoes, lima beans, whole-grain cereals in diet
• To take as directed; to continue with follow-up exams, blood work

P

QUEtiapine (Rx)

(kwe-tie′a-peen)

SEROquel, SEROquel XR

Func. class.: Antipsychotic, atypical

Chem. class.: Dibenzothiazepine

Do not confuse:

QUEtiapine/OLANZapine

SEROquel/Serzone/SINEquan

ACTION: Functions as an antagonist at multiple neurotransmitter receptors in the brain, including $5HT_{1A}$, $5HT_2$, dopamine D_1, D_2, H_1, and adrenergic α_1, α_2 receptors

USES: Bipolar disorder, bipolar I disorder, depression, mania, schizophrenia, borderline personality disorder

CONTRAINDICATIONS: Hypersensitivity, breastfeeding

Precautions: Pregnancy, geriatric patients, hepatic/cardiac disease, breast cancer, long-term use, seizures, QT prolongation, brain tumor, hematologic disease, torsades de pointes, cataracts, dehydration, abrupt discontinuation

Black Box Warning: Children, suicidal ideation, increased mortality in elderly patients with dementia-related psychosis

DOSAGE AND ROUTES

Bipolar disorder, depressed phase, monotherapy in acute management:

• **Adult: PO** (Regular release and extended release) 50 mg/day on day 1, 100 mg/day on day 2, 200 mg/day on day 3, then 300 mg/day on day 4. Max 300 mg/day. All doses given at bedtime

Bipolar disorder, maintenance, in combination with lithium or divalproex

• **Adult: PO** (Regular-release tablets) 400-800 mg/day divided bid, max 800 mg/day; (ext-rel tablets) 400-800 mg/day in the evening, max 800 mg/day. Periodically reassess for need and appropriate dose for maintenance treatment

• **Geriatric, debilitated, or at risk for hypotension: PO** 25 mg bid, titrate upward slowly; **ext rel** 50 mg in evening, max 800 mg/day

• **Child ≥10 yr/adolescent: PO** 25 mg bid day 1, 50 mg bid day 2, 100 mg bid day 3, 150 mg bid day 4, 200 mg bid beginning day 5, max 600 mg/day; **ext rel** 50 mg day 1, 100 mg day 2, 200 mg day 3, 300 mg day 4, 400 mg day 5, give in evening

Schizophrenia

• **Adult: PO** (not at risk for hypotension) 25 mg bid on day 1, increase by 25-50 mg divided 2 to 3× on day 2 and day 3 to a target of 300-400 mg/day in divided doses by day 4, further dosage adjustment can be made in 25-50 mg bid increments, max 800 mg/day; **(XR)** 300 mg/day in PM, range 400-800 mg/day, max 800 mg/day

• **Adolescent 13-17 yr: PO** 25 mg bid on day 1, 50 mg bid on day 2, 100 mg bid on day 3, 150 mg bid on day 4, 200 mg bid on day 5; **ext rel** 50 mg on day 1, then 100 mg on day 2, 200 mg on day 3, 300 mg on day 4, 400 mg on day 5

• **Geriatric: PO EXT REL** 50 mg/day may increase in 50 mg/day increments

Depressive disorder

• **Adult: PO EXT REL** 50 mg/day in PM on days 1, 2; on day 3, give 150 mg in PM

• **Geriatric, debilitated or at risk for hypotension: PO EXT REL** 50 mg on day 1 and 2, may increase by 50 mg/day based on response

Available forms: Tabs 25, 50, 100, 200, 300, 400 mg; ext rel tab 50, 150, 200, 300, 400 mg

Administer:

• Reduced dose to geriatric patients

• Avoid use of CNS depressants

• Store in tight, light-resistant container

• If there is a wk or more absence of therapy, initiate at beginning dose

• **Immediate release:** without regard to meals

• **Ext rel:** without food or with light meal ≤300 calories; swallow whole; do not split, crush, chew; can switch from immediate release to extended release by giving total daily dose daily

SIDE EFFECTS

CNS: EPS, pseudoparkinsonism, akathisia, dystonia, tardive dyskinesia; *drowsiness,* insomnia, agitation, anxiety, *headache,* seizures, neuroleptic malignant syndrome, *dizziness,* dystonia, restless legs

CV: Orthostatic hypotension, tachycardia, QT prolongation, CV disease, Parkinson's disease, cardiomyopathy, myocarditis

ENDO: SIADH, hyperglycemia

GI: *Pancreatitis, nausea, anorexia, constipation,* abdominal pain, dry mouth

HEMA: Leukopenia, agranulocytosis

INTEG: Rash, DRESS

META: Hyponatremia

MISC: Asthenia, back pain, fever, ear pain

MS: Rhabdomyolysis

RESP: Rhinitis

SYST: Stevens-Johnson syndrome, anaphylaxis

PHARMACOKINETICS

Extensively metabolized by liver, half-life ≥6 hr, peak 1½ hr, ext rel 6 hr, inhibits P450 CYP3A4 enzyme system, 83% protein binding, excretion: <1% unchanged urine

INTERACTIONS

Increase: QT prolongation—class IA/III antidysrhythmics, some phenothiazines, β-agonists, local anesthetics, tricyclics, haloperidol, methadone, chloroquine, clarithromycin, droperidol, erythromycin, pentamidine, macrolides (clarithromycin)

Increase: CNS depression—alcohol, opioid analgesics, sedative/hypnotics, antihistamines

Increase: hypotension—alcohol, antihypertensives

Increase: QUEtiapine clearance, decrease QUEtiapine effect—phenytoin, thioridazine, barbiturates, glucocorticoids, carBAMazepine, rifampin

Increase: neurotoxicity—lithium

Increase: QUEtiapine action—fluconazole, itraconazole, ketoconazole (CYP3A4 inhibitors)

Increase: effects of erythromycin

Decrease: QUEtiapine clearance—cimetidine

Decrease: effects of DOPamine agonists, levodopa, LORazepam

Drug/Lab Test

Increase: cholesterol, triglycerides, LFTs, glucose

Decrease: thyroid tests, WBC

NURSING CONSIDERATIONS

Assess:

• **CV status:** QT prolongation, tachycardia, orthostatic B/P

Black Box Warning: Assess mental status before initial administration, AIMS assessment; affect, orientation, LOC, reflexes, gait, coordination, sleep pattern disturbances; suicidal thoughts/behaviors (child/young adult); dementia (geriatric patients)

Black Box Warning: Not to be used in child <10 yr (imm rel) or <18 yr (ext rel)

Black Box Warning: **Suicide:** restrict amount of product given; usually suicidal thoughts/behaviors occur early during treatment and among children/adolescents/young adults

• Baseline blood glucose, LFTs, neurologic function, ophthalmologic exam, weight, monitor glucose often in diabetes mellitus, thyroid function tests, serum electrolytes/creatinine/lipid profile/prolactin

• B/P standing, lying; pulse, respirations; determine q4hr during initial treatment; establish baseline before starting treatment; report drops of 30 mm Hg; watch for ECG changes

• Dizziness, faintness, palpitations, tachycardia on rising

• **EPS:** including akathisia (inability to sit still, no pattern to movements), tardive dyskinesia (bizarre movements of jaw, mouth, tongue, extremities), pseudoparkinsonism (rigidity, tremors, pill rolling, shuffling gait)

• **Serious rash:** assess for Stevens-Johnson syndrome, discontinue product; may cause rash, fever, joint pain, lesions

• **Pancreatitis:** assess for nausea, vomiting, severe abdominal pain

• **Neuroleptic malignant syndrome:** hyperthermia, increased CPK, altered mental status, muscle rigidity, seizures, tachycardia, diaphoresis, hypo/hypertension, fatigue; notify prescriber immediately if symptoms occur

• Constipation, urinary retention daily; if these occur, increase bulk, water in diet

• Supervised ambulation until patient stabilized on medication; do not involve patient in strenuous exercise program because fainting possible; patient should not stand still for long period of time

• **DRESS:** Fever, hepatitis, swelling of face, myositis, monitor eosinophils that may be elevated, discontinue

• **Hyperprolactinemia:** sexual dysfunction, menstrual changes

• **Beers:** avoid in older adults except for schizophrenia, bipolar disorder, or short-term use as an antiemetic for chemotherapy; increased risk for stroke

• **Pregnancy/breastfeeding:** use only if benefits outweigh fetal risk; pregnant women taking product should enroll in the National Pregnancy Registry for Atypical Antipsychotics, 1-866-961-2388; EPS may develop in the infant; breastfeeding isn't recommended, excreted in breast milk

Evaluate:

• Therapeutic response: decrease in emotional excitement, hallucinations, delusions, paranoia; reorganization of patterns of thought, speech

Teach patient/family:

• Not to become overheated, to drink plenty of fluids

• To rise slowly to prevent orthostatic hypotension

• To take medication only as prescribed; not to crush, chew ext rel product; not to use with alcohol; to take regular tabs without regard to food or only a light meal <300 calories, ext rel without food; not to use other products unless approved by prescriber; not to discontinue abruptly

• That follow-up is necessary, including LFTs, blood glucose, neurologic, cholesterol profile, weight

• If drowsiness occurs, to avoid hazardous activities such as driving; not to stand quickly, may be worse during first few days of dose change

• To avoid use of OTC, herbals, supplements meds unless directed by prescriber

• To notify prescriber if pregnancy is planned, suspected; not to breastfeed

• To notify prescriber immediately of fever, difficulty breathing, fatigue, sore throat, rash, bleeding

Black Box Warning: Suicide: to notify prescriber of suicidal thoughts/behaviors, primarily among children/adolescents/young adults, or worsening depression, severe anxiety, panic attacks, insomnia

• To have eye exam before treatment and yearly; cataracts may occur

• To notify providers before surgery

---

quinapril (Rx)

(kwin′a-pril)

Accupril ✦

Func. class.: Antihypertensive
Chem. class.: Angiotensin-converting enzyme (ACE) inhibitor

Do not confuse:
Accupril/Aciphex

ACTION: Selectively suppresses renin-angiotensin-aldosterone system; inhibits ACE, prevents conversion of angiotensin I to angiotensin II; results in dilation of arterial, venous vessels

USES: Hypertension, alone or in combination with thiazide diuretics; systolic HF

CONTRAINDICATIONS: Children, hypersensitivity to ACE inhibitors, angioedema

Black Box Warning: Pregnancy

Precautions: Breastfeeding, geriatric patients, impaired renal/hepatic function, dialysis patients, hypovolemia, blood

---

dyscrasias, bilateral renal stenosis, cough, hyperkalemia, aortic stenosis, ☜ African descent

DOSAGE AND ROUTES
Hypertension
• **Adult: PO** 10-20 mg/day initially, then 20-80 mg/day divided bid or daily (monotherapy); start at 5 mg/day (with diuretics), titrate ≥2 wk up to 80 mg/day
• **Geriatric: PO** 10 mg/day, titrate to desired response (monotherapy); start at 2.5 mg/day (with diuretics)
Heart failure
• **Adult: PO** 5 mg bid, may increase weekly until 20-40 mg/day in 2 divided doses
Renal dose
• **Adult: PO** CCr 61-89 mL/min 10 mg daily (hypertension), 5 mg bid (heart failure); CCr 30-60 mL/min, 5 mg/day initially; CCr 10-29 mL/min, 2.5 mg/day initially
Available forms: Tabs 5, 10, 20, 40 mg
Administer:
• Tabs may be crushed if necessary
• Store in airtight container at room temperature
• Do not use with high-fat meal, decreases absorption

SIDE EFFECTS
CNS: *Headache, dizziness, fatigue,* somnolence, depression, malaise, nervousness, vertigo, syncope
CV: *Hypotension,* postural hypotension, syncope, palpitations, *angina pectoris,* MI, tachycardia, vasodilation, chest pain
GI: *Nausea,* diarrhea, constipation, *vomiting,* gastritis, GI hemorrhage, dry mouth
GU: Increased BUN, creatinine; decreased libido, impotence
INTEG: Angioedema, rash, sweating, photosensitivity, pruritus
META: Hyperkalemia
MISC: Back pain, amblyopia
MS: Myalgia
RESP: *Dry cough,* pharyngitis, dyspnea

PHARMACOKINETICS
Bioavailability ≥60%, onset <1 hr, peak 1-2 hr, duration 24 hr, protein binding 97%, half-life 2 hr, metabolized by liver (active metabolite quinaprilat), metabolites excreted in urine (60%)/feces (37%)

INTERACTIONS
Increase: hyperkalemia—vasodilators, hydrALAZINE, prazosin, potassium-sparing diuretics, sympathomimetics, potassium supplements, ACE/angiotensin II receptor antagonists; aliskiren (diabetic patients)
Increase: hypotension—diuretics, other antihypertensives, ganglionic blockers, adrenergic blockers, phenothiazines, nitrates, acute alcohol ingestion
Increase: toxicity of lithium
Decrease: absorption of tetracycline, quinolone antibiotics
Decrease: hypotensive effect of quinapril—NSAIDs
Drug/Herb
Increase: risk of cough—capsaicin
Decrease: antihypertensive effect—ma huang
Drug/Food
Hyperkalemia: do not use with potassium-containing salt substitutes; read label carefully
Drug/Lab Test
Increase: potassium, creatinine, BUN, LFTs

NURSING CONSIDERATIONS
Assess:
• **Hypertension:** B/P, orthostatic hypotension, syncope; monitor B/P before giving and after 2 hr; African-American patients are more resistant to antihypertension effect
• **Heart failure:** edema in feet, legs daily; weight daily
• **Collagen-vascular disease:** blood studies: neutrophils, decreased platelets; WBC with differential at baseline, periodically, q3mo; if neutrophils <1000/mm³, discontinue treatment
• Renal studies: protein, BUN, creatinine; watch for increased levels; may indicate nephrotic syndrome
• For dry cough: notify provider, product may need to be discontinued

---

Side effects: *italics* = common; red = life-threatening

• Baselines of hepatic studies before therapy, periodically; increased LFTs; uric acid, glucose may be increased
• Potassium levels; hyperkalemia rare
• **Allergic reactions:** angioedema, rash, fever, pruritus, urticaria, swelling of eyes/face/throat/neck, SOB, difficulty breathing; product should be discontinued; angioedema is more common in African-American patients

Black Box Warning: Do not use in pregnancy, breastfeeding

Evaluate:
• Therapeutic response: decrease in B/P
Teach patient/family:
• Not to discontinue product abruptly
• Not to use OTC products (cough, cold, allergy); not to use salt substitutes containing potassium unless directed by prescriber, to avoid high-fat meal at same time as product
• To comply with dosage schedule, even if feeling better
• To rise slowly to sitting or standing position to minimize orthostatic hypotension, to report excessive perspiration, dehydration, vomiting, diarrhea; may lead to fall in B/P; maintain adequate hydration
• To notify prescriber of mouth sores, sore throat, fever, swelling of hands/feet, irregular heartbeat, chest pain, persistent dry cough
• That product may cause dizziness, fainting, light-headedness; may occur during first few days of therapy
• That product may cause skin rash, impaired taste perception
• How to take B/P, normal readings for age group

Black Box Warning: **Pregnancy:** to report if pregnancy is planned or suspected; not to breastfeed

TREATMENT OF OVERDOSE: 0.9% NaCl IV infusion

⚠ HIGH ALERT

quiNIDine gluconate (Rx)
(kwin´i-deen)
quiNIDine sulfate (Rx)
Func. class.: Antidysrhythmic (Class IA)
Chem. class.: QuiNINE dextroisomer

Do not confuse:
quiNIDine/quiNINE

ACTION: Prolongs duration of action potential and effective refractory period, thus decreasing myocardial excitability; anticholinergic properties

USES: Atrial fibrillation, PAT, ventricular tachycardia, atrial flutter, Wolff-Parkinson-White syndrome; PVST, malaria/IV quiNIDine gluconate
Unlabeled uses: Singultus (hiccups)

CONTRAINDICATIONS: Hypersensitivity, idiosyncratic response, digoxin toxicity, blood dyscrasias, myasthenia gravis, AV block
Precautions: Pregnancy, breastfeeding, children, geriatric patients, electrolyte imbalance, renal/hepatic disease, HF, respiratory depression, bradycardia, hypotension, syncope

Black Box Warning: Cardiac arrhythmias, MI

DOSAGE AND ROUTES
QuiNIDine gluconate
• **Adult: PO** (ext rel) 324-648 mg q8-12hr; **IM** 600 mg, then 400 mg q2hr; **IV** give 16 mg/min
Severe *Plasmodium falciparum* malaria
• **Adult: IV** 10 mg/kg/dose over 1-2 hr, then **IV INF** of 0.02 mg/kg/min for ≥24 hr
QuiNIDine sulfate
PVST/WPW/atrial fibrillation/flutter
• **Adult: PO** 200-300 mg q6-8hr × 5-8 doses; may increase daily until sinus rhythm

---

restored; max 4 g/day given only after digitalization; maintenance 200-300 mg tid-qid or **EXT REL** 300-600 mg q8-12hr

Hiccups (unlabeled)

• **Adult: PO** 200 mg qid

Available forms: *Gluconate:* ext rel tabs 324 mg; inj gluconate 80 mg/mL; *sulfate:* tabs 200, 300 mg; sus rel tabs 300 mg

Administer:

• AV node blocker (digoxin) before starting quinidine to avoid increased ventricular rate

PO route

• Do not break, crush, chew ext rel products

• With full glass of water or with food; GI upset occurs

• Sus rel forms not interchangeable

• Do not use with grapefruit juice

IM route

• IM inj in deltoid; aspirate to avoid intravascular administration; IM route not recommended

Intermittent IV INFUSION route

• After diluting 800 mg/50 mL D_5W (16 mg/mL); give ≤1 mg/min, use infusion pump; quiNIDine absorbed by PVC tubing, minimize length

Y-site compatibilities: Alfentanil, amikacin, anidulafungin, argatroban, arsenic trioxide, ascorbic acid, asparaginase, atenolol, atracurium, atropine, benztropine, bleomycin, bumetanide, buprenorphine, butorphanol, calcium gluconate, caspofungin, chlorproMAZINE, cimetidine, CISplatin, cyanocobalamin, cycloSPORINE, DACTINomycin, digoxin, diltiaZEM, diphenhydrAMINE, DOBUTamine, DOCEtaxel, DOPamine, doxycycline, enalaprilat, ePHEDrine, EPINEPHrine, epoetin alfa, erythromycin, esmolol, etoposide, famotidine, fenoldopam, fentaNYL, fluconazole, fludarabine, gatifloxacin, gemcitabine, gentamicin, glycopyrrolate, granisetron, HYDROmorphone, IDArubicin, imipenem-cilastatin, irinotecan, isoproterenol, labetalol, lidocaine, linezolid, LORazepam, magnesium sulfate, mannitol, mechlorethamine, meperidine, metaraminol, methoxamine, methyldopate, metoclopramide, metoprolol, metroNIDAZOLE, miconazole, milrinone, mitoXANTRONE, morphine, multiple vitamins, mycophenolate, nalbuphine, naloxone, nesiritide, netilmicin, nitroglycerin, norepinephrine, octreotide, ondansetron, oxaliplatin, PACLitaxel, palonosetron, pamidronate, pancuronium, papaverine, pentamidine, pentazocine, phenylephrine, phytonadione, polymyxin B, potassium chloride, procainamide, prochlorperazine, promethazine, propranolol, protamine, pyridoxine, ranitidine, ritodrine, succinylcholine, SUFentanil, tacrolimus, teniposide, theophylline, thiamine, thiotepa, tirofiban, tobramycin, tolazoline, trimethoprim, urokinase, vancomycin, vasopressin, verapamil, vinorelbine, voriconazole, zoledronic acid

SIDE EFFECTS

CNS: *Headache, dizziness,* involuntary movement, confusion, psychosis, restlessness, irritability, syncope, excitement, depression, ataxia

CV: Hypotension, *bradycardia,* PVCs, heart block, CV collapse, arrest, torsades de pointes, widening QRS complex, ventricular tachycardia

EENT: Cinchonism: tinnitus, blurred vision, hearing loss, mydriasis, disturbed color vision

GI: Nausea, vomiting, anorexia, abdominal pain, *diarrhea,* hepatotoxicity

HEMA: Thrombocytopenia, hemolytic anemia, agranulocytosis, hypoprothrombinemia

INTEG: Rash, urticaria, angioedema, swelling, photosensitivity, flushing with severe pruritus

RESP: Dyspnea, respiratory depression

PHARMACOKINETICS

PO: (sulfate) peak 1-6 hr, duration 6-8 hr, (sulfate ER) peak 4 hr, duration 8-12 hr; (gluconate PO) peak 3-4 hr, duration 6-8 hr, half-life 6-7 hr (prolonged in geriatric patients, cirrhosis, HF), metabolized in liver, excreted unchanged (10%-50%) by kidneys, protein bound (80%-90%)

Q

INTERACTIONS

• Additive vagolytic effect: anticholinergic blockers

Increase: cardiac depression: other antidysrhythmics, phenothiazines, reserpine

Increase: effects of neuromuscular blockers, digoxin, warfarin, tricyclics, propranolol

Increase: QT prolongation—macrolides, quinolones, tricyclics, procainamide, antipsychotics

Increase: quiNIDine effects—cimetidine, sodium bicarbonate, carbonic anhydrase inhibitors, antacids, hydroxide suspensions, amiodarone, verapamil, NIFEdipine, protease inhibitors

Decrease: quiNIDine effects—barbiturates, phenytoin, rifampin, sucralfate, cholinergics

Drug/Herb

Increase: quiNIDine effect—hawthorn, licorice

Drug/Food

• Delayed absorption, decreased metabolism: grapefruit juice

Drug/Lab Test

Decrease: platelets, Hgb, granulocytes

NURSING CONSIDERATIONS

Assess:

• Monitor ECG, B/P, pulse continuously during IV, baseline, and periodically (PO) to determine increased PR or QRS segments, QT interval; discontinue product or reduce dose

• Blood levels (therapeutic level 2-5 mcg/mL), CBC, LFTs

• **For cinchonism:** tinnitus, headache, nausea, dizziness, fever, vertigo, tremors; may lead to hearing loss

Black Box Warning: Cardiac toxicity: asystole, ventricular dysrhythmias, widening QRS, torsades de pointes

• CNS effects: dizziness, confusion, psychosis, paresthesias, seizures; product should be discontinued

• **Hepatotoxicity:** monitor LFTs for first 1-2 mo of treatment

• **Pregnancy/breastfeeding:** use only if clearly needed; avoid use in breastfeeding, excreted in breast milk

Evaluate:

• Therapeutic response: decreased dysrhythmias

Teach patient/family:

• That if dizziness, drowsiness occurs, to avoid driving or hazardous activities

• To use sunglasses; product may cause sensitivity to light

• To carry emergency ID stating disease, medication use

• How to take pulse; when to notify prescriber

• To avoid all products unless approved by prescriber

• Not to crush, chew ext rel product

• Not to use grapefruit juice with this product

• **QuiNIDine toxicity (cinchonism):** to report immediately visual changes, nausea, headache, ringing in the ears

• To report diarrhea, anorexia, decreased B/P

RABEprazole (Rx)

(rah-bep'rah-zole)

Aciphex, Aciphex Sprinkle, Pariet ✦

Func. class.: Antiulcer, proton pump inhibitor

Chem. class.: Benzimidazole

Do not confuse:

Aciphex/Aricept/Accupril

RABEprazole/ARIPiprazole

ACTION: Suppresses gastric secretion by inhibiting hydrogen/potassium ATPase enzyme system in the gastric parietal cells; characterized as a gastric acid pump inhibitor because it blocks the final step of acid production

USES: Gastroesophageal reflux disease (GERD), severe erosive esophagitis, poorly responsive systemic GERD, pathologic hypersecretory conditions (Zollinger-Ellison syndrome, systemic mastocytosis, multiple endocrine adenomas); treatment of active duodenal ulcers with/without antiinfectives for *Helicobacter pylori;* daytime, nighttime heartburn

Unlabeled uses: Gastric ulcer, heartburn, *H. pylori* eradication in children

CONTRAINDICATIONS: Hypersensitivity to this product or proton pump inhibitors (PPIs)

Precautions: Pregnancy, breastfeeding, children, ⚕ Asian patients, diarrhea, geriatric patients, gastric cancer, hepatic/GI disease, IBS, osteoporosis, pseudomembranous colitis, ulcerative colitis, vit B₁₂ deficiency

DOSAGE AND ROUTES

Healing of duodenal ulcers

• **Adult: PO** 20 mg/day × ≤4 wk; to be taken after breakfast

Healing of erosive esophagitis or ulcerative GERD

• **Adult: PO** 20 mg/day × 4-8 wk; may use an additional course

• **Adolescent and child ≥12 yr: PO** 20 mg/day up to 8 wk

• **Child 1-11 yr (≥15 kg): PO** (sprinkle) 10 mg daily up to 12 wk

• **Child 1-11 yr (<15 kg): PO** 5 mg daily up to 12 wk; may increase to 10 mg daily if needed

H. pylori eradication

• **Adult: PO** 20 mg bid × 7 days with amoxicillin 1 g bid × 7 days with clarithromycin 500 mg bid × 7 days

Pathologic hypersecretory conditions

• **Adult: PO** 60 mg/day; may increase to 120 mg in 2 divided doses

Gastric ulcer (unlabeled)

• **Adult: PO** 20 mg/day after AM meal × 3-6 wk

Dyspepsia/heartburn (unlabeled)

• **Adult: PO** 20 mg/day × ≤14 days

Available forms: Del rel tabs 20 mg; del rel caps 5, 10 mg

Administer:

PO route

• Do not break, crush, chew del-rel tab; after breakfast daily with full glass of water, without regard to food

• **Delayed-release capsule:** open, use on spoonful of applesauce or liquid, give dose immediately (within 15 min), ½ hr before a meal; do not crush, chew delayed-release product

SIDE EFFECTS

CNS: *Headache, dizziness*

EENT: Tinnitus, taste perversion

GI: *Diarrhea, abdominal pain, vomiting, nausea, constipation, flatulence, acid regurgitation,* abdominal swelling, anorexia, hepatitis, hepatic encephalopathy, *Clostridium difficile*-associated diarrhea

MS: Back pain, arthralgia, myalgia, osteoporosis, fractures

MISC: Infection

PHARMACOKINETICS

Eliminated in urine as metabolites and in feces, half-life 1-2 hr, metabolized by CYP2C19 ⚕ enzyme system, protein binding 96.3%

R

INTERACTIONS

Increase: bleeding risk—warfarin, clopidogrel

Increase: serum levels of RABEprazole—benzodiazepines, phenytoin, clarithromycin, antacids, other proton pump inhibitors, H₂ blockers

Increase: levels of—digoxin, nelfinavir/omeprazole, methotrexate

Decrease: levels of RABEprazole—sucralfate, calcium carbonate, vit B₁₂

Decrease: levels of ketoconazole, itraconazole, iron salts, atazanavir/ritonavir, ampicillin, cycloSPORINE, protease inhibitors

Drug/Herb

Decrease: RABEprazole—St. John's wort

Drug/Lab Test

Decrease: magnesium

NURSING CONSIDERATIONS

Assess:

• GI system: bowel sounds, abdomen for pain, swelling, anorexia, emesis/stool for occult blood

• *Clostridium difficile–associated diarrhea:* may occur with most antibiotic therapy; watery diarrhea, abdominal pain, fever; may occur several weeks after treatment concludes

• **Vit B₁₂/cyanocobalamin deficiency/hypomagnesemia:** may occur several weeks after treatment concludes; use magnesium, vit B₁₂, cyanocobalamin supplement; if severe, discontinuation of product may be needed. Assess for low magnesium level: tremors, muscle soreness, spasms, anxiety, change in heart rate, palpitations

• Hepatic studies: AST, ALT, alk phos during treatment; CBC with differential periodically

• CBC with differential before, periodically during treatment; blood dyscrasias may occur (rare)

• Obtain susceptibility testing if *H. pylori* treatment is ineffective; another anti-infective may be needed

• **Osteoporosis/fractures:** may occur with prolonged use (1 yr or longer) of high dose, usually in those ≥50 yr; make sure adequate vitamin D, calcium are taken

• **Beers:** avoid scheduled use >8 wk in older adults unless for high-risk patients

Evaluate:

• Therapeutic response: absence of epigastric pain, swelling, fullness; decreased symptoms of GERD after 4-8 wk

Teach patient/family:

• CDAD To report severe diarrhea or black, tarry stools; product may have to be discontinued

• To avoid hazardous activities because dizziness, drowsiness may occur

• To avoid alcohol, salicylates, NSAIDs because they may cause GI irritation; to avoid other OTC, herbal products unless approved by prescriber

• That osteoporosis and fractures are more common in those who take the product >1 yr

• To use as directed for length of time prescribed; to take missed dose when remembered; not to double dose; to take del-rel tab whole, do not cut, break; that cap should be opened and sprinkled on food (applesauce) to take within 15 min of being sprinkled and 30 min before meal; to take the tablet form for ulcers after meal, for *H. pylori* with morning/evening meals

• To notify prescriber if pregnancy is planned, suspected

RARELY USED

radioactive iodine (sodium iodide) ¹³¹I (Rx)

Func. class.: Antithyroid
Chem. class.: Radiopharmaceutical

USES: *High dose:* Thyroid cancer, hyperthyroidism
Low dose: Visualization to determine thyroid cancer, diagnostic aid for thyroid function studies

CONTRAINDICATIONS: Pregnancy, breastfeeding, age <30 yr, recent MI, large nodular goiter, vomiting/diarrhea, acute hyperthyroidism, use of thyroid products

DOSAGE AND ROUTES
Thyroid cancer
• **Adult: PO** 50-150 mCi; may repeat, depending on clinical status
Hyperthyroidism
• **Adult: PO** 4-10 mCi, depending on serum thyroxine level

---

raloxifene (Rx)
(ral-ox'ih-feen)
Evista
Func. class.: Bone resorption inhibitor
Chem. class.: Hormone modifier, selective estrogen receptor modulator (SERM)

ACTION: Tissue-selective estrogen agonist/antagonist; agonist activity in bone and on lipid metabolism; antagonist activity on breast and uterus; reduces resorption of bone and decreases bone turnover

USES: Prevention, treatment of osteoporosis in postmenopausal women; breast cancer prophylaxis in postmenopausal women with osteoporosis or in postmenopausal women at high risk for developing the disease; invasive breast cancer risk reduction
Unlabeled uses: Uterine leiomyomata in postmenopausal women with osteoporosis or in postmenopausal women who are at high risk for developing the disease

CONTRAINDICATIONS: Pregnancy, breastfeeding, hypersensitivity

Black Box Warning: Women with active or history of venous thromboembolic events

Precautions: CV/hepatic disease, cervical/uterine cancer, elevated triglycerides, pulmonary embolism

Black Box Warning: Stroke

DOSAGE AND ROUTES
• **Adult postmenopausal women: PO** 60 mg/day, max 60 mg/day
Available forms: Tabs 60 mg
Administer:
• PO: without regard to meals, give with vit D
• Add calcium supplement if inadequate
• Do not use during immobilization or prolonged bedrest

SIDE EFFECTS
CNS: Insomnia, depression, migraines
CV: Hot flashes, peripheral edema, thromboembolism, stroke, fever, chest pain
EENT: Pharyngitis, sinusitis, laryngitis
GI: *Nausea,* vomiting, diarrhea, dyspepsia, abdominal pain, gastroenteritis
GU: Vaginitis, leukorrhea, cystitis, UTI, vaginal bleeding
INTEG: Rash, sweating
META: Weight gain, peripheral edema
MS: Arthralgia, myalgia, *leg cramps,* arthritis
RESP: Increased cough

PHARMACOKINETICS
Duration 24 hr, elimination half-life 28-32 hr; excreted in feces, breast milk; highly bound to plasma proteins

INTERACTIONS
• Administer cautiously with other highly protein-bound products, (ibuprofen, diazePAM, naproxen, systemic estrogens)
Decrease: action of anticoagulants, dessicated thyroid, levothyroxine, liotrix
Decrease: action of raloxifene—ampicillin, bile acid sequestrants
Drug/Food
Decrease: raloxifene, effect of—soy
Drug/Lab Test
Increase: triglycerides

NURSING CONSIDERATIONS
Assess:

Black Box Warning: History of stroke, TIA, thrombosis, atrial fibrillation, hypertension, smoking; venous thrombosis may occur; avoid prolonged sitting; discontinue 3 days before surgery, other immobilization; mortality is increased after stroke

R

Side effects: *italics* = common; red = life-threatening

• Bone density test at baseline, throughout treatment, bone-specific alk phos, osteocalcin

Pregnancy/breastfeeding: do not use in pregnancy/breastfeeding

Evaluate:

• Therapeutic response: prevention, treatment of osteoporosis in postmenopausal women; prevention of breast cancer in postmenopausal women with osteoporosis or in those who are at high risk for developing the disease

Teach patient/family:

> **Black Box Warning:** To discontinue product 72 hr before prolonged bedrest; to avoid staying in one position for long periods, to report possible blood clots immediately, usually during first few months of therapy

• To take calcium supplements, vit D if intake is inadequate
• To increase exercise using weights
• To stop smoking; to decrease alcohol consumption
• That product does not help to control hot flashes; hot flashes may be increased, as these are a common side effect
• To report fever, acute migraine, insomnia, emotional distress; urinary tract infection, vaginal burning/itching; swelling, warmth, pain in calves; uterine bleeding, abnormal breast changes
• To notify prescriber if pregnancy is planned or suspected; not to use in pregnancy, breastfeeding
• Provide product package insert and discuss with patient

---

raltegravir (Rx)
(ral-teg'ra-vir)
Isentress, Isentress HD
Func. class.: Antiretroviral
Chem. class.: HIV integrase strand transfer inhibitor (ISTIs)

ACTION: Inhibits catalytic activity of HIV integrase, which is an HIV-encoded enzyme needed for replication

USES: HIV in combination with other antiretrovirals

CONTRAINDICATIONS: Breastfeeding, hypersensitivity

Precautions: Pregnancy, children, geriatric patients, hepatic disease, immune reconstitution syndrome, hepatitis, antimicrobial resistance, lactase deficiency

DOSAGE AND ROUTES
Human immunodeficiency virus (HIV) infection in combination with other antiretroviral agents

• **Adult: PO** (400-mg film-coated tablet) 400 mg bid. During coadministration with rifampin, recommended dosage is 800 mg bid
• **Adolescent/child ≥25 kg: PO** (400-mg film-coated tablet) 400 mg bid
• **Adolescent/child** (weight-based dosage): **PO** (chewable tablets) **≥40 kg,** 300 mg bid; **28-39 kg,** 200 mg bid; **20-27 kg,** 150 mg bid; **14-19 kg,** 100 mg bid; **11-13 kg,** 75 mg bid
• **Child: PO** (powder for suspension) **14-19 kg,** 100 mg (5 mL) bid; **11-13 kg,** 80 mg (4 mL) bid; **≥4 wk of age and 8-10 kg,** 60 mg (3 mL) bid; **≥4 wk and 6-7 kg,** 40 mg (2 mL) bid; **≥4 wk and 4-5 kg,** 30 mg (1.5 mL) bid; **≥4 wk and 3 kg,** 20 mg (1 mL) bid
High-dose regimen
• **Adult: PO** (600-mg film-coated tablet) 1200 mg (2 × 600 mg)/day. Coadministration with rifAMPin is not recommended
• **Adolescent/child ≥40 kg: PO** (600 mg film-coated tablet) 1200 mg (2 × 600 mg)/day. Coadministration with rifampin is not recommended

Available forms: Tabs 400, 600 mg; chew tabs 25, 100 mg; granules for oral suspension 100 mg/packet

Administer:
PO route

• Tablets and chew tablets are not interchangeable
• Chew tabs should be chewed or swallowed whole
• Do not break, crush, chew regular tabs
• May give without regard to meals, with 8 oz of water

• Store at room temperature
Oral suspension: Open foil, use 5 mL of water in provided measuring cup, close cup, swirl, do not turn upside down, use oral syringe to administer, use within 30 min, discard any remaining suspension

SIDE EFFECTS

CNS: *Fatigue*, fever, *dizziness, headache,* asthenia, suicidal ideation, insomnia
CV: MI
GI: *Nausea,* vomiting, diarrhea, abdominal pain, asthenia, gastritis, hepatitis
GU: Acute renal failure
HEMA: Anemia, neutropenia
INTEG: Rash, urticaria, pruritus, pain or phlebitis at IV site, unusual sweating, alopecia, Stevens-Johnson syndrome, toxic epidermal necrolysis
META: Hyperamylasemia, hyperglycemia, lipodystrophy
MS: Myopathy, rhabdomyolysis
SYST: Immune reconstitution syndrome

PHARMACOKINETICS

Max absorption 3 hr if taken on an empty stomach; half-life 9 hr; metabolized in the liver by uridine diphosphate glucuronosyltransferase ⊘ₐₓ (UGTA1A enzyme system); excreted in feces 51%, urine 32%

INTERACTIONS

Increase: raltegravir effect—proton pump inhibitors, H₂ blockers; UGT1A1 inhibitors (atazanavir)
Increase: rhabdomyolysis, myopathy, elevated CPK—fibric acid derivatives, HMG-CoA reductase inhibitors
Decrease: raltegravir levels—rifAMPin, efavirenz, tenofovir, tipranavir/ritonavir

Drug/Lab Test
Increase: AST, ALT, GGT, total bilirubin, alk phos, amylase/lipase, CK, serum glucose, total/HDL/LDL cholesterol
Decrease: Hgb, platelets, ANC

NURSING CONSIDERATIONS
Assess:

• **HIV infection:** CD4, T-cell count, plasma HIV RNA, viral load; resistance testing before therapy, at treatment failure

• **Rhabdomyolysis:** assess for muscle pain, darkening of urine, increased CPK; product should be discontinued
• Skin eruptions: rash, urticaria, itching
• **Suicidal thoughts/behaviors:** monitor for depression; more common in those with mental illness
• **Immune reconstitution syndrome,** usually during initial phase of treatment; may give antiinfective before starting; opportunistic infections or autoimmune disorders may occur
• **Stevens-Johnson syndrome:** Skin eruptions: rash, urticaria, itching
• Monitor total/HDL/LDL cholesterol, blood glucose, LFTs, serum bilirubin (total and direct), baseline and periodically (all may be elevated); pregnancy test, CBC with differential, hepatitis serology, plasma hepatitis C, RNA, urinalysis, baseline and periodically
• **Pregnancy/breastfeeding:** use only if benefits outweigh fetal risk, pregnant women taking this product should enroll in the Antiretroviral Pregnancy Registry, 1-800-258-4263; do not breastfeed

Evaluate:
• Therapeutic response: improvement in CD4 counts, T-cell counts, viral load
• Decreased progression of AIDs, HIV

Teach patient/family:
• To take as prescribed; if dose missed, to take as soon as remembered up to 1 hr before next dose; not to double dose; not to share with others
• That sexual partners need to be told that patient has HIV; that product does not cure infection, just controls symptoms; that it does not prevent infecting others
• To report sore throat, fever, fatigue (may indicate immune reconstitution syndrome)
• That product must be taken in equal intervals 2×/day to maintain blood levels for duration of therapy
• To notify prescriber immediately of suicidal thoughts/behaviors
• **Pregnancy:** to notify prescriber if pregnancy is planned or suspected; not to breastfeed

R

• To continue with follow-up exams, blood work
• To report rash, muscle pain immediately

> ⚠ **HIGH ALERT**

ramelteon (Rx)

(rah-mel′tee-on)

Rozerem

Func. class.: Sedative/hypnotic, antianxiety

Chem. class.: Melatonin receptor agonist

Do not confuse:
Rozerem/Razadine

ACTION: Binds selectively to melatonin receptors (MT_1, MT_2); thought to be involved in circadian rhythms and in the normal sleep/wake cycle

USES: Insomnia (difficulty with sleep onset)

CONTRAINDICATIONS: Breastfeeding, children, infants, hypersensitivity
Precautions: Pregnancy, hepatic disease, alcoholism, COPD, seizure disorder, sleep apnea, suicidal ideation, angioedema, depression, sleep-related behaviors (sleepwalking), schizophrenia, bipolar disorder; alcohol intoxication, hepatic encephalopathy

DOSAGE AND ROUTES

• **Adult: PO** 8 mg within 30 min of bedtime
Hepatic dose
• Do not use with severe hepatic disease; use with caution for mild to moderate hepatic disease
Available forms: Tabs 8 mg
Administer:
• Within 30 min of bedtime for sleeplessness; on empty stomach for fast onset, do not give within 1 hr of high-fat foods
• Do not break, crush, chew tabs; swallow whole
• Store in tight container in cool environment

SIDE EFFECTS

CNS: Dizziness, somnolence, fatigue, headache, worsening insomnia, depression, complex sleep-related reactions (sleep driving, sleep eating), suicidal thoughts/behaviors
GI: Nausea, diarrhea, dysgeusia, vomiting
SYST: Severe allergic reactions, angioedema

PHARMACOKINETICS

Absorbed rapidly; peak ½-1½ hr; protein binding 82%; rapid first-pass metabolism via liver by CYP1A2; 84% excreted in urine, 4% in feces; half-life 2-5 hr metabolite

INTERACTIONS

• **Possible toxicity:** antiretroviral protease inhibitors
Increase: ramelteon effect, toxicity—alcohol; CYP1A2 inhibitors, azole antifungals (ketoconazole, fluconazole), fluvoxaMINE, anxiolytics, sedatives, hypnotics, barbiturates, ciprofloxacin, strong CYP2C9 inhibitors, strong CYP3A4 inhibitors, opioids
Decrease: effect of ramelteon—strong CYP inducer (rifAMPin)
Drug/Food
• Prolonged absorption, sleep onset reduced: high-fat/heavy meal
Drug/Lab
Increase: protein level
Decrease: testosterone level

NURSING CONSIDERATIONS
Assess:
• **Severe hypersensitive reactions:** assess for angioedema (facial swelling); product should be discontinued
• **Sleep characteristics:** type of sleep problem: falling asleep, staying asleep; complex sleep disorders (sleep walking/driving/eating) after taking product
• Mental status: mood, sensorium, affect, memory (long, short term), suicidal ideation
• LFTs: before treatment, periodically
• **Beers:** avoid use in older adults with a high risk of delirium; delirium might be induced or worsened

---

• **Pregnancy/breastfeeding:** use only if benefits outweigh fetal risk, may be fetal toxic; cautious use in breastfeeding, excretion is unknown

Evaluate:

• Therapeutic response: ability to sleep at night, decreased amount of early morning awakening

Teach patient/family:

• To avoid driving, other activities requiring alertness until product stabilized; drowsiness may continue the next day

• To avoid alcohol ingestion, CNS depressants

• About alternative measures to improve sleep: reading, exercise several hr before bedtime, warm bath, warm milk, TV, self-hypnosis, deep breathing

• To report if pregnancy is planned or suspected; to avoid breastfeeding

• To take product within 30 min before going to bed

• Not to ingest a high-fat/heavy meal before taking product

• To report cessation of menses, galactorrhea (women), decreased libido, infertility, worsening of insomnia, behavioral changes, severe allergic reactions, suicidal thoughts/behaviors, if insomnia gets worse, swelling of face, tongue, trouble breathing

• Med guide should be given to patient and reviewed

---

ramipril (Rx)

(ra-mi′pril)

Altace

Func. class.: Antihypertensive

Chem. class.: Angiotensin-converting enzyme inhibitor (ACE)

Do not confuse:
ramipril/enalapril
Altace/alteplase

ACTION: Selectively suppresses renin-angiotensin-aldosterone system; inhibits ACE, prevents conversion of angiotensin I to angiotensin II; results in dilation of arterial, venous vessels

USES: Hypertension, alone or in combination with thiazide diuretics; HF (post-MI), reduction in risk for MI, stroke, death from CV disorders

Unlabeled uses: Proteinuria due to diabetic nephropathy

CONTRAINDICATIONS: Breastfeeding, children, hypersensitivity to ACE inhibitors, history of ACE inhibitor–induced angioedema

> **Black Box Warning:** Pregnancy

Precautions: Geriatric patients, impaired renal/hepatic function, dialysis patients, hypovolemia, blood dyscrasias, HF, renal artery stenosis, cough, African descent, aortic stenosis

DOSAGE AND ROUTES

Hypertension

• **Adult: PO** 2.5 mg/day initially, then 2.5-20 mg/day divided bid or daily

HF post-MI

• **Adult: PO** 1.25-2.5 mg bid; may increase to 5 mg bid

Reduction in risk for MI, stroke, death

• **Adult: PO** 2.5 mg/day × 7 days, then 5 mg/day × 21 days, then may increase to 10 mg/day

Renal dose

• **Adult: PO** CCr <40 mL/min, reduce by 50%, titrate upward to max 5 mg/day

Proteinuria due to diabetic nephropathy (unlabeled)

• **Adult: PO** 2.5 mg/day up to 20 mg/day

Available forms: Caps 1.25, 2.5, 5, 10 mg

Administer:

• Without regard to meals

• Swallow cap or tablet whole

• Caps can be opened, added to food; mixture is stable for 24 hr at room temperature, 48 hr refrigerated

• Store in tight container at ≤86° F (30° C)

SIDE EFFECTS

CNS: *Headache, dizziness,* anxiety, insomnia, paresthesia, *fatigue,* depression, malaise, vertigo, syncope

R

Side effects: *italics* = common; red = life-threatening

CV: *Hypotension,* chest pain, palpitations, angina, syncope, dysrhythmia, heart failure, MI

GI: *Nausea,* constipation, vomiting, anorexia, diarrhea, abdominal pain

GU: Proteinuria, increased BUN, creatinine, impotence

INTEG: Rash, sweating, photosensitivity, pruritus

META: *Hyperkalemia*

MS: Arthralgia, arthritis, myalgia

RESP: *Dry cough,* dyspnea

PHARMACOKINETICS

Bioavailability >50%-60%, onset 1-2 hr, peak 1-3 hr, duration 24 hr, protein binding 73%, half-life 13-17 hr, metabolized by liver (metabolites excreted in urine, feces)

INTERACTIONS

• Do not use with aliskiren in moderate-severe renal disease

Increase: hyperkalemia—potassium-sparing diuretics, potassium supplement, angiotensin II receptor agonists

Increase: hypotension—diuretics, other antihypertensives, ganglionic blockers, adrenergic blockers, nitrates, acute alcohol ingestion

Increase: toxicity—vasodilators, hydrALAZINE, prazosin, potassium-sparing diuretics, sympathomimetics, potassium supplements

Increase: serum levels of lithium

Decrease: absorption—antacids

Decrease: antihypertensive effect—indomethacin, NSAIDs, salicylates

Drug/Herb

Increase: antihypertensive effect—hawthorn

Decrease: antihypertensive effect—ephedra

Drug/Food

Increase: hyperkalemia—potassium salt substitutes; avoid use

Drug/Lab Test

Increase: LFTs, BUN, creatinine, glucose, potassium

Decrease: RBC, Hgb, platelets

NURSING CONSIDERATIONS

Assess:

• **Hypertension:** monitor B/P baseline and regularly, orthostatic hypotension, syncope

• **Heart failure:** edema in feet, legs daily; weight daily

• **Collagen-vascular disease (SLE, scleroderma):** neutrophils, decreased platelets; WBC with differential at baseline, periodically; if neutrophils <1000/mm³, discontinue treatment

• **Renal disease:** protein, BUN, creatinine, potassium, sodium at baseline, periodically; increased levels may indicate nephrotic syndrome; renal symptoms: polyuria, oliguria, urinary frequency, dysuria

• **Serious allergic reactions: angioedema, Stevens-Johnson syndrome,** rash, fever, pruritus, urticaria; product should be discontinued if antihistamines fail to help

• Monitor electrolytes baseline and periodically; potassium may be increased

> **Black Box Warning: Pregnancy:** identify if pregnant or if pregnancy is planned or suspected; if pregnant, discontinue product; do not use in pregnancy/breastfeeding; can cause injury or death to developing fetus

• For dry cough; notify prescriber as product may need to be discontinued

Evaluate:

• Therapeutic response: decrease in B/P; HF

Teach patient/family:

• Not to discontinue product abruptly; to comply with dosage schedule, even if feeling better

• Not to use OTC products (cough, cold, allergy), herbals, supplements unless directed by prescriber; not to use salt substitutes containing potassium without consulting prescriber

• To rise slowly to sitting or standing position to minimize orthostatic hypotension

• To notify prescriber of mouth sores, sore throat, fever, swelling of hands or feet, irregular heartbeat, chest pain

• To report excessive perspiration, dehydration, vomiting, diarrhea; may lead to fall in B/P; to maintain hydration

• That product may cause dizziness, fainting, light-headedness; that these may occur during first few days of therapy; to avoid hazardous activities until response is known

• That product may cause skin rash, impaired perspiration
• How to take B/P, normal readings for age group
• To report dry cough to provider

Black Box Warning: To inform prescriber if pregnancy is planned or suspected; not to breastfeed

TREATMENT OF OVERDOSE: 0.9% NaCl IV infusion, hemodialysis

---

ranibizumab (Rx)

(ran-ih-biz′oo-mab)
Lucentis
Func. class.: Ophthalmic
Chem. class.: Selective vascular endothelial growth factor antagonist

---

ACTION: Binds to receptor-binding site of active forms of vascular endothelial growth factor A (VEGF-A), ◆◈ which causes angiogenesis and cell proliferation

USES: Age-related macular degeneration (neovascular) (wet), macular edema after retinal vein occlusion (RVO), diabetic macular edema

CONTRAINDICATIONS: Hypersensitivity, ocular infections
Precautions: Pregnancy, breastfeeding, children, retinal detachment, increased intraocular pressure

DOSAGE AND ROUTES
Macular degeneration/macular edema after retinal vein occlusion (RVO)
• **Adult: INTRAVITREAL** 0.5 mg (0.05 mL) of 10 mg/mL product monthly or 0.5 mg monthly ×4 mo, then 0.5 mg q3mo
Diabetic macular edema
• **Adult: INTRAVITREAL** 0.3 mg of 6 mg/mL product q28day

Available forms: Sol for inj 6 mg/mL, 10 mg/mL
Administer:
• By ophthalmologist via intravitreal injection using adequate anesthesia; use 19-gauge filter
• Store in refrigerator; do not freeze
• Protect from light

SIDE EFFECTS
CNS: Dizziness, headache, peripheral neuropathy
EENT: Blepharitis, cataract, conjunctival hemorrhage/hyperemia, detachment of retinal pigment epithelium, dry eye, irritation/pain in eye, visual impairment, vitreous floaters, ocular infection
GI: Constipation, nausea
MISC: Hypertension, UTI, thromboembolism, nonocular bleeding, anemia, arthralgia
RESP: Bronchitis, cough, sinusitis, URI
INTEG: Impaired wound healing

PHARMACOKINETICS
Elimination half-life 9 days, peak 1 day

INTERACTIONS
Increase: severe inflammation—verteporfin photodynamic therapy (PDT)

NURSING CONSIDERATIONS
Assess:
• **Eye changes:** redness; sensitivity to light, vision change; increased intraocular pressure change; report infection to ophthalmologist immediately, complete procedure with anesthesia and antibiotic before use, check perfusion of optic nerve after use
• **Hypersensitivity:** monitor for inflammation
Evaluate:
• Therapeutic response: prevention of increasing macular degeneration
Teach patient/family:
• If eye becomes red, sensitive to light, painful, or if there is a change in vision, to seek immediate care from ophthalmologist
• About reason for treatment, expected results; that product is injected into the eye, an anesthetic will be used

R

Side effects: *italics* = common; red = life-threatening

---

raNITIdine (Rx, otc)
(ra-nit′i-deen)
Acid Reducer ✦, Zantac, Zantac
75, Zantac 150, Zantac 300
Func. class.: H₂-Histamine receptor
antagonist

Do not confuse:
raNITIdine/amantadine/riMANTAdine
Zantac/Xanax/Zofran/ZyrTEC

ACTION: Inhibits histamine at H₂-
receptor site in parietal cells, which
inhibits gastric acid secretion

USES: Duodenal ulcer, Zollinger-
Ellison syndrome, gastric ulcers, hypersecretory conditions, gastroesophageal
reflux disease, stress ulcers, erosive esophagitis (maintenance), active duodenal
ulcers with *Helicobacter pylori* in
combination with clarithromycin, systemic
mastocytosis, multiple endocrine adenoma syndrome, heartburn
Unlabeled uses: Prevention of aspiration pneumonitis, upper GI bleeding,
angioedema, gastritis, urticaria, NSAID-
induced ulcer prophylaxis

CONTRAINDICATIONS: Hypersensitivity
Precautions: Pregnancy, breastfeeding,
child <12 yr, renal/hepatic disease

DOSAGE AND ROUTES
Duodenal ulcer
• **Adult:** PO 150 mg bid or 300 mg/day
after PM meal or at bedtime; maintenance
150 mg at bedtime
• **Infant/child:** PO 2-4 mg/kg bid, max
300 mg/day
Zollinger-Ellison syndrome
• **Adult:** PO 150 mg bid, may increase if
needed up to 6 g/day in those with severe
disease
Gastric ulcer
• **Adult:** PO 150 mg bid × 6 wk, then
150 mg at bedtime
• **Infant/child:** PO 2-4 mg/kg bid, max
300 mg/day

GERD
• **Adult:** PO 150 mg bid
Erosive esophagitis
• **Adult:** PO 150 mg qid for up to 12 wk
• **Child ≥1 mo:** PO 5-10 mg/kg/day in
2-3 divided doses
Renal dose
• **Adult:** PO CCr <50 mL/min, give 50%
of dose or extend dosing interval
**NSAID-induced ulcer prophylaxis
(unlabeled)**
• **Adult:** PO 150 mg bid
**Stress gastritis prophylaxis
(unlabeled)**
• **Adult:** IM/INT IV INFUSION 50 mg
q6-8hr or **CONT IV INFUSION** 6.25 mg/
hr (150 mg/24 hr)
**Severe, acute urticaria/angioedema
(unlabeled)**
• **Adult:** INT IV INFUSION 50 mg with
H₁-blocker
Available forms: Tabs 75, 150, 300 mg;
sol for inj 25 mg/mL; caps 150, 300 mg;
syr 15 mg/mL
Administer:
PO route
• Antacids 1 hr before or 1 hr after ra-
NITIdine
• Without regard to meals
• Store at room temperature
• Give q day dose at bedtime
IM route
• No dilution needed; inject in large
muscle mass, aspirate
Direct IV route
• Dilute to max 2.5 mg/mL (50 mg/20 mL)
using 0.9% NaCl (nonpreserved) or D₅W,
give dose over ≥5 min (max 4 mg/mL)
Intermittent IV INFUSION route
• Dilute to max 0.5 mg/mL with D₅W, NS,
give over 15-20 min (5-7 mL/min); pre-
mixed ready-to-use bags as 1 mg/mL (50
mg/50 mL), infusion over 15-20 min
Continuous 24-hr IV INFUSION route
• **Adult:** dilute 150 mg/250 mL of D₅W
or NS; run over 24 hr (6.25 mg/hr or as
directed); use infusion device; use within
48 hr; *Zollinger-Ellison syndrome:* dilute in D₅W, NS; max concentration 2.5
mg/mL, use infusion device

Y-site compatibilities: Acyclovir, aldesleukin, alemtuzumab, alfentanil, allopurinol, amifostine, amikacin, aminophylline, amphotericin B liposome, amsacrine, anikinra, anidulafungin, ascorbic acid, atracurium, atropine, aztreonam, bivalirudin, bumetanide, buprenorphine, butorphanol, calcium chloride/gluconate, CARBOplatin, ceFAZolin, cefepime, cefonicid, cefoperazone, cefotaxme, cefoTEtan, cefOXitin, cefTAZidime, ceftizoxime, cefTRIAXone, cefuroxime, chloramphenicol, chlorproMAZINE, cimetidine, ciprofloxacin, cisatracurium, CISplatin, clindamycin, cyanocobalamin, cyclophosphamide, cycloSPORINE, cytarabine, DACTINomycin, DAPTOmycin, dexamethasone, dexmedetomidine, digoxin, diltiazem, DOBUTamine, DOCEtaxel, DOPamine, doripenem, doxacurium, doxapram, DOXOrubicin, DOXOrubicin liposome, doxycycline, enalaprilat, ePHEDrine, EPINEPHrine, epirubicin, epoetin alfa, ertapenem, erythromycin, esmolol, etoposide, etoposide phosphate, famotidine, fenoldopam, fentaNYL, filgrastim, fluconazole, fludarabine, fluorouracil, folic acid, foscarnet, furosemide, ganciclovir, gemcitabine, gentamicin, glycopyrrolate, granisetron, heparin, hydrocortisone, HYDROmorphone, IDArubicin, ifosfamide, imipenem/cilastatin, inamrinone, indomethacin, isoproterenol, ketorolac, labetalol, levofloxacin, lidocaine, linezolid, LORazepam, magnesium sulfate, mannitol, mechlorethamine, melphalan, meperidine, metaraminol, methotrexate, methoxamine, methyldopate, methylPREDNISolone, metoclopramide, metoprolol, metroNIDAZOLE, midazolam, milrinone, mitoXANtrone, morphine, multivitamin, nalbuphine, naloxone, nesiritide, niCARdipine, nitroglycerin, nitroprusside, norepinephrine, octreotide, ondansetron, oxacillin, oxaliplatin, oxytocin, PACLitaxel, palonosetron, pancuronium, papaverine, PEMEtrexed, penicillin G, pentamidine, pentazocine, PENTobarbital, PHENobarbital, phentolamine, phenylephrine, phytonadione, piperacillin/tazobactam, potassium chloride, procainamide, prochlorperazine, promethazine, propofol, propranolol, protamine, pyridoxine, remifentanil, riTUXimab, rocuronium, sargramostim, sodium acetate/bicarbonate, succinylcholine, SUFentanil, tacrolimus, teniposide, theophylline, thiamine, thiopental, thiotepa, ticarcillin/clavulanate, tigecycline, tirofiban, tobramycin, tolazoline, trastuzumab, trimethaphan, urokinase, vancomycin, vecuronium, vinCRIStine, vinorelbine, warfarin, zidovudine, zoledronic acid

SIDE EFFECTS

CNS: Headache, dizziness, confusion, agitation, depression; hallucination (geriatric patients)
EENT: Blurred vision
GI: Constipation, abdominal pain, diarrhea, nausea, vomiting, hepatotoxicity
INTEG: Anaphylaxis, angioedema, burning at injection site

PHARMACOKINETICS

PO: Peak 2-3 hr; duration 8-12 hr; metabolized by liver; excreted in urine (30% unchanged, PO), breast milk; half-life 2-3 hr; protein binding 15%

INTERACTIONS

Increase: effect of pramipexole, procainamide, trospium, triazolam, calcium channel blockers, memantine, saquinavir, adefovir
Increase: GI obstruction risk—NIFEdipine ext rel products
Increase: toxicity—sulfonylureas, procainamide, benzodiazepines, calcium channel blockers
Decrease: absorption of raNITIdine—antacids, anticholinergics
Decrease: warfarin clearance—warfarin
Decrease: effects of cephalosporins, iron salts, ketoconazole, itraconazole, atazanavir, delavirdine
Increase: GI obstruction risk—NIFEdipine ext rel products
Drug/Lab Test
Increase: AST, ALT, creatinine
False positive: urine protein (Multistix)

NURSING CONSIDERATIONS
Assess:
• **GI complaints:** nausea, vomiting, diarrhea, cramps, abdominal discomfort, jaundice; report immediately

• I&O ratio, BUN, creatinine, LFTs, serum, stool guaiac before, periodically during therapy

• For vitamin B_{12} deficiency if product is taken long term, >2 yr

• **Beers:** avoid in older adults with delirium or at high risk for delirium; may induce delirium or make it worse; report confusion

Evaluate:
• Therapeutic response: decreased abdominal pain, heartburn, healing of ulcers, absence of gastroesophageal reflux

Teach patient/family:
• To avoid driving, other hazardous activities until stabilized on product

• That product must be continued for prescribed time to be effective

• Not to take maximum OTC daily dose for >2 wk

• To take once-daily dose before bedtime

• To report immediately coffee-ground emesis, black tarry stools, abdominal pain, cramping

---

ranolazine (Rx)
(ruh-no'luh-zeen)
Ranexa
Func. class.: Antianginal
Chem. class.: Piperazine derivative

ACTION: Antianginal, antiischemic; unknown, may work by inhibiting portal fatty-acid oxidation

USES: Chronic stable angina pectoris; use in patients who have not responded to other treatment options; should be used in combination with other antianginals such as amLODIPine, β-blockers, nitrates
Unlabeled uses: Unstable angina

CONTRAINDICATIONS: Preexisting QT prolongation, hepatic disease (Child-Pugh class A, B, C), hypersensitivity, hypokalemia, renal failure, torsades de pointes, ventricular dysrhythmia, ventricular tachycardia, hepatic cirrhosis
Precautions: Pregnancy, breastfeeding, children, geriatric patients, hypotension, renal disease, females at risk for torsades de pointes

DOSAGE AND ROUTES
Chronic angina
• **Adult:** PO 500 mg bid, increased to 1000 mg bid based on response; max 1000 mg bid; limit to 500 mg bid in those taking moderate CYP3A4 inhibitors
Available forms: Ext rel tabs 500, 1000 mg
Administer:
• **Ext rel tabs:** do not break, crush, chew tabs; take product as prescribed; do not double or skip dose

• Use in combination with H_2 blocker, metroNIDAZOLE, proton pump inhibitor, and clarithromycin for *H. pylori*

• Without regard to meals, bid; do not use with grapefruit juice or grapefruit

SIDE EFFECTS
CNS: *Headache, dizziness,* hallucinations
CV: Palpitations, QT prolongation, orthostatic hypotension
EENT: Tinnitus
GI: Nausea, vomiting, constipation, dry mouth
MISC: Peripheral edema
RESP: Dyspnea

PHARMACOKINETICS
Absorption varied; peak 2-5 hr; half-life 7 hr; extensively metabolized by the liver (CYP3A and less by CYP2D6); excreted in urine (75%), feces (25%); protein binding 62%

INTERACTIONS
Increase: ranolazine action—diltiaZEM, ketoconazole, macrolide antibiotics, dofetilide, PARoxetine, protease inhibitors, quiNIDine, sotalol, thioridazine, verapamil, ziprasidone, avoid using together
Increase: action of digoxin, simvastatin

Increase: ranolazine absorption, toxicity—antiretroviral protease inhibitors

Increase: QT prolongation and torsades de pointes—class IA/III antidysrhythmics, arsenic trioxide, chloroquine, droperidol, haloperidol, methadone, pentamidine, chlorproMAZINE, mesoridazine, thioridazine, pimozide; CYP3A4 inhibitors (ketoconazole, fluconazole, itraconazole, IV miconazole, voriconazole, diltiaZEM, verapamil)

Drug/Food

• Do not use with grapefruit, grapefruit juice

Drug/Herb

Decrease: ranolazine level—St. John's wort, don't use together

NURSING CONSIDERATIONS
Assess:

• **Angina:** characteristics of pain (intensity, location, duration, alleviating/precipitating factors)

• **QT prolongation:** ECG for QT prolongation, ejection fraction; assess for chest pain, palpitations, dyspnea; torsades de pointes may occur

• Cardiac status: B/P, pulse, respirations

• LFTs, serum creatinine/BUN (in those with CCr <60 mL/min), magnesium, potassium before treatment, periodically; if BUN and creatinine increase significantly, discontinue product

• **Pregnancy/breastfeeding:** use only if benefits outweigh fetal risk; do not breastfeed, excretion unknown

Evaluate:

• Therapeutic response: decreased anginal pain, attacks

Teach patient/family:

• To avoid hazardous activities until stabilized on product, dizziness no longer a problem

• To avoid OTC drugs, grapefruit juice, products prolonging QTc (quiNIDine, dofetilide, sotalol, erythromycin, thioridazine, ziprasidone or protease inhibitors, diltiaZEM, ketoconazole, macrolide antibiotics, verapamil) unless directed by prescriber; to notify prescriber of palpitations, fainting

• To comply with all areas of medical regimen

• To take as directed; not to skip dose, double doses

• Not to chew or crush; not to use with grapefruit juice

• To notify all health care providers of product use

• To notify prescriber of dizziness, edema, dyspnea

• For acute angina, to take other products prescribed; this product does not decrease acute attack

---

rasagiline (Rx)

(ra-sa'ji-leen)

Azilect

Func. class.: Antiparkinson agent

Chem. class.: MAOI, type B

Do not confuse:

Azilect/Aricept

ACTION: Inhibits MAOI type B at recommended doses; may increase DOPamine levels

USES: Idiopathic Parkinson's disease monotherapy or with levodopa

CONTRAINDICATIONS: Breastfeeding; hypersensitivity to this product, MAOIs; pheochromocytoma

Precautions: Pregnancy, children, psychiatric disorders, moderate to severe hepatic disorders

DOSAGE AND ROUTES
Parkinson disease
Monotherapy

• **Adult: PO** 1 mg/day

Adjunctive therapy

• **Adult: PO** 0.5 mg/day, may increase 1 mg/day; change of levodopa dose for adjunct therapy; reduced levodopa dose may be needed

Hepatic dose

• **Adult: PO** 0.5 mg for mild hepatic disease

Concomitant ciprofloxacin, other CYP1A2 inhibitors

• **Adult: PO** 0.5 mg; plasma concentrations of rasagiline may double

R

Side effects: *italics* = common; red = life-threatening

Available forms: Tabs 0.5, 1 mg
Administer:

• With meals to prevent nausea; continuing therapy usually reduces or eliminates nausea; do not give with foods/liquids containing large amounts of tyramine

• Reduce dose of carbidopa/levodopa cautiously

• Renal failure: in dialysis, increase dose slowly

SIDE EFFECTS
Monotherapy

CNS: Drowsiness, hallucinations, depression, headache, malaise, paresthesia, vertigo, syncope
CV: Angina, hypertensive crisis (ingestion of tyramine products), orthostatic hypotension
GI: *Nausea,* diarrhea, dry mouth, dyspepsia
GU: Impotence, decreased libido
HEMA: Leukopenia
INTEG: Alopecia, skin cancers
MISC: Conjunctivitis, fever, flu syndrome, neck pain, allergic reaction, alopecia
MS: Arthralgia, arthritis, dyskinesia
RESP: Rhinitis

PHARMACOKINETICS

Onset, peak, duration unknown; 35%-40% absorbed; protein binding >88%-94%; metabolized by CYP1A2 in liver; excreted by kidneys <1%, half-life 1.3 hr

INTERACTIONS

• Do not give with meperidine, other analgesics because serious reactions (including coma and death) may occur; do not give with sympathomimetics

Increase: levels of rasagiline up to 2-fold—ciprofloxacin, CYP1A2 inhibitors (atazanavir, mexiletine, taurine)

Increase: severe CNS toxicity with antidepressants (tricyclics, SSRIs, SNRIs, mirtazapine, cyclobenzaprine)

Increase: hypertensive crisis—MAOIs

Drug/Herb

• Do not give with St. John's wort, yohimbe

Drug/Food

• Do not give with foods/liquids that have large amounts of tyramine (cured meats, aged cheese)

Drug/Lab Test
Increase: LFTs
Decrease: WBCs

NURSING CONSIDERATIONS
Assess:

• **Parkinson symptoms:** tremors, ataxia, muscle weakness and rigidity at baseline, periodically; increased dyskinesia, postural hypotension if used in combination with levodopa

• **Mental status:** hallucinations, confusion; notify prescriber

• **Hypertensive crisis:** severe headache, blurred vision, seizures, chest pain, difficulty thinking, nausea, vomiting, signs of stroke; any unexplained severe headache should be considered to be hypertensive crisis

• **Melanoma:** periodic skin exams by a dermatologist for possible skin cancer

• Cardiac status: B/P, ECG periodically; orthostatic hypotension during 2 months of treatment during beginning treatment

• **Tyramine products:** foods, other medications may lead to hypertensive crisis (tachycardia, bradycardia, chest pain, nausea, vomiting, sweating, dilated pupils)

• Drowsiness, daytime sleepiness or falling asleep, may need to be discontinued

• **Serotonin syndrome:** agitation, coma, tachycardia, hyperreflexia, nausea, vomiting, diarrhea; may be precipitated in those taking SSRIs, SNRIs

• **Pregnancy/breastfeeding:** use only if benefits outweigh fetal risk; cautious use in breastfeeding, excretion unknown
Evaluate:

• Therapeutic response: improved symptoms in patients with Parkinson's disease
Teach patient/family:

• To change positions slowly to prevent orthostatic hypotension

• To avoid hazardous activities until stabilized on product; that dizziness can occur

• To rinse mouth frequently; to use sugarless gum to alleviate dry mouth

• To take as prescribed; not to miss dose or double doses; to take missed dose as soon as remembered if several hours before next dose

• To prevent hypertensive crisis by avoiding high-tyramine foods (>150 mg), give list to patient
• To avoid CNS depressants, alcohol
• To notify all providers of product use; to avoid elective surgery, other procedures involving CNS depressants
• Check skin periodically for possible skin cancer, higher evidence in Parkinson disease

---

⚠ HIGH ALERT

rasburicase (Rx)

(rass-burr'i-case)
Elitek, Fasturtec ✦
Func. class.: Enzyme
Chem. class.: Recombinant urate-oxidase enzyme

ACTION: Catalyzes enzymatic oxidation of uric acid into an inactive and soluble metabolite (allantoin)

USES: To reduce uric acid levels in patients with leukemia, lymphoma, or solid tumor malignancies who are receiving chemotherapy

CONTRAINDICATIONS: Hypersensitivity

Black Box Warning: ⚠ G6PD deficiency (Mediterranean, African descent), hemolytic reactions, methemoglobinemia reactions to product

Precautions: Pregnancy, breastfeeding, children <2 yr, anemia, acute bronchospasm, angina, atony, African-American and Mediterranean patients, hypotension

Black Box Warning: **Anaphylaxis**, interference with uric acid measurements

DOSAGE AND ROUTES
• **Adult/adolescent/infant:** IV INFUSION 0.2 mg/kg as single daily dose × 5 days
Available forms: Powder for inj 1.5, 7.5 mg/vial

Administer:
Intermittent IV INFUSION route
• Determine number of vials that are needed based on weight, concentration required
• Reconstitute with diluent provided, add 1 mL of diluent/each vial, swirl, withdraw amount needed, mix with NS to final volume of 50 mL, use within 24 hr, give over 30 min, do not use filter, use different line; if not possible, flush with ≥15 mL of saline before, after use
• Chemotherapy started 4-24 hr after 1st dose

SIDE EFFECTS
CNS: *Headache*, fever
CV: Chest pain, hypotension
GI: *Nausea, vomiting, anorexia, diarrhea, abdominal pain, constipation, dyspepsia, mucositis*
HEMA: Neutropenia with fever, hemolysis, methemoglobinemia
INTEG: *Rash*
MISC: Edema
SYST: Anaphylaxis, hemolysis, sepsis

PHARMACOKINETICS
Half-life 16-21 hr, duration up to 12 hr

INTERACTIONS
Drug/Lab Test

Black Box Warning: **Interference:** uric acid

R

NURSING CONSIDERATIONS
Assess:
• Blood studies: BUN, serum uric acid, urine creatinine clearance, electrolytes, CBC with differential before, during therapy
• Monitor temperature; fever may indicate beginning of infection; no rectal temperatures

Black Box Warning: **Anaphylaxis:** dyspnea, urticaria, flushing, wheezing, swelling of lips, tongue, throat; have emergency equipment nearby

⚠ Black Box Warning: **G6PD deficiency, hemolytic reactions, methemoglobinemia**; these patients should not be given this product; screen patients who are at higher risk for these disorders

---

Side effects: *italics* = common; red = life-threatening

Black Box Warning: Altered uric acid measurements: for accurate results, collect blood in prechilled tubes with heparin, place tubes on ice, test within 4 hr

• GI symptoms: frequency of stools, cramping; if severe diarrhea occurs, fluid, electrolytes may need to be given
Evaluate:
• Therapeutic response: decreased uric acid levels in children when antineoplastics causing high uric acid levels used
Teach patient/family:
• About the reason for therapy, expected results
• **Pregnancy/breastfeeding:** identify if pregnancy is planned or suspected or if breastfeeding

---

⚠ HIGH ALERT

regorafenib
(re′goe-raf′e-nib)
Stivarga
Func. class.: Antineoplastic; multikinase inhibitor
Chem. class.: Signal transduction inhibitor (STI)

ACTION: Inhibits tyrosine kinase in patients with colorectal cancer

USES: Metastatic colorectal cancer in those who have received fluoropyrimidine, oxaliplatin, irinotecan-based chemotherapy, an anti-VEGF therapy; and an anti-EGFR therapy if *KRAS* wild type

CONTRAINDICATIONS: Pregnancy
Precautions: Breastfeeding, children, geriatric patients, cardiac/renal/hepatic/dental disease, fistula, GI bleeding or perforation, bone marrow suppression, infection, wound dehiscence, thrombocytopenia, neutropenia, immunosuppression

Black Box Warning: Hepatic disease

DOSAGE AND ROUTES
• **Adult:** PO 160 mg/day with a low-fat breakfast × 21 days of a 28-day cycle, cycles may be repeated
Available forms: Tabs 40 mg
Administer:
• Store at 77° F (25° C)
• Give at the same time each day with a low-fat breakfast that contains less than 30% fat such as 2 slices of white toast with 1 tbsp of low-fat margarine and 1 tbsp of jelly, and 8 oz of skim milk; or 1 cup of cereal, 8 oz of skim milk, 1 slice of toast with jam, apple juice, and 1 cup of coffee or tea
• Swallow tablets whole
• If a dose is missed, take as soon as possible that day; do not take 2 doses on the same day
• **Hand-foot skin reaction:** Reduce to 120 mg (grade 2 palmar-plantar erythrodysesthesia); hold if grade 2 toxicity does not improve in ≤7 days or recurs; hold for ≥7 days in grade 3 toxicity; reduce to 80 mg for recurrent grade 2 toxicity; discontinue if 80 mg is not tolerated
• **Hypertension:** Hold in grade 2 hypertension
Other severe toxicity (except hepatotoxicity)
• Hold until toxicity resolves in grade 3 or 4 toxicity; consider the risk/benefits of continuing therapy in grade 4 toxicity, reduce dosage to 120 mg; if grade 3 or 4 toxicity recurs, hold until toxicity resolves, then reduce to 80 mg; discontinue in those who do not tolerate 80-mg dose
• **Hepatic dose:** Baseline mild (Child-Pugh class A) or moderate (Child-Pugh class B): no change; baseline severe hepatic impairment (Child-Pugh class C): use not recommended; AST/ALT elevations during therapy; For grade 3 AST/ALT level elevations, hold dose; if therapy is continued, reduce to 120 mg after levels recover; discontinue in those with AST/ALT >20 × ULN; AST/ALT >3 × ULN and bilirubin >2 × ULN; recurrence of AST/ALT >5 × ULN despite a reduction to 120 mg

SIDE EFFECTS
CNS: Headache, tremor
CV: Hypertensive crisis, MI

EENT: Blurred vision, conjunctivitis

GI: Hepatotoxicity, GI hemorrhage, diarrhea, GI perforation, xerostomia

HEMA: Neutropenia, thrombocytopenia, bleeding

INTEG: Rash, alopecia

META: Hypokalemia

MISC: Fatigue, decreased weight, hand-foot syndrome, hypothyroidism

PHARMACOKINETICS

Protein binding 99%, metabolized by CYP3A4, UGT1A0, half-life 14-58 hr

INTERACTIONS

Increase: regorafenib concentrations—CYP3A4 inhibitors (ketoconazole, itraconazole, erythromycin, clarithromycin)

Increase: plasma concentrations of simvastatin, calcium channel blockers, ergots

Increase: plasma concentration of warfarin; avoid use with warfarin; use low-molecular-weight anticoagulants instead

Decrease: regorafenib concentrations—CYP3A4 inducers (dexamethasone, phenytoin, carBAMazepine, rifAMPin, PHENobarbital)

Drug/Food

Increase: regorafenib effect—grapefruit juice; avoid use while taking product

Drug/Herb

Decrease: imatinib concentration—St. John's wort

NURSING CONSIDERATIONS
Assess:

> Black Box Warning: **Hepatic disease:** fatal hepatotoxicity can occur; obtain LFTs baseline and at least every 2 wk × 2 mo, then monthly

• Assess any wounds for wound healing; report wound dehiscence, stop medication, notify prescriber

• **Fatal bleeding:** from GI, respiratory, GU tracts; permanently discontinue in those with severe bleeding

• **Palmar-plantar erythrodysesthesia (hand-foot syndrome):** more common in those previously treated; reddening, swelling, numbness, desquamation on palms, soles

• **GI perforation/fistula:** discontinue if this occurs; assess for pain in epigastric area, dyspepsia, flatulence, fever, chills

• **Hypertension/hypertensive crisis:** hypertension usually occurs in the first cycle in those with preexisting hypertension; do not start treatment until B/P is controlled; monitor B/P every wk × 6 wk, then at start of each cycle or more often if needed; temporarily or permanently discontinue for severe uncontrolled hypertension

• **Pregnancy/breastfeeding:** identify whether patient is pregnant or if pregnancy is planned; identify contraception type in both men and women; do not use in pregnancy, breastfeeding

Evaluate:

• Therapeutic response: decrease in spread or size of tumor

Teach patient/family:

• To report adverse reactions immediately: bleeding, rash

• About reason for treatment, expected results

• That effect on male fertility is unknown

• To take at the same time of day with low-fat food; not to use grapefruit juice; to take missed dose on same day; not to take multiple doses on the same day; to keep original container

• To report immediately **hepatic effect** (yellowing skin, eyes, nausea, vomiting, dark urine), **increased B/P** (severe headache), **GI perforation/fistula** (dyspepsia, flatulence, fever, chills, epigastric pain)

• **Pregnancy/breastfeeding:** not to use in pregnancy; to report if pregnancy is suspected or if breastfeeding; for men and women to use contraception during and for 2 mo after termination of treatment

R

> **⚠ HIGH ALERT**
>
> ## remifentanil (Rx)
> (rem-ih-fin′ta-nill)
>
> Ultiva
> *Func. class.:* Opiate agonist analgesic
> *Chem. class.:* μ-Opioid agonist
>
> **Controlled Substance Schedule II**

ACTION: Inhibits ascending pain pathways in limbic system, thalamus, midbrain, hypothalamus

USES: In combination with other products for general anesthesia to provide analgesia

CONTRAINDICATIONS: Hypersensitivity

Precautions: Pregnancy, breastfeeding, children <12 yr, geriatric patients, increased intracranial pressure, acute MI, severe heart disease, GI/renal/hepatic disease, asthma, respiratory conditions, seizure disorders, bradyarrhythmias

Black Box Warning: Potential for overdose or poisoning, substance abuse

DOSAGE AND ROUTES
• **Adult:** IV induction 0.5-1 mcg/kg/min with hypnotic or volatile agent; maintenance with isoflurane or propofol 0.25 mcg/kg/min (range 0.05-2 mcg/kg/min); **CONT INFUSION** 0.025-0.2 mcg/kg/min
• **Child 1-12 yr: CONT IV INFUSION** 0.25 mcg/kg/min with isoflurane
• **Full-term neonate and infant up to 2 mo: CONT IV INFUSION** 0.4 mcg/kg/min with nitrous oxide
Available forms: Powder for inj lyophilized 1, 2, 5 mg
Administer:
• Add 1 mL diluent per mg remifentanil
• Shake well; further dilute to a final concentration of 20, 25, 50, or 250 mcg/mL
• Store in light-resistant area at room temperature
• Interruption of infusion results in rapid reversal (no residual opioid effect within 5-10 min)
Direct IV route
• To be used only during maintenance of general anesthesia; inject into tubing close to venous cannula; give to nonintubated patients over 30-60 sec
Continuous IV INFUSION route
• Use infusion device, max 16 hr; do not use same tubing as blood, do not admix

Y-site compatibilities: Acyclovir, alfentanil, amikacin, aminophylline, ampicillin, ampicillin/sulbactam, aztreonam, bumetanide, buprenorphine, butorphanol, calcium gluconate, ceFAZolin, cefepine, cefotaxime, cefoTEtan, cefOXitin, cefTAZidime, ceftizoxime, cefTRIAXone, cefuroxime, cimetidine, ciprofloxacin, cisatracurium, clindamycin, dexamethasone, digoxin, diltiazem, diphenhydrAMINE, DOBUTamine, DOPamine, doxacurium, doxycycline, droperidol, enalaprilat, EPINEPHrine, esmolol, famotidine, fentaNYL, fluconazole, furosemide, ganciclovir, gatifloxacin, gentamicin, haloperidol, heparin, hydrocortisone sodium succinate, HYDROmorphone, hydrOXYzine, imipenem-cilastatin, inamrinone, isoproterenol, ketorolac, lidocaine, LORazepam, magnesium sulfate, mannitol, meperidine, methylPREDNISolone sodium succinate, metoclopramide, metroNIDAZOLE, midazolam, morphine, nalbuphine, nitroglycerin, norepinephrine, ondansetron, phenylephrine, piperacillin, potassium chloride, procainamide, prochlorperazine, promethazine, raNITIdine, SUFentanil, theophylline, thiopental, ticarcillin/clavulanate, tobramycin, vancomycin, zidovudine

Solution compatibilities: D$_5$W, 0.45% NaCl, LR, D$_5$LR, 0.9% NaCl

SIDE EFFECTS
CNS: Drowsiness, *dizziness,* confusion, *headache,* sedation, euphoria, delirium, agitation, anxiety
CV: Palpitations, *bradycardia,* change in B/P, facial flushing, syncope, asystole
EENT: Tinnitus, blurred vision, miosis, diplopia
GI: *Nausea, vomiting,* anorexia, constipation, cramps, dry mouth
GU: Urinary retention, dysuria
INTEG: Rash, urticaria, bruising, flushing, diaphoresis, pruritus
MS: Rigidity
RESP: Respiratory depression, apnea

PHARMACOKINETICS
70% protein binding, terminal half-life 3-10 min, excreted in urine; onset: 1-3 min

INTERACTIONS

Increase: respiratory depression, hypotension, profound sedation: alcohol, sedatives, hypnotics, other CNS depressants; antihistamines, phenothiazines, MAOIs

Drug/Herb

Increase: CNS depression—kava

NURSING CONSIDERATIONS

Assess:

• I&O ratio; check for decreasing output; may indicate urinary retention, especially in geriatric patients

• CNS changes; dizziness, drowsiness, hallucinations, euphoria, LOC, pupil reaction

• GI status: nausea, vomiting, anorexia, constipation

• Allergic reactions: rash, urticaria

Black Box Warning: **Substance abuse:** assess patients for risks of addiction, abuse, or misuse before drug initiation, and monitor those who receive opioids for the development of these behaviors, conditions; also assess for depression or other mental illness in the patient or family members

Black Box Warning: **Potential for overdose or poisoning:** there is a significant potential; proper patient selection and counseling are needed before use; keep out of reach of children, pets; accidental overdose and death may occur

• **Respiratory dysfunction:** respiratory depression, character, rate, rhythm; notify prescriber if respirations <12/min; CV status; bradycardia, syncope

• **Pregnancy/breastfeeding:** use only if benefits outweigh fetal risk; avoid use in breastfeeding, excretion unknown

Evaluate:

• Therapeutic response: maintenance of anesthesia

Teach patient/family:

• Reason for product, expected results

⚠ HIGH ALERT

repaglinide (Rx)

(re-pag'lih'nide)

Gluconorm ✦, Prandin

Func. class.: Antidiabetic
Chem. class.: Meglitinide

Do not confuse:
Prandin/Avandia

ACTION: Causes functioning β-cells in pancreas to release insulin, thereby leading to a drop in blood glucose levels; closes ATP-dependent potassium channels in the β-cell membrane; this leads to the opening of calcium channels; increased calcium influx induces insulin secretion

USES: Type 2 diabetes mellitus

CONTRAINDICATIONS: Hypersensitivity to meglitinides; diabetic ketoacidosis, type 1 diabetes

Precautions: Pregnancy, breastfeeding, children, geriatric patients, thyroid/cardiac disease, severe renal/hepatic disease, severe hypoglycemic reactions

DOSAGE AND ROUTES

• **Adult:** PO 0.5-4 mg with each meal, max 16 mg/day; adjust at weekly intervals; oral hypoglycemic–naive patients or patients with A1c <8% should start with 0.5 mg with each meal

Renal/hepatic dose

• **Adult:** PO CCr 20-39 mL/min, 0.5 mg/day; titrate upward cautiously

Available forms: Tabs 0.5, 1, 2 mg

Administer:

• Up to 15-30 min before meals; 2, 3, or 4×/day preprandially

• Skip dose if meal skipped; add dose if meal added

• Store in tight container at room temperature

• May be added to metFORMIN for better control

SIDE EFFECTS

CNS: *Headache, weakness,* paresthesia
CV: Angina

EENT: Tinnitus, sinusitis
ENDO: Hypoglycemia
GI: Nausea, vomiting, diarrhea, constipation, dyspepsia, pancreatitis
INTEG: Rash, allergic reactions
MISC: Chest pain, UTI, allergy
MS: Back pains, arthralgia
RESP: URI, sinusitis, rhinitis, bronchitis

PHARMACOKINETICS

Completely absorbed by GI route; onset 30 min; peak 1 hr; duration <4 hr; half-life 1 hr; metabolized in liver by CYP3A4; excreted in urine, feces (metabolites); crosses placenta; 98% protein bound

INTERACTIONS

• Do not use with gemfibrozil, isophane insulin (NPH)

Increase: repaglinide effect—CYP3A4, OATP101, CYP2C9 inhibitors
Increase: in both—levonorgestrel/ethinyl estradiol
Increase: repaglinide metabolism—CYP3A4 inducers: rifAMPin, barbiturates, carBAMazepine
Increase: repaglinide effect—NSAIDs, salicylates, sulfonamides, chloramphenicol, MAOIs, coumarins, β-blockers, probenecid, gemfibrozil, simvastatin, fenofibrate, deferasirox
Decrease: repaglinide metabolism—CYP3A4 inhibitors: antifungals (ketoconazole, miconazole), erythromycin, macrolides
Decrease: repaglinide action—calcium channel blockers, corticosteroids, oral contraceptives, thiazide diuretics, thyroid preparations, estrogens, phenothiazines, phenytoin, rifAMPin, isoniazid, PHENobarbital, sympathomimetics

Drug/Herb
Increase: antidiabetic effect—garlic, chromium, horse chestnut

Drug/Food
Decrease: repaglinide level; give before meals
Decrease: repaglinide metabolism—grapefruit juice

Drug/Lab Test
Increase/decrease: glucose

NURSING CONSIDERATIONS
Assess:

• **Hypo/hyperglycemic reaction,** which can occur soon after meals: dizziness, weakness, headache, tremors, anxiety, tachycardia, hunger, sweating, abdominal pain, A1c, fasting, postprandial glucose during treatment

• **Pregnancy/breastfeeding:** use only if benefits outweigh fetal risk, usually insulin is used in pregnancy; do not breastfeed, excretion unknown

Evaluate:
• Therapeutic response: decrease in polyuria, polydipsia, polyphagia; clear sensorium; absence of dizziness; stable gait; blood glucose, A1c improvement

Teach family/patient:
• About technique for blood glucose monitoring; how to use blood glucose meter
• About the symptoms of hypo/hyperglycemia, what to do about each
• That product must be continued on daily basis; about the consequences of discontinuing product abruptly
• To avoid OTC medications unless ordered by prescriber; not to use alcohol
• That diabetes is a lifelong illness; that product will not cure disease
• That all food included in diet plan must be eaten to prevent hypoglycemia; that if a meal is omitted, dose should be omitted; to have glucagon emergency kit available; to take repaglinide 15-30 min before meals 2, 3, or 4×/day; to carry emergency ID

TREATMENT OF OVERDOSE:
Glucose 25 g IV via dextrose 50% solution, 50 mL or 1 mg glucagon

---

RARELY USED

reslizumab
(res-liz' ue- mab)
Cinqair ✦
Func. class.: Respiratory antiinflammatory agent

USES: For add-on maintenance treatment of severe asthma of eosinophilic phenotype

---

CONTRAINDICATIONS: Hypersensitivity

DOSAGE AND ROUTES
• **Adult: IV INFUSION** 3 mg/kg q4wk; discontinue the infusion immediately if a severe systemic reaction, including anaphylaxis, occurs

retapamulin (topical)
(re-te-pam'you-lin)
Altabax
Func. class.: Topical antiinfective
Chem. class.: Pleuromutilin

ACTION: Antibacterial activity results from inhibition of protein synthesis

USES: For the treatment of impetigo

CONTRAINDICATIONS: Hypersensitivity to this product
Precautions: Children

DOSAGE AND ROUTES
• **Adult/child ≥9 mo: TOP** apply to affected area bid × 5 days
Available forms: Topical ointment 1%
Administer:
Topical route
• Do not use skin products near the eyes, nose, or mouth
• Wash hands before and after use
• **Ointment:** Apply a thin film to the cleansed affected area and massage gently into affected areas

SIDE EFFECTS
INTEG: Pruritus, irritation, headache, diarrhea, nausea

NURSING CONSIDERATIONS
Assess:
• **Allergic reaction:** hypersensitivity, product may need to be discontinued
• **Infection:** number of lesions, severity of impetigo
Evaluate:
• Therapeutic response: decreased lesions, infection in impetigo

Teach patient/family:
Topical route
• Not to use skin products near the eyes, nose, or mouth
• To wash hands before and after use
• **Ointment:** to apply a thin film to the cleansed affected area

revefenacin
(rev' e-fen' a-sin)
Yupelri
Func. class.: Respiratory muscarinic antagonists—long-acting

ACTION: In airways, it exhibits pharmacological effects through inhibition of the M3 receptor at the smooth muscle, leading to bronchodilation

USES: Maintenance treatment of those with COPD

CONTRAINDICATIONS: Hypersensitivity
Precautions: Acute/paradoxical bronchospasm, acutely deteriorating COPD, acute symptoms, other anticholinergics, breastfeeding, cardiac disease, children, closed-angle glaucoma, dementia, driving or hazardous tasks, geriatric patients, hepatic disease, ocular exposure, pregnancy, prostatic hypertrophy, urinary retention/obstruction

DOSAGE AND ROUTES
• **Adult: INH** 1 175-mcg vial (3 mL) once daily, by oral inhalation only
Available forms: 175 mcg/3 mL sol for inhalation
Administer
Oral inhalation route
• Give by oral inhalation via nebulizer only; do not swallow, no dilution necessary, single-dose vials are ready-to-use
• Remove the unit-dose vial from the foil pouch only immediately before use; product should be colorless; discard if the solution is not colorless
• Do not mix with other drugs

R

• Give the inhalation solution via a standard jet nebulizer connected to an air compressor; give over 8 min
• Discard the vial and any residual solution after use

SIDE EFFECTS
CNS: Headache
RESP: Cough, nasopharyngitis, upper respiratory tract infection
MS: Back pain

PHARMACOKINETICS
Extensively distributed to tissues, primarily metabolized via hydrolysis to a metabolite, half-life of active metabolite 22-70 hr, excreted 54% feces, 27% urine

INTERACTIONS
Increase: anticholinergic effect—other anticholinergics; avoid coadministration
Increase: revefenacin effect—OATP1B1, OATP1B3 inhibitors (rifampicin, cyclosporine); avoid coadministration

NURSING CONSIDERATIONS
Assess
• **Respiratory status:** lung sounds, pulse, B/P before and after product is given; note wheezing, shortness of breath, cough; monitor pulmonary function tests baseline and periodically
• **Pregnancy/breastfeeding:** no well-controlled studies; animal studies showed no evidence of fetal harm; anticholinergics suppress lactation
Evaluate:
• Therapeutic response: prevention or relief of the symptoms of COPD
Teach patient/family
• To contact health care provider if symptoms are not relieved or if shortness of breath continues or if bronchospasm occurs
• To notify health care provider of all OTC preparations, other medications, herbs, and supplements taken; not to start or stop products without approval of provider
• Not to swallow during nebulization
• That pulmonary function tests will be monitored periodically
• **Pregnancy/breastfeeding:** to inform health care provider if pregnancy is planned or suspected, or if breastfeeding

---

RARELY USED

Rh$_o$(D) immune globulin standard dose IM (Rx)
HyperRHO S/D Full Dose, RhoGAM
Rh$_o$(D) immune globulin microdose IM (Rx)
HyperRHO S/D mini-Dose, MICRhoGAM, Mini-Gamulin R, Rho(D) immune globulin microdose (IM, IV) Rhophylac
Rh$_o$(D) immune globulin IV (Rx)
WinRho SDF
Func. class.: Immune globulins

ACTION: Suppresses immune response of nonsensitized Rh$_o$(D or D^u)-negative patients who are exposed to Rh$_o$(D or D^u)-positive blood

USES: Prevention of isoimmunization in Rh-negative women given Rh-positive blood after abortions, miscarriages, amniocentesis; chronic idiopathic thrombocytopenia purpura (Rhophylac)

CONTRAINDICATIONS: Previous immunization with this product, Rh$_o$(O)-positive/D^u-positive patient

Black Box Warning: Hemolysis

Precautions: Pregnancy

Black Box Warning: Requires a specialized setting

DOSAGE AND ROUTES
Rho (D) Immune globulin (for IM Only)
• **Adult: IM before delivery HyperRHO S/D Full Dose, RhoGam** 1 vial standard dose (300 mcg) at 26-28 wk; **after delivery** 1 vial standard dose (300 mcg) within 72 hr of delivery

---

Pregnancy termination (<13 wk gestation)
• **Adult:** IM HyperRho Minidose, MicroRhoGAM 1 vial microdose (50 mcg) within 72 hr of termination

Pregnancy termination (>13 wk gestation)
• **Adult:** IM HyperRHO S/D Full Dose, RhoGam 1 vial standard dose (300 mcg) within 72 hr of termination

Massive fetomaternal hemorrhage (>15 mL)
• **Adult:** IM RhoGam 20 mcg/mL of Rho(D) positive fetal RBCs

Transfusion accident
• **Adult:** IM Hyper Rho Full Dose, RhoGam (Rh –positive blood given (volume) × Hct of donor blood)/15 will be the number of vial needed (standard dose), round to next whole vial

Rho(D) Immune Globulin IV (for IV/IM use)
• **Adult:** IM/IV WinRho SDF, 1500 IU (300 mcg) at 28 wk; **after delivery** 1 vial, **after delivery** 600 IU (120 mcg) within 72 hr of delivery

Termination of pregnancy, amniocentesis
• **Adult:** IM/IV WinRho SDF 600 IU (120 mcg) with 72 hr

Amniocentesis, chorionic villus sampling
• **Adult:** IM/IV WinRho SDF (<34 wk gestation) 1500 IU (300 mcg) repeat q12wk during pregnancy

Massive fetomaternal hemorrhage (>15 mL)/transfusion accident
• **Adult:** IM WinRho SDF 6000 IU (1200 mcg) repeat q12hr until total dose given by amount of blood loss; **IM WinRho SDF** 3000 IU (600 mcg) repeat q8hr until total dose is given by amount of blood loss

Immune thrombocytopenic purpura (ITP)
• **Adult and child:** IV WinRho SDF 250 IU (50 mcg)/kg, if HGB <10g/dL use 25-40 mcg (125-200 IU), dosing determined by clinical response

Available forms: IM MICRhoGAM, HyperRho S/D: **Minidose** 50 mcg/vial;

300 mcg/vial **standard dose**; IM/IV 600 IU (120 mcg)/vial, 1500 IU (300 mcg)/vial 2500 IU (500 mcg)/vial, 5000 IU (1000 mcg)/vial, 15,000 IU (3000 mcg)/vial; prefilled syringe 1500 IU (300 mcg/2 mL)

Administer:
• Store in refrigerator
• HyperRHO S/D, MICRhoGAM, RhoGAM given by IM only; do not give IV
• Do not confuse different types
• Inspect for particulate matter; do not use if particulate matter present
• Reconstitute/dilution: no reconstitution or dilution needed for HyperRHO SD; MICRhoGAM, RhoGAM, or liquid formulation of WinRho SDF

IM route
• Use aseptic technique, observe for 20 min after administration
• Bring Rhophylac to room temperature before use
• Inject into deltoid muscle of upper arm or anterolateral portion of upper thigh; do not inject into gluteal muscle
• If dose calculated requires multiple vials or syringes, use different sites at same time

IV route
• Use aseptic technique
• WinRho SDF: remove entire contents of vial to obtain calculated dose; if partial vial required for dosage calculation, withdraw entire vial contents to ensure correct calculation; infuse correct calculated dose over 3-5 min; do not infuse with other fluids, products
• Rhophylac: bring to room temperature; infuse by slow IV; observe for 20 min

SIDE EFFECTS
CNS: Lethargy, dizziness, headache
CV: Hypo/hypertension
INTEG: Irritation at inj site, fever
MISC: Infection, ARDS, anaphylaxis, pulmonary edema, DIC
MS: Myalgia, arthralgia
HEMA: Anemia, DIC, intravascular hemolysis

INTERACTIONS
Decrease: antibody response—live virus vaccines (measles, mumps, rubella)

Side effects: *italics* = common; red = life-threatening

NURSING CONSIDERATIONS
Assess:

• Allergies, reactions to immunizations; previous immunization with product

• **Intravascular hemolysis:** back pain, chills, hemoglobinuria, renal insufficiency; usually when WinRho SDF is given in those with immune thrombocytopenia purpura

• Type, crossmatch mother and newborn's cord blood; if mother Rh$_0$ (D)-negative, D^u-negative and newborn Rh$_0$ (D)-positive, product should be given

Evaluate:

• Rh$_0$(D) sensitivity in transfusion error, prevention of erythroblastosis fetalis for normal vision

Teach patient/family:

• How product works; that product must be given after subsequent deliveries if subsequent babies are Rh-positive

• To report immediately: shaking, fever, chills, dark urine, swelling of hands or feet, back pain, SOB (intravascular hemolysis)

---

ribociclib
(rye-boe-sye′-klib)
Kisqali
Func. class.: Antineoplastic
Chem. class.: Protein kinase inhibitors

ACTION: A cyclin-dependent kinase (CDK) 4 and 6 inhibitor. Regulates cell-cycle progression through phosphorylation of the retinoblastoma protein. The combination of ribociclib and an antiestrogen such as letrozole inhibited tumor growth more than either agent alone

USES: For the initial endocrine-based treatment of hormone receptor (HR)-positive, HER2-negative advanced or metastatic breast cancer in combination with an aromatase inhibitor in postmenopausal women

CONTRAINDICATIONS: Hypersensitivity

Precautions: Breastfeeding, contraception requirements, hepatic disease, hepatotoxicity, infertility, neutropenia, pregnancy, pregnancy testing, reproductive risk, thromboembolic disease

DOSAGE AND ROUTES
Hormone receptor (HR)-positive, HER2-negative advanced or metastatic breast cancer in combination with an aromatase inhibitor in postmenopausal women

• **Adult:** 600 mg/day on days 1 to 21, followed by 7 days of rest, in combination with letrozole (2.5 mg daily) or another aromatase inhibitor on days 1 to 28; repeat cycle q28days

Therapeutic drug monitoring
Neutropenia

• **ANC ≥1000 cells/mm^3 (grade ≤2):** no change

• **ANC 500 cells/mm^3 to 999 cells/mm^3 (grade 3):** hold. For the first occurrence of grade 3 neutropenia, resume at original dose level when the ANC returns to ≥1000 cells/mm^3 (grade ≤2); for recurrent grade 3 neutropenia, resume at next lower dose level (reduce 600 mg to 400 mg; reduce 400 mg to 200 mg). If further dose reduction below 200 mg per day is required, discontinue

• **ANC 500 cells/mm^3 to 999 cells/mm^3 (grade 3 neutropenia) with single episode of fever >38.3° C or >38° C for >1 hr and/or concurrent infection:** hold; resume at the next lower dose level when ANC returns to ≥1000 cells/mm^3 (grade 2 or less) (reduce 600 mg to 400 mg; reduce 400 mg to 200 mg). If further dose reduction below 200 mg per day is required, discontinue

QT prolongation

• **QTcF 481-500 msec and no serious arrhythmia:** hold; monitor ECG frequently. For the first occurrence, resume at the same dose when QTcF prolongation resolves to ≤480 msec; for a recurrence of QTcF >480 msec, resume at the next lower dose level (reduce 600 mg to 400 mg; reduce 400 mg to 200 mg). If

---

further dose reduction below 200 mg/day is required, discontinue

• **QTcF >500 msec and no serious arrhythmia:** repeat ECG. If the QTcF >500 msec on at least 2 separate ECGs at the same visit, hold; monitor ECG more frequently. Resume at the next lower dose level (reduce 600 mg to 400 mg; reduce 400 mg to 200 mg) when QTcF prolongation resolves to ≤480 msec. If further dose reduction below 200 mg/day is required, discontinue

Hepatic dose

• **Mild hepatic impairment (Child-Pugh A):** no change; **moderate to severe hepatic impairment (Child-Pugh B or C):** reduce starting dose to 400 mg/day
• **AST/ALT >ULN to 3× ULN (grade 1); total bilirubin <2× ULN:** no change
• **AST/ALT 3.01–5× ULN (grade 2); total bilirubin <2× ULN:** if baseline hepatic impairment was grade 2, continue; monitor LFTs more frequently. If baseline was grade 0 or 1, hold. For the first occurrence of grade 2 hepatotoxicity, resume treatment at original dose when AST/ALT resolve to less than or equal to baseline. For recurrent grade 2 hepatotoxicity, resume at next lower dose level (reduce 600 mg to 400 mg; reduce 400 mg to 200 mg), monitor LFTs more frequently. If further dose reduction below 200 mg/day is required, discontinue
• **AST/ALT >3× ULN (grade >2); total bilirubin >2× ULN (irrespective of baseline; in the absence of cholestasis):** discontinue
• **AST/ALT 5.01–20× ULN (grade 3); total bilirubin <2× ULN:** hold. For first occurrence of grade 3 hepatotoxicity, resume at the next lower dose level when AST/ALT recover to less than or equal to baseline grade (reduce 600 mg to 400 mg; reduce 400 mg to 200 mg). Monitor LFTs more frequently. If further dose reduction below 200 mg/day is required, discontinue. Discontinue for recurrent grade 3 hepatotoxicity
• **AST/ALT >20× ULN (grade 4); total bilirubin <2× ULN:** discontinue

Nephrotoxicity dosage adjustments
• **Serum creatinine (SCr) ≤3× ULN or glomerular filtration rate (GFR) ≥25% of the lower limit of normal (LLN) (grade 1 or 2):** no change
• **SCr 3.01 × ULN or GFR <25% of LLN (chronic dialysis not indicated) (grade 3):** hold. For first occurrence of a grade 3, resume at the original dose grade ≤1; for a recurrent grade 3, resume at the next lower dose level (reduce 600 mg to 400 mg; reduce 400 mg to 200 mg). If further dose reduction below 200 mg per day is required, discontinue
• **SCr >6× ULN or requiring chronic dialysis or renal transplant (grade 4):** discontinue

Administer:

• Take ribociclib and letrozole at the same time every day, preferably in the morning
• Swallow tablets whole; do not chew, crush, or split. Do not take if broken, cracked
• If a dose is missed, or if the patient vomits, do not replace the missed dose. Resume with the next scheduled daily dose

SIDE EFFECTS

GI: Diarrhea, *abdominal pain, anorexia, nausea, vomiting, constipation, stomatitis, weight loss*
CNS: *Fatigue, headache, insomnia*
MS: *Back pain*
INTEG: *Rash, alopecia*
HEMA: Leukemia, neutropenia
MISC: Infection

PHARMACOKINETICS

Protein binding 70%; half-life 29.7-54.7 hr; fecal excretion 97.1%; extensively metabolized (CYP3A4); unchanged drug 17% and 12% in feces and urine, respectively; peak 1-4 hr

INTERACTIONS

Increase: QT prolongation—drugs known to prolong QT interval; avoid concomitant use
Increase: ribociclib effect—strong or moderate CYP3A4 inhibitors; avoid concomitant use; if cannot be avoided, reduce dose

R

Side effects: *italics* = common; red = life-threatening

Decrease: ribociclib effect—strong or moderate CYP3A4 inducers; avoid concomitant use

Drug/Lab Test
Increase: LFTs

Drug/Food
• Avoid use with pomegranates, pomegranate juice, grapefruit, and grapefruit juice

NURSING CONSIDERATIONS
Assess:
• **Hepatotoxicity,** including elevated transaminases with or without an elevation in total bilirubin; may occur in combination therapy with ribociclib plus letrozole. Usually grade ≥3 was 57 days. Monitor LFTs baseline, q2wk for the first 2 cycles, before the next 4 cycles, and then as needed. A dose interruption, reduction, or discontinuation of therapy may be necessary.

• **Bone marrow suppression:** onset of grade ≥2 neutropenia was 16 days. Monitor CBC baseline, q2wk for the first 2 cycles, before the next 4 cycles, and then as needed. A dose interruption, reduction, or discontinuation of therapy may be needed in those with an absolute neutrophil count (ANC) <1000 cells/mm^3

• **Long QT syndrome:** avoid use in long QT syndrome, uncontrolled or significant cardiac disease (cardiac arrhythmias, recent MI, heart failure, unstable angina, bradycardia or bradyarrhythmias, electrolyte imbalance (hypomagnesemia, hypokalemia, hypocalcemia), with products causing prolonged QT interval or that strongly inhibit CYP3A4. Females, geriatric patients, and patients with diabetes mellitus, thyroid disease, malnutrition, alcoholism, or hepatic disease may also be at increased risk for QT prolongation. Assess ECG before starting therapy; do not start product if QTcF >450 msec. Repeat ECG at day 14 of first cycle, at the beginning of second cycle, and then as needed; prolongation of the QTcF interval may require interruption of therapy, dose reduction, or discontinuation of therapy. Monitor serum electrolytes (potassium, calcium, phosphorous, and magnesium) baseline, at the beginning of the first 6 cycles, and as needed; correct electrolyte imbalances before starting product

• **Pregnancy/breastfeeding:** avoid use by females of reproductive potential during treatment and for at least 3 wk after last dose; can cause fetal harm or death; discontinue breastfeeding during treatment and for 3 wk after final dose; presence in breast milk unknown. Obtain pregnancy test before starting treatment

Evaluate
• Therapeutic outcome: decrease in size of cancerous tumor

Teach patient/family:
• **Pregnancy/breastfeeding:** not to use drug in pregnancy, breastfeeding; contraception should be used during treatment and for at least 3 wk after last dose

• **Hepatotoxicity:** patient should report immediately yellowing of skin or eyes, dark urine

• **QT prolongation:** signs and symptoms of QT prolongation (irregular or rapid heartbeat, fainting). To notify health care provider immediately if any of these occur

• **Neutropenia:** to immediately notify health care provider if a fever occurs; usually may occur with an infection

• **Drug interactions:** to avoid pomegranates, pomegranate juice, grapefruit, and grapefruit juice; that all OTC or prescription medications, herbals, and supplements should be approved by provider

• **Alopecia:** that hair is often lost; make suggestions for wigs, scarves to make patient feel more comfortable about hair loss

---

riboflavin (vit B₂) (otc)
(rye′boh-flay-vin)
Func. class.: Vit B₂, water soluble

ACTION: Needed for respiratory reactions by catalyzing proteins

USES: Vit B$_2$ deficiency or polyneuritis; cheilosis adjunct with thiamine
Unlabeled uses: Migraine prophylaxis

CONTRAINDICATIONS
None known
Precautions: Pregnancy

DOSAGE AND ROUTES
Deficiency
• **Adult: PO** 5-30 mg/day
• **Child ≥12 yr: PO** 3-10 mg/day, then 0.6 mg/1000 calories ingested
RDA
• **Adult: PO** (males) 1.3 mg, (females) 1.1 mg
Migraine prophylaxis (unlabeled)
• **Adult: PO** 400 mg/day × 3 mo
Available forms: Tabs 5, 10, 25, 50, 100, 250 mg
Administer:
• With food for better absorption
• Store in airtight, light-resistant container

SIDE EFFECTS
GU: Yellow discoloration of urine

PHARMACOKINETICS
Half-life 65-85 min, 60% protein bound, unused amounts excreted in urine (unchanged)

INTERACTIONS
Increase: riboflavin need—alcohol, probenecid, tricyclics, phenothiazines
Decrease: action of tetracyclines
Drug/Lab Test
• May cause false elevations of urinary catecholamines

NURSING CONSIDERATIONS
Assess:
• Nutritional status: liver, eggs, dairy products, yeast, whole grains, green vegetables
Evaluate:
• Therapeutic response: absence of headache, GI problems, cheilosis, skin lesions, depression; burning, itchy eyes; anemia
Teach patient/family:
• That urine may turn bright yellow
• About the addition of needed foods rich in riboflavin
• To avoid alcohol

RARELY USED

rifabutin (Rx)
(riff'a-byoo-ten)
Mycobutin
Func. class.: Antimycobacterial agent
Chem. class.: Rifamycin S derivative

Do not confuse:
rifabutin/rifAMPin/rifapentine

ACTION: Inhibits DNA-dependent RNA polymerase in susceptible strains of *Escherichia coli* and *Bacillus subtilis;* mechanism of action against *Mycobacterium avium* unknown

USES: Prevention of *M. avium* complex (MAC) in patients with advanced HIV infection
Unlabeled uses: *Helicobacter pylori* that has not responded to other treatment

CONTRAINDICATIONS: Hypersensitivity, active TB, WBC <1000/mm^3 or platelet count <50,000/mm^3
Precautions: Pregnancy, breastfeeding, children, hepatic disease, blood dyscrasias

DOSAGE AND ROUTES
• **Adult: PO** 300 mg/day (may take as 150 mg bid); max 600 mg/day
Renal dose
• **Adult: PO** CCr <30 mL/min, reduce by 50%
Available forms: Caps 150 mg
Administer:
• With food if GI upset occurs; better to take on empty stomach 1 hr before or 2 hr after meals; high-fat foods slow absorption; may take in 2 divided doses, may open capsule, mix with applesauce if unable to swallow whole cap
• Antiemetic if vomiting occurs
• After C&S completed; monthly to detect resistance

SIDE EFFECTS
CNS: *Headache,* fatigue, anxiety, confusion, insomnia

Side effects: *italics* = common; red = life-threatening

GI: *Nausea, vomiting, anorexia, diarrhea,* heartburn, hepatitis, discolored saliva, CDAD

GU: *Discolored urine*

HEMA: Hemolytic anemia, eosinophilia, thrombocytopenia, leukopenia

INTEG: *Rash*

MISC: Flulike symptoms, shortness of breath, chest pressure

MS: Asthenia, arthralgia, myalgia

PHARMACOKINETICS

53% absorbed, peak 2-3 hr, duration >24 hr, half-life 45 hr, metabolized in liver (active/inactive metabolites), excreted in urine primarily as metabolites

INTERACTIONS

Increase: levels of rifabutin—ritonavir

Decrease: action of amprenavir, anticoagulants, β-blockers, barbiturates, busPIRone, clofibrate, corticosteroids, cycloSPORINE, dapsone, delavirdine, disopyramide, doxycycline, efavirenz, estrogens, fluconazole, indinavir, ketoconazole, losartan, nelfinavir, nevirapine, oral contraceptives, phenytoin, quiNIDine, saquinavir, sulfonylureas, theophylline, tricyclic antidepressants, zidovudine, zolpidem

Drug/Food

• High-fat diet decreases absorption

Drug/Lab Test

Interference: folate level, vit B_{12}, BSP, gallbladder studies

NURSING CONSIDERATIONS

Assess:

• **Acute TB:** chest x-ray, sputum culture, blood culture, biopsy of lymph nodes, PPD; product should not be given for active TB

• CBC for neutropenia, thrombocytopenia, eosinophilia

• **CDAD:** diarrhea, abdominal pain/cramping, fever, bloody stools; report immediately; may occur several weeks after discontinuing treatment

• Signs of anemia: Hct, Hgb, fatigue

• **Hepatotoxicity:** ALT, AST, bilirubin; assess weekly for decreased appetite, jaundice, dark urine, fatigue

• Renal status before, each mo: BUN, creatinine, output, specific gravity, urinalysis

Evaluate:

• Therapeutic response: not used for active TB because of risk for development of resistance to rifAMPin; culture negative

Teach patient/family:

• That patients using oral contraceptives should consider using nonhormonal methods of birth control, may decrease effect; to notify prescriber if pregnancy planned, suspected

• That compliance with dosage schedule, duration necessary

• That scheduled appointments must be kept because relapse may occur

• That urine, feces, saliva, sputum, sweat, tears may be colored red-orange; that soft contact lenses may be permanently stained

• **To report flulike symptoms:** excessive fatigue, anorexia, vomiting, sore throat; unusual bleeding, yellowish discoloration of skin, eyes; myositis: muscle or bone pain; diarrhea, fever, abdominal cramping, bloody stools

---

rifAMPin (Rx)

(rif'am-pin)

Rifadin, Rofact ✦

Func. class.: Antitubercular

Chem. class.: Rifamycin B derivative

Do not confuse:
rifAMPin/rifabutin/rifAXIMin

ACTION: Inhibits DNA-dependent polymerase, decreases tubercle bacilli replication

USES: Pulmonary TB, meningococcal carriers (prevention)

Unlabeled uses: Endocarditis, *Haemophilus influenzae* type B prophylaxis, Hansen's disease, *Mycobacterium avium* complex (MAC), orthopedic device–related infection, pruritus

CONTRAINDICATIONS: Hypersensitivity to this product, rifamycins; active *Neisseria meningitidis* infection

---

Precautions: Pregnancy, breastfeeding, children <5 yr, hepatic disease, blood dyscrasias

DOSAGE AND ROUTES
Tuberculosis
• **Adult: PO/IV** Max 600 mg/day as single dose 1 hr before meals or 2 hr after meals or 10 mg/kg/day 5 days/wk or 2-3×/wk
• **Child >5 yr: PO/IV** 10-20 mg/kg/day as single dose 1 hr before meals or 2 hr after meals, max 600 mg/day with other antituberculars
• **6-mo regimen:** 2 mo treatment of isoniazid, rifAMPin, pyrazinamide, and possibly streptomycin or ethambutol, then rifAMPin and isoniazid 3-4 mo
• **9-mo regimen:** rifAMPin and isoniazid supplemented with pyrazinamide, streptomycin, or ethambutol
Meningococcal carriers
• **Adult: PO/IV** 600 mg bid × 2 days, max 600 mg/dose
• **Child >5 yr: PO/IV** 10-20 mg/kg × 2 days, max 600 mg/dose
• **Infant 3 mo-1 yr: PO** 5 mg/kg bid × 2 days
Prevention of *H. influenzae* type B infection (unlabeled)
• **Adult: PO** 600 mg/day × 4 days
• **Child: PO** 20 mg/kg/day × 4 days
• **Neonates: PO** 10 mg/kg/day × 4 days
MAC (unlabeled)
• **Adult: PO/IV** 600 mg/day used with ≥3 other active microbials
• **Child: PO/IV** 10-20 mg/kg/day used with ≥3 other active microbials
Endocarditis with prosthetic valves (unlabeled)
• **Adult: PO** 300 mg q8hr with gentamicin and vancomycin
• **Child: PO** 20 mg/kg/day in 2 divided doses with gentamicin and vancomycin, max 900 mg/day
Available forms: Caps 150, 300 mg; powder for inj 600 mg/vial
Administer:
• After C&S completed; monthly to detect resistance
• Do not give IM, SUBCUT

PO route
• On empty stomach, 1 hr before or 2 hr after meals with full glass of water; give with other products for TB
• Antiemetic if vomiting occurs
• Capsules may be opened, mixed with applesauce or jelly
Intermittent IV INFUSION route
• After diluting each 600 mg/10 mL of sterile water for inj (60 mg/mL), swirl, withdraw dose, and dilute in 100 mL or 500 mL of D$_5$W given as infusion over 3 hr; if diluted in 100 mL, give over $^1/_2$ hr; do not admix with other sol or products

Y-site compatibilities: amiodarone, bumetanide, midazolam, pantoprazole, vancomycin

SIDE EFFECTS
CNS: Headache, fatigue, anxiety, drowsiness, confusion
EENT: Visual disturbances
GI: *Nausea, vomiting, anorexia, diarrhea,* CDAD, *heartburn,* sore mouth and tongue, pancreatitis, increased LFTs
GU: Hematuria, acute renal failure, hemoglobinuria
HEMA: Hemolytic anemia, eosinophilia, thrombocytopenia, leukopenia
INTEG: Rash, pruritus, urticaria
MISC: Flulike symptoms, menstrual disturbances, edema, SOB, Stevens-Johnson syndrome, toxic epidermal necrolysis, angioedema, anaphylaxis, DRESS
MS: Ataxia, weakness
MISC: Staining of teeth, contact lens; coloring of urine, sweat, tears

PHARMACOKINETICS
PO: Peak 1-4 hr, half-life 1-5 hr, metabolized in liver (active/inactive metabolites), excreted in urine as free product (30% crosses placenta) and in breast milk

INTERACTIONS
Do not use with protease inhibitors
Increase: hepatotoxicity—isoniazid, alcohol, ketoconazole, pyrazinamide
Decrease: action of acetaminophen, alcohol, anticoagulants, antidiabetics,

β-blockers, barbiturates, benzodiazepines, chloramphenicol, clofibrate, corticosteroids, cycloSPORINE, dapsone, digoxin, doxycycline, haloperidol, hormones, imidazole antifungals, NIFEdipine, oral contraceptives, phenytoin, protease inhibitors, theophylline, verapamil, zidovudine

Increase: LFTs
Decrease: Hgb
Drug/Lab Test
Increase: alk phosphatase, ALT, AST, uric acid, bilirubin, eosinophils
Interference: folate level, vit B_{12}

NURSING CONSIDERATIONS
Assess:
• **Infection:** sputum culture, lung sounds, characteristics of sputum, susceptibility tests baseline and periodically to determine effectiveness and resistance
• Signs of anemia: Hct, Hgb, fatigue
• Hepatic function monthly: ALT, AST, bilirubin, decreased appetite, jaundice, dark urine, fatigue
• Renal status before, each mo: BUN, creatinine, output, specific gravity, urinalysis
• **Serious skin reactions:** fever, sore throat, fatigue, ulcers; lesions in mouth, lips, rash; can be fatal
• **CDAD:** diarrhea, fever, abdominal pain/cramping, bloody stools; product should be discontinued, prescriber notified
• **DRESS:** Rash, fever, large lymph nodes, discontinue product if these occur
• To take on an empty stomach 1 hr before or 2 hr after food
Evaluate:
• Therapeutic response: decreased symptoms of TB, culture negative
Teach patient/family:
• That compliance with dosage schedule, duration necessary
• That scheduled appointments must be kept because relapse may occur
• To avoid alcohol because hepatotoxicity may occur
• That urine, feces, saliva, sputum, sweat, tears may be colored red-orange; that soft contact lenses may be permanently stained

• **To report flulike symptoms:** excessive fatigue, anorexia, vomiting, sore throat; unusual bleeding; yellowish discoloration of skin, eyes; diarrhea with pus, mucus, blood
• To use nonhormonal form of birth control; to notify prescriber if pregnancy is planned, suspected; not to breastfeed

---

rifapentine (Rx)
(riff'ah-pen-teen)
Priftin
Func. class.: Antitubercular
Chem. class.: Rifamycin derivative

Do not confuse:
rifapentine/rifAMPin/rifabutin

ACTION: Inhibits DNA-dependent polymerase, decreases tubercle bacilli replication

USES: Pulmonary TB; must be used with at least one other antitubercular agent

CONTRAINDICATIONS: Hypersensitivity to rifamycins, porphyria
Precautions: Pregnancy, breastfeeding, children <12 yr, geriatric patients, hepatic disease, blood dyscrasias, HIV

DOSAGE AND ROUTES
Intensive phase
• **Adult/adolescent >12 yr: PO** 600 mg (four 150-mg tabs) 2×/wk with an interval of 72 hr between doses × 2 mo; must be given with at least 1 other antitubercular agent
Continuation phase
• **Adult/adolescent >12 yr: PO** 600 mg weekly × 4 mo in combination with isoniazid or other appropriate antitubercular product
Available forms: Tabs 150 mg
Administer:
• May give with food for GI upset; use other products for TB
• Antiemetic if vomiting occurs
• After C&S completed; monthly to detect resistance

SIDE EFFECTS

CNS: Headache, fatigue, anxiety, dizziness

EENT: Visual disturbances

GI: *Nausea, vomiting, anorexia, diarrhea,* bilirubinemia, hepatitis, increased ALT, AST, *heartburn,* pancreatitis, CDAD

GU: Hematuria, pyuria, proteinuria, urinary casts, urine discoloration

HEMA: Thrombocytopenia, leukopenia, neutropenia, lymphopenia, anemia, leukocytosis, purpura, hematoma

INTEG: Rash, pruritus, urticaria, acne

MISC: Increased B/P

MS: Gout, arthrosis

PHARMACOKINETICS

Peak 5-6 hr; half-life 13 hr; metabolized in liver (active/inactive metabolites); excreted in urine, feces, breast milk; protein binding 97%; steady state 10 days; CYP450 3A4, 2C8/9 inducer

INTERACTIONS

• Do not use with protease inhibitors

Decrease: action of amitriptyline, anticoagulants, antidiabetics, barbiturates, β-blockers, chloramphenicol, clarithromycin, clofibrate, corticosteroids, cycloSPORINE, dapsone, delavirdine, diazePAM, digoxin, diltiaZEM, disopyramide, doxycycline, fentaNYL, fluconazole, haloperidol, indinavir, itraconazole, ketoconazole, methadone, mexiletine, nelfinavir, NIFEdipine, nortriptyline, oral contraceptives, phenothiazines, phenytoin, progestins, quiNIDine, quiNINE, ritonavir, saquinavir, sildenafil, tacrolimus, theophylline, thyroid preparations, tocainide, verapamil, warfarin, zidovudine

Drug/Food

Increase: absorption with food

Drug/Lab Test

Increase: LFTs, platelets

Decrease: Hgb, WBC

Interference: folate level, vit B_{12}

NURSING CONSIDERATIONS

Assess:

• Baselines of CBC, AST, ALT, bilirubin, platelets

• **Infection:** sputum culture, lung sounds

• Signs of anemia: Hct, Hgb, fatigue

• Hepatic studies monthly: ALT, AST, bilirubin; decreased appetite, jaundice, dark urine, fatigue

• Renal status monthly: BUN, creatinine, output, specific gravity, urinalysis

• **CDAD:** diarrhea, fever, abdominal pain/cramping, bloody diarrhea; discontinue if present, notify prescriber

Evaluate:

• Therapeutic response: decreased symptoms of TB, culture negative

Teach patient/family:

• That compliance with dosage schedule, duration necessary

• That scheduled appointments must be kept because relapse may occur

• That urine, feces, saliva, sputum, sweat, tears may be colored red-orange; that soft contact lenses, dentures may be permanently stained

• **Pregnancy/breastfeeding:** to use alternative method of contraception; that oral contraceptive action may be decreased; to notify prescriber if pregnancy is planned, suspected; to avoid breastfeeding

• **To report flulike symptoms:** excessive fatigue, anorexia, vomiting, sore throat; unusual bleeding, yellowish discoloration of skin, eyes; diarrhea with pus, mucus, blood

---

rifAXIMin (Rx)

(rif-ax'i-min)

Xifaxan, Zaxine ✦

Func. class.: Antiinfective—miscellaneous

Chem. class.: Analog of rifAMPin

Do not confuse:

rifAXIMin/rifAMPin

ACTION: Binds to bacterial-DNA–dependent RNA polymerase, thereby inhibiting bacterial RNA synthesis

USES: Traveler's diarrhea in those ≥12 yr caused by *E. coli,* hepatic encephalopathy, irritable bowel syndrome

Unlabeled uses: Crohn's disease, diverticulitis

Side effects: *italics* = common; red = life-threatening

CONTRAINDICATIONS: Hypersensitivity to product, rifamycins; diarrhea with fever, blood in stool

Precautions: Pregnancy, breastfeeding, children, geriatric patients

DOSAGE AND ROUTES
Traveler's diarrhea
• **Adult/child ≥12 yr: PO** 200 mg tid × 3 days without regard to meals
Hepatic encephalopathy
• **Adult: PO** 550 mg bid
Irritable bowel syndrome
• **Adult: PO** 550 mg tid × 14 days, may give another two courses if recurrence
Crohn's disease (unlabeled)
• **Adult: PO** 200 mg tid × 16 wk
Diverticulitis (unlabeled)
• **Adult: PO** 400 mg bid with mesalamine 800 mg tid × 7 days, then 7 days/mo
Available forms: Tabs 200, 550 mg
Administer:
• Without regard to food

SIDE EFFECTS
CNS: Abnormal dreams, dizziness, insomnia, *headache,* fatigue, depression
CV: Hypotension, chest pain, peripheral edema, ascites
GI: *Abdominal pain, constipation, defecation urgency, flatulence, nausea, rectal tenesmus,* vomiting, ascites, CDAD
GU: Proteinuria, polyuria, increased urinary frequency
MISC: *Pyrexia,* motion sickness, tinnitus, rash, photosensitivity, exfoliative dermatitis
MS: Arthralgia, muscle pain, myalgia
RESP: Dyspnea, cough, pharyngitis

PHARMACOKINETICS
Low systemic absorption, distribution to GI tract, half-life 1.8-4.5 hr, excreted in feces, peak 1-4 hr

INTERACTIONS
Increase: effect of—afatinib
Increase: levels—P-glycoprotein inhibitors
Drug/Lab Test
Increase: LFTs, potassium
Decrease: blood glucose, sodium

NURSING CONSIDERATIONS
Assess:
• GI symptoms: amount, character of diarrhea; abdominal pain, nausea, vomiting, blood in stool; do not use in those with blood in stool, increased temperature with diarrhea
• Overgrowth of infection, CDAD
• **Pregnancy/breastfeeding:** do not use in 1st trimester; use only if benefits outweigh fetal risk; do not breastfeed, excretion unknown
Evaluate:
• Therapeutic response: absence of infection
Teach patient/family:
• To discontinue rifAXIMin, notify prescriber if diarrhea persists >24-48 hr, if diarrhea worsens, or if blood in stools and fever present
• To avoid hazardous activities if dizziness occurs
• To notify prescriber if pregnancy is planned, suspected
• That headache, rash, insomnia, abnormal dreams, tinnitus may occur
• To take without regard to food
• To take as directed, consume all of the product prescribed

---

rilpivirine
Edurant
Func. class.: Antiretroviral
Chem. class.: Nonnucleoside transcriptase inhibitors (NNTIs)

ACTION: Inhibits HIV-1 reverse transcriptase; unlike nucleoside reverse transcriptase inhibitors (NRTIs), it does not compete for binding nor does it require phosphorylation to be active; binds directly to a site on reverse transcriptase, causing disruption of the enzyme's active site and thereby blocking RNA-dependent and DNA-dependent DNA polymerase activities

USES: HIV in combination with other antiretrovirals

CONTRAINDICATIONS: Hypersensitivity

Precautions: Pregnancy, breastfeeding, neonates, infants, children, adolescents <18 yr, immune reconstitution syndrome, antimicrobial resistance, pancreatitis, coinfection hepatitis B or C and HIV, hepatic disease, depression, suicidal ideation, QT prolongation, torsades de pointes, hyperlipidemia, hypertriglyceridemia, hypercholesterolemia, immune reconstitution syndrome

DOSAGE AND ROUTES

• **Adult/child ≥12 yr and ≥35 kg: PO** 25 mg/day with a meal; if used with rifabutin, increase rilpivirine dose to 50 mg/day

Available forms: Tab 25 mg

Administer:

• Give with other antiretroviral agents; in antiretroviral treatment-naive adults, rilpivirine is used as an alternative to efavirenz in NNRTI-based treatment regimens; potential rilpivirine-based treatment regimens combine rilpivirine with either tenofovir plus emtricitabine or lamiVUDine; or abacavir plus emtricitabine or lamiVUDine; or zidovudine plus emtricitabine or lamiVUDine

• Give with a meal

• Store at room temperature away from heat and moisture

SIDE EFFECTS

CNS: Depressed mood, dizziness, drowsiness

GI: Hepatotoxicity

INTEG: Drug reaction with eosinophilia and systemic symptoms (DRESS)

MISC: Immune reconstitution syndrome

PHARMACOKINETICS: Protein binding (99.7%) to albumin; metabolism via oxidation CYP3A; half-life 50 hr, excretion feces (85%), 25% excreted unchanged; urine (6.1%); peak 4-5 hr; increased effect 40% (food), decreased effect 50% (high protein drink)

INTERACTIONS

Increase: rilpivirine effect—CYP3A4 inhibitors (delavirdine, efavirenz, darunavir, tipranavir, atazanavir, fosamprenavir, indinavir, nelfinavir, aldesleukin IL-2, amiodarone aprepitant, basiliximab, boceprevir, bromocriptine, chloramphenicol, clarithromycin, conivaptan, danazol, dalfopristin, dasatinib, diltiaZEM, dronedarone, erythromycin, ethinyl estradiol, fluconazole, FLUoxetine, fluvoxaMINE, fosaprepitant, imatinib, isoniazid, itraconazole, ketoconazole, lanreotide, lapatinib, nefazodone, niCARdipine, octreotide, posaconazole, quiNINE, ranolazine, rifaximin, tamoxifen, telaprevir, telithromycin, troleandomycin, verapamil, voriconazole, zafirlukast)

• **Increase:** QT prolongation—class IA/III antidysrhythmics, some phenothiazines, β-agonists, local anesthetics, tricyclics, chloroquine, droperidol, haloperidol, pentamidine; CYP3A4 inhibitors (amiodarone, clarithromycin, erythromycin, telithromycin, troleandomycin, arsenic trioxide); CYP3A4 substrates (methadone, pimozide, QUEtiapine, quiNIDine, risperiDONE, ziprasidone, lopinavir, saquinavir, fluconazole, posaconazole, dasatinib, dronedarone, lapatinib, octreotide, ranolazine, citalopram, abarelix, alfuzosin, amoxapine, apomorphine, artemether, lumefantrine, asenapine, ofloxacin, ciprofloxacin, cloZAPine, cyclobenzaprine, dolasetron, eriBULin, flecainide, gatifloxacin, gemifloxacin, halogenated anesthetics, iloperidone, levoFLOXacin, maprotiline, mefloquine, moxifloxacin, nilotinib, norfloxacin, OLANZapine, ondansetron, paliperidone, palonosetron, QUEtiapine)

Increase: rilpivirine adverse reactions, fungal infections—fluconazole, voriconazole

Decrease: rilpivirine effect, treatment failure—CYP3A4 inducers (phenytoin, fosphenytoin, barbiturates, OXcarbazepine, carBAMazepine, rifabutin, rifAMPin, rifapentine, dexamethasone) efavirenz, nevirapine, ritonavir; aminoglutethimide, bexarotene, bosentan, griseofulvin, metyraPONE, modafinil, flutamide, nafcillin, pioglitazone, primidone, topiramate; proton pump inhibitors (PPIs)

Decrease: rilpivirine effect, treatment failure—H₂ receptor antagonists (cimetidine, famotidine, nizatidine, raNITIdine), give 12 hr before or 4 hr after rilpivirine

Decrease: rilpivirine effect—antacids, use >2 hr before or 4 hr after rilpivirine

Drug/Herb

Decreased effect—St. John's wort, do not use together

Drug/Food

Increase: adverse reactions—grapefruit juice

NURSING CONSIDERATIONS
Assess:

• **HIV:** Assess symptoms of HIV including opportunistic infections before and during treatment; some may be life-threatening; monitor plasma HIV RNA, CD4+, CD8+ cell counts, serum β-2 microglobulin, serum ICD+24 antigen levels; treatment failures occur more frequently in those with baseline HIV-1 RNA concentrations >100,000 copies/mL than in patients with concentrations <100,000 copies/mL; monitor serum cholesterol, lipid panel; assess for redistribution of body fat

• Antiretroviral drug resistance testing before initiation of therapy in antiretroviral treatment-naive patients

• For adults and adolescents, initiation of antiretroviral therapy is recommended in any patient with a history of an AIDS-defining infection; with a CD4 ≤500/mm³; who is pregnant; who has HIV-associated nephropathy; or who is being treated for hepatitis B (HBV) infection. Only delay treatment for resistance testing

• **Hepatic disease:** monitor for elevated hepatic enzymes (>2.5 × ULN); grade 3 and 4 may be higher in patients coinfected with hepatitis B or C

• **DRESS:** may occur in 2-8 wk, skin eruptions, eosinophilia, lymphadenopathy, fever, inflammation of internal organs; if these occur, stop product, report immediately; systemic steroids are usually given

• **Pregnancy/breastfeeding:** use only if benefits outweigh fetal risk; enroll pregnant women taking this product in the Antiretroviral Pregnancy Registry, 1-800-258-4263; do not breastfeed, excretion unknown

Teach patient/family:

• That product is not a cure but controls symptoms; that continuing use is required

• That product must be taken in combination with other prescribed products; that if dose is missed, not to take if next dose is within 12 hr

• To discuss all products taken, including OTC, Rx, herbals, supplements, as there are many interactions

• To immediately report if pregnancy is suspected; not to breastfeed

• To report immediately mood changes and depression

• To report hypersensitivity reactions

• That dizziness may occur, not to drive until response is known

---

RARELY USED

riluzole (Rx)
(rill'you-zole)
Rilutek
Func. class.: ALS agent
Chem. class.: Benzathiazole

USES: Amyotropic lateral sclerosis (ALS)

CONTRAINDICATIONS: Hypersensitivity

DOSAGE AND ROUTES
• **Adult: PO** 50 mg q12hr; take 1 hr before or 2 hr after meals

---

rimexolone ophthalmic
See Appendix B

---

risedronate (Rx)
(rih-sed'roh-nate)
Actonel, Atelvia, Actonel DR ✦
Func. class.: Bone resorption inhibitor
Chem. class.: Bisphosphonate

Do not confuse:
Actonel/Actos

ACTION: Inhibits bone resorption, absorbs calcium phosphate crystal in bone, and may directly block dissolution of hydroxyapatite crystals of bone

USES: Paget's disease; prevention, treatment of osteoporosis in postmenopausal women; glucocorticoid-induced osteoporosis; osteoporosis in men
Unlabeled uses: Osteolytic metastases

CONTRAINDICATIONS: Hypersensitivity to bisphosphonates, inability to stand or sit upright for ≥30 min, esophageal stricture, achalasia, hypocalcemia
Precautions: Pregnancy, breastfeeding, children, renal disease, active upper GI disorders, dental disease, hyperparathyroidism, infection, vit D deficiency, coagulopathy, chemotherapy, asthma

DOSAGE AND ROUTES
Paget's disease (Actonel)
• **Adult:** PO 30 mg/day × 2 mo; patients with Paget's disease should receive calcium and vit D if dietary intake lacking; if relapse occurs, retreatment advised
Treatment/prevention of postmenopausal osteoporosis
• **Adult:** PO 5 mg/day or 35 mg/wk or 75 mg/day × 2 consecutive days 2× monthly or 150 mg/mo
Glucocorticoid osteoporosis
• **Adult:** PO 5 mg/day
Osteoporosis in men
• **Adult:** PO 35 mg/wk
Osteolytic metastases (unlabeled)
• **Adult:** PO 30 mg/day × 6 mo
Renal dose
• **Adult:** PO CCr <30 mL/min, avoid use
Available forms: Tabs 5, 30, 150 mg; tab, weekly 35 mg
Administer:
• For 2 mo to be effective for Paget's disease
• With a full glass of water; patient should be in upright position for $^1/_2$ hr; swallow whole; do not crush, break, chew, give del rel tablet in AM after breakfast, only use with food (del rel)
• Supplemental calcium and vit D for Paget's disease if instructed by prescriber

• Give daily ≥30 min before meals or give weekly
• Store in cool environment, out of direct sunlight

SIDE EFFECTS
CNS: Dizziness, headache, depression, asthenia, dizziness, insomnia, *weakness*
CV: *Chest pain,* hypertension, atrial fibrillation
GI: *Abdominal pain, diarrhea, nausea,* constipation, esophagitis
MISC: Rash, UTI, pharyngitis, hypocalcemia, hypophosphatemia, increase PTH
MS: Osteonecrosis of the jaw, severe muscle/joint/bone pain, fractures
SYST: Angioedema

PHARMACOKINETICS
Rapidly cleared from circulation, taken up mainly by bones (50%), eliminated primarily through kidneys, absorption decreased by food, terminal half-life 23 hr, delayed release 560 hr

INTERACTIONS
Increase: GI irritation—NSAIDs, salicylates
Decrease: absorption of risedronate—aluminum, calcium, iron, magnesium salts, antacids
Decrease: absorption of del rel risedronate H₂ antagonists, proton pump inhibitors, do not use together
Drug/Food
Decrease: bioavailability—take $^1/_2$ hr before food or drinks other than water
Drug/Lab Test
Decrease: calcium, phosphorus

NURSING CONSIDERATIONS
Assess:
• **Paget's disease:** headache, bone pain, increased head circumference
• **Osteoporosis:** in men or postmenopausal women; bone density study before and periodically during treatment
• Phosphate, alk phos, calcium; creatinine, BUN (renal disease)
• **Hypocalcemia:** paresthesia, twitching, laryngospasm, Chvostek's/Trousseau's signs
• **Serious skin reactions:** angioedema

Side effects: *italics* = common; red = life-threatening

• **Dental health:** provide antiinfectives for dental extraction; cover with antiinfectives before dental extraction
• For atrial fibrillation
• **Pregnancy/breastfeeding:** use only if benefits outweigh fetal risk; do not breastfeed, excretion unknown

Evaluate:
• Therapeutic response: increased bone mass, absence of fractures

Teach patient/family:
• To sit upright for $1/2$ hr after dose to prevent irritation
• To notify prescriber immediately if difficulty swallowing, severe heartburn, or pain in chest
• To comply with diet, vitamin/mineral supplements
• To notify prescriber if pregnancy is suspected or if breastfeeding
• To maintain good oral hygiene
• To notify all health care providers of use
• That musculoskeletal pain may occur within a few days/mo after starting but usually resolves; use acetaminophen
• To exercise regularly; to avoid alcohol, tobacco

---

risperiDONE (Rx)

(ris-pehr'ih-dohn)

RisperDAL, RisperDAL Consta, RisperDAL M-TAB

Func. class.: Antipsychotic
Chem. class.: Benzisoxazole derivative

Do not confuse:
RisperDAL/reserpine

ACTION: Unknown; may be mediated through both dopamine type 2 (D_2) and serotonin type 2 ($5\text{-}HT_2$) antagonism

USES: Irritability associated with autism, bipolar disorder, mania, schizophrenia
Unlabeled uses: Acute psychosis, agitation, ADHD, dementia, psychotic depression, Tourette's syndrome

CONTRAINDICATIONS: Hypersensitivity, breastfeeding

Precautions: Pregnancy, children, geriatric patients, cardiac/renal/hepatic disease, breast cancer, Parkinson's disease, CNS depression, brain tumor, dehydration, diabetes, hematologic disease, seizure disorders, abrupt discontinuation, suicidal ideation, phenylketonuria

Black Box Warning: Increased mortality in elderly patients with dementia-related psychosis

DOSAGE AND ROUTES
• **Adult:** PO 2 mg/day as single dose or in 2 divided doses, adjust dose at intervals of ≥24 hr and 1-2 mg/day as tolerated to 4-8 mg/day; **IM** establish dosing with **PO** before **IM** 25 mg q2wk, may increase to max 50 mg q2wk
• **Adolescent:** PO 0.5 mg/day in AM or PM, adjust dose at intervals of ≥24 hr and 0.5-1 mg/day as tolerated to 3 mg/day
• **Geriatric:** PO 0.5 mg daily-bid, increase by 1 mg/wk; **IM** 25 mg q2wk

Hepatic/renal dose
• **Adult:** PO 0.5 mg bid, increase by 0.5 mg bid, increase to 1.5 mg bid at intervals ≥1 wk

Available forms: Tabs 0.25, 0.5, 1, 2, 3, 4 mg; oral sol 1 mg/mL; orally disintegrating tabs 0.25, 0.5, 1, 2, 3, 4 mg; long-acting inj kit (Risperdal Consta) 12.5, 25, 37.5, 50 mg

Administer:
• Reduced dose in geriatric patients
• Anticholinergic agent on order from prescriber, to be used for EPS
• Avoid use with CNS depressants
• Conventional tabs: give without regard to meals
• **Oral disintegrating tab** (Risperdal M-TAB): do not open blister pack until ready to use; tear at perforation; bend; peel back foil; do not push tab through foil; remove from pack and place product on patient's tongue; tab disintegrates in seconds and can be swallowed with/without liquids, do not split or chew
• **Oral sol:** May dilute 3-4 oz of beverage, measure dose using calibrated pipette;

not compatible with tea, cola; compatible with water, coffee, orange juice, low-fat milk

IM route

Preparation

• Only use diluent and needle provided

• Allow to come to room temperature for 30 min

• Remove colored cap from the vial without removing the gray rubber stopper; wipe top of stopper with an alcohol wipe

• Peel back the blister pouch and remove the Vial Access Device by holding between the white Luer cap and the skirt; do not touch the spike tip at any time

• Place the vial on a hard surface and hold the base; orient the Vial Access Device vertically over the vial so that the spike tip is at the center of the vial's rubber stopper

• With a straight downward push, press the spike tip of the Vial Access Device through the center of the vial's rubber stopper until the device securely snaps onto the vial top

• Hold the base of the vial and swab the syringe connection point (blue circle) of the Vial Access Device with an alcohol wipe and allow to dry before attaching the syringe

• While holding the white collar of the syringe, insert and press the syringe tip into the blue circle of the Vial Access Device and twist clockwise

• Inject the entire contents of the syringe containing the diluent into the vial

• Shake the vial vigorously; suspension should appear uniform, thick, and milky colored, and all the powder is dispersed in liquid; the microspheres will be visible in liquid, but no dry microspheres remain

• Invert completely and slowly withdraw the contents of the suspension from the vial into the syringe; tear the section of the vial label at the perforation and apply the detached label to the syringe

• While holding the white collar of the syringe, unscrew the syringe from the Vial Access Device, then discard both the vial and the Vial Access Device appropriately

• Select the appropriate color-coded needle provided with the kit; they are not interchangeable; do not use the needle intended for gluteal injection for deltoid injection, and vice versa

• Peel the blister pouch of the Needle-Pro safety device open halfway; grasp the transparent needle using the pouch, attach the Luer connection of the orange Needle-Pro to the syringe with an easy clockwise twisting motion

• While holding the white collar of the syringe, grasp the transparent needle sheath and seat the needle firmly on the orange Needle-Pro device with a push and a clockwise twist

• Pull the transparent needle sheath straight away from the needle

• Resuspension is necessary before administration

• Only for IM; do not give IV

• Remove air bubbles

• Inject the entire contents of the syringe into the upper outer quadrant of the gluteal or deltoid muscle; inject immediately after reconstitution; gluteal injections should be alternated between the two buttocks

• After the injection is complete, press the needle into the orange Needle-Pro safety device

• Do not store the vial after reconstitution or the suspension will settle

• Do not combine 2 different dosage strengths of RisperDAL Consta in a single administration

• The dose pack device is for single use only

Stability after reconstitution:

Once in suspension, the product may remain at room temperature; use within 6 hr

SIDE EFFECTS

CNS: *EPS, pseudoparkinsonism, akathisia, dystonia, tardive dyskinesia; drowsiness, insomnia, agitation, anxiety, headache,* seizures, neuroleptic malignant syndrome, dizziness, suicidal ideation, head titubation (shaking)

CV: Orthostatic hypotension, tachycardia, heart failure, sudden death (geriatric patients), AV block

R

Side effects: *italics* = common; red = life-threatening

EENT: Blurred vision, tinnitus

GI: *Nausea,* vomiting, *anorexia, constipation,* jaundice, weight gain

GU: Hyperprolactinemia, gynecomastia, dysuria

HEMA: Neutropenia, granulocytopenia

MISC: Renal artery occlusion; hyperprolactinemia (child)

MS: Rhabdomyolysis

RESP: Rhinitis, sinusitis, upper respiratory infection, cough

PHARMACOKINETICS

PO: Extensively metabolized by liver to major active metabolite, ⚕ determined by poor metabolizer or average metabolizers; plasma protein binding 90%, peak 1-2 hr, excreted 90% in urine, terminal half-life 3-24 hr

INTERACTIONS

Increase: seizures—traMADol

Increase: possible death in dementia-related psychosis: furosemide

Increase: sedation—other CNS depressants, alcohol

Increase: serotonin syndrome, neuroleptic malignant syndrome—CYP2D6 inhibitors (SSRIs, SNRIs)

Increase: EPS—other antipsychotics

Increase: risperiDONE excretion—carBAMazepine

Increase: QT prolongation—class IA/III antidysrhythmics, some phenothiazines, β-agonists, local anesthetics, tricyclics, haloperidol, methadone, chloroquine, clarithromycin, droperidol, erythromycin, pentamidine, thioridazine, ziprasidone

Increase: risperiDONE levels—acetylcholinesterase inhibitors, CYP2D6 inhibitors, SSRIs, valproic acid, verapamil

Decrease: risperiDONE action—CYP2D6 inducers (carBAMazepine, barbiturates, phenytoins, rifAMPin)

Decrease: levodopa effect—levodopa

Drug/Herb

Decrease: risperiDONE effect—echinacea

Drug/Lab Test

Increase: prolactin levels, blood, glucose, lipids

NURSING CONSIDERATIONS

Assess:

• **Suicidal thoughts/behaviors:** often when depression is lessened; mental status before initial administration

• Thyroid function test, blood glucose, serum electrolytes/prolactin/lipid profile, bilirubin, creatinine, weight, pregnancy test, CBC, LFTs, AIMS assessment, baseline and periodically

• Affect, orientation, LOC, reflexes, gait, coordination, sleep pattern disturbances

• **QT prolongation:** B/P standing, lying; pulse, respirations; take these q4hr during initial treatment; establish baseline before starting treatment; report drops of 30 mm Hg; watch for ECG changes

• Dizziness, faintness, palpitations, tachycardia on rising

• **EPS:** akathisia, tardive dyskinesia (bizarre movements of the jaw, mouth, tongue, extremities), pseudoparkinsonism (rigidity, tremors, pill rolling, shuffling gait)

• **Serious reactions in geriatric patient:** fatal pneumonia, heart failure, sudden death, dementia

• **Neuroleptic malignant syndrome:** hyperthermia, increased CPK, altered mental status, muscle rigidity, seizures, change in B/P, fatigue, tachycardia

• Constipation, urinary retention daily; if these occur, increase bulk, water in diet

• Decreased stimuli by dimming lights, avoiding loud noises

• Supervised ambulation until patient stabilized on medication; do not involve patient in strenuous exercise program because fainting is possible; patient should not stand still for a long time

• Increased fluids to prevent constipation

• Store in tight, light-resistant container (PO); unopened vials in refrigerator, protect from light; do not freeze

• **Beers:** avoid use in older adults except for schizophrenia, bipolar disorder, or as a short-term antiemetic in chemotherapy

• **Pregnancy/breastfeeding:** use only if benefits outweigh fetal risk; EPS may occur in neonate; enroll pregnant women in the National Pregnancy Registry for Atypical Antipsychotics, 1-866-961-2388; do not breastfeed, excreted in breast milk

Evaluate:

• Therapeutic response: decrease in emotional excitement, hallucinations, delusions, paranoia; reorganization of patterns of thought, speech

Teach patient/family:

• That orthostatic hypotension may occur; to rise from sitting or lying position gradually

• To avoid abrupt withdrawal of product because EPS may result; product should be withdrawn slowly

• To avoid OTC preparations (cough, hay fever, cold) unless approved by prescriber; that serious product interactions may occur; to avoid use of alcohol because increased drowsiness may occur

• To avoid hazardous activities if drowsy or dizzy

• To comply with product regimen

• To report impaired vision, tremors, muscle twitching

• That heat stroke may occur in hot weather; to take extra precautions to stay cool; to avoid hot tubs, hot showers, tub baths

• To use contraception; to inform prescriber if pregnancy is planned or suspected; not to breastfeed

• To notify provider of suicidal thoughts/behaviors

TREATMENT OF OVERDOSE:
Lavage if orally ingested; provide airway; *do not induce vomiting*

---

ritonavir (Rx)

(ri-toe′na-veer)

Norvir

Func. class.: Antiretroviral
Chem. class.: Protease inhibitor

Do not confuse:
ritonavir/Retrovir

ACTION: Inhibits human immunodeficiency virus (HIV-1) protease and prevents maturation of the infectious virus

USES: HIV-1 in combination with at least 2 other antiretrovirals

CONTRAINDICATIONS: Hypersensitivity

> **Black Box Warning:** Coadministration with other drugs

Precautions: Pregnancy, breastfeeding, hepatic disease, pancreatitis, diabetes, hemophilia, AV block, hypercholesterolemia, immune reconstitution syndrome, neonates, cardiomyopathy, immune reconstitution syndrome, infants 1-6 mo (overdose)

DOSAGE AND ROUTES

• **Adult/adolescent >16 yr: PO** 600 mg bid; if nausea occurs, begin at $1/2$ dose and gradually increase, max 1200 mg/day in divided doses

• **Adolescent ≤16 yr/child/infant: PO** 250 mg/m² bid; increase by 50 mg/m² bid q2-3days, to a maintenance of 350-400 mg bid; max 600 mg bid

Available forms: Caps 100 mg; oral sol 80 mg/mL; tab 100 mg

Administer:

Tablet/capsule

• Take with food, swallow whole; do not crush, break, chew

• When switching from cap to tab, more GI symptoms may occur, will lessen over time

• Use dosage titration to minimize side effects

• Store caps in refrigerator

• **Oral sol:** shake well, use calibrated measuring device

• Mix liquid formulation with chocolate milk or liquid nutritional supplement to improve taste

• **Overdose:** infants, children, 43.2% alcohol, 26.57% propylene glycol oral sol, calculate total amount of alcohol, propylene glycol from all products given

SIDE EFFECTS

CNS: *Paresthesia, headache,* seizures, fever, dizziness, insomnia, asthenia, intracranial bleeding

---

Side effects: *italics* = common; red = life-threatening

CV: QT, PR interval prolongation

GI: *Diarrhea,* buccal mucosa ulceration, *abdominal pain, nausea, taste perversion,* dry mouth, *vomiting, anorexia,* pancreatitis, pseudomembranous colitis, hepatitis

INTEG: Rash

MISC: Asthenia, angioedema, anaphylaxis, Stevens-Johnson syndrome, increase lipids, lipodystrophy, toxic epidermal necrolysis, immune reconstitution syndrome

MS: Pain, rhabdomyolysis, myalgia

HEMA: Leukopenia, thrombocytopenia

PHARMACOKINETICS

Well absorbed, 98% protein binding, hepatic metabolism, peak 2-4 hr, terminal half-life 3-5 hr

INTERACTIONS

Black Box Warning: Increase: toxicity—amiodarone, astemizole, azole antifungals, benzodiazepines, buPROPion, CISapride, cloZAPine, desipramine, dihydroergotamine, encainide, ergotamine, flecainide, HMG-CoA reductase inhibitors, interleukins, meperidine, midazolam, pimozide, piroxicam, propafenone, propoxyphene, quiNIDine, ranolazine, saquinavir, terfenadine, triazolam, zolpidem; CYP2D6 inhibitors

Black Box Warning: Increase: QT prolongation—class IA/III antidysrhythmics, some phenothiazines, β-agonists, local anesthetics, tricyclics, haloperidol, chloroquine, droperidol, pentamidine, CYP3A4 inhibitors (amiodarone, clarithromycin, dasatinib, erythromycin, telithromycin, troleandomycin), arsenic trioxide, CYP3A4 substrates (methadone, pimozide, QUEtiapine, quiNIDine, risperiDONE, ziprasidone)

Increase: ritonavir levels—fluconazole

Increase: level of both products—clarithromycin, ddI

Increase: levels of—bosentan

Decrease: ritonavir levels—rifamycins, nevirapine, barbiturates, phenytoin

Decrease: levels of anticoagulants, atovaquone, divalproex, ethinyl estradiol, lamoTRIgine, phenytoin, sulfamethoxazole, theophylline, voriconazole, zidovudine

Drug/Herb

Decrease: ritonavir levels—St. John's wort; avoid concurrent use

• Avoid use with red yeast rice

Drug/Lab Test

Increase: AST, ALT, K, CK, cholesterol, GGT, triglycerides, uric acid

Decrease: Hct, Hgb, RBC, neutrophils, WBC

NURSING CONSIDERATIONS

Assess:

• **HIV:** viral load, CD4 at baseline, throughout therapy; blood glucose, plasma HIV RNA, serum cholesterol/lipid profile; resistance testing before starting therapy and after treatment failure

• **Immune reconstitution syndrome:** may occur with combination therapy; may develop inflammatory response with opportunistic infection (MAC, Graves' disease, Guillain-Barré syndrome, TB, PCP); may occur during initial treatment or months after

• Signs of anemia, anemia

• Hepatic studies: ALT, AST in those with hepatic disease, monitor q3mo

• Bowel pattern before, during treatment; if severe abdominal pain with bleeding occurs, discontinue product; monitor hydration

• Skin eruptions; rash

• **Rhabdomyolysis:** muscle pain, increased CPK, weakness, swelling of affected muscles, dark urine; if these occur and if confirmed by CPK, product should be discontinued

• **QT prolongation:** ECG for QT prolongation, ejection fraction; assess for chest pain, palpitations, dyspnea

• **Serious skin disorders:** Stevens-Johnson syndrome, angioedema, anaphylaxis, toxic epidermal necrolysis

• **Pregnancy/breastfeeding:** use only if benefits outweigh fetal risk; enroll pregnant women in the Antiretroviral Pregnancy Registry, 1-800-258-4263; do not breastfeed

Evaluate:
• Therapeutic response: improvement in HIV symptoms; improving viral load, CD4+ T cells

Teach patient/family:
• To take as prescribed; if dose is missed, to take as soon as remembered up to 1 hr before next dose; not to double dose
• That product not a cure for HIV; that opportunistic infections may continue to be acquired
• That redistribution of body fat or accumulation of body fat may occur
• That others may continue to contract HIV from patient

> Black Box Warning: To avoid OTC, prescription medications, herbs, supplements unless approved by prescriber; not to use St. John's wort because it decreases product's effect

• That regular follow-up exams and blood work will be required

---

⚠ HIGH ALERT

riTUXimab (Rx)
(rih-tuks′ih-mab)
Rituxan
Func. class.: Antineoplastic—miscellaneous; DMARDs
Chem. class.: Murine/human monoclonal antibody

ACTION: Directed against the CD20 antigen that is found on malignant B lymphocytes; CD20 regulates a portion of cell-cycle initiation/differentiation

USES: ✱ Non-Hodgkin's lymphoma (CD20+, B-cell), bulky disease (tumors >10 cm), rheumatoid arthritis, Wegener's granulomatosis, microscopic polyangiitis
Unlabeled uses: Acquired blood factor deficiency, acute lymphocytic leukemia (ALL), Burkitt's lymphoma, chronic lymphocytic leukemia (CLL), hemolytic anemia, human herpesvirus 8, mantle cell lymphoma (MCL), multicentric Castleman's disease, peripheral blood stem cell (PBSC) mobilization, refractory pemphigus vulgaris, relapsing/remitting MS, ITP with dexamethasone, steroid refractory chronic graft-versus-host disease

CONTRAINDICATIONS: Hypersensitivity, murine proteins
Precautions: Pregnancy, breastfeeding, children, geriatric patients, pulmonary/cardiac/renal conditions

> Black Box Warning: Exfoliative dermatitis, infusion-related reactions, progressive multifocal leukoencephalopathy, hepatitis B exacerbation

DOSAGE AND ROUTES
Relapsed or refractory low-grade or follicular, CD20+, B-cell non-Hodgkin's lymphoma (NHL)
• **Adult: IV** 375 mg/m^2/wk × 4 doses, may re-treat with 4 more doses of 375 mg/m^2/wk
First-line treatment of follicular, CD20+, B-cell NHL in combination with chemotherapy
• **Adult: IV** 375 mg/m^2 on day 1 of each cycle for up to 8 cycles; may be given with cyclophosphamide **IV** 750 mg/m^2 on day 1, vinCRIStine **IV** 1.4 mg/m^2 (max 2 mg) on day 1, and predniSONE 40 mg/m^2/day **PO** on days 1-5
Single-agent maintenance therapy
• **Adult: IV** 375 mg/m^2 every 8 wk × 12 doses as maintenance therapy starting 8 wk after the completion of induction chemotherapy with 8 doses of riTUXimab with 6-8 cycles of cyclophosphamide, vinCRIStine, and predniSONE; 4-6 cycles of cyclophosphamide, DOXOrubicin, vinCRIStine, and predniSONE
Component of the Zevalin (ibritumomab tiuxetan) regimen
• **Adult: IV** As a required component of the ibritumomab regimen; riTUXimab 250 mg/m^2 given within 4 hr before administration of Yttrium-90 ibritumomab that may occur on day 7, 8, or 9

R

First-line treatment of diffuse large B-cell, CD20+ NHL
• **Adult 18-59 yr:** IV 375 mg/m^2 on day 1 of each cycle for up to 8 infusions

Single-agent maintenance therapy in patients with low-grade, CD20+, B-cell NHL
• **Adult:** IV 375 mg/m^2/wk × 4 wk repeated q6mo × 2 yr (total of 16 doses) as maintenance therapy starting 4 wk after the completion of first-line chemotherapy with 6-8 cycles of cyclophosphamide, vinCRIStine, and predniSONE (CVP)

GPA/MPA
• **Adult:** IV 375 mg/m^2 weekly × 4 wk

Rheumatoid arthritis
• **Adult:** IV infusion 1000 mg initially, the other dose in 2 wk

Available forms: Inj 10 mg/mL (100 mg/10 mL, 500 mg/50 mL)

Administer:
Rheumatoid arthritis:
  Give methylPREDNISolone 100 mg or similar product 30 min before infusion to decrease reactions

Intermittent IV INFUSION route
• Hold antihypertensives 12 hr before administration
• After diluting to final concentration of 1-4 mg/mL; use 0.9% NaCl, D$_5$W, gently invert bag to mix; do not mix with other products; give 50 mg/hr initially; if no reaction, increase rate by 50 mg/hr to max 400 mg/hr
• Store vials at 36° F-40° F; protect vials from direct sunlight; infusion sol is stable at 36° F-46° F × 24 hr and at room temperature for another 12 hr

Y-site compatibilities: Acyclovir, amifostine, amikacin, aminophylline, ampicillin, ampicillin/sulbactam, aztreonam, bleomycin, bumetanide, buprenorphine, busulfan, butorphanol, calcium gluconate, CARBOplatin, carmustine, ceFAZolin, cefoperazone, cefotaxime, cefoTEtan, cefOXitin, cefTAZidime, ceftizoxime, cefTRIAXone, cefuroxime, chlorproMAZINE, cimetidine, CISplatin, clindamycin, cyclophosphamide, cytarabine, DACTINomycin, DAUNOrubicin hydrochloride, dexamethasone, dexrazoxane, digoxin, diphenhydrAMINE, DOBUTamine, DOCEtaxel, DOPamine, DOXOrubicin liposome, doxycycline, droperidol, enalaprilat, etoposide phosphate, famotidine, fentaNYL, filgrastim, floxuridine, fluconazole, fludarabine, fluorouracil, ganciclovir, gemcitabine, gentamicin, granisetron, haloperidol, heparin, hydrocortisone, HYDROmorphone, IDArubicin, ifosfamide, imipenem/cilastatin, irinotecan, leucovorin, levorphanol, LORazepam, magnesium sulfate, mannitol, meperidine, mesna, methotrexate, methylPREDNISolone, metoclopramide, metroNIDAZOLE, mitoMYcin, mitoXANTRONE, morphine, nalbuphine, netilmicin, PACLitaxel, pentamidine, piperacillin/tazobactam, plicamycin, potassium chloride, prochlorperazine, promethazine, ranitidine, sargramostim, streptozocin, teniposide, theophylline, thiotepa, ticarcillin/clavulanate, tobramycin, trimethoprim/sulfamethoxazole, trimethobenzamide, vinBLAStine, vinCRIStine, vinorelbine, zidovudine

SIDE EFFECTS
CNS: Life-threatening brain infection (progressive multifocal leukoencephalopathy)

CV: Cardiac dysrhythmias, heart failure, hypertension, MI, supraventricular tachycardia, angina

GI: *Nausea, vomiting, anorexia,* GI obstruction/perforation

GU: Renal failure

HEMA: Leukopenia, neutropenia, thrombocytopenia, anemia

INTEG: *Irritation at site, rash,* fatal mucocutaneous infections (rare)

MISC: *Fever,* chills, asthenia, *headache,* angioedema, hypotension, myalgia, bronchospasm, ARDs

SYST: Toxic epidermal necrolysis, tumor lysis syndrome, Stevens-Johnson syndrome, exfoliative dermatitis

META: Hyperkalemia, hypocalcemia, hyperphosphatemia

PHARMACOKINETICS
Half-life varies, binds to CD20 sites or lymphoma cells

INTERACTIONS

Increase: hypotension—antihypertensives, separate by 12 hr

Increase: nephrotoxicity—CISplatin, avoid concurrent use; if used, monitor renal status

Increase: bleeding—anticoagulant

• Avoid with vaccines, toxoids

NURSING CONSIDERATIONS
Assess:

Black Box Warning: Fatal infusion reaction: hypoxia, pulmonary infiltrates, ARDS, MI, ventricular fibrillation, cardiogenic shock; most fatal reactions occur with 1st infusion; potentially fatal

Black Box Warning: Severe mucocutaneous reactions: Stevens-Johnson syndrome, lichenoid dermatitis, toxic epidermal lysis; occur 1-13 wk after product given, discontinue treatment immediately

Black Box Warning: Tumor lysis syndrome: acute renal failure requiring hemodialysis, hyperkalemia, hypocalcemia, hyperuricemia, hyperphosphatemia; allopurinol and adequate hydration may be needed

Black Box Warning: Multifocal leukoencephalopathy: confusion, dizziness, lethargy, hemiparesis; monitor periodically

• **Bone marrow suppression:** CBC, differential, platelet count weekly; withhold product if WBC is <3500/mm^3 or platelet count <100,000/mm^3; notify prescriber of results; product should be discontinued

• ECG, serum creatinine/BUN, electrolytes, uric acid; correct electrolyte imbalances before use; hyperkalemia, hypocalcemia, hyperphosphatemia often occur

• GI symptoms: frequency of stools, abdominal pain, perforation/obstruction may occur

• **Infection:** fever, increased temperature, flulike symptoms in those with Wegener's granulomatosis and microscopic polyangiitis in those using DMARDs

Black Box Warning: Hepatitis B exacerbation: fulminant hepatitis, hepatic failure, death may occur during or following treatment; screen all patients for HBV infection (HBV/HBsAg and anti-HB$_c$ titers) before use; monitor those with current or prior HBV for signs of hepatitis or for HBV reactivation for several months after therapy; if reactivation occurs, discontinue product

• **Pregnancy/breastfeeding:** use only if benefits outweigh fetal risk; contraception should be used; enroll pregnant women in the Mother To Baby Autoimmune Diseases in Pregnancy Study, 1-877-311-8972 (patients with RA); do not breastfeed, excretion unknown

Evaluate:

• Therapeutic response: prevention of increasing cancer progression

Teach patient/family:

• To avoid use with vaccines, toxoids

• To use contraception during and for up to 12 mo after therapy

• To report to prescriber possible infection (cough, fever, chills, sore throat), renal issues (painful urination, back/side pain), bleeding (gums, stools, urine, bruising, emesis, fatigue)

• To avoid OTC products

• To avoid crowds, those with known infections

• To increase fluid intake

⚠ HIGH ALERT

rivaroxaban

Xarelto

Func. class.: Anticoagulant
Chem. class.: Factor Xa inhibitor

ACTION: A novel oral anticoagulant that selectively and potently inhibits coagulation factor Xa

---

Side effects: *italics* = common; red = life-threatening

USES: For deep venous thrombosis (DVT) prophylaxis/treatment, pulmonary embolism (PE), in patients undergoing knee or hip replacement surgery; for stroke prophylaxis and systemic embolism prophylaxis in patients with nonvalvular atrial fibrillation

CONTRAINDICATIONS
Severe hypersensitivity

Black Box Warning: Active bleeding

Precautions: Pregnancy, breastfeeding, neonates, infants, children, adolescents, geriatric patients, moderate or severe hepatic disease (Child-Pugh Class B or C), hepatic disease associated with coagulopathy, creatinine clearance <30 mL/min for use as DVT prophylaxis and <15 mL/min for stroke and systemic embolism prophylaxis in nonvalvular atrial fibrillation, dental procedures, aneurysm, diabetes retinopathy, diverticulitis, endocarditis, GI bleeding, hypertension, obstetric delivery, peptic ulcer disease, stroke, surgery

Black Box Warning: Abrupt discontinuation, epidermal/spinal anesthesia

Patients, especially those with dental disease, should be instructed in proper oral hygiene, including caution in use of regular toothbrushes, dental floss, toothpicks

DOSAGE AND ROUTES
DVT prophylaxis (knee or hip replacement)
• **Adult: PO** 10 mg/day × 12 days after knee replacement surgery or × 35 days after hip replacement; administer the initial dose ≥6-10 hr after surgery once hemostasis has been established
DVT/PE treatment/reduction of risk
• **Adult: PO** 15 mg bid with food × 21 days, then 20 mg daily for a total of 6 mo, may continue after 6 mo to reduce risk
Stroke prophylaxis and systemic embolism prophylaxis (with nonvalvular atrial fibrillation)
• **Adult: PO** 20 mg/day with evening meal (CrCl >50 mL/min)

Converting from warfarin to rivaroxaban
• Discontinue warfarin and start rivaroxaban when INR is <3
Converting from another anticoagulant other than warfarin to rivaroxaban
• Start rivaroxaban 0-2 hr before the next scheduled evening administration of anticoagulant (omit that dose of anticoagulant); for continuous infusion of unfractionated heparin, stop the infusion and initiate rivaroxaban simultaneously
Converting from rivaroxaban to another anticoagulant with rapid onset (not warfarin)
• Discontinue rivaroxaban and give the first dose of the other anticoagulant (oral or parenteral) at the time that the next dose of rivaroxaban would have been administered
Hepatic dose
• **Adult: PO** Child-Pugh class B or C: avoid use
Renal dose
• **Adult: PO** (nonvalvular atrial fibrillation) CCr 15-50 mL/min 15 mg daily; CCr <15 mL/min avoid use; (treatment/prophylaxis of DVT/pulmonary embolism) CCr <30 mL/min avoid use

Available forms: Tabs 10, 15, 20 mg
Administer:
• **For DVT prophylaxis:** give daily without regard to food; give initial dose ≥6-10 hr after surgery when hemostasis has been established
• **For stroke/systemic embolism prophylaxis:** give daily with evening meal
• If dose is not given at correct time, give as soon as possible on the same day
• 15-, 20-mg tabs should be taken with food; for those unable to swallow whole, tabs may be crushed, mixed with applesauce; immediately following administration, instruct to eat; crushed tabs are stable in applesauce for up to 4 hr
• 10-mg tab can be taken without regard to food; all doses ≥15 mg should be given with food
Nasogastric (NG) tube or gastric feeding tube:
• Confirm gastric placement of tube

• Crush 15- or 20-mg tab, suspend in 50 mL of water, and administer via NG or gastric feeding tube

• To minimize reduced absorption, avoid administration distal to the stomach

• Enteral feeding should immediately follow administration of a crushed dose

• Crushed tabs are stable in water for up to 4 hr

Missed doses

• Patients receiving 15 mg twice daily should take their missed dose immediately to ensure intake of 30 mg per day; two 15-mg tabs may be taken at once followed by the regular 15 mg twice daily dose the next day

• For patients receiving once-daily dosing, take the missed dose as soon as it is remembered

• Store at room temperature

SIDE EFFECTS

GI: Increased hepatic enzymes, hyperbilirubinemia, jaundice, nausea, cholestasis, cytolytic hepatitis

HEMA: Bleeding, intracranial bleeding, epidural hematoma, GI bleeding, retinal hemorrhage, adrenal bleeding, retroperitoneal hemorrhage, cerebral hemorrhage, subdural hematoma, epidural hematoma, hemiparesis, thrombocytopenia

INTEG: Pruritus, blister, hypersensitivity, anaphylactic reaction, anaphylactic shock

SYST: Stevens-Johnson syndrome

PHARMACOKINETICS

Bioavailability 80%-100%, protein binding (92%-95%) albumin, excreted in urine 66% (36% unchanged, 30% metabolites), 28% in feces (7% unchanged, 21% metabolites), unchanged drug excreted in urine (via active tubular secretion, glomerular filtration); terminal elimination half-life 5-9 hr, peak 2-4 hr; increased effect in hepatic/renal disease, Japanese patients, increased terminal half-life in geriatric patients

INTERACTIONS

Increase: rivaroxaban effect, possible bleeding—ketoconazole itraconazole, ritonavir, lopinavir/ritonavir; conivaptan, clarithromycin, erythromycin, salicylates, NSAIDs, other anticoagulants, thrombolytics, platelet inhibitors, niCARdipine, fluconazole

Decrease: rivaroxaban effect—carBAMazepine, phenytoin, rifAMPin

Increase: rivaroxaban effect in renal impairment—telithromycin, darunavir, miFEPRIStone, nelfinavir, pantoprazole, posaconazole, saquinavir, tamoxifen, lapatinib, azithromycin, diltiaZEM, verapamil, quiNIDine, ranolazine, dronedarone, amiodarone, felodipine

Drug/Herb

Decrease: rivaroxaban effect—St. John's wort

Drug/Food

Increase: rivaroxaban effect in renal disease—grapefruit juice

NURSING CONSIDERATIONS
Assess:

Black Box Warning: **Bleeding:** monitor for bleeding, including bleeding during dental procedures (easy bruising, blood in urine, stools, emesis, sputum, epistaxis); there is no specific antidote

Black Box Warning: **Abrupt discontinuation:** avoid abrupt discontinuation unless an alternative anticoagulant in those with atrial fibrillation; discontinuing puts patients at an increased risk of thrombotic events; if product must be discontinued for reasons other than pathological bleeding, consider administering another anticoagulant

Black Box Warning: **Epidural/spinal anesthesia:** epidural or spinal hematomas that result in long-term or permanent paralysis may occur in patients who have received anticoagulants and are receiving neuraxial anesthesia or undergoing spinal puncture; epidural catheter should not be removed <18 hr after the last dose of rivaroxaban; do not administer the next rivaroxaban dose <6 hr after the catheter removal; delay rivaroxaban administration for 24 hr if traumatic puncture occurs; monitor for neuro changes

• **Hepatic/renal disease:** increase in effect of product in hepatic disease (Child-Pugh class B or C), hepatic disease with coagulopathy; renal failure/severe renal impairment (creatinine clearance <30 mL/min in DVT prophylaxis and <15 mL/min for stroke or systemic embolism prophylaxis in nonvalvular atrial fibrillation); product should be discontinued in acute renal failure; reduce dose in those with atrial fibrillation and CrCl 15-50 mL/min; monitor renal function periodically (creatinine clearance, BUN)

• **Beers:** avoid use in older adults with CCr <30 mL/min; reduce dose in CCr 30-50 mL/min

• **Pregnancy/breastfeeding:** use only if benefits outweigh fetal risk; do not breastfeed, excretion unknown; pregnancy-related hemorrhage may occur

Evaluate:

• Prevention of DVT, stroke, and systemic embolism

Teach patient/family:

• To report if pregnancy is planned or suspected; not to breastfeed

Black Box Warning: To report bleeding (bruising, blood in urine, stools, sputum, emesis, heavy menstrual flow); use soft toothbrush, electric shaver

• To inform all health care providers of use; to report to prescriber all products used; to take all medication for the duration, exactly as prescribed to prevent clots; to notify prescriber if unable to take so that a different anticoagulant may be used

Black Box Warning: To avoid abrupt discontinuation without another blood thinner

• To report numbness of extremities, weakness, tingling, contact prescriber immediately (neuraxial anesthesia, spinal puncture)

rivastigmine (Rx)

(riv-as-tig′mine)
Exelon, Exelon Patch
Func. class.: Anti-Alzheimer agent
Chem. class.: Cholinesterase inhibitor

ACTION: Potent, selective inhibitor of brain acetylcholinesterase (AChE) and butyrylcholinesterase (BChE)

USES: Mild to severe Alzheimer's dementia, mild to moderate Parkinson's disease dementia (PDD)

Unlabeled uses: Vascular dementia, dementia with Lewy bodies, Pick's disease

CONTRAINDICATIONS: Hypersensitivity to this product, other carbamates

Precautions: Pregnancy, breastfeeding, children, respiratory/cardiac/renal/hepatic disease, seizure disorder, peptic ulcer, urinary obstruction, asthma, increased intracranial pressure, surgery, GI bleeding, jaundice

DOSAGE AND ROUTES

• **Adult:** PO 1.5 mg bid with food; after ≥4 wk, may increase to 3 mg bid; may increase to 4.5 mg bid and thereafter 6 mg bid, max 12 mg/day; **TRANSDERMAL** apply 4.6 mg/24 hr/day, after ≥4 wk may increase to 9.5 mg/24 hr/day; max 13.3 mg/24 hr; for those using 6-12 mg/day **PO** and switching to transdermal use one 9.5 mg/24 hr daily, for those using <6 mg/day **PO** and switching to transdermal use one 4.6 mg/24 hr daily

Available forms: Caps 1.5, 3, 4.5, 6 mg; transdermal patch 4.6, 9.5, 13.3 mg/24 hr

Administer:

• With meals; take with morning and evening meal even though absorption may be decreased

• If adverse reactions cause intolerance, discontinue treatment for several doses; restart at same or next lower dosage level

• If treatment is interrupted for more than several days, treatment should be initiated with lowest daily dose and titrated as indicated previously

Transdermal route

• Once a day to hairless, clean, dry skin, not in an area that clothing will rub; rotate sites daily; do not apply to same site more than once q14days; remove liner; apply firmly; may be used during bathing, swimming; avoid excess sunlight or external heat such as saunas; each 5-cm^2 patch contains 9 mg base, rate of 4.6 mg/24 hr, each 10-cm^2 patch 18 mg base, rate of 9.5 mg/24 hr

SIDE EFFECTS

CV: QT prolongation, AV block, cardiac arrest, angina, MI, palpitations, bradycardia

CNS: *Tremors, confusion, insomnia,* psychosis, hallucination, depression, dizziness, headache, anxiety, somnolence, fatigue, syncope, EPS, exacerbation of Parkinson's disease

GI: *Nausea, vomiting, anorexia, abdominal distress, flatulence,* diarrhea, constipation, dyspepsia, colitis, eructation, fecal incontinence, GI bleeding/obstruction, GERD, gastritis, pancreatitis

MISC: Urinary tract infection, asthenia, increased sweating, hypertension, flulike symptoms, weight change

PHARMACOKINETICS

Rapidly and completely absorbed; peak 1 hr, metabolized to decarbamylated metabolite; half-life 1.5 hr; excreted via kidneys (metabolites); clearance lowered in geriatric patients, hepatic disease and increased with nicotine use; 40% protein binding

INTERACTIONS

Increase: synergistic effect—cholinergic agonists, other cholinesterase inhibitors
Increase: metabolism—nicotine
Increase: GI effects—NSAIDs
Decrease: rivastigmine effect—anticholinergics, sedating H$_1$ blockers, tricyclics, phenothiazines

NURSING CONSIDERATIONS

Assess:

• Hepatic studies: AST, ALT, alk phos, LDH, bilirubin, CBC

• **Severe GI effects:** nausea, vomiting, anorexia, weight loss, diarrhea, GI bleeding

• B/P, heart rate, respiration during initial treatment; hypo/hypertension should be reported

• **Cognitive/mental status:** affect, mood, behavioral changes, depression, insomnia; complete suicide assessment

• Assistance with ambulation during beginning therapy; dizziness may occur

• **Beers:** avoid use in older adults; increased risk of orthostatic hypotension or bradycardia

• **Pregnancy/breastfeeding:** use only if clearly needed; do not breastfeed, excretion unknown

Evaluate:

• Therapeutic response: improved mood/cognition

Teach patient/family:

• How to apply **transdermal** product, to fold in half and throw away, not to get in eyes, to wash hands after application; not to use heating pad, sauna, tanning bed

• To notify prescriber of severe GI effects

• That product may cause dizziness, anorexia, weight loss

• That effect may take weeks or months; not to discontinue abruptly

• To notify prescriber if pregnancy is planned or suspected

• To give with food in AM, PM if using oral tablet

• To notify prescriber of history of low heart rate, sick sinus syndrome, risk of bradycardia

• How to take B/P, pulse at home

• To report nausea, vomiting, diarrhea

• To inform prescriber of all products taken

R

---

rizatriptan (Rx)

(rye-zah-trip′tan)

Maxalt, Maxalt-MLT

Func. class.: Migraine agent

Chem. class.: 5-HT$_{1D}$ receptor agonist, abortive agent-triptan

---

Side effects: *italics* = common; red = life-threatening

ACTION: Binds selectively to the vascular 5-HT$_{1B/1D}$ receptor subtype; exerts antimigraine effect; causes vasoconstriction of the cranial arteries

USES: Acute treatment of migraine

CONTRAINDICATIONS: Angina pectoris, history of MI, documented silent ischemia, Prinzmetal's angina, ischemic heart disease, concurrent ergotamine-containing preparations, uncontrolled hypertension, hypersensitivity, basilar or hemiplegic migraine
Precautions: Pregnancy, breastfeeding, children, geriatric patients, postmenopausal women, men >40 yr, risk factors for CAD, hypercholesterolemia, obesity, diabetes, impaired renal/hepatic function

DOSAGE AND ROUTES
• **Adult:** PO 5-10 mg single dose, redosing separated by ≥2 hr, max 30 mg/24 hr; use 5 mg for patient receiving propranolol, max 15 mg/24 hr
Available forms: Tabs (Maxalt) 5, 10 mg; orally disintegrating tabs (Maxalt-MLT) 5, 10 mg
Administer:
• **Orally disintegrating tab:** do not open blister until use; peel blister open with dry hands; place tab on patient's tongue, where it will dissolve, and have patient swallow with saliva (contains phenylalanine)
• Not to be used for more than 3-4 times per month

SIDE EFFECTS
CNS: *Dizziness, drowsiness, headache, fatigue,* warm/cold sensations, flushing
CV: MI, ventricular fibrillation, ventricular tachycardia, coronary artery vasospasm, palpitations, hypertension, peripheral vascular ischemia, ECG changes
ENDO: Hot flashes, mild increase in growth hormone
GI: *Nausea,* dry mouth, diarrhea, abdominal pain, ischemic colitis
RESP: Chest tightness, pressure, dyspnea

PHARMACOKINETICS
Onset of pain relief 10 min-2 hr; peak 1-1$\frac{1}{2}$ hr; duration 14-16 hr; 14% plasma protein binding; metabolized in liver (metabolite); excreted in urine (82%), feces (12%); half-life 2-3 hr

INTERACTIONS
Weakness, hyperreflexia, incoordination: SSRIs
Increase: levels of sibutramine
Increase: rizatriptan action—cimetidine, oral contraceptives, MAOIs, nonselective MAOI (type A and B), isocarboxazid, pargyline, phenelzine, propranolol, tranylcypromine
Increase: vasospastic effects—ergot, ergot derivatives, other 5-HT receptor agonists
Drug/Herb
Serotonin syndrome: St. John's wort

NURSING CONSIDERATIONS
Assess:
• **Migraine symptoms:** visual disturbances, aura, intensity, nausea, vomiting, photophobia
• Stress level, activity, recreation, coping mechanisms
• Neurologic status: LOC, blurring vision, nausea, vomiting, tingling in extremities preceding headache
• **Ingestion of tyramine foods** (pickled products, beer, wine, aged cheese), food additives, preservatives, colorings, artificial sweeteners, chocolate, caffeine, which may precipitate these types of headaches
• Renal status: urine output
• Quiet, calm environment with decreased stimulation: noise, bright light, excessive talking
• **Pregnancy/breastfeeding:** use only if benefits outweigh fetal risk; enroll in the registry, 1-800-986-8999; cautious use in breastfeeding, excretion unknown
Evaluate:
• Therapeutic response: decrease in frequency, severity of headache
Teach patient/family:
• **About use of orally disintegrating tab:** instruct patient not to open blister until use, to peel blister open with dry hands, to place tab on tongue, where it will dissolve, and to swallow with saliva (contains phenylalanine)

• To report any side effects to prescriber
• To use alternative contraception while taking product if oral contraceptives are being used
• That product does not prevent or reduce number of migraines; if 1st dose does not relieve pain, do not use more, notify prescriber; to avoid use in acute headache, use of agent >10 days a month due to the risk of medication overuse headaches

---

roflumilast
Daliresp
Func. class.: Respiratory antiinflammatory agent
Chem. class.: Phosphodiesterase-4 (PDE4) inhibitor

ACTION: Roflumilast (and the active metabolite roflumilast N-oxide) selectively inhibit phosphodiesterase-4 (PDE4); not a bronchodilator; inhibition of the PDE4 enzyme blocks the hydrolyses and inactivation of cyclic adenosine monophosphate (cAMP), resulting in intracellular cAMP accumulation; decreases inflammatory activity, PDE4 inhibition may affect migration and actions of proinflammatory cells (neutrophils, other leukocytes, T-lymphocytes, monocytes, macrophages, fibroblasts)

USES: For the prevention of COPD exacerbations in patients with severe COPD associated with chronic bronchitis and a history of exacerbations

CONTRAINDICATIONS: *Moderate to severe hepatic disease* (Child-Pugh B or C)
Precautions: Pregnancy, breastfeeding, neonates, infants, children, adolescents, acute bronchospasm, anxiety, insomnia, depression, suicidal ideation or behavior

DOSAGE AND ROUTES
• **Adult: PO** 500 mcg/day
Available forms: Tabs 500 mcg

Administer:
PO route
• Give without regard to meals
• Store at room temperature

SIDE EFFECTS
CNS: Insomnia, anxiety, depression, headache, dizziness, tremors, suicidal ideation
EENT: Rhinitis, sinusitis
GI: *Weight loss, diarrhea, nausea,* anorexia, abdominal pain, dyspepsia, gastritis, vomiting
GU: Urinary tract infection
MS: Back pain, muscle cramps/spasm
SYST: Infections, influenza

PHARMACOKINETICS
80% absolute bioavailability; protein binding 99% (roflumilast); 97% (N-oxide metabolite); low penetration across the blood–brain barrier; extensively metabolized (liver); metabolism by CYP3A4 and CYP1A2 produces active metabolite N-oxide; half-life parent drug 17 hr, metabolite 30; steady state 4 days (parent drug), 6 days (metabolite); 70% excreted in urine; parent drug peak 1 hr (range, 0.5-2 hr), metabolite peak 8 hr (range, 4-13 hr); contraindicated in moderate to severe hepatic impairment; use with caution in patients with mild hepatic impairment

INTERACTIONS
Increase: roflumilast effect—CYP3A4/CYP1A2 inhibitors (enoxacin, cimetidine, delavirdine, indinavir, isoniazid, itraconazole, dalfopristin, quinupristin, tipranavir)
Increase: roflumilast effect—oral contraceptives (gestodene and ethinyl estradiol)
Decrease: roflumilast effect—CYP3A4 inducers (rifAMPin, barbiturates, carBAMazepine, phenytoin, erythromycin, ketoconazole, fluvoxaMINE, alcohol, etravirine, ritonavir, bexarotene, rifabutin, OXcarbazepine, nevirapine, modafinil, metyraPONE, PHENobarbital, bosentan, dexamethasone)
Altered effect of: fosamprenavir

R

Drug/Herb

Decrease: roflumilast effect—St. John's wort

NURSING CONSIDERATIONS
Assess:

• Lung sounds and respiratory function baseline and periodically thereafter

• Behavioral changes including mood, depression, suicidal thoughts/behaviors

• Liver function tests baseline and periodically thereafter; if increases in liver function studies occur, product should be discontinued

• Weight; weight loss is common

• **Pregnancy/breastfeeding:** use only if benefits outweigh fetal risk; do not breastfeed, excreted in breast milk

Evaluate:

• Decreasing exacerbations in COPD

Teach patient/family:

• To take product as directed; not to skip or double doses; to take missed doses as soon as remembered unless almost time for next dose

• Not to use OTC or other products without prescriber approval; not to discontinue other respiratory products unless approved by prescriber

• Not to be used for acute bronchospasm but may be continued during acute asthma attacks

• Suicidal thoughts/behaviors: to notify prescriber of worsening depression or suicidal thoughts/behaviors

---

RARELY USED

romiPLOStim (Rx)
(roe-mi-ploe´stim)

Nplate

Func. class.: Hematopoietin

Chem. class.: Thrombopoietin receptor agonist

USES: Chronic idiopathic thrombocytopenic purpura in patients who have had an insufficient response to corticosteroids, immunoglobulins, or splenectomy

CONTRAINDICATIONS: Hypersensitivity to this product or mannitol

DOSAGE AND ROUTES
Thrombocytopenia in chronic idiopathic thrombocytopenic purpura (ITP)

• **Adult:** SUBCUT 1 mcg/kg/wk (based on actual body weight); increase the weekly dosage by 1 mcg/kg until platelet count ≥50,000/mm³; 10 mcg/kg/wk max

---

rOPINIRole (Rx)
(roh-pin´ih-role)

Requip, Requip XL

Func. class.: Antiparkinson agent

Chem. class.: DOPamine-receptor agonist, nonergot

Do not confuse:
rOPINIRole/risperiDONE

ACTION: Selective agonist for D_2 receptors (presynaptic/postsynaptic sites); binding at D_3 receptor contributes to antiparkinson effects

USES: Parkinson's disease, restless legs syndrome (RLS)

CONTRAINDICATIONS: Hypersensitivity

Precautions: Pregnancy, dysrhythmias, affective disorder, psychosis, cardiac/renal/hepatic disease

DOSAGE AND ROUTES
Parkinson's disease

• **Adult:** **PO (regular release)** Initially, 0.25 mg tid × 1 wk; gradually titrate at weekly intervals: **Week 2**, 0.5 mg tid; **Week 3**, 0.75 mg tid; **Week 4**, 1 mg tid; **After week 4**, may increase by 1.5 mg/day each week, max 9 mg/day total dosage, and then by 3 mg/day each week, max 24 mg/day

• **PO (ext rel)** Initially, 2 mg/day × 1-2 wk, may increase by mg/day at intervals ≥1 wk based upon response; max 24 mg/day; if significant interruption of therapy occurs, retitration may be necessary

---

Conversion from immediate-release to extended-release tablets

- **Adult: PO** currently taking 0.75-2.25 mg/day imm rel: give 2 mg/day ext rel
- **PO** currently taking 3-4.5 mg/day imm rel: give 4 mg/day ext rel
- **PO** currently taking 6 mg/day imm rel: give 6 mg/day ext rel
- **PO** currently taking 7.5-9 mg/day imm rel: give 8 mg/day ext rel
- **PO** currently taking 12 mg/day imm rel: give 12 mg/day ext rel
- **PO** currently taking 15-18 mg/day imm rel: give 16 mg/day ext rel
- **PO** currently taking 21 mg/day imm rel: give 20 mg/day ext rel
- **PO** currently taking 24 mg/day imm rel: give 24 mg/day ext rel

Restless legs syndrome

- **Adult: PO (reg rel)** Initially, 0.25 mg every day 1-3 hr before bedtime; days 3-7, may increase to 0.5 mg every day; at the beginning of wk 2 (day 8), the dosage may be increased to 1 mg every day × 1 wk; weeks 3-6, dosage may be titrated up by 0.5 mg each wk (from 1.5-3 mg over the 5-wk period) as needed to achieve desired effect; wk 7, may increase dosage to 4 mg/day; dosage is titrated based on clinical response; give all doses 1-3 hr before bedtime

Available forms: Tabs 0.25, 0.5, 1, 2, 3, 4, 5 mg; ext rel tab 2, 4, 6, 8, 12 mg

Administer:

- Product until NPO before surgery
- Adjust dosage to patient response; taper when discontinuing
- With meals to reduce nausea
- **Extended release:** do not chew, crush, or divide
- Testing for diabetes mellitus, acromegaly if patient receiving long-term therapy

SIDE EFFECTS

CNS: *Agitation, insomnia,* psychosis, hallucination, dystonia, depression, dizziness, somnolence, sleep attacks, impulse control disorders

CV: *Orthostatic hypotension,* tachycardia, hypo/hypertension, syncope, palpitations

EENT: Blurred vision

GI: *Nausea, vomiting, anorexia, dry mouth,* constipation, dyspepsia, flatulence

GU: Impotence, urinary frequency

HEMA: Hemolytic anemia, leukopenia, agranulocytosis

INTEG: Rash, sweating

RESP: Pharyngitis, rhinitis, sinusitis, bronchitis, dyspnea

PHARMACOKINETICS

Peak 1-2 hr, half-life 6 hr, extensively metabolized by liver by P450 CYP1A2 enzyme system, protein binding 40%

INTERACTIONS

Increase: rOPINIRole effect—cimetidine, ciprofloxacin, diltiaZEM, enoxacin, erythromycin, fluvoxaMINE, mexiletine, norfloxacin, tacrine, digoxin, theophylline, ʟ-dopa

Decrease: rOPINIRole effects—butyrophenones, metoclopramide, phenothiazines, thioxanthenes

NURSING CONSIDERATIONS

Assess:

- **Parkinsonism:** akinesia, tremors, staggering gait, muscle rigidity, drooling
- B/P, respirations during initial treatment; hypo/hypertension should be reported
- **Sleep attacks:** drowsiness, falling asleep without warning even during hazardous activities
- Mental status: affect, mood, behavioral changes, depression; complete suicide assessment; worsening of symptoms in restless legs syndrome
- **Pregnancy/breastfeeding:** use only if benefits outweigh fetal risk; avoid breastfeeding, excretion unknown

Evaluate:

- Therapeutic response: improvement in movement disorder

Teach patient/family:

- To notify prescriber if pregnancy is planned or suspected, or if breastfeeding
- To take with food to prevent nausea
- To report hallucinations, confusion (usually in geriatric patients)

Side effects: *italics* = common; red = life-threatening

• That therapeutic effects may take several weeks to a few months

• To change positions slowly to prevent orthostatic hypotension

• To report any suspicious skin lesions; that dermatologic or skin examinations should be performed regularly due to risk of melanoma in Parkinson's patients

• To use product exactly as prescribed; that if product is discontinued abruptly, parkinsonian crisis may occur; that product will be titrated weekly

• That drowsiness, sleep attacks may occur; to avoid driving, other hazardous activities until response known

• To avoid alcohol, CNS depressants, cough and cold products

• To notify prescriber if unusual urges occur

⚠ HIGH ALERT

rosiglitazone (Rx)

(ros-ih-glit'ah-zone)

Avandia

Func. class.: Antidiabetic, oral
Chem. class.: Thiazolidinedione

Do not confuse:
rosiglitazone/pioglitazone
Avandia/Prandin

ACTION: Improves insulin resistance by hepatic glucose metabolism, insulin receptor kinase activity, insulin receptor phosphorylation

USES: Type 2 diabetes mellitus, alone or in combination with sulfonylureas, metformin, insulin

CONTRAINDICATIONS: Breast-feeding, children, hypersensitivity to thiazolidindiones, diabetic ketoacidosis, jaundice

Black Box Warning: NYHA III, IV acute heart failure, heart failure

Precautions: Pregnancy, geriatric patients, thyroid disease, renal/hepatic disease, MI, heart failure class I, II NYHA

DOSAGE AND ROUTES

• **Adult: PO** 4 mg/day or in 2 divided doses, may increase to 8 mg/day or in 2 divided doses after 12 wk; may be added to metFORMIN, sulfonylurea for adult dose

Available forms: Tabs 2, 4, 8 mg
Administer:

• Conversion from other oral hypoglycemic agents if needed; change may be made without gradual dosage change; monitor blood glucose during conversion

• Store in tight container in cool environment

PO route

• Once or in 2 divided doses, without regard to food

• Tabs crushed and mixed with food or fluids for patients with difficulty swallowing

SIDE EFFECTS

CNS: Fatigue, *headache*

CV: MI, HF, death (geriatric patients)

ENDO: Hypo/hyperglycemia

GI: Weight gain, hepatotoxicity, increase total LDL, HDL cholesterol; decrease free fatty acids, diarrhea

MISC: Accidental injury, URI, sinusitis, anemia, back pain, diarrhea, edema, bone fractures (female), pulmonary/macular/peripheral edema

SYST: Anaphylaxis, Stevens-Johnson syndrome

PHARMACOKINETICS

Maximal reductions in fasting blood sugar after 6-12 wk; protein binding 99.8%; excreted in urine, feces; elimination half-life 3-4 hr; may be excreted in breast milk

INTERACTIONS

Increase: hypoglycemia—gemfibrozil, fluvoxaMINE, ketoconazole, trimethoprim; monitor glucose

• Avoid concurrent use with insulin, nitrates

• May increase or decrease level: CYP2C5 inducer/inhibitors

Drug/Herb

Increase: antidiabetic effect—garlic, horse chestnut

Drug/Lab Test
Increase: ALT, HDL, LDL, total cholesterol, blood glucose
Decrease: Hgb/Hct

NURSING CONSIDERATIONS
Assess:

Black Box Warning: HF/MI: dyspnea, crackles, edema, weight gain ≥5 lb, jugular venous distention; may need to change dose or discontinue product; do not use in acute coronary syndrome, NYHA Class III/IV heart failure

• Hypoglycemic reactions (sweating, weakness, dizziness, anxiety, tremors, hunger), hyperglycemic reactions soon after meals
• **Systemic reactions:** anaphylaxis, Stevens-Johnson syndrome
• **Hepatotoxicity:** LFTs periodically, AST, ALT (if ALT >2.5 × ULN, do not use product)
• Fasting blood sugar, A1c, plasma lipids/lipoproteins, B/P, body weight during treatment
• To use product provider/patient must be enrolled in the Avandia-Rosiglitazone Medicines Access Program
• **Beers:** avoid in older adults; may promote fluid retention or exacerbate heart failure
• **Pregnancy/breastfeeding:** use only if benefits outweigh fetal risk, usually insulin is used in pregnancy; do not breastfeed, excretion unknown

Evaluate:
• Therapeutic response: decrease in polyuria, polydipsia, polyphagia; clear sensorium; absence of dizziness; stable gait; blood glucose, A1c improvement

Teach patient/family:
• To monitor blood glucose; that periodic liver function tests mandatory; to report edema, weight gain
• About the symptoms of hypo/hyperglycemia, what to do about each; that these symptoms are more likely to occur in those using insulin

• That product must be continued on daily basis; about the consequences of discontinuing the product abruptly
• To avoid OTC medications, herbal preparations, nitrates, or insulin unless approved by prescriber
• That diabetes is lifelong; that product is not a cure, only controls symptoms
• That all food included in diet plan must be eaten to prevent hypoglycemia
• To carry emergency ID and glucagon emergency kit
• To report symptoms of hepatic dysfunction (nausea, vomiting, abdominal pain, fatigue, anorexia, dark urine, jaundice) immediately; to report macular edema (change in vision)
• That 2 wk is needed to see reduction in blood glucose level and 2-3 mo needed to see full effect of product
• To notify prescriber if oral contraceptives are used
• Not to use if breastfeeding; may be secreted in breast milk
• That a medication guide should be dispensed with each prescription/refill

---

rosuvastatin (Rx)
(roe-soo′va-sta-tin)
Crestor
Func. class.: Antilipemic
Chem. class.: HMG-CoA reductase inhibitor

R

ACTION: Inhibits HMG-CoA reductase enzyme, which reduces cholesterol synthesis

USES: As an adjunct for primary hypercholesterolemia (types IIa, IIb) and mixed dyslipidemia, elevated serum triglycerides, homozygous/heterozygous familial hypercholesterolemia (FH), slowing of atherosclerosis, CV disease prophylaxis, MI, stroke prophylaxis (normal LDL)

CONTRAINDICATIONS: Pregnancy, breastfeeding, hypersensitivity, active hepatic disease

---

Side effects: *italics* = common; red = life-threatening

Precautions: Children <10 yr, geriatric patients, past hepatic disease, alcoholism, severe acute infections, trauma, hypotension, uncontrolled seizure disorders, severe metabolic disorders, electrolyte imbalances, severe renal impairment, hypothyroidism, Asian patients

DOSAGE AND ROUTES

Hypercholesterolemia, hyperlipoproteinemia, and/or hypertriglyceridemia

• **Adult:** PO 10 mg/day as usual starting dose; 5 mg/day in those requiring less aggressive LDL cholesterol reductions, in patients with CrCl <30 mL/min, or in patients at higher risk for myopathy

Homozygous familial hypercholesterolemia (HoFH)

• **Adult:** PO 20 mg/day as usual starting dose

• **Adolescent/child 7-17 yr:** PO 20 mg/day

Heterozygous familial hypercholesterolemia (HeFH)

• **Adolescent/child 10-17 yr:** PO 5-20 mg/day; individualize based on therapy goal; adjust dose q4wk or more

• **Child 8-9 yr:** PO 5-10 mg/day; individualize based on therapy goal; adjust dose q4wk or more

For slowing the progression of atherosclerosis (e.g., carotid, coronary)

• **Adult:** PO 10 mg/day as usual starting dose; initially 5 mg/day in those requiring less aggressive LDL cholesterol reductions, in patients with CCr <30 mL/min, or in patients at higher risk for myopathy

Primary prevention of cardiovascular disease

• **Adult:** PO 10-20 mg/day as usual starting dose; range 5-40 mg/day

Renal dose

• **Adult:** PO CCr <30 mL/min, initially, 5 mg/day in those not receiving dialysis; **max** 10 mg/day

Available forms

Tabs 5, 10, 20, 40 mg

Administer

• May be taken at any time of day, with/without food

• Store in cool environment in airtight, light-resistant container

SIDE EFFECTS

CNS: *Headache, dizziness,* insomnia, paresthesia, confusion

GI: *Nausea, constipation, abdominal pain, flatus, diarrhea, dyspepsia, heartburn,* kidney failure, liver dysfunction, vomiting

HEMA: Thrombocytopenia, hemolytic anemia, leukopenia

INTEG: *Rash, pruritus*

MS: *Asthenia, muscle cramps, arthritis, arthralgia, myalgia,* myositis, rhabdomyolysis; leg, shoulder, or localized pain

PHARMACOKINETICS

Peak 3-5 hr, minimal live metabolism (about 10%), 88% protein bound, excreted primarily in feces (90%), crosses placenta, half-life 19 hr, not dialyzable

INTERACTIONS

Increase: hepatotoxicity—alcohol

Increase: myalgia, myositis, rhabdomyolysis—cycloSPORINE, gemfibrozil, niacin, clofibrate, azole antifungals, antiretroviral protease inhibitors, fibric acid derivatives

Increase: bleeding risk—warfarin

Drug/Lab Test

Increase: LFTs

NURSING CONSIDERATIONS

Assess:

• Diet; obtain diet history including fat, cholesterol in diet

• Fasting cholesterol, LDL, HDL, triglycerides at baseline and q4-6wk, then periodically

• Liver function: LFTs at baseline, then if clinically indicated; AST, ALT, LFTs may increase

• Renal function in patients with compromised renal system: BUN, creatinine, I&O ratio

• **Rhabdomyolysis:** muscle pain, tenderness, obtain CPK; if these occur, product may need to be discontinued; for patients with Asian ancestry: increased blood levels, rhabdomyolysis

- **Pregnancy/breastfeeding:** do not use in pregnancy, breastfeeding

Evaluate:

- Therapeutic response: decreased LDL, cholesterol, triglycerides, increased HDL, slowing CAD

Teach patient/family:

- To report suspected pregnancy; to use contraception while taking product; not to breastfeed

- To report weakness, muscle tenderness, pain, fever, liver injury (jaundice, anorexia, abdominal pain)

- That blood work and follow-up exams will be necessary during treatment

- To report severe GI symptoms, dizziness, headache, muscle pain, weakness

- That previously prescribed regimen will continue: low-cholesterol diet, exercise program, smoking cessation

---

⚠ HIGH ALERT

rucaparib
(roo-kap′ a-rib)

Rubraca

Func. class.: Antineoplastic

Chem. class.: Poly (ADP-ribose) polymerase (PARP) inhibitor

ACTION: Inhibits poly (ADP-ribose) polymerase (PARP) enzymes; inhibition of PARP enzyme activity results in increased PARP-DNA complexes, causing DNA damage, apoptosis, and cell death

USES: BRCA mutation–positive (germline and/or somatic) epithelial ovarian, fallopian tube, or primary peritoneal cancer in patients who have received 2 or more prior chemotherapy regimens, as monotherapy

CONTRAINDICATIONS:
Hypersensitivity

Precautions: Breastfeeding, contraceptive requirements, leukemia, myelodysplastic syndrome (MDS), pregnancy, pregnancy testing, reproductive risk

DOSAGE AND ROUTES
BRCA mutation–positive epithelial ovarian, fallopian tube, or primary peritoneal cancer

- **Adult: PO** 600 mg bid; continue until disease progression or severe toxicity

Dose adjustments for treatment-related toxicities

- First dose reduction: 500 mg bid; second dose reduction: 400 mg bid; third dose reduction: 300 mg bid

Hematologic toxicity

- **Grade ≥1 hematologic toxicity:** hold and monitor CBC weekly. When toxicity resolves to grade ≤1, therapy may be resumed

Available forms: Tabs 200 mg, 300 mg

SIDE EFFECTS
CNS: Fatigue, dizziness, fever, asthenia

GI: *Nausea, vomiting, constipation, anorexia, abdominal pain, diarrhea,* dysgeusia

HEMA: Anemia, thrombocytopenia, neutropenia, febrile neutropenia, myelodysplastic syndrome (MDS)/acute myeloid leukemia

INTEG: *Pruritus, rash,* photosensitivity, hand-foot syndrome

RESP: Dyspnea

PHARMACOKINETICS
70% protein binding, peak 1.9 hr, half-life 17-19 hr, metabolized by CYP2D6 (major) and CYP3A4, CYP1A2 (minor)

INTERACTIONS
None known.

Drug/Lab:

Increase: AST, ALT, cholesterol

Decrease: ANC, Hb, platelets

NURSING CONSIDERATIONS
Assess:

- **Myelodysplastic syndrome (MDS)/ acute myeloid leukemia (AML):** monitor for signs and symptoms of MDS/AML; monitor CBC baseline and monthly; do not start until prior hematologic toxicity resolves to grade ≤1. For prolonged hematologic toxicity (>4 wk), hold therapy or reduce dose and check a CBC weekly until recovery; discontinue if a diagnosis of MDS or AML occurs

---

Side effects: *italics* = common; red = life-threatening

• **Pregnancy/breastfeeding:** assess use of effective contraception during treatment and for 6 mo after last dose; pregnancy testing should be done before use; can cause fetal harm or death; do not breastfeed during treatment and for 2 wk after the final dose

• Monitor AST/ALT, cholesterol, creatinine; all may be elevated

Evaluate:

• Therapeutic response: decrease in growth, spread of ovarian cancer

Teach patient/family:

• To notify prescriber of all OTC, Rx, and herbal products taken; not to start new products without prescriber approval

• **Pregnancy/breastfeeding:** that product can cause fetal harm or death; that pregnancy testing should be done before use; to use effective contraception during treatment and for 6 mo after final dose; not to breastfeed during treatment or for 2 wk after final dose;

• **Myelodysplastic syndrome (MDS)/ acute myeloid leukemia (AML):** to report weakness, fatigue, bruising, bleeding, trouble breathing, blood in urine, stool, emesis; that continuing blood work will be needed

• **Photosensitivity:** to wear protective clothing, sunscreen or to stay out of sun to prevent burns

---

RARELY USED

rufinamide (Rx)

(roo-fin′a-mide)

Banzel

Func. class.: Anticonvulsant
Chem. class.: Triazole derivative

USES: Lennox-Gastaut syndrome
Unlabeled uses: Partial seizures

CONTRAINDICATIONS: Hypersensitivity, familial short QT syndrome

DOSAGE AND ROUTES

• **Adult: PO** 400-800 mg/day divided bid; increase by 400-800 mg/day q2days to 3200 mg/day

• **Child 1 to <17 yr: PO** 10 mg/kg/day divided equally bid; increase by 10 mg/kg/day every other day to 45 mg/kg/day or 3200 mg/day, whichever is less

---

safinamide
(sa-fin'-a-mide)

Xadago

Func. class.: Antiparkinson agent
Chem. class.: MAO type B inhibitor

ACTION: The precise mechanism of action of safinamide in treating "off" episodes in Parkinson's disease is unknown; however, one mechanism may be related to its MAO-B inhibitory activity, which causes an increase in DOPamine levels centrally. The elevated DOPamine levels and subsequent increased dopaminergic activity are likely to mediate the beneficial effects of safinamide

USES: For adjunctive treatment to levodopa-carbidopa therapy in patients with Parkinson's disease experiencing "off" episodes

CONTRAINDICATIONS: Hypersensitivity, MAOI therapy

Precautions: Abrupt discontinuation, alcoholism, breastfeeding, pregnancy, cataracts, use with CNS depressants, dental work, diabetic retinopathy, hypertension, hepatic disease, impulse control problems, psychosis, schizophrenia, surgery, uveitis

DOSAGE AND ROUTES
• **Adult: PO** Initially, 50 mg/day. May increase after 2 wk to 100 mg/day based on need and tolerability. Max 100 mg/day
Available forms: Tabs 50, 100 mg

Administer:
• Give at same time each day; may be given with or without food
• If a dose is missed, take the next dose at the usual time on the following day
• Food and drug interactions with safinamide can be serious. Patients should avoid foods/beverages containing large amounts of tyramine

SIDE EFFECTS
CNS: Drowsiness, dyskinesia, insomnia, impulse control symptoms, neuroleptic malignant syndrome, psychosis, serotonin syndrome
CV: Orthostatic hypotension
MISC: Cough, dyspepsia, cataracts

PHARMACOKINETICS
Not highly protein bound, excreted via kidneys 5% (unchanged), 76% recovered in the urine; half-life 20-26 hr, peak 2-3 hr; inhibits intestinal breast cancer resistance protein (BCRP)

INTERACTIONS
• **Increase:** severe somnolence—anxiolytics, sedatives, hypnotics, barbiturates, ALPRAZolam, clonazePAM, zolpidem, zaleplon; avoid using together
• **Increase:** hypertension, hypertensive crisis—MAOIs, linezolid; do not use within 14 days of these products
• **Increase:** serotonin syndrome—meperidine, some other opioids; SNRIs; tricyclic antidepressants and other cyclic antidepressants; triazolopyridine antidepressants; cyclobenzaprine; stimulants (methylphenidate, amphetamines), dextromethorphan; use the lowest dose of safinamide
• **Decrease:** safinamide effects—atypical antipsychotics

NURSING CONSIDERATIONS
Assess:
• **Parkinson's disease:** assess for changes before and during treatment; tremors, pin-rolling, movement, balance, anxiety, drooling, depression, delusions, hallucinations, insomnia, shuffling gait; decreasing of "off" periods
• **Mental status:** affect, depression, mood, complete suicide assessment
• **Hypertension:** may cause hypertension, exacerbate preexisting hypertension, or cause hypertensive crisis. Monitor for new-onset hypertension or hypertension that is not adequately controlled after starting product; adjust dose if elevations in B/P are sustained, do not exceed max dose; monitor for hypertension if coadministered with sympathomimetics (prescription or nonprescription nasal, oral, and ophthalmic decongestants, cold preparations)

S

• **Drug interactions:** review before use; there are many serious reactions

• **Impulse control:** inquire periodically about new or worsening impulse control symptoms (gambling, increased sexual urges, binge eating, intense urges to spend money, or other intense urges); if these occur, dose reduction or discontinuation may be needed

• **Hepatic disease:** monitor LFTs baseline and periodically in those with hepatic disease

• **Neuroleptic malignant syndrome-like symptoms:** elevated temperature, muscular rigidity, altered consciousness, and autonomic instability; may occur with rapid dose reduction

• **Serotonin syndrome:** nausea, vomiting, sedation, dizziness, diaphoresis (sweating), facial flushing, mental status changes, myoclonus, restlessness, shivering, and hypertension. If serotonin syndrome occurs, any serotonergic agents should be discontinued

• **Pregnancy/breastfeeding:** may cause fetal harm; use in pregnancy only if the potential benefit outweighs fetal risk; do not use in breastfeeding, serious adverse reactions may occur

Teach patient/family:

• **Impulse control:** that symptoms (gambling, increased sexual urges, binge eating, intense urges to spend money, or other intense urges) may occur; to report to provider

• **Pregnancy/breastfeeding:** to report if pregnancy is planned or suspected or if breastfeeding

• Not to drive or engage in hazardous activities until effect of product is known; drowsiness may occur

• To take B/P regularly

• To change position slowly to prevent orthostatic hypotension

• To use product as prescribed; if discontinued abruptly, neuroleptic malignant syndrome-like symptoms may occur; to taper gradually; to take at same time of day; to take with levodopa-carbidopa

• To use physical activity to maintain mobility, lessen spasms

• **Serotonin syndrome:** to report dry, hot skin, fever, agitation, delirium, diarrhea; to avoid use with other serotonergic products

• To avoid use of tyramine-containing products; give list to patient

---

salicylic acid topical
See Appendix B

---

salmeterol (Rx)

(sal-met′er-ole)

Serevent Diskhaler Disk, Serevent Diskus

Func. class.: β_2-Adrenergic agonist (long acting), bronchodilator

ACTION: Causes bronchodilation by action on β_2 (pulmonary) receptors by increasing levels of cAMP, which relaxes smooth muscle with little effect on heart rate; maintains improvement in FEV from 3 to 12 hr; prevents nocturnal asthma symptoms

USES: Prevention of exercise-induced bronchospasm, COPD, asthma

CONTRAINDICATIONS: Hypersensitivity to sympathomimetics, tachydysrhythmias, severe cardiac disease, monotherapy treatment of asthma

Precautions: Pregnancy, breastfeeding, cardiac disorders, hyperthyroidism, diabetes mellitus, hypertension, closed-angle glaucoma, seizures, acute asthma, as a substitute to corticosteroids, QT prolongation

Black Box Warning: Asthma-related death, children <4 yr

DOSAGE AND ROUTES

• **Adult/child ≥4 yr: Asthma INH** 50 mcg (1 inhalation as dry powder) q12hr; **exercise-induced bronchospasm** 50 mcg (1 inhalation) $^1/_2$-1 hr before exercise

---

Available forms: Inhalation powder 50 mcg/blister
Administer:
• Gum, sips of water for dry mouth
• Use $1/2$ hr before exercise for exercise-induced bronchospasm prevention, do not use additional doses if using bid
• Use this medication before other medications, allow at least 1 min between other inhaled products
• Do not use spacer with this product
• Store in foil pouch; do not expose to temperature >86° F (30° C); discard 6 wk after removal from foil pouch

SIDE EFFECTS

CNS: *Tremors, anxiety,* insomnia, headache
CV: Palpitations, tachycardia
EENT: Dry nose, irritation of nose and throat
GI: Nausea, vomiting, abdominal pain
MS: Muscle cramps
RESP: Paradoxical bronchospasm, cough, asthma-related death

PHARMACOKINETICS

INH: Onset 30-50 min; peak 4 hr; duration 12 hr; metabolized in liver; excreted in urine, breast milk; crosses placenta, blood-brain barrier; protein binding 94%-98%; terminal half-life 3-5 hr

INTERACTIONS

Increase: CV effect—CYP3A4 inhibitors (itraconazole, ketoconazole, nelfinavir, nefazodone, saquinavir), avoid using together
Increase: action of aerosol bronchodilators
Increase: action of salmeterol—tricyclics, MAOIs
Decrease: salmeterol action—other β-blockers

NURSING CONSIDERATIONS

Assess:
• **Respiratory function:** vital capacity, forced expiratory volume, ABGs, lung sounds, heart rate and rhythm baseline and periodically
• **Paradoxical bronchospasm:** dyspnea, wheezing, chest tightness; do not use in bronchospasm

Black Box Warning: Children should not use this product as monotherapy for asthma; use only with persistent asthma in those whose symptoms are not well controlled with a long-term asthma product; after product controls asthma, use another bronchodilator

• **Hypersensitivity:** assess for rash, urticaria; rarely leads to anaphylaxis, angioedema

Black Box Warning: **Asthma-related death:** long-acting beta agonists have been associated with an increased risk of severe asthma exacerbations and asthma-related death. If wheezing worsens and cannot be relieved during an acute asthma attack, patients should be instructed to seek immediate medical attention. Avoid use of single-ingredient long-acting beta agonists for asthma in all age groups; increases the risk of asthma-related events, asthma-related hospitalization, asthma-related intubation, and asthma-related death. Do not use in those with significantly worsening or acutely deteriorating asthma, which may be a life-threatening condition

• **Pregnancy/breastfeeding:** use only if benefits outweigh fetal risk; cautious use in breastfeeding, excretion unknown
Evaluate:
• Therapeutic response: absence of dyspnea, wheezing
Teach patient/family:

Black Box Warning: **Asthma-related deaths:** to seek medical attention immediately for serious asthma attack; death may be greater in black patients

• Not to use for acute bronchospasm; never to exhale into Diskus; to hold level, keep mouthpiece dry
• Not to use OTC medications, extra stimulation may occur

S

Side effects: *italics* = common; red = life-threatening

- If using to prevent exercise-induced bronchospasm, to use ½-1 hr before exercise
- Review package insert with patient
- To avoid getting powder in eyes
- To avoid smoking, smoke-filled rooms, persons with respiratory infections
- Not for treatment of acute exacerbation; a fast-acting β-blocker should be used instead
- To immediately report dyspnea after use if ≥1 canister is used in 2 mo time
- To notify prescriber if >4 inhalations are needed or if product is no longer working
- To take other products as prescribed
- To notify prescriber if pregnancy is suspected or if breastfeeding

TREATMENT OF OVERDOSE: β₂-Adrenergic blocker

⚠ HIGH ALERT

sargramostim (GM-CSF) (Rx)

(sar-gram′oh-stim)

Leukine, GM-CSF

Func. class.: Biologic modifier, hematopoietic agent

Chem. class.: Granulocyte macrophage colony-stimulating factor (GM-CSF)

Do not confuse:
Leukine/leucovorin/Leukeran

ACTION: Stimulates proliferation and differentiation of hematopoietic progenitor cells (granulocytes, macrophages)

USES: Acceleration of myeloid recovery in patients with non–Hodgkin's lymphoma, acute lymphoblastic leukemia, acute myelogenous leukemia, autologous bone marrow transplantation in Hodgkin's disease; bone marrow transplantation failure or engraftment delay, mobilization and transplant of peripheral blood progenitor cells (PBPCs)

Unlabeled uses: Aplastic anemia, Crohn's disease, ganciclovir- or zidovudine-induced neutropenia, malignant melanoma, myelodysplastic syndrome (MDS)

CONTRAINDICATIONS: Neonates; hypersensitivity to GM-CSF, benzyl alcohol, yeast products; excessive leukemic myeloid blast in bone marrow, peripheral blood

Precautions: Pregnancy, breastfeeding, children; lung/cardiac/renal/hepatic disease; pleural, pericardial effusions, peripheral edema, leukocytosis, mannitol hypersensitivity, hepatic/renal disease

DOSAGE AND ROUTES
Myeloid recovery in Hodgkin's disease, non-Hodgkin's lymphoma, acute lymphocytic leukemia
- **Adult:** IV 250 mcg/m²/day over a 2-hr period beginning 2-4 hr after infusion of bone marrow and not <24 hr after last dose of chemotherapy or radiotherapy
- **Child (unlabeled):** SUBCUT/IV 250 mcg/m²/day beginning 2-4 hr after infusion of bone marrow and not <24 hr after last dose of chemotherapy

Acceleration of myeloid recovery
- **Adult:** IV 250 mcg/m²/day × 14 days; give over 2 hr; may repeat in 7 days; may repeat 500 mcg/m²/day × 14 days after another 7 days if no improvement

Mobilization of PBPCs
- **Adult:** CONT IV 250 mcg/m²/24 hr or SUBCUT q day; continue through collection

After PBPC transplantation
- **Adult:** CONT IV 250 mcg/m²/day until ANC >1500 cells/mm³

Aplastic anemia (unlabeled)
- **Adult:** SUBCUT 250-500 mcg/day or 5 mcg/kg/day × 14-90 days, used with erythropoietin or immunosuppressive therapy

Available forms: Powder for inj lyophilized 250 mcg; sol for inj 500 mcg/mL

Administer:
- Store in refrigerator; do not freeze

SUBCUT route
- No further dilution of reconstituted sol is needed; take care not to inject intradermally

Intermittent IV INFUSION route
• After reconstituting with 1 mL sterile water for inj without preservative; do not reenter vial; discard unused portion; direct reconstitution sol at side of vial; rotate contents; do not shake
• Dilute in 0.9% NaCl inj to prepare IV infusion; if final concentration is <10 mcg/mL, add human albumin to make final concentration of 0.1% to NaCl before adding sargramostim to prevent adsorption; for a final concentration of 0.1% albumin, add 1 mg human albumin/1 mL 0.9% NaCl inj run over 2 hr (**bone marrow transplant or failure of graft**); over 4 hr (**chemotherapy for AML**); over 24 hr as cont infusion (**PBPCs**); give within 6 hr after reconstitution

Y-site compatibilities: Amikacin, aminophylline, aztreonam, bleomycin, butorphanol, calcium gluconate, CARBOplatin, carmustine, ceFAZolin, cefepime, cefotaxime, cefoTEtan, ceftizoxime, cefTRIAXone, cefuroxime, cimetidine, CISplatin, clindamycin, cyclophosphamide, cycloSPORINE, cytarabine, dacarbazine, DACTINomycin, dexamethasone, diphenhydrAMINE, DOPamine, DOXOrubicin, doxycycline, droperidol, etoposide, famotidine, fentaNYL, floxuridine, fluconazole, fluorouracil, furosemide, gentamicin, granisetron, heparin, IDArubicin, ifosfamide, immune globulin, magnesium sulfate, mannitol, mechlorethamine, meperidine, mesna, methotrexate, metoclopramide, metroNIDAZOLE, minocycline, mitoXANTRONE, netilmicin, pentostatin, piperacillin/tazobactam, potassium chloride, prochlorperazine, promethazine, ranitidine, teniposide, ticarcillin, ticarcillin-clavulanate, trimethoprim-sulfamethoxazole, vinBLAStine, vinCRIStine, zidovudine

SIDE EFFECTS

CNS: Fever, malaise, CNS disorder, weakness, chills, dizziness, syncope, headache
CV: Transient supraventricular tachycardia, peripheral edema, pericardial effusion, hypotension, tachycardia
GI: Nausea, vomiting, diarrhea, anorexia, GI hemorrhage, stomatitis, liver damage, hyperbilirubinemia
GU: Urinary tract disorder, abnormal kidney function
HEMA: Blood dyscrasias, hemorrhage
INTEG: Alopecia, rash, peripheral edema
MS: Bone pain, myalgia
RESP: Dyspnea

PHARMACOKINETICS
Half-life elimination: IV 60 min, SUBCUT 2-3 hr; detected within 5 min after administration, peak 2 hr

INTERACTIONS
Increase: myeloproliferation—lithium, corticosteroids
Drug/Lab Test
Increase: bilirubin, BUN, creatinine, eosinophils, LFTs, leukocytes

NURSING CONSIDERATIONS
Assess:
• **Blood studies:** CBC, differential count before treatment, 2× weekly; leukocytosis may occur (WBC >50,000 cells/mm³, ANC >20,000 cells/mm³), platelets; if ANC >20,000/mm³ or 10,000/mm³ after nadir has occurred or platelets >500,000/mm³, reduce dose by ½ or discontinue; if blast cells occur, discontinue
• Renal, hepatic studies before treatment: BUN, creatinine, urinalysis; AST, ALT, alk phos; 2× weekly monitoring is needed in renal/hepatic disease
• **Hypersensitivity,** rashes, local inj-site reactions; usually transient
• Body weight, hydration status; increased fluid retention in cardiac disease; pulmonary function
• **Constitutional symptoms:** asthenia, chills, fever, headache, malaise
• Myalgia, arthralgia in legs, feet; use analgesics, antipyretics
• **Gasping syndrome in neonates:** due to benzyl alcohol hypersensitivity, do not use
• **Pregnancy/breastfeeding:** use only if clearly needed; cautious use in breastfeeding, excretion unknown
Evaluate:
• Therapeutic response: WBC and differential recovery

S

Teach patient/family:
• That bone pain may occur with use of the product and is normal
• To report excessive diarrhea, B/P increase, or respiratory symptoms to health care provider immediately
• To review all aspects of product use

---

sarilumab

(sar-il' ue-mab)

Kevzara

Func. class.: Antirheumatic, immunosuppressive

Chem. class.: Interleukin antagonist, monoclonal antibody

ACTION: Inhibits interleukin-6 (IL-6) receptors by binding to them, antiinflammatory action and a reduction in C-reactive protein

USES: Treatment of moderately to severely active rheumatoid arthritis in patients who have had an inadequate response or intolerance to one or more disease-modifying antirheumatic drugs (DMARDs); used as monotherapy or in combination with methotrexate or DMARDs

CONTRAINDICATIONS: Hypersensitivity, active infections, active severe hepatic disease, ANC <2000/mm³, platelets <150,000/mm³

Precautions: Chronic/recurrent infections, corticosteroid therapy, diabetes mellitus, TB, diverticulitis, risk of GI perforation, hepatic disease (Child-Pugh B), severe renal disease, pregnancy, lactation, children, geriatric patients, HIV, neoplastic disease

> **Black Box Warning:** Infection

DOSAGE AND ROUTES
• **Adult:** SUBCUT 200 mg q2wk

Dosage modifications for neutropenia, thrombocytopenia, or elevated liver enzymes
• Neutrophil count (ANC) 500 to 1000/mm³: Hold and restart when ANC >1000 cells/mm³; <500/mm³: Discontinue
• Platelets 50,000 to 100,000/mm³: Hold and restart when platelets >100,000/mm³; <50,000/mm³: Repeat test; discontinue if confirmed
• AST/ALT: If above the upper limit of normal (ULN), consider dose modification
Available forms: Sol for SUBCUT inj 150 mg/1.14 mL, 200 mg/1.14 mL single-use prefilled syringes or prefilled pen
Administer:
SUBCUT route
• A TB test before use; do not start therapy if patient has latent TB, treat first
• Visually inspect for particulate matter and discoloration before use; product is clear and colorless to pale yellow
• Allow to sit at room temperature for 30 min
• Inject full amount of the syringe
• Do not rub the injection site
• Dispose of used syringe or pen properly. Do not recap after use. Do not reuse the pen or syringe
• Rotate injection sites with each injection
• **Storage:** Use within 14 days after being taken out of the refrigerator

SIDE EFFECTS
GI: GI perforation
GU: UTI
HEMA: Thrombocytopenia, neutropenia, leukopenia
INTEG: Injection site reactions, rash, pruritus
MISC: Infections (TB), hypersensitivity, immunosuppression, malignancy
RESP: URI, dyspnea

PHARMACOKINETICS
Peak 2-4 days, duration 28-43 days depending on dose, half-life 150-mg dose is 8 days, 200-mg dose 10 days

---

INTERACTIONS

• **Increase:** immunosuppression, infections—DMARDs, TNF antagonists, corticosteroids, live virus vaccines

• **Altered effect:** CYP450 substrates (cyclosporine, atorvastatin, lovastatin, theophylline, warfarin, hormonal contraceptives); monitor substrate levels

NURSING CONSIDERATIONS

Assess

• **Infection:** flulike symptoms, fever, dyspnea, inflammation of wounds; perform TB test before starting treatment

• **Reactivation of viral herpes zoster:** blisters, rash; hepatitis B: dark urine, jaundice, clay-colored stools, weakness, fatigue, anorexia, nausea, vomiting, abdominal pain; immediately report any of these symptoms

• **Blood studies:** AST, ALT at baseline, 4 wk and 8 wk after starting therapy, and q3mo thereafter; lipid levels: at baseline, 4 wk and 8 wk after starting treatment, and q6mo thereafter; platelets at baseline, 4 wk and 8 wk after starting therapy, and q3mo thereafter; neutrophils: at baseline, 4 wk and 8 wk after starting therapy, and q3mo thereafter

Evaluate:

• Therapeutic response: slowing progression of rheumatoid arthritis

Teach patient/family:

• The reason for therapy and expected result

• The correct technique for subcut injection and proper disposal of syringes; to review the Medication Guide

• **Infection:** to report immediately fever, flulike symptoms, cough, blood in emesis, urine, stools; hypersensitivity: rash, itching

• **Pregnancy/breastfeeding:** to notify prescriber if pregnancy is planned or suspected or if breastfeeding; that pregnant women should enroll in the pregnancy registry at 1-877-311-8972

• To avoid live virus vaccines while taking this product; that vaccinations should be brought up-to-date before treatment

• To avoid OTC, herbal products or supplements without consent of prescriber; to discuss with all prescribers all medications and products taken

---

⚠ **HIGH ALERT**

SAXagliptin (Rx)

(sax-a-glip′tin)

Onglyza

Func. class.: Antidiabetic, oral

Chem. class.: Dipeptidyl-peptidase-4 inhibitor (DPP-4 inhibitor)

Do not confuse:
SAXagliptin/SITaGLIPtin

ACTION: Slows the inactivation of incretin hormones; improves glucose homeostasis, improves glucose-dependent insulin synthesis, lowers glucagon secretions, and slows gastric emptying time

USES: In adults, type 2 diabetes mellitus as monotherapy or in combination with other antidiabetic agents

CONTRAINDICATIONS: Hypersensitivity, angioedema, serious rash, type 1 diabetes, ketoacidosis

Precautions: Pregnancy, geriatric patients, GI obstruction, surgery, thyroid/renal/hepatic disease, trauma, diabetic, heart failure

DOSAGE AND ROUTES

• **Adult: PO** 2.5-5 mg; may use with other antidiabetic agents other than insulin; if used with insulin, a lower dose may be needed; max 2.5 mg with strong 3A4-5 inhibitors

Renal dose

• **Adult: PO** CCr ≤50 mL/min, 2.5 mg daily; **hemodialysis:** 2.5 mg/day after hemodialysis

Available forms: Tabs 2.5, 5 mg

Administer:

PO route

• May be taken with/without food

• Do not break or cut tabs

• Conversion from other antidiabetic agents; change may be made with gradual dosage change

S

• Store in tight containers at room temperature

SIDE EFFECTS
CNS: *Headache*
ENDO: Hypoglycemia (renal impairment)
GI: *Nausea, vomiting,* abdominal pain, pancreatitis
INTEG: Urticaria, angioedema, anaphylaxis
CV: Edema, HF
EENT: Sinusitis

PHARMACOKINETICS
Rapidly absorbed, metabolized by liver—CYP3A4, excreted by the kidneys (unchanged 24%), half-life 2.5 hr, 3.1 hr metabolite, peak 2 hr, duration 24 hr

INTERACTIONS
Increase: hypoglycemia—androgens, insulins, β-blockers, cimetidine, corticosteroids, salicylates, MAOIs, fibric acid derivatives, FLUoxetine, insulin, sulfonylureas, ACE inhibitors; strong CYP3A4/5 inhibitors; dosage reduction may be needed

Drug/Herb
Increase: antidiabetic effect—garlic, horse chestnut

Drug/Lab Test
Decrease: lymphocytes, glucose

NURSING CONSIDERATIONS
Assess:
• **Hypoglycemic reactions** (sweating, weakness, dizziness, anxiety, tremors, hunger); monitor blood glucose, HbA1c
• **Renal studies:** BUN, creatinine during treatment
• **Heart failure:** history of risk factors for heart failure; use cautiously in these patients
• **Pancreatitis:** abdominal pain, nausea; discontinue product immediately; previous pancreatitis may be a contributing factor
• **Pregnancy/breastfeeding:** use only if clearly needed, usually insulin is used in pregnancy; cautious use in breastfeeding, excretion unknown
Evaluate:
• Therapeutic response: decrease in polyuria, polydipsia, polyphagia; clear sensorium; absence of dizziness; stable gait, blood glucose at normal level
Teach patient/family:
• To perform regular self-monitoring of blood glucose using blood-glucose meter
• About the symptoms of hypo/hyperglycemia; what to do about each
• That product must be continued on daily basis; about consequences of discontinuing product abruptly
• To avoid OTC medications, alcohol, digoxin, exenatide, insulins, nateglinide, repaglinide, and other products that lower blood glucose unless approved by prescriber
• That diabetes is lifelong; that this product is not a cure, only controls symptoms
• That all food included in diet plan must be eaten to prevent hypo/hyperglycemia
• To carry emergency ID
• To take product without regard to food
• To notify prescriber when surgery, trauma, stress occurs because dose may need to be adjusted or insulin used
• **Pancreatitis:** to immediately report and stop product if severe abdominal pain with vomiting occurs
• **Hypersensitivity:** to immediately get medical assistance and stop product if itching, rash, swelling of face, tongue occurs

RARELY USED

scopolamine (Rx)
(skoe-pol′a-meen)
Transderm Scop
Func. class.: Cholinergic blocker
Chem. class.: Belladonna alkaloid

USES: Preoperatively to produce amnesia, sedation and to decrease secretions; motion sickness, parkinsonian symptoms

CONTRAINDICATIONS: Hypersensitivity, closed-angle glaucoma, myasthenia gravis, GI/GU obstruction, hypersensitivity to belladonna, barbiturates

DOSAGE AND ROUTES
Motion sickness
• **Adult: TD** 1 patch 4 hr before travel and q3days

Preoperatively
• **Adult:** **IM/IV/SUBCUT** 0.32-0.65 mg; **TD** apply 1 patch PM before surgery or 1 hr before C-section
Nausea and vomiting
• **Adult:** **SUBCUT** 0.6-1 mg
• **Child:** **SUBCUT** 0.006 mg/kg; max 0.3 mg/dose

RARELY USED

secnidazole
Solosec
Func. class.: Antiinfective

USES: Bacterial vaginosis

DOSAGE AND ROUTES
• **Adult:** **PO** 2 g as a single dose

---

secukinumab (Rx)
(sek'-ue-kin'-ue-mab)
Cosentyx
Func. class.: Immune response modifier
Chem. class.: Monoclonal antibody

ACTION: Interleukin (IL)-12, IL-23 antagonist

USES: Plaque psoriasis, ankylosing spondylitis, psoriatic arthritis

CONTRAINDICATIONS: Hypersensitivity, active TB
Precautions: Pregnancy, breastfeeding, Crohn's disease, infection, latex hypersensitivity, vaccination

DOSAGE AND ROUTES
Ankylosing spondylitis
• **Adult:** **SUBCUT** 150 mg at weeks 0, 1, 2, 3, and 4 and q4wk thereafter, or 150 mg **SUBCUT** q4wk
Psoriatic arthritis
• **Adult:** **SUBCUT** 150 mg at weeks 0, 1, 2, 3, and 4 and q4wk thereafter; may give with or without methotrexate; may consider dose of 300 mg if active disease persists, or 150 mg **SUBCUT** q4wk; may give with or without methotrexate; may consider a dose of 300 mg if active disease persists
Psoriatic arthritis with plaque psoriasis:
• **Adult:** **SUBCUT** Initially, 300 mg (2 injections of 150 mg) at weeks 0, 1, 2, 3, and 4; **Maintenance:** 300 mg (2 injections of 150 mg) q4wk
Available forms: Solution for injection 150 mg/mL (pen, prefilled syringe), 2-pack and single
Administer:
• Visually inspect for particulate matter or discoloration; solution should be slightly yellow and may contain a few small translucent or white particles; do not use if discolored, cloudy, or if foreign particulate matter is present; do not shake
• Use a 27-G, 0.5-inch needle
• May be administered SUBCUT into upper arm, abdomen, or thigh; rotate injection sites
• Use by SUBCUT injection only
• Those with latex hypersensitivity should not handle cap of injection
SUBCUT injection:
• Patients may use the prefilled syringe or Sensoready pen after proper training; the lyophilized powder is for health care provider use only
• Each 300-mg dose is used as 2 SUBCUT injections of 150 mg
• Do not administer where skin is tender, bruised, erythematous, indurated, or affected by psoriasis
• **Reconstitution of lyophilized powder:** allow to warm to room temperature for 15-30 min, use 1 mL sterile water for injection to reconstitute, rotate, do not shake or invert vial, allow to stand for 10 min, again rotate vial, allow to stand for another 5 min (150 mg/mL)
• Storage: use immediately or refrigerate for up to 24 hr. Do not freeze. If refrigerated, allow reconstituted solution to reach room temperature (15-30 min) before administration

S

Side effects: *italics* = common; red = life-threatening

• **Preparation for use of prefilled syringe or Sensoready pen:** remove prefilled syringe or Sensoready pen from refrigerator and allow 15-30 min to reach room temperature
• Storage: the prefilled syringe or Sensoready should be used within 1 hr

SIDE EFFECTS

EENT: Ocular infections, sinusitis, oral ulceration, rhinitis
GI: Diarrhea
HEMA: Bleeding
INTEG: *Injection-site reaction,* urticaria
SYST: Serious infections, anaphylaxis, antibody formation, candidiasis
RESP: URI

PHARMACOKINETICS

Maximum serum concentration: 13.5 days after a single 45-mg SUBCUT dose, 7 days after a single 90-mg SUBCUT dose; half-life 14.9-45.6 days

INTERACTIONS

• Do not give concurrently with vaccines; immunizations should be brought up-to-date before treatment
• Avoid use with immunosuppressives
Drug/Lab tests
Increase: LFTs

NURSING CONSIDERATIONS
Assess:

• **TB:** TB testing should be done before starting treatment
• For injection-site pain, swelling
• Bring immunizations up-to-date before starting treatment
• **Infection:** monitor for fever, sore throat, cough; do not use during active infections
• **Malignancy:** skin cancer may occur, especially in older patients who have used ultraviolet treatments with immunosuppressants
• **Pregnancy/breastfeeding:** use only if benefits outweigh fetal risk; cautious use in breastfeeding, excretion unknown
Evaluate:
• Therapeutic response: decreased plaque psoriasis
Teach patient/family:

• That product must be continued for prescribed time to be effective; to use as prescribed
• Not to receive live vaccinations during treatment; that vaccinations should be brought up-to-date before use of this product
• To notify prescriber of possible infection (upper respiratory or other) or allergic reactions
• To report to provider the presence of inflammatory bowel disease, persistent diarrhea; product can cause inflammatory bowel disease
• To report latex allergy; prefilled injection device (Sensoready) may contain latex
• Not to use pen if fluid contains particulate; to use within 1 hr of removing from refrigerator
• Injection techniques and disposal of equipment; not to reuse needles, syringes; to rotate injection sites with each dose; not to inject into bruised or damaged skin

---

selegiline (Rx)
(se-le′ji-leen)
Eldepryl, Emsam, Zelapar
Func. class.: Antiparkinson agent, antidepressant
Chem. class.: MAOI, type B

Do not confuse:
selegiline/Salagen
Zelapar/ZyPREXA

ACTION: Increased dopaminergic activity by inhibition of MAO type B activity; not fully understood

USES: Adjunct management of Parkinson's disease for patients being treated with levodopa/carbidopa who had poor response to therapy; depression (transdermal)
Unlabeled uses: Alzheimer's disease

CONTRAINDICATIONS:
Children/adolescents (suicide/hypertensive crisis), hypersensitivity, breastfeeding, MAOIs

Precautions: Pregnancy, abrupt discontinuation, alcoholism, ambient temperature increase, behavioral changes, bipolar disorders, driving or operating machinery, geriatrics, heating pad, hepatic disease, hypertension, hypotension, melanoma, phenylketonuria, psychosis, renal disease, sunlight exposure

DOSAGE AND ROUTES
• **Adult:** PO 5 mg bid given with levodopa/carbidopa in divided doses, after 2-3 days, begin to reduce dose of levodopa/carbidopa 10%-30%; **ORAL DISINTEGRATING** 1.25 mg (1 tab) × 6 wk or more initially, then 2.5 mg (2 tabs) dissolved on tongue daily before breakfast; max 2.5 mg/day; **TRANSDERMAL** (depression) 6 mg/24 hr initially, increase by 3 mg/24 hr at ≥2 wk, up to 12 mg/24 hr if needed

Alzheimer's disease (unlabeled)
• **Adult:** PO 5 mg bid AM, PM

Available forms: Tabs 5 mg; caps 5 mg; oral disintegrating tabs 1.25 mg; transdermal 6 mg/24 hr (20 mg/20 cm^2), 9 mg/24 hr (30 mg/30 cm^2), 12 mg/24 hr (40 mg/40 cm^2)

Administer:
PO route
• Do not use in children due to risk for hypertensive crisis
• Product until NPO before surgery
• Adjust dosage to response
• With meals; limit protein taken with product
• Dosing bid in AM and afternoon; avoid PM or bedtime dosing
• At doses of <10 mg/day because of risks associated with nonselective inhibition of MAO
• **Oral disintegrating tab:** peel back foil; remove tab; do not push through foil; place tab on tongue; allow to dissolve; swallow with saliva; no fluids 5 min before or after use; avoid using >2.5 mg/day, hypertensive crisis is more common

Transdermal route (depression)
• Apply to dry intact skin on upper torso, upper thigh, or outer surface of upper arm q24hr

• When using 9 mg/24 hr or 12 mg/24 hr, specific manufacturer's recommendation for tyramine intake must be followed to prevent hypertensive crisis

SIDE EFFECTS
CNS: Increased tremors, tardive dyskinesia, dystonic symptoms, hallucinations, *dizziness,* mood changes, nightmares, delusions, serotonin syndrome, headache, migraine, confusion, anxiety, suicide in child/adolescent, suicidal ideation in adults
CV: Orthostatic hypotension, angina pectoris, hypertensive crisis (children)
EENT: Tinnitus
GI: Nausea, weight loss, vomiting, flatulence
GU: Slow urination, nocturia, prostatic hypertrophy, urinary hesitation, retention, frequency, sexual dysfunction
INTEG: Increased sweating, melanoma, acne, pruritus; site reactions (transdermal)
RESP: Asthma, SOB

PHARMACOKINETICS
PO peak ½-2 hr, orally disintegrating tab 10-15 min, TD 2 wk; rapidly metabolized (active metabolites: *N*-desmethyldeprenyl, amphetamine, methamphetamine); metabolites excreted in urine; half-life 10 hr, orally disintegrating tab 1.3 hr, transdermal 18-25 hr; protein binding up to 85%

INTERACTIONS
• **Fatal interaction:** opioids (especially meperidine); do not administer together
• **Serotonin syndrome (confusion, seizures, fever, hypertension, agitation; death):** FLUoxetine, PARoxetine, sertraline, fluvoxaMINE (discontinue 5 wk before selegiline treatment); do not use together
Increase: side effects of levodopa/carbidopa

S

Increase: unusual behavior, psychosis — dextromethorphan
Increase: hypotension—antihypertensives
Drug/Lab Test
Decrease: VMA
False positive: urine ketones, urine glucose
False negative: urine glucose (glucose oxidase)
False increase: uric acid, urine protein

NURSING CONSIDERATIONS
Assess:
• **Parkinson's symptoms:** decreased rigidity, unsteady gait, weakness, tremors
• Cardiac status: tachycardia/bradycardia; B/P, respiration throughout treatment

> **Black Box Warning: Depression:** affect, mood, behavioral changes, depression; perform suicide assessment on all patients; suicidal ideation may occur

• **Opioids:** if patient has received, do not administer selegiline; fatal reactions have occurred
• **Orthostatic hypotension:** may occur during first few months of treatment, usually in patients >60 yr
Evaluate:
• Therapeutic response: decrease in akathisia, improved mood
Teach patient/family:
• To change positions slowly to prevent orthostatic hypotension
• **Hypertensive crisis:** to notify prescriber immediately of nausea, vomiting, sweating, agitation, change in mental status, headache, chest pain
• **Serotonin syndrome:** to report twitching, sweating, shivering, diarrhea to prescriber immediately
• To use product exactly as prescribed; that if discontinued abruptly, parkinsonian crisis may occur
• To use during the day to prevent insomnia
• To avoid heating pads, hot tubs when using transdermal products
• To avoid hazardous activities until response is known

• To avoid foods high in tyramine: cheese, pickled products, wine, beer, large amounts of caffeine as per manufacturer

> **Black Box Warning: Suicidal ideation:** to report change in symptoms, worsening depression, or suicidal thoughts, behaviors; treatment may need to be changed

• Not to exceed recommended dose of 10 mg (PO) because this might precipitate hypertensive crisis; to report severe headache, other unusual symptoms
• Pregnancy: to report if pregnancy is planned or suspected; not to breastfeed

TREATMENT OF OVERDOSE:
IV fluids for hypertension, IV dilute pressure agent for B/P titration

selenium topical
See Appendix B

RARELY USED

semaglutide
Ozempic
Func. class.: Antidiabetic

USES: For the treatment of type II diabetes

DOSAGE AND ROUTES
Type 2 diabetes mellitus in combination with diet and exercise
• **Adult:** SUBCUT Initially, 0.25 mg q7days (weekly); give at any time of day, with or without meals; after 4 wk increase dose to 0.5 mg weekly

sertraline (Rx)
(ser'tra-leen)
Zoloft
Func. class.: Antidepressant
Chem. class.: SSRI

Do not confuse:
Zoloft/Zocor

ACTION: Inhibits serotonin reuptake in CNS; increases action of serotonin; does not affect dopamine, norepinephrine

USES: Major depressive disorder, obsessive-compulsive disorder (OCD), posttraumatic stress disorder (PTSD), panic disorder, social anxiety disorder, premenstrual dysphoric disorder (PMDD)
Unlabeled uses: Generalized anxiety disorder

CONTRAINDICATIONS: Hypersensitivity to this product or SSRIs
Precautions: Pregnancy, breastfeeding, geriatric patients, renal/hepatic disease, epilepsy, recent MI, latex sensitivity (dropper of oral concentration)

Black Box Warning: Children, suicidal ideation

DOSAGE AND ROUTES
Major depression/OCD
• **Adult/geriatric patient/adolescent (unlabeled):** PO 25-50 mg/day; may increase to max of 200 mg/day; do not change dose at intervals of <1 wk; administer daily in AM or PM
• **Child 6-12 yr (unlabeled):** PO 25 mg/day, increase by 25-50 mg/wk
PTSD/social anxiety disorder/panic disorder
• **Adult:** PO 25 mg/day, may increase by 50 mg/day after 7 days, range 50-200 mg
Premenstrual dysphoric disorder
• **Adult:** PO 50-150 mg nightly
Hepatic dose
• **Adult:** PO use lower dose or less frequent dosing intervals
Available forms: Tabs 25, 50, 100 mg; concentrate 20 mg/mL; capsules 25 ✤, 50 ✤, 100 mg ✤
Administer:
• Store at room temperature; do not freeze
• Increased fluids, bulk in diet for constipation, urinary retention
• With food, milk for GI symptoms

• Tablets crushed if patient is unable to swallow medication whole
• Sugarless gum, hard candy, frequent sips of water for dry mouth
• **Oral concentration:** dilute before use with 4 oz ($^1/_2$ cup) of water, orange juice, ginger ale, or lemon/lime soda; do not mix with other liquids
• Avoid use with other CNS depressants
• Dropper contains latex

SIDE EFFECTS
CNS: *Insomnia, agitation, dizziness, headache, fatigue,* confusion, gait abnormality (geriatric patients), neuroleptic malignant syndrome–like reaction, serotonin syndrome, suicidal ideation, anxiety, drowsiness
CV: Palpitations, chest pain
EENT: Vision abnormalities, yawning, tinnitus, intraocular pressure
ENDO: SIADH (geriatric patients); diabetes mellitus
GI: *Diarrhea, nausea, constipation, anorexia, dry mouth,* dyspepsia, *vomiting, flatulence,* weight gain/loss
GU: *Male sexual dysfunction,* menstrual disorders, urinary frequency
INTEG: Increased sweating, rash, hot flashes
MISC: Hyponatremia, neonatal abstinence syndrome

PHARMACOKINETICS
PO: Peak 4.5-8.4 hr; protein binding 98%; distribution to tissues, half-life 26 hr; extensively metabolized; metabolite excreted in urine, bile; weak inhibitor of CYP3A4, moderate inhibitor of CYP2D6

INTERACTIONS
• Altered lithium levels: lithium
• Disulfiram reaction: disulfiram and oral concentration due to alcohol content
Fatal reactions: MAOIs, pimozide; avoid use within 2 wk
Increase: sertraline levels—cimetidine, warfarin, other highly protein-bound products
Increase: effects of antidepressants (tricyclics), diazepam, TOLBUTamide,

S

warfarin, benzodiazepines, SUMAtriptan, phenytoin, cloZAPine

Increase: bleeding risk—anticoagulants, NSAIDs, thrombolytic, platelet inhibitors, salicylates

Increase: serotonin syndrome, neuroleptic malignant syndrome—SSRIs, SNRIs, serotonin-receptor agonists, tricyclics, cyclobenzeprine, sibutramine, traZODone, busPIRone, linezolid, traMADol; avoid concurrent use

Drug/Herb

Increase: SSRI, serotonin syndrome—St. John's wort, SAM-e, tryptophan; do not use together

Increase: CNS effect—kava, valerian

Drug/Lab Test

Increase: AST, ALT

False positive: urine screen for benzodiazepines

NURSING CONSIDERATIONS
Assess:

Black Box Warning: **Depression/OCD/ PTSD:** mood, sensorium, affect, suicidal tendencies (child/young adult), increase in psychiatric symptoms, depression, panic attacks, OCD, PTSD, social anxiety disorder; symptoms usually occur in first few months of treatment

• **Premenstrual dysphoric disorder:** emotional lability, sad, hopelessness, insomnia, anxiety, food cravings, breast pain/tenderness
• **Serotonin syndrome** (hyperthermia, hypertension, rigidity, delirium, coma, myoclonus) or **neuroleptic malignant syndrome–like reaction** (muscle cramps, fever, unstable B/P, agitation, tremors, mental changes)
• **Bleeding (platelet serotonin depletion):** GI bleeding, ecchymoses, epistaxis, hematomas, petechiae, hemorrhage
• LFTs, thyroid function tests, growth rate, weight at baseline and periodically
• **Hypotension:** B/P (lying/standing), pulse q4hr; if systolic B/P drops 20 mm Hg, hold product, notify prescriber; VS q4hr in patients with CV disease
• Weight weekly; appetite may decrease with product

• Urinary retention, constipation, especially in geriatric patients
• Alcohol consumption; hold dose until morning
• **Beers:** avoid in older adults unless safer alternatives are unavailable; may cause ataxia, impaired psychomotor function
• **Pregnancy/breastfeeding:** use only if benefits outweigh fetal risk; serious complications may occur in neonates; cautious use in breastfeeding, excretion unknown

Evaluate:
• Therapeutic response: significant improvement in depression, OCD, PTSD, PMDD

Teach patient/family:
• That therapeutic effect may take ≥1 wk
• To use caution when driving, performing other activities requiring alertness because drowsiness, dizziness, blurred vision may occur
• Not to discontinue medication quickly after long-term use; may cause nausea, headache, malaise
• To avoid alcohol
• May be taken without regard to food
• That follow-up exams will be needed
• **Serotonin syndrome:** agitation, nausea, vomiting, diarrhea, twitching, sweating, shivering; report to prescriber immediately

Black Box Warning: **Suicidal ideation:** that suicidal thoughts/behaviors may occur in children/adolescents; to notify prescriber immediately if suicidal thoughts, panic attacks, severe anxiety occur

• To notify prescriber if pregnant or if planning to become pregnant, or if breastfeeding

sildenafil (Rx)
(sil-den'a-fill)
Revatio, Viagra
Func. class.: Erectile agent, antihypertensive, pulmonary vasodilator
Chem. class.: Phosphodiesterase type-5 inhibitor

Do not confuse:
Viagra/Allegra

ACTION: Enhances the effect of nitric oxide (NO) by inhibiting phosphodiesterase type 5 (PDE5), which is necessary for degrading cGMP in the corpus cavernosum

USES: Treatment of erectile dysfunction (Viagra), improvement in exercise ability, pulmonary hypertension (Revatio)
Unlabeled uses: Sexual dysfunction (women); altitude sickness, Raynaud's disease

CONTRAINDICATIONS: Hypersensitivity to this product or nitrates
Precautions: Pregnancy, anatomical penile deformities, sickle cell anemia, leukemia, multiple myeloma, retinitis pigmentosa, bleeding disorders, active peptic ulceration, CV/renal/hepatic disease, multiproduct antihypertensive regimens, geriatric patients

DOSAGE AND ROUTES
Erectile dysfunction (Viagra only)
• **Adult male <65 yr: PO** 50 mg 1 hr before sexual activity; may be increased to 100 mg or decreased to 25 mg; max frequency 1×/day; use with alpha blockers: space 50-100 mg dose ≥4 hr of alpha blocker
• **Adult ≥65 yr (male): PO** 25 mg as needed about 1 hr before sexual activity
Renal/hepatic dose
• **Adult: PO** (Child-Pugh A, B) 25 mg, take 1 hr before sexual activity; max 1×/day; CCr <30 mL/min, 25 mg starting dose
Pulmonary hypertension (Revatio only)
• **Adult: PO** 20 mg tid; take 4-6 hr apart; **IV BOL** 10 mg tid
Pulmonary hypertension induced by altitude sickness (unlabeled)
• **Adult: PO** 40 mg 6-8 hr after arriving at 14,272 ft, then 40 mg tid × 6 days
Anorgasmy in antidepressant therapy/sexual dysfunction in women (unlabeled)
• **Adult: PO** 50 mg 60-90 min before sexual activity

Available forms: Tabs (Viagra), 25, 50, 100 mg; ; tabs (Revatio) 25 mg; sol for inj 10 mg/12.5 mL; powder for oral suspension 10 mg/mL (Revatio)
Administer:
• **Erectile dysfunction:** give approximately 1 hr before sexual activity; do not use more than 1×/day; give on empty stomach for better absorption
• **Pulmonary hypertension:** give 3×/day, 4-6 hr apart
IV Push Route
• Give undiluted, check that solution is not discolored or precipitate is present, give tid

SIDE EFFECTS
CNS: *Headache, flushing, dizziness,* transient global amnesia, seizures
CV: MI, sudden death, CV collapse, TIAs, ventricular dysrhythmias, CV hemorrhage
MISC.: *Dyspepsia, nasal congestion, UTI, abnormal vision, diarrhea, rash,* nonarteritic ischemic optic neuropathy, hearing loss, priapism, sickle cell crisis

PHARMACOKINETICS
Rapidly absorbed; bioavailability 40%; metabolized by P45 CYP3A4, 2C9 in the liver (active metabolites); terminal half-life 4 hr; peak 15-30 min; reduced absorption with high-fat meal; excreted in feces, urine

INTERACTIONS
Do not use with nitrates, riociguat; fatal fall in B/P

Increase: sildenafil levels—cimetidine, erythromycin, ketoconazole, itraconazole, antiretroviral protease inhibitors, tacrolimus
Decrease: sildenafil levels—CYP450 inducers, rifampin, barbiturates, bosentan, carBAMazepine, dexamethasone, phenytoin, nevirapine, rifabutin, troglitazone; antacids
Decrease: B/P—α-blockers, alcohol, amLODIPine, angiotensin II receptor blockers
Drug/Food
Increase: product effect—grapefruit
Decrease: absorption—high-fat meal

S

Side effects: *italics* = common; red = life-threatening

NURSING CONSIDERATIONS
Assess:

• **For erectile dysfunction before use (Viagra):** question about any failure to achieve erection or failure to maintain intercourse, anorgasmia

• **Phosphodiesterase type 5 inhibitors with lopinavir/ritonavir (Kaletra):** assess for hypotension, visual changes, prolonged erection, syncope; give only 25 mg q48hr and monitor for adverse reactions

• **Vision loss:** any severe loss of vision while taking this or any similar products; products should not be used

• Use of organic nitrates that should not be used with this product

• **MI, sudden death, CV collapse:** those with an MI within 6 mo, resting hypotension <90/50, resting hypertension >170/100, fluid depletion should use this product cautiously; may occur right after sexual activity to days afterward

• **Sickle cell crisis (vasoocclusive crisis):** when used for pulmonary hypertension; may require hospitalization

• **Pulmonary hypertension:** Cardiac status, hemodynamic parameters, exercise tolerance in pulmonary hypertension: B/P, pulse (Revatio)

Evaluate:

• Therapeutic response: decreasing pulmonary hypertension/improved exercise tolerance (Revatio); ability to perform sexually (male) (Viagra)

Teach patient/family:

• That product does not protect against sexually transmitted diseases, including HIV

• That product absorption is reduced with a high-fat meal, to take on empty stomach for faster action; to take 30 min to 4 hr before sexual activity; peak is 2 hr

• That product should not be used with nitrates or soluble guanylate cyclase stimulators (riociguat) (PAH)

• That tabs may be split

• To notify prescriber immediately and to stop taking product if vision/hearing loss occurs or erection lasts >4 hr

• Do not use more than 100 mg in 24 hr

• To use only as directed

• That color vision may be altered

• **About cardiac risk:** usually in cardiac disease

• **Pregnancy/breastfeeding:** not indicated for women (Viagra), unknown in PAH, cautious use in breastfeeding (Revatio)

---

silodosin (Rx)

(si-lo'do-seen)

Rapaflo

Func. class.: Selective α_1-adrenergic blocker, BPH agent

Chem. class.: Sulfamoylphenethylamine derivative

ACTION: Binds preferentially to α_{1A}-adrenoceptor subtype located mainly in the prostate

USES: Symptoms of benign prostatic hyperplasia (BPH)

CONTRAINDICATIONS: Hypersensitivity, renal failure, hepatic disease
Precautions: Pregnancy, breastfeeding, children, females, geriatric patients, renal/hepatic disease, hypotension, ocular surgery, orthostatic hypotension, prostate cancer, syncope

DOSAGE AND ROUTES

• **Adult: PO** 8 mg/day with meal; max 8 mg/day

Renal dose

• **Adult: PO** CCr 30-49 mL/min, 4 mg/day; CCr <30 mL/min, not recommended

Available forms: Cap 4, 8 mg

Administer:

• Give with meal at same time each day

• Cap may be opened and sprinkled on applesauce, if unable to swallow, use water after applesauce

• Store at room temperature; protect from light and moisture

SIDE EFFECTS

CNS: *Dizziness, headache,* insomnia

CV: Orthostatic hypotension

EENT: Nasal congestion
GI: Diarrhea
GU: *Abnormal ejaculation*, urinary incontinence
INTEG: Rash, pruritus, allergic reactions

PHARMACOKINETICS
Decreased absorption with high-fat/high-calorie meal, half-life 13.3 hr of metabolite 24 hr, metabolized in liver extensively by CYP3A4, UGT2B7, excreted via urine, feces (55%) extensively protein bound (97%), onset rapid, peak up to 24 hr, duration up to 24 hr

INTERACTIONS
Increase: silodosin effect—CYP3A4 inhibitors (clarithromycin, itraconazole, ritonavir, antiretroviral protease inhibitors, aprepitant, chloramphenicol, conivaptan, dalfopristin, danazol, delavirdine, efavirenz, fosaprepitant, fluconazole, fluvoxaMINE, imatinib, isoniazid, miFEPRIStone, nefazodone, tamoxifen, telithromycin, troleandomycin, voriconazole, zileuton, zafirlukast); P-gb inhibitors
Drug/Food
Increase: silodosin effect—grapefruit juice
Drug Lab/Test
Increase: LFTs

NURSING CONSIDERATIONS
Assess:
• **Prostatic hyperplasia:** change in urinary patterns at baseline and throughout treatment; testing for prostate cancer before administration is recommended
• BUN, uric acid, urodynamic studies (urinary flow rates, residual volume), CCr; contraindicated in CCr <30 mL/min; I&O ratios, weight daily, edema, report weight gain or edema
• B/P (sitting, standing) during initial treatment; monitor for orthostatic hypotension; increased risk in elderly >65 yr
• **Pregnancy/breastfeeding:** not indicated for women
Evaluate:
• Therapeutic response: decreased symptoms of BPH

Teach patient/family
• Not to drive or operate machinery until effect is known; orthostatic hypotension occasionally occurs after first dose
• Not to use with grapefruit juice
• To take with same meal each day; contents of capsule may be sprinkled on room-temperature applesauce if consumed within 5 min; follow with 8 oz cool water

⚠ HIGH ALERT

RARELY USED

siltuximab
(sil-tux'-i-mab)
Sylvant ✿
Func. class.: Antineoplastic: immune response modifier

USES: Multicentric Castleman disease (MCD) patients who are HIV-negative and human herpesvirus-8 (HHV-8)–negative

CONTRAINDICATIONS: Hypersensitivity

DOSAGE AND ROUTES
• **Adult: IV** 11 mg/kg over 1 hr q3wk until treatment failure

silver nitrate 1% ophthalmic
See Appendix B

silver nitrate 1% sulfacetamide sodium ophthalmic
See Appendix B

silver sulfADIAZINE topical
See Appendix B

RARELY USED

simethicone (OTC, Rx)

(si-meth′i-kone)

Barriere ♣, Gas Relief ♣, Gas-Relief, Gas-X, Mylanta Gas Relief, Mylanta Gas, Mylicon, Ovol ♣, Phazyme

Func. class.: Antiflatulent

USES: Flatulence
Unlabeled uses: Dyspepsia

CONTRAINDICATIONS: Hypersensitivity, GI obstruction/perforation

DOSAGE AND ROUTES
• **Adult and child >12 yr: PO** 40-125 mg after meals and at bedtime prn, max 500 mg/day, 750 mg/day chewable
• **Child 2-12 yr: PO** 40-50 mg after meals and at bedtime prn, max 240 mg/day
• **Child <2 yr: PO** 20 mg qid prn

---

simvastatin (Rx)

(sim-va-sta′tin)

Zocor

Chem. class.: HMG-CoA reductase inhibitor

Do not confuse:
Zocor/Cozaar/Zoloft

ACTION: Inhibits HMG-CoA reductase enzyme, which reduces cholesterol synthesis

USES: As an adjunct for primary hypercholesterolemia (types IIa, IIb), isolated hypertriglyceridemia (Fredrickson type IV), and type III hyperlipoproteinemia, CAD, heterozygous familial hypercholesterolemia; MI/stroke prophylaxis

CONTRAINDICATIONS: Pregnancy, breastfeeding, hypersensitivity, active hepatic disease
Precautions: Past hepatic disease, alcoholism, severe acute infections, trauma, severe metabolic disorders, electrolyte imbalances, Chinese patients

DOSAGE AND ROUTES
• **Adult: PO** 20-40 mg/day in PM initially; usual range 5-40 mg/day in PM, max 40 mg/day for most patients, max 80 mg/day for patients taking 80 mg/day chronically without myopathy; dosage adjustments may be made in ≥4-wk intervals; those taking verapamil and amiodarone max 20 mg/day; max <80 mg for Chinese patients taking lipid-modifying niacin doses
• **Child/adolescent ≥10 yr including girls ≥1 yr postmenarche: PO** 10 mg in PM, range 10-40 mg/day
With diltiaZEM/verapamil/dronedarone
• **Adult: PO** 5-10 mg in PM, max 10 mg/day
With amiodarone, amoLODIPine, ranolazine
• **Adult: PO** 5-20 mg daily in evening, max 20 mg/day
Heterozygous familial hypercholesterolemia
• **Adult: PO** 40 mg daily in evening, make dosage adjustments q4wk
Heterozygous familial hypercholesterolemia in boys and postmenarchal girls
• **Child 10-17 yr: PO** 10 mg/day in the evening, max 40 mg/day
Renal dose
• **Adult: PO** 5 mg/day in the evening (severe renal disease)
Available forms: Tabs 5, 10, 20, 40, 80 mg
Administer:
• Discontinuing use before surgery is recommended in renal failure; restart afterward
• Avoid grapefruit juice
• Total daily dose in evening
• Store in cool environment in tight container protected from light

SIDE EFFECTS
CNS: Headache, cognitive impairment
GI: Nausea, constipation, diarrhea, dyspepsia, flatus, abdominal pain, liver dysfunction, pancreatitis, hyperglycemia
INTEG: Rash, pruritus

♣ Canada only

🧬 Genetic warning

MS: Muscle cramps, *myalgia*, myositis, rhabdomyolysis, myopathy
RESP: Upper respiratory tract infection

PHARMACOKINETICS

Metabolized in liver (active metabolites); >98% protein bound; excreted primarily in bile, feces (60%), kidneys (15%); peak 1-2 hr; half-life 3 hr

INTERACTIONS

Do not use with cycloSPORINE, gemfibrozil
Increase: effects of warfarin
Increase: rhabdomyolysis, myalgia; do not use concurrently—CYP3A4 inhibitors, niacin, erythromycin, clofibrate, clarithromycin, ketoconazole, itraconazole, protease inhibitors, macrolide antibiotics, danazol, delavirdine, nefazodone, verapamil, diltiaZEM, amiodarone, azole antifungals, telithromycin, voriconazole
Increase: simvastatin effect—ATP1B1 inhibitors
Increase: serum level of digoxin
Drug/Herb
Increase: effect—red yeast rice, kava, eucalyptus
Decrease: effect—St. John's wort
Drug/Food
Increase: simvastatin level—grapefruit juice (large amounts)
Drug/Lab Test
Increase: CK, LFTs, HbA1c, ALT, AST

NURSING CONSIDERATIONS
Assess:
• **Diet history:** fat consumption; baseline and lipid profile: LDL, HDL, TG, cholesterol
• Hepatic studies at baseline, if clinically indicated; AST, ALT may increase
• **Rhabdomyolysis:** muscle tenderness, increased CPK levels (10 × ULN); therapy should be discontinued, more likely in those receiving >80 mg/day, first year of treatment, those ≥65 yr, females
• **Chinese patients:** avoid high doses (80 mg) if taking niacin >1 g/day due to increased risk of myopathies
• Renal studies in patients with compromised renal systems: BUN, I&O ratio, creatinine

• **Pregnancy/breastfeeding:** do not use in pregnancy, breastfeeding
Evaluate:
• Therapeutic response: decrease in LDL, total cholesterol, triglycerides; increase in HDL; slowing CAD
Teach patient/family:
• That blood work, follow-up exams will be necessary during treatment
• To report severe GI symptoms, headache
• That previously prescribed regimen will continue: low-cholesterol diet, exercise program, smoking cessation
• To take in evening, avoid using grapefruit juice
• To report muscle pain, weakness, abdominal pain, dark urine, yellowing of skin, eyes, memory loss
• This product may affect blood sugar levels in diabetes
• That compliance is needed for positive results, not to skip or double doses
• To notify prescriber if pregnancy is suspected or planned; not to breastfeed

---

⚠ HIGH ALERT

sirolimus (Rx)
(seer-oh-lie′mus)
Rapamune
Func. class.: Immunosuppressant
Chem. class.: Macrolide

S

ACTION: Produces immunosuppression by inhibiting T-lymphocyte activation and proliferation

USES: Organ transplants to prevent rejection; recommended use is with cycloSPORINE and corticosteroids

CONTRAINDICATIONS: Breastfeeding, hypersensitivity to this product, components of product
Precautions: Pregnancy, children <13 yr, severe cardiac/renal/hepatic disease; diabetes mellitus, hyperkalemia, hyperuricemia, hypertension, interstitial lung disease, hyperlipidemia, soya lecithin hypersensitivity

---

Side effects: *italics* = common; red = life-threatening

Black Box Warning: Lymphomas, infection, other malignancies, liver transplant, lung transplant; requires a specialized setting; requires an experienced clinician

Black Box Warning: Only those experienced in immunosuppressant therapy and transplant should use this drug; must use in a specialized care setting with adequate medical equipment

DOSAGE AND ROUTES
Kidney transplant
• **Adult/adolescent ≥40 kg:** PO 2 mg/day with 6 mg loading dose
• **Child >13 yr weighing <40 kg (88 lb):** PO 1 mg/m^2/day, 3 mg/m^2 loading dose
Hepatic dose
• Adult/child ≥13 yr/<40 kg: PO reduce by 33% for maintenance dose (mild to moderate hepatic impairment); reduce by 50% for maintenance dose (severe hepatic impairment)
Lymphangioleimyotosis
Adult: PO 2 mg daily trough level (whole blood) after 10-20 days, titrate to 5-15 ng/mL, then monitor trough q3mo
Available forms: Oral sol 1 mg/mL; tabs 0.5 mg, 1 mg, 2 mg
Administer:
• Prophylaxis for *Pneumocystis jiroveci* pneumonia for 1 yr after transplantation; prophylaxis for CMV is recommended for 90 days after transplantation in those at increased risk for CMV
• All medications PO if possible; avoid IM inj; bleeding may occur
• For 3 days before transplant surgery; patients should be placed in protective isolation; give at same time of day; give 4 hr after cycloSPORINE oral sol or caps; do not give with grapefruit juice
• Use amber oral dose syringe and withdraw amount of oral sol needed; empty dose into plastic/glass container holding 60 mL of water/orange juice; stir vigorously and have patient drink at once; refill container with additional 120 mL water/orange juice; stir vigorously and have patient drink at once; if using a pouch, squeeze entire contents into container; follow above directions
• Store protected from light, refrigerate; stable for 30 days after opening (sol)
• Do not crush, chew; store tabs at room temperature

SIDE EFFECTS
CNS: *Tremors, headache, insomnia, paresthesia,* chills, fever, progressive multifocal leukoencephalopathy (PML)
CV: Hypertension, *atrial fibrillation, HF,* hypotension, palpitation, tachycardia, peripheral edema, thrombosis
EENT: Blurred vision, photophobia
GI: Nausea, vomiting, diarrhea, constipation, hepatotoxicity, CDAD
GU: UTIs, albuminuria, hematuria, proteinuria, renal failure, nephrotic syndrome, increased creatinine, amenorrhea
HEMA: Anemia, leukopenia, thrombocytopenia
INTEG: *Rash, acne,* photosensitivity
META: Hyperglycemia, increased creatinine, edema, hypercholesterolemia, *hyperlipemia,* hypophosphatemia, weight gain, hypo/hyperkalemia, hyperuricemia, hypomagnesemia, hypertriglyceridemia
MS: Arthralgia
RESP: Pleural effusion, atelectasis, *dyspnea,* pneumonitis, pulmonary embolism/fibrosis, pulmonary hypertension, interstitial lung disease
SYST: Lymphoma, exfoliative dermatitis

PHARMACOKINETICS
Rapidly absorbed; peak 1 hr single dose, 2 hr multiple dosing; protein binding 92%; distribution to major organs, extensively metabolized by CYP3A4 excretion 91% feces, half-life 57-63 hr

INTERACTIONS
Increase: angioedema—ACE inhibitors, angiotensin II–receptor antagonists, cephalosporins, iodine-containing radiopaque contrast media, neuromuscular blockers, NSAIDs, penicillins, salicylates, thrombolytics
Increase: blood levels—antifungals, calcium channel blockers, cimetidine, danazol,

erythromycin, cycloSPORINE, meto-
clopramide, bromocriptine, HIV-protease
inhibitors
Decrease: blood levels—carBAMaze-
pine, PHENobarbital, phenytoin, rifamy-
cin, rifapentine
Decrease: effect of vaccines
Drug/Herb
• St. John's wort: may decrease the effect
of sirolimus
Drug/Food
• Alters bioavailability; use consistently
with/without food; do not use with grape-
fruit juice
Drug/Lab Test
Increase: LFTs, alk phos, lipids, triglycer-
ides, total cholesterol, BUN, creatinine,
LDH, phosphate
Decrease: platelets, sodium
Increase or decrease: magnesium, glu-
cose, calcium

NURSING CONSIDERATIONS
Assess:
• Blood levels in patients who may have
altered metabolism, trough level ≥15 ng/
mL is associated with increased adverse
reactions; monitor trough concentrations
in all patients
• Creatinine/BUN, CBC, serum potassium
• **Lipid profile:** cholesterol, triglycerides;
lipid-lowering agent may be needed

Black Box Warning: **Infection:** immunosuppression may lead to susceptibility to
infection

Black Box Warning: **Neoplastic disease:** lymphoma, skin cancer may occur;
limit UV exposure; use protective clothing, sunscreen

Black Box Warning: **Liver/lung transplant:** not recommended; mortality and
graft loss may occur

• **High risk:** those with Banff grade 3
acute rejection or vascular rejection before
cycloSPORINE withdrawal, dialysis dependent, creatinine >4.5 mg/dL, African

descent, re-transplants, multiorgan transplant, high panel of reactive antibodies
• **Pulmonary fibrosis, pulmonary effusion, pneumonitis:** dyspnea, cough, hypoxia; some fatal cases have occurred
• **Wound dehiscence and anastomotic
disruption:** wound, vascular, airway, ure-
teral, biliary, inhibition of growth factors;
do not combine with corticosteroids, not
recommended in lung or liver transplant
• **Anaphylaxis, angioedema, exfoliative dermatitis:** more common when
given with ACE inhibitors; do not use if a
hypersensitivity reaction occurs
• **Bone marrow suppression:** Hgb,
WBC, platelets during treatment each
mo; if leukocytes <3000/mm³ or platelets
<100,000/mm³, product should be discon-
tinued or reduced; decreased hemoglobin
level
• **Hepatotoxicity:** alk phos, AST, ALT, amylase, bilirubin, dark urine, jaundice, itching, light-colored stools; product should
be discontinued
• **Pregnancy/breastfeeding:** avoid use
in pregnancy; obtain pregnancy test at
baseline; use effective form of contraception, continue for 12 wk after discontinuing product; notify prescriber if pregnancy
occurs; unknown breastfeeding effects;
weigh benefits, risks with prescriber
Evaluate:
• Therapeutic response: absence of graft
rejection; immunosuppression with autoimmune disorders
Teach patient/family:
• To report fever, rash, severe diarrhea,
chills, sore throat, fatigue; serious infections may occur; clay-colored stools,
cramping (hepatotoxicity); fever, chills,
sore throat (infection)
• To avoid crowds, persons with known
infections to reduce risk for infection
• To use sunscreen, protective clothing
to prevent burns, skin cancer
• Not to use with grapefruit juice
• To avoid live virus vaccines during
treatment
• That lifelong use will be required to
prevent rejection
• That continuing follow-up exams and
blood work will be required

Side effects: *italics* = common; red = life-threatening

• To take with or without regard to food, at same time, consistently
• Take 4 hr after oral cycloSPORINE when used for renal transplant
• **Pregnancy/breastfeeding:** to use contraception before, during, for 12 wk after product discontinued; to avoid breastfeeding

---

⚠ HIGH ALERT

sitaGLIPtin (Rx)

(sit-a-glip′tin)

Januvia

Func. class.: Antidiabetic, oral

Chem. class.: Dipeptidyl-peptidase-4 inhibitor (DPP-4 inhibitor)

ACTION: Slows the inactivation of incretin hormones; improves glucose homeostasis, improves glucose-dependent insulin secretion, lowers glucagon secretions, and slows gastric emptying time

USES: Type 2 diabetes mellitus as monotherapy or in combination with other antidiabetic agents

CONTRAINDICATIONS: Angioedema, diabetic ketoacidosis (DKA)
Precautions: Pregnancy, geriatric patients, GI obstruction, surgery, thyroid/renal/hepatic disease, trauma, breastfeeding, pancreatitis, hypercortisolism, hyperglycemia, hyperthyroidism, hypoglycemia, ileus, pituitary insufficiency, surgery, type 1 diabetes mellitus, diabetic ketoacidosis, adrenal insufficiency, burns

DOSAGE AND ROUTES
• **Adult:** PO 100 mg/day; lower dose may be needed when used with a sulfonylurea or insulin
Renal dose
• **Adult:** PO CCr 30-50 mL/min, 50 mg daily; CCr <30 mL/min, 25 mg daily
Available forms: Tabs 25, 50, 100 mg
Administer:
• May be taken with/without food
• Do not split, crush, chew; swallow whole

• Conversion from other antidiabetic agents: change may be made with gradual dosage change
• Store in tight container at room temperature

SIDE EFFECTS
CNS: *Headache*
ENDO: Hypoglycemia
GI: *Nausea, vomiting,* abdominal pain, diarrhea, pancreatitis, constipation
GU: Acute renal failure
MISC: *Peripheral edema, upper respiratory infection*
SYST: Anaphylaxis, Stevens-Johnson syndrome, angioedema

PHARMACOKINETICS
Rapidly absorbed, excreted by the kidneys (unchanged 79%), half-life 12.4 hr, peak 1-4 hr, duration up to 24 hr

INTERACTIONS
Increase: levels of digoxin
Increase: hypoglycemia—antidiabetics, chloroquine, hydroxychloroquine
Drug/Herb
Increase: antidiabetic effect—garlic, green tea, horse chestnut
Drug/Lab Test
Increase: creatinine, LFTs

NURSING CONSIDERATIONS
Assess:
• **Hypoglycemic reactions:** sweating, weakness, dizziness, anxiety, tremors, hunger; hyperglycemic reactions soon after meals
• **Serious skin reactions:** swelling of face, mouth, lips; dyspnea; wheezing
• **Pancreatitis:** severe abdominal pain, nausea, vomiting; discontinue product, monitor amylase, lipase
• **Renal studies:** BUN, creatinine during treatment, especially in geriatric patients or those with renal disease
• Glycosylated hemoglobin A1c; monitor blood glucose (BG) as needed
Evaluate:
• Therapeutic response: decrease in polyuria, polydipsia, polyphagia; clear sensorium; absence of dizziness; stable gait, blood glucose, A1c improvement

---

Teach patient/family:

• To perform regular self-monitoring of blood glucose using blood-glucose meter

• About the symptoms of hypo/hyperglycemia; what to do about each; to carry emergency ID

• To report severe joint pain immediately; may have a late onset

• That product must be continued on daily basis; about consequences of discontinuing product abruptly; to continue health regimen (diet, exercise)

• To avoid OTC medications, alcohol, digoxin, exenatide, insulins, nateglinide, repaglinide, and other products that lower blood glucose unless approved by prescriber

• That diabetes is a lifelong illness; that product is not a cure, only controls symptoms

• That all food included in diet plan must be eaten to prevent hypo/hyperglycemia

• To immediately notify prescriber of hypersensitivity reactions (rash, swelling of face, trouble breathing)

• To notify prescriber if pregnancy is planned, suspected

---

sodium bicarbonate (Rx, OTC)

Baking soda Bell-Ans, Neut, Soda mint ✦

Func. class.: Alkalinizer
Chem. class.: NaHCO$_3$

ACTION: Orally neutralizes gastric acid, which forms water, NaCl, CO_2; increases plasma bicarbonate, which buffers H^+ ion concentration; reverses acidosis IV

USES: Acidosis (metabolic), cardiac arrest, alkalinization (systemic/urinary), antacid, salicylate poisoning
Unlabeled uses: Contrast media nephrotoxicity prevention

CONTRAINDICATIONS: Metabolic/respiratory alkalosis, hypochloremia, hypocalcemia

Precautions: Pregnancy, children, HF, cirrhosis, toxemia, renal disease, hypertension, hypokalemia, breastfeeding, hypernatremia, Bartter's syndrome, Cushing syndrome, hyperaldosteronism

DOSAGE AND ROUTES
Acidosis, metabolic (not associated with cardiac arrest)
• **Adult/child: IV INFUSION** 2-5 mEq/kg over 4-8 hr depending on CO_2, pH, ABGs
Cardiac arrest
• **Adult/child: IV BOL** 1 mEq/kg of 7.5% or 8.4% sol, then 0.5 mEq/kg q10min, then doses based on ABGs
• **Infant: IV** 1 mEq/kg over several min (use only the 0.5 mEq/mL [4.2%] sol for inj)
Alkalinization of urine
• **Adult: PO** 325 mg to 2 g qid or 48 mEq (4 g), then 12-24 mEq q4hr
• **Child: PO** 84-840 mg/kg/day (1-10 mEq/kg) in divided doses q4-6hr
Antacid
• **Adult: PO** 300 mg to 2 g chewed, taken with water daily-qid
Available forms: Tabs 300, 325, 600, 650 mg; inj 4.2%, 5%, 7.5%, 8.4%
Administer:
PO route
• Chew antacid tablets and drink 8 oz water
• Do not take antacid with milk because milk-alkali syndrome may result
Direct IV route
• Use for cardiac emergencies, not used often in cardiac arrest
• Use ampules or prefilled syringes only; give by rapid bolus dose; flush with NS before, after use
Continuous IV INFUSION route
• Diluted in an equal amount of compatible sol given 2-5 mEq/kg over 4-8 hr, max 50 mEq/hr; slower rate in children
• Extravasation with IV administration (tissue sloughing, ulceration, necrosis)

Y-site compatibilities: Acyclovir, amifostine, asparaginase, aztreonam, bivalirudin, bumetanide, ceFAZolin, cefepime, cefTAZidime, ceftizoxime, cefTRIAXone, chloramphenicol, cimetidine, cladribine,

S

---

clindamycin, cyclophosphamide, cycloSPO-RINE, cytarabine, DAPTOmycin, DAUNOrubicin, dexamethasone sodium phosphate, dexmedetomidine, digoxin, DOCEtaxel, DOXOrubicin, enalaprilat, ertapenem, erythromycin, esmolol, etoposide, etoposide phosphate, famotidine, fentaNYL, filgrastim, fluconazole, fludarabine, furosemide, gallium nitrate, gemcitabine, gentamicin, granisetron, heparin, hydrocortisone sodium succinate, ifosfamide, indomethacin, insulin, ketorolac, labetalol, levoFLOXacin, lidocaine, linezolid, LORazepam, magnesium sulfate, melphalan, mesna, meperidine, methylPREDNISolone sodium succinate, metoclopramide, metoprolol, metroNIDAZOLE, milrinone, morphine, nafcillin, nitroglycerin, nitroprusside, PACLitaxel, palonosetron, pantoprazole, PEMEtrexed, penicillin G potassium, phenylephrine, phytonadione, piperacillin/tazobactam, potassium chloride, procainamide, propranolol, propofol, protamine, raNITIdine, remifentanil, tacrolimus, teniposide, thiotepa, ticarcillin/clavulanate, tirofiban, tobramycin, tolazoline, vasopressin, vit B complex with C, voriconazole

SIDE EFFECTS

CNS: Irritability, headache, confusion, stimulation, tremors, *twitching, hyperreflexia*, tetany, weakness, seizures of alkalosis

CV: Irregular pulse, cardiac arrest, water retention, edema, weight gain

GI: Flatulence, *belching, distention*

META: *Metabolic alkalosis*

MS: Muscular twitching, tetany, irritability

PHARMACOKINETICS

PO: Onset rapid, duration 10 min

IV: Onset 15 min, duration 1-2 hr, excreted in urine

INTERACTIONS

Increase: effects—amphetamines, mecamylamine, quiNINE, quiNIDine, pseudoephedrine, flecainide, anorexiants, sympathomimetics

Increase: sodium and decrease potassium—corticosteroids

Decrease: effects—lithium, chlorproPAMIDE, barbiturates, salicylates, benzodiazepines, ketoconazole, corticosteroids

Drug/Lab Test

Increase: sodium, lactate

Decrease: potassium

NURSING CONSIDERATIONS

Assess:

• Respiratory and pulse rate, rhythm, depth, lung sounds; notify prescriber of abnormalities

• **Fluid balance** (I&O, weight daily, edema); notify prescriber of fluid overload; assess for edema, crackles, shortness of breath

• Electrolytes, blood pH, PO_2, HCO_3^- during treatment; ABGs frequently during emergencies

• Weight daily with initial therapy

• **Alkalosis:** irritability, confusion, twitching, hyperreflexia stimulation, slow respirations, cyanosis, irregular pulse

• **Milk-alkali syndrome:** confusion, headache, nausea, vomiting, anorexia, urinary stones, hypercalcemia

• For GI perforation secondary to carbon dioxide in GI tract; may lead to perforation if ulcer is severe enough

• **Pregnancy/breastfeeding:** use as an antacid is considered unsafe; may breastfeed

Evaluate:

• Therapeutic response: ABGs, electrolytes, blood pH, HCO_3^- WNL

Teach patient/family:

• Not to take antacid with milk because milk-alkali syndrome may result; not to use antacid for >2 wk

• To notify prescriber if indigestion accompanied by chest pain; trouble breathing; diarrhea; dark, tarry stools; vomit that looks like coffee grounds; swelling of feet/ankles

• About sodium-restricted diet; to avoid use of baking soda for indigestion

---

sodium polystyrene sulfonate (Rx)

(po-lee-stye′reen)

Kalexate, Kayexalate, ✦, Kionex, SPS

Func. class.: Potassium-removing resin

Chem. class.: Cation exchange resin

ACTION: Removes potassium by exchanging sodium for potassium in body, primarily in large intestine

USES: Hyperkalemia in conjunction with other measures

CONTRAINDICATIONS: Hypersensitivity to saccharin or parabens that may be in some products, GI obstruction, neonate (reduced gut motility)

Precautions: Pregnancy, geriatric patients, renal failure, HF, severe edema, severe hypertension, sodium restriction, constipation, GI bleeding, hypocalcemia

DOSAGE AND ROUTES

• **Adult:** PO 15 g daily-qid; **RECT** enema 30-50 g q1-2hr initially prn, then q6hr prn

• **Child (unlabeled):** PO 1 g/kg q6hr prn; **RECT** 1 g/kg q2-6hr prn

Available forms: Powder for susp 453.6 g, 454 g; oral susp 15 g/60 mL

Administer:

PO route

• **Powdered resin:** Each dose of the powdered resin is usually given orally as a suspension in water or in a syrup; the amount of fluid ranges from 20 to 100 mL, depending on the dosage, or 3-4 mL/g of resin; suspensions should be freshly prepared and not stored for >24 hr; the powder should not be mixed with foods or liquids that contain a large amount of potassium (bananas or orange juice)

Rectal route

• Precede retention enema with a cleansing enema

• Instruct patient to lie down on left side with lower leg extended and the upper leg flexed for support, or place the patient in the knee-chest position; gently insert a soft, large (28 Fr) rubber tube into the rectum for a distance of about 20 cm; the tip should be well into the sigmoid colon; tape the tube in place; suspend the sodium polystyrene sulfonate powdered resin in 100 mL of an aqueous vehicle (water or sorbitol) that has been warmed to body temperature and introduce through the tube by gravity; the particles should be kept suspended by stirring the suspension during administration; alternatively, 120-180 mL of a commercially available suspension may be administered as a retention enema after the suspension has been warmed to body temperature; following administration, flush the tube with 50-100 mL of fluid and clamp the tube and leave in place; the suspension should be retained in the colon for at least 30-60 min or for several hours, if possible

• After several hours have passed, administer a cleansing enema using a non–sodium-containing solution at body temperature; up to 2 quarts of fluid may be necessary; drain fluid through a Y-tube connection; observe the drainage if sorbitol was used

SIDE EFFECTS

GI: Constipation, *anorexia, nausea, vomiting, diarrhea* (sorbitol), fecal impaction, gastric irritation

META: Hypocalcemia, hypokalemia, hypomagnesemia, sodium retention

INTERACTIONS

Increase: hypokalemia—loop diuretics, cardiac glycosides

Increase: metabolic alkalosis—magnesium/calcium antacids

Increase: colonic necrosis—sorbitol; do not use concurrently

Decrease: effect of—lithium, thyroid hormones

NURSING CONSIDERATIONS

Assess:

• **Hyperkalemia:** confusion, dyspnea, weakness, dysrhythmias; ECG for spiked

S

T waves, depressed ST segments, prolonged QT and widening QRS complex
• Bowel function daily; note consistency of stools, times/day
• **Hypotension:** confusion, irritability, muscular pain, weakness
• **Electrolytes:** serum potassium, calcium, magnesium, sodium; acid-base balance
• I&O ratio, weight daily; crackles, dyspnea, jugular venous distention, edema
• **Digoxin toxicity** (nausea, vomiting, blurred vision, anorexia, dysrhythmias) in those receiving digoxin
Evaluate:
• Therapeutic response: potassium level 3.5-5 mg/dL
Teach patient/family:
• About reason for medication and expected results
• To follow a low-potassium diet, provide sample diet
• To avoid laxatives, antacids, electrolyte-based products unless approved by prescriber

---

sofosbuvir
(soe-fos′bue-vir)
Sovaldi
Func. class.: Antiviral, antihepatitis agent
Chem. class.: Nucleotide analog polymerase inhibitor

ACTION: Inhibits hepatitis C virus RNA polymerase by incorporating the polymerase into the viral RNA; also acts as a chain terminator

USES: Chronic hepatitis C (genotypes 1, 2, 3, 4) with compensated liver disease

CONTRAINDICATIONS: Hypersensitivity, pregnancy in combination; male-mediated teratogenicity
Precautions: Breastfeeding, children, hepatic/renal disease

Black Box Warning: Hepatitis B exacerbation

DOSAGE AND ROUTES
Chronic hepatitis C
Genotype 1, 4
• **Adult: PO** 400 mg daily with peginterferon alfa and ribavirin ×12 wk; may consider use for genotype 1 with only ribavirin ×24 wk
Chronic hepatitis C
Genotype 2
• **Adult: PO** 400 mg daily with ribavirin ×12 wk
Chronic hepatitis C
Genotype 3
• **Adult: PO** 400 mg daily with ribavirin or daclatasvir ×24 wk
Chronic hepatitis C with hepatocellular carcinoma in those waiting for liver transplant
• **Adult: PO** 400 mg daily with ribavirin ×48 wk or until transplant
Available forms: Tabs 400 mg
Administer:
• By mouth without regard to food
• Do not use as monotherapy
• Do not crush, break tabs

SIDE EFFECTS
CNS: Headache, chills, weakness, fatigue, fever, insomnia
GI: Diarrhea, hyperbilirubinemia
MISC: Rash, pruritus, neutropenia, anemia, myalgia

PHARMACOKINETICS
PO: Peak $1/2$-2 hr, excreted by kidneys 80%, 61%-65% protein binding; half-life 0.4-27 hr

INTERACTIONS
Decrease: sofosbuvir-P-glycoprotein (P-gp) inducers (carBAMazepine, PHENobarbital, phenytoin, rifAMPin); OXcarbazepine, rifabutin, rifapentine, tipranavir; avoid concurrent use
Increase: bradycardia—amiodarone; avoid using together
Increase: sofosbuvir level—carvedilol, cobicistat
Drug/Herb
Decrease: sofosbuvir level—St. John's wort; do not use together

---

NURSING CONSIDERATIONS
Assess:

• Heart rate, B/P; severe bradycardia may occur with amiodarone used concurrently
• Serum HCV-RNA baseline and periodically
• Severe renal disease/GFR <30 mL/min/1.73 m^2: monitor BUN, creatinine
• Closer monitoring in geriatric patients; may develop renal, cardiac symptoms more rapidly
• **HBV reactivation:** test is required before beginning therapy; monitor throughout, monitor coinfected patients closely

Black Box Warning: **Hepatitis B exacerbation:** monitor HBsAg, HBV DNA, hepatic enzymes, bilirubin

• **Pregnancy:** if planned or suspected; if pregnant, call the Antiretroviral Pregnancy Registry, 1-800-258-4263; obtain pregnancy test before starting treatment; women who have HIV-1 and HCV who are taking antiretrovirals also should enroll with the registry

Evaluate:
• Therapeutic response: decreased symptoms of chronic hepatitis C

Teach patient/family:
• That optimal duration of treatment is unknown; that product is not a cure; that transmission may still occur
• To avoid use with other medications unless approved by prescriber
• Not to stop abruptly unless directed; worsening of hepatitis may occur, not to use alone, keep in original container
• **Pregnancy/breastfeeding:** to notify prescriber if pregnancy is planned or suspected; to use two forms of reliable contraception; to avoid breastfeeding

Black Box Warning: **Hepatitis B exacerbation:** to notify prescriber immediately of liver toxicity, yellow eyes or skin, fatigue, weakness, loss of appetite, nausea/vomiting, light-colored stools

---

sofosbuvir/velpatasvir
(soe-fos' bue-vir / vel-pat' as-vir)
Epclusa
Func. class.: Antiviral, antihepatitis agent

ACTION: Sofosbuvir: A nucleotide prodrug that prevents hepatitis C viral (HCV) replication by inhibiting the activity of HCV NS5B RNA polymerase. It undergoes intracellular metabolism to form an active uridine analog triphosphate. Hepatitis C virus NS5B RNA polymerase incorporates this metabolite into the viral RNA, where it acts as a chain terminator. It does not inhibit human DNA or RNA polymerase, nor does it block mitochondrial RNA polymerase
Velpatasvir: Inhibits the HCV NS5A protein, which is required for viral replication

USES: Treatment of chronic hepatitis C infection, including genotypes 1, 2, 3, 4, 5, and 6, in those without cirrhosis and in patients with compensated cirrhosis (Child-Pugh A); treatment of chronic hepatitis C infection in patients with decompensated cirrhosis (Child-Pugh B or C)

CONTRAINDICATIONS: Hypersensitivity
Precautions: Breastfeeding, hepatitis C and HIV coinfection, male-mediated teratogenicity, pregnancy, renal failure/impairment

Black Box Warning: Hepatitis B exacerbation

DOSAGE AND ROUTES
Chronic hepatitis C infection in patients without cirrhosis and in patients with compensated cirrhosis (Child-Pugh A)
• **Adult: PO** 1 tablet (400 mg sofosbuvir; 100 mg velpatasvir) qday × 12 wk

---

Side effects: *italics* = common; red = life-threatening

Chronic hepatitis C infection in patients with decompensated cirrhosis (Child-Pugh B or C)

- **Adult:** PO 1 tablet (400 mg sofosbuvir; 100 mg velpatasvir) qday plus ribavirin × 12 wk. The dose of ribavirin is based on weight as follows: <75 kg give 500 mg bid; ≥75 kg give 600 mg bid

Available forms: Tabs 400 mg sofosbuvir-100 mg velpatasvir

Administer:

- Take without regard to food
- If given with ribavirin, take ribavirin with food

SIDE EFFECTS

CNS: *Fatigue, headache,* insomnia, depression, irritability, asthenia
GI: *Nausea, diarrhea*
INTEG: Rash
META: Hyperbilirubinemia
HEMA: Anemia

PHARMACOKINETICS

- **Sofosbuvir:** 61 to 65% protein binding, converted in the liver from the nucleotide prodrug to active nucleoside analog triphosphate; elimination via kidneys 80%, feces 14%, expired air 2.5%, terminal elimination half-life of 25 hr, peak 0.5-1 hr, high-fat meal increases bioavailability
- **Velpatasvir:** 99.5% protein binding, metabolized by CYP2B6, CYP2C8, and CYP3A4, excretion in bile 77% of the parent drug, 95% feces, 0.4% urine, terminal elimination half-life 15 hr, peak 3 hr, increased by high-fat meal

INTERACTIONS

Increase: velpatasvir level—CYP3A4 inhibitors (aldesleukin, aliskiren, amLODIPine, clarithromycin, aprepitant, fosaprepitant, atazanavir, bromocriptine, chloramphenicol, ciprofloxacin, cycloSPORINE, delavirdine, dasatinib, danazol, darunavir, diltiaZEM, dronedarone, erythromycin, fluconazole, FLUoxetine, fluvoxaMINE, idelalisib, imatinib, indinavir, isavuconazonium, amprenavir, bocenavir, ketoconazole, itraconazole, dalfopristin/quinupristin, ritonavir, tipranavir, isoniazid, miconazole), P-gp inhibitors

Increase: bradycardia—amiodarone; avoid using together
Increase: myopathy, rhabdomyolysis—atorvastatin
Increase: sofosbuvir level—carvedilol, cobicistat
Increase: effect of both products—clarithromycin, azithromycin, boceprevir, canagliflozin, carvedilol, crizotinib
Decrease: velpatasvir level—CYP3A4 inducers (armodafinil, barbiturates, bexarotene, bosentan, carBAMazepine, dexamethasone, efavirenz, enzalutamide, eslicarbazepine, ethanol, etravirine, felbamate, flutamide, griseofulvin, lesinurad, modafinil, nafcillin, nevirapine, rifAMPin, rifapentine, rifabutin, phenytoin, PHENobarbital, pioglitazone, primadone); antacids, PPIs separate by 4 hr
Decrease: sofosbuvir level—P-glycoprotein (P-gp) inducers (carBAMazepine, PHENobarbital, phenytoin, rifAMPin); OXcarbazepine, rifabutin, rifapentine, tipranavir; avoid concurrent use
Decrease: levels of—ritonavir

Drug/Herb

Decrease: sofosbuvir level—St. John's wort; do not use together

NURSING CONSIDERATIONS
Assess

Black Box Warning: Hepatitis B exacerbation: monitor serum HCV-RNA baseline and periodically, continue to monitor co-infected patients during and after treatment for clinical and laboratory signs of hepatitis B exacerbation (HBsAg, HBV DNA, hepatic enzymes, bilirubin), assess for signs of liver toxicity (yellow eyes or skin, fatigue, weakness, loss of appetite, nausea, vomiting, or light-colored stools); to decrease the risk of reactivating an HBV infection, screen all potential recipients for evidence of current or prior HBV infection by testing HBsAg and anti-HBc concentrations. For those patients whose screening reveals serologic evidence of HBV infection, a baseline HBV DNA concentration should be obtained before starting sofosbuvir/velpatasvir; monitor LFTs

• Heart rate, B/P; severe bradycardia may occur with amiodarone used concurrently

• Severe renal disease/GFR <30 mL/min/1.73 m^2; monitor BUN, creatinine

• Closer monitoring in geriatric patients; may develop renal, cardiac symptoms more rapidly

Anemia:

• monitor Hgb/Hct if anemia is suspected

• **Pregnancy/breastfeeding:** the use of sofosbuvir/velpatasvir in combination with ribavirin is contraindicated in pregnant women and in the male partners of women who are pregnant; birth defects and/or death of the fetus may result. May cause male-mediated teratogenicity and is contraindicated for use during pregnancy, in females who may become pregnant, or in men whose female partners are pregnant. Patients and their partners are required to use two reliable forms of effective contraception during treatment and for 6 mo after use of these combination therapies. Females must also undergo a pregnancy test immediately before initiation of therapy, monthly during therapy, and for 6 mo post-therapy. To monitor maternal-fetal outcomes of pregnancies in female patients and female partners of male patients exposed to ribavirin during treatment and for 6 mo following cessation of treatment, health care providers are encouraged to report any cases to the Ribavirin Pregnancy Registry, 800-593-2214. For patients who are also infected with HIV and taking concomitant antiretrovirals, an Antiretroviral Pregnancy Registry is available at 800-258-4263; do not breastfeed

Evaluate:

• Decreased symptoms of chronic hepatitis C

Teach Patient/Family:

• That optimal duration of treatment is unknown; that product is not a cure, that transmission to others may still occur

• To avoid use with other products unless approved by prescriber

• Not to stop abruptly unless directed, worsening of hepatitis may occur; to keep in original container

• **Pregnancy/breastfeeding:** teach patients that they and their partners are required to use two reliable forms of effective contraception during treatment and for 6 mo after use of these combination therapies; that pregnancy tests are needed immediately before initiation of therapy, monthly during therapy, and for 6 mo post-therapy; not to breastfeed

Black Box Warning: Hepatitis exacerbation: report to provider immediately signs of liver toxicity (yellow eyes or skin, fatigue, weakness, loss of appetite, nausea, vomiting, or light-colored stools)

---

solifenacin (Rx)

(sol-i-fen′a-sin)

VESIcare

Func. class.: Urinary antispasmodic, anticholinergic

Chem. class.: Antimuscarinic

Do not confuse:
Vesicare/Vesanoid

ACTION: Relaxes smooth muscles in urinary tract by inhibiting acetylcholine at postganglionic sites

USES: Overactive bladder (urinary frequency, urgency, incontinence)

CONTRAINDICATIONS: Hypersensitivity, uncontrolled closed-angle glaucoma, urinary retention, gastric retention
Precautions: Pregnancy, breastfeeding, children, geriatric patients, renal/hepatic disease, controlled closed-angle glaucoma, bladder outflow obstruction, GI obstruction, decreased GI motility, history of QT prolongation

DOSAGE AND ROUTES

• **Adult: PO** 5 mg/day, max 10 mg/day
Renal/hepatic dose

• **Adult: PO** (Child-Pugh B) max 5 mg/day; CCr ≤30 mL/min, 5 mg/day

---

Side effects: *italics* = common; red = life-threatening

Available forms: Tabs 5, 10 mg
Administer:
PO route
• Without regard to meals
• Swallow product whole with water, liquid

SIDE EFFECTS

CNS: *Dizziness,* headache, confusion, depression, drowsiness
CV: Palpitations, sinus tachycardia
EENT: *Vision abnormalities*
GI: *Nausea, anorexia,* abdominal pain, *constipation, dry mouth*
INTEG: Angioedema

PHARMACOKINETICS

90% absorbed; 98% protein bound; extensively metabolized by CYP3A4; excreted in urine 69% (metabolites), feces 22%; half-life 45-68 hr; peak 4-8 hr, duration up to 24 hr

INTERACTIONS

Increase: QT prolongation—Class IA, III antidysrhythmias
Increase: CNS depression—sedatives, hypnotics, benzodiazepines, opioids
Increase: effects—CYP3A4 inhibitors (ketoconazole, clarithromycin, diclofenac, doxycycline, erythromycin, isoniazid, nefazodone, propofol, protease inhibitors, verapamil), max dose 5 mg
Decrease: effects—CYP3A4 inducers (carBAMazepine, nevirapine, PHENobarbital, phenytoin)
Drug/Herb
Decrease: effects—St. John's wort
Drug/Food
Increase: effect—grapefruit juice
Drug/Lab Test
Increase: LFTs

NURSING CONSIDERATIONS

Assess:
• **Urinary patterns:** distention, nocturia, frequency, urgency, incontinence
• **Allergic reactions:** rash
• Angioedema of the face, lips, tongue, larynx
• **Pregnancy/breastfeeding:** use only if benefits outweigh fetal risk; do not breastfeed, excretion unknown

Evaluate:
• Therapeutic response: decreasing dysuria, frequency, nocturia, incontinence
Teach patient/family:
• To avoid hazardous activities because dizziness may occur
• That constipation, blurred vision may occur; to notify prescriber if abdominal pain with constipation occurs
• To take without regard to food
• To swallow tab whole; do not split, crush, chew
• To call prescriber if severe abdominal pain or constipation lasts for ≥3 days
• That heat prostration may occur if used in hot environment, sweating is decreased
• About **anticholinergic effects:** blurred vision, constipation, urinary retention, hyperthermia

---

⚠ **HIGH ALERT**

somatropin (Rx)
(soe-ma-troe′pin)
Genotropin, Humatrope, Norditropin, Norditropin Flexpro, Nutropin, Nutropin AQ, Omnitrope, Saizen, Serostim, Zorbtive, Zomacton
Func. class.: Pituitary hormone
Chem. class.: Growth hormone

Do not confuse:
somatropin/SUMAtriptan/somatrem

ACTION: Stimulates growth; somatropin is similar to natural growth hormone; both preparations were developed with the use of recombinant DNA

USES: Pituitary growth hormone deficiency (hypopituitary dwarfism), children with human growth hormone deficiency/growth failure, AIDS wasting syndrome, cachexia, adults with somatropin deficiency syndrome (SDS), short stature in Noonan syndrome, SHOX deficiency, Turner's syndrome, Prader-Willi syndrome

CONTRAINDICATIONS: Hypersensitivity to benzyl alcohol, creosol, closed epiphyses, intracranial lesions, acute respiratory failure, Prader-Willi syndrome with obesity, trauma

Precautions: Pregnancy, breastfeeding, newborn, geriatric patients, diabetes mellitus, hypothyroidism, prolonged treatment in adults, scoliosis, sleep apnea, chemotherapy, respiratory disease, glycerin hypersensitivity (with formulations that contain these products)

DOSAGE AND ROUTES
Genotropin
• **Child:** SUBCUT 0.16-0.24 mg/kg/wk divided in 6 or 7 daily inj; give in abdomen, thigh, buttocks
• **Adult:** SUBCUT 0.04-0.08 mg/kg/wk divided in 6-7 daily doses

Humatrope
• **Adult:** IM 0.006 international units/kg/day, max 0.0125 units/kg/day
• **Child:** SUBCUT/IM 0.18 mg/kg divided into equal doses either on 3 alternate days or 6×/wk, max weekly dose 0.3 mg/kg

Nutropin/Nutropin AQ (growth hormone deficiency)
• **Child:** SUBCUT 0.3 mg/kg/wk

Serostim
• **Adult:** SUBCUT at bedtime >55 kg, 6 mg; >45-55 kg, 5 mg; 35-45 kg, 4 mg

Norditropin
• **Child:** SUBCUT 0.024-0.034 mg/kg 6-7×/wk

Replacement of GH in GH deficiency
• **Adult:** SUBCUT (Saizen) 0.005 mg/kg/day; may increase after 4 wk to max 0.01 mg/kg/day

Available forms: Powder for inj (lyophilized) 1.5 mg (4 international units/mL), 4 mg (12 international units/vial), 5 mg (13 international units/vial), 5 mg (15 international units/vial) rDNA origin, 5.8 mg (15 international units/mL), 6 mg (18 international units/mL), 8 mg (24 international units/vial), 10 mg (26 international units/vial); inj 10 mg (30 international units/vial), 5 mg/1.5 mL, 10 mg/1.5 mL, 15 mg/1.5 mL

Administer:
• Give IM or subcut; do not use IV
• Discontinue therapy if final height is achieved or epiphyseal fusion occurs
• Visually inspect parenteral products for particulate matter and discoloration

Reconstitution and storage
Genotropin
• Powder, filled in a two-chamber cartridge with the active substance in the front chamber and the diluent in the rear chamber; available in a 5-mg cartridge (green tip) and a 12-mg cartridge (purple tip); the 5- and 12-mg cartridges may be used with the Genotropin Pen or the Genotropin Mixer; also in various doses ranging from 0.2 mg to 2 mg, in single use, auto-mix devices called Genotropin Miniquicks
• **Cartridges:** store cartridges refrigerated before reconstitution, do not freeze; protect from light; a reconstitution device supplied is used to mix the powder and the diluent; after the powder and diluent are mixed, gently tip the cartridge upside down a few times until powder is dissolved; *do not shake*; if solution is cloudy, do not use; following reconstitution, the 5-mg cartridge contains 5 mg/mL; the 12-mg cartridge contains 12 mg/mL; 5-mg and 12-mg cartridges contain overfill; the cartridges contain diluent with preservative (m-cresol) and may be stored refrigerated ≤28 days after reconstitution; do not use the 5-mg and 12-mg cartridges in patients with m-cresol hypersensitivity
• **Genotropin Miniquicks:** after dispensing but before reconstitution, store at ≤77° ≤3 mo; a reconstitution device is supplied; this product contains a diluent with no preservative, refrigerate after reconstitution and use within 24 hr; use the reconstituted solution only once and discard any remaining

Humatrope
• Before reconstitution, store refrigerated
• **Vials:** reconstitute each 5-mg vial with 1.5-5 mL of the diluent (contains m-cresol as a preservative) or bacteriostatic

S

Side effects: *italics* = common; red = life-threatening

water for injection (contains benzyl alcohol as a preservative); direct the liquid against the glass vial wall; swirl until contents are dissolved; do not shake; if the solution is cloudy, do not use; small, colorless particles may be present after refrigeration; vials reconstituted with the diluent or bacteriostatic water are stable for 14 days when refrigerated; for vials reconstituted with sterile water, use the vial only once and discard if not used immediately, refrigerate and use within 24 hr; avoid freezing

• **Cartridges:** reconstitute cartridges using *only* the supplied diluent syringe; the cartridges are designed for use only with the Humatrope injection device; once reconstituted, the cartridges are stable for up to 28 days when stored refrigerated; store the injection device without the needle attached; avoid freezing reconstituted solutions

Norditropin

• Do not use reconstituted solution if it is cloudy or contains particulate matter
• Before use, store refrigerated
• Reconstitution of the cartridges is not required; the cartridge is intended for use only with the NordiPen injector; a prefilled, disposable pen, NordiFlex Pen injector, is also available; each cartridge size (5 mg, 10 mg, or 15 mg per 1.5-mL cartridge)
• After a cartridge has been inserted into the NordiPen injector or once a NordiFlex pen is in use, the pen should be stored refrigerated and used within 4 wk; alternatively, the 5-mg and 10-mg cartridges may be stored in the pen at room temperature, no higher than 77°, for up to 3 wk; NovoFine needles are recommended for administration; wipe the stopper of the pen cartridge with rubbing alcohol

Nutropin

• Before reconstitution, store refrigerated
• Reconstitute each 5-mg vial with 1-5 mL bacteriostatic water for injection (benzyl alcohol preserved) and each 10-mg vial with 1-10 mL of bacterio-

static water for injection (benzyl alcohol preserved); if using for newborns, reconstitute with sterile water for injection; direct the liquid against the glass vial wall; swirl vial; do not shake; if the solution is cloudy after reconstitution or refrigeration, do not use; small, colorless particles may be present after refrigeration

• Solutions reconstituted with bacteriostatic water for injection are stable for 14 days refrigerated
• Solutions reconstituted with sterile water for injection should be used immediately and only once; discard any unused portions; avoid freezing reconstituted solutions

Nutropin AQ

• Does not require reconstitution; solution should be clear; small, colorless particles may be present after refrigeration; allow vial or pen cartridge to come to room temperature, and gently swirl; if solution is cloudy, do not use
• **Vials:** before inserting needle, wipe the vial septum with rubbing alcohol or antiseptic solution; use syringes with small enough volume that the prescribed dose may be drawn from the vial with reasonable accuracy
• **Pen cartridge:** intended for use only with Nutropin AQ Pen; each pen and cartridge are color coded to ensure accurate placement of the 10-mg or 20-mg cartridge into the appropriate pen; wipe septum of pen cartridge with rubbing alcohol or antiseptic solution; follow the directions provided in the Nutropin AQ Pen Instructions for Use; the Nutropin AQ 10 pen allows administration of a minimum 0.1-mg dose to a maximum 4-mg dose, in 0.1-mg increments; the Nutropin AQ 20 pen allows administration of a minimum 0.2-mg dose to a maximum 8-mg dose, in 0.2-mg increments
• **Prefilled device:** a prefilled multidose, dial-a-dose device is available in 3 strengths; administer using disposable needles; follow the directions provided in the Nutropin AQ NuSpin Instructions for Use

---

• After initial use, products are stable for 28 days refrigerated; avoid freezing; protect from light

Omnitrope

• Before reconstitution, store vials refrigerated; store in the carton; Omnitrope is sensitive to light

• **Vials:** reconstitute the vial with diluent provided; swirl the vial gently, but do not shake; if the solution is cloudy after reconstitution, the contents must not be injected; after reconstitution, the 1.5-mg vial may be refrigerated ≤24 hr; the 1.5-mg vial does not contain a preservative and should only be used once; discard any remaining solution; the 5.8-mg vial diluent contains benzyl alcohol as a preservative; after reconstitution, the contents must be used within 3 wk; after the first injection, store the 5.8-mg vial in the carton, to protect from light, in the refrigerator; avoid freezing

• **Omnitrope Pen 5 cartridge:** each 5-mg cartridge must be inserted into the Omnitrope Pen 5 delivery system; follow the directions provided in the Omnitrope Instructions for Use; the cartridge contains benzyl alcohol as a preservative; after the first use, store refrigerated ≤28 days; protect from light, avoid freezing

• **Omnitrope Pen 10 cartridge:** each 10-mg cartridge must be inserted into the Omnitrope Pen 10 delivery system; follow the directions provided in the Omnitrope Instructions for Use; after the first use, store refrigerated ≤28 days; protect from light, avoid freezing

Saizen

• Before reconstitution, store at room temperature

• **Vials:** reconstitute each 5-mg vial with 1-3 mL bacteriostatic water for injection; reconstitute each 8.8-mg vial with 2-3 mL bacteriostatic water for injection (benzyl alcohol preserved); swirl vial with a gentle rotary motion until contents are dissolved completely; do not shake; the solution should be clear; if it is cloudy immediately after reconstitution or refrigeration, do not use; small colorless particles may be present after

refrigeration; after reconstitution, store vials mixed with bacteriostatic water for injection refrigerated and use within 14 days; for vials mixed with sterile water for injection, the solution should be used immediately, and any unused portion should be discarded; avoid freezing

• **Cartridges:** available in 4-mg and 8.8-mg click.easy® cartridges for use in a compatible injection device; a reconstitution device supplied by the manufacturer is used to mix the Saizen with accompanying diluent containing metacresol; cartridges reconstituted with the diluent containing metacresol are stable under refrigeration for ≤21 days; avoid freezing

Serostim

• Before reconstitution, store vials and diluent at room temperature (15-30° C; 59-86° F)

• **Vials:** reconstitute the 5-mg or 6-mg vials with 0.5-1 mL of supplied diluent (sterile water for injection); reconstitute the 4-mg vial with 0.5-1 mL of bacteriostatic water for injection (benzyl alcohol preserved) and the 8.8-mg vial with 1-2 mL of bacteriostatic water for injection (benzyl alcohol preserved); swirl vial; do not shake; the solution should be clear; if it is cloudy immediately after reconstitution or refrigeration, do not use; small colorless particles may be present after refrigeration; if reconstituted with sterile water for injection, use within 24 hr; if reconstituted with bacteriostatic water for injection (benzyl alcohol preserved), the solution is stable for up to 14 days under refrigeration (2-8° C or 36-46° F); avoid freezing

• **Cartridges:** available in 8.8-mg click.easy® cartridges for use in a compatible injection device; a reconstitution device is supplied by the manufacturer and is used to mix the Serostim with accompanying diluent containing metacresol; after reconstitution, cartridges are stable under refrigeration for ≤21 days; avoid freezing

Serostim LQ

• Before use, store refrigerated

• Available in 6-mg single-use cartridges that do not require reconstitution;

S

administer using sterile disposable syringes and needles

• Bring to room temperature before use; discard single-use cartridge after use, even if some drug remains; discard cartridges after the expiration date stated on the product; do not freeze; protect from light

Zomacton (formerly Tev-Tropin)

• Before reconstitution, store refrigerated
• Reconstitute each 5-mg vial with 1-5 mL bacteriostatic 0.9% sodium chloride (benzyl alcohol preserved) for injection; swirl vial; do not shake; the solution should be clear; if it is cloudy immediately after reconstitution, do not inject; small, colorless particles may be present after refrigeration; when administering to newborns, reconstitute with sterile normal saline for injection that is unpreserved
• Solution reconstituted with bacteriostatic 0.9% sodium chloride is stable for 14 days when stored refrigerated; solution reconstituted with sterile normal saline should be used only once; discard any remaining solution; avoid freezing

Valtropin

• Before dispensing, store vials and diluent refrigerated; after dispensing to patients, may be stored at or below 77° F for up to 3 mo
• Reconstitute each 5-mg vial with the entire contents of the accompanying diluent, which contains metacresol as a preservative; swirl vial; do not shake; the solution should be clear, if it is cloudy or contains particulate matter immediately after reconstitution or after refrigeration, do not inject; the final concentration is 3.33 mg/mL
• After reconstitution with the provided diluent, solutions may be stored refrigerated for up to 14 days; after reconstitution with sterile water for injection, use only one dose of Valtropin per vial and discard the unused portion if not used immediately

Zorbtive

• Unreconstituted vials of drug and diluent may be stored at room temperature until expiration date

• Reconstitute each vial of 4 mg, 5 mg, or 6 mg with 0.5-1 mL sterile water for injection, USP; reconstitute each 8.8 mg with 1-2 mL bacteriostatic water for injection (0.9% benzyl alcohol preserved); in newborns or patients with a benzyl alcohol hypersensitivity, sterile water for injection may be used; swirl vial; do not shake; the solution should be clear; if it is cloudy after reconstitution or refrigeration, do not use; small colorless particles may be present after refrigeration
• After reconstitution with sterile water for injection, use the solution immediately and discard any unused portion; when using bacteriostatic water for injection, reconstituted solutions are stable for up to 14 days refrigerated; avoid freezing

IM route

• Inject deeply into a large muscle; aspirate before injection; rotate injection sites daily

SUBCUT route

• Volumes >1 mL of reconstituted solution are not recommended; do not inject intradermally
• Allow refrigerated solutions to come to room temperature before injection
• Subcutaneous injections may be given in the thigh, buttocks, or abdomen; rotate injection sites daily

SIDE EFFECTS

CNS: Headache, growth of intracranial tumor, fever, aggressive behavior
ENDO: Hyperglycemia, ketosis, hypothyroidism, thyroid hormone replacement may be needed
GI: Nausea, vomiting, pancreatitis
GU: *Hypercalciuria*
INTEG: Rash, urticaria, pain; inflammation at inj site, hematoma
MS: Tissue swelling, joint and muscle pain
SYST: Antibodies to growth hormone

PHARMACOKINETICS

Half-life 15-60 min, duration 7 days, metabolized in liver

INTERACTIONS

Increase: epiphyseal closure—androgens, thyroid hormones

Decrease: growth—glucocorticosteroids

Decrease: insulin, antidiabetic effect—dosage adjustment may be needed

Drug/Lab Test

Increase: glucose, urine glucose

Decrease: glucose, thyroid hormones

NURSING CONSIDERATIONS

Assess:

• Signs/symptoms of diabetes

• Growth hormone antibodies if patient fails to respond to therapy

• Thyroid function tests: T_3, T_4, TSH to identify hypothyroidism

• **Allergic reaction:** rash, itching, fever, nausea, wheezing

• **Hypercalciuria:** urinary stones; groin, flank pain; nausea, vomiting, urinary frequency, hematuria, chills

• Growth rate, bone age of child at intervals during treatment

• **Respiratory infection:** in those with Prader-Willi syndrome, may have sleep apnea, upper airway obstruction; discontinue if obstruction occurs

• Rapid growth: assess for slipped capital femoral epiphysis; may also occur in endocrine disorders

• Monitor ophthalmologic status baseline and periodically; intracranial hypertension may occur

• **Beers:** avoid in older adults except as hormone replacement following pituitary gland removal

• **Pregnancy/breastfeeding:** effects unknown; cautious use in breastfeeding

Evaluate:

• Therapeutic response: growth in children

Teach patient/family:

• That treatment may continue for years; that regular assessments are required

• To maintain a growth record; to report knee/hip pain or limping

• That treatment is very expensive

• About subcut injection; to rotate injection site to avoid tissue atrophy; not to shake medication; to report peripheral edema, swelling to the provider

---

⚠ HIGH ALERT

RARELY USED

sonidegib
(soe′-ni-deg′-ib)
Odomzo ✦
Func. class.: Antineoplastic

USES: Locally advanced basal cell carcinoma that has recurred after surgery or radiation therapy or in those who are not candidates for surgery or radiation therapy

CONTRAINDICATIONS: Hypersensitivity

Black Box Warning: Pregnancy, intrauterine fetal death, contraceptive requirement

DOSAGE AND ROUTES

• **Adult:** PO 200 mg daily until disease progression or unacceptable toxicity; take on an empty stomach ≥1 hr before or 2 hr after a meal. Avoid use with strong CYP3A inhibitors or strong and moderate CYP3A inducers

---

⚠ HIGH ALERT

sotalol (Rx)
(sot′ah-lahl)
Betapace, Betapace AF, Rylosol
✦, Sorine, Sotylize
Func. class.: Antidysrhythmic group III
Chem. class.: Nonselective β-blocker

Do not confuse:
sotalol/Sudafed

ACTION: Blockade of β_1- and β_2-receptors leads to antidysrhythmic effect, prolongs action potential in myocardial fibers without affecting conduction, prolongs QT interval, no effect on QRS duration

S

USES: Life-threatening ventricular dysrhythmias; Betapace AF: to maintain sinus rhythm with symptomatic atrial fibrillation/flutter

Unlabeled uses: Atrial fibrillation prophylaxis, cardiac surgery, PSVT, Wolff-Parkinson-White (WPW) syndrome

CONTRAINDICATIONS: Hypersensitivity to β-blockers, cardiogenic shock, heart block (2nd/3rd degree), sinus bradycardia, HF, bronchial asthma, CCr <40 mL/min, hypokalemia

Black Box Warning: Congenital or acquired long QT syndrome

Precautions: Pregnancy, breastfeeding, major surgery, diabetes mellitus, renal/thyroid disease, COPD, well-compensated heart failure, CAD, nonallergic bronchospasm, electrolyte disturbances, bradycardia, peripheral vascular disease

Black Box Warning: Cardiac dysrhythmias, torsades de pointes, ventricular dysrhythmias, ventricular fibrillation; requires a specialized care setting

DOSAGE AND ROUTES
Atrial fibrillation/atrial flutter
• **Adult: PO** Initially, 80 mg bid; may increase in increments of 80 mg/day q3days if QTc is <500 msec; 320 mg/day; **IV** Initially, 75 mg bid; may increase by 75 mg/day q3days if the QTc is <500 msec; max 300 mg/day

Life-threatening tachycardia
• **Adult: PO** Initially, 80 mg bid; may increase by 80 mg/day q3days if the QTc is <500 msec to 160-320 mg/day. 480-640 mg/day may be used in refractory life-threatening arrhythmias; **IV** Initially, 75 mg bid; may increase by 75 mg/day q3days if the QTc is <500 msec to 150-300 mg/day. 550-600 mg/day may be used in refractory life-threatening arrhythmias

• **Adolescent/child 6-17 yr (unlabeled): PO** Initially, 30 mg/m²/dose tid titrated up as needed at intervals of ≥36 hr (**max** 60 mg/m²/dose tid)

Renal dose
• **Betapace/Betapace AF and Sorine (both for ventricular arrhythmies)**
• **Adult:** CCr ≥60 mL/min: no change; CCr 30-59 mL/min: extend dosage interval to q24hr. Dose may be titrated after at least 5 doses; CCr 10-29 mL/min: extend dosage interval to 36-48 hr according to clinical response. Dose may be titrated after at least 5 doses; CCr <10 mL/min: individualize

Betapace/Betapace AF (for atrial fibrillation/atrial flutter), Sotylize, and intravenous (IV) sotalol
• **Adult:** CCr ≥60 mL/min: no change; CCr 40-59 mL/min: extend dosage interval to q24hr. Dose may be titrated after at least 5 doses; CCr <40 mL/min: use is contraindicated

Available forms: Tabs 80, 120, 160, 240 mg; (Betapace AF) 80, 120, 160 mg; inj 150 mg/10 mL (15 mg/mL)

Administer:
PO route
• Before, at bedtime; tab may be crushed or swallowed whole; give 1 hr before or 2 hr after meals
• Reduced dosage in renal dysfunction
• Betapace and Betapace AF are not interchangeable
• Do not give within 2 hr of antacids
• Store in dry area at room temperature; do not freeze

IV route
• Dilute to vol of either 120 mL or 300 mL with D₅W, LR
• **75-mg dose:** withdraw 6 mL sotalol inj (90 mg), add 114 mL diluent to make 120 mL (0.75 mg/mL); or withdraw 6 mL sotalol inj (90 mg), add 294 mL diluent to make 300 mL (0.3 mg/mL)
• **112.5-mg dose:** withdraw 9 mL sotalol inj (135 mL), add 111 mL diluent to make 120 mL (1.125 mg/mL); or withdraw 9 mL sotalol (135 mg), add 291 mL diluent to make 300 mL (0.45 mg/mL)
• **150-mg dose:** withdraw 12 mL of sotalol (180 mg), add 108 mL diluent to make 120 mL (1.5 mg/mL); or withdraw 12 mL sotalol (180 mg), add 288 mL diluent to make 300 mL (0.6 mg/mL)
• Use infusion pump and infuse 100 or 250 mL over 5 hr at a constant rate

SIDE EFFECTS

CNS: Dizziness, mental changes, drowsiness, fatigue, headache, depression, anxiety, paresthesia, insomnia, decreased concentration

CV: Prodysarrhythmia, prolonged QT, orthostatic hypotension, HF, ventricular dysrhythmias, AV block, palpitations, torsades de pointes; life-threatening ventricular dysrhythmias (Betapace AF)

EENT: Tinnitus, visual changes

GI: Nausea, vomiting, diarrhea, dry mouth, constipation, anorexia

GU: Impotence, dysuria

INTEG: Rash, alopecia, urticaria, pruritus, fever, diaphoresis

MS: Arthralgia, muscle cramps

RESP: Bronchospasm, wheezing

PHARMACOKINETICS

PO: Onset 1-2 hr, peak 2-4 hr, duration 8-12 hr; **IV:** onset 5-10 min, peak/duration unknown; half-life 12 hr, excreted unchanged in urine, crosses placenta, excreted in breast milk, protein binding 0%

INTERACTIONS

Black Box Warning: **Increase:** QT prolongation—class IA/III antidysrhythmics, some phenothiazines, β agonists, local anesthetics, tricyclics, haloperidol, chloroquine, droperidol, pentamidine; CYP3A4 inhibitors (amiodarone, clarithromycin, erythromycin, telithromycin, troleandomycin), arsenic trioxide; CYP3A4 substrates (methadone, pimozide, QUEtiapine, quiNIDine, risperiDONE, ziprasidone)

Increase: hypoglycemia effect—insulin

Increase: effects of lidocaine

Increase: hypotension—diuretics, other antihypertensives, nitroglycerin

Decrease: β-blocker effects—sympathomimetics

Decrease: bronchodilating effects of theophylline, β₂-agonists

Decrease: hypoglycemic effects of sulfonylureas

Drug/Lab Test

False increase: urinary catecholamines

Interference: glucose, insulin tolerance tests

Drug/Herb

• Do not use with hawthorn

NURSING CONSIDERATIONS

Assess:

• I&O, weight daily; edema in feet, legs daily

• B/P, pulse q4hr; note rate, rhythm, quality

• Potassium, magnesium levels

Black Box Warning: Requires a specialized care setting: for a minimum of at least 3 days on maintenance dose with continuous ECG monitoring; calculate creatinine clearance before dosing

Black Box Warning: **Cardiogenic shock, acute pulmonary edema:** do not use, effect can further depress cardiac output

Black Box Warning: **QT syndrome:** apical/radial pulse before administration: notify prescriber of any significant changes; monitor ECG continuously (Betapace AF); use QT interval to determine patient eligibility; baseline QT must be ≤450 msec, if ≥500 msec, frequency or dosage must be decreased or drug discontinued

• Baselines of renal studies before therapy begins

• **Abrupt discontinuation:** do not discontinue abruptly, taper over 1-2 wk

• Dose should be adjusted slowly, with at least 3 days between changes; monitor ECG for QT interval

• Monitor electrolytes (hypokalemia, hypomagnesemia); may increase dysrhythmias

• **Pregnancy/breastfeeding:** use only if benefits outweigh fetal risk; do not breastfeed, excreted in breast milk

Evaluate:

• Therapeutic response: absence of life-threatening dysrhythmias

S

Side effects: *italics* = common; red = life-threatening

Teach patient/family:
• Not to discontinue product abruptly; to taper over 2 wk or may precipitate angina; to take exactly as prescribed

• Not to use antacids or OTC products containing α-adrenergic stimulants (nasal decongestants, OTC cold preparations) unless directed by prescriber

• To report bradycardia, dizziness, confusion, depression, fever

• To take pulse at home; advise patient when to notify prescriber

• To avoid alcohol, smoking, sodium intake

• To carry emergency ID to identify product being taken, allergies

• To avoid hazardous activities if dizziness present

• To report symptoms of HF, including difficulty breathing, especially on exertion or when lying down; night cough, swelling of extremities

• To wear support hose to minimize effects of orthostatic hypotension

• To monitor blood glucose if diabetic

• That hospitalization will be required for ≥3 days

---

spironolactone (Rx)

(speer'on-oh-lak'tone)

Aldactone ♣

Func. class.: Potassium-sparing diuretic

Chem. class.: Aldosterone antagonist

Do not confuse:
Aldactone/Aldactazide

ACTION: Competes with aldosterone at receptor sites in distal tubule, thereby resulting in the excretion of sodium chloride and water and the retention of potassium and phosphate

USES: Edema of HF, hypertension, diuretic-induced hypokalemia, primary hyperaldosteronism (diagnosis, short-term treatment, long-term treatment), edema of nephrotic syndrome, cirrhosis of liver with ascites

Unlabeled uses: HF

CONTRAINDICATIONS: Hypersensitivity, anuria, severe renal disease, hyperkalemia

Precautions: Breastfeeding, dehydration, hepatic disease, renal impairment, electrolyte imbalances, metabolic acidosis, gynecomastia, pregnancy

> Black Box Warning: Secondary malignancy

DOSAGE AND ROUTES
Edema/hypertension
• **Adult:** PO 25-100 mg/day in 1-2 divided doses

Heart failure (unlabeled)
• **Adult:** PO 12.5-25 mg/day; max 50 mg/day

Edema
• **Child:** PO 1.5-3.3 mg/kg/day as single dose or in divided doses

Hypertension
• **Child (unlabeled):** PO 1.5-3.3 mg/kg/day in divided doses

Hypokalemia
• **Adult:** PO 25-100 mg/day; if **PO**, potassium supplements must not be used

Primary hyperaldosteronism diagnosis
• **Adult:** PO 400 mg/day × 4 days or 4 wk depending on test, then 100-400 mg/day maintenance

Edema (nephrotic syndrome, HF, hepatic disease)
• **Adult:** PO 100 mg/day given as single dose or in divided doses, titrate to response

• **Child:** PO 1.5-3.3 mg/kg/day or 60 mg/m²/day given daily or in 2-4 divided doses

Renal dose
• **Adult:** PO CCr 10-50 mL/min, give dose q12-24hr; CCr <10 mL/min, avoid use

Available forms: Tabs 25, 50, 100 mg

Administer:
• In AM to avoid interference with sleep
• With food; if nausea occurs, absorption may be decreased slightly
• Effect may take 2 wk

SIDE EFFECTS
CNS: *Headache,* confusion, drowsiness, lethargy, ataxia

ELECT: Hyperchloremic metabolic acidosis, hyperkalemia, hyponatremia
ENDO: Impotence, gynecomastia, irregular menses, amenorrhea, postmenopausal bleeding, hirsutism, deepening voice, breast pain
GI: *Diarrhea*, cramps, bleeding, gastritis, *vomiting*, anorexia, nausea, hepatocellular toxicity
HEMA: Agranulocytosis
INTEG: *Rash, pruritus,* urticaria

PHARMACOKINETICS

Onset 24-48 hr, peak 48-72 hr, metabolized in liver, excreted in urine, crosses placenta, protein binding >90%, terminal half-life 10-35 hr

INTERACTIONS

Increase: action of antihypertensives, digoxin, lithium
Increase: hyperchloremic acidosis in cirrhosis—cholestyramine
Increase: hyperkalemia—potassium-sparing diuretics, potassium products, ACE inhibitors, salt substitutes, angiotensin II receptor antagonists
Decrease: effect of anticoagulants, monitor INR/PT
Decrease: effect of spironolactone—ASA, NSAIDs
Drug/Food
Increase: hyperkalemia—potassium-rich foods, potassium salt substitutes
Drug/Herb
Increase: hypotension—hawthorn, horse chestnut
Decrease: antihypertensive effect—ephedra
Increase: severe photosensitivity—St. John's wort
Increase: BUN, potassium
Decrease: sodium, magnesium
Drug/Lab Test
Interference: 17-OHCS, 17-KS, radioimmunoassay, digoxin assay

NURSING CONSIDERATIONS
Assess:
• **Hypokalemia:** polyuria, polydipsia; dysrhythmias, including a U wave on ECG

• **Hyperkalemia:** weakness, fatigue, dyspnea, dysrhythmias, confusion, fatigue
• Electrolytes (sodium, chloride, potassium), BUN, serum creatinine, ABGs, CBC; potassium must be checked within 3 days, 1 wk, 1 mo × 3, then q3mo; recheck after starting products that alter potassium
• **HF assessment daily:** weight, I&O to determine fluid loss; effect of product may be decreased if used daily; ECG periodically with long-term therapy, breath sounds, edema, B/P
• Signs of metabolic acidosis: drowsiness, restlessness
• Confusion, especially in geriatric patients; take safety precautions if needed
• **Hydration:** skin turgor, thirst, dry mucous membranes

Black Box Warning: **Secondary malignancy:** assess periodically

• **Beers:** avoid in older adults with heart failure or CCr <30 mL/min
• **Pregnancy/breastfeeding:** use only if benefits outweigh fetal risk; fetal harm has occurred; do not breastfeed, excreted in breast milk
Evaluate:
• Therapeutic response: improvement in edema of feet, legs, sacral area daily if medication is being used in HF
Teach patient/family:
• To avoid foods with high potassium content: oranges, bananas, salt substitutes, dried apricots, dates; to avoid potassium salt substitutes
• That drowsiness, ataxia, mental confusion may occur; to observe caution when driving
• To notify prescriber of cramps, diarrhea, lethargy, thirst, headache, skin rash, menstrual abnormalities, deepening voice, breast enlargement
• To take in AM to prevent sleeplessness
• To avoid hazardous activities until reaction is known
• To notify prescriber if pregnancy is planned or suspected; not to breastfeed

S

TREATMENT OF OVERDOSE: Lavage if taken orally; monitor electrolytes, administer IV fluids, monitor hydration, renal, CV status

---

stavudine (d4T) (Rx)

(sta´vyoo-deen)

Zerit

Func. class.: Antiretroviral
Chem. class.: Nucleoside reverse transcriptase inhibitor (NRTI)

Do not confuse:
Zerit/ZyrTEC

ACTION: Prevents replication of HIV by the inhibition of the enzyme reverse transcriptase; causes DNA chain termination

USES: Treatment of HIV-1 in combination with other antiretrovirals

CONTRAINDICATIONS: Hypersensitivity to this product or zidovudine; didanosine, zalcitabine; severe peripheral neuropathy
Precautions: Breastfeeding, advanced HIV infection, bone marrow suppression, renal disease, peripheral neuropathy, osteoporosis, obesity

Black Box Warning: Pregnancy, hepatic disease, pancreatitis, lactic acidosis

DOSAGE AND ROUTES
- **Adult >60 kg: PO** 40 mg q12hr
- **Adult <60 kg: PO** 30 mg q12hr
- **Child <30 kg: PO** 1 mg/kg q12hr
- **Child ≥30 kg, ≤60 kg: PO** 30 mg q12hr
- **Child >60 kg: PO** 40 mg q12hr

Renal dose
- Adult: PO CCr 26-50 mL/min, reduce by 50%, give q12hr; CCr 10-25 mL/min, reduce by 50%, give q24hr

Available forms: Caps 15, 20, 30, 40 mg; powder for oral sol 1 mg/mL
Administer:
- With/without meals; absorption does not appear to be lowered when taken with food
- Use after hemodialysis
- Every 12 hr around the clock
- Shake suspension well before using

SIDE EFFECTS
CNS: *Peripheral neuropathy,* insomnia, anxiety, depression, dizziness, confusion, *headache,* chills/fever, malaise, neuropathy
CV: Chest pain, vasodilation, hypertension
EENT: Conjunctivitis, abnormal vision
GI: Hepatotoxicity, *diarrhea, nausea, vomiting,* anorexia, dyspepsia, constipation, stomatitis, pancreatitis
HEMA: Bone marrow suppression, leukopenia, macrocytosis
INTEG: *Rash,* sweating, pruritus, benign neoplasms
MISC: Lactic acidosis, asthenia, lipodystrophy
MS: Myalgia, arthralgia
RESP: Dyspnea, pneumonia, asthma

PHARMACOKINETICS
Excreted in urine, breast milk; peak 1 hr; half-life: elimination 1-1.6 hr

INTERACTIONS
Increase: myelosuppression—other myelosuppressants
Increase: peripheral neuropathy—lithium, dapsone, chloramphenicol didanosine, ethambutol, hydrALAZINE, phenytoin, vinCRIStine, zalcitabine
Increase: stavudine levels—probenecid
Decrease: stavudine effect—methadone, zidovudine

NURSING CONSIDERATIONS
Assess:

Black Box Warning: **Lactic acidosis and severe hepatomegaly with steatosis:** death may result; monitor LFTs

Black Box Warning: **Pancreatitis:** severe upper abdominal pain, radiating to back, nausea, vomiting usually when used in combination with didanosine

- Blood studies: WBC, differential, RBC, Hct, Hgb, platelets, serum amylase,

lipase, blood glucose, plasma hepatitis C RNA, pregnancy test, serum cholesterol, serum lipids, hepatitis serology, baseline and periodically
• Renal tests: urinalysis, protein, blood, serum creatinine
• Lipoatrophy/lipodystrophy during treatment
• Bowel pattern before, during treatment
• Weakness, tremors, confusion, dizziness; product may have to be decreased, discontinued
• Viral load, CD4 counts, plasma HIV RNA at baseline and throughout treatment
• **Peripheral neuropathy:** tingling, pain in extremities; discontinue product, may not resolve after treatment is discontinued
• **Pregnancy/breastfeeding:** use only if benefits outweigh fetal risk; register patient in the Antiretroviral Pregnancy Registry, 1-800-258-4263; do not breastfeed

Evaluate:
• Therapeutic response: decreased symptoms of HIV

Teach patient/family:
• **About the signs of peripheral neuropathy:** burning, weakness, pain, prickling feeling in extremities
• That product should not be given with antineoplastics
• That product is not a cure for AIDS but will control symptoms
• To notify prescriber if sore throat, swollen lymph nodes, malaise, fever occur; that other products may be needed to prevent other infections
• That, even with use of product, patient may pass AIDS virus to others
• That follow-up visits are necessary; that serious toxicity may occur; that blood counts must be done q2wk
• That serious product interactions may occur if other medications are ingested; to see prescriber before taking chloramphenicol, dapsone, CISplatin, didanosine, ethambutol, lithium, antifungals, antineoplastics
• To notify prescriber if pregnancy is planned or suspected; that fatal lactic acidosis may occur; to avoid breastfeeding
• That product may cause fainting or dizziness

---

stiripentol
(stir-i-pen′ tol)
Diacomit
Func. class.: Anticonvulsant—miscellaneous

ACTION: Several possible mechanisms of action, including effects on the gamma-aminobutyric acid (GABA) A receptor and novel inhibition of lactate dehydrogenase

USES: Seizures associated with Dravet syndrome in patients taking clobazam

CONTRAINDICATIONS: Hypersensitivity
Precautions: Abrupt discontinuation, breastfeeding, children, depression, driving or operating machinery, growth inhibition, hepatic disease, neutropenia, PKU, pregnancy, renal disease, suicidal ideation, thrombocytopenia

DOSAGE AND ROUTES
• **Adult/adolescent/child 12-17 yr: PO** 50 mg/kg/day in 2 or 3 divided doses; round to nearest possible dosage, which is usually within 50 to 150 mg of the recommended 50 mg/kg/day. Max 3000 mg/day
Available forms: Caps 250, 500 mg
Administer:
• Use seizure precautions
• Give during a meal, swallow whole with glass of water; do not break or open capsules
• Take missed doses as soon as possible; if it is almost time for the next dose, take only that dose, do not take double doses

SIDE EFFECTS
CNS: Suicidal ideation, depression, drowsiness, dizziness, ataxia, tremor, agitation, fatigue, insomnia, fever
GI: Anorexia, weight loss or gain, nausea, vomiting

HEMA: Neutropenia, thrombocytopenia
MISC: Infection, hypersalivation

Side effects: *italics* = common; red = life-threatening

PHARMACOKINETICS
Protein binding 99%, half-life 4.5-15 hr, peak 2-3 hr

INTERACTIONS
None known

NURSING CONSIDERATIONS
Assess:
• Monitor weight for increase or decrease; nausea, vomiting, anorexia; closely monitor growth rate, weight in pediatric patients
• **Depression, suicidal ideation:** assess for depression, suicidal thoughts and behaviors any time during treatment; monitor mental status (orientation, mood, behavior) often during treatment
• **Pregnancy/breastfeeding:** encourage pregnant patients to enroll in the North American Antiepileptic Drug (NAAED) Pregnancy Registry by calling 1-888-233-2334; no data on breastfeeding
• Monitor CBC baseline and periodically during treatment; significant neutropenia and thrombocytopenia may occur
Evaluate:
• Therapeutic response: lessening amount and duration of seizures with minimal sedation
Teach patient/family:
• To take only as prescribed, not to skip or double doses, to take at the same times of the day
• To notify all professional health care providers of products used, including OTC, Rx, herbals, and supplements; not to change products unless approved by prescriber
• To notify health care providers before surgery of product use
• **Depression, suicidal thoughts/behaviors:** that suicidal thoughts and behaviors that may increase with use of this product
• **Pregnancy/breastfeeding:** to inform health care provider if pregnancy is planned or suspected or if breastfeeding
• To avoid driving or hazardous activities until reaction is known; dizziness, drowsiness may occur; resume driving only with prescriber clearance

• That exams and blood work will be needed throughout treatment
• To report excessive sedation, severe nausea/vomiting, depression, suicidal thoughts and behaviors

⚠ **HIGH ALERT**

succinylcholine (Rx)
(suk-sin-ill-koe'leen)
Anectine, Quelicin
Func. class.: Neuromuscular blocker (depolarizing, ultra short)

ACTION: Inhibits transmission of nerve impulses by binding with cholinergic receptor sites, thus antagonizing action of acetylcholine; causes release of histamine

USES: Facilitation of endotracheal intubation, skeletal muscle relaxation during orthopedic manipulations

CONTRAINDICATIONS: Hypersensitivity, malignant hyperthermia, trauma
Precautions: Pregnancy, breastfeeding, geriatric or debilitated patients, cardiac disease, severe burns, fractures (fasciculations may increase damage), electrolyte imbalances, dehydration, neuromuscular/respiratory/cardiac/renal/hepatic disease, collagen diseases, glaucoma, eye surgery, hyperkalemia

Black Box Warning: Children <2 yr, myopathy, rhabdomyolysis

DOSAGE AND ROUTES
• **Adult:** IV 0.3-1.1 mg/kg, max 150 mg, maintenance 0.04-0.07 mg/kg q5-10min as needed; **CONT IV INFUSION** dilute to concentration of 1-2 mg/mL in D_5W or NS 10-100 mcg/kg/min
• **Child:** IV initially 1-2 mg/kg; **CONT IV INFUSION** not recommended
Available forms: Inj 20, 50, 100 mg/mL; powder for inj 100, 500 mg/vial, 1 g/vial

Administer:
• Give IV or IM; only experienced clinicians familiar with the use of neuromuscular blocking drugs should administer or supervise the use of this product
• Visually inspect parenteral products for particulate matter and discoloration before use
• Monitor heart rate and mechanical ventilator status during use
• Store in refrigerator, powder at room temperature; close tightly

IM route
• Recommended for infants and other patients in whom a suitable vein is not accessible
• Inject into a large muscle, preferably high into the deltoid muscle; aspirate before injection

Rapid IV injection route
• Owing to tachyphylaxis and prolonged apnea, this method is not recommended for prolonged procedures; rapid IV injection of succinylcholine can result in profound bradycardia or asystole in pediatric patients; as with adults, the risk increases with repeated doses; pretreatment with atropine may be needed
• No dilution of injection solution is necessary
• Inject rapidly IV over 10-30 sec

Continuous IV infusion route
• Not recommended for infants and children owing to risk of malignant hyperthermia
• This route is preferred for long surgical procedures owing to possible tachyphylaxis and prolonged apnea associated with administration of repeated fractional doses
• Dilute succinylcholine to a concentration of 1-2 mg/mL with D₅W, D₅NS, NS, or 1/6 M sodium lactate injection; 1 g of the powder for injection or 20 mL of a 50-mg/mL solution may be added to 1 L or 500 mL of diluent to give solutions containing 1 or 2 mg/mL, respectively; alternatively, 500 mg of the powder for injection or 10 mL of a 50 mg/mL solution may be added to 500 mL or 250 mL of diluent to give solutions containing 1 or 2 mg/mL, respectively

• Infuse IV at a rate of 2.5 mg/min (range = 0.5-10 mg/min); adjust rate based on patient's response and requirements

Y-site compatibilities: Etomidate, heparin, potassium chloride, propofol, vit B/C

SIDE EFFECTS

CV: Bradycardia, *tachycardia; increased, decreased B/P;* sinus arrest, dysrhythmias, edema
EENT: Increased secretions, intraocular pressure
HEMA: Myoglobulinemia
INTEG: Rash, flushing, pruritus, urticaria
MS: Weakness, muscle pain, fasciculations, prolonged relaxation, myalgia, rhabdomyolysis
RESP: Prolonged apnea, bronchospasm, cyanosis, respiratory depression, wheezing, dyspnea
SYST: Anaphylaxis, angioedema

PHARMACOKINETICS
Hydrolyzed in blood, excreted in urine (active/inactive metabolites)
IM: Onset 2-3 min, duration 10-30 min
IV: Onset 1 min, peak 2-3 min, duration 6-10 min

INTERACTIONS
Increase: dysrhythmias: theophylline
Increase: neuromuscular blockade—aminoglycosides, β-blockers, cardiac glycosides, clindamycin, lincomycin, procainamide, quiNIDine, local anesthetics, polymyxin antibiotics, lithium, opioids, thiazides, enflurane, isoflurane, magnesium salts, oxytocin

Drug/Herb
• Blocks succinylcholine: melatonin

NURSING CONSIDERATIONS
Assess:
• Electrolyte imbalances (potassium, magnesium); may lead to increased action of product
• VS (B/P, pulse, respirations, airway) until fully recovered; rate, depth, pattern of respirations, strength of hand grip
• I&O ratio; check for urinary retention, frequency, hesitancy

S

Side effects: *italics* = common; red = life-threatening

• **Recovery:** decreased paralysis of face, diaphragm, leg, arm, rest of body
• **Allergic reactions:** rash, fever, respiratory distress, pruritus; product should be discontinued

> **Black Box Warning: Myopathy, rhabdomyolysis:** in pediatric patients (rare)

• Assess temperature for malignant hyperthermia, previous reactions to anesthesia or paralytics
• Reassurance if communication is difficult during recovery from neuromuscular blockade; postoperative stiffness is normal, soon subsides
• **Pregnancy/breastfeeding:** use only if clearly needed; cautious use in breastfeeding, excretion unknown

Evaluate:
• Therapeutic response: paralysis of jaw, eyelid, head, neck, rest of body

Teach patient/family
• Reason for product, expected results

---

sucralfate (Rx)
(soo-kral′fate)
Carafate, Sulcrate ♦
Func. class.: Protectant, antiulcer
Chem. class.: Aluminum hydroxide, sulfated sucrose

ACTION: Forms a complex that adheres to ulcer site, adsorbs pepsin

USES: Duodenal ulcer, oral mucositis, stomatitis after radiation of head and neck
Unlabeled uses: Gastric/aphthous ulcers, gastroesophageal reflux, NSAID-induced ulcer prophylaxis, proctitis, stomatitis, stress gastritis prophylaxis, *C. difficile*

CONTRAINDICATIONS: Hypersensitivity
Precautions: Pregnancy, breastfeeding, children, renal failure; hypoglycemia (diabetics)

DOSAGE AND ROUTES
Duodenal ulcers
• **Adult: PO** 1 g qid 1 hr before meals, at bedtime

• **Child: PO** 40-80 mg/kg/day divided
Aphthous ulcer/stomatitis (unlabeled)
• **Adult: PO** 5-10 mL (500 mg-1 g) swished in mouth for several min; spit or swallow qid
Gastric ulcer/NSAID-induced ulcer prophylaxis/esophagitis/GERD (unlabeled)
• **Adult: PO** 1 g qid, 1 hr before meals and at bedtime
Available forms: Tabs 1 g; oral susp 1 g/10 mL
Administer:
PO route
• Do not crush or chew tabs; tabs may be broken or dissolved in water
• Do not take antacids 30 min before or after sucralfate
• On an empty stomach 1 hr before meals or other medications and at bedtime
• Store at room temperature
Side effects
GI: *Dry mouth, constipation*

PHARMACOKINETICS
PO: Duration up to 6 hr

INTERACTIONS
Decrease: action of tetracyclines, phenytoin, fat-soluble vitamins, digoxin, ketoconazole, theophylline
Decrease: absorption of fluoroquinolones
Decrease: absorption of sucralfate—antacids, cimetidine, raNITIdine

NURSING CONSIDERATIONS
Assess:
• **GI symptoms:** abdominal pain, blood in stools
• **Hypoglycemia:** may occur in patients with diabetes mellitus; monitor blood glucose carefully
Evaluate:
• Therapeutic response: absence of pain, GI complaints
Teach patient/family:
• To take on empty stomach
• To take full course of therapy; not to use for >8 wk; to avoid smoking
• To avoid antacids, milk, alkaline water within 1 hr of this product

---

Ⓖⓔⓧ Genetic warning

• To increase fluids, bulk, exercise to lessen constipation

sulfamethoxazole-trimethoprim (Rx)

(sul-fa-meth-ox'a-zole–trye-meth'oh-prim)

Bactrim, Bactrim DS, Septra, Septra DS, SMZ/TMP, Protrin DF, Trisulfa DS ✿, Trisulfa S ✿

Func. class.: Antiinfective
Chem. class.: Sulfonamide—miscellaneous

ACTION: Sulfamethoxazole (SMZ) interferes with the bacterial biosynthesis of proteins by competitive antagonism of PABA when adequate levels are maintained; trimethoprim (TMP) blocks the synthesis of tetrahydrofolic acid; the combination blocks 2 consecutive steps in the bacterial synthesis of essential nucleic acids and protein

USES: UTI, otitis media, acute and chronic prostatitis, shigellosis, chancroid, traveler's diarrhea, *Enterobacter* sp., *Escherichia coli, Haemophilus influenzae (beta-lactamase negative), Haemophilus influenzae (beta-lactamase positive), Klebsiella* sp., *Morganella morganii, Pneumocystis carinii, Pneumocystis jiroveci, Proteus mirabilis, Proteus* sp., *Proteus vulgaris, Shigella flexneri, Shigella sonnei, Streptococcus pneumoniae;* **may also be effective for** *Acinetobacter baumannii, Actinomadura madurae, Actinomadura pelletieri, Bordetella pertussis, Burkholderia pseudomallei, Cyclospora cayetanensis, Haemophilus ducreyi, Isospora belli, Klebsiella granulomatis, Legionella micdadei, Legionella pneumophila, Listeria monocytogenes, Moraxella catarrhalis, Neisseria gonorrhoeae, Nocardia asteroides, Nocardia brasiliensis, Nocardia otitidiscaviarum, Pediculus capitis, Plasmodium falciparum, Providencia* sp., *Salmonella* sp., *Serratia* sp., *Shigella* sp., *Staphylococcus aureus (MRSA), Staphylococcus aureus (MSSA), Staphylococcus epidermidis, Stenotrophomonas maltophilia, Streptococcus pyogenes* (group A beta-hemolytic streptococci), *Streptomyces somaliensis, Toxoplasma gondii, Vibrio cholerae,* viridans streptococci, *Yersinia enterocolitica*

CONTRAINDICATIONS: Breast-feeding, infants <2 mo; hypersensitivity to trimethoprim or sulfonamides; pregnancy at term, megaloblastic anemia, CCr <15 mL/min

Precautions: Pregnancy, geriatric patients, infants, renal disease, G6PD deficiency, impaired hepatic/renal function, possible folate deficiency, severe allergy, bronchial asthma, UV exposure, porphyria, hyperkalemia, hypothyroidism

DOSAGE AND ROUTES
Based on TMP content
Most infections
• **Adult/child >2 mo:** PO/IV 6-12 mg TMP/kg/day divided q12hr
UTI
• **Adult:** PO 160 mg TMP q12hr × 10-14 days
• **Child:** PO 8 mg/kg TMP/day in 2 divided doses q12hr (treatment): 2 mg/kg/day (prophylaxis)
Otitis media
• **Child:** PO 8 mg/kg TMP/day in 2 divided doses q12hr × 10 days
Chronic bronchitis
• **Adult:** PO 160 mg TMP q12hr × 10-14 days
Serious infections/*Pneumocystis jiroveci* pneumonitis
• **Adult/child:** PO 15-20 mg/kg TMP daily in 4 divided doses q6hr × 14-21 days; **IV** 15-20 mg/kg/day (based on TMP) in 3-4 divided doses for ≤14 days
Renal dose
• **Adult:** PO CCr >30 mL/min, usual dose; CCr 15-30 mL/min, give 50% of usual dose; CCr <15 mL/min, not recommended
Available forms: Tabs 20 mg TMP/100 SMX ✿, 80 mg trimethoprim/400 mg

S

sulfamethoxazole, 160 mg trimethoprim/800 mg sulfamethoxazole; susp 40 mg-200 mg/5 mL, 160 mg-800 mg/20 mL; IV 16 mg/80 mg/mL

Administer:
PO route
• Medication after C&S; repeat C&S after full course of medication
• With resuscitative equipment, EPINEPHrine available; severe allergic reactions may occur
• Without regard to meals
• With full glass of water to maintain adequate hydration; increase fluids to 2 L/day to decrease crystallization in kidneys
• Store in tight, light-resistant container at room temperature

Intermittent IV INFUSION route
• After diluting 5 mL of product/125 mL D₅W, run over 1-1¹/₂ hr, if using Septra ADD-Vantage vials dilute each 10-mL vial in ADD-Vantage diluent containers containing 250 mL of D₅W, infuse over 60-90 min, change site q48-72hr

Y-site compatibilities: Acyclovir, aldesleukin, allopurinol, amifostine, amphotericin B cholesteryl, atracurium, aztreonam, cefepime, cyclophosphamide, diltiaZEM, DOXOrubicin liposome, enalaprilat, esmolol, filgrastim, fludarabine, gallium, granisetron, HYDROmorphone, labetalol, LORazepam, magnesium sulfate, melphalan, meperidine, morphine, pancuronium, perphenazine, piperacillin/tazobactam, remifentanil, sargramostim, tacrolimus, teniposide, thiotepa, vecuronium, zidovudine

SIDE EFFECTS
CNS: Headache, insomnia, hallucinations, depression, vertigo, fatigue, anxiety, seizures, drug fever, chills, aseptic meningitis
CV: Allergic myocarditis
EENT: Tinnitus
GI: *Nausea, vomiting, abdominal pain,* stomatitis, hepatitis, glossitis, pancreatitis, diarrhea, enterocolitis, anorexia, pseudomembranous colitis
GU: Renal failure, toxic nephrosis; increased BUN, creatinine; crystalluria
HEMA: Leukopenia, neutropenia, thrombocytopenia, agranulocytosis, hemolytic anemia, hypoprothrombinemia, Henoch-Schönlein purpura, methemoglobinemia, eosinophilia
INTEG: Rash, dermatitis, urticaria, Stevens-Johnson syndrome, erythema, photosensitivity, pain, inflammation at inj site, toxic epidermal necrolysis, erythema multiforme
RESP: Cough, SOB
SYST: Anaphylaxis, SLE

PHARMACOKINETICS
PO: Rapidly absorbed; peak 1-4 hr; half-life 8-13 hr; excreted in urine (metabolites and unchanged), breast milk; crosses placenta; 68% bound to plasma proteins; TMP achieves high levels in prostatic tissue and fluid

INTERACTIONS
Increase: thrombocytopenia—thiazide diuretics
Increase: potassium levels—potassium-sparing diuretics, potassium supplements
Increase: hypoglycemic response—sulfonylurea agents
Increase: anticoagulant effects—oral anticoagulants
Increase: levels of dofetilide
Increase: crystalluria—methenamine
Increase: bone marrow depressant effects—methotrexate
Decrease: hepatic clearance of phenytoin, CYP2C9, CYP3A4 inducers
Decrease: response—cycloSPORINE
Drug/Lab Test
Increase: creatinine, bilirubin
Decrease: Hgb, platelets

NURSING CONSIDERATIONS
Assess:
• I&O ratio; note color, character, pH of urine if product administered for UTI
• Renal studies: BUN, creatinine, urinalysis with long-term therapy
• Type of infection; obtain C&S before starting therapy
• Blood dyscrasias, skin rash, fever, sore throat, bruising, bleeding, fatigue, joint pain
• **Allergic reaction:** rash, dermatitis, urticaria, pruritus, dyspnea, bronchospasm; product should be discontinued at 1st sign of rash; AIDS patients more susceptible, identify if patient has a sulfa allergy

Pregnancy/breastfeeding: use only if benefits outweigh fetal risk, may be harmful to fetus, do not breastfeed

Evaluate:

• Therapeutic response: absence of pain, fever; C&S negative

Teach patient/family:

• To take each oral dose with full glass of water to prevent crystalluria; to drink 8-10 glasses of water/day; to take product on an empty stomach 1 hr before meals, 2 hr after meals, not to treat diarrhea with OTC product, to notify health care professional if diarrhea lasts more than 2 days

• To complete full course of treatment to prevent superinfection

• To avoid sunlight; to use sunscreen to prevent burns

• To avoid OTC medications (aspirin, vit C) unless directed by prescriber

• To notify prescriber if skin rash, sore throat, fever, mouth sores, unusual bruising, bleeding occur; to notify prescriber of CNS effects: anxiety, depression, hallucinations, seizures

---

sulfaSALAzine (Rx)

(sul-fa-sal′a-zeen)

Azulfidine, Azulfidine EN-tabs, Salazopyrin ✦

Func. class.: GI antiinflammatory, antirheumatic (DMARD)

Chem. class.: Sulfonamide

Do not confuse:

sulfaSALAzine/sulfiSOXAZOLE

ACTION: Prodrug to deliver sulfapyridine and 5-aminosalicylic acid to colon; antiinflammatory in connective tissue also

USES: Ulcerative colitis; RA; juvenile RA (Azulfidine EN-tabs)

Unlabeled uses: Crohn's disease

CONTRAINDICATIONS: Pregnancy at term, children <2 yr; hypersensitivity to sulfonamides or salicylates; intestinal, urinary obstruction; porphyria

Precautions: Pregnancy, breastfeeding, impaired renal/hepatic function, severe allergy, bronchial asthma, megaloblastic anemia

DOSAGE AND ROUTES

Ulcerative colitis

• **Adult:** PO 3-4 g/day in divided doses; maintenance 2 g/day in divided doses q6hr

• **Child ≥2 yr:** PO 40-60 mg/kg/day in 4-6 divided doses, then 30 mg/kg/day in 4 doses, max 2 g/day

Rheumatoid arthritis

• **Adult:** PO 0.5-1 g/day, then increase daily dose by 500 mg/wk to 2 g/day in 2-3 divided doses

Juvenile rheumatoid arthritis

• **Child ≥6 yr:** PO 30-50 mg/kg/24 hr in 2 divided doses

Renal dose

• Modify dose based on renal impairment, response

Crohn's disease (unlabeled)

• **Adult:** PO 1 g/15 kg, max 5 g/day

Available forms: Tabs 500 mg; oral susp 250 mg/5 mL; del rel tabs 500 mg

Administer:

• Do not break, crush, chew del rel tabs

• With full glass of water to maintain adequate hydration; increase fluids to 2 L/day to decrease crystallization in kidneys

• Total daily dose in evenly spaced doses and after meals to help minimize GI intolerance

• Store in tight, light-resistant container at room temperature

SIDE EFFECTS

CNS: Headache, neuropathy

GI: *Nausea, vomiting, abdominal pain,* stomatitis, hepatitis, glossitis, pancreatitis, diarrhea

GU: Orange-colored urine

HEMA: Leukopenia, neutropenia, thrombocytopenia, agranulocytosis, hemolytic anemia

INTEG: Rash, dermatitis, urticaria, Stevens-Johnson syndrome, erythema, photosensitivity

SYST: Anaphylaxis

PHARMACOKINETICS

PO: Partially absorbed; peak $1^1/_2$-6 hr; duration 6-12 hr; half-life 6 hr; excreted in urine as sulfaSALAzine (15%),

S

Side effects: *italics* = common; red = life-threatening

sulfapyridine (60%), 5-aminosalicylic acid, metabolites (20%-33%); excreted in breast milk; crosses placenta

INTERACTIONS

Increase: leukopenia risk—thiopurines (azaTHIOprine, mercaptopurine)
Increase: hypoglycemic response—oral hypoglycemics
Increase: anticoagulant effects—oral anticoagulants
Decrease: effect of cycloSPORINE, digoxin, folic acid
Decrease: renal excretion of methotrexate
Drug/Food
Decrease: iron/folic acid absorption
Drug/Lab Test
False positive: urinary glucose test

NURSING CONSIDERATIONS
Assess:
• **Ulcerative colitis, proctitis, other inflammatory bowel disease:** character, amount, consistency of stools; abdominal pain, cramping, blood, mucus
• **Rheumatoid arthritis:** assess mobility, joint swelling, pain, ability to complete activities of daily living
• Renal studies: BUN, creatinine, urinalysis (long-term therapy)
• **Blood dyscrasias:** skin rash, fever, sore throat, bruising, bleeding, fatigue, joint pain; monitor CBC before therapy and q3mo
• **Allergic reaction:** rash, dermatitis, urticaria, pruritus, dyspnea, bronchospasm; identify sulfa, salicylate allergy
• **Pregnancy/breastfeeding:** use only if clearly needed; cautious use in breastfeeding, excreted in breast milk
Evaluate:
• Therapeutic response: absence of fever, mucus in stools, pain in joints
Teach patient/family:
• To take each oral dose with full glass of water to prevent crystalluria
• That contact lenses, urine, skin may be yellow-orange
• To avoid sunlight or use sunscreen to prevent burns

• To notify prescriber of skin rash, sore throat, fever, mouth sores, unusual bruising, bleeding
• That decreased sperm production may occur; that it resolves after completion of medication
• To notify prescriber if enteric-coated tablets are seen in stool; discontinue if present

---

SUMAtriptan (Rx)
(soo-ma-trip′tan)
ALSUMA Auto-injector, Imitrex, Imitrex DF ✦
Imitrex STAT-Dose, Sumavel DosePro, Onzetra Xsail, Zembrance SymTouch
Func. class.: Antimigraine agent
Chem. class.: 5-HT₁B/D receptor agonist, abortive agent, triptan

Do not confuse:
SUMAtriptan/somatropin

ACTION: Binds selectively to the vascular 5-HT₁B/D receptor subtype; exerts antimigraine effect; causes vasoconstriction in cranial arteries

USES: Acute treatment of migraine with/without aura and cluster headache

CONTRAINDICATIONS: Angina pectoris, history of MI, documented silent ischemia, Prinzmetal's angina, ischemic heart disease, IV use, concurrent ergotamine-containing preparations, uncontrolled hypertension, hypersensitivity, basilar or hemiplegic migraine
Precautions: Pregnancy, breastfeeding, children <18 yr, geriatric patients, postmenopausal women, men >40 yr, risk factors for CAD, hypercholesterolemia, obesity, diabetes, impaired renal/hepatic function, overuse

DOSAGE AND ROUTES
• **Adult:** SUBCUT ≤6 mg; may repeat in 1 hr; max 12 mg/24 hr; **PO** 25 mg with fluids, if no relief in 2 hr, give another

---

dose, max 200 mg/day; **NASAL** single dose of 5, 10, or 20 mg in 1 nostril, may repeat in 2 hr, max 40 mg/24 hr; 1 puff each nostril q2hr; **nasal powder** 11 mg in each nostril may repeat after 2 hr

Hepatic dose

• **Adult: PO** 25 mg; if no response after 2 hr, give ≤50 mg

Available forms: Inj 4, 6 mg/0.5 mL; tabs 25, 50, 100 mg; nasal spray 5 mg/100 mcl-U; dose spray device 20 mg/100 mcl-U

Administer:

PO route

• Swallow tabs whole; do not break, crush, or chew

• Take tabs with fluids as soon as symptoms appear; may take a 2nd dose >4 hr; max 200 mg/24 hr

SUBCUT route

• SUBCUT only just below the skin; avoid IM or IV administration; use only for actual migraine attack

• Give 1st dose supervised by medical staff to patients with coronary artery disease or those at risk for CAD

Nasal route

• May give as 2 sprays of 5 mg in 1 nostril or 1 spray in each nostril (10 mg)

Nasal powder: fully press and release button, insert into nostril with tight seal, rotate mouthpiece to place in mouth, blow forcefully to deliver powder, discard nosepiece repeat

SIDE EFFECTS

CNS: *Tingling, hot sensation, burning, feeling of pressure, tightness, numbness, dizziness, sedation,* headache, anxiety, fatigue, cold sensation

CV: *Flushing,* MI, hypo/hypertension

EENT: Throat, mouth, nasal discomfort; vision changes

GI: Abdominal discomfort

INTEG: Inj-site reaction, sweating

MS: *Weakness, neck stiffness,* myalgia

RESP: Chest tightness, pressure

PHARMACOKINETICS

Onset of pain relief 10 min-2 hr, peak 2-4 hr, duration 24 hr; nasal onset 60 min, peak 2 hr; 10%-20% protein binding;

metabolized in liver (metabolite); excreted in urine, feces; nasal spray half-life 2 hr

INTERACTIONS

Increase: vasospastic effects: ergot, ergot derivatives

Increase: serotonin syndrome—SSRIs, SNRIs, serotonin-receptor agonists, sibutramine

Increase: SUMAtriptan effect—MAOIs

Drug/Herb

• **Increase:** serotonin syndrome: SAMe, St. John's wort

NURSING CONSIDERATIONS

Assess:

• **Migraine:** type of pain, aura; alleviating, aggravating factors; sensitivity to light, noise

• Increase: **serotonin syndrome:** delirium, coma, agitation, diaphoresis, hypertension, fever, tremors; may resemble neuroleptic malignant syndrome in patients taking SSRIs, SNRIs

• B/P; signs, symptoms of coronary vasospasms, ECG

• Tingling, hot sensation, burning, feeling of pressure, numbness, flushing, inj-site reaction

• Stress level, activity, recreation, coping mechanisms

• Neurologic status: LOC, blurring vision, nausea, vomiting, tingling in extremities preceding headache

• Ingestion of tyramine foods (pickled products, beer, wine, aged cheese), food additives, preservatives, colorings, artificial sweeteners, chocolate, caffeine, which may precipitate these types of headaches

• Renal function, urinary output

• Quiet, calm environment with decreased stimuli: noise, bright light, excessive talking

• **Pregnancy/breastfeeding:** use only if benefits outweigh fetal risk; avoid breastfeeding

Evaluate:

• Therapeutic response: decrease in frequency, severity of migraine

Teach patient/family:

• To report chest pain, tightness; sudden, severe abdominal pain; swelling of

S

eyelids, face, lips; skin rash to prescriber immediately

• To notify prescriber if pregnancy is planned or suspected; to use contraception while taking product

• **Risk of medication overuse:** do not use for abortive headache treatments more than 10 days/month (ergotamines, triptans, opioids or combinations)

• **Nasal spray:** to use 1 spray in 1 nostril; may repeat if headache returns; not to repeat if pain continues after 1st dose

• To have a dark, quiet environment

• To avoid hazardous activities if dizziness, drowsiness occur

• To avoid alcohol; may increase headache

• To use SUBCUT inj technique, nasal route if prescribed

• That product does not reduce number of migraines; to be used for acute migraine; to use as symptoms occur

• **Nasal powder:** Use in each nostril using nosepiece and mouthpiece

• **SUBCUT:** provide pamphlet from manufacturer, review with patient

---

⚠ HIGH ALERT

SUNItinib (Rx)

(soo-nit′-in-ib)

Sutent

Func. class.: Antineoplastic—miscellaneous

Chem. class.: Protein-tyrosine kinase inhibitor

ACTION: Inhibits multiple receptor tyrosine kinases (RTKs); some are responsible for tumor growth

USES: Gastrointestinal stromal tumors (GIST) after disease progression or intolerance to imatinib; advanced renal carcinoma, pancreatic neuroendocrine tumors (pNET) in patients with unresectable locally advanced/metastatic disease

CONTRAINDICATIONS: Pregnancy, breastfeeding, hypersensitivity

Precautions: Children, geriatric patients, active infections, QT prolongation, torsades de pointes, stroke, heart failure

---

Black Box Warning: Hepatotoxicty

DOSAGE AND ROUTES
Gastrointestinal stromal tumors (GIST)/renal cell cancer

• **Adult:** PO 50 mg/day × 4 wk, then 2 wk off; may increase or decrease dose by 12.5 mg; if administered with CYP3A4 inducers, give 87.5 mg/day; if given with CYP3A4 inhibitors, give 37.5 mg/day

Pancreatic neuroendocrine (pNET)

• **Adult:** PO 37.5 mg daily continuously, increase or decrease by 12.5 mg based on tolerance, avoid potent CYP3A4 inhibitors/inducers; if used with CYP3A4 inhibitors, decrease SUNItinib dose to minimum of 25 mg/day; if used with CYP3A4 inducers, increase SUNItinib to max 62.5 mg/day

Available forms: Caps 12.5, 25, 37.5, 50 mg

Administer:

• With meal and large glass of water to decrease GI symptoms

• Store at 25° C (77° F)

SIDE EFFECTS

CNS: Headache, dizziness, insomnia, fatigue, reversible posterior leukoencephalopathy syndrome (RPLS)

CV: Hypertension, left ventricular dysfunction, QT prolongation, torsades de pointes, thrombotic microangiopathy, cardiac arrest, thromboembolism

ENDO: Hypo/hyperthyroidism

GI: *Nausea,* hepatotoxicity, vomiting, dyspepsia, *anorexia, abdominal pain,* altered taste, *constipation,* stomatitis, mucositis, pancreatitis, diarrhea, GI bleeding/perforation

GU: Nephrotic syndrome

HEMA: Neutropenia, thrombocytopenia, hemolytic anemia, leukopenia

INTEG: *Rash, yellow skin discoloration,* depigmentation of hair or skin, alopecia, necrotizing fasciitis, pyoderma gangrenosum

---

MS: Pain, arthralgia, myalgia, *myopathy*, rhabdomyolysis
RESP: Cough, dyspnea, *pulmonary embolism*
SYST: Bleeding, electrolyte abnormalities, hand-foot syndrome, *serious infection*, *tumor lysis syndrome*

PHARMACOKINETICS

Protein binding 95%; metabolized by CYP3A4; excreted in feces, small amount in urine; peak levels 6-12 hr; half-life 40-60 hr (SUNItinib); active metabolite 80-110 hr

INTERACTIONS

Increase: microangiopathic hemolytic anemia—bevacizumab; avoid concurrent use
Increase: QT prolongation—class IA/III antidysrhythmics, some phenothiazines, β agonists, local anesthetics, tricyclics, haloperidol, chloroquine, droperidol, pentamidine; CYP3A4 inhibitors (amiodarone, clarithromycin, erythromycin, telithromycin, troleandomycin), arsenic trioxide; CYP3A4 substrates (methadone, pimozide, QUEtiapine, quiNIDine, risperiDONE, ziprasidone)
Increase: hepatotoxicity—acetaminophen
Increase: plasma concentrations of simvastatin, calcium channel blockers, warfarin; avoid use with warfarin, use low-molecular-weight anticoagulants instead
Decrease: SUNItinib concentrations—dexamethasone, phenytoin, carBAMazepine, rifAMPin, PHENobarbital
Drug/Herb
Decrease: SUNItinib concentration—St. John's wort
Drug/Food
Increase: plasma concentrations—grapefruit juice

NURSING CONSIDERATIONS
Assess:

• ANC and platelets; if ANC <1 × 10⁹/L and/or platelets <50 × 10⁹/L, stop until ANC >1.5 × 10⁹/L and platelets >75 × 10⁹/L; if ANC <0.5 × 10⁹/L and/or platelets <10 × 10⁹/L, reduce dosage by 200 mg; if cytopenia continues, reduce dosage by another 100 mg; if cytopenia continues for 4 wk, stop product until ANC ≥1 × 10⁹/L
• **CV status:** hypertension, QT prolongation can occur; monitor left ventricular

ejection fraction (LVEF), MUGA at baseline, periodically; ECG
• **Renal toxicity:** if bilirubin >3 × IULN, withhold SUNItinib until bilirubin levels return to <1.5 × IULN; electrolytes

> **Black Box Warning: Hepatotoxicity:**
> monitor LFTs before treatment, monthly;
> if liver transaminases >5 × IULN, withhold SUNItinib until transaminase levels
> return to <2.5 × IULN

• **Nephrotic syndrome:** monitor urinalysis and proteinuria
• **Hand-foot syndrome:** redness, swelling, numbness, desquamation on palms and soles of the feet may occur days to months after use; if these occur, product should be discontinued
• **HF:** adrenal insufficiency in those experiencing trauma
• **QT prolongation:** those taking CYP3A4 inhibitors, those with sinus bradycardia, cardiac disease or electrolyte disturbances are at greater risk; monitor electrolytes, especially magnesium, potassium; monitor ECG
• **Osteonecrosis of the jaw:** dental disease or use of bisphosphonates may increase risk; invasive dental procedures should be avoided
• **Tumor lysis syndrome:** usually in renal cell carcinoma or GI stromal tumor; may be fatal, monitor for hyperkalemia, severe muscle weakness, hypocalcemia, hyperphosphatemia, myopathy, hyperuricemia; monitor serum electrolytes before each dose
• Bleeding: epistaxis; rectal, gingival, upper GI, genital, wound bleeding; tumor-related hemorrhage may occur rapidly
• Nutritious diet with iron, vitamin supplement, low fiber, few dairy products
• **Pregnancy/breastfeeding:** do not use in pregnancy, breastfeeding
Evaluate:
• Therapeutic response: decrease in size of tumor
Teach patient/family:
• **To report adverse reactions immediately:** SOB, bleeding
• About reason for treatment, expected result

Side effects: *italics* = common; red = life-threatening

S

• That many adverse reactions may occur: high B/P, bleeding, mouth swelling, taste change, skin discoloration, depigmentation of hair/skin
• To avoid persons with known upper respiratory infections; that immunosuppression is common
• To avoid grapefruit juice
• To report if pregnancy is planned or suspected or if breastfeeding

---

⚠ HIGH ALERT

suvorexant
(soo'voe-rex'ant)

Belsomra

Func. class.: Psychotropic—sedative/hypnotic, anxiolytic

Chem. class.: Orexin receptor antagonist

Controlled Substance Schedule IV

ACTION: Suvorexant alters the signaling of neurotransmitters called orexins, which are responsible for regulating the sleep-wake cycle

USES: The treatment of insomnia characterized by difficulties with sleep onset and/or sleep maintenance

CONTRAINDICATIONS: Narcolepsy, hypersensitivity
Precautions: Preexisting respiratory disease, COPD, breastfeeding, pregnancy, labor, geriatrics, hepatic disease, sleep apnea, substance abuse, alcohol use, suicidal ideation, mental changes, depression

DOSAGE AND ROUTES
• **Adult: PO** 10 mg every night within 30 min of going to bed, and with ≥7 hr remaining before the planned time of awakening, may increase to maximum 20 mg every night
Available forms: Tabs 5, 10, 15, 20 mg
Administer:
• Give 30 min before bedtime

• Effect may be delayed if taken with food, take on empty stomach for faster effect

SIDE EFFECTS
CNS: Amnesia, suicidal ideation, anxiety, dizziness, drowsiness, hallucinations, headache, memory impairment, sleep paralysis
GI: Diarrhea

PHARMACOKINETICS
High protein binding, peak 2 hr, half-life 12 hr, excreted by feces (66%), urine (23%)

INTERACTIONS
Avoid use with CYP3A inhibitors
Increase: effects of both products—CNS depressants
Decrease: suvorexant effect—CYP3A inducers
Drug/Herb:
Increase: suvorexant effect—kava, valerian, melatonin

NURSING CONSIDERATIONS
Assess:
• **Sleeping patterns:** waking in the night, inability to fall asleep or stay asleep, amnesia
• **Beers:** avoid in older adults with delirium or at high risk for delirium
• **Pregnancy/breastfeeding:** use only if benefits outweigh fetal risk; cautious use in breastfeeding, excretion unknown
Evaluate:
• Therapeutic response: normalized sleeping patterns
Teach patient/family:
• To use on an empty stomach for faster effect
• To report immediately suicidal thoughts/behaviors or if depression worsens
• To avoid use with other products unless approved by prescriber
• To notify provider if pregnancy is planned or suspected, or if breastfeeding
• That complex sleep behaviors may occur (sleep driving, sleep eating)
• That daytime drowsiness or dizziness may occur; to avoid hazardous activities until response is known
• To avoid grapefruit juice

---

tacrolimus (Rx) (PO, IV)

(tak-row'lim-us)

Advagraf ✦, Envarsus ER,
Astagraf XL, Prograf

tacrolimus (topical) (Rx)

Protopic

Func. class.: Immunosuppressant
Chem. class.: Macrolide

Do not confuse:
Prograf/PROzac

ACTION: Produces immunosuppression by inhibiting T-lymphocytes

USES: Organ transplants to prevent rejection; **topical:** atopic dermatitis

CONTRAINDICATIONS: Children <2 yr (topical); hypersensitivity to this product or to some kinds of castor oil (IV); long-term use (topical)

Precautions: Pregnancy, breastfeeding, severe renal/hepatic disease, diabetes mellitus, hyperkalemia, hyperuricemia, hypertension, acute bronchospasm, African-American patients, heart failure, seizures, QT prolongation

Black Box Warning: Children <12, lymphomas, infection, neoplastic disease, neonates, infants, requires a specialized setting, requires an experienced clinician; liver transplant (ext rel)

DOSAGE AND ROUTES—NTI
Kidney transplant rejection prophylaxis

• **Adult: IV** 0.03-0.05 mg/kg/day as **CONT INFUSION,** may begin within 24 hr of transplantation, delay until renal function has recovered; **PO** 0.2 mg/kg/day in 2 divided doses q12hr with aza-THIOprine and corticosteroids, may give first dose within 24 hr of transplantation, delay until renal function has recovered; **EXT REL CAPS** 0.1 mg/kg daily preoperatively on empty stomach, 1st dose 12 hr before reperfusion and 0.2 mg/kg once daily postoperatively,

1st dose within 12 hr of reperfusion but ≥4 hr after preoperative dose in combination with mycophenolate and corticosteroids

Liver transplant rejection prophylaxis

• **Adult: PO** 0.1-0.15 mg/kg/day in 2 divided doses q12hr; give no sooner than 6 hr after transplantation; **IV** 0.03-0.05 mg/kg/day as **CONT INFUSION;** give no sooner than 6 hr after transplantation

Heart transplant rejection prophylaxis

• **Adult: PO** 0.075 mg/kg/day in 2 divided doses q12hr; give no sooner than 6 hr after transplantation; **IV** 0.01 mg/kg/day as **CONT INFUSION;** give no sooner than 6 hr after transplantation

Atopic dermatitis

• **Adult: TOP** use 0.03% or 0.1% ointment; apply bid × 7 days after clearing of signs

• **Child ≥2-15 yr: TOP** 0.03% ointment; apply bid × 7 days after clearing of signs

Graft-versus-host disease (orphan drug)

• **Adult/adolescent: IV** 0.1 mg/kg/day in 2 divided doses given with other immunosuppressants or **PO** 0.3 mg/kg/day in 2 divided doses

• **Child: CONT IV INFUSION** 0.1 mg/kg/day

Lung transplant rejection (unlabeled)

• **Adult: PO** 0.15 mg/kg/day, maintain 12-hr trough, whole blood concentration 1-1.5 ng/mL

Available forms: Inj 5 mg/mL; caps 0.5, 1, 5 mg; ext rel cap (Astagraf XL) 0.5, 1, 3, 5 mg; ointment 0.03%, 0.1%; ext rel cap (Envarsus XR) 0.75, 1.4 mg

Administer
PO route
Conventional immediate-release capsules

• Give consistently with or without food

Extended-release capsules (Astagraf XL)

• Take in the AM, preferably on an empty stomach at least 1 hr before a meal or at least 2 hr after a meal

---

Side effects: *italics* = common; red = life-threatening

- Swallow whole; do not chew, divide, or crush capsules
- Do not administer with an alcoholic beverage
- If a dose is missed up to 14 hr from the scheduled time, take the dose; if a dose is missed at >14 hr from the scheduled time, skip the dose and take the next dose at the regularly scheduled time

Extended-release tablets (Envarsus XR)

- Take in the AM, preferably on an empty stomach at least 1 hr before a meal or at least 2 hr after a meal
- Swallow whole; do not chew, divide, or crush capsules
- Do not administer with an alcoholic beverage
- If a dose is missed up to 15 hr from the scheduled time, take the dose; if a dose is missed at >15 hr from the scheduled time, skip the dose and take the next dose at the regularly scheduled time

Topical route

- Apply thin layers to affected skin only; rub in gently
- Do not use occlusive dressings
- Use on small area of skin
- Topical ointment carries risk of developing cancer; use only when other options have failed

IV route

- Visually inspect for particulate matter and discoloration before use
- Because of the risk of hypersensitivity reactions, IV use should be reserved for those who cannot take tacrolimus orally. Oral therapy should replace IV therapy as soon as possible
- Observe patients for 30 min after beginning the infusion and frequently thereafter for possible hypersensitivity reactions
- Due to chemical instability, tacrolimus should not be mixed or infused with solutions with a pH of 9 or more (acyclovir or ganciclovir)

Dilution

- The concentrate for injection must be diluted with NS or D_5W injection to a final concentration between 0.004 mg/mL and 0.02 mg/mL

- Prepare solutions in polyethylene or glass containers to allow storage for 24 hr; do not use polyvinyl chloride (PVC) containers because stability is decreased and the polyoxyl 60 hydrogenated castor oil in the formulation may leach phthalates from PVC containers

Continuous IV infusion

- Give through non-PVC tubing to minimize the potential for drug adsorption onto the tubing
- Infuse the required daily dose of the diluted IV solution over 24 hr

Y-site compatibilities: Alemtuzumab, alfentanil, amifostine, amikacin, aminophylline, amiodarone, amphotericin B colloidal, amphotericin B liposome, anidulafungin, argatroban, atracurium, aztreonam, benztropine, bivalirudin, bleomycin, bumetanide, buprenorphine, busulfan, butorphanol, calcium acetate/chloride/gluconate, CARBOplatin, carmustine, caspofungin, ceFAZolin, cefoperazone, cefotaxime, cefoTEtan, cefOXitin, cefTAZidime, ceftizoxime, cefTRIAXone, cefuroxime, chloramphenicol, chlorproMAZINE, cimetidine, ciprofloxacin, cisatracurium, CISplatin, clindamycin, cyclophosphamide, cycloSPORINE, cytarabine, DACTINomycin, DAPTOmycin, dexamethasone, dexmedetomidine, dexrazoxane, digoxin, diltiaZEM, diphenhydrAMINE, DOBUTamine, DOCEtaxel, dolasetron, DOPamine, doripenem, doxacurium, DOXOrubicin hydrochloride, doxycycline, droperidol, enalaprilat, ePHEDrine, EPINEPHrine, epiRUBicin, ertapenem, erythromycin, esmolol, etoposide, etoposide phosphate, famotidine, fenoldopam, fentaNYL, fluconazole, fludarabine, foscarnet, fosphenytoin, gemcitabine, gentamicin, glycopyrrolate, granisetron, haloperidol, heparin, hydrALAZINE, hydrocortisone, HYDROmorphone, IDArubicin, ifosfamide, imipenem/cilastatin, inamrinone, insulin, isoproterenol, ketorolac, labetalol, leucovorin, levoFLOXacin, levorphanol, lidocaine, linezolid, LORazepam, magnesium sulfate, mannitol, mechlorethamine, meperidine, meropenem, mesna, metaraminol, methotrexate, methyldopate, methylPREDNISolone, metoclopramide, metoprolol, metroNIDAZOLE, micafungin, midazolam, milrinone, mitoMYcin, mitoXANTRONE, mivacurium, morphine, multivitamins, nafcillin, nalbuphine, naloxone, nesiritide, niCARdipine, nitroglycerin, nitroprusside, norepinephrine, octreotide, ondansetron, oxacillin, oxaliplatin, oxytocin, PACLitaxel, palonosetron, pancuronium, PEMEtrexed, penicillin G, pentamidine, pentazocine, perphenazine, phentolamine, phenylephrine, piperacillin/tazobactam, potassium chloride/phosphates, procainamide, prochlorperazine, promethazine, propranolol, quinupristin/dalfopristin, raNITIdine, remifentanil, rocuronium, sodium acetate/bicarbonate/phosphates, streptozocin, succinylcholine, SUFentanil, teniposide, theophylline, thiotepa, ticarcillin/clavulanate, tigecycline, tirofiban, tobramycin, tolazoline, trimethobenzamide, vancomycin, vasopressin, vecuronium, verapamil, vinCRIStine, vinorelbine, voriconazole, zidovudine, zoledronic acid

SIDE EFFECTS

CNS: *Tremors, headache,* insomnia, paresthesia, chills, fever, seizures, BK virus–associated nephropathy, coma, posttransplant lymphoproliferative disorder (PTLD)

CV: Hypertension, myocardial hypertrophy, prolonged QTc, cardiomyopathy

EENT: Blurred vision, photophobia

GI: Nausea, vomiting, diarrhea, constipation, GI bleeding, GI perforation

GU: UTIs, albuminuria, hematuria, proteinuria, renal failure, hemolytic uremic syndrome

HEMA: Anemia, leukocytosis, thrombocytopenia, purpura

INTEG: Rash, flushing, itching, alopecia

META: Hyperglycemia, hyperuricemia, hypokalemia, hypomagnesemia, hyperkalemia

MS: Back pain, muscle spasms

RESP: Pleural effusion, atelectasis, dyspnea, interstitial lung disease

SYST: Anaphylaxis, infection, malignancy

PHARMACOKINETICS

PO: Extensively metabolized, half-life 10 hr, 75% protein binding

INTERACTIONS

Increase: QT prolongation—class IA/III antidysrhythmics, some phenothiazines, β agonists, local anesthetics, tricyclics, haloperidol, chloroquine, droperidol, pentamidine; CYP3A4 inhibitors (amiodarone, clarithromycin, erythromycin, telithromycin, troleandomycin), arsenic trioxide; CYP3A4 substrates (methadone, pimozide, QUEtiapine, quiNIDine, risperiDONE, ziprasidone); do not use together

Increase: toxicity—aminoglycosides, CISplatin, cycloSPORINE

Increase: blood levels—antifungals, calcium channel blockers, cimetidine, danazol, mycophenolate, mofetil

Decrease: blood levels—carBAMazepine, PHENobarbital, phenytoin, rifamycin

Decrease: effect of live virus vaccines

Drug/Herb

Decrease: immunosuppression—astragalus, echinacea, melatonin, ginseng, St. John's wort

Drug/Food

Increase: effect—grapefruit juice

Decreased absorption: food

Drug/Lab Test

Increase: glucose, BUN, creatinine

Increase or decrease: LFTs, potassium

Decrease: magnesium, Hgb, platelets

NURSING CONSIDERATIONS
Assess:

• **Blood studies:** Hgb, WBC, platelets during treatment monthly; if leukocytes <3000/mm^3 or platelets <100,000/mm^3, product should be discontinued or reduced; decreased hemoglobin level may indicate bone marrow suppression

• **Hepatic studies:** alk phos, AST, ALT, amylase, bilirubin; for hepatotoxicity: dark urine, jaundice, itching, light-colored stools; product should be discontinued

• **Atopic dermatitis:** Check lesions baseline and during treatment

• Assess for castor oil allergy (HCO-60); do not use if present

• Serum creatinine/BUN, serum electrolytes, lipid profile, serum tacrolimus concentration

T

Side effects: *italics* = common; red = life-threatening

• **Anaphylaxis:** rash, pruritus, wheezing, laryngeal edema; stop infusion, initiate emergency procedures

• **QT prolongation:** ECG, ejection fraction; assess for chest pain, palpitations, dyspnea

• **PTLD:** Malaise, fever, weight loss, night sweats, decreased appetite can be fatal, allogenic hematopoietic stem cell transplant (HSCT) may be required

• **Blood level monitoring:** maintain tacrolimus whole blood (7-20 ng/mL) then 5-15 ng/mL for 1 yr in kidney transplant; 1-3 mo maintain whole blood at 8-20 ng/mL, then 6-18 ng/mL 3-18 mo after transplant (heart)

Black Box Warning: **Liver transplant:** ext rel product should not be used because of increased female mortality rate

Black Box Warning: **Specialized care setting, experienced clinician:** this product should only be used when equipped and staffed with adequate supportive medical services and by those experienced in immunosuppressive therapy and organ transplantation

Black Box Warning: **Children, infants, neonates:** not approved use of ointment in those <2 yr, ext rel in those <16 yr; not approved for pediatric kidney/heart transplant

• **Pregnancy/breastfeeding:** use only if benefits outweigh fetal risk; do not breastfeed, excretion unknown

Evaluate:

• Therapeutic response: absence of graft rejection; immunosuppression in patients with autoimmune disorders

Teach patient/family:

PO route

• To report fever, rash, severe diarrhea, chills, sore throat, fatigue; that serious infections may occur; to report clay-colored stools, cramping (hepatotoxicity), nephrotoxicity, signs of diabetes mellitus

• To avoid exposure to natural or artificial sunlight

• Not to breastfeed while taking product

• That repeated lab tests will be needed during treatment

• To avoid vaccines

• Not to use with alcohol, grapefruit, grapefruit juice

• **Organ rejection:** B/P, provide treatment for hypertension to help prevent rejection

Black Box Warning: To report symptoms of lymphoma, skin cancer; to avoid crowds, persons with known infections to reduce risk for infection; to avoid eating raw shellfish

Topical route

• To stop using topical product when atopic dermatitis is resolved; not to use >6 wk if symptoms do not improve; not to shower or swim after applying

• To report if pregnancy is planned or suspected

---

tadalafil (Rx)

(tah-dal′a-fil)

Adcirca, Cialis

Func. class.: Impotence agent

Chem. class.: Phosphodiesterase type 5 inhibitor

ACTION: Inhibits phosphodiesterase type 5 (PDE5); enhances erectile function by increasing the amount of cGMP, which causes smooth muscle relaxation and increased blood flow into the corpus cavernosum; improves erectile function for up to 36 hr

USES: Treatment of erectile dysfunction (Cialis), benign prostatic hyperplasia (BPH) with or without erectile dysfunction, pulmonary arterial hypertension (PAH) (Adcirca only)

Unlabeled uses: Sexual dysfunction in males receiving antidepressants

CONTRAINDICATIONS: Newborns, children, women, hypersensitivity, patients taking organic nitrates either regularly and/or intermittently, patients

---

taking any α-adrenergic antagonist other than 0.4 mg once-daily tamsulosin

Precautions: Pregnancy, anatomic penile deformities, sickle cell anemia, leukemia, multiple myeloma, CV/renal/hepatic disease, bleeding disorders, active peptic ulcer, prolonged erection

DOSAGE AND ROUTES
Erectile dysfunction
• **Adult: PO** (Cialis) 10 mg taken before sexual activity; dose may be reduced to 5 mg or increased to max 20 mg; usual max dosing frequency is 1×/day; once-daily dosing 2.5 mg/day at same time each day

BPH
• **Adult: PO** 5 mg daily at the same time every day

For improvement in exercise ability in patients with WHO Group I pulmonary hypertension (Adcirca)
• **Adult: PO** 40 mg (two 20-mg tablets) daily with or without food

Concomitant administration with ketoconazole, itraconazole, ritonavir
• **Adult: PO** max 10 mg q72hr

Renal dose
• **Adult: PO** CCr 51-80 mL/min: no adjustment for erectile dysfunction, 20 mg/day initially for pulmonary hypertension; CCr 31-50 mL/min, 5 mg/day, max 10 mg q48hr; CCr <30 mL/min, max 5 mg q72hr

Hepatic dose
• **Adult: PO** (Child-Pugh A, B) max 10 mg/day or 20 mg/day (pulmonary hypertension) max 40 mg/day; (Child-Pugh C) not recommended

Male sexual dysfunction (from antidepressants) (unlabeled)
• **Adult: PO** (Cialis) 10-20 mg before sexual activity

Available forms: Tabs (Cialis) 2.5, 5, 10, 20 mg; tabs (Adcirca) 20 mg
Administer:
• Product should not be used with nitrates in any form
• **Sexual dysfunction:** give before sexual activity; do not use more than 1×/day
• **Pulmonary hypertension:** give Adcirca with/without meals

SIDE EFFECTS
CNS: *Headache, flushing, dizziness,* seizures, transient global amnesia
CV: Hypotension, QT prolongation
INTEG: Stevens-Johnson syndrome, exfoliative dermatitis, urticaria
MISC: Back pain/myalgia, *dyspepsia, nasal congestion, UTI,* blurred vision, changes in color vision, *diarrhea,* pruritus, priapism, nonarteritic ischemic optic neuropathy (NAION), hearing loss

PHARMACOKINETICS
Rapidly absorbed; metabolized by liver by CYP3A4; terminal half-life 17.5 hr; peak $^1/_2$-6 hr; excreted primarily as metabolites in feces, urine; excreted 61% in feces, 36% in urine; 94% protein bound; rate and extent of absorption not influenced by food

INTERACTIONS
Do not use with nitrates because of unsafe drop in B/P, which could result in MI or stroke
Increase: tadalafil levels—itraconazole, ketoconazole, ritonavir (although not studied, may also include other HIV protease inhibitors)
Decrease: B/P—alcohol, α-blockers, amLODIPine, angiotensin II receptor blockers, enalapril
Decrease: effects of tadalafil—bosentan, antacids
Drug/Food
Increase: tadalafil effect—grapefruit

T

NURSING CONSIDERATIONS
Assess:
• **Cialis:** underlying cause of erectile dysfunction before treatment; use of organic nitrates that should not be used with this product; any severe loss of vision while taking this or any similar products

BPH: urinary hesitancy, poor stream, dribbling baseline and periodically

• **Adcirca:** hemodynamic parameters to exercise tolerance at baseline and periodically

Side effects: *italics* = common; red = life-threatening

• **Pregnancy/breastfeeding:** use only if clearly needed (Adcirca only); Cialis is not indicated for women; not used in breastfeeding

• **Beers:** use with caution in older adults; may exacerbate syncope; monitor frequently for syncope

Evaluate:

• Therapeutic response: ability to engage in sexual intercourse, improvement in exercise ability in pulmonary hypertension

Teach patient/family:

• To take 1 hr before sexual activity

• Not to drink large amounts of alcohol

• To discuss with provider all OTC, Rx, herbals, supplements taken

• That product does not protect against sexually transmitted diseases, including HIV

• That product has no effect in the absence of sexual stimulation; to seek medical help if erection lasts >4 hr

• To notify physician about all medicines, vitamins, herbs being taken, especially ritonavir, indinavir, ketoconazole, itraconazole, erythromycin, nitrates, α-blockers; that tadalafil is contraindicated for use with α-blockers except 0.4 mg/day tamsulosin

• To notify prescriber immediately and to stop taking product if vision, hearing loss occurs or if erection lasts >4 hr or if chest pain occurs

---

tafenoquine

(ta fen′ oh-kwin)

Krintafel, Arakoda

Func. class.: Antimalarial

Chem. class.: 8-aminoquinoline

ACTION: Activity against the pre-erythrocytic liver stages of the parasite prevents the development of the erythrocytic forms, which are responsible for malarial relapse; may inhibit hematin polymerization, inducing apoptotic-like death of the parasite

USES: Prevention of relapse of *Plasmodium vivax* malaria in those receiving antimalarial therapy for acute *P. vivax* infection (Krintafel); for malaria prophylaxis (Arakoda)

CONTRAINDICATIONS:

Hypersensitivity to this product or iodoquinol or primaquine, G6PD deficiency, psychosis

Precautions: Breastfeeding, contraception requirements, hepatic disease, methemoglobin reductase deficiency, pregnancy, pregnancy testing, psychiatric events, renal disease, reproductive risk

DOSAGE AND ROUTES

Prevention of relapse of *Plasmodium vivax* malaria

• **Adult/adolescent ≥16 yr: PO** 300 mg as a single dose on the first or second day of the antimalarial therapy (chloroquine)

For malaria prophylaxis (Arakoda)

• **Adult: PO** 200 mg daily for 3 days before travel as loading dose, then 200 mg weekly starting 7 days after the last loading dose, continuing during travel to malarious area as maintenance, then 200 mg once at 7 days after the last maintenance dose in the wk after exit from malarious area; may be given for ≤6 mo of continuous dosing

Administer:

• Give with food

• Swallow tablets whole. Do not break, crush, or chew

• If vomiting occurs within 1 hr after dosing, repeat the dose; do not attempt to redose more than once (prevention of relapse single-dose therapy)

• **Storage:** at room temperature in original container, protect from moisture

SIDE EFFECTS

CNS: Dizziness, headache, anxiety, abnormal dreams, insomnia, somnolence

EENT: Vortex keratopathy, photophobia

GI: Nausea, vomiting

HEMA: Decreased Hgb

INTEG: Angioedema, urticaria

PHARMACOKINETICS
Protein binding 99.5%, peak 12-15 hr, half-life 12-15 days (Krintafel). Affected cytochrome P450 isoenzymes and drug transporters: OCT2, MATE-1, MATE2-K

INTERACTIONS
• Avoid use with MATE (multidrug and toxin extrusion substrates) and OCT2 (organic cation transporter-2) (dofetilide, metformin); if these products must be given, monitor for toxicity

Drug/Lab:
Increase: methemoglobin, ALT, creatinine

NURSING CONSIDERATIONS
Assess
• **Malaria symptoms:** anemia, jaundice, diarrhea, sweating, vomiting, fast heart rate, low B/P; report symptoms to health care provider
• **Methemoglobinemia:** monitor for increased methemoglobin; report immediately shortness of breath, cyanosis, mental status changes; O₂ and methylene blue may be given
• **Psychiatric effects:** serious psychiatric adverse reactions have been observed in patients with a previous history of psychiatric conditions at doses higher than the approved dose; the effects may occur during or after treatment.
• **Hypersensitivity reactions:** serious hypersensitivity reactions (angioedema) may occur; these reactions may occur during or after conclusion of therapy
• **Pregnancy/breastfeeding:** avoid use in pregnancy, a pregnancy test is required in all females of reproductive potential, adequate contraception is required during and for 3 mo after last dose; infant should be tested for G6PD deficiency before breastfeeding

Evaluate:
• Therapeutic response: prevention of relapse or prevention of malaria

Teach patient/family:
• **Pregnancy/breastfeeding:** not to use during pregnancy; adequate contraception should be used during and for 3 mo after last dose; infant should have a lab test performed before breastfeeding
• To swallow tablets whole, not to split or cut; to take with food
• To report immediately dark urine or lips as these may be symptoms of hemolytic anemia
• To use sunglasses in bright light to prevent photophobia

---

talazoparib
(tal′ a-zoe′ pa-rib)
Talzenna
Func. class.: Antineoplastic
Chem. class.: Poly (ADP-ribose) polymerase (PARP) inhibitors

ACTION: An inhibitor of poly (ADP-ribose) polymerase (PARP) enzymes (PARP1 and PARP2). These enzymes play a role in DNA repair. Cytotoxicity may involve inhibition of PARP enzymatic activity and increased formation of PARP-DNA complexes, resulting in DNA damage, decreased cell proliferation, and apoptosis.

USES: Deleterious/suspected deleterious germline BRCA-mutated (gBRCAm), HER2-negative locally advanced or metastatic breast cancer

CONTRAINDICATIONS:
Hypersensitivity
Precautions: Anemia, bone marrow suppression, breastfeeding, contraception requirements, infertility, leukemia, leukopenia, male-mediated teratogenicity, myelodysplastic syndrome, neutropenia, new primary malignancy, pregnancy, pregnancy testing, reproductive risk, thrombocytopenia

DOSAGE AND ROUTES
• **Adult: PO** 1 mg daily until disease progression or unacceptable toxicity

Renal dose
• **Adult: PO** Moderate renal impairment (CrCL 30-59 mL/min): 0.75 mg daily

---

Hematologic toxicity dose
• Do not start until patient has adequately recovered from hematologic toxicity caused by previous therapy
• Hemoglobin <8 g/dL: Hold, monitor blood counts weekly. When Hgb recovers to ≥9 g/dL, reduce daily dose by 0.25 mg and resume
• Neutrophil count <1000 cells/mm³: Hold, monitor blood counts weekly. When neutrophils recover to ≥1500 cells/mm³, reduce daily dose by 0.25 mg and resume
• Platelet count <50,000 cells/mm³: Hold, monitor blood counts weekly. When platelets recover to ≥75,000 cells/mm³, reduce daily dose by 0.25 mg and resume

Nonhematologic toxicity dose
• **Grade 3 or 4**: Hold; when toxicity resolves to grade ≤1, consider reducing dose by 0.25 mg and resuming
Available forms: Caps 0.25 mg, 1 mg
Administer:
• Swallow capsules whole; do not open or dissolve
• May be taken with or without food
• If patient vomits or misses a dose, an additional dose should not be taken; take the next dose at regularly scheduled time
• **Storage:** At room temperature

SIDE EFFECTS
CNS: Fatigue, headache, dizziness
GI: Nausea, vomiting, diarrhea, anorexia, abdominal pain
HEMA: Anemia, neutropenia, thrombocytopenia
META: Hyperglycemia, hypocalcemia,
MISC: New primary malignancy, leukemia, MDS/AML

PHARMACOKINETICS
74% protein binding, metabolized in liver, excretion in urine 68.7%, 19.8 % in feces

INTERACTIONS
• **Increase:** effect of talazoparib—P-gp inhibitors (amiodarone, carvedilol, clarithromycin, itraconazole, verapamil); monitor for potential increased adverse reactions

• **Increase:** effect of talazoparib—BCRP inhibitors; monitor for potential increased adverse reactions when coadministering

Drug/Lab:
• **Increase:** glucose, ALT, AST, alk phos
• **Decrease:** hemoglobin, platelets, neutrophils, lymphocytes, leukocytes, calcium

NURSING CONSIDERATIONS
Assess:
• Monitor CBC with differential baseline and monthly; serum creatinine; do not start until patient has recovered from hematologic toxicities from other chemotherapy
• **Pregnancy/breastfeeding:** obtain pregnancy test in females of reproductive potential before use; fetal harm may occur when used in pregnant women; advise females of reproductive potential to use effective contraception during treatment and for at least 7 mo after the last dose; male patients with female partners of reproductive potential or pregnant partners should use effective contraception during treatment and for at least 4 mo following the last dose; based on animal studies, fertility may be impaired in males of reproductive potential

Evaluate:
• Therapeutic response: decreased growth, spread of breast cancer

Teach patient/family:
• **MDS/AML:** to report to health care provider if feeling tired or experiencing symptoms of weakness, fever, weight loss, frequent infections, bruising, bleeding easily, breathlessness, blood in urine or stool
• **Myelosuppression:** that product may cause anemia, leukopenia/neutropenia, and/or thrombocytopenia; that frequent lab testing will be required
• To take daily with or without food; that if a dose is missed, to take next normal dose at the usual time; to swallow each capsule whole; that capsules must not be opened or dissolved
• **Pregnancy/breastfeeding:** to notify health care provider if pregnant or plan-

ning to become pregnant; that product carries risk to fetus and potential loss of pregnancy; that females of reproductive potential must use effective contraception during treatment and for ≥7 mo after last dose; not to breastfeed during treatment or for ≥1 mo after receiving the last dose; that male patients with female partners of reproductive potential or who are pregnant should use effective contraception during treatment and for at least 4 mo after receiving the last dose

• To notify health care provider of nausea, vomiting to obtain options to lessen these side effects

• To notify health care provider of all Rx, OTC, herbals or supplements taken; not to add or change medications unless approved by provider

---

⚠ HIGH ALERT

tamoxifen (Rx)
(ta-mox'i-fen)
Nolvadex-D ✽, Tamofen ✽,
Tamone ✽, Tamoplex ✽
Func. class.: Antineoplastic
Chem. class.: Antiestrogen hormone

ACTION: Inhibits cell division by binding to cytoplasmic estrogen receptors; resembles normal cell complex but inhibits DNA synthesis and estrogen response of target tissue

USES: Advanced breast carcinoma not responsive to other therapy in estrogen-receptor–positive patients (usually postmenopausal), prevention of breast cancer, after breast surgery/radiation for ductal carcinoma in situ
Unlabeled uses: Mastalgia, to reduce pain/size of gynecomastia

CONTRAINDICATIONS: Pregnancy, breastfeeding, hypersensitivity

Black Box Warning: Thromboembolic disease, endometrial cancer, stroke

Precautions: Women of childbearing age, leukopenia, thrombocytopenia, cataracts

Black Box Warning: Uterine cancer

DOSAGE AND ROUTES
Breast cancer (men/women)
• **Adult:** PO 20-40 mg/day for 5 yr; doses >20 mg/day, divide AM/PM
High risk for breast cancer
• **Adult:** PO 20 mg/day × 5 yr
Ductal carcinoma in situ (DCIS)
• **Adult:** PO 20 mg/day × 5 yr
Mastalgia/gynecomastia in men with prostate cancer (unlabeled)
• **Adult (male):** PO 20 mg/day for ≤1 yr
Available forms: Tabs 10, 20 mg; oral solution 10 mg/5 mL
Administer:
• Do not break, crush, or chew tabs
• Antacid before oral agent; give product after evening meal, before bedtime; give with food or fluids for GI symptoms
• Antiemetic 30-60 min before product to prevent vomiting
• Store in light-resistant container at room temperature
Oral solution: Use calibrated container, dose >20 mg/day should be divided morning and evening, may be used with food for gastric irritation

SIDE EFFECTS
CNS: *Hot flashes, headache, light-headedness,* depression, mood changes, stroke
CV: Chest pain, stroke, fluid retention, flushing
EENT: Blurred vision (high doses)
GI: *Nausea, vomiting,* altered taste
GU: Vaginal bleeding, uterine malignancies, *altered menses, amenorrhea*
HEMA: Thrombocytopenia, leukopenia, DVT
INTEG: *Rash,* alopecia
META: Hypercalcemia
RESP: Pulmonary embolism

PHARMACOKINETICS
PO: Peak 4-7 hr, half-life 7 days (1 wk terminal), metabolized in liver, excreted primarily in feces

---

Side effects: *italics* = common; red = life-threatening

INTERACTIONS

Increase: risk for death from breast cancer—PARoxetine

Increase: bleeding—anticoagulants

Increase: tamoxifen levels—bromocriptine

Increase: thromboembolic events—cytotoxics

Increase: toxicity—CYP3A4 inhibitors (aprepitant, antiretroviral protease inhibitors, clarithromycin, danazol, delavirdine, diltiaZEM, erythromycin, fluconazole, FLUoxetine, fluvoxaMINE, imatinib, ketoconazole, mibefradil, nefazodone, telithromycin, voriconazole)

Decrease: tamoxifen levels—aminoglutethimide, rifamycin

Decrease: letrozole levels—letrozole

Decrease: tamoxifen effect—CYP3A4 inducers (barbiturates, bosentan, carBAMazepine, efavirenz, phenytoins, nevirapine, rifabutin, rifampin)

Decrease: tamoxifen effects—CYP2D6 inhibitors (antidepressants)

Drug/Herb

• Avoid use with St. John's wort, dong quai, black cohosh

Drug/Lab Test

Increase: serum calcium, T_4, AST, ALT, cholesterol, triglycerides, BUN

NURSING CONSIDERATIONS
Assess:

• CBC, differential, platelet count baseline and periodically notify prescriber; breast exam, mammogram, pregnancy test, bone mineral density, LFTs, serum calcium, serum lipid profile, periodic eye exams (cataracts, retinopathy), pap smear

Black Box Warning: **Bleeding** q8hr: hematuria, guaiac, bruising, petechiae, mucosa, or orifices

• Effects of alopecia on body image; discuss feelings about body changes

Black Box Warning: Uterine malignancies, symptoms of stroke, pulmonary embolism that may occur in women with ductal carcinoma in situ (DCIS) and women at high risk for breast cancer; monitor gynecologic exams periodically

• **Severe allergic reactions:** rash, pruritus, urticaria, purpuric skin lesions, itching, flushing

• **Bone pain:** may give analgesics; pain usually transient

• **Pregnancy/breastfeeding:** do not use in pregnancy, breastfeeding

Evaluate:

• Therapeutic response: decreased tumor size, spread of malignancy

Teach patient/family:

• **About risk of stroke and PE:** to seek medical attention immediately in case of blurred vision, headache, weakness on one side of the body (stroke signs); or chest pain, fainting, sweating, difficulty breathing (PE)

• To report any complaints, side effects to prescriber; that use may be 5 yr

• To increase fluids to 2 L/day unless contraindicated

• To wear sunscreen, protective clothing, sunglasses

• That vaginal bleeding, pruritus, hot flashes are reversible after discontinuing treatment

• To immediately report decreased visual acuity, which may be irreversible; about need for routine eye exams; that care providers should be told about tamoxifen therapy

• To report vaginal bleeding immediately

• That tumor flare—increase in size of tumor, increase in bone pain—may occur and will subside rapidly; that analgesics may be taken for pain

• That hair may be lost during treatment; that a wig or hairpiece may make patient feel better; that new hair may be different in color, texture

• To use nonhormonal contraception during and for 2 mo after discontinuing treat, that premenopausal women must use mechanical birth control because ovulation may be induced

---

tamsulosin (Rx)

(tam-sue-lo′sen)

Flomax

Func. class.: Selective α_1-peripheral adrenergic blocker, BPH agent

Chem. class.: Sulfamoylphenethyl-amine derivative

Do not confuse:

Tamsulosin/tacrolimus

ACTION: Binds preferentially to α_{1A}-adrenoceptor subtype, which is located mainly in the prostate

USES: Symptoms of benign prostatic hyperplasia (BPH)

CONTRAINDICATIONS: Hypersensitivity

Precautions: Pregnancy, breastfeeding, children, hepatic disease, CAD, severe renal disease, prostate cancer; cataract surgery (floppy iris syndrome)

DOSAGE AND ROUTES

• **Adult: PO** 0.4 mg/day increasing to 0.8 mg/day if required after 2-4 wk

Available forms: Caps 0.4 mg

Administer:

• Without regard to food

• Swallow caps whole; do not break, crush, or chew

• Give $^1/_2$ hr after same meal each day

• If treatment is interrupted for several days, restart at lowest dose (0.4 mg/day)

• Store in tight container in cool environment

SIDE EFFECTS

CNS: *Dizziness, headache,* asthenia, insomnia

CV: Chest pain, orthostatic hypotension

EENT: Amblyopia, floppy iris syndrome

GI: Nausea, diarrhea, dysgeusia

GU: Decreased libido, abnormal ejaculation, priapism

INTEG: Rash, pruritus, urticaria

MS: Back pain

RESP: Rhinitis, pharyngitis, cough

SYST: Angioedema

PHARMACOKINETICS

Peak 4-5 hr, duration 9-15 hr, half-life 9-13 hr, metabolized in liver, excreted via urine, extensively protein bound (98%)

INTERACTIONS

Increase: B/P—prazosin, terazosin, doxazosin, α-blockers, vardenafil

Increase: toxicity—cimetidine

NURSING CONSIDERATIONS

Assess:

• **Prostatic hyperplasia:** change in urinary patterns at baseline and throughout treatment; I&O ratios, weight daily; edema; report weight gain or edema

• **Orthostatic hypotension:** monitor B/P, standing, sitting

• **Pregnancy/breastfeeding:** not to be used for women

Evaluate:

• Therapeutic response: decreased symptoms of benign prostatic hyperplasia

Teach patient/family:

• Not to drive or operate machinery for 4 hr after 1st dose or after dosage increase

• To continue to take even if feeling better

• To advise providers of all products, herbs taken

• To make position changes slowly because orthostatic hypotension may occur

• To take $^1/_2$ hr after same meal each day

• To teach about priapism (rare)

• Not to crush, break, chew

• That decreased ejaculate or absence may occur; resolves after discontinuing product

---

⚠ HIGH ALERT

tapentadol (Rx)

(ta-pen′ta-dol)

Nucynta, Nucynta ER, Nucynta IR

Func. class.: Analgesic, misc.

Chem. class.: µ-Opioid receptor agonist

Controlled Substance Schedule II

Side effects: *italics* = common; red = life-threatening

ACTION: Centrally acting synthetic analgesic; μ-opioid agonist activity is thought to result in analgesia; inhibits norepinephrine uptake

USES: Moderate to severe pain, diabetic peripheral neuropathy

CONTRAINDICATIONS: Hypersensitivity, asthma, ileus, respiratory depression

Black Box Warning: Respiratory depression

Precautions: Pregnancy, breastfeeding, children <18 yr, increased intracranial pressure, MI (acute), severe heart disease, respiratory depression, renal/hepatic disease, GI obstruction, ulcerative colitis, sleep apnea, seizure disorder

Black Box Warning: Accidental exposure, avoid ethanol, substance abuse, neonatal opioid withdrawal syndrome, potential for overdose, poisoning, coadministration with other CNS depressants

DOSAGE AND ROUTES
• **Adult:** PO 50-100 mg q4-6hr, may give 2nd dose ≥1 hr after 1st dose, max 700 mg on day 1, max 600 mg/day thereafter; ext rel 50 mg q12hr (opioid-naive), titrate to 50 mg/dose bid q3days, max 250 mg q12hr

Hepatic disease
• **Adult:** PO Immediate rel 50 mg q8hr, may titrate to response; ext rel 50 mg daily, max 100 mg/day

Available forms: Tabs 50, 75, 100 mg; tabs ext rel 50, 100, 150, 200, 250 mg; oral solution 20 mg/mL

Administer:
• With antiemetic if nausea, vomiting occur
• When pain is beginning to return; determine dosage interval by response
• Do not crush, chew, break ext rel product, or use with alcohol
• Preferred analgesic in those with altered cytochrome P450 or mild hepatic, mild to moderate renal disease

• Store in light-resistant area at room temperature

Black Box Warning: These products have high potential for overdose, poisoning; may be fatal because of respiratory depression

• **Oral solution:** measure using calibrated syringe

SIDE EFFECTS
CNS: *Drowsiness, dizziness, confusion, headache, euphoria,* hallucinations, restlessness, syncope, anxiety, flushing, psychological dependence, insomnia, lethargy, tremors, seizures
CV: Palpitations, bradycardia, hypo/hypertension, orthostatic hypotension, sinus tachycardia
GI: *Nausea, vomiting, anorexia, constipation, cramps,* gastritis, dyspepsia, biliary spasms
GU: Urinary retention/frequency
INTEG: *Rash,* urticaria, diaphoresis, pruritus
RESP: Respiratory depression, cough
SYST: Anaphylaxis, infection, serotonin syndrome

PHARMACOKINETICS
Bioavailability 32%, extensively metabolized by liver, excreted in urine 99%, terminal half-life 4 hr, protein binding 20%

INTERACTIONS

Black Box Warning: **Increase:** effects with other CNS depressants—alcohol, opioids, sedative/hypnotics, antipsychotics, skeletal muscle relaxants

Increase: toxicity—MAOIs
Increase: serotonin syndrome—SSRIs, SNRIs, serotonin-receptor agonists, tricyclics

Black Box Warning: Do not use with alcohol; fatal overdose may occur

Drug/Herb
Increase: sedative effect—kava, St. John's wort, valerian

NURSING CONSIDERATIONS
Assess:
• **Pain:** intensity, location, type, characteristics; need for pain medication by pain/sedation scoring; physical dependence

• I&O ratio; check for decreasing output; may indicate urinary retention

• CNS changes: dizziness, drowsiness, hallucinations, euphoria, LOC, pupil reaction

• **Serotonin syndrome:** increased heart rate, shivering, sweating, dilated pupils, tremors, high B/P, hyperthermia, headache, confusion; if these occur, stop product, administer serotonin antagonist if needed

• **Seizures:** history of seizures increased with SSRIs, SNRIs, tricyclic antidepressants

• Allergic reactions: rash, urticaria, anaphylaxis

Black Box Warning: **Addiction risk, previous substance abuse:** assess before using ext rel product; some may crush ext rel product and snort, inject product that is dissolved

Black Box Warning: **Accidental exposure:** identify if alcohol has been used before giving this product; may be fatal if used with tapentadol; keep from pets, children; avoid coadministration with other CNS depressants

Black Box Warning: **Respiratory dysfunction:** respiratory depression, character, rate, rhythm; notify prescriber if respirations are <10/min; B/P, pulse

Black Box Warning: **Neonatal opioid withdrawal syndrome:** may be fatal; monitor neonates for irritability, hyperactivity, abnormal sleep pattern, high-pitched crying, tremors, vomiting, diarrhea, failure to gain weight

• **Pregnancy/breastfeeding:** use only if benefits outweigh fetal risk, including neonatal opioid withdrawal syndrome; do not breastfeed, excretion unknown

Evaluate:
• Therapeutic response: decrease in pain
Teach patient/family:
• To report any symptoms of CNS changes, allergic reactions, seizures, serotonin syndrome

• That physical dependency may result from extended use

• That withdrawal symptoms may occur: nausea, vomiting, cramps, fever, faintness, anorexia

• To avoid CNS depressants, alcohol

• To avoid driving, operating machinery if drowsiness, dizziness occur

• To change positions slowly to decrease orthostatic hypotension

• Teach patient to take as directed, not to double doses, if breakthrough pain occurs, notify provider, do not discontinue abruptly, gradually taper

• **Seizures:** Teach patient that if seizure occurs, discontinue, notify provider

• Not to drive or perform other hazardous activities until response is known

• **Orthostatic hypertension:** To rise slowly to prevent orthostatic hypertension

• **Serotonin syndrome:** Teach patient symptoms of serotonin syndrome and when to contact provider

• To discuss with provider all OTC, Rx, herbals, supplements taken

Black Box Warning: Not to use with alcohol; may be fatal

• To notify prescriber if pregnancy is planned or suspected, or if breast feeding

T

RARELY USED

tasimelteon
(tas-i-mel′tee-on)
Hetlioz
Func. class.: Anxiolytic/sedative/hypnotics

USES: Sleep-wake disorder in the blind

CONTRAINDICATIONS: Hypersensitivity

Side effects: *italics* = common; red = life-threatening

DOSAGE AND ROUTES
• **Adult:** PO 20 mg before bedtime at the same time every night; take without food

---

tavaborole topical
See Appendix B

---

teduglutide
(te'due-gloo'tide)
Gattex
Func. class.: Functional GI disorder agent
Chem. class.: Recombinant glucagon-like peptide-2 analog

USES: Short bowel syndrome, dependent on parenteral support

DOSAGE AND ROUTES
• **Adult:** SUBCUT 0.05 mg/kg daily

---

telavancin (Rx)
(tel-a-van'sin)
Vibativ
Func. class.: Antiinfective, miscellaneous
Chem. class.: Lipoglycopeptide

ACTION: Inhibits bacterial cell-wall synthesis, disrupts cell membrane integrity, blocks glycopeptides

USES: Skin/skin-structure infections caused by *Enterococcus faecalis, E. faecium, Staphylococcus aureus* (MRSA), *S. aureus* (MSSA), *S. epidermidis, S. haemolyticus, Streptococcus agalactiae* (group B), *S. dysgalactiae, S. pyogenes* (group A β-tremolytic), *S. anginosus, S. intermedius, S. constellatus,* nosocomial pneumonia caused by susceptible gram-positive bacteria
Unlabeled uses: Bacteremia

CONTRAINDICATIONS: Hypersensitivity
Precautions: Breastfeeding, children, geriatric patients, renal disease, antimicrobial resistance, diabetes mellitus, diarrhea, GI disease, heart failure, hypertension, pseudomembranous colitis, QT prolongation, vancomycin hypersensitivity

Black Box Warning: Pregnancy, renal disease

DOSAGE AND ROUTES
Complicated skin/skin-structure infections
• **Adult:** IV INFUSION 10 mg/kg over 60 min q24hr × 7-14 days
Nosocomial pneumonia
• **Adult:** IV INFUSION 10 mg/kg q24hr × 7-21 days
Renal dose
• **Adult:** IV CCr 30-50 mL/min 7.5 mg/kg q24hr; CCr 10-29 mL/min 10 mg/kg q48hr
Available forms: Lyophilized powder for inj 250, 750 mg
Administer:
• Use only for susceptible organisms to prevent drug-resistant bacteria
• Antihistamine if red man syndrome occurs: decreased B/P; flushing of neck, face
• Avoid IM, subcut use
Intermittent IV INFUSION route
• After reconstitution with 15 mL D$_5$W sterile water for inj; 0.9% NaCl (15 mg/mL) 250-mg vial; add 45 mL to 750-mg vial (15 mg/mL) for dose of 150-800 mg; further dilute with 100-250 mL of compatible sol; for dose <150 mg or >800 mg, further dilute to concentration of 0.6-8 mg/mL with compatible sol; give over 60 min; reconstituted or diluted sol is stable for 4 hr room temperature, 7 hr refrigerated; avoid rapid IV; may cause red man syndrome

Y-site compatibility: Amphotericin B lipid complex (Abelcet), ampicillin-sulbactam, azithromycin, calcium gluconate, caspofungin, cefepime, cefTAZidime, cefTRIAXone, ciprofloxacin,

---

dexamethasone, diltiaZEM, DOBUTamine, DOPamine, doripenem, doxycycline, ertapenem, famotidine, fluconazole, gentamicin, hydrocortisone, labetalol, magnesium sulfate, mannitol, meropenem, metoclopramide, milrinone, norepinephrine, ondansetron, pantoprazole, phenylephrine, piperacillin-tazobactam, potassium chloride/phosphates, raNITIdine, sodium bicarbonate, sodium phosphates, tigecycline, tobramycin, vasopressin

SIDE EFFECTS

CNS: Anxiety, chills, flushing, headache, insomnia, dizziness
CV: QT prolongation, irregular heartbeat
EENT: Hearing loss
GI: Nausea, vomiting, CDAD, abdominal pain, constipation, diarrhea, metallic/soapy taste
GU: Nephrotoxicity, *increased BUN, creatinine,* renal failure, foamy urine
HEMA: Leukopenia, eosinophilia, anemia, thrombocytopenia
INTEG: Chills, fever, rash, thrombophlebitis at inj site; urticaria, pruritus, necrosis (red man syndrome)
SYST: Anaphylaxis, superinfection

PHARMACOKINETICS

Onset rapid, half-life 8-9 hr, excreted in urine (76%), protein binding 90%, hepatic metabolism

INTERACTIONS

Increase: otoxicity or nephrotoxicity—aminoglycosides, cephalosporins, colistin, polymyxin, bacitracin, CISplatin, amphotericin B, nondepolarizing muscle relaxants, cidofovir, tacrolimus, IV pentamidine, acyclovir, adefovir, cycloSPORINE, foscarnet, ganciclovir, pamidronate, streptozocin, zoledronic acid, NSAIDs, salicylates, ACE inhibitors
Increase: QT prolongation—class IA, III antidysrhythmics; some phenothiazines; chloroquine, clarithromycin, droperidol, dronedarone, erythromycin, haloperidol, methadone, pimozide, ziprasidone
Drug/Lab Test
False increase: INR, PT, PTT

NURSING CONSIDERATIONS
Assess:

• **Infection:** WBC, urine, stools, sputum, characteristics of wound throughout treatment, C&S

Black Box Warning: **Nephrotoxicity:** I&O ratio; report hematuria, oliguria; monitor BUN, CCr, avoid in those with CCr ≤50 mL/min; more common in those with diabetes, HF, hypertension, geriatric patients, renal disease

• **CDAD:** monitor for diarrhea, fever, blood in stools, abdominal pain; may happen several wk after therapy ends, report to prescriber immediately
• **Anaphylaxis:** monitor for rash, itching, wheezing, laryngeal edema; discontinue and notify prescriber immediately; emergency equipment and EPINEPHrine should be nearby
• Auditory function during, after treatment; hearing loss; ringing, roaring in ears; product should be discontinued
• B/P during administration; sudden drop may indicate red man syndrome; also flushing, pruritus, rash, use slow IV infusion to prevent
• Respiratory status: rate, character, wheezing, tightness in chest
• Adequate intake of fluids (2 L/day) to prevent nephrotoxicity

Black Box Warning: **Pregnancy:** obtain a pregnancy test before use; if a woman has taken this product during pregnancy, the national registry should be notified

Evaluate:
• Therapeutic response: negative culture
Teach patient/family:
• About all aspects of product therapy; that culture may be taken after completed course of medication
• To notify prescriber if infection continues
• That bitter taste, nausea, vomiting, headache may occur
• To report sore throat, fever, fatigue; could indicate superinfection; diarrhea (CDAD); hearing loss; rash, wheezing,

---

Side effects: *italics* = common; red = life-threatening

tightness of chest, itching, tightening of throat (anaphylaxis)

Black Box Warning: To use contraception while taking this product; not to breastfeed; to notify prescriber if pregnancy is planned or suspected

---

telbivudine (Rx)

(tel-bi·vyoo-deen)

Sebivo ✤, Tyzeka

Func. class.: Antiretroviral
Chem. class.: Nucleoside reverse transcriptase inhibitor (NRTI)

ACTION: Inhibits replication of HBV DNA polymerase, which inhibits HBV replication

USES: Treatment of chronic hepatitis B

CONTRAINDICATIONS: Hypersensitivity, breastfeeding
Precautions: Pregnancy, children, severe renal disease, anemia, organ transplant, dialysis, HIV, obesity, alcoholism; Hispanic or African descendants (safety not established)

Black Box Warning: Impaired hepatic function, lactic acidosis

DOSAGE AND ROUTES
• **Adult and adolescent >16 yr: PO** 600 mg/day; max 600 mg/day
Renal dose
• **Adult: PO** CCr 30-49 mL/min, 600 mg tab q48hr or 400 mg oral sol daily; CCr <30 mL/min (not requiring dialysis), 600 mg tab q72hr or 200 mg oral sol daily
Available forms: Tabs 600 mg
Administer:
• With/without food with a full glass of water
• Store at room temperature

SIDE EFFECTS
CNS: *Fever, headache, malaise,* weakness, *dizziness, insomnia*
EENT: Taste change, hearing loss, photophobia

GI: *Nausea, vomiting, diarrhea, anorexia,* abdominal pain, hepatomegaly, hepatotoxicity
INTEG: *Rash*
MISC: Lactic acidosis
MS: Myalgia, arthralgia, muscle cramps
RESP: Cough

PHARMACOKINETICS
Excreted by kidneys (unchanged), steady state 5-7 days, protein binding 3.3%, terminal half-life 40-49 hr, peak 1-4 hr

INTERACTIONS
Altered telbivudine levels: any agent altering renal function
• Do not use with pegylated interferon α-2a
Increase: myopathy risk possible—HMG-CoA reductase inhibitors, fibric acid derivatives, penicillAMINE, zidovudine, cycloSPORINE, erythromycin, niacin, azole antifungals, corticosteroids, hydrochloroquine

NURSING CONSIDERATIONS
Assess:

Black Box Warning: **Hepatotoxicity:** LFTs, hepatitis B serology, creatine kinase, periodically, monitor HBV DNA after 24 wk; if viral suppression incomplete (≥300 copies/mL), start alternate therapy; monitor HBV DNA q6mo

Black Box Warning: **Lactic acidosis:** obtain baseline liver function tests; if elevated, discontinue treatment; discontinue even if liver function tests normal but lactic acidosis, hepatomegaly present; may be fatal

• **Pregnancy/breastfeeding:** use only if benefits outweigh fetal risk; register patients in the Antiretroviral Pregnancy Registry, 1-800-258-4263; do not breastfeed, excreted in breast milk
Evaluate:
• Therapeutic response: decreasing hepatitis B serology
Teach patient/family:
• That GI complaints and insomnia may resolve after 3-4 wk of treatment
• That follow-up visits must be continued

• That serious product interactions may occur if OTC products are ingested; to check with prescriber before taking

• That product may cause dizziness; to avoid hazardous activities until response is known

• To report symptoms of cough, difficulty sleeping, excessive headache, muscle pain/weakness

• To report progressive liver dysfunction: light-colored stools, dark urine, poor appetite, nausea, yellowing of skin, eyes

• That product will not cure HBV, and precautions should be taken to protect others

---

telmisartan (Rx)

(tel-mih-sar′tan)

Micardis

Func. class.: Antihypertensive

Chem. class.: Angiotensin II receptor (Type AT$_1$) antagonist

---

ACTION: Blocks the vasoconstricting and aldosterone-secreting effects of angiotensin II; selectively blocks the binding of angiotensin II to the AT$_1$ receptor found in tissues

USES: Hypertension, alone or in combination; stroke, MI prophylaxis (>55 yr) in patients unable to take ACE inhibitors

Unlabeled uses: Heart failure, proteinuria in diabetic nephropathy

CONTRAINDICATIONS: Hypersensitivity

Black Box Warning: Pregnancy

Precautions: Pregnancy, breastfeeding, children, geriatric patients; hypersensitivity to ACE inhibitors; renal/hepatic disease, renal artery stenosis, dialysis, HF, hyperkalemia, hypotension, hypovolemia, African descent

DOSAGE AND ROUTES

Hypertension

• **Adult: PO** 40 mg/day; range 20-80 mg/day

Stroke, MI prophylaxis

• **Adult >55 yr: PO** 80 mg/day

Available forms: Tabs 20, 40, 80 mg

Administer:

• Without regard to meals

• Increased dose to African-American patients or consider alternative agent; B/P response may be reduced

• Do not remove from blister pack until ready to use

SIDE EFFECTS

CNS: Dizziness, insomnia, *anxiety,* headache, fatigue, syncope

GI: Diarrhea, dyspepsia, *anorexia, vomiting*

META: Hyperkalemia

MS: Myalgia, pain

RESP: *Cough, upper respiratory infection,* sinusitis, pharyngitis

SYST: Angioedema

PHARMACOKINETICS

Onset of antihypertensive activity 3 hr, peak 0.5-1 hr, extensively metabolized, terminal half-life 24 hr, protein binding 99.5%, excreted in feces >97%, B/P response is less in African-American patients

INTERACTIONS

Increase: digoxin peak/trough concentrations—digoxin

Increase: antihypertensive action—diuretics, other antihypertensives, NSAIDs

Increase: hyperkalemia—potassium-sparing diuretics, potassium salt substitutes, ACE inhibitors

Decrease: antihypertensive effect—NSAIDs, salicylates

Drug/Lab Test

Increase: LFTs

NURSING CONSIDERATIONS

Assess:

Black Box Warning: **Pregnancy/breastfeeding:** if pregnancy test is positive, stop treatment; can cause death to fetus; do not breastfeed

• B/P, pulse standing, lying; note rate, rhythm, quality; if severe hypotension occurs, place in supine position; usually

T

Side effects: *italics* = common; red = life-threatening

occurs during first few weeks of treatment

• Baselines of renal, hepatic, electrolyte studies before therapy begins

• **Heart failure:** edema in feet, legs daily; jugular venous distention; dyspnea, crackles; weight increase >5 lb per week

Evaluate:

• Therapeutic response: decreased B/P

Teach patient/family:

• To comply with dosage schedule, even if feeling better; to take at same time of day; that therapeutic effect may take 2-4 wk

• To notify prescriber immediately of mouth sores, fever, swelling of hands or feet, swelling of face or lips, irregular heartbeat, chest pain, decreased urine output

• Not to stop abruptly; increased B/P will occur

• That excessive perspiration, dehydration, vomiting, diarrhea may lead to fall in blood pressure; to consult prescriber if these occur

• That product may cause dizziness, fainting, light-headedness; to avoid hazardous activities until response is known

Black Box Warning: To notify prescriber if pregnancy is planned or suspected; do not use in pregnancy, breastfeeding

• To notify prescriber of all prescriptions, OTC products, and supplements taken; to rise slowly from sitting to prevent drop in B/P

• **Overdose:** dizziness, bradycardia, or tachycardia

---

telotristat
(tel-oh'tri-stat)
Xermelo
Func. class.: Antidiarrheal
Chem. class.: Tryptophan hydroxylase inhibitor

Do not confuse:
Xermelo/Xarelto

ACTION: Reduces serotonin production; this decreases stools in carcinoid syndrome

USES: Carcinoid syndrome diarrhea; used with somatostatin analogue (SSA) when SSA alone does not control symptoms

CONTRAINDICATIONS:
Hypersensitivity

Precautions: Abdominal pain, breastfeeding, constipation, GI perforation/obstruction, pregnancy

DOSAGE AND ROUTES
• **Adult:** PO 250 mg tid

SIDE EFFECTS
CNS: Headache, depression, fever
CV: Peripheral edema
GI: Nausea, constipation, flatulence, anorexia, abdominal pain

PHARMACOKINETICS
Peak 0.5-2 hr, half-life 0.6 hr, 99% plasma protein binding, excreted in urine (93.2%), affected by CYP3A4, P-glycoprotein (P-gp)

INTERACTIONS
Decrease: effect of—CYP3A4 substrates; monitor for ineffective results; dose of CYP3A4 may need to be increased
Decrease: effect of—octreotide; give short-acting octreotide 30-60 min after telotristat
Increase: telotristat effect—P-glycoprotein (P-gp) products
Drug/Lab
Increase: ALT, AST, alk phos

NURSING CONSIDERATIONS
Assess:
• **Stools:** volume, color, characteristics, frequency; bowel pattern before product; rebound constipation, abdominal pain; discontinue if abdominal pain or constipation is severe
• **Pregnancy/breastfeeding:** use only if benefits outweigh fetal risk, not studied in pregnancy; breastfeeding not recommended, effects unknown

Evaluate:
• Therapeutic response: decreased diarrhea without abdominal pain or severe constipation

Teach Patient/Family:
• To take with food
• That if dose is missed, do not double; take regular dose at next scheduled time
• **Pregnancy/breastfeeding:** to contact health care provider if pregnancy is suspected or planned, or if breastfeeding
• To discontinue and notify health care provider if abdominal pain or severe constipation occurs

---

⚠ **HIGH ALERT**

temazepam (Rx)
(te-maz′e-pam)
Restoril
Func. class.: Sedative/hypnotic
Chem. class.: Benzodiazepine, short to intermediate acting

Controlled Substance Schedule IV (USA), Schedule F (Canada)

Do not confuse:
Restoril/RisperDAL

ACTION: Produces CNS depression at limbic, thalamic, hypothalamic levels of the CNS; may be mediated by neurotransmitter γ-aminobutyric acid (GABA); results are sedation, hypnosis, skeletal muscle relaxation, anticonvulsant activity, anxiolytic action

USES: Insomnia, short-term treatment (generally 7-10 days)

CONTRAINDICATIONS: Pregnancy, breastfeeding, hypersensitivity to benzodiazepines

Precautions: Children <15 yr, geriatric patients, anemia, renal/hepatic disease, suicidal individuals, drug abuse, psychosis, acute closed-angle glaucoma, seizure disorders, angioedema, sleep-related behaviors (sleepwalking), intermittent porphyria, COPD, dementia, myasthenia gravis

Black Box Warning: Coadministration with other CNS depressants

DOSAGE AND ROUTES
• **Adult: PO** 7.5 to 30 mg at bedtime
• **Geriatric: PO** 7.5 mg at bedtime
Available forms: Caps 7.5, 15, 22.5, 30 mg

Administer:
• 15-30 min before bedtime for sleeplessness
• Without regard to food

Black Box Warning: Avoid use with CNS depressants; serious CNS depression may result

• Store in tight container in cool environment

SIDE EFFECTS
CNS: *Lethargy, drowsiness, daytime sedation,* dizziness, confusion, lightheadedness, headache, anxiety, irritability, complex sleep-related reactions (sleep driving, sleep eating), fatigue
CV: Chest pain, pulse changes, hypotension
EENT: Blurred vision
GI: Nausea, vomiting, diarrhea, heartburn, abdominal pain, constipation, anorexia
SYST: Severe allergic reactions

PHARMACOKINETICS
Onset 30 min, peak 1-2 hr, duration 6-8 hr, half-life 10-20 hr, metabolized by liver, excreted by kidneys, crosses placenta, excreted in breast milk, 98% protein binding

INTERACTIONS
Increase: effects of cimetidine, disulfiram, oral contraceptives

Black Box Warning: Increase: action of both products—alcohol, CNS depressants

Increase: effect of temazepam—probenecid
Decrease: effect of antacids, theophylline, rifAMPin

Side effects: *italics* = common; red = life-threatening

Drug/Herb
Increase: CNS depression—hops, kava, valerian, chamomile, skullcap
Drug/Food
Decrease: temazepam effect—caffeine
Drug/Lab Test
Increase: ALT, AST

NURSING CONSIDERATIONS
Assess:
• Mental status: mood, sensorium, affect, memory (long, short), orientation
• **Type of sleep problem:** falling asleep, staying asleep, baseline, periodically
• **Dependency:** restrict amount given to patient, assess for physical/psychological dependency; high-level risk for abuse
• Assistance with ambulation after receiving dose
• **Beers:** avoid in older adults; increased sensitivity to benzodiazepines and decreased metabolism; may cause delirium
Evaluate:
• Therapeutic response: ability to sleep at night, decreased early morning awakening if taking product for insomnia
Teach patient/family:
• To avoid driving, other activities requiring alertness until stabilized; may cause dizziness, drowsiness

Black Box Warning: To avoid alcohol ingestion, other CNS depressants

• That effects may take 2 nights for benefits to be noticed
• To take as directed; not to increase dose unless approved by prescriber
• To limit to 7-10 days of continuous use
• About alternative measures to improve sleep: reading, exercise several hours before bedtime, warm bath, warm milk, TV, self-hypnosis, deep breathing
• Not to discontinue abruptly, withdraw gradually
• That complex sleep-related behaviors may occur: sleep driving/eating/walking
• That hangover, memory impairment are common in geriatric patients but less common than with barbiturates
• To notify prescriber if pregnancy is planned or suspected; to use contracep-

tion while taking this product; not to use in pregnancy; to use caution in breast-feeding, excretion unknown

TREATMENT OF OVERDOSE:
Lavage; monitor electrolytes, VS

⚠ HIGH ALERT

temozolomide (Rx)
(tem-oh-zole′oh-mide)
Temodar
Func. class.: Antineoplastic-alkylating agent
Chem. class.: Imidazotetrazine derivative

ACTION: Prodrug that undergoes conversion to MTIC; MTIC action prevents DNA transcription

USES: Anaplastic astrocytoma with relapse, glioblastoma multiforme, malignant glioma
Unlabeled uses: Metastatic melanoma

CONTRAINDICATIONS: Pregnancy, breastfeeding; hypersensitivity to this product, carbazine, or gelatin
Precautions: Geriatric patients, radiation therapy, renal/hepatic disease, bone marrow suppression, infection, myelosuppression

DOSAGE AND ROUTES
Glioblastoma multiforme
• **Adult: PO/IV** 75 mg/m^2/day × 42 days with focal radiotherapy, then maintenance of 6 cycles; maintenance dose: 150 mg/m^2 on days 1-5 of a 28-day cycle
Refractory anaplastic astrocytoma
• **Adult: IV** 150 mg/m^2/day over 90 min on days 1-5 q28days, may increase to 200 mg/m^2/day on days 1-5 q28days if hematologic parameters permit
Available forms: Caps 5, 20, 100, 140, 180, 250 mg; powder for inj 100 mg
Administer:
PO route
• Do not break, crush, chew, open caps

• Antiemetic 30-60 min before product to prevent vomiting
• Caps 1 at a time with 8 oz of water at same time of day
• Fluids IV or PO before chemotherapy to hydrate patient
• If caps accidentally damaged, do not allow contact with skin or inhale
• Use proper procedures for handling/ disposing of chemotherapy products
• Give on empty stomach at bedtime to prevent nausea/vomiting
• Store in light-resistant container in a dry area

IV route
• Bring vial to room temperature; discard if cloudy
• Inject 41 mL sterile water for inj into vial (2.5 mg/mL)
• Gently swirl; do not shake

Intermittent IV INFUSION route
• Withdraw up to 40 mL from each vial to make total dose; transfer to empty 250-mL PVC infusion bag; flush before and after infusion
• Run over 90 min
• Use reconstituted sol within 14 hr, including infusion time
• Do not admix

SIDE EFFECTS

CNS: Seizures, *hemiparesis, dizziness, poor coordination, amnesia, insomnia, paresthesia, somnolence, paresis, ataxia, anxiety, dysphagia, depression, confusion*
GI: *Nausea, anorexia, vomiting,* abdominal pain, constipation
GU: Urinary incontinence, UTI, frequency
HEMA: Thrombocytopenia, leukopenia, anemia, myelosuppression, neutropenia
INTEG: *Rash, pruritus*
MISC: Headache, fatigue, asthenia, fever, edema, back pain, weight increase, diplopia
RESP: URI, pharyngitis, sinusitis, coughing
SYST: Anaphylaxis, secondary malignancy

PHARMACOKINETICS

Absorption complete, rapid; crosses blood-brain barrier; excreted in urine, feces; half-life 1.8 hr; peak 1 hr

INTERACTIONS

Increase: myelosuppression—radiation, other antineoplastics
Increase: bleeding risk—NSAIDs, anticoagulants, platelet inhibitors, thrombolytics
Decrease: antibody reaction—live virus vaccines, toxoids
Decrease: action of digoxin
Drug/Food
Decrease: drug absorption
Drug/Lab Test
Decrease: Hgb, platelets, WBC, neutrophils

NURSING CONSIDERATIONS
Assess:
• CBC on day 22 (21 days after 1st dose), CBC weekly until recovery if ANC is <1.5 $\times 10^9$/L and platelets <100 $\times 10^9$/L; do not administer to patients who do not tolerate 100 mg/m^2; myelosuppression usually occurs late during the treatment cycle
• Seizures throughout treatment; mental status
• Monitor temperature; may indicate beginning infection
• Hepatic studies before, during therapy (bilirubin, AST, ALT, LDH), as needed or monthly
• Bleeding: hematuria, guaiac, bruising, petechiae, mucosa or orifices
• **Pregnancy/breastfeeding:** do not use in pregnancy, breastfeeding
Evaluate:
• Therapeutic response: decreased tumor size, spread of malignancy
Teach patient/family:
• To report signs of infection: fever, sore throat, flulike symptoms
• To report signs of anemia: fatigue, headache, faintness, SOB, irritability
• To report bleeding; to avoid use of razors, commercial mouthwash
• To notify prescriber if pregnancy is planned or suspected; not to breastfeed

T

Side effects: *italics* = common; red = life-threatening

RARELY USED

temsirolimus (Rx)
(tem-sir-oh'li-mus)
Torisel
Func. class.: Biologic response modifier
Chem. class.: Kinase inhibitor, mTOR antagonist

USES: Renal cell carcinoma

CONTRAINDICATIONS: Pregnancy, breastfeeding; hypersensitivity to this product or to sirolimus; polysorbate 80
Precautions: Children <13 yr, females, severe pulmonary/renal/hepatic disease (bilirubin >1-1.5 × ULN or AST >ULN but bilirubin ≤ULN), diabetes mellitus, hyperkalemia, hyperuricemia, hypertension, bone marrow suppression, hypertriglyceridemia/hyperlipidemia, surgery, brain tumors

DOSAGE AND ROUTES
• **Adult:** IV 25 mg over 30-60 min weekly; treat until disease progression or severe toxicity occurs
Hepatic dose
• **Adult:** IV (mild impairment) bilirubin >1-1.5×ULN or AST >ULN but bilirubin ≤ULN: reduce to 15 mg/wk; moderate or severe impairment, do not use

▲ HIGH ALERT

tenecteplase (TNK-tPA) (Rx)
(ten-ek'ta-place)
TNKase
Func. class.: Thrombolytic
Chem. class.: Tissue plasminogen activator

Do not confuse:
TNKase/Activase

ACTION: Activates conversion of plasminogen to plasmin (fibrinolysin): plasmin breaks down clots (fibrin), fibrinogen, factors V, VII; occlusion of venous access lines

USES: Acute myocardial infarction, coronary artery thrombosis

CONTRAINDICATIONS: Hypersensitivity, arteriovenous malformation, aneurysm, active bleeding, intracranial/intraspinal surgery or trauma within 2 mo, CNS neoplasms, severe hypertension, severe renal/hepatic disease, history of CVA, increased ICP/stroke
Precautions: Pregnancy, breastfeeding, children, geriatric patients, arterial emboli from left side of heart, hypocoagulation, subacute bacterial endocarditis, rheumatic valvular disease, cerebral embolism/thrombosis/hemorrhage, intraarterial diagnostic procedure or surgery (10 days), recent major surgery, dysrhythmias, hypertension

DOSAGE AND ROUTES
Total dose, max 50 mg based on patient's weight
• **Adult <60 kg: IV BOL** 30 mg, give over 5 sec
• **Adult ≥60-<70 kg: IV BOL** 35 mg, give over 5 sec
• **Adult ≥70-<80 kg: IV BOL** 40 mg, give over 5 sec
• **Adult ≥80-<90 kg: IV BOL** 45 mg, give over 5 sec
• **Adult ≥90 kg: IV BOL** 50 mg, give over 5 sec, max 50 mg total dose
Available forms: Powder for inj, lyophilized 50 mg
Administer:
Intermittent IV INFUSION route
• As soon as thrombi are identified; not useful for thrombi >1 wk old
• Cryoprecipitate or fresh frozen plasma if bleeding occurs
• Heparin after fibrinogen level >100 mg/dL; heparin infusion to increase PTT to 1.5-2× baseline for 3-7 days; IV heparin with loading dose is recommended
• Aseptically withdraw 10 mL of sterile water for inj from diluent vial; use red cannula syringe-filling device; inject all contents of syringe into product vial; direct into powder, swirl, withdraw correct

dose; discard any unused sol; stand shield with dose vertically on flat surface and passively recap red cannula; remove entire shield assembly by twisting counterclockwise; give by IV BOL
• IV therapy: use upper-extremity vessel that is accessible to manual compression
• If product not used immediately, refrigerate; use within 8 hr; not compatible with dextrose; flush dextrose-containing lines with saline before and after administration

SIDE EFFECTS

CV: Dysrhythmias, hypotension, pulmonary edema, pulmonary embolism, cardiogenic shock, cardiac arrest, heart failure, myocardial reinfarction, myocardial rupture, tamponade, pericarditis, pericardial effusion, thrombosis, CVA
HEMA: Decreased Hct, bleeding
INTEG: Rash, urticaria, phlebitis at IV infusion site, itching, flushing
SYST: GI, GU, intracranial, retroperitoneal bleeding, surface bleeding, anaphylaxis

PHARMACOKINETICS

IV: Onset immediate, half-life 20-24 min, metabolized by liver

INTERACTIONS

Increase: bleeding—aspirin, indomethacin, phenylbutazone, anticoagulants, antithrombolytics, glycoprotein IIb/IIIa inhibitors, dipyridamole, clopidogrel, ticlopidine, NSAIDs, cefamandole, cefoperazone, cefoTEtan, SSRIs, SNRIs
Drug/Herb
Increase: risk of bleeding—feverfew, garlic, ginger, ginkgo, green tea, horse chestnut
Drug/Lab Test
Increase: INR, PT, PTT

NURSING CONSIDERATIONS
Assess:
• **Allergy:** fever, rash, itching, chills; mild reaction may be treated with antihistamines
• Cholesterol embolism, blue-toe syndrome, renal failure, MI, cerebral/spinal cord/bowel/retinal infarction, hypertension; can be fatal

• **Bleeding during 1st hr of treatment;** hematuria, hematemesis, bleeding from mucous membranes, epistaxis, ecchymosis; may require tranfusion (rare), continue to assess for bleeding for 24 hr
• **AVM, recent surgery, actual bleeding:** assess for contraindications before use
• **Studies to be monitored:** Hct, platelets, PTT, PT, TT, aPTT before starting therapy; PT or aPTT must be <2× control before starting therapy; PTT or PT q3-4hr during treatment; also monitor CPK, ECG, fibrin degradation products (FDPs), fibrinogen, INR
• Hypersensitive reactions: fever, rash, dyspnea; product should be discontinued
• VS, B/P, pulse, respirations, neurologic signs, temperature at least q4hr; temperature >104° F (40° C) indicates internal bleeding; systolic pressure increase >25 mm Hg should be reported to prescriber
• Neurologic changes that may indicate intracranial bleeding; if suspected, a CT scan should be performed
• **Retroperitoneal bleeding:** back pain, leg weakness, diminished pulses
• Bed rest during entire course of treatment
• Avoidance of venous or arterial puncture, inj, rectal temperature, any invasive treatment, if possible; if arterial puncture is needed, use upper extremity, use pressure dressing for at least 30 min, monitor closely
• Treatment of fever with acetaminophen or aspirin
• Pressure for 30 sec to minor bleeding sites; inform prescriber if this does not attain hemostasis; apply pressure dressing
• **Pregnancy/breasfeeding:** use only if benefits outweigh fetal risk; cautious use in breastfeeding, excretion unknown
Evaluate:
• Therapeutic response: resolution of MI
Teach patient/family:
• About proper dental care to avoid bleeding
• To notify prescriber immediately of sudden, severe headache
• To notify prescriber of bleeding; hypersensitivity; fast, slow, or uneven heart rate; feeling of faintness; blood in urine, stools; nosebleeds

Side effects: *italics* = common; red = life-threatening

tenofovir (Rx)

(ten-oh-foh′veer)

Viread

Func. class.: Antiretroviral

Chem. class.: Nucleoside reverse transcriptase inhibitor (NRTI)

ACTION: Inhibits replication of HIV virus by competing with the natural substrate and then incorporating into cellular DNA by viral reverse transcriptase, thereby terminating cellular DNA chain

USES: HIV-1 infection with at least 2 other antiretrovirals, hepatitis B

CONTRAINDICATIONS: Hypersensitivity

Black Box Warning: Lactic acidosis

Precautions: Pregnancy, breastfeeding, children, geriatric patients, renal disease, CCr <60 mL/min, osteoporosis, immune reconstitution syndrome

Black Box Warning: Hepatic disease, hepatitis

DOSAGE AND ROUTES
Human immunodeficiency virus (HIV) infection

• **Adult/adolescent/child weighing ≥35 kg: PO** Tablet: 300 mg once daily; Oral powder 300 mg/day (7.5 scoops) with 2-4 oz soft food

• **Adolescent/child weighing 28-34 kg: PO** Tablet: 250 mg/day

• **Child ≥2 yr and weighing 22-27 kg: PO** Tablet: 200 mg/day

• **Child ≥2 yr and weighing 17-21 kg: PO** Tablet: 150 mg/day

• **Child/adolescent ≥2 yr and weighing <35 kg: PO** Oral powder: 8 mg/kg/dose daily with 2-4 oz soft food. Round dose to nearest 20-mg increment

Renal dose (tenofovir DF)

• **Adult: PO** CCr 30-49 mL/min, 300 mg q48hr; CCr 10-29 mL/min, 300 mg q72-96hr; CCr <10 mL/min, not recommended

Renal dose (tenofovir alafenamide)

• **Adult: PO** CCr <15 mL/min: not recommended

Available forms: Tabs 150, 200, 250, 300 mg; oral powder 40 mg/scoop

Administer:

• Without regard to food

• Store at 25° C (77° F)

• **Oral powder:** use scoop provided, mix powder into 2-4 oz ($^1/_4$-$^1/_2$ cup) of applesauce, yogurt, do not mix with liquid, product will not mix, product is bitter, use immediately after mixing, clean scoop

SIDE EFFECTS

CNS: *Headache, asthenia*

GI: *Nausea, vomiting, diarrhea,* anorexia, *flatulence, abdominal pain,* pancreatitis

GU: Renal failure, renal tubular acidosis/necrosis, Fanconi's syndrome

HEMA: Neutropenia, osteopenia

INTEG: *Rash,* angioedema

META: Lactic acidosis, hypokalemia, hypophosphatemia

MS: Arthralgia, myalgia, decreased bone mineral density

SYST: Lipodystrophy

PHARMACOKINETICS

Rapidly absorbed, distributed to extravascular space, excreted unchanged in urine 70%-80%, terminal half-life 17 hr, peak 1-2 hr

INTERACTIONS

Increase: tenofovir level—cidofovir, acyclovir, valACYclovir, ganciclovir, valGANciclovir

Increase: level of didanosine when given with tenofovir

Increase: tenofovir level—any product that decreases renal function

NURSING CONSIDERATIONS
Assess:

• Viral load, CD4+ T-cell count, plasma HIV RNA, serum creatinine/BUN/phosphate

• Resistance testing at start of therapy and at treatment failure

---

Black Box Warning: Hepatitis exacerbations: monitor hepatic studies: AST, ALT, bilirubin; amylase, lipase, triglycerides baseline and periodically during treatment, after treatment, assess for exacerbations for 6 mo after last dose

• **Bone, renal toxicity**: if bone abnormalities are suspected, obtain tests; serum phosphorus, creatinine

Black Box Warning: Lactic acidosis, severe hepatomegaly with steatosis, Fanconi's syndrome: obtain baseline liver function tests; if elevated, discontinue treatment; discontinue even if liver function tests normal but lactic acidosis, hepatomegaly present; may be fatal

• **Pregnancy/breastfeeding:** use only if clearly needed; register patients in the Antiretroviral Pregnancy Registry, 1-800-258-4263; do not breastfeed

Evaluate:

• Therapeutic response: decrease in signs, symptoms of HIV

Teach patient/family:

• To take without regard to food

• That GI complaints resolve after 3-4 wk of treatment

• Not to breastfeed while taking this product

• That product must be taken daily even if patient feels better

• That follow-up visits must be continued because serious toxicity may occur; that blood counts must be done q2wk

• That product will control symptoms but is not a cure for HIV; that patient is still infectious, may pass HIV virus on to others

• To discuss with provider all OTC, Rx, herbals, supplements taken

• **Hepatotoxicity:** To notify provider of yellow skin, eyes, dark urine, clay-colored stools, nausea, abdominal pain

• That other products may be necessary to prevent other infections

• If used for prophylaxis (PREP): does not prevent sexually transmitted infections; use appropriate barrier protection and safe sex practices

• That changes in body fat distribution, usually in the breasts, neck, and back, may occur

Black Box Warning: To notify prescriber of symptoms of lactic acidosis (nausea, vomiting, weakness, abdominal pain)

---

terazosin (Rx)

(ter-ay′zoe-sin)

Hytrin ✖

Func. class.: Antihypertensive
Chem. class.: α-Adrenergic blocker

ACTION: Decreases total vascular resistance, which is responsible for a decrease in B/P; this occurs by the blockade of α_1-adrenoreceptors

USES: Hypertension, as a single agent or in combination with diuretics or β-blockers; BPH

CONTRAINDICATIONS: Hypersensitivity

Precautions: Pregnancy, breastfeeding, children, prostate cancer, syncope

DOSAGE AND ROUTES

Hypertension

• **Adult: PO** 1 mg at bedtime, may increase dose slowly to desired response; max 20 mg/day divided q12hr

Benign prostatic hyperplasia

• **Adult: PO** 1 mg at bedtime, gradually increase up to 5-10 mg; max 20 mg divided q12hr

Available forms: Caps 1, 2, 5, 10 mg

Administer:

• Give dose at bedtime; patient should not operate machinery because fainting may occur

• If treatment is interrupted for several days, restart with initial dose

• Without regard to food; feeding tube: place cap in 60 mL of warm tap water; stir until liquid spills from ruptured shell (5 min); stir until cap dissolves; draw solution into oral syringe; give through feeding tube; flush with water

• Store at room temperature

T

Side effects: *italics* = common; red = life-threatening

SIDE EFFECTS

CNS: *Dizziness, headache, drowsiness,* anxiety, depression, vertigo, weakness, fatigue, syncope

CV: *Palpitations, orthostatic hypotension,* tachycardia, *edema,* rebound hypertension

EENT: Blurred vision, epistaxis, tinnitus, dry mouth, red sclera, nasal congestion, sinusitis

GI: *Nausea,* vomiting, diarrhea, constipation, abdominal pain

GU: Urinary frequency, incontinence, impotence, priapism

RESP: Dyspnea, cough, pharyngitis, nasal congestion

PHARMACOKINETICS

Half-life 9-12 hr; protein binding 90%-94%; metabolized in liver; excreted in urine, feces, peak 2-3 hr, onset 15 min, duration 24 hr

INTERACTIONS

Increase: hypotensive effects—β-blockers, nitroglycerin, verapamil, other antihypertensives, alcohol, phosphodiesterase (PDE5) inhibitors (vardenafil, tadalafil, sildenafil)

Decrease: hypotensive effects—estrogens, NSAIDs, sympathomimetics, salicylates

Drug/Herb

Increase: antihypertensive effect—hawthorn

Decrease: antihypertensive effect—ephedra

Drug/Lab Test

Decrease: Hgb, WBC, platelets, albumin

NURSING CONSIDERATIONS

Assess:

• **BPH:** urinary patterns (hesitancy, frequency, change in stream, dribbling, dysuria, urgency)

• **Hypertension:** crackles, dyspnea, orthopnea q30min; orthostatic B/P, pulse, jugular venous distention q4hr; weight daily, I&O

• BUN, uric acid if patient receiving long-term therapy

• **Beers:** avoid use in older adults as antihypertensive; high risk of orthostatic hypotension

• **Pregnancy/breastfeeding:** use only if benefits outweigh fetal risk; cautious use in breastfeeding, excretion unknown

Evaluate:

• Therapeutic response: decreased B/P, edema in feet, legs; decreased symptoms of BPH

Teach patient/family:

• That fainting occasionally occurs after 1st dose; not to drive or operate machinery for 4 hr after 1st dose or after an increase in dose; to take 1st dose at bedtime

• To rise slowly from sitting or lying position

• Not to discontinue abruptly; if doses have been missed for several days, notify prescriber; dose may need to be retitrated

• Not to drink alcohol

• **Hypertension:** to continue with regimen, including diet, exercise

---

terbinafine oral (Rx)

(ter-bin′a-feen)

Lamisil, Lamisil AT

Func. class.: Antifungal

Chem. class.: Synthetic allylamine derivative

Do not confuse:

terbinafine/terbutaline

LamISIL/LaMICtal

ACTION: Interferes with cell-membrane permeability of fungi such as *Trichophyton rubrum, Trichophyton mentagrophytes, Trichophyton tonsurans, Epidermophyton floccosum, Microsporum canis, Microsporum audouinii, Microsporum gypseum, Candida;* broad-spectrum antifungal

USES: (Oral) onychomycosis of toenail or fingernail due to dermatophytes, tinea capitis/corporis/cruris/pedis/versicolor

Unlabeled uses: Cutaneous candidiasis

CONTRAINDICATIONS: Hypersensitivity

Precautions: Pregnancy, breastfeeding, children, chronic/active hepatic disease,

⚠Ⓖⓡ Genetic warning

renal disease GFR ≤50 mL/min, immunosuppression

DOSAGE AND ROUTES
• **Adult: PO** 250 mg/day × 6 wk (fingernail); × 12 wk (toenail)
Available forms: Tabs 250 mg; oral granules 125, 187.5 mg
Administer:
• **PO:** without regard to food
• Store at <25° C (77° F); protect from light
• **Granules:** take with food; sprinkle packet contents on pudding or nonacidic soft food; swallow without chewing; do not use fruit-based foods

SIDE EFFECTS
CNS: Depression
EENT: Tinnitus, hearing impairment
GI: Diarrhea, dyspepsia, vertigo, abdominal pain, nausea, hepatitis
HEMA: Neutropenia
INTEG: Rash, pruritus, urticaria, Stevens-Johnson syndrome, photosensitivity
MISC: Headache, hepatic enzyme changes, taste, visual/olfactory disturbance

PHARMACOKINETICS
Peak 1-2 hr, >99% protein binding, half-life 36 hr

INTERACTIONS
Increase: levels of dextromethorphan
Increase: terbinafine clearance—rifAMPin
Increase: clearance of cycloSPORINE
Decrease: terbinafine clearance—cimetidine
Decrease: metabolism of—CYP2D6 (antidysrhythmics IC, III, amoxapine, atomoxetine, cloZAPine)
Drug/Herb
• Side effects: cola nut, guarana, yerba maté, tea (black, green), coffee
Drug/Lab Test
Increase: LFTs

NURSING CONSIDERATIONS
Assess:
• Hepatic studies (ALT, AST) before beginning treatment; do not use in presence of hepatic disease

• CBC in treatment >6 wk
• Continuing infection: increased size, number of lesions
• **Pregnancy/breastfeeding:** avoid during pregnancy and breastfeeding
Evaluate:
• Therapeutic response: decrease in size, number of lesions
Teach patient/family:
• That treatment may take 12 wk (toenail), 6 wk (fingernail)
• To notify prescriber of nausea, vomiting, fatigue, jaundice, dark urine, clay-colored stool, RUQ pain; may indicate hepatic dysfunction
• To take without regard to meals; granules may be sprinkled on soft food but not chewed; do not mix with fruit-based products
• To report vision changes immediately

---

terbinafine topical
See Appendix B

---

terbutaline (Rx)
(ter-byoo'ta-leen)
Func. class.: Selective β2-agonist; bronchodilator
Chem. class.: Catecholamine

ACTION: Relaxes bronchial smooth muscle by direct action on β2-adrenergic receptors through the accumulation of cAMP at β-adrenergic receptor sites; bronchodilation, diuresis, CNS, cardiac stimulation occur; relaxes uterine smooth muscle

USES: Bronchospasm
Unlabeled uses: Premature labor, nonresponsive status asthmaticus in children (IV)

CONTRAINDICATIONS: Hypersensitivity to sympathomimetics, closed-angle glaucoma, tachydysrhythmias
Precautions: Pregnancy, breastfeeding, geriatric patients, cardiac disorders,

hyperthyroidism, diabetes mellitus, prostatic hypertension, hypertension, seizure disorder

> **Black Box Warning:** Labor

DOSAGE AND ROUTES
Bronchospasm
• **Adult/child ≥12 yr: PO** 2.5-5 mg q8hr; **SUBCUT** 0.25 mg q15-30min, max 0.5 mg in 4 hr
• **Child 6-11 yr (unlabeled): PO** 0.05 mg/kg q8hr, may increase slowly
Renal dose
• **Adult: PO** CCr 10-50 mL/min, 50% of dose; CCr <10 mL/min, avoid use
Tocolytic (preterm labor) (unlabeled)
• **Adult: SUBCUT** 0.25 mg q20min to 6 hr, hold if pulse >120 bpm
Available forms: Tabs 2.5, 5 mg; inj 1 mg/mL
Administer:
• With food; may be crushed
• 2 hr before bedtime to avoid sleeplessness

IV route (unlabeled)
• Only used if subcut is ineffective
• IV after diluting each 5 mg/1 L D$_5$W for infusion
• IV, run 5 mcg/min; may increase 5 mcg q10min, titrate to response; after $^1/_2$-1 hr, taper dose by 5 mcg; switch to PO as soon as possible
• Store at room temperature; do not use discolored sol

Y-site compatibilities: Insulin (regular)

SIDE EFFECTS
CNS: Tremors, anxiety, insomnia, headache, dizziness, stimulation
CV: Palpitations, tachycardia, hypertension, dysrhythmias, cardiac arrest, QT prolongation
GI: Nausea, vomiting
META: Hypokalemia, hyperglycemia
RESP: Paradoxical bronchospasm, dyspnea

PHARMACOKINETICS
PO: Onset $^1/_2$ hr, peak 1-2 hr, duration 4-8 hr, half-life 3.4 hr

SUBCUT: Onset 6-15 min, peak $^1/_2$-1 hr, duration 1$^1/_2$-4 hr, half-life 5.7 hr

INTERACTIONS
Increase: hypertensive crisis—MAOIs
Increase: effects of both products—other sympathomimetics
Decrease: action—β-blockers; do not use together
Drug/Herb
Increase: effect—green tea (large amounts), guarana

NURSING CONSIDERATIONS
Assess:
• **Respiratory function:** vital capacity, forced expiratory volume, ABGs, B/P, pulse, respiratory pattern, lung sounds, sputum before and after treatment
• Tolerance in patients receiving long-term therapy; dose may have to be changed; monitor for rebound bronchospasm
• **Paradoxical bronchospasm:** dyspnea, wheezing; keep emergency equipment nearby

> **Black Box Warning: Labor:** maternal heart rate, B/P, contraction, fetal heart rate; can inhibit uterine contractions, labor; monitor for hypoglycemia; do not use injectable product for prevention or treatment over 72 hr in preterm labor; do not use oral product for preterm labor; avoid in breastfeeding

• Increase in fluids of >2 L/day
Evaluate:
• Therapeutic response: absence of dyspnea, wheezing
Teach patient/family:
• Not to use OTC medications because extra stimulation may occur
• About all aspects of product; to avoid smoking, smoke-filled rooms, persons with respiratory infections
• To increase fluids by >2 L/day; to allow 15 min between inhalation of product and inhaled product containing steroid
• To take on time; if missed, not to make up after 1 hr; to wait until next dose

terconazole vaginal antifungal
See Appendix B

---

teriflunomide
(ter'i-floo'noe-mide)
Aubagio
Func. class.: Multiple sclerosis agent
Chem. class.: Pyrimidine synthesis inhibitor

ACTION: Antiproliferative effects including peripheral T- and B-lymphocytes, might reduce inflammatory demyelination

USES: Reduction of the frequency of relapses or remitting MS

CONTRAINDICATIONS: Hypersensitivity

Black Box Warning: Pregnancy

Precautions: Breastfeeding, alcoholism, diabetes mellitus, eosinophilic pneumonia, hepatitis, jaundice, male-mediated teratogenicity, pneumonitis, pulmonary disease/fibrosis, sarcoidosis, TB, vaccination

Black Box Warning: Hepatic disease, contraception requirements, male-mediated teratogenicity

DOSAGE AND ROUTES
Adult: PO 7 or 14 mg/day
Available forms: Tabs 7, 14 mg
Administer:
PO route
• May be taken without regard to food

SIDE EFFECTS
CNS: Anxiety, headache
CV: Palpitations, hypertension, MI
EENT: Blurred vision, conjunctivitis, sinusitis
GI: Nausea, vomiting, diarrhea, cystitis

HEMA: Leukopenia, lymphopenia, neutropenia
INTEG: Acne vulgaris, alopecia, pruritus
META: Weight loss
MISC: Infection, cystitis, Stevens-Johnson syndrome

PHARMACOKINETICS
Protein binding >99%, median half-life 18-19 days, peak 1-4 hr

INTERACTIONS
• Do not use with leflunomide, live virus vaccines
Increase: teriflunomide effect—cycloSPORINE, eltrombopag, gefitinib

Black Box Warning: **Increase:** hepatotoxicity—methotrexate, HMG-CoA reductase inhibitors

Increase: hematologic toxicity—zidovudine
Increase: effect of—oral contraceptives, repaglinide, pioglitazone, rosiglitazone, PACLitaxel, naproxen, topotecan, bosentan, furosemide
Decrease: effect of—warfarin, alosetron, DULoxetine, theophylline, tiZANidine, quiNINE, tamoxifen, bendamustine, rasagiline, rOPINIRole, selegiline, propafenone, mexiletine, lidocaine, anagrelide, cloZAPine, cinacalcet, caffeine; monitor closely
Decrease: effect of teriflunomide—cholestyramine

NURSING CONSIDERATIONS
Assess:
• CNS symptoms: anxiety, confusion, vertigo
• GI status: diarrhea, vomiting, abdominal pain
• Cardiac status: tachycardia, palpitations, vasodilation, chest pain; monitor B/P
• **Stevens-Johnson syndrome, toxic epidermal necrolysis:** Assess for fever, blisters, aches, fatigue, if these occur, stop product immediately
• **Hepatotoxicity:** Monitor LFTs after 6 mo or less of treatment, and monthly after start of treatment, do not use if ALT >2X ULN, discontinue if >3X ULN, monitor bilirubin

Side effects: *italics* = common; red = life-threatening

- **Blood dyscrasias:** Monitor CBC, platelets 6 mo before use and periodically, monitor for infection, monitor INR

Black Box Warning: Pregnancy: do not start treatment until pregnancy is ruled out; this product should not be used during pregnancy or for 2 yr after stopping the drug; those wishing to become pregnant must discontinue the product and undergo an accelerated elimination procedure with verification of teriflunomide plasma level <0.02 mg/L; do not use in breastfeeding

Evaluate:
- Therapeutic response: decreased symptoms of MS

Teach patient/family:
- That blurred vision can occur
- That hair may be lost, that a wig or hairpiece may be used
- Not to change dosing or stop taking without advice of prescriber
- To report skin changes, rashes immediately
- To avoid live virus vaccines; that updated vaccines should be done before use
- To report signs, symptoms of infection
- Teach patient to take as directed, provide "Medication Guide"
- Teach patient to notify provider of nausea, vomiting, loss of appetite, dark urine, yellow eyes or skin

Black Box Warning: To notify prescriber if pregnancy is planned or suspected; do not use in pregnancy or breastfeeding

---

teriparatide (Rx)
(tah-ree-par'ah-tide)
Forteo
Func. class.: Parathyroid hormone (rDNA)
Chem. class.: Teriparatide

ACTION: Contains human recombinant parathyroid hormone to stimulate new bone growth

USES: Postmenopausal women with osteoporosis, men with primary or hypogonadal osteoporosis who are at high risk for fracture, glucocorticoid-induced osteoporosis
Unlabeled uses: Hypoparathyroidism

CONTRAINDICATIONS: Hypersensitivity, increased baseline risk for osteosarcoma (Paget's disease, open epiphyses; previous bone radiation), bone metastases, history of skeletal malignancies, other metabolic bone diseases, preexisting hypercalcemia
Precautions: Pregnancy, breastfeeding, children, urolithiasis, hypotension, use >2 yr, cardiac disease

Black Box Warning: Secondary malignancy (osteogenic sarcoma)

DOSAGE AND ROUTES
- **Adult: SUBCUT** 20 mcg/day up to 2 yr
Available forms: Prefilled pen delivery device (delivers 20 mcg/day)
Administer:
SUBCUT route
- Give by SUBCUT using disposable pen only; inject in thigh or abdomen; lightly pinch fold of skin; insert needle; release skin; inject at 90-degree angle over 5 sec; rotate inj sites
- Have patient sit or lie down; orthostatic hypotension may occur
- Protect from freezing, light; refrigerate pen
- Store refrigerated; do not freeze; may be used for 28 days after first inj

SIDE EFFECTS
CNS: Dizziness, headache, insomnia, depression, vertigo
CV: Hypertension, angina, syncope
GI: Nausea, diarrhea, dyspepsia, vomiting, constipation
INTEG: Rash, sweating
MISC: Pain, asthenia, hyperuricemia
MS: Arthralgia, leg cramps, back/leg pain, weakness, osteosarcoma (rare)
RESP: Rhinitis, cough, pharyngitis, pneumonia, dyspnea

PHARMACOKINETICS

SUBCUT: Extensively and rapidly absorbed, metabolized by liver, excreted by kidneys, terminal half-life 1 hr, onset rapid, peak $^1/_2$ hr, duration 3 hr

INTERACTIONS

Increase: digoxin toxicity: digoxin
Increase: urinary calcium excretion; dose may need to be adjusted
Drug/Lab Test
Increase: calcium, uric acid, urinary calcium
Decrease: phosphorous, magnesium

NURSING CONSIDERATIONS
Assess:

> Black Box Warning: **Secondary malignancy:** osteosarcoma, dependent on length of treatment; those at higher risk for osteosarcoma should not use this product

• Uric acid, magnesium, creatinine, BUN, urine pH, vit D, phosphate for normal serum levels; serum calcium may be transiently increased after dosing (max at 4-6 hr after dose)
• Bone pain, headache, fatigue, changes in LOC, leg cramps
• **Signs of persistent hypercalcemia:** nausea, vomiting, constipation, lethargy, muscle weakness
• Nutritional status: diet for sources of vit D (milk, some seafood), calcium (dairy products, dark green vegetables), phosphates (dairy products)
• **Pregnancy/breastfeeding:** use only if benefits outweigh fetal risk; not to be used in pregnant females; do not breastfeed
Evaluate:
• Therapeutic response: increased bone mineral density
Teach patient/family:
• About the symptoms of hypercalcemia
• About foods rich in calcium, vit D
• How to use delivery device, dispose of needles; not to share pen with others; to use at same time of day
• To sit or lie down if dizziness or fast heartbeat occurs after 1st few doses
• To rotate administration sites
• To store pen in refrigerator; pen may be used for 28 days

---

tesamorelin

Egrifta

Func. class.: Pituitary hormone, growth hormone modifiers

ACTION: Binds to growth hormone (GH) releasing factor receptors on the pituitary somatotroph cells; binding stimulates the production, release of endogenous GH

USES: Treatment of excess abdominal fat in HIV-infected patients with lipodystrophy

CONTRAINDICATIONS: Hypersensitivity to this product or mannitol, neoplastic disease, pregnancy, disruption of the hypothalamic-pituitary axis (hypothalamic-pituitary-adrenal [HPA] suppression) due to hypophysectomy, hypopituitarism, pituitary tumor/surgery, radiation therapy of the head or head trauma, IV/IM administration
Precautions: Breastfeeding, CABG, diabetes, diabetic retinopathy, edema, geriatric patients, children, infants, adolescents

DOSAGE AND ROUTES
• **Adult: SUBCUT** 2 mg/day
Available forms: Powder for injection 1 mg
Administer:
Subcut route:
• Visually inspect parenteral products for particulate matter and discoloration before use
• To reconstitute, use 2 1-mg vials, inject 2.1 mL sterile water for inj into the first 1-mg vial; use syringe with needle already attached; to avoid foaming, push plunger in slowly with needle on a slight angle and gently roll vial for 30 sec until mixed; do not shake; withdraw 2.1 mL of the reconstituted sol and add to second 1-mg vial; roll, do not shake
• To administer, take syringe out of vial, place needle cap on its side against a clean flat surface, do not touch needle, hold syringe and slide needle into cap, push cap all the way or until it snaps shut; do not touch cap until it covers needle completely; remove needle, insert

Side effects: *italics* = common; red = life-threatening

a 0.5-inch 27-G safety injection needle onto syringe; use immediately; inject subcut into abdomen; avoid scar tissues, bruises, or navel; rotate inj sites in abdomen; slowly push plunger down until all sol has been injected

• Use a piece of sterile gauze to rub the inj site clean; if bleeding, apply pressure to site with gauze for 30 sec; if bleeding continues, apply a bandage to site

• Properly dispose of used syringe, needles, vial, and sterile water for injection bottle

SIDE EFFECTS

CNS: Depression, peripheral neuropathy paresthesias, hypoesthesia, flushing, night sweats, insomnia, headache

CV: Hypertension, edema, peripheral edema

GI: Nausea, vomiting, upper abdominal pain, dyspepsia, diarrhea, constipation

INTEG: Pruritus, urticaria, rash, flushing, injection site reactions

MS: Arthralgia, joint swelling, stiffness, myalgias, carpal tunnel syndrome

RESP: Upper respiratory tract infection

SYST: Secondary malignancy

META: Hypercalcemia, hyperuricemia

PHARMACOKINETICS

Half-life 26 min in healthy patients, 38 min in those with HIV infection; peak 0.15 hr

INTERACTIONS

Decrease: effect of—simvastatin, ritonavir, cortisone, predniSONE

NURSING CONSIDERATIONS

Assess:

• **Lipodystrophy:** sunken cheeks, thinning arms and legs, fat accumulation in the abdomen, jaws, and back of neck; after treatment these should lessen

• Monitor for edema, joint pains, carpal tunnel syndrome, therapy may need to be discontinued

• Monitor glycosylated hemoglobin A1c (HbA1c), serum IGF-1 concentrations, ophthalmologic exam

• **Beers:** avoid in older adults except as hormone replacement following pituitary gland removal; may cause edema, arthralgia

• **Pregnancy/breastfeeding:** do not use in pregnancy, breastfeeding

Evaluate:

• Decreasing lipodystrophy in HIV patients

Teach Patient/Family:

• That body fat distribution should change

• That lab exams will be needed

• About injection technique and preferred injection sites; to avoid bruised, scarred, or broken skin

• About expectations; the product is not indicated for weight-loss management

• **Hypersensitivity:** To report rash, swelling of face, trouble breathing immediately

• **Fluid retention:** To report edema, joint pain

---

testosterone buccal (Rx)

Striant

testosterone cypionate (Rx)

Depo-Testosterone

testosterone enanthate (Rx)

Delatestryl

testosterone gel (Rx)

AndroGel, FORTESTA, Testim, Vogelxo

testosterone nasal gel

Natesto

testosterone pellets (Rx)

Testopel

testosterone transdermal (Rx)

Androderm

testosterone undecanoate

Jatenzo

Func. class.: Androgenic anabolic steroid

Chem. class.: Halogenated testosterone derivative

Controlled Substance Schedule III

Do not confuse:
Testoderm/Testoderm TTS

ACTION: Increases weight by building body tissue; increases potassium, phosphorus, chloride, nitrogen levels, bone development

USES: Female breast cancer, hypogonadism, eunuchoidism, male climacteric, oligospermia, impotence, vulvar dystrophies, low testosterone levels, delayed male puberty (inj)
Unlabeled uses: Weight loss in AIDS patients, andropause, anemia, cryptorchidism, lichen sclerosus, microphallus, transsexualism

CONTRAINDICATIONS: Pregnancy, breastfeeding, severe cardiac/renal/hepatic disease, hypersensitivity, genital bleeding (rare), male breast/prostate cancer
Precautions: Diabetes mellitus, CV disease, MI, urinary tract disorders, prostate cancer, hypercalcemia

Black Box Warning: Children, accidental exposure, pulmonary oil microembolism, risk of serious hypersensitivity reactions or anaphylaxis

DOSAGE AND ROUTES
Replacement
• **Adult: IM (enanthate or cypionate)** 50-400 mg q2-4wk; **TOPICAL SOL (Axiron)** 60 mg (2 pump actuations); apply each ᴀᴍ
• **Adult (male)/child: SUBCUT (pellets)** 150-450 mg (2-6 pellets) inserted q3-6mo
• **Adult: TRANSDERMAL (Testoderm, Androderm)** 4-6 mg applied q24hr; **GEL (AndroGel)** 1% 5 mg applied q24hr, once daily; 1.62% 40.5 mg (2 pump actuations) every ᴀᴍ; topical sol **(Axiron)** 30 mg/actuation; **BUCCAL** 1 buccal system (30 mg) to the gum region q12hr before meals/ᴘᴍ; **NASAL GEL** 1 pump actuation in each nostril tid
Breast cancer
• **Adult: IM** 200-400 mg q2-4wk (cypionate or enanthate)

Delayed male puberty
• **Child >12 yr: IM** ≤100 mg/mo for ≤6 mo
Available forms: Enanthate: inj 200 mg/mL; **cypionate:** inj 100, 200 mg/mL; pellets 75 mg; **transdermal** 2, 4 mg/24 hr; **gel** 1%, 1.62%, 10 mg/actuation; **buccal system** 30 mg; **topical sol** 30 mg/actuation; **nasal gel** 5.5 mg/actuation
Administer:
• Titrated dose; use lowest effective dose
• IM inj deep into upper outer quadrant of gluteal muscle
• **Transdermal patches:** Testoderm to skin of scrotum; Androderm to skin of back, upper arms, thighs, abdomen; area must be dry shaved; may be reapplied after bathing, swimming
• **Gel:** products not interchangeable; dosage and administration for AndroGel 1% differs from that of AndroGel 1.62%; apply daily to clean, dry area on shoulders, upper arms, or abdomen; women, children should not touch treated skin
Buccal system route
• Do not chew or swallow buccal system
• Rotate sites; place above incisor tooth on either side of mouth
• Open packet; place rounded side of surface against gum and hold firmly in place with finger over lip for 30 sec; if product falls off, replace with new system; discard in trash can away from children or pets
Topical solution route
• Using the provided applicator, apply to clean, dry intact skin of the axilla at the same time each morning; do not apply to any other part of the body; allow to dry; if an antiperspirant or deodorant is used, apply at least 2 min before applying the solution; the pump must be primed before the first use by fully depressing the pump mechanism 3×; discard any solution that is released during the priming; to dispense, position the nozzle over the applicator cup and depress the pump once fully; with the applicator upright, place it up into the axilla and wipe steadily down and up into the axilla; do not use fingers or hand to rub the solution; if multiple applications are necessary for the required dose, alternate ap-

Side effects: *italics* = common; red = life-threatening

plication between the left and right axilla; when repeat application to the same axilla is necessary, allow the solution to dry completely before the next application; after use, rinse the applicator under running water and pat dry with tissue; wash hands with soap and water

• Following application, allow the site to dry before putting on clothing

• Direct contact of the medicated skin with the skin of another person can result in the transfer of residual testosterone and absorption by the other person; to reduce accidental transfer, the patient should cover the application site(s) with clothing (e.g., a T-shirt) after the solution has dried; the application site should be washed with soap and water before any skin-to-skin contact regardless of the length of time since application; in the case of direct contact, the other person should wash the area of contact with soap and water

• Be advised that the topical solution is flammable; fire, flame, and smoking should be avoided during use

• Advise patients to avoid swimming or washing the application site until 2 hr following application

SIDE EFFECTS

CNS: Dizziness, headache, fatigue, tremors, paresthesias, flushing, sweating, anxiety, lability, insomnia, carpal tunnel syndrome

CV: Increased B/P

EENT: Conjunctival edema, nasal congestion

ENDO: Abnormal glucose tolerance test

GI: Nausea, vomiting, constipation, weight gain, cholestatic jaundice

GU: Hematuria, amenorrhea, vaginitis, decreased libido, decreased breast size, clitoral hypertrophy, testicular atrophy, gynecomastia, large prostate

HEMA: Polycythemia

INTEG: Rash, acneiform lesions, oily hair/skin, flushing, sweating, acne vulgaris, alopecia, hirsutism

MS: Cramps, spasms

PHARMACOKINETICS

PO: Metabolized in liver; excreted in urine, breast milk; crosses placenta

INTERACTIONS

• Edema: ACTH, adrenal steroids, buPROPion

Increase: effects of oxyphenbutazone

Increase: PT—anticoagulants

Decrease: glucose levels—may alter need for oral antidiabetics, insulin

Drug/Lab Test

Increase: serum cholesterol, blood glucose, urine glucose

Decrease: serum calcium, serum potassium, T_4, T_3, thyroid ^{131}I uptake test, urine 17-OHCS, 17-KS, PBI

NURSING CONSIDERATIONS

Assess:

• Weight daily; notify prescriber if weekly weight gain >5 lb

• B/P q4hr, Hgb/HCT

• I&O ratio; be alert for decreasing urinary output, increasing edema

• Growth rate, bone age in children; growth rate may be uneven (linear/bone growth) with extended use

• Electrolytes: potassium, sodium, chlorine, calcium; cholesterol

• Hepatic studies: ALT, AST, bilirubin

• Edema, hypertension, cardiac symptoms, jaundice

Black Box Warning: **Anaphylaxis:** usually with testosterone undecanoate (Aveed) oil for injection; may occur after any injection, observe for 30 min after each use; this product is contraindicated in those with castor oil, benzyl alcohol, benzoic acid hypersensitivity

Black Box Warning: **Accidental exposure** in children has occurred with topical product after contact with application site, with clothing; wash hands with soap, water

Black Box Warning: Pulmonary oil microembolism: occurs immediately after 1000 mg IM injected of testosterone undecanoate; symptoms include cough, dyspnea, chest pain, dizziness, throat tightening; some events resolve with supportive measures after a few minutes, some require emergency measures

• **Mental status:** affect, mood, behavioral changes, aggression
• **Signs of masculinization in female:** increased libido, deepening of voice, decreased breast tissue, enlarged clitoris, menstrual irregularities; **male:** gynecomastia, impotence, testicular atrophy
• **Hypercalcemia:** lethargy, polyuria, polydipsia, nausea, vomiting, constipation; product may have to be decreased
• **Hypoglycemia** in diabetic patients; oral antidiabetic action is increased
• Diet with increased calories, protein; decrease sodium if edema occurs
• **Pregnancy/breastfeeding:** do not use in pregnancy, breastfeeding
• **Beers:** avoid in older adults unless indicated for confirmed hypogonadism with clinical symptoms; potential for cardiac problems; do not use in prostate cancer
Evaluate:
• Therapeutic response: 4-6 wk in osteoporosis
Teach patient/family:
• That product must be combined with complete health plan: diet, rest, exercise
• To notify prescriber if therapeutic response decreases, if edema occurs
• About changes in sex characteristics: priapism, gynecomastia, increased libido
• That women should report menstrual irregularities, voice changes, acne, facial hair growth; if pregnancy is planned or suspected, or if breastfeeding
• That course of 1-3 mo is necessary for response with breast cancer
• About the proper application of patches and how to use gel, IM injection, buccal system, intranasal gel; about SUB-CUT implant complications

• **Nasal:** Teach patient to report nasal bleeding, irritation, pain
• **Topical:** Teach patient to avoid contact with area that has been treated, to wash area before contact
• **Buccal:** Teach patient how to administer buccal tab to gum
• **Transdermal:** Advise patient to notify provider of virilization in females

---

tetracaine ophthalmic
See Appendix B

---

tetracaine topical
See Appendix B

---

tetracycline (Rx)
(tet-ra-sye′kleen)
Func. class.: Broad-spectrum antiinfective
Chem. class.: Tetracycline

ACTION: Inhibits protein synthesis and phosphorylation in microorganisms; bacteriostatic

USES: Syphilis, *Chlamydia trachomatis,* gonorrhea, lymphogranuloma venereum; uncommon gram-positive, gram-negative organisms; rickettsial infections

CONTRAINDICATIONS: Pregnancy, breastfeeding, children <8 yr, hypersensitivity to tetracyclines
Precautions: Renal/hepatic disease, UV exposure

DOSAGE AND ROUTES
Susceptible gram-positive/gram-negative infections
• **Adult:** PO 250-500 mg q6hr
• **Child >8 yr:** PO 25-50 mg/kg/day in divided doses q6hr

T

Side effects: *italics* = common; red = life-threatening

Chlamydia trachomatis
• **Adult: PO** 500 mg qid × 7 days
Syphilis
• **Adult and adolescent: PO** 500 mg qid × 2 wk; if syphilis duration >1 yr, must treat 28 days
Brucellosis
• **Adult: PO** 500 mg q6hr × 3 wk with **IM** 1 g streptomycin bid × 1st wk, then daily × 2nd wk
Urethral, endocervical, rectal infections *(C. trachomatis)*
• **Adult: PO** 500 mg qid × 7 days
Acne
• **Adult/adolescent: PO** 250 mg q6hr, then 125-500 mg/day or every other day
Renal dose
• **Adult: PO** CCr 51-90 mL/min, give dose q8-12hr; CCr 10-50 mL/min, give dose q12-24hr; CCr <10 mL/min, give dose q24hr
Available forms: Caps 250, 500 mg
Administer:
• After C&S obtained, therapy may start before results are received
• 2 hr before or after iron products; 1 hr after antacid products
• Should be given on empty stomach (1 hr before or 2 hr after meals)
• Store in tight, light-resistant container at room temperature

SIDE EFFECTS
CNS: Fever, headache, paresthesia
CV: Pericarditis
EENT: Dysphagia, glossitis, decreased calcification, discoloration of deciduous teeth, oral candidiasis, oral ulcers
GI: *Nausea,* abdominal pain, *vomiting, diarrhea,* anorexia, enterocolitis, hepatotoxicity, flatulence, abdominal cramps, epigastric burning, stomatitis, hepatitis, CDAD
GU: *Increased BUN,* azotemia, acute renal failure
HEMA: Eosinophilia, neutropenia, thrombocytopenia, leukocytosis, hemolytic anemia
INTEG: *Rash, urticaria, photosensitivity, increased pigmentation,* exfoliative dermatitis, **pruritus,** angioedema, Stevens-Johnson syndrome

MISC: Increased intracranial pressure, candidiasis

PHARMACOKINETICS
PO: Peak 2-3 hr; duration 6 hr; half-life 6-12 hr; excreted in urine, breast milk; crosses placenta; 65% protein bound

INTERACTIONS
Fatal nephrotoxicity: methoxyflurane; do not use together
Increase: Pseudotumor cerebi—ISOtretinoin; avoid concurrent use
Increase: effect of warfarin—digoxin
Decrease: hormonal contraceptive (possible but unlikely); use additional contraception
Decrease: effect of tetracycline—antacids, sodium bicarbonate, alkali products, iron, cimetidine
Decrease: effect of penicillins
Drug/Herb
• Photosensitivity: dong quai
Drug/Food
Decrease: tetracycline effect—dairy products
Drug/Lab Test
Increase: BUN, LFTs

NURSING CONSIDERATIONS
Assess:
• **CDAD:** diarrhea, abdominal pain, fever, fatigue, anorexia; possible anemia, elevated WBC count, low serum albumin; stop product; usually either vancomycin or IV metroNIDAZOLE is given
• Signs of anemia: Hct, Hgb, fatigue
• I&O ratio
• Blood studies: PT, CBC, AST, ALT, BUN, creatinine if on prolonged therapy
• **Allergic reactions:** rash, itching, pruritus
• **Serious skin reactions:** angioedema, Stevens-Johnson syndrome, exfoliative dermatitis; report immediately after stopping product
• Nausea, vomiting, diarrhea; administer antiemetic, antacids as ordered
• **Superinfection:** fever, malaise, redness, pain, swelling, drainage, perineal itching, diarrhea, changes in cough or sputum if on prolonged therapy

• **Pregnancy/breastfeeding:** do not use in pregnancy, toxic to fetus; do not breastfeed, excreted in breast milk

Evaluate:

• Therapeutic response: absence of lesions, negative C&S, resolution of infection, prevention of malaria

Teach patient/family:

• To avoid sun exposure; that sunscreen does not seem to decrease photosensitivity

• That all prescribed medication must be taken to prevent superinfection

• To avoid milk products, antacids or to separate by 2 hr; to take with full glass of water; to take 1 hr before bedtime to prevent esophageal ulceration

• That tooth discoloration may occur, especially in children; not to use in child <8 yr, may cause bone formation abnormalities

• To notify prescriber immediately of diarrhea with pus, mucus, fever, abdominal pain

• To notify prescriber if pregnancy is planned or suspected

• Not to use outdated products; Fanconi's syndrome (nephrotoxicity) may occur

---

tetrahydrozoline nasal agent
See Appendix B

---

tetrahydrozoline ophthalmic
See Appendix B

RARELY USED

tezacaftor/ivacaflor
Symdeko
Func. class.: Respiratory agent, cystic fibrosis agent

USES: Cystic fibrosis (CF) in patients who are homozygous for the F508del mutation or have at least 1 mutation in the CFTR gene that is responsive to tezacaftor/ivacaflor

CONTRAINDICATIONS: None

DOSAGE AND ROUTES

• **Adult: PO** 1 tablet (tezacaftor 100 mg/ivacaftor 150 mg) AM and 1 tablet (ivacaftor 150 mg) PM, 12 hr apart and given with fat-containing food

• **Adolescent/child 12-17 yr: PO** 1 tablet (tezacaftor 100 mg/ivacaftor 150 mg) AM and 1 tablet (ivacaftor 150 mg) PM,12 hr apart and given with fat-containing food

---

thiamine (vit B₁) (PO-OTC; IV, IM-Rx)
Vitamin B₁
Func. class.: Vit B₁
Chem. class.: Water soluble

Do not confuse:
thiamine/Tenormin

ACTION: Needed for pyruvate metabolism, carbohydrate metabolism

USES: Vit B_1 deficiency or polyneuritis, cheilosis adjunct with thiamine beriberi, Wernicke-Korsakoff syndrome, pellagra, metabolic disorders, alcoholism

CONTRAINDICATIONS: Hypersensitivity
Precautions: Pregnancy

DOSAGE AND ROUTES
RDA

• **Adult: PO** (males) 1.2-1.5 mg; (females) 1.1 mg; (pregnancy) 1.4 mg; (breastfeeding) 1.4 mg

• **Child 9-13 yr: PO** 0.9 mg

• **Child 4-8 yr: PO** 0.6 mg

• **Child 1-3 yr: PO** 0.5 mg

• **Infant 7 mo-1 yr: PO** 0.3 mg

• **Neonate/infant ≤6 mo: PO** 0.2 mg

Beriberi

• **Adult: PO** 5-30 mg daily or in 3 divided doses × 1 mo; **IM/IV** 5-30 mg daily or in 3 divided doses, then convert to **PO**

T

• **Infant/child:** PO 10-50 mg daily × 2 wk, then 5-10 mg daily × 1 mo; **IV/IM** 10-25 mg/day × 2 wk, then 5-10 mg daily × 1 mo

Wernicke-Korsakoff syndrome

• **Adult:** IV 100 mg, then 50-100 mg every day

Available forms: Tabs 50, 100, 250, 500 mg; inj 100 mg/mL; enteric-coated tabs 20 mg

Administer:

IM route

• By IM inj; rotate sites if pain and inflammation occur; do not mix with alkaline sol; Z-track to minimize pain

Direct IV route

• Undiluted at 100 mg/mL over 5 min

Continuous IV INFUSION route

• Diluted in compatible IV sol

Y-site compatibilities: Famotidine

SIDE EFFECTS

CNS: Weakness, restlessness
CV: Collapse, pulmonary edema, hypotension
EENT: Tightness of throat
GI: Hemorrhage, *nausea, diarrhea*
INTEG: Angioneurotic edema, cyanosis, sweating, warmth
SYST: Anaphylaxis

PHARMACOKINETICS

PO/INJ: Unused amounts excreted in urine (unchanged)

NURSING CONSIDERATIONS

Assess:

• **Anaphylaxis (IV only):** swelling of face, eyes, lips, throat, wheezing
• **Thiamine deficiency:** anorexia, weakness/pain, depression, confusion, blurred vision, tachycardia
• **Nutritional status:** yeast, beef, liver, whole or enriched grains, legumes
• Application of cold to help decrease injection site pain
• **Pregnancy/breastfeeding:** considered compatible with pregnancy, breastfeeding

Evaluate:

• Therapeutic response: absence of nausea, vomiting, anorexia, insomnia, tachycardia, paresthesias, depression, muscle weakness

Teach patient/family:

• About the necessary foods to be included in diet: yeast, beef, liver, legumes, whole grains

---

RARELY USED

thioridazine (Rx)

(thye-or-rid′a-zeen)
Func. class.: Antipsychotic (typical)
Chem. class.: Phenothiazine piperidine

ACTION: Depresses cerebral cortex, hypothalamus, limbic system, which control activity, aggression; blocks neurotransmission produced by DOPamine at synapse; exhibits strong α-adrenergic and anticholinergic blocking action; mechanism for antipsychotic effects is unclear

USES: Psychotic disorders, schizophrenia, behavioral problems in children, anxiety, major depressive disorders, organic brain syndrome

Unlabeled uses: Behavioral symptoms associated with dementia in geriatric patients

CONTRAINDICATIONS: Children <2 yr, hypersensitivity, coma, CNS depression

Black Box Warning: QT prolongation, cardiac dysrhythmias

DOSAGE AND ROUTES

Psychosis

• **Adult:** PO 25-100 mg tid, max 800 mg/day; dose gradually increased to desired response, then reduced to minimum maintenance

Depression/behavioral problems/ organic brain syndrome

• **Adult:** PO 25 mg tid, range from 10 mg bid-qid to 50 mg tid-qid, max 800 mg/day for short period

---

• **Geriatric:** PO 10-25 mg daily-tid, increase 4-7 days by 10-25 mg to desired dose, max 800 mg/day for short period
• **Child 2-12 yr:** PO 0.5-3 mg/kg/day in divided doses, max 3 mg/kg/day

RARELY USED

thyroid USP (desiccated) (Rx)
(thye'roid)
Armour Thyroid, Bio-Throid, Nature Thyroid, NP Thyroid
Func. class.: Thyroid hormone
Chem. class.: Active thyroid hormone in natural state and ratio

USES: Hypothyroidism, cretinism (juvenile hypothyroidism), myxedema

CONTRAINDICATIONS: Adrenal insufficiency, MI, thyrotoxicosis, porcine protein hypersensitivity

Black Box Warning: Obesity treatment

DOSAGE AND ROUTES
Hypothyroidism
• **Adult:** PO 30 mg/day, increased by 15 mg/mo until desired response; maintenance dose 60-120 mg/day
• **Geriatric:** PO 7.5-15 mg/day, increase dose q6-8wk until desired response
Cretinism/juvenile hypothyroidism
• **Child:** PO 15 mg/day, then 30 mg/day after 2 wk, then 60 mg/day after another 2 wk; maintenance dose 60-180 mg/day
Myxedema
• **Adult:** PO 15 mg/day, double dose q2wk, maintenance 60-180 mg/day

tiaGABine (Rx)
(tie-ah-ga'been)
Gabitril
Func. class.: Anticonvulsant

Do not confuse:
tiaGABine/tiZANidine

ACTION: Inhibits reuptake and metabolism of GABA, may increase seizure threshold; structurally similar to GABA; tiaGABine binding sites in neocortex, hippocampus

USES: Adjunct treatment of partial seizures in adults and children ≥12 yr

CONTRAINDICATIONS: Hypersensitivity
Precautions: Pregnancy, breastfeeding, children <12 yr, geriatric patients, renal/hepatic disease, suicidal thoughts/behaviors, status epilepticus, mania, bipolar disorder, abrupt discontinuation, depression

DOSAGE AND ROUTES
• **Adult (those receiving an enzyme-inducing antiepileptic product):** PO 4 mg/day in divided doses, may increase by 4-8 mg/wk until desired response, max 56 mg/day
• **Child 12-18 yr:** PO 4 mg/day, may increase by 4 mg at beginning of wk 2; may increase by 4-8 mg/wk until desired response; max 32 mg/day
Hepatic dose
• **Adult:** PO reduce dose or increase dosing interval
Available forms: Tabs 2, 4, 12, 16 mg
Administer:
• Store at room temperature, away from heat and light
• Use with food

SIDE EFFECTS
CNS: *Dizziness, anxiety,* somnolence, ataxia, confusion, *asthenia,* unsteady gait, depression, suicidal ideation, seizures, tremors, hostility, EEG changes, insomnia
CV: Vasodilation, tachycardia, hypertension
ENDO: Goiter, hypothyroidism
GI: Nausea, vomiting, diarrhea, increased appetite
INTEG: Pruritus, rash, Stevens-Johnson syndrome, alopecia, hyperhidrosis
MS: Myalgia
RESP: Pharyngitis, coughing

T

Side effects: *italics* = common; red = life-threatening

PHARMACOKINETICS

Absorption >95%; peak 45 min; protein binding 96%; metabolized in the liver via CYP3A4; half-life 7-9 hr without enzyme inducers, 2-5 hr with enzyme inducers

INTERACTIONS

• Lower doses may be needed when used with valproate

Increase: CNS depression—CNS depressants, alcohol

Decrease: tiaGABine effect—sevelamer

Decrease: effect—carBAMazepine, PHENobarbital, phenytoin, primidone

Drug/Food

Decrease: rate of absorption—high-fat meal

NURSING CONSIDERATIONS

Assess:

• Hepatic studies: ALT, AST, bilirubin at baseline and periodically

• Seizures: location, duration, presence of aura; assess for weakness

• Withdraw gradually to prevent seizures

• May cause status epilepticus and unexplained death

• Mental status: mood, sensorium, affect, behavioral changes, suicidal thoughts/behaviors; if mental status changes, notify prescriber; hypomania may be present before suicide attempt

• Assistance with ambulation during early part of treatment; dizziness occurs

• **Seizure precautions:** padded side rails; move objects that may harm patient

• **Pregnancy/breastfeeding:** use only if benefits outweigh fetal risks, may be fetal toxic; pregnant women should enroll in the North American Antiepileptic Drug Pregnancy Registry at 1-888-233-2334; avoid breastfeeding, likely to be excreted in breast milk

• **Beers:** avoid in older adults unless safer alternatives are unavailable; may cause ataxia, impaired psychomotor function

Evaluate:

• Therapeutic response: decreased seizure activity; document on patient's chart

Teach patient/family:

• To carry emergency ID stating patient's name, products taken, condition, prescriber's name and phone number

• To avoid driving, other activities that require alertness, until response is known

• Not to discontinue medication quickly after long-term use

• To take with food

• To notify prescriber if pregnancy is planned or suspected; to avoid breastfeeding

• To report suicidal thoughts, behaviors immediately

⚠ HIGH ALERT

ticagrelor

Brilinta

Func. class.: Platelet inhibitor

Chem. class.: ADP receptor antagonist

Do not confuse:
Brilinta/Brintellix

ACTION: Reversibly binds to the platelet receptor, preventing platelet activation

USES: Arterial thromboembolism prophylaxis in acute coronary syndrome (ACS) (unstable angina, acute MI), including in patients undergoing percutaneous coronary intervention (PCI)

CONTRAINDICATIONS: Hypersensitivity, severe hepatic disease

Black Box Warning: Bleeding, intracranial bleeding

Precautions: Pregnancy, breastfeeding, infants, neonates, children, GI bleeding, hepatic disease, abrupt discontinuation

Black Box Warning: Coronary artery bypass graft surgery (CABG), surgery, abrupt discontinuation, aspirin coadministration

DOSAGE AND ROUTES

• **Adult:** PO loading dose 180 mg with aspirin (usually 325 mg PO); then give

---

90 mg bid with aspirin 75-100 mg/day, do not give maintenance doses of aspirin >100 mg/day

Available forms: Tab 60, 90 mg

Administer:

PO route

- May be taken without regard to food
- Discontinue 5-7 days before surgery
- May be crushed (90 mg tab) and mixed with purified water, 100 mL (PO) or 50 mL (NG); ensure entire dose is given by flushing mortar, syringe, NG tube with 2 additional 50 mL of water
- Store at room temperature, in original container in dry place

SIDE EFFECTS

CNS: Headache, dizziness, fatigue

CV: Hypertension, hypotension, chest pain, atrial fibrillation, bradyarrhythmias, syncope, ventricular pauses

GI: Nausea, diarrhea

HEMA: Serious, fatal bleeding

MISC: Back pain, hyperuricemia, gynecomastia

RESP: Dyspnea, cough

PHARMACOKINETICS

Absolute bioavailability 36%, protein binding (>99%), metabolism by CYP3A4, weak P-glycoprotein substrates and inhibitors, elimination for product and metabolite are hepatic and biliary, 84% excreted in feces, 16% in urine, half-life is 7 hr for ticagrelor, 9 hr for metabolite, maximum inhibition of platelet aggregation (IPA) effect 2 hr, maintained ≥8 hr, peak 1.5 hr product, 2.5 hr metabolite

INTERACTIONS

Black Box Warning: **Increase:** bleeding risk—CYP3A4 inhibitors (ketoconazole, itraconazole, voriconazole, clarithromycin, telithromycin, nefazodone, ritonavir, lopinavir, ritonavir, saquinavir, nelfinavir, indinavir, atazanavir, delavirdine, isoniazid, dalfopristin, quinupristin, tipranavir)

Decrease: ticagrelor action—CYP3A4 inducers (rifAMPin, dexamethasone, phenytoin, carBAMazepine, PHENobarbital)

Increase: effect of—simvastatin, lovastatin

Increase: bleeding risk—NSAIDs, anticoagulants, platelet inhibitors

Increase or decrease: digoxin

Drug/Lab Test

Increase: serum creatinine

NURSING CONSIDERATIONS

Assess:

- **Thromboembolism:** Monitor CBC with differential with platelet count baseline and periodically during treatment

Black Box Warning: **Bleeding:** assess for bleeding that may occur when aspirin is combined with this product; some bleeding can be fatal, usually aspirin doses >100 mg/day; watch for frank bleeding, hypotension; avoid with active bleeding, history of intracranial hemorrhage

Black Box Warning: **CABG:** do not use in those undergoing CABG; discontinue ≥5 days before surgery

Black Box Warning: **Aspirin coadministration:** use with 75-100 mg of aspirin/day, avoid higher doses; ticagrelor efficacy is decreased with aspirin >1000 mg/day

Black Box Warning: **Abrupt discontinuation:** do not discontinue abruptly; may increase risk for MI, stent thrombosis, death

- **Pregnancy/breastfeeding:** use only if benefits outweigh fetal risk, may be fetal toxic; do not breastfeed, excretion unknown

Evaluate:

- Prevention of thromboembolism

Teach patient/family:

- To take only as prescribed; not to skip or double doses; if a dose is missed, to take next dose at scheduled time

Black Box Warning: To notify prescriber of chills, fever, bruising, bleeding; not to use aspirin >100 mg/day

---

• Not to use any prescription, OTC products, herbs without approval of prescriber; products with aspirin, NSAIDs may cause bleeding; to be taken with aspirin; prescriber will order, do not alter dose
• To notify all health care providers of product use
• That product can be taken without regard to meals
• That it may take longer for bleeding to stop
• To notify prescriber if pregnancy is planned or suspected, not to breastfeed

---

ticarcillin/clavulanate (Rx)

Func. class.: Broad-spectrum antiinfective
Chem. class.: Extended-spectrum penicillin, β-lactamase inhibitor

---

ACTION: Interferes with cell-wall replication of susceptible organisms; osmotically unstable cell-wall swells, bursts from osmotic pressure; clavulanate inhibits β-lactamase and protects against enzymatic degradation of ticarcillin

USES: Respiratory, soft-tissue, and urinary tract infections; bacterial septicemia; effective for gram-positive cocci *(Staphylococcus aureus, Streptococcus faecalis, Streptococcus pneumoniae),* gram-negative cocci *(Neisseria gonorrhoeae),* gram-positive bacilli *(Clostridium perfringens, Clostridium tetani),* gram-negative bacilli *(Bacteroides, Fusobacterium nucleatum, Escherichia coli, Proteus mirabilis, Salmonella, Morganella morganii, Proteus rettgeri, Enterobacter, Pseudomonas aeruginosa, Serratia);* and *Peptococcus, Peptostreptococcus,* and *Eubacterium*

CONTRAINDICATIONS: Neonates, hypersensitivity to penicillins
Precautions: Pregnancy, hypersensitivity to cephalosporins, renal disease

DOSAGE AND ROUTES
Systemic/urinary tract infections, moderate/severe infections
• **Adult ≥60 kg: IV INFUSION** 3.1 g q4-6hr
• **Adult <60 kg: IV INFUSION** 200-300 mg/kg/day q4-6hr
• **Child >60 kg: IV INFUSION** 3.1 g q4-6hr
• **Child <60 kg: IV INFUSION** 200-300 mg/kg/day q4hr
• **Full-term neonates/infants <3 mo (unlabeled): IV** 50 mg/kg q4hr for severe infections; **IV** 50 mg/kg q6hr for mild to moderate infections

Mild to moderate infections
• **Child ≥60 kg: IV INFUSION** 3.1 g q6hr
• **Child <60 kg: IV INFUSION** 200 mg/kg/day q6hr
Renal dose
• **Adult: IV INFUSION** loading dose 3.1 g; CCr 60 mL/min, 3.1 g q4hr; CCr 30-59 mL/min, 2 g q4hr; CCr 10-29 mL/min, 2 g q8hr; CCr <10 mL/min, 2 g q12hr; CCr <10 mL/min with hepatic dysfunction, 2 g q24hr

Available forms: Inj 3 g ticarcillin, 0.1 g clavulanate; IV infusion 3 g ticarcillin, 0.1 g clavulanate; powder for inj 3 g ticarcillin, 0.1 g clavulanate
Administer:
• Product after C&S, give ≥q1hr before bactericidal antiinfectives, change IV site q48hr
Intermittent IV INFUSION route
• After diluting ≤3.1 g/13 mL of sterile water or NaCl (200 mg/mL), shake; may further dilute in ≥50-100 mL NS, D₅W, or LR sol and run over ¹/₂ hr
• Store reconstituted sol 12-24 hr at room temperature, or 3-7 days refrigerated

Y-site compatibilities: Allopurinol, amifostine, amikacin, anidulafungin, atropine, aztreonam, bivalirudin, bumetanide, ceFAZolin, cefepime, cefotaxime, cefOXitin, cefTAZidime, ceftizoxime, cefTRIAXone, cefuroxime, chloramphenicol, cimetidine, clindamycin, cyclophosphamide, cycloSPORINE, dexamethasone, dexmedetomidine, digoxin, diltiaZEM, diphenhydrAMINE, DOCEtaxel, DOPamine, DOXOrubicin liposome, doxycycline, enalaprilat, EPINEPHrine, esmolol, etoposide phosphate, famotidine, fenoldopam, filgrastim, fluconazole, furosemide, gemcitabine, gentamicin, granisetron, heparin, hydrocortisone, HYDROmorphone, imipenem/cilastatin, insulin, isoproterenol, labetalol, levoFLOXacin, lidocaine, linezolid, LORazepam, melphalan, meperidine, methylPREDNISolone, metoclopramide, metoprolol, metroNIDAZOLE, milrinone, morphine, nitroglycerin, nitroprusside, norepinephrine, ondansetron, palonosetron, pantoprazole, PEMEtrexed, penicillin G potassium, perphenazine, phenylephrine, procainamide, propofol, propranolol, raNITIdine, remifentanil, sargramostim, sodium bicarbonate, tacrolimus, teniposide, theophylline, thiotepa, tirofiban, tobramycin, vasopressin, verapamil, vinorelbine, voriconazole

SIDE EFFECTS

CNS: Anxiety, seizures, confusion, drowsiness
GI: *Nausea, vomiting, diarrhea;* increased AST, ALT; abdominal pain, glossitis, colitis, CDAD, hepatotoxicity
HEMA: Anemia, increased bleeding time, bone marrow depression, granulocytopenia
INTEG: Rash, urticaria, toxic epidermal necrolysis, pain at injection site
META: Hypokalemia, hypernatremia
SYST: Anaphylaxis, Stevens-Johnson syndrome, overgrowth of organisms

PHARMACOKINETICS

IV: Peak 30-45 min, duration 4 hr, half-life 64-68 min, excreted in urine

INTERACTIONS

Increase: bleeding—anticoagulants
Increase: methotrexate level—methotrexate
Increase: ticarcillin concentrations—probenecid, sulfipyrazone
Decrease: antimicrobial effect of ticarcillin—tetracyclines, aminoglycosides IV, chloramphenicol, macrolides, sulfonamides

Decrease: effect—oral contraceptives, erythromycin
Drug/Lab Test
False positive: urine glucose, urine protein, Coombs' test
Increase: LFTs, sodium, eosinophils, INR bleeding time, uric acid, bilirubin, BUN, creatinine, alk phos, LDH
Decrease: Hgb, potassium, platelets, WBC, granulocytes

NURSING CONSIDERATIONS
Assess:
• **Infection:** WBC, wound, temperature, sputum, urine, baseline and periodically
• **CDAD:** diarrhea, abdominal pain, fever, fatigue, anorexia; possible anemia, elevated WBC count, low serum albumin; stop product; usually either vancomycin or IV metroNIDAZOLE is given
• **Serious skin reactions:** Stevens-Johnson syndrome, toxic epidermal necrolysis; anaphylaxis: wheezing, rash, laryngeal edema; have emergency equipment nearby
• Hepatic studies: AST, ALT
• Blood studies: WBC, RBC, Hct, Hgb, bleeding time, platelets, baseline and periodically
• Renal studies: BUN, creatinine, sodium, potassium
• Skin eruptions after administration of penicillin to 1 wk after discontinuing product
• EPINEPHrine, suction, tracheostomy set, endotracheal intubation equipment
Evaluate:
• Therapeutic response: resolution of infection
Teach patient/family:
• To report persistent diarrhea with blood, pus, mucus, or fever
• That culture may be taken after completed course of medication
• To report sore throat, fever, fatigue (may indicate superinfection); CNS effects (anxiety, depression, hallucinations, seizures)
• To wear or carry emergency ID if allergic to penicillins
• To use alternative birth control method instead of hormonal

T

Side effects: *italics* = common; red = life-threatening

TREATMENT OF OVERDOSE: Withdraw product, maintain airway, administer EPINEPHrine, O₂, IV corticosteroids for anaphylaxis

> ### ⚠ HIGH ALERT
> ### RARELY USED
>
> ### ticlopidine (Rx)
> (tye-cloe′pi-deen)
> *Func. class.:* Platelet aggregation inhibitor
> *Chem. class.:* Thienopyridine compound

USES: Reducing the risk for stroke in high-risk patients

CONTRAINDICATIONS: Hypersensitivity, severe hepatic disease, active bleeding, coagulopathy

Black Box Warning: Agranulocytosis, neutropenia, thrombocytopenia, thrombotic thrombocytopenic purpura (TTP)

Black Box Warning: Anemia, hematologic disease

DOSAGE AND ROUTES
• **Adult:** PO 250 mg bid with food

tigecycline (Rx)
(tye-ge-sye′kleen)
Tygacil
Func. class.: Broad-spectrum antiinfective
Chem. class.: Glycylcyclines

ACTION: Inhibits protein synthesis and phosphorylation in microorganisms; bacteriostatic structurally similar to the tetracyclines

USES: Complicated skin/skin-structure infections (*Escherichia coli, Enterococcus faecalis* [vancomycin-susceptible only], *Staphylococcus aureus, Streptococcus agalactiae, S. anginosus* group, *S. pyogenes, Bacteroides fragilis*); complicated intraabdominal infections (*Citrobacter freundii, Enterobacter cloacae, E. coli, Klebsiella oxytoca, K. pneumoniae, E. faecalis* [vancomycin-susceptible only], *S. aureus* [methicillin-susceptible only], *S. anginosus* group, *B. fragilis, Bacteroides thetaiotaomicron, B. uniformis, B. vulgatus, Clostridium perfringens, Peptostreptococcus micros*); community-acquired pneumonia

CONTRAINDICATIONS: Pregnancy, breastfeeding, children <18 yr, hypersensitivity to tigecycline
Precautions: Renal/hepatic disease, hypersensitivity to tetracyclines, ventilator-associated/hospital-acquired pneumonias

Black Box Warning: Infection

DOSAGE AND ROUTES
• **Adult:** IV 100 mg then 50 mg q12hr, IV INFUSION given over 30-60 min q12hr; given for 5-14 days, depending on infection
Hepatic dose
• **Adult:** IV (Child-Pugh C) 100 mg, then 25 mg q12hr
Available forms: Powder for inj, lyophilized 50 mg
Administer:
• Tigecycline allergy test before using; obtain C&S, do not begin treatment before results or if susceptible organism is strongly suspected
Intermittent IV INFUSION route
• Reconstitute each vial with 5.3 mL of 0.9% NaCl or D₅ (10 mg/mL); swirl to dissolve; immediately withdraw 5 mL of reconstituted sol and add to 100-mL IV bag for infusion (1 mg/mL); may be yellow or orange; if not, sol should be discarded; do not give if particulate matter is present, use a dedicated IV line or Y-site, flush with NS before and after use, give over ½ hr

- Store in tight, light-resistant container at room temperature, diluted sol at room temperature for up to 24 hr, 6 hr in vial, and remaining time in IV bag, ≤48 hr refrigerated

Y-site compatibilities: Acyclovir, alfentanil, allopurinol, amifostine, amikacin, aminocaproic acid, aminophylline, amphotericin B liposome, ampicillin, ampicillin/sulbactam, argatroban, azithromycin, aztreonam, bivalirudin, bumetanide, buprenorphine, butorphanol, calcium chloride/gluconate, CARBOplatin, carmustine, caspofungin, ceFAZolin, cefepime, cefotaxime, cefoTEtan, cefOXitin, cefTAZidime, ceftizoxime, cefTRIAXone, cefuroxime, cimetidine, ciprofloxacin, cisatracurium, CISplatin, clindamycin, cyclophosphamide, cycloSPORINE, cytarabine, dacarbazine, DACTINomycin, DAPTOmycin, DAUNOrubicin hydrochloride, dexamethasone, dexmedetomidine, dexrazoxane, digoxin, diltiaZEM, diphenhydrAMINE, DOBUTamine, DOCEtaxel, dolasetron, DOPamine, doripenem, DOXOrubicin hydrochloride, DOXOrubicin liposome, droperidol, enalaprilat, EPINEPHrine, eptifibatide, ertapenem, erythromycin, esmolol, etoposide, etoposide phosphate, famotidine, fenoldopam, fentaNYL, fluconazole, fludarabine, fluorouracil, foscarnet, fosphenytoin, furosemide, ganciclovir, gemcitabine, gentamicin, glycopyrrolate, granisetron, haloperidol, heparin, hydrocortisone, HYDROmorphone, ifosfamide, imipenem/cilastatin, insulin, irinotecan, isoproterenol, ketorolac, labetalol, lansoprazole, lepirudin, leucovorin, levoFLOXacin, lidocaine, linezolid, LORazepam, magnesium sulfate, mannitol, mechlorethamine, melphalan, meperidine, meropenem, mesna, methohexital, methotrexate, methyldopa, metoclopramide, metoprolol, metroNIDAZOLE, midazolam, milrinone, mitoMYcin, mitoXANTRONE, morphine, moxifloxacin, mycophenolate, nafcillin, nalbuphine, naloxone, nesiritide, nitroglycerin, nitroprusside, norepinephrine, octreotide, ondansetron, oxaliplatin, oxytocin, PACLitaxel, palonosetron, pamidronate, pancuronium, pantoprazole, PEMEtrexed, pemtamidine, pentazocin, PENTobarbital, PHENobarbital, phenylephrine, piperacillin/tazobactam, potassium acetate/chloride/phosphate, procainamide, prochlorperazine, promethazine, propofol, propranolol, raNITIdine, remifentanil, rocuronium, sodium acetate/bicarbonate/phosphate, streptozocin, succinylcholine, SUFentanil, tacrolimus, teniposide, theophylline, thiopental, thiotepa, ticarcillin/clavulanate, tirofiban, tobramycin, topotecan, trimethoprim/sulfamethoxazole, vancomycin, vasopressin, vecuronium, vinBLAStine, vinCRIStine, vinorelbine, zidovudine, zoledronic acid

SIDE EFFECTS
CNS: Headache, dizziness, insomnia
CV: Hypo/hypertension, phlebitis
EENT: Tooth discoloration
GI: *Nausea, vomiting, diarrhea,* anorexia, constipation, dyspepsia, abdominal pain, hepatotoxicity, hepatic failure, pseudomembranous colitis
HEMA: Anemia, leukocytosis, thrombocytopenia
INTEG: *Rash,* pruritus, sweating, photosensitivity
META: Increased ALT, AST, BUN, lactic acid, alk phos, amylase; hyperglycemia, hypokalemia, hypoproteinemia, bilirubinemia
MISC: Back pain, fever, abnormal healing, abdominal pain, abscess, asthenia, infection, pain, peripheral edema, local reactions
RESP: Cough, dyspnea
SYST: Anaphylaxis

PHARMACOKINETICS
Not extensively metabolized, 22% of unchanged product excreted in urine, terminal half-life 42 hr, primarily biliary excreted, protein binding 71%-89%

INTERACTIONS
Increase: effect of warfarin
Decrease: effect of oral contraceptives

T

Side effects: *italics* = common; red = life-threatening

Drug/Lab Test
Increase: amylase, LFTs, alk phos, BUN, creatinine, LDH, WBC, INR, PTT, PT
Decrease: potassium, calcium, sodium, Hgb/Hct, platelets

NURSING CONSIDERATIONS
Assess:

Black Box Warning: Increased mortality risk: use only with confirmation of strongly suspected bacterial infection; do not use as a prophylactic

• **Pseudomembranous colitis:** diarrhea, abdominal pain, fever, fatigue, anorexia; possible anemia, elevated WBC level, low serum albumin; stop product; usually either vancomycin or IV metroNIDAZOLE is given
• Signs of anemia: Hct, Hgb, fatigue
• Blood studies: PT, CBC, AST, ALT, BUN creatinine
• **Allergic reactions:** rash, itching, pruritus, angioedema
• **Serious allergic skin reactions:** Stevens-Johnson anaphylaxis
• Nausea, vomiting, diarrhea; administer antiemetic, antacids as ordered
• **Toxicity:** pseudotumor cerebri, photosensitivity, antianabolic actions (azotemia, BUN, hypophosphatemia, metabolic acidosis); tigecycline is structurally similar to tetracycline; pancreatitis, hyperamylasemia (may be fatal); if these occur, discontinue, improvement usually occurs after product is discontinued
• **Overgrowth of infection:** fever, malaise, redness, pain, swelling, drainage, perineal itching, diarrhea, changes in cough or sputum
• **Pregnancy/breastfeeding:** do not use in pregnancy or breastfeeding; may cause fetal harm
Evaluate:
• Therapeutic response: decreased temperature, absence of lesions, negative C&S
Teach patient/family:
• To avoid sun exposure; sunscreen does not seem to decrease photosensitivity
• To avoid pregnancy while taking this product; fetal harm may occur; to avoid breastfeeding

• To report infection, increase in temperature; to report burning, pain at inj site
• To report diarrhea, fatigue, abdominal pain, severe nausea, vomiting

---

⚠ HIGH ALERT

timolol (Rx)
(tye′moe-lole)
Apo-Timol ✦, Novo-Timol ✦
Func. class.: Antihypertensive
Chem. class.: Nonselective β-blocker

ACTION: Competitively blocks stimulation of β-adrenergic receptor within vascular smooth muscle (decreases rate of SA node discharge, increases recovery time); slows conduction of AV node and decreases heart rate, which decreases O_2 consumption in myocardium; also decreases renin-aldosterone-angiotensin system; at high doses, inhibits $β_2$-receptors in bronchial system

USES: Mild to moderate hypertension, migraine prophylaxis, to decrease mortality after MI
Unlabeled uses: Tremors, angina pectoris

CONTRAINDICATIONS: Hypersensitivity to β-blockers, cardiogenic shock, heart block (2nd/3rd degree), sinus bradycardia, HF, cardiac failure, severe COPD, asthma
Precautions: Pregnancy, breastfeeding, major surgery, diabetes mellitus, COPD, well-compensated heart failure, nonallergic bronchospasm, peripheral vascular disease, thyroid/renal/hepatic disease

Black Box Warning: Abrupt discontinuation

DOSAGE AND ROUTES
Hypertension
• **Adult:** PO 10 mg bid or 20 mg/day, may increase by 10 mg q7days, max 60 mg/day

• **Geriatric patients:** PO initiate dose cautiously

Myocardial infarction

• **Adult:** PO 10 mg bid beginning 1-4 wk after MI for ≥2 yr

Migraine headache prevention

• **Adult:** PO 10 mg bid or 20 mg/day; may increase to 30 mg/day, 20 mg in AM, 10 mg in PM; discontinue if not effective after 8 wk

Available forms: Tabs 5, 10, 20 mg

Administer:

• PO before or immediately after meals, at bedtime; tab may be crushed or swallowed whole

• Reduced dosage in renal dysfunction

• Store at room temperature; do not freeze

SIDE EFFECTS

CNS: *Insomnia, dizziness,* hallucinations, anxiety, fatigue, depression, headache

CV: Hypotension, bradycardia, HF, edema, chest pain, claudication, angina, AV block, ventricular dysrhythmias

EENT: *Visual changes;* sore throat; *double vision;* dry, burning eyes

GI: *Nausea,* vomiting, ischemic colitis, diarrhea, *abdominal pain,* mesenteric arterial thrombosis, flatulence, constipation

GU: Impotence, urinary frequency

HEMA: Agranulocytosis, thrombocytopenia, purpura

INTEG: Rash, alopecia, pruritus, fever

META: Hypoglycemia

MUSC: *Joint pain, muscle pain*

RESP: Bronchospasm, *dyspnea,* cough, crackles, nasal stuffiness

PHARMACOKINETICS

Peak 1-2 hr; half-life 4 hr; metabolized by liver; excreted in urine, breast milk; protein binding <10%

INTERACTIONS

Increase: hypotension, bradycardia—hydrALAZINE, methyldopa, prazosin, anticholinergics, alcohol, reserpine, nitrates

Increase: effects of β-blockers, calcium channel blockers

Decrease: antihypertensive effects—NSAIDs, sympathomimetics, thyroid, salicylates

Decrease: hypoglycemic effects—insulin, sulfonylureas

Decrease: bronchodilation—theophyllines

Drug/Lab Test

Increase: renal, hepatic studies, uric acid

Interference: glucose, insulin tolerance test

NURSING CONSIDERATIONS

Assess:

> Black Box Warning: **Abrupt discontinuation:** may result in myocardial ischemia, MI, severe hypotension, ventricular dysrhythmias in those with preexisting cardiovascular disease

• **Headaches:** location, severity, duration, frequency at baseline and throughout treatment

• I&O, weight daily, edema in feet, legs daily

• B/P during initial treatment, periodically thereafter, pulse q4hr; note rate, rhythm, quality

• Apical/radial pulse before administration; notify prescriber of any significant changes

• Baselines of renal, hepatic studies before therapy begins

• Edema in feet, legs daily

• **Pregnancy/breastfeeding:** use only if benefits outweigh fetal risk, do not breastfeed, excreted in breast milk

Evaluate:

• Therapeutic response: decreased B/P after 1-2 wk

Teach patient/family:

• To take before or immediately after meals

> Black Box Warning: Not to discontinue product abruptly; to taper over 2 wk; may precipitate angina

• Not to use OTC products containing α-adrenergic stimulants (nasal decongestants, cold preparations) unless directed by prescriber

• To report bradycardia, dizziness, confusion, depression, fever, sore throat, SOB to prescriber

---

Side effects: *italics* = common; red = life-threatening

• Product masks hypoglycemia; monitor blood sugar

• To take pulse at home; when to notify prescriber

• To avoid alcohol, smoking, sodium intake

• To comply with weight control, dietary adjustments, modified exercise program

• To carry emergency ID to identify product, allergies

• To avoid hazardous activities if dizziness is present

• To report symptoms of HF: difficulty breathing, especially on exertion or when lying down; night cough; swelling of extremities

• To take medication at bedtime; to wear support hose to minimize effect of orthostatic hypotension

TREATMENT OF OVERDOSE: Lavage, IV atropine for bradycardia, IV theophylline for bronchospasm, digoxin, O_2, diuretic for cardiac failure, hemodialysis; administer vasopressor (norepinephrine)

---

timolol (ophthalmic)

(tie-moe′lol)

Betimol, Istalol, Timoptic, Timoptic-XE

Func. class.: Antiglaucoma

Chem. class.: β-Blocker

ACTION: Can decrease aqueous humor and increase outflows

USES: Treatment of chronic open-angle glaucoma and ocular hypertension

CONTRAINDICATIONS: Hypersensitivity, AV block, heart failure, bradycardia, sick sinus syndrome, asthma

Precautions: Abrupt discontinuation, pregnancy, breastfeeding, children, COPD, depression, diabetes mellitus, myasthenia gravis, hyperthyroidism, pulmonary disease, angle-closure glaucoma

DOSAGE AND ROUTES

• **Adult:** instill 1 drop in each affected eye bid (0.25% solution) initially; if no

response, 1 drop in each affected eye bid (0.5% solution) or 1 drop of gel in each affected eye daily

Available forms: Ophthalmic solution 0.25, 0.5%; ophthalmic gel 0.25%, 0.5%

Administer:

• For ophthalmic use only

• Do not touch the tip of the dropper to the eye, fingertips, or other surface to prevent contamination

• Wash hands before and after use

• Tilt head back slightly and pull the lower eyelid down with the index finger to form a pouch; squeeze the prescribed number of drops into the pouch; close eyes to spread drops; to avoid excessive systemic absorption, apply finger pressure on the lacrimal sac for 1-2 min after use

• If >1 topical ophthalmic drug product is being used, the drugs should be administered at least 5 min apart

• Administer other topically applied ophthalmic medications at least 10 min before timolol gel-forming solution

• To avoid contamination or the spread of infection, do not use dropper for more than one person

• Some products contain the preservative benzalkonium chloride, which can be absorbed by soft contact lenses; remove contact lenses before administration of the solution; lenses may be reinserted 15 min after administration

• Decreased intraocular pressure can take several weeks, monitor IOP after a month

SIDE EFFECTS

CNS: *Insomnia,* headache, *dizziness,* anxiety, depression, headache, nightmares, *fatigue*

CV: Palpitations, heart failure, hypotension

EENT: Eye stinging/burning, tearing, photophobia, visual disturbances

GI: Nausea, dry mouth

RESP: Bronchospasm

PHARMACOKINETICS

Onset 30 min, peak 1-2 hr, duration 12-24 hr

INTERACTIONS

Increase: β-blocking effect—oral β-blockers

Increase: intraocular pressure reduction—topical miotics, dipivefrin, EPINEPHrine, carbonic anhydrase inhibitors; this may be beneficial

Increase: B/P, severe—when abruptly stopping cloNIDine

Increase: depression of AV nodal conduction, bradycardia, or hypotension—adenosine, cardiac glycosides, disopyramide, other antiarrhythmics, class 1C antiarrhythmic drugs (flecainide, propafenone, moricizine, encainide, quiNIDine, calcium-channel blockers, or drugs that significantly depress AV nodal conduction)

Increase: AV block nodal conduction, induce AV block—high doses of procainamide

Increase: antihypertensive effect—other antihypertensives

NURSING CONSIDERATIONS
Assess:
• **Systemic absorption:** when used in the eye, systemic absorption is common with the same adverse reactions and interactions
• Glaucoma: monitor intraocular pressure
• **Pregnancy/breastfeeding:** use only if benefits outweigh fetal risks; do not breastfeed, excreted in breast milk
Evaluate:
• Decreasing intraocular pressure
Teach patient/family:
• That product is for ophthalmic use only
• Not to touch the tip of the dropper to the eye, fingertips, or other surface to prevent contamination
• To wash hands before and after use
• To tilt the head back slightly and pull the lower eyelid down with the index finger to form a pouch; squeeze the prescribed number of drops into the pouch; close eyes to spread drops
• To apply finger pressure on the lacrimal sac for 1-2 min following use to prevent excessive systemic absorption
• To administer drugs at least 5 min apart if more than one topical ophthalmic drug product is being used

• To administer other topically applied ophthalmic medications at least 10 min before timolol gel-forming solution
• To not use dropper for more than one person to avoid contamination or the spread of infection
• That some products contain the preservative benzalkonium chloride, which may be absorbed by soft contact lenses; to remove contact lenses before administration of the solution; that lenses may be reinserted 15 min after administration

---

⚠ HIGH ALERT

tinidazole (Rx)
(tye-ni′da-zole)
Tindamax
Func. class.: Antiprotozoal
Chem. class.: Nitroimidazole derivative

ACTION: Interferes with DNA/RNA synthesis in protozoa

USES: Amebiasis, giardiasis, trichomoniasis

Unlabeled uses: *Bacteroides* sp., *Clostridium* sp., *Eubacterium* sp., *Fusobacterium* sp., *Peptococcus* sp., *Peptostreptococcus* sp., gingivitis, urethritis, *Veillonella* sp.

CONTRAINDICATIONS: Pregnancy, breastfeeding; hypersensitivity to this product or nitroimidazole derivative
Precautions: Children, geriatric patients, hepatic disease, CNS depression, blood dyscrasias, candidiasis, seizures, viral infection, alcoholism, pregnancy

Black Box Warning: Secondary malignancy

DOSAGE AND ROUTES
Intestinal amebiasis/amebic involvement of the liver
• **Adult: PO** 2 g daily × 3 days
• **Child ≥3 yr/adolescent: PO** 50 mg/kg/day × 3 days, max 2 g/day

---

Giardiasis
• **Adult: PO** 2 g as a single dose
• **Child ≥3 yr: PO** 50 mg/kg as a single dose, max 2 g
Trichomoniasis
• **Adult: PO** 2 g as a single dose
Bacterial vaginosis
• **Adult (nonpregnant woman): PO** 2 g/day × 2 days with food or 1 g/day × 5 days with food
Available forms: Tabs 250, 500 mg
Administer:
• Tabs can be crushed and mixed with artificial cherry syrup for children
• With food to increase plasma concentrations, minimize epigastric distress and other GI effects

SIDE EFFECTS

CNS: *Dizziness, headache,* seizures, *peripheral neuropathy,* malaise, fatigue
GI: *Nausea, vomiting,* anorexia, increased AST/ALT, constipation, abdominal pain, indigestion, altered taste
HEMA: Leukopenia, neutropenia
INTEG: Pruritus, urticaria, *rash,* oral candidiasis
SYST: Angioedema, cramping

PHARMACOKINETICS

Peak $1\frac{1}{2}$ hr; metabolized extensively in liver; excreted unchanged (20%-25%) in urine, (12%) feces; half-life 12-14 hr; crosses blood-brain barrier

INTERACTIONS

• Do not use within 2 wk of disulfiram
Increase: tinidazole action—CYP3A4 inhibitors (cimetidine, ketoconazole): increased action of tinidazole
Increase: action of anticoagulants, cyclo-SPORINE, tacrolimus, fluorouracil, hydantoins, lithium
Decrease: tinidazole action—CYP3A4 inducers (PHENobarbital, rifampin, phenytoin); cholestyramine, oxytetracycline: decreased action of tinidazole
Drug/Herb
Increase or decrease: tinidazole level—St. John's wort
Drug/Lab Test
Increase: triglycerides, LDH, AST/ALT, glucose
Decrease: WBCs

NURSING CONSIDERATIONS
Assess:
• **Giardiasis:** obtain 3 stool samples several days apart beginning q3-4wk after treatment
• **Amebic liver abscess:** monitor CBC, ESR, amebic gel diffusion test, ultrasound; also total and differential leukocyte count

Black Box Warning: Secondary malignancy: avoid unnecessary use

• Signs of infection, anemia
• Bowel pattern before, during treatment
• **Pregnancy/breastfeeding:** contraindicated during first trimester; do not breastfeed
Evaluate:
• Therapeutic response: decrease in infection as evidenced by negative culture
Teach patient/family:
• To take with food to increase plasma concentrations, minimize epigastric distress and other GI effects; not to use alcoholic beverages during or for 3 days after treatment
• **Trichomoniasis:** that all partners should be notified and treated at the same time
• To avoid alcohol; may cause disulfiram reaction
• To avoid doing hazardous activities until reaction is known
• That product causes unpleasant taste
• Not to use OTC, Rx, or herbal products unless approved by prescriber

---

tioconazole vaginal antifungal
See Appendix B

---

tiotropium (Rx)
(ty-oh′tro-pee-um)
Spiriva HandiHaler, Spiriva Respimat
Func. class.: Anticholinergic, bronchodilator
Chem. class.: Synthetic quaternary ammonium compound

Do not confuse:
Spiriva/Inspra/Apidra

ACTION: Inhibits interaction of acetylcholine at receptor sites on the bronchial smooth muscle, thereby resulting in decreased cGMP and bronchodilation

USES: COPD; for the long-term treatment and once-daily maintenance of bronchospasm associated with COPD, including chronic bronchitis and emphysema

CONTRAINDICATIONS: Hypersensitivity to this product, atropine, or its derivatives

Precautions: Pregnancy, breastfeeding, children, geriatric patients, closed-angle glaucoma, prostatic hypertrophy, bladder neck obstruction, renal disease

DOSAGE AND ROUTES
• **Adult:** INH content of 1 cap/day (18 mcg) using HandiHaler inhalation device or 2 INH (spray) (2.5 mcg each) daily
Available forms: Powder for INH 18 mcg in blister packs containing 6 caps with inhaler; 30 caps with inhaler; spray inhaler (Respimat) 2.5 mcg/spray
Administer:
Inhalation route (caps)
• Caps are for INH only; do not swallow
• Immediately before administration, peel back foil until cap is visible and to "stop" line; remove cap from blister cavity; open dust cap of HandiHaler by pulling upward, then open mouthpiece; place cap in center chamber; firmly close mouthpiece until it clicks, leaving dust cap open
• When finished taking dose, remove used capsule and dispose of it; close mouthpiece and dust cap; store
• Rinse mouth after use
Inhalation route (spray)
• Insert cartridge into inhaler, prime inhaler, must reprime once if not used for >3 days, if not used for >21 days, prime until aerosol is visible, and 3 more times

SIDE EFFECTS
CNS: Depression, paresthesia
CV: Chest pain, increased heart rate

EENT: Dry mouth, blurred vision, glaucoma
GI: Vomiting, abdominal pain, constipation, dyspepsia
GU: Urinary difficulty, urinary retention, UTI
INTEG: Rash, angioedema
MISC: Candidiasis, flulike syndrome, herpes zoster, infections, angina pectoris
MS: Arthritis, myalgic leg/skeletal pain
RESP: *Cough, sinusitis, upper respiratory tract infection*, epistaxis, pharyngitis

PHARMACOKINETICS
Half-life 5-6 days in animals, does not cross blood-brain barrier, very little metabolized in the liver, excreted in urine, 72% protein binding

INTERACTIONS
• Anticholinergics: avoid use with other anticholinergics
Drug/Lab Test
Increase: cholesterol, glucose

NURSING CONSIDERATIONS
Assess:
• **Respiratory status:** oral thrush, dyspnea, rate, breath sounds before and during treatment; pulmonary function tests at baseline and periodically; upper respiratory infections, cough, sinusitis
• Tolerance over long-term therapy; dose may have to be increased or changed
• Patient's ability to use HandiHaler
• **Pregnancy/breastfeeding:** use only if benefits outweigh fetal risk, cautious use in breastfeeding, unlikely to cause harm in the infant
Evaluate:
• Therapeutic response: ability to breathe easier
Teach patient/family:
• Signs of closed-angle glaucoma (eye pain, blurred vision, visual halos)
• That product is used for long-term maintenance, not for immediate relief of breathing problems; that effect takes 20 min, lasts 24 hr
• To avoid getting the powder in the eyes; may cause blurred vision and pupil dilation

T

• To breathe out completely; not to breathe into mouthpiece at any time
• To hold HandiHaler with mouthpiece upward; to press button in once, completely, and release; this allows for medication to be released
• To raise device to mouth and close lips tightly around mouthpiece
• With head upright, to breathe in slowly and deeply, but allow the cap to vibrate; to breathe until the lungs fill; to hold breath and remove mouthpiece; to resume normal breathing
• To rinse mouth after use; to use hard candy or regular oral hygiene to reduce dry mouth
• To report immediately blurred vision, eye pain, halos
• To keep caps in sealed blisters before use; to store at room temperature

---

tipranavir (Rx)
(ti-pran′a-veer)
Aptivus
Func. class.: Antiretroviral
Chem. class.: Protease inhibitor

ACTION: Inhibits human immunodeficiency virus (HIV) protease, thereby preventing the maturation of the virus

USES: HIV in combination with other antiretrovirals

CONTRAINDICATIONS: Hypersensitivity
Precautions: Pregnancy, breastfeeding, children, renal disease, history of renal stones, sulfa allergy, hemophilia, diabetes mellitus, pancreatitis, alcoholism, immune reconstitution syndrome, surgery, trauma, infection

Black Box Warning: Intracranial bleeding, hepatitis, hepatic disease (Child-Pugh B, C)

DOSAGE AND ROUTES
• **Adult: PO** 500 mg coadministered with ritonavir 200 mg bid with food

• **Adolescent and child ≥2 yr: PO** 14 mg/kg given with ritonavir 6 mg/kg bid or 375 mg/m² given with ritonavir 150 mg/m² bid, max 500 mg with ritonavir 200 mg bid
Available forms: Caps 250 mg
Administer:
• Not to be used in those who are treatment-naive
• Swallow cap whole; do not break, crush, chew; store caps in refrigerator before use; after opening, store at room temperature; use within 60 days
• After meals
• In equal intervals around the clock to maintain blood levels

SIDE EFFECTS
CNS: *Headache, insomnia,* dizziness, somnolence, fatigue, *fever,* intracranial bleeding
GI: *Diarrhea, abdominal pain, nausea, vomiting,* anorexia, dry mouth, hepatitis B or C, pancreatitis, fatalities when given with ritonavir
GU: Nephrolithiasis
INTEG: *Rash,* urticaria, lipodystrophy, serious rash
MS: Pain
OTHER: Asthenia, insulin-resistant hyperglycemia, *hyperlipidemia,* ketoacidosis

PHARMACOKINETICS
Terminal half-life 6 hr, peak 3 hr, plasma protein binding 99.9%, steady state 7-10 days, metabolism CYP3A4, 80% fecal excretion

INTERACTIONS
Life-threatening dysrhythmias: amiodarone, astemizole, cisapride, ergots, flecainide, midazolam, pimozide, propafenone, quiNIDine, rifabutin, rifAMPin, terfenadine, triazolam
Increase: myopathy, rhabdomyolysis—HMG-CoA reductase inhibitors (lovastatin, simvastatin)
Increase: tipranavir levels—ketoconazole, delavirdine, itraconazole
Increase: levels of both products—clarithromycin, zidovudine
Increase: levels of tipranavir—oral contraception

Decrease: tipranavir levels—rifamycins, fluconazole, nevirapine, efavirenz
Drug/Herb
Decrease: tipranavir levels—St. John's wort; avoid concurrent use
Drug/Food
Decrease: tipranavir absorption—grapefruit juice; high-fat, high-protein foods
Drug/Lab Test
Increase: AST/ALT, cholesterol, blood glucose, amylase, lipase, triglycerides

NURSING CONSIDERATIONS
Assess:
• Signs of infection, anemia; presence of other sexually transmitted diseases

Black Box Warning: Hepatitis, pancreatitis: ALT, AST; total bilirubin, amylase; all may be elevated, discontinue in those with hepatic insufficiency or hepatitis or AST/ALT 10 × upper limit or AST/ALT 5-10 × ULN and total bilirubin 2.5 × ULN; assess for anorexia, nausea, jaundice, hepatomegaly, clay-colored stools

• **HIV:** Viral load, CD4, plasma HIV RNA, serum cholesterol profile, serum triglycerides during treatment
• Bowel pattern before, during treatment; if severe abdominal pain with bleeding occurs, product should be discontinued; monitor hydration
• **Serious rash:** if serious rash occurs, product should be discontinued
• **Immune reconstitution syndrome:** has been reported with combination antiretroviral therapy, patients may develop pain (MAC, CMV, PcP, TB) and autoimmune disease months after treatment

Black Box Warning: Intracranial bleeding: more common in those with trauma, surgery, or those taking antiplatelets or anticoagulants; assess for headache, nausea, vomiting, seizures, confusion, inability to speak, can be fatal

• Cushingoid symptoms: buffalo hump, facial/peripheral wasting, breast enlargement, central obesity

• **Pregnancy/breastfeeding:** use only if benefits outweigh fetal risk; enroll pregnant women in the Antiretroviral Pregnancy Registry, 1-800-258-4263; do not breastfeed
Evaluate:
• Therapeutic response: improving CD4 counts, viral load
Teach patient/family:
• To take as prescribed; if dose is missed, to take as soon as remembered up to 1 hr before next dose; not to double dose; that this product must be taken with other antivirals
• That product must be taken in equal intervals around the clock to maintain blood levels for duration of therapy
• That hyperglycemia may occur; to watch for increased thirst, weight loss, hunger, dry, itchy skin; to notify prescriber
• That product does not cure AIDS, only controls symptoms; not to donate blood
• That redistribution of body fat may occur
• Not to use with other products unless approved by prescriber, many drug interactions
• That product must be taken in combination with ritonavir
• To stop product and notify prescriber if anorexia, nausea, vomiting, yellowing of skin or eyes, clay-colored stools, fatigue, pain in upper abdomen

⚠ HIGH ALERT

T

tirofiban (Rx)
(tie-roh-fee′ban)
Aggrastat
Func. class.: Antiplatelet
Chem. class.: Glycoprotein IIb/IIIa inhibitor

Do not confuse:
Aggrastat/argatroban

ACTION: Antagonist of platelet glycoprotein (GP) IIb/IIIa receptor that prevents binding of fibrinogen and von

---

Side effects: *italics* = common; red = life-threatening

Willebrand's factor, which inhibits platelet aggregation

USES: Acute coronary syndrome in combination with heparin

CONTRAINDICATIONS: Hypersensitivity, active internal bleeding, stroke, major surgery, severe trauma within 30 days, intracranial neoplasm, aneurysm, hemorrhage, acute pericarditis, platelets <100,000/mm³, history of thrombocytopenia, coagulopathy, systolic B/P >180 mm Hg or diastolic B/P >110 mm Hg

Precautions: Pregnancy, breastfeeding, children, geriatric patients, renal disease, bleeding tendencies, hypertension, platelets <150,000/mm³

DOSAGE AND ROUTES
• **Adult:** IV 25 mcg/kg within 5 min, then 0.15 mcg/kg/min for up to 18 hr after
Renal dose
• **Adult:** IV CCr <60 mL/min, 25 mcg/kg, then 0.075 mcg/kg/min
Available forms: Inj 50 mL vials; inj premixed bag 50 mcg/mL in 100, 250 mL
Administer:
Intermittent IV INFUSION route
• Discontinue no less than 2-4 hr before CABG
• Do not use if particulates are present
• Dilute inj: withdraw and discard 100 mL from 500-mL bag of sterile 0.9% NaCl or D₅W and replace this vol with 100 mL of tirofiban inj from 2 vials
• Tirofiban inj for sol is premixed in containers of 500 mL 0.9% NaCl (50 mg/mL), infuse over 30 min
• Minimize other arterial/venous punctures, IM inj, catheter use, intubation to reduce bleeding risk
• Discard unused solution after 24 hr from start of infusion

Y-site compatibilities: Acyclovir, alfentanil, allopurinol, amifostine, amikacin, aminocaproic acid, aminophylline, amiodarone, ampicillin, ampicillin/sulbactam, anidulafungin, argatroban, arsenic trioxide, atracurium, atropine, azithromycin, aztreonam, bivalirudin, bleomycin, bumetanide, buprenorphine, butorphanol, calcium chloride/gluconate, capreomycin, CARBOplatin, carmustine, caspofungin, ceFAZolin, cefepime, cefotaxime, cefoTEtan, cefOXitin, cefTAZidime, ceftizoxime, cefTRIAXone, cefuroxime, chloramphenicol, chlorproMAZINE, cimetidine, ciprofloxacin, cisatracurium, CISplatin, clindamycin, cyclophosphamide, cycloSPORINE, cytarabine, DACTINomycin, DAPTOmycin, dexamethasone, dexmedetomidine, dexrazoxane, digoxin, diltiaZEM, diphenhydrAMINE, DOBUTamine, DOCEtaxel, dolasetron, DOPamine, doxacurium, DOXOrubicin, DOXOrubicin liposome, doxycycline, droperidol, enalaprilat, ePHEDrine, EPINEPHrine, epiRUBicin, eptifibatide, ertapenem, erythromycin, esmolol, etoposide, etoposide phosphate, famotidine, fenoldopam, fentaNYL, fluconazole, fludarabine, fluorouracil, foscarnet, fosphenytoin, furosemide, ganciclovir, gemcitabine, gentamicin, glycopyrrolate, granisetron, haloperidol, heparin, hydrALAZINE, hydrocortisone, HYDROmorphone, IDArubicin, ifosfamide, imipenem/cilastatin, insulin, irinotecan, isoproterenol, ketorolac, labetalol, leucovorin, lidocaine, linezolid, LORazepam, magnesium sulfate, mannitol, mechlorethamine, melphalan, meperidine, meropenem, mesna, methylhexital, methotrexate, methyldopate, methylPREDNISolone, metoclopramide, metoprolol, metroNIDAZOLE, midazolam, milrinone, mitoXANTRONE, morphine, mycophenolate, nafcillin, nalbuphine, naloxone, nesiritide, niCARdipine, nitroglycerin, nitroprusside, norepinephrine, octreotide, ondansetron, oxaliplatin, oxytocin, PACLitaxel, palonosetron, pamidronate, pancuronium, pantoprazole, PEMEtrexed, PENTobarbital, PHENobarbital, phentolamine, phenylephrine, piperacillin/tazobactam, potassium acetate, potassium chloride/phosphates, procainamide, prochlorperazine, promethazine, propranolol, quinupristin/ dalfopristin, raNITIdine, remifentanil, rocuronium, sodium acetate/bicarbonate, streptozocin, succinylcholine, SUFentanil, tacrolimus, teniposide, theophylline, thiopental, thiotepa, ticarcillin/clavulanate, tigecycline, tobramycin, topotecan, vancomycin, vasopressin, vecuronium, verapamil, vinBLAStine, vinCRIStine, vinorelbine, voriconazole, zidovudine, zoledronic acid

SIDE EFFECTS

CNS: Dizziness, headache
CV: Bradycardia, hypotension
GI: Nausea, vomiting
HEMA: Bleeding, thrombocytopenia
INTEG: *Rash*
MISC: Dissection, edema, pain in legs/pelvis, sweating
SYST: Anaphylaxis

PHARMOCOKINETICS

Half-life 2 hr; excretion via urine, feces; plasma clearance 20%-25% lower in geriatric patients with CAD; renal insufficiency decreases plasma clearance

INTERACTIONS

Increase: bleeding—aspirin, heparin, NSAIDs, abciximab, eptifibatide, clopidogrel, ticlopidine, dipyridamole, cefamandole, cefoTEtan, cefoperazone, valproic acid, heparins, thrombin inhibitors, SSRIs, SNRIs
Increase: tirofiban clearance—levothyroxine, omeprazole
Drug/Lab
Decrease: platelets, Hct, Hgb

NURSING CONSIDERATIONS
Assess:

• **Bleeding:** platelet counts, Hct, Hgb before treatment, within 6 hr of loading dose, and at least daily thereafter; watch for bleeding from puncture sites, catheters, or in stools, urine; discontinue if platelets <100,000/mm³; if platelets <90,000/mm³ additional platelet counts should be performed to exclude pseudo-thrombocytopenia; if thrombocytopenia is confirmed, tirofiban and heparin should be discontinued

• Assess for contraindications to therapy: recent major surgery, active bleeding, peptic ulcer disease, trauma within 30 days

• **Pregnancy/breastfeeding:** do not use unless clearly needed; do not breastfeed, excretion unknown

Evaluate:

• Therapeutic response: treatment of acute coronary syndrome

Teach patient/family:

• That it is necessary to quit smoking to prevent excessive vasoconstriction

• About signs, symptoms of bleeding and low platelets; report bleeding (blood in stool/urine); use mechanical razors, soft-bristle toothbrush

• That there are many product and herbal interactions; do not use unless approved by prescriber

---

⚠ HIGH ALERT

RARELY USED

tisagenlecleucel
(TIH-suh-jen-LEK-loo-sel)
Kymriah
Func. class.: Antineoplastic

USES: For the treatment of refractory B-cell precursor acute lymphoblastic leukemia

DOSAGE AND ROUTES

• **Adult ≤25 yr/adolescent/child/infant/neonate: IV (>50 kg):** Infuse a single dose of $0.1\text{-}2.5 \times 10^8$ CAR-positive viable T cells (non–weight-based); **(≤50 kg):** Infuse a single dose of $0.2\text{-}5 \times 10^6$ CAR-positive viable T cells per kg of body weight. Give at 2-14 days after the completion of lymphocyte depletion with fludarabine and cyclophosphamide

tiZANidine (Rx)

(ti-za′nih-deen)

Zanaflex

Func. class.: Skeletal muscle relaxant, α_2-adrenergic agonist

Chem. class.: Imidazoline

Do not confuse:

tiZANidine/tiaGABine

ACTION: Increases presynaptic inhibition of motor neurons and reduces spasticity by α_2-adrenergic agonism

USES: Acute/intermittent management of increased muscle tone associated with spasticity, symptoms of MS

Unlabeled uses: Tension headache, low back pain, trigeminal neuralgia

CONTRAINDICATIONS: Hypersensitivity

Precautions: Pregnancy, breastfeeding, children, geriatric patients, hypotension, renal/hepatic disease

DOSAGE AND ROUTES

• **Adult: PO** 8 mg q6-8hr, max 36 mg/24 hr

Renal dose

• **Adult: PO** CCr <25 mL/min, start with lower dose

Available forms: Tabs 2, 4 mg; caps 2, 4, 6 mg

Administer

• Consistently either with/without food; food may affect absorption

• Titrate doses carefully

• Avoid use with other CNS depressants

• Caps, tabs are equivalent if used on empty stomach

SIDE EFFECTS

CNS: Somnolence, dizziness, speech disorder, dyskinesia, nervousness, hallucination, psychosis

CV: Hypotension, bradycardia

GI: Dry mouth, vomiting, increased ALT, abnormal LFTs, constipation

OTHER: Blurred vision, urinary frequency, pharyngitis, rhinitis, tremors, rash, muscle weakness

PHARMACOKINETICS

Completely absorbed, widely distributed, peak 1-2 hr, duration 3-6 hr, half-life 2.5 hr, protein binding 30%, metabolized by liver; excreted in urine, feces

INTERACTIONS

Increase: CNS depression—alcohol, other CNS depressants, opioids; do not use together unless absolutely needed

Increase: tiZANidine levels—other CYP1A2 inhibitors (acyclovir, amiodarone, famotidine, mexiletine, enoxacin, norfloxacin, propafenone, tacrine, verapamil, zileuton, oral contraceptives, ciprofloxacin), fluvoxaMINE; avoid concurrent use

Increase: hypotension—antihypertensives

Increase: effect of rasagiline

Decrease: absorption of acetaminophen; monitor effect

Drug/Herb

Increase: CNS depression—kava, St. John's wort

Drug/Lab Test

Increase: alk phos, AST, ALT

NURSING CONSIDERATIONS

Assess:

• **Muscle spasticity** at baseline and throughout treatment

• **Hypotension:** gradual dosage increase should lessen hypotensive effects; have patient rise slowly from supine to upright; watch those patients receiving antihypertensives for increased effects

• Increased sedation, dizziness, hallucinations, psychosis; product may need to be discontinued

• Vision by ophthalmic exam; corneal opacities may occur

• Hepatic studies: baseline, at 1 mo after therapeutic dose is achieved and if clinically indicated during treatment and periodically thereafter

• **Pregnancy/breastfeeding:** use only if benefits outweigh fetal risk; no well-controlled studies; cautious use in breastfeeding, excretion unknown

• **Beers:** avoid in older men; may cause urinary retention

Evaluate:

• Therapeutic response: decreased muscle spasticity

🍁 Canada only   ✷⊙℞ Genetic warning

Teach patient/family:

• To rise slowly from lying or sitting to upright position to prevent orthostatic hypotension

• To ask for assistance if dizziness, sedation occur; to avoid drinking alcohol; to avoid operating machinery, driving until effects known

• To discontinue gradually

• To avoid hazardous activities until reaction is known

• Not to use other products unless approved by prescriber; to avoid use with other CNS depressants, opioids; to get medical assistance if adverse reaction occurs

• To use gum, lozenges for dry mouth

• To report vision changes, hallucinations immediately to prescriber

• To always take consistently either with food or without food; effects may be altered by taking differently

---

tobramycin (Rx)

(toe-bra-mye′sin)

Aktob, Bethkis, TOBI, TOBI Podhaler

Func. class.: Antiinfective

Chem. class.: Aminoglycoside

ACTION: Interferes with protein synthesis in bacterial cell by binding to ribosomal subunits, thereby causing inaccurate peptide sequences to form in protein chain causing bacterial death

USES: Severe systemic infections of CNS, respiratory, GI, urinary tract, bone, skin, soft tissues; cystic fibrosis (nebulizer) for *Acinetobacter calcoaceticus, Citrobacter* sp., *Enterobacter aerogenes, Enterobacter* sp., *Enterococcus* sp., *Escherichia coli, Haemophilus aegyptius, Haemophilus influenzae* (beta-lactamase negative), *Haemophilus influenzae* (beta-lactamase positive), *Klebsiella pneumoniae, Klebsiella* sp., *Moraxella lacunata, Morganella morganii, Neisseria* sp., *Proteus mirabilis, Proteus vulgaris, Providencia* sp., *Pseudomonas aeruginosa, Serratia* sp., *Staphylococcus aureus* (MSSA), *Staphylococcus epidermidis, Staphylococcus* sp., *Streptococcus pneumoniae, Streptococcus* sp.; may also be used for the following: *Acinetobacter* sp., *Aeromonas* sp., *Bacillus anthracis, Salmonella* sp., *Shigella* sp.

Unlabeled uses: Endocarditis, febrile neutropenia, surgical infection prophylaxis

CONTRAINDICATIONS: Hypersensitivity to aminoglycosides

Black Box Warning: Pregnancy, severe renal disease

Precautions: Breastfeeding, geriatric patients, neonates, mild renal disease, myasthenia gravis, Parkinson's disease

Black Box Warning: Hearing deficits, neuromuscular disease

DOSAGE AND ROUTES
Serious infection

• **Adult: IM/IV** 3 mg/kg/day in divided doses q8hr; may give up to 6 mg/kg/day in divided doses q8-12hr; once-daily dosing (pulse dosing) (unlabeled) **IV** 5-7 mg/kg, dosing intervals determined using nomogram, based on random levels drawn 8-12 hr after 1st dose

• **Child ≥6 yr: NEB** 300 mg bid in repeating cycles of 28 days on/28 days off of product; give **INH** over 10-15 min using a handheld PARI LC PLUS reusable nebulizer with DeVilbiss Pulmo-Aide compressor

• **Neonate <1 wk: IM/IV** ≤4 mg/kg/day divided q12hr

Cystic fibrosis with *Pseudomonas aeruginosa*

• **Child: IM/IV** 6-7.5 mg/kg/day in 3-4 equal divided doses

---

Side effects: *italics* = common; red = life-threatening

Renal dose

Conventional dosing:

• Multiply the serum creatinine (mg/100 mL) by 6 to determine the dosing; to decrease the dose, divide the standard dose by the serum creatinine (mg/100 mL) to determine the lower recommended dose

Available forms: Inj 10, 40 mg/mL; powder for inj 1.2 g; neb sol 300 mg/5 mL; powder for inh 28 mg

Administer:

• After obtaining specimen for C&S; begin treatment before results

• Product in evenly spaced doses to maintain blood level; separate aminoglycosides and penicillins by ≥1 hr

• Use only on susceptible organisms to prevent development of product-resistant bacteria

IM route

• IM inj in large muscle mass; rotate inj sites, aspirate

• Draw peak 1 hr after dose, trough right before next dose; absorption erratic

Inhalation route: (TOBI Podhaler)

• Use with Podhaler device; do not swallow caps; use device for 7 days, then discard

• Keep caps in blister pack until ready to use; administer other inhaled products or chest physiotherapy before

• While holding base of Podhaler device, unscrew lid, stand upright, unscrew mouthpiece; while holding body, tear blister card in half lengthwise along precut lines, peel back foil, place cap in chamber at top of device, reattach mouthpiece and tighten; with mouthpiece pointed down, press blue button down with thumb, release, exhale completely, place mouth over mouthpiece, close lips, inhale with single breath, hold 5 sec, exhale normally away from device; after a few normal breaths, repeat, unscrew mouthpiece, and remove cap; cap should be empty; repeat process 3 more times (total 4 caps); after use, reattach mouthpiece and wipe with clean, dry cloth

Intermittent IV INFUSION route

• Visually inspect sol; do not use if discolored or particulate is present

• **Vantage vials** are for IV only and only for exactly 60 or 80 mg

• Diluted in 50-100 mL 0.9% NaCl, D_5W (D_{10}W, Ringer's, LR); infuse over 20-60 min; volume for pediatric patients needs to be sufficient to allow for 20-60 min infusion

Y-site compatibilities: Acyclovir, aldesleukin, alfentanil, alprostadil, amifostine, aminophylline, amiodarone, amsacrine, anidulafungin, ascorbic acid, atracurium, atropine, aztreonam, bivalirudin, bretylium, bumetanide, buprenorphine, butorphanol, calcium chloride/gluconate, CARBOplatin, caspofungin, chloramphenicol, cimetidine, ciprofloxacin, cisatracurium, CISplatin, clindamycin, cyanocobalamin, cyclophosphamide, cycloSPORINE, cytarabine, DACTINomycin, DAPTOmycin, dexmedetomidine, digoxin, diltiaZEM, diphenhydrAMINE, DOBUTamine, DOCEtaxel, DOPamine, doripenem, doxacurium, DOXOrubicin hydrochloride, DOXOrubicin liposome, doxycycline, enalaprilat, ePHEDrine, EPINEPHrine, epiRUBicin, epoetin alfa, ertapenem, esmolol, etoposide, etoposide phosphate, famotidine, fenoldopam, fentaNYL, filgrastim, fluconazole, fludarabine, fluorouracil, foscarnet, furosemide, gemcitabine, gentamicin, glycopyrrolate, granisetron, HYDROmorphone, ifosfamide, imipenem/cilastatin, isoproterenol, ketorolac, labetalol, levoFLOXacin, lidocaine, linezolid

LORazepam, magnesium sulfate, mannitol, mechlorethamine, melphalan, meperidine, metaraminol, metaraminol, methicillin, methotrexate, methoxamine, methyldopate, methylPREDNISolone, metoclopramide, metoprolol, metroNIDAZOLE, miconazole, midazolam, milrinone, minocycline, mitoXANTRONE, morphine, moxalactam, multiple vitamins, nafcillin, nalbuphine, naloxone, niCARdipine, nitroglycerin, nitroprusside, norepinephrine, octreotide, ondansetron, oxaliplatin, oxytocin, PACLitaxel, palonosetron, pantoprazole, papaverine, penicillin G, pentazocine, perphenazine, PHENobarbital, phentolamine, phenylephrine, phytonadione, potassium chloride, procainamide, prochlorperazine, promethazine, propranolol, protamine, pyridoxime, quinupristin/dalfopristin, raNITIdine, remifentanil, riTUXimab, rocuronium, sodium acetate/bicarbonate, succinylcholine, SUFentanil, tacrolimus, teniposide, theophylline, thiamine, thiotepa, ticarcillin/clavulanate, tigecycline, tirofiban, tolazoline, trastuzumab, trimethaphan, urokinase, vancomycin, vasopressin, vecuronium, verapamil, vinCRIStine, vinorelbine, voriconazole, zidovudine

SIDE EFFECTS

CNS: Confusion, depression, numbness, tremors, seizures, muscle twitching, neurotoxicity, dizziness, vertigo
CV: Hypo/hypertension, palpitation
EENT: Ototoxicity, deafness, visual disturbances, tinnitus
GI: *Nausea, vomiting, anorexia;* increased ALT, AST, bilirubin, hepatomegaly, hepatic necrosis, splenomegaly
GU: Oliguria, hematuria, renal damage, azotemia, renal failure, nephrotoxicity

HEMA: Agranulocytosis, thrombocytopenia, leukopenia, eosinophilia, anemia
INTEG: *Rash,* burning, urticaria, dermatitis, alopecia

PHARMACOKINETICS
Plasma half-life 2-3 hr, prolonged in neonates; not metabolized; excreted unchanged in urine; crosses placental barrier; poor penetration into CSF
IM: Onset rapid, peak 1 hr, duration 8 hr
IV: Onset immediate, peak 30 min, duration 8 hr

INTERACTIONS

Black Box Warning: **Increase:** ototoxicity, neurotoxicity, nephrotoxicity—other aminoglycosides, amphotericin B, polymyxin, vancomycin, ethacrynic acid, furosemide, mannitol, methoxyflurane, CISplatin, cephalosporins, bacitracin, acyclovir, penicillins, cidofovir

Drug/Lab Test
Increase: eosinophils, BUN, creatinine, AST, ALT, LDH, alk phos, glucose
Decrease: potassium, calcium, sodium, magnesium, WBC, granulocytes, platelets

NURSING CONSIDERATIONS
Assess:
• Weight before treatment; dosage is usually based on ideal body weight but may be calculated on actual body weight
• I&O ratio, urinalysis daily for proteinuria, cells, casts; report sudden change in urine output
• VS during infusion; watch for hypotension, change in pulse
• IV site for thrombophlebitis, including pain, redness, swelling; change site if needed; apply warm compresses to discontinued site

T

Black Box Warning: **Serum amino-glycoside concentration;** serum peak drawn at 30-60 min after IV infusion or 60 min after IM inj, trough drawn just before next dose, peak 4-10 mcg/mL, trough 0.5-2 mcg/mL, increased level may lead to serious toxicity

Black Box Warning: **Renal impairment:** CCr, BUN, serum creatinine; lower dosage should be given in renal impairment (CCr <80 mL/min); monitor electrolytes: potassium, sodium, chloride, magnesium monthly if patient receiving long-term therapy

Black Box Warning: **Deafness by audiometric testing;** ringing, roaring in ears; vertigo; assess hearing before, during, after treatment

• **Overgrowth of infection:** fever, malaise, redness, pain, swelling, perineal itching, diarrhea, stomatitis, change in cough, sputum
• **Vestibular dysfunction:** nausea, vomiting, dizziness, headache; product should be discontinued if severe
• Adequate fluids of 2-3 L/day unless contraindicated to prevent irritation of tubules

Black Box Warning: **Pregnancy:** identify if pregnancy is planned or suspected; do not use in pregnancy, breastfeeding

Evaluate:
• Therapeutic response: absence of fever, draining wounds, negative C&S after treatment
Teach patient/family:
• To promptly report headache, dizziness, symptoms of overgrowth of infection, renal impairment

Black Box Warning: To report loss of hearing; ringing, roaring in ears; feeling of fullness in head

Black Box Warning: To notify prescriber if pregnancy is planned or suspected; not to use in pregnancy, breastfeeding

• To avoid hazardous activities until response is known
Nebulizer
• To use other therapies first, then tobramycin, not to use if cloudy or contains particulates

TREATMENT OF OVERDOSE: Hemodialysis; monitor serum levels of product

tobramycin ophthalmic
See Appendix B

tocilizumab (Rx)
(toe'si-liz'oo-mab)
Actemra
Func. class.: DMARDs (disease-modifying antirheumatoid drugs)/ tumor necrosis factor (TNF) modifier

ACTION: Interleukin-6 (IL-6) receptor inhibiting monoclonal antibody

USES: Rheumatoid arthritis, active systemic juvenile idiopathic arthritis

CONTRAINDICATIONS: Hypersensitivity
Precautions: Breastfeeding, pregnancy; risk for GI perforation, active hepatic disease, severe neutropenia/thrombocytopenia, demyelinating disorders

Black Box Warning: Invasive fungal infection, active TB

DOSAGE AND ROUTES
Moderate-severe rheumatoid arthritis
• **Adult: IV** 4 mg/kg over 1 hr q4wk, may increase to 8 mg/kg q4wk based on clinical response, max dose 800 mg/infu-

sion; do not initiate if ANC <2000/mm³, platelets <100,000/mm³

• **Adult <100 kg: SUBCUT** 162 mg every other wk (monotherapy or in combination); increase to 162 mg weekly based on response

• **Adult ≥100 kg: SUBCUT** 162 mg weekly (monotherapy or in combination)

Juvenile idiopathic arthritis

• **Child ≥2 yr/adolescent ≥30 kg: IV** 8 mg/kg over 1 hr q2wk

• **Child ≥2 yr/adolescent <30 kg: IV** 10 mg/kg over 1 hr q2wk

Polyarticular juvenile idiopathic arthritis (PJIA)

• **Child ≥2 yr and weighing ≥30 kg: IV INFUSION** 8 mg/kg over 1 hr q4wk

• **Child ≥2 yr and weighing <30 kg: IV INFUSION** 10 mg/kg over 1 hr q4wk

Therapeutic drug monitoring

• Before initiation of treatment, check ANC, platelet count, and liver function tests (ALT/AST concentrations). In adults, not recommended for use in those with ANC <2,000/mm³, platelet count <100,000/mm³, or ALT or AST >1.5 × ULN

Hepatic dose

• **Adult patients with rheumatoid arthritis or giant cell arteritis with hepatic impairment**

Do not initiate treatment with tocilizumab if baseline AST/ALT is >1.5× ULN. However, patients with severe or life-threatening CRS frequently have elevated ALT or AST; the decision to administer tocilizumab should take into account the potential benefit of treating the CRS vs. risks of short-term treatment with tocilizumab

Hepatic enzyme elevations occurring during treatment:

• AST and/or ALT from 1-3× ULN: dose modify concomitant DMARDs, if appropriate. For persistent increases of transaminases in this range, reduce IV tocilizumab dose to 4 mg/kg or reduce SUBCUT dosing interval to every other week, or interrupt tocilizumab dosing until AST/

ALT have normalized. For SUBCUT dosing, once ALT/AST have normalized, resume at every other week dosing and increase to once weekly as clinically appropriate

• AST and/or ALT >3× and up to 5× ULN, confirmed by repeat testing: Interrupt tocilizumab dosing until AST/ALT is <3× ULN. Then, if appropriate, dose modify concomitant DMARDs. For persistent increases of transaminases 3× ULN or less, reduce IV tocilizumab dose to 4 mg/kg, or reduce SUBCUT dosing interval to every other week, or interrupt tocilizumab until AST/ALT have normalized. For SUBCUT dosing, once ALT/AST have normalized, resume at every other week dosing and increase to once weekly as clinically appropriate. For persistent increases >3× ULN, discontinue tocilizumab

• AST and/or ALT >5× ULN: discontinue tocilizumab

Available forms: Sol for inj 20 mg/mL; prefilled syringes 162 mg/0.9 mL

Administer:

SUBCUT route

• Remove syringe, allow to warm for 30 min at room temperature. Do not warm in any other way

• Use injection site such as the front of thigh, outer area of upper arm, or the abdomen except for the 2-inch area around the navel. Do not inject into moles; scars; or areas where skin is tender, bruised, red, hard, or not intact. Rotate injection sites with each injection. Inject at >1 inch from the last area injected

• Remove the needle cap immediately before injection, and gently pinch a cleaned area of skin. Using a dartlike motion, insert the needle at a 45- or 90-degree angle to the skin. Release the pinched skin, and gently push the plunger all the way down to inject the full amount in the prefilled syringe (0.9 mL), which provides 162 mg of product

T

Side effects: *italics* = common; red = life-threatening

Intermittent IV INFUSION route

• Visually inspect for particulate matter, discoloration before administration; should be colorless to pale yellow liquid
• From 100-mL infusion bag or bottle, withdraw vol of 0.9% sodium chloride inj equal to vol of tocilizumab sol required for patient's dose
• Slowly add tocilizumab from each vial into infusion bag or bottle; gently invert bag to avoid foaming; fully diluted sols are compatible with polypropylene, polyethylene, polyvinyl chloride infusion bags and polypropylene, polyethylene, glass infusion bottles
• Fully diluted sol for infusion may be stored refrigerated or at room temperature for ≤24 hr and should be protected from light; do not use unused product remaining in vials; no preservatives
• Allow the fully diluted sol to reach room temperature before infusion
• Give over 60 minutes with infusion set; do not administer as IV push or bolus
• Do not infuse concomitantly in same IV line with other drugs

SIDE EFFECTS

CNS: Headache, dizziness
CV: Hypertension
GI: Perforation, abdominal pain, gastritis, mouth ulcerations
HEMA: Neutropenia, thrombocytopenia
INTEG: Rash, infusion reactions
RESP: Upper respiratory infections, nasopharyngitis, bronchitis
SYST: Serious infections, anaphylaxis, infusion-related reactions, anti-tocilizumab antibody formation, secondary malignancy

INTERACTIONS

Decrease: product level—cycloSPORINE, theophylline, warfarin

• Do not give with live virus vaccines
• Avoid use with TNF modifiers, DMARDs, immunosuppressives due to increased risk of infection

PHARMACOKINETICS

Half-life approx 6 days with single dose, approx 11 days with multiple (steady-state) doses

NURSING CONSIDERATIONS
Assess:

• **Rheumatoid arthritis:** ROM, pain, stiffness at baseline q1-2wk
• Blood studies: CBC with differential, LFTs, platelet count, serum lipid profile at baseline and periodically; LFTS 1-3 × ULN reduce dose, if 3-5 × ULN interrupt; platelets 50,000-100,000/mm³ interrupt until platelets are >100,000/mm³ then reduce at lower dose

Black Box Warning: **Infection** before treatment and periodically; obtain TB screening before beginning treatment, invasive fungal infections; discontinue if infection occurs during administration; may use antituberculosis therapy before tocilizumab in past history of latent or active TB when adequate course of treatment cannot be confirmed and those with a negative TB with risk factors for infections

• **Anaphylaxis:** Assess for rash, facial swelling, dyspnea, antihistamine, corticosteroids, emergency equipment should be available
• **Fungal infection:** Assess for flulike symptoms, dyspnea, may lead to shock, notify provider immediately
• **Secondary malignancy:** assess for malignancy periodically
• **Pregnancy/breastfeeding:** use only if benefits outweigh fetal risk; pregnant patients should enroll in the MotherToBaby Autoimmune Diseases in Pregnancy Registry; do not breastfeed, excretion unknown

Evaluate:

• Therapeutic response: ability to move more easily with less pain

Teach patient/family:

• That this treatment must continue unless safety or effectiveness is an issue
• About reason for use and expected results
• To avoid live vaccines; to bring immunizations up-to-date before treatment

Black Box Warning: To report signs, symptoms of infection, including TB and hepatitis B; to avoid others with infections

• To notify prescriber if pregnancy or suspected pregnancy; not to use if breastfeeding; to consider using a non-hormonal contraceptive because contraception may be decreased

tofacitinib

(toe′fa-sye′ti-nib)

Xeljanz, Xeljanz XR

Func. class.: Antirheumatic agent (disease modifying), immunomodulator/biologic DMARD

Chem. class.: Janus kinase inhibitor

ACTION: Affects the signaling pathway of Janus kinase

USES: Rheumatoid arthritis (moderately to severely active) in those who have taken methotrexate with inadequate response or intolerance

CONTRAINDICATIONS: Hypersensitivity

Precautions: Pregnancy, breastfeeding, neonates, infants, children, geriatric patients, neoplastic disease, ulcerative colitis, neutropenia, peptic ulcer disease, active infections, risk of lymphomas/leukemias, TB, posttransplant lymphoproliferative disorder (PTLD), kidney disease, diabetes mellitus, HIV, hypercholesterolemia, herpes virus infection reactivation, Asian patients

Black Box Warning: Infection, secondary malignancy

DOSAGE AND ROUTES
Psoriatic arthritis

• **Adult: PO** 5 mg bid with a DMARD if receiving potent CYP3A4 inhibitor, 5 mg/day if receiving moderate CYP3A4 inhibitor and 2C19 inhibitors; **EXT REL** 11 mg/day with a DMARD

Moderate to severe rheumatoid arthritis

• **Adult: PO** 5 mg bid with or without methotrexate or a DMARD; **EXT REL** 11 mg/day

Ulcerative colitis

• **Adult: PO** 10 mg bid × 8 wk or more, then 5 or 10 mg bid (immediate release)

Available forms: Tabs 5 mg; ext rel tab 11 mg

Administer:

PO route

• Without regard to food

SIDE EFFECTS

CNS: Headache, paresthesias, insomnia, fatigue

CV: Hypertension

GI: Abdominal pain, nausea, liver damage, dyspepsia, vomiting, diarrhea, gastritis, GI perforation, steatosis

HEMA: Anemia, lymphocytosis, lymphopenia, neutropenia

INTEG: Rash, pruritus

MISC: Increased cancer risk, risk of infection (TB, invasive fungal infections, other opportunistic infections), may be fatal, posttransplant lymphoproliferative disorder (PTLD)

PHARMACOKINETICS

Bioavailability 70%, protein binding 40% (albumin), metabolism mediated by CYP3A4, half-life 3 hr, peak 0.5-1 hr

INTERACTIONS

Black Box Warning: Do not use with TNF modifiers, vaccines, potent immunosuppressants, other biologic DMARDS; serious infections may occur

Increase: tofacinib effect—CYP3A4 inhibitors (amprenavir, boceprevir, delavirdine, ketoconazole, indinavir, itraconazole, dalfopristin/quinupristin, ritonavir, tipranavir, fluconazole, isoniazid, miconazole)

Decrease: tofacinib effect—CYP3A4 inducers (rifAMPin, rifapentine, rifabutin, primidone, phenytoin, PHENobarbital, nevirapine, nafcillin, modafinil, griseofulvin, etravirine, efavirenz, barbiturates, bexarotene, bosentan, carBAMazepine, enzalutamide, dexamethasone)

Drug/Lab Test

Increase: LFTs, cholesterol

Decrease: neutrophils, lymphocytes, Hct, Hgb

NURSING CONSIDERATIONS

Assess:

• Monitor lipid profile, Hct/Hgb, WBC, LFTs

• **RA:** Pain, stiffness, ROM, swelling of joints before, during treatment

Black Box Warning: **Active infection, including localized infection:** evaluate and test patients for latent or active TB before use; treat with antimycobacterials before use of product; this product increases the risk of serious including fatal infections (pulmonary or extrapulmonary TB; invasive fungal infections; and bacterial, viral, and opportunistic infections); during and after use, monitor for infection including TB in those who tested negative for latent TB before use; if a serious infection develops, interrupt receipt until the infection is controlled, reactivation of viral infections is higher in Asian patients

Black Box Warning: **Secondary malignancy:** lymphoma and other malignancies have been noted with product use

• **Epstein-Barr virus–associated posttransplant lymphoproliferative disorder (PTLD):** in kidney transplant patients when used with this product and immunosuppressives

• **Liver disease:** not recommended in severe liver disease, impairment; dose modification is needed with moderate liver impairment, monitor LFTs

• **GI perforation:** assess in those with diverticulitis, peptic ulcer disease, or ulcerative colitis

Black Box Warning: **Immunosuppression:** obtain neutrophil and lymphocyte counts before use; do not start the product in lymphocyte count <500 cells/mm³ or ANC <1000 cells/mm³; for ANC >1000 cells/mm³, monitor neutrophil counts after 4-8 wk and every 3 mo thereafter; lymphocyte count >500 cells/mm³, monitor lymphocyte counts every 3 mo

• **Anemia:** determine Hgb, do not start in Hgb <9 g/dL; in Hgb ≥9 g/dL, monitor Hgb after 4-8 wk and every 3 mo thereafter

• **Pregnancy/breastfeeding:** use during pregnancy only if the potential benefit justifies the potential risk to the fetus; if pregnancy occurs, enrollment in the pregnancy registry is encouraged by calling 1-877-311-8972; discontinue product or breastfeeding; serious adverse reactions can occur in nursing infants

Black Box Warning: Neoplastic disease (lymphomas/leukemias)

Evaluate:

• Therapeutic response: decreased inflammation, pain in joints, decreased joint destruction

Teach patient/family:

• Not to take any live virus vaccines during treatment; vaccines should be brought up-to-date before starting treatment

• To report signs of infection, allergic reaction

• **Pregnancy:** to report if pregnancy is planned or suspected; not to breastfeed

tolcapone (Rx)

(toll'cah'pone)

Tasmar

Func. class.: Antiparkinson agent
Chem. class.: COMT inhibitor

ACTION: Inhibits COMT; used as adjunct to levodopa/carbidopa therapy

USES: Parkinson's disease

CONTRAINDICATIONS: Hypersensitivity, rhabdomyolysis
Precautions: Pregnancy, breastfeeding, cardiac/renal disease, hypertension, asthma, history of rhabdomyolysis

Black Box Warning: Hepatic disease

DOSAGE AND ROUTES

• **Adult: PO** 100-200 mg tid with levodopa/carbidopa therapy; max 600 mg/day, discontinue if no benefit after 3 wk
Available forms: Tabs 100, 200 mg
Administer:

• Only to be used if levodopa/carbidopa does not provide satisfactory results
• Give without regard to food

SIDE EFFECTS

CNS: Dystonia, dyskinesia, dreaming, *fatigue, headache, confusion,* psychosis, hallucination, dizziness, sleep disorders
CV: *Orthostatic hypotension,* chest pain, hypotension
EENT: Cataract, eye inflammation
GI: *Nausea, vomiting, anorexia, abdominal distress,* diarrhea, constipation, fatal hepatic failure, increased LFTs
GU: UTI, urine discoloration, uterine tumor, micturition disorder, hematuria
HEMA: Hemolytic anemia, leukopenia, agranulocytosis
INTEG: Sweating, alopecia
MS: Rhabdomyolysis

PHARMACOKINETICS

Rapidly absorbed, peak 2 hr, protein binding 99%, extensively metabolized, half-life 2-3 hr, excreted in urine (60%)/feces (40%)

INTERACTIONS

Increase: CNS depression—CNS depressant

• May influence pharmacokinetics of α-methyldopa, DOBUTamine, apomorphine, isoproterenol
• Inhibition of normal catecholamine metabolism: MAOIs; MAO-B inhibitor may be used

NURSING CONSIDERATIONS
Assess:

Black Box Warning: **Hepatic disease:** AST, ALT, alk phos, LDH, bilirubin, CBC; monitor ALT, AST q2wk × 1 yr, then q4wk × 6 mo, then q8wk thereafter; if LFTs elevated, product should not be used, if no improvement in 3 wk, discontinue; do not use in hepatic disease

• Involuntary movements of parkinsonism: akinesia, tremors, staggering gait, muscle rigidity, drooling
• B/P, respiration during initial treatment; hypo/hypertension should be reported
• Mental status: affect, mood, behavioral changes, avoid use in those with dystonia
Evaluate:
• Therapeutic response: decrease in akathisia, increased mood
Teach patient/family:
• To change positions slowly to prevent orthostatic hypotension
• That urine, sweat may change color
• That food taken within 1 hr before meals or 2 hr after meals decreases action of product by 20%; may be taken without regard to food
• To notify prescriber if pregnancy is planned or suspected
• That CNS changes may occur, hallucinations, involuntary movement
• To avoid hazardous activities until reaction is known; dizziness may occur
• To notify prescriber of poor impulse control, urges to gamble, spend money (rare)

T

Side effects: *italics* = common; red = life-threatening

• To report diarrhea, nausea, vomiting, anorexia; that nausea may occur at beginning of treatment

---

tolnaftate topical
See Appendix B

---

tolterodine (Rx)
(toll-tehr'oh-deen)
Detrol, Detrol LA
Func. class.: Overactive bladder product
Chem. class.: Muscarinic receptor antagonist

ACTION: Relaxes smooth muscles in urinary tract by inhibiting acetylcholine at postganglionic sites

USES: Overactive bladder (urinary frequency, urgency), urinary incontinence

CONTRAINDICATIONS: Hypersensitivity, uncontrolled closed-angle glaucoma, urinary retention, gastric retention
Precautions: Pregnancy, breastfeeding, children, renal disease, controlled closed-angle glaucoma, bladder obstruction, QT prolongation, decreased GI motility

DOSAGE AND ROUTES
Overactive bladder
• **Adult and geriatric: PO** 2 mg bid; may decrease to 1 mg bid; **EXT REL** 4 mg/day, may decrease to 2 mg/day if needed, max 4 mg/day
Hepatic/renal dose
• **Adult: PO** 1 mg bid (50% dose) or **EXT REL** 2 mg/day; CCr ≤30 mL/min, reduce by 50%

CYP3A4 inhibitor dose
• **Adult: PO** 1 mg bid; **EXT REL** 2 mg/day
Available forms: Tabs 1, 2 mg; ext rel caps 2, 4 mg
Administer:
• Whole; take with liquids; do not crush, chew, or break ext rel product; without regard to meals

SIDE EFFECTS
CNS: Anxiety, paresthesia, fatigue, *dizziness, headache;* increasing dementia, memory impairment
CV: Chest pain, hypertension, QT prolongation
EENT: Vision abnormalities, xerophthalmia
GI: *Nausea, vomiting, anorexia,* abdominal pain, constipation, dry mouth, dyspepsia
GU: Dysuria, urinary retention, frequency, UTI
INTEG: Rash, pruritus
RESP: Bronchitis, cough, pharyngitis, upper respiratory tract infection
SYST: Angioedema, Stevens-Johnson syndrome

PHARMACOKINETICS
Rapidly absorbed; highly protein bound; extensively metabolized by CYP2D6; a portion of the population may be poor metabolizers; excreted in urine, feces half-life 2-3.7 hr

INTERACTIONS
• Do not use in those with known hypersensitivity to fesoterodine
• **Increase:** QT prolongation—class IA/III antidysrhythmics, some phenothiazines, β-agonists, local anesthetics, tricyclics, haloperidol, methadone, chloroquine, clarithromycin, droperidol, erythromycin, pentamidine
Increase: action of tolterodine—antiretroviral protease inhibitors, macrolide antiinfectives, azole antifungals
Increase: anticholinergic effect—antimuscarinics
Increase: urinary frequency—diuretics
Drug/Food
• Food increases bioavailability of tolterodine
Drug/Lab
Increase: LFTs, bilirubin

NURSING CONSIDERATIONS
Assess:

• **Urinary patterns:** distention, nocturia, frequency, urgency, incontinence, residual urine

• **Serious skin disorders:** angioedema, Stevens-Johnson syndrome; allergic reactions: rash; if this occurs, product should be discontinued; usually occurs in first few doses

• **QT prolongation:** ECG, ejection fraction; assess for chest pain, palpitations, dyspnea; may be compounded in those taking class IA/III dysrhythmics

Black Box Warning: Fatal hepatic injury: increased LFTs, bilirubin during first 18 mo of therapy in those with autosomal dominant polycystic kidney disease; assess for fatigue, anorexia, right upper abdominal pain, dark urine, jaundice; if these occur, discontinue product and do not restart if cause is liver injury

• **Beers:** avoid in older adults with delirium or at high risk for delirium; monitor for confusion, delirium frequently

Evaluate:

• Decreasing dysuria, frequency, nocturia, incontinence

Teach patient/family:

• To avoid hazardous activities; dizziness may occur

• Not to drink liquids before bedtime; to swallow ext rel product whole

• About the importance of bladder maintenance

• Not to breastfeed; to notify prescriber if pregnancy is planned or suspected

• To report signs of infection, skin effects, shortness of breath, urinary retention

---

tolvaptan (Rx)
(tole-vap′tan)

Jinarc ✦, Samsca

Func. class.: Antihypertensive

Chem. class.: Vasopressin receptor antagonist, V2

ACTION: Arginine vasopressin (AVP) antagonist with affinity for V2 receptors; level of circulating AVP in circulating blood is critical for the regulation of water and the electrolyte balance, and it is usually elevated with euvolemic/hypervolemic hyponatremia

USES: Hypervolemic/euvolemic hyponatremia with heart failure, cirrhosis, SIADH

CONTRAINDICATIONS: Hypersensitivity, hypovolemia, anuria

Precautions: Pregnancy, breastfeeding, children, dehydration, geriatric patients, hyperkalemia, autosomal dominant PKD, malnutrition, alcoholism, hepatic disease

Black Box Warning: Osmotic demyelination syndrome; requires a specialized care setting

DOSAGE AND ROUTES

• **Adult: PO** 15 mg daily; after 24 hr, may increase to 30 mg daily; max 60 mg/day max 30 days

Available forms: Tabs 15, 30 mg

Administer:

• PO with/without food

• Avoid fluid restriction for first 24 hr

• Initiate in hospital setting

• Do not use with grapefruit, grapefruit juice

SIDE EFFECTS

CNS: Fever, dizziness

CV: Ventricular fibrillation, DIC, stroke, thrombosis

GI: *Nausea,* vomiting, *constipation,* colitis, hepatic injury

GU: Polyuria

HEMA: Bleeding

META: *Dehydration, hyperglycemia,* hyperkalemia, hypernatremia

MS: Rhabdomyolysis

RESP: Respiratory depression, pulmonary embolism

T

Side effects: *italics* = common; red = life-threatening

PHARMACOKINETICS

Peak 2-4 hr, protein binding 99%, metabolized by CYP3A4, terminal half-life 12 hr

INTERACTIONS

Increase: concentrations of tolvaptan—CYP3A4 inhibitors (efavirenz, fosamprenavir, quiNINE); P-gp inhibitors (cycloSPORINE, azithromycin, mefloquine, palperidone, propafenone, quiNIDine, testosterone)

Decrease: concentration of tolvaptan—CYP3A4 inducers (carBAMazepine, dexamethasone, etravirine, flutamide, griseofulvin, metyraPONE, modafinil, nafcillin, nevirapine, OXcarbazepine, phenytoin, rifAMPin, rifabutin, rifapentine, topiramate)

Drug/Herb

Decrease: tolvaptan effect—CYP3A4 inducer (St. John's wort)

Drug/Food

• Grapefruit/grapefruit juice; do not use together

NURSING CONSIDERATIONS

Assess:

• Renal, hepatic function

Black Box Warning: **Osmotic demyelination syndrome:** frequent sodium vol status; overly rapid correction of sodium concentration (>12 mEq/L per 24 hr); may occur in alcoholism, severe malnutrition, advanced liver disease, syndrome of inappropriate antidiuretic hormone; correct sodium levels slowly, may result in dysarthria, mutism, dysphagia, coma, seizure, death

• CV status: ventricular fibrillation, hypertension; monitor B/P, pulse
• Monitor electrolytes (sodium, potassium)

Black Box Warning: **Specialized care setting:** needed so that neurologic status and sodium can be monitored

• **Liver injury:** fatigue, abdominal pain, dark urine, clay-colored stools, jaundice
• **Pregnancy/breastfeeding:** use only if benefits outweigh fetal risk; do not breastfeed

Evaluate:

• Therapeutic response: correction of serum sodium levels

Teach patient/family:

• About administration procedure and expected results; that product will be used for ≤30 days

• To report difficulty swallowing, speaking, seizures, dizziness, drowsiness; embolism may be the cause

• To drink fluid in response to thirst
• Not to use grapefruit juice
• To notify prescriber before using other products

• To report right upper abdominal pain, nausea, vomiting, anorexia, dark urine, yellowing of skin, eyes (hepatic injury)

• That product will be started or restarted in the hospital when monitoring is possible

• To avoid pregnancy, breastfeeding while taking this product

---

topiramate (Rx)

(toh-pire′ah-mate)

Qudexy XR, Topamax, Topamax Sprinkle, Trokendi XR

Func. class.: Anticonvulsant—miscellaneous

Chem. class.: Monosaccharide derivative

Do not confuse:

Topamax/Toprol XL

ACTION: May prevent seizure spread as opposed to an elevation of seizure threshold, increases GABA activity

USES: Partial seizures in adults and children 2-16 yr old; tonic-clonic seizures; seizures with Lennox-Gastaut syndrome; migraine prophylaxis

Unlabeled uses: Infantile spasms, bipolar disorder, alcohol dependence, absence seizures, neuropathic pain, cluster headaches, mania, bulimia nervosa

CONTRAINDICATIONS: Hypersensitivity, metabolic acidosis, pregnancy

Precautions: Breastfeeding, children, renal/hepatic disease, acute myopia, secondary closed-angle glaucoma, behavioral disorders, COPD, dialysis, encephalopathy, status asthmaticus, status epilepticus, surgery, paresthesias, maculopathy, nephrolithiasis

DOSAGE AND ROUTES
Adjunctive therapy for seizures
• **Adult/adolescent/child ≥10 yr: PO** 25-50 mg/day initially, titrate by 25-50 mg/wk, up to 200-400 mg/day in 2 divided doses

• **Adult/adolescent/child ≥10 yr: PO** (Qudexy XR, Trokendi XR) 50 mg daily, increase by 50 mg weekly during wk 2, 3, 4, increase by 100 mg weekly, wk 5, 6, final dose 400 mg daily

• **Child 2-9 yr: PO** week 1: 25 mg in PM, then 25 mg bid if tolerated (week 2), then increase by 25-50 mg/day each week as tolerated over 5- to 7-wk titration period, maintenance given in 2 divided doses; <11 kg, minimum 150 mg/day, max 250 mg/day; 12-22 kg, minimum 200 mg/day, max 300 mg/day; 23-31 kg, minimum 200 mg/day, max 350 mg/day; 32-38 kg, minimum 250 mg/day, max 350 mg/day; >38 kg, minimum 250 mg/day, max 400 mg/day; Qudexy XR 25 mg daily at night, may increase to 50 mg wk 2, if tolerated, increase by 25-50 mg each wk over 5- to 7-wk titration period, max dose based on weight

• **Child ≤11 kg: PO** Qudexy XR minimum 150 mg daily, max 250 mg daily
• **Child 12-22 kg:** minimum 200 mg daily, max 300 mg daily
• **Child 23-31 kg:** minimum 200 mg daily, max 350 mg daily
• **Child 32-38 kg:** minimum 250 mg daily, max 350 mg daily
• **Child >38 kg:** minimum 250 mg daily, max 400 mg daily
Migraine prophylaxis
• **Adult: PO** 25 mg/day initially, increase by 25 mg/day/wk up to 100 mg/day in 2 divided doses
Renal dose
• **Adult: PO** CCr <70 mL/min, give $^1/_2$ dose

Atonic/atypical absence/myoclonic seizures (unlabeled)
• **Adult/adolescent >16 yr: PO** 50 mg/day, titrate slowly by 50 mg/wk to 100-300 mg tid
• **Child 2-16 yr: PO** 0.5-1 mg/kg, max 25 mg, initially daily × 7 days, then increase by 0.5-1 mg/kg/day weekly up to 3-6 mg/kg/day in divided doses
Refractory infantile spasms (unlabeled)
• **Child: PO** 25 mg/day, may increase by 25 mg q2-3days until spasms controlled, max 24 mg/kg/day
Alcoholism (unlabeled)
• **Adult: PO** 25 mg/day, titrated to max 300 mg/day in divided doses
Neuropathic pain (unlabeled)
• **Adult: PO** 12.5-25 mg daily or bid × 4 wk, then double dose q4wk to max 100-200 mg/day in divided doses
Bipolar disorder (unlabeled)
• **Adult: PO** 25 mg/day, then increase by 25-mg increments to 200 mg/day

Available forms: Tabs 25, 50, 100, 200 mg; sprinkle caps 15, 25 mg; ext rel caps 25, 50, 100, 200 mg; ext rel cap (sprinkles 24 hr) 25, 50, 100, 150, 200 mg
Administer:
• Swallow tabs whole; do not break, crush, or chew tabs; very bitter
• May take without regard to meals
• Sprinkle cap can be given whole or opened and sprinkled on soft food; do not chew, drink water after sprinkle
• Store at room temperature away from heat, light

SIDE EFFECTS
CNS: *Dizziness, fatigue,* cognitive disorders, insomnia, *anxiety,* depression, paresthesia, *memory loss, tremors,* motor retardation, suicidal ideation, poor balance, ataxia
CV: Flushing, chest pain
EENT: Diplopia, *vision abnormality*
GI: Diarrhea, *anorexia, nausea, dyspepsia,* abdominal pain, constipation, dry mouth, pancreatitis
GU: Breast pain, dysmenorrhea, menstrual disorder
INTEG: Rash, alopecia

T

Side effects: *italics* = common; red = life-threatening

MISC: Weight loss, leukopenia, metabolic acidosis, increased body temperature; unexplained death (epilepsy)
RESP: Upper respiratory tract infection, pharyngitis, sinusitis

PHARMACOKINETICS
Well absorbed, peak 2 hr, terminal half-life 19-25 hr, excreted in urine (55%-97% unchanged), crosses placenta, excreted in breast milk, protein binding (9%-17%), steady state 4 days

INTERACTIONS
Increase: renal stones—carbonic anhydrase inhibitors
Increase: effect of amitriptyline
Increase: CNS depression—alcohol, CNS depressants
Increase: topiramate levels—metFORMIN, hydroCHLOROthiazide, lamoTRIgine
Decrease: levels of hormonal contraceptives, estrogen, digoxin, valproic acid, lithium, risperiDONE
Decrease: topiramate levels—phenytoin, carBAMazepine, valproic acid, probenecid

NURSING CONSIDERATIONS
Assess:
• **Seizures:** location, type, duration, aura; **seizure precautions:** padded side rails; move objects that may harm patient
• **Bipolar disorder:** mood, behavior, activity
• Renal studies: urinalysis, BUN, urine creatinine, electrolytes q3mo; symptoms of renal colic
• Hepatic studies: ALT, AST, bilirubin if patient receiving long-term treatment
• CBC during long-term therapy (anemia); serum bicarbonate (metabolic acidosis)
• **Migraines:** pain location, duration; alleviating factors
• Mental status: mood, sensorium, affect, behavioral changes, suicidal thoughts/behaviors; if mental status changes, notify prescriber

• Body weight, perception of body image; eating disorders may occur or be exacerbated, especially in adolescents; evidence of cognitive disorder
• Assistance with ambulation during early part of treatment; dizziness occurs
• **Pregnancy/breastfeeding:** use only if benefits outweigh fetal risk, birth defects have occurred; pregnant patients should register with the Antiepileptic Drug Pregnancy Registry, 1-888-233-2334; may decrease effectiveness of hormonal contraceptives; cautious use in breastfeeding, excretion unknown
• **Beers:** avoid in older adults unless safer alternative is unavailable; may cause ataxia, impaired psychomotor function
Evaluate:
• Therapeutic response: decreased seizure activity
Teach patient/family:
• To carry emergency ID stating patient's name, products taken, condition, prescriber's name, and phone number
• To avoid driving, other activities that require alertness, until response is known
• Not to discontinue medication quickly after long-term use; do not restart without close supervision if several doses are missed; to follow prescriber's directions closely
• To notify prescriber immediately of blurred vision, periorbital pain; that vision loss may occur
• To maintain adequate fluid intake
• About administration procedure and expected results
• To use nonhormonal contraceptive; that effect of oral contraceptives is decreased
• To drink plenty of fluids to prevent kidney stones
• May need to increase amount of food consumed; weight loss may occur
• To swallow ext rel product whole
• That minor hair loss may occur; to report to prescriber if severe

> **▲ HIGH ALERT**

topotecan (Rx)

(toh-poh-tee′kan)

Hycamtin

Func. class.: Antineoplastic, natural; topoisomerase inhibitor

Chem. class.: Camptothecin analog

ACTION: Antitumor product with topoisomerase-I–inhibitory activity; topoisomerase I relieves torsional strain in DNA by causing single-strand breaks; also causes double-strand DNA damage

USES: Metastatic ovarian cancer after failure of traditional chemotherapy; relapsed small-cell lung cancer; cervical cancer

Unlabeled uses: Non–small-cell lung cancer (NSCLC), rhabdomyosarcoma

CONTRAINDICATIONS: Pregnancy, breastfeeding, hypersensitivity, severe bone marrow depression

> **Black Box Warning:** Neutropenia, bone marrow suppression

Precautions: Children, renal disease, gelatin hypersensitivity, anemia, contraceptive requirements, dehydration, diarrhea, extravasation, herpes, infertility, neutropenia, pulmonary fibrosis, varicella

DOSAGE AND ROUTES

Metastatic carcinoma of the ovary

• **Adult:** IV INFUSION 1.5 mg/m^2 over 30 min daily × 5 days starting on day 1 of 21-day course × 4 courses

Persistent cervical cancer

• **Adult:** IV INFUSION 0.75 mg/m^2 on days 1, 2, 3 then 50 mg/m^2 cisplatin IV on day 1 then repeat q21days; adjust for toxicity

Relapsed small-cell lung cancer

• **Adult:** PO 2.3 mg/m^2/day × 5 days then repeat q21days

Hematologic toxicity

• Do not administer subsequent courses until neutrophils recover to >1000 cells/mm^3, platelets to >100,000 cells/mm^3, and hemoglobin to >9 g/dL

Neutropenia

• Single agent IV (ANC <500 cells/mm^3): Reduce dose of topotecan to 1.25 mg/m^2. Alternatively, granulocyte-colony stimulating factor (G-CSF) may be administered, starting at least 24 hr after last dose of topotecan

• Single agent PO (ANC <500 cells/mm^3 for ≥7 days, or ANC 500–1000 cells/mm^3 lasting beyond day 21): Reduce dose of topotecan to 1.9 mg/m^2/day, with subsequent dose reductions by 0.4 mg/m^2/day if necessary

Thrombocytopenia

• Single agent IV (platelets <25,000 cells/mm^3 in the previous cycle): Reduce dose to 1.25 mg/m^2

• Single agent PO (platelets <25,000 cells/mm^3): Reduce dose to 1.9 mg/m^2/day, with subsequent dose reductions by 0.4 mg/m^2/day if necessary

• In combination with CISplatin IV (platelets <25,000 cells/mm^3 in the previous cycle): Reduce dose to 0.6 mg/m^2, and further to 0.45 mg/m^2 if necessary

Neutropenic fever

• Single agent PO (ANC <500 cells/mm^3 associated with fever or infection): Reduce to 1.9 mg/m^2/day, with subsequent dose reductions by 0.4 mg/m^2/day if necessary

T

• In combination with CISplatin **IV** (ANC <1000 cells/mm³ with temperature ≥38° C or 100.4° F): Reduce dose to 0.6 mg/m², and further to 0.45 mg/m² if necessary. Alternatively, G-CSF may be given, starting at least 24 hr after last dose

Diarrhea (grade 3 or 4)

• Single agent **PO:** Hold; when diarrhea resolves to grade ≤1, resume at 1.9 mg/m²/day, with subsequent dose reductions by 0.4 mg/m²/day if necessary

Renal dose

• **Adult: PO** CCr ≥50 mL/min: No change; CCr 30-49 mL/min: Reduce dose to 1.5 mg/m²/day; dose may be increased by 0.4 mg/m²/day after the first course if no severe hematologic or gastrointestinal toxicities occur; CCr <30 mL/min: Reduce dose to 0.6 mg/m²/day; dose may be increased by 0.4 mg/m²/day after the first course if no severe hematologic or gastrointestinal toxicities occur

• **Adult: IV** CCr 40-60 mL/min: No change; CCr 20-39 mL/min: Reduce dose to 0.75 mg/m²; CCr <20 mL/min: unknown

Available forms

• Lyophilized powder for inj 4 mg; caps 0.25, 1 mg

Administer:

• Store caps in refrigerator; IV INFUSION unopened at room temperature; protect both from light

PO route

• Do not break, crush, chew, or open caps; protect from light

• Take without regard to food

Intermittent IV INFUSION route

• Visually inspect for particulate matter and discoloration before use

• Reconstitute each 4-mg vial with 4 mL sterile water for injection; use immediately; no preservative

• Withdraw the appropriate volume of the reconstituted solution; dilute further; dilute in 0.9% NaCl or D₅W before administration

• The reconstituted solution is yellow or yellow-green

• Topotecan injection diluted for infusion is stable at room temperature with normal light for 24 hr

• Infuse over 30 min

SIDE EFFECTS

CNS: Arthralgia, *asthenia, headache,* myalgia, *pain,* weakness

GI: *Abdominal pain, constipation,* diarrhea, obstruction, *nausea,* stomatitis, *vomiting;* increased ALT, AST; anorexia

HEMA: Neutropenia, leukopenia, thrombocytopenia, anemia, sepsis

INTEG: *Total alopecia*

RESP: Dyspnea, cough, interstitial lung disease

PHARMACOKINETICS

Rapidly and completely absorbed, excreted in urine and feces as metabolites, half-life 2.8 hr, 7%-35% bound to plasma proteins, PO Peak 1-2 hr

INTERACTIONS

• Avoid use with P-glycoprotein, breast cancer resistance protein inhibitors (amiodarone, clarithromycin, diltiaZEM, erythromycin, indinavir), quiNIDine, testosterone, verapamil, tamoxifen, itraconazole, mefloquine, RU-486, niCARdipine, vaccines, toxoids

Increase: myelosuppression when used with CISplatin

Increase: bleeding risk—NSAIDs, anticoagulants, thrombolytics, platelet inhibitors

Drug/Food

• Avoid use with grapefruit juice

NURSING CONSIDERATIONS

Assess:

• Hepatic studies: AST, ALT, alk phos, which may be elevated; creatinine, BUN

Black Box Warning: **Bone marrow suppression:** CBC, differential, platelet count weekly; withhold product if WBC is <3500/mm³ or platelet count is <100,000/mm³; notify prescriber of results; product should be discontinued

• **Pregnancy/breastfeeding:** do not use in pregnancy or breastfeeding, can cause fetal harm; use contraception during and for ≥1 mo after final dose (female), during and for 3 mo after final dose (males); may cause infertility in both males/females

• Buccal cavity for dryness, sores or ulcerations, white patches, oral pain, bleeding, dysphagia

- **Interstitial lung disease (ILD):** fever, cough, dyspnea, hypoxia; may be fatal
- Increased fluid intake to 2-3 L/day to prevent dehydration unless contraindicated

Evaluate:
- Therapeutic response: decreased tumor size, spread of malignancy

Teach patient/family:
- That total alopecia may occur; that hair grows back but is different in color and texture
- To avoid foods with citric acid, hot temperature, or rough texture if stomatitis is present; to drink adequate fluids
- To report stomatitis and any bleeding, white spots, ulcerations in mouth; to examine mouth daily; to report symptoms

Black Box Warning: To report signs of anemia: fatigue, headache, faintness, SOB, irritability

- Rinsing of mouth tid-qid with water, club soda; brushing of teeth bid-tid with soft brush or cotton-tipped applicator for stomatitis; to use unwaxed dental floss
- To use effective contraception during treatment and for 6 mo after; that males should use contraception during and for 3 mo after final dose; not to breastfeed
- To avoid OTC products without approval of prescriber
- To avoid driving or other activities requiring alertness
- To avoid vaccines, toxoids
- Not to crush, chew capsules
- Not to retake dose if vomiting occurs; to notify prescriber

---

RARELY USED

toremifene (Rx)
(tor-em'ih-feen)
Fareston
Func. class.: Antineoplastic
Chem. class.: Antiestrogen hormone

USES: Advanced breast carcinoma not responsive to other therapy in estrogen receptor–positive patients (usually postmenopausal)

CONTRAINDICATIONS: Pregnancy, hypersensitivity, history of thromboembolism

Black Box Warning: QT prolongation

DOSAGE AND ROUTES
- **Adult: PO** 60 mg/day

---

torsemide (Rx)
(tor'suh-mide)
Demadex
Func. class.: Loop diuretic
Chem. class.: Sulfonamide derivative

ACTION: Acts on loop of Henle by inhibiting absorption of chloride, sodium, water

USES: Treatment of hypertension and edema with HF, ascites

CONTRAINDICATIONS: Infants, hypersensitivity to sulfonamides, anuria
Precautions: Pregnancy, breastfeeding, diabetes mellitus, dehydration, severe renal disease, electrolyte depletion, hypovolemia, syncope, ventricular dysrhythmias

DOSAGE AND ROUTES
HF diuresis
- **Adult: PO** 10-20 mg/day, may increase as needed, max 200 mg/day

Diuresis in chronic renal failure
- **Adult: PO** 20 mg/day, may increase to 200 mg/day

Hepatic cirrhosis
- **Adult: PO** 5-10 mg/day, may increase as needed, max 40 mg/day

Hypertension
- **Adult: PO** 5 mg/day, may increase to 10 mg/day

Available forms: Tabs 5, 10, 20, 100 mg

Administer:

PO route

• In AM to avoid interference with sleep if using product as diuretic

• With food or milk if nausea occurs; absorption may be decreased slightly

SIDE EFFECTS

CNS: *Headache, dizziness,* asthenia, insomnia, nervousness

CV: Orthostatic hypotension, chest pain, ECG changes, circulatory collapse, ventricular tachycardia, edema

EENT: *Loss of hearing,* ear pain, tinnitus, blurred vision

ELECT: *Hypokalemia, hypochloremic alkalosis, hyponatremia,* metabolic alkalosis

ENDO: *Hyperglycemia, hyperuricemia*

GI: *Nausea,* diarrhea, dyspepsia, cramps, constipation

GU: *Polyuria,* renal failure, glycosuria

INTEG: *Rash,* photosensitivity, pruritus

MS: Cramps, stiffness

RESP: Rhinitis, cough increase

PHARMACOKINETICS

PO: Rapidly absorbed; duration 6 hr; excreted in breast milk; crosses placenta; half-life 3.5 hr; protein binding 97%-99%, cleared through hepatic metabolism

INTERACTIONS

Increase: toxicity—lithium, nondepolarizing skeletal muscle relaxants, digoxin

Increase: action of antihypertensives, oral anticoagulants, nitrates; cautious use

Increase: ototoxicity—aminoglycosides, CISplatin, vancomycin; cautious use

Decrease: antihypertensive effect of torsemide—indomethacin, carBAMazepine, PHENobarbital, phenytoin, rifAMPin, NSAIDs

Decrease: hypoglycemic effect—antidiabetics; monitor blood glucose levels often

Drug/Herb

• Severe photosensitivity: St. John's wort

Drug/Lab Test

Increase: BUN, creatinine, uric acid, blood glucose, cholesterol

Decrease: potassium, magnesium, chloride sodium

NURSING CONSIDERATIONS

Assess:

• **Heart failure:** B/P lying, standing; postural hypotension may occur; weight, I&O daily to determine fluid loss; effect of product may be decreased if used daily

• Hearing when giving high doses

• **Sulfa allergy:** determine before using product

• Electrolytes: potassium, sodium, chlorine; include blood glucose, CBC, blood pH, ABGs, uric acid; calcium, magnesium, potassium supplements may be required

• Blood glucose of diabetic patients, glycosuria

• **Renal failure:** monitor urinalysis, BUN, CCr

• **Hyperuricemia:** exacerbation of gout may occur

• **Metabolic alkalosis:** drowsiness, restlessness

• **Hypokalemia:** postural hypotension, malaise, fatigue, tachycardia, leg cramps, weakness

• Rashes, temperature elevation daily

• Confusion, especially in geriatric patients; take safety precautions if needed

• **Pregnancy/breastfeeding:** use only if clearly needed, no well-controlled studies; cautious use in breastfeeding

• **Beers:** use with caution in older adults; may exacerbate or cause SIADH or hyponatremia; monitor sodium levels frequently

Evaluate:

• Therapeutic response: improvement in edema of feet, legs, sacral area daily if medication is being used with HF

Teach patient/family:

• To rise slowly from lying, sitting position

• To recognize adverse reactions: muscle cramps, weakness, nausea, dizziness, tinnitus

---

- To take with food or milk for GI symptoms; to limit alcohol use
- To take early during the day to prevent nocturia
- To use sunscreen, protective clothing to prevent sunburn
- To notify prescriber if pregnancy is planned or suspected
- To report tinnitus immediately; may indicate toxicity
- Not to use any OTC medications, herbal products before approved by prescriber

TREATMENT OF OVERDOSE:
Lavage if taken orally; monitor electrolytes; administer dextrose in saline; monitor hydration, CV, renal status

---

⚠ HIGH ALERT

traMADol (Rx)
(tram′a-dole)
ConZip, Durela ✦, Raliva ✦, Tridural ✦, Ultram, Ultram ER, Zytram ✦
Func. class.: Analgesic—miscellaneous

Controlled Substance Schedule IV

Do not confuse:
traMADol/traZODone
Ultram/lithium

ACTION: Binds to μ-opioid receptors, inhibits reuptake of norepinephrine, serotonin

USES: Management of moderate to severe pain, chronic pain
Unlabeled uses: Restless legs syndrome (RLS), postoperative shivering, arthralgia/myalgia, bone/dental/neuropathic pain, headache, osteoarthritis

CONTRAINDICATIONS: Hypersensitivity, acute intoxication with any CNS depressant, alcohol, asthma, children, adenoidectomy, GI obstruction ileus, MAOIs

Black Box Warning: Respiratory depression

Precautions: Pregnancy, breastfeeding, geriatric patients, seizure disorder, renal/hepatic disease, head trauma, increased intracranial pressure, acute abdominal condition, drug abuse, depression, suicidal ideation, abrupt discontinuation, constipation

Black Box Warning: Coadministration with other CNS depressants, neonatal opioid withdrawal syndrome

DOSAGE AND ROUTES
Mild to moderate pain
- **Adult: PO** 25 mg daily, titrate by 25 mg ≥3 days to 100 mg/day (25 mg qid), then may increase by 50 mg ≥3 days to 200 mg (50 mg qid), then 50-100 mg q4-6hr, max 400 mg/day, use caution in geriatric patients
- **Geriatric >75 years: PO** <300 mg/day in divided doses

Moderate to severe chronic pain
- **Adult: PO-ER** (Ultram ER) 100 mg daily, titrate upward q5days in 100-mg increments, max 300 mg/day; (Ryzolt) 100 mg, titrate upward q2-3days in 100-mg increments, max 300 mg/day; products are not interchangeable

Renal dose
- **Adult: PO** CCr <30 mL/min, give regular dose q12hr, max 200 mg/day; do not use ext rel tab

Hepatic dose
- **Adult: PO** (Child-Pugh C) 50 mg q12hr; do not use ext rel tab

Restless legs syndrome (RLS) (unlabeled)
- **Adult: PO** 50-150 mg/day × 15-24 mo
Available forms: Tabs 50 mg; ext rel tab 100, 200, 300 mg
Administer:
- Some ext rel products (Ultram ER) are not interchangeable
- Do not break, crush, or chew ext rel product
- With antiemetic for nausea, vomiting

Side effects: *italics* = common; red = life-threatening

• When pain is beginning to return; determine dosage interval by patient response

• With or without food; ER: always give with food, or always give on empty stomach

• Store in cool environment; protected from sunlight

SIDE EFFECTS

CNS: Dizziness, CNS stimulation, somnolence, headache, anxiety, confusion, euphoria, seizures, hallucinations, sedation, neuroleptic malignant syndrome–like reactions

CV: Vasodilation, orthostatic hypotension, tachycardia, hypertension, abnormal ECG

EENT: Visual disturbances

GI: Nausea, constipation, vomiting, dry mouth, diarrhea, abdominal pain, anorexia, flatulence, GI bleeding

GU: Urinary retention/frequency, menopausal symptoms, dysuria, menstrual disorder

INTEG: Pruritus, rash, urticaria, vesicles, flushing

SYST: Anaphylaxis, Stevens-Johnson syndrome, toxic epidermal necrolysis, serotonin syndrome

PHARMACOKINETICS

Rapidly and almost completely absorbed, steady state 2 days, peak 1.5 hr, duration 6 hr, half-life 7.9-8.8 hr (PO), 8-10 hr (ext rel), may cross blood-brain barrier, extensively metabolized, 30% excreted in urine as unchanged product, protein binding 20%

INTERACTIONS

• Inhibition of norepinephrine and serotonin reuptake: MAOIs; use together with caution

Black Box Warning: **Increase:** CNS depression—alcohol, sedatives, hypnotics, opiates

Increase: serotonin syndrome—SSRIs, SNRIs, serotonin-receptor agonists

Increase: traMADol levels—CYP3A4 inhibitors (aprepitant, antiretroviral protease inhibitors, clarithromycin, danazol, delavirdine, diltiaZEM, erythromycin, fluconazole, FLUoxetine, fluvoxaMINE, imatinib, ketoconazole, mibefradil, nefazodone, telithromycin, voriconazole)

Decrease: traMADol effects—CYP3A4 inducers (barbiturates, bosentan, carBAMazepine, efavirenz, phenytoins, nevirapine, rifabutin, rifAMPin)

Decrease: levels of traMADol—carBAMazepine

Drug/Herb

• Avoid use with St. John's wort

Increase: CNS depression—chamomile, hops, kava, skullcap, valerian

Drug/Lab Test

Increase: creatinine, hepatic enzymes

Decrease: Hgb

NURSING CONSIDERATIONS

Assess:

• **Pain:** location, type, character; give before pain becomes extreme

Black Box Warning: **Respiratory depression:** withhold if respirations <12/min; may be compounded by use of other CNS depressants

Black Box Warning: **Neonatal opioid withdrawal syndrome:** prolonged use of opioids in the mother may result in withdrawal effects in the neonate; can be fatal; assess for irritability, hyperactivity, abnormal sleep pattern, high-pitched cry, tremor, vomiting, diarrhea, failure to gain weight in the neonate

• I&O ratio: check for decreasing output; may indicate urinary retention

• Need for product; dependency

• Bowel pattern; for constipation; increase fluids, bulk in diet

• CNS changes: dizziness, drowsiness, hallucinations, euphoria, LOC, pupil reaction; avoid use with other CNS depressants

• **Hypersensitivity:** usually after beginning treatment

- Increased side effects in renal/hepatic disease
- **Serotonin syndrome, neuroleptic malignant syndrome:** increased heart rate, shivering, sweating, dilated pupils, tremors, high B/P, hyperthermia, headache, confusion; if these occur, stop product, administer serotonin antagonist if needed
- Assistance with ambulation
- Safety measures: side rails, night-light, call bell within easy reach
- **Pregnancy/breastfeeding:** use only if benefits outweigh fetal risk, no well-controlled studies; do not use in labor/delivery; do not breastfeed
- **Beers:** avoid in older adults; may lower seizure threshold; monitor for seizures frequently in those with a seizure disorder

Evaluate:
- Therapeutic response: decrease in pain

Teach patient/family:
- Before taking, to inform health care provider of any history of head injury; seizures; liver, kidney, thyroid problems; problems in urinating; pancreas or gallbladder problems; abuse of street or prescription drugs; alcohol addiction; or mental health problems
- Not to take other prescription medications, OTC products, vitamins, or herbal supplements without approval from health care provider
- To take exactly as prescribed by health care provider; not to take more than prescribed dose and not to take >8 tablets/day. If dose is missed, to take the next dose at usual time
- To notify health care provider if the prescribed dose does not control pain
- Not to stop product abruptly if taking regularly without talking to health care provider
- Not to drive or operate heavy machinery until effects of product are known; may cause dizziness or light-headedness
- Not to drink alcohol or use a prescription or OTC product that contains alcohol
- To notify health care provider of severe constipation, nausea, sleepiness, vomiting, tiredness, headache, dizziness, abdominal pain
- To get emergency medical help for difficulty in breathing, shortness of breath, fast heartbeat, chest pain, swelling of face, tongue, or throat, extreme drowsiness, light-headedness when changing positions, feeling faint, agitation, high body temperature, trouble walking, stiff muscles, or mental changes such as confusion
- To notify health care provider if pregnancy is planned or suspected. Prolonged use during pregnancy can cause withdrawal symptoms in neonate that could be life threatening if not recognized and treated. Do not breastfeed

---

⚠ HIGH ALERT

RARELY USED

trametinib
(tra-me′ti-nib)
MeKinist
Func. class.: Antineoplastic biologic response modifiers
Chem. class.: Signal transduction inhibitors (STIs), tyrosine kinase inhibitor

USES: Unresectable or metastatic BRAD V600E or BRAF V600K mutated malignant melanoma

CONTRAINDICATIONS: Pregnancy, hypersensitivity

DOSAGE AND ROUTES
Unresectable or metastatic malignant melanoma
- **Adult: PO** 2 mg daily; may be used in combination with dacarbazine or PACLitaxel in those with BRAF V600E

Unresectable or metastatic malignant melanoma
• **Adult: PO** 2 mg daily with dabrafenib 150 mg q12hr until disease progression, take both at same time

Management of treatment-related toxicity
Cutaneous toxicity:
• **Grade 2 rash:** reduce dose by 0.5 mg (e.g., 2 mg/day to 1.5 mg/day) or discontinue in patients who are receiving trametinib 1 mg/day; in patients with an intolerable grade 2 rash that does not improve within 3 wk of a dosage reduction, withhold trametinib for up to 3 wk; if the rash is improved within 3 wk, resume therapy at a lower dose (reduce the previous dose by 0.5 mg); discontinue in patients who are receiving trametinib 1 mg/day; if the rash does not improve within 3 wk, permanently discontinue
• **Grade 3 or 4 rash:** withhold for up to 3 wk; if the rash is improved within 3 wk, resume at a lower dose (reduce the previous dose by 0.5 mg); discontinue in patients who are receiving trametinib 1 mg/day; if the rash does not improve within 3 wk, permanently discontinue therapy

Cardiac toxicity:
• **Asymptomatic cardiac toxicity and an absolute decrease in LVEF of ≥10% from baseline and is below institutional lower limits of normal (LLN) from pretreatment value:** withhold for up to 4 wk; if the LVEF is improved within 4 wk, resume at a lower dose (reduce the previous dose by 0.5 mg); discontinue in patients who are receiving 1 mg/day; if the LVEF does not improve to normal within 4 wk, permanently discontinue
• **Symptomatic HF or an absolute decrease in LVEF of >20% from baseline and is below institutional LLN:** permanently discontinue

Ocular toxicity:
• **Grade 2 or 3 retinal pigment epithelial detachment (RPED):** withhold for up to 3 wk; if the RPED improves to grade 1 or less within 3 wk, resume at a lower dose (reduce the previous dose by 0.5 mg); discontinue therapy in patients who are receiving 1 mg/day; if the RPED does not improve to at least grade 1 within 3 wk, permanently discontinue
• **Retinal vein occlusion:** permanently discontinue therapy

Pulmonary toxicity
• **Interstitial lung disease/pneumonitis:** permanently discontinue

Other toxicity:
• **Grade 3 toxicity:** withhold for up to 3 wk: if the toxicity improves to grade 1 or less within 3 wk, resume at a lower dose (reduce the previous dose by 0.5 mg); discontinue in patients who are receiving 1 mg/day; if the toxicity does not improve to at least grade 1 within 3 wk, permanently discontinue
• **Grade 4 toxicity:** permanently discontinue

RARELY USED

trandolapril (Rx)
(tran-doe'la-prill)
Func. class.: Antihypertensive
Chem. class.: Angiotension-converting enzyme inhibitor

USES: Hypertension, heart failure, left ventricular dysfunction post MI

CONTRAINDICATIONS: Breastfeeding, hypersensitivity, history of angioedema

Black Box Warning: Pregnancy

DOSAGE AND ROUTES
Hypertension
• **Adult: PO** 1 mg/day; 2 mg/day in African Americans; make dosage adjustment ≥1 wk; max 8 mg/day

Heart failure, left ventricular dysfunction post MI
• **Adult: PO** 1 mg/day, titrate upward to 4 mg/day if tolerated, continue for 2-4 yr

Renal/hepatic dose
• **Adult: PO** CCr <30 mL/min or hepatic disease, 0.5 mg/day

---

A HIGH ALERT

trastuzumab (Rx)
(tras-tuz'uh-mab)
Herceptin
Func. class.: Antineoplastic—miscellaneous
Chem. class.: Humanized monoclonal antibody

ACTION: DNA-derived monoclonal antibody selectively binds to extracellular portion of human epidermal growth factor receptor 2; it inhibits the proliferation of cancer cells

USES: Breast cancer; metastatic with overexpression of *Θσ* HER2, early breast cancer (adjuvant, neoadjuvant), gastric cancer; previously untreated HER2 overexpressing metastatic gastric or gastroesophageal junction adenocarcinoma with CISplatin, 5-fluorouracil, or capecitabine

CONTRAINDICATIONS: Hypersensitivity to this product, Chinese hamster ovary cell protein
Precautions: Breastfeeding, children, geriatric patients, pulmonary disease, anemia, leukopenia

Black Box Warning: Respiratory distress syndrome, respiratory insufficiency, infusion-related reactions, cardiomyopathy, contraception requirement, pregnancy, pulmonary toxicity

DOSAGE AND ROUTES
HER2-positive, node-positive or node-negative (ER/PR negative) in combination (AC-TH)
• **Adult: IV** 4 mg/kg over 90 min on day 1, then 2 mg/kg over 30 min q wk for a total of 12 wk, with PACLitaxel (either 80 mg/m² **IV** wk or 175 mg/m² q3wk) beginning on day 1 for a total of 4 cycles (12 wk). On week 13, begin trastuzumab 6 mg/kg over 30-90 min q3wk as monotherapy for a total of 52 wk of trastuzumab therapy; begin PACLitaxel plus trastuzumab after the completion of 4 cycles of AC chemotherapy (doxorubicin 60 mg/m² **IV** and cyclophosphamide 600 mg/m² **IV** q21days)
HER2-positive, node-positive or node-negative (ER/PR negative) in combination (AC-TH)
• **Adult: IV** 4 mg/kg over 90 min on day 1, then 2 mg/kg over 30 min weekly (total of 12 wk), with DOCEtaxel 100 mg/m² **IV** q21days beginning on day 1 for a total of 4 cycles (12 wk). On week 13, begin trastuzumab 6 mg/kg **IV** over 30-90 min q3wk as monotherapy for a total of 52 wk of trastuzumab therapy. Begin DOCEtaxel plus trastuzumab after the completion of 4 cycles of AC chemotherapy (doxorubicin 60 mg/m² **IV** and cyclophosphamide 600 mg/m² **IV** q21days)
HER2-positive, node-positive or node-negative (ER/PR negative) in combination (TCH)
• **Adult: IV** 4 mg/kg over 90 min on day 1, then 2 mg/kg over 30 min weekly

T

(total of 18 wk), with DOCEtaxel 75 mg/m² IV followed by CARBOplatin AUC 6 IV over 30-60 min beginning on day 1, q3wk, for a total of 6 cycles (18 wk). On week 19, begin trastuzumab 6 mg/kg IV over 30-90 min q3wk as monotherapy (52 wk of trastuzumab)

HER2-positive, node-positive or node-negative (ER/PR negative) monotherapy

• **Adult:** IV 8 mg/kg over 90 min on day 1, followed by 6 mg/kg IV over 30-90 min q21days (total of 52 wk)

Available forms: Lyophilized powder 150, 440 mg

Administer:

• Acetaminophen as ordered to alleviate fever and headache

Intermittent IV INFUSION route

• Use cytotoxic handling procedures; avoid treatment >1 yr

• After reconstituting vial with 20 mL bacteriostatic water for inj, 1.1% benzyl alcohol preserved (supplied) to yield 21 mg/mL; mark date on vial 28 days from reconstitution date; if patient is allergic to benzyl alcohol, reconstitute with sterile water for inj; use immediately; infuse over 90 min; q3wk give 8 mg/kg loading dose over 90 min; subsequent 6 mg/kg dose may be given over 30-60 min

• Do not mix or dilute with other products or dextrose sol

SIDE EFFECTS

CNS: *Dizziness, numbness, paresthesias,* depression, *insomnia,* neuropathy, peripheral neuritis

CV: Tachycardia, heart failure

GI: Nausea, vomiting, *anorexia, diarrhea,* abdominal pain, hepatotoxicity, dysgeusia

HEMA: *Anemia,* leukopenia

INTEG: Rash, acne, herpes simplex

META: Edema, peripheral edema

MISC: *Flulike symptoms; fever, headache, chills*

MS: Arthralgia, *bone pain*

RESP: *Cough, dyspnea, pharyngitis, rhinitis,* sinusitis, pneumonia, pulmonary edema/fibrosis, acute respiratory distress syndrome (ARDS)

SYST: Anaphylaxis, angioedema

PHARMACOKINETICS

Half-life 1-32 days, 97% washout by 7 mo after end of treatment

Drug/Lab

Decrease: WBCs

INTERACTIONS

Increase: bleeding risk—warfarin

Increase: cardiomyopathy—anthracyclines, cyclophosphamide; avoid use

Decrease: immune response—vaccines, toxoids

NURSING CONSIDERATIONS

Assess:

• CBC, HER2 overexpression

Black Box Warning: HF, other cardiac symptoms: dyspnea, coughing; gallop; obtain full cardiac workup, including ECG, before and q3mo during treatment and q6mo for ≥2 yr after adjuvant treatment (LVEF, MUGA or ECHO); monitor for clinical deterioration in those with decreased LVEF

- Symptoms of infection; may be masked by product
- CNS reaction: LOC, mental status, dizziness, confusion
- Hypersensitivity reactions, anaphylaxis

Black Box Warning: Infusion reactions that may be fatal: fever, chills, nausea, vomiting, pain, headache, dizziness, hypotension; discontinue product

- **Pulmonary toxicity:** dyspnea, interstitial pneumonitis, pulmonary hypertension, ARDS; can occur after infusion reaction, those with lung disease may have more severe toxicity
- **Benzyl alcohol hypersensitivity:** reconstitute with Sterile Water for Injection, USP; discard any unused portion
- **Hamster protein hypersensitivity** (Chinese hamster ovary cell hypersensitivity): increased risk of severe allergic reactions
- **Pregnancy/breastfeeding:** fetal harm may occur if given during pregnancy or within 7 mo of conception; monitoring for oligohydramnios is recommended. If oligohydramnios occurs, fetal testing should be done that is appropriate for gestational age and is consistent with community standards of care. Encourage these women to enroll in the MotHER Pregnancy Registry, 1-800-690-6720 or http://www.motherpregnancyregistry.com. Effective contraception should be used during and for at least 7 mo after treatment; females of reproductive potential should undergo pregnancy testing before use. Women who become pregnant while receiving or within 7 mo of the last dose should be apprised of potential hazard to the fetus. Unknown whether product is excreted into breast milk; advise women to discontinue breastfeeding during treatment and for 7 mo after last dose

Evaluate:
- Therapeutic response: decrease in size of tumors

Teach patient/family:
- To take acetaminophen for fever
- To avoid hazardous tasks because confusion, dizziness may occur

- To report signs of infection: sore throat, fever, diarrhea, vomiting
- That emotional lability is common; to notify prescriber if severe or incapacitating

Black Box Warning: Pregnancy/breast-feeding: to use contraception while taking this product and for 7 mo after last dose; not to breastfeed during and for 7 mo after treatment

Black Box Warning: To report pain at infusion site, usually with first dose

Black Box Warning: Cardiomyopathy: to report cough, swelling in extremities, shortness of breath; may occur during or after completion of treatment

---

travoprost ophthalmic
See Appendix B

---

traZODone (Rx)
(tray´zoe-done)
Oleptro ✦, Trazorel ✦
Func. class.: Antidepressant—miscellaneous
Chem. class.: Triazolopyridine

Do not confuse:
traZODone/traMADol

ACTION: Selectively inhibits serotonin uptake by brain; potentiates behavioral changes

USES: Depression
Unlabeled uses: Anxiety, insomnia, chronic pain

CONTRAINDICATIONS: Hypersensitivity to tricyclics
Precautions: Pregnancy, suicidal patients, severe depression, increased intraocular pressure, closed-angle

T

---

glaucoma, urinary retention, cardiac/hepatic disease, hyperthyroidism, electroshock therapy, elective surgery, bleeding, abrupt discontinuation, bipolar disorder, breastfeeding, dehydration, hyponatremia, hypovolemia, recovery phase of MI, seizure disorders, prostatic hypertrophy, family history of long QT

> **Black Box Warning:** Suicidal ideation in children/adolescents

DOSAGE AND ROUTES
Depression
• **Adult: PO** 150 mg/day in divided doses, may increase by 50 mg/day q3-4days, max 400 mg/day (outpatient), 600 mg/day (inpatient); **EXT REL** 150 mg in PM, may increase gradually by 75 mg/day q3days, max 375 mg/day
• **Child 6-18 yr (unlabeled): PO** 1.5-2 mg/kg/day in divided doses, may increase q3-4days up to 6 mg/kg/day or 400 mg/day, whichever is less
• **Geriatric: PO** 25-50 mg at bedtime, increase by 25-50 mg q3-7days to desired dose, usually 75-150 mg/day
Alcoholism (unlabeled)
• **Adult: PO** 50-100 mg/day
Panic disorder (unlabeled)
• **Adult: PO** 150 mg in divided doses, may increase by 50 mg/day q3-4days
Available forms: Tabs 50, 100, 150, 300 mg; ext rel tabs 150, 300 mg
Administer:
• Increased fluids, bulk in diet if constipation occurs, especially in geriatric patients
• With food, milk for GI symptoms
• Dosage at bedtime for oversedation during day; may take entire dose at bedtime; geriatric patients may not tolerate daily dosing
• Avoid use of CNS depressants
• Do not crush, break, chew ext rel product
• Store in tight, light-resistant container at room temperature

SIDE EFFECTS
CNS: *Dizziness, drowsiness,* confusion, headache, anxiety, tremors, stimulation, weakness, insomnia, nightmares, EPS (geriatric patients), increase in psychiatric symptoms, suicide in children/adolescents
CV: *Orthostatic hypotension, ECG changes, tachycardia,* hypertension, palpitations
EENT: *Blurred vision,* tinnitus, mydriasis
GI: *Diarrhea, dry mouth,* nausea, vomiting, paralytic ileus, increased appetite, cramps, epigastric distress, jaundice, hepatitis, stomatitis, constipation
GU: *Urinary retention,* acute renal failure, priapism
HEMA: Agranulocytosis, thrombocytopenia, eosinophilia, leukopenia
INTEG: Rash, urticaria, sweating, pruritus, photosensitivity

PHARMACOKINETICS
Peak 1 hr without food, 2 hr with food; metabolized by liver (CYP3A4); excreted by kidneys, in feces; half-life 4.4-7.5 hr

INTERACTIONS
Hyperpyretic crisis, seizures, hypertensive episode: MAOIs; do not use within 14 days of traZODone
Increase: toxicity, serotonin syndrome—FLUoxetine, nefazodone, other SSRIs, SNRIs, linezolid; methylene blue (IV)
Increase: effects of direct-acting sympathomimetics (EPINEPHrine), alcohol, barbiturates, benzodiazepines, CNS depressants, digoxin, phenytoin, carBAMazepine
Increase: effects of traZODone—CYP3A4, 2D6 inhibitors (phenothiazines, protease inhibitors, azole antifungals)
Increase or decrease: effects of warfarin
Decrease: effects of guanethidine, cloNIDine, indirect-acting sympathomimetics (ePHEDrine)
Drug/Herb
Increase: serotonin syndrome—SAM-e, St. John's wort
Increase: CNS depression—hops, kava, lavender, valerian
Drug/Lab Test
Increase: LFTs
Decrease: Hgb

NURSING CONSIDERATIONS

Assess: B/P lying, standing; pulse q4hr; if systolic B/P drops 20 mm Hg, hold product, notify prescriber; take vital signs q4hr in patients with CV disease

• Blood studies: CBC, leukocytes, differential

• Hepatic studies: AST, ALT, bilirubin

• Weight weekly; appetite may increase with product

• ECG for flattening of T wave, bundle branch block, AV block, dysrhythmias in cardiac patients

• EPS, primarily in geriatric patients: rigidity, dystonia, akathisia

Black Box Warning: Mental status changes: mood, sensorium, affect, suicidal tendencies, increase in psychiatric symptoms, depression, panic; observe for suicidal behaviors in children/adolescents, not approved for children; if worsening depression occurs, product may need to be tapered as rapidly as possible, without abrupt discontinuation

• Urinary retention, constipation; constipation most likely in children

• Alcohol consumption; hold dose until morning

• **Serotonin syndrome, neuroleptic malignant syndrome:** increased heart rate, shivering, sweating, dilated pupils, tremors, high B/P, hyperthermia, headache, confusion; if these occur, stop product, administer serotonin antagonist if needed

• **Pregnancy/breastfeeding:** use only if benefits outweigh fetal risk; no well-controlled studies; cautious use in breastfeeding, excreted in breast milk

Evaluate:

• Therapeutic response: decreased depression

Teach patient/family:

• That therapeutic effects may take 2-3 wk; to take ext rel product before bedtime; not to crush, chew ext rel product

• To use caution when driving, performing other activities requiring alertness because of drowsiness, dizziness, blurred vision

• To avoid alcohol ingestion

• Not to discontinue medication quickly after long-term use; may cause nausea, headache, malaise

• To report urinary retention, priapism >4 hr immediately

• To wear sunscreen or large hat because photosensitivity occurs

Black Box Warning: That suicidal thoughts/behaviors may occur (adolescents/children); to notify health care professional if there is an increase in depression, agitation

• To notify prescriber if pregnancy is planned or suspected; to avoid breastfeeding

• To rise slowly to prevent dizziness

TREATMENT OF OVERDOSE:
ECG monitoring; lavage; administer anticonvulsant, atropine for bradycardia

---

treprostinil (Rx)
(treh-prah′stin-ill)
Remodulin, Tyvaso, Orenitram
Func. class.: Antihypertensive, vasodilators
Chem. class.: Tricyclic benzidine prostacyclin analog

ACTION: Direct vasodilation of pulmonary, systemic arterial vascular beds; inhibition of platelet aggregation

USES: Pulmonary arterial hypertension (PAH) NYHA class II through IV

Unlabeled uses: Pulmonary arterial hypertension in children/adolescents, pediatric patients transitioning from epoprostenol to treprostinil, claudication

CONTRAINDICATIONS: Hypersensitivity to this product, other prostacyclin analogs

Precautions: Pregnancy, breastfeeding, children, geriatric patients, past renal/hepatic disease, thromboembolic disease, abrupt discontinuation, IV administration

DOSAGE AND ROUTES
Pulmonary arterial hypertension
• **Adult: SUBCUT CONT INFUSION/IV CONT INFUSION** Initially, 1.25 ng/kg/min. If not tolerated, reduce to 0.625 ng/kg/min. Increase dose by increments ≤1.25 ng/kg/min per wk × first 4 wk, then no greater than 2.5 ng/kg/min per wk; **ORAL INH:** Initially, 3 breaths (18 mcg) inhaled via the Tyvaso Inhalation System qid 4 hr apart during waking hours; **PO:** 0.25 mg q12hr or 0.125 mg q8hr, increase by 0.25 or 0.5 mg bid or 0.125 mg tid q3-4days as tolerated

• **Adult taking gemfibrozil (or other strong CYP2C8 inhibitor): PO** 0.125 mg q12hr, increase by 0.125 mg bid q3-4days, as tolerated

For patients transitioning from IV or SUBCUT to PO
• **Adult: PO** For patients already receiving IV or **SUBCUT**, use the following equation to estimate a comparable total daily dose of **PO:** Total daily PO dose = 0.0072 × IV or SUBCUT dose (ng/kg/min) × Weight (kg). Reduce dose of IV or SUBCUT by up to 30 ng/kg/min per day while simultaneously increasing dose of PO up to 6 mg/day (2 mg PO tid), if tolerated

Hepatic dose
• **Adult: SUBCUT INFUSION** 0.625 ng/kg ideal body weight/min; increase cautiously

Available forms: Inj 1, 2.5, 5, 10 mg/mL; neb sol 1.74 mg/2.9 mL; ext rel tab 0.125, 0.25, 2.5 mg

Administer:
• Sudden decreased doses, abrupt withdrawal may worsen pulmonary arterial hypertension symptoms

PO route
• Give with food
• Swallow tablets whole; use only intact tablets

Injectable route
• Visually inspect for particulate matter and discoloration before use
• Administer injection by continuous SUBCUT infusion as the preferred route. May be administered by continuous IV infusion in those who do not tolerate continuous SUBCUT (severe injection site pain or reaction)
• Have immediate access to a backup infusion pump and infusion sets. Avoid abrupt discontinuation of the infusion. If temporary cessation is necessary for less than a few hours, the infusion can be restarted at the previously used dose and rate; if the infusion is stopped for longer than a few hours, retitration may be necessary

• The infusion pump used should be: small and lightweight; adjustable to approximately 0.002 mL/hr; have alarms for occlusion, end of infusion and low battery, programming error and motor malfunctions; accurate to +/− 6% of the programmed rate; positive-pressure driven. The reservoir should be made of polyvinyl chloride, polypropylene, or glass
• **Opened vials:** A single vial should be used ≤30 days after the initial entry into the vial

CONTINUOUS IV route
• Given via a surgically placed central venous catheter via an ambulatory infusion pump. A peripheral IV cannula, placed into a large vein, may be used temporarily; use of a peripheral vein for more than a few hours may increase the risk of thrombophlebitis
• Infusion sets with an in-line 0.22- or 0.2-micron pore size filter should be used

IV infusion preparation
• May be diluted with Remodulin sterile diluent for injection or similar approved high-pH glycine diluents (sterile diluent for Flolan or sterile diluent for epoprostenol sodium), sterile water for injection, or 0.9% NaCl for injection
• The concentration of diluted treprostinil should be calculated using the following formula: diluted concentration = [dose (ng/kg/min) × weight (kg) × 0.00006] / IV infusion rate (mL/hr)
• Typical ambulatory infusion pump reservoirs have volumes of 50 or 100 mL.

The IV infusion rate is predetermined based on the volume of the reservoir with a desired infusion length of 48 hr (i.e., for a 50-mL reservoir, the infusion rate would be 1 mL/hr; for a 100-mL reservoir, the infusion rate would be 2 mL/hr)
• The reservoir should be filled with the calculated volume and a sufficient amount of diluent to achieve the total volume of the reservoir
• Once diluted with any diluent, may be given for 48 hr at 40° C
• **Storage:** If diluted with sterile water for injection or 0.9% NaCl, store up to 4 hr at room temperature or 24 hr if refrigerated. If diluted with an approved high-pH glycine diluent (sterile diluent for Remodulin, Flolan, or epoprostenol sodium), it may be stored for 14 days at room temperature at concentrations as low as 0.004 mg/mL

SUBCUT continuous infusion
• Give via a self-inserted SUBCUT catheter using an ambulatory infusion pump designed for subcutaneous drug delivery
SUBCUT infusion preparation
• Further dilution is NOT required before continuous SUBCUT use
• Do not mix or co-infuse with other medications
• The SUBCUT infusion rate can be calculated using the following formula: SUBCUT infusion rate = [dose (ng/kg/min) × weight (kg) × 0.00006] / treprostinil vial strength (mg/mL)

• During SUBCUT use, a single reservoir (syringe) of product can be given ≤72 hr at a max temperature of 37° C (98.6° F)

Oral inhalation administration

• Must be used only with the Tyvaso Inhalation System

• Avoid skin or eye contact with solution. Do not take PO

• Have access to a backup Optineb-ir device to avoid interruptions in therapy

• Do not mix with other medications in the Optineb-ir device

• One ampule contains a volume for all 4 treatment sessions in a single day

SIDE EFFECTS

CNS: Dizziness, headache, syncope

CV: Vasodilation, *hypotension, edema,* right ventricular heart failure

GI: Nausea, *diarrhea*

INTEG: *Rash,* pruritus

OTHER: Jaw pain, cough, throat irritation

SYST: Infusion-site reactions, pain; increased risk for infection

PHARMACOKINETICS

Metabolized by liver; excreted in urine, feces; terminal half-life 2-4 hr; 90% protein binding

INTERACTIONS

• Excessive hypotension: diuretics, antihypertensives, vasodilators, MAOIs, β-blockers, calcium channel blockers

Increase: bleeding tendencies—anticoagulants, aspirin, NSAIDs, thrombin inhibitors, SSRIs

NURSING CONSIDERATIONS

Assess:

• Avoid abrupt discontinuation

• **Hypertension:** monitor B/P, baseline and periodically

• Hepatic studies: AST, ALT, bilirubin, creatinine with long-term therapy

• Blood studies: CBC; CBC q2wk × 3 mo, Hct, Hgb, PT with long-term therapy, ABGs

• Bleeding time at baseline, throughout treatment; levels may be 2-5× normal limit

• **Beers:** use with caution in older adults; may exacerbate episodes of syncope; monitor frequently

• **Pregnancy/breastfeeding:** use only if clearly needed, no well-controlled studies; cautious use in breastfeeding, excretion unknown

Evaluate:

• Therapeutic response: decreased pulmonary arterial hypertension (PAH)

Teach patient/family:

• That blood work will be necessary during treatment; that treatment may last for years

• To report side effects such as diarrhea, skin rashes

• That therapy will be needed for prolonged periods of time, sometimes years

• To use aseptic technique for preparation, administration of treprostinil to prevent infection

• That there are many product, herbal interactions

• **Tablet:** to take with food; not to crush or chew tablets, not to skip doses

• **Subcut:** about injection technique; to rotate injection sites; to avoid irritated, scarred, or bruised skin

• **Inhalation:** to avoid contact of solution with skin or eyes; to wash hands after handling inhaler; to follow directions for use in package insert

• How to use inhaled solution; how to care for equipment

• About signs, symptoms of bleeding; blood in urine, stools

tretinoin (vit A acid, retinoic acid) (Rx)

(tret′i-noyn)

Avita, Renova, Retin-A, Retin-A Micro, Stieva-A ✦

Func. class.: Vit A acid, acne product; antineoplastic (miscellaneous)

Chem. class.: Tretinoin derivative

ACTION: (Topical) Decreases cohesiveness of follicular epithelium, decreases microcomedone formation; (PO) induces maturation of acute promyelocytic leukemia, exact action is unknown

USES: (Topical) Acne vulgaris (grades 1-3); (PO) acute promyelocytic leukemia, facial wrinkles, photoaging

Unlabeled uses: Acne rosacea, actinic keratosis, ichthyosis, Kaposi's sarcoma, keloids, keratosis follicularis, melasma

CONTRAINDICATIONS: Hypersensitivity to retinoids or sensitivity to parabens

Black Box Warning: Pregnancy (PO)

Precautions: Pregnancy (topical), breastfeeding, eczema, sunburn, sun exposure

Black Box Warning: Rapid-evolving leukocytosis, respiratory compromise, acute promyelocytic leukemia differentiation syndrome, requires a specialized care setting, experienced clinician

DOSAGE AND ROUTES

• **Adult/child:** TOP cleanse area, apply 0.025%-0.1% cream or 0.05% liquid gel at bedtime, cover lightly

Promyelocytic leukemia

• **Adult:** PO 45 mg/m²/day given as 2 evenly divided doses until remission, discontinue treatment 30 days after remission or 90 days after start of treatment, whichever is first

Available forms: Cream 0.01%, 0.02%, 0.025%, 0.05%, 0.1%; gel 0.01%, 0.025%, 0.04%, 0.05%, 0.1%; liquid 0.05%; caps 10 mg

Administer:

Topical route

• Once daily before bedtime; cover area lightly using gauze; use gloves to apply

• Store at room temperature

• Handwashing after application

SIDE EFFECTS

PO route

CNS: *Headache, fever, sweating,* fatigue

CV: Cardiac dysrhythmias, pericardial effusion

GI: *Nausea, vomiting,* hemorrhage, *abdominal pain, diarrhea, constipation, dyspepsia, distention, hepatitis*

Topical route

INTEG: Rash, stinging, warmth, redness, erythema, blistering, crusting, peeling, contact dermatitis, hypo/hyperpigmentation, dry skin, pruritus, scaly skin, retinoic acid syndrome (RAS)

META: Hypercholesterolemia, hypertriglyceridemia

RESP: Pneumonia, upper respiratory tract disease

PHARMACOKINETICS

PO: Terminal half-life 0.5-2 hr

TOPICAL: Poor systemic absorption

INTERACTIONS

• Use with caution: medicated, abrasive soaps; cleansers that have a drying effect; products with high concentration of alcohol astringents (topical)

Increase: peeling—medication containing agents such as sulfur, benzoyl peroxide, resorcinol, salicylic acid (topical)

Increase: plasma concentrations of tretinoin—ketoconazole (PO)

Increase: ICP, risk of pseudotumor cerebri—tetracyclines; do not use together

Increase: photosensitivity—retinoids, quinolones, phenothiazines, sulfonamides, sulfonylureas, thiazide diuretics

T

Increase: thrombotic complications—aminocaproic acid, aprotinin, tranexamic acid

Drug/Lab Test
Increase: AST, ALT

NURSING CONSIDERATIONS
Assess:
Topical route
• Area of body involved, what helps or aggravates condition; cysts, dryness, itching; lesions may worsen at beginning of treatment

PO route
• Hepatic function, coagulation, hematologic parameters; also cholesterol, triglycerides
• **Pregnancy/breastfeeding:** do not use PO in pregnancy, breastfeeding

Evaluate:
• Therapeutic response: decrease in size, number of lesions

Teach patient/family:
Topical route
• To avoid application on normal skin; to avoid getting cream in eyes, nose, other mucous membranes; not to use product on areas with cuts, scrapes
• To use cream/gel by applying a thin layer to affected skin; to rub gently; to use liquid by applying with fingertip or cotton swab
• To avoid sunlight, sunlamps; to use protective clothing, sunscreen
• That treatment may cause warmth, stinging; that dryness, peeling will occur
• That cosmetics may be used over product; not to use shaving lotions
• That rash may occur during first 1-3 wk of therapy
• That product does not cure condition, only relieves symptoms
• That therapeutic results may be seen in 2-3 wk but may not be optimal until after 6 wk

PO route

Black Box Warning: To notify prescriber if pregnancy is planned or suspected

---

tretinoin topical
See Appendix B

---

triamcinolone (ophthalmic)
See Appendix B

---

triamcinolone (Rx)
(trye-am-sin′oh-lone)
Aristospan, Kenalog-10, Kenalog-40, Tac-3, Triesence
Func. class.: Corticosteroid, synthetic
Chem. class.: Glucocorticoid, intermediate acting

ACTION: Decreases inflammation by suppression of migration of polymorphonuclear leukocytes, fibroblasts; reversal of increased capillary permeability and lysosomal stabilization

USES: Severe inflammation, immunosuppression, neoplasms, asthma (steroid dependent); collagen, respiratory, dermatologic/rheumatic disorders

CONTRAINDICATIONS: Hypersensitivity, neonatal prematurity; epidural/intrathecal administration (triamcinolone acetonide injections [Kenalog]), systemic fungal infections
Precautions: Pregnancy, breastfeeding, diabetes mellitus, glaucoma, osteoporosis, seizure disorders, ulcerative colitis, HF, myasthenia gravis, renal disease, esophagitis, peptic ulcer, acne, cataracts, coagulopathy, head trauma, children <2 yr, psychosis, idiopathic thrombocytopenia, acute glomerulonephritis, amebiasis, fungal infections, nonasthmatic bronchial disease, AIDS, TB, adrenal insufficiency, acute bronchospasm, acne rosacea, Cushing syndrome, acute MI, thromboembolism

---

DOSAGE AND ROUTES

• **Adult:** IM (acetonide) 40-80 mg q4wk; intraarticular (hexacetonide) 2-20 mg q3-4wk

• **Child:** IM acetonide 40 mg q4wk or 30-200 mcg/kg (1-6.25 mg/m^2) q1-7days (acetonide) 40-80 mg q4wk; intraarticular (hexacetonide) 2-20 mg q3-4wk

Available forms: Inj 3, 10, 40 mg/mL acetonide; inj 20, 5 mg/mL hexacetonide

Administer:

IM route

• After shaking susp (parenteral)

• Titrated dose; use lowest effective dose

• IM inj deep in large muscle mass; rotate sites; avoid deltoid; use 21-G needle

• Avoid SUBCUT administration, may damage tissue

SIDE EFFECTS

CNS: *Depression,* headache, mood changes

CV: *Hypertension,* circulatory collapse, embolism, tachycardia, edema

EENT: Fungal infections, increased intraocular pressure, blurred vision

GI: *Diarrhea, nausea, abdominal distention,* GI hemorrhage, *increased appetite,* pancreatitis

HEMA: Thrombocytopenia

INTEG: Acne, poor wound healing, ecchymosis, petechiae

MS: Fractures, osteoporosis, weakness

PHARMACOKINETICS

PO/IM: Peak 1-2 hr, half-life 2-5 hr

INTERACTIONS

Increase: side effects—alcohol, salicylates, indomethacin, amphotericin B, digoxin, cycloSPORINE, diuretics, quinolones

Increase: action of triamcinolone—salicylates, estrogens, indomethacin, oral contraceptives, ketoconazole, macrolide antiinfectives, carBAMazepine

Decrease: action of triamcinolone—cholestyramine, colestipol, barbiturates, rifAMPin, ePHEDrine, phenytoin, theophylline

Decrease: effects of anticoagulants, anticonvulsants, antidiabetics, ambenonium, neostigmine, isoniazid, toxoids, vaccines, anticholinesterases, salicylates, somatrem

Drug/Herb

• Hypokalemia: aloe, cascara, senna

Drug/Lab Test

Increase: cholesterol, sodium, blood glucose, uric acid, calcium, urine glucose

Decrease: calcium, potassium, T$_4$, T$_3$, thyroid ^{131}I uptake test, urine 17-OHCS, 17-KS, PBI

False negative: skin allergy tests

NURSING CONSIDERATIONS

Assess:

• Potassium, blood glucose, urine glucose while patient receiving long-term therapy; hypokalemia and hyperglycemia

• Weight daily; notify prescriber if weekly gain of >5 lb

• B/P, pulse; notify prescriber if chest pain occurs

• I&O ratio; be alert for decreasing urinary output, increasing edema

• Plasma cortisol levels during long-term therapy (normal level: 138-635 nmol/L SI units when drawn at 8 AM)

• **Infection:** increased temperature, WBC even after withdrawal of medication; product masks infection

• Potassium depletion: paresthesias, fatigue, nausea, vomiting, depression, polyuria, dysrhythmias, weakness

• Edema, hypertension, cardiac symptoms

• Mental status: affect, mood, behavioral changes, aggression

• Assistance with ambulation for patient with bone-tissue disease to prevent fractures

• **Beers:** avoid in older adults with delirium or at high risk for delirium; monitor for confusion, delirium

• **Pregnancy/breastfeeding:** use only if benefits outweigh fetal risk, cleft lip/palate has occurred (1st trimester); cautious use in breastfeeding, excreted in breast milk

T

Evaluate:

• Therapeutic response: ease of respirations, decreased inflammation

Teach patient/family:

• That emergency ID as corticosteroid user should be carried; not to discontinue abruptly, taper dose

• To notify prescriber if therapeutic response decreases; that dosage adjustment may be needed

• To avoid OTC products: salicylates, alcohol in cough products, cold preparations unless directed by prescriber; to avoid live vaccines

• About cushingoid symptoms

• **About the symptoms of adrenal insufficiency:** nausea, anorexia, fatigue, dizziness, dyspnea, weakness, joint pain

---

triamcinolone nasal agent
See Appendix B

---

triamcinolone (topical)
(try-am-sin′oh-lone)
Kenalog, Triderm
Func. class.: Corticosteroid, topical

ACTION: Crosses cell membrane to attach to receptors to decrease inflammation, itching; inhibits multiple inflammatory cytokines

USES: Inflammation/itching in corticosteroid-responsive dermatoses on the skin or inflammation in the mouth

CONTRAINDICATIONS: Hypersensitivity, use on face or ear canal, infections

Precautions: Pregnancy, breastfeeding, children

DOSAGE AND ROUTES

• Apply to the affected areas bid-qid

Available forms: Aerosol 0.2 mg; paste (dental) 0.1%; lotion, cream, ointment 0.025%; ointment 0.05%; lotion, cream, ointment 0.1%; ointment, cream 0.5%

Administer:

Topical route

• May be used with occlusive dressings

• **Cream/ointment/lotion:** apply sparingly in a thin film and rub gently into the cleansed, slightly moist affected area; may use gloves to apply cream/ointment/lotion

• **Paste:** apply without rubbing, press into lesion until film develops

• **Spray:** spray a small amount of preparation onto the lesion

SIDE EFFECTS

ENDO: HPA axis suppression, Cushing's syndrome

INTEG: Burning, folliculitis, pruritus, dermatitis, hypopigmentation

META: Hyperglycemia; glycosuria

PHARMACOKINETICS
Absorption varies

INTERACTIONS
Increase: blood glucose

NURSING CONSIDERATIONS

Assess:

• Skin reactions: burning, pruritus, folliculitis, mouth lesions

Evaluate:

• Decreasing itching, inflammation on the skin, decreasing mouth lesions

Teach patient/family:

• How to use each product

• That long-term use may cause thinning skin, loss of fat tissue; avoid long-term use

---

triamcinolone (topical-oral) (Rx, OTC)
(trye-am-sin′oh-lone)
Kenalog in Orabase, Oralone Dental
Func. class.: Topical anesthetic
Chem. class.: Synthetic fluorinated adrenal corticosteroid

ACTION: Binds with steroid receptors, decreases inflammation

USES: Oral pain

CONTRAINDICATIONS: Hypersensitivity, application to large areas; presence of fungal, viral, or bacterial infections of mouth or throat
Precautions: Pregnancy, children <6 yr, sepsis, denuded skin, geriatric patients

DOSAGE AND ROUTES
• **Adult: TOP** Press $1/4$ inch into affected area until film appears, repeat bid-tid
Available forms: Paste 0.1%
Administer:
• After cleansing oral cavity after meals

SIDE EFFECTS
INTEG: Rash, irritation, sensitization

NURSING CONSIDERATIONS
Assess:
• Allergy: rash, irritation, reddening, swelling
• Infection: if affected area is infected, do not apply
Evaluate:
• Therapeutic response: absence of pain in affected area
Teach patient/family:
• To report rash, irritation, redness, swelling
• How to apply paste

⚠ HIGH ALERT

triazolam (Rx)
(trye-ay′zoe-lam)
Halcion
Func. class.: Sedative-hypnotic, antianxiety
Chem. class.: Benzodiazepine, short acting

Controlled Substance Schedule IV (USA), Targeted (CDSA IV) (Canada)

Do not confuse:
Halcion/Haldol/halcinonide

ACTION: Produces CNS depression at limbic, thalamic, hypothalamic levels of CNS; may be mediated by neurotransmitter γ-aminobutyric acid (GABA); results are sedation, hypnosis, skeletal muscle relaxation, anticonvulsant activity, anxiolytic action

USES: Insomnia, sedative/hypnotic

CONTRAINDICATIONS: Pregnancy, breastfeeding, hypersensitivity to benzodiazepines
Precautions: Children <15 yr, geriatric patients, anemia, renal/hepatic disease, suicidal individuals, drug abuse, psychosis, acute closed-angle glaucoma, seizure disorders, angioedema, respiratory disease, depression, sleep-related behaviors (sleep walking), intermittent porphyria, myasthenia gravis, Parkinson's disease

Black Box Warning: Coadministration with other CNS depressants, respiratory depression

DOSAGE AND ROUTES
• **Adult: PO** 0.125-0.5 mg at bedtime, max 0.5 mg/day
• **Geriatric: PO** 0.0625-0.125 mg at bedtime, max 0.25 mg/day
Available forms: Tabs 0.125, 0.25 mg
Administer:
• After trying conservative measures for insomnia
• $1/2$ hr before bedtime for sleeplessness
• On empty stomach for fast onset; may be taken with food if GI symptoms occur
• Avoid use with CNS depressants; serious CNS depression may result

SIDE EFFECTS
CNS: *Headache, lethargy, drowsiness, daytime sedation,* dizziness, confusion, light-headedness, anxiety, irritability, amnesia, poor coordination, complex sleep-related reactions: sleep driving, sleep eating
CV: Chest pain, pulse changes, ECG changes

T

GI: Nausea, vomiting, diarrhea, heartburn, abdominal pain, constipation, hepatic injury
SYST: Severe allergic reactions

PHARMACOKINETICS
Onset 15-30 min, duration 6-8 hr, metabolized by liver, excreted by kidneys (inactive metabolites), crosses placenta, excreted in breast milk, half-life 1.5-5.5 hr

INTERACTIONS
• Smoking may decrease hypnotic effect
Increase: triazolam levels—CYP3A4 inhibitors, protease inhibitors
Increase: effects of cimetidine, disulfiram, erythromycin, clarithromycin, probenecid, isoniazid, oral contraceptives; do not use concurrently

Black Box Warning: **Increase:** action of both products—alcohol, CNS depressants

Decrease: effect of antacids, theophylline, rifAMPin
Drug/Herb
Increase: CNS depression—chamomile, hops, kava, lavender, valerian
Drug/Food
• Grapefruit may increase action; avoid concurrent use
Drug/Lab Test
Increase: ALT, AST, serum bilirubin
Decrease: RAI uptake
False increase: urinary 17-OHCS

NURSING CONSIDERATIONS
Assess:
• **Severe allergic reactions:** may occur during any use

Black Box Warning: Respiratory depression: may occur more frequently with coadministration of other CNS depressants; monitor respirations often

• Blood studies: Hct, Hgb, RBC if blood dyscrasias suspected (rare)
• Hepatic studies: AST, ALT, bilirubin if hepatic damage has occurred

• Mental status: mood, sensorium, affect, memory (long, short term), insomnia, withdrawal symptoms, excessive sedation, impaired coordination
• Blood dyscrasias: fever, sore throat, bruising, rash, jaundice, epistaxis (rare)
• Type of sleep problem: falling asleep, staying asleep
• Assistance with ambulation after receiving dose
• **Pregnancy/breastfeeding:** do not use in pregnancy; not recommended in breastfeeding
• **Beers:** avoid use in older adults; increased sensitivity to benzodiazepines and decreased metabolism; may cause or worsen delirium
Evaluate:
• Therapeutic response: ability to sleep at night, decreased amount of early morning awakening if taking product for insomnia
Teach patient/family:
• To use reliable contraception
• That dependence is possible after long-term use
• To avoid driving, other activities requiring alertness until product is stabilized

Black Box Warning: To avoid alcohol ingestion, sedatives, hypnotics

• That effects may take 2 nights for benefits to be noticed; that product is for short-term use only; to use for 7-10 continuous nights
• About alternative measures to improve sleep: reading, exercise several hours before bedtime, warm bath, warm milk, TV, self-hypnosis, deep breathing
• That complex sleep-related behaviors (sleep eating/driving) may occur
• That hangover is common in geriatric patients but less common than with barbiturates; that rebound insomnia may occur for 1-2 nights after discontinuing product; to discontinue by decreasing dose by 50% q2nights until 0.125 mg for 2 nights, then stop

---

TREATMENT OF OVERDOSE:
Lavage; monitor electrolytes, VS

---

trifluridine ophthalmic
See Appendix B

RARELY USED

trimethobenzamide (Rx)
(trye-meth-oh-ben′za-mide)
Tigan
Func. class.: Antiemetic, anticholinergic
Chem. class.: Ethanolamine derivative

USES: Nausea, vomiting

CONTRAINDICATIONS: Children (parenterally), hypersensitivity to opioids, shock

DOSAGE AND ROUTES
Nausea/vomiting
• **Adult:** IM 200 mg 3-4×/day; PO 300 mg 3-4×/day
Postoperative
• **Adult:** IM 200 mg followed by 2nd dose 1 hr later
Renal dose
• **Adult:** IM CCr 15-30 mL/min, give 50% of dose

---

trospium (Rx)
(trose′pee-um)
Sanctura ✦, Trosec ✦
Func. class.: Anticholinergic, urinary antispasmodic
Chem. class.: Muscarinic receptor antagonist

ACTION: Relaxes smooth muscles in bladder by inhibiting acetylcholine effect on muscarinic receptors

USES: Overactive bladder (urinary frequency, urgency)

CONTRAINDICATIONS: Hypersensitivity, uncontrolled closed-angle glaucoma, urinary retention, gastric retention, myasthenia gravis
Precautions: Pregnancy, breastfeeding, children, geriatric patients, renal/hepatic disease, controlled closed-angle glaucoma, ulcerative colitis, intestinal atony, bladder outflow obstruction

DOSAGE AND ROUTES
• **Adult <75 yr:** PO 20 mg bid 1 hr before meals or on empty stomach; **EXT REL** 60 mg in AM
• **Geriatric ≥75 yr:** PO titrate down to 20 mg/day based on response and tolerance
Renal dose
• **Adult:** PO CCr <30 mL/min, 20 mg/day at bedtime, ext rel product not recommended

Available forms: Tabs 20 mg; caps ext rel 60 mg
Administer:
• 1 hr before meals or on empty stomach (reg rel), in AM (ext rel) ≥1 hr before meal

SIDE EFFECTS
CNS: Fatigue, dizziness, headache, confusion
CV: Tachycardia
EENT: Dry eyes, vision abnormalities
GI: Flatulence, abdominal pain, *constipation, dry mouth,* dyspepsia
GU: Urinary retention, UTI
INTEG: Dry skin, angioedema
MISC: Heat stroke, fever

PHARMACOKINETICS
Rapidly absorbed (10%); peak 5-6 hr; protein bound (50%-85%); extensively metabolized; excreted in urine, feces; excreted in urine by active tubular secretion; half-life 20 hr

INTERACTIONS
Increase: drowsiness—CNS depressants, alcohol
Increase or decrease: trospium effect—products excreted by active renal secretion (aMILoride, digoxin, morphine), metFORMIN, quiNIDine, procainamide,

T

Side effects: *italics* = common; red = life-threatening

raNITIdine, tenofovir, triamterene, vancomycin

Drug/Food

Decrease: absorption—high-fat meal

NURSING CONSIDERATIONS

Assess:

• **Urinary patterns:** I&O ratio, CCr baseline and periodically, post-void residual distention, nocturia, frequency, urgency, incontinence, voiding patterns

• **Pregnancy/breastfeeding:** use only if benefits outweigh fetal risk; cautious use in breastfeeding, excreted in breast milk

• **Beers:** avoid in older adults with delirium or at high risk for delirium

Evaluate:

• Therapeutic response: correction of urinary status: absence of dysuria, frequency, nocturia, incontinence

Teach patient/family:

• To avoid hazardous activities because dizziness may occur

• That alcohol may increase drowsiness

• About anticholinergic effects that may occur

• That overheating may occur with strenuous exercise

• To avoid all other products unless approved by prescriber

• To use hard candy for dry mouth (most common side effect)

undecylenic acid topical
See Appendix B

unoprostone ophthalmic
See Appendix B

ustekinumab (Rx)
(us'te-kin'ue-mab)
Stelara
Func. class.: Immune response modifier, antipsoriatic agent
Chem. class.: Monoclonal antibody

ACTION: Interleukin (IL)-12, IL-23 antagonist, binds to an interleukin protein, decreases inflammation

USES: Plaque psoriasis, psoriatic arthritis

CONTRAINDICATIONS: Hypersensitivity, sepsis, active infections
Precautions: Pregnancy, breastfeeding, children ≤18 yr, geriatric patients, surgery, TB, diabetes mellitus, immunosuppression

DOSAGE AND ROUTES
Moderate to severe plaque psoriasis
• **Adult ≥100 kg with plaque psoriasis:** SUBCUT 90 mg, repeat in 4 wk, then 90 mg q12wk starting wk 16
• **Adult <100 kg without plaque psoriasis:** SUBCUT 45 mg, repeat in 4 wk, then 45 mg q12wk starting wk 16
Psoriatic arthritis with moderate to severe plaque psoriasis (monotherapy or methotrexate combination)
• **Adult ≥100 kg:** SUBCUT 90 mg, repeat in 4 wk, then q12wk maintenance
Crohn's disease
• **Adult (weight-based dosing):** IV single induction dose **>85 kg,** 520 mg; **>55–85 kg,** 390 mg; **≤55 kg,** 260 mg; **maintenance:** 90 mg SUBCUT q8wk, starting 8 wk after induction dose

Available forms: Solutions for inj 45 mg/0.5 mL, 90 mg/mL single use
Administer:
• Do not shake the prefilled syringe or vial, as irreparable damage to the product may occur
• Visually inspect for particulate matter and discoloration before use; solution should be colorless to slightly yellow and may contain a few small translucent or white particles. Do not use if discolored, cloudy, or if foreign particulate matter is present
IV route
• **Preparation:** use an IV infusion only for the induction treatment of Crohn's disease
• Each vial is for single use only
• Calculate the dose and number of vials needed based on patient weight; each 26-mL vial contains 130 mg of product
• Withdraw and discard a volume of the 0.9% sodium chloride injection from a 250-mL infusion bag equal to the volume of needed product to be added
• Withdraw 26 mL of product from each vial needed and add it to the 250-mL infusion bag. The final volume in the infusion bag should be 250 mL
• Gently mix; do not shake
• **Storage:** diluted solution must be used within 4 hr (no preservative). If administration is not immediate, store for up to 4 hr at room temperature up to 25°C (77°F). Do not freeze; discard unused portion
IV infusion route
• Give the diluted product over ≥1 hr
• Use only an infusion set with an in-line, sterile, nonpyrogenic, low protein-binding filter (pore size 0.2 micron)
• Do not infuse concomitantly in the same intravenous line with other agents

SUBCUT route Only an individual trained in subcut drug delivery should give the injection. A patient who is properly trained in injection technique may self-inject using the prefilled syringe or vial if his/her prescriber deems the action appropriate. However, the first injection needs to be under the supervision of a qualified health care professional

U

Side effects: *italics* = common; red = life-threatening

• Injection sites include the front part of the middle thigh, the gluteal or abdominal region, and the outer area of the upper arm
• Do not give where skin is tender, bruised, red, or indurated
• Rotate injection sites. If a second injection is needed because two 45-mg vials or prefilled syringes are used for a 90-mg dose, repeat the injection process with new materials, and use a different injection site
• For the vial, use a 27-gauge, 0.5-inch needle to withdraw the dose
• Gently pinch the cleaned area of skin and insert the needle at about a 45-degree angle subcutaneously; do not rub the injection site; slight bleeding may occur
• For the prefilled syringe, hold the syringe body and pull off the needle cover. The needle cover of the prefilled syringe contains latex. Persons allergic to natural rubber or latex should not handle the cover of the prefilled syringe
• Gently pinch the cleaned area of skin and insert the needle at about a 45-degree angle subcutaneously
• Do not rub the injection site; slight bleeding may occur. The needle safety guard will be activated once the pressure on the plunger head is released; do not touch the needle guard activation clips to prevent premature activation of the needle safety guard
• Each single-use vial or single-use prefilled syringe contains 45 mg/0.5 mL or 90 mg/mL of product; no preservatives are present; discard unused portion.

SIDE EFFECTS
CNS: Headache, leukoencephalopathy, depression, dizziness, fatigue
HEMA: Bleeding
INTEG: *Inj-site reaction,* pruritus, skin irritation, erythema
SYST: Serious infections, malignancies
MS: Myalgia, back pain
RESP: URI

PHARMACOKINETICS
Maximum serum concentration: 13.5 days after a single 45-mg subcut dose, 7 days after a single 90-mg subcut dose; half-life 14.9-45.6 days

INTERACTIONS
• Do not give concurrently with vaccines; immunizations should be brought up-to-date before treatment
• Avoid use with immunosuppressives

NURSING CONSIDERATIONS
Assess:
• Bring immunizations up-to-date before starting treatment; do not administer live vaccines during treatment and for 3 mo after treatment ends
• Infection: monitor for fever, sore throat, cough; do not use during active infections
• **Malignancy:** skin cancer may occur, especially in older patients who have used ultraviolet treatments with immunosuppressants
• **TB:** TB testing should be done before starting treatment
• For inj-site pain, swelling
• **Pregnancy/breastfeeding:** pregnant patients should enroll in the Stelara pregnancy registry, 1-877-311-8972; use only if benefits outweigh fetal risk; cautious use in breastfeeding, excretion unknown
Evaluate:
• Therapeutic response: decreased plaque psoriasis
Teach patient/family:
• That product must be continued for prescribed time to be effective; to use as prescribed
• Not to receive live vaccinations during treatment
• To notify prescriber of possible infection (upper respiratory or other) or allergic reactions
• Injection techniques and disposal of equipment; not to reuse needles, syringes
• That follow-up will be needed

valACYclovir (Rx)

(val-a-sye′kloh-vir)

Valtrex
Func. class.: Antiviral
Chem. class.: Synthetic purine
nucleoside analog

Do not confuse:
valACYclovir/valGANciclovir
Valtrex/Valcyte

ACTION: Interferes with DNA synthesis by conversion to acyclovir, thereby causing decreased viral replication, time of lesional healing

USES: Treatment or suppression of herpes zoster (shingles), genital herpes, herpes labialis (cold sores), varicella, varicella zoster

CONTRAINDICATIONS: Hypersensitivity to this product or acyclovir, valGANciclovir
Precautions: Pregnancy, breastfeeding, geriatric patients, hepatic/renal disease, electrolyte imbalance, dehydration, penciclovir, famciclovir, ganciclovir, hypersensitivity, varicella

DOSAGE AND ROUTES
Herpes zoster (shingles)
• **Adult: PO** 1 g tid × 1 wk
Genital herpes (suppressive, initial)
• **Adult: PO** 1 g bid × 10 days initially
Genital herpes (recurrent episodes)
• **Adult: PO** 500 mg bid × 3 days
Genital herpes (suppressive therapy)
• **Adult: PO** 1 g/day with normal immune function; 500 mg/day for those with ≤9 recurrences/yr; 500 mg bid for HIV-infected patients with CD4 count ≥100
Reduction of transmission
• **Adult: PO** 500 mg/day for source partner
Herpes labialis
• **Adult: PO** 2 g bid × 1 day at 1st sign of lesions

Varicella (chickenpox) in immunocompetent patients
• **Adolescent and child ≥2 yr: PO** 20 mg/kg/dose tid × 5 days, max 3 g/day; start at 1st sign, preferably within 24 hr of rash
Renal dose
• **Adult: PO** CCr 30-49 mL/min, 1 g q12hr **(for regimens 1 g q8hr)**; 1 g q12hr × 1 day **(herpes labialis)**; CCr 10-29 mL/min, 1 g q24hr **(genital herpes/herpes zoster)**; 500 mg q24hr **(recurrent genital herpes)**; CCr <10 mL/min, 500 mg q24hr **(genital herpes/herpes zoster)**, 500 mg q24hr **(recurrent genital herpes)**
Available forms: Tabs 500 mg, 1 g
Administer:
• As soon as possible (herpes labialis, genital herpes); within 24 hr of rash (varicella)
• Within 72 hr of outbreak (herpes zoster), within 24 hr (chickenpox)
• Without regard to food
• Caps may be made into susp by pharmacy
• Store at room temperature; protect from light, moisture

SIDE EFFECTS
CNS: Tremors, lethargy, *dizziness, headache,* weakness, depression, hallucinations, seizures, encephalopathy
GU: Crystalluria, renal failure
ENDO: *Dysmenorrhea*
GI: *Nausea,* vomiting, diarrhea, abdominal pain, constipation, *increased AST*
HEMA: Thrombocytopenic purpura, hemolytic uremic syndrome
INTEG: *Rash*
MISC: Dehydration

PHARMACOKINETICS
Onset unknown, Peak 1.5-2.5 hr, duration up to 24 hr; half-life $2^{1}/_{2}$-$3^{1}/_{2}$ hr; converted to acyclovir in intestine, liver; crosses placenta, enters breast milk; excreted in urine primarily as acyclovir; protein binding 13.5%-17.9%

INTERACTIONS
Increase: blood levels of valACYclovir—cimetidine, probenecid; only significant with renal disease

---

Side effects: *italics* = common; red = life-threatening

Drug/Lab Test
Increase: LFTs, creatinine
Decrease: WBC, platelets

NURSING CONSIDERATIONS
Assess:
• **Infection:** characteristics of lesions; therapy should be started at 1st sign or symptom of herpes; most effective within 72 hr of outbreak
• Thrombocytopenic purpura, hemolytic uremic syndrome; may be fatal
• C&S before product therapy; product may be taken as soon as culture is taken; repeat C&S after treatment; determine presence of other sexually transmitted diseases
• Bowel pattern before, during treatment
• Skin eruptions: rash
• Allergies before treatment, reaction to each medication
• **Pregnancy/breastfeeding:** use only if benefits outweigh fetal risk; cautious use in breastfeeding, excreted in breast milk
Evaluate:
• Therapeutic response: absence of itching, painful lesions; crusting and healed lesions
Teach patient/family:
• To take as prescribed; if dose is missed, to take as soon as remembered up to 2 hr before next dose; not to double dose; to take without regard to meals
• That product may be taken orally before infection occurs; that product should be taken when itching or pain occurs, usually before eruptions
• To discuss all Rx, OTC, herbal supplements taken with health care professional
• That adequate hydration is needed to prevent crystalluria
• Pregnancy/breastfeeding: Identify if pregnancy is planned or suspected or if breastfeeding
• That partners need to be told that patient has herpes because they can become infected; that condoms must be worn to prevent reinfections
• That product does not cure infection, just controls symptoms; that product does not prevent infection of others
• To report CNS changes (tremors, weakness, lethargy, hallucinations, seizures) immediately

---

RARELY USED

valbenazine
(val-ben´-a-zeen)
Ingrezza
Func. class.: CNS agent; monoamine depletor

USES: For the treatment of tardive dyskinesia

DOSAGE AND ROUTES
• **Adult: PO** Initially, 40 mg daily; after 1 wk, increase to 80 mg daily. Continuation of 40 mg daily may be considered for some patients

---

valGANciclovir (Rx)
(val-gan-sy´kloh-veer)
Valcyte
Func. class.: Antiviral
Chem. class.: Synthetic nucleoside

Do not confuse:
valGANciclovir/valACYclovir
Valcyte/Valtrex

ACTION: Metabolized to ganciclovir; inhibits replication of human cytomegalovirus in vivo and in vitro by selective inhibition of viral DNA synthesis

USES: Cytomegalovirus (CMV) retinitis in immunocompromised persons, including those with AIDS, after indirect ophthalmoscopy confirms diagnosis; prevention of CMV with transplantation; prevention of CMV in at-risk patient going through transplant (kidney, heart, pancreas)
Unlabeled uses: Colitis, Epstein-Barr virus, esophagitis, herpes simplex type 1, 2; human herpesvirus 6, 8; multicentric Castleman's disease, varicella-zoster virus

CONTRAINDICATIONS: Breastfeeding, hypersensitivity to ganciclovir, valACYclovir; absolute neutrophil count

---

<500/mm³; platelet count <25,000/mm³; hemodialysis; liver transplantation
Precautions: Children, geriatric patients, renal function impairment; hypersensitivity to acyclovir, penciclovir, famciclovir

Black Box Warning: Preexisting cytopenias, secondary malignancy, infertility, anemia, pregnancy

DOSAGE AND ROUTES
Treatment of CMV
• **Adult and adolescent: PO** induction 900 mg bid × 21 days with food; maintenance 900 mg/day with food
Transplant (CMV prophylaxis)
• **Adult/adolescent >16 yr: PO** 900 mg/day with food starting 10 days before transplantation until day 100 after transplantation (Kidney/pancreas/heart); continue for 200 days (kidney)
• **Infant ≥4 mo/child/adolescent ≤16 yr: PO** give within 10 days of heart/kidney transplant; calculate dose as 7 × BSA × CCr, give as single daily dose
Renal dose
• **Adult: PO** CCr ≥60 mL/min, same as above; CCr 40-59 mL/min, 450 mg bid for 21 days, then 450 mg/day; CCr 25-39 mL/min, 450 mg/day, then 450 mg q2days; CCr 10-24 mL/min, 450 mg q2days, then 450 mg 2×/week
Available forms: Tabs 450 mg, powder for oral sol 50 mg/mL
Administer:
PO tab
• With food for better absorption; avoid getting product on skin, wash hands if contact with skin; do not break, crush, or chew
Oral solution
• Oral with food
• Measure 9 mL purified water in graduated cylinder, shake bottle to loosen powder, add ½ liquid, shake well, add remaining water, shake; remove child-resistant cap and push bottle adapter into neck of bottle, close with cap, give using dispenser provided

• Store liquid in refrigerator; do not freeze; throw away any unused after 49 days

SIDE EFFECTS
CNS: *Fever,* chills, *confusion,* dizziness, *headache, insomnia,* psychosis, tremors, *paresthesia, weakness,* seizures
EENT: Retinal detachment with CMV retinitis
GI: *Nausea, vomiting, anorexia, diarrhea, abdominal pain*
GU: Hematuria, increased creatinine, BUN
HEMA: Thrombocytopenia, irreversible neutropenia, anemia, pancytopenia
INTEG: *Rash,* alopecia, *pruritus,* urticaria, pain at site, phlebitis, Stevens-Johnson syndrome
MISC: Local and systemic infections, sepsis

PHARMACOKINETICS
60% absorbed in GI tract, peak 1-3 hr, duration up to 24 hr. Metabolized to ganciclovir, which has a half-life of 3-4½ hr; excreted by kidneys (unchanged); crosses blood-brain barrier, CSF

INTERACTIONS
Increase: Severe granulocytopenia: immunosuppressants, zidovudine, antineoplastics, radiation; do not use together
Increase: toxicity—dapsone, pentamidine, flucytosine, vinCRIStine, vinBLAStine, adriamycin, DOXOrubicin, amphotericin B, trimethoprim-sulfamethoxazole combinations or other nucleoside analogs, cycloSPORINE
Increase: effect of both drugs—mycophenolate
Increase: seizures—imipenem-cilastatin
Increase: effect of didanosine; monitor for adverse effects, toxicity
Decrease: renal clearance of valGANciclovir—probenecid
Drug/Food
Increase: absorption—high-fat meal
Drug/Lab Test
Increase: creatinine, BUN

Decrease: RBC/WBC, Hct/Hgb

NURSING CONSIDERATIONS
Assess:

• CMV retinitis: determine diagnosis by ophthalmoscopy before beginning treatment, culture may be used, negative results do not confirm that CMV retinitis is not present, use ophthalmoscopy q2wk during treatment

Black Box Warning: Leukopenia/ neutropenia/thrombocytopenia: WBCs, platelets q2days during 2×/day dosing, then q1wk, do not use if ANC <500 mm³, platelets <25,000/mm³, Hgb <8 g/ dL; leukopenia with daily WBC count in patients with prior leukopenia with other nucleoside analogs or for whom leukopenia counts are <1000 cells/mm³ at start of treatment

Black Box Warning: Malignancy: monitor for malignancy, avoid accidental exposure of broken, crushed tabs, powder; if these were in contact with skin, wash well with soap and water

• Serum creatinine or CCr, BUN ≥q2wk, I&O, and increase in fluid intake

Black Box Warning: Pregnancy/breastfeeding: Considered potentially teratogenic; adequate contraception should be used; do not breastfeed

Evaluate:
• Therapeutic response: decreased symptoms of CMV
Teach patient/family:
• That product does not cure condition; that regular ophthalmologic q1mo and blood tests are necessary
• That major toxicities may necessitate discontinuing product
• To take with food, avoid high-fat meals
• **Blood dyscrasias:** bruising, bleeding, petechiae; seizures, dizziness; to avoid driving, hazardous activities
• To use sunscreen to prevent burns

Black Box Warning: Pregnancy/breastfeeding: To use contraception during treatment; that infertility may occur; that men should use barrier contraception for 90 days after treatment; not to breastfeed

---

valproate (Rx)
(val′proh-ate)
Depacon
valproic acid (Rx)
(val′proh-ik)
DepaKene ✦
divalproex sodium (Rx)
(dye-val′proh-ex)
Depakote, Depakote ER, Depakote Sprinkle, Epival ✦
Func. class.: Anticonvulsant, vascular headache suppressant
Chem. class.: Carboxylic acid derivative

ACTION: Increases levels of γ-aminobutyric acid (GABA) in the brain, which decreases seizure activity

USES: Simple (petit mal), complex (petit mal), absence, mixed seizures; manic episodes associated with bipolar disorder, prophylaxis of migraine, adjunct for schizophrenia, tardive dyskinesia, aggression in children with ADHD, organic brain syndrome, mania, migraines; tonic-clonic (grand mal), myoclonic seizures
Unlabeled uses: Rectal for seizures (valproic acid)

CONTRAINDICATIONS: Hypersensitivity, urea cycle disorders, mitochondrial disease, hepatic disease
Precautions: Breastfeeding, geriatric patients, abrupt discontinuation, carnitine deficiency, coagulopathy, depression, diarrhea, encephalopathy, head trauma, organic brain syndrome, HIV, renal disease, suicidal ideation, surgery, thrombocytopenia

---

Black Box Warning: Children <2 yr, contraception requirements, hepatotoxicity, pancreatitis, pregnancy

DOSAGE AND ROUTES
Simple absence seizures, complex absence seizures, or complex partial seizures
• **Adult/adolescent/child ≥10 yr: PO/IV** Initially, 10-15 mg/kg/day; increase by 5-10 mg/kg/day qwk, max 60 mg/kg/day; **rectal enema** 17-20 mg/kg, then 10-15 mg/kg/dose q8hr dilute 1:1 with water
Acute mania
• **Adult: PO** (delayed-release divalproex [Depakote] or delayed-release valproic acid [Stavzor]): Initially, 750 mg/day in divided doses, then increase as rapidly as possible to the lowest effective dose, max 60 mg/kg/day; **PO** (extended-release divalproex [Depakote ER]): Initially, 25 mg/kg/day, increase as rapidly as possible to achieve the desired clinical effect
For migraine prophylaxis
• **Adult ≤65 yr: PO** (delayed-release divalproex [Depakote] or delayed-release valproic acid [Stavzor]): Initially, 250 mg bid, titrate as needed up to a max 500 mg bid; **PO** (extended-release divalproex; Depakote ER): Initially, 500 mg/day × 1 wk, then increasing to 1000 mg/day, max 1000 mg/day
Available forms: *Valproate:* inj 100 mg/mL; *valproic acid:* caps 250, 500 ♣ mg; oral solution 250 mg/5 mL; *divalproex:* gastro-resistant tabs 125, 250, 500 mg; ext rel tabs 250, 500 mg; sprinkle cap 125 mg
Administer:
PO route
• Do not confuse different forms
• Swallow tabs or caps whole; do not break, crush, or chew ext rel tabs
• Sprinkle cap contents on food
• Oral solution alone; do not dilute with carbonated beverage; do not give oral solution to patients with sodium restrictions, shake before use; may mix with foods or other liquids, as taste is bitter
• Give with food or milk to decrease GI symptoms

IV Infusion route
• Dilute dose with ≥50 mL D_5W, NS, LR (2 mg/mL)
• Run over 60 min (20 mg/min)

• **Y-site compatibilities:** cefepime, ceftazadime, cloxacillin, naloxone

SIDE EFFECTS
CNS: *Sedation, drowsiness,* dizziness, headache, depression, behavioral changes, tremors, aggression, weakness, coma, suicidal ideation, hypothermia
CV: Peripheral edema
EENT: Visual disturbances, taste perversion
GI: *Nausea, vomiting, constipation, diarrhea, dyspepsia,* anorexia, pancreatitis, stomatitis, weight gain, dry mouth, hepatotoxicity
HEMA: Thrombocytopenia, leukopenia
INTEG: *Rash,* alopecia, photosensitivity, dry skin, DRESS
META: Hyperammonemia, SIADH

PHARMACOKINETICS
Absorption complete (IV) well (PO); distribution widely, crosses blood-brain barrier. Metabolized by liver; excreted by kidneys, in breast milk; crosses placenta; half-life 6-16 hr; 90% protein binding; **PO:** Peak 4 hr (regular rel); 4-17 hr (ext rel)

INTERACTIONS
Increase: valproic acid toxicity level—erythromycin, felbamate, salicylates, NSAIDs, rifampin, carBAMazepine, cimetidine
Increase: CNS depression—alcohol, opioids, barbiturates, antihistamines, MAOIs, sedative/hypnotics, tricyclics
Increase: action of, possible toxicity—phenytoin, carBAMazepine, ethosuximide, barbiturates, zidovudine, LORazepam, rufinamide, lamoTRIgine
Increase: bleeding—warfarin
Decrease: seizure threshold—tricyclics
Decrease: valproate levels—carBAMazepine, cholestyramine, estrogen, hormonal contraceptives, neuropenem, phenobarbital, phenytoin, rifAMPin
Drug/Lab Test
False positive: ketones, urine
Interference: thyroid function tests
Increase: LFTs, bleeding time, ammonia

Decrease: sodium

NURSING CONSIDERATIONS
Assess:
• **Seizure disorder:** location, aura, activity, duration; seizure precautions should be in place
• **Mental status:** bipolar disorder: mood, activity, sleeping/eating, behavior; suicidal thoughts/behaviors
• **Migraines:** frequency, intensity, alleviating factors
• Blood studies: Hct, Hgb, RBC, serum folate, PT/PTT, serum ammonia, platelets, vit D if patient receiving long-term therapy

Black Box Warning: **Hepatotoxicity:** AST, ALT, bilirubin, ammonia baseline and periodically during 6 mo or more, discontinue if hyperammonemia occurs; hepatic failure has occurred; monitor for fever, anorexia, vomiting, lethargy, jaundice of skin, eyes that may occur during treatment; those with organic brain disorders, mental retardation, children <2 yr are at greater risk

• **DRESS:** eosinophilia, changes in lab work, fever, rash, lymphadenopathy if present and condition confirmed, discontinue immediately, do not restart
• **Suicidal thoughts/behaviors:** usually occurs during beginning of therapy, limit amount of product that is given to the patient
• **Hyperammonemic encephalopathy:** can be fatal in those with urea cycle disorders (UCD); lethargy, confusion, coma, CV, respiratory changes; discontinue
• **Trough/peak:** serum blood levels: therapeutic level 50-125 mcg/mL, during seizures

Black Box Warning: **Pancreatitis:** may be fatal; report immediately nausea, vomiting, anorexia, abdominal pain; may occur anytime during treatment or for several months/years after discontinuing treatment

• **Beers:** avoid in older adults unless safer alternative is unavailable; ataxia, impaired psychomotor function may occur

Black Box Warning: **Pregnancy/breastfeeding:** do not use in pregnancy (migraine prophylaxis), use only in pregnancy (epilepsy, manic episodes) if other alternatives are unavailable; major malformations may occur; enroll pregnant patients in the North American Antiepileptic Drug Pregnancy Registry, 888-233-2334; cautious use in breastfeeding, excreted in breast milk

Evaluate:
• Therapeutic response: decreased seizures

Teach patient/family:
• That physical dependency may result from extended use
• To avoid driving, other activities that require alertness
• To drink plenty of fluids
• To discuss all OTC, Rx, herbals, supplements taken with health care professional
• Not to discontinue medication quickly after long-term use because seizures may result, to take as directed, not to skip, double doses

Black Box Warning: To report visual disturbances, rash, diarrhea, abdominal pain, light-colored stools, jaundice, protracted vomiting, weakness to prescriber

• **DRESS:** to report fever, swelling of lymph glands, rash
• **Hepatotoxicity:** to report immediately, anorexia, nausea, vomiting, abdominal pain, fever
• That continuing follow-up exams and blood work will be needed
• To carry an emergency ID with condition, medications taken
• **Overdose symptoms:** Heart block, coma

• To report immediately suicidal thoughts/behaviors

valsartan (Rx)

(val'sahr-tan)

Diovan

Func. class.: Antihypertensive

Chem. class.: Angiotensin II receptor antagonist (Type AT_1)

Do not confuse:

Diovan/Zyban

ACTION: Blocks the vasoconstrictor and aldosterone-secreting effects of angiotensin II; selectively blocks the binding of angiotensin II to the AT_1 receptor found in tissues

USES: Hypertension, alone or in combination in patients >6 yr, HF, post MI with left ventricular dysfunction/failure in stable patients

CONTRAINDICATIONS: Hypersensitivity, severe hepatic disease, bilateral renal artery stenosis

Precautions: Breastfeeding, children, geriatric patients, hypersensitivity to ACE inhibitors; HF, hypertrophic cardiomyopathy, aortic/mitral valve stenosis, CAD, angioedema, renal/hepatic disease, hyperkalemia, hypovolemia, African descent

DOSAGE AND ROUTES

Hypertension (alone or in combination)

• **Adult: PO** 80 or 160 mg/day alone or in combination with other antihypertensives, may increase to 320 mg/day

• **Geriatric: PO** adjust on clinical response; may start with lower dose

• **Child and adolescent 6-16 yr: PO** 1.3 mg/kg/dose daily, max 40 mg/day, initially adjust based on clinical response, max 2.7 mg/kg/day

Heart failure, classes II to IV

• **Adult: PO** 40 mg bid, up to 160 mg bid

Post MI

• **Adult: PO** 20 mg bid as early as 12 hr post MI, may be titrated within 7 days to 40 mg bid, then titrate to maintenance of 160 mg bid

Available forms: Tabs 40, 80, 160, 320 mg

Administer:

• Without regard to meals

SIDE EFFECTS

CNS: *Dizziness, insomnia,* drowsiness, vertigo, headache, fatigue

CV: Angina pectoris, 2nd-degree AV block, cerebrovascular accident, hypotension, MI, *dysrhythmias*

EENT: Conjunctivitis

GI: *Diarrhea,* abdominal pain, nausea, hepatotoxicity

GU: Impotence, nephrotoxicity, renal failure

HEMA: *Anemia,* neutropenia

META: Hyperkalemia

MISC: Vasculitis, angioedema

MS: Cramps, myalgia, pain, stiffness

RESP: *Cough*

PHARMACOKINETICS

Onset up to 2 hr; peak 2-4 hr; duration 24 hr; extensively metabolized; protein binding 95%; half-life 6 hr; excreted in feces, urine, breast milk

INTERACTIONS

• Do not use with aliskiren

Increase: effects of lithium, antidiabetics

Increase: hyperkalemia—potassium-sparing diuretics, potassium supplements, ACE inhibitors, cycloSPORINE

Increase: valsartan level—rifampin, ritonavir, gemfibrozil, telithromycin

Decrease: antihypertensive effects—NSAIDs, salicylates

Drug/Herb

Increase: antihypertensive effect—garlic, hawthorn

V

Side effects: *italics* = common; red = life-threatening

Decrease: antihypertensive effect—ephedra, ma huang
Drug/Food
Increase: hyperkalemia—salt substitutes with potasssium

NURSING CONSIDERATIONS
Assess:
- B/P, pulse q4hr lying, sitting, standing; note rate, rhythm, quality periodically
- Blood studies; BUN, creatinine, LFTs, potassium, total/direct bilirubin before treatment
- **Angioedema:** facial swelling; SOB; edema in feet, legs daily
- Skin turgor, dryness of mucous membranes for hydration status; correct volume depletion before initiating therapy

Black Box Warning: **Pregnancy/breastfeeding:** Do not use in pregnancy, may cause fetal death; do not breastfeed

Evaluate:
- Therapeutic response: decreased B/P
Teach patient/family:
- To comply with dosage schedule, even if feeling better; that, if dose is missed, to take it as soon as possible unless it is within 1 hr of next dose
- To notify prescriber of fever, swelling of hands or feet, irregular heartbeat, chest pain, dizziness, persistent cough
- That excessive perspiration, dehydration, diarrhea may lead to fall in blood pressure; to consult prescriber if these occur; to maintain hydration
- That product may cause dizziness, fainting, light-headedness; to rise slowly to sitting or standing position to minimize orthostatic hypotension; to take B/P readings
- To avoid potassium supplements and foods, salt substitutes

Black Box Warning: Not to take product if pregnant or breastfeeding

- **Overdose symptoms:** bradycardia or tachycardia, circulatory collapse

vancomycin (Rx)
(van-koe-mye′sin)
Vancocin
Func. class.: Antiinfective—miscellaneous
Chem. class.: Tricyclic glycopeptide

ACTION: Inhibits bacterial cell-wall synthesis, blocks glycopeptides

USES: *Actinomyces* sp., *Bacillus* sp., *Clostridium difficile, Clostridium* sp., *Enterococcus faecalis, Enterococcus faecium, Enterococcus* sp., *Lactobacillus* sp., *Listeria monocytogenes, Staphylococcus aureus* (MRSA), *Staphylococcus aureus* (MSSA), *Staphylococcus epidermidis, Staphylococcus* sp., *Streptococcus agalactiae* (Group B), *Streptococcus bovis, Streptococcus pneumoniae, Streptococcus pyogenes* (group A beta-hemolytic streptococci), viridans streptococci; may be effective against *Corynebacterium jeikeium, Corynebacterium* sp., pseudomembranous colitis, staphylococcal enterocolitis, endocarditis prophylaxis for dental procedures, bacteremia, joint/bone infections, osteomyelitis, pneumonia, septicemia

CONTRAINDICATIONS: Hypersensitivity to this product or corn
Precautions: Pregnancy, breastfeeding, neonates, geriatric patients, renal disease, hearing loss

DOSAGE AND ROUTES
Serious systemic infections
- **Adult:** IV 500 mg q6-8hr or 1 g q12hr or 15-20 mg/kg q12hr
- **Child:** IV 40-60 mg/kg/day divided q6-8hr
- **Neonate:** IV 15 mg/kg initially, then 10 mg/kg q8-24hr
CDAD
- **Adult:** PO 125 mg qid × 10-14 days
- **Child:** PO (unlabeled) 40 mg/kg/day divided q6hr × 7-10 days, max 2 g/day

Staphylococcal endocarditis prophylaxis
• **Adult: IV** 2 g divided (500 mg q6hr, or 1 g q12hr)
• **Child: IV** 20 mg/kg over 1 hr given 1 hr before procedure

Staphylococcal enterocolitis
• **Adult: IV PO** 500-2000 mg/day in 3-4 divided doses × 7-10 days
•**Child PO:** 40mg/kg/day in 3-4 divided doses X 7-10 days, max 2000mg/day

Renal dose
• **Adult: IV** 15-20 mg/kg loading dose in seriously ill; individualize all other doses

Available forms: Cap 125, 250 mg; powder for inj 500 mg, 1, 5, 10 g; dextrose sol for inj 500 mg/100 mL, 750 mg/150 mL, 1 g/200 mL

Administer:
• Use only for susceptible organisms to prevent product-resistant bacteria
• Antihistamine if red-man syndrome occurs: decreased B/P, flushing of neck, face; stop or slow infusion
• Dose based on serum concentration

IT route
• Dilute with preservative-free normal saline (1-5 mg/mL), give into ventricular cerebrospinal fluid
• **PO:** without regard to food, swallow whole (used only for *Clostridium difficile, staphylococcal enterocolitis*)
• Use calibrated measuring device for liquid
• IV form may be used NG after diluting in 30 mL water
• Store at room temperature for ≤2 wk after reconstitution

Intermittent IV INFUSION route
• After reconstitution with 10 mL sterile water for inj (500 mg/10 mL); further dilution is needed for IV, 500 mg/100 mL 0.9% NaCl, D₅W given as intermittent infusion over 1 hr; decrease rate of infusion if red-man syndrome occurs

Continuous IV INFUSION route (unlabeled)
• May infuse 1-2 g in volume to give over 24 hr if intermittent IV route cannot be used

• A central line may be considered for long-term therapy, assess peripheral lines for phlebitis

Y-site compatibilities: Acetylcysteine, acyclovir, alatrofloxacin, aldesleukin, alemtuzumab, alfentanil, allopurinol, alprostadil, amifostine, amikacin, amino acids injection, aminocaproic acid, amiodarone, amoxicillin-clavulanate, amsacrine, anidulafungin, argatroban, ascorbic acid injection, atenolol, atracurium, atropine, azithromycin, benztropine, bleomycin, bretylium, bumetanide, buprenorphine, butorphanol, calcium chloride/gluconate, CARBOplatin, carmustine, caspofungin, cefpirome, chlorproMAZINE, cimetidine, ciprofloxacin, cisatracurium, CISplatin, clarithromycin, clindamycin, codeine, cyanocobalamin, cyclophosphamide, cycloSPORINE, cytarabine, DACTINomycin, DAUNOrubicin liposome, dexamethasone, dexmedetomidine, dexrazoxane, digoxin, diltiazem, diphenhydrAMINE, DOBUTamine, DOCEtaxel, dolasetron, DOPamine, doripenem, doxacurium, doxapram, DOXOrubicin, DOXOrubicin liposomal, doxycycline, enalaprilat, ePHEDrine, EPINEPHrine, epirubicin, eptifibatide, ertapenem, erythromycin, esmolol, etoposide, etoposide phosphate, famotidine, fenoldopam, fentaNYL, filgrastim, fluconazole, fludarabine, folic acid (as sodium salt), gallium, gemcitabine, gentamicin, glycopyrrolate, granisetron, HYDROmorphone, hydrOXYzine, ifosfamide, insulin (regular), irinotecan, isoproterenol, isosorbide, ketamine, labetalol, lactated Ringer's injection, lepirudin, levofloxacin, lidocaine, linezolid, LORazepam, magnesium sulfate, mannitol, mechlorethamine, melphalan, meperidine, meropenem, metaraminol, methyldopate, metoclopramide, metoprolol, metroNIDAZOLE, midazolam, milrinone, minocycline, mitoXANtrone, morphine, multiple vitamins injection, mycophenolate, nalbuphine, naloxone, nesiritide, netilmicin, niCARdipine, nitroglycerin, nitroprusside, norepinephrine, octreotide, ofloxacin, ondansetron, oxacillin, oxaliplatin, oxytocin, PACLitaxel

V

(solvent/surfactant), palonosetron, pamidronate, pancuronium, papaverine, PEMEtrexed, penicillin G potassium/sodium, pentamidine, pentazocine, PENTobarbital, perphenazine, PHENobarbital, phentolamine, phenylephrine, phytonadione, piritramide, polymyxin B, potassium acetate/chloride, procainamide, prochlorperazine, promethazine, propranolol, protamine, pyridoxine, quiNIDine, ranitidine, remifentanil, rifampin, Ringer's injection, riTUXimab, sodium acetate/bicarbonate/citrate, succinylcholine, SUFentanil, tacrolimus, teniposide, thiamine, thiotepa, tigecycline, tirofiban, TNA (3-in-1), tobramycin, tolazoline, TPN (2-in-1), trastuzumab, urapidil, vasopressin, vecuronium, verapamil, vinBLAStine, vinCRIStine, vinorelbine, voriconazole, zidovudine, zoledronic acid

SIDE EFFECTS

CNS: Headache
CV: Hypotension, peripheral edema
EENT: *Ototoxicity*
GI: Nausea, CDAD
GU: Nephrotoxicity
HEMA: Leukopenia, eosinophilia
INTEG: Chills, fever, rash, thrombophlebitis at inj site (red-man syndrome), skin/subcutaneous tissue disorders
MS: Back pain
SYST: Anaphylaxis, superinfection

PHARMACOKINETICS

Widely distributed, crosses placenta, penetration in CSF (20%-30%)
PO: Absorption poor
IV: Onset rapid, peak 1 hr, half-life 4-8 hr, excreted in urine (active form)

INTERACTIONS

Increase: neuromuscular effects—nondepolarizing muscle relaxants
Drug/Lab Test
Increase: BUN/creatinine, eosinophils
Decrease: WBC

NURSING CONSIDERATIONS
Assess:
• **Infection:** WBC, urine, stools, sputum, characteristics of wound throughout treatment; obtain C&S before starting treatment,

may start treatment before results are received
• **Nephrotoxicity:** I&O ratio; report hematuria, oliguria; nephrotoxicity may occur; BUN, creatinine
• Serum levels: peak 1 hr after 1-hr infusion 25-40 mg/L, trough before next dose 5-10 mg/L, especially in renal disease; no trough levels are needed for oral form
• **CDAD:** watery or bloody diarrhea, abdominal cramps, fever, pus, mucus, nausea, dehydration; discontinue immediately
• Auditory function during, after treatment; hearing loss, ringing, roaring in ears; product should be discontinued
• B/P during administration; sudden drop may indicate red-man syndrome
• Skin eruptions
• **Red-man syndrome:** flushing of neck, face, upper body, arms, back, may lead to anaphylaxis; slow IV infusion to >1 hr
• EPINEPHrine, suction, tracheostomy set, endotracheal intubation equipment on unit; anaphylaxis may occur
• Adequate intake of fluids (2 L/day) to prevent nephrotoxicity
Evaluate:
• Therapeutic response: absence of fever, sore throat; negative culture
Teach patient/family:
• About all aspects of product therapy; about the need to complete entire course of medication to ensure organism death (7-10 days); that culture may be taken after completed course of medication
• To report sore throat, fever, fatigue; could indicate superinfection
• That product must be taken in equal intervals around the clock to maintain blood levels
• That labs will need to be regularly monitored with IV infusion
• To notify prescriber if there is no change in 72-96 hr
• That antiinfectives must be taken before dental/medical invasive procedures in rheumatic heart disease
• **Pregnancy/breastfeeding:** identify if pregnancy is planned or suspected or if breastfeeding

---

vardenafil (Rx)

(var-den'a-fil)

Levitra, Staxyn

Func. class.: Erectile dysfunction agent

Chem. class.: Phosphodiesterase type 5 inhibitor

ACTION: Inhibits phosphodiesterase type 5 (PDE5), enhances erectile function by increasing the amount of cGMP, which in turn causes smooth muscle relaxation and increased blood flow into the corpus cavernosum

USES: Treatment of erectile dysfunction

CONTRAINDICATIONS: Hypersensitivity, coadministration of α-blockers or nitrates, renal failure, congenital or acquired QT prolongation

Precautions: Pregnancy; not indicated for women, children, or newborns; hepatic impairment, retinitis pigmentosa, anatomical penile deformities, sickle cell anemia, leukemia, multiple myeloma, bleeding disorders, active peptic ulceration, CV/renal disease

DOSAGE AND ROUTES

Levitra

• **Adult: PO** 10 mg taken 1 hr before sexual activity; dose may be reduced to 5 mg or increased to max 20 mg; max dosing frequency once daily; orally disintegrating tab 10 mg 60 min before sexual activity; do not use with potent CYP3A4 inhibitors

• **Geriatric >65 yr: PO** 5 mg initially, titrated as needed/tolerated

Hepatic dose

• **Adult: PO** (Child-Pugh B) 5 mg, max 10 mg/day

Concomitant medications

• Ritonavir, max 2.5 mg q72hr; for indinavir, ketoconazole 400 mg/day and itraconazole 400 mg/day, max 2.5 mg/day; for ketoconazole 200 mg/day, itraconazole 200 mg/day and erythromycin max 5 mg/day

Staxyn

• **Adult: PO** 10 mg 1 hr before sexual activity, max 10 mg/24 hr

Available forms: Tabs 2.5, 5, 10, 20 mg; orally disintegrating tab 10 mg

Administer:

• Approximately 1 hr before sexual activity; do not use more than once daily; orally disintegrating tabs are not interchangeable with film-coated tabs

• Without regard to food; avoid taking with high-fat meal

• **Oral disintegrating tab:** place on tongue immediately after opening blister pack, allow to dissolve, do not use water

SIDE EFFECTS

CNS: *Headache, flushing, dizziness, insomnia*

EENT: Diminished vision, hearing loss

GU: Abnormal ejaculation, priapism

GI: Nausea

MISC: Flulike symptoms

PHARMACOKINETICS

Rapidly absorbed, bioavailability 15%, protein binding 95%, metabolized by liver by CYP3A4, distribution semen, terminal half-life 4-5 hr, onset 20 min, peak $1/_2$-$1^1/_2$ hr, duration <5 hr, reduced absorption with high-fat meal, primarily excreted in feces (91%-95%)

INTERACTIONS

• Do not use with nitrates because of unsafe decrease in B/P, which could result in MI or stroke

• **Serious dysrhythmias:** class IA/III antiarrhythmics, clarithromycin, droperidol, procainamide, quiNIDine, quinolones; do not use concurrently

Increase: hypotension—α-blockers, protease inhibitors, metoprolol, NIFEdipine, alcohol, amLODIPine, angiotensin II receptor blockers; do not use concurrently

Increase: vardenafil levels—erythromycin, azole antifungals (ketoconazole, itraconazole), cimetidine

Drug/Food

Decrease: absorption—high-fat meal

V

Side effects: *italics* = common; red = life-threatening

Increase: vardenafil level—grapefruit juice; avoid concurrent use
Drug/Lab Test
Increase: CK

NURSING CONSIDERATIONS
Assess:

• Erectile dysfunction and cause before treatment
• Any severe loss of vision while taking this or similar products; products should not be used
• Use of organic nitrates, which should not be used with this product
• **Pregnancy/breastfeeding:** not used in women
Teach patient/family:
• That product does not protect against STDs, including HIV
• That product absorption is reduced with high-fat meal
• That product should not be used with nitrates in any form; to inform physician of all medications being taken
• That product has no effect in the absence of sexual stimulation; that patient should seek immediate medical attention if erections last >4 hr
• To notify prescriber immediately and stop taking product if vision loss occurs
• To take 1 hr before sexual activity and only once per day
• To notify prescriber of all OTC, prescription, and herbal products taken

---

varenicline (Rx)
(var-e-ni′kleen)
Champix ✦, Chantix
Func. class.: Smoking cessation agent
Chem. class.: Nicotine receptor agonist

ACTION: Partial agonist for nicotine receptors; partially activates receptors to help curb cravings; occupies receptors to prevent nicotine binding

USES: Adjunct to psychosocial interventions for tobacco cessation (smoking)

CONTRAINDICATIONS: Hypersensitivity, eating disorders
Precautions: Pregnancy, breastfeeding, children <18 yr, geriatric patients, renal disease, recent MI, angioedema, bipolar disorder, depression, schizophrenia, suicidal ideation

DOSAGE AND ROUTES
• **Adult: PO** therapy should begin 1 wk before smoking stop date (i.e., take product plus tobacco for 7 days); titrate for 1 wk; days 1 through 3, 0.5 mg/day; days 4 through 7, 0.5 mg bid; day 8 through end of treatment, 1 mg bid; treatment is for 12 wk and may be repeated for another 12 wk
Renal dose
• **Adult: PO** CCr ≤50 mL/min, titrate to max 0.5 mg bid
Available forms: Tabs 0.5, 1 mg
Administer:
• Do not break, crush, or chew tabs
• Increased fluids, bulk in diet if constipation occurs
• After eating with a full glass of water
• Sugarless gum, hard candy, frequent sips of water for dry mouth

SIDE EFFECTS
CNS: Headache, agitation, dizziness, insomnia, abnormal dreams, fatigue, malaise, behavioral changes, depression, homicidal ideation, suicidal ideation, amnesia, hallucinations, hostility, mania, psychosis, tremors, seizures, stroke
CV: Dysrhythmias, MI
EENT: *Blurred vision*
GI: *Nausea, vomiting, dry mouth,* increased/decreased appetite, *constipation,* flatulence, GERD, diarrhea, gingivitis, dyspepsia, enterocolitis
GU: Erectile dysfunction, urinary frequency, menstrual irregularities
INTEG: Rash, pruritus, angioedema, Stevens-Johnson syndrome, flushing, dermatitis
MS: *Back pain,* myalgia, *arthralgia*
HEMA: Anemia

PHARMACOKINETICS

Elimination half-life 24 hr; metabolism minimal; 93% excreted unchanged in urine; steady state 4 days, onset 4 days, peak 3-4 hr

NURSING CONSIDERATIONS

Assess:

• **Smoking history:** motivation for smoking cessation, years used, amount each day; smoking cessation after 12 wk; if progress not made, product may be used for additional 12 wk

• Renal function in geriatric patients; cardiac status in cardiac disease

• **Neuropsychiatric symptoms:** mood, sensorium, affect; behavioral changes, agitation, depression, suicidal ideation; suicide has occurred; possible worsening of depression, schizophrenia, bipolar disorder, risk is increased in adolescents

• **Angioedema, Stevens-Johnson syndrome:** rash during treatment; discontinue if rash, fever, fatigue, joint pain, lesions occur

• Risk of hypotension: take B/P baseline and periodically

• **Pregnancy/breastfeeding:** use only if benefits outweigh fetal risk, no well-controlled studies

Evaluate:

• Therapeutic response: smoking cessation

Teach patient/family:

• To set a date to quit smoking and to initiate treatment 1 wk before that date

• That treatment for smoking cessation lasts 12 wk and that another 12 wk may be required

• To use caution when driving, performing other activities requiring alertness; blurred vision may occur

• How to titrate product

• Not to use with nicotine patches unless directed by prescriber; may increase B/P

• That vivid dreams, insomnia may occur during beginning of treatment, but usually subside

• To notify prescriber of all OTC, prescription, or herbal products used

• To notify prescriber immediately of change in thought/behavior (suicidal ideation, hostility, depression); stop product

• Not to drive or operate machinery until effects are known

• To notify prescriber if pregnancy is planned or suspected or if breastfeeding

---

⚠ HIGH ALERT

vasopressin (Rx)

(vay-soe-press′in)

Vasostrict

Func. class.: Pituitary hormone
Chem. class.: Lysine vasopressin

ACTION: Promotes the reabsorption of water via action on the renal tubular epithelium; causes vasoconstriction

USES: Diabetes insipidus (nonnephrogenic/nonpsychogenic), hypotension, shock, septic shock, postcardiotomy cardiogenic shock

Unlabeled uses: bleeding, esophageal varices, cardiac arrest

CONTRAINDICATIONS: Hypersensitivity, chronic nephritis

Precautions: Pregnancy, breastfeeding, CAD, asthma, vascular/renal disease, migraines, seizures

DOSAGE AND ROUTES

Diabetes insipidus

• **Adult: IM/SUBCUT** 5-10 units bid-qid as needed; **CONT IV INFUSION** 0.0005 units/kg/hr (0.5 milliunit/kg/hr), double dose q30min as needed

• **Child: IM/SUBCUT** 2.5-10 units bid-qid as needed

Hypotension in septic shock

• **Adult: IV** 0.01 units/min, titrate by 0.005 units/min q10-15min until B/P target is achieved, to max 0.07 units/min after target B/P of 8 hr without use of catecholamines; taper 0.005 units/min q1hr to maintain B/P

V

GI hemorrhage (unlabeled)
• **Adult:** IV 0.2-0.4 units/min, titrate, max 0.8 units/min
Available forms: Sol for inj 20 units/mL
Administer
Direct IV route
• During adult CPR, resuscitation drugs may be administered intravenously by bolus injection into a peripheral vein, followed by an injection of 20 mL IV fluid; elevate the extremity for 10-20 sec

Continuous IV INFUSION route
• Dilute 2.5 or 5 mg/500 mL respectively of 0.9% NaCL or D$_5$W to 0.1 or 1 unit/mL in NS or D$_5$W. 1 unit/mL is suggested for those with fluid restrictions.
• Discard unused solution after 18 hr at room temperature or 24 hr under refrigeration

IM route
• Inject deeply into a large muscle; aspirate prior to injection to avoid injection into a blood vessel

SUBCUT route:
• Inject SUBCUT, taking care not to inject intradermally

SIDE EFFECTS
CNS: Headache, lethargy, flushing, vertigo
CV: Chest pain, MI
GI: Nausea, heartburn, cramps, vomiting, flatus
MISC: urticaria

PHARMACOKINETICS
IM: Onset 1 hr; duration 3-8 hr; **IV** duration 60 min; half-life 15 min; metabolized in liver, kidneys; excreted in urine

INTERACTIONS
Increase: antidiuretic effect—tricyclics, SSRIs, carBAMazepine, chloropromide, fludrocortisone, clofibrate
Decrease: antidiuretic effect—lithium, demeclocycline, chlorpropamide, cyclophosphamide, enalapril, felbamate, haloperidol, pentamine

NURSING CONSIDERATIONS
Assess:
• Pulse, B/P, ECG periodically during treatment; if using for CPR, monitor continuously
• **Diabetes insipidus:** I&O ratio, weight daily; fluid/electrolyte balance, urine specific gravity; check for extreme thirst, poor skin turgor, dilute urine, large urine volume
• **Water intoxication:** lethargy, behavioral changes, disorientation, neuromuscular excitability
• Small doses may precipitate coronary adverse effects; keep emergency equipment nearby
• **Pregnancy/breastfeeding:** use only if benefits outweigh fetal risk; breastfeeding women should pump and discard milk for 1½ hr after receiving product

Evaluate:
• Therapeutic response: absence of severe thirst, decreased urine output, osmolality

Teach patient/family:
• To measure and record I&O
• To avoid herbals, supplements, all OTC medications unless approved by prescriber

---

vedolizumab
(ve′-doe-liz′ue-mab)
Entyvio
Func. class.: GI antiinflammatory
Chem class.: Integrin receptor antagonist

ACTION: A specific integrin receptor antagonist that inhibits the migration of specific memory T-lymphocytes across the endothelium into inflamed gastrointestinal parenchymal tissue. The action reduces the chronic inflammatory process present in both ulcerative colitis and Crohn's disease

USES: For moderately to severely active ulcerative colitis/Crohn's disease to reduce signs and symptoms, and to induce

---

and maintain clinical remission in patients who have an inadequate response to conventional therapy

CONTRAINDICATIONS: Hypersensitivity

Precautions: Hepatic disease, infections, progressive multifocal leukoencephalopathy (PML), pregnancy, breastfeeding, live vaccines, TB, human antichimeric antibody (HACA)

DOSAGE AND ROUTES

• **Adult: IV INFUSION** 300 mg 30 min at weeks 0, 2, and 6 as induction therapy, then 300 mg q8wk, continue if response occurs by week 14

Available forms: Powder for injection 300-mg/20-mL vial

Administer:

• Full response is usually observed by 6 wk; those who do not respond by week 14 are unlikely to respond

• Give as IV infusion only, do not use as an IV push or bolus

• Make sure all immunizations are up to date

• Reconstitute with 4.8 mL of sterile water for injection, using a syringe with a 21- to 25-gauge needle

• Insert the syringe needle into the vial and direct the stream of sterile water for injection to the glass wall of the vial, gently swirl the solution for 15 sec, do not shake

• Allow the solution to stand for up to 20 min at room temperature to allow for reconstitution and for any foam to settle

• Once dissolved, product should be clear or opalescent, colorless to light brownish yellow, and free of visible particulates. Discard if discolored or if foreign particles are present

• Before withdrawing solution from vial, gently invert vial 3 times. Withdraw 5 mL (300 mg) of reconstituted product using a 21- to 25-gauge needle. Discard remaining product

• Add the 5 mL (300 mg) of reconstituted product to 250 mL of sterile 0.9% sodium chloride and gently mix infusion bag. Do not mix with other medications.

Administer solution as soon as possible; if necessary, may be stored for up to 4 hr refrigerated, do not freeze. Infuse over 30 min; after infusion, flush line with 30 mL of sterile 0.9% sodium chloride injection. Discard any unused infusion solution

SIDE EFFECTS

CNS: *Headache*, fatigue, dizziness
GI: Nausea, vomiting
MISC: Rash, pruritus, infusion-related reactions
MS: *Arthralgia*, back pain
RESP: Cough
SYST: Anaphylaxis, progressive multifocal leukoencephalopathy (PML), increased infection risk

PHARMACOKENETICS

Absorption complete, onset up to 6 wk, duration up to 8 wk, half-life 25 days

INTERACTIONS

Increase: infection risk—immunosuppressives, natalizumab, antineoplastics
Do not use with tumor necrosis factor (TNF) modifiers

Decrease: immune response—vaccines, toxoids

NURSING CONSIDERATIONS

Assess:

• **Ulcerative colitis/Crohn's disease:** monitor symptoms before and after treatment

• **Hypersensitivity:** swelling of lips, tongue, throat, face; rash; wheezing; hypertension; if serious reactions occur, discontinue product

• **Liver dysfunction:** elevated hepatic enzymes, jaundice, malaise, nausea, vomiting, abdominal pain, and anorexia are predictive of severe liver injury that may be fatal or may require a liver transplant in some patients; if hepatic dysfunction is suspected, discontinue

• **Tuberculosis (TB) latent/active:** obtain TB skin test both before and during treatment; do not give in active infection such as influenza or sepsis

• **Progressive multifocal leukoencephalopathy (PML):** increased weakness on one side of the body or clumsiness of

V

limbs, visual disturbance, and changes in thinking, memory, and orientation leading to confusion and personality changes; severe disability or death can come over weeks or months

Evaluate:

• Therapeutic response: lessening of ulcerative colitis and Crohn's disease

Teach patient/family:

• About the symptoms of infection and to report to health care provider immediately

• To report allergic reactions, PML; teach symptoms

• Not to use live virus vaccines while taking this product; to bring vaccinations up-to-date before starting this product

• The reason for product, expected result

• Risk of infection is increased, to notify health care professional of fever, chills, trouble breathing

• To discuss with health care professional all Rx, OTC, herbals, supplements taken

• To report planned or suspected pregnancy, or if breastfeeding; if pregnant, call 877-825-3327 to enroll in the Entyvia Pregnancy Registry

---

⚠ HIGH ALERT

vemurafenib

Zelboraf

Func. class.: Antineoplastic
Chem class.: Kinase inhibitor

ACTION: Inhibitor of some mutated forms of BRAF serine threonine kinase, thereby blocking cellular proliferation in melanoma cells with the mutation; inhibits other kinases including CRAF, ARAF, wild-type BRAF, SRMA, ACK1, MAP4H5, and FGR; potent adenosine triphosphate-competitive inhibitor of RAFs, with a modest preference for mutant BRAF and CRAF compared with wild-type BRAF

USES: Unresectable or metastatic malignant melanoma with V600E mutation of the BRAF gene

Precautions: Pregnancy, breastfeeding, children, infants, neonates, hepatic disease, QT prolongation, secondary malignancy, torsades de pointes, hypokalemia, hypomagnesemia, sunlight exposure

DOSAGE AND ROUTES

• **Adult: PO** 960 mg (4 tabs) bid about q12hr, continue until unacceptable toxicity or disease progression, if strong CYP3A4 inducers are used increase dose to 1200 mg (5 tablets)

Dose adjustments for toxicity due to adverse reactions or QTc prolongation

Grade 1 or tolerable grade 2: no dosage change; **intolerable grade 2 or grade 3 (1st episode):** interrupt treatment until toxicity resolves to grade ≤1, when resuming, reduce dosage to 720 mg (3 tabs) bid; **grade 2 or grade 3 (2nd episode):** interrupt treatment until toxicity resolves to grade ≤1, when resuming, reduce dose to 480 mg (2 tabs) bid; **grade 2 or grade 3 (3rd episode):** discontinue treatment permanently; **grade 4 (1st episode):** discontinue permanently or interrupt until toxicity resolves to grade ≤1, when resuming, reduce dose to 480 mg (2 tabs) bid; **grade 4 (2nd episode):** discontinue permanently

Available forms: Tabs 240 mg

Administer:

• Continue until disease progresses or unacceptable toxicity occurs

• Missed doses can be taken up to 4 hr before the next dose is due; take about 12 hr apart, take without regard to meals

• Swallow whole with a full glass of water; do not crush or chew

• Store at room temperature in original container

SIDE EFFECTS

CNS: *Fatigue*, fever, headache, dizziness, peripheral neuropathy, *weakness*

CV: QT prolongation, atrial fibrillation, torsades de pointes

---

EENT: Uveitis, blurred vision, iritis, photophobia

GI: Nausea, diarrhea, dysgeusia, hepatotoxicity

INTEG: *Alopecia, pruritus,* hyperkeratosis, *maculopapular rash,* actinic keratosis, *xerosis/dry skin,* papular rash, palmar-plantar erythrodysesthesia (hand and foot syndrome), *photosensitivity*

MS: *Arthralgia, myalgias,* extremity pain, musculoskeletal pain, back pain, arthritis

GU: *Acute tubular necrosis, interstitial nephritis*

SYST: Secondary malignancy, anaphylaxis, Stevens-Johnson syndrome, toxic epidermal necrolysis, drug reaction with eosinophilia, anaphylaxis

PHARMACOKINETICS

>99% protein binding (albumin and alpha-1 acid glycoprotein), an inhibitor of CYP1A2, 2A6, 2C9, 2C19, 2D6, 3A4/5 CYP1A2 inhibitor, a weak CYP2D6 inhibitor, and a CYP3A4 inducer; elimination 94% in feces, 1% in urine, half-life 57 hr, Peak 3 hr, duration up to 12 hr

INTERACTIONS

Increase: vemurafenib effect—CYP3A4/CYP1A2 inhibitors (enoxacin, cimetidine, delavirdine, indinavir, isoniazid, itraconazole, dalfopristin, quinupristin, tipranavir)

Increase: QT prolongation, torsades de pointes—arsenic trioxide, certain phenothiazines (chlorproMAZINE, mesoridazine, thioridazine), grepafloxacin, pentamidine, probucol, sparfloxacin, troleandomycin, class IA antiarrhythmics (disopyramide, procainamide, quiNIDine), class III antiarrhythmics (amiodarone, dofetilide, ibutilide, sotalol), clarithromycin, ziprasidone, pimozide, haloperidol, halofantrine, quiNIDine, chloroquine, dronedarone, droperidol, erythromycin, methadone, posaconazole, propafenone, saquinavir, abarelix, amoxapine, apomorphine, asenapine, β-agonists, ofloxacin, eribulin, ezogabine, flecainide, gatifloxacin, gemifloxacin, halogenated anesthetics, iloperidone, levofloxacin, local anesthetics, magnesium sulfate, potassium sulfate, sodium, maprotiline, moxifloxacin, nilotinib, norfloxacin, ciprofloxacin, OLANZapine, paliperidone, some phenothiazines (fluPHENAZine, perphenazine, prochlorperazine, trifluoperazine), telavancin, tetrabenazine, tricyclic antidepressants, venlafaxine, vorinostat, citalopram, alfuzosin, cloZAPine, cyclobenzaprine, dolasetron, palonosetron, QUEtiapine, rilpivirine, SUNItinib, tacrolimus, vardenafil, indacaterol, dasatinib, fluconazole, lapatinib, lopinavir/ritonavir, mefloquine, octreotide, ondansetron, ranolazine, risperiDONE, telithromycin, vemurafenib

Decrease: vemurafenib effect—CYP3A4 inducers (rifampin, barbiturates, carBAMazepine, phenytoin, erythromycin, ketoconazole, fluvoxaMINE, alcohol, etravirine, ritonavir, bexarotene, rifabutin, OXcarbazepine, nevirapine, modafinil, metyraPONE)

Drug/Lab Test:

Increase: serum creatinine, LFTs, alkaline phosphatase, bilirubin

NURSING CONSIDERATIONS

Assess:

• **Hepatotoxicity:** liver function test (LFT) abnormalities, altered bilirubin levels may occur; monitor LFTs and bilirubin levels before treatment, then monthly; more frequent testing is needed in those with grade 2 or greater toxicities; laboratory alterations should be managed with dose reduction, treatment interruption, or discontinuation

• **QT prolongation:** avoid in patients with QT prolongation; monitor ECG and electrolytes in those with heart failure, bradycardia, electrolyte imbalance (hypokalemia, hypomagnesemia), or those who are taking concomitant medications known to prolong the QT interval; treatment interruption, dosage adjustment, treatment discontinuation may be needed in those who develop QT prolongation

• Serum electrolytes, CCr, bilirubin, ECG

• **BRAF testing:** obtain testing before use; do not use in wild-type BRAF; confirm BRAF V600E mutation

V

Side effects: *italics* = common; red = life-threatening

• **Skin reactions:** assess for skin reaction
• **Pregnancy/breastfeeding:** identify whether pregnancy is planned or suspected; do not use in pregnancy; avoid breastfeeding
Evaluate:
• Decreased spread of malignancy
Teach patient/family:
• That missed doses can be taken up to 4 hr before the next dose is due to maintain the twice-daily regimen; that if vomiting occurs, do not retake dose, take next dose as scheduled
• To notify prescriber of new skin lesions
• To avoid sun exposure; to wear sunscreen, protective clothing
• **Hepatotoxicity:** To notify health care professional of yellow skin, eyes, dark urine, clay-colored stool, nausea/vomiting, pain in right side of abdomen
• **Allergic reactions:** To report rash, trouble breathing, swelling of face, lips, blisters
• To discuss with health care professional all RX, OTC, herbals, supplements taken
• **Pregnancy:** to use reliable contraception; that both women and men of childbearing age should use adequate contraceptive methods during therapy and for at least 90 days after completing treatment

RARELY USED

venetoclax
(veh-neh′toh-klax)
Venclexta ✦
Func. class.: Antineoplastic, signal transduction inhibitor

USES: Treatment of CLL in patients with a 17p deletion who have received at least 1 prior therapy

CONTRAINDICATIONS:
Hypersensitivity, pregnancy

DOSAGE AND ROUTES
• **Adult: PO** Initially, 20 mg/day × 7 days, increase dose qwk × 5 wk: wk 2,

50 mg/day; wk 3, 100 mg/day; wk 4, 200 mg/day; wk 5 and beyond, 400 mg/day. Continue therapy until disease progression. A dose reduction and/or therapy interruption may be necessary in patients who develop toxicity

venlafaxine (Rx)
(ven-la-fax′een)
Effexor XR
Func. class.: Antidepressant—SNRI
Chem. class.: SNRI

ACTION: Potent inhibitor of neuronal serotonin and norepinephrine uptake, weak inhibitor of dopamine; no muscarinic, histaminergic, or α-adrenergic receptors in vitro

USES: Prevention/treatment of major depression; depression at the end of life; long-term treatment of general anxiety disorder, panic disorder, social anxiety disorder (Effexor XR only)
Unlabeled uses: Hot flashes, premenstrual dysphoric disorder (PMDD), headache, neuropathic pain, fibromyalgia, diabetic neuropathy

CONTRAINDICATIONS: Hypersensitivity, MAOIs
Precautions: Pregnancy, breastfeeding, geriatric patients, mania, hypertension, seizure disorder, recent MI, cardiac/renal/hepatic disease, eosinophilic pneumonia, desvenlafaxine hypersensitivity, bipolar disorder, interstitial lung disease

Black Box Warning: Children, suicidal ideation

DOSAGE AND ROUTES
Major Depression
• **Adult: PO** 75 mg/day in 2-3 divided doses; taken with food, may be increased to 150 mg/day; if needed, may be further increased to 225 mg/day; increments of 75 mg/day at intervals of ≥4 days; some hospi-

talized patients may require up to 375 mg/day in 3 divided doses; **EXT REL** 37.5-75 mg PO daily, max 225 mg/day; give XR daily

Anxiety disorders
• **Adult: PO** 75 mg/day or 37.5 mg/day × 4-7 days initially, max 225 mg/day

Renal dose
• **Adult: PO** CCr 10-70 mL/min, reduce dose by 25%-50%; CCr <10 mL/min, reduce dose by 50%

Hepatic dose
• **Adult: PO** moderate impairment, 50% of dose

Hot flashes (unlabeled)
• **Adult (male, prostate cancer): PO** 12.5 mg bid × 4 wk; **females** 37.5-75 mg/day

Neuropathic pain, diabetic neuropathy, headache, fibromyalgia (unlabeled)
• **Adult: PO** 37.5-75 mg/day, max 75 mg bid (regular rel) or 150 mg/day (ext rel)

Premenstrual dysphoric disorder (PMDD) (unlabeled)
• **Adult female: PO** 50-200 mg/day, start at 50 mg/day for 1st cycle, titrate upward

Available forms: Tabs scored 25, 37.5, 50, 75, 100 mg; ext rel cap (Effexor XR) 37.5, 75, 150 mg, 225 mg

Administer:
• With food, milk for GI symptoms; do not crush, chew caps; caps can be opened and contents sprinkled on applesauce, given with full glass of water, use immediately
• Sugarless gum, hard candy, frequent sips of water for dry mouth
• Avoid use with CNS depressants
• Give in small amounts because of suicide potential, especially at beginning of therapy
• Store in tight container at room temperature; do not freeze

SIDE EFFECTS

CNS: Emotional lability, *dizziness, weakness,* headache, hallucinations, insomnia, anxiety, suicidal ideation in children/adolescents, seizures, neuroleptic malignant syndrome–like reaction, *anxiety, abnormal dreams, paresthesia*

CV: Hypertension, chest pain, tachycardia, change in QTc interval, increased cholesterol, extrasystoles, syncope

EENT: *Abnormal vision,* taste, *ear pain*

GI: *Dysphagia, eructation, nausea,* anorexia, dry mouth, colitis, gastritis, gingivitis, *constipation,* stomatitis, stomach and mouth ulceration, *abdominal pain, vomiting, weight loss*

GU: *Anorgasmia,* abnormal ejaculation, urinary frequency, decreased libido, impotence, menstrual changes, *impaired urination*

INTEG: *Ecchymosis,* dry skin, photosensitivity, sweating, Stevens-Johnson syndrome; angioedema (ext rel)

META: *Peripheral edema, weight loss*

PHARMACOKINETICS

Well absorbed; extensively metabolized in liver by CYP2D6 to active metabolite, some are poor metabolizers ⚕; 87% of product recovered in urine; 27% protein binding; half-life 5, 11 hr (active metabolite), respectively, onset up to 14 days, peak up to 4 wk

INTERACTIONS

Hyperthermia, rigidity, rapid fluctuations of vital signs, mental status changes, neuroleptic malignant syndrome: MAOIs

Increase: bleeding risk—salicylates, NSAIDs, platelet inhibitors, anticoagulants

Increase: venlafaxine effect—cimetidine

Increase: CNS depression—alcohol, opioids, antihistamines, sedative/hypnotics

Increase: levels of cloZAPine, desipramine, haloperidol, warfarin

Increase: serotonin syndrome—sibutramine, SUMAtriptan, traZODone, traMADol, SSRIs, serotonin receptor agonist, linezolid, methylene blue, tryptophan

Decrease: effect of indinavir

Decrease: venlafaxine effect—cyproheptadine

Drug/Herb
• **Serotonin syndrome:** St. John's wort, tryptophan

Increase: CNS depression—chamomile, hops, kava, valerian

Drug/Lab Test
Increase: alk phos, bilirubin, AST, ALT, BUN, creatinine, serum cholesterol, CPK, LDH

False positive: amphetamines, phencyclidine

V

Side effects: *italics* = common; red = life-threatening

NURSING CONSIDERATIONS
Assess:

Black Box Warning: Mental status: mood, sensorium, affect, increase in psychiatric symptoms, depression, panic; assess for suicidal ideation in children/ adolescents and in early treatment

• B/P lying, standing; pulse q4hr; if systolic B/P drops 20 mm Hg, hold product, notify prescriber; take VS q4hr in patients with CV disease
• **Bleeding:** GI, ecchymosis, epistaxis, hematomas, petechiae, hemorrhage
• Blood studies: CBC, differential, leukocytes, cardiac enzymes if patient is receiving long-term therapy
• Hepatic studies: AST, ALT, bilirubin
• Weight weekly; weight loss or gain; appetite may increase; peripheral edema may occur; monitor cholesterol
• **Withdrawal symptoms:** flulike symptoms, headache, nervousness, agitation, nausea, vomiting, muscle pain, weakness; not usual unless product is discontinued abruptly
• **Serotonin syndrome, neuroleptic malignant syndrome:** increased heart rate, shivering, sweating, dilated pupils, tremors, high B/P, hyperthermia, headache, confusion; if these occur, stop product, administer serotonin antagonist if needed; usually worse if given with linezolid, methylene blue, tryptophan
• Assistance with ambulation during beginning therapy because drowsiness, dizziness occur
• **Beers:** use with caution in older adults; may exacerbate or cause syndrome of inappropriate antidiuretic hormone secretion (SIADH)
• **Pregnancy/breastfeeding:** use only if benefits outweigh fetal risk; use in late 3rd trimester has resulted in neonatal complications; do not breastfeed, excreted in breast milk
Evaluate:
• Therapeutic response: decreased depression, anxiety; increased well-being

Teach patient/family:
• To notify prescriber of rash, hives, allergic reactions, bleeding
• To use with caution when driving, performing other activities requiring alertness because of drowsiness, dizziness, blurred vision

Black Box Warning: That worsening of symptoms, suicidal thoughts/behaviors may occur in children or young adults; discuss with family members

• To avoid alcohol ingestion
• Not to discontinue medication abruptly after long-term use; may cause nausea, headache, malaise; taper over 14 days
• To wear sunscreen or large hat because photosensitivity occurs
• To avoid pregnancy or breastfeeding while taking this product; birth defects have occurred when used in the 3rd trimester
• To monitor B/P for new hypertension or if patient has history of hypertension
• **Serotonin syndrome, neuroleptic malignant syndrome:** to report immediately shivering, sweating, tremors, fever, dilated pupils
• To take as prescribed, contents of capsule may be sprinkled on applesauce if unable to swallow whole

TREATMENT OF OVERDOSE:
ECG monitoring; lavage; administer anticonvulsant; may require whole-bowel irrigation for ext rel product

---

⚠ HIGH ALERT

verapamil (Rx)
(ver-ap′a-mill)
Calan, Calan SR, Covera-HS ♣, Isoptin SR, Tarka ♣, Verelan, Verelan PM
Func. class.: Calcium channel blocker; antihypertensive; antianginal, antidysrhythmic (class IV)
Chem. class.: Diphenylalkylamine

ACTION: Inhibits calcium ion influx across cell membrane during cardiac depolarization; produces relaxation of coronary vascular smooth muscle; dilates coronary arteries; decreases SA/AV node conduction; dilates peripheral arteries

USES: Chronic stable, vasospastic, unstable angina; dysrhythmias, hypertension, supraventricular tachycardia, atrial flutter or fibrillation

Unlabeled uses: Prevention of migraine headaches, claudication, mania

CONTRAINDICATIONS: Sick sinus syndrome, 2nd-/3rd-degree heart block, hypotension <90 mm Hg systolic, cardiogenic shock, severe HF, Lown-Ganong-Levine syndrome, Wolff-Parkinson-White syndrome

Precautions: Pregnancy, breastfeeding, children, geriatric patients, HF, hypotension, hepatic injury, renal disease, concomitant β-blocker therapy

DOSAGE AND ROUTES
Angina
• **Adult: PO** 80-120 mg tid, increase weekly, max 480 mg/day
Dysrhythmias
• **Adult: PO** 240-480 mg/day in 3-4 divided doses in digitalized patients
• **Adult: IV BOL** 5-10 mg (0.075-0.15 mg/kg) over 2 min, may repeat 10 mg (0.15 mg/kg) ¹/₂ hr after 1st dose
• **Child 1-15 yr: IV BOL** 0.1-0.3 mg/kg over 2 min, repeat in 30 min, max 5 mg in single dose
• **Child 0-1 yr: IV BOL** 0.1-0.2 mg/kg over 2 min, may repeat after 30 min
Hypertension
• **Adult: PO** 80 mg tid, may titrate upward; **EXT REL** 120-240 mg/day as single dose, may increase to 240-480 mg/day
Hepatic disease/geriatric patients/ compromised ventricular function
• **Adult: PO** 40 mg tid initially, increase as tolerated
Claudication due to PVD (unlabeled)
• **Adult: PO** 120-480 mg/day in divided doses

Mania (unlabeled)
• **Adult: PO** 160-320 mg/day in divided doses, may be given with lithium
Migraine prophylaxis (unlabeled)
• **Adult: PO** 80 mg tid
Available forms: Tabs 40, 80, 120 mg; ext rel tabs 120, 180, 240 mg; inj 2.5 mg/mL in ampules, syringes, vials; ext rel caps 100, 200, 240, 300 mg
Administer:
PO route
• **Reg rel:** Give without regard to food, give with meals or milk to prevent gastric upset
Ext rel route
• Do not crush or chew ext rel products; Verelan caps may be opened and contents sprinkled on food; do not dissolve chew cap contents
• Before meals, at bedtime; give ext rel product with food
Direct IV route
• Undiluted through Y-tube or 3-way stopcock of compatible sol; give over 2 min or 3 min for geriatric patients, with continuous ECG and B/P monitoring, discard unused solution
• Do not use IV with IV β-blockers; may cause AV nodal blockade

Y-site compatibilities: Alfentanil, amikacin, argatroban, ascorbic acid, atracurium, atropine, aztreonam, bivalirudin, bumetanide, buprenorphine, butorphanol, calcium chloride/gluconate, CARBOplatin, caspofungin, ceFAZolin, cefonicid, cefotaxime, cefoTEtan, cefOXitin, ceftizoxime, cefTRIAXone, cefuroxime, chlorproMAZINE, cimetidine, ciprofloxacin, clindamycin, cyanocobalamin, cyclophosphamide, cycloSPORINE, cytarabine, DACTINomycin, DAPTOmycin, dexamethasone, dexmedetomidine, digoxin, diltiazem, diphenhydrAMINE, DOBUTamine, DOCEtaxel, DOPamine, doxacurium, DOXOrubicin hydrochloride, doxycycline, enalaprilat, ePHEDrine, EPINEPHrine, epirubicin, epoetin alfa, eptifibatide, erythromycin, esmolol, etoposide, etoposide phosphate, famotidine, fenoldopam, fentaNYL, fluconazole, fludarabine, gemcitabine, gentamicin, glycopyrrolate, granisetron, heparin, hydrALAZINE, hydrocortisone, HYDRO-morphone, ifosfamide, imipenem/cilastatin, inamrinone, insulin, isoproterenol, ketorolac, labetalol, levoFLOXacin, lidocaine, linezolid, LORazepam, magnesium sulfate, mannitol, mechlorethamine, meperidine, metaraminol, methotrexate, methoxamine, methyldopate, methylPREDNISolone, metoclopramide, metoprolol, metroNIDAZOLE, miconazole, midazolam, milrinone, mitoXANtrone, morphine, multivitamins, nalbuphine, naloxone, nesiritide, nitroglycerin, nitroprusside, norepinephrine, octreotide, ondansetron, oxaliplatin, oxytocin, PACLitaxel, palonosetron, papaverine, PEMEtrexed, penicillin G, pentamidine, pentazocine, phentolamine, phenylephrine, phytonadione, piperacillin/tazobactam, potassium chloride, procainamide, prochlorperazine, promethazine, propranolol, protamine, pyridoxime, quinupristin/dalfopristin, ranitidine, rocuronium, sodium acetate, succinylcholine, SUFentanil, tacrolimus, teniposide, theophylline, thiamine, ticarcillin/clavulanate, tirofiban, tobramycin, tolazoline, trimethaphan, urokinase, vancomycin, vasopressin, vecuronium, vinCRIStine, vinorelbine, voriconazole

SIDE EFFECTS

CNS: *Headache, drowsiness,* dizziness, anxiety, depression, weakness, insomnia, confusion, light-headedness, asthenia, fatigue
CV: *Edema,* HF, bradycardia, hypotension, palpitations, AV block, dysrhythmias
GI: *Nausea,* diarrhea, gastric upset, *constipation,* increased LFTs
GU: Impotence, gynecomastia, nocturia, polyuria
HEMA: Bruising, petechiae, bleeding
EENT: Blurred vision, tinnitus, equilibrium change, epistaxis
RESP: Cough
INTEG: Rash, bruising
MISC: Gingival hyperplasia
SYST: Stevens-Johnson syndrome

PHARMACOKINETICS

Metabolized by liver by CYP3A4, excreted in urine (70% as metabolites), protein binding 90%

PO: Onset variable; peak 3-4 hr; duration 17-24 hr; half-life 4 min, 3-12 hr
IV: Onset 3 min, peak 3-5 min, duration 10-20 min

INTERACTIONS

Increase: hypotension—prazosin, quiNIDine, fentaNYL, other antihypertensives, nitrates
Increase: effects of verapamil—β-blockers, cimetidine, clarithromycin, erythromycin, monitor for CV effects
Increase: levels of digoxin, theophylline, cycloSPORINE, carBAMazepine, nondepolarizing muscle relaxants
Decrease: effects of lithium
Decrease: antihypertensive effects—NSAIDs
Drug/Food
Increase: hypotensive effects—grapefruit juice
Drug/Herb
Increase: verapamil effect—ginseng, ginkgo
Increase: hypertension—ephedra (ma huang)
Decrease: verapamil effect—St. John's wort
Drug/Lab Test
Increase: AST, ALT, alk phos, BUN, creatinine, serum cholesterol

NURSING CONSIDERATIONS
Assess:
• **Cardiac status:** B/P, pulse, respiration, ECG intervals (PR, QRS, QT); notify prescriber if pulse <50 bpm, systolic B/P <90 mm Hg
• **HF:** I&O ratios, weight daily; crackles, weight gain, dyspnea, jugular venous distention
• Renal, hepatic studies during long-term treatment, serum potassium periodically
• **Stevens-Johnson syndrome:** rash with fever, fatigue, joint pain, lesions; discontinue immediately
• **Pregnancy/breastfeeding:** use only if benefit outweighs fetal risk; avoid breastfeeding
• **Beers:** avoid use in older adults; may cause fluid retention or exacerbate heart failure

Evaluate:
• Therapeutic response: decreased anginal pain, decreased B/P, dysrhythmias
Teach patient/family:
• To increase fluids, fiber to counteract constipation
• How to take pulse, B/P before taking product; to keep record or graph
• To avoid hazardous activities until stabilized on product, dizziness no longer a problem
• To limit caffeine consumption; to avoid alcohol products
• To avoid OTC or grapefruit products unless directed by prescriber
• To comply with all areas of medical regimen: diet, exercise, stress reduction, product therapy
• To change positions slowly to prevent syncope
• Not to discontinue abruptly; chest pain may occur
• To report chest pain, palpitations, irregular heartbeats, swelling of extremities, skin irritation, rash, tremors, weakness
• To notify prescriber if pregnancy is planned; to avoid breastfeeding

TREATMENT OF OVERDOSE: Defibrillation, atropine for AV block, vasopressor for hypotension, IV calcium

---

vigabatrin (Rx)
(vye-ga´ba-trin)
Sabril
Func. class.: Anticonvulsant
Chem. class.: GABA transaminase inhibitor

ACTION: May inhibit reuptake and metabolism of GABA; may increase seizure threshold; structurally similar to GABA

USES: Adjunct treatment of partial seizures in adults and children ≥12 yr, infantile spasm

CONTRAINDICATIONS: Hypersensitivity to this product

Precautions: Pregnancy, breastfeeding, children <2 yr, geriatric patients, renal/hepatic disease, suicidal thoughts/behaviors, abrupt discontinuation

Black Box Warning: Visual disturbance; requires an experienced clinician

DOSAGE AND ROUTES
Partial seizures
• **Adult/child ≥16 yr/child 10-16 yr >60 kg: PO** 500 mg bid, titrate in 500-mg increments at weekly intervals up to 1.5 g bid
Infantile spasm
• **Infant >1 mo/child ≤2 yr: PO** 50 mg/kg/day in 2 divided doses, titrate in increments of 25 to 50 mg/kg/day q3days, max 150 mg/kg/day
Renal dose
• **Adult: PO** CCr 50-80 mL/min, reduce dose by 25%; CCr 30-49 mL/min, reduce dose by 50%; CCr 10-29 mL/min, reduce dose by 75%
Available forms: Tabs 500 mg; powder for oral solution 500 mg
Administer:
PO route (tab)
• Give without regard to meals
PO route (oral sol)
• Reconstitute immediately before using
• Empty contents of appropriate number of packets into clean cup
• For each packet, dissolve 10 mL water, concentration 50 mg/mL; do not use other liquids
• Stir until dissolved, sol should be clear
• Use calibrated oral syringe to measure correct dosage
• Discard any unused sol
• Store at room temperature

SIDE EFFECTS
CNS: Headache, memory impairment, *dizziness*, irritability, lethargy, malignant hyperthermia, insomnia, suicidal ideation
CV: Edema
EENT: Visual impairment

Side effects: *italics* = common; red = life-threatening

GI: Nausea, vomiting, diarrhea, increased appetite, abdominal pain, GI bleeding, hemorrhoids, weight gain, constipation
GU: Impotence, dysmenorrhea
HEMA: Anemia
INTEG: Pruritus, rash
RESP: Coughing, respiratory depression, pulmonary embolism

PHARMACOKINETICS
Absorption >95%, no protein binding, widely distributed, not metabolized, excretion in urine 80% parent drug, excretion slowed in renal disease, peak 2 hr, half-life 7.5 hr

INTERACTIONS
Increase: CNS depression—CNS depressants
Increase: Serious ophthalmic effects (glaucoma, retinopathy): azaTHIOprine, chloroquine, corticosteroids, deferoxamine, ethambutol, hydroxychloroquine, interferons, loxapine, mecasermin, rh-IGF-1, pentostatin, phenothiazine, phosphodiesterase inhibitors, tamoxifen, thiothixene; avoid concurrent use
Drug/Lab Test
Decrease: ALT/AST

NURSING CONSIDERATIONS
Assess:

Black Box Warning: **Visual impairment:** Prescribers must be registered with the SHARE program due to risk of permanent vision loss; if no clinical response in 2-4 wk of pediatric patients or 3 mo in adults discontinue, provide vision assessment before and after ≤4 wk at least q3mo, and 3-6 mo after stopping product

• Renal studies: urinalysis, BUN, urine creatinine q3mo in those with renal disease
• Hepatic studies: ALT, AST, bilirubin
• Description of seizures: location, duration, presence of aura
• Mental status: mood, sensorium, affect, behavioral changes; if mental status changes, notify prescriber

• Assistance with ambulation during early part of treatment; dizziness occurs
• Seizure precautions: padded side rails; move objects that may harm patient
• **Pregnancy/breastfeeding:** use only if benefits outweigh fetal risk; pregnant patients should enroll in the North American Antiepileptic Drug Pregnancy Registry, 1-888-233-2334; do not breastfeed, excreted in breast milk
Evaluate:
• Therapeutic response: decreased seizure activity
• **Beers:** avoid in older adults unless safer alternatives are unavailable; may cause ataxia, impaired psychomotor function
Teach patient/family:
• To carry emergency ID stating patient's name, products taken, condition, prescriber's name and phone number
• To avoid driving, other activities that require alertness
• Not to discontinue medication quickly after long-term use
• To notify prescriber if pregnancy is planned or suspected
• To report suicidal thoughts/behaviors immediately
• To avoid alcohol; drowsiness, dizziness may occur

Black Box Warning: That drug may cause vision impairment; that regular exams will be needed; to notify prescriber at once if loss of vision occurs

• To notify prescriber if pregnancy is planned or suspected; not to breastfeed

vilazodone (Rx)
(vil-az′oh-done)
Viibryd
Func. class.: Antidepressant
Chem. class.: SSRI, benzofuran

ACTION: Novel antidepressant unrelated to other antidepressants, enhances serotonergic action by a dual mechanism

USES: Major depression

CONTRAINDICATIONS:
Concomitant use of MAO inhibitors or within 14 days after discontinuing MAO inhibitor or within 14 days after discontinuing vilazodone

Precautions: Pregnancy, labor, infants, geriatric patients, abrupt discontinuation, bipolar disorder, bleeding, operating machinery, ECT, hepatic disease, hyponatremia, hypovolemia, substance abuse, history of seizures, serotonin syndrome, neuroleptic malignant syndrome; use with serotonin precursors or serotonergic drugs; suicidal ideation, worsening depression or behavior

Black Box Warning: Children, suicidal ideation

DOSAGE AND ROUTES
Major depressive disorder
• **Adult:** PO 10 mg × 7 days, then 20 mg × 7 days, then 40 mg/day; if taking potent CYP3A4 inhibitor, max 20 mg/day; potent CYP3A4 inducer increase dose up to double may be needed, max 80 mg/day

Available forms: Tabs 10, 20, 40 mg
Administer:
• With food to increase absorption
• Do not use within 2 wk of MAOIs
• Store at room temperature, away from moisture, heat

SIDE EFFECTS
CNS: Restlessness, dizziness, drowsiness, fatigue, mania, insomnia, migraine, neuroleptic malignant syndrome–like reaction, paresthesias, seizures, suicidal ideation, tremors, night sweats, dream disorders
CV: Palpitations, ventricular extrasystole
EENT: Cataracts, blurred vision
GI: *Nausea*, vomiting, flatulence, *diarrhea, xerostomia*, altered taste, gastroenteritis, increased appetite
GU: Decreased libido, ejaculation disorder, increased frequency of urination, sexual dysfunction
HEMA: Bleeding, decreased platelets
INTEG: Sweating
MS: Arthralgia

SYST: Neonatal abstinence syndrome, withdrawal, serotonin syndrome

INTERACTIONS
Do not use within 2 wk of MAO inhibitors, linezolid, or methylene blue

Increase: serotonin syndrome—SSRIs, SNRIs, serotonin receptor agonists, selegiline, busPIRone, dextromethorphan, ergots, fenfluramine, dexfluramine, lithium, meperidine, fentaNYL, methylphenidate, dexmethylphenidate, metoclopramide, mirtazapine, nefazodone, pentazocine, phenothiazines, haloperidol, loxapine, thiothixene, molindone, amphetamines

Increase: bleeding—anticoagulants, thrombolytics, platelet inhibitors, salicylates, NSAIDs

Increase: vilazodone levels—CYP3A4 inhibitors (ketoconazole, erythromycin, efavirenz, dronedarone, clarithromycin and others)

Decrease: vilazodone effect—CYP3A4 inducers (carBAMazepine)

Drug/Food
• Avoid use with grapefruit juice
Drug/Herb
Increase: serotonin syndrome—St. John's wort
Drug/Lab Test
Decrease: sodium

PHARMACOKINETICS
Protein binding 96%-99%, metabolized by liver by CYP3A4 (major) and CYP2C19 and CYP2D (minor) and non-CYP pathways, peak 4-5 hr, half-life 25 hr

NURSING CONSIDERATIONS
Assess:

Black Box Warning: Mental status: orientation, mood, behavior initially and periodically; initiate suicide precautions if indicated; history of seizures, mania

• Renal/hepatic status: hyponatremia (confusion, weakness, headache); monitor serum sodium
• **Abrupt discontinuation:** do not discontinue abruptly, taper, monitor for symptoms of withdrawal; if intolerable, re-

V

---

sume previous dose and decrease more slowly

• **Serotonin syndrome:** nausea, vomiting, sedation, sweating, facial flushing, high B/P; discontinue product, notify prescriber

• **Neuroleptic malignant syndrome:** fever, change in mental status, seizures, rigidity; discontinue product, notify prescriber immediately

• **Pregnancy/breastfeeding:** use only if benefits outweigh fetal risk; if used in 3rd trimester, fetal complications may occur; avoid breastfeeding, excreted in breast milk

Evaluate:
• Therapeutic response: remission of depressive symptoms, decreased anxiety

Teach patient/family:
• To take as directed, with food, not to double dose, follow-up will be needed

• To avoid abrupt discontinuation unless approved by prescriber

• Not to drive or operate machinery until effects are known

• Not to use other products unless approved by prescriber, do not use alcohol

• **To contact prescriber regarding the following:** allergic reactions; personality changes (aggression, anxiety, anger, hostility); extreme sleepiness or drowsiness; feeling confused, nervous, restless, or clumsy; numbness, tingling, or burning pain in hands, arms, legs, or feet; tremors; unusual behavior or thoughts about hurting oneself

Black Box Warning: **Suicidal thoughts/ behaviors:** discuss with family the possibility of suicidal thoughts/behaviors and that prescriber should be notified immediately if these occur

• To notify prescriber if pregnancy is planned or suspected; to avoid breastfeeding

---

⚠ HIGH ALERT

vinBLAStine (VLB) (Rx)
(vin-blast′een)
Func. class.: Antineoplastic
Chem. class.: Vinca alkaloid

Do not confuse:
vinBLAStine/vinCRIStine/vinorelbine

ACTION: Inhibits mitotic activity, arrests cell cycle at metaphase; inhibits RNA synthesis, blocks cellular use of glutamic acid needed for purine synthesis; vesicant

USES: Breast, testicular cancer, lymphomas, neuroblastoma; Hodgkin's/ non-Hodgkin's lymphoma; mycosis fungoides, histiocytosis, Kaposi's sarcoma, Langerhans cell histiocytosis
Unlabeled uses: Lung, bladder, prostate cancer; desmoid tumor, malignant melanoma

CONTRAINDICATIONS: Pregnancy, breastfeeding, infants, hypersensitivity, leukopenia, granulocytopenia, bone marrow suppression, infection
Precautions: Renal/hepatic disease, tumor lysis syndrome

Black Box Warning: Extravasation, intrathecal use

DOSAGE AND ROUTES
Doses vary greatly
Breast cancer
• **Adult: IV** 4.5 mg/m^2 on day 1 of every 21 days in combination with DOXOrubicin and thiotepa
Hodgkin's disease
• **Adult: IV** 6 mg/m^2 on days 1 and 15 of every 28 days with DOXOrubicin, bleomycin, dacarbazine (ABVD regimen)
• **Child: IV** 2.5-6 mg/m^2/day once q1-2wk × 3-6 wk, max weekly dose 12.5 mg/m^2

Available forms: Inj, powder 10 mg for 10 mL IV; sol for inj 1 mg/mL
Administer:

Black Box Warning: Extravasation: aspirate, give hyaluronidase 150 units/mL in 1 mL NaCl, through IV catheter or subcut in circular pattern around extravasated site, warm compress for extravasation for vesicant activity treatment

Black Box Warning: Do not administer intrathecally; fatal

IV inj route
• After diluting 10 mg/10 mL NaCl; give through Y-tube or 3-way stopcock or directly over 1 min
Intermittent IV INFUSION route
• Further dilute in 50-100 mL of NS, infuse over 15-30 min

Y-site compatibilities: Acyclovir, alemtuzumab, alfentanil, allopurinol sodium, amifostine, amikacin, aminophylline, amiodarone, amphotericin B cholesteryl (Amphotec); amphotericin B lipid complex (Abelcet); ampicillin, ampicillin-sulbactam, anidulafungin, argatroban, arsenic trioxide, atenolol, atracurium, aztreonam, bivalirudin, bleomycin, bretylium, bumetanide, buprenorphine, busulfan, butorphanol, calcium chloride/gluconate, capreomycin, carboplatin, carmustine, caspofungin, cefazolin, cefoperazone, cefotaxime, cefotetan, cefOXitin, cefTAZidime, ceftazidime (ʟ-arginine), ceftizoxime, cefTRIAXone, cefuroxime, chloramphenicol sodium succinate, chlorproMAZINE, cimetidine, ciprofloxacin, cisatracurium, cisplatin, clindamycin, codeine, cyclophosphamide, cycloSPORINE, dacarbazine, DACTINomycin, DAPTOmycin, DAUNOrubicin, dexamethasone, dexmedetomidine, dexrazoxane, digoxin, diltiaZEM, diphenhydrAMINE, DOBUTamine, DOCEtaxel, dolasetron, DOPamine, DOXOrubicin, DOXOrubicin liposomal, doxycycline, droperidol, enalaprilat, ePHEDrine, EPINEPHrine, epiRUBicin, ertapenem, erythromycin, esmolol, etoposide, famotidine, fenoldopam, fentaNYL, filgrastim, fluconazole, fludarabine, fluorouracil, foscarnet, fosphenytoin, gallium, ganciclovir, garenoxacin, gatifloxacin, gemcitabine, gentamicin, glycopyrrolate, granisetron, haloperidol, heparin, hydrALAZINE, hydrocortisone, HYDROmorphone, hydrOXYzine, IDArubicin, ifosfamide, imipenem-cilastatin, inamrinone, insulin (regular), irinotecan, isoproterenol, ketorolac, labetalol, lepirudin, leucovorin, levoFLOXacin, levorphanol, lidocaine, linezolid, LORazepam, magnesium sulfate, mannitol, mechlorethamine, melphalan, meperidine, meropenem, mesna, metaraminol, methadone, methohexital, methotrexate, methyldopate, metoclopramide, metoprolol, metroNIDAZOLE, midazolam, milrinone, minocycline, mitoMYcin, mitoXANTRONE, morphine, moxifloxacin, nafcillin, nalbuphine, naloxone, nesiritide, nitroglycerin, nitroprusside, norepinephrine, octreotide, ofloxacin, ondansetron, oxaliplatin, PACLitaxel, palonosetron, pamidronate, pancuronium, PEMEtrexed, pentamidine, pentazocine, PENTobarbital, PHENobarbital, phentolamine, phenylephrine, piperacillin, piperacillin-tazobactam, polymyxin B, potassium acetate/chloride/phosphates, procainamide, prochlorperazine, promethazine, propranolol, quiNIDine, quinupristin-dalfopristin, raNITIdine, remifentanil, riTUXimab, sargramostim, sodium acetate/bicarbonate/phosphates, succinylcholine, SUFentanil, sulfamethoxazole-trimethoprim, tacrolimus, teniposide, theophylline, thiopental, thiotepa, ticarcillin, ticarcillin-clavulanate, tigecycline, tirofiban, tobramycin, tolazoline, topotecan, trastuzumab, trimethobenzamide, vancomycin, vasopressin, vecuronium, verapamil, vinCRIStine, vinorelbine, voriconazole, zidovudine, zoledronic acid.

V

SIDE EFFECTS
CNS: Paresthesias, peripheral neuropathy, depression, headache, seizures, malaise
CV: Tachycardia, orthostatic hypo/hypertension
GI: *Nausea, vomiting,* ileus, *anorexia, stomatitis, constipation,* abdominal

---

Side effects: *italics* = common; red = life-threatening

pain, GI/rectal bleeding, hepatotoxicity, pharyngitis

GU: Urinary retention, renal failure, hyperuricemia

HEMA: Thrombocytopenia, leukopenia, myelosuppression, agranulocytosis, granulocytosis, aplastic anemia, neutropenia, pancytopenia

INTEG: *Rash, alopecia,* photosensitivity, extravasation, tissue necrosis

META: SIADH

RESP: Fibrosis, pulmonary infiltrate, bronchospasm

SYST: Tumor lysis syndrome (TLS)

PHARMACOKINETICS
Half-life (triphasic) <5 min, 50-155 min, 23-85 hr; metabolized in liver; excreted in urine, feces; crosses blood-brain barrier

INTERACTIONS
Increase: synergism—bleomycin
• Do not use with radiation
Increase: bleeding risk—NSAIDs, anticoagulants, thrombolytics, antiplatelets
Increase: toxicity, bone marrow suppression—antineoplastics
Increase: action of methotrexate
Increase: adverse reactions—live virus vaccines
Increase: toxicity—CYP3A4 inhibitors (aprepitant, antiretroviral protease inhibitors, clarithromycin, danazol, delavirdine, diltiaZEM, erythromycin, fluconazole, FLUoxetine, fluvoxaMINE, imatinib, ketoconazole, mibefradil, nefazodone, telithromycin, voriconazole)
Decrease: vinBLAStine effect—CYP3A4 inducers (barbiturates, bosentan, carBAMazepine, efavirenz, phenytoins, nevirapine, rifabutin, rifAMPin)

Drug/Herb
• Avoid use with St. John's wort

Drug/Lab Test
Increase: uric acid, bilirubin
Decrease: Hgb, platelets, WBC

NURSING CONSIDERATIONS
Assess:
• B/P baseline and during use
• CBC, differential, platelet count weekly; withhold product if WBC is <2000/mm^3 or

platelet count is <75,000/mm^3; notify prescriber; RBC, Hct, Hgb may be decreased, nadir occurs on days 4-10 (leukopenia) and continues for another 1-2 wk

• **Tumor lysis syndrome:** monitor for hyperkalemia, hyperphosphatemia, hyperuricemia; usually occurs with leukemia, lymphoma; alkalinization of the urine, allopurinol should be used to prevent urate nephropathy; monitor electrolytes and renal function (BUN, uric acid, urine CCR)

• **Hepatitis:** transient hepatitis may occur with continuous IV

• Bleeding: hematuria, guaiac, bruising, petechiae, mucosa or orifices

• **Bronchospasm:** can be life-threatening; usually occurs when giving mitoMYcin

• Effects of alopecia on body image; discuss feelings about body changes

• Sensitivity of feet/hands, which precedes neuropathy

• Jaundiced skin, sclera; dark urine, clay-colored stools, itchy skin, abdominal pain, fever, diarrhea

• Buccal cavity q8hr for dryness, sores, ulcerations, white patches, oral pain, bleeding, dysphagia

> Black Box Warning: **Extravasation:** local irritation, pain, burning, discoloration at IV site

• **Symptoms indicating severe allergic reaction:** rash, pruritus, urticaria, purpuric skin lesions, itching, flushing
• Increased fluid intake to 2-3 L/day to prevent urate deposits, calculi formation
• **Pregnancy/breastfeeding:** do not use in pregnancy; do not breastfeed

Evaluate:
• Therapeutic response: decreased tumor size, spread of malignancy

Teach patient/family:
• Brushing of teeth bid-tid with soft brush or cotton-tipped applicator for stomatitis; to use unwaxed dental floss
• To report any bleeding, white spots, ulcerations in mouth to prescriber; to examine mouth daily

---

- To report any changes in breathing or coughing; to avoid exposure to persons with infection
- That hair may be lost during treatment; that a wig or hairpiece may make patient feel better; that new hair may be different in color, texture
- To report change in gait or numbness in extremities; may indicate neuropathy
- To avoid foods with citric acid, hot temperature, or rough texture
- To wear sunscreen, protective clothing, sunglasses
- To avoid receiving vaccinations
- **Infection:** to report sore throat, flulike symptoms; to avoid persons with known infections
- **Pregnancy:** not to breastfeed; that product may cause male infertility; to notify prescriber if pregnancy is planned or suspected

---

⚠ HIGH ALERT

vinCRIStine (VCR) (Rx)

(vin-kris'teen)
Func. class.: Antineoplastic—miscellaneous
Chem. class.: Vinca alkaloid

Do not confuse:
vinCRIStine/vinBLAStine/vinorelbine

ACTION: Inhibits mitotic activity, arrests cell cycle at metaphase; inhibits RNA synthesis, blocks cellular use of glutamic acid needed for purine synthesis; vesicant

USES: Lymphomas, neuroblastoma, Hodgkin's disease, acute lymphoblastic and other leukemias, rhabdomyosarcoma, Wilms' tumor, non-Hodgkin's lymphoma, malignant glioma, soft-tissue sarcoma; liposomal: Philadelphia chromosome—negative ALL in second or greater relapse or that has progressed after ≥2 antileukemia therapies

Unlabeled uses: Lung, breast, colorectal, head/neck, osteogenic sarcomas;

small-cell lung cancer, trophoblastic disease

CONTRAINDICATIONS: Pregnancy, breastfeeding, infants, hypersensitivity, radiation therapy

Black Box Warning: Intrathecal use

Precautions: Renal/hepatic disease, hypertension, neuromuscular disease

Black Box Warning: Extravasation

DOSAGE AND ROUTES
- **Adult: IV** 0.4-1.4 mg/m²/wk, max 2 mg
- **Child: IV** 1-2 mg/m²/wk, max 2 mg
Available forms: Inj 1 mg/mL
Administer:

Black Box Warning: Do not give intrathecally; fatal

IV route
- After diluting with diluent provided or 1 mg/10 mL sterile water or NaCl; give through Y-tube or 3-way stopcock or directly over 1 min; do not use 5-mg vial for single doses

Black Box Warning: Hyaluronidase 150 units/mL in 1 mL NaCl; apply warm compress for extravasation

Y-site compatibilities: Acyclovir, alemtuzumab, alfentanil, allopurinol, amifostine, amikacin, aminocaproic acid, aminophylline, amiodarone, amphotericin B cholesteryl, amphotericin B lipid complex, amphotericin B liposome, ampicillin, ampicillin-sulbactam, anidulafungin, argatroban, arsenic trioxide, asparaginase, atenolol, atracurium, azithromycin, aztreonam, bivalirudin, bleomycin, bumetanide, buprenorphine, butorphanol, calcium chloride/gluconate, capreomycin, CARBOplatin, carmustine, caspofungin, ceFAZolin, cefoperazone, cefoTEtan, cefOXitin, cefTAZidime, ceftizoxime, cefTRIAXone, cefuroxime, chlorproMAZINE, cimetidine, ciprofloxacin, cisatracurium, CISplatin, cladribine, clindamycin, codeine, cyclophosphamide, cycloSPORINE, cytarabine, D_5W-dextrose 5%, dacarbazine, DACTINomycin, DAPTOmycin, DAUNOrubicin, DAUNOrubicin citrate liposome, dexamethasone, dexmedetomidine, dexrazoxane, digoxin, diltiazem, diphenhydrAMINE, DOBUTamine, DOCEtaxel, dolasetron, DOPamine, doxacurium, doxapram, DOXOrubicin, DOXOrubicin liposomal, doxycycline, droperidol, enalaprilat, ePHEDrine, EPINEPHrine, epiRUBicin, ertapenem, erythromycin, esmolol, etoposide, famotidine, fenoldopam, fentaNYL, filgrastim, fluconazole, fludarabine, fluorouracil, foscarnet, fosphenytoin, gallium, ganciclovir, garenoxacin, gatifloxacin, gemcitabine, gentamicin, granisetron, haloperidol, heparin, hydrocortisone sodium phosphate/succinate, HYDROmorphone, hydrOXYzine, ifosfamide, imipenem-cilastatin, inamrinone, insulin (regular), isoproterenol, ketorolac, labetalol, lepirudin, leucovorin, levoFLOXacin, levorphanol, lidocaine, linezolid, LORazepam, magnesium sulfate, mannitol, mechlorethamine, melphalan, meperidine, meropenem, mesna, methadone, methohexital, methotrexate, methylPREDNISolone, metoclopramide, metoprolol, metroNIDAZOLE, midazolam, milrinone, minocycline, mitoMYcin, mitoXANtrone, mivacurium, morphine, moxifloxacin, nalbuphine, naloxone, nesiritide, niCARdipine, nitroglycerin, nitroprusside, norepinephrine, octreotide, ondansetron, oxaliplatin, PACLitaxel (solvent/surfactant), palonosetron, pamidronate, pancuronium, PEMEtrexed, pentamidine, pentazocine, PENTobarbital, PHENobarbital, phenylephrine, piperacillin, piperacillin–tazobactam, potassium acetate/chloride/phosphates, procainamide, prochlorperazine, promethazine, propranolol, quinupristin-dalfopristin, ranitidine, remifentanil, riTUXimab, rocuronium, sargramostim, sodium acetate/phosphates, succinylcholine, SUFentanil, sulfamethoxazole-trimethoprim, tacrolimus, teniposide, theophylline, thiopental, thiotepa, ticarcillin, ticarcillin-clavulanate, tigecycline, tirofiban, tobramycin, topotecan, trastuzumab, trimethobenzamide, vancomycin, vasopressin, vecuronium, verapamil, vinBLAStine, vinorelbine, voriconazole, zidovudine, zoledronic acid

SIDE EFFECTS

CNS: *Decreased reflexes, numbness, weakness, motor difficulties,* CNS depression, cranial nerve paralysis, seizures, peripheral neuropathy

CV: Orthostatic hypotension

EENT: *Diplopia*

GI: *Nausea, vomiting, anorexia, stomatitis, constipation,* paralytic ileus, *abdominal pain,* hepatotoxicity

GU: Renal tubular obstruction

HEMA: Thrombocytopenia, leukopenia, myelosuppression, anemia

INTEG: *Alopecia,* extravasation

SYST: Tumor lysis syndrome (TLS)

PHARMACOKINETICS

Half-life (triphasic) <5 min, 50-155 min, 23-85 hr; metabolized in liver; excreted in bile, feces; crosses placental, blood-brain barrier

INTERACTIONS

Decrease: immune response—vaccines toxoids

Decrease: digoxin level—digoxin

Decrease: vinCRIStine effect—CYP3A4 inducers (barbiturates, bosentan, carBAMazepine, efavirenz, phenytoins, nevirapine, rifabutin, rifAMPin)

• Do not use with radiation

• **Acute pulmonary reactions:** mitoMYcin C

• **Increase:** toxicity—CYP3A4 inhibitor (aprepitant, antiretroviral protease inhibitors, clarithromycin, danazol, delavirdine, diltiaZEM, erythromycin, fluconazole, FLUoxetine, fluvoxaMINE, imatinib, ketoconazole, mibefradil, nefazodone, telithromycin, voriconazole)

Drug/Herb

• Avoid use with St. John's wort

Drug/Lab Test
Increase: uric acid
Decrease: Hgb, WBC, platelets, sodium

NURSING CONSIDERATIONS
Assess:
• CBC, differential, platelet count before each dose; withhold product if WBC is <4000/mm^3 or platelet count is <75,000/mm^3; notify prescriber; RBC, Hct, Hgb; may be decreased, nadir occurs on day 4-10 (leukopenia); continues for another 1-2 wk
• **Bronchospasm:** more common with mitoMYcin
• Hepatic studies before, during therapy (bilirubin, AST, ALT, LDH) as needed or monthly
• Sensitivity of feet/hands, which precedes neuropathy
• **Tumor lysis syndrome:** hyperkalemia, hyperphosphatemia, hyperuricemia, hypocalcemia; more common in leukemia, lymphoma; use alkalinization of urine with allopurinol, monitor electrolytes, renal function (BUN, urine, CCR, uric acid)

Black Box Warning: Extravasation: pain, swelling, poor blood return; if extravasation occurs, local inj of hyaluronidase and moderate heat to area may help disperse product

• **Pregnancy/breastfeeding:** do not use in pregnancy, breastfeeding
Intrathecal administration
• **Bleeding:** hematuria, guaiac, bruising, petechiae, mucosa or orifices q8hr
• Effects of alopecia on body image; discuss feelings about body changes
• Buccal cavity q8hr for dryness, sores, ulcerations, white patches, oral pain, bleeding, dysphagia
• Symptoms indicating severe allergic reaction: rash, pruritus, urticaria, purpuric skin lesions, itching, flushing
Evaluate:
• Therapeutic response: decreased tumor size, spread of malignancy
Teach patient/family:
• To brush teeth bid-tid with soft brush or cotton-tipped applicator for stomatitis; to use unwaxed dental floss

• To report change in gait or numbness in extremities; may indicate neuropathy
• To report any bleeding, white spots, or ulcerations in mouth to prescriber; to examine mouth daily
• To increase bulk, fluids, exercise to prevent constipation
• **Infection:** to report sore throat, fever, flulike symptoms; to avoid persons with known infection
• To avoid vaccinations
• That hair may be lost; that hair will grow back but with different texture, color
• **Pregnancy/breastfeeding:** to notify prescriber if pregnancy is planned or suspected; to use effective contraception during and for 2 mo after therapy; not to breastfeed

vinCRIStine liposomal (Rx)
Marqibo
Func. class.: Antineoplastic—miscellaneous
Chem. class.: Vinca alkaloid

Do not confuse:
vinCRIStine/vinBLAStine/vinorelbine

ACTION: Inhibits mitotic activity, arrests cell cycle at metaphase; inhibits RNA synthesis, blocks cellular use of glutamic acid needed for purine synthesis; vesicant

USES: Lymphomas, neuroblastoma, Hodgkin's disease, acute lymphoblastic and other leukemias, rhabdomyosarcoma, Wilms' tumor, non-Hodgkin's lymphoma, malignant glioma, soft-tissue sarcoma; liposomal: Philadelphia chromosome–negative ALL in second or greater relapse or that has progressed after ≥2 antileukemia therapies
Unlabeled uses: Lung, breast, colorectal, head/neck, osteogenic sarcomas; small-cell lung cancer, trophoblastic disease

CONTRAINDICATIONS:
Pregnancy, breastfeeding, infants, hypersensitivity, radiation therapy

V

Side effects: *italics* = common; red = life-threatening

Precautions: Renal/hepatic disease, hypertension, neuromuscular disease

DOSAGE AND ROUTES
• **Adult:** IV 2.25 mg/m^2 over 1 hr q7days
Available forms: Liposomal 5 mg/31 mL injection kit

Administer:
IV route
• Use safety cabinet and 60-90 min to prepare; manufacturer provides needed equipment, do not use in-line filters, do not admix; usually prepared in the pharmacy; please consult manufacturer for preparation
Intravenous Infusion
• Administer diluted solution IV over 1 hr; finish infusion within 12 hr after starting the preparation

Y-site compatibilities Acyclovir, alemtuzumab, alfentanil, allopurinol, amifostine, amikacin, aminocaproic acid, aminophylline, amiodarone, amphotericin B cholesteryl, amphotericin B lipid complex, amphotericin B liposome, ampicillin, ampicillin-sulbactam, anidulafungin, argatroban, arsenic trioxide, asparaginase, atenolol, atracurium, azithromycin, aztreonam, bivalirudin, bleomycin, bumetanide, buprenorphine, butorphanol, calcium chloride/gluconate, capreomycin, CARBOplatin, carmustine, caspofungin, ceFAZolin, cefoperazone, cefoTEtan, cefOXitin, cefTAZidime, ceftizoxime, cefTRIAXone, cefuroxime, chlorproMAZINE, cimetidine, ciprofloxacin, cisatracurium, CISplatin, cladribine, clindamycin, codeine,

cyclophosphamide, cycloSPORINE, cytarabine, D$_5$W-dextrose 5%, dacarbazine, DACTINomycin, DAPTOmycin, DAUNOrubicin, DAUNOrubicin citrate liposome, dexrazoxane, digoxin, diltiazem, diphenhydrAMINE, DOBUTamine, DOCEtaxel, dolasetron, DOPamine, doxacurium, doxapram, DOXOrubicin, DOXOrubicin liposomal, doxycycline, droperidol, enalaprilat, ePHEDrine, EPINEPHrine, epirubicin, ertapenem, erythromycin, esmolol, etoposide, famotidine, fenoldopam, fentaNYL, filgrastim, fluconazole, fludarabine, fluorouracil, foscarnet, fosphenytoin, gallium, ganciclovir, garenoxacin, gatifloxacin, gemcitabine, gentamicin, granisetron, haloperidol, heparin, hydrocortisone sodium phosphate/succinate, HYDROmorphone, hydrOXYzine, ifosfamide, imipenem-cilastatin, inamrinone, insulin, regular, isoproterenol, ketorolac, labetalol, lepirudin, leucovorin, levofloxacin, levorphanol, lidocaine, linezolid, LORazepam, magnesium sulfate, mannitol, mechlorethamine, melphalan, meperidine, meropenem, mesna, methadone, methohexital, methotrexate, methylPREDNISolone, metoclopramide, metoprolol, metroNIDAZOLE, midazolam, milrinone, minocycline, mitoMYcin, mitoXANtrone, mivacurium, morphine, moxifloxacin, nalbuphine, naloxone, nesiritide, niCARdipine, nitroglycerin, nitroprusside, norepinephrine, octreotide, ondansetron, oxaliplatin, PACLitaxel (solvent/surfactant), palonosetron, pamidronate, pancuronium, PEMEtrexed, pentamidine, pentazocine, PENTobarbital, PHENobarbital, phenylephrine, piperacillin, piperacillin-tazobactam, potassium acetate/chloride/phosphates, procainamide, prochlorperazine, promethazine, propranolol, quinupristin-dalfopristin, ranitidine, remifentanil, riTUXimab, rocuronium, sargramostim, sodium acetate/phosphates, succinylcholine, SUFentanil, sulfamethoxazole-trimethoprim, tacrolimus, teniposide, theophylline, thiopental, thiotepa, ticarcillin, ticarcillin-clavulanate, tigecycline, tirofiban, tobramycin, topotecan, trastuzumab, trimethobenzamide, vancomycin, vasopressin, vecuronium, verapamil, vinBLAStine, vinorelbine, voriconazole, zidovudine, zoledronic acid

SIDE EFFECTS

CNS: *Decreased reflexes, numbness, weakness, motor difficulties,* CNS depression, cranial nerve paralysis, seizures, peripheral neuropathy

CV: Orthostatic hypotension

EENT: *Diplopia*

GI: *Nausea, vomiting, anorexia, stomatitis, constipation,* paralytic ileus, *abdominal pain,* hepatotoxicity

GU: Renal tubular obstruction

HEMA: Thrombocytopenia, leukopenia, myelosuppression, anemia

INTEG: *Alopecia,* extravasation

SYST: Tumor lysis syndrome (TLS)

PHARMACOKINETICS

Half-life (triphasic) <5 min, 50-155 min, 23-85 hr; metabolized in liver; excreted in bile, feces; crosses placental, blood-brain barrier

INTERACTIONS

Decrease: immune response—vaccines, toxoids

Decrease: digoxin level—digoxin

Decrease: vinCRIStine effect—CYP3A4 inducers (barbiturates, bosentan, carBAMazepine, efavirenz, phenytoins, nevirapine, rifabutin, rifampin)

• Do not use with radiation

• **Acute pulmonary reactions:** mitoMYcin C

Increase: toxicity—CYP3A4 inhibitors (aprepitant, antiretroviral protease inhibitors, clarithromycin, danazol, delavirdine, diltiaZEM, erythromycin, fluconazole, FLUoxetine, fluvoxaMINE, imatinib, ketoconazole, mibefradil, nefazodone, telithromycin, voriconazole)

Drug/Herb

• Avoid use with St. John's wort

Drug/Lab Test

Increase: uric acid

Decrease: Hgb, WBC, platelets, sodium

NURSING CONSIDERATIONS

Assess:

• CBC, differential, platelet count before each dose; withhold product if WBC

is <4000/mm^3 or platelet count is <75,000/mm^3; notify prescriber; RBC, Hct, Hgb may be decreased

• **Bronchospasm:** more common with mitoMYcin

• Hepatic studies before, during therapy (bilirubin, AST, ALT, LDH) as needed or monthly

• Sensitivity of feet/hands, which precedes neuropathy

• **Tumor lysis syndrome:** hyperkalemia, hyperphosphatemia, hyperuricemia, hypocalcemia; more common in leukemia, lymphoma; use alkalinization of urine with allopurinol, monitor electrolytes, renal function (BUN, urine, CCR, uric acid)

Black Box Warning: **Extravasation:** pain, swelling, poor blood return; if extravasation occurs, local inj of hyaluronidase and moderate heat to area may help disperse product

• **Bleeding:** hematuria, guaiac, bruising, petechiae, mucosa or orifices q8hr

• Effects of alopecia on body image; discuss feelings about body changes

• Buccal cavity q8hr for dryness, sores, ulcerations, white patches, oral pain, bleeding, dysphagia

• Symptoms indicating severe allergic reaction: rash, pruritus, urticaria, purpuric skin lesions, itching, flushing

• Brushing of teeth bid-tid with soft brush or cotton-tipped applicator for stomatitis; use unwaxed dental floss

Evaluate:

• Therapeutic response: decreased tumor size, spread of malignancy

Teach patient/family:

• To report change in gait or numbness in extremities; may indicate neuropathy

• To report any bleeding, white spots, or ulcerations in mouth to prescriber; to examine mouth daily

• To increase bulk, fluids, exercise to prevent constipation

• **Infection:** to report sore throat, fever, flulike symptoms; to avoid persons with known infection

• To avoid vaccinations

Side effects: *italics* = common; red = life-threatening

• That hair may be lost; that hair will grow back but with different texture, color
• **Pregnancy:** to notify prescriber if pregnancy is planned or suspected
• To use effective contraception during and for 2 mo after therapy; to avoid breastfeeding

---

⚠ HIGH ALERT

vinorelbine (Rx)

(vi-nor′el-bine)

Navelbine

Func. class.: Antineoplastic—miscellaneous

Chem. class.: Semisynthetic vinca alkaloid

ACTION: Inhibits mitotic spindle activity, arrests cell cycle at metaphase; inhibits RNA synthesis, blocks cellular use of glutamic acid needed for purine synthesis; vesicant

USES: Unresectable advanced non–small-cell lung cancer (NSCLC) stage IV; may be used alone or in combination with CISplatin for stage III or IV NSCLC

Unlabeled uses: Hodgkin's disease, breast/ovarian/head/neck cancer, desmoid tumor

CONTRAINDICATIONS: Pregnancy, breastfeeding, infants, hypersensitivity, granulocyte count <1000 cells/mm³ pretreatment

Black Box Warning: Severe neutropenia, intrathecal administration

Precautions: Children, geriatric patients, renal/hepatic/pulmonary/neurologic disease, anemia, bone marrow suppression, severe neutropenia, intrathecal administration, extravasation

Black Box Warning: Extravasation

DOSAGE AND ROUTES
• **Adult:** IV 30 mg/m²/wk

• **ANC 1000-1499/mm³:** give 50% of dose; <1000/mm³, hold dose; <1000/mm³ × 3 wk, discontinue
Hepatic dose
• **Adult:** IV total bilirubin 2.1-3 mg/dL 15 mg/m²/wk; total bilirubin ≥3 mg/dL 7.5 mg/m²/day

Available forms: Inj 10 mg/mL
Administer:

Black Box Warning: Do not give intrathecally, fatal; syringes with this product should be labeled "Warning, for IV use only, fatal if given intrathecally"

Intermittent IV INFUSION route
• Dilute to 0.5-2 mg/mL with 0.9% NaCl, 0.45% NaCl, D₅W, D₅/0.45% NaCl, LR, Ringer's sol, give over 6-10 min into Y-site or central line, flush line

Black Box Warning: **Extravasation:** stop infusion, give hyaluronidase 150 units/mL in 1 mL NaCl through IV catheter or subcut in circular pattern around site, warm compress for extravasation for vesicant activity treatment

Continuous IV INFUSION route
• 40 mg/m² q3wk after IV bol of 8 mg/m²; may be given in combination with DOXOrubicin, fluorouracil, CISplatin

Y-site compatibilities: Amikacin, aztreonam, bleomycin, bumetanide, buprenorphine, butorphanol, calcium gluconate, CARBOplatin, carmustine, cefotaxime, cefTAZidime, ceftizoxime, chlorproMAZINE, cimetidine, CISplatin, clindamycin, cyclophosphamide, cytarabine, dacarbazine, DACTINomycin, DAUNOrubicin, dexamethasone, diphenhydrAMINE, DOXOrubicin, DOXOrubicin liposome, doxycycline, droperidol, enalaprilat, etoposide, famotidine, filgrastim, floxuridine, fluconazole, fludarabine, gallium, gentamicin, granisetron, haloperidol, heparin, hydrocortisone, HYDROmorphone, hydrOXYzine, IDArubicin, ifosfamide, imipenem-cilastatin,

---

LORazepam, mannitol, mechlorethamine, melphalan, meperidine, mesna, methotrexate, metoclopramide, metroNIDAZOLE, minocycline, mitoXANtrone, morphine, nalbuphine, netilmicin, ondansetron, plicamycin, streptozocin, teniposide, ticarcillin, ticarcillin-clavulanate, tobramycin, vancomycin, vinBLAStine, vinCRIStine, zidovudine

SIDE EFFECTS

CNS: Paresthesias, peripheral neuropathy, depression, headache, seizures, weakness, jaw pain, asthenia
CV: Chest pain
GI: *Nausea, vomiting,* ileus, *anorexia, stomatitis,* constipation, abdominal pain, *diarrhea,* hepatotoxicity, GI obstruction/perforation
HEMA: Neutropenia, anemia, thrombocytopenia, granulocytopenia
INTEG: *Rash, alopecia,* photosensitivity, inj site reaction, necrosis
META: SIADH
MS: Myalgia
RESP: SOB, dyspnea, pulmonary edema, acute bronchospasm, acute respiratory distress syndrome (ARDS)

PHARMACOKINETICS

Half-life 27-43 hr; peak 1-2 hr; highly bound to platelets, lymphocytes; metabolized in liver; excreted in feces; small amount unchanged in kidneys

INTERACTIONS

Increase: bleeding risk—NSAIDs, anticoagulants
Increase: toxicity—CYP3A4 inhibitors (aprepitant, antiretroviral protease inhibitors, clarithromycin, danazol, delavirdine, diltiaZEM, erythromycin, fluconazole, FLUoxetine, fluvoxaMINE, imatinib, ketoconazole, mibefradil, nefazodone, telithromycin, voriconazole)
Decrease: vinorelbine effect—CYP3A4 inducers (barbiturates, bosentan, carBAMazepine, efavirenz, phenytoins, nevirapine, rifabutin, rifampin)
Drug/Herb
• Avoid use with St. John's wort

Drug/Lab Test
Increase: LFTs, bilirubin
Decrease: Hgb, WBC, platelets

NURSING CONSIDERATIONS
Assess:
• B/P (baseline) during administration

> **Black Box Warning: Bone marrow suppression:** CBC, differential, platelet count before each dose; withhold product if WBC is <4000/mm³ or platelet count is <75,000/mm³; notify prescriber of results; recovery will take 3 wk

• **Bronchospasm:** more common with mitoMYcin; also dyspnea, wheezing; may be treated with oxygen, bronchodilators, corticosteroids, especially if there is underlying pulmonary disease
• **Neurologic status:** paresthesia, peripheral neuropathy, weakness; these may occur even after termination of treatment
• Renal studies: BUN, serum uric acid, urine CCr before, during therapy; I&O ratio; report fall in urine output to <30 mL/hr; decreased hyperuricemia
• **Infection,** cold, fever, sore throat; notify prescriber if these occur; effects of alopecia on body image
• **Bleeding:** hematuria, guaiac, bruising, petechiae, mucosa or orifices, no rectal temperatures; avoid IM inj; apply pressure to venipuncture sites
• Hepatic function tests: AST, ALT, bilirubin, LDH
• **Severe allergic reactions:** rash, pruritus, urticaria, itching, flushing, bronchospasm, hypotension; EPINEPHrine and crash cart should be nearby
• **Pregnancy:** determine pregnancy before starting treatment; do not use in pregnancy; do not breastfeed
Evaluate:
• Therapeutic response: decreased tumor size, spread of malignancy
Teach patient/family:
• To report change in gait or numbness in extremities, continuing constipation; may indicate neurotoxicity

V

• To brush teeth bid-tid with soft brush or cotton-tipped applicator for stomatitis; to use unwaxed dental floss

• To examine mouth daily for bleeding, white spots, ulcerations; to notify prescriber

• **Infection:** report sore throat, fever, flulike symptoms

• To avoid crowds, people with infections, vaccinations, OTC products

• **Pregnancy:** to notify prescriber if pregnancy is planned or suspected; to use effective contraception during treatment and for ≥2 mo after product is discontinued; not to breastfeed

• That hair may be lost; that hair will grow back but with different texture, color

---

⚠ HIGH ALERT

vismodegib
(vis′moe-deg′ib)

Erivedge

Func. class.: Antineoplastic biologic response modifier

Chem. class.: Signal transduction inhibitor (STI)

ACTION: A hedgehog (Hh) signaling pathway inhibitor

USES: Patients who have metastatic basal cell carcinoma, locally advanced, that has recurred after surgery and who are not candidates for surgery/radiation

CONTRAINDICATIONS: Hypersensitivity, breastfeeding

Black Box Warning: Intrauterine fetal death, male-mediated teratogenicity, pregnancy

Precautions: Children, blood donation

DOSAGE AND ROUTES
• **Adult:** PO 150 mg/day

Available forms: Cap 150 mg
Administer:
• Give without regard to food
• Swallow whole, do not open or crush caps
• If a dose is missed, do not take additional dose, take at usual time
• Store at 77° F (25° C)

SIDE EFFECTS
GI: *Nausea, vomiting, dysgeusia, constipation, anorexia, diarrhea*
GU: Amenorrhea, azotemia
INTEG: *Alopecia*
META: Hyponatremia
MISC: *Fatigue, decreased weight*
MS: *Arthralgia*

PHARMACOKINETICS
Protein binding >99%, elimination half-life 4 days

INTERACTIONS
Increase: vismodegib effect—osimertinib
Increase: effect of sofosbuvir, velpatasvir, topotecan
Increase: INR levels—warfarin; increase INR monitoring

NURSING CONSIDERATIONS
Assess:

Black Box Warning: **Pregnancy:** Verify pregnancy status of all women within 7 days before starting therapy; effective contraception is needed during and for 24 mo after treatment; men receiving this product should use condoms with spermicide (even after vasectomy) during sexual intercourse with female partners and for 2 mo after the last dose; semen donation is contraindicated during treatment and for 3 mo after treatment; report exposure during pregnancy to the Genentech Adverse Event Line at 1-888-835-2555

Evaluate:
• Therapeutic response: decreased spread of tumor
Teach patient/family:

Black Box Warning: Pregnancy: Teach patients to notify their providers immediately if pregnancy is suspected (or in a female partner for male patients); effective contraception is needed during and for 7 mo after treatment; men receiving this product should use condoms with spermicide (even after vasectomy) during sexual intercourse with female partners and for 2 mo after the last dose; if product is used during pregnancy or if the patient becomes pregnant during use, the woman (or female partner for male patients) should be apprised of the potential hazard to the fetus; encourage exposed women (either directly or through seminal fluid) to participate in the ERIVEDGE pregnancy pharmacovigilance program

• About reason for treatment, expected results
• That if dose is missed, do not take, but resume scheduled doses; to swallow whole, not to crush or chew
• Not to donate blood during therapy or for ≥ 24 mo after conclusion of product
• **Amenorrhea:** it is unknown if reversible after completion of treatment

---

vitamin A (Rx, PO-OTC, Rx-IM)

Aquasol A, Vitamin A
Func. class.: Vitamin, fat soluble
Chem. class.: Retinol

ACTION: Needed for normal bone, tooth development; visual dark adaptation; skin disease; mucosa tissue repair; assists with production of adrenal steroids, cholesterol, RNA

USES: Vit A deficiency

CONTRAINDICATIONS: Pregnancy (IM), hypersensitivity to vit A, malabsorption syndrome, hypervitaminosis A, IV administration

Precautions: Pregnancy (PO), breastfeeding, impaired renal function, children, hepatic disease, infants, alcoholism, hepatitis

DOSAGE AND ROUTES
• **Adult and child >8 yr:** PO 100,000-500,000 international units/day × 3 days then 50,000 international units/day × 2 wk; dose based on severity of deficiency; maintenance 10,000-20,000 international units for 2 mo
• **Child 1-8 yr:** IM 5000-15,000 international units/day × 10 days
• **Infant <1 yr:** IM 5000-15,000 international units/day × 10 days
Maintenance
• **Child 4-8 yr:** IM 15,000 international units/day × 2 mo
• **Child <4 yr:** IM 10,000 international units/day × 2 mo
Available forms: Caps 10,000, 25,000, 50,000 international units; drops 5000 international units; inj 50,000 international units/mL; tabs 10,000, 25,000, 50,000 international units
Administer:
PO route
• With food (PO) for better absorption
• Do not administer IV because of risk of anaphylactic shock; IM only
• Oral preparations not indicated for vit A deficiency in those with malabsorption syndrome
• Store in tight, light-resistant container
IM route
• Give deep in large muscle mass; do not use deltoid muscle for administration of >1 mL

SIDE EFFECTS
CNS: Headache, increased intracranial pressure, intracranial hypertension, lethargy, malaise
EENT: Gingivitis, papilledema, exophthalmos, inflammation of tongue and lips
GI: Nausea, vomiting, anorexia, abdominal pain, jaundice
INTEG: Drying of skin, pruritus, increased pigmentation, night sweats, alopecia

V

META: Hypomenorrhea, hypercalcemia
MS: Arthralgia, retarded growth, hard areas on bone

PHARMACOKINETICS
Stored in liver, kidneys, fat; excreted (metabolites) in urine, feces

INTERACTIONS
Increase: levels of vit A—corticosteroids, oral contraceptives
Decrease: absorption of vit A—mineral oil, cholestyramine, colestipol
Drug/Lab Test
False increase: bilirubin, serum cholesterol

NURSING CONSIDERATIONS
Assess:
• Nutritional status: yellow and dark green vegetables, yellow/orange fruits, vit A–fortified foods, liver, egg yolks
• **Vit A deficiency:** decreased growth; night blindness; dry, brittle nails; hair loss; urinary stones; increased infection; hyperkeratosis of skin; drying of cornea
• **Pregnancy/breastfeeding:** do not use IM in pregnancy, fetal complications may occur; breastfeeding is considered safe at recommended dietary levels
Evaluate:
• Therapeutic response: increased growth rate, weight; absence of dry skin and mucous membranes, night blindness
Teach patient/family:
• That if dose is missed, it should be omitted
• That ophthalmic exams may be required periodically throughout therapy
• Not to use mineral oil while taking this product
• To notify prescriber of nausea, vomiting, lip cracking, loss of hair, headache
• Not to take more than prescribed amount

TREATMENT OF OVERDOSE:
Discontinue product

---

vitamin C (ascorbic acid) (OTC, Rx)
(a-skor'bic)
Func. class.: Vit C—water-soluble vitamin

ACTION: Wound healing, collagen synthesis, antioxidant, carbohydrate metabolism

USES: Vit C deficiency, scurvy; delayed wound, bone healing; chronic disease; urine acidification; before gastrectomy; dietary supplement
Unlabeled uses: Common cold prevention

CONTRAINDICATIONS: Tartrazine, sulfite sensitivity; G6PD deficiency
Precautions: Pregnancy, gout, diabetes, renal calculi (large doses)

DOSAGE AND ROUTES
Dietary supplementation
• **Adult:** PO 50-500 mg/day
• **Child 14-18 yr:** PO 65 mg (female), 75 mg (male)
• **Child 9-13 yr:** PO 45 mg/day
• **Child 4-8 yr:** PO 25 mg/day
• **Child 1-3 yr:** PO 15 mg/day
• **Infant:** PO 40-50 mg/day
Scurvy
• **Adult:** PO/SUBCUT/IM/IV 100-250 mg/day × 2 wk, then 50 mg or more daily
• **Child:** PO/SUBCUT/IM/IV 100-300 mg/day × 2 wk, then 35 mg or more daily
Wound healing/chronic disease/ fracture (may be given with zinc)
• **Adult:** SUBCUT/IM/IV/PO 200-500 mg/day for 1-2 mo
• **Child:** SUBCUT/IM/IV/PO 100-200 mg added doses for 1-2 mo
Urine acidification
• **Adult:** PO 4-12 g/day in divided doses
• **Child:** PO 500 mg q6-8hr
Available forms: Tabs 25, 50, 100, 250, 500, 1000, 1500 mg; effervescent tabs 1000 mg; chewable tabs 100, 250,

---

500 mg; timed-release tabs 500, 750, 1000, 1500 mg; timed-release caps 500 mg; crys 4 g/tsp; powder 4 g/tsp; liq 35 mg/0.6 mL; sol 100 mg/mL; syr 20 mg/mL, 500 mg/5 mL; inj SUBCUT, IM, IV 100, 250, 500 mg/mL

Administer:
PO route
• Do not crush or chew ext rel tabs or caps
• Caps may be opened and contents mixed with jelly
IV, direct route
• 100 mg undiluted by direct IV over at least 1 min; rapid infusion may cause fainting
Intermittent IV INFUSION route
• Diluted with D₅W, D₅NaCl, NS, LR, Ringer's, sodium lactate and given over 15 min

Syringe compatibilities: Metoclopramide, aminophylline, theophylline
Y-site compatibilities: Warfarin

SIDE EFFECTS
CNS: Headache, insomnia, dizziness, fatigue, flushing
GI: Nausea, vomiting, diarrhea, anorexia, heartburn, cramps
GU: Polyuria, urine acidification, oxalate/urate renal stones, dysuria
HEMA: Hemolytic anemia in patients with G6PD
INTEG: Inflammation at inj site

PHARMACOKINETICS
PO/INJ: Readily absorbed PO, metabolized in liver; unused amounts excreted in urine (unchanged), metabolites; crosses placenta, breast milk

INTERACTIONS
Drug/Lab Test
False negative: occult blood, urine bilirubin, leukocyte determination

NURSING CONSIDERATIONS
Assess:
• I&O ratio; urine pH (acidification)
• Ascorbic acid levels throughout treatment if continued deficiency is suspected
• Nutritional status: citrus fruits, vegetables

• Inj sites for inflammation
• Thrombophlebitis if receiving large dose
• **Pregnancy/breastfeeding:** use only recommended dietary allowances in pregnancy, breastfeeding

Evaluate:
• Therapeutic response: absence of anorexia, irritability, pallor, joint pain, hyperkeratosis, petechiae, poor wound healing

Teach patient/family:
• Necessary foods to include in diet, such as citrus fruits
• That smoking decreases vit C levels; not to exceed prescribed dose; that excesses will be excreted in urine, except when taking timed-release forms

---

vitamin E (OTC)
Aquasol E
Func. class.: Vit E
Chem. class.: Fat soluble

ACTION: Needed for digestion and metabolism of polyunsaturated fats; decreases platelet aggregation, blood clot formation; promotes normal growth and development of muscle tissue, prostaglandin synthesis

USES: Vit E deficiency, impaired fat absorption, hemolytic anemia in premature neonates, prevention of retrolental fibroplasia, sickle cell anemia, supplement for malabsorption syndrome

CONTRAINDICATIONS: IV use in infants
Precautions: Pregnancy, anemia, breastfeeding, hypoprothrombinemia

DOSAGE AND ROUTES
Deficiency
• **Adult: PO** 60-75 units/day
• **Child: PO** 1 unit/kg/day (malabsorption)
Prevention of deficiency
• **Adult: PO** 30 units/day; **TOP** apply to affected areas

V

• **Infant: PO** 5 units/day

Available forms: Caps 100, 200, 400, 500, 600, 1000 units; tabs 100, 200, 400 units; drops 15 mg/0.3 mL; chew tabs 400 units; ointment; cream; lotion; oil

Administer:

PO route

• Administer with or after meals
• Chew chewable tabs well
• Sol may be dropped in mouth or mixed with food
• Store in tight, light-resistant container

Topical route

• To moisturize dry skin

SIDE EFFECTS

CNS: Headache, fatigue
CV: Increased risk for thrombophlebitis
EENT: Blurred vision
GI: Nausea, cramps, diarrhea
GU: Gonadal dysfunction
INTEG: Sterile abscess, contact dermatitis
META: Altered metabolism of hormones (thyroid, pituitary, adrenal), altered immunity
MS: Weakness

PHARMACOKINETICS

PO: Metabolized in liver, excreted in bile

INTERACTIONS

Increase: action of oral anticoagulants
Decrease: absorption—cholestyramine, colestipol, mineral oil, sucralfate

NURSING CONSIDERATIONS

Assess:

• Nutritional status: wheat germ; dark green, leafy vegetables; nuts; eggs; liver; vegetable oils; dairy products; cereals
• **Pregnancy/breastfeeding:** use only recommended dietary allowances in pregnancy, breastfeeding

Evaluate:

• Therapeutic response: absence of hemolytic anemia, adequate vit E levels, improvement in skin lesions, decreased edema

Teach patient/family:

• About the necessary foods for diet
• To omit dose if missed
• To avoid vitamin supplements unless directed by prescriber

⚠ HIGH ALERT

vorapaxar
(vor′a-pax′ar)
Zontivity
Func. class.: Platelet inhibitor

ACTION: Antagonizes the protease-activated receptor-1 (PAR-1) expressed on platelets

USES: Secondary myocardial infarction prophylaxis or stroke prophylaxis or thrombosis prophylaxis for reduction of thrombotic cardiovascular events in patients with a history of myocardial infarction or with peripheral arterial disease

CONTRAINDICATIONS:

Black Box Warning: Bleeding, intracranial bleeding, stroke

Precautions: Breastfeeding, coronary artery bypass graft surgery (CABG), geriatric patients, hepatic disease, labor, obstetric delivery, pregnancy, renal impairment, surgery

DOSAGE AND ROUTES

• **Adult: PO** 2.08 mg once daily with aspirin and/or clopidogrel

Available forms: Tab 2.08 mg

Administer:

• May be administered without regard to food

SIDE EFFECTS

HEMA: Bleeding
CNS: Depression, intracranial bleeding
EENT: Retinal changes
INTEG: Rash

PHARMACOKINETICS

Within 1 week of treatment reaches ≥80% inhibition of thrombin receptor, half-life is 8 days, protein binding 99%, primarily eliminated feces; peak 1 hr

INTERACTIONS

Increase: bleeding risk—anticoagulants, aspirin, NSAIDs, other platelet inhibitors, SSRIs, rifampin, SNRIs, thrombolytics, ethyl estradiol, calcium channel blockers

Decrease: vorapaxar effect—CYP3A inducers (carBAMazepine, phenytoin, rifAMPin)

Increase: vorapaxor effect—CYP3A4 inhibitors (clarithromycin, indinavir, itraconazole, ketoconazole, nefazodone, nelfinavir, posaconazole, ritonavir, saquinavir, teleprivir)

Drug/Herb

Decrease: vorapaxar level—St. John's wort; avoid concurrent use

NURSING CONSIDERATIONS
Assess:

> **Black Box Warning:** For bleeding, including intracranial bleeding and stroke during treatment; bleeding should be suspected in any patient presenting with hypotension who has recently undergone surgery, coronary angiography, percutaneous coronary intervention (PCI), or CABG; avoid products that increase bleeding risk (salicylates, NSAIDs, SSRIs, SNRIs); avoid use in liver failure

• **Pregnancy/breastfeeding:** use only if benefits outweigh fetal risk; do not breastfeed, excretion unknown

Evaluate:

• Therapeutic response: absence of MI, stroke

Teach patient/family:

• To report any unusual bruising, bleeding to prescriber; that it may take longer to stop bleeding; that no true antidote exists and that there is an increased bleeding risk for 4 wk after last dose

• To take without regard to food

• To inform all providers that this product is being used; not to use OTC, prescription, or herbal products without approval of prescriber

• Not to breastfeed; to report if pregnancy is planned or suspected

• To take as prescribed with aspirin or clopidogrel; not to use alone; not to discontinue without prescriber approval

---

voriconazole (Rx)

(vohr-i-kahn′a-zol)

Vfend

Func. class.: Antifungal, systemic
Chem. class.: Triazole derivative

Do not confuse:
Vfend/Venofer

ACTION: Inhibits fungal CYP450-mediation demethylation; needed for biosynthesis; causes leakage from cell membrane

USES: Invasive aspergillosis, serious fungal infections (*Candida* sp., *Scedosporium apiospermum, Fusarium* sp., *Monosporium apiospermum*)

Unlabeled uses: *Acremonium* sp., *Blastomyces dermatitidis, Coccidioides immitis, Cryptococcus neoformans,* febrile neutropenia, fungal keratitis, *Histoplasma capsulatum,* oropharyngeal candidiasis, *Rhodotorula* sp., *Scedosporium* sp., cutaneous aspergillosis, candidemia (premature neonates), fungal infections in children ≥12 yr

CONTRAINDICATIONS: Pregnancy, breastfeeding, children, hypersensitivity, severe bone marrow depression, severe hepatic disease

Precautions: Renal disease (IV); patients of Asian/African descent; cardiomyopathy, cholestasis, chemotherapy, lactase deficiency, visual disturbances, renal failure, pancreatitis, QT prolongation, hypokalemia; ventricular dysrhythmias, torsades de pointes

V

DOSAGE AND ROUTES
Esophageal candidiasis
• **Adult/geriatric/child ≥12 yr and ≥40 kg: PO/IV** 200 mg q12hr; **<40 kg,** 100 mg q12hr
Candidemia of the skin, kidney, bladder wall, abdomen (nonneutropenic patients)
• **Adult/child ≥12 yr: IV** loading dose 6 mg/kg q12hr × 24 hr, then 3-4 mg/kg q12hr × ≥14 days and ≥7 days after resolution of symptoms; **PO** after loading dose **>40 kg** 200 mg q12hr × ≥14 days and ≥7 days after resolution of symptoms; **<40 kg** 100 mg q12hr × ≥14 days and ≥7 days after resolution of symptoms
Invasive aspergillosis
• **Adult/adolescent: IV** 6 mg/kg q12hr (loading dose), then 4 mg/kg q12hr, may reduce to 3 mg/kg q12hr if intolerable
• **Child ≥12 yr: IV** 6 mg/kg q12hr, then 4 mg/kg q12hr
CNS blastomycosis/blastomycosis meningitis (unlabeled)
• **Adult: PO** 200-400 mg bid × at least 12 mo and until resolution of CSF abnormalities
Renal dose
• **Adult: PO** CCr <50 mL/min, use orally only
Hepatic dose
• **Adult: PO/IV** (Child-Pugh Class A or B) standard loading dose, then 50% of maintenance dose; (Child-Pugh class C) avoid use

Available forms: Tabs 50, 200 mg; powder for inj, lyophilized 200 mg, powder for oral susp 45 g (40 mg/mL after reconstitution)
Administer:
PO route
• Oral susp: tap bottle; add 46 mL of water to bottle; shake well; remove cap; push bottle adapter into neck of bottle; replace cap; write expiration date (14 days); shake well before each use; administer using only oral dispenser supplied, 1 hr before or after meals; tabs and susp may be interchanged

• Store at room temperature (powder, tabs)
Intermittent IV INFUSION route
• Product only after C&S confirms organism and product needed to treat condition; make sure product used only in life-threatening infections
• Reconstitute powder with 19 mL water for inj to 10 mg/mL; shake until dissolved; infuse over 1-2 hr at concentration of ≤5 mg/mL; do not admix with other products, 4.2% sodium bicarbonate infusion

Y-site compatibilities: Acyclovir, alfentanil, allopurinol, amifostine, amikacin, aminocaproic acid, aminophylline, amiodarone, amphotericin B liposome, ampicillin, ampicillin/sulbactam, anidulafungin, azithromycin, aztreonam, bivalirudin, bleomycin, bumetanide, buprenorphine, butorphanol, calcium acetate/chloride/gluconate, CARBOplatin, carmustine, caspofungin, ceFAZolin, cefotaxime, cefoTEtan, cefOXitin, cefTAZidime, ceftizoxime, cefTRIAXone, chloramphenicol, chlorproMAZINE, cimetidine, ciprofloxacin, cisatracurium, CISplatin, clindamycin, cyclophosphamide, cytarabine, dacarbazine, DACTINomycin, DAPTOmycin, DAUNOrubicin, dexamethasone, dexmedetomidine, dexrazoxane, digoxin, diltiaZEM, diphenhydrAMINE, DOBUTamine, DOCEtaxel, dolasetron, DOPamine, doripenem, doxacurium, doxycycline, droperidol, enalaprilat, ePHEDrine, EPINEPHrine, epirubicin, ertapenem, erythromycin, esmolol, etoposide, etoposide phosphate, famotidine, fenoldopam, fentaNYL, fluconazole, fludarabine, fluorouracil, foscarnet, fosphenytoin, furosemide, ganciclovir, gemcitabine, gentamicin, glycopyrrolate, granisetron, haloperidol, heparin, hydrALAZINE, hydrocortisone, ifosfamide, imipenem/cilastatin, inamrinone, insulin, irinotecan, isoproterenol, ketorolac, labetalol, leucovorin, levoFLOXacin, lidocaine, linezolid, LORazepam, magnesium sulfate, mannitol, mechlorethamine, melphalan, meperidine, meropenem, mesna, metaraminol, methohexital, methotrexate, methyldopate, methylPREDNISolone, metoclopramide, metoprolol, metroNIDAZOLE, midazolam, milrinone, mitoMYcin, morphine, nafcillin, nalbuphine, naloxone, niCARdipine, nitroglycerin, norepinephrine, octreotide, ondansetron, oxaliplatin, oxytocin, PAClitaxel, pamidronate, pancuronium, pentamidine, pentazocine, PENTobarbital, PHENobarbital, phentolamine, phenylephrine, piperacillin/tazobactam, potassium chloride/phosphates, procainamide, promethazine, propranolol, quinupristin/dalfopristin, remifentanil, rocuronium, sodium acetate/bicarbonate/phosphates, streptozocin, succinylcholine, SUFentanil, tacrolimus, teniposide, theophylline, thiotepa, ticarcillin/clavulanate, tirofiban, tobramycin, topotecan, trimethobenzamide, trimethoprim/sulfamethoxazole, vancomycin, vasopressin, vecuronium, verapamil, vinBLAStine, vinCRIStine, vinorelbine, zidovudine

SIDE EFFECTS

CNS: *Headache,* paresthesias, peripheral neuropathy, *hallucinations,* psychosis, EPS, depression, Guillain-Barré syndrome, insomnia, suicidal ideation, dizziness, fever

CV: Tachycardia, hypo/hypertension, vasodilation, atrial arrhythmias, atrial fibrillation, AV block, bradycardia, HF, MI, QT prolongation, torsades de pointes, peripheral edema

EENT: *Blurred vision,* eye hemorrhage, visual disturbances

GI: *Nausea, vomiting, anorexia, diarrhea,* cramps, hemorrhagic gastroenteritis, acute hepatic failure, hepatitis, intestinal perforation, pancreatitis

GU: *Hypokalemia,* azotemia, renal tubular necrosis, permanent renal impairment, anuria, oliguria

HEMA: Anemia, eosinophilia, hypomagnesemia, thrombocytopenia, leukopenia, pancytopenia

INTEG: *Burning, irritation,* pain, necrosis at inj site with extravasation, dermatitis, *rash,* photosensitivity

MISC: Respiratory disorder

SYST: Stevens-Johnson syndrome, toxic epidermal necrolysis, sepsis; melanoma, photosensitivity reactions

PHARMACOKINETICS

By CYP3A4, CYP2C9 enzymes; max serum concentration 1-2 hr after dosing; eliminated via hepatic metabolism; protein binding 58%; elimination half-life 6 hr (dose dependent)

INTERACTIONS

Increase: effects of benzodiazepines, calcium channel blockers, cycloSPORINE, ergots, HMG-CoA reductase inhibitors, pimozide, quiNIDine, prednisoLONE, sirolimus, sulfonylureas, tacrolimus, vinca alkaloids, warfarin, rifabutin, proton pump inhibitors, NNRTIs, protease inhibitors, phenytoin

Increase: nephrotoxicity—other nephrotoxic antibiotics (aminoglycosides, CISplatin, vancomycin, cycloSPORINE, polymyxin B)

Increase: hypokalemia—corticosteroids, digoxin, skeletal muscle relaxants, thiazides

Increase: QT prolongation—class IA/III antidysrhythmics, some phenothiazines, β agonists, local anesthetics, tricyclics, haloperidol, chloroquine, droperidol, pentamidine; CYP3A4 inhibitors (amiodarone, clarithromycin, erythromycin, telithromycin, troleandomycin), arsenic trioxide; CYP3A4 substrates (methadone, pimozide, QUEtiapine, quiNIDine, risperiDONE, ziprasidone)

Drug/Herb
• Do not use with St. John's wort

Drug/Food
• Avoid use with high-fat meals, take 1 hr before or after meal

Drug/Lab Test
Increase: AST/ALT, alk phos, creatinine, bilirubin
Decrease: Hgb/Hct, platelets, WBC

NURSING CONSIDERATIONS
Assess:
• VS q15-30min during first infusion; note changes in pulse, B/P

V

• I&O ratio; watch for decreasing urinary output, change in specific gravity; discontinue product to prevent permanent damage to renal tubules
• Blood studies: CBC, potassium, sodium, calcium, magnesium, q2wk; BUN, creatinine weekly
• Weight weekly; if weight increases >2 lb/wk, edema is present; renal damage should be considered
• **Renal toxicity:** increasing BUN, serum creatinine; if BUN is >40 mg/dL or if serum creatinine >3 mg/dL, product may be discontinued or dosage reduced
• **Hepatotoxicity:** increasing AST, ALT, alk phos, bilirubin, baseline and periodically
• **Allergic reaction:** dermatitis, rash; product should be discontinued, antihistamines (mild reaction) or EPINEPHrine (severe reaction) administered
• **Hypokalemia:** anorexia, drowsiness, weakness, decreased reflexes, dizziness, increased urinary output, increased thirst, paresthesias
• **Ototoxicity:** tinnitus (ringing, roaring in ears), vertigo, loss of hearing (rare); visual disturbance
• **QT prolongation:** ECG, ejection fraction; assess for chest pain, palpitations, dyspnea
• **Pregnancy/breastfeeding:** do not use in pregnancy, may cause fetal harm; do not breastfeed

Evaluate:
• Therapeutic response: decreased fever, malaise, rash, negative C&S for infecting organism

Teach patient/family:
• That long-term therapy may be needed to clear infection (2 wk-3 mo, depending on type of infection)
• To notify prescriber of bleeding, bruising, soft-tissue swelling, dark urine, persistent nausea or diarrhea, headache, rash, yellow skin/eyes
• Take 1 hr before or after meal (PO)
• Not to drive at night because of vision changes

• Avoid strong, direct sunlight
• Women of childbearing age should use effective contraceptive

---

vortioxetine
(vor'tye-ox'e-teen)
Brintellix
Func. class.: Antidepressant
Chem. class.: Serotonin modulator

Do not confuse:
Brintellix/ Brilinta

ACTION: Reuptake inhibition at the serotonin transporter and agonist, or antagonist effects at serotonin receptors

USES: Major depressive disorder in adults

CONTRAINDICATIONS: Hypersensitivity, MAOI therapy
Precautions: Pregnancy, breastfeeding, seizure disorder, bipolar disorder, hyponatremia, hypovolemia, abrupt discontinuation, anticoagulant therapy, bleeding, closed-angle glaucoma, geriatric patients, hepatic disease

Black Box Warning: Children, suicidal ideation

DOSAGE AND ROUTES
• **Adult:** PO 10 mg/day, may start with 5 mg/day initially, increase to 20 mg/day as tolerated, max 20 mg/day; poor metabolizers of CYP2D6 max 10 mg/day
Available forms: Tabs 5, 10, 20 mg
Administer: Without regard to food

SIDE EFFECTS
CNS: Flushing, mania, serotonin syndrome, vertigo, dizziness, suicidal attempts
GI: *Nausea, diarrhea*, dyspnea, constipation, vomiting, flatulence
GU: Impotence, *ejaculation/orgasm dysfunction*
INTEG: Pruritus

SYST: Serotonin syndrome, neonatal abstinence syndrome, angioedema, pulmonary hypertension of the newborn, SIADH

PHARMACOKINETICS
Protein binding 98%, excreted in urine (59%), feces (26%)

INTERACTIONS
Increase: effect of tricyclics; use cautiously

Increase: serotonin syndrome—serotonin receptor agonists, SSRIs, traMADol, lithium, MAOIs, traZODone, SNRIs (venlafaxine, DULoxetine)

Increase: bleeding risk—NSAIDs, salicylates, thrombolytics, anticoagulants, antiplatelets

Increase: CNS effects—barbiturates, sedative/hypnotics, other CNS depressants

Decrease: vortioxetine levels—carBAMazepine

Drug/Herb:

Increase: serotonin syndrome—St. John's wort

NURSING CONSIDERATIONS
Assess:

Black Box Warning: Mental status: mood, sensorium, affect, suicidal tendencies, increase in psychiatric symptoms, depression, panic

• **Serotonin syndrome:** increased heart rate, sweating, dilated pupils, tremors, twitching, hyperthermia, agitation

• Alcohol consumption; if alcohol is consumed, hold dose until AM

• **Sexual dysfunction:** impotence

• **Pregnancy/breastfeeding:** use only if benefits outweigh fetal risk; do not breastfeed

Evaluate:

• Therapeutic response: decreased depression

Teach patient/family:

• That therapeutic effect may take several wk

• That decrease in libido or impotence may occur

• To use caution when driving, performing other activities that require alertness because of drowsiness, dizziness, blurred vision; to report signs, symptoms of bleeding

• To avoid alcohol, other CNS depressants

Black Box Warning: That suicidal ideas, behaviors may occur in children or young adults

• To notify prescriber if pregnant, planning to become pregnant, or breastfeeding

Black Box Warning: About the effects of serotonin syndrome: nausea/vomiting, tremors; if symptoms occur, to discontinue immediately, notify prescriber

V

⚠ HIGH ALERT

warfarin (Rx)
(war·far·in)

Coumadin ✦, Jantoven
Func. class.: Anticoagulant
Chem. class.: Coumarin derivative

Do not confuse:
Coumadin/Cardura/Avandia
Jantoven/Janumet/Januvia

ACTION: Interferes with blood clotting by indirect means; depresses hepatic synthesis of vit K–dependent coagulation factors (II, VII, IX, X)

USES: Antiphospholipid antibody syndrome, arterial thromboembolism prophylaxis, DVT, MI prophylaxis, after MI, stroke prophylaxis, thrombosis prophylaxis, pulmonary embolism

CONTRAINDICATIONS: Pregnancy, breastfeeding, hypersensitivity, hemophilia, leukemia with bleeding, peptic ulcer disease, thrombocytopenic purpura, hepatic disease (severe), malignant hypertension, subacute bacterial endocarditis, acute nephritis, blood dyscrasias, eclampsia, preeclampsia, hemorrhagic tendencies; surgery of CNS, eye; traumatic surgery with large open surface, bleeding tendencies of GI/GU/respiratory tract, stroke, aneurysms, pericardial effusion, spinal puncture, major regional/lumbar block anesthesia

Black Box Warning: Bleeding

Precautions: Geriatric patients, alcoholism, HF, debilitated patients, trauma, indwelling catheters, severe hypertension, active infections, protein C deficiency, polycythemia vera, vasculitis, severe diabetes, ⚠ Asian patients (CYP2C9), protein C, S deficiency or VKORC1 AA genotype

DOSAGE AND ROUTES–NTI
• **Adult: PO** 2-5 mg/day × 2-4 days, then titrated to INR/PT

• **Adolescent/child/infant: PO** 0.2 mg/kg/day × 2 days titrated to INR, max 10 mg
Available forms: Tabs 1, 2, 2.5, 3, 4, 5, 6, 7.5, 10 mg
Administer:
PO route
• Obtain coagulation studies—INR, PT—before use; INR level should be 2.0-3.0
• At same time each day to maintain steady blood levels without regard to food; food decreases rate but not extent of absorption; do not change brands
• Tabs whole or crushed
• Avoiding all IM inj that may cause bleeding
• Store in tight container

SIDE EFFECTS
GI: Nausea, cramps, calciphylaxis
GU: Hematuria
HEMA: Hemorrhage, agranulocytosis, leukopenia, eosinophilia, anemia, ecchymosis, petechiae
INTEG: *Rash,* dermal necrosis
MISC: Fever
MS: Bone fractures
SYST: Anaphylaxis, coma, cholesterol, microembolism, exfoliative dermatitis, purple toe syndrome

PHARMACOKINETICS
PO: Onset 12-24 hr, peak $1^1/_2$-4 days, duration 3-5 days, effective half-life 20-60 hr; metabolized in liver; excreted in urine, feces (active/inactive metabolites); crosses placenta, 99% bound to plasma proteins

INTERACTIONS
Increase: warfarin action—allopurinol, amiodarone, azithromycin, chloral hydrate, chloramphenicol, cimetidine, clofibrate, cotrimoxazole, COX-2 selective inhibitors, dextrothyroxine, diflunisal, disulfiram, erythromycin, ethacrynic acids, furosemide, glucagon, heparin, HMG-CoA reductase inhibitors, indomethacin, isoniazid, levoFLOXacin, mefenamic acid, metroNIDAZOLE, miFEPRIStone, NSAIDs, oxyphenbutazone, penicillins, phenylbutazone, quiNIDine, quinolone antiinfectives,

RU-486, salicylates, sulfinpyrazone, sulfonamides, sulindac, SSRIs, steroids, thrombolytics, thyroid, tricyclics

Increase/decrease: effectiveness—assess for use of products that may increase or decrease effect

Increase: toxicity—oral sulfonylureas, phenytoin

Decrease: warfarin action—aprepitant, azaTHIOprine, barbiturates, bile acid sequestrants, bosentan, carBAMazepine, dicloxacillin, estrogens, ethchlorvynol, factor IX/VIIa, griseofulvin, nafcillin, oral contraceptives, phenytoin, rifAMPin, sucralfate, sulfaSALAzine, vit K, vit K foods

Drug/Herb

Increase: risk for bleeding—anise, chamomile, dong quai, evening primrose, feverfew, garlic, ginger, ginkgo, ginseng, horse chestnut, licorice, melatonin, red yeast rice, saw palmetto

Decrease: anticoagulant effect—coenzyme Q10, St. John's wort

Drug/Lab Test

Increase: T_3 uptake, LFTs, INR, PT, PTT

NURSING CONSIDERATIONS
Assess:

Black Box Warning: Blood studies (Hct, PT, platelets, occult blood in stools) q3mo; INR: in hospital daily after 2nd or 3rd dose; when in therapeutic range (2-3) for 2 consecutive days, monitor 2-3× wk for 1-2 wk, then less frequently, depending on stability of INR results; *Outpatient:* monitor every few days until stable dose, then periodically thereafter, depending on stability of INR results, usually at least monthly

• Geriatric/pediatric patients more often; adverse reactions may occur at lower therapeutic ranges

Black Box Warning: **Bleeding:** bleeding gums, petechiae, ecchymosis, black tarry stools, hematuria, occult bleeding (cerebral, intraabdominal; fatal hemorrhage can occur; do not use in uncontrolled bleeding

• Fever, skin rash, urticaria

• **Pregnancy/breastfeeding:** do not use in pregnancy; use effective contraception during and for 1 mo after final dose; cautious use in breastfeeding

Evaluate:

• Therapeutic response: decrease in deep venous thrombosis, absence of pulmonary embolism

Teach patient/family:

• To avoid OTC preparations that may cause serious product interactions unless directed by prescriber; to avoid alcohol, herbs, supplements

• To carry emergency ID identifying product taken

• About the importance of compliance with exams and doses

Black Box Warning: **Bleeding:** to report any signs of bleeding: gums, nosebleed, under skin, urine, stools; to use soft-bristle toothbrush to avoid bleeding gums; to use electric razor

• To avoid hazardous activities (e.g., football, hockey, skiing), dangerous work

• To inform all health care providers of anticoagulant intake

• To take exactly as prescribed; dosage changes are common for desired effect, not to skip, double doses, take missed dose when remembered

• To eat a diet that is not varied; several foods contain vitamin K and can alter warfarin effect

• To report to prescriber fever, rash, trouble breathing

• That continuing follow-up exams and lab work will be needed

TREATMENT OF OVERDOSE: W
Administer vit K, fresh frozen plasma, prothrombin complex concentrate

zafirlukast (Rx)

(za-feer′loo-cast)

Accolate

Func. class.: Bronchodilator

Chem. class.: Leukotriene receptor antagonist

Do not confuse:

Accolate/Accupril/Aclovate

ACTION: Antagonizes the contractile action of leukotrienes (LTD_4, LTE_4) in airway smooth muscle; inhibits broncho-constriction caused by antigens

USES: Prophylaxis and chronic treatment of asthma in adults/children >5 yr

Unlabeled uses: Allergic rhinitis

CONTRAINDICATIONS: Hypersensitivity, hepatic encephalopathy

Precautions: Pregnancy, breastfeeding, children, geriatric patients, hepatic disease, Churg-Strauss syndrome, acute bronchospasm

DOSAGE AND ROUTES

- **Adult/child ≥12 yr:** PO 20 mg bid
- **Child 5-11 yr:** PO 10 mg bid

Available forms: Tabs 10, 20 mg

Administer:

- 1 hr before or 2 hr after meals; absorption may be decreased if given with food

SIDE EFFECTS

CNS: Headache, dizziness, suicidal ideation, insomnia, fever

GI: Nausea, diarrhea, abdominal pain, vomiting, dyspepsia, hepatic failure, hepatitis

HEMA: Agranulocytosis

OTHER: Infections, pain, asthenia, myalgia, fever, increased ALT, urticaria, rash, angioedema

PHARMACOKINETICS

Rapidly absorbed, peak 3 hr, 99% protein binding (albumin), extensively metabolized, inhibits CYP2C9 and 3A4 enzyme systems, excreted in feces, clearance reduced in geriatric patients, hepatic impairment, half-life 10 hr

INTERACTIONS

Increase: plasma levels of zafirlukast—aspirin

Increase: PT—warfarin

Decrease: plasma levels of zafirlukast—erythromycin, theophylline

Drug/Food

Decrease: bioavailability

NURSING CONSIDERATIONS

Assess:

- **Adult patients carefully for symptoms of Churg-Strauss syndrome** (rare), including eosinophilia, vasculitic rash, worsening pulmonary symptoms, cardiac complications, neuropathy; may be caused by reducing oral corticosteroids
- Respiratory rate, rhythm, depth; auscultate lung fields bilaterally; notify prescriber of abnormalities; not to be used for acute bronchospasm in acute asthma
- **Hepatic/renal/pancreatic/visual function:** monitor liver function tests
- **Pregnancy/breastfeeding:** use only if clearly needed; do not breastfeed, excreted in breast milk

Evaluate:

- Therapeutic response: ability to breathe more easily

Teach patient/family:

- To check OTC medications, current prescription medications that may increase stimulation, do not stop other asthma medications unless instructed to do so
- To avoid hazardous activities because dizziness may occur
- That if GI upset occurs, to take product with 8 oz water; to take 1-2 hr after a meal; to avoid taking with food if possible because absorption may be decreased
- To notify prescriber of nausea, vomiting, diarrhea, abdominal pain, fatigue, jaundice, anorexia, flulike symptoms (hepatic dysfunction)
- Not to use for acute asthma episodes
- Not to take if breastfeeding
- To take even if symptom free

A HIGH ALERT

zaleplon (Rx)
(zal'eh-plon)
Sonata
Func. class.: Hypnotic, nonbarbiturate
Chem. class.: Pyrazolopyrimidine

Controlled Substance Schedule IV

Do not confuse:
Sonata/Soriatane

ACTION: Binds selectively to omega-1 receptor of the $GABA_A$ receptor complex; results are sedation, hypnosis, skeletal muscle relaxation, anticonvulsant activity, anxiolytic action

USES: Insomnia (short-term treatment)

CONTRAINDICATIONS: Hypersensitivity, severe hepatic disease
Precautions: Pregnancy, breastfeeding, children <15 yr, geriatric patients, respiratory/renal/hepatic disease, psychosis, angioedema, depression, sleep-related behaviors (sleep walking), Asian descent, CNS depression

DOSAGE AND ROUTES
• **Adult: PO** 10 mg at bedtime; may increase dose to 20 mg at bedtime if needed; 5 mg may be used in low-weight persons
• **Geriatric/hepatic dose: PO** 5 mg at bedtime; may increase if needed
Available forms: Caps 5, 10 mg
Administer:
• Immediately before bedtime for sleeplessness
• On empty stomach for fast onset
• Store in tight container in cool environment

SIDE EFFECTS
CNS: *Lethargy, drowsiness, daytime sedation,* dizziness, confusion, anxiety, amnesia, depersonalization, hallucinations, hyperesthesia, paresthesia, somnolence, tremors, vertigo, complex sleep-related reactions: sleep driving, sleep eating
CV: Chest pain, peripheral edema

EENT: Vision change, ear/eye pain, hyperacusis, parosmia
GI: Nausea, abdominal pain, constipation, anorexia, colitis, dyspepsia, dry mouth
MISC: Asthenia, fever, headache, myalgia, dysmenorrhea
MS: Myalgia, back pain, arthritis
RESP: Bronchitis
SYST: Severe allergic reactions

PHARMACOKINETICS
Rapid onset, metabolized by liver extensively, excreted by kidneys (inactive metabolites), half-life 1 hr, onset, peak 1 hr, duration 3-4 hr

INTERACTIONS
Increase: effect of zaleplon—cimetidine
Decrease: zaleplon bioavailability—CYP3A4 inducers
Drug/Food
• Prolonged absorption, sleep onset reduced: high-fat/heavy meal

NURSING CONSIDERATIONS
Assess:
• Mental status: mood, sensorium, affect, memory (long, short term), excessive sedation, impaired coordination
• **Sleep disorder:** type of sleep problem: falling asleep, staying asleep; monitor for complex sleep disorders
• **Beers:** avoid in older adults with delirium or at high risk for delirium; potential for worsening or inducing delirium
Evaluate:
• Therapeutic response: ability to sleep at night, decreased amount of early morning awakening
Teach patient/family:
• To avoid driving or other activities requiring alertness until product is stabilized
• To avoid alcohol ingestion
• That product may cause memory problems, dependence (if used for longer periods of time), changes in behavior/thinking, complex sleep-related behaviors (sleep eating/driving)
• That product is for short-term use only
• To take immediately before going to bed

Z

Side effects: *italics* = common; red = life-threatening

• Not to ingest a high-fat/heavy meal before taking

• **Pregnancy/breastfeeding:** Identify if pregnancy is planned or suspected or if breastfeeding

---

zanamivir (Rx)

(zan′ah-mih-veer)

Relenza

Func. class.: Antiviral

Chem. class.: Neuraminidase inhibitor

ACTION: Inhibits neuraminidase enzyme needed for influenza virus replication

USES: Treatment of influenza types A and B for patients who have been symptomatic for ≤2 days, seasonal influenza prophylaxis

CONTRAINDICATIONS: Hypersensitivity

Precautions: Pregnancy, breastfeeding, children <7 yr, geriatric patients, respiratory disease, angioedema, milk protein hypersensitivity, Reye's syndrome

DOSAGE AND ROUTES

Treatment of influenza A and B

• **Adult/child >7 yr: INH** 2 inhalations (two 5-mg blisters) q12hr × 5 days; on the 1st day, 2 doses should be taken with at least 2 hr between doses

Prophylaxis of influenza A and B

• **Adult/child >5 yr: INH** 10 mg (2 inhalations) daily × 28 days

Available forms: Blisters of powder for inhalation: 5 mg

Administer:

• Within 2 days of symptoms of influenza; continue for 5 days

• Give patient Patient's Instructions for Use, review all points before using delivery system

• Do not use as nebulized sol or in mechanical ventilation

• Store in tight, dry container

SIDE EFFECTS

CNS: *Headache, dizziness,* seizures, fatigue; self-injury, delirium (child)

EENT: Ear, nose, throat infections, throat discomfort

GI: *Nausea, vomiting,* diarrhea

RESP: Nasal symptoms, cough, sinusitis, bronchitis, bronchospasm

SYST: Angioedema

PHARMACOKINETICS

Half-life $2^1/_2$-5 hr, not metabolized, excreted in urine unchanged

INTERACTIONS

• May decrease intranasal influenzae vaccine; separate by ≥48 hr; do not restart antiviral products for ≥2 wk

NURSING CONSIDERATIONS

Assess:

• **Influenza:** headache, joint aches/pain, fever, cough, sore throat, baseline and periodically through treatment; used only in those who are symptomatic ≤2 days

• Skin eruptions, photosensitivity after administration of product

• Respiratory status: rate, character, wheezing, tightness in chest

• Allergies before initiation of treatment, reaction to each medication; avoid use in those who are lactose intolerant

• Signs of infection

• **Pregnancy/breastfeeding:** use only if benefits outweigh fetal risk; avoid use in breastfeeding

Evaluate:

• Therapeutic response: absence of fever, malaise, cough, dyspnea with infection

Teach patient/family:

• That product does not reduce transmission risk of influenza to others

• That patients with asthma or COPD should carry a fast-acting inhaled bronchodilator because bronchospasm may occur; to use scheduled inhaled bronchodilators before using product

• To avoid hazardous activities if dizziness occurs

• To use as directed, finish all medication

• To avoid use if pregnant or breastfeeding

---

zidovudine (Rx)

(zye-doe′-vue-deen)

Novo-AZT ✤, Retrovir

Func. class.: Antiretroviral

Chem. class.: Nucleoside reverse transcriptase inhibitor (NRTI)

Do not confuse:

Retrovir/ritonavir

ACTION: Inhibits replication of HIV-1 virus by incorporating into cellular DNA by viral reverse transcriptase, thereby terminating the cellular DNA chain

USES: Used in combination with at least 2 other antiretrovirals for HIV-1 infection

Unlabeled uses: Epstein-Barr virus, hepatitis B, human T-lymphotropic virus type I (HTLV-I), thrombocytopenia

CONTRAINDICATIONS: Hypersensitivity

Precautions: Pregnancy, breastfeeding, children, granulocyte count <1000/mm^3 or Hgb <9.5 g/dL, severe renal disease, obesity

Black Box Warning: Hepatotoxicity, anemia, lactic acidosis, myopathy, neutropenia

DOSAGE AND ROUTES

For the treatment of human immunodeficiency virus (HIV) infection in combination with other antiretroviral agents

• **Adult: PO** 300 mg bid or 200 mg tid; **IV INFUSION** 1 mg/kg over 1 hr q4hr around the clock (total daily dose: 6 mg/kg/day). Initiate oral therapy as soon as possible. Monotherapy with zidovudine is not recommended for treatment of HIV

• **Adolescent/child ≥30 kg: PO** 300 mg bid (preferred) or 200 mg tid

• **Child/infant 9-29 kg: PO** 9 mg/kg bid (preferred) or 6 mg/kg tid

• **Child/infant 4-8 kg: PO** 12 mg/kg bid (preferred) or 8 mg/kg tid

• **Neonate ≥35 wk gestational age (unlabeled): PO** Initially, 4 mg/kg bid; increase to 12 mg/kg bid after 4 wk of age

• **Neonate 30-34 wk gestational age (unlabeled): PO** Initially, 2 mg/kg bid; increase to 3 mg/kg bid at 2 wk of age, then increase to 12 mg/kg bid after 6-8 wk of age·

• **Neonate <30 wk gestational age: PO** Initially, 2 mg/kg bid; increase to 3 mg/kg bid at 4 wk of age, then increase to 12 mg/kg bid after 8-10 wk of age

For perinatal human immunodeficiency virus (HIV) prophylaxis

• **Pregnant females (intrapartum): IV INFUSION** 2 mg/kg over 1 hr, followed by 1 mg/kg/hr **IV CONT INFUSION** until clamping of the umbilical cord

• **Neonate ≥35 wk gestational age: IV** 3 mg/kg q12hr beginning as soon as possible after birth (preferably within 6-12 hr); increase to 9 mg/kg q12hr after 4 wk of age

Renal dose

• **Adult: PO** CCr ≥15 mL/min: no change; CCr <15 mL/min, 100 mg q8hr or 300 mg/day

• **Pediatric patients: PO** GFR ≥10 mL/min/1.73 m^2: no change; GFR <10 mL/min/1.73 m^2: reduce dose by 50%

• Latex is in vial stopper

Available forms: Caps 100; tabs 300 mg; inj 10 mg/mL; oral syr

Administer:

• By mouth; capsules should be swallowed whole

• Trimethoprim-sulfamethoxazole, pyrimethamine, or acyclovir as ordered to prevent opportunistic infections; if these products are given, watch for neurotoxicity

• Store in cool environment; protect from light

Intermittent IV INFUSION route

• After diluting each 1 mg/0.25 mL or more D$_5$W to ≤4 mg/mL; give over 1 hr

• Protect unopened product from light; use diluted sol within 24 hr room temperature, 48 hr refrigerated, do not use discolored solutions

Y-site compatibilities: Acyclovir, alemtuzumab, allopurinol, amifostine, amikacin, amphotericin B, amphotericin B cholesteryl, anidulafungin, argatroban, aztreonam, cefepime, cefTAZidime, cefTRIAXone, cimetidine, cisatracurium, clindamycin,

Z

dexamethasone, DOBUTamine, DOPamine, DOXOrubicin liposome, erythromycin, filgrastim, fluconazole, fludarabine, gentamicin, granisetron, heparin, imipenem-cilastatin, LORazepam, melphalan, metoclopramide, morphine, nafcillin, ondansetron, oxacillin, PACLitaxel, pentamidine, phenylephrine, piperacillin, piperacillin-tazobactam, potassium chloride, raNITIdine, remifentanil, sargramostim, tacrolimus, teniposide, thiotepa, tobramycin, trimethoprim-sulfamethoxazole, trimetrexate, vancomycin, vinorelbine, zoledronic acid

SIDE EFFECTS

CNS: *Fever, headache, malaise,* diaphoresis, *dizziness, insomnia,* paresthesia, somnolence, chills, tremors, twitching, anxiety, confusion, depression, lability, vertigo, loss of mental acuity, seizures, malaise
EENT: Taste change, hearing loss, photophobia
GI: *Nausea, vomiting, diarrhea, anorexia,* cramps, *dyspepsia, constipation,* dysphagia, *flatulence,* rectal bleeding, mouth ulcer, abdominal pain, hepatomegaly
GU: Dysuria, polyuria, urinary frequency, hesitancy
HEMA: Granulocytopenia, anemia
INTEG: *Rash,* acne, pruritus, urticaria
MS: Myalgia, arthralgia, muscle spasm
RESP: Dyspnea, cough, wheezing
SYST: Lactic acidosis

PHARMACOKINETICS

PO: Rapidly absorbed from GI tract, peak $1/_2$-$1^1/_2$ hr; IV peak infusions end; metabolized in liver (inactive metabolites), excreted by kidneys, protein binding 38%, half-life $1/_2$-3 hr

INTERACTIONS

Increase: bone marrow depression—antineoplastics, radiation, ganciclovir, valGANciclovir, trimethoprim-sulfamethoxazole
Increase: zidovudine level—methadone, atovaquone, fluconazole, probenecid, trimethoprim, valproic acid; may need to reduce zidovudine dose
Increase: toxicity-fluconazole, probenecid

Decrease: zidovudine levels—clarithromycin, interferons, NRTIs, DOXOrubicin, ribavirin, stavudine; avoid concurrent use

Drug/Lab Test
Decrease: platelets, granulocytes
Increase: LFTs, amylase, CPK

NURSING CONSIDERATIONS

Assess:
• **HIV:** monitor for symptoms of HIV, baseline and throughout treatment
• Blood dyscrasias (anemia, granulocytopenia): bruising, fatigue, bleeding, poor healing

Black Box Warning: **Bone marrow suppression:** blood counts q2wk; watch for decreasing granulocytes, Hgb; if low, therapy may have to be discontinued and restarted after hematologic recovery; blood transfusions may be required; viral load, CD4 counts, LFTs, plasma HIV RNA, serum creatinine/BUN at baseline and throughout treatment

Black Box Warning: **Lactic acidosis, severe hepatomegaly with steatosis:** Obtain baseline liver function tests; if elevated, discontinue treatment; discontinue even if liver function tests are normal but lactic acidosis, hepatomegaly are present; may be fatal; more common in females

• Monitor lipid profile, blood glucose, hepatitis B serology, plasma hepatitis C RNA, serum cholesterol, pregnancy test, urinalysis, serum lipase, amylase
• **Pregnancy/breastfeeding:** register pregnant patients at the Antiretroviral Pregnancy Registry, 1-800-258-4263; do not breastfeed, excreted in breast milk
Evaluate:
• Therapeutic response: decreased viral load, increased CD4 counts, decreased symptoms of HIV
Teach patient/family:
• That GI complaints and insomnia resolve after 3-4 wk of treatment
• **HIV:** That repeat testing in 4-6 wk is needed due to risk of false positive if used in newborn

- That product is not a cure for AIDS but will control symptoms; that compliance with treatment is required
- To notify prescriber of sore throat, swollen lymph nodes, malaise, fever, shortness of breath because other infections may occur; to avoid crowds or people with known infections
- That patient is still infective, may pass AIDS virus on to others
- That follow-up visits must be continued because serious toxicity may occur; that blood counts must be done q2wk; that blood transfusions may be needed for severe anemia
- That product must be taken bid or tid around the clock to prevent variations in blood levels
- That serious product interactions may occur if OTC products are ingested; to check with prescriber before taking aspirin, acetaminophen, indomethacin
- That other products may be necessary to prevent other infections
- That product may cause fainting or dizziness; to avoid driving or other hazardous tasks until response is known
- That redistribution of body fat may occur
- Not to breastfeed during treatment

---

zinc (Rx, OTC)

Galzin

Func. class.: Trace element; nutritional supplement

ACTION: Needed for adequate healing, bone and joint development (23% zinc)

USES: Prevention of zinc deficiency, adjunct to vit A therapy
Unlabeled uses: Wound healing
Precautions: Pregnancy, parenteral; breastfeeding, neonates, hypocupremia, neonatal prematurity, renal disease

DOSAGE AND ROUTES
Dietary supplement (elemental zinc)
- **Adult/adolescent/pregnant female:** PO 11-13 mg/day
- **Adult/lactating female:** PO 12-14 mg/day × 12 mo

- **Adult/adolescent male ≥14 yr:** PO 11 mg/day
- **Adult female ≥19 yr:** PO 8 mg/day
- **Adolescent female ≥14 yr:** PO 9 mg/day
- **Child 9-13 yr:** PO 8 mg/day
- **Child 4-8 yr:** PO 5 mg/day
- **Child 1-3 yr:** PO 3 mg/day
- **Infant 7-12 mo:** PO 3 mg/day
- **Infant birth to 6 mo:** PO 2 mg/day (adequate intake)

Nutritional supplement (IV)
- **Adult:** 2.5-4 mg/day; may increase by 2 mg/day if needed
- **Child 1-5 yr:** IV 50 mcg/kg/day

Wound healing
- **Adult:** PO 50 mg tid until healed (elemental zinc)

Available forms: Tabs 66, 110, 220 mg; inj 1 mg/mL, 5 mg/mL; caps 25, 50 mg
Administer:
- With meals to decrease gastric upset; avoid dairy products

SIDE EFFECTS
GI: Nausea, vomiting, cramps, heartburn, ulcer formation
OVERDOSE: Diarrhea, rash, dehydration, restlessness

INTERACTIONS
Decrease: absorption of fluoroquinolones—tetracyclines
Drug/Food
Decrease: absorption of PO zinc—dairy products, caffeine

NURSING CONSIDERATIONS
Assess:
- **Zinc deficiency:** poor wound healing, absence of taste, smell, slowing growth
- Alkaline phosphatase, HDL monthly in long-term therapy
- Zinc levels during treatment, CBC
- **Pregnancy/breastfeeding:** use only if benefits outweigh fetal risk (IV); considered safe in breastfeeding
Evaluate:
- Therapeutic response: absence of zinc deficiency
Teach patient/family:
- That element must be taken for 2-3 mo to be effective

Z

Side effects: *italics* = common; red = life-threatening

• To immediately report nausea, diarrhea, rash, severe vomiting, restlessness, abdominal pain, tarry stools

---

ziprasidone (Rx)

(zi-praz'ih-dohn)

Geodon, Zeldox ✦

Func. class.: Antipsychotic/neuroleptic
Chem. class.: Benzisoxazole derivative

ACTION: Unknown; may be mediated through both dopamine type 2 (D_2) and serotonin type 2 (5-HT_2) antagonism

USES: Schizophrenia, acute agitation, acute psychosis, bipolar disorder, mania, psychotic depression

CONTRAINDICATIONS: Breastfeeding, hypersensitivity, acute MI, heart failure, QT prolongation

Precautions: Pregnancy, children, geriatric patients, cardiac/renal/hepatic disease, breast cancer, diabetes, seizure disorders, AV block, CNS depression, abrupt discontinuation, agranulocytosis, ambient temperature increase, suicidal ideation, torsades de pointes, strenuous exercise

> **Black Box Warning:** Increased mortality in geriatric patients with dementia-related psychosis

DOSAGE AND ROUTES
Schizophrenia
• **Adult: PO** 20 mg bid with food, adjust dosage every 2 days upward to max of 80 mg bid; **IM** 10-20 mg; may give 10 mg q2hr; doses of 20 mg may be given q4hr; max 40 mg/day (acute episodes); switch to **PO** as soon as possible
Bipolar disorder
• **Adult: PO** 40 mg bid with food; on day 2 increase to 60 or 80 mg bid, then adjust to response; maintenance as adjunct to lithium/valproate 40-80 mg bid
Available forms: Caps 20, 40, 60, 80 mg; inj 20 mg/mL single-dose vials

Administer:
PO route
• Take cap whole and with food, with plenty of fluid at same time of day
• Reduced dose in geriatric patients
• Anticholinergic agent on order from prescriber to be used for EPS
• Store in tight, light-resistant container
IM route
• Add 1.2 mL sterile water for inj to vial; shake vigorously until dissolved; do not admix; give only IM; give deeply in large muscle; do not mix with other products, do not use if particulates are present, keep patient recumbent for 30 min after injection
• Do not give over 3 consecutive days
• Store injection at room temperature, protect from light, after reconstituting may be stored at room temperature × 24 hr, 7 days refrigerated

SIDE EFFECTS
CNS: *EPS, pseudoparkinsonism, akathisia, dystonia, tardive dyskinesia; drowsiness, insomnia, agitation, anxiety, headache,* seizures, neuroleptic malignant syndrome, dizziness, tremors, facial droop
CV: Orthostatic hypotension, tachycardia, prolonged QT/QTc, hypertension, sudden death, heart failure (geriatric patients), torsades de pointes
HEMA: Agranulocytosis
EENT: Blurred vision, diplopia
ENDO: Hypoglycemia
GI: *Nausea,* vomiting, *anorexia, constipation,* jaundice, weight gain, diarrhea, dry mouth, abdominal pain
GU: Priapism
INTEG: Rash, injection-site pain, sweating, DRESS, Steven's Johnson Syndrome
RESP: Infection, cough

PHARMACOKINETICS
IM: Peak 60 min
PO: Peak 6-8 hr, Extensively metabolized by liver to major active metabolite, plasma protein binding 99%, half-life 7 hr

INTERACTIONS
Increase: Respiratory depression-opioids, avoid concurrent use

---

Increase: Ziprasidone level-CYP3A4 inhibitors (Ketoconazole, itraconazole); dose may need to be reduced

Increase: QT prolongation—class IA/III antidysrhythmics, some phenothiazines, β-agonists, local anesthetics, tricyclics, haloperidol, methadone, chloroquine, clarithromycin, droperidol, erythromycin, pentamidine, moxifloxacin

Increase: sedation—other CNS depressants, alcohol

Increase: EPS, possible neurotoxicity—other antipsychotics, lithium

Increase: ziprasidone excretion—carBAMazepine, barbiturates, phenytoin, rifAMPin

Increase: hypotension—antihypertensives, monitor B/P

Increase: serotonin syndrome, neuroleptic malignant syndrome—SSRIs, SNRIs

Decrease: ziprasidone effect—carbamazepine

NURSING CONSIDERATIONS
Assess:

• Mental status before initial administration, AIMS assessment

> **Black Box Warning:** Assess geriatric patient with dementia closely; heart failure, sudden death have occurred; this product is not approved for the treatment of dementia-related psychosis in the elderly

• **DRESS:** rash, fever, swollen lymph nodes, product should be discontinued
• Steven's Johnson Syndrome: rash with fever, aches, blisters, swelling of face, discontinue product immediately
• **Seizures:** Seizures in those with seizure disorders, provide seizure precautions, seizure threshold is lowered
• Bilirubin, CBC, LFTs, fasting blood glucose, cholesterol profile; potassium, magnesium when taken with loop/thiazide diuretics monthly
• Urinalysis before, during prolonged therapy
• B/P standing and lying; also pulse, respirations; take these q4hr during initial treatment; establish baseline before starting treatment; report drops of 30 mm Hg; watch for ECG changes; QT

prolongation may occur; discontinue product if QTc >500 msec
• Dizziness, faintness, palpitations, tachycardia on rising; metabolic changes, weight gain
• **EPS,** including akathisia (inability to sit still, no pattern to movements), tardive dyskinesia (bizarre movements of the jaw, mouth, tongue, extremities), pseudoparkinsonism (rigidity, tremors, pill rolling, shuffling gait)
• **Neuroleptic malignant syndrome, serotonin syndrome:** hyperthermia, increased CPK, altered mental status, muscle rigidity
• Constipation, urinary retention daily; if these occur, increase bulk and water in diet
• Supervised ambulation until patient is stabilized on medication; do not involve patient in strenuous exercise program because fainting is possible; patient should not stand still for a long time
• Increased fluids to prevent constipation
• **Beers:** avoid use in older adults except for schizophrenia, bipolar disorder, or short term as an antiemetic during chemotherapy; increased risk of stroke and cognitive decline
• **Pregnancy/breastfeeding:** use only if benefits outweigh fetal risk, may cause EPS in the neonate, enroll pregnant women in the Atypical Antipsychotic Pregnancy Registry, 1-866-961-2388; avoid breastfeeding, excretion unknown

Evaluate:
• Therapeutic response: decrease in emotional excitement, hallucinations, delusions, paranoia; reorganization of patterns of thought, speech

Teach patient/family:
• That orthostatic hypotension may occur; to rise from sitting or lying position gradually
• To avoid hot tubs, hot showers, tub baths because hypotension may occur
• To avoid abrupt withdrawal of product because EPS may result; that product should be withdrawn slowly
• To avoid OTC preparations (cough, hay fever, cold), herbals, supplements unless approved by prescriber because serious product interactions may occur; to avoid use with alcohol because increased drowsiness may occur

Z

Side effects: *italics* = common; red = life-threatening

- To avoid hazardous activities if drowsy or dizzy
- To report impaired vision, tremors, muscle twitching
- That continuing follow up exams will be needed
- In hot weather, that heat stroke may occur; to take extra precautions to stay cool, take adequate liquids

TREATMENT OF OVERDOSE:
Lavage if orally ingested; provide airway; *do not induce vomiting*

⚠ HIGH ALERT

ziv-aflibercept
(ziv-a-flih′ber-sept)

Zaltrap

Func. class.: Antineoplastic
Chem. class.: Signal transduction inhibitor (STI), fusion protein

---

ACTION: An angiogenesis inhibitor, a fusion protein that binds to vascular endothelial growth factors ⋇⊕⋇ (VEGF-A, VEGF-B) and placental growth factor 1 and 2

USES: Metastatic colorectal cancer that is resistant or has progressed after an oxaliplatin-containing regimen in combination with 5-fluorouracil, leucovorin, irinotecan (FOLFIRI)

CONTRAINDICATIONS: Hypersensitivity

Precautions: Infertility, male-mediated teratogenicity, encephalopathy, hypertension, dental work, breastfeeding, children, neonates, geriatric patients, infection, neutropenia, pregnancy

> **Black Box Warning:** Bleeding, GI bleeding/perforation, intracranial bleeding, surgery

DOSAGE AND ROUTES
- **Adult:** IV 4 mg/kg over 1 hr on day 1 every 2 wk in combination with the FOLFIRI regimen (irinotecan 180 mg/m² over 90 min on day 1 with dl-racemic leucovorin

400 mg/m² over 2 hr) (infused at the same time, in same Y-line; then on day 1 by 5-fluorouracil 400 mg/m² as a bolus, then 2400 mg/m² as a 46-hr cont IV infusion)

Available forms: Solution for injection 100 mg/4 mL; 200 mg/8 mL

Administer:
- Give before FOLFIRI chemotherapy; visually inspect for particulate matter and discoloration before use

Dilution and preparation
- Withdraw the calculated dose; add to 0.9% sodium chloride or dextrose 5% solution to 0.6-8 mg/mL; use polyvinyl chloride (PVC) infusion bags containing bis (2-ethylhexyl) phthalate (DHEP) or polyolefin infusion bags; do not re-enter the vial after first puncture; discard any unused portion; do not mix or combine with other drugs in the same infusion bag; the diluted solution may be stored refrigerated for ≤4 hr; discard any unused portion in the infusion bag

IV infusion
- Give diluted solution over 1 hr using a 0.2-micron polyethersulfone filter; do not use nylon or polyvinylidene fluoride (PVDF) filters; do not give IV push or bolus; do not mix or combine with other drugs in the same IV line; give using an infusion set made of one of the following: PVC containing DEHP, DEHP-free PVC containing trioctyl-trimellitate (TOTM), polypropylene, polyethylene-lined PVC, or polyurethane
- **Dosage adjustments for recurrent or severe hypertension:** Hold until B/P is controlled and then permanently reduce dose to 2 mg/kg; discontinue in hypertensive crisis or hypertensive encephalopathy
- **Dosage adjustments for proteinuria (2 g/24 hr):** Hold until proteinuria is <2 g/24 hr; if proteinuria recurs, hold therapy until proteinuria is <2 g/24 hr, then reduce to 2 mg/kg; discontinue in nephrotic syndrome or thrombotic microangiopathy

SIDE EFFECTS
CNS: Intracranial bleeding, *headache,* *dizziness,* reversible posterior leukoencephalopathy
CV: Hypertensive crisis, hypertension stroke

GI: Nausea, hepatotoxicity, dyspepsia, GI hemorrhage, *abdominal pain*, GI perforation

GU: Proteinuria, hematuria

HEMA: Neutropenia, leukopenia

INTEG: Rash, pruritus, alopecia, hypersensitivity, *anorexia, diarrhea, palmar-plantar erythrodysesthesia*

MISC: Fatigue, epistaxis, night sweats, decreased weight, flulike symptoms, infection

RESP: Dyspnea, pulmonary embolism

PHARMACOKINETICS
Half-life 6 days

NURSING CONSIDERATIONS
Assess:

Black Box Warning: **Severe bleeding:** GI bleeding, intracranial bleeding, and pulmonary hemorrhage/hemoptysis may be fatal; monitor patients for signs and symptoms of bleeding

Black Box Warning: **GI perforation:** some cases are fatal; monitor patients for signs and symptoms of GI perforation; discontinue therapy if GI perforation develops

• **Poor wound healing:** hold ≥4 wk before elective surgery; after major surgery, do not restart for ≥4 wk and until the surgical wound is entirely healed

• **Severe hypertension/hypertensive crisis:** usually occurs within the first 2 cycles (grade 3 or 4 hypertension); monitor B/P every 2 wk or more often if needed; treatment with antihypertensives may be needed; product may need to be discontinued

• **Severe proteinuria/nephrotic syndrome/thrombotic microangiopathy (TMA):** monitor urine protein by dipstick analysis and urinary protein-to-creatinine ratio (UPCR); obtain a 24-hr urine collection for a UPCR >1; for proteinuria of 2 g/24 hr, temporarily hold doses until proteinuria is <2 g/24 hr; if proteinuria recurs, hold doses until proteinuria is <2 g/24 hr, then permanently reduce; discontinue in nephrotic syndrome or TMA

• **Febrile neutropenia, neutropenic infection/sepsis:** monitor CBC with differential at baseline and before each cycle; hold FOLFIRI until the neutrophil count is ≥1.5 × 10⁹/L
• **Geriatric toxicity:** assess for diarrhea, dizziness, asthenia, weight loss, and dehydration that can indicate toxicity

Evaluate:
• Therapeutic response: decrease in spread of size of tumor

Teach patient/family:
• **Pregnancy/breastfeeding:** that highly effective contraception should be used during and up to 3 mo after the last dose in all patients of reproductive potential; infertility and male-mediated teratogenicity can occur; infertility is reversible within 18 wk after stopping product; do not breastfeed
• About reason for treatment, expected results

Black Box Warning: Notify prescriber immediately of bleeding, severe abdominal pain, poor wound healing

---

zoledronic acid (Rx)
(zoh'leh-drah'nick ass'id)
Aclasta ✢ Reclast, Zometa
Func. class.: Bone-resorption inhibitor
Chem. class.: Bisphosphonate

Do not confuse:
Zometa/Zoframil/Zoladex

ACTION: Potent inhibitor of osteoclastic bone resorption; inhibits osteoclastic activity, skeletal calcium release caused by stimulating factors released by tumors; reduction of abnormal bone resorption is responsible for therapeutic effect with hypercalcemia; may directly block dissolution of hydroxyapatite bone crystals

USES: Moderate to severe hypercalcemia associated with malignancy; multiple myeloma; bone metastases from solid tumors (used with antineoplastics); active Paget's disease;

Z

---

osteoporosis, glucocorticoid-induced osteoporosis, osteoporosis prophylaxis in postmenopausal women

CONTRAINDICATIONS: Pregnancy, breastfeeding; hypersensitivity to this product or bisphosphonates; hypocalcemia
Precautions: Children, geriatric patients, renal dysfunction, asthmatic patients, acute bronchospasm, anemia, chemotherapy, coagulopathy, dehydration, dental disease, diabetes mellitus, renal disease, electrolyte imbalance, hypertension, hypovolemia, infection, multiple myeloma, phosphate hypersensitivity

DOSAGE AND ROUTES
Hypercalcemia of malignancy
• **Adult: IV INFUSION** 4 mg, given as single infusion over ≥15 min; may retreat with 4 mg if serum calcium does not return to normal within 1 wk
Multiple myeloma/metastatic bone lesions
• **Adult: IV INFUSION** 4 mg, give over 15 min q3-4wk
Osteoporosis
• **Adult: IV INFUSION** 5 mg over ≥15 min q12mo
Active Paget's disease
• **Adult: IV INFUSION** 5 mg over ≥15 min
Osteoporosis prophylaxis (Reclast), postmenopausal women
• **Adult: IV INFUSION** 5 mg every other year
Osteoporosis prophylaxis (Reclast) when taking systemic glucocorticoids
• **Adult: IV** 5 mg every yr
Renal dose
• **Adult: IV INFUSION** CCr 50-60 mL/min, 3.5 mg; CCr 40-49 mL/min, 3.3 mg; CCr 30-39 mL/min, 3 mg; CCr <30 mL/min, do not use
Early breast cancer (unlabeled)
• **Adult: IV** 4 mg q6mo with goserelin 3.6 mg **SUBCUT** monthly and tamoxifen 20 mg daily or anastrozole 1 mg daily for 3 yr
Available forms: (Zometa) sol for inj 4 mg/5 mL; (Reclast) inj 5 mg/100 mL
Administer:
• Saline hydration must be performed before administration; urine output

should be 2 L/day during treatment; do not overhydrate patient
• Sol reconstituted with sterile water may be stored under refrigeration for up to 24 hr
• Acetaminophen before and for 72 hr after to decrease pain
• **Fluid volume status:** encourage additional fluid intake or give bolus before use
IV route
Zometa
• Administer after reconstituting by adding 5 mL of sterile water for inj to each vial then add to ≥100 mL of sterile 0.9% NaCl, D₅W; run over ≥15 min
• Administer in separate IV line from all other products
Reclast
• No further dilution required
• Infuse over ≥15 min at constant rate; max 5 mg

SIDE EFFECTS
CNS: Dizziness, headache, anxiety, confusion, insomnia, agitation
CV: Hypotension, leg edema, atrial fibrillation, chest pain
GI: Abdominal pain, anorexia, constipation, nausea, diarrhea, vomiting, taste change
GU: UTI, possible reduced renal function, renal damage
META: Anemia, hypokalemia, hypomagnesemia, hypophosphatemia, hypocalcemia, increased serum creatinine
MISC: Fever, chills, flulike symptoms
MS: Severe bone pain, arthralgias, myalgias, osteonecrosis of jaw
INTEG: Steven's Johnson Syndrome Toxic epidermal necrolysis

PHARMACOKINETICS
Rapidly cleared from circulation, taken up mainly by bones, not metabolized, eliminated primarily by kidneys, approximately 50% eliminated in urine within 24 hr, max effect 7 days; terminal half-life 167 hr, protein binding 22%

INTERACTIONS
• Hypomagnesemia, hypokalemia: digoxin
Decrease: effect of zoledronic acid—calcium, vit D

• Do not mix with calcium-containing infusion sol such as lactated Ringer's sol

Increase: nephrotoxicity—aminoglycosides, NSAIDs, radiopaque contrast agents

Drug/Lab Test

Increase: creatinine

Decrease: calcium, phosphorus, magnesium, potassium, Hct/Hgb, RBC, platelets, WBC

NURSING CONSIDERATIONS
Assess:

• Renal tests, calcium, phosphate, magnesium, potassium; creatinine, BUN; if creatinine elevated, hold treatment

• **Pregnancy/breastfeeding:** do not use in pregnancy, breastfeeding

• **Hypocalcemia:** paresthesia, twitching, laryngospasm; Chvostek's/Trousseau's signs

• **Dental status:** dental health may be required before starting this product; assess mouth for sores, dental caries, gingivitis; a professional dental exam should be done; cover with antiinfectives for dental extraction

• Atrial fibrillation

• **Skeletal survey:** bone fractures may occur; use fall prevention strategies

• I&O, repeat status screening before use in renal disease

Evaluate:

• Therapeutic response: decreased calcium levels, increased bone density

Teach patient/family:

• To report hypercalcemic relapse: nausea, vomiting, bone pain, thirst

• To continue with dietary recommendations, including calcium and vit D; to take a multiple vitamin daily as well as 500 mg of calcium, 400 international units vit D with multiple myeloma

• If nausea or vomiting occurs, to eat small, frequent meals, to use lozenges or chewing gum

• If bone pain occurs, to notify prescriber to obtain analgesics

• That oral health—repair of dental caries, treatment of gingivitis—may be required before starting product in high-risk patients

• To report ocular infection or eye pain immediately

• That musculoskeletal pain and weakness may occur

• To continue good oral hygiene, to have regular checkups; to report mouth sores or jaw pain (osteonecrosis of the jaw)

• Use, expected results of product

ZOLMitriptan (Rx)

(zole-mih-trip′tan)

Zomig, Zomig-ZMT

Func. class.: Migraine agent, abortive

Chem. class.: 5-HT$_{1B}$/5HT$_{1D}$ receptor agonist (triptan)

ACTION: Binds selectively to the vascular 5-HT$_{1B}$/5HT$_{1D}$ receptor subtype, exerts antimigraine effect; causes vasoconstriction in cranial arteries

USES: Acute treatment of migraine with/without aura

CONTRAINDICATIONS: Angina pectoris, history of MI, documented silent ischemia, ischemic heart disease, uncontrolled hypertension, hypersensitivity, basilar or hemiplegic migraine, risk of CV events

Precautions: Pregnancy, breastfeeding, children, postmenopausal women, men >40 yr, geriatric patients, risk factors for CAD, hypercholesterolemia, obesity, diabetes, impaired renal/hepatic function

DOSAGE AND ROUTES

• **Adult: PO** start at ≤2.5 mg (tab may be broken), may repeat after 2 hr, max single dose 5 mg, max 10 mg/24 hr; **NASAL** 1 spray in 1 nostril at onset of migraine, repeat in 2 hr if no relief

Available forms: Tabs 2.5, 5 mg; orally disintegrating tabs 2.5, 5 mg; nasal spray 2.5, 5 mg

Administer:

PO route

• Take with fluids as soon as symptoms of migraine occur

• Not approved for more than 3-4 uses in a month

Z

Side effects: *italics* = common; red = life-threatening

- **Orally disintegrating tab:** do not crush or chew; allow to dissolve on tongue

Nasal Route

- Blow nose before use
- Remove top, insert in nostril, hold other nostril shut
- Press on plunger while breathing
- Discard for single use only

SIDE EFFECTS

CNS: *Tingling, hot sensation, burning, feeling of pressure, tightness, numbness, dizziness, sedation*
CV: Palpitations, chest pain
GI: Abdominal discomfort, nausea, dry mouth, dyspepsia, dysphagia
MISC: Odd taste (spray)
MS: *Weakness, neck stiffness,* myalgia
RESP: Chest tightness, pressure

PHARMACOKINETICS

Duration $2-3^{1}/_{2}$ hr; 25% plasma protein binding; half-life $3-3^{1}/_{2}$ hr; metabolized in liver (metabolite); excreted in urine (60-80%), feces (20-40%)

INTERACTIONS

- **Extended vasospastic effects:** ergot, ergot derivatives
- Do not use within 2 wk of MAOIs
- **Weakness, hyperreflexia, incoordination:** SSRIs (FLUoxetine, fluvoxaMINE, PARoxetine, sertraline), SNRI
Increase: half-life of ZOLMitriptan—cimetidine, oral contraceptives
Increase: ZOLMitriptan levels—sibutramine

Drug/Herb
- **Serotonin syndrome:** SAM-e, St. John's wort

Drug/Lab Test
Increase: alk phos

NURSING CONSIDERATIONS
Assess:

- Tingling, hot sensation, burning, feeling of pressure, numbness, flushing
- Neurologic status: LOC, blurring vision, nausea, vomiting, tingling in extremities preceding headache
- Ingestion of tyramine foods (pickled products, beer, wine, aged cheese), food additives, preservatives, colorings, artifi-

cal sweeteners, chocolate, caffeine, which may precipitate these types of headaches, use over 10 day/month may lead to exacerbation of headache
- **Serotonin syndrome** if also taking SSRI, SNRI
- **Pregnancy/breastfeeding:** use only if benefits outweigh fetal risk; may cause harm, death to fetus; do not breastfeed, excreted in breast milk

Evaluate:
- Therapeutic response: decrease in frequency, severity of headache

Teach patient/family:
- To report any side effects to prescriber
- To use contraception while taking product
- That product does not prevent or reduce number of migraines; not to use for other headaches
- To report chest pain, rash, swelling of face
- Not to double doses; if second dose is needed, wait at least 2 hr; disintegrating dosage form—do not split, break, alter; to remove from blister pack immediately before taking

---

⚠ **HIGH ALERT**

zolpidem (Rx)
(zole′pih-dem)
Ambien, Ambien CR, Edluar, ,
Sublinox ✦, Zolpimist,
Intermezzo
Func. class.: Sedative/hypnotic
Chem. class.: Imidazopyridine

**Controlled Substance
Schedule IV**

Do not confuse:
Ambren/Abilify/Ativan/Zolipidem/lorazepam/Zalepton/zolmitroptan

ACTION: Produces CNS depression at limbic, thalamic, hypothalamic levels of CNS; may be mediated by neurotransmitter γ-aminobutyric acid (GABA); results are sedation, hypnosis, skeletal muscle relaxation, anticonvulsant activity, anxiolytic action

---

USES: Insomnia, short-term treatment; insomnia with difficulty of sleep onset/maintenance (ext rel)

Unlabeled uses: Head trauma

CONTRAINDICATIONS: Hypersensitivity to benzodiazepines

Precautions: Pregnancy, breastfeeding, children <18 yr, geriatric patients, anemia, hepatic disease, suicidal individuals, drug abuse, seizure disorders, angioedema, depression, respiratory disease, sleep apnea, sleep-related behaviors (sleepwalking), myasthenia gravis, pulmonary disease, next-morning impairments; females (lower dose needed)

DOSAGE AND ROUTES

• **Adult: PO** 5 mg (women), 5-10 mg (men) at bedtime × 7-10 days only; total max dose 10 mg; **EXT REL** 6.25 (women), 6.25-12.5 mg (men) immediately before bedtime, may be useful for ≤24 wk in people 18-64 yr with primary insomnia, max 12.5 mg/day; **oral spray** (Zolpimist) 5 mg (women), 5-10 mg (men) immediately before bedtime, max 10 mg/day; **SL** (Edluar) 5 mg (women), 5-10 mg (men) just before bedtime

• **Geriatric: PO** 5 mg at bedtime; **EXT REL** 6.25 mg; **SL** 5 mg at bedtime

Available forms: Tabs 5, 10 mg; ext rel tabs 6.25, 12.5 mg; SL: 1.75, 3.5, 5, 10 mg; oral spray 5 mg/spray

Administer:

PO route

• Do not break, crush, or chew ext rel

• Take with full glass of water

• $\frac{1}{2}$-1 hr before bedtime (PO); right before retiring (ext rel)

• On empty stomach for fast onset; may be taken with food if GI symptoms occur

• Store in tight container in cool environment

Spray route

• Prime before first use or if pump is not used for ≥14 days

• Do not use spray with or after a meal

Sublingual route

• Separate blister pack at perforation; peel paper and push product through; place product under tongue; allow to dissolve before swallowing; do not take with water

SIDE EFFECTS

CNS: Headache, lethargy, drowsiness, daytime sedation, dizziness, confusion, light-headedness, anxiety, irritability, amnesia, poor coordination, complex sleep-related reactions (sleep driving, sleep eating), depression, somnolence, suicidal ideation, abnormal thinking/behavioral changes

CV: Chest pain, palpitations

GI: Nausea, vomiting, diarrhea, heartburn, abdominal pain, constipation

HEMA: Leukopenia, granulocytopenia (rare)

MISC: Myalgia

SYST: Severe allergic reactions, angioedema, anaphylaxis

PHARMACOKINETICS

PO: Onset up to 1.5 hr, metabolized by liver, excreted by kidneys (inactive metabolites), crosses placenta, excreted in breast milk, half-life 2-3 hr

INTERACTIONS

Increase: action of both products—alcohol, CNS depressants

Increase or decrease: zolpidem levels—CYP3A4 inhibitors/inducers

Decrease: zolpidem effect—rifamycins

Drug/Herb

Chamomile, Kava, Valerian

St. John's Wort: Increased-action

NURSING CONSIDERATIONS

Assess:

• **Mental status:** mood, sensorium, affect, memory (long, short term), excessive sedation, impaired coordination, suicidal thoughts/behaviors

• Blood dyscrasias: fever, sore throat, bruising, rash, jaundice, epistaxis (rare)

• Type of sleep problem: falling asleep, staying asleep

• **Pregnancy/breastfeeding:** use only if benefits outweigh fetal risk, may cause fetal harm; cautious use in breastfeeding

• **Beers:** avoid in older adults; CNS effects occur

Z

Side effects: *italics* = common; red = life-threatening

Evaluate:

• Therapeutic response: ability to sleep at night, decreased amount of early morning awakening if taking product for insomnia

Teach patient/family:

• That dependence is possible after long-term use

• That complex sleep-related behaviors may occur (sleep driving/eating)

• To avoid driving or other activities requiring alertness until dosage is stabilized

• To avoid alcohol ingestion

• That effects may take 2 nights for benefits to be noticed; next-morning impairment may occur

• Not to use during pregnancy, breastfeeding

• That hangover is common in geriatric patients but less common than with barbiturates; that rebound insomnia may occur for 1-2 nights after discontinuing product; not to discontinue abruptly; to taper

• Not to crush, chew, break ext rel tabs

• To prime spray pump before using

TREATMENT OF OVERDOSE:
Lavage; monitor electrolytes, VS

---

zonisamide (Rx)
(zone-is'a-mide)
Zonegran
Func. class.: Anticonvulsant
Chem. class.: Sulfonamides

ACTION: May act through action at sodium and calcium channels, but exact action is unknown; serotonergic action

USES: Adjunctive therapy for partial seizures

CONTRAINDICATIONS: Hypersensitivity to this product or sulfonamides
Precautions: Pregnancy, breastfeeding, children <16 yr, geriatric patients, allergies, renal/hepatic disease; psychiatric condition, hepatic failure, pulmonary disease, suicidal ideation

DOSAGE AND ROUTES
• **Adult/child >16 yr:** 100 mg/day, may increase after 2 wk to 200 mg/day, may increase q2wk, max dose 600 mg/day
Available forms: Caps 25, 50, 100 mg
Administer:
• Without regard to food; swallow whole

SIDE EFFECTS
CNS: Dizziness, insomnia, paresthesias, depression, fatigue, headache, confusion, somnolence, agitation, irritability, speech disturbance, suicidal ideation, seizures, status epilepticus
EENT: Diplopia, verbal difficulty, speech abnormalities, taste perversion, amblyopia, pharyngitis, rhinitis, tinnitus, nystagmus
GI: Nausea, constipation, anorexia, weight loss, diarrhea, dyspepsia, dry mouth, abdominal pain
GU: Kidney stones
HEMA: Aplastic anemia, granulocytopenia (rare); ecchymosis
INTEG: Rash, pruritus
MISC: Flulike symptoms
SYST: Stevens-Johnson syndrome, metabolic acidosis

PHARMACOKINETICS
Peak 2-6 hr, half-life in RBCs 105 hr, metabolized by liver, excreted by kidneys, protein binding 40%

INTERACTIONS
Decrease: half-life of zonisamide—carBAMazepine, phenytoin, PHENobarbital
Altered product levels: CYP3A4 inhibitors/inducers
Increase: CNS depression—alcohol
Drug/Herb
Increase: effect of this product—St John's wort
Drug/Food
• Do not use with grapefruit
Drug/Lab Test
Increase: BUN, creatinine

NURSING CONSIDERATIONS
Assess:
• **Seizures:** duration, type, intensity, precipitating factors

---

• Renal function: albumin concentration, BUN, urinalysis, creatinine, serum bicarbonate at baseline and periodically
• **Mental status:** mood, sensorium, affect, memory (long-, short-term), **suicidal thoughts/behaviors**
• **Stevens-Johnson syndrome, aplastic anemia, fulminant hepatic necrosis;** may cause death; monitor for rashes and hypersensitivity reactions
• Obtain bicarbonate before treatment/periodically; metabolic acidosis may occur in children
• **Beers:** avoid in older adults unless safer alternative is unavailable; may cause ataxia, impaired psychomotor function
• **Pregnancy/breastfeeding:** use only if benefits outweigh fetal risk, may cause fetal harm; pregnant women should enroll in the North American Antiepileptic Drug Pregnancy Registry, 1-888-233-2334; do not breastfeed, excreted in breast milk

Evaluate:
• Therapeutic response: decrease in severity of seizures

Teach patient/family:
• Not to discontinue product abruptly because seizures may occur
• To avoid hazardous activities until stabilized on product
• To carry emergency ID stating product use
• To notify prescriber of rash immediately; to notify prescriber of back pain, abdominal pain, blood in urine; to increase fluid intake to reduce risk of kidney stones
• To notify prescriber if pregnancy is planned, suspected
• To avoid grapefruit
• To notify prescriber of sore throat, fever, easy bruising
• To report suicidal thoughts, behaviors immediately

Appendix A

aclidinium/ formoterol (Rx)

Duaklir Pressair

Func. class.: Respiratory agent
Chem. class.: Respiratory corticosteroid; long-acting β_2 agonist; respiratory long-acting muscarinic antagonist

USES: Maintenance treatment of chronic obstructive pulmonary disease (COPD)

CONTRAINDICATIONS: Hypersensitivity.

DOSAGE AND ROUTES
• **Adult: INH** 1 inhalation (400 mcg aclidinium and 12 mcg formoterol per actuation) inhaled bid (morning and evening). Max: 1 INH bid.

alpelisib

(al-peh-lih′-sib)

Piqray

Func. class.: Antineoplastic
Chem. class.: Small molecule antineoplastic phosphatidylinositol-3-kinase (PI3K) inhibitors

ACTION: In breast cancer cell lines, inhibits the phosphorylation of PI3K downstream targets, including Akt, and showed activity in cell lines harboring a *PI3KCA* mutation.

USES: Hormone receptor (HR)–positive, *HER2*–negative, *PIK3CA*-mutated, advanced or metastatic breast cancer in men and postmenopausal women after progression on or after an endocrine-based regimen, in combination with fulvestrant

CONTRAINDICATIONS: Hypersensitivity, pregnancy
Precautions: Breast feeding, chronic lung disorders, contraceptive requirement, diabetes mellitus, diarrhea, hyperglycemia, infertility, interstitial lung disease, male mediated teratogenicity

DOSAGE AND ROUTES
Males and postmenopausal females: PO 300 mg PO q day with food, in combination with fulvestrant (500 mg IM on days 1, 15, 29 and monthly thereafter) until disease progression or unacceptable toxicity.
Available forms: Tabs 200, 250, 300 mg
Administer:
• Give with food at approximately the same time each day.
• Do not crush, chew, or split; do not use any tablet that is broken, cracked, or otherwise not intact.
• If a dose is missed, it can be taken with food within 9 hrs after the time it is usually taken. After more than 9 hr, skip the dose for that day and resume dosing on the following day at the usual time.
• If vomiting occurs, do not administer an additional dose on that day. Resume dosing the following day at the usual time.

SIDE EFFECTS
CNS: *Fever, headache*
ENDO: Hypoglycemia, hyperglycemia
INTEG: *Rash, pruritus*
GU: Renal dysfunction
GI: *Nausea, vomiting, diarrhea, abdominal pain, anorexia, weight loss*
SYST: Infection, anaphylaxis, Stevens-Johnson syndrome

PHARMACOKINETICS
89% protein binding, half-life 8-9 hr; 81% excreted in feces (36% unchanged, 32% as metabolite), 14% excreted in urine (2% unchanged, 7.1% metabolite);

affected by CYP2C9, CYP3A4, BCRP; peak 2-4 hr

INTERACTIONS

Avoid use with CYP3A4 inhibitors, inducers, substrates

Drug/Lab Test
Increase: LFTs

NURSING CONSIDERATIONS
Assess:

• **Diabetes mellitus:** Fasting blood glucose and hemoglobin A1c (HbA1c) should be monitored before starting treatment and any antidiabetic treatment change; continue to monitor blood glucose weekly for the first 2 wk, then q4wk; monitor HbA1c q3mo.

• **Severe diarrhea:** May use with antidiarrheal medication (loperamide). An interruption of therapy, dose reduction, or discontinuation of therapy may be necessary.

• **Severe hypersensitivity reactions (anaphylaxis and anaphylactic shock):** Monitor for severe hypersensitivity reactions (dyspnea, flushing, rash, fever, or tachycardia); permanently discontinue if this occurs.

• **Pregnancy/breastfeeding:** Do not use in pregnancy/breastfeeding. Obtain pregnancy testing before use.

Evaluate:

• Therapeutic response: Decreased disease progression in breast cancer.

Teach patient/family:

• **Pregnancy/breastfeeding:** To report planned or suspected pregnancy; to use effective contraception during treatment and for at least 1 mo after the last dose; to avoid breastfeeding

• To report new or worsening side effects
• To take tabs whole, not to crush or chew; to take with food

• Preexisting chronic lung disease (CLD); severe pneumonitis/interstitial lung disease: Advise patients to immediately report any new or worsening respiratory symptoms (hypoxia, cough, dyspnea)

• Diarrhea: Teach patients to begin antidiarrheal treatment, increase oral fluids, and notify their health care provider if diarrhea occurs

---

bremelanotide injection (Rx)

(bre′ me-lan′ oh-tide)

Vyleesi

Func. class.: Sexual dysfunction agent

Chem. class.: Melanocortin receptor agonists

ACTION: Nonselectively activates several receptor subtypes. The mechanism is unknown. It may activate selected brain pathways involved in normal sexual responses

USES: Premenopausal women with acquired, generalized hypoactive sexual desire disorder

CONTRAINDICATIONS: Hypersensitivity, men, postmenopausal women, cardiac disease

Precautions: Pregnancy, breastfeeding, contraception requirement, geriatric, hepatic disease, hypertension, renal dysfunction, skin hyperpigmentation

DOSAGE AND ROUTES

• **Adult premenopausal women:** SUBCUT 1.75 mg as needed, at least 45 minutes before anticipated sexual activity; max: 1 dose/ 24 hr

Available forms: Autoinjector solution for injection 1.75 mg/0.3 mL

Administer:
SUBCUT Route

• Visually inspect parenteral products for particulate matter and discoloration before use. Do not use injections that are unusually cloudy, discolored, or contain particulate, injection is clear and colorless

• Inject subcut into the abdomen or thigh. Do not administer within 2 inches around the umbilicus or where the skin is tender, bruised, red, hard, thick, or scaly

• The dose is administered at least 45 minutes before anticipated sexual activity

• Not to be used more than 1 dose/24 hr. No more than 8 doses/month

---

Side effects: *italics* = common; red = life-threatening

• Discard the used autoinjector in a sharps container after use

SIDE EFFECTS
CNS: *Flushing, headache*
INTEG: *Injection site reactions*
GI: *Nausea,* hepatitis
GU: Hot flashes
CV: Hypertension

PHARMACOKINETICS
21% binds to human serum protein, half-life 1.9 to 4 hr; metabolism involves multiple hydrolyses of the amide bond of the cyclic peptide; excreted 64.8% urine, 22.8% feces

INTERACTIONS
Decreased: effect of naltrexone; do not use together

NURSING CONSIDERATIONS
Assess:
• **Sexual arousal:** Identify characteristics of lack of sexual arousal, length of time, other treatments administered in the past
• **Hypertension/cardiac disease:** Monitor B/P before starting treatment and periodically ensure blood pressure is well controlled
• **Nausea/vomiting:** Is a common side effect, may require an antiemetic; product may need to be discontinued for persistent or severe nausea or antiemetic therapy initiated for those patients who are bothered by nausea
• **Skin hyperpigmentation:** May be more common in those with darker skin and with daily dosing, more common on face, gingiva, and breast; may be permanent
• **Severe hepatic/renal disease (Child-Pugh C; score 10 to 15) or severe renal impairment (eGFR less than 30 mL/min/1.73 m2):** May have an increase in severity of adverse reactions as a result of increased drug exposure
• **Pregnancy/breastfeeding:** Contraception requirements are advised; females of child-bearing potential should be counseled regarding appropriate methods of contraception while on therapy; discontinue if pregnancy is suspected; pregnant women are encouraged to call the Bremelanotide

Pregnancy Exposure Registry at (877) 411-2510; avoid breastfeeding—no data are available regarding safety
Evaluate:
• Therapeutic response
• Sexual arousal
Teach patient/family:
• **Sexual arousal:** Report if product has resolved lack of sexual arousal
• **Hypertension/cardiac disease:** Teach patient that B/P will be evaluated periodically.
• **Nausea/vomiting:** Teach patient to report nausea and vomiting, may require an antiemetic
• **Skin hyperpigmentation:** Teach patient to report skin hyperpigmentation; product may need to be discontinued
Train the patient on the use of the autoinjector, to read the manufacturer-provided instructions for use
• **Pregnancy/breastfeeding:** Counsel patients on need for contraception; females of child-bearing potential should be counseled regarding appropriate methods of contraception while on therapy; advise patient to discontinue if pregnancy is suspected; pregnant women are encouraged to call the Bremelanotide Pregnancy Exposure Registry at (877) 411-2510; avoid breastfeeding

---

brexanolone (Rx)
(REMS)
(brek-san' oh-lone)
Zulresso
Func. class.: Antidepressants
Chem. class.: GABA Modulator

ACTION: Not fully known but thought to be related to its positive modulation of γ-aminobutyric acid A (GABA-A) receptors; GABA is a major inhibitory neurotransmitter in the brain

USES: Postpartum depression

CONTRAINDICATIONS: Hypersensitivity
Precautions: Abrupt discontinuation, driving or hazardous activities, breastfeeding, coadministration with other CNS

depressants, alcohol use, hypoxia, pregnancy, renal failure, suicidal ideation

> **Black Box Warning:** CNS depression, loss of consciousness; requires a specialized setting

DOSAGE AND ROUTES
Adult Females Continuous IV: Give over a total of 60 hr (2.5 days) as follows: 0 to 4 hr: initiate with a dose of 30 mcg/kg/hr; 4 to 24 hr: increase dose to 60 mcg/kg/hr; 24 to 52 hr: increase dose to 90 mcg/kg/hr; 52 to 56 hr: decrease dose to 60 mcg/kg/hr; 56 to 60 hr: decrease dose to 30 mcg/kg/hr

Available forms: Solution for injection 100 mg/20 mL

Administer:
• The vials require dilution
• Visually inspect product; vial should be clear, colorless without particulate matter and discoloration; do not use discolored vials or vials with particulate matter
• 5 infusion bags will be required for the 60-hr infusion; additional bags will be needed for those ≥90 kg
• Prepare and store in a polyolefin, non-DEHP, nonlatex bag only; do not use in-line filter
• Dilute in the infusion bag immediately after the initial puncture of the vial
• Withdraw 20 mL of product from the vial and place in the infusion bag; dilute with 40 mL of Sterile Water for Injection, and further dilute with 40 mL of 0.9% Sodium Chloride Injection (total volume of 100 mL) to achieve a target concentration of 1 mg/mL
• Immediately place the infusion bag in refrigerator until use
• Give as a continuous IV infusion over a total of 60 hr (2.5 days) via a dedicated line; do not inject other medications into the infusion bag or admix
• Use a programmable peristaltic infusion pump, prime infusion sets with admixture before inserting into the pump and connecting to the venous catheter
• A healthcare provider must be available on site to continuously monitor
• Initiate treatment early enough during the day to allow for recognition of excessive sedation

• After the product is diluted, it can be stored in infusion bags under refrigerated conditions for up to 96 hr
• Each diluted product can be used for up to 12 hr of infusion time at room temperature; discard any unused after 12 hr of infusion

SIDE EFFECTS
CNS: Sedation, drowsiness, loss of consciousness, suicidal ideation
CV: Tachycardia
RESP: Hypoxia
INTEG: Injection site reaction

PHARMACOKINETICS
Extensive distribution into tissues, protein binding >99%, extensively metabolized by non-CYP pathways including keto-reduction, glucuronidation, and sulfation; half-life 9 hr; excreted as metabolites in feces (47%) and urine (42%); less than 1% of the drug is excreted as unchanged

INTERACTIONS
None known

NURSING CONSIDERATIONS
Assess:
• Monitor for hypoxia using continuous pulse oximetry with an alarm; if hypoxia occurs, discontinue and do not reinitiate

> **Black Box Warning:** Assess for excessive sedation q2hr during planned, non-sleep periods, and stop the infusion if excessive sedation occurs until the symptom resolves; thereafter, the infusion may be resumed at the same or lower dose

• Available only through the Zulresso risk Evaluation and Mitigation Strategy (Zulresso REMS) program; risks of serious adverse outcomes (excessive sedation or sudden loss/alteration of consciousness)

> **Black Box Warning:** Requires a specialized care setting; healthcare settings must be certified in the REMS program); for further information, including a list of certified healthcare facilities, visit www.zulressorems.com or call 1-844-472-4379

• **Suicidal ideation:** Assess for suicidal thoughts and behavior; more common in young adults

Evaluate:

• Therapeutic response: decrease in postpartum depression, improved mood

Teach patient/family:

• Reason for product and expected result
• To discuss all Rx, OTC, herbals and supplements with healthcare provider
• To report pain, inflammation at injection site
• **Excessive sedation and sudden loss of consciousness:** excessive sedation or loss of consciousness can occur; checking q2hr for these symptoms will be required; if these occur, tell your healthcare provider
• A family member or caregiver needs to help care for you and your children during the infusion
• Not to drive or engage in hazardous tasks while sleepiness occurs
• Not to use alcohol or other CNS depressants
• **Pregnancy/breastfeeding:** to identify if pregnancy is planned or suspected or if breastfeeding; if pregnant, register with the National Pregnancy Registry for Antidepressants at 1-844-405-6185 or visit https://womensmentalhealth.org/clinical-and-research-programs/pregnancyregistry/antidepressants/

---

caplacizumab (Rx)
(kap' luh-sih'-zoo-mab)
Cablivi
Func. class.: Hematologic agent

USES: Acquired thrombotic thrombocytopenia purpura (aTTP), in combination with plasma exchange and immunosuppressive therapy

CONTRAINDICATIONS
Hypersensitivity

DOSAGE AND ROUTES

• **Adult:** IV 11 mg once at least 15 min before plasma exchange on the first day of treatment (initial dose); subcut 11 mg daily starting after the completion of plasma exchange on day 1 and continuing for 30 days after the last daily plasma exchange; treatment may be extended for a maximum of 28 days after the initial treatment (maintenance dose)

---

cladribine (Rx)
(klad'-dri-been)
Leustatin, Mavenclad
Func. class.: Multiple sclerosis agent/ antineoplastic
Chem. class.: Purine nucleoside antimetabolite

ACTION: May be lymphocyte depletion through cytotoxic effects on B and T lymphocytes through impairment of DNA synthesis

USES: Relapsing multiple sclerosis, active hairy-cell leukemia

CONTRAINDICATIONS: Breastfeeding, HIV, TB

Black Box Warning: Pregnancy

Precautions:
Contraceptive requirements, hepatic disease, infection, renal disease, progressive multifocal, leukoencephalopathy, neonates, premature

Black Box Warning: Bone marrow suppression, neurotoxicity, nephrotoxicity, new primary malignancy, reproductive risk; requires an experienced clinician

DOSAGE AND ROUTES

Relapsing forms of multiple sclerosis

Adults: PO 1.75 mg/kg per treatment course divided into 2 cycles and given as divided doses of 1 or 2 tablets daily over 4 or 5 days for each cycle with second cycle starting 23 to 27 days after the last dose of first cycle; give a second course at least 43 wk after the last dose of the first course, second cycle for a cumulative dosage of 3.5 mg/kg; max: 20 mg (2 tablets)/cycle day.

Active hairy-cell leukemia (orphan drug)
Adults:

Continuous Infusion

0.09 mg/kg/day × 7 days

Available forms: Tablet 10 mg, solution for injection 1 mg/mL

Administer:

• Follow cytotoxic handling and disposal procedures

• Separate all other products by ≥3 hr during the 4- or 5-day treatment cycles

PO Route

• Use dry hands; wash hands after use; avoid prolonged contact with skin

If a tablet is left on a surface, broken or fragmented, wash the area with water

Take without regard to meals; swallow whole with water immediately after removal from blister; do not chew

IV Route

• Visually inspect for particulate matter and discoloration before use; a precipitate may occur during the exposure of injection to low temperatures; it may be resolubilized by allowing the solution to warm naturally to room temperature and by shaking vigorously; do not heat or microwave the solution

• Use aseptic technique; does not contain preservative

• The concentrate for injection must be diluted before use; do not use Dextrose 5% Injection, or benzyl alcohol in neonates; do not admix

Daily IV infusion:

• Add the calculated single daily dose of the concentrate through a sterile 0.22-micrometer disposable hydrophilic syringe filter to a polyvinyl chloride infusion bag containing 500 mL of 0.9% Sodium Chloride Injection; prepare each solution daily; discard any unused portion; vials are for single-use only; once solutions are diluted, promptly administer or store at 2° to 8° C for no more than 8 hr before the start of administration

• Infuse continuously over 24 hr

• Admixtures are stable for at least 24 hr at room temperature under normal room fluorescent light in Baxter Viaflex PVC infusion containers

Seven-day IV infusion:

• Calculate the dose for a 7-day period and withdraw from the concentrate for injection; dilute in bacteriostatic 0.9% Sodium Chloride Injection containing benzyl alcohol as a preservative; to minimize the risk of microbial contamination, first the calculated 7-day dose and then the amount of diluent needed to bring the total volume to 100 mL should be passed through a sterile 0.22-micrometer disposable hydrophilic syringe filter as each solution is being added to the infusion reservoir; after completing solution preparation, clamp off the line, disconnect, and discard the filter; aseptically aspirate air bubbles from the reservoir as necessary using the syringe and a dry second sterile filter or a sterile vent filter assembly; reclamp the line, and discard the syringe and filter assembly

• Discard any unused portion of injection; vials are for single-use only; once solutions are diluted, promptly administer or store at 2 to 8° C for no more than 8 hr before the start of administration

• Solutions prepared for individuals weighing more than 85 kg may have reduced preservative effectiveness because of greater dilution of the benzyl alcohol; admixtures for the 7-day infusion have demonstrated acceptable chemical and physical stability for at least 7 days in the SIMS Deltec Medication Cassette Reservoir

• Infuse continuously over 7 days

SIDE EFFECTS
CNS: *Fatigue, fever, headache,* neurotoxicity
HEMA: *Anemia, neutropenia, thrombocytopenia, lymphopenia*
GI: *Nausea*
GU: Nephrotoxicity
INTEG: *Rash*

PHARMACOKINETICS
Protein binding is 20%; crosses the blood-brain barrier; half-life 1 day; a substrate of breast cancer resistance protein (BCRP),

---

Side effects: *italics* = common; red = life-threatening

P-glycoprotein (P-gp), equilibrative nucleoside transporter 1 (ENT1), and concentrative nucleoside transporter 3 (CNT3); inhibition of BCRP in the GI tract may increase oral bioavailability and systemic exposure; potent ENT1 or CNT3 inhibition may alter intracellular distribution and renal elimination; PO product effect is decreased by a high-fat meal

INTERACTIONS

• Do not use with live virus vaccines
• Duplicate effects: immunosupressives, avoid using together
• Antiviral and antiretroviral drugs: avoid concomitant use
• BCRP or ENT/CNT inhibitors: may alter bioavailability; avoid using together

NURSING CONSIDERATIONS
Assess:

• **Progressive multifocal leukoencephalopathy (PML):** Assess for new or worsening neurologic, cognitive, or behavioral signs or symptoms, irreversible paraparesis and quadriparesis; may be more common in those who received continuous infusion at high doses (4 to 9 times the recommended dose for hairy cell leukemia)

Black Box Warning: Bone marrow suppression: Assess for neutropenia, anemia, thrombocytopenia; usually reversible and appears to be dose dependent; during the first 2 weeks after treatment initiation, mean platelet count, absolute neutrophil count (ANC) and HGB declined, and then increased with normalization of mean counts by day 15, week 5, and week 8; monitor hematologic parameters especially during the first 4 to 8 weeks after treatment

Black Box Warning: Secondary malignancies: Monitor for secondary malignancies

Black Box Warning: Pregnancy/breastfeeding: Assess if pregnancy is planned or suspected or if breastfeeding.

Evaluate:
Therapeutic response
Decrease in spread of malignancy
Teach patient/family:
If a dose is missed, take the missed dose on the following day and extend the number of days in that treatment cycle; if 2 consecutive doses are missed, extend the treatment cycle by 2 days

Black Box Warning: Pregnancy/breastfeeding: Advise females of reproductive potential to use effective contraception during treatment with PO product and for at least 6 months after the last dose in each treatment course; instruct women who are using systemic hormonal contraceptives to add a barrier method during PO product and for at least 4 wk after the last treatment; advise male patients of reproductive potential to take precautions to prevent pregnancy of their partner during PO treatment and for at least 6 months after the last dose in each treatment course; highly effective contraception is recommended during treatment with IV product

---

darolutamide (Rx)
(dar′-oh-loo′-tuh-mide)
Nubeqa
Func. class.: Antineoplastic-hormone

ACTION: Competitively inhibits androgen binding, AR nuclear translocation, and androgen receptor-mediated transcription

USES: Nonmetastatic castration-resistant prostate cancer

DOSAGE AND ROUTES
• **Adults: PO**
600 mg bid until disease progression or unacceptable toxicity
Administer:
• Patient should be receiving a gonadotropin-releasing hormone (GnRH) analog or has had a bilateral orchiectomy

• Give with food
• Have the patient swallow the tablet whole; do not crush or chew
• If a dose is missed, it should be taken as soon as the patient remembers before the next scheduled dose; do not take 2 doses at the same time if a dose is missed

SIDE EFFECTS
CNS: Fatigue
GI: Elevated LFTs, hyperbilirubinemia, diarrhea, nausea
GU: Hot flashes
HEMA: Neutropenia, anemia
MS: MS pain
CV: Hyper-hypotension, *heart failure*
Integ: Rash

PHARMACOKINETICS
Use with food increases bioavailability by 2- to 2.5-fold increase; protein binding (albumin) is 92% for darolutamide and 99.8% for the active metabolite, keto-darolutamide; half-life 20 hr, 63.4% excreted in the urine, 32.4% in the feces (30% unchanged); metabolized by CYP3A4, UGT1A9, and UGT1A1, a BCRP inhibitor, inhibits OATP1B1 and OATP1B3l

INTERACTIONS
Avoid use with CYP3A4, UGT1A9, UGT1A1

NURSING CONSIDERATIONS
Assess:
• **Prostate cancer:** decreasing signs/ symptoms of prostate cancer
• **Hepatic/renal disease:** monitor for hepatic and renal involvement
• **Pregnancy:** males with female partners of reproductive potential should avoid pregnancy and use effective contraception during and for at least 1 wk after treatment
Evaluate:
Therapeutic response: decreased progression of prostate cancer
Teach patient/family:
• **Pregnancy:** patients with female partners of reproductive potential should avoid pregnancy and use effective contraception during and for at least 1 wk after treatment; there is a possibility of infertility

---

diroximel
(dye-rox' i-mel)
Vumerity
Func. class.: MS agent

USES: Relapsing multiple sclerosis

CONTRAINDICATIONS
Hypersensitivity

DOSAGE AND ROUTES
• **Adults: PO** 231 mg bid for 7 days, then increase to 462 mg bid

---

dolutegravir/lamivudine
(doe-loo-leg' ra-vir la-mi' vyoo-deen)
Dovato
Func. class.: Antiretroviral/antiviral
Chem. class.: INST/NRTI

ACTION: Dolutegravir; lamivudine is active against infections caused by human immunodeficiency virus type 1 (HIV-1). Lamivudine is a nucleoside analog that works by inhibiting HIV reverse transcriptase, while dolutegravir works by inhibiting the catalytic activity of HIV integrase

USES: HIV-1 infection in adults

CONTRAINDICATIONS: Hypersensitivity
Precautions: Alcoholism, autoimmune disease, bone fractures, breastfeeding, children, depression, females, Graves' disease, Guillain-Barré syndrome, hepatic disease, hepatitis, hepatitis B and HIV coinfection, hepatitis C and HIV coinfection, hepatomegaly, HIV resistance, hypercholesterolemia, hyperlipidemia, hypertriglyceridemia, hypophosphatemia, immune reconstitution syndrome, lactic acidosis, obesity, osteomalacia, osteoporosis, pregnancy, renal failure, renal impairment, serious rash, suicidal ideation, torsades de pointes

---

Side effects: *italics* = common; red = life-threatening

Black Box Warning: Hepatitis B exacerbation, hepatotoxicity

DOSAGE AND ROUTES
Adults: who are treatment-naïve **PO** One tablet (50 mg dolutegravir; 300 mg lamivudine) q day
Available forms: Tablet 50 mg-300 mg
Administer:
• Give without regard to food.
• During coadministration with carbamazepine or rifampin, the dolutegravir dose needs to be increased to 50 mg BID; add 50 mg/day of dolutegravir (separated by 12 hours from dolutegravir; lamivudine) should be given
• Avoid use in treatment-experienced patients and in patients with known substitutions associated with resistance to dolutegravir or lamivudine
• Do not use within 2 hrs before or 6 hrs after iron or calcium supplement. If coadministration is unavoidable, give the supplement and dolutegravir; lamivudine with food.
• Do not use within 2 hrs before or 6 hrs after antacids, laxatives, or other medicines that contain aluminum, magnesium, sucralfate, or buffered medicines
• Admixtures are stable for at least 24 hr at room temperature under normal room fluorescent light in Baxter Viaflex PVC infusion containers

SIDE EFFECTS
CNS: *Headache,* abnormal dreams, *depression, dizziness, insomnia,* neuropathy, paresthesia, asthenia, fatigue, drowsiness
GI: *Nausea, vomiting, anorexia, diarrhea, abdominal pain, dyspepsia* hepatomegaly with stenosis (may be fatal), hyperbilirubinemia, hypercholesterolemia, pancreatitis
GU: Glomerulonephritis membranous/mesangial **proliferative**
INTEG: *Rash,* skin discoloration
MS: *Arthralgia, myalgia,* rhabdomyolysis
RESP: Cough
SYST: *Change in body fat distribution,* lactic acidosis

PHARMACOKINETICS
• **Lamivudine:** 36% bound to plasma protein, the parent drug is not metabolized, with most of the oral dose (approximately 70%) being excreted unchanged in the urine by active organic cationic secretion. Half-life is 13 to 19 hrs
• **Dolutegravir:** 99% protein binding, metabolism occurs via UDP-glucuronosyltransferase (UGT)1A1 (major) and by the hepatic isoenzyme CYP3A (minor), half-life 14 hrs, 53% excreted unchanged in the feces, urine excretion 31%

INTERACTIONS
Increased level:
• CYP3A4 inhibitors (aldesleukin IL-2, amiodarone, aprepitant, atazanavir, basiliximab, boceprevir, bromocriptine, chloramphenicol, clarithromycin, conivaptan, danazol, dalfopristin, darunavir, dasatinib, delavirdine, diltiazem, dronedarone, efavirenz, erythromycin, ethinyl estradiol, fluconazole, fluoxetine, fluvoxamine, fosamprenavir, fosaprepitant, imatinib, indinavir, isoniazid, itraconazole, ketoconazole, lanreotide, lapatinib, miconazole, nefazodone, nelfinavir, nicardipine, octreotide, posaconazole, quinine, ranolazine, rifaximin, tamoxifen, telaprevir, telithromycin, tipranavir, troleandomycin, verapamil, voriconazole, zafirlukast)
Increased: metformin
Increased: dofetilide, coadministration is contraindicated
Decrease: dolutegravir-carbamazepine, rifampin, an additional dolutegravir 50-mg dose should be taken,
Decrease: dolutegravir-oxcarbazepine Phenytoin Phenobarbital, avoid coadministration
Drug/Herb
Decrease: dolutegravir-oxcarbazepine Phenytoin Phenobarbital, avoid coadministration
Drug/lab test
Increased: AST/ALT, amylase, bilirubin, CK, glucose, lipase
Decrease: Neutrophils

NURSING CONSIDERATIONS
Assess:

• **HIV infection:** Assess symptoms of HIV, including opportunistic infections, before and during treatment, some may be life threatening; monitor plasma CD4+, CD8 cell counts, serum beta-2 microglobulin, serum antigen levels, treatment failures occur more often in those with baseline HIV-1 RNA concentrations <100,000 copies/ml than in those <100,000 copies/ml; monitor blood glucose, CBC with differential, serum cholesterol, lipid panel

Black Box Warning: **Hepatotoxicity/ lactic acidosis:** Monitor hepatitis B serology, LFTs, plasma hepatitis C RNA, lactic acidosis levels. If lab reports confirm these conditions, discontinue product. More common in females or those who are overweight. Avoid use in alcoholism

• **Pregnancy:** Obtain pregnancy testing before use; Hepatitis B exacerbation: Those with coexisting HBV and HIV infections who discontinue this product may experience severe acute hepatitis B exacerbation with some cases resulting in hepatic decompensation and hepatic failure.
• Patients coinfected with HBV and HIV who discontinue this product should have transaminase concentrations monitored q6wk for the first 3 mo, and q3-6 mo thereafter.
• Resumption of anti–hepatitis B treatment may be required. For patients who refuse a fully suppressive antiretroviral regimen but still require treatment for HBV, consider 48 wk of peginterferon alfa; do not administer HIV-active medications in the absence
• Periodically monitor serum bilirubin (total and direct), serum creatinine, urinalysis, LFTs, amylase, lipase

Evaluate

• **Therapeutic response:** Improvement in CD4, HIV RNC counts, decreasing signs and symptoms of HIV

Teach patient/family

• That hepatitis and HIV coinfected patients should avoid consuming alcohol; offer vaccinations against hepatitis A/ hepatitis B as appropriate
• That GI complaints resolve after 2-3 wk of treatment
• To report suspected or planned pregnancy, not to breastfeed, Instruct mothers with HIV-1 infection not to breastfeed because HIV-1 can be passed to the baby in the breast milk, inform patients that there is an antiretroviral pregnancy registry to monitor fetal outcomes
• To take at the same time of day to maintain blood level, not to crush, break, or chew
• That product controls the symptoms of HIV but does not cure, that patient is still able to infect others, that other products may be necessary to prevent other infections
• **Lactic acidosis:** To notify prescriber of fatigue, muscle aches/pains, abdominal pain, difficulty breathing, nausea, vomiting, change in heart rhythm

Black Box Warning: **Hepatotoxicity:** To notify prescriber of dark urine, yellowing skin or eyes, clay-colored stools, anorexia, nausea, vomiting .

• Discuss with provider all Rx, OTC, herbs and supplements taken as there are many drug interactions
• **Immune Reconstitution Syndrome** Advise patients to inform their healthcare provider immediately of any signs and symptoms of infection as inflammation from previous infection may occur
• Instruct patients that if they miss a dose, to take it as soon as they remember, not to double their next dose or take more than the prescribed dose

entrectinib (Rx)
(en-trex' tih-nib)

Rozlytrek

Func. class.: Antineoplastic orphan drug
Chem. class.: tyrosine kinase ROS1 inhibitor, tropomyosin receptor kinase (TRK) inhibitor

USES: ROS1-positive non–small cell lung cancer and NTRK gene fusion–positive solid tumors

CONTRAINDICATIONS
Hypersensitivity, pregnancy, breastfeeding

DOSAGE AND ROUTES
• **Adult:** PO 600 mg daily until disease progression or unacceptable toxicity

---

erdafitinib (Rx)
(er'-duh-fih'-tih-nib)

Balversa

Func. class.: Antineoplastic-kinase inhibitor

Chem. class.: Fibroblast growth factor receptor (FGFR) inhibitors

---

ACTION: Inhibits the enzymatic activity of FGFR1, FGFR2, FGFR3, and FGFR4

USES: Locally advanced or metastatic urothelial carcinoma

DOSAGE AND ROUTES
• **Adult:** PO 8 mg daily initially; after 14 to 21 days of treatment, increase dose to 9 mg daily if serum phosphate level is <5.5 mg/dL and there are no ocular disorders or grade 2 or higher adverse reactions; continue treatment until disease progression or unacceptable toxicity

Available forms:
Tabs 3, 4, 5 mg

Administer:
• Swallow tablets whole, with or without food
• If vomiting occurs, do not replace the dose; the next dose should be taken the next day
• If a dose is missed, it can be taken as soon as possible on the same day; do not take extra tablets to make up for the missed dose; resume the regular daily schedule on the next day

SIDE EFFECTS
GI: Abdominal pain, nausea, vomiting, anorexia, constipation, diarrhea

CNS: Fatigue, fever

EENT: Stomatitis, blurred vision, retinal detachment

INTEG: Rash, nail discoloration

META: Hyperglycemia, hyper-hypophosphatemia, hypomagnesemia, hyponatremia, hypoalbuminemia

HEMA: Leukopenia, anemia, thrombocytopenia

SYST: Infection

PHARMACOKINETICS
99.8% protein bound to α-1-acid glycoprotein; half-life 59 hr; 69% excreted in feces (19% unchanged) and 19% in urine (13% unchanged), metabolized by CYP2C9 (39%) and CYP3A4 (20%); an inhibitor of OCT2; peak 2.5 hr

INTERACTIONS
Avoid use with CYP3A4 inducers, inhibitors

NURSING CONSIDERATIONS
Assess:
• **Ocular disease:** Provide dry eye prophylaxis with ocular demulcents as needed; perform monthly ophthalmologic examinations during the first 4 months of treatment and every 3 months thereafter, and urgently at any time for visual disturbance; examinations should include an assessment of visual acuity, slit-lamp examination, fundoscopy, and optical coherence tomography; an interruption of therapy, discontinuation of therapy, or dose reduction may be necessary for ocular adverse reactions
• **Infection:** Assess for infection (fever, flulike symptoms)
• Avoid coadministration with agents that alter serum phosphate levels before the initial dose increase period (days 14 to 21); monitor phosphate levels monthly for hyperphosphatemia and follow dose modification guidelines when required; in patients with hyperphosphatemia, restrict phosphate intake to 600 to 800 mg daily; if serum phosphate is >7 mg/dL, consider adding an oral phosphate binder until the serum phosphate level returns to less than 5.5 mg/dL

• **Pregnancy/breastfeeding:** Pregnancy should be avoided during and for at least 1 month after the last dose; obtain pregnancy testing before use

Evaluate:

• Therapeutic response: decreased progression of cancer

Teach patient/family:

• About the reproductive risk and contraception requirements during treatment; men with female partners of reproductive potential should also use effective contraception during treatment and for 1 month after the last dose; not to breastfeed during and for 1 month after last dose

• Ophthalmic examinations will be needed periodically

---

esketamine (Rx)

(es- ket′-a- meen)

Spravato nasal spray

Func. class.: Antidepressant
Chem. class.: Augmentation agent
Controlled substance III

ACTION: Noncompetitively blocks the NMDA receptor, which is an ionotropic glutamate receptor; mechanism of action for antidepressant effect is unknown; however, the activity on NMDA receptors may be responsible for both the therapeutic and the adverse psychiatric effects

USES: Treatment-resistant depression in adults with an oral antidepressant

CONTRAINDICATIONS

Aneurysm, arteriovenous malformation, intracranial bleeding, ketamine hypersensitivity

Precautions:

Alcoholism, breastfeeding, cardiac disease, cerebrovascular disease, coadministration with other CNS depressants, driving or operating machinery, encephalopathy, geriatrics, hepatic disease, hypertension, hypertensive crisis, loss of consciousness, pregnancy, psychosis, schizophrenia

Black Box Warning: Children, CNS depression, dissociation, requires a specialized care setting, substance abuse, suicidal ideation

DOSAGE AND ROUTES

Adults: NASAL INDUCTION PHASE: On day 1, give 56 mg; for subsequent doses during wk 1 through 4, give 56 mg or 84 mg twice weekly; use two devices for the 56-mg dose and 3 devices for the 84-mg dose with a 5-min rest between use of each device; **MAINTENANCE PHASE:** During wk 5 through 8, give 56 mg or 84 mg weekly; during wk 9 and thereafter, give 56 mg or 84 mg q2wks or weekly.

Available forms: Nasal spray 56, 84 dose kit

Administer: Nasal Route

• Must be given under the direct supervision of a healthcare provider and including a supervised postadministration observation

• Each device contains 28 mg; use 2 devices for a 56-mg dose and 3 devices for an 84-mg dose with a 5-min rest between use of each device

• To prevent loss of medication, do not prime the device before use

• During and after use at each treatment session, observe the patient for at least 2 hr until the patient is safe to leave

• Assess B/P before use; if baseline B/P > 140 mm Hg systolic or >90 mm Hg diastolic, do not use if an increase in B/P or intracranial pressure poses a serious risk

• Reassess B/P about 40 min after dosing and subsequently as clinically indicated; if B/P is decreasing and the patient appears clinically stable for at least 2 hr, the patient may be discharged at the end of the post-dose monitoring period; if not, continue to monitor.

• Because of the potential for drug-induced nausea and vomiting, advise patients to avoid food for at least 2 hr before use and avoid liquids at least 30 min before administration

• Patients requiring a nasal corticosteroid or nasal decongestant on dosing day

---

Side effects: *italics* = common; red = life-threatening

should use these at least 1 hr before receiving this product

• If treatment sessions are missed and there is a worsening of depression symptoms, consider returning to the previous dosing schedule

SIDE EFFECTS

CNS: Anxiety, dissociation, drowsiness, dizziness, headache, vertigo, dependence, impaired cognition, hallucinations, confusion, lethargy, suicidal ideation

CV: Hypertension hypertensive crisis

GI: Nausea

PHARMACOKINETICS

Primarily metabolized to noresketamine, the active metabolite, by CYP2B6 and CYP3A4 and to a lesser extent by CYP2C9 and CYP2C19; noresketamine is metabolized by CYP-dependent pathways and metabolism occurs through glucuronidation; elimination is biphasic, with a rapid decline for the initial 2-4 hr and a mean terminal half-life 7-12 hr; elimination of the metabolite is also biphasic, 4 hr and a terminal half-life of 8 hr; metabolites are excreted in urine (78%) and feces (2%); bioavailability 48%; peak 20-40 min

INTERACTIONS

Black Box Warning: Increased: CNS depression, other CNS depressants—do not use together

Black Box Warning: Increased: sedation, B/P, MAOIs, psychostimulants—do not use together

NURSING CONSIDERATIONS
Assess

Black Box Warning: **Dissociation:** Monitor patient for at least 2 hr after each treatment session, then provide an assessment to determine when the patient is stable and ready to leave the healthcare setting; special care is needed with those with schizophrenia

Black Box Warning: **Substance abuse:** Monitor for signs of abuse or dependence; physical dependence has been reported with prolonged use of ketamine; withdrawal symptoms of ketamine include craving, fatigue, poor appetite, anxiety

Black Box Warning: **Suicidal ideation:** behaviors should be closely monitored during treatment; consider changing the therapeutic regimen, including the discontinuation of esketamine and/or the concurrent oral antidepressant, in patients with worsening of depression or emergent suicidality

Evaluate

• Therapeutic response: decreasing depression

Teach patient/family:

Black Box Warning: **Suicidal ideation:** Teach family members or caregivers to monitor for changes in behavior and to alert the healthcare provider if such behaviors occur

Black Box Warning: **CNS depression:** Tell your healthcare provider about all the Rx, OTC, vit and herbal supplements used, not to use with other CNS depressants unless discussed with healthcare provider

• Before use instruct patients not to engage in potentially hazardous activities (driving, operating heavy machinery), until the next day after a restful sleep

HOW TO USE:

• **Step 1:** Instruct patient to blow nose before the first device use only; confirm the required number of devices (56 mg = 2 devices; 84 mg = 3 devices)

• **Step 2:** Check expiration date; peel blister and remove device; do not prime the device—this will cause loss of medication; ensure that the indicator on the device shows 2 green dots; give device to patient

• **Step 3:** Instruct patient to hold device with thumb gently supporting but not pressing the plunger as shown in the product labeling; patient should recline head at about 45 degrees during administration to keep medication in nose

• **Step 4:** Instruct patient to insert tip straight into the first nostril; the nose rest should touch the skin between the nostrils; close the opposite nostril; breathe in through nose while pushing plunger all the way up until it stops; sniff gently after spraying to keep medication inside nose; switch hands to insert tip into the second nostril; repeat steps to deliver second spray

• **Step 5:** After administration is complete, take the device from the patient; check that indicator on device shows no green dots; if green dot remains, have patient spray again into the second nostril. Instruct patient to rest comfortably (preferably semi-reclined) for 5 min after each device; if liquid drips out, dab nose with a tissue; DO NOT blow nose

• If a second device is required, ensure a 5-min waiting period before use to allow medication from first device to be absorbed

• **Pregnancy/breastfeeding:** Identify if pregnancy is planned or suspected or if breastfeeding; if patient is pregnant, she should register with the National Pregnancy Registry for Antidepressants online at https://womensmentalhealth.org/clinical-and-research-programs/pregnancyregistry/antidepressants/ or by calling 1-844-405-6185

fam-trastuzumab deruxtecan-nxki

Enhertu
Func. class.: Antineoplastic, *HER2*-directed antibody

USES: *HER2* breast cancer

DOSAGE AND ROUTES
Adult:
Intermittent IV Infusion
5.4 mg/kg once q3wk (21-day cycle) until disease progression or unacceptable toxicity

CONTRAINDICATIONS
Hypersensitivity

fedratinib (Rx)
(fed-ra′ ti-nib)
Inrebic
Func. class.: Orphan drug

USES: Intermediate-2 or high-risk primary or secondary (post–polycythemia vera or post–essential thrombocythemia) myelofibrosis; orphan drug

CONTRAINDICATIONS
Hypersensitivity, encephalopathy, thiamine deficiency

DOSAGE AND ROUTES
• **Adults:** PO 400 mg daily in patients with a baseline platelet count of 50×10^9 cells/L or greater

istradefylline (Rx)
(iz-tra′ de-fye′ leen)
Nourianz
Func. class.: Anti-Parkinson agent
Chem. class.: Adenosine receptor antagonist

ACTION: Adenosine A_{2A} receptor antagonist that acts through a nondopaminergic mechanism to improve motor function

USES: Adjuvant treatment in patients with Parkinson's disease experiencing "off" episodes

CONTRAINDICATIONS
Hypersensitivity

Side effects: *italics* = common; red = life-threatening

Precautions:
Behavioral changes, breastfeeding, children, contraception requirements, dyskinesia, geriatric, hepatic disease, impulse control symptoms, infants, pregnancy, psychosis, reproductive risk, tobacco smoking

DOSAGE AND ROUTES
Adults PO 20 mg daily; adjust dose based on response and tolerability; max: 40 mg daily; 20 or more cigarettes, 40 mg daily
Available forms: Tabs 20, 40 mg
Administer: May give without regard to meals

SIDE EFFECTS
CNS: *Dyskinesia*, psychosis, dizziness, hallucinations, insomnia
GI: Nausea, constipation

PHARMACOKINETICS
• Protein binding 98%, metabolized by CYP1A1, CYP3A4, with a minor contribution from CYP1A2, CYP2B6, CYP2C8, CYP2C9, CYP2C18, and CYP2D6 metabolites 39% and excreted urine (39%), feces (48%); half-life 83 hr; dosage modifications are needed in heavy smoking; peak 4 hr (fasting), increased with high-fat meal

INTERACTIONS
Increased: istradefylline effect—strong CYP3A4 Inhibitors (ketoconazole, itraconazole, clarithromycin); max 20 mg daily
Decreased: istradefylline effect—strong CYP3A4 Inducers (carBAMazepine, rifAMPin, phenytoin, St. John's wort); avoid using together
Drug: herb
Decreased: istradefylline effect—St. John's wort; avoid using together

NURSING CONSIDERATIONS
Assess:
• **Parkinson's disease:** Assess for decreasing "off" episodes, tremors usually first appearing in hands/foot while at rest, slow movement, rigidity, postural instability, problems with speech and voice, incontinence, difficulty swallowing, inability to start movements or continue repeated movement, excessive sweating, constipation, dry skin, mood changes
• **Dyskinesia:** Assess for grimacing, eye blinking, lip smacking, repetitive movements, these should lessen with treatment
• **Hallucinations/psychosis/ impulse control/compulsive behaviors:** Assess for these effects, and if present, decreased dose or discontinuation of treatment may be needed
• Monitor LFTs in hepatic disease
Evaluate:
• Therapeutic response: decreasing symptoms of Parkinson's disease
Teach patient/family:
• To identify if tobacco is used and, if so, how much per day; dosage change may be needed
• To identify all Rx, OTC, herbals, supplements that are used and discuss with healthcare provider
• **Pregnancy/breastfeeding:** Identify if pregnancy is planned or suspected or if breastfeeding, use in pregnancy is not recommended; adequate contraception should be used in women of childbearing

---

lasmiditan
(las-mid′ i- tan)
Reyvow
Func. class.: Antimigraine

USES: Migraine with or without aura in adults

CONTRAINDICATIONS
Hypersensitivity

DOSAGE AND ROUTES
• **Adults:** PO 50, 100, or 200 mg as a single dose; max: 1 dose in 24 hr

---

lefamulin (Rx)
(le-FAM ue-lin)
Xenleta
Func. class.: Antiinfective
Chem. class.: Pleuromutilin antibiotics

ACTION: May be bacteriostatic or bactericidal depending on the organism; inhibits bacterial protein synthesis through interactions (hydrogen bonds, hydrophobic interactions, and Van der Waals forces) in rRNA of the 50S subunit

USES: Treatment of community acquired bacterial pneumonia caused by *Chlamydophila pneumoniae, Haemophilus influenzae (β-lactamase negative), Haemophilus influenzae (β-lactamase positive), Haemophilus parainfluenzae, Legionella pneumophila, Moraxella catarrhalis, Mycoplasma pneumoniae, Staphylococcus aureus* (MRSA), *Staphylococcus aureus* (MSSA), *Streptococcus agalactiae* (group B streptococci), *Streptococcus anginosus, Streptococcus mitis, Streptococcus pneumoniae, Streptococcus pyogenes* (group A β-hemolytic streptococci), *Streptococcus salivarius*

CONTRAINDICATIONS

Hypersensitivity to this product or pleuromutilin antibiotics; use with CYP3A4 substrates

Precautions:

Alcoholism, bradycardia, breastfeeding, cardiac disease, contraception requirements, CAD, diabetes mellitus, dialysis, diarrhea, geriatrics, hepatic disease, hypertension, hypocalcemia, hypokalemia, hypomagnesemia, long QT syndrome, renal failure, reproductive risk, thyroid disease, torsades de pointes, ventricular dysrhythmias

DOSAGE AND ROUTES

• **Adults: PO** 600 mg q12hr × 5 days; IV 150 mg q12hr × 5-7 days

Hepatic dose

• **Adults: IV** Give over 60 min q24hr (Child-Pugh Class C); PO not recommended for patients with moderate (Child-Pugh Class B) or severe (Child-Pugh Class C)

Available forms:

Tablet 600 mg; solution for injection 150 mg/15 mL (10 mg/mL)

Administer:

PO route

• If a dose is missed, give the dose as soon as possible and anytime up to 8 hr before the next scheduled dose; if less than 8 hr remain before the next scheduled dose, do not give the missed dose, and resume dosing at the next scheduled dose

• Administer at least 1 hour before a meal or 2 hr after a meal

• Swallow tablet whole with 6 to 8 ounces of water; do not crush or divide tablets

• **Intermittent IV route** Visually inspect for particulate matter and discoloration prior to use, do not use if present

Dilution: Dilute the entire 15 mL vial into the supplied diluent bag; mix thoroughly; do not use the diluent bag in series connections, do not admix

Storage: Store up to 24 hr at room temperature and up to 48 hr when refrigerated at 2° to 8° C (36° to 46° F)

• Infuse over 60 min

SIDE EFFECTS

GI: Nausea, diarrhea, CDAD, vomiting
CNS: Insomnia, headache
META: Hypokalemia

PHARMACOKINETICS

Protein binding 94.8% to 97.1%, metabolized by CYP3A4; excreted urine 15.5% (9.6%-14.1% unchanged) after IV, 5.3% (unchanged after PO, excreted feces 77.3% (4.2%-9.1% unchanged) after IV and 88.5% (7.8%-24.8% unchanged) after PO; half-life is 3-20 hr; is a CYP3A4 and P-glycoprotein (P-gp) substrate; inhibits CYP2C8, breast cancer resistance protein (BCRP), and MATE1; PO peak 0.88-2 hr

INTERACTIONS

Decreased: Lefamulin effect—strong or moderate CYP3A inducers or P-gp inducers; avoid using together; if used, monitor for reduced effect

Increased: lefamulin effect—strong CYP3A inhibitors or P-gp inhibitors; avoid using together; if used together, monitor for adverse reactions.

Increased: QT interval—CYP3A substrates; do not use together

NURSING CONSIDERATIONS
Assess:
• **Pneumonia:** Assess for signs of pneumonia
• QT prolongation: Assess for QT prolongation

Evaluate:
Therapeutic response: decreasing symptoms of pneumonia, culture negative

Teach patient/family:
• Advise patients to take at least 1 hr before a meal or 2 hr after a meal and should be swallowed whole with water (6-8 ounces); do not crush or divide
• That nausea/vomiting is common
• That serious allergic reactions may occur and require immediate attention
• To take exactly as directed, not to skip doses or not complete the full course of therapy
• **CDAD, diarrhea:** Assess for diarrhea that is watery or has mucous, with or without fever, stomach cramps that may occur up to 2 months after final dose
• **Pregnancy/breastfeeding:** Identify if pregnancy is planned or suspect, or if breastfeeding, pregnancy testing will be needed before use; use adequate contraception during use and for 2 days after final dose; not to be used in pregnancy; if used inadvertently during pregnancy or if a patient becomes pregnant while receiving product, report exposure by calling 1-855-5NABRIVA to enroll; if breastfeeding, pump and discard milk for the duration of treatment and for 2 days after the final dose

---

lumateperone
(Luma-tep´-erone)

Caplyta
Func. class.: Antimigraine

USES: Schizophrenia

DOSAGE AND ROUTES
• **Adult: PO** 42 mg/day

CONTRAINDICATIONS
Hypersensitivity

Black Box Warning: Dementia-related psychosis

---

nintedanib (Rx)
(nin-ted´ a- nib)

Ofev
Func. class.: Interstitial lung disease agent
Chem. class.: Idiopathic pulmonary fibrosis agent

ACTION: Inhibitor of multiple receptor tyrosine kinases (RTK), including platelet-derived growth factor receptor (PDGFR) α and β, fibroblast growth factor receptor (FGFR), vascular endothelial growth factor receptor, and Fms-like tyrosine kinase 3 (FLT3); competitively binds to the ATP binding these receptors, blocking intracellular signaling and inhibiting proliferation, migration, and transformation of fibroblasts

USES: Systemic sclerosis–associated interstitial lung disease; idiopathic pulmonary fibrosis (IPF) (orphan drug)

CONTRAINDICATIONS
Hypersensitivity

DOSAGE AND ROUTES
• **Adults PO** 150 mg q12hr
Available forms: Capsule 100, 150 mg
Administer:
• Give with food
• Administer capsules whole with liquid; do not chew or crush

SIDE EFFECTS
GI: Abdominal pain, anorexia, diarrhea, nausea, vomiting, weight loss, pancreatitis
CNS: Fatigue
INTEG: Skin ulcer
CV: Hypertensive crisis, stroke, cardiomyopathy

PHARMACOKINETICS

Protein binding 97.8%, with serum albumin excretion biliary/feces 90%; metabolized to an active metabolite BIBF 1202, then glucuronidated to the inactive metabolite BIBF 1202 glucuronide by UGT1A1, UGT1A7, UGT1A8, and UGT1A10; half-life 9.5 hr; food increases exposure by 20% and delays peak from 2 hr to 3.98 hr

INTERACTIONS

Increased: nintedanib exposure—P-glycoprotein (P-gp) and CYP3A4 inhibitors (ketoconazole, erythromycin), monitor patients closely for tolerability

Increased: bleeding risk—anticoagulants; monitor patients on full anticoagulation therapy closely for bleeding and adjust as needed

Decreased: nintedanib exposure—P-gp and CYP3A4 inducer (rifAMPin, carBAMazepine, phenytoin, St. John's wort)

NURSING CONSIDERATIONS

Assess:

• **Interstitial lung disease:** dyspnea, dry, hacking cough, fatigue, anorexia, bleeding in the lungs

• Obtain LFTs and a pregnancy test (females) baseline and thereafter if needed

Evaluate:

• **Therapeutic response:** decreased dyspnea, cough

Teach patient/family:

• That if a dose is missed, take the next dose at the next scheduled time; do not take 2 doses at the same time

• That abdominal pain, loss of appetite, nausea, vomiting, diarrhea are common

• **Pregnancy/breastfeeding:** Teach patient about pregnancy prevention and planning; verify the pregnancy status of females of reproductive potential before treatment and during treatment as appropriate; contraception is necessary during and for 3 months after last dose; use a barrier method with hormonal contraceptives if taken; discuss that reduced fertility in females may occur; breastfeeding is not recommended

---

pexidartinib (Rx)

(pex′-i-dar′-ti-nib)

Turalio

Func. class.: Antineoplastic-orphan drug

Chem. class.: Colony stimulating factor-1 receptor (CSF-1R) inhibitor

USES: Symptomatic tenosynovial giant cell tumor

CONTRAINDICATIONS

Hypersensitivity, pregnancy, breastfeeding

Black Box Warning: Hepatotoxicity

DOSAGE AND ROUTES

• **Adults: PO** 400 mg bid on an empty stomach until disease progression

---

pitolisant (Rx)

(pi-tol′ i sant)

Wakix

Func. class.: Narcolepsy agent

Chem. class.: Histamine receptor modulator

ACTION: Selective antagonist/inverse agonist of the histamine-3 (H3) receptor; activation of histaminergic neurons increases histamine release, which promotes wakefulness, attention, and memory; regulates the release of other neurotransmitters involved in wake promotion, including dopamine, noradrenaline, and acetylcholine

USES: Excessive daytime sleepiness in adults with narcolepsy

CONTRAINDICATIONS

Hypersensitivity, severe hepatic disease

PRECAUTIONS

Alcoholism, bradycardia, CAD, cardiac disease, children, breastfeeding, contraception requirement, diabetes mellitus, females, geriatrics, heart failure, hepatic

---

Side effects: *italics* = common; red = life-threatening

disease, hypertension, hypocalcemia, hypokalemia, hypomagnesemia, long QT syndrome, MI, malnutrition, poor metabolizers, pregnancy, QT prolongation, renal disease, thyroid disease

DOSAGE AND ROUTES
• **Adults PO** Initially, 8.9 mg daily in the morning on awakening for 1 wk; then increase to 17.8 mg daily for 1 wk; after that, the dose may be adjusted based on efficacy response and tolerability; max: 35.6 mg/day; limit to 17.8 mg/day in CYP2D6 poor metabolizers; up to 8 wks may be necessary

Available forms: Tablets 4.45, 17.8 mg
Administer:
• Give each dose in the morning on patient wakening

SIDE EFFECTS
CNS: *Headache, insomnia, anxiety,* hallucinations, irritability, cataplexy
GI: *Nausea,* abdominal pain, anorexia, dry mouth
INTEG: Rash
RESP: URI
MS: MS pain
CV: Increased heart rate

PHARMACOKINETICS
Protein binding is 91%-96%, metabolized by CYP2D6 and to a lesser extent by CYP3A4; inactive metabolites are further metabolized or conjugated with glycine or glucuronic acid, excreted 90% urine (<2% unchanged), 2.3% feces; half-life 7.5-24.2 hours, absorption 90%; peak 2-5 hr; increased in hepatic/renal disease

INTERACTIONS
Increased: cardiac dysrhythmia risk—drugs that prolong the QT interval (class Ia, III antidysrhythmics); avoid using together
Increased: pitolisant effect—CYP2D6 inhibitors (buPROPion, PARoxetine, FLUoxetine); reduce dose by half
Decreased: pitolisant effect—CYP3A4 inducers (carBAMazepine, phenytoin, rifAMPin); increase dose to double
Decreased: pitolisant effect—histamine-1 receptor antagonists (diphenhydrAMINE, imipramine, clomiPRAMINE); avoid using together

Decreased: CYP3A4 substrates (midazolam, hormonal contraceptives, cycloSPORINE)—use alterative contraception

NURSING CONSIDERATIONS
Assess:
• **Narcolepsy:** assess for trouble staying awake baseline and after 1 wk, 2 wk
• **Hepatic/renal disease:** monitor LFTs, serum bilirubin, BUN, creatinine baseline and periodically
Evaluate:
• **Therapeutic response:** ability to stay awake
Teach patient/family:
• If a dose is missed, skip the missed dose and administer the next dose the following day in the morning on wakening
• Report to healthcare provider if inability to stay awake continues
• **Pregnancy/breastfeeding:** identify if pregnancy is planned to suspected; if using hormonal contraceptives, an alternative method should be used during and for 21 days after last dose; do not use in pregnancy; encourage to enroll in the WAKIX pregnancy registry if patient becomes pregnant; to enroll or obtain information from the registry, call 1-800-833-7460; present in breast milk

---

pretomanid (Rx)
(pree-toh´ mah-nid)
Pretomanid*
*Both trade and generic the same name
Func. class.: Antimycobacterial
Chem. class.: Nitroimidazooxazine

ACTION: Kills actively replicating *Mycobacterium tuberculosis* by inhibiting mycolic acid biosynthesis, thereby blocking cell wall production

USES: Drug-resistant TB

CONTRAINDICATIONS
Hypersensitivity

PRECAUTIONS
Breastfeeding, hepatic disease, myelosuppression, pregnancy, QT prolongation, infertility

DOSAGE AND ROUTES

• **Adult PO Pretomanid** Tablet 200 mg daily × 26 ws; **bedaquiline** 400 mg PO daily × 2 wk, then 200 mg 3 times per wk, with at least 48 hr between doses, X 24 weeks (total of 26 wk); **linezolid** 1,200 mg PO daily × 26 wk, with adjustments to 600 mg daily and further reduction to 300 mg daily or interruption of dosing for known linezolid adverse reactions of myelosuppression, peripheral neuropathy, and optic neuropathy

Available forms: Tablets 200 mg

Administer:

• Take the combination with food, swallow whole with water

• If the combination is interrupted for safety reasons, missed doses can be made up at the end of the treatment; doses of linezolid alone missed because of linezolid adverse reactions should not be made up

• Combination may be extended beyond 26 wk if needed

SIDE EFFECTS

CNS: Peripheral neuropathy, headache, insomnia

CV: QT prolongation, hypertension

GI: Nausea, vomiting, anorexia, abdominal pain, weight loss, diarrhea, constipation, gastritis, dyspepsia

INTEG: Acne, rash, pruritus, dry skin

RESP: Lower respiratory tract infection, cough, pleuritic pain

HEMA: Thrombocytopenia, neutropenia, anemia

META: Hypoglycemia

MS: MS pain

EENT: Visual impairment, increased hyperamylasemia hemoptysis, hyperlipasemia

PHARMACOKINETICS

Protein binding 86.4%, metabolized by multiple reductive and oxidative pathways; 53% excreted in urine, 38% in feces, as metabolites; half-life 16.9-17.4 hr; CYP3A4 is responsible for 20% of the metabolism; pretomanid significantly inhibits organic anion transporter-3 (OAT3) transporter

INTERACTIONS

Decreased: pretomanid effect—strong or moderate CYP3A4 inducers (rifAMPin, efavirenz); avoid using together

Increased: effect of OAT3 substrates—monitor for adverse reactions; dosage reduction for OAT3 substrate drugs may be needed

Increased: AST/ALT,   bilirubin, γ-glutamyltransferase

NURSING CONSIDERATIONS

Assess:

• **Hepatotoxicity:** assess for fatigue, anorexia, nausea, jaundice, clay-colored stools, dark urine, liver tenderness, and hepatomegaly; obtain LFTs baseline, at 2 wk, monthly; if new or worsening hepatic dysfunction occurs, test for viral hepatitis and discontinue other hepatotoxic medications; interrupt treatment with the entire regimen if ALT/AST are accompanied by total bilirubin elevation >2× ULN or ALT/AST >8× ULN or ALT/AST >5× ULN and continue >2 wk

• **Myelosuppression:** assess for anemia (may be fatal), leukopenia, thrombocytopenia, pancytopenia; monitor CBC baseline, 2 wk, monthly; decreasing or interrupting dosing may be needed in worsening myelosuppression

• **Peripheral/optic neuropathy, peripheral neuropathy:** monitor visual function; if an impairment occurs, interrupt dosing and obtain ophthalmologic testing

• **QT prolongation:** obtain an ECG baseline, and ≤2, 12, 24 wk; obtain serum potassium, calcium, and magnesium at baseline and correct if abnormal; continue to monitor if QT prolongation occurs; may occur more often in a history of torsades des pointes, congenital long QT syndrome, hypothyroidism, bradydysrhythmia, uncompensated HF or serum calcium, magnesium, or potassium levels less than lower limits of normal

• **Lactic acidosis:** assess for recurrent nausea or vomiting; if this occurs, evaluate immediately bicarbonate and lactic acid levels and possible interruption of combination

---

Side effects: *italics* = common; red = life-threatening

Evaluate:

Therapeutic response: TB cultures negative

Teach patient/family:

• To report fatigue, vomiting, anorexia, nausea, jaundice, clay-colored stools, dark urine, liver tenderness, and visual impairment immediately

• To swallow whole with water; that all products must be taken as a combination regimen

• **Pregnancy/breastfeeding:** to report if pregnancy is planned or suspected: not to be used in pregnancy or breastfeeding

---

ramucirumab
(ra-mue-sir′ ue-mab)

Cyramza

Func. class.: Antineoplastic

Chem. class.: Vascular endothelial growth factor antagonist

ACTION: Binds to vascular endothelial growth factor receptor 2 (VEGFR2; kinase insert domain-containing receptor; KDR), preventing the binding of ligands; as a result, ramucirumab inhibits its ligand-induced proliferation and migration of human endothelial cells

USES: Advanced or metastatic gastric or gastroesophageal junction adenocarcinoma with disease progression on or after fluoropyrimidine- or platinum-containing chemotherapy, as monotherapy or in combination with paclitaxel, for the treatment of metastatic NSCLC with disease progression on or after platinum-based chemotherapy, in combination with docetaxel, for the treatment of metastatic colorectal cancer (mCRC) in patients with disease progression on or after prior therapy with bevacizumab, oxaliplatin, and a fluoropyrimidine, in combination with irinotecan, folinic acid (leucovorin), and fluorouracil (FOLFIRI) for the treatment of advanced hepatocellular cancer in patients with α-fetoprotein (AFP) ≥400 ng/mL and who have previously been treated with sorafenib

CONTRAINDICATIONS

Hypersensitivity, pregnancy, breastfeeding

Precautions: Anticoagulant therapy, bleeding, cirrhosis, MI, contraception requirements, GI perforation, hepatic disease, human antihuman antibody (HAHA), hypertension, hypothyroidism, infusion related reactions, renal disease, stroke, surgery

DOSAGE AND ROUTES

Gastric cancer or gastroesophageal junction adenocarcinoma

• **Adults IV infusion** 8 mg/kg over 60 min q2wk until disease progression or unacceptable toxicity; if first infusion is tolerated, all subsequent infusions may be administered over 30 min

NSCLC

• **Adults IV infusion** 10 mg/kg over 60 min with docetaxel (75 mg/m2 IV) on day 1, q21days until disease progression or unacceptable toxicity

mCRC

• **Adults IV** 8 mg/kg IV over 60 min on day 1 before FOLFIRI use, q2wk until disease progression or unacceptable toxicity; FOLFIRI consists of irinotecan 180 mg/m2 IV over 90 min and folinic acid (leucovorin) 400 mg/m2 given over 120 min on day 1, followed by fluorouracil 400 mg/m2 IV bolus over 2-4 min on day 1, followed by fluorouracil 2,400 mg/m2 by continuous IV infusion over 46-48 hr; if first infusion is tolerated, all subsequent infusions may be given over 30 min

Hepatocellular cancer

• **Adults IV Infusion** 8 mg/kg over 60 min q2wk until disease progression or unacceptable toxicity; if first infusion is tolerated, all subsequent infusions may be administered over 30 min

Hepatic dose

• Adults IV

Mild to moderate hepatic impairment (Child-Pugh A; total bilirubin 1.1-3 times ULN and any AST, OR or total bilirubin within ULN and AST greater than ULN): no change; Severe hepatic impairment (Child-Pugh B or C): Use only if the potential benefits outweigh the risks

Available forms: Injection 10 mg/mL single-dose vial
Administer: Intermittent IV infusion route
Intermittent IV infusion route
• Use cytotoxic handling precautions
• Premedicate with an IV histamine-1 (H1) receptor antagonist (diphenhydramine); for patients who have had a prior grade 1 or 2 infusion-related reaction, premedicate with an H1-receptor antagonist, dexamethasone (or equivalent), and acetaminophen before each infusion
• Dilute with normal saline to a final volume of 250 mL; invert to mix; do not shake; stable for 4 hr at room temperature
• Inspect for particles and discoloration before using
• Use a protein-sparing 0.22-micron filter; use separate line; flush with normal saline after use
• Do not admix with other solutions or medications
• Store vials in refrigerator; protect from light, do not freeze

SIDE EFFECTS
CNS: Headache, fatigue, RPLS
CV: Hypertension, arterial thromboembolic events, hemorrhage
EENT: Epistaxis
GI: Intestinal obstruction, diarrhea
GU: Proteinuria
HEMA: Neutropenia, anemia
RESP: Lower respiratory tract infection, cough, pleuritic pain
INTEG: Rash
Misc.: Hypothyroidism, hyponatremia, IRR, antibody formation, infusion site reactions, poor wound healing

PHARMACOKINETICS
Increased bleeding risk: anticoagulants, NSAIDs, antiplatelets

INTERACTIONS
Increased: urine protein
Decreased: RBCs, serum sodium

NURSING CONSIDERATIONS
Assess
• **Bleeding/hemorrhage:** assess for GI bleeding; perforation (severe abdominal pain, nausea, vomiting, fever) may be fatal; discontinue and do not restarts if this occurs
• **Poor wound healing:** assess all wounds for changes, avoid use if present
• **Hypertension:** monitor B/P frequently, at least q2wk; if hypertension occurs, withhold until controlled
• **RPLS:** assess for hypertension, blurred vision, impaired consciousness, seizures, headache; may be confirmed with MRI; discontinue and do not restart if confirmed
• **ATE:** assess for serious cardiac events, including MI, stroke; discontinue permanently if these occur
• **Pregnancy/breastfeeding:** do not use in pregnancy; women should use adequate contraception during and for ≥3 months after last dose; if childbearing potential, do not breastfeed

Evaluate:
• **Therapeutic response:** decreased progression of cancer

Teach patient/family:
• **Bleeding:** teach patient that bleeding may occur, to contact provider for bleeding
• **Poor wound healing:** teach patient to report wound changes, to discuss with all providers use of product
• **Hypertension:** teach patient to monitor B/P frequently, at least q2wk; if high or if headache is present, notify provider
• **RPLS:** assess for hypertension, blurred vision, impaired consciousness, seizures, headache; may be confirmed with MRI; discontinue and do not restart if confirmed
• **Pregnancy/breastfeeding:** identify if pregnancy is planned or suspected; teach not use in pregnancy, to use adequate contraception during and for ≥3 months after last dose; if childbearing potential, do not breastfeed; product may impair fertility

---

ravulizumab
(rav´-yoo-liz´-yoo-mab)
Ultomiris
Func. class.: Monoclonal antibody

USES: Atypical hemolytic uremic syndrome in adults and pediatrics

CONTRAINDICATIONS
Hypersensitivity

DOSAGE AND ROUTES
Treat for at least 6 months
• **Adults ≥ 100 kg: IV** 3,000 mg load, then 3,600 mg q8wk starting 2 wk after loading dose
• **Adults 60 to 99 kg: IV** 2,700 mg load, then 3,300 mg q8wk starting 2 wk after loading dose
• **Adults 40 to 59 kg: IV** 2,400 mg load, then 3,000 mg q8wk starting 2 wk after loading dose
• **Adults 40 to 59 kg: IV** 2,400 mg load, then 3,000 mg q8wk starting 2 wk after loading dose
• **Adolescents ≥ 100 kg: IV** 3,000 mg load, then 3,600 mg q8wk starting 2 wk after the loading dose
• **Children and adolescents 60 to 99 kg: IV** 2,700 mg load, then 3,300 mg q8wk starting 2 wk after loading dose
• **Children and adolescents 40 to 59 kg: IV** 2,400 mg load, then 3,000 mg q8wk starting 2 wk after loading dose
• **Children and adolescents 30 to 39 kg: IV** 1,200 mg load, then 2,700 mg qy 8 wk starting 2 wk after loading dose
• **Children 20 to 29 kg: IV** 900 mg load, then 2,100 mg q8wk starting 2 wk after the loading dose
• **Infants and children 10 to 19 kg: IV** 600 mg load, then 600 mg q4wk starting 2 wk after loading dose
• **Infants and children 5 to 9 kg: IV** 600 mg load, then 300 mg q4wk starting 2 wk after loading dose.

---

risankizumab (Rx)
(ris′ an- kiz′ ue- mab)
Skyrizi
Func. class.: Systemic antipsoriasis agents

ACTION: A humanized immunoglobulin G1 (IgG1) monoclonal antibody that selectively binds to the p19 subunit of human interleukin-23 (IL-23), thereby inhibiting its interaction with the IL-23 receptor; human IL-23 is a naturally occurring cytokine involved in inflammatory and immune responses; by blocking IL-23 from binding to its receptor, prevents the release of proinflammatory cytokines and chemokines

USES: Moderate to severe plaque psoriasis

CONTRAINDICATIONS
Hypersensitivity
Precautions:
Pregnancy, breastfeeding, TB, infection, immunosuppression

DOSAGE AND ROUTES
• **Adult: SUBCUT** 150 mg (two 75-mg injections) at wk 0, 4, and q12wk thereafter
Available forms: Prefilled syringe solution for injection 75 mg/0.83 mL 2-pack
Administer:
Subcut route
• Keep in the original carton to protect from light until time of use
• Do not shake the carton or prefilled syringe
• Before use, allow to reach room temperature out of direct sunlight (15-30 min); do not use other methods to speed warming process
• Visually inspect parenteral products for particulate matter and discoloration; solution should be clear to slightly opalescent, colorless to slightly yellow; solution may contain a few translucent white particles
• Do not use if solution contains large particles or is cloudy or discolored; solution has been frozen; syringe has been dropped or damaged; syringe tray seal is broken or missing
• Only an individual trained in subcut drug delivery should administer the injection; an adult who is properly trained in injection technique may self-inject; the first injection needs to be under the supervision of a qualified healthcare professional

• Wash and dry hands

• Select an injection site (right or left thigh, abdomen at least 2 inches from the navel) and wipe with an alcohol swab; do not inject into skin that is tender, bruised, red, hard, or affected by psoriasis; do not inject into a scar or stretch mark; administer injections at different sites at least 1 inch apart

• Removed needle cover from the 1st prefilled syringe

• With 1 hand, gently pinch cleaned injection site; use the other hand to insert needle at a 45-degree angle using a quick short movement

• Slowly push plunger until all the solution is injected

• Pull needle out of skin; release plunger and allow prefilled syringe to move up until the entire needle is covered by needle guard

• Apply cotton ball or gauze pad over injection site for 10 sec; do not rub injection site

• To obtain the full dose, repeat the injection process using 2nd prefilled syringe; select and cleanse an alternative injection site that is at least 1 inch away from first site; do not inject into the same site as the 1st syringe

• If a dose is missed, administer as soon as possible; then resume dosing at the regularly scheduled time

SIDE EFFECTS

CNS: *Headache,* fatigue, asthenia
EENT: *Sinusitis*
INTEG: *Inj site reaction*
MISC: Flulike symptoms, antibody development to this drug; *risk of infection* (TB, invasive fungal infections, other opportunistic infections)

PHARMACOKINETICS
Bioavailability 89%, peak 3-14 days

INTERACTIONS
Avoid use with live virus vaccines

NURSING CONSIDERATIONS
Assess:

• **Plaque psoriasis:** red, raised, inflamed patches of skin, whitish-silver scales or plaques on the red patches; dry skin

that may crack and bleed; soreness around patches; itching and burning sensations around patches; thick, pitted nails; painful, swollen joints

• For inj site pain, swelling, redness—usually occur after 2 inj (4-5 days); use cold compress to relieve pain/swelling

• **Infections** (fever, flulike symptoms, dyspnea, change in urination, redness/swelling around any wounds): stop treatment if present; some serious infections including sepsis may occur; patients with active infections should not be started on this product

• Latent TB before therapy; treat before starting this product

• **Pregnancy/breastfeeding:** use only if clearly needed; no well-controlled studies; cautious use in breastfeeding, no data

Evaluate

• Therapeutic response: decreasing plaques, painful, swollen joints

Teach patient/family:

• About self-administration if appropriate: inj should be made in thigh, abdomen, upper arm; rotate sites at least 1 inch from old site; do not inject in areas that are bruised, red, hard

• To refrigerate in container that product was received in; to dispose of needles and equipment as instructed

• That if medication is not taken when due, inject dose as soon as remembered and inject next dose as scheduled

• Not to take any live virus vaccines during treatment

• To report signs of infection, allergic reaction, or TB, immediately

---

selinexor
(sel-ih-nex'-or)
Xpovio
Func. class.: Antineoplastic
Chem class.: Small molecule antineoplastic nuclear export inhibitor

USES: Multiple myeloma in those who have received at least 4 prior therapies and who are refractory to at least 2 proteasome inhibitors, at least 2 immunomodulatory agents, and an anti-CD38 monoclonal antibody, in combination with dexamethasone

CONTRAINDICATIONS
Hypersensitivity, pregnancy, breastfeeding

DOSAGE AND ROUTES
• **Adult: PO** 80 mg in combination with dexamethasone 20 mg orally on days 1 and 3 of each week; repeat weekly until disease progression or unacceptable toxicity

---

solriamfetol (Rx)
(sol' ri- am' fe-tol)
Sunosi
Func. class.: Narcolepsy agent
Chem. class.: Dopamine norepinephrine reuptake inhibitor
Controlled substance IV

ACTION: Unknown, action may be due to its inhibitor of a dopamine and norepinephrine reuptake

USES: Excessive daytime sleepiness due to narcolepsy or obstructive sleep apnea

CONTRAINDICATIONS: Hypersensitivity, MAOIs
Precautions:
Alcoholism, bipolar disorder, cardiac disease, breastfeeding, diabetes mellitus, geriatrics, heart failure, hepatic disease, hypertension, MI, pregnancy, renal disease, schizophrenia, stroke, substance abuse, valvular heart disease, ventricular dysfunction

DOSAGE AND ROUTES
Narcolepsy
Adults: PO Initially, 75 mg daily on awakening; may increase to 150 mg after ≥3 days; max 150 mg/day Obstructive sleep apnea
• **Adults: PO** Initially, 37.5 mg daily on awakening; double the dose at intervals of at least 3 days if needed; max 150 mg/day

Renal dose
Adult: PO 37.5 mg/day; may increase to 75 mg/day after ≥7 days
Available forms: Tablet 75, 150 mg
Administer:
• Without regard to food
• Take on awakening; avoid within 9 hr of bedtime

SIDE EFFECTS
CNS: *Insomnia, anxiety, headache,* dizziness
CV: Palpitations, chest discomfort
GI: *Anorexia, nausea, dry mouth, constipation,* abdominal pain
INTEG: Hyperhidrosis

PHARMACOKINETICS
Protein binding <20%, minimally metabolized; half-life 7.1 hr, increased in renal disease; excreted 95% unchanged, peak 1.2-3 hr

INTERACTIONS
Increased: hypertensive reaction—MAOIs; do not use within 14 days
Use caution when using dopaminergic agents or drugs that increase B/P or heart rate

NURSING CONSIDERATIONS
Assess:
• **Narcolepsy:** assess for trouble staying awake baseline and after 1 wk, 2 wk
• B/P and heart rate baseline and periodically; hypertension should be treated before starting this product
• Psychiatric symptoms: assess for symptoms baseline and periodically; those with renal disease may be at higher risk
• Abuse: assess for those with a recent history of drug abuse, especially alcohol, amphetamines, cocaine, methylphenidate; watch for drug-seeking behaviors
Evaluate:
• Therapeutic response: ability to stay awake
Teach patient/family:
• To discuss all Rx, OTC, herbs, and supplements taken and if taking an MAOI

• That if a dose is missed, skip missed dose and administer the next dose the following day in the morning on wakening

• To report to healthcare provider if inability to stay awake continues or if you develop anxiety, agitation, irritability problems sleeping

• **Pregnancy/breastfeeding:** identify if pregnancy is planned to suspected, encourage to enroll in the pregnancy registry if she becomes pregnant; to enroll or obtain information from the registry, online at www.SunosiPregnancyRegistry.com or by calling 1-877-283-6220; present in breast milk

---

tenapanor
(ten-a′ pa- nor)
Ibsrela
Func. class.: IBS agent

USES: Irritable bowel syndrome with constipation in adults

CONTRAINDICATIONS
Hypersensitivity, GI obstruction

DOSAGE AND ROUTES
• **Adult: PO** 50 mg bid immediately before breakfast or the first meal of the day and immediately before dinner

---

ubrogepant
Ubrelvy
Func. class.: Calcitonin gene–related peptide (CGRP) receptor antagonist

USES: Acute migraine

DOSAGE AND ROUTES
• **Adult: PO** 50 or 100 mg; If needed, may take second dose at least 2 hr after initial dose; max: 200 mg/24 hr

CONTRAINDICATIONS
Hypersensitivity, strong CYP3A4 inhibitors

---

upadacitinib (Rx)
(Ue-pad′ a-sye′ ti-nib)
Rinvoq
Func. class.: Immunomodulating agent
Chem. class.: Janus associated kinase (JAK) inhibitor

ACTION: Oral JAK inhibitor; Janus kinase, a tyrosine kinase enzyme that transmit signals arising from cytokine or growth factor–receptor interactions on the cellular membrane to influence cellular processes of immune cell function and hematopoiesis

USES: Treatment of rheumatoid arthritis

CONTRAINDICATIONS
Hypersensitivity
Precautions: AIDS, anemia, breastfeeding, children, contraception requirements, corticosteroid use, diverticulitis, geriatrics, GI perforation, hepatic disease, hepatitis B exacerbation, herpes, HIV, neutropenia, pregnancy, pregnancy testing, vaccination

> Black Box Warning: Infection, new primary malignancy, thrombosis

DOSAGE AND ROUTES
• **Adults: PO** 15 mg daily with or without methotrexate or other nonbiologic DMARDs
Available forms: Extended release tablet 15 mg
Administer:
• Give with or without food
• Swallow whole; do not split, crush or chew

NURSING CONSIDERATIONS
Assess:
• **RA:** pain, stiffness, ROM, swelling of joints before, during treatment
• Infections (fever, flulike symptoms, dyspnea, change in urination, redness/

---

swelling around any wounds)—stop treatment if present

Black Box Warning: Some serious infections including sepsis may occur, may be fatal; patients with active infections should not be started on this product

Black Box Warning: Thrombosis (DVT, PE, arterial thrombosis): Assess for symptoms and treat immediately, some have been fatal

May reactivate hepatitis B in chronic carriers; may be fatal

Black Box Warning: Latent TB before therapy; treat before starting this product

Blood dyscrasias: CBC, differential periodically

Black Box Warning: Neoplastic disease (lymphomas/leukemia) monitor for these and skin cancer

• **Pregnancy/breastfeeding:** use only if clearly needed, no well-controlled studies; cautious use in breastfeeding, excreted in breast milk

Evaluate:

• Therapeutic response: decreased inflammation, pain in joints, decreased joint destruction

Teach patient/family:

• Not to take any live virus vaccines during treatment

• To report signs of infection, TB immediately

Appendix B

Ophthalmic, Nasal, Topical, and Otic Products

OPHTHALMIC PRODUCTS

ANESTHETICS
lidocaine (Rx)
(lye'doe-kane)
Akten
proparacaine (Rx)
(proe-par'a-kane)
Diocaine ✤
tetracaine (Rx)
(tet'ra-kane)
TetraVisc
ANTIHISTAMINES
alcaftadine
(al-caf'tah-deen)
Lastacaft
azelastine (Rx)
(ay-zell'ah-steen)
emedastine (Rx)
(ee-med'a-steen)
Emadine
epinastine (Rx)
(ep-een-as'teen)
Elestat
ketotifen (Rx, OTC)
(kee-toh-tif'en)
Claritin Eye, Zaditor
levocabastine (Rx)
(lee-voh-cab'ah-steen)
Livostin

olopatadine (Rx)
(oh-loh-pat'ah-deen)
Patanase, Pataday, Patanol, Pazeo
ANTIINFECTIVES
azithromycin (Rx)
(ay-zi-thro-my'sin)
AzaSite
besifloxacin (Rx)
(be'si-flox'a-sin)
Besivance
ciprofloxacin (Rx)
(sip-ro-floks'a-sin)
Ciloxan
erythromycin (Rx)
(er-ith-roe-mye'sin)
ganciclovir (Rx)
(gan-sye'kloe-vir)
Zirgan
gatifloxacin (Rx)
(gat-ih-floks'ah-sin)
Zymaxid
gentamicin (Rx)
(jen-ta-mye'sin)
Gentak
levofloxacin (Rx)
(lee-voh-flock'sah-sin)
moxifloxacin (Rx)
(mox-i-flox'a-sin)
Moxeza, Vigamox

natamycin (Rx)
(nat-a-mye'sin)

Natacyn

ofloxacin (Rx)
(oh-floks'a-sin)

Ocuflox

silver nitrate 1% (Rx)
silver nitrate
sulfacetamide sodium (Rx)
(sul-fa-seet'a-mide)

Bleph-10

tobramycin (Rx)
(toe-bra-mye'sin)

Tobrex

trifluridine (Rx)
(trye-floor'i-deen)

Viroptic

β-ADRENERGIC BLOCKERS
betaxolol (Rx)
(beh-tax'oh-lole)

Betoptic

carteolol (Rx)
(kar-tee'oh-lole)

levobetaxolol (Rx)
(lee-voh-beh-tax'oh-lohl)

Betaxon

levobunolol (Rx)
(lee-voe-byoo'no-lole)

Betagen

metipranolol (Rx)
(met-ee-pran'oh-lole)

timolol (Rx)
(tym'moe-lole)

Betimol, Timoptic

CARBONIC ANHYDRASE INHIBITORS
brinzolamide (Rx)
(brin-zoh'la-mide)

Azopt

dorzolamide (Rx)
(dor-zol'a-mide)

Trusopt

CHOLINERGICS (Direct-acting)
acetylcholine (Rx)
(ah-see-til-koe'leen)

Miochol-E

carbachol (Rx)
(kar'ba-kole)

Isopto Carbachol

pilocarpine (Rx)
(pye-loe-kar'peen)

Isopto Carpine

CHOLINESTERASE INHIBITORS
physostigmine (Rx)
(fi-zoe-stig'meen)

CORTICOSTEROIDS
dexamethasone (Rx)
(dex-a-meth'a-sone)

Dexycu, Dextenza, Maxidex

fluorometholone (Rx)
(flure-oh-meth'oh-lone)

Flarex, FML, FML Forte, FML S.O.P.

loteprednol (Rx)
(loe-tee-pred-nole)

Alrex, Inveltys, Lotemax

prednisoLONE (Rx)
(pred-niss'oh-lone)

Econopred Plus, Omnipred, Pred-Forte, Pred Mild

rimexolone (Rx)
(ri-mex'a-lone)
Vexol

MYDRIATICS

atropine (Rx)
(a'troe-peen)

cyclopentolate (Rx)
(sye-kloe-pen'toe-late)
Cyclogyl

homatropine (Rx)
(home-a'troe-peen)

phenylephrine (OTC)
(fen-ill-ef'rin)

NONSTEROIDAL ANTI-INFLAMMATORIES

bromfenac (Rx)
(brome'fen-ak)
BromSite, Prolensa

diclofenac (Rx)
(dye-kloe'fen-ak)

flurbiprofen (Rx)
(flure-bi'pro-fen)
Ocufen

ketorolac (Rx)
(kee-toe'role-ak)
Acular, Acuvail

nepafenac (Rx)
(ne-pa-fen'ak)
Ilevro, Nevanac

SYMPATHOMIMETICS

apraclonidine (Rx)
(a-pra-klon'i-deen)
Iopidine

brimonidine (Rx)
(brem-on'i-dine)
Alphagan P

latanoprostene bunod (Rx)
(la-tan-oh-pros'teen bu'nod)
Vyzulta

OPHTHALMIC DECONGESTANTS/VASOCONSTRICTORS

lodoxamide
(loe-dox'ah-mide)
Alomide

naphazoline (Rx, OTC)
(naf-az'oh-leen)
AK-Con ✤, All Clear Eye Drops ✤, All Clear AR Maximum Strength Ophthalmic Solution ✤, CVS Maximum Redness Relief Eye Drops, CVS Redness Relief Lubricant Eye Drops

tetrahydrozoline (OTC)
(tet-ra-hye-dro'zoe-leen)
Opti-Clear, Visine Original

MISCELLANEOUS OPHTHALMICS

bimatoprost (Rx)
(bih-mat'o-prost)
Latisse, Lumigan

cyclosporine
(sye'kloe-spor-een)
Cequa

latanoprost (Rx)
(la-tan'oh-prost)
Xalatan, Xelpros

travoprost (Rx)
(tra'voe-prost)
Travatan

unoprostone (Rx)
(yoo-noe-pros'tone)
Rescula

β-ADRENERGIC BLOCKERS

ACTION: Reduces production of aqueous humor by unknown mechanism

USES: Ocular hypertension, chronic open-angle glaucoma

ANESTHETICS

ACTION: Decreases ion permeability by stabilizing neuronal membrane

USES: Cataract extraction, tonometry, gonioscopy, removal of foreign objects, corneal suture removal, glaucoma surgery (ophthalmic); pruritus, sunburn, toothache, sore throat, cold sores, oral pain, rectal pain and irritation, control of gagging (topical)

ANTIINFECTIVES

ACTION: Inhibits folic acid synthesis by preventing PABA use, which is necessary for bacterial growth

USES: Conjunctivitis, superficial eye infections, corneal ulcers, prophylaxis against infection after removal of foreign matter from the eye

ANTIINFLAMMATORIES

ACTION: Decreases inflammation, resulting in decreased pain, photophobia, hyperemia, cellular infiltration

USES: Inflammation of eye, eyelids, conjunctiva, cornea; uveitis, iridocyclitis, allergic conditions, burns, foreign bodies, postoperatively in cataract

CARBONIC ANHYDRASE INHIBITOR

ACTION: Converted to epINEPHrine, which decreases aqueous production and increases outflow

USES: Open-angle glaucoma, ocular hypertension

DIRECT-ACTING MIOTIC

ACTION: Acts directly on cholinergic receptor sites; induces miosis, spasm of accommodation, fall in intraocular pressure, caused by stimulation of ciliary, pupillary sphincter muscles, which leads to pulling away of iris from filtration angle, resulting in increased outflow of aqueous humor

USES: Primary glaucoma, early stages of wide-angle glaucoma (less useful in advanced stages), chronic open-angle glaucoma, acute closed-angle glaucoma before emergency surgery; also neutralizes mydriatics used during eye exam; may be used alternately with mydriatics to break adhesions between iris and lens

CONTRAINDICATIONS: Hypersensitivity

Precautions: Pregnancy, breastfeeding, children, aphakia, hypersensitivity to carbonic anhydrase inhibitors, sulfonamides, thiazide diuretics, ocular inhibitors, renal/hepatic insufficiency

Administer
• Storage at room temperature away from light

ADVERSE EFFECTS
CNS: Headache
CV: Hypertension, tachycardia, dysrhythmias
EENT: Burning, stinging
GI: Bitter taste

NURSING CONSIDERATIONS
Assess
• Monitor ophthalmic exams and intraocular pressure readings
• Monitor blood counts; renal/hepatic function tests and serum electrolytes during long-term treatment

Teach patient/family
• Teach how to instill drops
• Advise patient that product may cause burning, itching, blurring, dryness of eye area

Evaluate

Positive therapeutic outcome
• Absence of increased intraocular pressure

NASAL AGENTS

NASAL ANTIHISTAMINES
olopatadine (Rx)
(oh-low-pat'uh-deen)

Patanase

NASAL DECONGESTANTS
azelastine (Rx)
(ay-zell'ah-steen)

Astepro

EPINEPHrine (OTC)
(ep-i-neff'rin)

Adrenalin Nasal Solution

oxymetazoline (OTC)
(ox-i-met-az'oh-leen)

12-Hour Nasal Decongestant, Afrin No Drip, Vicks QlearQuil, Vicks Sinex

phenylephrine (OTC)
(fen-ill-eff'rin)

4-Way Nasal Spray, Neo-Synephrine

tetrahydrozoline (OTC)
(tet-ra-hye-dro'zoe-leen)

Tyzine, Tyzine Pediatric

NASAL STEROIDS
beclomethasone (Rx)
(be-kloe-meth'a-sone)

Beconase AQ Nasal, Qnasl

budesonide (Rx)
(byoo-des'oh-nide)

Rhinocort Allergy, Rhinocort Aqua

flunisolide (Rx)
(floo-niss'oh-lide)

fluticasone (Rx)
(floo-tic'a-son)

Flonase

triamcinolone (Rx)
(trye-am-sin'oh-lone)

Nasal Allergy 24 HR Nasal Spray, Nasacort

NONSTEROIDAL ANTIINFLAMMATORY
ketorolac (Rx)
(kee'toe-role-ak)

Sprix

ACTION: Produces vasoconstriction (rapid, long acting) of arterioles, thereby decreasing fluid exudation, mucosal engorgement by stimulation of α-adrenergic receptors in vascular smooth muscle

Therapeutic outcome: Absence of nasal congestion

USES: Nasal congestion

CONTRAINDICATIONS: Hypersensitivity to sympathomimetic amines

Precautions: Pregnancy, children <6 yr, geriatric patients, diabetes, CV disease, hypertension, hyperthyroidism, increased ICP, prostatic hypertrophy, glaucoma

Administer
• Have patient tilt head back, squeeze bulb to create a vacuum, and draw correct amount of sol into dropper; insert 2 gtt of sol into nostril; repeat in other nostril
• Store in light-resistant container; do not expose to high temperature or let sol come into contact with aluminum
• Give for <4 consecutive days
• Provide environmental humidification to decrease nasal congestion, dryness

ADVERSE EFFECTS
CNS: Anxiety, restlessness, tremors, weakness, insomnia, dizziness, fever, headache
EENT: Irritation, burning, sneezing, stinging, dryness, rebound congestion
GI: Nausea, vomiting, anorexia
INTEG: Contact dermatitis

NURSING CONSIDERATIONS
Assess
• Assess for redness, swelling, pain in nasal passages before, during treatment

---

Side effects: *italics* = common; red = life-threatening

• Assess for systemic absorption; hypertension, tachycardia; notify prescriber; systemic absorption occurs at high doses or after prolonged use

Teach patient/family
• Advise patient that stinging may occur for several applications; drying of mucosa may be decreased by environmental humidification
• Caution patient to notify prescriber if irregular pulse, insomnia, dizziness, or tremors occur
• Teach patient proper administration to avoid systemic absorption
• Advise patient to rinse dropper with very hot water to prevent contamination

Evaluate
Positive therapeutic outcome
• Decreased nasal congestion

TOPICAL GLUCOCORTICOIDS

alclometasone (Rx)
(al-kloe-met'a-sone)
Aclovate

amcinonide
(am-sin'oh-nide)
Cyclocert 🍁

betamethasone (Rx)
(bay-ta-meth'a-sone)
Beben 🍁, Betacort 🍁, Beta Derm 🍁, Betanate, Betnovate 🍁, Celestoderm 🍁, Del-Beta, Luxiq, Sernivo

betamethasone (augmented) (Rx)
(bay-ta-meth'a-sone)
Diprolene AF

clobetasol (Rx)
(kloe-bay'ta-sol)
Clobex, Clodan, Cormax, Dermovate 🍁, Impoyz, Olux E, Olux Topical Foam, Temovate

desonide (Rx)
(dess'oh-nide)
Desocort 🍁, Desonate, DesOwen, LoKara, Tridesilon, Verdeso Foam 🍁

desoximetasone (Rx)
(dess-ox-i-met'a-sone)
Desoxi 🍁, Topicort

diflorasone
(dye-flor'a-sone)
fluocinolone (Rx)
(floo-oh-sin'oh-lone)
Capex 🍁, Derma-Smoothe/FS, Fluoderm 🍁, Synalar

flurandrenolide (Rx)
(flure-an-dren'oh-lide)
Cordran, Drenison 1/4 🍁, Drenison Tape 🍁

fluticasone (Rx)
(floo-tik'a-sone)
Cutivate

halcinonide (Rx)
(hal-sin'oh-nide)
Halog

hydrocortisone (Rx)
(hye-droe-kor'ti-sone)
Ala-Cort, Ala-Scalp, Anusol HC, Barriere-HC 🍁, CaldeCORT, Cortacet 🍁, Cortalo, Cortate 🍁, Cortef 🍁, Corticreme 🍁, Cortifoam, Cortoderm 🍁, Hyderm 🍁, Instacort, Nutracort, Sarna HC 🍁, Synacort, Texacort, Topiderm HC, Uremol HC 🍁

triamcinolone (Rx)
(trye-am-sin'oh-lone)
Aristocort C 🍁, Aristocort R 🍁, Kenalog, Triaderm 🍁, Triderm

ACTION: Antipruritic, antiinflammatory

Therapeutic outcome: Decreased itching, inflammation

USES: Psoriasis, eczema, contact dermatitis, pruritus; usually reserved for severe dermatoses that have not responded to less potent formulation

CONTRAINDICATIONS: Hypersensitivity, viral infections, fungal infections

Precautions: Pregnancy

DOSAGE AND ROUTES
Adult and child: Apply to affected area

Administer
• Apply only to affected areas; do not get in eyes
• Apply and leave site uncovered or lightly covered; occlusive dressing is not recommended—systemic absorption may occur
• Use only on dermatoses; do not use on weeping, denuded, or infected area
• Cleanse area before application of product
• Continue treatment for a few days after area has cleared
• Store at room temperature

ADVERSE EFFECTS
INTEG: *Acne, atrophy, epidermal thinning, purpura, striae*

NURSING CONSIDERATIONS
Assess
• Monitor temp; if fever develops, product should be discontinued
• Monitor for systemic absorption, increased temp, inflammation, irritation

Teach patient/family
• Teach patient to avoid sunlight on affected area; burns may occur
• Teach patient to limit treatment to 14 days

Evaluate
Positive therapeutic outcome
• Absence of severe itching, patches on skin, flaking

TOPICAL ANTIFUNGALS

clotrimazole (OTC)
(kloe-trye'ma-zole)
Alevazol, Antifungal, Anti-Fungal, Canesten ♦, Clotrimaderm ♦, Lotrimin AF, Neo-zol ♦

econazole (OTC)
(ee-kon'a-zole)
Ecostatin ♦, Ecoza

efinaconazole
(ef-in-a-kon'a-zole)
Jublia

ketoconazole (OTC)
(kee-toe-kon'a-zole)
Extina, Ketoderm ♦, Nizoral, Nizoral A-D, Xolegel

luliconazole
(loo-li-kon'a-zole)
Luzu

miconazole (OTC)
(mye-kon'a-zole)
Fungold, Lotrimin AF, Micatin, Micozole ♦, Zeasorb-AF

naftifine
(naff'ti-feen)
Naftin

nystatin (OTC)
(nye-stat'in)
Nyaderm ♦, Nystop

oxiconazole
(ox-i-kon'a-zole)
Oxistat

sulconazole
(sul-kon'a-zole)
Exelderm

tavaborole
(ta'va-bor'ole)
Kerydin

terbinafine (OTC)
(ter-bin'a-feen)
Lamisil AF
tolnaftate (OTC)
(tole-naf'tate)
Absorbine Junior ✦, Flexitol ✦,
Fungicure ✦, Lamicill AF,
Pitrex ✦, Podactin, Proclearz ✦,
Tinactin
undecylenic acid (OTC)
(un-deh-sih-len'ik)

ACTION: Interferes with fungal cell membrane permeability

Therapeutic outcome: Absence of itching and white patches of the skin

USES: Tinea cruris, tinea pedis, diaper rash, minor skin irritations; amphotericin B is used for *Candida* infections

CONTRAINDICATIONS: Hypersensitivity

Precautions: Pregnancy, breastfeeding, children

DOSAGE AND ROUTES
Massage into affected area, surrounding area daily or bid, continue for 7-14 days, max 4 wk

Administer
• Apply to affected area, surrounding area; do not cover with occlusive dressings
• Store below 30° C (86° F)

ADVERSE EFFECTS
INTEG: Burning, stinging, dryness, itching, local irritation

NURSING CONSIDERATIONS
Assess
• Assess skin for fungal infections: peeling, dryness, itching before, throughout treatment
• Assess for continuing infection; increased size, number of lesions

Teach patient/family
• Instruct to apply with glove to prevent further infection; not to cover with occlusive dressings
• Teach patient that long-term therapy may be needed to clear infection (2 wk-6 mo depending on organism); compliance is needed even after feeling better
• Teach patient proper hygiene: handwashing technique, nail care, use of concomitant top agents if prescribed
• Caution patient to avoid use of OTC creams, ointments, lotions unless directed by prescriber
• Instruct patient to use medical asepsis (hand washing) before, after each application; to change socks and shoes once a day during treatment of tinea pedis
• Advise patient to report to health care prescriber if infection persists or recurs; if blisters, burning, oozing, swelling occur
• Caution patient to avoid alcohol because nausea, vomiting, hypertension may occur
• Caution patient to use sunscreen or avoid direct sunlight to prevent photosensitivity
• Advise patient to notify prescriber of sore throat, fever, skin rash, which may indicate overgrowth of organisms

Evaluate

Positive therapeutic outcome
• Decrease in size, number of lesions

> **TOPICAL
> ANTIINFECTIVES**
>
> **azelaic acid (Rx)**
> (a-zuh-lay'ic)
> Azelex, Finacea
> **bacitracin (OTC)**
> (bass-i-tray'sin)
> Bacitin ✦
> **clindamycin (Rx)**
> (klin-da-my'sin)
> Cleocin T, Clindacin ETZ,
> Clindacin-P, Clindagel,
> Clindamax, Evocin

erythromycin (Rx, OTC)
(er-ith-roe-mye'sin)
Emgel, Emcin Clear, Ery, Erygel

gentamicin (Rx)
(jen-ta-mye'sin)

mafenide (Rx)
(ma'fe-nide)
Sulfamylon

metronidazole (Rx)
(met-roh-nye'da-zole)
MetroGel, MetroCream,
MetroLotion, Nydamax,
Noritate, Rosaden

mupirocin (Rx)
(myoo-peer'oh-sin)
Bactroban, Centany

retapamulin (Rx)
(re-tap'a-mue'lin)
Altabax

salicylic acid (Rx)
(sal'i-sil'ik)
Bensal HP, Compound W,
Demarest, Freeze Zone,
Keralyt, Salmaz, Salvax,
UltraSal-ER, Xalex

silver sulfADIAZINE (Rx)
(sul-fa-dye'a-zeen)
Flamazine ♣, Silvadene, SSD,
Thermazene

tretinoin (Rx)
(treh'tih-noyn)
Altreno, Atralin, Avita, Complex A,
Refissa, Retin-A, Tretin-X, Renova

CONTRAINDICATIONS: Hypersensitivity, large areas, burns, ulcerations

Precautions: Pregnancy, breastfeeding, impaired renal function, perforated eardrum

Administer
• Apply enough medication to cover lesions completely
• Apply after cleansing with soap, water before each application; dry well
• Apply to less than 20% of body surface area when patient has impaired renal function
• Store at room temperature in dry place

ADVERSE EFFECTS
INTEG: Rash, *urticaria, scaling, redness*

NURSING CONSIDERATIONS
Assess
• Assess for allergic reaction: burning, stinging, swelling, redness
• Assess for signs of nephrotoxicity or ototoxicity

Evaluate

Positive therapeutic outcome
• Decrease in size, number of lesions

> **TOPICAL ANTIVIRALS**

acyclovir (Rx)
(ay-sye'kloe-ver)
Zovirax Topical
penciclovir (Rx)
(pen-sye'kloe-ver)
Denavir

ACTION: Interferes with bacterial protein synthesis

Therapeutic outcome: Resolution of infection

USES: Skin infections, minor burns, wounds, skin grafts, primary pyodermas, otitis externa

ACTION: Interferes with viral DNA replication

Therapeutic outcome: Resolution of infection

USES: Simple mucocutaneous herpes simplex, in immunocompromised clients with initial herpes genitalis

Side effects: *italics* = common; red = life-threatening

CONTRAINDICATIONS: Hypersensitivity

Precautions: Pregnancy, breast-feeding

Administer
• Apply with finger cot or rubber glove to prevent further infection
• Apply enough medication to cover lesions completely
• Apply after cleansing with soap, water before each application; dry well
• Store at room temperature in dry place

ADVERSE EFFECTS
INTEG: Rash, urticaria, stinging, burning, pruritus, vulvitis

NURSING CONSIDERATIONS
Assess
• Assess for allergic reaction: burning, stinging, swelling, redness, rash, vulvitis, pruritus
• Assess for signs of nephrotoxicity or ototoxicity

Teach patient/family
• Teach patient not to use in eyes or when there is no evidence of infection
• Advise patient to apply with glove to prevent further infection
• Advise patient to avoid use of OTC creams, ointments, lotions unless directed by prescriber
• Advise patient to use medical asepsis (hand washing) before, after each application and to avoid contact with eyes
• Advise patient to adhere strictly to prescribed regimen to maximize successful treatment outcome
• Advise patient to begin taking product when symptoms arise

Evaluate

Positive therapeutic outcome
• Decrease in size, number of lesions

TOPICAL ANESTHETICS

benzocaine (OTC)
(ben'zoe-kane)
Americaine Anesthetic, Anbesol Maximum Strength
dibucaine (OTC)
(dye'byoo-kane)
Nupercainal
lidocaine (Rx, OTC)
(lye'doe-kane)
Astero, ClindaEze, EnovaRx, Glydo, Lidomar, LidoRx, Zilactin-L
pramoxine (OTC)
(pra-mox'een)
Prax, Proctofoam, Sarna
tetracaine (OTC, Rx)
(tet'ra-cane)
Pontocaine, Viractin

ACTION: Inhibits conduction of nerve impulses from sensory nerves

Therapeutic outcome: Decreasing inflammation, itching, pain

USES: Oral irritation, sore throat, toothache, cold sore, canker sore, sunburn, minor cuts, insect bites, pain, itching

CONTRAINDICATIONS: Hypersensitivity, infants <1 yr, application to large areas

Precautions: Pregnancy, children <6 yr, sepsis, denuded skin

DOSAGE AND ROUTES
Adult and child: TOP apply qid as needed; RECT insert tid and after each BM

Administer
• Store in tight, light-resistant container; do not freeze, puncture, or incinerate aerosol container

---

ADVERSE EFFECTS
INTEG: Rash, irritation, sensitization

NURSING CONSIDERATIONS
Assess
• Assess pain: location, duration, characteristics before, after administration
• Assess for infection: redness, drainage, inflammation; this product should not be used until infection is treated

Teach Patient/Family
• Teach patient to avoid contact with eyes
• Teach patient not to use for prolonged periods: use for <1 wk; if condition remains, prescriber should be contacted

Evaluate

Positive therapeutic outcome
• Decreased redness, swelling, pain

TOPICAL MISCELLANEOUS

docosanol (OTC)
(doh-koh'sah-nohl)
Abreva
pimecrolimus (Rx)
(pim-eh-kroh-ly'mus)
Elidel
oxymetazoline (Rx)
(ox-ee'meh-taz-oh-lin)
Rhofade

ACTION: Docosanol unknown; pimecrolimus may bind with macrophilin and inhibit calcium-dependent phosphatase

Therapeutic outcome: Decreased redness, swelling, pain

USES: Docosanol applied to fever blisters to promote more rapid healing; pimecrolimus used to treat mild to moderate atopic dermatitis in nonimmunocompromised patients ≥2 yr who are unresponsive to other treatment

CONTRAINDICATIONS: Hypersensitivity

Precautions: Pregnancy, breastfeeding, dermal infections

DOSAGE AND ROUTES
Docosanol
Adult: TOP rub into blisters 5 ×/day until healing occurs

Pimecrolimus
Adult and child ≥2 yr: TOP apply thin layer 2 ×/day and rub in; use as long as needed

Administer
• Apply to skin, rub in gently

ADVERSE EFFECTS
Docosanol
NONE known

Pimecrolimus
INTEG: Burning

NURSING CONSIDERATIONS
Assess
• Assess skin condition (color, pain, inflammation) before, after administration
• Assess for signs and symptoms of skin infections (redness, draining lesions); if present, avoid use of product (pimecrolimus)

Teach patient/family
• Advise patient to avoid contact between medication and eyes
• Instruct patient to discontinue use of product when condition clears

Evaluate

Positive therapeutic outcome
• Decreased inflammation, redness

VAGINAL ANTIFUNGALS

butoconazole (OTC)
(byoo-toh-kone'ah-zole)
Gynazol-1, Mycelex- 3

Side effects: *italics* = common; red = life-threatening

clotrimazole (OTC)
(kloe-trye'ma-zole)
Canesten ✤, Clotriamaderm ✤,
Gyne-Lotrimin 3, Mycelex-7

miconazole (OTC)
(mye-kon'a-zole)
Monistat 1, Monistat 3, Monistat
7, Vagistat-3

terconazole (OTC)
(ter-kone'ah-zole)
Terazol 7, Tetrazol 3

tioconazole (OTC)
(tye-oh-kone'ah-zole)
1-Day, Monistat 1 Day,
Vagistat-1

ACTION: Interferes with fungal DNA replication; binds sterols in fungal cell membranes, which increases permeability, leaking of nutrients

Therapeutic outcome: Fungistatic/ fungicidal against susceptible organisms: *Candida* only

USES: Vaginal, vulval, vulvovaginal candidiasis (moniliasis)

CONTRAINDICATIONS: Hypersensitivity

Precautions: Pregnancy, breastfeeding, children <2 yr

Administer
Topical route
• Administer one full applicator every night high into the vagina
• Store at room temperature in dry place

ADVERSE EFFECTS
GU: Vulvovaginal burning, itching, pelvic cramps
INTEG: Rash, urticaria, stinging, burning
MISC: *Headache*, body pain

NURSING CONSIDERATIONS
Assess
• Assess for allergic reaction: burning, stinging, itching, discharge, soreness

Teach patient/family
• Instruct patient in asepsis (hand washing) before, after each application
• Teach patient to apply with applicator only; to avoid use of any other vaginal product unless directed by prescriber; sanitary napkin may prevent soiling of undergarments
• Instruct patient to abstain from sexual intercourse until treatment is completed; reinfection and irritation may occur
• Advise patient to notify prescriber if symptoms persist

Evaluate

Positive therapeutic outcome
• Decrease in itching or white discharge (vaginal)

**OTIC
ANTIINFECTIVES**

ciprofloxacin (Rx)
(sip'roe-flox'a-sin)
Cetraxal, Otiprio

ACTION: Inhibits protein synthesis in susceptible microorganisms

USES: Ear infection (external), short-term use

CONTRAINDICATIONS: Hypersensitivity, perforated eardrum

Precautions: Pregnancy

Administer
• After removing impacted cerumen by irrigation
• After cleaning stopper with alcohol
• After restraining child if necessary
• After warming sol to body temp

ADVERSE EFFECTS
EENT: Itching, irritation in ear
INTEG: Rash, urticaria

NURSING CONSIDERATIONS
Assess
• Assess for redness, swelling, fever, pain in ear, which indicates superinfection

Teach patient/family
• Teach patient correct method of instillation using aseptic technique, including not touching dropper to ear
• Inform patient that dizziness may occur after instillation

Evaluate

Positive therapeutic outcome
• Decreased ear pain

Appendix C Vaccines and Toxoids

GENERIC NAME	TRADE NAME	USES	DOSAGE AND ROUTES	CONTRAINDICATIONS
anthrax vaccine	BioThrax	Pre-/postexposure prophylaxis	**Preexposure** Adult: SUBCUT 0.5 mL at 0, 2, 4 wk, then 0.5 mL at 6, 12, 18 mo **Postexposure** Adult: SUBCUT 0.5 mL 0, 2, 4 wk, with antibiotics	Hypersensitivity
BCG vaccine	TICE BCG	TB exposure	Adult and child ≥1 mo: 0.2-0.3 mL Child <1 mo: Reduce dose by 50% using 2 mL of sterile water after reconstituting	Hypersensitivity, hypogamma-globulinemia, positive TB test, burns
dengue tatravalent vaccine, live	Dengvaxia	Prevention of dengue disease	Child 9-16 yr SUBCUT 0.5 mL × 3 doses, 6 mo apart at mo 1, 6, 12	Hypersensitivity
diphtheria and tetanus toxoids, adsorbed	Tenivac	Induces antitoxins to provide immunity to diphtheria and tetanus	Adult and child ≥7 yr: IM (adult strength) 0.5 mL q4-8wk × 2 doses, then 3rd dose 6-12 mo after 2nd dose, booster IM 0.5 mL q10yr Child 1-6 yr: IM (pediatric strength) 0.5 mL q4wk × 2 doses, booster 6-12 mo after 2nd dose Infant 6 wk-1 yr: IM (pediatric strength) 0.5 mL q4wk × 3 doses, booster 6-12 mo after 3rd dose	Hypersensitivity to mercury; thimerosal; immunocompromised patients; radiation; corticosteroids; acute illness
diphtheria and tetanus toxoids and whole-cell pertussis vaccine (DPT, DTP)	DTwP, Tri-Immunol	Prevention of diphtheria, tetanus, pertussis	Doses vary Check product information	Hypersensitivity, active infection, poliomyelitis outbreak, immunosuppression, febrile illness
diphtheria and tetanus toxoids and acellular pertussis vaccine	Adacel, Boostrix, Daptacel, Infanrix	Prevention of diphtheria, tetanus, pertussis	Doses vary Check product information	Hypersensitivity, active infection, poliomyelitis outbreak, immunosuppression, febrile illness
diphtheria, tetanus, pertussis, haemophilus, polio IPV	Pentacel	Immunity to diphtheria, tetanus, pertussis, haemophilus, polio IPV	Infant >6 wk and child ≤5 yr: IM 0.5 mL at 2, 4, 6, and 15-18 mo	Hypersensitivity, polio outbreak, acute infection, immunosuppression
diphtheria, tetanus, pertussis, polio vaccine IPV	Kinrix, Quadracel	Immunity to diphtheria, tetanus, pertussis, polio vaccine IPV	Child: IM 0.5 mL.	Hypersensitivity, polio outbreak, acute infection, immunosuppression

GENERIC NAME	TRADE NAME	USES	DOSAGE AND ROUTES	CONTRAINDICATIONS
ebola zaire vaccine, live	Ervebo		1 mL (single-dose vial) once	Hypersensitivity
H1N1 influenza A (swine flu) virus vaccine	Influenza A (H1N1)	Immunity to H1N1	Adult <50 yr, adolescent, child ≥2 yr: Intranasal 1 dose (roughly 0.1 mL) into each nostril; child 2-9 repeat dose ≥4 wk later Adult, adolescent, child ≥3 yr: IM 0.5 mL as a single dose; child 3-9 yr repeat dose ≥4 wk later (Sanofi) (CSL); child 4-9 yr repeat dose ≥4 wk later (Novartis); infants ≥6 mo, child <36 mo: IM 0.25 mL, repeat in 4 wk (Sanofi) Adult: IM 0.5 mL as a single dose (GSK)	Hypersensitivity, febrile illness, active infection
haemophilus b conjugate vaccine, diphtheria CRM₁₉₇ protein conjugate (HbOC)	HibTITER	Polysaccharide immunization of children 2-6 yr against *H. tn-fluenzae* b, conjugate	**HibTITER (IM only)** Child: IM 0.5 mL. Child 2-6 mo: 0.5 mL q2mo × 3 inj	
haemophilus b conjugate vaccine, meningococcal protein conjugate (PRP-OMP)	PedvaxHIB	Immunization of child 2, 4, 6 mo	Child 7-11 mo: Previously unvaccinated 0.5 mL q2mo inj Child 12-14 mo: Previously unvaccinated 0.5 mL × 1 inj **PedvaxHIB (IM only)** Child 2-14 mo: 0.5 mL × 2 inj at 2, 4 mo of age (6 mo dose not needed), then booster at 12-18 mo against invasive disease Child ≥15 mo: Previously unvaccinated 0.5 mL inj	
hepatitis A vaccine, inactivated	Havrix, VAQTA	Active immunization against hepatitis A virus	Adult: IM 1440 EL units (Havrix) or 50 units (VAQTA) as a single dose; booster dose is the same given at 6, 12 mo Child 2-18 yr: IM 720 EL units (Havrix) or 25 units (VAQTA) as a single dose, booster dose is the same given at 6, 12 mo	Hypersensitivity
hepatitis B vaccine, recombinant	Engerix-B, Recombivax HB	Immunization against all subtypes of hepatitis B virus	Varies widely	Hypersensitivity to this vaccine or yeast
human papillomavirus recombinant vaccine, quadrivalent	Gardasil	Prevention of HPV types 6, 11, 16, 18, cervical cancer, genital warts, precancerous dysplastic lesions, anal cancer/anal intraepithelial neoplasia	Adult up to 26 yr and child >9 yr to 26 yr: IM give as 3 separate doses; 1st dose is elected; 2nd dose 2 mo after 1st dose; 3rd dose 6 mo after 1st dose	Child <9 yr, pregnancy, breastfeeding, geriatric patients, active disease, hypersensitivity

influenza virus vaccine	Afluria, FluMist, Fluvirin, Fluzone	Prevention of seasonal influenza	Adult and child >12 yr: IM 0.5 mL in 1 dose Adult 18-64 yr: ID 0.1 mL as a single dose Child 3-12 yr: IM 0.5 mL, repeat in 1 mo (split) unless 1978-1985 vaccine was given; also given nasal Child 6 mo to 3 yr: IM 0.25 mL, repeat in 1 mo (split) unless 1978-1985 vaccine was given; also given nasal	Hypersensitivity, active infection, chicken egg allergy; Guillain-Barré syndrome, active neurologic disorders
Japanese encephalitis virus vaccine, inactivated	Ixiaro	Active immunity against Japanese encephalitis (JE)	Adult and child >3 yr: SUBCUT 0.5 mL (deltoid), then 0.5 mL 28 days later. Give the second dose ≥1 wk before potential exposure Child ≥2 mo to <3 yr: IM 0.25 mL (anterolateral aspect of the thigh or deltoid for children 1-2 yr with adequate muscle mass), then 0.25 mL 28 days later	Hypersensitivity to murine, thimerosal; allergic reactions to previous dose
measles, mumps, and rubella vaccine, live	M-M-R-II	Prevention of measles, mumps, rubella	Adult: SUBCUT 1 vial; 2 vials separated by 1 mo, in person born after 1957 Child >15 mo and adult: SUBCUT 0.5 mL.	Hypersensitivity, blood dyscrasias, anemia, active infection, immunosuppression; egg, chicken allergy; pregnancy, febrile illness, neomycin allergy, neoplasms
measles, mumps, rubella, varicella	ProQuad	Immunity to measles, mumps, rubella, varicella	Child: SUBCUT 0.5 mL.	Hypersensitivity to eggs, neomycin, cancer, radiation, corticosteroids, blood dyscrasias, active untreated TB
meningococcal polysaccharide vaccine	Menomune-A/C	Prophylaxis to meningococcal meningitis	Adult and child >2 yr: SUBCUT 0.5 mL	Hypersensitivity to thimerosal, pregnancy, acute illness
pneumococcal 7-valent conjugate vaccine	Prevnar	Immunity against *Streptococcus pneumoniae*	Child: IM 0.5 mL × 3 doses (7-11 mo); × 2 doses (12-23 mo); × 1 dose >2-9 yr	Hypersensitivity to diphtheria toxoid or this product
pneumococcal vaccine, polyvalent	Pneumovax 23	Pneumococcal immunization	Adult and child >2 yr: IM/SUBCUT 0.5 mL	Hypersensitivity, Hodgkin's disease, ARDS
poliovirus vaccine (IPV)	IPOL	Prevention of polio	Adult and child >2 yr: PO 0.5 mL, given q8wk × 2 doses, then 0.5 mL ½-1 yr after dose 2 Infant: PO 0.5 mL at 2, 4, 18 mo; booster at 4-6 yr; may also be given: IPV at 2, 4 mo, then TOPV at 12-18 mo, booster at 4-6 yr	Hypersensitivity, active infection, allergy to neomycin/streptomycin, immunosuppression, vomiting, diarrhea
rabies vaccine, human diploid cell (HDCV)	Imovax, RabAvert	Active immunity to rabies	**Preexposure** Adult and child: IM 1 mL day 0, 7, 21, or 28 (total 4 doses) **Postexposure** Adult and child: IM 1 mL on day 0, 3, 7, 14, 28 (total 5 doses)	No contraindications

GENERIC NAME	TRADE NAME	USES	DOSAGE AND ROUTES	CONTRAINDICATIONS
rotovirus	RotaTeq, Rotarix	Prevents rotovirus	Infant: PO 3 doses given between 6 and 32 wk of age; 1st dose between 6-12 wk of age; 2nd and 3rd doses q4-10wk	Hypersensitivity to this product or latex, immunocompromised, blood products given within 6 wk, lymphatic disorders
smallpox and monkeypox vaccine, live, nonreplicating	Jynneos	Prevention of smallpox and monkeypox disease	Adult: SUBCUT 0.5 mL × 2 doses, 4 wk apart	Hypersensitivity
tetanus toxoid, adsorbed	No trade name	Tetanus toxoid: Used for prophylactic treatment of wounds	Adult and child: IM 0.5 mL q4-6wk × 2 doses, then 0.5 mL 1 yr after dose 2 (adsorbed); SUBCUT/IM 0.5 mL q4-8wk × 3 doses, then 0.5 mL ½-1 yr after dose 3, booster dose 0.5 mL q10yr	Hypersensitivity, active infection, poliomyelitis outbreak, immunosuppression
typhoid vaccine, parenteral typhoid vaccine, oral	Typhim Vi Vivotif Berna Vaccine	Active immunity to typhoid fever	Adult: PO 1 cap 1 hr before meals × 4 doses, booster q5yr Adult and child >10 yr: SUBCUT 0.5 mL, repeat in 4 wk, booster q3yr Child 6 mo-10 yr: SUBCUT 0.25 mL, repeat in 4 wk, booster q3yr	Parenteral: Systemic or allergic reaction, acute respiratory or other acute infection, intensive physical exercise in high temperatures Oral: Hypersensitivity; acute febrile illness, suppressive or antibiotic products
typhoid Vi polysaccharide vaccine	Typhim Vi	Active immunity to typhoid fever	Adult and child ≥2 yr: IM 0.5 mL as a single dose, reimmunize q2yr 0.5 mL IM, if needed	Hypersensitivity, chronic typhoid carriers
varicella-zoster virus vaccine	Varivax, Zostavax	Prevention of varicella zoster (chickenpox)	Adult and child ≥13 yr: SUBCUT 0.5 mL, 2nd dose SUBCUT 0.5 mL 4-8 wk later	Hypersensitivity to neomycin; blood dyscrasias, immunosuppression, active untreated TB, acute illness, pregnancy, diseases of lymphatic system
yellow fever vaccine	YF-Vax	Active immunity to yellow fever	Adult and child ≥9 mo: SUBCUT 0.5 mL deeply, booster q10yr Child 6-9 mo: same as above if exposed	Hypersensitivity to egg or chicken embryo protein, pregnancy, child <6 mo, immunodeficiency
zoster vaccine recombinant, adjuvanted	Shingrix	Prevention of herpes zoster (shingles)	Adult: IM 2 doses (0.5 mL each) at 0 and 2 to 6 months	History of severe allergic reaction (e.g., anaphylaxis) to any component of the vaccine or after a previous dose

Appendix D

Recent FDA Drug Approvals

GENERIC	TRADE	USE
fam-trastuzumab deruxtecan-nxki	Enhertu	Breast Cancer
enfortumab vedotin-ejfv	Padcev	Urothelial Carcinoma
lemborexant	Dayvigo	Insomnia
levamlodipine	Conjupri	Hypertension

Index

Drug names and/or monographs denoted with an asterisk are found on your Evolve Resources at http://evolve.elsevier.com/nursingdrugupdates/Skidmore/NDR

Entries can be identified as follows: DISEASES/DISORDERS, *DRUG CATEGORIES*, generic names, Trade Names.

Entries can be identified as follows: DISEASES/DISORDERS, *DRUG CATEGORIES*, generic names,
Trade Names.

INDEX

Entries can be identified as follows: DISEASES/DISORDERS, *DRUG CATEGORIES*, generic names,
Trade Names.

Entries can be identified as follows: DISEASES/DISORDERS, *DRUG CATEGORIES*, generic names, Trade Names.

Entries can be identified as follows: DISEASES/DISORDERS, *DRUG CATEGORIES*, generic names, Trade Names.

Entries can be identified as follows: DISEASES/DISORDERS, *DRUG CATEGORIES*, generic names, Trade Names.

Entries can be identified as follows: DISEASES/DISORDERS, *DRUG CATEGORIES*, generic names,
Trade Names.

Entries can be identified as follows: DISEASES/DISORDERS, *DRUG CATEGORIES*, generic names,
Trade Names.

Entries can be identified as follows: DISEASES/DISORDERS, *DRUG CATEGORIES*, generic names,
Trade Names.

Entries can be identified as follows: DISEASES/DISORDERS, *DRUG CATEGORIES*, generic names, Trade Names.

Entries can be identified as follows: DISEASES/DISORDERS, *DRUG CATEGORIES*, generic names,
Trade Names.

Entries can be identified as follows: DISEASES/DISORDERS, *DRUG CATEGORIES*, generic names,
Trade Names.

Entries can be identified as follows: DISEASES/DISORDERS, *DRUG CATEGORIES*, generic names, Trade Names.

Entries can be identified as follows: DISEASES/DISORDERS, *DRUG CATEGORIES*, generic names, Trade Names.

Entries can be identified as follows: DISEASES/DISORDERS, *DRUG CATEGORIES*, generic names, Trade Names.

Entries can be identified as follows: DISEASES/DISORDERS, *DRUG CATEGORIES*, generic names,
Trade Names.

INDEX

Entries can be identified as follows: DISEASES/DISORDERS, *DRUG CATEGORIES*, generic names, Trade Names.

Entries can be identified as follows: DISEASES/DISORDERS, *DRUG CATEGORIES*, generic names,
Trade Names.

INDEX

Entries can be identified as follows: DISEASES/DISORDERS, *DRUG CATEGORIES*, generic names,
Trade Names.

Entries can be identified as follows: DISEASES/DISORDERS, *DRUG CATEGORIES*, generic names, Trade Names.

INDEX

Entries can be identified as follows: DISEASES/DISORDERS, *DRUG CATEGORIES*, generic names,
Trade Names.

Entries can be identified as follows: DISEASES/DISORDERS, *DRUG CATEGORIES*, generic names, Trade Names.

Entries can be identified as follows: DISEASES/DISORDERS, *DRUG CATEGORIES*, generic names, Trade Names.

INDEX

Entries can be identified as follows: DISEASES/DISORDERS, *DRUG CATEGORIES*, generic names,
Trade Names.

Entries can be identified as follows: DISEASES/DISORDERS, *DRUG CATEGORIES*, generic names, Trade Names.

Entries can be identified as follows: DISEASES/DISORDERS, *DRUG CATEGORIES*, generic names,
Trade Names.

Entries can be identified as follows: DISEASES/DISORDERS, *DRUG CATEGORIES*, generic names,
Trade Names.

INDEX

Entries can be identified as follows: DISEASES/DISORDERS, *DRUG CATEGORIES*, generic names,
Trade Names.

Entries can be identified as follows: DISEASES/DISORDERS, *DRUG CATEGORIES*, generic names,
Trade Names.

Entries can be identified as follows: DISEASES/DISORDERS, *DRUG CATEGORIES*, generic names, Trade Names.

Entries can be identified as follows: DISEASES/DISORDERS, *DRUG CATEGORIES*, generic names, Trade Names.

Entries can be identified as follows: DISEASES/DISORDERS, *DRUG CATEGORIES*, generic names, Trade Names.

INDEX

Entries can be identified as follows: DISEASES/DISORDERS, *DRUG CATEGORIES*, generic names, Trade Names.

INDEX

Entries can be identified as follows: DISEASES/DISORDERS, *DRUG CATEGORIES*, generic names,
Trade Names.

Entries can be identified as follows: DISEASES/DISORDERS, *DRUG CATEGORIES*, generic names,
Trade Names.

INDEX

Entries can be identified as follows: DISEASES/DISORDERS, *DRUG CATEGORIES*, generic names, Trade Names.

Entries can be identified as follows: DISEASES/DISORDERS, *DRUG CATEGORIES*, generic names,
Trade Names.

Entries can be identified as follows: DISEASES/DISORDERS, *DRUG CATEGORIES*, generic names,
Trade Names.

Entries can be identified as follows: DISEASES/DISORDERS, *DRUG CATEGORIES*, generic names, Trade Names.

Entries can be identified as follows: DISEASES/DISORDERS, *DRUG CATEGORIES*, generic names,
Trade Names.

Entries can be identified as follows: DISEASES/DISORDERS, *DRUG CATEGORIES*, generic names, Trade Names.

Entries can be identified as follows: DISEASES/DISORDERS, *DRUG CATEGORIES*, generic names, Trade Names.

Entries can be identified as follows: DISEASES/DISORDERS, *DRUG CATEGORIES*, generic names,
Trade Names.

Entries can be identified as follows: DISEASES/DISORDERS, *DRUG CATEGORIES*, generic names, Trade Names.

Entries can be identified as follows: DISEASES/DISORDERS, *DRUG CATEGORIES*, generic names,
Trade Names.

Entries can be identified as follows: DISEASES/DISORDERS, *DRUG CATEGORIES*, generic names,
Trade Names.

Entries can be identified as follows: DISEASES/DISORDERS, *DRUG CATEGORIES*, generic names, Trade Names.

INDEX

Entries can be identified as follows: DISEASES/DISORDERS, *DRUG CATEGORIES*, generic names,
Trade Names.

Entries can be identified as follows: DISEASES/DISORDERS, *DRUG CATEGORIES*, generic names, Trade Names.

Entries can be identified as follows: DISEASES/DISORDERS, *DRUG CATEGORIES*, generic names, Trade Names.

Entries can be identified as follows: DISEASES/DISORDERS, *DRUG CATEGORIES*, generic names,
Trade Names.

Entries can be identified as follows: DISEASES/DISORDERS, *DRUG CATEGORIES*, generic names,
Trade Names.

Entries can be identified as follows: DISEASES/DISORDERS, *DRUG CATEGORIES*, generic names,
Trade Names.

INDEX

Entries can be identified as follows: DISEASES/DISORDERS, *DRUG CATEGORIES*, generic names,
Trade Names.

Entries can be identified as follows: DISEASES/DISORDERS, *DRUG CATEGORIES*, generic names, Trade Names.

Formulas

Surface area rule:

$$\text{Child dose} = \frac{\text{Surface area (m}^2)}{1.73 \text{ m}^2} \times \text{Adult dose}$$

Calculating strength of a solution:

$$\textit{Solution Strength:} \quad \textit{Desired Solution:}$$
$$\frac{x}{100} = \frac{\text{Amount of drug desired}}{\text{Amount of finished solution}}$$

Calculating flow rate for IV:

$$\text{Rate of flow} = \frac{\text{Amount of fluid} \times \text{Administration set calibration}}{\text{Running time}}$$

$$\frac{x}{1} = \frac{\text{(mL) (gtt/min)}}{\text{min}}$$

Calculation of medication dosages:

Formula method:

$$\frac{\text{Amount ordered}}{\text{Amount on hand}} \times \text{Vehicle} = \text{Number of tablets, capsules, or amount of liquid}$$

Vehicle is the drug form or amount of liquid containing the dosage. Amounts used in calculation by formula must be in same system.

Ratio–proportion method:

tablet:tablet in mg on hand::x tablet order in mg
$$\quad\quad\quad\quad \text{Know or have::Want to know or order}$$
Multiply means and extremes, divide both sides by known amount to get x. Amounts used in equation must be in same system.

Dimensional analysis method:

$$\text{Order in mg} \times \frac{1 \text{ tablet or capsule}}{\text{What 1 tablet or capsule is in mg}}$$
$$= \text{Tablets or capsules to be given}$$

If amounts are in different systems:

$$\text{Order in mg} \times \frac{1 \text{ tablet or capsule}}{\text{What 1 tablet or capsule is in g}} \times \frac{1}{1000 \text{ mg}}$$
$$= \text{Tablets or capsules to be given}$$

Temperature conversion:

$$= C \times \tfrac{9}{5} + 32$$
$$= \tfrac{5}{9} (F - 32)$$

Nomogram for calculation of body surface area

Place a straight edge from the patient's height in the left column to the patient's weight in the right column. The point of intersection on the body surface area column indicates the body surface area (BSA). (Reproduced in Behrman RE, Kliegman RM, Jenson HB: *Nelson textbook of pediatrics,* ed 18, Philadelphia, 2011, WB Saunders; Nomogram modified from data of E. Boyd by CD West.)

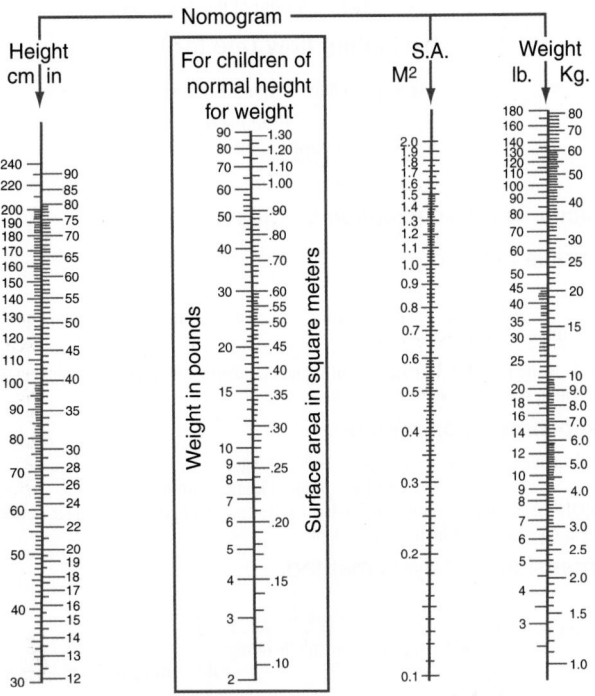

Alternative (Mosteller's formula):

$$\text{Surface area (m}^2) = \sqrt{\frac{\text{Height (cm)} \times \text{Weight (kg)}}{3600}}$$

Antitoxins and antivenins

GENERIC NAME	TRADE NAME	USES	DOSAGE AND ROUTES	CONTRAINDICATIONS
Black widow spider antivenin (*Lactrodectus mactans*)	No trade name	Black widow spider bite	Adult and child: IM 2.5 ml, 2nd dose may be given if severe; give in anterolateral thigh, obtain test for sensitivity before inj	Hypersensitivity to this product or horse serum
Crotalidae antivenom, polyvalent	No trade name	Rattlesnake bite	Adult and child: IV 20-150 ml depending on seriousness of bite, may give additional doses based on response	Hypersensitivity
Diphtheria antitoxin, equine	No trade name	Diphtheria	Adult and child: IM/slow IV 20,000-120,000 units, may give additional doses after 24 hr	Hypersensitivity
Micrurus fulvius antivenin	No trade name	East/Texas coral snake bite	Adult and child: IV 30-50 ml, give through running IV line of normal saline, give 1st 1-2 ml over 4-5 min, watch for allergic reaction	Hypersensitivity
Scorpion antivenin (centruroides sculpturatus equine)	Anascorp	Scorpion stings	Adult and child: IV 3 vial/50 ml NS given over 10 min, may give other doses 1 vial/50 ml NS over 10 min q30-60min	N/A

Abbreviations

ABG	arterial blood gas	**GVHD**	graft-versus-host disease
ADA	American Diabetes Association	**H₂**	histamine$_2$
ADH	antidiuretic hormone	**hCG**	human chorionic gonadotropin
ALT	alanine aminotransferase	**Hct**	hematocrit
ANA	antinuclear antibody	**HDCV**	human diploid cell rabies vaccine
APLA	antiphospholipid antibody syndrome	**Hgb**	hemoglobin
APTT	activated partial thromboplastin time	**H & H**	hematocrit and hemoglobin
ASA	acetylsalicylic acid, aspirin	**5-HIAA**	5-hydroxyindoleacetic acid
AST	aspartate aminotransferase (SGOT)	**HIV**	human immunodeficiency virus (AIDS)
AV	atrioventricular	**HR**	heart rate
bid	twice a day	**IBD**	inflammatory bowel disease
BPH	benign prostatic hypertrophy	**IC**	intracardiac
BPM	beats per minute	**ICP**	intracranial pressure
BUN	blood urea nitrogen	**ID**	intradermal
CAD	coronary artery disease	**IgG**	immunoglobulin G
CBC	complete blood cell count	**IM**	intramuscular
CCr	creatinine clearance	**INF**	infusion
CHF	congestive heart failure	**INH**	inhalation
CNS	central nervous system	**inj**	injection
CONT	continuous	**I&O**	intake and output
COPD	chronic obstructive pulmonary disease	**INT**	intermittent
CPAP	continuous positive airway pressure	**IPPB**	intermittent positive-pressure breathing
CPK	creatine phosphokinase	**IT**	intrathecal
CPS	carbamoyl phosphate synthetase	**ITP**	idiopathic thrombocytopenic purpura
C&S	culture and sensitivity	**IUD**	intrauterine device
CSF	cerebrospinal fluid	**IV**	intravenous
CTCL	cutaneous T-cell lymphoma	**IVP**	intravenous pyelogram
CV	cardiovascular	**K**	potassium
CVA	cerebrovascular accident	**LDH**	lactic dehydrogenase
CVP	central venous pressure	**LE**	lupus erythematosus
D&C	dilatation and curettage	**LFT**	liver function test
DIC	diffuse intravascular coagulation	**LH**	luteinizing hormone
DIR INF	direct infusion	**LOC**	level of consciousness
D₅W	5% glucose in distilled water	**LR**	lactated Ringer's solution
DVT	deep vein thrombosis	**LT**	leukotriene
ECG	electrocardiogram (EKG)	**m**	minim
EDTA	ethylenediamine tetraacetic acid	**m²**	square meter
EEG	electroencephalogram	**MAC**	monitored anesthesia care
EPS	extrapyramidal symptom	**MAOI**	monoamine oxidase inhibitor
ESR	erythrocyte sedimentation rate	**mcg**	microgram
EXT REL	extended release	**mEq**	milliequivalent
FBS	fasting blood sugar	**mg**	milligram
FHT	fetal heart tones	**MI**	myocardial infarction
FSH	follicle-stimulating hormone	**ml**	milliliter
GABA	γ-aminobutyric acid	**mm**	millimeter
GPC	giant papillary conjunctivitis	**mo**	month
gr	grain	**Na**	sodium
GT	glucose tolerance test	**ng**	nanogram
GU	genitourinary	**NGU**	non-gonococcal urethritis